MW01008546

NEINSTEIN'S

Adolescent
and Young Adult
Health Care

A Practical Guide

NEINSTEIN'S
Adolescent and Young Adult Health Care

A Practical Guide

7TH EDITION ///

Editor-in-Chief
Debra K. Katzman, MD, FRCPC
Professor of Pediatrics, Department of Pediatrics, Division
   of Adolescent Medicine
The Hospital for Sick Children and University of Toronto
Toronto, Ontario
Canada

Senior Associate Editor
Catherine M. Gordon, MD, MS
Professor of Pediatrics
Senior Faculty, USDA/ARS Children's Nutrition Research
   Center
Baylor College of Medicine
Houston, Texas

Associate Editors
S. Todd Callahan, MD, MPH
Professor of Pediatrics
Director, Division of Adolescent and Young Adult Health
Monroe Carell Jr. Children's Hospital at Vanderbilt
Vanderbilt University Medical Center
Nashville, Tennessee

Alain Joffe, MD, MPH
Former Director, Adolescent Medicine
Johns Hopkins Medical Institutions
Former Director, Student Health and Wellness Center
Johns Hopkins University
Baltimore, Maryland

Susan L. Rosenthal, PhD, ABPP
Professor of Medical Psychology (in Pediatrics and
   Psychiatry)
Vice Chair, Faculty Development, Department of Pediatrics
Columbia University Irving Medical Center-Vagelos College
   of Physicians and Surgeons
New York, New York

Maria Trent, MD, MPH
Bloomberg Endowed Professor of American Health
Professor of Pediatrics, Public Health, and Nursing
Director, Division of Adolescent/Young Adult Medicine
Senior Associate Dean of Diversity and Inclusive
   Excellence for Johns Hopkins Medicine
Johns Hopkins University Schools of Medicine, Public
   Health, and Nursing
Baltimore, Maryland

Richard J. Chung, MD
Professor of Pediatrics
Professor in Medicine
Director of Adolescent and Young Adult Health
Duke University School of Medicine
Durham, North Carolina

. Wolters Kluwer

Philadelphia • Baltimore • New York • London
Buenos Aires • Hong Kong • Sydney • Tokyo

Acquisitions Editor: James P. Sherman
Development Editors: Thomas Celona and Maria M. McAvey
Editorial Coordinator: Nancy Dickson
Marketing Manager: Kirsten Watrud
Production Project Manager: Kirstin Johnson
Design Manager: Stephen Druding
Manufacturing Coordinator: Beth Welsh
Prepress Vendor: Aptara, Inc.

Seventh Edition

Copyright © 2023

Copyright © 2016 by Lippincott Williams & Wilkins, a Wolters Kluwer business (sixth edition). © 2008 by Lippincott Williams & Wilkins, a Wolters Kluwer business (fifth edition). © 2002 by Lippincott Williams & Wilkins (fourth edition). © 1996 by Williams & Wilkins (third edition). © 1991 by Urban & Schwarzenberg (second edition). © 1984 by Urban & Schwarzenberg (first edition). All rights reserved. This book is protected by copyright. No part of this book may be reproduced or transmitted in any form or by any means, including as photocopies or scanned-in or other electronic copies, or utilized by any information storage and retrieval system without written permission from the copyright owner, except for brief quotations embodied in critical articles and reviews. Materials appearing in this book prepared by individuals as part of their official duties as U.S. government employees are not covered by the above-mentioned copyright. To request permission, please contact Wolters Kluwer at Two Commerce Square, 2001 Market Street, Philadelphia, PA 19103, via email at permissions@lww.com, or via our website at shop.lww.com (products and services).

9 8 7 6 5 4 3 2 1

Printed in Mexico

Library of Congress Cataloging-in-Publication Data

Names: Katzman, Debra, editor.
Title: Neinstein's adolescent and young adult health care : a practical
    guide / editor-in-chief, Debra K. Katzman ; senior associate editor,
    Catherine M. Gordon ; associate editors, S. Todd Callahan, Alain Joffe,
    Susan L. Rosenthal, Maria Trent, Richard J. Chung.
Other titles: Adolescent and young adult health care
Description: Seventh edition. | Philadelphia : Wolters Kluwer, [2023] |
    Includes bibliographical references and index.
Identifiers: LCCN 2022031467 (print) | LCCN 2022031468 (ebook) | ISBN
    9781975160296 (hardback) | ISBN 9781975160319 (ebook)
Subjects: MESH: Adolescent Health | Adolescent Medicine | Young Adult. |
    Handbook | BISAC: MEDICAL / Pediatrics
Classification: LCC RJ550 (print) | LCC RJ550 (ebook) | NLM WS 39 | DDC
    616.00835–dc23/eng/20220826
LC record available at https://lccn.loc.gov/2022031467
LC ebook record available at https://lccn.loc.gov/2022031468

This work is provided "as is," and the publisher disclaims any and all warranties, express or implied, including any warranties as to accuracy, comprehensiveness, or currency of the content of this work.

This work is no substitute for individual patient assessment based upon healthcare professionals' examination of each patient and consideration of, among other things, age, weight, gender, current or prior medical conditions, medication history, laboratory data and other factors unique to the patient. The publisher does not provide medical advice or guidance and this work is merely a reference tool. Healthcare professionals, and not the publisher, are solely responsible for the use of this work including all medical judgments and for any resulting diagnosis and treatments.

Given continuous, rapid advances in medical science and health information, independent professional verification of medical diagnoses, indications, appropriate pharmaceutical selections and dosages, and treatment options should be made and healthcare professionals should consult a variety of sources. When prescribing medication, healthcare professionals are advised to consult the product information sheet (the manufacturer's package insert) accompanying each drug to verify, among other things, conditions of use, warnings and side effects and identify any changes in dosage schedule or contraindications, particularly if the medication to be administered is new, infrequently used or has a narrow therapeutic range. To the maximum extent permitted under applicable law, no responsibility is assumed by the publisher for any injury and/or damage to persons or property, as a matter of products liability, negligence law or otherwise, or from any reference to or use by any person of this work.

QUADM0123

This book is dedicated to the memory of Lawrence S. Neinstein, our treasured colleague and mentor, who demonstrated a passion for teaching and a dedication to the health of adolescents and young adults (AYAs) and their families.

Contributors

Matthew C. Aalsma, PhD
Professor of Psychology and Pediatrics
Director, Adolescent Behavioral Health
  Research Program
Department of Pediatrics
Indiana University School of Medicine
Indianapolis, Indiana

William P. Adelman, MD
Adjunct Professor of Pediatrics
The Children's Hospital of Philadelphia,
  Division of Adolescent Medicine
Executive Director, Student Health and
  Counseling
Perelman School of Medicine at the
  University of Pennsylvania
Philadelphia, Pennsylvania

Mark E. Alexander, MD
Associate Professor, Harvard Medical
  School
Cardiac Electrophysiologist and Director of
  Exercise Physiology
Vice Chair, Institutional Review Board
Arrhythmia Service, Department of
  Cardiology
Boston Children's Hospital
Boston, Massachusetts

Rachel H. Alinsky, MD, MPH
Assistant Professor of Pediatrics
Johns Hopkins University School of
  Medicine
Baltimore, Maryland

Louise Ashwell, MSW
Research Manager
The Haven, King's College Hospital NHS
  Foundation Trust
London, United Kingdom

**Colette (Coco) Auerswald, MD,
MS, FSAHM**
Professor, Community Health Sciences
Martin Sisters Chair in Medical Research
  and Public Health
Co-Director, I4Y (Innovations for Youth)
Faculty Lead, Youth and Allies Against
  Homelessness
UC Berkeley School of Public Health
Berkeley, California

Romina Loreley Barral, MD, MsCR
Associate Professor, Department of Pediatrics
School of Medicine, University of Missouri
Kansas City, Missouri
Research Assistant Professor, Department
  of Pediatrics
University of Kansas Medical Center
Kansas City, Kansas
Attending Physician, Division of
  Adolescent Medicine
Children's Mercy Hospital Kansas City
Kansas City, Missouri

Teresa A. Batteiger, MD, MS
Assistant Professor of Medicine,
  Department of Medicine
Division of Infectious Diseases, Indiana
  University School of Medicine
Indianapolis, Indiana

Michael A. Beasley, MD
Instructor of Orthopaedics, Harvard
  Medical School
Division of Sports Medicine, Boston
  Children's Hospital
Boston, Massachusetts

Jonathon J. Beckmeyer, PhD
Assistant Professor, School of Counseling
  and Well-Being
West Virginia University
Morgantown, West Virginia

**Meera S. Beharry, MD, FAAP,
FSAHM**
Clinical Associate Professor, Department
  of Medical Education
College of Medicine, Texas A&M University
Affiliate Medical Associate Professor,
  Department of Clinical Medicine, CUNY
  School of Medicine at the City of
  College of New York
New York
Treasurer, International Association of
  Adolescent Health
Owner and Lead Physician, Healthy
  Horizons Hebiatrics, PLLC
Fort Pierce, Florida

Marvin E. Belzer, MD
Professor of Clinical Pediatrics
Keck School of Medicine of USC
Children's Hospital Los Angeles
Los Angeles, California

Heather M. Bernard, MD
Clinical Instructor, Department of
  Pediatrics, Harvard Medical School
Attending Physician, Department of General
  Pediatrics, Boston Children's Hospital
Boston, Massachusetts

William R. Betts, PhD
Director of Counseling and Health
  Services
Ball State University
Muncie, Indiana

Rebecca M. Beyda, MD, MS
Clinical Associate Professor, Pediatrics &
  Adolescent Medicine
Adolescent Medicine Fellowship Director
McGovern Medical School at Houston
Houston, Texas

Joshua S. Borus, MD, MPH
Assistant Professor of Pediatrics, Harvard
  Medical School
Physician, Division of Adolescent/Young
  Adult Medicine, Boston Children's
  Hospital
Boston, Massachusetts

Terrill Bravender, MD, MPH
David Rosen Professor of Adolescent
  Medicine, Professor of Pediatrics
  and Psychiatry, Division Director of
  Adolescent Medicine
Department of Pediatrics
C.S. Mott Children's Hospital, University of
  Michigan
Ann Arbor, Michigan

Paula K. Braverman, MD
Professor of Pediatrics, Department of
  Pediatrics
UMass Chan Medical School-Baystate
Division Chief, Adolescent Medicine,
  Department of Pediatrics
Baystate Children's Hospital
Springfield, Massachusetts

Lauren Bretz, MD, MEd
Assistant Professor, Pediatric Adolescent
  and Sports Medicine, Baylor College of
  Medicine
Adolescent Medicine, Texas Children's
  Hospital
Houston, Texas

**Cora Collette Breuner, MD,
MPH, FAAP**
Professor, Department of Pediatrics,
  Adolescent Medicine Division
Adjunct Professor, Orthopedics and Sports
  Medicine
Seattle Children's Hospital, University of
  Washington
Seattle, Washington

Jeremi M. Carswell, MD
Professor of Pediatrics, Harvard Medical
    School
Director, Gender Multispecialty Program
Staff, Division of Endocrinology
Boston Children's Hospital
Boston, Massachusetts

Emma G. Carter, MD
Assistant Professor of Pediatric Neurology,
    Department of Pediatrics
Vanderbilt University
Pediatric Epileptologist
Monroe Carell Jr. Children's Hospital at
    Vanderbilt
Nashville, Tennessee

Mariam R. Chacko, MD
Distinguished Professor Emeritus
Department of Pediatrics
Division of Adolescent Medicine & Sports
    Medicine
Baylor College of Medicine
Texas Children's Hospital
Houston, Texas

Joanne E. Cox, MD
Associate Professor of Pediatrics,
    Department of Pediatrics, Harvard
    Medical School
Associate Chief, Division of General
    Pediatrics, Boston Children's Hospital
Boston, Massachusetts

LaKeshia N. Craig, MD
Adolescent Medicine Fellow
Division of Adolescent and Transition
    MedicineCincinnati Children's Hospital
    Medical Center
Cincinnati, Ohio

Nancy Crimmins, MD
Associate Professor, Pediatric
    Endocrinology, University of Cincinnati
Associate Professor, Pediatric
    Endocrinology, Cincinnati Children's
    Hospital Medical Center
Cincinnati, Ohio

Lawrence J. D'Angelo, MD, MPH
Professor of Pediatrics, Medicine, and
    Epidemiology
George Washington University
Emeritus Chief, Division of Adolescent and
    Young Adult Medicine
Children's National Hospital
Washington, DC

Diana D. Deister, MS, MD
Instructor in Psychiatry, Department of
    Psychiatry & Behavioral Sciences
Boston Children's Hospital, Harvard
    Medical School
Assistant in Medicine, Developmental
    Medicine Center
Boston Children's Hospital
Boston, Massachusetts

Allyson L. Dir, PhD
Assistant Professor of Psychiatry
Department of Psychiatry
Indiana University School of Medicine
Indianapolis, Indiana

**Amy Desrochers DiVasta, MD,
MMSc**
Associate Professor, Harvard Medical
    School
Director, Young Women's Health Research
Co-Director, Adolescent Long-Acting
    Reversible Contraception (LARC)
    Program
Division of Adolescent/Young Adult Medicine
Department of Pediatrics
Boston Children's Hospital
Boston, Massachusetts

Toni Eimicke, CPNP
Pediatric Nurse Practitioner, Pediatric
    Endocrinology
Maine Medical Center
Portland, Maine

Abigail English, JD
Director, Center for Adolescent Health &
    the Law
Chapel Hill, North Carolina

Ashlee LaFontaine Enzinger, MD
Clinical Assistant Professor, Department of
    Orthopedics and Rehabilitation, Division
    of Sports Medicine Clinical
Assistant Professor, Department of
    Pediatrics, General Pediatrics
University of Iowa Hospitals and Clinics
Cedar Rapids, Iowa

Lisa Fedina, PhD, MSW
Assistant Professor
University of Michigan School of Social
    Work
Ann Arbor, Michigan

**Errol L. Fields, MD, PhD, MPH,
FAAP**
Assistant Professor of Pediatrics,
    Department of Pediatrics
Division of Adolescent/Young Adult
    Medicine, Johns Hopkins School of
    Medicine
Baltimore, Maryland

Shannon Fitzgerald, MD, MPH
Instructor, Department of Pediatrics,
    Harvard Medical School
Attending, Division of Adolescent and
    Young Adult Medicine, Boston Children's
    Hospital
Boston, Massachusetts

Amy Fleischman, MD, MMSc
Assistant Professor, Harvard Medical
    School
Attending Physician, Director of Clinical
    Operations, Endocrinology, Boston
    Children's Hospital
Boston, Massachusetts

Joseph T. Flynn, MD, MS
Dr. Robert O. Hickman Endowed Chair in
    Pediatric Nephrology
Professor of Pediatrics, University of
    Washington
Chief, Division of Nephrology, Seattle
    Children's Hospital
Seattle, Washington

Michelle Forcier, MD, MPH
Professor of Pediatrics, Assistant Dean of
    Admissions, Office of Medical Education
Alpert School of Medicine
Brown University
Providence, Rhode Island

Melanie A. Gold, DO, DMQ
Professor of Pediatrics and Population &
    Family Health
Columbia University Irving Medical Center
Medical Director, School-Based Health
    Centers, New York-Presbyterian
New York, New York

Neville H. Golden, MD
The Marron and Mary Elizabeth Kendrick
    Professor of Pediatrics, Department of
    Pediatrics
Stanford University School of Medicine
Chief, Division of Adolescent Medicine,
    Department of Pediatrics
Lucile Packard Children's Hospital Stanford
Stanford, California

Kassandra Gonzalez, JD
People's Community Clinic
Austin, Texas

Holly C. Gooding, MD, MSc
Medical Director, Adolescent Medicine,
    Children's Healthcare of Atlanta
Associate Professor of Pediatrics, Emory
    University School of Medicine

Catherine M. Gordon, MD, MS
Professor of Pediatrics and Senior Faculty
USDA/ARS Children's Nutrition Research
    Center
Baylor College of Medicine
Houston, Texas

Kevin M. Gray, MD
Professor of Psychiatry and Behavioral
Sciences and Assistant Vice President for
    Advancing Research Partnerships
Medical University of South Carolina
    Charleston, South Carolina

Rebecca Gudeman, JD, MPA
Senior Director, Health
National Center for Youth Law
Oakland, California

Scott E. Hadland, MD, MPH, MS
Chief, Division of Adolescent and Young
    Adult Medicine
MassGeneral Hospital for Children and
    Harvard Medical School
Boston, Massachusetts

Jillian R. Hagerman, DO
Kaiser Permanente Adolescent Medicine
Tacoma, Washington

Tamara S. Hannon, MD, MS
Professor, Pediatrics, Indiana University
    School of Medicine
Director, Pediatric Diabetes Program
Riley Hospital for Children
Indiana University Health
Indianapolis, Indiana

Scott B. Harpin, PhD, MPH, RN, FSHAM
Associate Professor & MCH Division Chair
College of Nursing, University of Colorado,
    Anschutz Medical Campus
Aurora, Colorado

Jacob C. Hartz, MD, MPH
Instructor, Department of Pediatrics,
    Harvard Medical School
Director of Preventive Cardiology,
    Department of Cardiology, Boston
    Children's Hospital
Boston, Massachusetts

Devon J. Hensel, MD, PhD
Department of Pediatrics, Indiana
    University School of Medicine
Department of Sociology, Indiana
    University–Purdue University
    Indianapolis
Indianapolis, Indiana

Todd I. Herrenkohl, PhD, MSW
Marion Elizabeth Blue Professor of
    Children and Families
University of Michigan School of Social
    Work
Ann Arbor, Michigan

Paula J. Adams Hillard, MD
Professor Emerita, Department of
    Obstetrics and Gynecology
Stanford University School of Medicine
Pediatric and Adolescent Gynecology,
    Lucile Packard Children's Hospital
    Stanford
Stanford, California

Jesse D. Hinckley, MD, PhD
Assistant Professor, Department of
    Psychiatry
Division of Addiction Research, Prevention
    & Treatment
University of Colorado School of Medicine
Aurora, Colorado

Lisa M. Horowitz, PhD, MPH
Senior Associate Scientist/Pediatric
    Psychologist
Office of the Clinical Director
National Institute of Mental Health, NIH
Bethesda, Maryland

Jill S. Huppert, MD, MPH
Physician scientist, Agency for Healthcare
    Research and Quality
Rockville, Maryland

James R. Jacobs, MD, PhD
Associate Professor, Department of
    Psychiatry and Behavioral Sciences and
    (by courtesy) Emergency Medicine
Associate Vice Provost and Executive
    Director, Vaden Health Services
Stanford University
Stanford, California

M. Susan Jay, MD
Professor of Pediatrics
Medical College of Wisconsin
Milwaukee, Wisconsin

Christine Johnston, MD, MPH
Associate Professor, Department of
    Medicine
Division of Allergy and Infectious
    Diseases, University of Washington
Seattle, Washington

James Kaferly, MD
Assistant Professor, Department of
    Pediatrics, University of Colorado School
    of Medicine
Aurora, Colorado
Assistant Professor, Department of
    Pediatrics, Denver Health and Hospital
    Authority
Denver, Colorado

Jessica A. Kahn, MD
Division Director, Professor
Division of Adolescent and Transition
    Medicine
Cincinnati Children's Hospital Medical
    Center
University of Cincinnati College of
    Medicine
Cincinnati, Ohio

Patricia E. Kapunan, MD, MPH
Assistant Professor
Department of Pediatrics
George Washington University School of
    Medicine & Health Sciences
Attending Physician
Division of Adolescent and Young Adult
    Medicine
Children's National Hospital
Washington, DC

Ashley Rowatt Karpinos, MD, MPH
Assistant Professor, Department of
    Medicine, Division of General Internal
    Medicine & Public Health, Section of
    Med-Peds
Assistant Professor, Department of
    Pediatrics, Division of General Pediatrics
Assistant Professor, Department of
    Orthopaedics, Division of Sports
    Medicine
Vanderbilt University Medical Center
Nashville, Tennessee

Debra K. Katzman, MD, FRCPC
Professor of Pediatrics, Department of
    Pediatrics, Division of Adolescent Medicine
The Hospital for Sick Children and University
    of Toronto
Toronto, Ontario
Canada

Ellen Stubbe Kester, PhD, CCC-SLP
Founder and President, Bilinguistics
Austin, Texas

Sari L. Kives, MD, FRCSC, MSc
Associate Professor
Hospital for Sick Children
University of Toronto
Toronto, Ontario, Canada

Michael R. Kohn, MBBS, FRACP, PhD
Professor of Medicine, Sydney University
Head, Adolescent and Young Adult
    Medicine
Westmead Hospital, Westmead
Sydney, Australia

Daphne J. Korczak, MD, MSc, FRCPC
Associate Professor of Psychiatry, Temerty
    Faculty of Medicine, University of
    Toronto
Associate Scientist, Neurosciences and
    Mental Health
Psychiatrist, Hospital for Sick Children
Toronto, Ontario, Canada

Chana B. Korenblum, BSc (Hons), MD, FRCPC
Assistant Professor, Departments of
    Pediatrics and Psychiatry
Temerty Faculty of Medicine, University of
    Toronto
Staff Physician, Department of Pediatrics,
    Division of Adolescent Medicine,
    The Hospital for Sick Children, and
    Department of Supportive Care,
    Princess Margaret Cancer
Centre, University Health Network
Toronto, Ontario, Canada

Faye Korich, MD, MHS
Assistant Professor of Clinical Pediatrics,
    Department of Pediatrics
Perelman School of Medicine at the
    University of Pennsylvania
Philadelphia, Pennsylvania

Martin A. Koyle, MD, MSc, MMgmt, FAAP, FACS, FRCSC, FRCS (Eng.)
Professor Emeritus, Temerty Faculty of
    Medicine, Department of Surgery &
    Institute of Health Policy, Management
    & Evaluation (IHPME)
University of Toronto
Toronto, Ontario, Canada

Daniel P. Krowchuk, MD, FAAP
Professor Emeritus of Pediatrics and
    Dermatology
Wake Forest School of Medicine
Winston-Salem, North Carolina

Sinduja Lakkunarajah, MD, MMHPE
Adolescent Medicine Faculty
Department of Pediatrics
Marshfield Clinic Health System
Marshfield, Wisconsin

Cecilia A. Larson, MD
Endocrinologist, Internal Medicine
Winchester Hospital
Winchester, Massachusetts

Sharon Levy, MD, MPH
Director, Adolescent Substance Use and
    Addiction Program
Boston Children's Hospital
Associate Professor of Pediatrics
Harvard Medical School
Boston, Massachusetts

Carol Lewis, MD
Professor of Pediatrics
Department of Pediatrics, Alpert Medical
    School of Brown University
Hasbro Children's Hospital
Providence, Rhode Island

Keith J. Loud, MDCM, MMSc, MMgmt
Chair, Department of Pediatrics,
    Dartmouth Geisel School of Medicine
Physician-in-Chief, Dartmouth Health
    Children's
Lebanon, New Hampshire

Jen Makrides, MD, MA, MHS
Assistant Professor, Division of Adolescent
    Medicine, The Medical College of
    Wisconsin
Children's Wisconsin
Milwaukee, Wisconsin

Renée Marquardt, MD
Senior Instructor, Department of
    Psychiatry, University of Colorado
Chief Medical Officer, Colorado
    Department of Human Services
Denver, Colorado

Bethany Marston, MD
Associate Professor of Pediatrics and
    Medicine
Division Director, Pediatric Rheumatology
Program Director, Rheumatology
    Fellowship
Department of Pediatrics, Pediatric
    Rheumatology and Department of
    Medicine, Allergy/Immunology and
    Rheumatology Divisions
University of Rochester
Strong Memorial Hospital/Golisano
    Children's Hospital
Rochester, New York

Tamara Itzel Martinez, MD
Assistant Professor, Department of Family
    Medicine, University of Colorado School
    of Medicine
Medical Staff, Department of Family
    Medicine, UCHealth University of
    Colorado Hospital
Denver, Colorado

Pamela A. Matson, PhD, MPH
Assistant Professor of Pediatrics,
    Department of Pediatrics, Johns
    Hopkins University School of Medicine
Baltimore, Maryland

William P. Meehan III, MD
Professor of Pediatrics, Harvard Medical
    School
Division of Sports Medicine, Boston
    Children's Hospital
Boston, Massachusetts

Matthew J. Meyers, MD, MPH
Assistant Clinical Professor of Pediatrics
Division of Adolescent and Young Adult
    Medicine
University of California, San Francisco
San Francisco, California

Elizabeth Miller, MD, PhD
Professor of Pediatrics, Public Health, and
    Clinical and Translational Science
University of Pittsburgh School of Medicine
Director, Division of Adolescent and Young
    Adult Medicine
UPMC Children's Hospital of Pittsburgh
Pittsburgh, Pennsylvania

Catherine Miller, MD
Clinical Assistant Professor, Adolescent
    Medicine Fellowship Program Director,
    Department of Pediatrics, Division of
    Adolescent Medicine, University of
    Michigan
C.S. Mott Children's Hospital
Ann Arbor, Michigan

Melissa Mirosh, MD, FRCSC (Obs/Gyne)
Clinical Assistant Professor, Department of
    Obstetrics and Gynecology
Cumming School of Medicine, University
    of Calgary
Cochrane, Alberta, Canada

Laurie A. P. Mitan, MD
Professor of Pediatrics, University of
    Cincinnati College of Medicine
Department of Pediatrics, Division of
    Adolescent and Transition Medicine,
    Cincinnati Children's Hospital Medical
    Center
Cincinnati, Ohio

Peter J. Mogayzel Jr, MD, PhD, MBA
Menowitz/Rosenstein Professor of
    Pediatric Respiratory Sciences
Johns Hopkins Hospital
Baltimore, Maryland

Suneeta Monga, MD, FRCPC
Associate Professor of Psychiatry, Temerty
    Faculty of Medicine, University of
    Toronto
Associate Psychiatrist-in-Chief, Hospital for
    Sick Children
Toronto, Ontario, Canada

Megan A. Moreno, MD, MSEd, MPH
Professor, Academic Division Chief:
    General Pediatrics and Adolescent
    Medicine, Vice Chair of Academic Affairs
Department of Pediatrics, University of
    Wisconsin-Madison
Adolescent Medicine Physician,
    Department of Pediatrics, UW Hospital
    and Clinics
Madison, Wisconsin

Anna-Barbara Moscicki, MD
Professor of Pediatrics
Chief, Adolescent and Young Adult
    Medicine
Associate Vice Chair of Clinical Research
Department of Pediatrics
University of California, Los Angeles
Los Angeles, California

Annabelle M. Mournet, BA
Intramural Research Training Award Fellow
Office of the Clinical Director
National Institute of Mental Health, NIH
Bethesda, Maryland

Niamh C. Murphy, MD, MRCPI, MRCOG
Consultant Obstetrician CHI at Temple
    Street/Paediatric and Adolescent
    Gynaecologist
Coombe Women and Infants University
    Hospital
Dublin, Ireland

Celia B. Neavel, MD, FSAHM, FAAFP
Affiliate Faculty, Population Health,
    The University of Texas at Austin Dell
    Medical School
Medical Director, Center for Adolescent
    Health, People's Community Clinic
Austin, Texas

Anita L. Nelson, MD
Professor & Chair, Obstetrics &
    Gynecology, Western University of
    Health Sciences
Pomona, California
Professor Emeritus, Obstetrics &
    Gynecology, University California Los
    Angeles (UCLA)
Clinical Professor, Obstetrics &
    Gynecology, University Southern
    California (USC)
Los Angeles, California

Christopher B. Oakley, MD
Co-Director, Johns Hopkins Headache
    Center
Assistant Professor of Neurology
Johns Hopkins University School of
    Medicine
Baltimore, Maryland

Johanna Olson-Kennedy, MD
Associate Professor of Clinical Pediatrics
Keck School of Medicine of the University
    of Southern California
Medical Director, The Center for
    Transyouth Health and Development
Children's Hospital Los Angeles
Los Angeles, California

Elizabeth M. Ozer, MA, PhD
Professor and Associate Vice Provost,
    Faculty Equity
Department of Pediatrics & Office of
    Diversity & Outreach
University of California, San Francisco
San Francisco, California

Anita K. Pai, MD
Assistant Professor, Department of
    Pediatrics, Vanderbilt University
Pediatric Transplant Hepatologist,
    Department of Pediatrics, Division of
    Gastroenterology, Hepatology, and
    Nutrition
Monroe Carell Jr Children's Hospital at
    Vanderbilt
Nashville, Tennessee

Maryland Pao, MD
Clinical Director
Office of the Clinical Director
National Institute of Mental Health, NIH
Bethesda, Maryland

Sarah Pitts, MD
Assistant Professor, Department of
    Pediatrics, Harvard Medical School
Director, Adolescent/Young Adult
    Fellowship Program and Co-Director,
    Long-acting Reversible Contraception
    (LARC) Program, Division of Adolescent/
    Young Adult Medicine, Boston Children's
    Hospital
Boston, Massachusetts

Laura Kester Prakash, MD, MPH
Associate Professor of Clinical Pediatrics,
    Department of Pediatrics
UC Davis School of Medicine
Sacramento, California

Judith J. Prochaska, PhD, MPH
Professor of Medicine, Department of
    Medicine
Stanford Prevention Research Center,
    Stanford University
Stanford, California

Mari Radzik, PhD
Assistant Professor of Clinical Pediatrics,
    KECK School of Medicine of USC
Clinical Psychologist—Program Area Lead
Division of Adolescent and Young Adult
    Medicine, Children's Hospital Los Angeles
Los Angeles, California

Maria H. Rahmandar, MD
Assistant Professor, Department of
    Pediatrics, Northwestern University
    Feinberg School of Medicine
Attending Physician, Division of
    Adolescent & Young Adult Medicine,
    Ann & Robert H. Lurie Children's
    Hospital of Chicago
Chicago, Illinois

Shilpa B. Reddy, MD
Assistant Professor of Pediatric Neurology,
    Department of Pediatrics, Vanderbilt
    University
Section Head, Pediatric Epilepsy and
    Pediatric Epileptologist, Monroe Carell
    Jr. Children's Hospital at Vanderbilt
Nashville, Tennessee

William Riccardelli, MD
Fellow in Addiction Medicine, Adolescent
    Substance Use and Addiction Program
Boston Children's Hospital
Boston, Massachusetts
Child, Adolescent & Adult Psychiatrist
Four Winds Hospital
Katonah, New York
Child & Adolescent Psychiatrist
Rockland Children's Psychiatric Center
Office of Mental Health—NY State
Orangeburg, New York

**Gabrielle Rigney, BPsych(Hons),
PhD**
Lecturer and Researcher, School of Health,
    Medical and Applied Sciences
Appleton Institute, Central Queensland
    University Australia
Adelaide, South Australia

Matthew B. Rivara, MD
Associate Professor of Medicine, Division
    of Nephrology
University of Washington
Seattle, Washington

Mary E. Romano, MD, MPH
Associate Professor, Adolescent/Young
    Adult Health, Vanderbilt University
    School of Medicine
Associate Professor, Adolescent/Young
    Adult Health, Vanderbilt University
    Medical Center
Nashville, Tennessee

Gwendolyn Rosen, MPH
Research Associate, Population and Family
    Health
Columbia University
New York, New York

Abby R. Rosenberg, MD, MS, MA
Associate Professor, Department of
    Pediatrics
Divisions of Hematology-Oncology, and
    Bioethics & Palliative Care, University of
    Washington School of Medicine
Director, Palliative Care and Resilience lab,
    Seattle Children's Research Institute
Director, Pediatrics at the Cambia Palliative
    Care Center of Excellence at the
    University of Washington
Director, Survivorship and Outcomes
    Research in the Seattle Children's
    Cancer and Blood Disorders Center
Seattle, Washington

Peter C. Rowe, MD
Professor, Department of Pediatrics, Johns
    Hopkins University School of Medicine
Director, Chronic Fatigue Clinic, Johns
    Hopkins Children's Center
Baltimore, Maryland

Gretchen J. Russo, RN, BSN, JD
Judicial and Legislative Administrator
Office of Children, Youth and Families
Colorado Department of Human Services
Denver, Colorado

Mandakini Sadhir, MD
Assistant Professor, Department of
    Pediatrics, Division of Adolescent
    Medicine
Interim Chief and Medical Director,
    Adolescent Medicine Clinic
Kentucky Children's Hospital
Lexington, Kentucky

**Renata Arrington Sanders, MD,
MPH, ScM**
Associate Professor, Department of
    Pediatrics, Division of Adolescent and
    Young Adult Medicine, Johns Hopkins
    School of Medicine
Associate Professor, Department of
    Pediatrics, Johns Hopkins Children's
    Center
Baltimore, Maryland

John S. Santelli, MD, MPH
Professor, Population and Family Health
    and Pediatrics
Columbia University
New York, New York

**Joana Dos Santos, MD, MHSc,
FRCPC**
Assistant Professor of Paediatrics,
    University of Toronto
Medical Urologist, Departments of
    Surgery and Paediatric Medicine
    (Cross-Appointed)
The Hospital for Sick Children
Toronto, Ontario, Canada

Susan M. Sawyer, MBBS, MD, FRACP
Geoff and Helen Handbury Chair of
  Adolescent Health, Department of
  Paediatrics
The University of Melbourne
Director, Centre for Adolescent Health,
  Royal Children's Hospital
Melbourne, Victoria, Australia

Wael N. Sayej, MD
Associate Professor of Pediatrics,
  Department of Pediatrics, UMass Chan
  Medical School-Baystate
Division Chief, Pediatric Gastroenterology
  and Nutrition, Department of Pediatrics,
  Baystate Children's Hospital
Springfield, Massachusetts

Holly Schroder, MD, MPH
Dartmouth Hitchcock Medical Center
Cheshire Medical Center, Family
  Medicine/Adolescent Medicine
Keene, New Hampshire

Christina Schutt, DO
Assistant Professor of Pediatrics
Program Director of Pediatric
  Rheumatology
Department of Pediatrics, Division of
  Pediatric Rheumatology
University of Rochester
Strong Memorial Hospital/Golisano
  Children's Hospital
Rochester, New York

Beth I. Schwartz, MD
Associate Professor of Obstetrics &
  Gynecology and Pediatrics, Sidney
  Kimmel Medical College at Thomas
  Jefferson University
Pediatric and Adolescent Gynecology,
  Department of Obstetrics & Gynecology,
  Thomas Jefferson University
Philadelphia, Pennsylvania
Division of Adolescent Medicine and
  Pediatric Gynecology, Nemours
  Children's Health
Wilmington, Delaware

Katherine Schwartz, JD, MPA
Assistant Research Professor of Pediatrics
Department of Pediatrics
Indiana University School of Medicine
Indianapolis, Indiana

Ellen M. Selkie, MD, MPH
Assistant Professor, Department of
  Pediatrics, University of Wisconsin
  School of Medicine and Public Health
Madison, Wisconsin

Susan M. Sawyer, MBBS, MD, FRACP
Geoff and Helen Handbury Chair of
  Adolescent Health, Department of
  Paediatrics, The University of Melbourne
Director, Centre for Adolescent Health,
  Royal Children's Hospital
Melbourne, Victoria, Australia

Sara Sherer, PhD
Associate Professor of Clinical Pediatrics,
  Department of Pediatrics, USC Keck
  School of Medicine
Director, Behavioral Services, Department
  of Pediatrics, Division of Adolescent
  and Young Adults Medicine, Children's
  Hospital Los Angeles
Los Angeles, California

Lydia A. Shrier, MD, MPH
Associate Professor of Pediatrics, Harvard
  Medical School
Research Director, Division of Adolescent/
  Young Adult Medicine
Co-Director, Center for Adolescent
  Behavioral Health Research
Boston Children's Hospital
Boston, Massachusetts

David M. Siegel, MD, MPH
Professor of Pediatrics, Emeritus
Golisano Children's Hospital
University of Rochester Medical Center
University of Rochester
Rochester, New York

Catherine Silva, MD, MHS
Assistant Professor, Department of
  Pediatrics, Division of Adolescent and
  Young Adult Medicine, Johns Hopkins
  School of Medicine
Assistant Professor, Department of
  Pediatrics, Johns Hopkins All Children's
  Hospital
St. Petersburg, Florida

Rebeccah L. Sokol, PhD, MSPH
Assistant Professor
University of Michigan School of Social
  Work
Ann Arbor, Michigan

Kristin M. W. Stackpole, MD
Clinical Staff Physician IV
The Center for Better Health and Nutrition,
  The Heart Institute
Cincinnati Children's Hospital Medical
  Center
Cincinnati, Ohio

Diane E. J. Stafford, MD
Clinical Professor of Pediatrics, Stanford
  University School of Medicine
Associate Chief, Division of Pediatric
  Endocrinology, Stanford Children's
  Health
Palo Alto, California

Cynthia J. Stein, MD, MPH
Assistant Professor of Orthopaedics,
  Harvard Medical School
Division of Sports Medicine, Boston
  Children's Hospital
Boston, Massachusetts

Lindsay C. Strowd, MD, FAAD
Associate Professor of Dermatology
Wake Forest University School of
  Medicine
Winston-Salem, North Carolina

Jonathan M. Swartz, MD, MMSc
Assistant Professor, Department of
  Pediatrics, Tufts University
Attending Physician, Division of Pediatric
  Endocrinology, Maine Medical Center
Portland, Maine

Heather Taussig, PhD
Professor, Graduate School of Social Work,
  University of Denver
Denver, Colorado
Adjunct Faculty, Kempe Center for the
  Prevention and Treatment of Child Abuse
  and Neglect, University of Colorado
  Anschutz Medical Campus
Aurora, Colorado

Alene Toulany, MD, MSc, FRCPC
Assistant Professor, Department of
  Paediatrics, University of Toronto
Adolescent Medicine Specialist Physician,
  The Hospital for Sick Children
Toronto, Ontario, Canada

Alison C. Tribble, MD, MSCE
Associate Professor of Pediatrics, Department
  of Pediatrics, Division of Pediatric Infectious
  Diseases, University of Michigan
C.S. Mott Children's Hospital
Ann Arbor, Michigan

Shamir Tuchman, MD, MPH
Medical Officer, Division of Pediatric and
  Maternal Health
The U.S. Food and Drug Administration
Silver Spring, Maryland

Sarah A. Van Orman, MD, MMM
Clinical Professor of Family Medicine
Division Health, College Health
Chief Health Officer, USC Student Health
Keck School of Medicine, University of
  Southern California
Los Angeles, California

Lori L. Vanscoy, MD
Assistant Professor, Pediatric Pulmonology
Johns Hopkins Hospital
Baltimore, Maryland

Gabriela Vargas, MD, MPH
Instructor in Pediatrics, Harvard Medical
  School
Attending Physician, Division of
  Adolescent/Young Adult Medicine,
  Boston Children's Hospital
Boston, Massachusetts

Russell M. Viner, CBE FMedSci
Professor, UCL Great Ormond Street
  Institute of Child Health
University College London
London, United Kingdom

Erin A. Vogel, PhD
Assistant Professor, TSET Health
  Promotion Research Center, Stephenson
  Cancer Center
University of Oklahoma Health Sciences
  Center
Oklahoma City, Oklahoma

Leslie R. Walker-Harding, MD
University of Washington Ford Morgan
  Endowed Professor and Chair
Department of Pediatrics
Seattle Children's Hospital Chief Academic
  Officer/Senior Vice President
Seattle, Washington

Joseph L. Ward, MBBS, PhD
NIHR Clinical Lecturer, UCL Great Ormond
  St. Institute of Child Health
University College London
London, United Kingdom

Curren W. Warf, MD, MSEd, FSAHM
Clinical Professor of Pediatrics (Retired),
  Department of Pediatrics
School of Medicine, University of British
  Columbia
Clinical Professor and Head (retired),
  Department of Pediatrics
Division of Adolescent Health and
  Medicine, British Columbia Children's
  Hospital
Berkeley, California

Jonathan D. Warus, MD
Assistant Professor of Clinical Pediatrics
Keck School of Medicine of USC
Children's Hospital Los Angeles
Los Angeles, California

Delma-Jean Watts, MD
Associate Professor of Pediatrics,
  Department of Pediatrics, Alpert Medical
  School of Brown University
Hasbro Children's Hospital
Providence, Rhode Island

Shelly K. Weiss, MD, FRCPC
Professor, Department of Pediatrics,
  University of Toronto
Division of Neurology, The Hospital for
  Sick Children
Toronto, Ontario, Canada

Merrill Weitzel, MD
Instructor, Department of Obstetrics and
  Gynecology and Reproductive Medicine,
  Harvard Medical School
Assistant in Gynecologic Surgery,
  Department of Surgery Division of
  Gynecology, Children's Hospital
Boston, Massachusetts

Elissa R. Weitzman, ScD, MSc
Associate Professor, Department of
  Pediatrics, Harvard Medical School
Associate Scientist, Division of Adolescent
  and Young Adult Medicine, Boston
  Children's Hospital
Boston, Massachusetts

Lea E. Widdice, MD
Associate Professor
Department of Pediatrics, University of
  Cincinnati College of Medicine
Division of Adolescent and Transition
  Medicine, Cincinnati Children's Hospital
  Medical Center
Cincinnati, Ohio

Constance M. Wiemann, PhD
Professor of Pediatrics, Director of
  Research
Department of Pediatrics
Division of Adolescent Medicine & Sports
  Medicine
Baylor College of Medicine
Texas Children's Hospital
Houston, Texas

Lauren E. Wisk, PhD
Assistant Professor, Division of General
  Internal Medicine and Health Services
  Research
David Geffen School of Medicine at the
  University of California Los Angeles
  (UCLA)
Los Angeles, California

Stavra A. Xanthakos
Professor of Pediatrics, Pediatrics,
  University of Cincinnati College of
  Medicine
Attending Physician, Division of
  Gastroenterology, Hepatology &
  Nutrition, Cincinnati Children's
Cincinnati, Ohio

Suellen Moli Yin, MD
Instructor in Pediatrics
Harvard Medical School
Attending Physician, Department of
  Cardiology
Boston Children's Hospital
Boston, Massachusetts

Foreword

I am extremely pleased and honored to write a foreword for the seventh edition of *Adolescent and Young Adult Health Care: A Practical Guide*. This accessible and comprehensive textbook continues to be a trusted resource that keeps adolescent and young adult (AYA)-serving professionals both in the United States and around the globe up to date on the ever evolving needs of AYAs. Adolescent and young adult health requires a broad range of skillsets and timely information in order to provide effective care. Recognizing this, Neinstein's textbook serves as an invaluable reference for not only medical providers, but any professional who works with AYAs.

The seventh edition builds on the practical, in-depth information from previous editions. Chapters on research and quality improvement provide useful and necessary information for better understanding the needs of AYAs, enhancing quality of care, and the continual growth and development of the AYA health field. This edition also adds a chapter on palliative care, death, and dying, reflecting this relatively new area of study's importance and necessity. In addition, a new section on providing health care to marginalized AYAs is essential and a critical addition as focus on health equity and justice for traditionally underserved populations (rightly) continues to increase.

There is a growing recognition that local health conditions both influence and are influenced by health conditions around the globe. This globalization of health is not a new phenomenon, but it has been powerfully exemplified by the global COVID-19 pandemic. COVID-19 is a primary transnational determinant of health and health equity today. Operating in an isolationist fashion will not work in the context of such a strong transnational determinant. It is likely that future innovations in AYA health care will be increasingly influenced by international practice and research. The section of Neinstein's textbook on global health will be very helpful to the understanding and application of AYA health in the global context.

As the world adolescents grow up in becomes more complex and interconnected, so must the field of AYA health. Today's AYAs must contend with the trifecta of the COVID-19 pandemic, resulting financial crisis, and continued racial reckoning. The intersectionality of their experiences and health care needs calls for an interdisciplinary AYA health workforce that understands the specific and evolving challenges they face, communicates clearly, and treats them with respect and compassion. No matter the specific ways that AYA health care responds to adolescents' changing experiences, however, it remains clear that Neinstein's textbook will continue to serve as the authoritative text for AYA clinicians to stay informed and up to date.

Angela Diaz, MD, PhD, MPH
Dean of Global Health, Social Justice, and Human Rights
Jean C. and James W. Crystal Professor, Department of Pediatrics,
Department of Global Health and Health Systems Design
and Department of Environmental Medicine and Public Health
Icahn School of Medicine at Mount Sinai
Director, Mount Sinai Adolescent Health Center (MSAHC)
New York, New York

For many years, Neinstein's textbook has been the major reference for those involved in the clinical care of adolescents and young adults (AYAs) and this seventh edition will not disappoint. Although primarily written for, and by, clinicians in the United States, it has also become the main textbook for those practicing AYA medicine elsewhere. It provides a comprehensive, up-to-date, evidence-based review of all the major conditions affecting the health of AYAs.

The previous edition introduced more information on the state of adolescent health at the population level. In this seventh edition, the new editor-in-chief, Professor Debra Katzman and her editorial team have added new chapters on research, quality improvement, palliative care and end of life, and health care for disenfranchised and marginalized AYAs. These new chapters address issues where AYA health practitioners face unique opportunities and challenges. For example, research with adolescents presents unparalleled opportunities to capitalize on the keenness of many AYAs to engage actively in the research process, but also presents special challenges such as when is parental consent required and how to maintain client confidentiality while respecting the rights of their parents or legal guardians.

This new edition builds on the previous six editions, but incorporates new findings from research and best practices and on guidance from the World Health Organization, the Centers for Disease Control and Prevention (CDC), and other authoritative sources.

Recent initiatives such as the Global Strategy for Women's, Children's and Adolescents Health,[1] the United Nations' Global Accelerated Action for the Health of Adolescents (AA-HA!) Guidance to Support Country Implementation,[2] the WHO Guideline on School Health Services[3] and the WHO-UNESCO Global Standards and Indicators for Health-Promoting Schools and Systems[4] are examples of the global priority being given to adolescent health and well-being and the increased resources that are now available to guide related policies and programs. To supplement these other resources, Neinstein's textbook provides detailed clinical guidance, situated within the context of the important developmental processes, that are happening rapidly within this age group.

The seventh edition of *Neinstein's Adolescent and Young Adult Health Care: A Practical Guide* constitutes an invaluable, well-organized resource to improve and update the competencies of AYA clinicians worldwide.

David A. Ross, MA, MSc, BMBCh, PhD
Extraordinary Professor of Epidemiology and Public Health,
Institute for Life Course Health Research, Department of Global
Health, Stellenbosch University, South Africa. Independent
consultant in adolescent health and well-being. Associate Editor,
Journal of Adolescent Health.

1. Every Woman, Every Child. The global strategy for women's, children's and adolescents' health (2016–2030). United Nations; 2016.
2. WHO/UNAIDS/UNESCO/UNFPA/UNICEF/UN Women/World Bank/PMNCH/EWEC 2017. Global AA-HA! (Accelerated Action for the Health of Adolescents). Guidance to Support Country Implementation. World Health Organization; 2017.
3. WHO, UNESCO. WHO guideline on school health services. World Health Organization; 2021.
4. WHO, UNESCO. Making every school a health-promoting school—Global standards and indicators. World Health Organization; 2021.

For decades *Neinstein's Adolescent and Young Adult Health Care: A Practical Guide* has been the preeminent source of evidence-based practical information for clinicians, educators, researchers, and learners on key topics related to AYA health, health conditions, and health care. The seventh edition of this comprehensive compendium continues this longstanding tradition of being an authoritative interdisciplinary source of clear, concise, and practical information for AYA clinicians and learners with its focus on fundamental issues related to AYA health, including pubertal and psychosocial development, nutrition and growth, chronic and other health conditions, psychosocial influences, and health behaviors. In addition to these foundational topics, this new edition provides insights into emerging issues that affect AYA health, including but not limited to the impact of the global COVID-19 pandemic on adolescents and young adults' mental and physical health, physical activity, and emotional well-being; the changing landscape of societal views on cannabis and the role that evolving laws and regulations have on AYAs' access, use, and misuse of cannabis; and the alarming and increasing rates of sexually transmitted infections and their sequelae have on AYAs' immediate and long-term sexual and reproductive health. This new edition also addresses the health needs and challenges that multiply marginalized, minoritized, and disenfranchised AYAs face including the intersecting effects of poverty, trauma, racism, and stigma. Importantly, the authors provide well-defined recommendations and suggest opportunities for intervening with and empowering young people using a strength-based approach that recognizes existing protective factors, which honors and builds resilience. To effectively address the complex issues surrounding AYA health requires an interdisciplinary team (e.g., medicine, nursing, public health, psychology, social work), multiple points of intervention (e.g., health care delivery, education, research), and a framework that guides the strategies used and addresses the interrelated social and structural determinants of health and health inequities. This textbook offers such a comprehensive perspective as evidenced by its diverse group of editors and contributing authors, the various disciplines represented, the range of topics covered, and the information provided, which touches every point along the health care continuum, including prevention and health care access, delivery, and treatment.

Cherrie B. Boyer, PhD, FSAHM
Professor
Associate Director for Research and Academic Affairs
Department of Pediatrics
Division of Adolescent and Young Adult Medicine
University of California, San Francisco

I am pleased to introduce the seventh edition of Larry *Neinstein's Adolescent and Young Adult Health Care: A Practical Guide*. This book's overview of medical, psychosocial, legal, and other adolescent health issues serves as a resource for clinicians and other professionals who care for young people. This new edition provides additional and welcome information on adolescent health research, quality improvement, service provision for historically underserved adolescents and young adults, and palliative care as well as death and dying.

As a pediatrician and adolescent medicine subspecialist, I am keenly aware of adolescence as a critical life stage in which clinicians can take crucial steps to improve health outcomes and reduce inequities. Adolescents experience physical, mental, emotional, and cognitive changes at the same time that they are developing a strong need for increased independence and autonomy. I feel strongly that health services for adolescents should be delivered in a manner that is comprehensive, equitable, and gender-affirming, and provided in youth-friendly settings where adolescents' ideas and preferences are heard and respected. This book is an important resource for everyone engaged in caring for adolescent patients.

Today's adolescents live in a complex and uncertain world in which technology has been a powerful driver of their experiences and will continue to affect their lives in ways that we cannot predict. Moreover, the COVID-19 pandemic has increased social isolation, experiences of fear and loss, and uncertainties and anxiety for all of us. We are just beginning to understand the impacts of COVID-19 on our youth's mental health from changes in routine, breaks in continuity of learning, missing significant life events, loss of security and safety, and having to cope with death and disease from an earlier stage. Understanding why some young people have thrived during this challenging time, while others have experienced increased psychological distress, is one of the many issues to be explored by further research. One specific example, is the development and worsening of eating disorders in adolescents during the COVID-19 pandemic. Ensuring access to affordable health care, including mental health services, is a critical component of enabling them to have a healthy future as adults.

This new edition will be a touchstone for all of us who are involved in adolescent health policy, research, and practice. It will have a prominent place on my bookshelf.

Rachel L. Levine, MD
Admiral, U.S. Public Health Service Commissioned Corps
Assistant Secretary for Health
U.S. Department of Health and Human Services

Preface

We are pleased to present the seventh edition of *Neinstein's Adolescent and Young Adult Health Care*. This edition is an extraordinary accomplishment for us as it is the first edition without the guiding hand of the founding editor-in-chief, Dr Lawrence S. Neinstein. Dr Neinstein passed away on April 27, 2016 at the age of 66 following a long battle with cancer. He was the editor-in-chief of his beloved textbook through six editions. During that time, *Neinstein's Adolescent and Young Adult Health Care* became the leading textbook on adolescent and young adult (AYA) health.

Dr Lawrence S. Neinstein was an inspiring mentor and teacher, compassionate doctor, extraordinary editor, and a loving husband, father, and grandfather. While he had extremely high standards and exquisite attention to detail, he was at the same time patient and kind. He was highly regarded as an expert on the health of AYAs. *Neinstein's Adolescent and Young Adult Health Care* has always been considered the "go-to" authoritative resource for comprehensive coverage of AYA health issues. For Dr Neinstein, this textbook was a labor of love. His goal for the textbook had always been that it be clinically relevant, practical to use, easy to read, and filled with resources to assist interdisciplinary clinicians in the care of AYAs, and ultimately, to improve the health and well-being of this population. In his final years, more than ever, Dr Neinstein was committed to creating a textbook that promoted teaching and learning about AYA health. As such, we have tried to honor Dr Neinstein's wishes in this seventh edition.

This book contains many new additions, as we continued to strive for it remaining both the most comprehensive textbook on AYA health and—as has been the case for the past 40 years—the one most utilized. This book has a focus on essential information with a goal of providing answers to clinical questions. The seventh edition is organized into 16 sections, including 85 chapters. All chapters include new information, the latest advances, and up-to-date clinical recommendations. New chapters have been added such as Palliative and End-of-Life Care, Quality Improvement Concepts in Adolescent Medicine and Young Adult Health, Research With and About Adolescents and Young Adults, Health Care for Minoritized, Disenfranchised, and Marginalized AYAs. Each chapter contains key illustrations, and comprehensive figures and tables to help the reader understand and remember important points. Websites, appropriate for teenagers, young adults, parents/caregivers, and professionals, are in both the text and reference section, and have been expanded to provide access to up-to-date information where relevant. The seventh edition also has both a print and a companion e-edition, designed to meet the needs of a wide variety of clinicians including pediatricians, family medicine practitioners, gynecologists, internists, psychiatrists, psychologists, nurses, nurse practitioners, physician assistants, medical students, residents, and fellows. The textbook is also ideal for a multitude of settings, including school-based health centers, college health centers, juvenile detention centers, pediatric emergency rooms, and other facilities that serve AYAs.

We are grateful for the expertise and collegiality of our associate editors, Drs S. Todd Callahan, Richard Chung, Alain Joffe, Susan Rosenthal, and Maria Trent. Our associate editors are among the most recognized and respected authorities in the field of AYA health care. They provide a wide range of expertise ranging from gynecology, reproductive endocrinology, mental health issues, and preventive health issues to substance use and sexually transmitted infections. They have been invaluable in continuing to raise the standards of this textbook. In addition to the associate editors, we have brought together the field's most influential authors in AYA health and health care to write these chapters and share their expertise. It has been a privilege to have the opportunity to work with this outstanding group of authors who have done an amazing job creating chapters that synthesize the most current scientific and clinical information to create a practical approach to caring for AYAs. We also wish to thank Nancy Dickson and Thomas Celona at WK who have superbly shepherded the production of the seventh edition.

Finally, we would also like to thank our families: the Katzman Zipursky family—Bob, Jonathan, Carolyn, Amy, and Adam—and the Gordon Bagley family—Bob, Benny, and Jack—for their understanding of the time and effort required to edit a book that attempts to maintain the tradition of Dr Lawrence S. Neinstein. We are grateful for the opportunity to have compiled the seventh edition and are excited about all that it has to offer. We have been privileged to learn so much from Dr Neinstein over the years. The past editions of Dr Neinstein's *Adolescent and Young Adult Health Care* have made a lasting, positive imprint on AYA health. We trust that the seventh edition will keep Dr Neinstein's memory alive and continue to be an important resource for our colleagues and trainees, and ultimately, continue to impact the lives of our patients and their families in a positive way.

Debra K. Katzman, MD, FRCPC
Editor-in-Chief, *Neinstein's Adolescent and Young Adult Health Care: A Practical Guide*

Catherine M. Gordon, MD, MS
Senior Associate Editor, *Neinstein's Adolescent and Young Adult Health Care: A Practical Guide*

Disclaimer

As we edited the seventh edition of Neinstein's, we tried at all times to be mindful that the choice and use of words matter as much when discussing health and health care as it does in other areas of life. To the best of our ability, and in keeping with the American Medical Association's style guide, we have tried to use language that is inclusive and respectful. It is a core value of Neinstein's to accurately capture the wide variety of experiences and perspectives of both our readers and the adolescent and young adult population. We also recognize that language is dynamic, changing as our community learns and evolves.

Family Dedication to Lawrence S. Neinstein

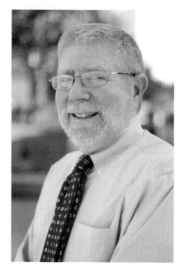

Lawrence S. Neinstein, MD, FACP

Founding Editor-in-Chief of *Adolescent and Young Adult Health Care: A Practical Guide*
1949–2016

Our dad and husband, Larry Neinstein, was a multi-talented and tireless man. Some remember him for bringing out his guitar and singing Bob Dylan's "Forever Young" as SAHM President at the 2007 annual meeting. Others remember him for his relentless focus and determination in creating the world-class Engemann Student Health Center at the University of Southern California. There are those who remember him for being a leader with high ethics and an uncompromising set of values. Still others remember him as their doctor, collaborator, or mentor who listened and cared deeply about equity in health care for adolescents and young adults. And many remember Larry Neinstein for his textbook *Adolescent Health Care: A Practical Guide*, also fondly referred to as *"Neinstein's."*

We are blessed to have memories of each of these aspects of our father and husband along with the more personal memories. He was our biggest supporter, always finding time to help us with a challenging school assignment, coach our sports teams, or work on Quicken to create a family budget. He was the quintessential "project man" capable of checking off multiple to-do lists to perfection, a travel agent for family and friends, and our personal human development teacher.

The first edition of Neinstein's *Adolescent Health Care: A Practical Guide* was written out by hand in 1984 on yellow legal pads by a caring and amazing young physician who was also a father to three young children. Five more editions followed under his keen eye and outstanding leadership. Sadly, Larry lost his battle with cancer in 2016. This seventh edition is now written with love and dedication by those who worked with Larry as colleagues and co-editors of the other editions, and who now carry on his legacy.

Training the next generation of clinicians, researchers, and teachers in adolescent and young adult health was Larry's passion. We hope the pieces of him that are preserved in this seventh edition provide the spark that supports you as you carry out this important work.

The Neinstein Family

Contents

Contributors   vii
Foreword   xv
Preface   xvii
Disclaimer   xix

PART I:	General Considerations in Adolescent and Young Adult Health

CHAPTER 1 Health of the World's Adolescents and Young Adults   2
Joseph L. Ward, John S. Santelli, Gwendolyn Rosen, Russell M. Viner

CHAPTER 2 Normal Physical Growth and Development   35
Jeremi M. Carswell, Diane E. J. Stafford

CHAPTER 3 Psychosocial Development in Normal Adolescents and Young Adults   45
Sara Sherer, Mari Radzik

CHAPTER 4 Office Visit, Interview Techniques, and Recommendations to Parents   50
Gabriela Vargas, Joshua S. Borus

CHAPTER 5 Preventive Health Care for Adolescents and Young Adults   58
Matthew J. Meyers, Elizabeth M. Ozer

CHAPTER 6 Nutrition   78
Michael R. Kohn

CHAPTER 7 Understanding Legal and Ethical Aspects of Care   85
Abigail English, Rebecca Gudeman

CHAPTER 8 Complementary and Integrative Medicine in Adolescents and Young Adults   90
Cora Collette Breuner

CHAPTER 9 Technology and Social Media   98
Megan A. Moreno, Ellen M. Selkie

CHAPTER 10 Chronic Health Conditions in Adolescents and Young Adults   105
Susan M. Sawyer

CHAPTER 11 Palliative Care and End of Life in Adolescents and Young Adults   112
Chana B. Korenblum, Abby R. Rosenberg

CHAPTER 12 Quality Improvement Concepts in Adolescent and Young Adult Health   118
Alene Toulany, Jill S. Huppert

CHAPTER 13 Research with and about Adolescents and Young Adults   127
Elissa R. Weitzman, Lauren E. Wisk

PART II:	Endocrine Disorders

CHAPTER 14 Abnormal Growth and Development   138
Toni Eimicke, Jonathan M. Swartz

CHAPTER 15 Thyroid Function and Disease in Adolescents and Young Adults   151
Cecilia A. Larson

CHAPTER 16   **Diabetes Mellitus   159**
Laura Kester Prakash, Tamara S. Hannon

PART III: **Cardiovascular and Pulmonary Disorders**

CHAPTER 17   **Cardiovascular Health and Cholesterol Disorders   168**
Holly C. Gooding, Jacob C. Hartz

CHAPTER 18   **Syncope, Vertigo, and Sudden Cardiac Arrest   179**
Amy Desrochers DiVasta, Mark E. Alexander

CHAPTER 19   **Heart Murmurs, Congenital Heart Disease, and Acquired Heart Disease   186**
Amy Desrochers DiVasta, Suellen Moli Yin, Mark E. Alexander

CHAPTER 20   **Systemic Hypertension   196**
Matthew B. Rivara, Joseph T. Flynn

CHAPTER 21   **Pulmonary Problems   204**
Lori L. Vanscoy, Peter J. Mogayzel Jr

PART IV: **Musculoskeletal Problems and Sport Medicine**

CHAPTER 22   **Common Musculoskeletal Problems   213**
Ashley Rowatt Karpinos, Keith J. Loud

CHAPTER 23   **Guidelines for Promoting Physical Activity and Sports Participation   229**
Ashley Rowatt Karpinos, Ashlee LaFontaine Enzinger

CHAPTER 24   **Concussion   249**
Michael A. Beasley, Cynthia J. Stein, William P. Meehan III

PART V: **Skin Disorders**

CHAPTER 25   **Acne   256**
Lindsay C. Strowd, Daniel P. Krowchuk

CHAPTER 26   **Miscellaneous Skin Conditions   263**
Lindsay C. Strowd, Daniel P. Krowchuk

PART VI: **Neurologic and Sleep Disorders**

CHAPTER 27   **Epilepsy   277**
Shilpa B. Reddy, Emma G. Carter

CHAPTER 28   **Headaches   286**
Christopher B. Oakley

CHAPTER 29   **Sleep Disorders   293**
Gabrielle Rigney, Shelly K. Weiss

PART VII: **Genitourinary Disorders**

CHAPTER 30   **Renal and Genitourinary Tract Infections in Adolescents and Young Adults   300**
Lawrence J. D'Angelo, Shamir Tuchman

CHAPTER 31   **Enuresis in Adolescents and Young Adults   306**
Joana Dos Santos, Martin A. Koyle

CHAPTER 32   **Asymptomatic Proteinuria and Hematuria   312**
Shamir Tuchman, Lawrence J. D'Angelo

PART VIII: Infectious Diseases

CHAPTER 33   **Infectious Mononucleosis   319**
Catherine Miller, Terrill Bravender

CHAPTER 34   **Infectious Respiratory Illnesses   324**
Terrill Bravender, Alison C. Tribble

CHAPTER 35   **Viral Hepatitis   331**
Mary E. Romano, Anita K. Pai

CHAPTER 36   **Human Immunodeficiency Virus Infections and Acquired Immunodeficiency Syndrome   341**
Jonathan D. Warus, Marvin E. Belzer

PART IX: Conditions Affecting Nutrition and Weight

CHAPTER 37   **Obesity   354**
Kristin M. W. Stackpole, Nancy Crimmins, Stavra A. Xanthakos

CHAPTER 38   **Feeding and Eating Disorders   362**
Debra K. Katzman, Neville H. Golden

PART X: Functional and Unexplained Medical Conditions

CHAPTER 39   **Chronic Noninflammatory Musculoskeletal Pain Disorders   375**
Christina Schutt, Bethany Marston, David M. Siegel

CHAPTER 40   **Fatigue and Myalgic Encephalomyelitis/Chronic Fatigue Syndrome   381**
Peter C. Rowe

CHAPTER 41   **Chronic Abdominal Pain   388**
Wael N. Sayej, Paula K. Braverman

PART XI: Sexuality and Contraception

CHAPTER 42   **Adolescent and Young Adult Sexuality   396**
Devon J. Hensel, Jonathon J. Beckmeyer

CHAPTER 43   **Sexual Minority Adolescents and Young Adults   401**
Jen Makrides, Errol L. Fields

CHAPTER 44   **Transgender Adolescents and Young Adults   408**
Johanna Olson-Kennedy

CHAPTER 45   **Adolescent and Young Adult Pregnancy and Parenting   413**
Joanne E. Cox, Heather M. Bernard

CHAPTER 46   **Contraception   422**
Romina Loreley Barral, Melanie A. Gold

CHAPTER 47   **Barrier Contraceptives and Spermicides   436**
Michelle Forcier

CHAPTER 48   **Contraceptive Pills, Patches, Rings, and Injections   449**
Anita L. Nelson

CHAPTER 49   **Long-Acting Reversible Contraception**   457
Michelle Forcier

PART XII: **Other Reproductive System and Breast Disorders**

CHAPTER 50   **Gynecologic Examination of the Adolescent and Young Adult**   468
Sarah Pitts, Merrill Weitzel

CHAPTER 51   **Normal Menstrual Physiology**   474
Sari L. Kives, Niamh C. Murphy

CHAPTER 52   **Dysmenorrhea and Premenstrual Disorders**   477
Paula K. Braverman

CHAPTER 53   **Abnormal Uterine Bleeding**   484
Beth I. Schwartz, Laurie A. P. Mitan

CHAPTER 54   **Amenorrhea, the Polycystic Ovary Syndrome, and Hirsutism**   488
Shannon Fitzgerald, Catherine M. Gordon, Amy Fleischman

CHAPTER 55   **Cervical Cancer Screening and Management of Abnormal Tests**   501
Anna-Barbara Moscicki

CHAPTER 56   **Vaginitis and Vaginosis**   507
Maria H. Rahmandar, Paula K. Braverman

CHAPTER 57   **Pelvic Masses**   514
Paula J. Adams Hillard

CHAPTER 58   **Ectopic Pregnancy**   525
Melissa Mirosh

CHAPTER 59   **Male Genitourinary Health and Disorders**   530
William P. Adelman

CHAPTER 60   **Breast Disorders and Gynecomastia**   539
Amy Desrochers DiVasta

PART XIII: **Sexually Transmitted Infections**

CHAPTER 61   **Overview of Sexually Transmitted Infections**   549
Lea E. Widdice

CHAPTER 62   **Neisseria Gonorrhoeae and Chlamydia Trachomatis**   555
Catherine Silva, Renata Arrington Sanders

CHAPTER 63   **Pelvic Inflammatory Disease**   563
Lydia A. Shrier

CHAPTER 64   **Syphilis**   569
Teresa A. Batteiger

CHAPTER 65   **Herpes Genitalis**   578
Christine Johnston

CHAPTER 66   **Human Papillomavirus Infection and Anogenital Warts**   584
LaKeshia N. Craig, Jessica A. Kahn

CHAPTER 67   Other Sexually Transmitted Infections Including Genital Ulcers, Pediculosis, Scabies, and Molluscum   591
Mandakini Sadhir, Sinduja Lakkunarajah, M. Susan Jay

PART XIV: Substance Use and Substance Use Disorders

CHAPTER 68   Adolescent and Young Adult Substance Use   602
Holly Schroder, Jillian R. Hagerman, Leslie R. Walker-Harding

CHAPTER 69   Alcohol   614
Rachel H. Alinsky, Scott E. Hadland

CHAPTER 70   Tobacco   622
Judith J. Prochaska, Erin A. Vogel

CHAPTER 71   Marijuana   633
Jesse D. Hinckley, Kevin M. Gray

CHAPTER 72   Psychoactive Substance Use   637
Diana D. Deister, Sharon Levy, William Riccardelli

CHAPTER 73   Approaches to Adolescent and Young Adult Substance Use   651
Sharon Levy, Elissa R. Weitzman, Tamara Itzel Martinez

PART XV: Mental Health

CHAPTER 74   Depression and Anxiety Disorders   660
Daphne J. Korczak, Suneeta Monga

CHAPTER 75   Suicide and Suicidal Behaviors in Adolescents and Young Adults   671
Lisa M. Horowitz, Annabelle M. Mournet, Maryland Pao

CHAPTER 76   Neurodevelopmental Differences and Disorders in Adolescents and Young Adults   676
Celia B. Neavel, Ellen Stubbe Kester, Kassandra Gonzalez

CHAPTER 77   Youth Violence   691
Todd I. Herrenkohl, Lisa Fedina, Rebeccah L. Sokol, Louise Ashwell

CHAPTER 78   Evaluating and Supporting Adolescents and Young Adults Who Have Experienced Sexual Violence   696
Constance M. Wiemann, Elizabeth Miller, Mariam R. Chacko

PART XVI: Special Populations

CHAPTER 79   College Health   706
Sarah A. Van Orman, James R. Jacobs

CHAPTER 80   Youth and Young Adults in the Military   717
Patricia E. Kapunan, William P. Adelman

CHAPTER 81   Youth Experiencing Homelessness   723
Meera S. Beharry, Lauren Bretz, Colette (Coco) Auerswald, Curren W. Warf

CHAPTER 82   Youth in and Emancipated from Out-of-Home Care   729
Heather Taussig, Scott B. Harpin, William R. Betts, Gretchen J. Russo, James Kaferly, Renée Marquardt

CHAPTER 83   Juvenile Detention and Incarcerated Youth and Young Adults   733
Matthew C. Aalsma, Allyson L. Dir, Rebecca M. Beyda, Katherine Schwartz

CHAPTER 84   **Immigrant Adolescents and Young Adults   738**
Carol Lewis, Delma-Jean Watts

CHAPTER 85   **Health Care for Minoritized, Disenfranchised, and Marginalized Adolescent and Young Adults   743**
Pamela A. Matson, Faye Korich

Index   751

General Considerations in Adolescent and Young Adult Health

CHAPTER 1

Health of the World's Adolescents and Young Adults

Joseph L. Ward
John S. Santelli
Gwendolyn Rosen
Russell M. Viner

KEY WORDS

- Adolescent-friendly care
- Demography
- Disability-adjusted life years (DALYs)
- Fertility
- Global health
- Health disparities
- Health status
- Life course
- Morbidity and mortality
- Social determinants of health
- Social transitions

INTRODUCTION

Adolescents and young adults (AYAs) comprise almost one-quarter (23%) of the world's population.[1] By 2025, a projected 1.3 billion adolescents (10 to 19 years) and 0.6 billion young adults (20 to 24 years) will inhabit the earth.[2] These AYAs will represent the largest cohort of young people in human history.[3] This "youth bulge," seen particularly in rapidly developing low- and middle-income countries (LMICs), has the potential to deliver a substantial economic and productivity dividend, as this increasingly better-educated generation of youth enters the workforce.

Adolescence and young adulthood have long been considered the healthiest times of life and have historically received little attention in terms of global health policy and financing. However, recently a wider recognition of AYA health has emerged including the influence of AYA health trajectories on future adult health and the health of the next generation.[4] Reflecting this, adolescents are increasingly included within global health strategies and initiatives, including within the United Nations (UN) Every Woman Every Child agenda, the *Countdown to 2030* collaboration to track progress toward the Sustainable Development Goals (SDGs), and the work of the Global Financing Facility.

However, there are ongoing concerns that health priorities in this age group are being neglected.[3] Globally, large numbers of deaths which occur among AYAs are avoidable, including those due to intentional and unintentional injuries, maternal mortality, and human immunodeficiency virus (HIV) infection.[5] Further, the rate of reduction in AYA mortality rates has lagged behind that of younger children in many regions of the world and is now higher than in children 1 to 4 years old in many high-, middle-, and some low-income countries.[6] Economic development and the sharp reduction in infectious diseases have resulted in improved child survival and created the "youth bulge" seen globally and in many LMICs. Yet, the same rapid social and economic change has often created adverse consequences for the health of AYAs. Indeed, AYA mortality from motor vehicle crashes (MVCs) and other transport injuries, suicide, substance use, and deaths due to violence is rising in many countries.[5]

Behaviors during this stage of the life course are critical determinants of current and future health. These behaviors are also profoundly shaped by social determinants, including poverty, socioeconomic disparities, access to education and employment, connectedness to schools and communities, and the influence of peers.[7,8] Five of the 10 major risk factors for poor lifelong health identified in the Global Burden of Disease (GBD) study 2019 largely originate during adolescent and young adult time period[9]; they are smoking, excess alcohol intake, obesity/overweight, poor diet, and physical inactivity.

Health issues among young adults (20 to 24 years) increasingly resemble those among adolescents (10 to 19 years), given intersecting social trends toward longer engagement in formal education and delays in marriage and childbearing.[1] Thus, these key social transitions of adolescence which once occurred in late adolescence now occur during the adult years. As a result, the time span from puberty to adult social and financial independence in developed countries has greatly increased. For example, gap from the median age at menarche to childbearing in the United States rose from 9.5 years for women born during 1940s to 15.5 years among those born in 1982.[10] This is a global phenomenon, with similar trends in high-income countries and LMICs.

This chapter addresses the health status of the world's AYAs. It begins with an integrated conceptual framework combining social determinants and life-course influences on the health of AYAs (Fig. 1.1).[4,7] The chapter then reviews global data on AYA mortality, morbidity, and health behaviors to characterize variations in AYA health and health determinants around the globe. Although a review of effective programs is beyond the scope of this chapter, we identify the health implications of our framework. The final part of this chapter reviews data sources that monitor the health of AYAs—over time and between nations—which can be used to inform specific policies and interventions to improve outcomes. Key terms used in this chapter are defined in Table 1.1.

SOCIAL DETERMINANTS

The World Health Organization (WHO) defines social determinants of health as "the conditions in which people are born, grow, live, work, and age."[2] Health services and health prevention often focus on individual-level risks and behaviors (see Chapters 4 and 5), while the social determinants approach recognizes the health impact of factors at family, peer group, school, community, national, and even global levels. As illustrated in the model shown in Figure 1.1, social determinants may have positive effects on resilience and health-enhancing behaviors as well as negative effects by increasing risk and harmful behaviors. Importantly, a social determinants framework can guide the development of health-enhancing policies and programs

Health Needs and Social Determinants

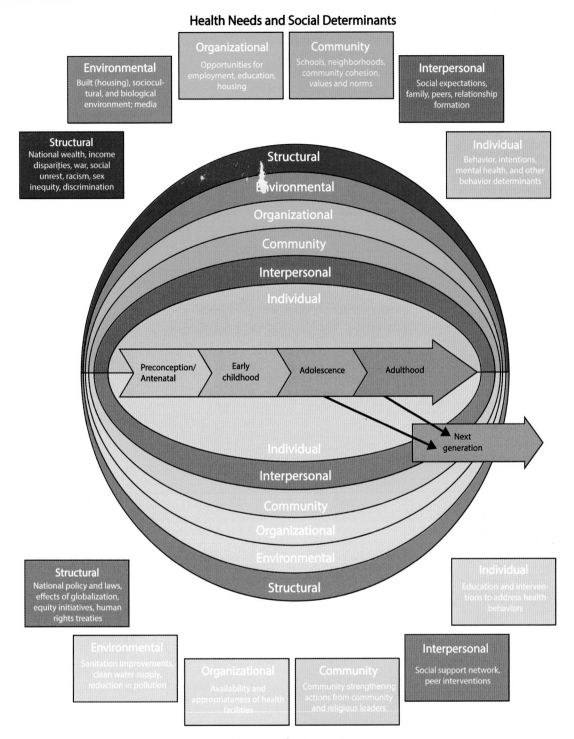

Actions and Interventions

FIGURE 1.1 Conceptual framework for social determinants of adolescent health and corresponding interventions from a life-course perspective. During the puberty and social role transitions of adolescence, health needs and health actions must reflect one another for optimal health. This investment in adolescent health results in a triple return on investment for adolescents, adults, and the next generation. Structural (or distal) factors include structural, environmental, and organizational determinants and corresponding interventions, while proximal factors include organizational, community, and interpersonal. Each layer of structural or proximal influence within adolescent's social context contains multiple touchpoints. The effect of social determinants on health needs and corresponding health actions is also influenced by exposure to both risk and preventative factors, as well as resiliency of the adolescent. (Adapted from World Health Organization. Health for the World's Adolescents: A Second Chance in the Second Decade. World Health Organization; 2014; adapted from Patton GC, Sawyer SM, Santelli JS, et al. Our future: a Lancet commission on adolescent health and wellbeing. *Lancet*. 2016;387(10036):2423–2478.)

TABLE 1.1	
Key Terms and Definitions for This Chapter	
Key Term	**Definition**
Adolescent fertility rate	Number of live births in a specified period of time in a population of females between 15 and 19 y of age[a]
Adolescent-friendly care	As developed by WHO, a framework for the delivery of health services to adolescents that addresses the five domains of equity, effectiveness, accessibility, acceptability, and appropriateness of care[b]
All-cause mortality	Death rate from all causes of death in a defined population within a specified period of time
Demographic dividend	A population's potential for economic growth following a demographic transition in which there is a shift toward more working-age people than dependents in the population. This economic growth hinges on structural factors such as sociopolitical climate[c]
Demographic transition	A country's shift from high birth and death rates to low fertility, low mortality, and longer life expectancy as a result of economic development[c]
Disability-adjusted life years (DALY)	A time-based measure of overall disease burden, calculated as the sum of the years of life lost due to premature mortality (YLLs) and years of life lost due to time lived in states (i.e., personal circumstances) of less than full health (YLDs)[d]
Disease-specific mortality	Death rate from a specific morbidity in a defined population within a specified period of time
Epidemiologic transition	Changes in patterns of mortality and morbidity as a population transitions from high mortality (high infant, maternal, and child mortality, famine, and infectious diseases) to lower mortality related to chronic and noncommunicable disease. The epidemiologic transition typically accompanies the demographic transitions
Fertility rate	Number of live births in a specified time period in a population of females between 15 and 44 y of age[e]
Global Burden of Disease (GBD) study	The most comprehensive, publicly available global observational epidemiologic study to date. The first GBD study of 1990 was commissioned by the World Bank and significantly impacted global health policy. GBD was then institutionalized by the World Health Organization (WHO); today it is led by Institute for Health Metrics and Evaluation (IHME) at the University of Washington with over 3,600 contributing researchers from more than 145 countries. This chapter references the 2019 report, the latest data at the time of publication. The 2019 study includes data from 204 countries and covers 369 diseases and injuries and 87 risk factors[f,g]
Health care transition	The process of changing from pediatric to adult-centered health care, including shifts in parent/caregiver involvement in an adolescent's care. This is often a period of disruption in health services for adolescents. Smooth transition processes have been shown to improve health outcomes
Incidence	New cases of a disease, injury, or events in a population within a specified period of time[h]
Life-course perspective	Body of evidence that health is influenced not only by current risk factors and social determinants, but also by factors from earlier in an individual's life. Adolescence is a key influential period in lifelong health trajectories
Migrant	A person who resides away from their usual residence, either within their home country or across international borders
Mortality rate	Number of deaths in a defined population (often by 100,000 population) within a specified period of time[i]
Not in education, employment, or training (NEET)	"Not in education, employment, or training." This umbrella terms refers to people who are not gaining experience in the workforce, not receiving an income, and not advancing their education or learning new skills[j]
Obesity and overweight	An abnormal or excessive fat accumulation that results in a risk to health. Body mass index (BMI) is the most common classification of weight class and is calculated by weight (kg) divided by height (meters) squared; BMI over 25 is classified as overweight and BMI over 30 is considered obese[k]
Organisation for Economic Co-Operation and Development (OECD) Countries	The 37 member countries of the OECD, an international organization working to establish international standards and solutions for social, economic, and environmental challenges
Prevalence	Current cases of a disease or injury in a population at a specified point in time[l]
Relative poverty	The share of people having less income than half the national median income (OECD definition)[m]
Social determinants of health	"The conditions in which people are born, grow, live, work, and age" that impact health status. For adolescents, these include structural factors (e.g., political, economic, education, and welfare systems) as well as proximal factors (e.g., peers, family, community, schools)[n]

TABLE 1.1

Key Terms and Definitions for This Chapter (*Continued*)

Key Term	Definition
Social transitions	A series of life-course transitions in the shift from childhood to adulthood. These include puberty, leaving school, entering the workforce, childbearing and marriage, and are influenced by the cultural norms of a particular time and place
Years lived with disability (YLDs)	Measure of years of healthy life lost due to disability or ill-health
Years of life lost from mortality (YLLs)	Measure of premature mortality that accounts for both frequency of deaths and the age at which death occurs

[a]World Health Organization. Global Health Observatory (GHO)—Adolescent Fertility. Accessed June 28, 2022. https://www.who.int/data/gho/indicator-metadata-registry/imr-details/3
[b]World Health Organization. Adolescent friendly health services: An agenda for change Geneva: World Health Organization, 2002.
[c]Das Gupta M, Engelman R, Levy J, et al., The Power of 1.8 Billion: Adolescents, Youth and the Transformation of the Future New York: United Nations Population Fund 2014.
[d]World Health Organization. Global Health Observatory—Disability-adjusted life years (DALYs). Accessed April 20, 2021. https://www.who.int/data/gho/indicator-metadata-registry/imr-details/158
[e]Centers for Disease Control and Prevention. Principles of Epidemiology in Public Health Practice, Third Edition. An Introduction to Applied Epidemiology and Biostatistics—Natality. Accessed April 20, 2021. https://www.cdc.gov/csels/dsepd/ss1978/lesson3/section4.html
[f]Institute for Health Metrics and Evaluation. About GBD. Accessed April 20, 2021. http://www.healthdata.org/gbd/about
[g]The Lancet. Global Burden of Disease. Accessed April 20, 2021. https://www.thelancet.com/gbd#searchContent
[h]Centers for Disease Control and Prevention. Principles of Epidemiology in Public Health Practice, Third Edition, An Introduction to Applied Epidemiology and Biostatistics—Morbidity. Accessed April 20, 2021. https://www.cdc.gov/csels/dsepd/ss1978/lesson3/section2.html
[i]Centers for Disease Control and Prevention. Principles of Epidemiology in Public Health Practice, Third Edition, An Introduction to Applied Epidemiology and Biostatistics—Mortality. Accessed April 20, 2021. https://www.cdc.gov/csels/dsepd/ss1978/lesson3/section3.html
[j]International Labour Office, Global Employment Trends for Youth 2020: Technology and the future of jobs. Geneva, Switzerland: International Labour Office, 2020.
[k]World Health Organization. Obesity and overweight. Accessed April 20, 2021. https://www.who.int/news-room/fact-sheets/detail/obesity-and-overweight
[l]Centers for Disease Control and Prevention. Principles of Epidemiology in Public Health Practice, Third Edition An Introduction to Applied Epidemiology and Biostatistics—Morbidity. Accessed April 20, 2021. https://www.cdc.gov/csels/dsepd/ss1978/lesson3/section2.html
[m]OECD. Crisis squeezes income and puts pressure on inequality and poverty. Accessed April 20, 2021. https://www.oecd.org/els/soc/OECD2013-Inequality-and-Poverty-8p.pdf
[n]World Health Organization, Closing the gap in a generation: Health equity through action on the social determinants of health. Geneva, 2008.

from efforts to reduce poverty, expand education opportunities, strengthen families and schools, reduce exposure to environmental and other risks, and provide health-enhancing role models.

The WHO Commission on the Social Determinants of Health[7] differentiates fundamental structural factors (e.g., political, economic, education, and welfare systems) and more proximal factors that influence the "circumstances of daily life." Proximal factors include social institutions (e.g., families, peers, and schools), food, housing, recreation, access to education and employment, and social and financial independence. The importance of various structural and proximal influences on AYA health is discussed below.

Structural Determinants of Health

Structural determinants of health include social policies and programs, economic policies, and politics that may create poor and unequal living conditions, which affect the health of populations. These structural determinants operate within countries, but increasingly operate between countries due to the effects of globalization and can explain much of the differences observed in poor health experienced by populations.

Income

National wealth and the distribution of income within countries are important determinants of many AYA health outcomes.

Globally, rising national income is associated with improvements in health status, with mortality and adolescent fertility far lower in high-income compared with low-income countries.

- In 2019, mortality rates per 100,000 population in 15- to 19-year-olds ranged from 23 in Denmark to 370 in Lesotho among males, and 12 in Japan to 248 in Lesotho among females (Fig. 1.2).[5]
- Adolescent fertility varies considerably between countries.[11] In 2019, the global fertility rate for 15- to 19-year-old females was 40 births per 1,000, but rates ranged from 1.4 in South Korea to 183 in Chad.[12] Fertility rates are profoundly influenced by structural determinants including national wealth, income inequalities, and expenditures on education; likewise, declines over time in adolescent fertility are shaped by structural determinants (Fig. 1.3).[11] The largest declines are occurring

in South Asia, Europe/Central Asia, and the Middle East/North Africa—regions with lower income inequalities (Figs. 1.4 and 1.5). National strategies to reduce adolescent fertility should include investments in economic development, job creation, and improvement and expansion of schooling—in addition to improving access to contraception.

- The strength of associations between national income and health appears to be weaker in adolescents than in young children.[13] Indeed, rapid economic growth can result in a transient increase in fatal and nonfatal injuries, of which adolescents are particularly vulnerable, as the introduction of safety legislation and appropriate infrastructure may lag behind rising demand for transportation.[13]
- Associations between national income and rates of injury and violence among AYAs are weaker than for other health outcomes, and rates of smoking among AYAs are higher in wealthier countries.[14]
- In contrast to national wealth, inequality in per capita income within a country appears to be equally damaging throughout the life course, and thus may be of greater relative importance to outcomes during adolescence.[13]
- The effect of income inequality within a country has a variable association between health outcomes. In one study, income inequality was positively associated with bullying, teenage pregnancy, HIV prevalence, and mortality outcomes for young people; however, no significant associations were found with smoking, violence, and injuries.[14]

Importantly, despite rising national wealth and improving health statistics within a country, health inequalities often persist.

- Inequality in household incomes is substantially higher in the United States compared to peer nations like those in Western Europe.
- Since the 1980s, the United States has had consistently higher poverty rates compared to peer high-income countries. Intergenerational economic mobility is also notably low, with more stagnation for Black populations compared to White populations.[8] This inequality is reflected in greater disparities in AYA health outcomes such as rates of teen pregnancy.

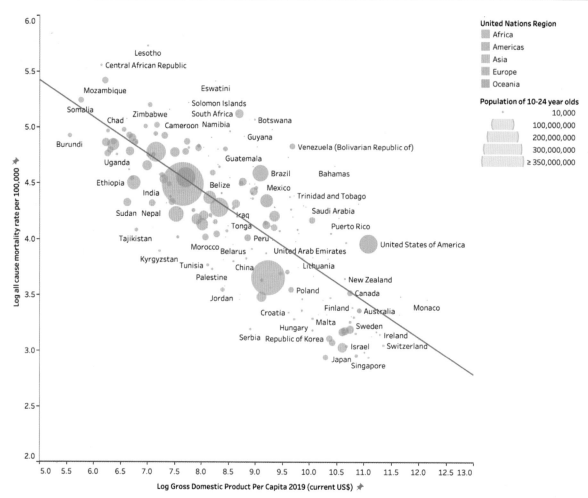

FIGURE 1.2 Mortality rate in 10- to 24-year-olds by Gross Domestic Product per capita. (Source: Data from Institute for Health Metrics Evaluation. Global Burden of Disease Study 2019, custom data acquired via website.)

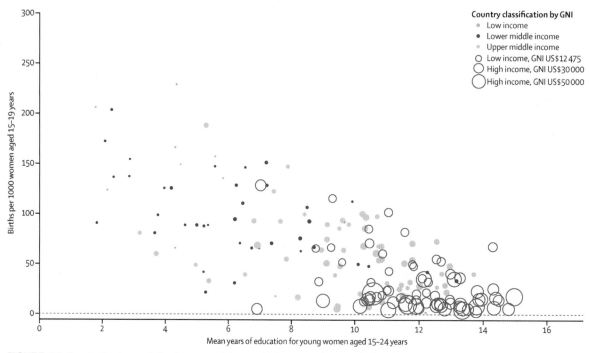

FIGURE 1.3 Country-level association between adolescent birth rates and years of education in 2010–2012. GNI, Gross national income defined as gross domestic product, plus net receipts from abroad of compensation of employees, property income, and net taxes less subsidies on production. (Source: Patton GC, Sawyer SM, Santelli JS, et al. Our future: a Lancet commission on adolescent health and wellbeing. *Lancet.* 2016;387(10036):2423–2478.)

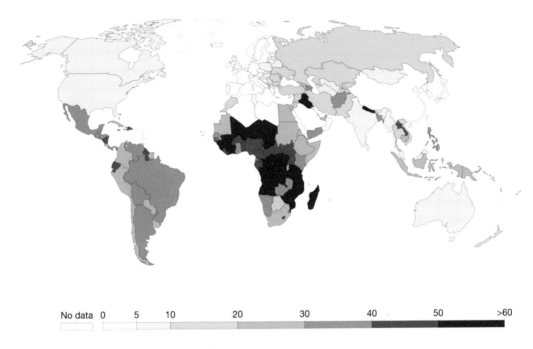

Adolescent birth rate in women aged 10-19 years, 2016

Number of livebirths per 1,000 women aged 10-19 years (defined as the adolescent fertility rate).

Our World in Data

No data   0   5   10   20   30   40   50   >60

Source: Institute for Health Metrics & Evaluation (IHME)   CC BY

FIGURE 1.4 Global map of adolescent birth rate in females aged 10 to 19 years, 2016. (Source: Global Burden of Disease Collaborative Network. Global Burden of Disease Study 2016 (GBD 2016) Health-related Sustainable Development Goals (SDG) Indicators 1990–2030. Seattle, United States: Institute for Health Metrics and Evaluation 2017. Published online at OurWorldInData.org. https://ourworldindata. org/grapher/adolescent-fertility-ihme)

- Understanding social gradients in AYA health requires analyzing relevant data on household income and other measures of socioeconomic status (SES). However, many countries, including the United States, do not routinely collect these data. The United States does routinely collect health data by race and ethnicity, although these data reflect the impact on health of racism, stigma, and discrimination, in addition to SES.

Education

Education has a powerful influence on health across the lifespan. The wealth of nations and of individual families influences access to education; therefore, education is also an indicator of social and economic empowerment. Financial insecurity and family instability may limit the opportunity for youth to continue education. Globally, rising educational attainment is associated with improved health status, among nations and among families within nations. Higher parental educational attainment is associated with improved child and adolescent health, and education is commonly perceived as a gateway to social advancement by families and political leaders.

Mechanisms through which education affects health outcomes are complex. Education is likely to bring increased earnings and access to resources, increase understanding of health, and increase one's willingness to adopt certain health behaviors now to reap health benefits in the future. These mechanisms independently improve health, but also affect the peer groups with whom young people spend time, further influencing outcomes. There are also direct effects of health education which occurs in schools, and prevention in participating in risky behaviors while in an education setting.[4]

- Although much of the focus on health benefits of education has been on primary education, higher rates of attendance in secondary education are associated with lower rates of injuries, teen births, HIV prevalence, and overall mortality.[4]
- The health effects are particularly marked among females, who are less likely to attend secondary school in some countries.
- Globally, there have been large increases in the number of young people in education, but improvements have slowed in recent years. United Nations Educational, Scientific and Cultural Organization (UNESCO) estimated that there were almost 200 million adolescents between 12 and 17 years old who were not in education in 2016. This is around 16% of 12- to 14-year-olds and 36% of 15- to 17-year-olds. There is also huge variation between regions, with the highest proportion of AYAs not in education in sub-Saharan Africa (SSA) at 36.6% of 12- to 14-year-olds, and 57.8% of 15- to 17-year-olds.[15]
- These differences are reflected in literacy rates in 15- to 24-year-olds. The United Nations International Children's Emergency Fund (UNICEF) estimates the global literacy rate of 15- to 24-year-olds to be more than 90%. However, in Nigeria, around a quarter of 15- to 24-year-olds are illiterate, and more than half of AYAs in Mali and Central African Republic are illiterate.[16]
- Associations between education and AYA health are also found in high-income countries. In the United States, educational gaps in life expectancy have widened over the past two decades. Over the course of the 2010s, those with a 4-year college degree experienced an increase in life expectancy while those without saw a decline. This trend was consistent among both Black and White Americans.[17]
- Among youth, connectedness to school, higher academic achievement, and school attendance are associated with lower rates of health-risk behaviors.[4]
- Educational and parenting support for young mothers significantly improves health outcomes of their children in adolescence (see Life-Course Perspective section).[13]

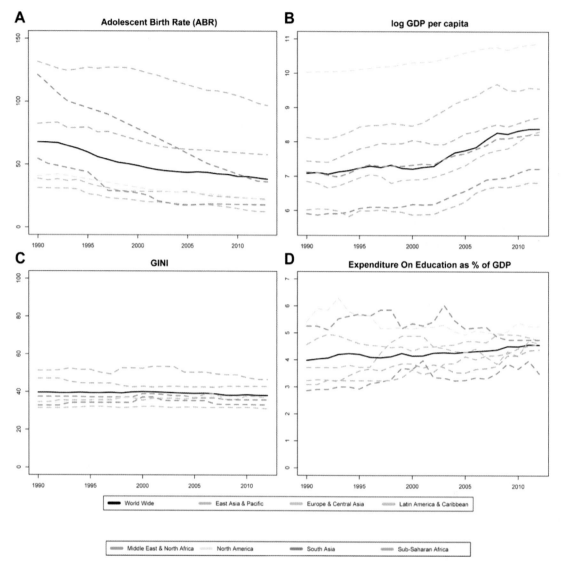

FIGURE 1.5 Worldwide and regional trends in median adolescent birth rate (**A**), log Gross Domestic Product (**B**), income inequalities (Gini index) (**C**), and expenditures on education as % of Gross Domestic Product (**D**), 1990–2012. GDP, Gross Domestic Product. (Source: Santelli JS, Song X, Garbers S, et al. Global trends in adolescent fertility, 1990–2012, in relation to national wealth, income inequalities, and educational expenditures. *J Adolesc Health.* 2017;60(2):161–168.)

Employment

Employment is a key determinant of AYA health and is closely linked with education. Globally, the International Labour Office estimates that 22.2% of young people aged 15 to 24 years were not in education, employment, or training (NEET) in 2019, and this percentage is predicted to increase in the coming years. Global estimates for females (31.1%) are almost double those for males (13.9%).[18] Adolescents and young adults in the United States who are identified as NEET more commonly report poor health status compared to AYAs who remain in school or employment.[19]

- Globally, young people aged 15 to 24 years are three times more likely to be unemployed than adults.[18]
- In the United States, unemployment rates among young adults are consistently around twice as high as the overall adult rate. In 2021, the unemployment rate for young adults (age 16 to 24 years) was between 13% and 18%, compared to under 8% for all other age groups.[20]
- Employment is an example of how indirect effects of the COVID-19 pandemic have disproportionally affected AYAs. Adolescents and young adults are more likely than older adults to work in sectors where restrictions have been introduced in many countries and

are at greater risk of losing employment and reporting reduced earnings during the pandemic.[5]

Migration

Another structural determinant of health is migration. There is no accepted definition for the term "migrant" under international law. The UN describes a migrant as a person who moves away from their usual place of residence, both temporarily or permanently, and both within a country or across international borders. Migration from rural to urban areas is common in LMICs. Adolescents and young adults may migrate for a variety of reasons, including seeking education or employment. Adolescents and young adults may be forced to migrate due to conflict, violence, persecution, or coercion. Migrant populations may be exposed to additional health risks because of the circumstances around their displacement, transit, and host country. These may compound inherent vulnerabilities of AYAs related to the physical, psychological, social, and educational transitions that occur during adolescence.

- Globally, in 2019, around 271 million people (3.5% of the world's population) lived outside their country of origin, of which around 40 million are aged 10 to 24 years (2.1% of total population).[21]

- Health needs and outcomes among migrant populations are varied. Studies of health outcomes for adult migrants suggest that some may be healthier than the general population (the "Healthy Migrant Effect"), although the evidence supporting this among AYAs is mixed.[22]
- Specific health risks of migrant AYAs are likely to include those related to mental health, nutrition, and infectious diseases, but will also include complexities of managing chronic non-communicable diseases.[22]
- Adolescents and young adults who are migrant workers may be exposed to increased occupational health risks and rates of both fatal and non-fatal injuries are higher in migrant compared with non-migrant populations.[22]
- Adolescents and young adults aged 15 to 19 years make up a large proportion of unaccompanied migrants, who face multiple increased health risks and are particularly vulnerable to unsafe employment, and sexual and physical violence.[22]
- Involuntary migration includes trafficking for sexual or labor exploitation.
- Migration from rural to urban settings may bring health risks and potential benefits to AYAs. In addition to potential economic benefits for AYAs and their families, there may be increased opportunities for education. However, separation from family support through migration can increase vulnerabilities, and rapid urbanization can increase health risks which are relevant to AYAs, including those related to injury, exposure to violence, hazardous substance use, and unsafe employment.[4]

War and Conflict

Conflict is likely to affect health outcomes among AYAs in many ways, although analyses exploring this are sparse. The effects of conflict are likely to include direct injuries and mental health sequelae, as well as indirect impacts resulting from forced displacement, and disruption of health services, food supply, housing, education, and employment opportunities.[23]

- The UN estimates that 82.4 million worldwide were forcibly displaced in 2020, of whom more than half were internally displaced. Approximately 12% of forcibly displaced people in 2020 were between 12 and 17 years old.[24]
- Specific health threats for AYAs related to conflict include increased vulnerability to sexual violence, early marriage, and exploitation.[23]
- Maternal mortality in conflict settings has been shown to increase, contributing to 10% of all conflict-attributable deaths in females in one analysis of armed conflicts in Africa.[25]
- Child soldiers are at particular risk. They are more likely to experience poor health outcomes than their peers, although education and family appear to confer a degree of protection.

Sex Inequality

Starting at puberty, sex is an increasingly important determinant of social roles, strongly influenced by cultural and religious factors. "Health outcomes by sex diverge throughout adolescence". Globally, females have a greater prevalence of poor self-reported health and psychological complaints, while males have "higher rates of injury, overweight/obesity, and overall mortality". At the country level, sex inequality (as measured by the UN's Sex Inequality Index) is an independent predictor of poor health outcomes for both sexes,[14] suggesting that sex inequality may be harmful for young males as well as young females.

Sexual orientation and gender identity is commonly established during adolescence.[4] Sexual minority youth, those who are lesbian, gay, bisexual, transgender, and queer or questioning (LGBTQ) about their sexual orientation and gender identity, frequently experience stigma and discrimination and are at risk for poor health outcomes. Poor mental health, including depression and suicide, may be a direct result of bullying and harassment

directed toward these AYAs. Efforts to improve the acceptance of diverse sexual identities within schools can diminish or eliminate the mental health disparities between LGBTQ adolescents and their straight peers.[26]

Racism

Racism is a social determinant of health that has a profound impact on the health status of children, AYAs, and their families.[27] Discrimination is pervasive within and across societies and can be based on skin color, physical characteristics or disabilities, language, religion, caste, sexual orientation and gender identity, national origin, and other physical or cultural characteristics. Discrimination affects various groups in specific communities. For example, in the United States, racism against persons of African origin has had a 400-year history beginning with chattel slavery, continuing through the Jim Crow era of legal and structural discrimination, and persists to this day exemplified by residential segregation, health disparities, and shootings of Black men by the police. Racism interacts with other social determinants such as education and income. For example, Hispanic and Black populations in the United States saw their life expectancy decrease between 2018 and 2020 by 3.88 and 3.25 years, respectively, while White populations only experienced a decrease of 1.36 years in the same period.[28]

Proximal Social Factors

More proximal determinants of health include the social institutions that directly influence AYAs. These include neighborhoods, schools, and families and encompass access to housing, education, recreation, food, and employment. These social factors have been shown to influence a wide variety of AYA health outcomes (see Fig. 1.1).

Neighborhood

Living in a poor neighborhood is associated with a range of adverse outcomes, including lower educational attainment, poorer mental health, and higher rates of teen pregnancy and youth violence. In addition to the structural effects of poverty described earlier, area-level deprivation is partly mediated through reduced social capital, which reduces resilience and opportunities available to AYAs.

School

Enjoyment and engagement with school (often described as school-connectedness) is associated with reduced substance use, better mental health, and a range of other health outcomes.[29] Schools can also play an important role in improving health, both through public health interventions (e.g., drug prevention programs and sex education) or through on-site health services, which have been shown to improve the quality of services young people receive and increase use of appropriate contraception.[30]

Families

While family influences are less dominant in AYAs than in early childhood, family connectedness and parental involvement remain important protective factors. Conversely, parental behaviors such as smoking, alcohol, and violence are all associated with higher rates of these behaviors among their children.

Orphanhood

Orphanhood (death of a parent or both parents) is associated with a variety of adverse physical and mental health and social consequences among adolescents including mental health distress, truncation of education, child marriage, and behavioral risk for HIV. Orphanhood is more common where adult mortality is higher (as in LMICs) and where HIV infection is prevalent, such as SSA. For example, UNICEF has estimated that between 1990 and 2015, 10.9 million children and adolescents (age 0 to 17 years) in SSA had lost one or both parents to HIV/acquired immunodeficiency syndrome

(AIDS).[31] The effect of the COVID-19 pandemic on orphanhood among adolescents may be considerable, with global estimates of more than 1 million children and adolescents experiencing the death of a primary parent/caregiver during the pandemic.[32]

Peers

The influence of peers becomes particularly important during early and middle adolescence.[29] Supportive peer relationships are associated with improved mental health outcomes, and so peer-led health interventions may offer an effective way to improve health behaviors. Peers can also negatively impact health. Unhealthy behaviors by peers increase the risk of adolescents experiencing adverse outcomes, including substance use, teenage pregnancy, and violent behavior.

New Media

Rapid growth in mobile phone and internet access among AYAs in both high- and low-income settings provides both challenges and opportunities relating to AYA health. Data from 2018 suggest more than 95% of adolescents in the United States own a smartphone, and almost half reported they are online "almost all the time."[33] Mobile phone use among AYAs is also common in middle- and low-income settings, where it is essential for both economic and social reasons.[34]

Implications for increased new media use and AYA health are complex. Studies have demonstrated the potential to use these platforms to provide health information and facilitate improvements in AYA health and well-being.[34] However, there are concerns regarding potential harms to AYAs associated with new media. For example, there is growing concern regarding the effect of frequent social media use on AYA mental health, although there is some evidence that these associations may be mediated by other factors including sleep disturbance and cyberbullying.[35]

🔵 LIFE-COURSE PERSPECTIVE

A life-course perspective is derived from an increasing body of evidence that health is influenced not only by current risk factors and social determinants, but also by factors from earlier in an individual's life. Adolescence is a critical period in lifelong health trajectories, with links both to prenatal and early childhood determinants and adult health outcomes.[36] For example:

- Micronutrient deficiencies in utero are associated with schizophrenia in adolescence,[37] and exposure to diethylstilbestrol in utero can cause vaginal cancer among AYA females.[8]
- Interventions in early childhood (such as Head Start programs to promote school readiness of infants, toddlers, and preschool-aged children in the United States) have been shown to reduce teenage pregnancy and criminal activity among adolescents.
- Adolescent smoking and sexual behaviors are associated with lung and genitourinary cancers in later life.[8] Thus, vaccines against the human papillomavirus given in adolescence prevent cancers occurring primarily among middle-aged adults.[38]

Adolescence is a sensitive period shaping lifelong trajectories in health and well-being.[14] While exploratory behavior is normal during adolescence and young adulthood, attitudes and habits acquired at this age often lead to lifelong health risks. Holistic interventions during this time may improve a wide range of health and other outcomes.[29]

Life-Course Transitions in Adolescence and Young Adulthood

Both social determinants and life-course factors interact with the intrinsic biologic, psychological, and social transitions that take place during adolescence. Biologic transitions are influenced by nutritional and environmental factors, with the age of puberty falling in rich countries during the 19th and early 20th century.

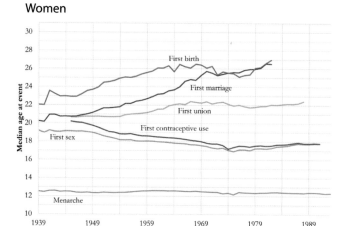

Women

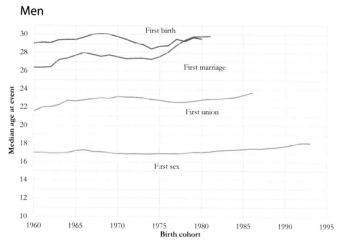

Men

FIGURE 1.6 Median ages at various reproductive events, U.S. birth cohorts. (Reprinted from Finer L, Philbin JM. Trends in ages at key reproductive transitions in the United States, 1951–2010. *Women's Health Issues*. 2014;24(3): e271–e279. With permission from Elsevier.) Footnote: Birth cohort notes a group of people born in a particular year (e.g., the median age of first birth was 23 years old for females born in 1944).

Subsequently, the timing of puberty has been stable in rich countries since the 1960s (Fig. 1.6). Epidemiologic and demographic transitions have resulted in the largest global cohort of adolescents in history, lower dependency ratios between children and elderly populations and those in the workforce, and shifts in other biologic and social transitions for adolescents.[4]

The World Bank describes five key aspects of the social transition from childhood to adulthood.[39]

- Learning for work and life
- Beginning to work
- Taking risks that impact health
- Forming families
- Transition into responsible and productive citizenship

Demographers have focused on life transitions related to family formation such as age at first sex, marriage, and childbearing and other social role transitions such as age at leaving education and entering workforce.[40] Medical practitioners have focused on the transition to adult medicine and learning to be responsible for one's own health care.

In the United States during the 1960s, 77% of females and 67% of males completed their education, left home, achieved financial independence, married, and had children by the age of 30. Between 2006 and 2015, the number of young people (ages 16 to 34) living with their parents increased while the number of those who had ever been married fell.[40] For females born between 1970 and 1980, the median age at first birth was between 25 and 27 years; for females born in the late 1970s, median age at first birth was earlier than the age at first marriage for the first time (see Fig. 1.6).[10] Young adults' experience of this process varies widely between different countries and cultures. Within the United States and globally, there have also been rapid changes in recent decades, influenced by diverse factors, including urbanization, migration, industrialization, and the rise of new media.

Health Correlates of Transitions to Adulthood

- Early parenthood is associated with health risks due to multiple factors including lack of resources and social support. Where early pregnancy violates community norms, these effects may be compounded by stigma and social isolation.
- Teenage mothers report poorer late-life health outcomes compared to older mothers.
- Education plays a large role in delaying motherhood.[41] In the United States, 40% of mothers with a bachelor's degree were 30 years or older at age of first birth. Comparatively, only 17% of mothers with a high school degree or less were over 30 years at age of first birth, and 62% were under 25 years of age.[42]
- Earlier transitions to financial autonomy, living independently, or intimate relationships are associated with poorer adult outcomes. In addition to higher rates of anxiety and poor health, the likelihood of other adverse outcomes increases with earlier transitions, including unhealthy substance use, criminal behavior, unemployment, divorce, and lower SES.
- Slow transition (defined as little or no transition to adult roles by age 24) is also associated with poor health outcomes, including increased criminal behavior and poor mental health.
- Similarly, very early adolescent transition to independent self-management of chronic conditions such as diabetes has been linked to poorer disease control outcomes; however, very late transition to self-management is also associated with poor outcomes.

DEMOGRAPHICS OF ADOLESCENTS AND YOUNG ADULTS

Global Overview

- The world now has the largest generation of AYAs in history—with a total population of 1.86 billion people aged 10 to 24 in 2019,[11] forecasted to reach 2 billion by 2030.[43]

- The countries with the largest adolescent populations are India (397 million), China (228 million), Pakistan (73 million), Nigeria (72 million), and Indonesia (68 million) (Figs. 1.7 to 1.20).[12]
- Globally, 89% of adolescents live in LMICs.[12]
- Rapid improvements in childhood survival have resulted in an increased proportion of youth as a percentage of the total population in many countries, particularly in rapidly developing countries. This can exacerbate youth unemployment, with too many workers for too few jobs.
- The region with highest growth in its AYA population is SSA, where numbers of adolescents are projected to overtake the numbers in South Asia and East Asia and Pacific Regions by 2025.[43]

Population Structure and Composition

- There is huge variation in population structures between countries. Globally, the proportion of the total population aged 10 to 24 years was 24% in 2019, but this ranges from around 15% in Europe and Central Asia, to over 30% in SSA. The range between specific countries is even wider; in the United Arab Emirates, the proportion of the total population aged 10 to 24 years is 11%, and in Equatorial Guinea, it is 37%.[12]
- Low replacement fertility and low rates of childhood mortality have produced a situation where some world regions currently have a greater number of AYAs than younger children. For every 10 children in the first decade of life in Europe, there are 10.1 young people in the second decade of life and 11.1 in the third decade.
- Conversely, data from SSA show continued high fertility and child mortality. For every 10 children in the first decade of life, there are 8.0 young people in the second decade and 5.8 in the third decade. Niger has the lowest ratio of AYAs to young children, with 6.5 young people in the second decade and 3.9 in the third decade for every 10 in the first.[12]
- The racial and ethnic composition of the AYA population is changing rapidly in many countries. For example, between 2000 and 2019 in the United States, the percentage of non-Hispanic White children under 18 decreased from 61% to 50%.[44] The child population in the United States is currently more diverse than its total population, driven by both immigration and the increase in interracial marriages.[45] Non-White populations are now spread more widely throughout the United States rather than living in concentrated areas, which was common in the past. Since 2010, an overwhelming majority (96%) of U.S. counties have reported a decline in their White population shares.[46]

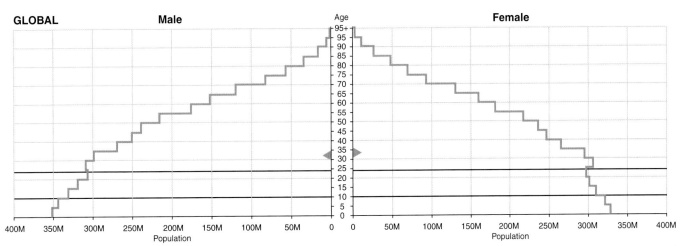

FIGURE 1.7 Population age structure, global, 2018. (Source: Modified from Institute for Health Metrics Evaluation. Used with permission. All rights reserved.) Footnote: *Triangle* corresponds to mean age of the population. *The space between the black lines* denotes adolescents and young adults.

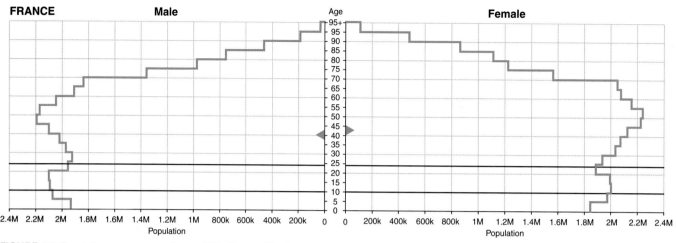

FIGURE 1.8 Population age structure, France, 2018. (Source: Modified from Institute for Health Metrics Evaluation. Used with permission. All rights reserved.) Footnote: *Triangle* corresponds to mean age of the population. *The space between the black lines* denotes adolescents and young adults.

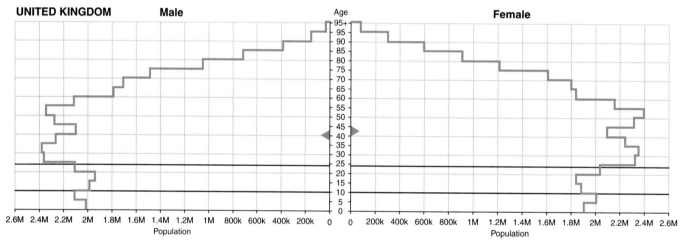

FIGURE 1.9 Population age structure, United Kingdom, 2018. (Source: Modified from Institute for Health Metrics Evaluation. Used with permission. All rights reserved.) Footnote: *Triangle* corresponds to mean age of the population. *The space between the black lines* denotes adolescents and young adults.

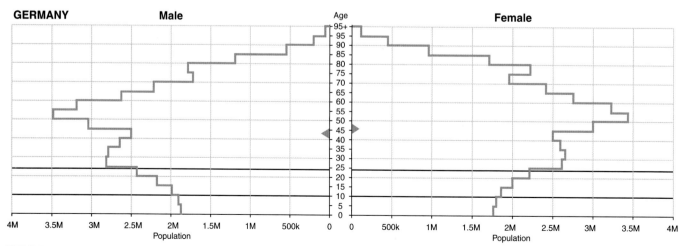

FIGURE 1.10 Population age structure, Germany, 2018. (Source: Modified from Institute for Health Metrics Evaluation. Used with permission. All rights reserved.) Footnote: *Triangle* corresponds to mean age of the population. *The space between the black lines* denotes adolescents and young adults.

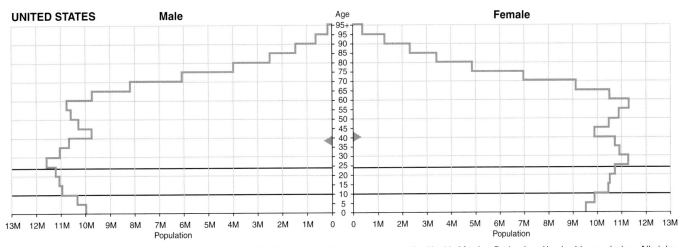

FIGURE 1.11 Population age structure, United States, 2018. (Source: Modified from Institute for Health Metrics Evaluation. Used with permission. All rights reserved.) Footnote: *Triangle* corresponds to mean age of the population. *The space between the black lines* denotes adolescents and young adults.

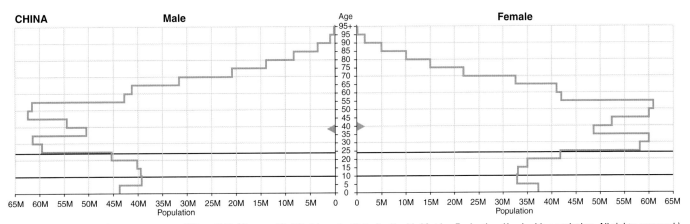

FIGURE 1.12 Population age structure, China, 2018. (Source: Modified from Institute for Health Metrics Evaluation. Used with permission. All rights reserved.) Footnote: *Triangle* corresponds to mean age of the population. *The space between the black lines* denotes adolescents and young adults.

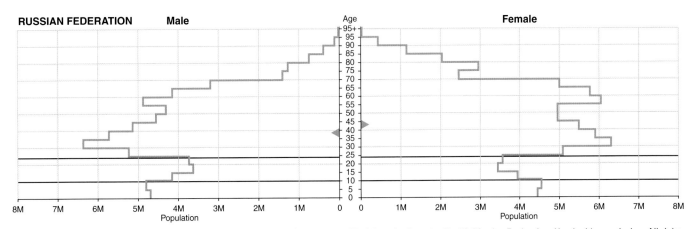

FIGURE 1.13 Population age structure, Russian Federation, 2018. (Source: Modified from Institute for Health Metrics Evaluation. Used with permission. All rights reserved.) Footnote: *Triangle* corresponds to mean age of the population. *The space between the black lines* denotes adolescents and young adults.

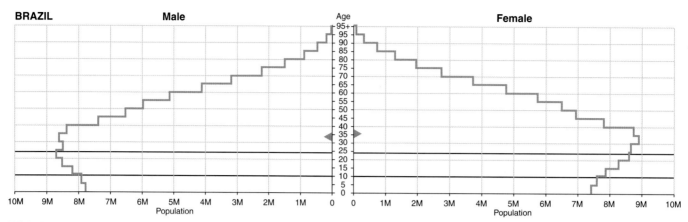

FIGURE 1.14 Population age structure, Brazil, 2018. (Source: Modified from Institute for Health Metrics Evaluation. Used with permission. All rights reserved.)
Footnote: *Triangle* corresponds to mean age of the population. *The space between the black lines* denotes adolescents and young adults.

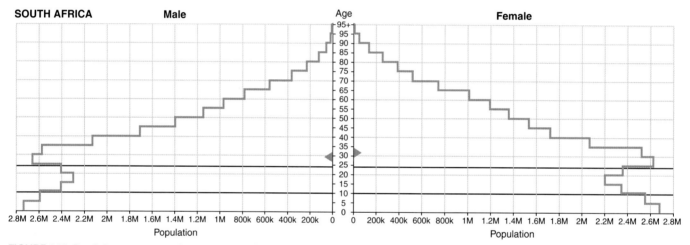

FIGURE 1.15 Population age structure, South Africa, 2018. (Source: Modified from Institute for Health Metrics Evaluation. Used with permission. All rights reserved.)
Footnote: *Triangle* corresponds to mean age of the population. *The space between the black lines* denotes adolescents and young adults.

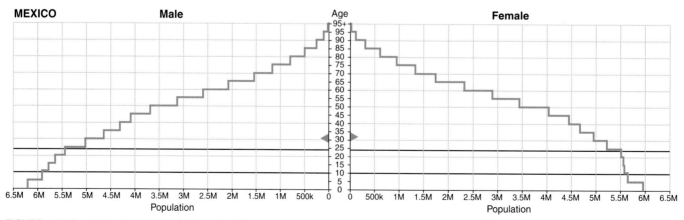

FIGURE 1.16 Population age structure, Mexico, 2018. (Source: Modified from Institute for Health Metrics Evaluation. Used with permission. All rights reserved.)
Footnote: *Triangle* corresponds to mean age of the population. *The space between the black lines* denotes adolescents and young adults.

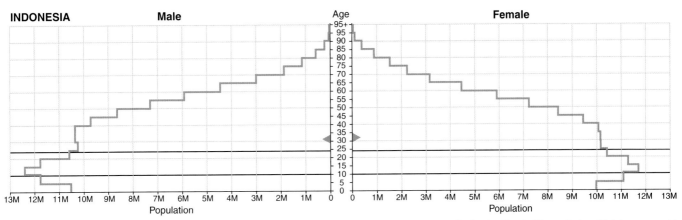

FIGURE 1.17 Population age structure, Indonesia, 2018. (Source: Modified from Institute for Health Metrics Evaluation. Used with permission. All rights reserved.)
Footnote: *Triangle* corresponds to mean age of the population. *The space between the black lines* denotes adolescents and young adults.

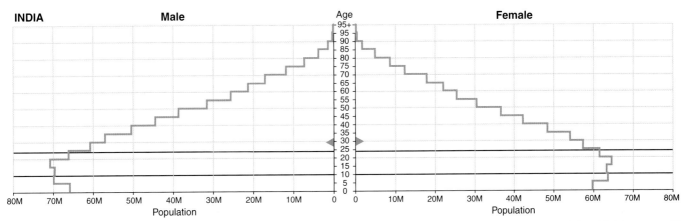

FIGURE 1.18 Population age structure, India, 2018. (Source: Modified from Institute for Health Metrics Evaluation. Used with permission. All rights reserved.)
Footnote: *Triangle* corresponds to mean age of the population. *The space between the black lines* denotes adolescents and young adults.

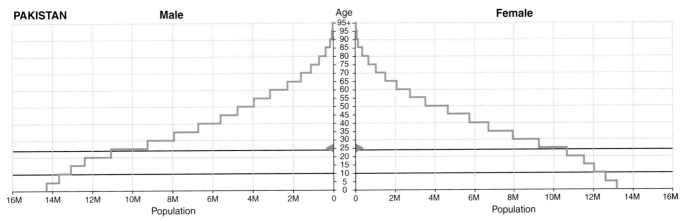

FIGURE 1.19 Population age structure, Pakistan, 2018. (Source: Modified from Institute for Health Metrics Evaluation. Used with permission. All rights reserved.)
Footnote: *Triangle* corresponds to mean age of the population. The *space between the black lines* denotes adolescents and young adults.

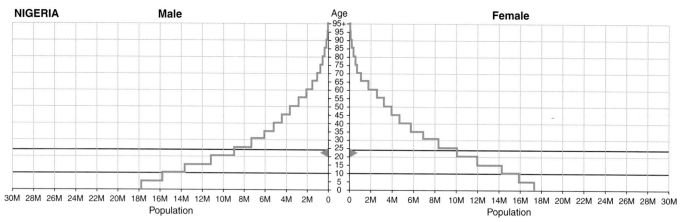

FIGURE 1.20 Population age structure, Nigeria, 2018. (Source: Modified from Institute for Health Metrics Evaluation. Used with permission. All rights reserved.)
Footnote: *Triangle* corresponds to mean age of the population. *The space between the black lines* denotes adolescents and young adults.

MORTALITY IN ADOLESCENTS AND YOUNG ADULTS

Global Mortality

Despite considerable global improvements in mortality among AYAs, numbers of deaths remain high, mainly from preventable causes. There is huge global variation in patterns of mortality by cause; injury, self-harm, and violence are common causes in all settings, but communicable and maternal causes remain leading causes in many middle- and low-income settings (Figs. 1.21 and 1.22; Table 1.2).

• Globally, an estimated 1.49 million deaths occurred among AYAs (10 to 24 years) in 2019.[5]

• Around 60% of these deaths occurred in males, with this proportion increasing with age. Mortality in adolescents is higher in males than females in all regions of the world except South Asia, where mortality is similar. The greatest difference in mortality in 2019 was in Latin America and the Caribbean, where the mortality rate among 15- to 24-year-olds was around three times higher in males than females, with that trend increasing over time. Differences in mortality between males and females are primarily driven by deaths due to violence and injuries, where outcomes among males are worse (Figs. 1.23 and 1.24).[5]

• Global reductions in mortality in AYAs have not matched those seen in young children. Among 1- to 4-year-olds, global mortality rates have declined by around 2.4% per year since 1990 in both males and females, compared to rates of decline in 15- to 19-year-olds of 1.3% in males and 1.6% in females.[5]

• Almost a quarter of deaths in 0- to 24-year-olds now occur during adolescence and young adulthood, with this proportion having doubled since 1950. Among high-income countries, this rises to more than one in two deaths.[5]

• Around a third of global deaths among 10- to 24-year-olds in 2019 were caused by transport injuries, unintentional injuries, or violence and conflict.[5]

• Mortality due to injuries among AYAs have decreased in all regions of the world in recent years but remain the leading cause of death in all regions except South Asia and SSA, where infectious diseases continue to predominate.

• Motor vehicle crashes and other transport injuries cause the greatest proportion of injury-related deaths in AYAs in all regions, except in Central and South American countries, where more injuries among young adult males were due to violence.

• Violence- and conflict-related mortality among AYAs have declined at a slower rate than other injury deaths and are increasing among males in many countries, particularly in Latin America and the Caribbean.

• Data on the number of global adolescent deaths attributable to domestic or sexual violence are sparse, although efforts to establish this are ongoing.[47] However, it is estimated that one-third of females experience intimate partner or nonpartner physical or sexual violence in their lifetime. Among adolescent females aged 15 to 19 years who have had partners, it is estimated that around a quarter have already experienced intimate partner violence.[48]

• Around 8% of global deaths among AYAs were due to self-harm in 2019 (120,000) and the percentage of AYAs who attempt suicide is much higher. Self-harm is now the leading cause of death in 15- to 24-year-olds in many regions of the world, with high-income countries and those in central and eastern Europe and central Asia particularly affected.[5]

• Mortality from communicable diseases among AYAs continues to fall rapidly, and in many regions of the world is a rare cause of death. Still, infectious diseases are a leading cause of death in South Asia among 10- to 14-year-olds, and in SSA this is the case throughout adolescence and young adulthood, particularly among females. Sexually transmitted infections (STIs) and HIV/AIDS have been the leading causes of mortality in SSA among females since the early 1990s in 15- to 24-year-olds, and since the early 2000s in 10- to 14-year-olds.[5]

• Similarly, there are low overall rates of mortality from nutritional disorders among AYAs, although nutrition is still a significant concern in certain populations and in some countries.

• Adolescents are at higher risk of maternal death than older females, particularly in low-to-middle income countries where the risk of maternal death is higher for girls under 15 than females in their 20s.[49] Unsafe abortion contributes considerably to maternal mortality. Across age groups, 55% of all abortions are considered safe (performed using a recommended method and by a trained clinician), 31% are less safe (meet either method or clinician criterion), and 14% are least safe (meeting no safe criteria). Adolescents are recognized as an at-risk group for complications due to unsafe abortion. In addition, an estimated 6.9 million females in the developing world are treated annually for complications related to unsafe abortions[50]; those cases, in addition to many who do not receive timely care, are associated with increased mortality risk.

• There continue to be significant improvements in maternal mortality globally. Still, in 2019, maternal mortality was among the top three causes of death for females aged 20 to 24 years in SSA, North Africa and the Middle East, and South Asia and was the highest in Latin America and the Caribbean[5] (Fig. 1.25).

TABLE 1.2

Definitions of Global Burden of Disease Causes

Broad Causes	Included Specific Causes
Cardiovascular diseases	Rheumatic and ischemic heart disease, stroke, hypertensive heart disease, nonrheumatic valve diseases, cardiomyopathy, atrial fibrillation, aortic aneurysm, peripheral artery, endocarditis, other cardiovascular disease
Chronic respiratory	Chronic Obstructive Pulmonary Disease (COPD), pneumoconiosis, asthma, interstitial lung disease, other chronic respiratory Neurologic disorders: Alzheimer disease, Parkinson disease, idiopathic epilepsy, multiple sclerosis, motor neuron disease, headache disorders, other neurologic causes
Diabetes and chronic kidney disease (CKD)	Diabetes, chronic kidney disease, acute glomerulonephritis
Enteric infections	Diarrheal disease, typhoid and paratyphoid, invasive non-typhoidal *Salmonella*, other intestinal infections Neglected tropical diseases and malaria: Malaria, Chagas disease, leishmaniasis, African trypanosomiasis, schistosomiasis, cysticercosis, cystic echinococcosis, lymphatic filariasis, onchocerciasis, trachoma, dengue, yellow fever, rabies, intestinal nematode, food-borne trematodiases, leprosy, ebola, zika virus, guinea worm
Human immunodeficiency virus/ acquired immunodeficiency syndrome and sexually transmitted infections (HIV/AIDS and STIs)	HIV/AIDS, syphilis, chlamydia, gonorrhea, trichomoniasis, genital herpes, and other sexually transmitted infections
Maternal and neonatal	Maternal hemorrhage, maternal sepsis, maternal hypertension, obstructed labor, maternal abortion miscarriage, ectopic pregnancy, maternal indirect, maternal late, maternal HIV, other maternal disorders, neonatal preterm birth, neonatal encephalopathy, neonatal sepsis, neonatal hemolytic, other neonatal causes
Mental disorders	Schizophrenia, depressive disorders, bipolar disorder, anxiety disorders, eating disorders, autism spectrum, attention deficit hyperactivity disorder (ADHD), conduct disorder, intellectual disability, other mental disorders Substance use: Alcohol and drug use disorders
Musculoskeletal disorders	Rheumatoid arthritis, osteoarthritis, low back pain, neck pain, gout, other musculoskeletal causes
Neoplasms	Over 20 different cancer diagnoses
Nutritional deficiencies	Protein-energy malnutrition, iodine deficiency, vitamin A deficiency, dietary iron deficiency, other nutritional causes
Other infectious diseases	Meningitis, encephalitis, diphtheria, whooping cough, tetanus, measles, varicella, acute hepatitis, other unspecified infectious diseases
Other noncommunicable diseases	Congenital defects, urinary diseases, gynecologic diseases, hemoglobinopathies, endo/metabolic/blood/immune, oral disorders, sudden infant death syndrome (SIDS)
Respiratory infections and tuberculosis (TB)	Lower and upper respiratory infections, tuberculosis, otitis media
Self-harm and violence	Self-harm, interpersonal violence, conflict and terror, execution and police
Sense organ disease	Blindness and vision loss, age-related hearing loss, other sense organ causes
Skin diseases	Dermatitis, psoriasis, bacterial skin, scabies, fungal skin diseases, viral skin diseases, acne vulgaris, alopecia areata, pruritus, urticaria, decubitus ulcer
Transport injuries	Road injuries (including pedestrian, cyclist, motor vehicle) and other transport injuries
Unintentional injury	Falls, drowning, fire and heat, poisonings, mechanical forces, adverse medical treatment, animal contact, foreign body, environmental heat and cold, nature disaster, and other unintentional injury

Source: Institute for Health Metrics Evaluation. Accessed September 15, 2021. http://www.healthdata.org/gbd/2019

Broad Causes

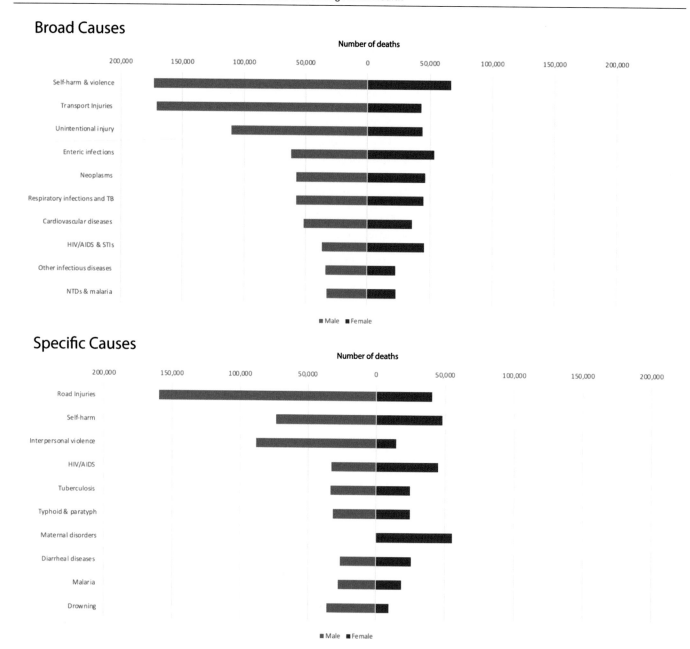

FIGURE 1.21 Top 10 causes of death among adolescents and young adults by sex, global, number of deaths 2019. TB, tuberculosis; HIV/AIDS, human immunodeficiency virus/acquired immunodeficiency syndrome; STIs, sexually transmitted infection; NTDs, neglected tropical diseases. (Source: Data from Institute for Health Metrics Evaluation. Global Burden of Disease Study 2019, custom data acquired via website.)

Mortality in the United States and Other High-Income Countries

- Mortality data for the United States and other high-income countries mirror global data, showing much smaller declines in age-specific mortality among AYAs than younger children.[5]
- As with global data, leading causes of death among AYAs in the United States and high-income countries also include transport and unintentional injuries and self-harm. There are also some important differences by age within AYAs: cancers are a more important cause of death among younger adolescents (10- to 14-year-olds), and unhealthy substance use a leading cause in older AYAs (15- to 24-year-olds).[5]
- Deaths due to substance use disorders in high-income countries have increased rapidly in the past 40 years among 15- to 24-year-olds, rising from around 1% of total deaths among 20- to 24-year-olds in 1980 to around 12% in 2019 in both sexes. Deaths due

to substance use are now the third-highest cause of mortality among males and fourth-highest among females.[5]
- The United States and countries within South and Central America and the Caribbean have the highest mortality rates due to violent deaths among AYAs within high-income countries (Fig. 1.26). According to WHO data from 2016, mortality rates in the United States due to firearms were higher than all other high-income and LMICs for whom data were available.[51]
- Suicide is the third most common cause of death among AYAs in the United States in 2019 and ranks highly in most other high-income countries. There is evidence that suicide is influenced by different factors among AYAs than older groups. Relative to older groups, suicide among young veterans were more likely to be associated with relationship problems or unhealthy use of alcohol and other substances. In contrast, suicide among older veterans was more strongly related to financial and medical concerns.

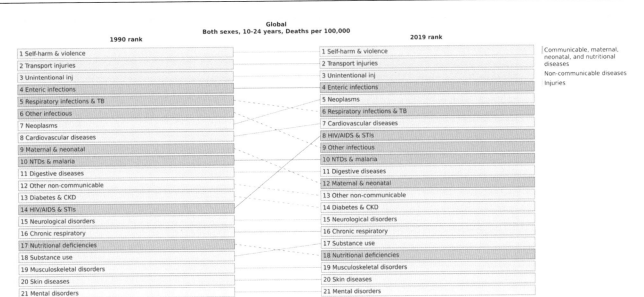

IHME

FIGURE 1.22 Top broad causes of adolescent mortality globally, 1990 versus 2019, mortality rate per 100,000. inj, injuries; TB, tuberculosis, NTDs, neglected tropical diseases; HIV/AIDS, human immunodeficiency virus/acquired immunodeficiency syndrome; STIs, sexually transmitted infections; CKD, chronic kidney disease. (Source: Institute for Health Metrics Evaluation. Used with permission. All rights reserved.)

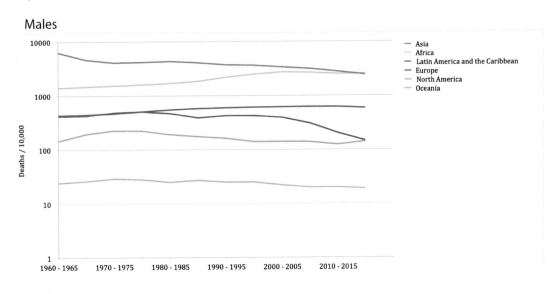

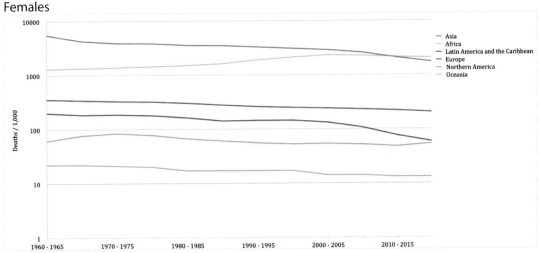

FIGURE 1.23 Trends in mortality rate per 100,000 1960 to 2020, ages 10 to 24, by continent. (Source: Data from United Nations, World Population Prospects. Department of Economic and Social Affairs Population Dynamics, 2019, custom data acquired via website.)

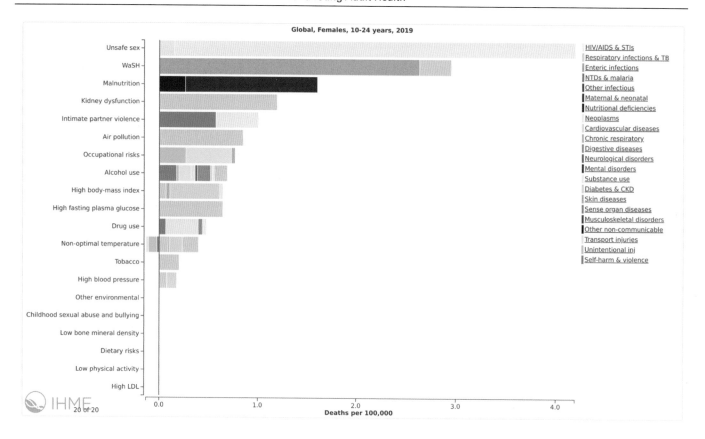

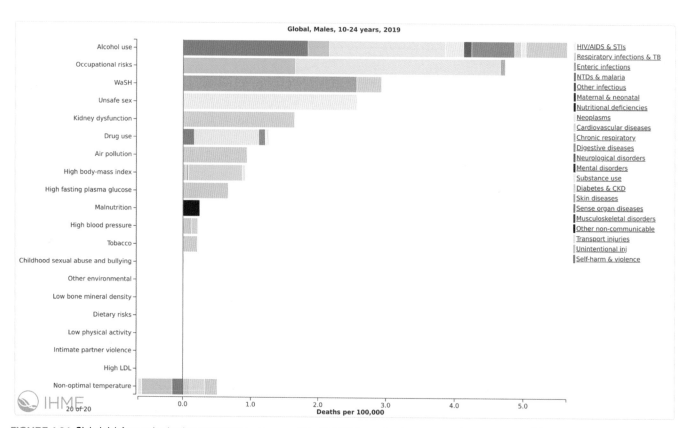

FIGURE 1.24 Global risk factors by deaths per 100,000, by sex, ages 10 to 24, 2019. Nonoptimal temperature is an aggregate of the mortality burden attributable to low and high temperatures. Note that heat-attributable nonoptimal temperature is associated with increased injury-related mortality and morbidity, and cold non-optimal temperature is associated with a protective effect. WaSH, water, sanitation, and hygiene; LDL, low-density lipoprotein; HIV/AIDS, human immunodeficiency virus/acquired immunodeficiency syndrome; STIs, sexually transmitted infections; TB, tuberculosis; NTDs, neglected tropical diseases; CKD, chronic kidney disease; inj, injuries. (Source: Institute for Health Metrics Evaluation. Used with permission. All rights reserved.)

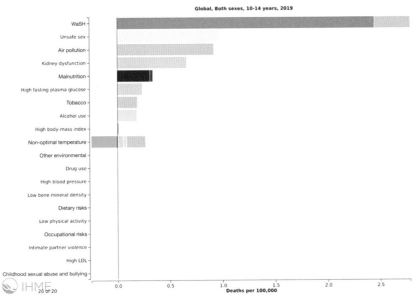

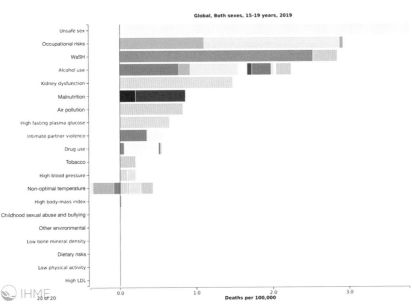

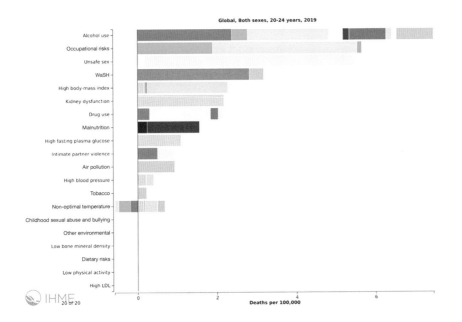

FIGURE 1.25 Global risk factors by deaths per 100,000, by age group, 2019. WaSH, water, sanitation, and hygiene; LDL, low-density lipoprotein; HIV/AIDS, human immunodeficiency virus/acquired immunodeficiency syndrome; STIs, sexually transmitted infections; TB, tuberculosis; NTDs, neglected tropical diseases; CKD, chronic kidney disease; inj, injuries. Nonoptimal temperature is an aggregate of the mortality burden attributable to low and high temperatures. (Source: Institute for Health Metrics Evaluation. Used with permission. All rights reserved.)

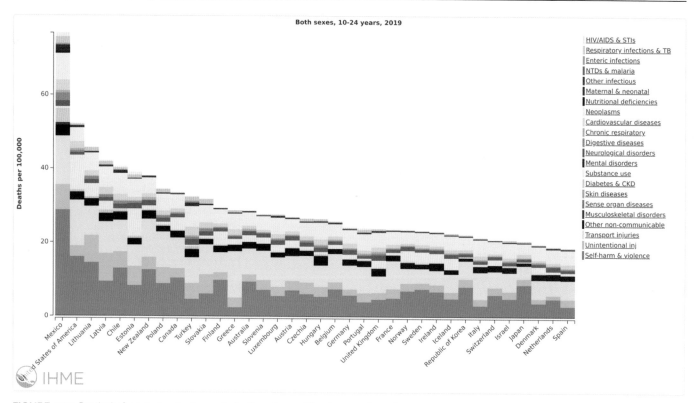

Both sexes, 10-24 years, 2019

HIV/AIDS & STIs
Respiratory infections & TB
Enteric infections
NTDs & malaria
Other infectious
Maternal & neonatal
Nutritional deficiencies
Neoplasms
Cardiovascular diseases
Chronic respiratory
Digestive diseases
Neurological disorders
Mental disorders
Substance use
Diabetes & CKD
Skin diseases
Sense organ diseases
Musculoskeletal disorders
Other non-communicable
Transport injuries
Unintentional inj
Self-harm & violence

FIGURE 1.26 Deaths in Organisation for Economic Co-Operation and Development Countries per 100,000 by country, both sexes, ages 10 to 24, 2019. HIV/AIDS, human immunodeficiency virus/acquired immunodeficiency syndrome; STIs, sexually transmitted infections; TB, tuberculosis; NTDs, neglected tropical diseases; CKD, chronic kidney disease; inj, injuries. (Source: Institute for Health Metrics Evaluation. Used with permission. All rights reserved.)

- Similarly, suicide in younger age groups is more commonly associated with impulsive and aggressive behaviors. The important role of impulsive behavior in AYA suicide reinforces the potential benefit of limiting access to firearms—around one in three firearms deaths among young people are self-inflicted.[52]

Differences in Mortality by Race and Ethnicity

- There are large subnational differences in AYA mortality, including by race and ethnicity. For example, in the United States, mortality rates are highest among Black AYAs (137 deaths/100,000 20- to 24-year-olds; 20.1 deaths/100,000 10- to 14-year-olds) and lowest among AYAs of Asian/Pacific Islander descent (39.5 and 9.6 deaths/100,000, respectively)[53] (**Table 1.3**).
- Among Black young adult males (age 20 to 24 years), homicide is by far the most common cause of death (93.2/100,000/year)—almost twice the rate of accidental deaths (49.4) and four times the rates of suicide (23.2).[53]
- In contrast, among White young adult females (age 20 to 24 years), accidents are the dominant cause of death (21.1/100,000), followed by suicide (6.2) and malignant neoplasms (3.0). Homicides are the fourth leading cause (2.4/100,000).[53]
- There were 3.8 deaths/100,000 due to homicides among Black males aged 10 to 14 years in the United States. For White males in this age group, the rate was 0.8/100,000.[53]

MORBIDITY

Overview of Global Morbidity

Years lived with disability (YLDs) and disability-adjusted life years (DALYs) are measures of disease burden due to nonfatal health outcomes, or morbidity, and allow comparison of the relative disease burden associated with different risk factors and disease categories. As with mortality, adolescence and young adulthood is a time of transition from childhood patterns of morbidity—dominated at a global level by nutritional deficiencies and infections (diarrhea, pneumonia)—to adult patterns with high levels of mental health, injuries, and violence.[54]

- Globally, the five leading causes of DALYs in AYAs aged 10 to 24 years in 2019 for males were road injuries, interpersonal violence, self-harm, headache, and depressive disorders. Among females, these were headaches, depressive disorders, anxiety, gynecologic disorders, and maternal disorders (Figs. 1.27 and 1.28). Patterns were similar among 15- to 19-year-olds and 20- to 24-year-olds, but among 10- to 14-year-olds, iron deficiency, conduct disorder, and some infectious causes were more important causes of morbidity (Fig. 1.29).[54]

Morbidity in the United States and Other High-Income Countries

- Figure 1.30 illustrates the relative contribution of leading risk factors to overall morbidity (expressed as DALYs per 100,000 population) globally, and in Organisation for Economic Co-Operation and Development (OECD) countries, in 2019.
- Among the high-income country group provided in the GBD study, the leading causes of DALYs in AYAs in 2019 in males were drug use disorders, road injuries, self-harm, low back pain, and depressive disorders in males; in females, these were depressive disorders, headache disorders, low back pain, anxiety disorders, and drug use disorders (Fig. 1.31).[54]
- About one in four adolescents in the United States have a chronic health condition such as obesity, asthma, or diabetes.[55] Prevalence of many chronic conditions increases throughout adolescence and young adulthood. Some conditions cause symptoms and influence quality of life in both short and long term. For example, diabetes is diagnosed in about 1% of 18- to 25-year-olds and 2% of 26- to 34-year-olds (although others

TABLE 1.3

Deaths by Age, Race, Ethnicity, Per 100,000 Population, United States, 2019

Race	Ethnicity	Age 10–14	Age 15–19	Age 20–24
American Indian or Alaska Native	Hispanic or Latino	Unreliable	16.8	21.2
	Not Hispanic or Latino	26.7	104.9	164.5
	Total	**15.8**	**64.6**	**101.3**
Asian or Pacific Islander	Hispanic or Latino	Unreliable	30.1	45.0
	Not Hispanic or Latino	9.8	26.9	39.2
	Total	**9.6**	**27.1**	**39.5**
Black or African American	Hispanic or Latino	6.0	24.4	45.2
	Not Hispanic or Latino	21.5	82.5	144.6
	Total	**20.1**	**77.6**	**137.0**
White	Hispanic or Latino	13.5	46.0	85.0
	Not Hispanic or Latino	15.0	43.0	84.0
	Total	**14.6**	**43.9**	**84.4**

Death rates are flagged as "Unreliable" when the rate is calculated with a numerator of 20 or less.
Source: Centers for Disease Control and Prevention, National Center for Health Statistics. Underlying Cause of Death 1999–2019 on CDC WONDER Online Database, released in 2020. Data are from the Multiple Cause of Death Files, 1999–2019, as compiled from data provided by the 57 vital statistics jurisdictions through the Vital Statistics Cooperative Program. Accessed on July 16, 2021. http://wonder.cdc.gov/ucd-icd10.html

have diabetes which is undiagnosed). In contrast, rates of other conditions, such as hypertension, increase during adolescence and young adulthood; however, the effects may not be noticed until later in life.[52]

Mental Health

- Approximately 20% of the world's adolescents are affected by mental health or behavioral problems. However, there is wide variation in estimates between countries, and some populations such as indigenous AYAs are at greater risk. Data availability on mental health prevalence for AYAs in low resource settings is poor.[56]
- The prevalence of psychiatric disorders increases through adolescence in both males and females, peaking in late adolescence for males and the late 20s for females.
- Mental health disorders contributed to around 12% of total DALYs in AYAs in 2019.[54]
- Half of lifetime cases of mental health disorders present by the age of 14 and 75% by the age of 24.[57]
- There is wide variation in age of onset of mental health conditions among AYAs. Median onset of impulse control disorders such as conduct disorder and attention deficit hyperactivity disorder is in mid-childhood and early adolescence (ages 7 to 15 years). This is similar to some anxiety disorders, but these have much wider variation in age of onset. Mood disorders and substance use disorders are rare before the mid-teens, but then rapidly increase during late adolescence and early adulthood. Psychotic disorders also increase in prevalence between ages 15 to 17 years, and the age of onset of schizophrenia is usually between ages 15 to 35 years, peaking in the early 20s (Fig. 1.32).[58]
- Mental health and hazardous substance use represent a substantial burden of health problems for AYAs and most mental disorders which persist to adulthood emerge in adolescence and

young adulthood. Unfortunately, mental health service provision is also weakest for this age group.[56]

Health Behaviors

Many of the leading risk factors for mortality and morbidity in adulthood are largely initiated during adolescence, including smoking and drinking alcohol, while others such as dietary risks and high body mass index are strongly determined by behaviors and attitudes acquired during this period.[54] Determinants of behaviors are often complex, with interacting effects of community, family, school, neighborhood, and peers, in addition to individual factors.[14] The U.S. National Academies of Sciences, Engineering, and Medicine estimates that 5 of the top 10 risk factors for total burden of disease in adults are initiated or shaped in adolescence.[29]

There are substantial gaps in available data on health behaviors for AYAs in many parts of the world. An important resource for data is the Health Behaviours in School-Aged Children (HBSC), which collects cross-sectional data on a wide range of health outcomes and behaviors in 11-, 13-, and 15-year-olds from 50 high- and middle-income countries across Europe and North America (although not currently in the United States). Data are collected every 4 years, with the latest survey including more than 200,000 adolescents providing a rich source of information on the health of AYAs. Data are collected on substance use, dietary habits, activity levels, as well as self-reported health and well-being.[59]

Substance Use: Smoking, Alcohol, and Other Drug Use

Substance use is commonly initiated during adolescence and peaks during young adulthood. In addition to direct health risks to AYAs, there are broader concerns that substance use may disrupt the multiple transitions which occur during adolescence, and that this increases susceptibility to later substance dependence.[60]

Broad Causes

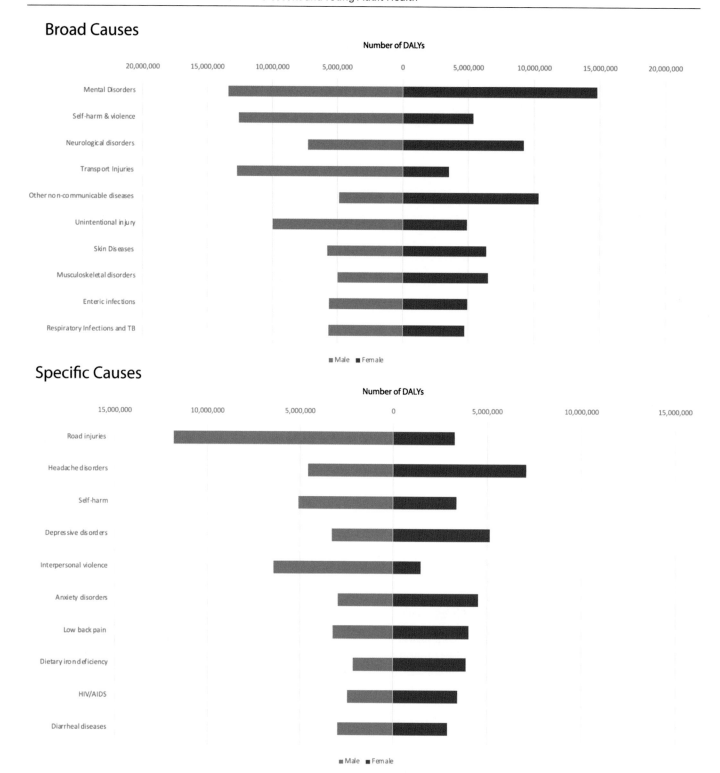

FIGURE 1.27 Top 10 causes of disability-adjusted life years among adolescents and young adults by sex, global, 2019. DALYs, disability-adjusted life years; TB, tuberculosis; HIV/AIDS, human immunodeficiency virus/acquired immunodeficiency syndrome. (Source: Data from Institute for Health Metrics Evaluation. Global Burden of Disease Study 2019, custom data acquired via website.)

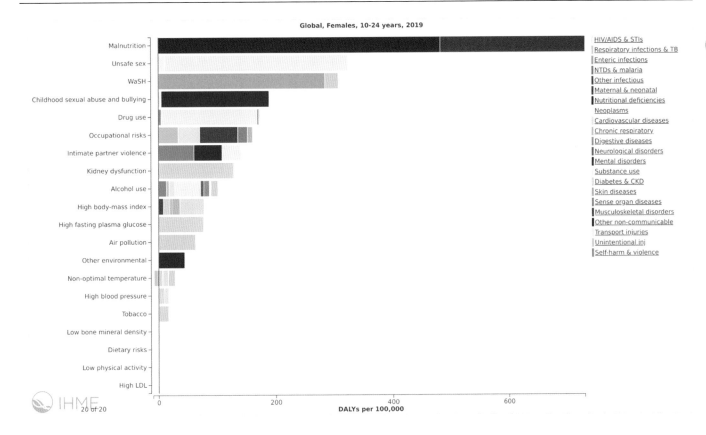

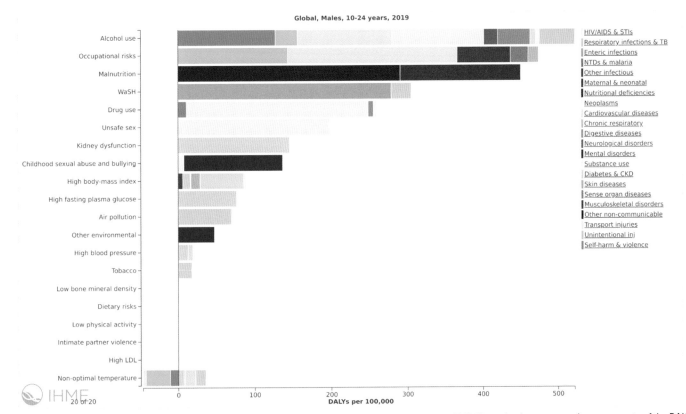

FIGURE 1.28 Global risk factor by disability-adjusted life years per 100,000, by sex, ages 10 to 24 years, 2019. Nonoptimal temperature is an aggregate of the DALY burden attributable to low and high temperatures. Note that heat-attributable nonoptimal temperature is associated with increased injury-related mortality and morbidity, and cold nonoptimal temperature is associated with a protective effect. DALYs, disability-adjusted life years; WaSH, water, sanitation, and hygiene; LDL, low-density lipoprotein; HIV/AIDS, human immunodeficiency virus/acquired immunodeficiency syndrome; STIs, sexually transmitted infections; TB, tuberculosis; NTDs, neglected tropical diseases; CKD, chronic kidney disease; inj, injuries. (Source: Institute for Health Metrics Evaluation. Used with permission. All rights reserved.)

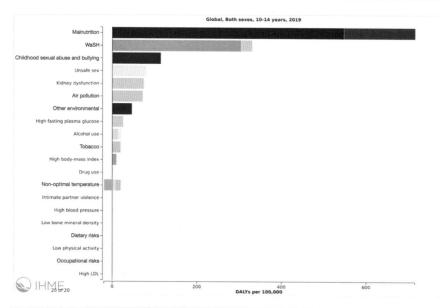

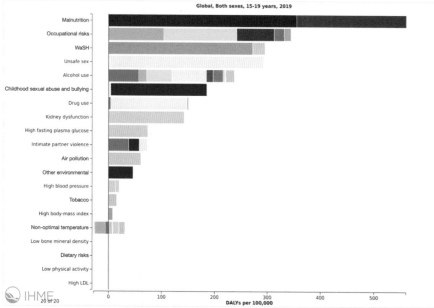

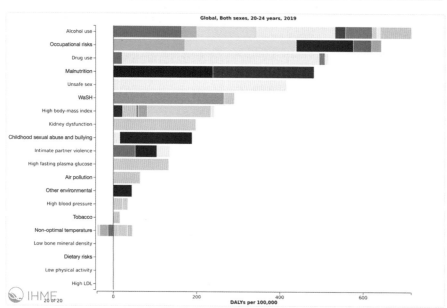

FIGURE 1.29 Global risk factors by disability-adjusted life years per 100,000, by age group, 2019. Nonoptimal temperature is an aggregate of the mortality burden attributable to low and high temperatures. Note that heat-attributable nonoptimal temperature is associated with increased injury-related mortality and morbidity, and cold nonoptimal temperature is associated with a protective effect. DALYs, disability-adjusted life years; WaSH, water, sanitation, and hygiene; LDL, low-density lipoprotein; HIV/AIDS, human immunodeficiency virus/acquired immunodeficiency syndrome; STIs, sexually transmitted infections; TB, tuberculosis; NTDs, neglected tropical diseases; CKD, chronic kidney disease; inj, injuries. (Source: Institute for Health Metrics Evaluation. Used with permission. All rights reserved.)

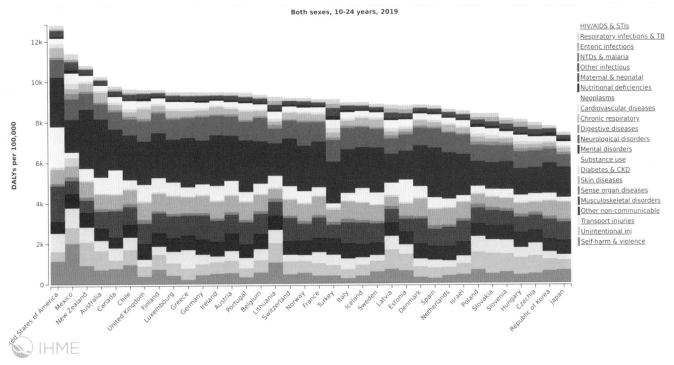

Both sexes, 10-24 years, 2019

HIV/AIDS & STIs
Respiratory infections & TB
Enteric infections
NTDs & malaria
Other infectious
Maternal & neonatal
Nutritional deficiencies
Neoplasms
Cardiovascular diseases
Chronic respiratory
Digestive diseases
Neurological disorders
Mental disorders
Substance use
Diabetes & CKD
Skin diseases
Sense organ diseases
Musculoskeletal disorders
Other non-communicable
Transport injuries
Unintentional inj
Self-harm & violence

IHME

FIGURE 1.30 Disability-adjusted life years per 100,000 among Organisation for Economic Co-Operation and Development Countries by country, both sexes, ages 10 to 24 years, 2019. DALYs, disability-adjusted life years; HIV/AIDS, human immunodeficiency virus/acquired immunodeficiency syndrome; STIs, sexually transmitted infections; TB, tuberculosis; NTDs, neglected tropical diseases; CKD, chronic kidney disease; inj, injuries. (Source: Institute for Health Metrics Evaluation. Used with permission. All rights reserved.)

There is a range of factors associated with substance use among AYAs, including contextual factors (laws and availability to AYAs), structural, familial, and individual markers of risk, and interpersonal factors. Populations of AYAs at particular risk of substance use include those with mental health problems, young offenders, the homeless, indigenous young people, and those who identify as LGBTQ.[60]

Smoking

- Recent analyses estimate that 82.6% of current smokers initiated between ages 14 and 25 years and 18.5% began regularly smoking before the age of 15.[61]
- In 2019, an estimated 155 million young people aged 15 to 24 years were tobacco smokers, with a global prevalence of 20.1% in males and 4.95% in females.[61]
- Prevalence of smoking among AYAs has continued to decline in many high- and middle-income countries but remains high in 15-year-olds in some countries according to the HBSC,[59] and has been increasing in some parts of the world.[61]
- Data from the HBSC estimate around a third of 15-year-olds have ever smoked, with 15% reported they have smoked in the past 30 days, rising to more than a quarter in Italy and some eastern European countries.[59]
- The prevalence of vaping among AYAs is increasing in many countries, including Canada and the United States. One survey of over 40,000 AYAs in the United States estimated the prevalence of vaping to have more than doubled between 2017 and 2019, with one in four students aged 17 to 18 years having vaped in the past 30 days.[62]

Alcohol and Illicit Drug Use

- There is striking similarity in terms of substance use initiation between countries. According to data from the World Mental Health Survey, median age of initiation of alcohol use is between 16 to 19 years, slightly younger than median age of initiation of both cannabis use (18 to 19 years) and cocaine (21 to 24 years).[63]

- Despite concern regarding so-called "gateway drugs," there is variation in patterns and order of substance use initiation among AYAs between and within countries.[60]
- Among AYAs surveyed for the HBSC, around one-third of 13-year-olds, and more than half of 15-year-olds had ever consumed alcohol. Around a third of 15-year-olds reported being drunk in the last 30 days.[59]
- Some studies suggest that early initiation of alcohol predicts future unhealthy alcohol use during adulthood, although the evidence for this is mixed, and robust studies exploring this association are needed.[64]
- Data from the HBSC estimate that 13% of 15-year-olds have ever used cannabis, with around 7% reporting use in the last 30 days. Prevalence varied greatly between countries, rising to more than a quarter of 15-year-olds in England, Switzerland, Canada, Italy, and Bulgaria.[59]

Obesity/Overweight, Physical Activity, and Nutrition

- Overall, one in five adolescents surveyed in the HBSC were living with overweight or obesity, with this proportion increasing in around a third of countries since 2014.[59]
- More affluent adolescents were less likely to report living with overweight/obesity than adolescents from more deprived backgrounds in half of the countries surveyed.[59]
- In the United States, 21.2% of AYAs aged 12 to 19 years are estimated to be living with obesity in 2017–2018, with higher rates in Black and Hispanic populations.[65]
- A recent analysis estimated 81% of adolescents aged 11 to 17 years globally do not meet WHO guidelines for levels of physical activity.[66]
- Although consumption of fruit and vegetables has increased in many countries, 48% of young people surveyed in 2017–2018 in the HBSC had eaten neither fruit nor vegetables every day.[59]
- Some developing countries are now seeing a "double nutrition" burden, where obesity is increasing alongside undernutrition.
- Globally, the prevalence of dietary iron deficiency among 10- to 24-year-olds is around 12% in 2019, rising to 25% of females in

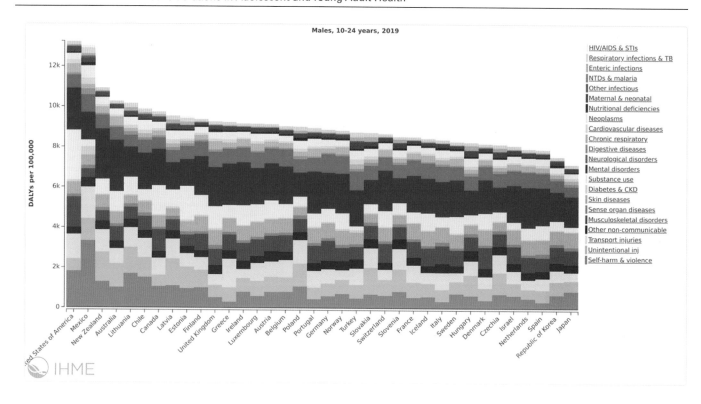

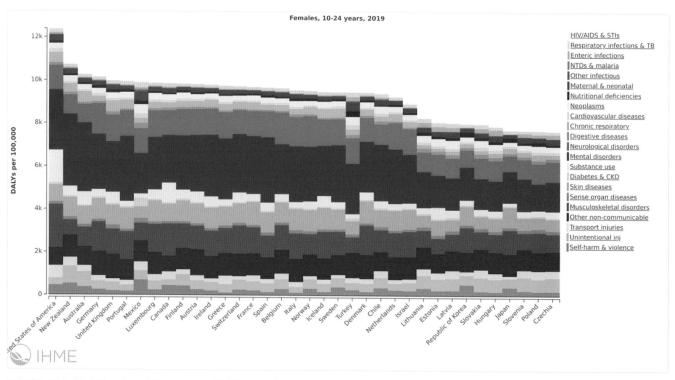

FIGURE 1.31 Disability-adjusted life years per 100,000 among Organisation for Economic Co-Operation and Development Countries by country, by sex, ages 10 to 24 years, 2019. DALYs, disability-adjusted life years; HIV/AIDS, human immunodeficiency virus/acquired immunodeficiency syndrome; STIs, sexually transmitted infections; TB, tuberculosis; NTDs, neglected tropical diseases; CKD, chronic kidney disease; inj, injuries. (Source: Institute for Health Metrics Evaluation. Used with permission. All rights reserved.)

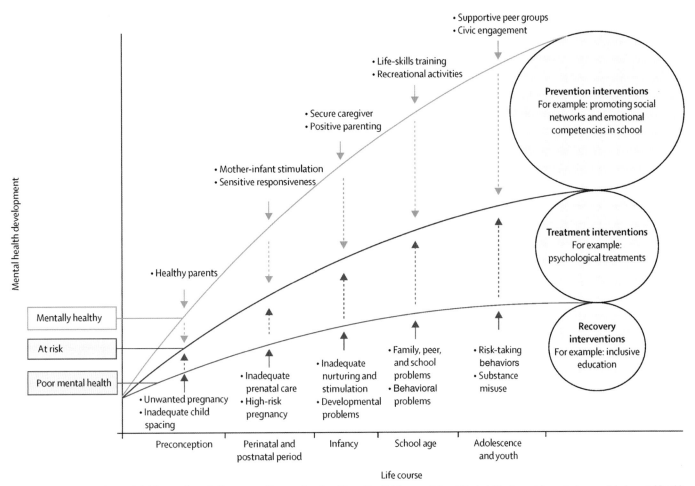

FIGURE 1.32 Protective and risk factors in early life course. (Source: Reprinted from Patel V, Saxena S, Lund C, et al. The Lancet Commission on global mental health and sustainable development. *Lancet.* 2018;392(10157):1553–1598. With permission from Elsevier.)

South Asia.[54] Underweight, anemia, and other nutritional deficiencies increase the health risks of pregnancy and childbirth for both mother and baby.[4]

Sexual and Reproductive Health

There are around 20 million pregnancies among AYA females (ages 15 to 19) each year in developing regions, of which around 50% are unintended. Over half of unintended pregnancies in 15- to 19-year-olds end in terminations, of which around two-thirds are thought to be unsafe. Improving access to modern contraception methods, safe abortion, and emergency obstetrical care among AYAs in these settings is likely to dramatically improve maternal health.[67]

- Globally, an estimated 20% of female AYAs marry before the age of 18 years.[16]
- The age of first sexual intercourse is increasing in most countries, although the proportion of AYAs having sex before the age of 15 years remains high in many countries in SSA.[68]
- Data from HBSC show one in four boys and one in seven girls aged 15 years report having had sex. Around a quarter of 15-year-olds reported not using either a condom or a contraceptive pill at last intercourse. There has also been a small decline in condom use between the 2014 and 2018 HBSC surveys.[59]
- Contraceptive methods may be used less effectively among adolescents: Sixty-two percent reported using a condom at last intercourse, of whom only two-thirds reported successful use.[52]
- Many countries have policies restricting access to contraception for AYAs, such as requiring parental consent or excluding provision to unmarried females.[4]

Sexually Transmitted Infections and Human Immunodeficiency Virus

- Adolescents and young adults are an important age group for prevention and treatment of STIs.
- In 2019, there were 460,000 new HIV infections among 10- to 24-year-olds (around a third of new infections globally), with most infections among female AYAs.[16]
- Around half of the 26 million new STIs in the United States in 2018 occurred in 15- to 24-year-olds, including two-thirds of all chlamydia infections. It has previously been estimated that a quarter of sexually active adolescent females in the United States have an STI.[55]
- Around 35,000 people in the United States were diagnosed with HIV in 2019, of whom around 7,000 were aged 13 to 24 years. New HIV infections among AYAs have been declining in recent years.[55]

HEALTH CARE UTILIZATION

Global Overview

High-quality health care services are an important determinant of AYA health and well-being. There is often a lack of reliable data regarding health care utilization among AYAs—either at a regional or country level, as many countries report health care statistics in very broad age ranges (e.g., 15- to 44-year-olds or 15- to 64-year-olds). Unmet health care needs in adolescence are associated with a range of poor health outcomes, including higher prevalence of physical and mental health symptoms, and higher rates of risk

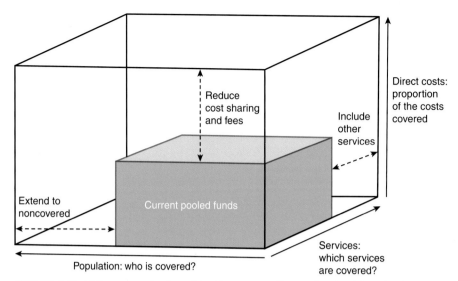

FIGURE 1.33 Adolescents and universal health coverage. (Source: Reprinted from Waddington C, Sambo C. Financing health care for adolescents: a necessary part of universal health coverage. *Bull World Health Organ.* 2015;93:57–59.)

behaviors. The WHO has advocated for universal access to health care among all age groups and in all countries, but there are growing concerns that health care needs of adolescents are not being adequately considered.[4] Three dimensions are important to consider as nations move toward universal health coverage: (1) the proportion of the population covered by pooled health financing arrangements; (2) the proportion of the costs covered, and (3) which services are covered (Fig. 1.33).[69]

- Health care services for AYAs need to incorporate the specific health priorities of this age group. The WHO guidance on providing adolescent-friendly health care highlights the importance of equity, effectiveness, accessibility, acceptability, and appropriateness of care.
- In a literature review of young people's perspectives on health care, domains that were highlighted by AYAs as important indicators of health care quality included: accessibility (location, affordability), staff attitude, age-appropriate environments, youth involvement, health outcomes, communication, and medical competency.[70]
- Adolescents and young adults are particularly vulnerable to catastrophic health costs, but barriers to health care access go beyond financial concerns and include concerns about the confidentiality or quality of the service offered, and transport and other practical problems. There are also legal barriers to accessing health care in many countries, particularly relating to sexual and reproductive health and contraception for unmarried AYAs.[4]
- In countries with universal access to health care, adolescence is a time of increasing health care utilization, and outside infancy, most health care contacts among children and young people are for AYAs.[71]
- Clinicians play an important part in ensuring health services are appropriately designed for AYAs, yet even in high-income settings, specific medical training in adolescent health is often not provided outside the United States, Canada, and Australia.[72]
- The United States is alone among developed nations in not providing universal health coverage. Health insurance in the United States is tied to employment or unemployment and poverty. Until the Affordable Care Act (ACA) was enacted in 2010, adolescents frequently lost health insurance and ready access to primary care services after age 18 years.[52] Prior to these health care reforms, young adults reported the lowest rates of insurance coverage of any age group.

- The number of uninsured AYAs decreased following passage of the ACA. Under these reforms, young adults are entitled to be covered by their parents' insurance until age 26 years. Young adults are also an important target group for the health insurance exchanges.

Defining and Improving the Quality of Adolescents and Young Adult Health and Health Promotion Services
Health Services

- Adolescence and young adulthood are often perceived as healthy times of life. Thus, services for AYAs are often a low priority and often do not meet the specific needs of this population.
- There is an increasing recognition and evidence base regarding the distinct health care needs and priorities of AYAs. In many cases, these needs are similar for AYAs across the world. For example, confidentiality and communications skills of clinicians are important in both the United States and low-income countries, although distinct cultural factors are present for each country.[4]
- Targeted age-appropriate health services can improve health outcomes in chronic conditions.
- For many conditions, outcomes worsen in early adulthood as independent management coincides with transition to adult services and geographic movement for study/work.
- Since the publication of the 2002 WHO Agenda for Change, there have been several policy efforts toward age-appropriate, adolescent-friendly health care.[4]
- Several quality frameworks and tools have been published to support professionals in improving the quality of service for AYAs. They include an Australian framework for AYA inpatient care,[73] European primary care and inpatient tools which have been endorsed by the WHO, and United States models like those for AYA mental health services and cancer care and follow-up.[52]

DATA SOURCES

Global trends in adolescent demographics, health behaviors, and health outcomes change from year to year. Below are key sources of multinational data used throughout this chapter, all of which update their online sources regularly for readers seeking the most recent statistics (**Tables 1.4** and **1.5**).

TABLE 1.4

Data Sources

Data Source	Brief Description	Source/Indicators	Link
Countdown to 2030	Global collaboration tracking progress of life-saving interventions for reproductive, maternal, newborn, child and adolescent health and nutrition	Collective of data from global, regional, and country institutions, United Nations (UN) agencies, World Bank and civil society organizations	https://www.countdown2030.org/
The Demographic and Health Surveys Program (DHS)	Collects and disseminates accurate, nationally representative data on health and population trends around the world	Facilitator of over 400 surveys in more than 90 countries on topics related to population trends, health, HIV, and nutrition	https://dhsprogram.com/
Eurostat	Statistical office of the European Union	Database on European Union (EU) economy, population and social conditions, industry, environment, science, technology, and more	https://ec.europa.eu/eurostat
Global Early Adolescent Study (GEAS)	Studies gender socialization in early adolescence on a global scale and its influence on health	Longitudinal study following 15,000 adolescents between 10 and 14 y old on five continents for up to 5 y	https://www.geastudy.org/
Guttmacher Institute	Research and policy organization with resources on the advancement of sexual and reproductive health worldwide	Sexual and reproductive health indicators (pregnancy, abortion, births) from the Guttmacher Institute and other trusted sources	https://data.guttmacher.org/regions
Healthy Behaviour in School-Aged Children (HBSC)	Cross-national study collecting data on young people's well-being, health behaviors and social environment	School-based surveys to children ages 11, 13, and 15 y old. Data collected every 4 y and includes 50 countries and regions across Europe and North America	http://www.hbsc.org/
Institute for Health Metrics and Evaluation (IHME)	Independent population health research center; home of the Global Burden of Disease (GBD) data among other projects	Comprehensive catalog of surveys, censuses, vital statistics, and other health-related data	http://www.healthdata.org/
The Organisation for Economic Co-Operation and Development (OECD)	International organization working to establish international standards and solutions for social, economic, and environmental challenges	Comparative socioeconomic data and analyses from 37 OECD member countries	https://data.oecd.org/
United Nations World Population Prospects	Population estimates and projections prepared by the Population Division of the Department of Economic and Social Affairs of the United Nations Secretariat	Demographic indicators for UN development groups, World Bank income groups, geographic regions, Sustainable Development Goals regions for selected periods between 1950 and 2100	https://population.un.org/wpp/
World Health Organization (WHO) Global Health Observatory	Health-related statistics for 194 WHO member states	Over 1,000 indicators on priority health topics, including global health estimates, mortality databases, progress toward health-related Sustainable Development Goals, and more	https://www.who.int/data/gho
Young Lives	International study illuminating drivers and impacts of child poverty	Qualitative longitudinal study including household child and school surveys; includes data from 12,000 children in four different countries (Ethiopia, India, Peru, Vietnam)	https://www.younglives.org.uk/

TABLE 1.5

Definitions and Data Availability for 12 Headline Indicators of Adolescent Health from the *Lancet* Commission on Adolescent Health and Well-Being

Headline Indicators	Data Source	Link	Countries Covered (*n* = 195)	Definition	Short Title
Health outcome					
DALYs due to communicable, maternal, and nutritional diseases in individuals aged 10–24 y	IHME	http://www.healthdata.org/	195 (100%)	DALYs per 100,000 adolescents due to communicable, maternal, and nutritional diseases in individuals aged 10–24 y	Group 1 DALYs
DALYs due to injury and violence in individuals aged 10–24 y	IHME	http://www.healthdata.org/	195 (100%)	DALYs per 100,000 adolescents due to injury and violence in individuals aged 10–24 y	Injury DALYs
DALYs due to noncommunicable diseases in individuals aged 10–24 y	IHME	http://www.healthdata.org/	195 (100%)	DALYs per 100,000 adolescents due to noncommunicable diseases in individuals aged 10–24 y	Noncommunicable disease DALYs
Health risks					
Daily smoking in individuals aged 10–24 y	IHME	http://www.healthdata.org/	195 (100%)	Prevalence of use of any smoked tobacco product in individuals aged 10–24 y	Daily tobacco
Binge drinking in the past 12 mo in individuals aged 15–19 y	IHME	http://www.healthdata.org/	195 (100%)	Prevalence of binge alcohol use (>48 g of alcohol for females, >60 g for males) in the past 12 mo for individuals aged 15–19 y	Binge drinking
Individuals aged 10–24 y who exceed WHO guidelines for overweight	IHME	http://www.healthdata.org/	195 (100%)	Prevalence of overweight and obesity (IOTF thresholds, age-specific and sex-specific thresholds, equivalent to a BMI ≥25 kg/m² at age 18 y) in individuals aged 10–24 y	Overweight and obesity
Prevalence of iron deficiency anemia in individuals aged 10–24 y	IHME	http://www.healthdata.org/	195 (100%)	Prevalence of anemia in individuals aged 10–24 y; for those aged 10–14 y hemoglobin <155 g/L; for those aged 15–24 y, <130 g/L for males, <120 g/L for nonpregnant females, and <110 g/L for pregnant females	Anemia
Social determinants of health					
Completing ≥12 y of education among individuals aged 20–24 y	Barro-Lee	http://www.barrolee.com/	143 (93%)	Proportion completing secondary school among individuals aged 20–24 y	Secondary education
Individuals aged 20–24 y who are NEET	International Labour Organization	https://www.ilo.org/global/lang--en/index.htm	123 (75%)	Proportion of individuals 15–24 y not in education, employment, or training	NEET
Annual birth rate per 1,000 adolescents aged 10–19 y	IHME	http://www.healthdata.org/	195 (100%)	Birth rate (livebirths per 1,000 population per year) in females aged 15–19 y	Adolescent livebirths
Marriage before age 18 y in females aged 20–24 y	Multiple Indicator Cluster Survey and Demographic and Health Survey	https://mics.unicef.org/	120 (62%)	Proportion of females aged 20–24 y in marriage or union before age 18 y	Child marriage
Females aged 15–24 y with met need for contraception	IHME	http://www.healthdata.org/	195 (100%)	Proportion of females aged 15–24 y whose demand for contraception is satisfied with a modern method	Demand for modern contraception satisfied

DALYs, disability-adjusted life years; IHME, Institute for Health Metrics and Evaluation; IOTF, World Obesity Federation; BMI, body mass index.

Source: Azzopardi PS, Hearps SJC, Francis KL, et al. Progress in adolescent health and wellbeing: tracking 12 headline indicators for 195 countries and territories, 1990 to 2016. *Lancet.* 2019;393(10176):1101–1118.

SUMMARY: HEALTH OF THE WORLD'S ADOLESCENTS AND YOUNG ADULTS

Investing in AYA health will not only improve outcomes for this age group, but will also affect future health trajectories for both adults and children, and will be an important determinant of future economic development.[4] Yet, economic and social changes threaten the health of AYAs in all countries. This chapter has reviewed specific challenges and opportunities relating to AYA health improvement that warrant the attention of professionals, researchers, policy makers, and other stakeholders. These include understanding the following: (1) complex web of social and other determinants to health outcomes, and how these operate in this age group; (2) ongoing shift in disease burden from early childhood to adolescence; (3) rapid demographic changes in many settings; (4) growth and impact of new media; and (5) need to adapt health systems to provide services for young people that reflect their specific health needs.

REFERENCES

1. Sawyer SM, Azzopardi PS, Wickremarathne D, et al. The age of adolescence. *Lancet Child Adolesc Health*. 2018;2(3):223–228.
2. United Nations. *World Population Prospects 2019 Data Booklet*. Department of Economic and Social Affairs, Population Division; 2019.
3. Azzopardi PS, Hearps SJC, Francis KL, et al. Progress in adolescent health and wellbeing: tracking 12 headline indicators for 195 countries and territories, 1990 to 2016. *Lancet*. 2019;393(10176):1101–1118.
4. Patton GC, Sawyer SM, Santelli JS, et al. Our future: a Lancet commission on adolescent health and wellbeing. *Lancet*. 2016;387(10036):2423–2478.
5. Ward JL, Azzopardi PS, Francis KL, et al. Global, regional, and national mortality among young people aged 10–24 years, 1950–2019: a systematic analysis for the Global Burden of Disease Study 2019. *The Lancet*. 2021;398(10311):1593–1618.
6. Viner RM, Coffey C, Mathers C, et al. 50-year mortality trends in children and young people: a study of 50 low-income, middle-income, and high-income countries. *Lancet*. 2011;377(9772):1162–1174.
7. World Health Organization. *Closing the Gap in a Generation: Health Equity Through Action on the Social Determinants of Health*. World Health Organization; 2008.
8. National Research Council (US), Institute of Medicine (US) Woolf SH, et al. eds. *U.S. Health in International Perspective: Shorter Lives, Poorer Health*. National Academies Press (US); 2013.
9. Bonnie RJ, Stroud C, Breiner H, eds. *Investing in the Health and Well-Being of Young Adults*. National Academies Press; 2015.
10. Finer L, Philbin JM. Trends in ages at key reproductive transitions in the United States, 1951–2010. *Womens Health Issues*. 2014;24(3):e271–e279.
11. Santelli JS, Song X, Garbers S, et al. Global trends in adolescent fertility, 1990–2012, in relation to national wealth, income inequalities, and educational expenditures. *J Adolesc Health*. 2017;60(2):161–168.
12. GBD 2019 Demographics Collaborators. Global age-sex-specific fertility, mortality, healthy life expectancy (HALE), and population estimates in 204 countries and territories, 1950–2019: a comprehensive demographic analysis for the Global Burden of Disease Study 2019. *The Lancet*. 2020;396(10258):1160–1203. doi:10.1016/S0140-6736(20)30977-6
13. Ward JL, Viner RM. The impact of income inequality and national wealth on child and adolescent mortality in low and middle-income countries. *BMC Public Health*. 2017;17(1):429.
14. Viner RM, Ozer EM, Denny S, et al. Adolescence and the social determinants of health. *Lancet*. 2012;379(9826):1641–1652.
15. UNESCO. *One in five children, adolescents and youth is out of school*. Accessed September 13, 2021. https://en.unesco.org/news/one-every-five-children-adolescents-and-youth-out-school-worldwide
16. UNICEF. *UNICEF Data: monitoring the situation of children and women*. Accessed February 17, 2021. https://data.unicef.org/
17. The Annie E. Casey Foundation, *2021 Kids Count Data Book: State Trends in Child Well-Being*. The Annie E Casey Foundation; 2021.
18. International Labour Office. Global employment trends for youth 2020: technology and the future of jobs: International Labour Office, 2020. https://www.ilo.org/wcmsp5/groups/public/—dgreports/—dcomm/—publ/documents/publication/wcms_737648.pdf
19. Chandler RF, Santos Lozada AR. Health status among NEET adolescents and young adults in the United States, 2016–2018. *SSM Popul Health*. 2021;14:100814.
20. US Department of Labor. *Unemployment rates*. Accessed September 13, 2021. https://www.dol.gov/agencies/wb/data/latest-annual-data/employment-rates
21. United Nations Department of Economic and Social Affairs Population Division. *International migrant stock 2019*. Accessed February 17, 2021. https://www.un.org/en/development/desa/population/migration/data/estimates2/estimatesmaps.asp?0t0
22. Abubakar I, Aldridge RW, Devakumar D, et al. The UCL–Lancet Commission on Migration and Health: the health of a world on the move. *Lancet*. 2018;392(10164):2606–2654.
23. Bendavid E, Boerma T, Akseer N, et al. The effects of armed conflict on the health of women and children. *Lancet*. 2021;397(10273):522–532.
24. United Nations High Comissioner for Refugees. *Figures at a glance*. Accessed July 6, 2021. https://www.unhcr.org/en-us/figures-at-a-glance.html
25. Wagner Z, Heft-Neal S, Wise PH, et al. Women and children living in areas of armed conflict in Africa: a geospatial analysis of mortality and orphanhood. *Lancet Glob Health*. 2019;7(12):e1622–e1631.
26. Hatzenbuehler ML, Birkett M, Van Wagenen A, et al. Protective school climates and reduced risk for suicide ideation in sexual minority youths. *Am J Public Health*. 2014;104(2):279–286.
27. Trent M, Dooley DG, Dougé J; Section on Adolescent Health, Council on Community Pediatrics, Committee on Adolescence. The impact of racism on child and adolescent health. *J Pediatr*. 2019;144(2):e20191765.
28. Woolf SH, Masters RK, Aron LY. Effect of the covid-19 pandemic in 2020 on life expectancy across populations in the USA and other high income countries: simulations of provisional mortality data. *BMJ*. 2021;373:n1343.
29. Institute of Medicine, National Research Council, Committee on the Science of Adolescence. *The Science of Adolescent Risk-Taking: Workshop Report*. The National Academies Press; 2011.
30. The Community Guide. *Health equity: school-based health centers*. Accessed September 13, 2021. https://www.thecommunityguide.org/findings/promoting-health-equity-through-education-programs-and-policies-school-based-health-centers
31. United Nations Children's Fund, For Every Child. *End AIDS: Seventh Stocktaking Report*. UNICEF; 2016.
32. Hillis SD, Unwin HJT, Chen Y, et al. Global minimum estimates for COVID-19 associated orphanhood and deaths of caregivers: a modelling study. *Lancet*. 2021;398:391–402.
33. Anderson M, Jiang J. *Teens, social media and technology 2018*. Accessed September 13, 2021. https://www.pewresearch.org/internet/2018/05/31/teens-social-media-technology-2018/
34. Kreniske P, Basmajian A, Nakyanjo N, et al. The promise and peril of mobile phones for youth in rural Uganda: multimethod study of implications for health and HIV. *J Med Internet Res*. 2021;23(2):e17837.
35. Viner RM, Gireesh A, Stiglic N, et al. Roles of cyberbullying, sleep, and physical activity in mediating the effects of social media use on mental health and wellbeing among young people in England: a secondary analysis of longitudinal data. *Lancet Child Adolesc Health*. 2019;3(10):685–696.
36. Viner RM, Ross D, Hardy R, et al. Life course epidemiology; recognising the importance of adolescence *J Epidemiol Community Health*. 2015;69:719–720.
37. Susser E, Hoek HW, Brown A. Neurodevelopmental disorders after prenatal famine: the story of the Dutch Famine Study. *Am J Epidemiol*. 1998;147(3):213–216.
38. Abbas KM, Van Zandvoort K, Brisson M, et al. Effects of updated demography, disability weights, and cervical cancer burden on estimates of human papillomavirus vaccination impact at the global, regional, and national levels: a PRIME modelling study. *Lancet Glob Health*. 2020;8(4):e536–e544.
39. World Bank. *World Development Report 2007: Development and the Next Generation*. World Bank; 2006.
40. Bauman K. *Mapping the transition to adulthood: a bird's-eye view of enrollment, employment, independence, and marriage*. Accessed September 13, 2021. https://www.census.gov/content/dam/Census/library/working-papers/2017/demo/SEHSD-WP2017-20.pdf
41. Angelini V, Mierau JO. Late-life health effects of teenage motherhood. *Demogr Res*. 2018;39(41):1081–1104.
42. Livingston G. *Pew Research Center: For most highly educated women, motherhood doesn't start until the 30s*. Accessed July 15, 2021. http://pewrsr.ch/1DIpIhX
43. Vollset SE, Goren E, Yuan CW, et al. Fertility, mortality, migration, and population scenarios for 195 countries and territories from 2017 to 2100: a forecasting analysis for the Global Burden of Disease Study. *Lancet*. 2020;396(10258):1285–1306.
44. The Annie E. Casey Foundation. *Child population by race in the United States*. Accessed September 13, 2021. https://datacenter.kidscount.org/data/tables/103-child-population-by-race#detailed/1/any/false/1729,133,11/68,69,67,12,70,66,71,72/424
45. The Annie E. Casey Foundation. *What the data say about race, ethnicity and American youth*. Accessed September 13, 2021. https://www.aecf.org/blog/what-the-data-say-about-race-ethnicity-and-american-youth
46. Frey WH. *Brookings Institute: six maps that reveal America's expanding racial diversity*. Accessed September 13, 2021. https://www.brookings.edu/research/americas-racial-diversity-in-six-maps/
47. Knaul FM, Bustreo F, Horton R, et al. Countering the pandemic of gender-based violence and maltreatment of young people: The Lancet Commission. *Lancet*. 2020;395(10218):98.
48. World Health Organization. *Violence Against Women Prevalence Estimates, 2018: Global, Regional and National Prevalence Estimates for Intimate Partner Violence Against Women and Global and Regional Prevalence Estimates for Non-Partner Sexual Violence Against Women*. World Health Organization; 2021.
49. UNFPA. *Adolescent pregnancy*. Accessed September 16, 2021. https://www.unfpa.org/adolescent-pregnancy#summery105866
50. Singh S, Remez L, Sedgh G, et al. *Abortion Worldwide 2017: Uneven Progress and Unequal Access*. Guttmacher Institute; 2018.
51. Cunningham RM, Walton MA, Carter PM. The major causes of death in children and adolescents in the United States. *N Engl J Med*. 2018;379(25):2468–2475.
52. National Research Council, Institute of Medicine, Board on Children. *Improving the Health, Safety, and Well-Being of Young Adults: Workshop Summary*. The National Academies Press; 2013.
53. CDC WONDER Online Database. *Underlying cause of death 1999–2019*. Accessed July 16, 2021. http://wonder.cdc.gov/ucd-icd10.html
54. GBD 2019 Diseases and Injuries Collaborators. Global burden of 369 diseases and injuries in 204 countries and territories, 1990–2019: a systematic analysis for the Global Burden of Disease Study 2019 [published correction appears in Lancet. 2020 November 14;396(10262):1562]. *The Lancet*. 2020;396(10258):1204–1222. doi:10.1016/S0140-6736(20)30925-9
55. Centers for Disease Control and Prevention. https://www.cdc.gov/
56. Patel V, Flisher AJ, Hetrick S, et al. Mental health of young people: a global public-health challenge. *Lancet*. 2007;369(9569):1302–1313.

57. Kessler RC, Angermeyer M, Anthony JC, et al. Lifetime prevalence and age-of-onset distributions of mental disorders in the World Health Organization's World Mental Health Survey Initiative. *World Psychiatry.* 2007;6(3):168.

58. Kessler RC, Amminger GP, Aguilar-Gaxiola S, et al. Age of onset of mental disorders: a review of recent literature. *Curr Opin Psychiatry.* 2007;20(4):359.

59. Inchley J, Currie D, Budisavljevic S, et al., eds. *Spotlight on Adolescent Health and Well-Being: Findings from the 2017/2018 Health Behaviour in School-Aged Children (HBSC) survey in Europe and Canada.* World Health Organization; 2020.

60. Degenhardt L, Stockings E, Patton G, et al. The increasing global health priority of substance use in young people. *Lancet Psychiatry.* 2016;3(3):251–264.

61. Reitsma MB, Flor LS, Mullany EC, et al. Spatial, temporal, and demographic patterns in prevalence of smoking tobacco use and initiation among young people in 204 countries and territories, 1990–2019. *Lancet Public Health.* 2021;6:e472–e481.

62. Miech R, Johnston L, O'Malley PM, et al. Trends in adolescent vaping, 2017–2019. *N Engl J Med.* 2019;381(15):1490–1491.

63. Degenhardt L, Chiu WT, Sampson N, et al. Toward a global view of alcohol, tobacco, cannabis, and cocaine use: findings from the WHO World Mental Health Surveys. *PLoS Med.* 2008;5(7):e141.

64. Maimaris W, McCambridge J. Age of first drinking and adult alcohol problems: systematic review of prospective cohort studies. *J Epidemiol Community Health.* 2014;68(3):268–274.

65. Fryar CD, Carroll MD, Afful J. *Prevalence of Overweight, Obesity, and Severe Obesity Among Children and Adolescents Aged 2–19 Years: United States, 1963–1965 Through 2017–2018.* NCHS Health E-Stats; 2020.

66. Guthold R, Stevens GA, Riley LM, et al. Global trends in insufficient physical activity among adolescents: a pooled analysis of 298 population-based surveys with 1.6 million participants. *Lancet Child Adolesc Health.* 2020;4(1):23–35.

67. Sully EA, Biddlecom A, Darroch JE, et al., *Adding it Up: Investing in Sexual and Reproductive Health 2019.* Guttmacher Institute; 2020.

68. Liang M, Simelane S, Fillo GF, et al. The state of adolescent sexual and reproductive health. *J Adolesc Health.* 2019;65(6):S3–S15.

69. Waddington C, Sambo C. Financing health care for adolescents: a necessary part of universal health coverage. *Bull World Health Organ.* 2015;93:57–59.

70. Ambresin AE, Bennett K, Patton GC, et al. Assessment of youth-friendly health care: a systematic review of indicators drawn from young people's perspectives. *J Adolesc Health.* 2013;52(6):670–681.

71. Hargreaves DS, Viner RM. Adolescent inpatient activity 1999–2010: analysis of English Hospital Episode Statistics data. *Arch Dis Child.* 2014;99(9):830–833.

72. Michaud P-A, Weber MW, Namazova-Baranova L, et al. Improving the quality of care delivered to adolescents in Europe: a time to invest. *Arch Dis Child.* 2019;104(3):214–216.

73. Sawyer SM, Ambresin AE, Bennett KE, et al. A measurement framework for quality health care for adolescents in hospital. *J Adolesc Health.* 2014;55(4):484–490.

📶 ADDITIONAL RESOURCES AND WEBSITES

Additional Resources and Websites for Clinicians:

The Future of Sex Education (FoSE) is a collaboration of Advocates for Youth, Answer, and SIECUS: Sex Ed for Social Change seeks to create a national dialogue about the future of sex education and to promote the institutionalization of comprehensive sexuality education in public schools. https://futureofsexed.org/

The Helping Adolescents Thrive (HAT) Initiative is a joint WHO-UNICEF effort to strengthen policies and programmes for the mental health of adolescents. Toolkits are available to promote and protect adolescent mental health and reduce self-harm and other risk behaviors. https://www.who.int/teams/mental-health-and-substance-use/promotion-prevention/who-unicef-helping-adolescents-thrive-programme

International Association for Adolescent Health (IAAH) is a multidisciplinary, non-government organization which aims to improve the health, development and well-being of 10- to 24-year-old adolescents and young adults, in every region of the world. IAAH's YouTube channel knowledge, skills, and experiences of and with those working in adolescent health. https://www.youtube.com/channel/UCwq54X-E5p1yrSGu9a80W-TQ

National Research Council (US), Institute of Medicine (US). In: Woolf SH, Aron L, eds. *U.S. Health in International Perspective: Shorter Lives, Poorer Health.* National Academies Press (US), 2013. https://www.ncbi.nlm.nih.gov/books/NBK115854/

Patton GC, Sawyer SM, Santelli JS, et al. Our future: a Lancet commission on adolescent health and wellbeing. *Lancet.* 2016;387(10036):2423–2478. https://www.thelancet.com/journals/lancet/article/PIIS0140-6736(16)00579-1/fulltext

Sawyer SM, Azzopardi PS, Wickremarathne D, et al. The age of adolescence. *Lancet Child Adolesc Health.* 2018;2(3):223–228. https://www.thelancet.com/journals/lanchi/article/PIIS2352-4642%2818%2930022-1/fulltext

Ward JL, Azzopardi PS, Francis KL, et al. Global, regional, and national mortality among young people aged 10–24 years, 1950–2019: a systematic analysis for the Global Burden of Disease Study 2019. *The Lancet.* 2021;398(10311):1593–618.

Additional Resources and Websites for Parents/Caregivers and Websites for Adolescents and Young Adults:

The Society for Adolescent Health and Medicine (SAHM) is a multidisciplinary organization committed to improving the physical and psychosocial health and well-being of all adolescents through advocacy, clinical care, health promotion, health service delivery, professional development, and research. Below are selected resources for parents and teenagers from their resource list, which can also be viewed in full here. https://www.adolescenthealth.org/Resources/Resources-for-Adolescents-and-Parents.aspx

AMAZE harnesses the power of digital media to provide young adolescents around the globe with medically accurate, age-appropriate, affirming, and honest sex education they can access directly online. AMAZE also gives parents, guardians, educators, and clinicians around the globe tools to communicate effectively with adolescents about sex and sexuality. https://amaze.org/

Bedsider is an online birth control support network for people between the ages of 18 to 29 operated by Power to Decide, the campaign to prevent unplanned pregnancy. Power to Decide works to ensure that every young person has the power to decide if, when, and under what circumstances to get pregnant—increasing their opportunity to pursue the future they want. https://www.bedsider.org/

Bright Futures is a national health promotion and prevention initiative led by the American Academy of Pediatrics and supported by the U.S. Department of Health and Human Services, Health Resources and Services Administration, and Maternal and Child Health Bureau. Bright Futures has resources on child and adolescent health for parents and children to explore together, as well as tip sheets for what parents can expect at a well visit. https://brightfutures.aap.org/materials-and-tools/family-materials/Pages/default.aspx

FamilyDoctor.org is a health information website from the American Academy of Family Physicians that provides information on puberty, sexuality, nutrition, fitness, and emotional well-being from family medicine perspective. https://familydoctor.org/

Go Ask Alice is the health question and answer Internet resource produced by Alice! Health Promotion at Columbia University. Adolescents can explore resources on sexuality, substances, nutrition, emotional health, and relationships, or submit their own questions. https://goaskalice.columbia.edu/

HealthyChildren.org is a parenting website backed by the American Academy of Pediatrics, committed to the attainment of optimal physical, mental, and social health and well-being for all infants, children, adolescents, and young adults. https://www.healthychildren.org/

Partnership to End Addiction is the leading organization dedicated to addiction prevention, treatment, and recovery, providing resources for parents to prevent and intervene in adolescent substance use. https://drugfree.org/

Planned Parenthood delivers vital reproductive health care, sex education, and information to millions of people worldwide. Their website features both teen-focused and parent resources on sex, puberty, physician visits, sexuality and gender identity, and more. https://www.plannedparenthood.org/learn

The Trevor Project is the leading national organization providing crisis intervention and suicide prevention services to lesbian, gay, bisexual, transgender, queer, and questioning (LGBTQ) young people under 25. https://www.thetrevorproject.org/

CHAPTER 2

Normal Physical Growth and Development °

Jeremi M. Carswell
Diane E. J. Stafford

KEY WORDS

- Adrenarche
- Gonadotropins
- Growth
- Growth hormone
- Puberty
- Sexual development
- Sexual maturity rating

INTRODUCTION

Accelerated growth, maturation of sexual characteristics, and the attainment of adult height and body proportions are the physical hallmarks of adolescence. Underlying these changes are the complicated activation and interplay of several hormonal axes that have been previously quiescent. This chapter provides an overview of the normal pubertal process and highlights the wide variation in the onset and duration of puberty in healthy adolescents and between birth-assigned male and female adolescents. Understanding these variations will provide the clinician a framework for differentiating normal variations from abnormal pubertal development. The focus of Chapter 14 is abnormalities in growth and pubertal development. Please note that in this text, we use the terms "female," "male," "girl," and "boy." While the term "birth-assigned" is not always used, it should be assumed that we are only discussing birth-assigned sex characteristics in this chapter.

ENDOCRINE AXES AFFECTING PUBERTAL MATURATION

Although there is activity and change in most hormonal systems during adolescence, the two that are primarily responsible for the physical changes of puberty are the hypothalamic–pituitary–gonadal (HPG) axis and the hypothalamic–pituitary–adrenal (HPA) axis.

Hypothalamic–Pituitary–Gonadal Axis

This axis is ultimately responsible for the release of estradiol and testosterone from the ovaries and testes, respectively, via the pituitary hormones, luteinizing hormone (LH), and follicle-stimulating hormone (FSH). This process originates with the release of gonadotropin-releasing hormone (GnRH) from the hypothalamic pulse generator that then signals the release of LH and FSH from the anterior pituitary. The mechanisms by which this system is activated are not completely understood, although it appears that it is released/inhibited by the central nervous system, which in turn enables a positive feedback loop that results in pubertal maturation (Fig. 2.1).

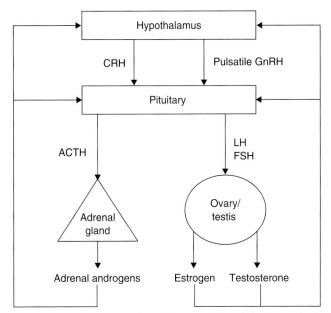

FIGURE 2.1 The hypothalamic–pituitary–gonadal and the hypothalamic–pituitary–adrenal axes. CRH, corticotropin-releasing hormone; GnRH, gonadotropin-releasing hormone; ACTH, adrenocorticotropic hormone; LH, luteinizing hormone; FSH, follicle-stimulating hormone.

Hypothalamic–Pituitary–Adrenal Axis

The products of HPA axis maturation in the context of puberty are the adrenal androgens, primarily dehydroepiandrosterone (DHEA) and its sulfate ester, dehydroepiandrosterone-sulfate (DHEA-S). These hormones exert their effects primarily by acting as precursors for the more potent androgens, testosterone, and dihydrotestosterone. It is important to recognize that production of these androgens is independent of the changes occurring in the HPG axis and that maturation may occur at different times.

MATURATION OF THE HYPOTHALAMIC–PITUITARY–GONADAL AXIS

Gonadal Steroids

Estrogen

Estradiol (E2) from the ovary accounts for most of the *circulating* estrogens, although there is a small amount of extraovarian conversion from androstenedione (to estrone) and testosterone (to estradiol). In addition to stimulating breast growth and maturation of the vaginal mucosa, estrogen has profound effects on the skeleton, being the primary hormone responsible for epiphysial closure. At higher doses, estrogen causes epiphyseal fusion and, therefore, termination of linear growth. The mechanism by which this occurs is thought to involve estrogen's stimulation of chondrogenesis on the epiphyseal growth plate.[1]

Testosterone

Although the testes represent the primary source of this hormone, a small amount is generated from the extratesticular conversion of the adrenal hormone androstenedione in both males and females. Testosterone is the primary hormone responsible for the voice change in males and attainment of male body habitus, but it is dihydrotestosterone, the product of conversion of testosterone by 5α-reductase, that causes phallic and prostate growth.

The Origins of Puberty: The Gonadotropin-Releasing Hormone Pulse Generator and the Influences of Genetics

Gonadotropin-Releasing Hormone Pulse Generator

The downstream release of gonadal steroids depends on the pulsatile hypothalamic release of GnRH. The exact triggers, as well as when they occur, are incompletely understood although three distinct changes are well characterized.

1. Nocturnal sleep-related augmentation of pulsatile LH secretion begins after the increased pulsatile release of GnRH.[2] The clinical implication of this is that LH levels must be measured in the early morning when assessing for biochemical evidence of early puberty.
2. The sensitivity of the hypothalamus and the pituitary to estradiol and testosterone decreases such that the gonadotropins, LH and FSH, begin to increase.
3. A positive feedback system develops in females, so that rising levels of estrogen trigger GnRH release, stimulating LH to initiate ovulation.

Kisspeptins and the KISS1/GPR54 System

Kisspeptins refer to a class of peptides encoded by the *KISS1/Kiss1* gene that act through the receptor, *GPR54*. These compounds appear to stimulate LH through GnRH at the hypothalamic level and are implicated as necessary for pubertal onset, as well as normal reproductive function.[3]

Leptin

This product of the *ob* gene produced by fat cells was initially thought to have a gateway role in pubertal development. It was discovered to play a key role in the regulation of appetite, food intake, and energy expenditure, providing a signal to the central nervous system regarding satiety and the amount of energy stored in adipose tissue.[4] With further investigation, its role has been identified as more modest; it appears that leptin is permissive for pubertal advancement at the hypothalamic level by modulation of the GnRH system, although it has also been shown to have effects at other levels of the HPG axis.[4]

Genetic Influences on the Timing of Puberty

While environmental factors can influence the timing of pubertal onset, there is a strong heritability component supported by both twin studies and parent/child correlation.[5] In addition to the KISS1/KISS1R/Kisspeptin system, other genes have been implicated in the timing of puberty. Both the Makorin RING finger protein 3 (MKRN3) and the delta-like noncanonical Notch ligand 1 (DLK1) genes are maternally imprinted and their dysfunction is associated with precocious puberty.[5] Large genome-wide association studies (GWAS) have also identified several alleles that have been associated with pubertal timing.[6]

⬤ PHYSICAL MANIFESTATIONS OF PUBERTY

What are commonly thought of as pubertal secondary sexual characteristics should be separated into gonadarche and adrenarche, arising from activation of the HPG axis and HPA axis, respectively. In birth-assigned females, gonadarche is represented by thelarche, or the onset of breast budding, and in birth-assigned males by testicular enlargement to 4 mL and above or 2.5 cm in the longest axis. Pubarche, or the growth of terminal sexual hair in birth-assigned girls, is mainly the result of adrenarche. In birth-assigned boys, both testicular and adrenal androgens contribute.

Sexual Maturity Rating Scales

Sexual maturity rating (SMR) scales (also called *Tanner staging*) as developed by Marshall and Tanner[7,8] allow for accurate classification of physical pubertal maturation. For both boys and girls, there are five stages categorizing secondary sexual characteristics (pubic hair and breast development in females, pubic hair and genitalia in males). These stages are described as follows and are shown in drawings in Figures 2.2 to 2.4.

Males (testicular volumes as measured by a Prader Orchidometer)
1. Genital stage 1 (G1): Prepubertal
   a. Testes: Volume, <4 mL, or long axis, ≤2.5 cm
   b. Phallus: Childlike
2. Genital stage 2 (G2)
   a. Testes: Volume, 4 to 8 mL, or long axis, 2.6 to 3.3 cm
   b. Scrotum: Reddened, thinner, and larger
   c. Phallus: No change
3. Genital stage 3 (G3)
   a. Testes: Volume, 10 to 15 mL, or long axis, 3.4 to 4.0 cm
   b. Scrotum: Greater enlargement
   c. Phallus: Increased length

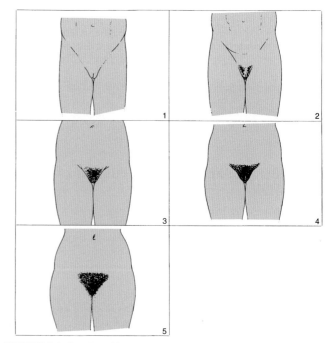

FIGURE 2.2 Female pubic hair development. SMR 1: Prepubertal; no pubic hair. SMR 2: Straight hair is extending along the labia and, between ratings 2 and 3, begins on the pubis. SMR 3: Pubic hair has increased in quantity, is darker, and is present in the typical female triangle but in smaller quantity. SMR 4: Pubic hair has increased in quantity, is darker, and is more dense, curled, and adult in distribution but less abundant. SMR 5: Abundant, adult-type pattern; hair may extend onto the medial aspect of the thighs. (From Daniel WA, Palshock BZ. A physician's guide to sexual maturity rating. *Patient Care.* 1979;30:122, with permission. Illustration by Paul Singh-Roy.)

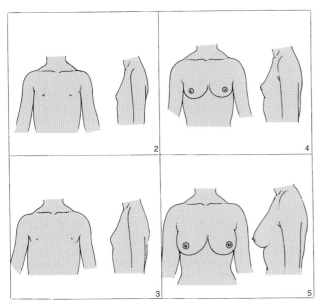

FIGURE 2.3 Female breast development. SMR 1, not shown: Prepubertal; elevations of papilla only. SMR 2: Breast buds appear; areola is slightly widened and projects as small mound. SMR 3: Enlargement of the entire breast with protrusion of the papilla or of the nipple. SMR 4: Enlargement of the breast and projection of areola and papilla as a secondary mound. SMR 5: Adult configuration of the breast with protrusion of the nipple; areola no longer projects separately from remainder of breast. (From Daniel WA, Paulshock BZ. A physician's guide to sexual maturity rating. *Patient Care.* 1979;30:122, with permission. Illustration by Paul Singh-Roy.)

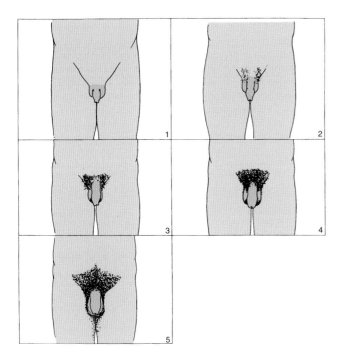

FIGURE 2.4 Male genital and pubic hair development. Ratings for pubic hair and for genital development can differ in a typical boy at any given time, because pubic hair and genitalia do not necessarily develop at the same rate. SMR 1: Prepubertal; no pubic hair. Genitalia unchanged from early childhood. SMR 2: Light, downy hair develops laterally and later becomes dark. Penis and testes may be slightly larger; scrotum becomes more textured. SMR 3: Pubic hair has extended across the pubis. Testes and scrotum are further enlarged; penis is larger, especially in length. SMR 4: More abundant pubic hair with curling. Genitalia resemble those of an adult; glans has become larger and broader, and scrotum is darker. SMR 5: Adult quantity and pattern of pubic hair, with hair present along the inner borders of the thighs. The testes and the scrotum are adult in size. (From Daniel WA, Paulshock BZ. A physician's guide to sexual maturity rating. *Patient Care.* 1979;30:122, with permission. Illustration by Paul Singh-Roy.)

4. Genital stage 4 (G4)
   a. Testes: Volume, 15 to 20 mL, or long axis, 4.1 to 4.5 cm
   b. Scrotum: Further enlargement and darkening
   c. Phallus: Increased length and circumference
5. Genital stage 5 (G5)
   a. Testes: Volume, >25 mL, or long axis, >4.5 cm
   b. Scrotum and phallus: Adult

Females
1. Breast stage 1 (B1)
   a. Breast: Prepubertal; no glandular tissue
   b. Areola and papilla: Areola conform to general chest line
2. Breast stage 2 (B2)
   a. Breast: Breast bud; small amount of glandular tissue
   b. Areola: Areola widens
3. Breast stage 3 (B3)
   a. Breast: Larger and more elevation; extends beyond areolar parameter
   b. Areola and papilla: Areola continues to enlarge but remains in contour with the breast
4. Breast stage 4 (B4)
   a. Breast: Larger and more elevation
   b. Areola and papilla: Areola and papilla form a mound projecting from the breast contour
5. Breast stage 5 (B5)
   a. Breast: Adult (size variable)
   b. Areola and papilla: Areola and breast in same plane, with papilla projecting above areola

Male and Female: Pubic hair
1. Pubic hair stage 1 (PH1)
   a. None
2. Pubic hair stage 2 (PH2)
   a. Small amount of long, slightly pigmented, downy hair along the base of the scrotum and phallus in the male or the labia majora in female; vellus hair versus sexual type hair (PH3)
3. Pubic hair stage 3 (PH3)
   a. Moderate amount of more curly, pigmented, and coarser hair, extending more laterally
4. Pubic hair stage 4 (PH4)
   a. Hair that resembles adult hair in coarseness and curliness but does not extend to medial surface of thighs
5. Pubic hair stage 5 (PH5)
   a. Adult type and quantity, extending to medial surface of thighs

Female Pubertal Changes

Events of Puberty

During puberty, the breasts develop and the ovaries, uterus, vagina, labia, and clitoris increase in size, with the uterus and ovaries increasing in size by approximately five- to sevenfold. Body composition changes, as girls accumulate fat mass at an average annual rate of 1.14 kg/year.[9]

Sequence

Often, the earliest physical sign of puberty in girls is thelarche, although few girls have pubic hair development as the first sign. On average, breast development starts at the age of 10 years for White girls and at 8.9 years for Black girls, according to a frequently cited large cross-sectional study.[10] The Breast Cancer and the Environment Research Program examined >1,200 girls longitudinally over 7 years in three urban areas and reported age at thelarche by both visual inspection, as well as palpation (in contrast to the Pediatric Research in Office Settings [PROS] study which employed only inspection); median age of thelarche (SMR B2) was 8.8 for Black girls, 9.3 years for Hispanic, and 9.7 years for Caucasian and Asian participants. Notably, higher body mass index (BMI) was associated with earlier attainment of SMR 2.[11] These physical findings, however, may be preceded by the growth spurt by approximately 1 year. As a result, the growth curve is an essential tool in the evaluation of precocious or delayed puberty. The average length of time for completion of puberty is 4 years, but can range from 1.5 to 8 years.

Menarche

Menarche usually occurs during SMR B3 or B4, and approximately 3.3 years after the growth spurt, or roughly 2 years after breast budding. The normal range for menarche varies from 9 to 15 years and is dependent on such factors as race, socioeconomic status, heredity, nutrition, and culture. It occurs later at higher altitudes, in rural areas, and in larger families. Body composition also influences age at menarche, although controversy exists on whether there is a necessary amount of adipose mass needed at the time of menarche.

While it is usually assumed that earlier menarche results in a shorter adult height and later puberty associated with a taller adult height, this is often not the case as the duration and intensity of the growth spurt provides a point of flex that results in similar adult heights.[12] On an average, girls grow 4 to 6 cm after menarche. The sequence of pubertal events in females is found in Figure 2.5. The age at menarche has gradually decreased during the last century. However, this trend has slowed significantly in the past few decades.

Several investigators have examined data from the Third National Health and Nutrition Examination Survey (NHANES III) conducted from 1988 to 1994.[5] One study[5] compared data from an earlier U.S. survey 25 years previous to the NHANES III data and found that the average age at menarche had declined only minimally (i.e., by approximately 2.5 months, from 12.8 to 12.5 years). Another study cited up to a 4-month decrease in age at menarche.[5] Review of all available data in 2008 suggested a trend toward earlier menarche in the United States between 1940 and 1994, but with a magnitude of change of 2.5 to 4 months, revealing questionable clinical significance.[5] All studies that have examined race have demonstrated that Black girls reach menarche the earliest, followed by Mexican American and White girls.

Age at Puberty

Although there are slight differences in the ages of onset, the trend is for earlier pubertal onset, but almost no change in the age at menarche. On an average, girls of Black descent appear to enter puberty earlier than their Hispanic and White counterparts. The large study from the PROS group sampled >17,000 White and Black girls from around the United States with the SMR method and found that the earliest signs of puberty are occurring earlier than previously described.[10] In that study, the mean ages at onset of breast development were 8.9 years for Black girls and 10 years for White girls. Pubic hair development started at 8.8 years for Black girls and at 10.5 years for White girls. Similarly, Black girls experienced menarche at 12.2 years, and White girls at 12.9 years.

Male Pubertal Changes

Events of Puberty

By the end of male puberty, the potential for reproduction is achieved. Internal and external genital organs increase in size, and body proportions change so that percentage of body fat actually declines[9] as opposed to the increase in females. Gynecomastia is a common issue in midpubertal boys that may cause significant concern (see Chapter 60). True gynecomastia is glandular development of at least 0.5 cm that is palpable. This may not be easily differentiated from pseudogynecomastia, which is an accumulation of fatty tissue.

Sequence

The earliest sign of physical pubertal development in approximately 98% of males is an increase in testicular volume to 4 mL or 2.5 cm in the long axis, although the first most noticeable event of male puberty is the growth of pubic hair. The growth spurt for boys is during mid- to late puberty, the time of rapidly rising testosterone levels. This contrasts with an early growth spurt in girls. This is also the time when the voice changes, axillary hair develops, and acne may appear. Ejaculation occurs usually at SMR G3, as does the first evidence of spermarche, but fertility is not usually attained until SMR G4. Facial hair growth typically starts approximately 3 years after pubic hair growth. The hair on the face, chest, back, and abdomen may continue throughout and beyond puberty into adulthood, the amount and distribution being quite variable and dependent on ethnicity and family patterns. The average length of time for completion of puberty is 3 years, but it can range from 2 to 5 years. The sequence of events for an average male is shown in the following text in Figure 2.6. Table 2.1 lists testicular volume by SMR.

Age at Puberty

NHANES III data for boys demonstrate a similar trend regarding the initiation of puberty, but no change from earlier studies

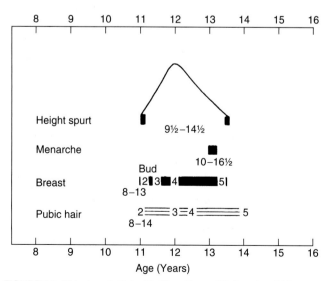

FIGURE 2.5 Biologic maturity in girls. (From Tanner JM. *Growth at Adolescence.* 2nd ed. Blackwell Scientific Publications, 1962, with permission. Copyright © 1962 by Blackwell Scientific Publications.)

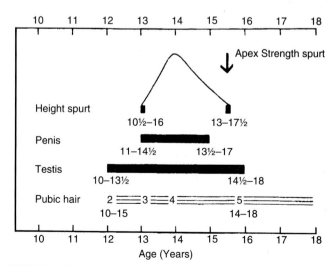

FIGURE 2.6 Biologic maturity in boys. (From Tanner JM. *Growth at Adolescence.* 2nd ed. Blackwell Scientific Publications, 1962, with permission. Copyright © 1962 by Blackwell Scientific Publications.)

TABLE 2.1
Testicular Volume by Sexual Maturity Rating (SMR)

	Volume (cm³)			
	Left Testis		Right Testis	
SMR[a]	Mean	SD	Mean	SD
1	4.8	2.8	5.2	3.9
2	6.4	3.2	7.1	3.9
3	14.6	6.5	14.8	6.1
4	19.8	6.2	20.4	6.8
5	28.3	8.5	30.2	9.6

[a]Mean of genital and pubic hair ratings.
Adapted from Daniel WA Jr, Feinstein RA, Howard-Peebles P, et al. Testicular volumes of adolescents. *J Pediatr.* 1982;101:1010.

with regard to the attainment of SMR 5.[13] Also, as with girls, there were noticeable differences noted among racial groups, with Black boys entering puberty the earliest, followed by White boys, then Mexican American boys. A more recent review of data from the PROS study found the mean ages for onset of genital development to be 10.14 years for non-Hispanic White boys, 9.14 years for Black boys, and 10.04 years for Hispanic boys,[14] generally consistent with NHANES data and earlier (age-wise) than previously reported.[7] However, as with girls, the age at completion of genital development is not significantly different from previous studies,[15-17] with White boys completing puberty at 15.9 years, Black boys at 15.7 years, and Mexican American boys at 14.9 years. The overall trend, therefore, is earlier entry with prolonged progression. The potential causes of this trend are not entirely known. It is clear, however, that precocious puberty in boys should always prompt further evaluation as this condition is associated with pathology more often than in girls. Further evaluation should be undertaken if there is evidence of signs and symptoms of pubertal development before the age of 9 years or out of context of family history.

In both sexes, consequences of earlier maturation with regard to teen behavior, sexual activity, and pregnancy need to be addressed with age-appropriate interventions during middle childhood and the preteen years. In addition, the lifetime health consequences of early sexual maturation merit further study.

ADRENARCHE

The increased secretion of androgens from the adrenals, called adrenarche, in the prepubertal and pubertal periods is independent of HPG changes. The two events are temporally related, with the increase in adrenal hormones preceding that of the gonadal sex steroids,[18] although the effects are evident later. It is important to note, however, that adrenal androgens are not necessary for pubertal development or the adolescent growth spurt. It is widely believed that adrenarche begins in midchildhood, at around the age of 6 years, and adrenal androgen levels continue to rise until the age of 20 to 30 years. Evidence, however, suggests that the rise of DHEA-S is a more gradual process and occurs as early as the preschool years.[19]

Physical Manifestations

Local conversion of DHEA-S to testosterone and then to dihydrotestosterone is responsible for hair growth in the androgen-dependent areas (face, chest, pubic area, axilla). Axillary and pubic areas are most sensitive to the effects of androgens, which is why these areas

are the first to develop sexual hair. In addition, local conversion of DHEA-S within the apocrine glands of the axillae causes body odor, and conversion within sebaceous glands is responsible for the development of acne.

THE GROWTH HORMONE AXIS AND PUBERTAL GROWTH

Growth Hormone Axis

Pituitary secretion of growth hormone (GH) is positively regulated by GH-releasing hormone (GHRH) and negatively by somatostatin. Growth hormone is released in a pulsatile manner, with maximum secretion at the onset of slow-wave sleep.

The effects of GH are primarily modulated through proteins called insulin-like growth factors (IGFs) and their binding proteins (BPs). The major mechanism for growth appears to be through stimulation of IGF-1 by GH, which affects bone growth. Measurement of IGF-1 and IGFBP-3 levels serves as a surrogate measure of GH production because of significant diurnal variation in GH levels. Serum IGF-1 levels increase with age and pubertal development (Fig. 2.7).

PHYSICAL GROWTH DURING PUBERTY

One of the most striking changes in adolescence is rapid growth velocity. This height spurt is dependent primarily on GH and the IGFs, but many other hormones may influence growth as well, especially the sex steroids. This is best illustrated by the example of the adolescent with isolated GH deficiency who grows throughout puberty but lacks a definitive growth spurt. Estrogens, and to a lesser extent, androgens, have a biphasic effect on the growth plate, stimulating bone formation early and inducing epiphyseal fusion late in puberty.[20] Premature or delayed puberty without prompt recognition and treatment may have marked effects on height.

Growth Hormone during Puberty

Most linear growth is dependent on GH and its feedback loop. Growth hormone secretion is increased by GHRH, and decreased by hypothalamic somatostatin (see Fig. 2.2). Growth hormone concentrations have been shown to double during the pubertal growth spurt. As with many hormones, GH is secreted in a pulsatile manner, with maximum rates at the onset of slow-wave sleep. It has been shown that the increased available GH is due to higher pulse amplitude and amount per pulse, as opposed to increased frequency or decreased clearance.[21] It is this pulsatile secretion which renders random GH testing unhelpful. Growth hormone exerts its effects through IGFs, mainly IGF-1 (or somatomedin-C) and IGF-2. Serum IGF-1 levels increase slowly and steadily during the prepubertal years, rise more steeply during puberty,[22] and remain elevated 1 to 2 years past the pubertal growth spurt. Insulin-like growth factor levels among males and females must be interpreted with regard to pubertal stage and age.

Height Velocity

Height velocity during the pubertal growth spurt is at its highest levels outside of infancy. It should be noted that when calculating height velocity, it is important to use an interval of 6 to 12 months, as height growth is greatest during the spring and summer months. Although males and females are roughly the same height upon entry into puberty, males emerge taller by 13 cm on average. This is primarily due to boys' 2-year lag behind girls in attainment of their peak height velocity, but a small amount of height may be accounted for by the higher peak velocity (Figs. 2.7 and 2.8). Girls gain their peak height velocity of 8.3 cm/year at an average age of 11.5 years and at SMR B2 to B3, whereas boys do not have their peak height velocity of 9.5 cm/year until the age of 13.5 years at SMR G3 to G4. Although there is great interindividual

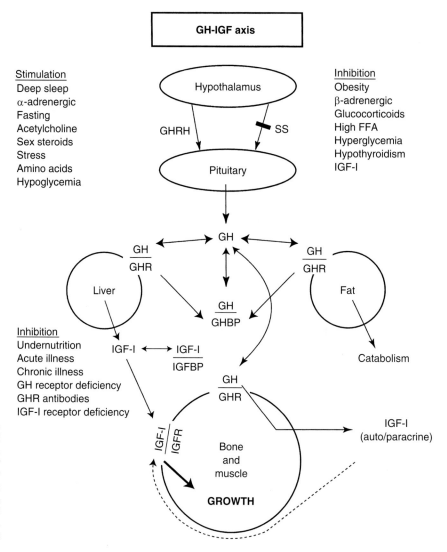

FIGURE 2.7 Simplified diagram of GH–IGF-1 axis involving hypophysiotropic hormones controlling pituitary GH release, circulating GHBP and its GH receptor source, IGF-1 and its largely GH-dependent BPs, and cellular responsiveness to GH and IGF-1 interacting with their specific receptors. FFA, free fatty acids; GHRH, growth hormone–releasing hormone. (From Rosenbloom AL, Guevara-Aguirre J, Rosenfeld RG, Pollock BH. Growth in growth hormone insensitivity. *Trends Endocrinol Metab.* 1994;5(7):296–303. doi: 10.1016/1043-2760(94)p3205-I. PMID: 18407222.)

variation for height, one trend is for the peak height velocity to be higher, but not more sustained, in those who mature early. Therefore, there may not be a difference in final height. There are also curves available for early and late maturers (Figs. 2.8 and 2.9).

Prediction of Final Height

Predicting final height is a difficult task, and it should be emphasized that the methods available provide a general estimate.

Midparental Target Height

One method of predicting a general range for adult height is by the average of parental heights, accounting for the height difference of 13 cm (or 5 inches) between males and females. This is referred to as the midparental target height. One standard deviation from midparental height is 2 inches. As a result, 4 inches around the midparental height is within two standard deviations of the mean.

For girls:

$$\frac{(\text{father's height} - 13 \text{ cm or 5 inches}) + \text{mother' height}}{2}$$

For boys:

$$\frac{(\text{mother's height} + 13 \text{ cm or 5 inches}) + \text{father's height}}{2}$$

Prediction Based on Bone Age

Skeletal maturation can be determined by comparing an x-ray of the adolescent's hand and wrist to standards of maturation in the normal population. Bone age is an index of physiologic maturation, providing an idea of the proportion of the total growth that has occurred. For example, if an adolescent is 15 years old and has a bone age of 12 years, there will be more potential growth than if the same adolescent's bone age were 15 years. The Bayley–Pinneau method uses the bone age to predict final height. This is based on obtaining a bone age (x-ray of the left hand and wrist) that is then matched to standards. Because sex steroids are known to cause bony maturation and epiphyseal fusion, this method is based on the percentage of final height as assessed by bone maturation. Various computer models have used these data to predict adult height. With these programs, basic information (e.g., height, weight, skeletal age) is entered and adult height is calculated using several methodologies, including that of Bayley and Pinneau. One such program can be found at http://www.bonexpert.com/adult-height-predictor. The use of skeletal age is discussed further in Chapter 14.

Genetic Influences on Growth

The use of midparental target height as a method of predicting the range of height for an individual recognizes the significant influence of inherited genetic factors in normal growth. In a given population, up to 90% of height variation may be attributed to a variety

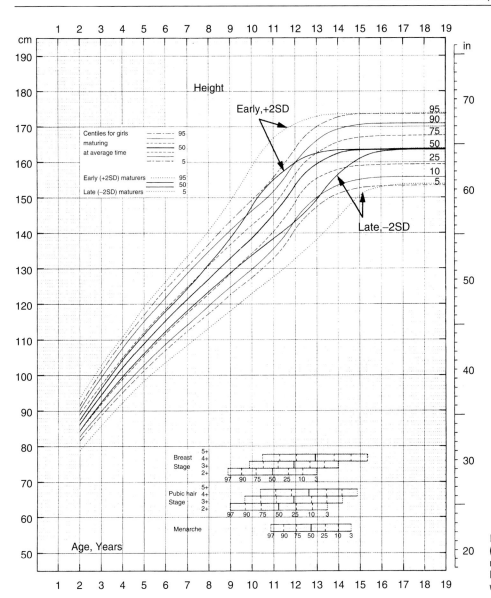

FIGURE 2.8 Height attained for American girls. (From Tanner JM, Davies PW. Clinical longitudinal standards for height and height velocity for North American children. *J Pediatr.* 1985;107:317, with permission.)

of inherited factors.[23] Genome-wide association studies have identified over 180 genetic loci that influence adult height, with many of these loci being connected in cellular pathways and associated with skeletal growth defects.[24] While some cases of short stature are due to specific single-gene mutations, most variations in growth and height are likely polygenic with an individual inheriting a variety of common variants that together explain their short stature.[25]

Weight Growth

1. Weight velocity increases and peaks during the adolescent growth spurt.
2. Pubertal weight gain accounts for approximately 50% of an individual's ideal body weight.
3. The onset of accelerated weight gain and the peak weight velocity (PWV) attained are highly variable. For example, normal weight gain during the year of PWV can vary from 4.6 to 10.6 kg in girls and from 5.8 to 13.2 kg in boys. Normal weight-for-age percentile curves are available through the Centers for Disease Control and Prevention (CDC) (www.cdc.gov/growthcharts/).

Pubertal Changes in Body Composition and Skeletal Mass

During childhood, boys and girls have relatively equal proportions of lean body mass, skeletal mass, and body fat. By the end

of puberty; however, males have 1.5 times more lean body mass and skeletal mass than females and females have double the fat mass. **Table 2.2** shows the effects of GH and the sex steroids on different aspects of body composition. The skeleton also undergoes epiphyseal maturation under the influence of estradiol and testosterone.

Lean Body Mass

1. Females: Lean body mass decreases from approximately 80% of body weight in early puberty to approximately 75% at maturity. The lean body mass increases in total amount, but decreases in percentage because adipose mass increases at a greater rate.
2. Males: Lean body mass increases from 80% to 85% to approximately 90% at maturity. This primarily reflects increased muscle mass from circulating androgens.

Skeletal Mass

Changes in bone mass, or bone mineral density (BMD), parallel the alterations in lean body mass, body size, and muscle strength. Major determinants of BMD are physical activity level, heredity, nutrition, endocrine function, and other lifestyle factors. The accretion of skeletal bone mass during puberty is critical. Peak bone mass is acquired by early adulthood, serving as the "bone

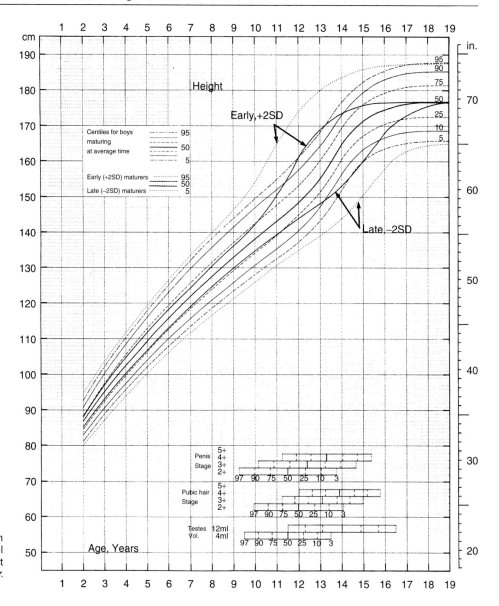

FIGURE 2.9 Height attained for American boys. (From Tanner JM, Davies PW. Clinical longitudinal standards for height and height velocity for North American children. *J Pediatr.* 1985;107:317, with permission.)

bank" for the remainder of life.[26] Bone mass is affected by the following:

1. Age at menarche: There is an inverse relation between the age at menarche and the risk of osteoporosis later in life, as demonstrated by epidemiologic studies.[27]
2. Nutrition: Much has been studied about the effects of calcium and vitamin D, with mixed results. Currently, there are no studies that have been able to separate the effects of vitamin D from the effects of calcium on skeletal accrual, although there is a consensus that adequate consumption of both of these nutrients is important for optimal bone mineral accrual.
3. Exercise: Weight-bearing physical activity during pre- and early puberty has been shown to improve bone strength, but results have been less promising regarding the effects of exercise on postmenarcheal girls.[28]

Body Mass Index

Body mass index increases with puberty, although it should be pointed out that BMI does not quantitate body composition. Body mass index varies with age, gender, and ethnicity. In children and adolescents, BMI must be compared using age-stratified standardized percentiles. Charts and tables for BMI, which should be tracked in all children and teenagers, can be obtained from the National Center for

Chronic Disease Prevention and Health Promotion of the CDC (www. cdc.gov/growthcharts/). There is a strong correlation between the timing of puberty and BMI: children with higher mean BMI mature earlier. Body mass index is determined by the following formula:

$$BMI = \text{Weight in kilograms} / (\text{height in meters})^2$$

or

$$BMI = (\text{Weight in kilograms} / \text{height in centimeters} / \text{height in centimeters}) \times 10,000$$

The BMI declines from birth and reaches a minimum between 4 and 6 years of age, before gradually increasing through adolescence and adulthood. The upward trend after the lowest point is referred to as the "adiposity rebound." Children with an earlier rebound are more likely to have an increased BMI.

Brain Maturation during Adolescence

Significant research in understanding brain development in adolescents and young adults (AYAs) is ongoing. This research has utilized new technologies (such as functional magnetic resonance imaging) that allow tracking of the growth of different regions of the brain, as well as investigating the connections within the brain. Some researchers are exploring the interactions between

TABLE 2.2
Primary Actions of GH and Sex Steroids on Body Composition[a]

	GH	Estradiol	Testosterone
Visceral fat[a,b]	↓↓	[c,d]	↓
Subcutaneous fat[a,e]	↓	↑	↓
Bone mineral[a,f]	↑	↑↑	↑↑
Muscle mass[a,e]	↑	[c]	↑↑
Extracellular water	↑ (acutely)	[c]	↑ (acutely)
Linear bone growth[a,e,f]	↑	↑↑	↑↑
Epiphyseal fusion[d,f]	[c]	↑↑	↑↑
Energy expenditure	↑	[c]	↑↑

GH, growth hormone.
[a]Possible synergy between somatotropic and gonadotropic signals.
[b]Nonaromatizable androgens also effectual.
[c]Limited or inconsistent data.
[d]Only in combination with a (synthetic) progestin.
[e]May differ in children and adults.
[f]Maximal effects require aromatization.
Adapted with permission from Veldhuis JD, Roemmich JN, Richmond EJ, et al. Endocrine control of body composition in infancy, childhood, and puberty. *Endocrine Rev.* 2005;26:114.

brain function, development, and behavior, while others have been investigating the sensitivity of the developing brain to effects of alcohol and other drugs. This research has resulted in some important new findings, including the discovery of significant changes in brain development even into the young adult years.

An understanding of brain development can assist in understanding the risk-taking behavior of AYAs. Brain development can play a significant role in these behaviors in conjunction with genetic makeup, childhood experiences, and environmental surroundings. Studies now indicate that the brain continues to develop in different ways and at different times into adolescence and young adulthood.

Developmental Stage
Early and Midadolescence
The brain undergoes significant growth and pruning. In general, this process moves from the back to front areas of the cerebral cortex.

Young Adulthood
Brain development that reflects sophisticated thinking and emotional regulation continues, but is not fully developed until mid-20s or sometimes later.[29] Of note, the brain is not fully mature at age 16, when many adolescents begin to drive, nor at age 18, the legal voting age, or at age 21, the legal drinking age. Rather, full maturity occurs at approximately age 25 in most individuals.

Area of the Brain
Prefrontal Cortex
Perhaps, the most widely studied areas for changes in young adulthood are in this brain region. The prefrontal cortex is associated with planning and problem solving. Two aspects affecting the efficiency of this functioning are as follows:
1. Myelination: Enhanced myelination of nerve fibers contributes to signals being transmitted more efficiently.
2. Synaptic pruning: The wild patches of connections resulting from nerve growth are pruned back. This again allows for signals to be transmitted more efficiently.

Executive Suite
The functions centering in the prefrontal cortex are sometimes called the "executive suite." This can include calibration of risk and reward, regulation of emotion, problem solving, self-evaluation, and long-term planning. This area may not be developed until the mid-20s.

Cerebellum
The cerebellum is involved in emotional processing; it is at adult volume in girls before 11 years of age, but not in boys.[30]

Connections among Regions
Connections between different parts of the brain are also critical and increase throughout childhood, adolescence, and young adulthood. This development allows the prefrontal cortex to communicate more fully and effectively with other parts of the brain, allowing enhanced planning, problem solving, and better control of emotions and impulses. In addition, these enhanced connections play an important role in growth of intellectual capacity and memory.

Brain Tissue
White Matter
The volume of white matter increases throughout childhood and adolescence.[29]

Gray Matter
This area of brain has an inverted U-shaped developmental curve overall.[31]

Rate of Development
It is clear that different parts of the brain mature at different rates. Overall, functional scans suggest that the parts of the brain that control basic functions, such as those controlling movement, mature first, while parts of the brain responsible for controlling impulses and planning ahead mature last.

While the brain of an adolescent or young adult may have a very high intellectual capacity and be "online," the areas of emotional and impulse control seem to reach maturity later. There is also the suggestion that the brain circuits involved in emotional responses are heightened in AYAs. These changes may relate to the risk-seeking behaviors and a tendency to act on impulse and without a regard for risk. In addition, some of these brain-based changes may even be involved in regulation of sleep and contribute to teens' preference for staying up late.

There continues to be much to learn and investigate with respect to the development of the human brain and relationships with behaviors and health. In addition, additional research is needed to examine the effects of environment, parenting, and alcohol and other substances on the developing brain. Some of this work may lead to answers about why so many symptoms of mental disorders first emerge during adolescence and young adulthood.

CONCERNS ABOUT GROWTH AND DEVELOPMENT

This chapter has discussed most of the features of normal adolescent growth and development. As essential as it is for the clinician to have a firm grasp of the facts of normal growth and development, a clear understanding and feeling for what these changes mean to the adolescent are also critically important. As their bodies change, adolescents develop tremendous concern about whether their bodies are "normal." The great variation in the timing of puberty, with resultant differences in physical maturity of similar-aged adolescents, serves to heighten teenagers' worries. Practitioners must be adept at detecting the adolescent's concerns about height, weight, pubic hair growth, or phallus size, for example, even if these concerns are not stated overtly in the initial complaint.

SUMMARY

The changes that occur during growth and puberty are a marvel of nature and a testimony to the intricacies and wonders of the human hormonal system. The clinician must understand these changes and the wide variations of normalcy. They must also be able to sense the profound effect these changes have on the adolescent, and be prepared to be a source of information, reassurance, and help if abnormalities are detected.

REFERENCES

1. Weise M, De-Levi S, Barnes KM, et al. Effects of estrogen on growth plate senescence and epiphyseal fusion. *Proc Natl Acad Sci U S A.* 2001;98(12): 6871–6876.
2. Marshall JC, Kelch RP. Gonadotropin-releasing hormone: role of pulsatile secretion in the regulation of reproduction. *N Engl J Med.* 1986;315(23):1459–1468.
3. Pinilla L, Aguilar E, Dieguez C, et al. Kisspeptins and reproduction: physiological roles and regulatory mechanisms. *Physiol Rev.* 2012;92(3):1235–1316.
4. Childs GV, Odle AK, MacNicol MC, et al. The importance of leptin to reproduction. *Endocrinology [Internet].* 2021;162(2):bqaa204. https://doi.org/10.1210/endocr/bqaa204
5. Roberts SA, Kaiser UB. Genetics in endocrinology: genetic etiologies of central precocious puberty and the role of imprinted genes. *Eur J Endocrinol.* 2020; 183(4):R107–R117.
6. Howard SR, Dunkel L. Delayed puberty—phenotypic diversity, molecular genetic mechanisms, and recent discoveries. *Endocr Rev.* 2019;40(5):1285–1317.
7. Marshall WA, Tanner JM. Variations in the pattern of pubertal changes in boys. *Arch Dis Child.* 1970;45(239):13–23.
8. Marshall WA, Tanner JM. Variations in pattern of pubertal changes in girls. *Arch Dis Child.* 1969;44(235):291–303.
9. Veldhuis JD, Roemmich JN, Richmond EJ, et al. Endocrine control of body composition in infancy, childhood, and puberty. *Endocr Rev.* 2005;26(1):114–146. doi: 10.1210/er.2003-0038. PMID: 15689575.
10. Herman-Giddens ME, Slora EJ, Wasserman RC, et al. Secondary sexual characteristics and menses in young girls seen in office practice: a study from the Pediatric Research in Office Settings network. *Pediatrics.* 1997;99(4):505–512.
11. Biro FM, Greenspan LC, Galvez MP, et al. Onset of breast development in a longitudinal cohort. *Pediatrics.* 2013;132(6):1019–1027.
12. Vizmanos B, Martí-Henneberg C, Clivillé R, et al. Age of pubertal onset affects the intensity and duration of pubertal growth peak but not final height. *Am J Hum Biol.* 2001;13(3):409–416.
13. Euling SY, Herman-Giddens ME, Lee PA, et al. Examination of US puberty-timing data from 1940 to 1994 for secular trends: panel findings. *Pediatrics.* 2008;121(Suppl 3):S172–S191.
14. Herman-Giddens ME, Steffes J, Harris D, et al. Secondary sexual characteristics in boys: data from the Pediatric Research in Office Settings Network. *Pediatrics.* 2012;130(5):e1058–1068.
15. Harlan WR, Grillo GP, Cornoni-Huntley J, et al. Secondary sex characteristics of boys 12 to 17 years of age: the U.S. Health Examination Survey. *J Pediatr.* 1979;95(2):293–297.
16. Lee PA. Normal ages of pubertal events among American males and females. *J Adolesc Health Care.* 1980;1(1):26–29.
17. Villarreal SF, Martorell R, Mendoza F. Sexual maturation of Mexican-American adolescents. *Am J Hum Biol.* 1989;1(1):87–95.
18. Ducharme JR, Forest MG, De Peretti E, et al. Plasma adrenal and gonadal sex steroids in human pubertal development. *J Clin Endocrinol Metab.* 1976;42(3):468–476.
19. Palmert MR, Hayden DL, Mansfield MJ, et al. The longitudinal study of adrenal maturation during gonadal suppression: evidence that adrenarche is a gradual process. *J Clin Endocrinol Metab.* 2001;86(9):4536–4542.
20. Vanderschueren D, Vandenput L, Boonen S, et al. Androgens and bone. *Endocr Rev.* 2004;25(3):389–425.
21. Martha PM Jr, Gorman KM, Blizzard RM, et al. Endogenous growth hormone secretion and clearance rates in normal boys, as determined by deconvolution analysis: relationship to age, pubertal status, and body mass. *J Clin Endocrinol Metab.* 1992;74(2):336–344.
22. Juul A, Bang P, Hertel NT, et al. Serum insulin-like growth factor-I in 1030 healthy children, adolescents, and adults: relation to age, sex, stage of puberty, testicular size, and body mass index. *J Clin Endocrinol Metab.* 1994;78(3):744–752.
23. Hirschhorn JN, Lettre G. Progress in genome-wide association studies of human height. *Horm Res.* 2009;71(Suppl 2):5–13.
24. Lango Allen H, Estrada K, Lettre G, et al. Hundreds of variants clustered in genomic loci and biological pathways affect human height. *Nature.* 2010;467(7317):832–838.
25. Dauber A, Rosenfeld RG, Hirschhorn JN. Genetic evaluation of short stature. *J Clin Endocrinol Metab.* 2014;99(9):3080–3092.
26. Gordon CM, Zemel BS, Wren TAL, et al. The determinants of peak bone mass. *J Pediatr.* 2016;180:261–269.
27. Sešelj M, Nahhas RW, Sherwood RJ, et al. The influence of age at menarche on cross-sectional geometry of bone in young adulthood. *Bone.* 2012;51(1):38–45.
28. MacKelvie KJ, Khan KM, McKay HA. Is there a critical period for bone response to weight-bearing exercise in children and adolescents? a systematic review. *Br J Sports Med.* 2002;36(4):250–257; discussion 257.
29. Lenroot RK, Gogtay N, Greenstein DK, et al. Sexual dimorphism of brain developmental trajectories during childhood and adolescence. *Neuroimage.* 2007;36(4): 1065–1073.
30. Caviness VS Jr, Kennedy DN, Richelme C, et al. The human brain age 7–11 years: a volumetric analysis based on magnetic resonance images. *Cereb Cortex.* 1996;6(5):726–736.
31. Giedd JN, Rapoport JL. Structural MRI of pediatric brain development: what have we learned and where are we going? *Neuron.* 2010;67(5):728–734.

📶 ADDITIONAL RESOURCES AND WEBSITES

Additional Resources and Websites for Clinicians:

Abbassi V. Growth and normal puberty. Pediatrics. 1998;102(Suppl 3): 507–511. https://pediatrics.aappublications.org/content/102/Supplement_3/507

Alotaibi MF. Physiology of puberty in boys and girls and pathological disorders affecting its onset. *J Adolesc.* 2019;71:63–71. doi: 10.1016/j.adolescence.2018.12.007. Epub 2019 January 14.

Puberty and Precocious Puberty, US Department of Health and Human Services, National Institutes of Health, https://www.nichd.nih.gov/health/topics/puberty

Rauber A. Growth and development. In: Walker HK, Hall WD, Hurst JW, eds. *Clinical Methods: The History, Physical, and Laboratory Examinations.* https://www.ncbi.nlm.nih.gov/books/NBK335/

Additional Resources and Websites for Parents/Caregivers:

American Academy of Pediatrics—https://www.healthychildren.org/English/ages-stages/gradeschool/puberty/Pages/default.aspx

Additional Resources and Websites for Adolescents and Young Adults:

The Stages of Puberty: Development in Girls and Boys—https://www.healthline.com/health/when-do-girls-stop-growing

CHAPTER 3

Psychosocial Development in Normal Adolescents and Young Adults

Sara Sherer

Mari Radzik

KEY WORDS

- Body image
- Cognitive development
- Early, middle, late adolescence
- Emerging adults
- Identity development
- Independence
- Peer group
- Psychosocial development
- Young adults

INTRODUCTION

This chapter provides a framework of the psychosocial developmental process of adolescents and young adults (AYAs). General considerations are reviewed, including a review of typical developmental phases. A review of the primary tasks for each of these phases includes a discussion of cognitive development, independence, body image, peer group, and identity development.

In terms of physical development, adolescence can be described as the period of life beginning with the appearance of secondary sexual characteristics and terminating with the cessation of somatic growth. Adolescence can also be viewed as a developmental biopsychosocial process that may start before the onset of puberty and last well beyond the termination of growth. Adolescence involves physical, psychological, emotional, and social growth and development, and each of these domains occurs at different rates. As such, the entire adolescence process is a period of increased vulnerability characterized by an ongoing process of transition and adjustment.[1-5]

Advances in neuroimaging techniques have led to a greater understanding of the structural and functional development of the AYA brain, and the cognitive processes during this period of life. Studies have demonstrated that changes in brain structure continue beyond adolescence, with the most dramatic growth occurring in the development of executive functioning, organization, decision making and planning, and response inhibition.[6,7] Understanding biologic changes in brain structure and function during adolescence and young adulthood has important implications for understanding behaviors (see Chapter 2).

Clinicians who integrate social determinants of health perspective with awareness of normal adolescent psychosocial development are well positioned to identify the various emotional and behavioral challenges that can affect the health and well-being of AYAs.[8,9]

THE PROCESS OF ADOLESCENCE

It is important to keep in mind that no outline of psychosocial development can adequately describe every AYA. Adolescents and young adults are not members of a homogeneous group, but a diverse group that displays wide variability in biologic, psychological, social, and emotional growth impacted by their environment.[10] Each AYA must meet their individual life demands, and respond to the opportunities and challenges they face in a unique and personal manner.[8-10]

The transition from childhood to adulthood is not a continuous, uniform, or synchronous process. In fact, biologic, social, emotional, and intellectual growth may be totally asynchronous.[5,11] In addition, psychosocial growth may be accented by frequent periods of regression.

Whereas adolescence has often been described as a period of extreme instability, most adolescents do not experience difficulties during this time, and can pass through unperturbed by the developmental process.[11] This ability to cope with the challenges of adolescence reflects a resiliency that is often overlooked, as challenging behaviors of adolescents are often the primary focus of attention.[12] Recent studies that focus attention on parenting AYAs find that difficulties are far less prevalent than previously thought.[11,12] Overall, there is no evidence that intractable and major conflict between parents and their adolescent children is a "normal" part of adolescence,[5,8,12] and in fact most AYAs and their parents enjoy healthy relationships as adults.[13,14]

Phases and Tasks of Adolescence

Adolescence and young adulthood can be conceptualized as four psychosocial developmental phases:

1. Early adolescence: approximate ages 10 to 13 years
2. Middle adolescence: approximate ages 14 to 17 years
3. Late adolescence: approximate ages 17 to 21 years
4. Young or "emerging" adults: approximate ages 18 to 25 years

By the end of adolescence, young adults strive toward independence from their parents/caregivers. Some have attained a psychosexual maturity along with the necessary skills and resources from family, education, and community to begin to support themselves in an emotionally, socially, and financially satisfying way.[13] Others may still need to be supported as they attain the necessary skills and resources to transition to adult independence.

Several tasks characterize the development of AYAs and are discussed in the following sections in conjunction with each developmental phase. These tasks include:

1. Expanding cognitive development that allows young people to think in new, more complex ways
2. Achieving independence from parents
3. Accepting one's body image
4. Adopting peer codes and lifestyles
5. Establishing self, sexual, vocational, social, and moral identities

EARLY ADOLESCENCE (APPROXIMATE AGES 10 TO 13)

Early adolescent psychosocial development is heralded by rapid physical changes with the onset of puberty. These physical changes engender self-absorption and initiate the adolescent's struggle for independence. The onset of puberty occurs 1 to 2 years earlier for girls than for boys (see Chapter 2). Concomitantly, psychosocial and emotional changes also occur 1 to 2 years earlier in girls.[15]

Cognitive Development

Early adolescent development is characterized by cognitive abilities dominated by concrete thinking, egocentrism, and impulsive behavior. Young adolescents may start showing improvements in reasoning, information processing, and developing expertise in their areas of interest.[6,7] The adolescent is at an early developmental stage in his or her abilities to long-range plan, see another's point of view and consider others' feelings.[7]

Movement toward Independence

Early adolescence is characterized by the beginning of the shift from dependence on parents/caregivers to independent behavior. Common events may include the following:
1. Increased ability to express oneself through speech
2. Search for new people to love in addition to parents/caregivers
3. Less interest in parental activities and more reluctance to accept parental advice or criticism; occasional rudeness; less idealization of the parent/caregiver
4. A gradual emotional separation from parents/caregivers, without the presence of a consistent alternative support group, can lead to behavioral changes (e.g., an increased interest in peers and a decrease in school performance).
5. Emotional lability (wide mood and behavior swings)

Body Image

Rapid physical changes lead the adolescent to be increasingly preoccupied with body image and the question of, "Am I normal?" Body image is a concept that changes with physical and psychosocial growth and development throughout adolescence and young adulthood. Youth show increased dissatisfaction with their body image from middle school which can persist into young adulthood. Weight dissatisfaction can lead to concerning health-compromising behaviors such as caloric restriction, dieting, binging, and purging (including excessive exercise, diuretics, diet pills, and laxatives). Dissatisfaction with body image may also lead to dieting and eating disorders.[16–18] The intense involvement of AYAs with social media and the exposure to its popular images may also impact the way adolescents view their bodies.

The early adolescent's concern with body image is characterized by the following four factors:
1. Preoccupation with self
2. Uncertainty and concerns about appearance and attractiveness
3. Frequent comparison of own body with those of others
4. Increased interest in sexual anatomy and physiology, including anxieties and questions regarding menstruation or nocturnal emissions, masturbation, and breast or penis size.

Peer Group

With the beginning of individuation from the family, the adolescent becomes more dependent on friends as a source of support.[19] The adolescent's peer group is characterized by the following:
1. Increasing focus on peers and an increase in solitary friendships with a member of the same gender. These idealized friendships may become intense; boys, for example, may become "comrades-in-arms" with sworn pacts and allegiances, and young teenage girls may develop deep crushes on others.

2. Strongly emotional, tender feelings toward peers. The peer group usually consists of nonromantic friendships, which may lead to opposite-, same-, or both-sex attractions, exploration, fears, and/or relationships.
3. Peer contact primarily with the same sex, with some contact of the opposite sex made in groups of friends.

Identity Development

Associated with a steady increase in the complexity of the adolescent's cognitive abilities is the initiation of identity development, which is the complex process by which AYAs come to know themselves as unique individuals. According to Piaget's[20] cognitive theory, this corresponds to the cognitive evolution from concrete thinking (concrete operational thoughts) to abstract thinking (formal operational thoughts). During this early stage, the adolescent is expected to achieve academically and to prepare for the future. This period of identity development is characterized by the following:
1. Young adolescents apply their developing cognitive skills to the process of self-exploration, leading to increased self-interest and fantasy. For example, the young adolescent may feel themselves constantly "onstage."
2. Frequent daydreaming, which is not only normal, but also an important component in identity development because it allows adolescents an avenue to explore, enact, problem solve, and recreate important aspects of their lives.
3. Setting unrealistic or idealistic (depending on the individual) vocational/academic goals.
4. Testing authority is a common behavior in adolescents as they attempt to better define who they are and is often a source of tension between the adolescents and adults in authority such as parents or teachers.
5. A need for greater privacy often realized by adolescents' attempts to have more private physical spaces (closing doors to room). Journaling or diary writing, and private social media/internet communications become more important.
6. Emergence of sexual feelings often relieved through masturbation or the telling of dirty jokes. Experimental curiosity, information seeking, and a lack of someone to discuss sexuality often drives adolescents to research via social media or the internet.[21]
7. Development of the adolescent's own value system, potentially leading to additional challenges to family and others.
8. Lack of impulse control and need for immediate gratification, which may result in dangerous risk-taking behavior.
9. Tendency to magnify one's personal situation (although adolescents often feel that they are continually onstage, conversely, they may also be convinced that they are alone and that their problems are unique).

MIDDLE ADOLESCENCE (APPROXIMATE AGES 14 TO 16)

Middle adolescence is characterized by an increased scope and intensity of affective expression and by the rise in importance of peer group values.

Cognitive Development

During middle adolescence, the capacity to think and plan more abstractly develops with higher-order abilities to anticipate or plan. Challenged by increasingly more complex academic and social tasks, adolescents become more efficient with abstract, multidimensional, planned, and hypothetical thinkers.[6,7] However, if confronted with highly stressful events, adolescents may regress to more concrete thinking typical of early adolescence.[22]

Moving toward Independence

Conflicts with parents/caregivers become more prevalent as the adolescents exhibit less interest in spending time with them and devote more their time to peers, in person or via social media and the internet.[14,19,22,23]

Body Image

Although most adolescents have experienced much of their pubertal changes, they continue to be preoccupied with their body image. All youth spend time focused on their physical appearance in order to "fit in" with their peer group. At the same time, adolescents are trying to develop their own unique style to achieve a satisfying and realistic body image. This developmental phase is associated with an increased risk for eating disorders.[16] In fact, anorexia nervosa has its peak onset in the mid- to late teenagers (15 to 19 years),[16] with a great prevalence of this disorder among girls, but boys are also affected (see Chapter 38).

Peer Group

The powerful role of peer groups is most apparent during middle adolescence.[19,22] Characteristics of this involvement include the following:

1. Intense involvement in the peer subculture
2. Conformity with peer values, codes, and dress, in an attempt to further separate from family
3. Peer groups expand to include romantic relationship, manifested by dating, sexual experimentation, and sexual activity
4. Involvement with clubs, team sports, gangs, and other groups of interest

Evidence suggests that during middle adolescence, friends are the primary source of influence on youths' behavior, but estimates of peer pressure are often overstated especially if an authoritative parenting style is employed.[12]

Adolescents' reactions to peer pressure are extremely varied. Some can be diverted from achieving educational and family goals, but many adolescents choose peer groups and are propelled by peer pressure to excel in school, sports, and other positive activities.[19]

Identity Development

As the young person's ability to abstract and to reason continues to increase, they are better able to view themselves as unique individuals with a new sense of individuality. The middle adolescent's identity development is characterized by the following:

1. Increased scope and openness of feelings, with a new ability to emphasize and examine the feelings of others
2. Increased intellectual ability and creativity
3. Realistic and aspirational vocational goals
4. A feeling of omnipotence and immortality, leading to risk-taking behaviors a factor in the high rate of accidents, suicidal behaviors, drug use, and risky sexual behaviors, resulting in pregnancies, and sexually transmitted diseases that become prevalent at this stage. At this developmental stage, these behaviors are enhanced in the presence of peers. Despite the fact that middle and late adolescents are often able to understand the risks involved in certain activities, in the presence of peers, and when emotionally aroused, they are more rewarded by the social stimuli associated with the peer group than by logical thinking.[19,22,24]

● LATE ADOLESCENCE (APPROXIMATE AGES 17 TO 21)

Late adolescence is characterized by the development of personal identity and separation. If all has proceeded well in early and middle adolescence, especially the presence of supportive parents/caregivers and peer groups, the adolescent will be well on their way to handling the tasks and responsibilities of adulthood.[13] If the previously mentioned tasks have not been achieved, then problems such as depression, suicidal tendencies, substance use,

or emotional disorders may develop or worsen with the increasing independence and responsibilities of young adulthood.[22,23,25]

Cognitive Development

During late adolescence, the ability to think more abstractly and to plan (i.e., career decisions) is more developed. Complex thinking processes rely less on self-centered concepts and more on advanced decision-making skills. At this point, adolescents may be able to make independent decisions about their life choices while weighing the costs and benefits more thoroughly.[22] During this time, the maturational brain processes are still developing (and will continue into emerging adulthood) and are often lagging behind in their ability to address the challenges reflected by arousal and emotional motivation brought on by pubertal maturation.[22,25]

Moving toward Independence

For most, late adolescence is a time of reduced restlessness and increased identity development. The older adolescent has grown to become a separate entity from their family and may begin to appreciate their parents'/caregivers' "values." Such an understanding may make it possible for the adolescent to seek and accept parental advice and guidance. However, it is not uncommon for some adolescents to be unable to or hesitant to accept the responsibilities of adulthood and to remain dependent on family and peers. Late adolescents often display the following:

1. A stronger personal identity
2. A greater ability to delay gratification
3. A better ability to solve problems and express ideas in words
4. A greater ability to make independent decisions and to compromise
5. A greater commitment to more stable interests

Body Image

The late adolescent has completed pubertal growth and development. However, body image issues may still be significant given the emphasis among peers and in the media. The emergence of disordered eating behaviors and eating disorders remain a significant problem.

Peer Group

As the late adolescent becomes more comfortable with their own identity and values, peer group values become less important. More time is spent in a relationship with one individual. Such relationships involve less experimentation and more sharing. The selection of a partner is based more on mutual understanding and enjoyment than on peer acceptance.

Identity Development

Identity development during late adolescence is characterized by the following:

1. The development of a rational and realistic conscience
2. The development of a sense of perspective, with the ability to delay gratification, compromise, and set limits
3. The development of practical vocational goals and the beginning of financial independence
4. The development of clearer sexual and gender identity
5. Further refinement of societal issues, moral, religious, and sexual values

● YOUNG OR "EMERGING" ADULTS (APPROXIMATE AGES 18 TO 25)

Although there is no specific definition of "young adulthood," it is described as a phase of the life that spans between late adolescence and early adulthood. It is a developmental period of exploration of possible life directions,[1,3,25,26] optimism, refined cognitive skills, and transition into adult roles.[3] Generally, young or "emerging" adulthood is the period between 18 and 25 years. A study of young people aged 18 to 29 years,[26] describes young adults as optimistic and encourages a more positive view of this developmental phase. The study also describes emerging adults as fairly well educated across all the demographic groups and ready for adult responsibilities.[26] However, research also demonstrates that this generational period is often the period when mental disorders that commonly arise during mid- to late adolescence evolve more fully and follow the young adult into later adulthood.[25] Recently, there appears to be a progressively increasing delay, or complexity, in attaining "traditional" life milestones, including completing school, leaving home, becoming financially independent, marrying, and having a child. In 1975, 77% of females and 65% of males at age 30 reached these life "milestones." In 2016, only 24% of young adults achieved all these goals.[26] Furthermore, cultural differences make for a complex picture of how young adults meet the challenges of adulthood.[27]

Cognitive Development

During emerging adulthood, brain development becomes more complex.[6,7] Brain imaging techniques reveal an extended period of maturation, especially in the frontal and parietal cortices, allowing for an increase in capacity for executive functioning (control and coordination of thought and behavior), the development of social cognition (what is perceived as important in the social world around the emerging adult), and perspective taking (taking on the viewpoint of another person)[6,7] (see Chapter 2). Emerging adults are therefore more successful in managing increased risk and the increased complexity of the adult world.[26] Toward the end of this stage, it is believed that the adolescent brain has fully matured.[26] Hence, by this period, a more complex cognitive facility is evident as emerging young adults manage to cope with the nuances of the social and emotional constructs impacting their lives.

Moving toward Independence

Moving away from home has a complex impact on the successful transition into adulthood. One study shows that an optimal and reasonable period of living with parents contributes to later psychological health.[13] Delayed transition to adulthood may help balance emotional health, while actual failure to fully transition to independent adulthood can become detrimental to the individual.[28,29] This study recognized that not leaving was often mitigated by social and financial difficulties but emphasized that emerging adults that experience a timely transition, fair better as adults.[29,23] The paths young adults take toward independence are unique and nonlinear; some move forward and backward on the path to adulthood. Further, while on the course toward adulthood, young adults utilize varied timeframes to navigate through the different developmental tasks. Emerging adulthood may involve refining plans, moving back into a parents' home, quitting a job, or returning to school.[25] Indeed, in a large study of parents of young adults, it was found that parents and their emerging adult children had positive relationships and most young adults stayed at their parents'/caregivers' homes while involved in attaining higher education.[25] This is especially true in more economically unstable situations and is highly impacted by the ethnic and racial background of the family.[26] Assessing the nature of the relationship between parents/caregivers and the young adult would help to understand if any stressors are present.

Body Image

As the adolescent moves into adulthood, earlier unresolved body image issues such as eating disorders or obesity may follow. Studies have shown that body image issues, disordered eating, and obesity established in adolescence may persist into the young adult years.[29,30] This raises the urgency for the clinician to assess and monitor health and wellness, body image, and eating behaviors during the earlier phases of adolescence to mitigate potential lasting issues.

Peer Group and Identity Development

Most AYAs use this stage to complete the tasks associated with peer group and identity issues discussed earlier. As young adults become more independent of peer groups, and more able to apply the advanced cognitive skills now available to them, they become more involved in mature intimate relationships, and may delve further into identity exploration to refine their personal identities. Young adults may seem unfocused when they try out various life possibilities. They may explore love and different levels of intimacy, seek work experiences that match possible occupational aspirations, try out different educational possibilities that may lead to different occupational futures, and consider a variety of world views reexamining earlier belief systems to develop their own set of values.[26] Consequently, as they move toward early adulthood, emerging adults are focused on refining their future goals and completing the pursuit of vocational goals, while taking greater responsibilities for their finances.[26]

🔵 SUMMARY

Successful attainment of adolescent developmental milestones across the globe is central to humankind's future.[8,9] Social determinants of health will impact development across the life span, but most AYAs progress through the psychosocial developmental trajectories outlined in this chapter successfully.[27] This brief overview is meant to inform the clinician of the typical scope of adolescent socioemotional development. The wealth of factors that impact AYAs are discussed throughout this book. Most importantly, an understanding of the intersectionality of social determinants and developmental pattern assists the clinician in evaluating the adolescent or young adult's psychosocial development and socioemotional needs; thus providing or linking to the supports needed to attain a successful move into adulthood.[8,27]

REFERENCES

1. Tanner JL, Arnett JJ. Presenting "emerging adulthood": what makes it developmentally distinctive. In: Arnett JJ, Kloep M, Hendry LB, Tanner JL, eds. *Debating Emerging Adulthood: Stage or Process?* Oxford University Press; 2011:13–30.
2. Mitchell KJ, Ybarra ML, Korchmaros JD, et al. Accessing sexual health information online: use, motivations and consequences for youth with different sexual orientations. *Health Educ Res.* 2014;29(1):147–157.
3. Arnett J, Schwab J. *The Clark University Poll of Young Adults: Striving, Struggling, Hopeful.* Clark University; 2012.
4. Jensen LA, Arnett JJ. Going global: new pathways for adolescents and emerging adults in a changing world. *J Soc Issues.* 2012;68(3):473–492.
5. Steinberg L. *Age of Opportunity: Lessons from the New Science of Adolescence.* Houghton Mifflin Harcourt; 2014.
6. Giedd JN. The amazing teen brain. *Scientific American.* 2015;312(6):32–37.
7. Giedd JN, Denker AH. The adolescent brain: insights from neuroimaging. In: Bourguignon JP, Carel JC, Christen Y, eds. *Brain Crosstalk in Puberty and Adolescence. Research and Perspectives in Endocrine Interactions*, vol 13, 2015. Springer, Cham. https://doi.org/10.1007/978-3-319-09168-6_7
8. Trent M, Dooley DG, Dougé J. The impact of racism on child and adolescent health. *Pediatrics.* 2019;144(2):e20191765.
9. Sukarieh M, Tannock S. *Youth Rising?: The Politics of Youth in the Global Economy.* Routledge; 2014.
10. Sawyer SM, Azzopardi PS, Wickremarathne D, et al. The age of adolescence. *Lancet Child Adolesc Health.* 2018;2(3):223–228.
11. Perry DG, Pauletti RE. Gender and adolescent development. *J Res Adolesc.* 2011;21(1):61–74.
12. Larzelere RE, Morris ASE, Harrist AW. *Authoritative Parenting: Synthesizing Nurturance and Discipline for Optimal Child Development.* American Psychological Association; 2013.
13. Johnson MD, Galambos NL. Paths to intimate relationship quality from parent–adolescent relations and mental health. *J Marriage Fam.* 2014;76(1):145–160.
14. Hoskins DH. Consequences of parenting on adolescent outcomes. *Societies.* 2014;4(3):506–531.
15. Neinstein L, Lu Y, Perez L, et al. *The New Adolescents: An Analysis of Health Conditions, Behaviors, Risks and Access to Services Among Emerging Young Adults.* University of Southern California; 2013.
16. van Hoeken D, Hoek HW. Review of the burden of eating disorders: mortality, disability, costs, quality of life, and family burden. *Curr Opin Psychiatry.* 2020;33(6):521.

17. Neumark-Sztainer D, Wall MM, Chen C, et al. Eating, activity, and weight-related problems from adolescence to adulthood. *Am J Prev Med.* 2018;55(2):133–141.

18. Neumark-Sztainer D, Wall M, Larson NI, et al. Dieting and disordered eating behaviors from adolescence to young adulthood: findings from a 10-year longitudinal study. *J Am Diet Assoc.* 2011;111(7):1004–1011.

19. Rambaran JA, Hopmeyer A, Schwartz D, et al. Academic functioning and peer influences: a short-term longitudinal study of network–behavior dynamics in middle adolescence. *Child Dev.* 2017;88(2):523–543.

20. Piaget J, Inhelder, B, Weaver H. *The Psychology of the Child.* Basic Books; 1969.

21. Simon L, Daneback K. Adolescents' use of the internet for sex education: a thematic and critical review of the literature. *Int J Sexual Health.* 2013;25(4):305–319.

22. Duell N, Steinberg L. Positive risk taking in adolescence. *Child Dev Perspect.* 2019; 13(1):48–52.

23. Pharo H, Sim C, Graham M, et al. Risky business: executive function, personality, and reckless behavior during adolescence and emerging adulthood. *Behav Neurosci.* 2011;125(6):970.

24. Adams SH, Knopf DK, Park MJ. Prevalence and treatment of mental health and substance use problems in the early emerging adult years in the United States: findings from the 2010 National Survey on drug use and health. *Emerg Adulthood.* 2014;2(3):163–172.

25. Arnett JJ, Žukauskienė R, Sugimura K. The new life stage of emerging adulthood at ages 18–29 years: Implications for mental health. *Lancet Psychiatry.* 2014;1(7):569–576.

26. Arnett JJ. New horizons in research on emerging and young adulthood. In: Booth A, Brown S, Landale N, Manning W, McHale S, eds. *Early Adulthood in a Family Context.* National Symposium on Family Issues, vol 2, 2012, Springer, New York, NY. https://doi.org/10.1007/978-1-4614-1436-0_15

27. Morone J. An integrative review of social determinants of health assessment and screening tools used in pediatrics. *J Pediatr Nurs.* 2017;37:22–28.

28. Jones PB. Adult mental health disorders and their age at onset. *Br J Psychiatry Suppl.* 2013;54:s5–s10.

29. Neinstein LS, Irwin CE Jr. Young adults remain worse off than adolescents. *J Adolesc Health.* 2013;53(5):559–561.

30. Vespa J. *The changing economics and demographics of young adulthood: 1975–2016.* US Department of Commerce, Economics and Statistics Administration, US Census Bureau, 2017.

ADDITIONAL RESOURCES AND WEBSITES

Additional Resources and Websites for Clinicians

American Academy of Child and Adolescent Psychiatry—professionals, parents and youth—http://www.aacap.org

The American Psychological Association's online resource center—https://www.apa.org/helpcenter

CDC—Adolescent and School Health—http://www.cdc.gov/healthyyouth/yrbs/pdf/us_overview_yrbs.pdf

Department of Health and Human Services—http://www.healthypeople.gov

Longitudinal Research from University of North Carolina—http://www.cpc.unc.edu/projects/addhealth

Society for the Study of Emerging Adulthood—professionals and parents—http://www.ssea.org/

Additional Resources and Websites for Parents/Caregivers

The ACT (Assets Coming Together) for Youth Center for Community Action—http://actforyouth.net/adolescence/toolkit/parents.cfm

American Psychological Association—Defining Racial and Ethnic Socialization (RES) Resources—https://www.apa.org/res/parent-resources

CHLA resources—https://www.chla.org/division-adolescent-and-young-adultmedicine-resources

https://youth.gov/ (formerly FindYouthInfo.gov) was created by the Interagency Working Group on Youth Programs (IWGYP), which is composed of representatives from 21 federal agencies that support programs and services focusing on youth. Resources and information—https://thementalhealthcoalition.org/

Web MD Health, search under "growth and development"—http://www.My.webmd.com

Additional Resources and Websites for Adolescents and Young Adults

BIPOC Mental Health Resources—https://thementalhealthcoalition.org/wp-content/uploads/2020/07/BIPOC-Mental-Health-Resources.pdf

Boston's Children's Hospital—https://youngmenshealthsite.org/

The Mental Health Coalition—https://thementalhealthcoalition.org/

National Alliance on Mental Illness—https://www.nami.org/Your-Journey/

Office on Women's Health—https://www.womenshealth.gov/

CHAPTER 4

Office Visit, Interview Techniques, and Recommendations to Parents

Gabriela Vargas

Joshua S. Borus

KEY WORDS

- Communication
- Confidentiality
- Health care transitions
- Interview techniques
- Parental advice
- Telehealth

INTRODUCTION

The skillful care of adolescent and young adult (AYA) patients requires competence that cannot be learned from a text alone. While we review principles and goals of management in this chapter, the art of relating to AYAs is improved only with practice and reflection. Both process and content of an interview are important, and one impacts the other. Adolescents and young adults are more likely to share concerns and information with a clinician if the clinician establishes rapport and trust.

GENERAL GUIDELINES FOR THE OFFICE VISIT

Comfort with Adolescents and Young Adults

While it may seem self-evident, effective care of AYAs requires the clinician to feel comfortable with and enjoy working with this population. Clinicians who are uncomfortable with critical issues related to the care of AYAs (i.e., contraception, sexual health, substance use, independence) should refer these patients to clinicians who are comfortable working with them.

There is significant overlap in the approach to AYAs, and as such these two populations are often grouped together in this chapter. However, there are some notable differences in the approach to the adolescent compared to the young adult based on chronologic and developmental age, especially with respect to consent, confidentiality, and privacy (see Chapter 7). We describe three approaches to the adolescent visit. Although these approaches translate well to the young adult population, we also review issues specific to young adults in more depth.

Meeting the Adolescent and Family: Initial Visit

The overarching goal of the AYA health visit is to improve outcomes for AYAs and help them establish good health practices as they move into adulthood. An important objective of the first visit is to build rapport with the patient and any parents/caregivers. Establishing the ground rules of the relationship, building trust, and focusing the visit on the adolescent's concerns are critical elements of the first visit. Confidentiality and its limits (see below) must be discussed, as well as giving practice and clinician contact information to both the adolescent and parent/caregiver.[1,2] This helps establish the adolescent as the principal participant in the visit while also recognizing the importance of the parent/caregiver role. Typically, one of three approaches outlined below is used to start the interview.

Start with Adolescent and Parent Together

Some clinicians prefer to start the interview with the adolescent and parent(s)/caregiver(s) together. How the adolescent and parent(s)/caregiver(s) interact with one another can provide insight into family dynamics and inform the clinician's strategy for addressing concerns during the visit. In addition, meeting together reinforces the importance of direct adolescent and parent/caregiver communication. After exchanging introductions, a verbal outline or "roadmap" of the visit should be provided to the patient and the parent(s)/caregiver(s). This is often a time to discuss medical history, family history, and social topics that are unlikely to be perceived as sensitive. Upon conclusion of this segment, the clinician then asks the parent(s)/caregiver(s) to leave the room while the remainder of the history is completed with the adolescent alone. The visit concludes with the clinician summarizing with everyone.

Start with Parent Alone

Some clinicians like to include separate time at the initial visit with parent(s)/caregiver(s) and then conduct the confidential interview with the adolescent. This option offers an opportunity for the parent(s)/caregiver(s) to express concerns about the adolescent in private. After greeting everyone, the clinician explains the order of the visit and explains the principles of confidentiality so that there is no confusion about the process or logistics of the visit. The clinician then meets with the parent(s)/caregiver(s) first, enabling them to express sensitive concerns at the beginning of the visit so that there is adequate time to address them. The clinician then meets with the adolescent alone to discuss the patient's concerns, obtain additional history, and conduct the physical examination. The visit concludes with the parents/clinician summarizing with everyone. Follow-up visits can start with a brief meeting with the parent(s)/caregivers alone if major issues persist, but should transition to one of the other types of visits described.

Start with Adolescent Alone

This approach allows the clinician to establish trust with and focus attention on the adolescent. After meeting with the adolescent privately, the adolescent and parent(s)/caregivers(s) meet with the clinician together to complete the visit. It is important for the adolescent to understand that their parent(s)/caregiver(s) will likely be asked about the patient's past medical history as well as any parent/caregiver concerns. Thus, confidentiality may need to be reviewed twice, once with adolescent alone and again when the parent/caregiver is present, so everyone understands the rules of the clinic.

Summarizing

The assessment usually concludes with a summary of the clinician's evaluation and management plan, including anticipatory guidance. Most of the discussion themes (e.g., concrete goals for eating healthier, resolution to get help from a teacher, details about medication use) can be done with the adolescent and parent/caregiver together, but sensitive concerns (e.g., discussion regarding safer sexual practices) should be discussed with the adolescent alone. The parent's/caregiver's role in this process diminishes as the adolescent matures into young adulthood.

The Young Adult Visit

Often, young adults come to medical visits alone, making these interactions more straightforward. However, when a family member is present with the young adult, it is essential (particularly when a chronic disease is being addressed) that there is a clear understanding that the young adult is in charge of their health care. Legal age requirements governing the definition of adulthood vary across the globe (see Chapter 7) relative to who has control of and rights to medical information. It is important for clinicians to understand the laws under which they practice. In most locales, the clinician will need written and verbal permission from the young adult to speak with a family member. Regardless, young adults should be given an opportunity to consent to having their family involved in the summary of nonconfidential issues or participate in a discussion about how the family can support the young adult in their health care.

Office Setup

Space

Adolescents and young adults prefer their own waiting room (or separate area) that is welcoming and developmentally appropriate. Some practices have separate blocks of time devoted to AYAs in an effort to create this type of environment. The examination room should include an examination table that has a curtain to promote a sense of privacy.

Clinic Staff

All clinic staff should have training on the developmental and health needs of AYAs. The clinic staff should adopt an AYA-friendly and nonjudgmental approach. Staff and receptionists should be familiar with issues such as confidentiality, crisis calls, and billing procedures. The staff should have flexible appointment booking procedures, including times to accept walk-in patients or a patient and their family who are in crisis. Every possible effort should be made to reduce wait times for AYAs.

Availability of Educational Materials

Age-appropriate magazines, hotline numbers, posters, websites, and health education brochures both welcome the patient and signal that the clinician is ready to talk about all topics, especially among youth who may be more reticent to discuss sensitive issues. Some practices place these materials in private places such as examination rooms and bathrooms to facilitate anonymous access.

Appointments

Ideally (though not feasible in some office settings), initial comprehensive visits should be given an hour in the schedule. Available after-school/early evening hours help AYAs to avoid missing school or work. A discussion about who is needed at the follow-up appointment (patient alone or both patient and family and/or partner) should occur at the end of each visit. Finally, the AYA should be asked about preferred methods of contact to confidentially review test results.

Billing for Sensitive Services in the United States

In the United States, billing for services that the AYA wishes to keep confidential is highly dependent on the patient's insurance.

The legal age of majority (18 years in most U.S. states) allows young adults to control their medical record. Insurance coverage currently allows parents to keep AYAs on their health care plan through age 26 years. Thus, when confidential services are billed to insurance, the AYA's parents are likely to receive an explanation of benefits that may undermine confidentially delivered health services. Using general symptoms for billing codes (e.g., dysuria or cervicitis rather than chlamydia), when appropriate, may be helpful in maintaining confidentiality in these circumstances.

When a practice has general screening rules, it is much easier to explain certain tests. For example, "Mrs. Jones, our clinic policy is to run a pregnancy test on all females with abdominal pain." Some practices elect to bill AYAs directly or write off the costs of certain diagnoses or tests to protect the patient, but this is not always possible. Other options include directing AYAs to obtain Medicaid coverage for conditions such as pregnancy, family planning, or substance use or offering to refer them to a health care setting that can provide low-cost or free confidential services.

Electronic Health Records

Patients should be aware that confidential details of care might be included in notes, letters, or electronic communication with other clinicians when appropriate. While there are benefits to electronic health records (EHRs), they also add complexity to documenting sensitive diagnoses, patient information, and lab results (see Chapters 7 and 9). As more clinicians embrace EHRs, the ease with which accessing patient data increases, as does the ease with which confidentiality can be broken. For example, an emergency department clinician sharing lab results with a patient and family may inadvertently reveal a positive screen for sexually transmitted infections or mistakenly disclose the AYA's use of birth control when showing them a computer screen. To protect AYAs' confidentiality when EHRs do not allow for sensitive information to remain confidential, it may be necessary to establish mechanisms or protocols so that sensitive diagnoses or topics are not disclosed to parents.[3] Patient portals and open notes provide health care access and transparency to AYAs, but also raise ethical and legal considerations regarding confidentiality.[4,5] The adolescent patient may be under pressure from a parent to allow unrestricted access to their record. Some strategies to improve protection of confidentiality in the EHR include creation of confidential diagnoses, fields, and/or medication sections that can only be accessed by the adolescent (see Chapters 7 and 9).

Interview Structure

It is not imperative to follow a rigidly prescribed format, but three central tasks must be addressed:
1. Introduction that puts the AYA at ease, presents a roadmap of the visit, and reviews concepts of confidentiality and limits
2. History that defines the patient's concerns/feelings and gathers other information (i.e., medical history and psychosocial assessment)
3. Summary discussion with the patient to review results of the examination, address concerns, answer questions, summarize nonconfidential issues with the parents/caregivers when appropriate, and establish an interval for follow-up

Previsit Questionnaires

Screening tools may help clinicians to increase delivery of preventive services and assess relevant social determinants of health. More clinicians are using written or electronic questionnaires to gather information which the AYA may complete at home or in the clinic. For mental health issues, the Patient Health Questionnaire (PHQ-9) is a validated depression screen for AYAs, and the Self-Report for Childhood Anxiety Related Disorders (SCARED) (see Chapter 74) has been validated as a screen for common anxiety disorders in adolescents. The American Academy of Pediatrics has developed questionnaires for early, middle, and late adolescents/young adults to screen for a variety of issues at each visit through the Bright Futures project.[6] These questionnaires may help prompt the AYA to consider important topics that they might want to address during the encounter. With increased use of social media, many AYAs find the computer a nonthreatening way to disclose personal information that can be reviewed and discussed during the clinical session. Importantly, answers to sensitive questions may not be accurate if the surveys are completed in public spaces, like waiting rooms.

Establish Rapport

Creating rapport is of paramount importance in the AYA patient–clinician relationship, and it may require more than one visit to establish. However, if rapport and trust are not built, subsequent visits will be less effective. Helpful ways to engage AYAs include the following:

1. Begin by introducing yourself with your preferred name and pronouns to the AYA and parent(s), if present. Address/shake hands with the patient first and ask how they would like to be addressed, including their preferred name and pronouns.
2. Invest a few minutes chatting informally about nonsensitive topics such as friends, school, or hobbies. This decreases tension and may provide insights into the patient's personality, mood, and how they conceptualize and articulate thoughts and feelings.
3. Let the AYA talk for a while on topics of interest to them.
4. Treat all of the patient's comments seriously.
5. Start with nonthreatening health questions such as a review of systems if the patient is tense or seems anxious.
6. Explore issues that concern the AYA. These issues may differ dramatically from concerns expressed by the parents (Table 4.1).

Ensure Confidentiality

Clinicians who care for AYAs must understand the concepts of confidential care and the limits of confidentiality. Clinicians need to know that limits of confidentiality vary across geographic areas, and they must be familiar with the local standards and laws that govern this core component of AYA care.[1,2,7]

It is the clinician's responsibility to explain confidentiality to the patient and parent(s)/caregiver(s). It is important that all parties understand the boundaries and exceptions to confidentiality. The patient should be made aware that if they are a danger to

---

TABLE 4.1

Interviewing Suggestions for AYAs

1. Shake hands with the AYA first.
2. Ask questions in context.
3. Focus initial history taking on the patient's complaints or problems.
4. Identify who has the problem (i.e., Is this problem the AYA's concern or the parent's?).
5. Talk in terms that the AYA will understand.
6. Highlight the positive.
7. Avoid lecturing and admonishing.
8. Take a neutral stance.
9. Usually, the less the interviewer says the better.
10. Avoid writing during the interview, especially during sensitive questioning.
11. Criticize the activity, not the AYA, and explain why you have concern.
12. Assess your own ability to listen. A clinician's difficulty in listening may be related to their own resentments or opinions of the adolescent's behavior.
13. When asking direct questions:
    a. Use less personal questions before more personal questions.
    b. Use open-ended questions.
    c. Avoid assumptions about gender and sexual preferences.

AYAs, adolescents and young adults.

---

themselves or a danger to others, the clinician will break confidentiality and report this information to the necessary parties. If the AYA is accompanied by a parent/caregiver to a clinic visit, the concept of confidentiality is best approached with the AYA and their parent/caregiver jointly.[8] This explanation may help the parents/caregivers feel more comfortable about allowing the AYA to meet with the clinician on their own. Discussing these complex concepts may also help dispel any conflicting beliefs the parent/caregiver has about confidentiality. For example, "Brian and Mrs. Jones, let me take a minute to review our clinic's confidentiality policy. We'll typically start our visits together so that everyone has a chance to raise topics for discussion. Then there will be a time when I speak with Brian alone. Brian, this is an opportunity to talk about anything you want or to ask questions and I'll have some questions for you as well. You should know that what we talk about in that setting stays between you (Brian) and the health care team *unless* I am concerned about you hurting yourself or someone else. Your family trusts me to help care for you, and they need to know that if you tell me that you are in danger, are a danger to someone else, or are a danger to yourself, we will let them know together. This is all about keeping you safe. Do you have any questions?" Ensuring confidential health care will foster a more open discussion about sensitive topics between AYAs and their clinicians.[7]

The clinician should make a reasonable effort to encourage the adolescent (and young adult, if appropriate) to involve parents/caregivers in health care decisions. Some AYAs may be more willing to discuss sensitive topics with their parents/caregivers in an environment where they feel safe and supported. For some AYAs, this may be the clinician's office. The clinician should be willing to help the AYA communicate with their family. Often, AYAs are willing to disclose sensitive information to their parents/caregivers, but may need help in framing the disclosure. It is often helpful when the clinician offers to facilitate a discussion that includes difficult topics.

Structure of the Social History

To structure the psychosocial history, many clinicians use the HEE-ADSSS (home, education/employment, eating, activities, drugs, sexuality, suicide/depression, safety) or SSHADESS (strengths, school, home, activities, drugs, emotions/eating/depression, sexuality, safety) screening frameworks (see Chapter 5).[9,10] The HEEADSSS approach moves from less personal to more personal questions for each topic, allowing the patient to become more comfortable as rapport is developed. The SSHADESS covers the same areas but emphasizes strengths first. While some patients may be uncomfortable with some of the social history questions at their initial visit, this approach allows each AYA to become familiar with important health topics that they may raise themselves and that their clinician is likely to raise at future encounters. This framework also allows the clinician to praise strengths or good decision making as well as comment on behaviors that may need to be addressed in order to promote health and wellness. Below are some sample questions for each category that apply to all AYAs. Many of these questions are open ended to facilitate greater communication between the patient and the clinician.

Home Where do you live? What's it like in your neighborhood? Who lives with you? Who is part of your family? How does everyone at home get along? Have there been recent changes?

Education/Employment Are you in school? What is the school like? Do you get extra support in any classes? What subjects do you do well in? Are there any favorite teachers/adults you can turn to for support? What do you want to do after finishing school? Do you have a job? What is the job like and how long do you plan to stay with it? What's next?

Eating Do you have any concerns about your body shape or size? Do you have meals with family, friends, or by yourself? What do you eat in a typical day? Do you snack in front of a screen? How much fast food do you consume? How many sugar-sweetened drinks, calcium-containing foods, or fruits and vegetables do you have in a day? Have you ever thrown up, restricted your intake, or taken diet pills or laxatives to control your weight? Do you take any nutritional supplements or vitamins?

Activities What do you do in your free time? What are you good at? What do you like to do for fun? Do you have a core set of friends? What do you do for physical activity? How much screen time do you get? Are you involved in groups or clubs?

Drugs Are there students at school who drink, smoke, or use other substances? Is there anybody at home who smokes, drinks, or uses other substances? Have you ever smoked cigarettes, electronic cigarettes, or cannabis? Have you ever drunk alcohol? Have you ever used prescription medicines that were not prescribed to you? Have you ever tried other substances? How often do you use these now? How do you pay for substances? In addition to these questions, there are a variety of validated, brief screening tools for substance use (see Chapters 68 to 73).

Sexuality How do you describe your gender? Everyone has a gender identity, some describe themselves as male, female, gender nonbinary, or gender fluid; how would you describe your gender identity? What pronouns would you like me to use? Are you in a relationship with anyone? Are you attracted to males, females, both, neither, or not sure? Have you had sex (clarify what sex is) or are you choosing to "hold off?" Do you have vaginal sex, meaning penis-in-vagina sex? Do you have anal sex, meaning penis-in-rectum/anus sex? How old were you when you first had sex? Have you had any problems with sex—is it what you thought it would be like? How many partners have you had? Whose decision is it to have sex? What are you using for protection? Do you know about emergency contraception and how to get it? Most AYAs masturbate—do you have any questions about masturbating? Have you ever been diagnosed with a sexually transmitted infection? Have you ever been pregnant or had an abortion?

Suicide/Depression How is your mood? Do you think you get frustrated or upset more than your friends? How is your sleep? How is your level of interest in regular activities? Do you feel guilty or anxious about things? What is your energy level like? Do you find it hard to concentrate? Have your eating habits changed? Have you ever thought about hurting yourself or killing yourself? Should I be worried about you?

Safety Do you feel safe at home, school, and in your neighborhood? Is there any bullying at school or online? Have you ever been hit, kicked, punched, or touched in an inappropriate way or against your will? How often do you wear a seatbelt while in a car?

Table 4.2 outlines some effective interviewing techniques that can be used in the assessment of an AYA patient.

Physical Examination

Typically, AYAs are examined alone, though some younger or developmentally delayed adolescents may wish to have a parent present. The clinician should describe aspects of the physical examination before actual assessment. If the examination will include evaluation of anorectal area, genital area, or the female breast, a chaperone is recommended. The decision for a chaperone should be a shared decision between the patient and clinician, and should include discussion of the patient's preferred gender of the chaperone. Male clinicians are strongly advised to use a chaperone (typically female) during genital or breast examination of all patients with female reproductive organs, and this seems to be standard practice.

TABLE 4.2

Interviewing Techniques for AYAs

Open-ended questions often facilitate communication	"What does your pain prevent you from doing?" or "Tell me more about the arguments with your mother" may uncover a richer response than "Does your pain stop you from playing sports?" or "Does it make you feel bad to argue with your mom?"
Restatement and summarization	This often clarifies a problem or encourages additional communication: "So what I'm hearing is you like Jim, but don't want to have sex with him. However, you're worried if you say no, he'll move on to someone else. Have I got it right or am I missing something?"
Clarification	The clinician should not be afraid to ask the patient for help decoding slang. It demonstrates interest, that they are willing to ask for help, and allows the patient to be an authority.
Insight questions	Some questioning should focus on gaining a global understanding of the AYAs. "What do you see yourself doing in a year?" or "How would your friends describe you?"
Reassuring questions	Providing context and normalizing sensitive subjects through reassuring statements may facilitate discussion. For example, "It is common for people your age to masturbate—it is completely normal. Do you masturbate?"
Support and empathy	Acknowledging the patient's feelings is crucial to all clinical encounters regardless of age. "I'm sorry you've had to deal with this—is there a way I can be helpful?" demonstrates the clinician's empathy and support.
Reflection responses	The reflection response mirrors the adolescent's feelings. Consider the following example: Clinician: How do you like school? Teen: I hate it. Clinician: You hate it? Teen: Yeah, my teachers always…

AYAs, adolescents and young adults.

While the converse should hold true, in practice, it is not unusual for female clinicians to examine patients with male reproductive organs without a chaperone if the patient agrees. Policies and laws regarding chaperones vary across geographic areas and institutions, as such clinicians must be familiar with local standards and laws. While completing the physical examination, the clinician has an excellent opportunity to reassure the patient about their growth and physical development. The physical examination provides an opportunity to educate the AYA about their changing body, especially for the younger adolescent. Pointing out normal findings may provide great relief to an unspoken concern, especially as it relates to the genital examination.

Closure

At the close of any visit, the clinician should:
1. Summarize the diagnosis and treatment for the AYA. Parents who accompany the patient may be included in the discussions of nonconfidential issues to provide support and assistance.
2. Discuss other resources available to the patient.

3. Allow time to address questions and concerns from the AYA and parent.
4. Schedule a follow-up appointment.
5. The clinician should inform the AYA about the clinician's office hours and availability should health concerns arise. The clinician should encourage the patient to contact the office for all their health care needs.

PRINCIPLES TO APPROACHING THE ADOLESCENT AND YOUNG ADULT PATIENT

Welcoming, Nonjudgmental Approach

It is imperative that clinicians create a welcoming, culturally appropriate, safe medical home for AYA patients of all races, ethnicities, gender identities, sexual orientation, abilities, immigration status, and other identities.[11] Clinicians should consider introducing themselves by their preferred name and pronouns.

Avoid a Surrogate Parent Role

Rather than being a surrogate parent, the clinician should function as a concerned adult who is nonjudgmental when asking questions, listening, and providing guidance.

Avoid a Peer Role

Most AYAs want a clinician who can be a sensitive and mature resource, rather than a friend. A lack of formality and a sense of humor may be inviting, but dressing and talking like a peer are not.

Sidestep Power Struggles

It is difficult to force adolescents and especially young adults into action. Avoiding power struggles, focusing on facts in a judgment-free way, and helping AYAs arrive at their own decision to make change in the clinical encounter are difficult, but much more effective in bringing about change. Motivational interviewing techniques, in which the clinician helps the AYA develop their own reasons to change behavior, facilitate change by emphasizing differences between desired goals and current behavior.[12]

Act as an Advocate

Clinicians should emphasize the patient's positive actions[10] and recognize that supporting the AYA does not mean endorsing the AYA's risky behavior.

Active Listening

It is important for the clinician to engage in active listening and acknowledge the concerns of the patient. Focusing on what the AYA communicates, understanding the patient's perspective, and refraining from giving advice without first getting permission will help earn the AYA's trust and provide the clinician with conversational opportunities to discuss health priorities.

Instill Responsibility

Encouraging the patient's personal responsibility for their health and health care can lead to improved outcomes. The clinician can be a willing coach but cannot make decisions for the AYA. Ultimately, the patient (often with the assistance of their family or support system) needs to commit to making decisions that will protect their health and safety.

Nonverbal Cues

It is important for the clinician to be aware of the patient's nonverbal interaction. Nonverbal communication such as facial expressions, gestures, eye contact, or posture provides important information and can help the clinician connect with their patient.

Behavioral Context

Exploring the thoughts, reasoning, and context behind a decision may change the way a clinician thinks about a patient's action. For example, a clinician might think differently about a patient with poorly controlled attention-deficit/hyperactivity disorder skipping class because of excessive frustration than a patient skipping class because of wanting to see friends who are also skipping class. In addition, younger adolescents are often concrete thinkers who may alter behavior if given alternative responses to a situation.

Hidden Agenda

Adolescents and young adults may be reluctant to disclose the real reason for a visit due to denial, embarrassment, or concerns about confidentiality. For example, a female adolescent may complain about vague abdominal pain instead of verbalizing concern for pregnancy or a male adolescent with chest pain may actually be concerned about gynecomastia. To reduce the AYA's hesitancy, clinicians should clearly express that they are open to all concerns and are interested in assisting the patient. Reassurance about variations of normal physical examination findings (i.e., "It looks like you have a small amount of tissue development under your nipple—I see this in a number of patients going through male puberty. This is completely normal, but sometimes guys are worried about it. Do you have any concerns?") and use of appropriate testing (i.e., "Sometimes patients with abdominal pain are worried that they might be pregnant. Is this something that you have thought about? We could do a simple test to help answer this question.") may make AYAs more comfortable inquiring about concerns that are sensitive.

Developmental Orientation

Clinicians must be sensitive to the developmental and behavioral trajectories of AYAs. Clinicians should be aware of the differences in cognitive processes, emotional maturity, and developmental tasks for each age and modify the interview approach around sensitive issues (i.e., body image, substance use, peer relationships, mental health, independence, sexual and reproductive health) so that it is developmentally appropriate for the AYA.

Special Interview Challenges

1. Garrulous patient: Overtalkative AYAs can often be directed by asking "I can see you like talking about this. Why?" or responding and then reframing the question with discrete answers. "It sounds like you've got some strong opinions about gym class. Tell me, do you exercise almost every day, a few times a week, or not at all?"
2. Quiet patient: Try to engage the quiet AYA by talking about anything—their T-shirt, their phone, a current event, or sports—to help break the silence.
3. Anxious patient: Reassurance is often helpful—"Sometimes it's difficult to talk about...."
4. Angry patient: Clarify how you can help the patient. "It sounds like talking about these issues is difficult—how can I help?"

Family Considerations and Social Determinants of Health

Family relationships are an important contributor to the AYA's development. For the clinician to optimally care for an AYA, they must understand the strengths, limitations, interactions, and stresses of the family and be willing to work with the entire family unit. Understanding the ability of the family to support and nurture the AYA's development is critical to providing effective care. Change in the AYA may be dependent on first initiating change within the family. Talking with parents or other family members (with the consent of the AYA) may help clarify past medical and family history, facilitate social support for the patient in complex treatment regimens,[13] and promote follow-up and referral care. Finally, the definition of family is likely to differ between individuals and over time, so an important element of the history is asking the AYA who they consider their family or support system.

In addition to family considerations, clinicians should understand the role of societal factors and constraints that impact AYAs.[14] Approximately 20% of U.S. adolescents live below the poverty level,[15] and economically disadvantaged AYAs rate their health status lower than those who are economically advantaged.[16]

Internal Considerations

Many practitioners recall their own experiences as an AYA to generate understanding and empathy for their patients. The clinician may wish to disclose some personal experience with the AYA about their own youth to bridge the gap between the clinician and the patient. However, there is a risk of making the patient feel uncomfortable. Clinician self-disclosure should be carefully considered before being used and should be solely motivated to help the patient.

Optimize Adolescent and Young Adult–Clinicians Communication

The patient's perception of their clinician's behavior contributes to their willingness to adhere to a treatment plan or to make a return visit.[17] Clinicians who demonstrate honesty, show respect, listen attentively, answer questions, affirm confidentiality, exchange information, and enhance satisfaction will increase the likelihood that the AYA will return for follow-up.[18]

⬤ RECOMMENDATIONS TO PARENTS OF ADOLESCENTS

Authoritative Parenting Style

Rothenberg and colleagues[19] have conducted extensive research that has examined the impact of parenting styles on a variety of adolescent outcomes. This research includes data from an economically and racially diverse group of adolescents and families from all over the world. A consistent finding in these studies is that parents who are identified as authoritative are more likely to have adolescent children with better health and social outcomes.

Authoritative parents:
1. are warm and loving
2. develop firm and consistent but not rigid family guidelines
3. foster a child's independence according to developmental stage. Independence helps a child develop a sense of self-direction. Failure to foster independence and decision making is associated with increasing levels of anxiety among adolescents.

Adolescents who have at least one parent with this parenting style demonstrated:
1. better academic performance
2. fewer mental health problems
3. fewer antisocial behaviors and diminished delinquency
4. higher self-esteem and self-reliance

General Suggestions

Other suggestions for parents about navigating the challenges of parenting AYAs include the following:
1. Listen and show interest in the AYA's activities.
2. Avoid power struggles if possible and solve conflicts using a collaborative approach.
3. Remain flexible.
4. Spend time together and create opportunities to have fun one-on-one.
5. Demonstrate trust.
6. Take opportunities to stress the positive when they arise.
7. Make resources available.
8. Ensure that standards and expectations are clear, but have some flexibility in how these are accomplished—for example, the time the trash is taken out does not matter as long as it is taken out in time for pick up.
9. Avoid minimizing problems while still giving perspective; conversely, do not overreact based on limited information.

Challenges of Adolescence

Parents should be aware of the developmental tasks (see Chapter 3) associated with adolescence as well as the impact of peers and technology (see Chapter 9) on the adolescent's social milieu. This will help parents understand what behaviors, feelings, and actions are normal and healthy during adolescence. Recognition and appreciation of normal adolescent behaviors can reduce conflict and difficulties between parents and their child.
1. Peers play an increasingly important role in an adolescent's life as they seek independence.
2. Parents must not overreact to rejection by the adolescent for a period of time. Parents should appreciate that most young people do not reject their parent's values and beliefs even as they may strive to be independent.
3. Adolescents need firm, fair, and explicit limits. Involvement of the adolescent in the limit-setting process is beneficial.
4. In addition to developing an authoritative parenting style, parents should be encouraged to be proactive about their adolescent's health and well-being. Parents should anticipate potential conflicts and prepare their child to deal with these conflicts by discussion, modeling, and reason. While substance use experimentation by adolescents is predictable, data suggest that adolescents with authoritative parents were less likely to smoke cigarettes, use marijuana, or binge drink than those with neglectful parents (defined as parents exhibiting neither warmth nor control).[20] In addition, adolescents with proactive parents were more likely to have received an annual health care visit, reported more frequent discussions about health, and placed a higher value on clinician discussions about health.[21]
5. Adolescents' sense of invulnerability adds to their willingness to expose themselves to risks.
6. The societal pressures of the 21st century present challenges as many families have less support than prior generations. Single parenting is more prevalent, extended families are less involved in care, and more families have no stay-at-home adult.
7. The lives of adolescents are increasingly influenced by media. Parents need to help adolescents be discerning consumers of media, recognizing that some media messages may be attempts to exploit youth and/or may promote unhealthy or unrealistic ideas in order to make a profit from the adolescent. In addition, it is important to help adolescents understand that online and social media platforms may: (1) be used to ridicule and bully (see Chapter 9), (2) result in a permanent "digital footprint" that leads to future embarrassment, and (3) convey inaccurate information.

Challenges of Young Adulthood
1. Young adults continue to work toward separation and individual identification. Parents should remember that the vast majority of young adults accept their parents' basic values.
2. Young adults typically seek to have a more equal relationship with parents even if they are not ready to be independent in all phases of their lives. This change in relationship will not occur instantaneously at the age of majority, but gradually over time.
3. Transitioning to adult health care, even when delayed into the mid-20s, may be difficult for the young adult.[22]

Establishing House Rules

House rules with AYAs should be clear, consistently enforced, and applied to all those living in the house. These should be discussed as a family and include the AYA in the decision-making process. Keeping the rules to a manageable number (5 to 10) and writing them down, especially for young adolescents, is also advised.

Health Care Transitions

The American Academy of Pediatrics, American Academy of Family Physicians, and American College of Physicians define health care transition as "the process of moving a child to an adult model of health care with or without a transfer to a new clinician."[23] While barriers to health care transition exist at the AYA, family, and clinician level, a successful transition is associated with improved health outcomes and health care engagement.[23,24] Clinicians should develop a structured transition process tailored to their patient population and clinic. Discussions and planning should begin years before actual transfer to an adult clinician and should occur annually or more often as appropriate. The discussion should also include health care proxies or guardianship as appropriate. Clinicians may consider using the six core elements of health care transition model, including: (1) transition policy; (2) transition tracking and monitoring; (3) transition readiness; (4) transition planning; (5) transfer and/or integration into adult-centered care; and (6) transition completion and ongoing care with adult clinician.[23,25]

Telehealth

Telemedicine is defined by the U.S. Centers for Medicare and Medicaid Services as a two-way audio-video interaction between a patient and a clinician or practitioner at a distant site.[26] The use of telemedicine has accelerated in the setting of the SARS-CoV-2 pandemic, and its use is now commonplace for many clinicians. While telemedicine does not replace the in-person visit, it can augment care when provided within the context of the medical home. Telemedicine can reduce barriers to care such as school/work absences, child-care issues, and transportation concerns while building patient–clinician rapport. During the pandemic, AYA practices have demonstrated the utility of telemedicine to address a range of care needs including primary care, acute visits, contraceptive care, gender-affirming care, eating disorder care, and substance use management.[27,28] The clinician may consider a hybrid model (both telemedicine and in-person visits) within their own clinical practice or in collaboration with local primary care clinicians when providing subspecialty care that requires an in-person physical examination and/or lab work.[27-29] As with in-person visits, confidentiality remains a critical component of telehealth visits. Clinicians should ask AYA patients about the presence of other people within the room. To help ensure confidentiality, clinicians may consider having the patient use headphones, answer yes or no to potentially sensitive questions, or use chat functions if available on their telehealth platforms. Finally, health care practices should work to address potential barriers to effective telemedicine, including assessing the patient's digital literacy and access to internet and audio-visual devices.[30]

◐ SUMMARY

Patient–clinician rapport is essential to the care of AYA patients whether during an in-person or telehealth visit. The principles of confidentiality and the psychosocial interview help provide a foundation for trust in the individual clinician, as well as the health care system.

◐ ACKNOWLEDGMENT

Supported in part by the Leadership Education in Adolescent Health Training grant #T71MC00009 from Maternal and Children Health Bureau, Health Resources and Services Administration.

REFERENCES

1. Guttmacher Institute. *An Overiew of Consent to Reproductive Health Services by Young People*. 2022. Accessed June 20, 2022. https://www.guttmacher.org/print/state-policy/explore/overview-minors-consent-law
2. Ford C, English A, Sigman G. Confidential health care for adolescents: position paper for the society for adolescent medicine. *J Adolesc Health*. 2004;35(2):160–167.
3. Gray SH, Pasternak RH, Gooding HC, et al; Society for Adolescent Health and Medicine. Recommendations for electronic health record use for delivery of adolescent health care. *J Adolesc Health*. 2014;54(4):487–490.
4. Carlson JL, Goldstein R, Buhr T, et al. Teenager, parent, and clinician perspectives on the electronic health record. *Pediatrics*. 2020;145(3):e20190193.
5. Bourgeois FC, DesRoches C, Bell SK. Ethical challenges raised by OpenNotes for pediatric and adolescent patients. *Pediatrics*. 2018;141(6):e20172745.
6. Bright futures. *Adolescence tools*. Accessed January 13, 2021. https://brightfutures.aap.org/materials-and-tools/tool-and-resource-kit/Pages/adolescence-tools.aspx
7. Ford CA, Millstein SG, Halpern-Felsher BL, et al. Influence of physician confidentiality assurances on adolescents' willingness to disclose information and seek future health care. A randomized controlled trial. *JAMA*. 1997;278(12):1029–1034.
8. Duncan RE, Vandeleur M, Derks A, et al. Confidentiality with adolescents in the medical setting: what do parents think? *J Adolesc Health*. 2011;49(4):428–430.
9. Klein DA, Goldenring JM, Adelman WP. HEADSSS 3.0: the psychosocial interview for adolescents updated for a new century fueled by media. *Contemp Pediatr*. 2014;31(4):16–28.
10. Ginsburg K. Viewing our adolescent patients through a positive lens. *Contemp Pediatr*. 2007;24:65–76.
11. Svetaz MV, Chulani V, West KJ, et al. Racism and its harmful effects on nondominant racial-ethnic youth and youth-serving providers: a call to action for organizational change. *J Adolesc Health*. 2018;63(2):257–261.
12. Naar-King S, Suarez M. *Motivational Interviewing with Adolescents and Young Adults*. Guilford Press; 2011.
13. Svetaz MV, Garcia-Huidobro D, Allen M. Parents and family matter: strategies for developing family-centered adolescent care within primary care practices. *Prim Care*. 2014;41(3):489–506.
14. Viner RM, Ozer EM, Denny S, et al. Adolescence and the social determinants of health. *Lancet* 2012;379(9826):1641–1652.
15. Baer TE, Gottlieb L, Sandel M. Addressing social determinants of health in the adolescent medical home. *Curr Opin Pediatr*. 2013;25(4):447–453.
16. Quon EC, McGrath JJ. Subjective socioeconomic status and adolescent health: a meta analysis. *Health Psychol*. 2014;33(5):433–447.
17. Ginsburg KR, Slap GB, Cnaan A, et al. Adolescents' perceptions of factors affecting their decisions to seek health care. *JAMA*. 1995;273(24):1913–1918.
18. van Staa A, Jedeloo S, van der Stege H; On Your Own Feet Research Group. "What we want": chronically ill adolescents' preferences and priorities for improving health care. *Patient Prefer Adherence*. 2011;5:291–305.
19. Rothenberg WA, Lansford JE, Bornstein MH, et al. Effects of parental warmth and behavioral control on adolescent externalizing and internalizing trajectories across cultures. *J Res Adolesc*. 2020;30(4):835–855.
20. Shakya HB, Chisakis NA, Fowler JH. Parental influence on substance use in adolescent social networks. *Arch Pediatr Adolesc Med*. 2012;166(12):1132–1139.
21. Rickert VI, Gilbert AL, Aalsma MC. Proactive parents are assets to the health and well-being of teens. *J Pediatr*. 2014;164(6):1390–1395.
22. Lemly DC, Weitzman ER, O'Hare K. Advancing healthcare transitions in the medical home: tools for providers, families and adolescents with special healthcare needs. *Curr Opin Pediatr*. 2013;25(4):439–446.
23. White PH, Colley WC, Transitions Clinical Report Authoring Group, American Academy of Pediatrics, American Academy of Family Physicians, American College of Physicians. Supporting the health care transition from adolescence to adulthood in the medical home. *Pediatrics*. 2018;142(5):e20182587.
24. Gabriel P, McManus M, Rogers K, et al. Outcome evidence for structured pediatric to adult health care transition interventions: a systematic review. *J Pediatr*. 2017;188:263–269.e15.
25. American Academy of Pediatrics, American Academy of Family Physicians, American College of Physicians, Transitions Clinical Report Authoring Group. Supporting the health care transition from adolescence to adulthood in the medical home. *Pediatrics*. 2011;128(1):182.
26. *Medicare Telemedicine Health Care Provider Fact Sheet* | CMS.gov. Accessed June 21, 2022, https://www.cms.gov/newsroom/fact-sheets/medicare-telemedicine-health-care-provider-fact-sheet
27. Barney A, Buckelew S, Mesheriakova V, et al. The COVID-19 pandemic and rapid implementation of adolescent and young adult telemedicine: challenges and opportunities for innovation. *J Adolesc Health*. 2020;67(2):164–171.
28. Wood SM, White K, Peebles R, et al. Outcomes of a rapid adolescent telehealth scale-up during the COVID-19 pandemic. *J Adolesc Health*. 2020;67(2):172–178.
29. North S. Telemedicine in the time of COVID and beyond. *J Adolesc Health*. 2020;67:145–146.
30. Nouri S, Khoong EC, Lyles CR, et al. Addressing equity in telemedicine for chronic disease management during the COVID-19 pandemic. *NEJM Catal Innov Care Deliv*. 2020.

ᯤ ADDITIONAL RESOURCES AND WEBSITES

Additional Resources and Websites for Clinicians:
American Academy of Pediatrics Clinical Resources—Adolescent Sexual Health—https://www.aap.org/en-us/advocacy-and-policy/aap-health-initiatives/adolescent-sexual-health/Pages/Caring-for-the-Adolescent-Patient.aspx
American Academy of Pediatrics Policy Statement on Chaperones—Committee on Practice and Ambulatory Medicine. Use of chaperones during the physical examination of the pediatric patient. *Pediatrics*. 2011;127(5):991–993.

Bright Futures/American Academy of Pediatrics Clinical Resources— https://brightfutures.aap.org/clinical-practice/Pages/default.aspx

Care of Transgender and Gender Diverse Youth in Primary Care—Rafferty JR, Donaldson AA, Forcier M. Primary Care Considerations for Transgender and Gender-Diverse Youth. *Pediatr Rev.* 2020;41(9):437–454.

Centers for Disease Control and Prevention—Adolescent and School Health— https://www.cdc.gov/healthyyouth/index.htm

Centers for Disease Control and Prevention—Sexually Transmitted Infections— https://www.cdc.gov/mmwr/volumes/70/rr/rr7004a1.htm?s_cid=rr7004a1_e&ACS TrackingID=USCDC_921-DM61908&ACSTrackingLabel=This%20Week%20in%20 MMWR%20-%20Vol.%2070%2C%20July%2023%2C%202021&deliveryName= USCDC_921-DM61908

Contemporary Pediatrics—HEEADSS 3.0 Psychosocial Interview—https://www. contemporarypediatrics.com/modern-medicine-feature-articles/heeadsss-30-psychosocial-interview-adolescents-updated-new-century-fueled-media

Digital Wellness Lab—Information and Webinars on Media Use—https://digitalwellness-lab.org/

Got Transition—Health Care Transition Resource—https://gottransition.org

Physicians for Reproductive Health—Adolescent Reproductive and Sexual Health Education Program (includes powerpoints and videos)—https://prh.org/arshep-ppts/

Society for Adolescent Health and Medicine—Resources and Virtual Chat Series— https://www.adolescenthealth.org/Resources.aspx

Additional Resources and Websites for Parents/Caregivers:

American Academy of Family Physicians—Informational Medical Website for Families—https://familydoctor.org

Bright Futures—Family-Centered Care Resource—https://brightfutures.aap.org/families/Pages/default.aspx

Digital Wellness Lab—Information and Webinars on Media Use— https://digitalwellnesslab.org/

Got Transition—Health Care Transition Resource for Parents and Caregivers— https://gottransition.org/parents-caregivers/

Society for Adolescent Health and Medicine—Resources for Adolescent and Parents— https://www.adolescenthealth.org/Resources/Resources-for-Adolescents-and-Parents.aspx

Substance Abuse and Mental Health Services Administration—Guidance for Parents on Discussing Substance Use with Their Child—https://www.samhsa.gov/talk-they-hear-you/parent-resources/why-you-should-talk-your-child

U.S. Department of Health and Human Services—Office of Population Affairs—Guide on adolescent development that provides guidance for parents and caregivers— https://opa.hhs.gov/adolescent-health/adolescent-development-explained

Young Men's Health Site—Informational Medical Website geared toward adolescents and young adults as well as caregivers—https://Youngmenshealthsite.org

Young Women's Health—Informational Medical Website geared toward adolescents and young adults as well as caregivers—https://Youngwomenshealth.org

Additional Resources and Websites for Adolescents and Young Adults:

Bedsider.org—Online Birth Control Support Network operated by Power to Decide, the campaign to prevent unplanned pregnancy—https://www.bedsider.org/

Digital Wellness Lab—Information and Webinars on Media Use—https://digitalwellness-lab.org/

Got Transition—Health Care Transition Resource for Youth and Young Adults— https://gottransition.org/youth-and-young-adults/

Society for Adolescent Health and Medicine—Resources for Adolescent and Parents— https://www.adolescenthealth.org/Resources/Resources-for-Adolescents-and-Parents.aspx

Young Men's Health Site—Informational Medical Website geared toward adolescents and young adults as well as caregivers—https://Youngmenshealthsite.org

Young Women's Health—Informational Medical Website geared toward adolescents and young adults as well as caregivers—https://Youngwomenshealth.org

Preventive Health Care for Adolescents and Young Adults

Matthew J. Meyers
Elizabeth M. Ozer

KEY WORDS

- Electronic health records
- Innovative technology
- Preventive care
- Preventive counseling
- Preventive health guidelines
- Risk behavior
- Screening and counseling

INTRODUCTION

Since the majority of adolescent and young adult (AYA) morbidity and mortality can be attributed to known preventable risk factors, preventive health care is the cornerstone of AYA Medicine. Behaviors initiated during adolescence, such as substance use, early sexual behavior, and risky driving, are responsible for the majority of deaths and disabling conditions in adolescence.[1,2] Motor vehicle deaths and homicide rates are highest during young adulthood as are rates of substance use, sexually transmitted infections (STIs), and mental health problems.[3] Unintentional injuries (including car crashes) account for the most deaths during adolescence and young adulthood, with suicide and homicide the second and third leading causes of death for AYAs, respectively.[2,4]

The psychosocial and developmental milieu of adolescence and young adulthood creates the potential for risk and vulnerability as well as developmental windows of opportunity.[5] A life course focus on AYA health is critical as AYA behaviors—shaped by biologic, emotional, and social determinants, including racism and discrimination—lay the foundation for future health behaviors and outcomes.[6]

The annual visit to a clinician offers an opportunity to improve the health of AYAs through preventive screening and counseling. Visits to a clinician should reinforce positive health behaviors, such as exercise and nutritious eating, and discourage health-risk behaviors such as those associated with unsafe sexual behaviors, unsafe driving, and use of tobacco or other drugs. Although the incidence of serious medical problems during adolescence and young adulthood is low, lifelong health habits are established during this time. It is therefore an ideal period for clinicians to invest time in health promotion and preventive services.

In this chapter, we review current best practices for preventive services for AYAs and highlight key aspects of preventive care, including preventive health guidelines, the health care delivery setting, the content of the visit, emerging areas of efficiency such as electronic health records (EHRs) and extending the reach of the clinician through innovative technology.

PREVENTIVE SERVICES FOR ADOLESCENTS AND YOUNG ADULTS

Clinical Guidelines for Preventive Services

Most AYAs visit primary care settings at least once a year; so primary care has been highlighted as an important setting for detection and early intervention for risk-taking behaviors and mental health issues in youth. Since many health problems during adolescence and young adulthood are preventable, primary care visits represent a key opportunity for preventive screening and intervention, with evidence supporting the efficacy of certain clinical preventive services.[1] Interventions during adolescence and young adulthood may have long-term implications because unhealthy behaviors tend to continue into middle and late adulthood, and are linked to preventable chronic conditions and premature deaths.[1,3]

Guidelines have been developed to help clinicians determine when and how to provide preventive services. The U.S. Preventive Services Task Force (USPSTF) offers evidence-based recommendations, generally based on large rigorous studies.[7] A broad consensus has emerged for comprehensive clinical preventive services for adolescents with the adoption of professional guidelines. The fourth and most recent edition of Bright Futures, a professional consensus document created jointly by the U.S. Health Resources and Services Administration's (HRSA's) Maternal and Child Health Bureau and the American Academy of Pediatrics (AAP), provides recommendations for the care of AYAs up to age 21 years.[8] Other professional organizations, such as the American College of Obstetrics and Gynecology (ACOG), offer additional recommendations; and the Advisory Committee on Immunization Practices (ACIP) of the Centers for Disease Control and Prevention (CDC) provides recommendations on immunizations.

Adolescents

In general, preventive health guidelines recommend that all adolescents have an annual, confidential visit to promote the receipt of preventive services.[9,10] During this visit, clinicians should provide screening, education, and counseling in a number of biomedical and sociobehavioral areas.[1] Adolescents should be screened for risky health behaviors, and strengths and competencies should be identified. The updated Bright Futures guidelines specifically encourage the promotion of positive youth development and recommend that clinicians focus on the strengths of the adolescent and their family in the annual visits.[8]

Health guidance should also be provided to parents to help them respond appropriately to the health needs of their adolescent child. This includes providing information about normative adolescent development, the signs and symptoms of disease and emotional distress, parenting behaviors that promote healthy adolescent adjustment, and methods to help adolescents avoid potentially harmful behaviors. Table 5.1 provides a summary of recommended clinical preventive services professional guidelines for adolescents up to age 18, with indication of guidelines supported by sufficient evidence to be recommended by the USPSTF.[11]

Young Adults

There are currently no specific guidelines developed for young adults regardless of the definition of age range for young adulthood.[12] The most comprehensive set of guidelines that intersect with the age group of 18 to 26 years is Bright Futures, which includes a focus on "late adolescence" (18 to 21 years).[8] However, when ages

TABLE 5.1

Summary of Clinical Preventive Services Guidelines for Adolescents up to Age 18 (CPSG-ADOL Summary)

Preventive Services	All (√)	At Risk (+)	Screening Test/Procedure and Other Notes
Nutrition/Exercise/Obesity			
Hypertension/blood pressure †	√		√ Bright Futures, *USPSTF insufficient evidence*
Obesity/BMI	√		**Screen ≥6 y; offer/refer to appropriate intervention**
Cholesterol level		+	√ Bright Futures, *USPSTF insufficient evidence*
Healthy diet and physical activity		+	√ Bright Futures, NHLBI
Dyslipidemia	√		√ Bright Futures recommends one screening each between ages 11 and 14, 15 and 17, and 18 and 21; *USPSTF insufficient evidence*
Substance use			
Alcohol (SBIRT)	√		√ Bright Futures, *USPSTF insufficient evidence*
Tobacco (SBIRT)	√		**Education and brief counseling to prevent initiation**
Substance use (SBIRT)	√		√ Bright Futures[a] and ACOG[b], *USPSTF insufficient evidence*
Mental health/depression			
Depression (screening and treatment) †	√		**Routinely screen for MDD ≥ age 12 with adequate systems for care are in place**
Suicide screening	√		√ Bright Futures and ACOG, *USPSTF insufficient evidence*
Safety/violence			
Family/partner violence	√		**Screen females of childbearing age**
Fighting	√		√ Bright Futures and ACOG
Helmets	√		√ Bright Futures and ACOG
Seat belts	√		√ Bright Futures and ACOG
Guns	√		√ Bright Futures and ACOG
Bullying	√		Bright Futures only
Reproductive health			
HIV	√	+	**Bright Futures and USPSTF recommend screening between ages 15–18; screen younger adolescents at increased risk**
STI (screening and counseling)		+	**Behavioral counseling for all sexually active adolescents**
Syphilis		+	**VDRL**
Gonorrhea (females) †		+	**NAATs; test if ≤24 and sexually active**
Chlamydia (females) †		+	**NAATs; test if ≤24 and sexually active**
Chlamydia and gonorrhea (male) †		+	√ Bright Futures, *USPSTF insufficient evidence*

(continued)

TABLE 5.1

Summary of Clinical Preventive Services Guidelines for Adolescents up to Age 18 (CPSG-ADOL Summary) (*Continued*)

Preventive Services	All (√)	At Risk (+)	Screening Test/Procedure and Other Notes
Birth control methods	√	+	√ ACOG, + Bright Futures
Pregnancy (counseling)		+	+ Bright Futures
Cancer screening			
Skin cancer (counseling)		+	**Counsel those aged 10–24 with fair skin on reducing UV exposure**
BRCA-related cancer		+	**Family history of breast, ovarian, tubal, or peritoneal cancer**
Infectious diseases including CDC immunization recommendations			
Td/Tdap	√		**1 dose Tdap, then Td booster every 10 y**
Human papillomavirus	√		**HPV vaccine for male and females up to age 26; 2–3 lifetime doses**
Varicella (live vaccine)	√		**2 lifetime doses at least 4 wks apart ᶜSee below**
Measles, mumps, rubella	√		**1 or 2 lifetime doses at least 4 wks apart**
Influenza	√		**1 dose annually**
Pneumococcal			**PCV13: 1 lifetime dose; PPSV23: 1–2 lifetime doses**
Hepatitis A	√		**Havrix or Vaqta: 2 doses; Twinrix (18+ y old): 3–4 doses**
Hepatitis B	√		**Recombivax HB (11–15 y old): 2 doses; Heplisav-B/Twinrix (18+ y old): 2–3 lifetime doses.**
Hepatitis C screening		+	**Anti-HCV antibody testing, polymerase chain reaction testing**
Meningococcal quadrivalent	√		**2 lifetime doses**
Serogroup B meningococcal		+	**MenB vaccine (2 or 3 dose series) to those 16–23 y old**

BMI, body mass index; SBIRT, Screening, Brief Intervention and Refer to Treatment; ACOG, American College of Obstetrics and Gynecology; USPSTF, United States Preventive Services Task Force; NHLBI, National Heart, Lung, Blood Institute; MDD, Major Depressive Disorder; VDRL, venereal disease research laboratory; NAAT, nucleic acid amplification test; HIV, Human Immunodeficiency Virus; STI, sexually transmitted infection.

Bold = US Preventive Services Task Force (USPSTF) A or B Recommendation or CDC recommendations for immunizations. *Current evidence is insufficient to assess the balance of benefits and harms of service.* √ = All adolescents + = Adolescents at risk. For more information, please view the appendix, and visit the official website.
ᵃunderline{Bright Futures}: recommendations are for annual visits, up to age 21.
ᵇunderline{American College of Obstetricians and Gynecologists} (ACOG) recommendations, up to age 26.
ᶜThe varicella vaccine should NOT be given to patients with these contraindications.
From National Adolescent and Young Adult Health Information Center. Summary of clinical preventive services guidelines for adolescents up to age 18. National Adolescent and Young Adult Health Information Center, University of California, San Francisco; 2020. http://nahic.ucsf.edu/resource_center/adolescent-guidelines/. Accessed June 20, 2022.

18 to 26 are "carved out" of guidelines from medical professional groups, there are recommendations that can inform care of young adults. Likewise, while the USPSTF issues recommendations for the pediatric population, including several specific to adolescents, no USPSTF recommendations are specific to young adults, though many include young adults within a broader age range.[12]

Table 5.2 provides a summary of clinical preventive services guidelines from medical professional groups that can inform the care of young adults aged 18 to 25 years in addition to the USPSTF recommendations.[13]

As shown in Table 5.2, many of the recommendations included in the Bright Futures guidelines for adolescents are supported by sufficient evidence to be recommended by the USPSTF for young adults over 18 years old, such as screening and counseling for tobacco and alcohol use, depression, body mass index (BMI), diet, and physical activity. However, there are areas in which Bright Futures recommends screening or counseling, but the USPSTF does not. These include:
• Screening and counseling for unhealthy drug use
• Screening for suicide

• Counseling for specific risks under the category of safety/violence

Although the recommendations of Bright Futures target AYAs aged 11 to 21 years, the evidence for screening is stronger in several areas for adults (≥18 years), including alcohol use, healthy diet, and physical activity. Thus, for late AYAs, there is greater consistency between the USPSTF guidelines and the Bright Futures guidelines. Table 5.3 displays a one-page clinician tool to facilitate the delivery of preventive care to AYAs. This summary highlights the USPSTF evidence-based recommendations for AYA care.

Preventive Services and Insurance Coverage in the United States

In the United States, the enactment of the Patient Protection and Affordable Care Act (ACA) of 2010 created the potential to improve AYA health by increasing health insurance coverage and by requiring that preventive health care be provided to AYAs. The ACA allows young adults to remain on their parent's health insurance plan until age 26, and these provisions helped expand coverage for adolescents and, especially, young adults. From 2010 to 2018, the

TABLE 5.2

Summary of Clinical Preventive Services Guidelines for Young Adults Ages 18–25

Preventive Services	All (√)	At Risk (+)	Screening Test/Procedure and Other Notes
Nutrition/Exercise/Obesity			
Hypertension/blood pressure	√		**Screen every 3–5 y with BP <130/85 mm Hg with no other risks**
Dyslipidemia screening	√		√ Bright Futures once between 18 and 21 y old; *USPSTF insufficient evidence*
Obesity/BMI	√		**(Weight [lb]/Height [in]) × 703**
Healthy diet and physical activity		+	**Intensive behavioral counseling**
Substance use			
Alcohol (screening and counseling)	√		**NIAA screening; AUDIT; √ Bright Futures**
Tobacco (screening and counseling) for nonpregnant adults	√		**5-A framework (Ask, Advise, Assess, Assist, Arrange); should undergo behavioral interventions**
Tobacco (screening and counseling) for pregnant females	√		**5-A framework (Ask, Advise, Assess, Assist, Arrange); should undergo behavioral interventions**
Unhealthy drug use (screening and counseling)	√		√ Bright Futures[a] and ACOG[b], *USPSTF insufficient evidence*
Mental health/depression			
Depression (screening and treatment)	√		**Screening instruments: PHQ, EPDS**
Suicide screening	√		√ Bright Futures and ACOG, *USPSTF insufficient evidence*
Safety/violence			
Family/partner violence	√		**HITS; OAS/OVAT; STaT; HARK; CTQ-SF; and WAST**
Fighting	√		√ Bright Futures and ACOG
Helmets	√		√ Bright Futures and ACOG
Seat belts	√		√ Bright Futures and ACOG
Guns	√		√ Bright Futures and ACOG
Bullying	√		Bright Futures only
Reproductive health			
HIV	√		**HIV screening**
STI (screening and counseling)		+	**High-intensity counseling interventions**
Syphilis		+	**RPR or VDRL followed by TPPA or FTA-ABS if first test result is positive**
Gonorrhea (females)		+	**NAATs; test if ≤24 and sexually active or if ≥25 and at increased risk**
Chlamydia (females)		+	**NAATs; test if ≤24 and sexually active or if ≥25 and at increased risk**
Chlamydia and gonorrhea (male)		+	√ Bright Futures, *USPSTF insufficient evidence*
Birth control methods	√	+	√ ACOG, + Bright Futures
Pregnancy (counseling)		+	+ Bright Futures
Folic acid		+	**Females planning/capable of pregnancy should take folic acid daily**

(*continued*)

TABLE 5.2

Summary of Clinical Preventive Services Guidelines for Young Adults Ages 18–25 (*Continued*)

Preventive Services	All (√)	At Risk (+)	Screening Test/Procedure and Other Notes
Cancer screening			
Cervical cancer		+	**Females aged ≥21: Cytology (pap smear) every 3 y**
Skin cancer (counseling)		+	**Counsel those aged 10–24 y with fair skin on reducing UV exposure**
Testicular cancer (self-clinician exam)	√		√ Bright Futures for all males 18–21, USPSTF recommends against
BRCA-related cancer		+	**Family history of breast, ovarian, tubal, or peritoneal cancer**
Infectious diseases including CDC immunization recommendations			
Td/Tdap	√		**1 dose Tdap, then Td booster every 10 y**
Human papillomavirus	√		**HPV vaccine for male and females up to age 26; 2–3 lifetime doses**
Varicella (live vaccine)	√		**2 lifetime doses at least 4 wks apart ᶜSee below**
Measles, mumps, rubella	√		**1 or 2 lifetime doses at least 4 wks apart**
Influenza	√		**1 dose annually**
Pneumococcal		+	**PCV13: 1 lifetime dose; PPSV23: 1–2 lifetime doses**
Hepatitis A	√		**Havrix or Vaqta: 2 doses; Twinrix (18+ y old): 3–4 doses**
Hepatitis B	√		**Recombivax HB (11–15 y old): 2 doses; Heplisav-B/Twinrix (18+ y old): 2–3 lifetime doses.**
Hepatitis C screening	√		**Anti-HCV antibody testing, polymerase chain reaction testing**
Meningococcal quadrivalent	√		**2 lifetime doses**
Serogroup B meningococcal		+	**MenB vaccine (2 or 3 dose series) to those 16–23 y old**

BMI, body mass index; ACOG, American College of Obstetrics and Gynecology; USPSTF, United States Preventive Services Task Force; VDRL, venereal disease research laboratory; NAAT, nucleic acid amplification test; HIV, Human Immunodeficiency Virus; STI, sexually transmitted infection.

Bold = US Preventive Services Task Force (USPSTF) A or B Recommendation or CDC recommendations for immunizations. *Current evidence is insufficient to assess the balance of benefits and harms of service.*√ = All adolescents + = Adolescents at risk. For more information, please view the appendix, and visit the official website.

ᵃBright Futures: recommendations are for annual visits, up to age 21.

ᵇAmerican College of Obstetricians and Gynecologists (ACOG) recommendations, up to age 26.

ᶜThe varicella vaccine should NOT be given to patients with these contraindications.

From National Adolescent and Young Adult Health Information Center. Summary of Clinical Preventive Services Guidelines for Adolescents up to Age 18. National Adolescent and Young Adult Health Information Center, University of California, San Francisco; 2020. http://nahic.ucsf.edu/resource_center/adolescent-guidelines/. Accessed June 20, 2022.

percentage of adolescents with insurance rose from 87% to 92%, and the percentage of young adults with insurance rose from 62% to 81%.[10]

The ACA includes specific provisions to improve the content of care and increase access to and use of preventive services. Most private health plans in the United States must cover annual well visits until age 21, and are required to cover a specified set of preventive services without cost sharing (copayments, deductibles, or coinsurance). As part of its preventive services mandate, the ACA requires that clinicians use professional guidelines, including (1) evidence-based services recommended by the USPSTF, (2) ACIP recommended immunizations, (3) services outlined in Bright Futures, and (4) Women's Preventive Health Services Guidelines issued by the U.S. federal government, which include many services relevant to AYAs. As a result of these provisions, data indicate a modest to moderate increase, with greatest gains for underserved youth, in receipt of preventive services for adolescents[14] and young adults[15] after ACA implementation.

In addition to the ACA, other factors influence the delivery of preventive health services for AYAs in the United States. For example, insurance companies often monitor and audit clinician performance on key aspects of preventive health care, including immunization rates and receipt of a periodic health examination. In some cases, receipt of individual preventive health services is also monitored. The Healthcare Effectiveness Data and Information Set (HEDIS), National Committee for Quality Assurance (NCQA) is a tool used by U.S. health plans to monitor clinician performance. Across all age groups, HEDIS includes 70 measures across five areas: effectiveness of care; access/availability of care; utilization; risk-adjusted utilization; and measures recorded using electronic clinical management systems. There are currently 10 HEDIS measures specific to the adolescent age group with an additional 20 measures that overlap with AYAs. Because many plans collect HEDIS data, and the measures are specifically defined, HEDIS makes it possible to compare the performance of health plans and clinicians.

Important safety net services also cover preventive services for AYAs who otherwise might not have access. The Department of Health and Human Services' Title X provides funds for comprehensive family planning services and other preventive health care. The Early and Periodic Screening, Diagnosis, and Treatment Program (EPSDT) is funded by Title V and administered by HRSA and the Maternal and Child Health Bureau. The Early and

TABLE 5.3

TABLE 5.3
Evidence-based Clinical Preventive Services for Adolescents and Young Adults

Adolescents 10–17 y	Young Adults 18–25 y
Substance use	
√ Education and counseling to prevent initiation of tobacco use	√ Alcohol screening and counseling √ Tobacco screening and cessation help √ Unhealthy drug use screening (when there are adequate systems in place to ensure accurate diagnosis, effective treatment, and follow-up)
Reproductive health	
√ Screening for HIV (everyone aged 15–17; <15 at increased risk) √ Screening for syphilis (anyone at increased risk) √ Screening for chlamydia and gonorrhea (sexually active females) √ STI behavioral counseling for all sexually active adolescents √ Folic acid supplementation for females who are planning or capable of becoming pregnant	√ Screening for HIV (everyone aged 18–65) √ Screening for syphilis (anyone at increased risk) √ Screening for chlamydia and gonorrhea (sexually active females 18–24; anyone at increased risk) √ Behavioral counseling for all who are at increased risk for STIs √ Folic acid supplementation for females who are planning or capable of becoming pregnant
Mental health	
√ Screening for depression (when there are adequate systems in place to ensure accurate diagnosis, effective treatment, and follow-up)	√ Screening for depression (when there are adequate systems in place to ensure accurate diagnosis, effective treatment, and follow-up)
Nutrition and exercise	
√ Obesity/BMI screening and referral	√ Obesity/BMI screening and referral √ Hypertension (≥18) √ Healthy diet and physical activity counseling for adults with cardiovascular disease risk factors
Cancer screening	
√ Skin cancer counseling for those with fair skin √ BRCA cancer screening for females with family history	√ Cervical cancer screening (≥21) √ Skin cancer counseling for those with fair skin (up to 24) √ BRCA cancer screening for females with family history
Safety and violence	
√ Intimate partner violence—screen females of reproductive age, refer those at risk to services	√ Intimate partner violence— screen females of reproductive age, refer those at risk to services
Immunizations	**Immunizations and infectious diseases**
CDC recommended immunizations	√ Screening for Hepatitis C (≥18) CDC recommended immunizations

BMI, body mass index; HIV, human immunodeficiency virus; STI, sexually transmitted infection.
√ Indicates A or B graded recommendations from the U.S. Preventive Services Task Force.

Periodic Screening, Diagnosis, and Treatment Program provides preventive (and other) services to children who are enrolled in Medicaid or who are uninsured. Some states have added additional programming to address the preventive services and family planning needs of uninsured AYAs, especially those seeking confidential care.

These services, while beneficial for increasing access for previously uninsured, are also helpful for maintaining confidentiality in certain circumstances. For example, many private U.S. insurance companies send an Explanation of Benefits (EOB), an itemization of services offered, to the primary insurance holder. Because U.S. AYAs are often insured through their parents' or caregivers' insurance, the EOB represents a means by which sensitive or confidential information can be inadvertently shared with parents or caregivers. Thus, health care systems should familiarize themselves with the resources in their community to provide sensitive confidential services.

Barriers to Providing Preventive Services

Health insurance coverage and clinical guidelines are important, but widespread implementation of preventive services for AYAs requires attention to many other factors. Current rates of screening and counseling for AYAs are lower than recommended, and there is inconsistency in screening across various risk areas. Research, utilizing both clinician and young adult report, shows that young adults receive preventive services at even lower rates than adolescents.[1,9,15–17] Barriers to delivering preventive services within busy clinical practices have been well documented, including clinician factors (attitudes, lack of training, skills, and/or confidence to deliver services) and external factors (time constraints, lack of appropriate screening tools, and lack of reimbursement for services).[1,12] Access to preventive health care may also be limited by other issues such as concerns over confidentiality and transportation.[17]

TABLE 5.4

Health Care Utilization, ages 10–25, by Age Group and Sex

Health Care	Adolescents (Ages 10–17)			Young Adults (Ages 18–25)		
	All	Females	Males	All	Females	Males
Any health care visit past year, 2018 [1]	89%	89%	89%	75%	84%	66%
Attended a preventive care visit within the past 12 mo, 2017 [2]	51%	51%	50%	33%	42%	25%

Sources: National Health Interview Survey. (2019). 2018 data release [Data set]. Centers for Disease Control and Prevention. https://www.cdc.gov/nchs/nhis/nhis_2018_data_release.htm. Accessed June 27, 2022; Agency for Healthcare Research and Quality. (2020). Medical expenditure panel survey 2017. U.S. Department of Health and Human Services. https://www.meps.ahrq.gov/mepsweb/. Accessed June 27, 2022.

Improving Preventive Services Delivery

Among the promising approaches to improving preventive service delivery for AYAs are offering alternate (and more convenient) locations for preventive services, policy changes that facilitate confidential care, using emerging technology for creating efficiencies for clinicians, AYA screening and promoting behavior change, and telehealth.[1,12]

Clinical Settings

Medical Clinic: To better serve AYAs, preventive services need to be available in a *wide range of health care settings* beyond clinicians' offices. As previously noted, AYAs have fewer well visits and receive fewer preventive services than recommended. This is particularly true for young adult males, who utilize fewer well-care preventive visits, receiving most of their care through acute care visits (Table 5.4). For this reason, acute care visits are an underutilized opportunity for the provision of preventive health screening and intervention.[10,16,18,19]

Community-Clinic Linkages: Linking health care systems with schools and community settings through school-based health centers, retail clinics, and community family planning clinics and other coordinated networks, is a promising strategy for increasing youth receipt of clinical preventive services. Studies show that school-based clinics increase delivery of preventive services with some model programs demonstrating effective increases across several health domains, including substance use, mental health, and reproductive health.[20] Retail clinics (stores or pharmacies) are a growing source of care for AYAs. Community-based family planning and public health clinics serve as an important safety net; and juvenile justice and child/family service agencies have successfully engaged underserved or hard-to-reach at-risk AYA populations.[1]

Telemedicine: Telemedicine provides a useful avenue to extend the reach of preventive care. With the rapid expansion of telemedicine services that occurred in 2020 and 2021 in response to the SARS-CoV-2 pandemic, clinics are well suited to integrate telemedicine services to reach patients who would be less likely to present for in-person services. Clinical concerns where physical examination is less critical are particularly amenable to telemedicine. These may include visits for substance use, medication management, eating disorder care, or mental health.[21]

Training and Screening Tools

Clinicians often cite inadequate training or insufficient confidence as a barrier to the provision of health services for AYAs. Clinician training and clinical decision-making supports, such as screening and charting tools, have been shown to reduce barriers and increase the delivery of preventive services to adolescents. These "training and tools" interventions have been evaluated across studies, usually in the context of a generalized approach (attempting to address multiple health behavior areas) but also in interventions targeting specific risk areas (e.g., substance use, tobacco use, and sexual health).[1] Examples include psychosocial screening assessments, and prompts and cues for clinicians. These tools have been integrated into patient charts, screening and charting forms, and office systems. A growing body of research is focused on the integration of technology to facilitate preventive service delivery using mobile devices, computerized behavioral screening, internet-based approaches, and tablet-based screening modules.[22]

DIGITAL HEALTH

Digital health refers to the use of information and communication technologies to help address health challenges and improve health. Connecting digital health technologies to clinical care is crucial for increasing the impact of these technologies on AYA clinical preventive services.[23]

The Electronic Health Record and Preventive Services

Because of their widespread adoption and potential to improve care quality, efficiency, and safety,[1] EHRs are increasingly important tools to facilitate and track preventive service delivery for individual patients and for entire patient populations. In the United States, the federal Meaningful Use Program delegated funds for institutions meeting core EHR technology requirements, thus most EHRs in the United States include a suite of features that can aid in the provision of preventive services for AYAs.

Challenges Related to Confidential Care

The provision of confidential care for adolescents seeking treatment for reproductive and mental health services is a well-established best practice. However, most EHRs are not designed to provide granular control of access to and release of information that facilitates the provision of confidential care for adolescents.[24] Institutions are left with a dilemma—make do with existing tools, or invest institutional resources in modifications of existing technology. To minimize the risk of unintended release of information, some institutions turn off key functionality of the EHR for adolescent patients such as the patient portal, social histories, after-visit summaries, and problem lists. Unfortunately, this strategy excludes adolescents from many of the benefits of the EHR and also compromises institutional participation in federal programs.

The role of optimizing the EHR to ensure confidentiality is contemporarily pertinent with the implementation of the 21st Century CURES ACT, a U.S. federal law which was passed in 2016. One of the main components of the law, a requirement that notes and labs be immediately viewable by patients and parents or caregivers, stands to challenge maintenance of confidentiality. Written into the law are a few exceptions including "Preventing Harm" and "Privacy," however, there are specific and narrow requirements that must be met to utilize these exceptions and block notes from being viewed by patients and parents. Thus, U.S. clinics providing confidential services to AYAs should be aware of the details of the law to ensure that confidentiality is maintained within the confines of the federal mandate.

Key Electronic Health Record Features for Adolescent and Young Adult Preventive Services

Summarized below are the various features of the EHR as they relate to AYAs, paying particular attention to confidential care challenges and opportunities where the EHR can be leveraged to improve care.

Previsit Questionnaires Automated screening offers several advantages to AYAs who may find it easier to disclose sensitive information electronically than to a clinician. Automated screening also saves time, and the information can be directly placed into the EHR. Automated screeners may be available separately from existing EHRs. Figures 5.1 and 5.2 show screen shots of the "Health e-Check" screening module that automates preventive health screening and allows for integration of adolescent responses into the EHR.[25] Previsit questionnaires can also be developed within an EHR either using provided tools or custom formats. Many EHRs have built-in validated screening tools (i.e., GAD-7, PHQ-9) that can be sent to patients through EHR messaging systems prior to a visit to allow the clinician to review those results in preparation for the clinical encounter. These previsit screeners/questionnaires can be completed just prior to the visit, or at home online before the visit.

Health Maintenance Most EHR systems offer both clinician and patient reminders when key health maintenance elements are due.

For example, annual flu vaccine alerts can be set to remind clinicians to order the vaccine. Institutions use these alerts for vaccine reminders, but they can also be used for other AYA preventive services, such as Papanicolaou (Pap) and chlamydia screening. This is especially helpful when the guidelines are complex and differ by age, gender, or prior health conditions. Electronic health records also offer the ability to create standard order sets for periodic health examinations to streamline and standardize the ordering of tests.

Population Health Management On a macrosystems level, EHRs may be used to determine rates of provision of preventive services on current patients in an individual practice. This type of population health management not only boosts receipt of preventive services, but also facilitates external reporting of health care effectiveness measures and internal quality control efforts.

Clinician Documentation Structured clinician templates for preventive services visits can increase clinician efficiency by listing the key components of the encounter assuring that required elements for billing and compliance are documented. Documentation in an EHR may be more efficient, because information can automatically populate using data from other areas of the health record. However, these same features can pose challenges for the protection of confidential health information. Special consideration is required so that information sharing does not undermine

Step 1: Adolescent completes survey on tablet.

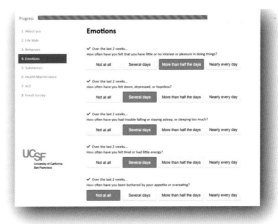

Step 2: Clinical report available to clinician within the EHR

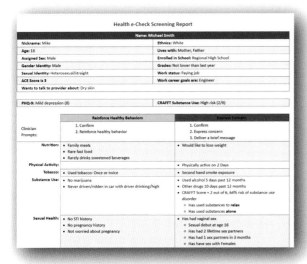

Step 3: Survey data imported to EHR Clinician may add or edit notes

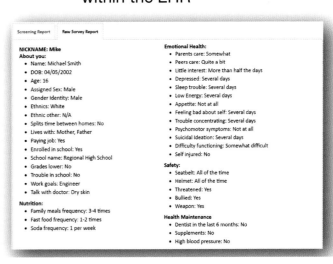

FIGURE 5.1 Health e-check EHR integration. (Source: Jasik CB, Berna M, Martin M, Ozer EM. Teen preferences for clinic-based behavior screens: who, where, when, and how? *J Adolesc Health.* 2016;59(6):722–724.)

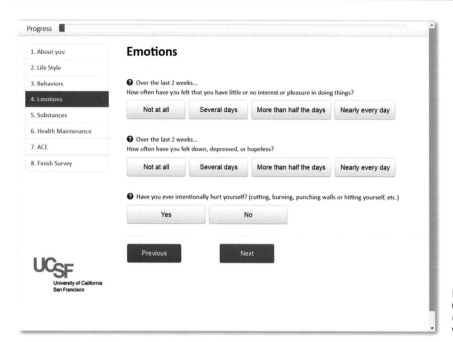

FIGURE 5.2 Health e-check: Emotional health items. (Jasik CB, Berna M, Martin M, Ozer EM. Teen preferences for clinic-based behavior screens: who, where, when, and how? *J Adolesc Health.* 2016;59(6):722–724.)

the patient's desire for confidentiality. For example, a prescription for birth control pills may appear on a shared medication list that will automatically appear in the notes of other clinicians. Further, information added to the sexual orientation/gender identity (SOGI) tab will be visible to all other clinicians who see that patient. To prevent unintended breaches in confidential care from a primary care visit, clinicians must be adept at using the tools to protect confidentiality built into the EHR.

Patient Portal The patient portal allows patients and/or parents to access personal health information online and to communicate with clinicians. Adolescents and young adults are uniquely suited to benefit from the patient portal given their ease with navigating digital technology. Despite their widespread adoption, institutions have historically excluded adolescents or only permitted access to parents due to lack of flexibility to allow differential access to adolescents and parents. However, the provision of telemedicine visits to AYAs during the SARS-CoV-2 pandemic required many institutions to rapidly enroll adolescents in patient portals in order to facilitate scheduling and clinical care.[21]

Extending the Preventive Reach of the Clinician Through Technology

Digital health technologies offer unique opportunities to improve engagement between health care systems and AYAs. High rates of acceptance and use of digital technology by AYAs, particularly on their mobile devices, facilitate the broad reach of digital platforms for preventive health at relatively low cost. Digital health technology also appears promising for reaching diverse AYA populations. Among digital health technology domains are social media, mobile Health (mHealth), wearable and digital devices, and games for health.[23] Considerable research and development activity has been leveraged because of the potential to improve AYA health, though additional research is needed to measure the impact. Challenges of new health technologies include issues in equitable access for AYAs, potential for bias, privacy and security concerns, and integration into clinical care.[22,23]

⬤ THE PREVENTIVE SERVICES VISIT

Caring for AYAs requires a different approach, format, and style than caring for children or adults; thus, it is not surprising that

many clinicians report barriers to, or lack of confidence in, caring for AYAs. The AYA preventive visit may potentially involve greater planning, sensitivity, expertise, and time than a visit with a younger child or adult. Most of the visit is spent taking a history or screening for health risks, so a comfortable space is needed in which to conduct the interview. A plan for including the parent or guardian in the visit is also needed.

Setting the Stage for Preventive Care

To provide effective preventive services, the office visit must be organized and structured in an appropriate way for AYAs. This includes the physical space, services available, staff training, and clinician training. The confidential psychosocial interview will be most successful if the environment is welcoming and the patient feels comfortable from the moment they enter the clinical space. This is particularly critical for the provision of care for transgender or nonbinary youth, and systems should be in place to ensure that patients are referred to by the correct name and pronouns.[26] Table 5.5 summarizes the key components for creating a friendly atmosphere for AYAs.[27]

Questionnaires and Screening Tools

To improve the efficiency of preventive care visits, screening questionnaires may be completed by the patient and/or parent prior to the visit. The standard previsit questionnaire for an AYA preventive services visit may assess health behaviors related to nutrition, physical activity, home life, education, substance use, mental health, sexual health, and exposure to violence. Bright Futures provides a previsit screening questionnaire for both adolescents and parents for use in primary care.[8] Clinicians may also want to conduct screening in a particular risk area, either among all patients or specifically for those who identify potential risk on general screens. Many clinics, programs, and practices elect to draw from these established questionnaires or create their own based on their knowledge of youth in their individual practices.

Two examples of domains in which specific screening tools can be helpful include mental health and substance use screening.

Depression screening: Depression is one area in which there are several options for standardized screening. The Patient Health Questionnaire (PHQ)-2, a short two-question tool validated for

CHAPTER 5 • Preventive Health Care for Adolescents and Young Adults

TABLE 5.5

Questions to Consider When Creating a Youth Friendly Environment

(?) Does your office/health center have...
- ☐ An atmosphere that is appealing to AYAs (pictures, posters, wallpaper)?
- ☐ Magazines that would interest AYAs and reflect their cultures and literacy levels?
- ☐ Appropriate-sized tables and chairs in your waiting and examination rooms (i.e., not for small children)?
- ☐ Private areas to complete forms and discuss reasons for visits?
- ☐ Facilities that comply with the Americans with Disabilities Act?
- ☐ Decorations that reflect the genders, sexual orientations, cultures, and ethnicities of your clients?

(?) Do you provide...
- ☐ Health education materials written for or by AYAs at the appropriate literacy level and in their first languages?
- ☐ Translation services appropriate for your patient population?
- ☐ A clearly posted office policy about confidentiality?
- ☐ After-school hours?
- ☐ Opportunities for parents and AYAs to speak separately with a clinician?
- ☐ Alternatives to written communications (i.e., phone calls, meetings, videos, audiotapes)?
- ☐ Health education materials in various locations, such as the waiting room, examination room, and bathroom, where teens would feel comfortable reading and taking them?
- ☐ Condoms?

(?) Does your staff...
- ☐ Greet AYAs in a courteous and friendly manner?
- ☐ Explain procedures and directions in an easy and understandable manner?
- ☐ Enjoy working with adolescents and their families?
- ☐ Have up-to-date knowledge about consent and confidentiality laws?
- ☐ Incorporate principles and practices that promote cultural and linguistic competence?
- ☐ Consider privacy concerns when adolescents check-in?
- ☐ Provide resource and referral information when there is a delay in scheduling a teen's appointment?

(?) When you speak to adolescents do you...
- ☐ Use nonjudgmental, jargon free, and gender-neutral language?
- ☐ Allow time to address their concerns and questions?
- ☐ Restate your name and explain your role and what you are doing?
- ☐ Ask gentle but direct questions?
- ☐ Offer options for another setting or clinician?
- ☐ Explain the purpose and costs for tests, procedures, and referrals?
- ☐ Keep in mind that their communication skills may not reflect their cognitive or problem-solving abilities?
- ☐ Ask for clarification and explanations?
- ☐ Listen?
- ☐ Congratulate them when they are making healthy choices and decisions?

(?) Are you aware...
- ☐ That your values may conflict with or be inconsistent with those of other cultural or religious groups?
- ☐ That age and gender soles may vary among different cultures?
- ☐ Of health care beliefs and acceptable behaviors, customs, and expectations of different geographic, religions, and ethnic groups?
- ☐ Of the socioeconomic and environmental risk factors that contribute to the major health problems among the diverse groups you serve?

AYA, adolescent and young adult.

screening of depressive symptoms in AYAs, can be used for initial screening for all patients seen in primary care (see Fig. 5.2). Should a PHQ-2 raise concern, a PHQ-9 can be utilized to further define the depressive symptoms in order to determine the need

for treatment (psychotherapy and medication). Further, a suicide screening tool such as the Columbia Suicide-Severity Rating Scale can be used to stratify suicide risk and determine the need for immediate intervention. In addition, a Generalized Anxiety Disorder scale (GAD)-7 can be used to systematically assess anxious symptoms and help to determine indications for psychotherapy and pharmacotherapy.

Substance use screening: The U.S. Substance Abuse and Mental Health Services Administration (SAMHSA) recommends universal substance use screening with a validated tool for all adolescent patients. The most common tools used in primary care with AYA patients are the Helping Patients Who Drink Too Much: A Clinician's Guide produced by the National Insitute on Alcohol Abuse and Alcoholism (NIAA), Screening to Brief Intervention (S2BI), Brief Screener for Alcohol, Tobacco, and other Drugs (BSTAD), Drug Abuse Screen Test (DAST) and CRAFFT 2.0. These tools were developed specifically for use in primary care settings to assess adolescent substance use, and create an objective, time-efficient measure to determine the need for further intervention. In addition, Screening, Brief Intervention, and Referral to Treatment (SBIRT), a primary care tool used to screen and intervene for substance use concerns, has been integrated into AAP recommendations. For more detail on this specific intervention and for its implementation, see the Chapter 73 on substance use and the SBIRT page on the AAP.[28]

Additional screening tools and toolkits can be found in ancillary resources at Bright Futures and at the National Adolescent and Young Adult Health Information Center (NAHIC) website.

History

As with any patient preventive visit history, essential domains include current health concerns, past medical history, family history, psychosocial history, and an age-appropriate review of systems. When preventive services are delivered during a visit made for another reason or health concern (e.g., sports physical, acute medical problem), it is important to make sure that the patient's concerns are fully addressed.

Past Medical History

Past medical history is best obtained from both the AYAs, and the parents when appropriate, and should include the following:
1. Childhood infections and illnesses
2. Prior hospitalizations and surgery
3. Significant injuries
4. Disabilities
5. Medications, including prescription medications, over-the-counter medications, complementary or alternative medications, vitamins, and nutritional supplements
6. Allergies
7. Immunization history
8. Developmental history, including prenatal, perinatal, and infancy history; peer relations; and school functioning
9. Mental health history, including a review of prior diagnoses, history of hospitalization or suicide attempt, outpatient counseling, medications, school interventions, or other current or historical mental health supports accessed

Family History

Often, for younger adolescents, information about family history is most accurately obtained from the parents. The family history should include the following:
1. Age and health status of family members
2. History of significant medical illnesses in the family, such as diabetes, cancer, heart disease, tuberculosis (TB), hypertension, or stroke
3. History of mental illness in the family, such as mood disorders, anxiety disorders, schizophrenia, or substance use

Developmental Assessment

A comprehensive developmental assessment is a core part of the evaluation of the AYAs and is necessary to help clinicians tailor preventive health screening and counseling.[8] Chapter 2 has a detailed review of adolescent growth and development. While age-based guidelines are useful, chronologic age does not always match developmental age. For example, a 15-year-old female patient who has the developmental progress of an early adolescent will require a different approach to preventive health counseling than a same-age peer in middle or late adolescence.

Psychosocial History

Given that the majority of morbidity and mortality among AYAs is related to behavioral risk factors, the core component of the preventive visit for these populations is the psychosocial/behavioral history. Typically, this history is completed in person, but it can be facilitated by structured questionnaires and electronic screening as mentioned above. Collateral information from parents/caregivers is helpful and should be obtained whenever possible. However, the majority of the psychosocial history should be completed with the AYA patient alone. One strategy to meet both of these goals is to complete the nonconfidential component with the parent/caregiver present. Once the nonconfidential portion is completed, the parent/caregiver should be excused from the room to complete the confidential portion with the patient alone.

The key to a successful psychosocial interview is building rapport with the patient and providing a comfortable and safe space (see Table 5.5). Adolescents are more likely to seek care for family planning, mental health, and substance use counseling if they know the care is confidential. Reassuring the adolescent that certain aspects of the interview can be kept confidential, as well as reviewing the circumstances under which information cannot be kept confidential, is helpful for establishing rapport and maintaining a therapeutic relationship. Clinicians within a practice should know the current local laws regarding confidential care and have a consistent approach to history taking, documentation, and billing to ensure that confidentiality is maintained. As significant morbidity and mortality in this age group can be attributed to issues related to mental health, substance use, and sexual and reproductive health, these domains should be universally and systematically addressed in all preventive health encounters with AYA patients. To accurately assess and counsel patients on sexual and reproductive health, each patient's gender identity, sexual orientation, and sexual behavior should be explored independently with gender-neutral language to prevent making cis-gender and heteronormative assumptions.

Chapter 3 summarizes the more commonly used structures for the psychosocial interview (the HEEADSSS and SHADES assessment). The key components of a complete psychosocial history that they share are summarized in Table 5.6.

Special Considerations for Patients Assigned-Female-at-Birth

For all patients who were assigned-female-at-birth (including transgender male and nonbinary patients), reproductive justice mandates that clinicians assess patients' individual desires around pregnancy without assuming that patients desire contraception. If contraception is desired, services should be comprehensive and noncoercive. When specific services such as long-acting reversible contraception (LARC) or pregnancy termination are unavailable at a particular clinic, clinicians should be aware of the resources in the community to ensure patients have access to those essential services should they desire.

Special Considerations for Male-Identifying Patients

As noted in Table 5.4, male-identifying AYA patients access preventive medical care at a much lower rate than their female-identifying

TABLE 5.6

The Adolescent/Young Adult Psychosocial History: A Summary

Home	Who lives at home? Does the teen split time between households?
Education/ employment	What grade are you in? Do you work? What are your plans for your future?
Eating	What did you eat yesterday? What did you drink yesterday? Is this typical? Do you skip meals? *Asses for disordered eating.* Are you happy with your current weight, trying to lose weight or trying to gain weight?
Activity	Do you have close friends? What do you do after school? Do you play sports?
Drugs	Have you ever smoked, drank alcohol, or done drugs? *Ask specifically about marijuana.* Do your friends use drugs? Do you ever drive, or ride with someone who has been drinking or using drugs? Do any of your family members use drugs or drink alcohol to excess?
Sexuality and gender	How do you see yourself, a guy, girl, neither, not sure, still figuring it out? Are you interested in guys, girls, nonbinary people, no one? Is there a term you feel comfortable with that describes your sexual orientation (gay, lesbian, straight, bi, pansexual, asexual, none of these? Have you ever had sex? *If yes,* what is the gender of your partners? What kind of sex are you having (oral, anal, vaginal)? How many partners have you had in your life? In the past 3 mo? What percentage of the time do you use condoms? *For birth-assigned females,* are you interested in having a baby now? If no, what do you use to prevent pregnancy? For *birth-assigned males,* have you ever gotten someone pregnant? Are you interested in having a baby now? If no, what are you using to prevent pregnancy? To all adolescents and young adults, have you ever had a sexually transmitted infection?
Suicide (mental health)	Do you ever feel sad, down, or hopeless? Do you feel lonely or bored? Have you ever felt so sad or down that you didn't think life was worth living? Have you ever cut yourself? Do you feel anxious?
Safety	Do you wear a helmet when riding a bike or a skateboard? Do you wear a seat belt when riding in a car? Do you have guns in your home? Do you carry a gun? Do you feel safe in your home, school, and community? Have you ever not felt safe? Do you have a history of sexual or physical abuse?

peers, particularly during the transition to adulthood. While the reasons for this are multifactorial, a contributing factor has been adherence to what has been described as conventional "masculine values", with lower health care utilization among young men with stronger masculine values.[19] Beliefs that young men should be independent, stoic, strong, and self-reliant may influence male-identifying patients and create a reticence to seek health care and/or share sexual or mental health concerns with clinicians. To optimize the likelihood of young men receiving appropriate care, a confidential, comprehensive, strengths-based psychosocial history is critical at any interaction with the medical system, not just preventive health care visits.

A report from a working group titled the "Male Training Center for Family Planning and Reproductive Health" established comprehensive preventive male sexual and reproductive health care guidelines to help meet the needs of young male-identifying patients.[29] One of the core recommendations includes a comprehensive assessment of sexual and reproductive health. Clinicians should assess all young men's desire for parenthood. If parenthood is not desired, clinicians should counsel patients on pregnancy prevention such as appropriate condom usage (with demonstration if necessary) and emergency contraception. In addition, the clinician should assess for healthy relationships and intimate partner violence.

Screening for substance use in the young male population should include not only alcohol, nicotine, cannabis, and illicit drug use, but also supplements and steroid use. Given that a large portion of the morbidity and mortality in young men is related to unintentional injuries and violence, an assessment of access to weapons, weapon ownership, exposure to violence, and safety practices to prevent unintentional injuries (driving under the influence, riding a bicycle without a helmet, etc.) is critical.

Special Considerations for Transgender, Gender Diverse, and Sexual Minority Youth

The needs of sexual and gender diverse youth overlap the needs of their cis-gender and heterosexual peers in many ways. However, clinicians should be aware of health disparities and unique medical needs in these communities. Research has shown that the youth in the Lesbian, Gay, Bisexual, Transgender, and Questioning (LGBTQ) communities have increased rates of mood and anxiety disorders, eating disorders, substance use, and suicide. Further, many of these AYAs experience bullying, family rejection, and interpersonal and structural stigma. Because of this, patients in the LGBTQ community may be reluctant to seek care, and hesitant to share their sexual orientation and gender identity when they do so. To ensure that patients feel comfortable seeking care, clinics should have visible materials demonstrating that they are an inclusive and welcoming space, and create practices to ensure that patients are greeted with their appropriate name, gender, and pronouns.

Clinicians should educate their clinic staff on sensitive and affirming approaches to providing care to the LGBTQ community, and also know the mental health, substance use, and gender-affirming resources in their community. If a clinician does not feel comfortable providing care to sexual minority or gender diverse youth, they should promptly refer to another clinician in their community with experience caring for LGBTQ youth.[26]

Review of Systems

The review of systems covers the following areas:
1. Vision: Trouble reading or watching television; vision correction
2. Hearing: Infections, trouble hearing, earaches
3. Dental: Prior care, pain, concerns (e.g., braces)
4. Head: Headaches, dizziness
5. Nose and throat: Frequent colds or sore throats, chronic rhinorrhea from allergies
6. Skin: Acne, moles, rashes, warts
7. Cardiovascular: Exercise intolerance, shortness of breath, chest pain, palpitations, syncope, and source of regular physical activity
8. Respiratory: Asthma, cough, sneezing, smoking, exposure to TB
9. Gastrointestinal: Abdominal pain, reflux, diarrhea, vomiting, bleeding, constipation
10. Genitourinary: Dysuria, bed-wetting, frequency, bleeding
11. Musculoskeletal: Limb pain, joint pain, or swelling
12. Central nervous system: Seizures, syncope
13. Menstrual: Menarche, frequency of menses, duration, menorrhagia or metrorrhagia, dysmenorrhea
14. Sexual: Sexual activity, contraception, pregnancy, abortions, STIs or STI symptoms

Measurements

Several key pieces of objective information are usually obtained and calculated by staff before the clinician evaluates the AYAs.

Height, Weight, and Body Mass Index Calculation

Yearly assessment of height, weight, and BMI calculation is essential to monitor adolescent growth and for early detection of malnutrition, eating disorders, overweight, and obesity. All values should be plotted on the growth chart, or referenced in the EHR, and interpreted in the context of prior trends (see Chapters 37 and 38 for the evaluation and management of AYAs with overweight/obesity and eating disorders, respectively).

Blood Pressure

Blood pressure should be measured with an appropriate cuff and if abnormal, remeasured manually after allowing the patient to sit for 5 minutes with their arm resting at their side. A diagnosis of hypertension is considered when the repeat blood pressure values on three separate visits (usually 2 weeks apart) are greater than the 95th percentile for age, gender, and height percentile using National High Blood Pressure Education Program Working Group tables, and can be further evaluated by 24-hour ambulatory continuous blood pressure monitoring. See Chapter 20 for additional information about the evaluation and management of hypertension in AYAs.

Other Vital Signs

Heart rate and temperature are also routinely measured. A high temperature could be a sign of current infection. A high heart rate could signal that the patient is in pain and/or, correlated with the history and physical, could be sign of a chronic health problem (i.e., hyperthyroidism, anemia). A heart rate below 50 or a temperature below 96 °F could be a sign of cardiac arrhythmia or malnutrition and should be correlated with the history and growth chart.

Vision Screening

Among 12- to 17-year-old adolescents, approximately 25% have visual acuity of 20/40 or greater requiring corrective lenses. As vision changes often occur in adolescence, vision screening should be performed at the time of their initial evaluation and every 2 to 3 years thereafter. This can be done with a standard Snellen chart or a similar test. To "pass" a line on the Snellen chart, the adolescent should view the chart with one eye covered and be able to read at least one-half of the letters on that line correctly. Referral should be made for vision <20/30 in either or both eyes.

Hearing Screening

There is increasing concern about threats to hearing due to earphone/headphone use. Every patient should have at least one hearing screen performed during adolescence. It is important that this test be performed in a quiet room to allow for detection of subtle defects. Screening examinations are usually conducted at frequencies of 1,000, 2,000, and 4,000 Hz at 20 dB. Referral for more comprehensive hearing testing is indicated if there is a failure to hear 1,000 or 2,000 Hz at 20 dB or 4,000 Hz at 25 dB. The more comprehensive threshold test evaluates for the lowest intensity of sound heard at frequencies of 250, 1,000, 2,000, and 4,000 Hz. Evaluation is indicated with a threshold of 25 dB at two or more frequencies or at 35 dB for any frequency.

Physical Examination

The physical examination allows the clinician to assess growth (weight, height, and BMI) and pubertal development and instruct the adolescent in methods of self-examination. The main elements of the physical examination are summarized below:

Skin

Check for evidence of acne, warts, fungal infections, and other lesions. Carefully inspect moles, especially in patients who are at particular risk for melanoma.

Teeth and Gums

Check for evidence of dental caries or gum infection. Look for signs of smokeless tobacco use. Enamel erosions are sometimes the first clue to the self-induced vomiting associated with some eating disorders.

Neck

Check for thyromegaly or adenopathy.

Cardiopulmonary

Check for heart murmurs or clicks.

Abdomen

Check for evidence of hepatosplenomegaly, tenderness, or masses.

Musculoskeletal

The musculoskeletal examination is especially important in adolescent athletes, in whom instabilities or other evidence of previous injury is the best predictor of future injury. In school-aged athletes, patients often present with a clearance form to participate in sports. Clinicians should know the specific examination techniques to accurately assess strength and range of motion in all muscle groups and joints. Additional assessment of overuse syndromes or osteochondrosis such as Osgood–Schlatter disease is indicated should patients report pain. Finally, assessment of scoliosis, particularly in premenarchal females, should be included as part of the musculoskeletal examination.

Neurologic

Test cranial nerves, strength, reflexes, and coordination.

Sexual Maturity Rating

The sexual maturity rating (SMR), discussed in Chapter 2, is the method by which pubertal development is evaluated and described. Because SMR is more reflective of physiology than age during adolescence, evaluation of SMR is important to provide context for many physical parameters (e.g., BMI, linear growth, menstruation, and gynecomastia) and laboratory values (e.g., hemoglobin) that are measured during the examination of an AYA patient.

Chest

Examine the chest for breast development in anyone birth-assigned female to determine SMR. In birth-assigned males, chest examination should be performed to identify gynecomastia which is present in approximately one-third of people who have gone through male natal puberty. See Chapter 60 for more details.

Genital Examination (for Birth-Assigned Male Patients)

Examine the penis, testicles, and pubic hair distribution. Assess testicular volume to determine SMR. Look for signs of varicocele, hydrocele, hernia, or STI. Retract the foreskin in uncircumcised patients.

Genital Examination (for Birth-Assigned Female Patients)

Assessment of pubic hair distribution may be helpful in staging sexual maturity, however, external genitalia examination or pelvic examination for birth-assigned females is indicated only for patients who have an active complaint such as pelvic pain, dyspareunia, or vaginal discharge.

Screening Tests

Universal screening: Guidelines currently recommend opt-out screening for dyslipidemia, human immunodeficiency virus (HIV), and Hepatitis C infection for all patients regardless of risk profile and cervical dysplasia screening for all birth-assigned female patients. Dyslipidemia screening is recommended once for all patients between ages 9 to 11 and again between ages 17 to 21. Human immunodeficiency virus screening is recommended once for all patients aged 15 to 18 years, and Hepatitis C screening is recommended for all adults aged 18 years and older at least once, except in settings where the prevalence is less than 0.1%. Cervical dysplasia screening recommendations vary by society. The American Cancer Society recommends primary human papillomavirus (HPV) test every 5 years for those aged 25 and older. If primary HPV testing is not available, screening may be done with either (1) a co-test that combines an HPV test with a Pap test every 5 years or (2) a Pap test alone every 3 years. According to the American College of Obstetrics and Gynecology, routine Pap smear screening is recommended starting at age 21 years. Considerations for repeating the aforementioned tests as well as additional screening tests are described in specific sections below.

Testing for Tuberculosis Infection

The most accessible screening test for TB is a purified protein derivative (PPD) tuberculin skin test. Placement of PPD should be considered based on an assessment of individual risk factors and recommendations of the local health department or school requirements. A PPD should be placed for patients with a known exposure to TB, immune deficiency or HIV, active symptoms, living or working in a high-risk congregate setting, or who were born or recently spent 1 month or more in a country with a high burden of TB (>20/100,000 population). Screening should be performed based on risk of exposure since last screen, and not based on lifetime risk. Tuberculosis blood antibody tests, called interferon-gamma release assays (IGRAs), are also available. Two IGRAs are currently approved in the United States: QuantiFERON and T-SPOT.

A positive test suggests that the patient has been infected with TB and further testing is needed to determine if the infection is latent or active. A negative test indicates that the patient does not have latent or active TB. Positivity is determined by risk factors for TB infection:

- 5-mm induration: Positive if the patient has a recent exposure to TB, HIV infection, is immunocompromised, or has a chest x-ray with cavitary lesions or other finding consistent with TB.
- 10-mm induration: Positive if the patient has a high risk for disseminated TB such as lymphoma, diabetes, renal failure, malnutrition, or high risk for exposure to TB such as living in a high prevalence area, homelessness, incarceration, or illicit drug use.
- All other patients are considered positive at 15 mm of induration.

The CDC recommends IGRAs over skin testing for patients who have received the bacille Calmette–Guérin (BCG) vaccine or who have had a difficult time returning for their PPD reading.

Hemoglobin or Hematocrit

A screening hemoglobin is only recommended if the nutrition screen is concerning for inadequate iron intake. Adolescents and young adults with a vegetarian, vegan, or restrictive diet should be screened for anemia.

Metabolic Testing

Metabolic testing includes a lipid profile, diabetes screen, and liver enzymes. Dyslipidemia is determined by the measurement of a fasting lipid panel—total cholesterol (TC), low-density lipoprotein (LDL), triglycerides, and high-density lipoprotein (HDL). A diabetes screen includes a fasting glucose and hemoglobin A1C, and liver enzymes (aspartate aminotransferase [AST] and alanine aminotransferase [ALT]) are useful for evaluating nonalcoholic fatty liver disease (NAFLD).

In addition to the universal screening guidelines for 11- to 13-year-olds and 17- to 21-year-olds outlined above, the 2011

National Heart, Lung, and Blood Institute Report and the AAP recommend dyslipidemia screening based on patient and family risk factors. Although the guidelines recommend fasting tests, random testing may be necessary for those in whom a fasting sample is unavailable. More detailed guidance for testing for dyslipidemia, diabetes, and nonalcoholic fatty liver is covered in other chapters in this text. Briefly, clinicians should consider screening tests for obese and overweight AYAs in the following cases:

1. Family history: Cardiovascular disease, hyperlipidemia, hypertension, stroke, obesity, or diabetes
2. Past medical history: Hypertension, diabetes/impaired fasting glucose, hyperlipidemia
3. BMI ≥85th percentile (if other risk factors are present), ≥95th percentile (all cases)

Labs should be repeated yearly for all youth with a BMI ≥95th percentile. The need for repeat testing is informed by the level of abnormality, progression of the obesity, and degree of engagement in lifestyle change. Regardless of the screening lab work, all youth with elevated BMI should be counseled on lifestyle modification to improve nutrition and exercise. As adolescents are growing, weight loss should not be the only goal, and conversations should focus on healthy behavior change rather than body weight or shape.

Gonorrhea and Chlamydia Screening

All sexually active AYAs should be screened annually for gonorrhea and chlamydia. Males who have sex with males (MSM) should be tested annually at all areas of sexual contact (pharyngeal, urethral, and rectal). Adults over 25 years old with high-risk sexual activity (multiple partners, transactional sex) should be tested annually. A combination test can be sent as a polymerase chain reaction test from a vaginal sample in females or a urine sample in males. With urine samples, a small volume of first-void collection is optimal. Urethral swabs are no longer necessary to screen males.

Screening for Other Sexually Transmitted Infections

Screening for HIV should be offered to all 15- to 18-year-olds once, and also any time that an AYA seeks STI screening. All MSM should be screened annually for HIV and syphilis, and Hepatitis B immunization status should be confirmed. Adolescents and young adults with HIV should be screened for syphilis annually, and pregnant females should be screened for syphilis at the first prenatal visit and again in the third trimester. Routine screening is not recommended for other STIs, and testing should be informed by the symptoms at presentation. When an AYA is diagnosed with one STI, he, she, or they should be screened for others. Syphilis serology should be considered in high-risk populations, or where syphilis is prevalent.

IMMUNIZATIONS

The timely provision of immunizations is a key component of AYA health care. Changing immunization schedules, inconsistent reporting of vaccines with transitions of care, and vaccine refusal may make this more complicated. With the advent of new requirements and vaccines, adolescents previously considered to be fully vaccinated can suddenly find themselves "behind." Some vaccines have waning efficacy and often require revaccination or boosters. Thus, clinicians should assess the vaccination status of AYAs at all preventive and urgent/acute care visits.

Recommended Vaccines

Figures 5.3 and 5.4 outline the CDC's recommended immunization schedule for AYAs. These guidelines are updated annually by the CDC and can be found at http://www.immunize.org/cdc/child-schedule.pdf. During adolescence, the vaccines that are typically given are those for meningococcus, HPV, and influenza.

Meningococcal Vaccine

Meningococcal disease usually presents as one of three syndromes: meningitis, bacteremia, or bacteremic pneumonia. *Neisseria meningitidis* serogroup B, C, and Y are the major causes of meningococcal disease in the United States. Each serogroup accounts for about one-third of disease; however, the proportion of diseases caused by each serogroup varies by age. About three-quarters of cases of disease among AYAs are caused by serogroups C, W, or Y. *Neisseria meningitidis* colonizes the nasopharyngeal mucosa and is transmitted by contact with respiratory tract secretions from those with disease or from asymptomatic carriers. Asymptomatic carriage rates are highest in the AYA population. Disease occurs infrequently as a result of nasopharyngeal colonization.

Currently, four meningococcal vaccines (MenACWY) have been licensed in the United States for the prevention of invasive diseases caused by serogroups A, C, W, and Y. Two vaccines targeting serogroup B have been approved by the U.S. Food and Drug Administration (FDA). In 2015, the ACIP recommended that the vaccine series be administered to certain groups of AYAs older than 10 years who are at increased risk for meningococcal disease, including AYAs with complement deficiencies, anatomic or functional asplenia, and those who work in labs with routine exposure to isolates of the bacteria, as well AYAs identified as being at increased risk because of a serogroup B meningococcal disease outbreak. Subsequently, the ACIP issued a permissive recommendation stating that the vaccine series may be administered to 16- to 23-year-old AYAs (preferred 16 to 18 years old) to provide short-term protection against serogroup B meningococcal disease.

Routine vaccination for adolescents against meningococcal disease has been recommended by the ACIP since 2005. The ACIP recommends routine immunization of all 11- to 18-year-old AYAs with MenACWY. A single dose should be given at 11 or 12 years, with a booster dose administered at age 16 years. If the adolescent does not receive the first dose until age 13 through 15 years, the booster dose should be administered at age 16 through 18 years. If the first dose is given after the 16th birthday, a booster dose is not needed unless the adolescent is at increased risk for meningococcal disease (anatomical or functional asplenia, complement component deficiency). The ACIP does not recommend routine administration of MenACWY to young adults over 19 years of age; however, the vaccine may be administered up to age 21 as catch-up for individuals who did not receive a dose after their 16th birthday. In addition, ACIP recommends that military recruits and first-year college students up to age 21 years living in residence halls receive at least one dose of MenACWY prior to college entry. Ideally, the timing of the most recent dose should occur on or after the 16th birthday. If the young adult has had only one dose of vaccine before the 16th birthday, a booster dose is recommended before college enrollment. Two doses of MenACWY at least 2 months apart are also recommended for adults with anatomical or functional asplenia, or persistent complement deficiencies. Human immunodeficiency virus infection is not an indication for routine vaccination.

Limited data suggest that the four MenACWY vaccine products can be used interchangeably; therefore, clinicians should administer the booster dose when indicated, regardless of the vaccine brand that was administered previously. Vaccination with MenACWY is contraindicated in those who have severe allergic reactions to any of its components (which include diphtheria and tetanus toxoid). No data are available on vaccination with MenACWY during pregnancy.

Human Papillomavirus

According to 2020 CDC data, approximately 72% of cervical cancer is related to HPV types 16 and 18 and an additional 16% is caused by HPV types 31, 33, 45, 52, and 58. About 90% of genital

These recommendations must be read with the notes that follow. For those who fall behind or start late, provide catch-up vaccination at the earliest opportunity as indicated by the green bars. To determine minimum intervals between doses, see the catch-up schedule (Table 2).

Vaccine	Birth	1 mo	2 mos	4 mos	6 mos	9 mos	12 mos	15 mos	18 mos	19–23 mos	2–3 yrs	4–6 yrs	7–10 yrs	11–12 yrs	13–15 yrs	16 yrs	17–18 yrs
Hepatitis B (HepB)	1st dose	←— 2nd dose —→			←———————— 3rd dose ————————→												
Rotavirus (RV): RV1 (2-dose series), RV5 (3-dose series)			1st dose	2nd dose	See Notes												
Diphtheria, tetanus, acellular pertussis (DTaP <7 yrs)			1st dose	2nd dose	3rd dose			←——— 4th dose ———→				5th dose					
Haemophilus influenzae type b (Hib)			1st dose	2nd dose	See Notes		3rd or 4th dose, See Notes										
Pneumococcal conjugate (PCV13)			1st dose	2nd dose	3rd dose		←—— 4th dose ——→										
Inactivated poliovirus (IPV <18 yrs)			1st dose	2nd dose	←———————— 3rd dose ————————→							4th dose					
Influenza (IIV4)					Annual vaccination 1 or 2 doses									Annual vaccination 1 dose only			
or																	
Influenza (LAIV4)											Annual vaccination 1 or 2 doses			Annual vaccination 1 dose only			
Measles, mumps, rubella (MMR)					See Notes		←— 1st dose —→					2nd dose					
Varicella (VAR)							←— 1st dose —→					2nd dose					
Hepatitis A (HepA)					See Notes		2-dose series, See Notes										
Tetanus, diphtheria, acellular pertussis (Tdap ≥7 yrs)														1 dose			
Human papillomavirus (HPV)														See Notes			
Meningococcal (MenACWY-D ≥9 mos, MenACWY-CRM ≥2 mos, MenACWY-TT ≥2years)								See Notes						1st dose		2nd dose	
Meningococcal B (MenB-4C, MenB-FHbp)															See Notes		
Pneumococcal polysaccharide (PPSV23)												See Notes					
Dengue (DEN4CYD; 9-16 yrs)														Seropositive in endemic areas only (See Notes)			

Range of recommended ages for all children	Range of recommended ages for catch-up vaccination	Range of recommended ages for certain high-risk groups	Recommended vaccination can begin in this age group	Recommended vaccination based on shared clinical decision-making	No recommendation/ not applicable

FIGURE 5.3 Recommended child and adolescent immunization schedule for ages 18 years or younger, US, 2022. (Source: Centers for Disease Control and Prevention (CDC). Recommended child and adolescent immunization schedule for ages 18 years or younger, US, 2022. Published 2022. Accessed June 20, 2022. https://www.cdc.gov/vaccines/schedules/downloads/child/0-18yrs-child-combined-schedule.pdf)

warts are related to types 6 and 11. In the United States, three vaccines against HPV have been recommended for AYAs, a bivalent vaccine (HPV2) (Cervarix, GlaxoSmithKline Inc.), a quadrivalent vaccine (HPV4) (Gardasil, Merck & Co.), and a 9-valent vaccine (HPV9) (Gardasil 9, Merck & Co.) (see Chapter 66). Each of the vaccines targets HPV types 16 and 18 (the most common HPV types implicated in cervical cancer). HPV4 and HPV9 also target HPV types 6 and 11 (the most common HPV types associated with genital warts) and HPV9 also targets HPV types 31, 33, 45, 52, and 58. The vaccines have been shown to be safe, highly immunogenic, and effective at preventing infections with HPV types 16 and/or 18 in randomized, double-blind, placebo-controlled trials.

Currently, ACIP recommends routine vaccination of all AYAs at age 11 or 12 years with either HPV2, HPV4, or HPV9. The series can be started as early as age 9 years at the discretion of the clinician. Vaccination is also recommended for AYA females aged 13 to 26 years who have not been vaccinated previously or who have not completed the series. Vaccination is not generally recommended for adults older than 26 years, however, 27- to 45-year-olds may get the vaccine after discussion with their clinician. For all males, ACIP recommends routine vaccination with HPV4 or HPV9 at age 11 or 12 years, but as early as age 9 years. Males, aged 13 to 21 years, who have not been vaccinated or who have not completed the three-dose series should also be vaccinated. Young adult males

aged 22 through 26 years may also be vaccinated. Ideally, vaccination should occur before the onset of sexual activity as the vaccine will not be effective against HPV subtypes that are acquired prior to vaccination. The dose series varies by age of first dose: for persons initiating vaccination before their 15th birthday, the recommended immunization schedule is two doses of HPV vaccine (at 0 and 6 to 12 months) and for persons initiating vaccination on or after their 15th birthday, or for persons with certain immunocompromising conditions, the recommended immunization schedule is three doses of HPV vaccine (at 0, 1 to 2, and 6 months).

Influenza

In the United States, two types of influenza vaccine are available, an inactivated vaccine and a live attenuated vaccine. Currently, both vaccine types are available as either trivalent (targeting three virus strains: two type A and one type B) or quadrivalent (targeting four virus strains: two type A and two type B), representing the strains most commonly found worldwide and predicted to be most likely to cause infections in the coming year. Vaccines are updated annually to reflect emerging virus serotypes. Influenza in AYAs is discussed in Chapter 34.

Annual influenza vaccine is recommended for all individuals older than 6 months of age who do not have contraindications to receipt of the vaccine. Influenza vaccine should be administered as soon as the vaccine becomes available each year. When vaccine supply is limited,

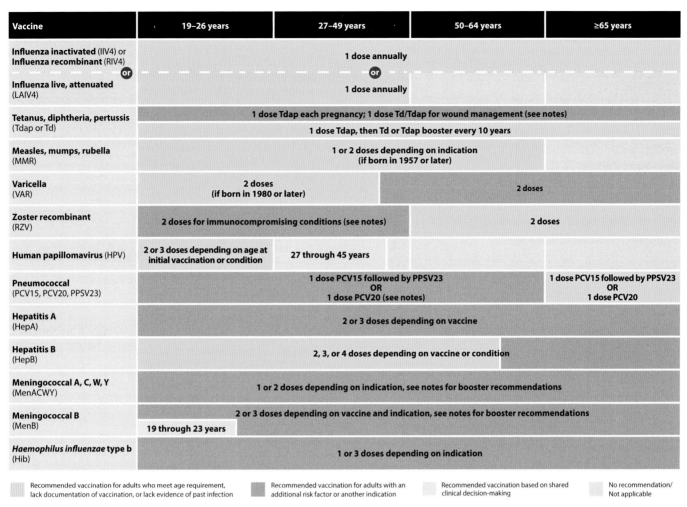

Vaccine	19–26 years	27–49 years	50–64 years	≥65 years
Influenza inactivated (IIV4) or **Influenza recombinant** (RIV4)	1 dose annually			
or				
Influenza live, attenuated (LAIV4)	1 dose annually			
Tetanus, diphtheria, pertussis (Tdap or Td)	1 dose Tdap each pregnancy; 1 dose Td/Tdap for wound management (see notes)			
	1 dose Tdap, then Td or Tdap booster every 10 years			
Measles, mumps, rubella (MMR)	1 or 2 doses depending on indication (if born in 1957 or later)			
Varicella (VAR)	2 doses (if born in 1980 or later)	2 doses		
Zoster recombinant (RZV)	2 doses for immunocompromising conditions (see notes)		2 doses	
Human papillomavirus (HPV)	2 or 3 doses depending on age at initial vaccination or condition	27 through 45 years		
Pneumococcal (PCV15, PCV20, PPSV23)		1 dose PCV15 followed by PPSV23 OR 1 dose PCV20 (see notes)		1 dose PCV15 followed by PPSV23 OR 1 dose PCV20
Hepatitis A (HepA)	2 or 3 doses depending on vaccine			
Hepatitis B (HepB)	2, 3, or 4 doses depending on vaccine or condition			
Meningococcal A, C, W, Y (MenACWY)	1 or 2 doses depending on indication, see notes for booster recommendations			
Meningococcal B (MenB)	2 or 3 doses depending on vaccine and indication, see notes for booster recommendations			
	19 through 23 years			
***Haemophilus influenzae* type b** (Hib)	1 or 3 doses depending on indication			

Recommended vaccination for adults who meet age requirement, lack documentation of vaccination, or lack evidence of past infection   Recommended vaccination for adults with an additional risk factor or another indication   Recommended vaccination based on shared clinical decision-making   No recommendation/Not applicable

FIGURE 5.4 Recommended adult immunization schedule by age group, US, 2022. (Source: Centers for Disease Control and Prevention (CDC). Recommended Adult Immunization Schedule by Age Group, US, 2022. Published 2022. Accessed June 20, 2022. https://www.cdc.gov/vaccines/schedules/downloads/adult/adult-combined-schedule.pdf)

priority should be given to AYAs with higher risk for influenza-related complications, including those with the following:

- Chronic pulmonary conditions (including asthma)
- Cardiovascular disease (with the exception of hypertension)
- Chronic renal, hepatic, neurologic, hematologic, or metabolic disorders
- Adolescents and young adults with immunosuppression (including those on immunosuppressing medication or who have HIV infection)
- Individuals who will be pregnant during influenza season
- Individuals on long-term aspirin therapy
- Residents of long-term care facilities
- American Indian/Alaskan natives
- Persons with morbid obesity (BMI ≥40 kg/m²)

Inactivated influenza vaccine is administered in the deltoid muscle. Only one dose is required for those older than 9 years. It is contraindicated in persons with anaphylactic reactions to eggs and should be delayed in those with significant febrile illnesses (but not in those with minor upper respiratory infections). A recombinant influenza vaccine has been approved for adults older than 18 years that contains no egg protein and can therefore be administered to adults with egg allergies.

Live, attenuated influenza vaccine (LAIV) is marketed in the United States as FluMist. It is administered intranasally and is indicated for healthy persons aged 5 to 49 years, including those who may have contact with high-risk groups. It is contraindicated in

individuals who are pregnant or immunosuppressed, and for those who are receiving aspirin or other salicylates (because of the association of Reye syndrome with wild-type influenza infection). Live, attenuated influenza vaccine is also contraindicated for AYAs with a history of Guillain–Barré syndrome within 6 weeks of previous influenza vaccination; hypersensitivity, including anaphylaxis, to eggs; or for those who have taken influenza antiviral medications in the previous 48 hours. Live, attenuated influenza vaccine should not be used in those who will have close contact with severely immunocompromised persons within 7 days of vaccination. While not strict contraindications, the safety of LAIV in persons with asthma, reactive airway disease, or other chronic conditions has not been established, and these conditions should be considered precautions for LAIV use. The LAIV is administered only through the intranasal route, 0.25 mL in each nostril. Only a single dose is required for those older than 9 years.

SARS-CoV-2 Vaccines

Three COVID-19 vaccines are currently approved under a Biologics License Application (BLA) or authorized under an Emergency Use Authorization by the U.S. FDA:

- Pfizer-BioNTech COVID-19 Vaccine/COMIRNATY
- Moderna COVID-19 Vaccine/SPIKEVAX
- Janssen (Johnson & Johnson) COVID-19 Vaccine

The Pfizer-BioNTech and Moderna vaccines are lipid nanoparticle-formulated, nucleoside-modified messenger ribonucleic acid (mRNA) vaccines encoding the prefusion spike glycoprotein of SARS-CoV-2, the virus that causes COVID-19. The Janssen COVID-19 Vaccine is a recombinant, replication-incompetent adenovirus type 26 (Ad26) vector encoding the stabilized prefusion spike glycoprotein of SARS-CoV-2. None of the currently FDA-approved or FDA-authorized COVID-19 vaccines are live-virus vaccines.

The vaccination schedule varies by age group and specific vaccine as follows. Of note, the CDC does not recommend mixing products for the primary series doses. Adults who are 18 years and older may get a different product for a booster than they received for their primary series. However, at the time of this publication, adolescent patients aged 12 to 17 years who received a Pfizer-BioNTech primary series, must get Pfizer-BioNTech for a booster.

Primary vaccine series for adults 18 and older:
- Pfizer-BioNTech vaccine: two doses given 3 to 8 weeks apart.
- Moderna vaccine: two doses given 4 to 8 weeks apart
- Janssen vaccine: one single dose

Booster vaccinations for adults 18 and older:
- For all adults: One booster, preferably of either Pfizer-BioNTech or Moderna COVID-19 vaccine, is recommended at least:
  - 5 months after completion of initial series of Pfizer-BioNTech or Moderna vaccine primary series
  - 2 months after completion of initial series of Janssen vaccine primary series
- For adults over 50 or anyone over 18 years old who are immunocompromised: An additional second booster of either Pfizer-BioNTech or Moderna COVID-19 vaccine is recommended at least 4 months after the first booster regardless of initial vaccine series.
- Adults aged 18 to 49 years who received a Janssen COVID-19 vaccine for both their primary dose and booster can choose to get a second booster of either Pfizer-BioNTech or Moderna COVID-19 vaccine at least 4 months after their first booster. However, at the time of writing this chapter, the second booster is not required to be considered up to date.

Primary vaccine series for adolescents aged 12 to 17:
- Pfizer-BioNTech: two doses given 3 to 8 weeks apart
- Moderna: two doses given 4 to 8 weeks apart

Booster vaccinations for patients aged 12 to17:
- For those who received the Pfizer-BioNTech COVID-19 primary vaccine series: One booster vaccination is recommended at least 5 months after the final dose in the primary series
- For those who received Moderna vaccine primary series: No booster is recommended at this time.

For all above referenced vaccination primary series and booster series, individuals are considered fully vaccinated 2 weeks after final dose in primary series and immediately after completion of the booster vaccine.

Specific prevaccination counseling:
All individuals should be informed of the benefit of COVID-19 vaccination in reducing the risk of severe outcomes from COVID-19 infection. Those receiving an mRNA vaccine (Pfizer Bio-NTech or Moderna), particularly males aged 12 to 39 years, should be informed of the rare risk of myocarditis and/or pericarditis following receipt of mRNA COVID-19 vaccines. Counseling should also include the need to seek care if symptoms of myocarditis or pericarditis occur after vaccination, particularly in the week following vaccination when symptoms are most likely to be present. Additionally, patients interested in receiving the Janssen COVID-19 vaccine should be informed of the risk and symptoms of thrombosis with thrombocytopenia syndrome (TTS), as well as the need to seek immediate medical care should symptoms develop after receiving Janssen vaccine.

Contraindications are limited and include:
- History of severe allergic reaction (e.g., anaphylaxis) after a previous dose or to a component of the COVID-19 vaccine
- A known diagnosed allergy to a component of the COVID-19 vaccine
- For the Janssen COVID-19 Vaccine, TTS syndrome following receipt of a previous Janssen COVID-19 Vaccine

Catch-Up Vaccines

Many adolescents may need catch-up vaccines for hepatitis A and varicella, and a tetanus and pertussis booster depending on prior vaccination status (see ancillary resources for further details). Adolescents who have been partially vaccinated should have their vaccination series completed without restarting the series. Likewise, adolescents who begin a vaccination series can complete it at any time after the vaccination process is interrupted, even if there has been a substantial delay between doses.

Consent for Vaccination

Since 1994, all clinicians in the United States who administer measles, mumps, rubella (MMR), polio, diphtheria and tetanus toxoids and pertussis (DTP), and tetanus-diphtheria (Td) vaccines have been required to distribute vaccine information sheets (VIS) each time a patient is vaccinated. The clinic should obtain consent from the patient and parent/guardian prior to any vaccine and provide the family with a VIS. This should also be noted in the medical record. Appropriate documentation of vaccination includes consent for vaccination, immunization type, date of administration, injection site, manufacturer and lot number of vaccine, and name and address of the clinician administering the vaccine.

Vaccine refusal by patients and their parents is becoming more common and has been associated with a rise in rates of measles, mumps, and pertussis in recent years. The AAP recommends responding to parent concerns, but also asking them to sign a waiver if they refuse recommended vaccines.

While laws for consent vary by location of practice, in some areas of the United States, AYAs can consent to HPV vaccination as a component of comprehensive sexual and reproductive health services. Practitioners should know the laws in their geographic area prior to administering HPV vaccine and other vaccines with respect to the need for parent/guardian consent.

Improving Vaccine Delivery

To improve vaccination rates, the ACIP has specifically addressed a variety of situations in which many practitioners or patients have chosen to defer or delay vaccination. Situations that specifically *do not* represent contraindications to vaccination include the following:

1. Reaction to a previous dose of DTP vaccine with only soreness, redness, or swelling
2. Mild acute illness with low-grade fever
3. Current antimicrobial therapy
4. Pregnancy of a household contact
5. Recent exposure to an infectious disease
6. Breast-feeding
7. History of nonspecific allergies
8. Allergy to penicillin or other antimicrobials except anaphylactic reactions to neomycin or streptomycin
9. Allergies to duck meat or duck feathers
10. Family history of seizures

In addition, "minor illnesses" such as mild upper respiratory tract infections, with or without low-grade fever, are not contraindications to vaccine administration. Delaying vaccine administration because of mild acute illness is unnecessary and leads to missed opportunities to protect AYAs from vaccine-preventable diseases.

Details on contraindications for each vaccine can be accessed through the ACIP. There are relatively few contraindications beyond prior history of anaphylaxis to vaccination, or encephalopathy within 7 days of vaccination. For live, attenuated vaccines only, contraindications include pregnancy and severe immunocompromised status.

PREVENTIVE HEALTH COUNSELING

After completing the patient evaluation, the clinician should provide anticipatory guidance regarding high-risk behavior, and support positive choices that the AYA is already making within a strength-based framework that helps AYAs recognize and employ their own strengths. This preventive health counseling portion of the examination should be done with the patient alone if confidential topics will be reviewed.

Approaches to Preventive Health Counseling

Preventive health counseling requires active listening, explicit questioning, and generating specific strategies in collaboration with the AYAs. Clinicians need to efficiently and effectively communicate simple key preventive health messages to their patients, ideally linking them to the patient's goals. Commonly used messages on a range of topics have been developed by Bright Futures, the Adolescent Health Working Group (AHWG), and other organizations, and a listing of resources and websites is available at the end of this chapter.

There are various approaches to preventive health counseling. One brief office-based intervention model, originally developed by the National Cancer Institute and recently modified by the USPSTF as a framework for behavioral counseling interventions, is the five A's approach:

1. **A**sk about the behavior.
2. **A**dvise a different course.
3. **A**ssess willingness to change.
4. **A**ssist in behavior change.
5. **A**rrange for follow-up.

A complementary approach originally developed for the American Medical Association's Guidelines for Adolescent Preventive Services (GAPS) offers a standardized method of assessment and intervention that embodies health education principles but remains practical for office practice. The mnemonic GAPS refers to Gather information, Assess further, Problem identification, and Specific Solutions. Table 5.7 from the AHWG summarizes the steps.

G (Gather Initial Information)

Obtain a complete psychosocial history (HEEADSSS or SHADES assessment) from the patient. This initial screening step may be facilitated by use of questionnaires, computers, or nonclinician personnel. If the initial screening does not identify increased risk, basic information and positive reinforcement of the healthy behavior should be offered. If increased health risk is identified, proceed to the next level.

A (Assess Further)

Assess the level and nature of risk in the particular area. Identify the seriousness of the problem by assessing the patient's knowledge and involvement, predisposing and protective factors, the availability of family and other support, and the self-perceived consequences for the patient's health and function (e.g., school, peer relationships). Specific interventions should be tailored to the risk assessment. For the patient at low risk, the provision of health information, a few targeted suggestions, and positive reinforcement about what the patient is already doing to stay healthy is often sufficient.[30] If the patient is at high risk, they probably need an in-depth evaluation that may be beyond the scope of a preventive services visit. If so, a return visit for more intensive intervention, or referral, is warranted. Patients who are at intermediate risk also require an explicit intervention (detailed in the following section). This can usually be done within the context of the preventive services visit.

P (Problem Identification)

This step involves working with the patient toward an agreement on the problem, helping the patient decide to make a change that seems attainable to them, and working with the patient to develop a specific plan for that change. The goal is to be "patient centered" in the approach—that is, to help the *patient* decide what is in their best interest, rather than assuming the patient will accept the clinician's view of the problem or behavior. Problem identification is an attempt to define the problem in terms that the patient recognizes

---

TABLE 5.7

Steps for Preventive Screening and Health Promotion

Negative	Positive		
Health Promotion • Reinforce positive behaviors • Provide health guidance	**Assess Further** • Degree of involvement • Psychosocial sexual and physical development • Knowledge about risk behaviors • Functional consequences to health, social performance, peer and family relationships • Support from family and others		
	If Positive, Assess Risk for Adverse Consequences...		
	Lower Risk for Adverse Consequences	**Moderate Risk for Adverse Consequences**	**Higher Risk for Adverse Consequences**
	Health Promotion • Reinforce positive behaviors • Provide health guidance	**Problem Identification** • Negotiate the problem • Determine readiness to change • Weigh the pros and cons • Identify opportunities and barriers **Solutions** • Negotiate the intervention(s) • Promote self-efficacy • Discuss strategies to overcome barriers • Develop a contract • Follow up	**Referral and Follow-Up**

Adapted from Simmons M, Shalwitz J, Pollock S, et al. *Adolescent Health Care 101: The Basics. Adolescent Health Working Group.* 2003.

(e.g., What is the difference between the way things are and the way I want them to be?).

When the AYA is engaging in risky health behavior, clinicians often attempt to impart health knowledge rather than engaging the patient and obtaining specific information. For example, imagine a clinical encounter in which a sexually active adolescent patient is asked about condom use. The patient responds that she uses condoms "sometimes." While a clinician might talk about the importance and health benefits of condom use, the patient's inconsistency with condom use may not be lack of knowledge but due to something else entirely—she cannot afford them, her partner refuses to use them, someone is allergic to latex, or there never seems to be a condom available when one is required. None of these potential barriers is likely to emerge if the clinician is too quick to intervene to educate on identified risky behaviors prior to asking the adolescent about her individual perspective and needs. Productive advice for this particular patient requires an understanding of her specific barriers to condom use. It is also important to move beyond focusing on barriers to condom usage and also assess the circumstances in which patients are able to use condoms (e.g., What What allows the patient to use a condom "some of the time"?).[31]

A focus on strengths can and should be integrated into risk reduction discussions, with a clinician reinforcing positive behavior and building on successful experiences. If a sexually active AYA is having difficulty regularly using condoms, he might be asked about when he was last able to use a condom, thereby shifting the emphasis to what circumstances enabled him to be successful. Likewise, if an AYA is consistently using a condom, he should receive positive reinforcement for the healthy and safe behavior.

If the patient does not agree that there is a problem with a specified behavior, look for areas of agreement and common ground. For example, a patient may not accept that their use of alcohol or cannabis is problematic, but may acknowledge that binge drinking puts them at risk or is getting in the way of some goal (e.g., disapproval from friends or a romantic interest, optimal sports performance, etc.). Any problem that poses an immediate threat to the patient's safety warrants an immediate intervention or referral even if the patient does not agree that it is a problem or is not fully prepared for change (i.e., driving under the influence or in the car with others who are).

S (Specific Solutions) Self-Efficacy, Support, Solving Problems, and "Shaking on a Contract"

Self-efficacy is assessed by asking the patient about their confidence to carry out the proposed plan. If the AYA is not sure that they can be successful, revisit perceived barriers and attempt to redefine specific solutions. The plans developed by the AYA should be concrete and achievable so that success becomes self-reinforcing. An overly ambitious plan may need to be modified.

Support in modifying behavior is important. Patients should be encouraged to identify people who can help them carry out their plan. Hopefully, they will be able to call on resources such as trusted adults or close friends. At times, AYAs may want advice on how best to recruit their support system. In addition to offering advice, the clinician may be helpful in facilitating the disclosure of information from patients to parents or others.

Solving problems includes assessing the barriers that the patient foresees and working with the AYA to develop specific strategies to overcome them. For example, if an adolescent recognizes that he will have difficulty not drinking at an upcoming party, he must have a plan for how to deal with that situation. It is usually most helpful if patients come up with their own solutions, identifying what has been helpful to them before and recognizing what they have been able to do to be successful.[31] The clinician can suggest modifications to the patient's solution, or suggest options that the AYA might not have considered.

"Shaking on a contract" and/or writing down or creating reminders in their phone about the agreed-upon plan is a crucial step. It serves as a tangible reinforcement of the proposed plan and implies some commitment on the patient's part. It is important to specify the actions agreed to and the time frame in which the actions are to be taken. Make sure that the AYA feels comfortable with the plan, feels ownership of it, and understands it. Including another party in the contract, such as a friend or parent when possible, may lead to better follow-through. Follow-up is critical and should be arranged in some form—a visit, telephone contact, or email—in the time frame agreed to in the contract.

HEALTH CARE TRANSITIONS

The transition from a family-centered pediatric approach to a patient-centered adult model of health care is often a critical time of medical vulnerability for AYAs accompanied by fewer primary care visits and marked increases in potentially preventable morbidity and mortality. Adolescents and young adults are at risk for negative health outcomes with respect to preventive health care and chronic condition management unless health care transitions (HCT) are carefully planned and supported. To create a systematic approach and facilitate the transition, the AAP, American Academy of Family Physicians, and American College of Physicians, collaboratively created a toolkit titled Got Transition.[32] Central to effective health care transition is the ongoing assessment of a young person's evolving ability to manage key aspects of their health care needs, a metric referred to as self-management or "transition readiness" starting at age 12 years. In the United States, the core components of transition readiness include the following health-related domains: understanding medical needs, navigating insurance coverage, financial considerations, prescription medication management, and scheduling appointments. The preventive health visit, and the time that it affords with the AYA alone, is an opportunity to engage AYAs in these discussions, ensuring that their perspectives are understood, and that transition planning is responsive to their social and developmental needs. Standardized readiness assessment questionnaires such as Transition Readiness Assessment Questionnaire (TRAQ) are useful tools to assess and track transition readiness across visits. While these readiness assessments are an integral component of transition planning with AYAs, it is important to note that it represents only one key component of the larger construct of a coordinated collaborative transition framework including clinicians, patients, and families. For more detail on the components of a comprehensive health care transition plan, please refer to the Six Core Elements of HCT, in the Got Transitions toolkit.

SUMMARY

As adolescence and young adulthood represents a period of relative physical health, the majority of morbidity and mortality in this age group stems from preventable risk factors. Thus, the preventive health care visit remains a cornerstone of AYA health care. While the transition through AYAs creates the potential for risk-taking behavior and medical vulnerability, it also provides developmental windows of opportunity for health promotion and the development of resilience. The clinical preventive services visit, as outlined in this chapter, provides a framework with which to structure a comprehensive approach to preventive health care aimed at reinforcing positive health behaviors to support resiliency and optimize health while also providing an integral touch point to identify and intervene to reduce risk behavior. Direct engagement of adolescents in their own health care is key to the preventive services visit, and care to this demographic should focus on the transition from adult-centered decision making to young adult autonomy in health care access and utilization. Finally, in addition to the traditional clinic-based encounter, connecting digital health technologies to clinical preventive care and the provision of services in a range of health care settings provides enhanced opportunities to improve AYA preventive health.

ACKNOWLEDGMENTS

This chapter is based on Chapter 5 from Neinstein's Adolescent and Young Adult Health Care 6th edition, authored by Carolyn Jasik and Elizabeth Ozer. The authors also wish to acknowledge David S. Rosen and Lawrence S. Neinstein for their contributions to previous versions of this chapter. This chapter was primarily supported by the Health Resources and Services Administration (HRSA) of the U.S. Department of Health and Human Services (HHS) under Cooperative Agreement number UA6MC27378, with supplemental support from HRSA MCHB award T71MC0003.

REFERENCES

1. Harris SK, Aalsma MC, Weitzman ER, et al. Research on clinical preventive services for adolescents and young adults: where are we and where do we need to go? *J Adolesc Health*. 2017;60(3):249–260.
2. National Center for Injury Prevention and Control, WISQARS. Fatal injury reports, national, regional and state, 1981–2018. The Centers for Disease Control and Prevention. Published 2020. Accessed March 25, 2021. https://webappa.cdc.gov/sasweb/ncipc/mortrate.html
3. Park MJ, Scott JT, Adams SH, et al. Adolescent and young adult health in the United States in the past decade: little improvement and young adults remain worse off than adolescents. *J Adolesc Health*. 2014;55(1):3–16.
4. Centers for Disease Control and Prevention (CDC). Injury prevention and control: data and statistics. WISQARS: leading causes of death [online database]. Published 2021. Updated February 11, 2021. Accessed March 31, 2021. https://www.cdc.gov/injury/wisqars/LeadingCauses.html
5. Giovanelli A, Ozer EM, Dahl RE. Leveraging technology to improve health in adolescence: a developmental science perspective. *J Adolesc Health*. 2020;67(2S):S7–S13.
6. Viner RM, Ozer EM, Denny S, et al. Adolescence and the social determinants of health. *Lancet*. 2012;379(9826):1641–1652.
7. US Preventive Services Task Force. Published recommendations. Updated July 6, 2020. Accessed March 31, 2021. https://www.uspreventiveservicestaskforce.org/uspstf/topic_search_results?topic_status=P&age_group%5B%5D=9&searchterm=
8. Hagan JF, Shaw JS, Duncan P. *Bright Futures: Guidelines for Health Supervision of Infants, Children, and Adolescents*, 4th ed.: American Academy of Pediatrics; 2017.
9. Adams SH, Park MJ, Twietmeyer L, et al. Increasing delivery of preventive services to adolescents and young adults: does the preventive visit help? *J Adolesc Health*. 2018;63(2):166–171.
10. Park MJ, Brindis CD, Irwin CE Jr. Health care policy for adolescents and young adults. In: Schulenburg J, ed. *American Psychological Association Handbook of Adolescent and Young Adult Development*. In press; 2021.
11. National Adolescent and Young Adult Health Information Center. Summary of clinical preventive services guidelines for adolescents up to age 18. *National Adolescent and Young Adult Health Information Center*, University of California, San Francisco. Published 2020. Accessed March 25, 2021. http://nahic.ucsf.edu/resource_center/adolescent-guidelines/
12. Ozer EM, Urquhart JT, Brindis CD, et al. Young adult preventive health care guidelines: there but can't be found. *Arch Pediatr Adolesc Med*. 2012;166(3):240–247.
13. National Adolescent and Young Adult Health Information Center. Summary of clinical preventive services guidelines for young adults ages 18–25. *National Adolescent and Young Adult Health Information Center*, University of California, San Francisco; Published 2020. Accessed March 25, 2021. https://nahic.ucsf.edu/resource_center/yaguidelines/
14. Adams SH, Park MJ, Twietmeyer L, et al. Association between adolescent preventive care and the role of the affordable care act. *JAMA Pediatr*. 2018;172(1):43–48.
15. Adams SH, Park MJ, Twietmeyer L, et al.. Young adult preventive healthcare: changes in receipt of care pre- to post-affordable care act. *J Adolesc Health*. 2019;64(6):763–769.
16. Callahan ST. Focus on preventive health care for young adults. *Arch Pediatr Adolesc Med*. 2012;166(3):289–290.
17. Institute of Medicine, National Research Council. *Investing in the Health and Well-Being of Young Adults*. The National Academies Press; 2014.
18. Fortuna RJ, Halterman JS, Pulcino T, et al. Delayed transition of care: a national study of visits to pediatricians by young adults. *Acad Pediatr*. 2012;12(5):405–411.
19. Bell DL, Breland DJ, Ott MA. Adolescent and young adult male health: a review. *Pediatrics*. 2013;132(3):535–546.
20. Tebb KP, Rodríguez F, Pollack LM, et al. Improving contraceptive use among latina adolescents: a cluster-randomized controlled trial evaluating an mhealth application, Health-E You/Salud iTu. *Contraception*. 2021;104(3):246–253.
21. Barney A, Buckelew S, Mesheriakova V, et al.. The COVID-19 pandemic and rapid implementation of adolescent and young adult telemedicine: challenges and opportunities for innovation. *J Adolesc Health*. 2020;67(2):164–171.
22. Ozer EM, Lester JC. Innovative digital technologies to improve adolescent and young adult health. *J Adolesc Health*. 2020;67(2S):S3.
23. Wong CA, Madanay F, Ozer EM, et al. Digital health technology to enhance adolescent and young adult clinical preventive services: affordances and challenges. *J Adolesc Health*. 2020;67(2S):S24–S33.
24. Society for Adolescent H, Medicine, Gray SH, et al. Recommendations for electronic health record use for delivery of adolescent health care. *J Adolesc Health*. 2014;54(4):487–490.
25. Jasik CB, Berna M, Martin M, et al. Teen preferences for clinic-based behavior screens: who, where, when, and how? *J Adolesc Health*. 2016;59(6):722–724.
26. Hadland SE, Yehia BR, Makadon HJ. Caring for lesbian, gay, bisexual, transgender, and questioning youth in inclusive and affirmative environments. *Pediatr Clin North Am*. 2016;63(6):955–969.
27. Simmons M, Shalwitz J, Pollock S, et al. *Adolescent Health Care 101: The Basics*. Adolescent Health Working Group; 2003.
28. Levy SJL, Williams JF, Committee on Substance Use and Prevention. Substance use screening, brief intervention, and referral to treatment. *Pediatrics*. 2016;138(1).
29. Marcell AV, The male training center for family planning and reproductive health. *Preventive Male Sexual and Reproductive Health Care: Recommendations for Clinical Practice*. Male Training Center for Family Planning and Reproductive Health and Office of Population Affairs; 2014.
30. Ozer EM, Adams SH, Orrell-Valente JK, et al. Does delivering preventive services in primary care reduce adolescent risky behavior? *J Adolesc Health*. 2011; 49(5):476–482.
31. Ozer MN. *Management of Persons With Chronic Neurological Illness*. Butterworth-Heinemann; 2000.
32. White PH, Cooley WC; Transitions Clinical Report Authoring Group; American Academy of Pediatrics; American Academy of Family Physicians; American College of Physicians. Supporting the Health Care Transition From Adolescence to Adulthood in the Medical Home. *Pediatrics*. 2018;142(5):e20182587.

ADDITIONAL RESOURCES AND WEBSITES

Additional Resources and Websites for Clinicians:

Adolescent Health Working Group (AHWG) Provider Resources—https://ahwg.org/provider-resources/

American Academy of Pediatrics. Adolescent Health Care: The Importance of Confidential Preventive Services—https://services.aap.org/en/news-room/campaigns-and-toolkits/adolescent-health-care/

Bright Futures/AAP Clinical Resources—https://www.aap.org/en/practice-management/bright-futures

CDC Advisory Committee on Immunization Practices (ACIP)—https://www.cdc.gov/vaccines/acip/recommendations.html

CDC Vaccination Information—https://www.cdc.gov/vaccines/index.html

Got Transitions Tool Kit—https://www.gottransition.org/

NAHIC Clinical Preventive Services Guidelines for Adolescents up to age 18—https://nahic.ucsf.edu/wp-content/uploads/2020/12/CPSG-ADOL-Supplement-September-2020.docx

National Adolescent Health Information Center (NAHIC)—https://nahic.ucsf.edu/

Society for Adolescent Health and Medicine (SAHM) Clinical Care Resources—https://www.adolescenthealth.org/Resources/Clinical-Care-Resources.aspx

Use of COVID-19 Vaccines in the United States. Centers for Disease Control and Prevention—https://www.cdc.gov/vaccines/covid-19/clinical-considerations/covid-19-vaccines-us.html. Accessed June 27, 2022.

U.S. Preventive Services Task Force—http://www.uspreventiveservicestaskforce.org/

Additional Resources and Websites for Parents/Caregivers:

Adolescent Health Working Group Parent Resources—https://ahwg.org/courses/resources-for-parents/

Bright Futures Parent Resources—https://brightfutures.aap.org/families/Pages/Resources-for-Families.aspx

Gender Spectrum Learn and Connect Parents and Families—https://genderspectrum.org/audiences/parents-and-family

HealthyChildren.Org (AAP)—https://www.healthychildren.org/english/ages-stages/teen/Pages/default.aspx

KidsHealth.org—https://kidshealth.org/en/parents/

SAHM Mental Health Resources for Parents—https://www.adolescenthealth.org/Resources/Clinical-Care-Resources/Mental-Health/Mental-Health-Resources-For-Parents-of-Adolescents.aspx

Teen Safe (Educational materials to prevent opioid use)—https://teen-safe.org/

UNITY—vaccination resources for parents—https://www.unity4teenvax.org/parents/

Additional Resources and Websites for Adolescents and Young Adults:

Adolescent Health Working Group Youth Resources—https://ahwg.org/youth-resources/

Center for Young Women's Health—https://youngwomenshealth.org/

Gender Spectrum, Learn and Connect Youth—https://genderspectrum.org/audiences/youth

Real Talk for Adolescents—https://realtalkwithdroffutt.org/index.html

SAHM Mental Health Resources for Youth—https://www.adolescenthealth.org/Resources/Clinical-Care-Resources/Mental-Health/Mental-Health-Resources-For-Parents-of-Adolescents.aspx

TeenHealth.org—https://kidshealth.org/en/teens/

The Truth Campaign—https://www.thetruth.com/

Truth (or nah!?)—https://www.truthornahsf.org/

UNITY—vaccination resources for AYAs—https://www.unity4teenvax.org/teens-and-young-adults/

Young Men's Health—https://youngmenshealthsite.org/

Nutrition

Michael R. Kohn

KEY WORDS

- Assessments
- Daily requirements
- Nutrition
- Special needs
- Therapy

INTRODUCTION

Nutrition is an essential component of adolescent and young adult (AYA) health care. Optimal nutrition assists in reaching the potential for physical growth, development, and the prevention of illness. Two important transformations occur during adolescence that change nutritional needs. Growth and changes in body composition are greater and more rapid than at any other time in life, except infancy. In general, there is also a significant change in the adolescent's eating habits and food consumption. Adolescents typically reduce regular breakfast consumption, increase consumption of prepared foods, snacks, fried foods, nutrient-poor foods, and sweetened beverages, and have a significant increase in portion size at each meal. This is associated with a decrease in the consumption of dairy products, fruits, and vegetables. Sodium intake is far in excess of recommended levels, whereas calcium and potassium intakes are below recommended levels.[1] The nutritional needs of young adults differ from both adolescents and the average population values.[2]

Clinicians should assess nutritional status and provide appropriate nutritional counseling as part of health supervision visits. The 2020–2025 Dietary Guidelines for Americans is a comprehensive resource for clinicians providing information on nutritional requirements and illustrations of healthy eating.[2] To assist AYAs and their families in making good nutritional choices, the U.S. Department of Agriculture (USDA) designed the plate graphic, MyPlate.[3] MyPlate includes sections for vegetables, fruits, grains, and foods high in protein. MyPlate's user-friendly, interactive website provides simple messages for AYAs and their families (Fig. 6.1).

POTENTIAL NUTRITIONAL PROBLEMS

The National Health and Nutrition Examination Survey (NHANES)[4] concluded that the highest prevalence of unsatisfactory nutritional status occurs in the adolescent age group. Of note, there were deficiencies noted in the intake of calcium, iron, riboflavin, thiamine, and vitamins A and C.

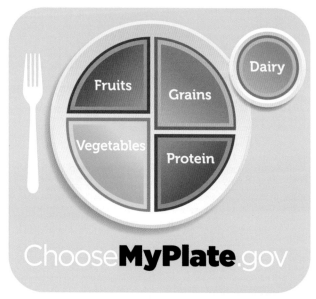

FIGURE 6.1 The My Plate site provides a range of healthy eating strategies and advice for professionals and consumers. (From the USDA Center for Nutrition Policy and Promotion's ChooseMyPlate.gov website.)

Risk Factors

1. Increased nutritional needs during adolescence are related to several factors.
   a. Adolescents gain 20% of their adult height.
   b. Adolescents gain at least 50% of their adult skeletal mass (i.e., peak bone mass).
   c. Caloric and protein requirements are maximal.
   d. Specific nutrient needs—for example, gender, chronic illness
2. Increased physical activities of AYAs make proper nutrition essential.
3. Eating habits of AYAs may contribute to nutritional problems.[5–8]
   a. Increasing autonomy during adolescence is associated with the adolescent making independent food choices and purchases.
   b. Missed meals are common, especially breakfast.
   c. High-energy snacks of low nutritional value are popular.
   d. Peer pressure leads to changes in a range of eating behaviors, including restrictive and overeating patterns, purging behaviors, and fad diets.

e. Positive role modeling is important in establishing an adolescent's food choices. The adolescent's family may exhibit poor eating habits, and meal preparation may be inadequate.

f. Social constraints on families may require multiple parents/caregivers, eating out, and fast-food consumption.

g. Inadequate financial resources to purchase food or to prepare nutritious meals

4. In AYAs, dietary choices contribute to an increased risk for cardiovascular disease.

a. Low fruit and vegetable consumption and high-sweetened beverage consumption are independently associated with the prevalence of metabolic syndrome in specific sex–ethnicity populations.

b. High-fiber diets may protect against obesity and cardiovascular disease by lowering insulin levels, among other factors.

5. Social media has an influence on AYAs' food choices.[9,10]

a. Exposure to image-related content may negatively impact body image and food choices in some healthy young people.

b. Young people exposed to unhealthy food images consume greater number of calories.

c. Social peers have been shown to influence a young person's food choices.

NUTRITIONAL ASSESSMENT

Assessing the nutrition of an adolescent or young adult should be part of a comprehensive health evaluation. This becomes even more important in AYAs who are identified as nutritionally at risk. Such young people include those with nutrition-related medical conditions, dietary deficiencies, or those with conditions that predispose them to inadequate nutrition. Nutritional assessment requires repeated measurements of nutritional status over time. Methods used in the nutritional assessment of adolescents include dietary and clinical evaluation, measurements of body composition, and obtaining laboratory data.

Dietary Data

There is a range of validated strategies used to obtain dietary data from AYAs. These include food records, 24-hour recall of all food consumed, food frequency questionnaires, and other questionnaires.[11]

An example of screening questions that are quick and easy to ask include the following:

1. How many meals do you usually eat in a day? Any snacks?
2. Tell me everything you have eaten in the past 24 hours.
3. Are there any foods that you have eliminated from your diet? If yes, why?
4. Are you on a diet?
5. Are you comfortable with your eating habits?
6. Do you ever eat in secret? Do you ever feel that you can't stop eating?
7. Have you recently lost or gained weight, or has your weight stayed the same?
8. Do you feel that your weight is too much, too little, or about right?
9. What is the most you have ever weighed, and what would you like to weigh?

Helpful screening questions for AYAs (followed by the associated sensitivity and specificity) for disordered eating in adolescence include the following[12]:

1. How many diets have you been on in the past year? (Two or three diets, 88% sensitivity and 63% specificity; four or five diets, 69% sensitivity and 86% specificity)
2. Do you feel that you should be dieting? (Often, 94% sensitivity and 67% specificity; usually, 87% sensitivity and 82% specificity)

3. Do you feel dissatisfied with your body size? (Often, 96% sensitivity and 61% specificity; usually, 88% sensitivity and 74% specificity)
4. Does your weight affect the way you feel about yourself? (Often, 97% sensitivity and 61% specificity; usually, 91% sensitivity and 74% specificity)

Each of these questions appears to have a very high correlation with the score on the Eating Attitudes Test (EAT-26) www.psychology-tools.com/test/eat-26. This screening test examines attitudes and behaviors regarding food, weight, and body image and has been validated for use in AYAs.

Clinical Signs of Nutritional Deficiencies

Please see Table 6.1.

Anthropometric Measurements

1. Weight and height: Weight-for-age and height-for-age charts can be obtained from the Centers for Disease Control and Prevention (CDC) on their website at http://www.cdc.gov/growthcharts/.
2. Body mass index is a useful screening tool, but it has its limitations (see Chapter 38).
3. Skinfold measurements and waist–hip ratio provide valuable information in a nutritional assessment. These measurements

TABLE 6.1

Clinical Manifestations of Nutritional Deficiency

Body Parts	Nutritional Deficiency	Clinical Manifestations of Deficiency
Skin	Iron	Pallor
	Vitamin A	Follicular hyperkeratosis
	Hyperlipidemia	Xanthoma
	Vitamin C	Petechiae
	Vitamin K, C, and folate	Bruising and purpura
Eyes	Riboflavin, niacin	Angular palpebritis
	Vitamin A	Night blindness
Lips	Riboflavin, niacin	Angular stomatitis
		Cheilosis
Tongue	Niacin, folic acid, vitamins B_6 and B_{12}	Glossitis
	Niacin, folic acid, vitamins B_6 and B_{12}, or iron	Papillary atrophy
	Zinc	Loss of taste and appetite
Gums	Vitamin C	Hypertrophy, bleeding
Teeth	Diet high in refined sugars	Cavities
Hair	Protein–energy malnutrition	Dry, dull, brittle
Neck	Iodine	Goiter
Nails	Malnutrition, iron, or calcium	Brittle with frayed borders
	Vitamin A	Concave or eggshell
	Vitamin C	Hangnails
Bones and Joints	Vitamin D	Rickets
	Vitamin C	Scurvy

can assist in quantifying obesity and have shown to have predictive value with respect to health outcomes such as cardiovascular disease and insulin resistance. They are not, however, currently recommended for clinical use because they require specific training to perform accurately.

Laboratory Tests

Laboratory tests helpful in assessing nutritional status include hemoglobin, hematocrit, ferritin, serum protein, albumin, and vitamins D, B_{12}, and folate.

Nutritional Requirements

Dietary reference intakes (DRIs) represent quantitative estimates of nutrients used to plan and evaluate diets for healthy people, including AYAs.[13] The DRIs are a set of four nutrient reference values that vary by age and sex and include the following:

1. Recommended dietary allowance (RDA): This is the dietary intake level that is sufficient to meet the nutrient requirements of almost all healthy individuals (97% to 98%) in the United States.
2. Adequate intake (AI): This is the value based on observed or experimentally determined approximations of nutrient intake by a group—used when RDA cannot be determined.
3. Estimated average requirement (EAR): This is the intake value that is estimated to meet the requirement defined by a specified indicator of adequacy in 50% of an age- and gender-specific group. At this level of intake, the remaining 50% of the specified group would not have its needs met.
4. Tolerable upper intake level (UL): This is the maximum level of daily nutrient intake that is unlikely to pose risks of adverse health effects to almost all individuals in the group for whom it is designed.

The DRIs cover the following groups of nutrients:
1. Calcium, vitamin D, phosphorus, magnesium, and fluoride
2. Folate and other B vitamins
3. Antioxidants (e.g., vitamin C, vitamin E, selenium)
4. Macronutrients (e.g., proteins, fats, carbohydrates)
5. Trace elements (e.g., iron, zinc)
6. Electrolytes and water
7. Other food components (e.g., fiber, phytoestrogens)

The requirements are reported to differ slightly in AYAs between 19 and 30 years of age.

Energy Requirements

Energy requirements are determined by basal metabolic rate, growth status, physical activity, and body composition. Energy requirements of adolescents vary depending on the timing of growth and pubertal development. As such, energy needs are based on height because it provides a better estimate of total daily caloric recommendations. Suggested caloric intakes are listed in **Table 6.2**.

Protein

Protein provides 4 kcal of energy in each gram. Protein requirements are based on the amount of protein needed to maintain existing lean body mass and the increase in additional lean body mass with growth and development. Protein requirements are highest during the peak height velocity. In the populations surveyed in the United States, most AYA diets exceed the RDA for protein.

Carbohydrates

Carbohydrates provide 4 kcal of energy in each gram. Carbohydrates should make up approximately 50% of the daily caloric intake. However, no more than 10% to 25% of calories should come from sweeteners (sucrose and high-fructose corn syrup). Nearly 12% of carbohydrates consumed by AYAs come from the added sweeteners in soft drinks.

Carbohydrate-containing foods include grain products, fruits, and vegetables. Approximately 25 to 35 g of fiber should be consumed daily. Fiber is found in whole grain foods, fruits, vegetables, legumes, nuts, and seeds.

Glycemic index (GI) classifies carbohydrate foods based on the effect on blood glucose. The GI represents the relative rise in the blood glucose level two hours after consuming that food. The index ranges from 0 to 100, with glucose or other reference standards being 100. Hence, the lower the GI, the lower the expected rise in blood sugar for a given food. In general, foods are classified into low GI (<40), moderate GI (40 to 70), and high GI (>70).

Alcohol provides 7 kcal of energy in each gram and can also be a significant source of calories with no nutritional benefits.

Fat

Fat provides 9 kcal of energy in each gram. Adolescents and young adults require dietary fat and essential fatty acids for many vital

TABLE 6.2

Recommended Dietary Allowances for Adolescents and Young Adults

Category	Male (y) 11–14	15–18	19–24	Female (y) 11–14	15–18	19–24	Pregnancy	Lactating (first 6 mo)	Lactating (second 6 mo)
Weight (kg)	45	66	72	46	55	58			
Height (cm)	157	176	177	157	163	164			
Energy (cal)	2,500	3,000	2,900	2,200	2,200	2,200	+300	+500	+500
Protein (g)	45	59	58	46	44	46	60	65	62
Minerals									
Iron (mg/d)	12	12	10	15	15	15	30	15	15
Zinc (mg/d)	15	15	15	12	12	12	15	19	16
Iodine (mcg/d)	150	150	150	150	150	150	175	200	200
Vitamins									
Vitamin A (IU)	10	10	10	10	10	10	10	10	10

Cal, calorie; g, grams; kg, kilogram; cm, centimeter.
Adapted from the U.S. Department of Health and Human Services—National Institute of Health. 2020. https://www.hc-sc.gc.ca/fn-an/alt_formats/hpfb-dgpsa/pdf/nutrition/dri_tables-eng.pdf

functions in the body. An AYA diet should contain no more than 30% of calories from fat. Most AYAs' total and saturated fat intake is greater than that recommended. For AYAs, trans fatty acid (TFA) intake should be reduced as much as possible because of its adverse effects on lipids and lipoproteins. The replacement of TFA with other saturated and unsaturated fatty acids in foods beneficially affects low-density lipoprotein cholesterol, the primary target for cardiovascular disease risk reduction.

Minerals

Iron There is an increased need for iron in both males and females during adolescence because of the rapid growth and increase in muscle mass and blood volume. In addition, AYA females require increase in iron because of menstrual losses. High-iron foods include lean meats, fish, and eggs. Nonheme iron present in plant sources is less bioavailable, but its absorption can be enhanced by concurrent intake of vitamin C.

Calcium Requirements for dietary calcium increase substantially during periods of peak velocity of growth and accrual of bone mineral content. Adolescents and young adults tend to eat a diet deficient in calcium. The DRI for calcium for 9- to 18-year-olds is 1,300 mg/day (Table 6.3). Many AYAs have inadequate calcium intake, in part due to the substitution of carbonated beverages for milk and increasing concern about lactose intolerance.

Those AYAs not taking in adequate calcium from food sources may need to take supplemental calcium such as calcium carbonate, citrate, lactate, or phosphate (absorption varies from 25% to 35%). In the context of normal vitamin D levels, optimal absorption of the calcium supplements occurs when no more than 500 mg/dose is taken with food. In addition to dairy products, calcium is found in tofu, salmon, sardines, dark green leafy vegetables, and calcium-fortified foods (such as orange juice; soy, almond, and rice milk; and some fortified breakfast cereals). Adequate levels of vitamin D are required for optimal calcium absorption from the intestine.

Zinc Zinc is needed for adequate growth, sexual maturation, and wound healing. The RDA for zinc is 8 mg/day for adolescents 9 to 13 years old and 9 mg/day and 11 mg/day for females and males 11 to 14 years old, respectively. Young adults have slightly decreased requirement. Good food sources of zinc include lean meats, seafood, eggs, and milk.

Vitamins

Vitamin requirements increase during adolescence, especially for vitamin B_{12}; folate; vitamins A, C, D, and E; thiamine; niacin; and riboflavin (see Table 6.3). It has been shown that supplements of antioxidant vitamins (A, C, E, and *b*-carotene) probably reduce the risk of cardiovascular disease and certain cancers, but there is no current recommendation to prescribe them routinely.

TABLE 6.3

Recommended Dietary Allowances (Light Face Type) and Adequate Intake (Bold Face Type) Values, by Age

Daily Amount	Male (y)			Female (y)			Pregnant (y)		Lactating (y)	
	9–13	14–18	19–30	9–13	14–18	19–30	<19	19–30	<19	19–30
Calcium (mg)	1,300	1,300	1,000	1,300	1,300	1,000	1,300	1,000	1,300	1,000
Phosphorus (mg)	1,250	1,250	700	1,250	1,250	700	1,250	700	1,250	700
Magnesium (mg)	240	410	400	1,250	1,250	700	1,250	700	1,250	700
Fluoride (mg)	2	3	4	2	3	3	3	3	3	3
Selenium (pg)	40	55	55	40	55	55	60	60	70	70
Vitamin C (mg)	45	75	90	45	65	75	80	85	115	120
Vitamin D (mcg)	5	5	5	5	5	5	5	5	5	5
Vitamin E (mg)	11	15	15	11	15	15	15	15	19	19
Thiamine (mg)	1.2	1.2	1.2	0.9	1.0	1.1	1.4	1.4	1.5	1.5
Riboflavin (mg)	0.9	1.3	1.3	0.9	1.0	1.1	1.4	1.4	1.6	1.6
Niacin (mg)	12	16	16	12	14	14	18	18	17	17
Vitamin B_6 (mg)	1.0	1.3	1.3	1.0	1.2	1.3	1.9	1.9	2.0	2.0
Folacin (mcg)	300	400	400	300	400	400	600	600	500	500
Vitamin B_{12} (mcg)	1.8	2.4	2.4	1.8	2.4	2.4	2.6	2.6	2.8	2.8
Pantothenic acid (B_5) (mg)	4	5	5	4	5	5	6	6	7	7
Biotin (mcg)	20	25	30	20	25	30	30	30	35	35
Choline (mg)	375	550	550	375	550	550	450	450	550	550

Adapted from the U.S. Department of Health and Human Services – National Institute of Health. 2020. https://www.hc-sc.gc.ca/fn-an/alt_formats/hpfb-dgpsa/pdf/nutrition/dri_tables-eng.pdf

🔴 GUIDELINES FOR NUTRITIONAL THERAPY

General Recommendations

1. Be aware of and sensitive to the family context, lifestyle, and cultural milieu.
2. Motivate lifestyle change by stressing the positive effects of dietary changes, for example, feeling good about oneself, feeling energetic.
3. Use the MyPlate Food Guide (see Fig. 6.1) to recommend the appropriate number of daily servings and quantity from each food group.
4. Recommend that AYAs participate in a regular exercise program for at least 30 minutes, at least 4 days of the week. Balance dietary energy intake with physical activity to maintain normal growth and development.
5. Simplify good nutrition concepts by recommending the following to AYAs and their families:
   • Maintain a healthy body weight.
   • Eat a wide variety of nutritious foods, including lean meat, fish, and poultry.
   • Limit solid fats (butter, margarine, shortening, lard) and choose foods low in saturated fat and TFA. Use more polyunsaturated fats.
   • Broil or bake instead of frying foods.
   • Use nonfat (skim) or low-fat milk and dairy products daily.
   • Eat plenty of vegetables, legumes, and fruits.
   • Eat plenty of cereals (including breads, rice, pasta, and noodles), preferably wholegrain.
   • Drink water instead of soft drinks or fruit drinks. Limit juice intake.
   • Eat meals and snacks regularly. Eating family meals is correlated with improved nutritional intake and reduces the likelihood that youth will develop eating disorders.[4,5]

Special Conditions

Vegetarian Diets

Adolescents and young adults may choose vegetarian diets because of ecologic, economic, religious, or philosophical beliefs. Adolescents and young adults who are vegetarians (but not choosing to be vegan) are likely to have an adequate nutritional intake. Nutritional counseling may be of benefit to ensure adequate intake of energy, protein, and micronutrients as well as to assess the need for micronutrient supplements.[14–16]

Types of Vegetarians[17]

Semivegetarians eat milk products and limited seafood and poultry but no red meat.
Lactovegetarians consume milk products but no eggs, meat, fish, or poultry.
Ovolactovegetarians consume milk products and eggs but no meat, fish, or poultry.
Vegans consume vegetable foods only and no foods of animal origin (i.e., no eggs, milk products, meat, fish, or poultry).
Fruitarians consume raw fruit and seeds only. Examples of such fruits include pineapple, mango, banana, avocado, apple, melon, orange, all kinds of berries, and the vegetable fruits such as tomato, cucumber, olives, and nuts.

Supplemental Needs of Vegetarians Potential nutritional issues with vegetarian diets include macronutrient and micronutrient deficiencies such as protein, fat, vitamin B_{12}, iron, zinc, calcium, and vitamin D.

Vitamins: Semivegetarians, lactovegetarians, and ovolactovegetarians have no need for supplements if attention is paid to dietary composition. Vegans may need supplemental iron, calcium, riboflavin, and vitamins B_{12} and D.

Protein: Adequate protein intake has been a traditional concern for vegetarians; however, vegetarians usually meet or exceed protein requirements (except for vegans). There is also mounting evidence that the practice of eating complementary proteins in the same meal is unnecessary. However, it is recommended that the day's meals supply all of them.

Minerals: There is no uniform need for supplements, but vegetarians are at increased risk for iron and zinc deficiencies. Vegetarians may need up to 50% more zinc in their diet since phytate (found in plants) and calcium hinder zinc absorption.

Lactose Intolerance

Adolescents and young adults with lactose intolerance are at risk of inadequate calcium intake. Some AYAs with lactose intolerance can tolerate small amounts of milk products, including aged cheese or yogurt with active cultures. There are many nondairy foods high in calcium, including green vegetables, such as broccoli and kale; fish with edible bones, such as salmon and sardines; calcium-fortified orange juice; and soy, almond, and rice milk. There are a variety of lactose-reduced/dairy-free products in the supermarket, including milk, butter, cottage cheese, ice cream, and processed cheese slices. Adolescents and young adults often find lactase enzyme replacement pills or liquid helpful (see Chapter 41).[18]

Pregnancy

Energy requirements are greater for pregnant compared with nonpregnant AYAs. Adolescents may require higher energy intake than young adults. As indicated in Table 6.2, pregnant adolescents should not consume less than 2,000 kcal/day and in many cases, their needs may be higher. The best gauge of adequate energy intake during pregnancy is satisfactory weight gain. Goals for weight gain are based on prepregnancy weight, height, age, stage of development, and usual eating patterns. Young pregnant females who are below an optimal weight are advised to gain more weight than females living with obesity.[19]

Folate is essential for nucleic acid synthesis and is required in greater amounts during pregnancy. Taking folic acid before and during early pregnancy can reduce the risk of spina bifida and other neural tube defects. Because these defects occur early in gestation, it is advised that females of childbearing age and those who can become pregnant consume 400 mcg/day of folic acid. The DRI for folate during pregnancy is 600 mcg/day. Good sources of folate include leafy dark green vegetables, legumes, citrus fruits and juices, peanuts, whole grains, and some fortified breakfast cereals.

The calcium recommendation during pregnancy is 1,300 mg/day for adolescents and 1,000 mg/day for young adults. Since most nonpregnant AYA females consume significantly less than the recommended amount of calcium, pregnant AYAs should either add calcium-rich foods to their diet or take calcium supplementation.

Dietary counseling can be one of the most important interventions for a pregnant AYA to ensure a healthy pregnancy and a healthy baby. Adolescents and young adults should be encouraged to obtain their nutrients from food. A low-dose vitamin–mineral supplement is recommended for pregnant adolescents who do not regularly consume a healthy diet. Adolescents and young adults should be counseled against dieting during pregnancy.

Athletes

Risk for Iron and Zinc Deficiency Both male and female AYA athletes are at risk for iron deficiency.[20] Athletes (especially menstruating females and those involved in endurance sports such as distance running) should be screened for low hemoglobin or hematocrit levels. Serum ferritin can be helpful in determining loss of iron stores and need for supplementation. A ferritin level of <16 mcg/L corresponds with depleted iron stores. For the athlete who is not anemic but has low iron stores (latent iron deficiency), 50 to 100 mg of elemental iron daily (ferrous gluconate 240 or 325 mg twice daily or ferrous sulfate 325 mg daily or twice daily) should be recommended. For the anemic athlete, 100 to 200 mg of elemental iron daily (ferrous gluconate 325 mg three times daily or ferrous sulfate 325 mg twice daily) should be given. Laboratory measurements should be repeated after 2 to 3 months to document response to therapy. Athletes with iron-deficiency anemia may also be zinc deficient. Education regarding good dietary sources of zinc and iron should be provided.[15,21]

Sodium and Potassium Athletes need increased intake of sodium and potassium. This requirement will generally be met as they increase their calorie intake.[22]

Calories The active athlete who engages in 2 hours/day of heavy exercise needs 800 to 1,700 extra calories/day beyond the recommended minimum for age, sex, height, and weight to maintain energy balance. The American Dietetic Association recommends the approximate distribution of calories should be carbohydrates, 55% to 60%; proteins, 12% to 15%; and fats, 25% to 30%.[23]

Hydration Attention must be given to hydration before and during activity.[24]
- Athletes should drink 10 to 16 oz (300 to 500 mL) of cold water 1 to 2 hours before exercise.
- Repeat 20 to 30 minutes before exercise.
- Drink 4 to 6 oz (300 to 500 mL) of cold water every 10 to 15 minutes during exercise.
- Cold fluids are preferable.
- Plain water can be used for exercise periods of <2 hours.
- Sports drinks may be used to provide carbohydrates for longer events. Fructose-containing solutions should be avoided since they are not as well absorbed as solutions with sucrose or glucose and can cause gastrointestinal upset.

Weight Restrictions Avoid any major weight restriction during the adolescent growth spurt. Alterations in diet to cause rapid weight gain or loss should be discouraged. Eating disorders are prevalent among athletes (largely female athletes), especially in those involved in running, solitary sports; swimming, diving, gymnastics, or dance (see Chapter 33). It is important to carefully explore issues related to body image, desired weight, and menstrual function in all athletes. Relative energy deficiency in sport (RED-S) is a condition of low energy availability and should be suspected in female and male athletes where dietary energy intake is insufficient to support the energy expended (see Chapter 38).

Carbohydrate Loading Diets that are chronically high in carbohydrates are not recommended. For optimal performance, the athlete should train lightly or rest 24 to 36 hours before competition. On the day of competition, the athlete may consider a high-carbohydrate, low-fat meal 3 to 6 hours before an event and an optional snack 1 to 2 hours before the event. Foods high in carbohydrates (60% to 70%) have also been recommended after competition to replace glycogen stores. A diet of 5,000 kcal/day that is only 45% carbohydrate is sufficient to restore muscle glycogen within 24 hours. An initial "depletion phase" consisting of vigorous workouts and low-carbohydrate eating before competition is also not recommended.[25]

Nutritional Supplements[26] The word "ergogenic" is derived from the Greek word ergon, which means "to increase work or potential for work." Anecdotal reports suggest that compounds such as bee pollen, caffeine, glycine, carnitine, lecithin, brewer's yeast, and gelatin improve strength or endurance. However, scientific research has failed to substantiate these claims.[27]

Adolescent and young adult athletes who are considering the use of nutritional supplements should be aware that the effects of long-term supplement use have not been studied. In addition, supplement use can be quite costly. Most athletes can maximize their performance through consistent, appropriate training and attention to adequate nutrition rather than relying on supplement use (http://www.drugfreesport.com/choices/supplements/). See Chapter 8 for further discussion on herbal therapies. Gains in muscle mass may best be sought by attempting to take advantage of timing of ingestion and composition of the proteins or amino acids ingested. Most athletes habitually ingest sufficient protein, therefore, recommending greater protein intakes does not appear warranted. Current literature suggests that it may be too simplistic to rely on recommendations of a particular commercial formulation, given the metabolic response is dependent on other factors, including the timing of ingestion in relation to exercise and/or other factors, such as the composition of ingested amino acids. Excessive protein intakes are unlikely to be advantageous. Nevertheless, the popularity of protein supplements in the form of powders and shakes continues for AYAs involved in physical training. There remains much to be studied about the optimal protein intake and long-term studies on the impact of different amounts of protein on performance variables, body composition, as well as the metabolic and molecular mechanisms relevant to physical performance.

Probiotics and Prebiotics[28] Probiotics are live microorganisms that, when administered in adequate amounts, may confer a health benefit on the host. Prebiotics are typically complex carbohydrates (such as inulin and other fructo-oligosaccharides) that microorganisms in the gastrointestinal tract use as metabolic fuel. Absorption and metabolism are altered through manipulation of the intestinal flora using these agents. Use of prebiotics and probiotics has been shown to modify symptoms in AYAs for conditions such as atopic dermatitis, antibiotic-associated diarrhea, irritable bowel syndrome, hypercholesterolemia, and obesity.

SUMMARY

Nutrition is an essential component of AYA health care. Optimal nutrition assists in reaching the potential for physical growth, development, and the prevention of illness. Healthy food choices vary with social circumstances and knowledge. Clinicians are in an optimal position to provide nutrition screening, assessment, and counseling to AYAs as a part of health supervision visits.

REFERENCES

1. Institute of Medicine. *Dietary Reference Intakes for Calcium and Vitamin D*. The National Academies Press; 2010. Appendix 7. Nutritional goals for age-sex groups based on dietary reference intakes and dietary guidelines recommendations. https://health.gov/our-work/food-nutrition/2015-2020-dietary-guidelines/guidelines/appendix-7/
2. https://www.dietaryguidelines.gov/sites/default/files/2020-12/Dietary_Guidelines_for_Americans_2020-2025.pdf
3. https://www.myplate.gov
4. https://www.cdc.gov/nchs/nhanes/index.htm
5. Larson N, MacLehose R, Fulkerson JA, et al. Eating breakfast and dinner together as a family: associations with sociodemographic characteristics and implications for diet quality and weight status. *J Acad Nutr Diet*. 2013;113(12):1601–1609.
6. Neumark-Sztainer D, Larson NI, Fulkerson JA, et al. Family meals and adolescents: what have we learned from Project EAT (Eating Among Teens)? *Public Health Nutr*. 2010;13(7):1113–1121. doi:10.1017/S1368980010000169
7. Anstine D, Grinenko D. Rapid screening for disordered eating in college aged females in the primary care setting. *J Adolesc Health*. 2000;26(5):338–342.
8. https://www.nede.com.au/NEDC-Resources/NEDC-Resources-GP.pdf
9. Hawkins LK, Farrow C, Thomas JM. Do perceived norms of social media users' eating habits and preferences predict our own food consumption and BMI? *Appetite*. 2020;149:104611. doi: 10.1016/j.appet.2020.104611. Epub 2020 Jan 18. PMID: 31958481.
10. Klassen KM, Douglass CH, Brennan L, et al. Social media use for nutrition outcomes in young adults: a mixed-methods systematic review. *Int J Behav Nutr Phys Act*. 2018;15(1):70. doi:10.1186/s12966-018-0696-y
11. https://epi.grants.cancer.gov/past-initiatives/assess_wc/review/agegroups/adolescents/validation.html?&url=/tools/children/review/agegroups/adolescents/validation.html
12. Gleaves DH, Pearson CA, Ambwani S, et al. Measuring eating disorder attitudes and behaviors: a reliability generalization study. *J Eat Disord*. 2014;2;6.
13. Dietary reference intakes definitions, and units with conversion tables. http://www.hc-sc.gc.ca/fn-an/alt_formats/hpfb-dgpsa/pdf/nutrition/dri_tables-eng.pdf
14. Winston JC, Health effects of vegan diets, *Am J Clin Nutr*. 2009;89(5):1627S–16 33S. https://doi.org/10.3945/ajcn.2009.26736N

15. Melina V, Craig W, Levin S. Position of the Academy of Nutrition and Dietetics: vegetarian diets. *J Acad Nutr Diet*. 2016;116(12):1970–1980. doi: 10.1016/j.jand.2016.09.025

16. Fassio F, Facioni MS, Guagnini F. Lactose maldigestion, malabsorption, and intolerance: a comprehensive review with a focus on current management and future perspectives. *Nutrients*. 2018;10(11):1599. doi:10.3390/nu10111599

17. http://www.vrg.org/

18. Yin J, Quinn S, Dwyer T, et al. Maternal diet, breastfeeding and adolescent body composition: a 16-year prospective study. *Eur J Clin Nutr*. 2012;66(12):1329–1334.

19. Marvin-Dowle K, Burley VJ, Soltani H. Nutrient intakes and nutritional biomarkers in pregnant adolescents: a systematic review of studies in developed countries. *BMC Pregnancy Childbirth*. 2016;16:268. https://doi.org/10.1186/s12884-016-1059-9

20. Vandevijvere S, Michels N, Verstraete S, et al. Intake and dietary sources of haem and non-haem iron among European adolescents and their association with iron status and different lifestyle and socio-economic factors. *Eur J Clin Nutr*. 2013;67(7):765.

21. Domellöf M, Thorsdottir I, Thorstensen K. Health effects of different dietary iron intakes: a systematic literature review for the 5th Nordic Nutrition Recommendations. *Food Nutr Res*. 2013;12;57.

22. Thomas DT, Erdman KA, Burke LM. American College of Sports Medicine joint position statement. Nutrition and athletic performance. *Med Sci Sports Exerc*. 2016;48(3):543–568. doi: 10.1249/MSS.0000000000000852

23. Sim A, Burns SF. Review: questionnaires as measures for low energy availability (LEA) and relative energy deficiency in sport (RED-S) in athletes. *J Eat Disord*. 2021;9(1):41. doi:10.1186/s40337-021-00396-7

24. https://www.usada.org/athletes/substances/nutrition/fluids-and-hydration/

25. Gonzalez JT, Betts JA. Dietary sugars, exercise and hepatic carbohydrate metabolism. *Proc Nutr Soc*. 2019;78(2):246–256. doi:10.1017/S0029665118002604

26. Peeling P, Binnie MJ, Goods PSR, et al. Evidence-based supplements for the enhancement of athletic performance. *Int J Sport Nutr Exerc Metab*. 2018;28(2):178–187. Accessed April 30, 2020. https://journals.humankinetics.com/view/journals/ijsnem/28/2/article-p178.xml

27. Buckman JF, Farris SG, Yusko DA. A national study of substance use behaviors among NCAA male athletes who use banned performance enhancing substances. *Drug Alcohol Depend*. 2013;131(1/2):50–55.

28. Salminen S, Collado MC, Endo A, et al. The International Scientific Association of Probiotics and Prebiotics (ISAPP) consensus statement on the definition and scope of postbiotics. *Nat Rev Gastroenterol Hepatol*. 2021;18(9):649–667. doi: 10.1038/s41575-021-00440-6. Epub 2021 May 4. PMID: 33948025

ADDITIONAL RESOURCES AND WEBSITES

Additional Resources and Websites for Clinicians:

Chau MM, Burgermaster M, Mamykina L. The use of social media in nutrition interventions for adolescents and young adults—a systematic review. *Int J Med Inform*. 2018;120: 77–91. doi: 10.1016/j.ijmedinf.2018.10.001

Dietary Guidelines for Americans, 2015–202, 8th ed.—https://health.gov/sites/default/files/2019-09/2015-2020_Dietary_Guidelines.pdf

Larson N, Neumark-Sztainer D. Adolescent nutrition. *Pediatr Rev*. 2009; 30(12): 494–496. doi: 10.1542/pir.30-12-494

Probiotics Fact Sheet for Health Professionals—https://ods.od.nih.gov/factsheets/Probiotics-HealthProfessional

Additional Resources and Websites for Parents/Caregivers:

American Academy of Pediatrics—A Teenager's Nutritional Needs—https://www.healthychildren.org/English/ages-stages/teen/nutrition/Pages/A-Teenagers-Nutritional-Needs.aspx

American Youth Academy—A Strategic Plan on Wellness Policies for Nutrition and Physical Activities 2021–2022—https://www.ayatampa.org/aya-wellness-policy.html

Healthy Eating During Adolescence—https://www.hopkinsmedicine.org/health/wellness-and-prevention/healthy-eating-during-adolescence

Additional Resources and Websites for Adolescents and Young Adults:

Duyff RL. *Academy of Nutrition and Dietetics Complete Food and Nutrition Guide*. 5th ed. Houghton Mifflin; 2017.

Resch E. *The Intuitive Eating Workbook for Teens: A Non-Diet, Body Positive Approach to Building a Healthy Relationship with Food*. Instant Help Books, An imprint of New Harbinger Publications, Inc.; 2019.

Slomin, J. *Sports Nutrition For Young Adults: A Game-Winning Guide to Maximize Performance*. Rockridge Press; 2020.

The Women's, The Royal Women's Hospital, Victoria Australia—Food and Nutrition for Adolescents—https://www.thewomens.org.au/health-information/staying-well/adolescent-girls/food-and-nutrition-for-adolescents

CHAPTER 7

Understanding Legal and Ethical Aspects of Care

Abigail English
Rebecca Gudeman

KEY WORDS

- Affordable Care Act (ACA)
- Confidentiality
- Consent
- Electronic health information (EHI)
- Ethics
- Family Educational Rights and Privacy Act (FERPA)
- Health Insurance Portability and Accountability Act (HIPAA)
- Law
- Payment
- Telehealth

INTRODUCTION

Clinicians treating adolescents and young adults (AYAs) must have a clear understanding of the legal framework within which care is provided. The laws differ based on age, legal status, and geography. This chapter discusses the legal framework in the United States. Application of laws related to consent, confidentiality, and payment may vary in different clinical settings and for different populations.

In the United States, the governing laws for young adults aged 18 years or older are typically the same as those for other adults. For minors—younger than age 18 years in almost all states—the laws may differ. The legal issues that arise most frequently fall into three specific areas:

1. Consent: Who is authorized to give consent for the minor's or young adult's care and whose consent is required?
2. Confidentiality: Who has the right to control the release of confidential information about the care, including medical records and electronic health information (EHI), and who has the right to receive such information?
3. Payment: Who is financially liable for payment and is there a source of insurance coverage or is public funding available that the AYA can access?

These issues of consent, confidentiality, and payment are handled differently depending on the setting and mechanism for delivering care; specialized settings, such as schools, and mechanisms, such as telehealth, warrant special attention.

LEGAL FRAMEWORK

An important aspect of the legal framework is that laws vary from state to state and change frequently. Interpretation and implementation of both federal and state laws also vary among health care sites and institutions. Therefore, it is essential for clinicians to be familiar with the applicable laws in their jurisdiction. Clinicians with questions about their obligations should consult legal counsel.

Constitutional Rights

Beginning more than 50 years ago, a series of U.S. Supreme Court decisions recognized that minors as well as adults have constitutional rights. These decisions delineated federal constitutional protections for minors related to due process in juvenile court, the death penalty, free speech, privacy, and other rights. Some subsequent Supreme Court decisions were more equivocal about the scope of minors' constitutional rights, and the future scope of those rights is not certain, but basic principles articulated in the early cases still stand at this time.

One area of frequent constitutional litigation with major implications for the rights of AYAs has been reproductive health care—abortion and contraception. In 1973, the Supreme Court decided *Roe v. Wade*, establishing federal constitutional protection for abortion, followed by a decision recognizing that minors have privacy rights and protecting their access to abortion.[1,2] Supreme Court decisions also provided constitutional protection for contraception for both adults and minors.[3–5] In 2022, in *Dobbs v. Jackson Women's Health Organization*, the Court upended the framework that had been in place for almost 50 years and overruled *Roe v. Wade*.[6] The *Dobbs* decision means that there is no longer a federal constitutional right to abortion. However, *Dobbs* does not mean that abortion is illegal or unconstitutional; it leaves the determination to the U.S. Congress and the states whether to ban abortion, impose restrictions, or affirmatively protect abortion access. As of July 2022, no federal statutes protect abortion or impose a ban, but numerous states have imposed partial or total bans while others have moved quickly to protect access to abortion.[7] In the absence of federal guideposts, state constitutional protections become important. Some state constitutions have an explicit right to privacy that has been interpreted to protect reproductive choice.[7] Other states are moving to add constitutional amendments that either restrict or protect abortion.[7] Thus, the landscape for abortion is evolving rapidly at the federal and state level, and clinicians should be aware of the specific status of abortion rights for AYAs in their state. The *Dobbs* decision did not overrule any of the cases establishing constitutional protection for contraception, but this is an issue of great importance for AYAs that should be monitored in the future.

State and Federal Laws

Most of the specific legal provisions that affect AYAs' access to health care are contained in state and federal statutes and regulations or in court decisions. These provisions cover a broad range of issues related to consent, confidentiality, and payment, and are critical in defining the parameters of what clinicians are legally permitted and required to do. Therefore, clinicians must develop a familiarity not only with the general constitutional principles that have evolved in recent decades but also with federal laws and state laws, including court decisions, that apply in their own states.

CONSENT

The law generally requires the consent of a parent before medical care can be provided to a minor but provides numerous exceptions. Often, someone other than a biologic or adoptive parent—such as a guardian, caretaker relative, foster parent, juvenile court, social worker, or probation officer—may be able to give consent in the place of the parent. State law typically dictates which adults may provide substitute consent. In emergency situations, care may be provided without prior consent to safeguard the life and health of the minor, or may be provided with the minor's consent, although typically parents must be notified as soon as possible thereafter. Other significant exceptions to the parent consent requirement typically authorize minors to consent for their own care based on either the type of services sought or the status of the minor.

All states have enacted one or more provisions that authorize minors to consent to certain health services.[8,9] These specific areas may include the following: contraceptive care; pregnancy-related care; diagnosis and treatment for sexually transmitted infections (STIs); diagnosis and treatment of either human immunodeficiency virus, or acquired immunodeficiency syndrome; diagnosis and treatment of reportable or communicable diseases; examination and treatment related to sexual assault; counseling and treatment related to substance use; and counseling and treatment for mental health issues. Few states have statutes covering all of these services. In many cases, the statutes contain minimum age requirements, which most frequently fall between the ages of 12 and 15 years.[8,9] The scope of covered services also may vary; for example, in some states, minors may consent to prevention, diagnosis, and treatment of STIs and in others only to diagnosis and treatment.

Similarly, all states have enacted one or more provisions that authorize minors who have attained a specific status to give consent for their own health care.[8,9] The groups of minors most frequently given this authority include minors who are legally emancipated by court order; living apart from their parents; married; in the armed services; or parents of a child.[8,9]

The Mature Minor Doctrine and Informed Consent

"Mature minor" is generally understood to mean a minor who exhibits the maturity to authorize their own health care. Even in the absence of a specific statute, "mature minors" may have the legal capacity to give consent for their own care. The basic criteria for determining whether a patient is capable of giving an informed consent are that the patient must be able to understand the risks and benefits of any proposed treatment or procedure and its alternatives and must be able to make a voluntary choice among the alternatives.[10] The "mature minor" doctrine has been recognized in statutes and in court decisions in a few states.[8]

Right to Refuse Treatment

Young adults with decision-making capacity are legally allowed to refuse medical care.[11] For minors, the right to consent to care may also encompass a right to refuse care. For example, a minor who has the right to choose an abortion also has the right to refuse an abortion. The issue becomes more complex when a minor refuses treatment that a parent or guardian has authorized. Some court decisions have addressed the issue in the context of potentially life-saving treatment and reached varying results, sometimes but not always allowing the minor to make the decision based on the mature minor rule.[12] A decades-old decision of the United States Supreme Court[13] granted minors some limited constitutional due process protections when they object to commitment to inpatient mental health facilities, leading to the enactment by many states of statutes establishing procedures for review of commitment when a minor objects. The issue may arise related to other medical care as well, such as use of psychotropic and other medications. In situations involving significant threats to life or health, where major disagreement exists between parents and a minor adolescent, legal counsel or an ethics review committee should be consulted.

Minors in State Custody and Consent

When minors are in state custody, either through the juvenile justice or child welfare system, questions often arise about who may consent for their health care. Minors typically retain their rights to consent to care under applicable minor consent laws even when in state custody. However, where parent consent is normally required, things can change. In some cases, when a minor is in state custody, the court, or state law, removes the right to consent from parents and appoints someone else to authorize health care for the minor. Even where parents retain the right to consent for their child's care, state law often authorizes others to consent for a minor's care in addition to a parent, either in general or in certain circumstances, such as emergencies. Laws may provide such authority to the court, social worker, foster parent, or probation officer. Clinicians treating a minor in state custody should not assume either that a parent can simply continue to consent for the minor's care or that a state custodian always has a right to consent.

Young Adults and Capacity to Consent

The law generally allows adults aged 18 years and older to consent to their own health care unless they lack the capacity to provide informed consent. "Capacity" is typically defined in state law and addressed by ethical principles, but generally, it means the capacity to understand the risks and benefits of a proposed treatment or procedure and its alternatives, and make a voluntary choice.[10] If a clinician believes that an adult patient does not have the capacity to consent either in a particular context or in general, state law typically provides alternative mechanisms to ensure patients receive appropriate and adequate health care. At the extreme, this may include asking a court to appoint a health care conservator to make medical decisions for the patient. Clinicians treating an adult who lacks capacity should not assume that a parent can simply continue to provide consent.

PRIVACY AND CONFIDENTIALITY

There are numerous reasons—grounded in both law and ethics—why it is important to maintain confidentiality in the delivery of health care services to AYAs. The confidentiality obligation has numerous sources in law and policy. They include the federal and state constitutions; federal statutes and regulations such as the rules issued under the Health Insurance Portability and Accountability Act (the HIPAA Privacy Rule and the HIPAA Security Rule),[14] Medicaid,[15] confidentiality regulations for Title X[16,17] and state family planning programs,[18] and federal substance use disorder confidentiality rules[19]; state statutes and regulations such as medical confidentiality and medical records laws, doctor–patient privilege statutes, professional licensing laws, and funding programs; court decisions; and professional ethical standards. Many health care professional organizations also have policy statements and codes of ethics that require confidentiality protections.[20,21]

In any given situation, one or several of the above laws and policies may apply depending upon the funding source, the location of service delivery, the type of clinician, and the type of service delivered. For this reason, clinicians must develop their own understanding of what is confidential and how to handle confidential information. In reviewing relevant confidentiality provisions, clinicians should look for what *may be* disclosed (based on their discretion and professional judgment), what *must be* disclosed, and what *may not be* disclosed, as confidentiality protections are rarely, if ever, absolute.

When an adolescent has requested privacy or a parent has requested access to information, and the clinician legally has discretion about whether to disclose, ethical principles—autonomy, nonmaleficence, beneficence, justice, confidentiality, and truth-telling—can provide useful guidance.

Confidentiality Protections for Adolescent Minors

Across the numerous confidentiality obligations, there are commonalities. In general, personal health information is confidential but *may be disclosed pursuant to an authorization* obtained from the patient or another appropriate person. Usually, when minors have the legal right to consent to their own care, they also have the right to control disclosure of confidential information about that care. This has been recognized in both state laws and in the federal HIPAA Privacy Rule and regulations for the Title X family planning and the substance use disorder programs.[14,16,19] Even when a minor has a general right to control disclosure of their own health information, there are a number of *circumstances in which disclosure over the objection of the minor must happen*—if a specific legal provision requires disclosure to parents; if a mandatory reporting obligation applies, as in the case of suspected physical or sexual abuse; or if the minor poses a severe danger to himself or herself or to others that ethical principles or legal provisions require to be reported. For example, the federal Title X family planning regulations include very strong confidentiality protections for AYAs but even those regulations require disclosure of otherwise confidential information to comply with mandatory reporting obligations.[16,17]

When the minor does not have the legal right to consent to care or to control disclosure, the release of confidential information usually must be authorized by the minor's parent or the person (or entity) with legal custody or guardianship. When parent authorization is necessary, it is still advisable—from an ethical perspective—for clinicians to seek the agreement of the minor to disclose confidential information and certainly, at minimum, to advise the minor at the outset of treatment of any limits to confidentiality.[20] There may be situations in which a clinician has concerns about releasing information to a parent or guardian even though the parent has a general right to that information. Most confidentiality laws include exceptions that allow the clinician to restrict parent authority to access or authorize disclosure of health records when the minor is a victim of abuse or is at risk.[8,14]

Clinicians can never promise absolute confidentiality to a minor patient, nor can they promise disclosure to a parent or guardian in all situations. Fortunately, in many circumstances, issues of confidentiality and disclosure can be resolved by discussion and informal agreement between a physician, the adolescent patient, and the parents, without reference to legal requirements.

The Health Insurance Portability and Accountability Act Privacy Rule

These federal medical confidentiality regulations apply to general health information and protect the health care information of both adolescent minors and young adults. States may adopt more protective confidentiality provisions but cannot waive the minimum protections established by the HIPAA Privacy Rule. Specifically, when minors are authorized to consent for their own health care and do so, the Rule treats them as "individuals" who are able to exercise rights over their own protected health information. Also, when parents have acceded to a confidentiality agreement between a minor and a clinician, the minor is considered an "individual" under the Rule.[22]

In general, the HIPAA Privacy Rule gives parents access to the health information of their unemancipated minor children, including adolescents. However, on the issue of when parents may have access to protected health information for minors who are considered "individuals" under the Rule and who have consented to their own care, it defers to "state and other applicable law."[22] Therefore, the laws that allow minors to consent for their own health care acquired increased significance with the advent of the HIPAA Privacy Rule. The Rule must also be understood in the broader context of other laws that affect disclosure of adolescents' confidential health information to their parents. Specifically, if state or other law explicitly requires information to be disclosed to a parent, the regulations allow a clinician to comply with that law and disclose the information. If state or other law explicitly permits, but does not require, information to be disclosed to a parent, the regulations allow a clinician to exercise discretion to disclose or not. If state or other law prohibits the disclosure of information to a parent without the consent of the minor, the regulations do not allow a clinician to disclose it without the minor's consent. If state or other

law is silent or unclear on the question, an entity covered by the Rule has discretion to determine whether to grant access to a parent to the protected health information, as long as the determination is made by a clinician exercising professional judgment.[22] The final provisions of the HIPAA Privacy Rule were issued in 2002. The federal government has the authority to revise and amend these regulations at any time. Indeed, in early 2021, modifications of the HIPAA Privacy Rule were proposed that would expand sharing of protected health information, including AYAs' information; in mid-2022 those modifications had not been finalized and were still pending.

Electronic Health Information, the Health Insurance Portability and Accountability Act Security Rule, and the 21st Century Cures Act

Two federal laws play an important role related to access to and confidentiality of EHI—the HIPAA Security Rule and the 21st Century Cures Act. Each impacts how health information technology (HIT) systems, including electronic health records (EHRs), should be designed, implemented, and used by clinicians and patients.

In addition to its Privacy Rule, HIPAA also contains a Security Rule. The regulations that make up the HIPAA Security Rule require covered entities, including clinicians, to ensure the confidentiality, integrity, and availability of all electronic personal health information (e-PHI) held by covered entities.[23] An important component of the HIPAA Security Rule is ensuring that EHI is accessible and useable *upon demand* by an authorized user and, at the same time, protected from access by unauthorized users. When minors are considered the "individual" with the right to control release of their own health information under the HIPAA Privacy Rule, they are authorized users for purposes of the HIPAA Security Rule. Among other things, the HIPAA Security Rule requires covered entities to implement reasonable and appropriate administrative, technical, and physical safeguards to achieve these ends. For example, the Rule includes some specific requirements regarding implementation of access control and identity authentication.[24] These regulations play a critical role in shaping how HIT systems are designed, implemented, and maintained.

In 2020, the Office of National Coordinator for Health Information Technology (ONC) issued a regulation (ONC Rule) implementing specific requirements of the 21st Century Cures Act.[25] This ONC Rule expands access to EHI for patients, including adolescent patients, and their proxies, who are usually their parents. The Rule also imposes a ban on information blocking, with the result that many forms of clinician notes and other EHI will be accessible via patient portals and other means. There are exceptions to the information blocking ban—including exceptions for privacy, preventing harm, and infeasibility—but even so, the Rule has major implications for the confidentiality of AYAs' health information.[25–27]

🔘 PAYMENT

There is an integral relationship among the legal provisions that pertain to consent, confidentiality, and payment in the delivery of health care services to AYAs. A source of payment is essential whether an AYA needs care on a confidential basis or not. Some of the state minor consent laws specify that if a minor is authorized to consent to care, it is the minor rather than the parent who is responsible for payment. In reality, however, few, if any, adolescents are able to pay for health care "out of pocket." Financing for the care is therefore an essential element of both confidentiality and access.

Some federal and state health care funding programs enable AYAs to obtain confidential care with little or no cost to them. Most notable is the federal Family Planning Program funded under Title X of the Public Health Services Act.[17] As significant a role as these programs play, they do not ensure access to the full array of comprehensive health services needed by AYAs. The financing available through insurance is therefore all the more important.

Since the enactment and implementation of the Affordable Care Act (ACA), beginning in 2010, millions of AYAs have been and will be covered by Medicaid or private health insurance, with young adults under age 26 years able to remain on a parent's private health insurance policy who would not otherwise have had coverage.[28] The ACA also expanded coverage for vulnerable groups of youth such as those exiting foster care, those in or leaving the juvenile or criminal justice system, and homeless youth.[29] The ACA requires health plans to cover without cost-sharing a wide range of preventive services—such as contraception, mental health, and substance use services—that are important for AYAs.[28]

For AYAs who are covered as dependents on a family policy, however, confidentiality can be compromised through the billing and health insurance claims process. A small number of states have begun to implement policies to enable covered dependents to receive confidential services without forfeiting payment by the insurer. Nevertheless, the limits on confidentiality that exist in the insurance arena remain a challenge that clinicians should be aware of and inform their AYA patients about.[30]

SPECIALIZED MECHANISMS AND SETTINGS FOR ADOLESCENT AND YOUNG ADULT CARE

The relevant areas of law for AYA services—consent, confidentiality, and payment—remain the same no matter where or how services are delivered. However, the legal rules can play out differently depending on the settings and the mechanism used to deliver care.

Providing Care through Telehealth

The legal framework for consent to treatment remains the same when services are being provided through telehealth. However, various legal and policy considerations affect implementation of telehealth for AYAs.[31] In some states, clinicians must obtain additional and separate consent in order to deliver care using telehealth technologies. In most cases, the individual or entity with authority to consent for care also has authority to consent to telehealth, but it is critical to review state laws and regulations to confirm. Similarly, the core confidentiality laws protecting the privacy of health information generated during a telehealth visit remain the same; however, clinicians must pay particular attention to the security rules regarding protection and transmission of EHI, as these rules may dictate which telehealth technologies can be used and how they must be implemented and maintained. When providing telehealth services, it is important to be aware that some insurers, including some public funding programs, treat, and sometimes reimburse for telehealth services differently than they do for in-person care. The use of telehealth also implicates ethics. Telehealth can be an important tool in expanding health care access to AYAs who may otherwise struggle to access care, and some AYAs feel safer and more comfortable receiving telehealth services than in-person care. On the other hand, telehealth also has limitations and may require changes to practice. For example, it is critical to consider both the safety and privacy of patients when services are being delivered to AYAs in shared living spaces.

Providing Health Care in School Settings

The legal framework for consent to treatment for AYAs remains the same when services are provided in a school setting; however, clinicians should be aware that different confidentiality rules may apply when delivering health care in either secondary schools or student health centers on college and university campuses. The HIPAA Privacy Rule typically controls release of health information created by clinicians but does not apply to some health records in school settings. The Family Educational Rights and Privacy Act (FERPA),[32] is a federal statute that controls the disclosure of the educational records of students at most primary, secondary, and postsecondary schools. Under FERPA, an "education record" can include health records created by a clinician employed or acting on behalf of a school or university. Thus, health records created by medical professionals employed by a school or university may be subject to FERPA rather

than HIPAA. For this reason, it is important for clinicians in school settings to understand which regulations apply to and control release of their patient information. Often, which regulation applies will be fact and situation specific. In light of the important ramifications, clinicians who provide care in school settings should consult with their legal counsel about whether their student health records are governed by HIPAA, FERPA, or state privacy laws.

ETHICAL PRINCIPLES AND ETHICAL CHALLENGES

Within the overall legal framework, application of the law is shaped by ethics and policy. Clinicians are bound to comply with certain ethical principles and with professional and employment policies. A fundamental principle in medicine is to do no harm, with roots in the Hippocratic Oath. Traditionally, along with the obligation to avoid doing harm, four principles of medical ethics have been identified as foundational guidance for health care practice—autonomy, nonmaleficence, beneficence, and justice[33,34]; two additional principles are embedded within the principle of autonomy—confidentiality and truth-telling.[35] The principle of justice encompasses considerations of equity that, along with confidentiality, are particularly important in the care of AYAs. Ethical principles provide additional context and guidance in application of the law to health care practice.

Clinicians who care for AYAs increasingly are experiencing ethical challenges as they strive to provide the highest quality care to their patients. Adhering to the foundational ethical principles is difficult when doing so conflicts with the law. More and more, laws are requiring medical practices, or imposing limitations, that clinicians may feel violate their ethical obligations.[36] Examples of these situations, often triggered by state laws, include the following: requirements to provide patients with inaccurate information; prohibitions on providing them medically accurate information; mandates to report medical care as abuse; mandates to report actions as child abuse in circumstances the clinician believes would be harmful to their patient; and bans on providing care that the clinician believes is essential for the health, safety, and well-being of their patient. These situations, sometimes exacerbated by ambiguities in the law, confront a clinician with the potential for severe legal consequences if they honor their ethical obligations, and the possibility of violating their ethical obligation to do no harm should they honor the law. Clinicians may wish to consult with their colleagues and legal counsel when such scenarios arise.

SUMMARY

Clinicians treating AYAs must have a clear understanding of the legal framework within which care is provided. The legal issues that arise most frequently fall into three specific areas—Consent: Who is authorized to give consent for the minor's or young adult's care and whose consent is required? Confidentiality: Who has the right to control the release of confidential information about the care, including medical records and EHI, and who has the right to receive such information? Payment: Who is financially liable for payment and is there a source of insurance coverage or is public funding available that the AYA can access? The laws differ based on age, legal status, and geography and may vary in different clinical settings and for different populations. This chapter discusses the legal framework for consent, confidentiality, and payment in the United States and notes where to find resources on state-specific law.

DISCLAIMER

Please note that this information does not represent legal advice. Clinicians are reminded that laws change and that statutes, regulations, and court decisions may be subject to differing interpretations. It is the responsibility of each clinician to be familiar with the current relevant laws that affect the health care of AYAs. In difficult cases involving legal issues, advice should be sought from someone with state-specific expertise. The information in this chapter applies to the United States. All clinicians should consult with their local legal counsel.

REFERENCES

1. Roe v. Wade, 410 U.S. 113 (1973).
2. Planned Parenthood of Central Missouri v. Danforth, 428 U.S. 52 (1976).
3. Griswold v. Connecticut, 381 U.S. 479 (1965).
4. Eisenstadt v. Baird, 405 U.S. 438 (1972).
5. Carey v. Populations Services International, 431 U.S. 678 (1977).
6. Dobbs v. Jackson Women's Health Organization, 597 U.S. ___ (2022).
7. Guttmacher Institute. Interactive Map: U.S. Abortion Policies and Access After Roe. https://states.guttmacher.org/policies/. Accessed July 31, 2022.
8. English A, Bass L, Boyle AD, et al. *State Minor Consent Laws: A Summary*. 3rd ed. Center for Adolescent Health & the Law; 2010.
9. Guttmacher Institute. *An overview of consent to reproductive health services by young people*. 2021. Accessed March 28, 2021. https://www.guttmacher.org/state-policy/explore/overview-minors-consent-law
10. Post LF, Blustein J, Dubler NN. *Handbook for Health Care Ethics Committees*. Johns Hopkins University Press; 2007.
11. Cooper S. Taking no for an answer: refusal of life-sustaining treatment. *Virtual Mentor*. 2010;12(6):444–449. Accessed March 28, 2021. https://journalofethics.ama-assn.org/article/taking-no-answer-refusal-life-sustaining-treatment/2010-06
12. Hartman RG. Adolescent autonomy: clarifying an ageless conundrum. *Hastings Law J*. 2000;51(6):1265–1362. Accessed March 28, 2021. https://repository.uchastings.edu/hastings_law_journal/vol51/iss6/4
13. Parham v. J.R., 442 U.S. 584 (1979).
14. 42 C.F.R. Parts 160 and 164, Subparts A and E.
15. 42 U.S.C. §§ 1396a(a)(7), 1396d(a)(4)(C).
16. 42 C.F.R. § 59.10.
17. Gudeman R, Madge S. *The Federal Title X Family Planning Program: Privacy and Access Rules for Adolescents*. Youth Law News; 2011. Accessed on March 28, 2021. https://youthlaw.org/publication/the-federal-title-x-family-planning-program-privacy-and-access-rules-for-adolescents1/
18. Guttmacher Institute. *Medicaid family planning eligibility expansions*. 2021. Accessed March 28, 2021. https://www.guttmacher.org/state-policy/explore/medicaid-family-planning-eligibility-expansions
19. 42 U.S.C. § 290dd-2; 42 C.F.R. § 2.
20. Ford CA, English A, Sigman G. Confidential health care for adolescents: position paper of the Society for Adolescent Medicine. *J Adolesc Health*. 2004;35(2):160–167.
21. AAP Committee on Adolescence. Achieving quality health services for adolescents. *Pediatrics*. 2016;138(2):e20161347.
22. English A, Ford CA. The HIPAA privacy rule and adolescents: legal questions and clinical challenges. *Perspect Sex Reprod Health*. 2004;36:80–86.
23. 45 C.F.R. Part 164, Subparts A and C.
24. 45 C.F.R. § 164.312.
25. 21st Century Cures Act: Interoperability, Information Blocking, and the ONC Health IT Certification Program. 85 Fed. Reg. 25642. 2020.
26. Carlson J, Goldstein R, Hoover K, et al. NASPAG/SAHM statement: the 21st Century Cures Act and adolescent confidentiality. *J Pediatr Adolesc Gynecol*. 2021;34(1):3–5.
27. English A, Ford CA. Adolescent consent and confidentiality: complexities in context of the 21st Century Cures Act. *Pediatrics*. 2022;149(6):e2022056414
28. English A. *The Patient Protection and Affordable Care Act of 2010: How Does it Help Adolescents and Young Adults*. Center for Adolescent Health & the Law; 2010. Accessed March 28, 2021. http://nahic.ucsf.edu/wp-content/uploads/2011/02/HCR_Issue_Brief_Aug2010_Final_Aug31.pdf
29. English A, Scott J, Park MJ. *Implementing the ACA: How Much Will it Help Vulnerable Adolescents & Young Adults?* Center for Adolescent Health & the Law; 2014. Accessed March 28, 2021. http://nahic.ucsf.edu/wp-content/uploads/2014/01/VulnerablePopulations_IB_Final.pdf
30. National Family Planning and Reproductive Health Association website. Confidentiality. Accessed March 21, 2021. https://www.nationalfamilyplanning.org/confidentiality
31. North S. Telemedicine in the time of COVID and beyond. *J Adolesc Health*. 2020;67(2):145–146. Published online 2020, June 27. doi: 10.1016/j.jadohealth.2020.05.024.
32. 20 U.S.C. § 1232g; 34 C.F.R. § 99.3.
33. Beauchamp TL, Childress JF. *Principles of Biomedical Ethics*. 8th ed. Oxford University Press; 2019.
34. President's Commission for the Study of Ethical Problems in Medicine and Biomedical and Behavioral Research, *Summing Up: Final Report on Studies of the Ethical and Legal Problems in Medicine and Biomedical and Behavioral Research*, Washington, D.C.; March 1983. Accessed August 1, 2022. https://repository.library.georgetown.edu/bitstream/handle/10822/559377/summing_up.pdf?sequence=4&isAllowed=y
35. Page K. The four principles: can they be measured and do they predict ethical decision making? *BMC Med Ethics*. 2012;13:10. Accessed March 28, 2021. http://www.biomedcentral.com/1472-6939/13/1/10
36. Chotiner I. What ethical health care looks like when abortion is criminalized: how can physicians meet their obligations to patients after Roe? *The New Yorker*. July 8, 2022. Accessed August 11, 2022. https://www.newyorker.com/news/q-and-a/ethical-health-care-after-roe

📶 ADDITIONAL RESOURCES AND WEBSITES

Additional Resources and Websites for Clinicians:

American Academy of Pediatrics (AAP)—http://www.aap.org. American Academy of Pediatrics is a membership organization committed to the optimal physical, mental, and social health and well-being of all infants, children, adolescents, and young adults. American Academy of Pediatrics includes on its website a broad array of position papers and policies that are relevant to legal issues in the health care of AYAs.

Center for Adolescent Health & the Law (CAHL)—http://www.cahl.org. Center for Adolescent Health & the Law is a national legal and policy organization that promotes the health of adolescents and young adults and their access to comprehensive health care. A CAHL publication, State Minor Consent Laws: A Summary, 3rd ed. (2010), contains detailed summaries and citations of the minor consent laws in all 50 U.S. states and the District of Columbia. The 4th edition will be issued in 2022.

Families USA—http://www.familiesusa.org. Families USA is a national nonprofit, nonpartisan organization dedicated to the achievement of high-quality, affordable health care for all Americans. Families USA's work focuses on four pillars: value, equity, coverage, and consumer experience.

Guttmacher Institute—http://www.guttmacher.org. The Guttmacher Institute is a national nonprofit organization that advances sexual and reproductive health worldwide through research, policy analysis, and public education. The website includes current reliable information, updated regularly, about the minor consent laws related to sexual and reproductive health in all U.S. states and the District of Columbia at https://www.guttmacher.org/united-states/teens/state-policies-teens.

Kaiser Family Foundation (KFF)—https://www.kff.org/. Kaiser Family Foundation is a nonprofit organization focusing on national health issues, as well as the U.S. role in global health policy. Kaiser Family Foundation serves as a nonpartisan source of facts, analysis, and journalism for policymakers, the media, the health policy community, and the public. The KFF website has many issue briefs and fact sheets relevant to legal issues for AYA health.

National Center for Youth Law (NCYL)—http://www.youthlaw.org. National Center for Youth Law is a national nonprofit law office that uses the law to ensure that children and adolescents have the resources, support, and opportunities they need for a fair start in life, including access to health and mental health care. National Center for Youth Law offers specific information about laws impacting adolescent health care in California at http://teenhealthlaw.org/.

National Family Planning and Reproductive Health Association (NFPRHA)—https://www.nationalfamilyplanning.org. National Family Planning and Reproductive Health Association is a membership organization that works to enhance the ability of nurse practitioners, doctors, and other health professionals to provide high-quality family planning care through training and advocacy. National Family Planning and Reproductive Health Association's website includes extensive information about confidentiality, including legal issues related to confidentiality and insurance, at https://www.nationalfamilyplanning.org/confidentiality.

National Health Law Program (NHeLP)—https://healthlaw.org. National Health Law Program is a national public interest law firm that seeks to improve health care for America's working and unemployed poor, minorities, the elderly, and people with disabilities, including children and adolescents.

Office for Civil Rights (OCR)—http://www.hhs.gov/ocr/hipaa. Office for Civil Rights is the agency in the U.S. Department of Health & Human Services charged with implementing the HIPAA Privacy and Security Rules. The OCR website has extensive Frequently Asked Questions (FAQs) about implementation of HIPAA.

Office of National Coordinator for Health Information Technology (ONC)—https://www.healthit.gov/. Office of National Coordinator for Health Information Technology is an agency in the U.S. Department of Health & Human Services. Office of National Coordinator for Health Information Technology is the principal federal entity charged with coordination of nationwide efforts to implement and use the most advanced health information technology and the electronic exchange of health information.

Society for Adolescent Health and Medicine (SAHM)—https://www.adolescenthealth.org/Advocacy/Position-Papers-Statements.aspx. Society for Adolescent Health and Medicine is a multidisciplinary organization committed to improving the physical and psychosocial health and well-being of all adolescents through advocacy, clinical care, health promotion, health service delivery, professional development, and research. Society for Adolescent Health and Medicine includes on its website numerous position papers and statements that are relevant to legal issues in the health care of adolescents.

Additional Resources and Websites for Parents/Caregivers:

American Academy of Pediatrics (AAP)—Parenting Website—https://healthychildren.org. The AAP Parenting Website has extensive resources for parents, including information about consent, confidentiality, and insurance.

Essential Health Access—"Talk with Your Kids"—https://www.talkwithyourkids.org/resources-parents/resources-parents.html. "Talk with Your Kids" has resources to help parents understand "sensitive service" health care as well as tips on how to open conversations with their children and key messages at different ages and stages about privacy, relationships, and sensitive health care.

Society for Adolescent Health and Medicine (SAHM)—https://www.adolescenthealth.org/Resources/Resources-for-Adolescents-and-Parents.aspx. Society for Adolescent Health and Medicine includes on its website several resources for parents and caregivers.

Additional Resources and Websites for Adolescents and Young Adults:

Advocates for Youth—http://www.advocatesforyouth.org/resources-tools/?_sft_type=policy-advocacy. Advocates for Youth works alongside young people in the United States and around the globe as they fight for sexual health, rights, and justice. Advocates for Youth website includes fact sheets on adolescent health law that can be relevant for young adults.

Guttmacher Institute—https://www.guttmacher.org/united-states/teens. The Guttmacher Institute is a national nonprofit organization that advances sexual and reproductive health worldwide through research, policy analysis, and public education. Their website includes information, updated regularly, about the minor consent laws in all states related to sexual and reproductive health.

National Center for Youth Law (NCYL)—http://teenhealthlaw.org/. National Center for Youth Law offers specific information about laws impacting adolescent health care in California.

Society for Adolescent Health and Medicine (SAHM)—https://www.adolescenthealth.org/Resources/Resources-for-Adolescents-and-Parents.aspx. Society for Adolescent Health and Medicine includes on its website resources for adolescents.

CHAPTER 8

Complementary and Integrative Medicine in Adolescents and Young Adults

Cora Collette Breuner

KEY WORDS

- Acupuncture
- Biofeedback
- Chiropractic
- Complementary and Integrative Medicine
- Herbal therapies
- Homeopathy
- Massage
- Mindfulness/Meditation
- Yoga

INTRODUCTION

Complementary and integrative medicine encompasses a wide spectrum of health practices and interventions that can be integrated into conventional medicine. Table 8.1 describes many, but not all of the modalities discussed in this chapter.[1]

Those who choose complementary and integrative approaches may be searching for a way to improve their general health, to alleviate symptoms associated with chronic illnesses, or to ameliorate adverse effects of conventional treatments. Complementary and integrative therapies most frequently used by adolescents and young adults (AYAs) include herbs, vitamins, supplements, chiropractic, homeopathy, massage, and acupuncture (Fig. 8.1). Medical conditions most frequently treated with complementary and integrative therapies include respiratory and gastrointestinal (GI) ailments, musculoskeletal and skin complaints, and chronic conditions such as cystic fibrosis, cancer, autism, and arthritis.[2,3]

The 2017 survey conducted by the National Center for Complementary and Integrative Health (NCCIH) and National Center for Health Statistics (NCHS) included substantially more questions focused on the use of complementary practices compared to previous surveys. Prevalence of use was consistent with previous surveys (12% to 25%), however, there was no information specific to AYAs. Further, more inclusive studies have found that many populations including Black, Indigenous, and people of color also utilize complementary and integrative therapies suggesting that all individuals should be routinely asked about complementary and integrative therapies at every health care visit.[4,5]

EDUCATION

Integrative medicine centers are a growing resource for patients, clinicians, and communities and are now embraced by many leading academic centers. Academic training in integrative medicine is a career option for trainees; as of 2021, there were 18 established integrative medicine fellowships. The American Board of Physician Specialties offered the first American Board of Integrative Medicine in November 2014, allowing those who have gone through Integrative Medicine fellowship training to become board certified and acknowledged as a subspecialty in the medical community.

RESEARCH

There are a number of excellent researchers in this field broadening the evidence in support of complementary and integrative therapies when indicated and safe.

The NCCIH is a primary funding source for research whose mission is to define, through rigorous scientific investigation, the usefulness and safety of complementary and integrative health interventions and their role in improving health and health care. The five objectives of NCCIH are the following:

1. Advance fundamental science and methods development
2. Advance research on the whole person and on the integration of complementary and conventional care
3. Foster research on health promotion and restoration, resilience, disease prevention, and symptom management
4. Enhance the complementary and integrative health research workforce
5. Provide objective evidence-based information on complementary and integrative health interventions[6]

TABLE 8.1

Commonly Used Complementary Products and Practices

Natural products
Herbs
Vitamins and minerals
Probiotics
Mind–body practices
Yoga
Meditation
Guided imagery
Clinical hypnosis
Massage therapy
Acupuncture
Relaxation techniques (breathing, progressive muscle relaxation)
Osteopathic manipulation
Chiropractic
Tai chi
Qigong
Feldenkrais method
Alexander technique
Other complementary health approaches
Traditional Chinese medicine
Ayurvedic medicine
Homeopathy
Naturopathy
Functional medicine

Adapted from the National Institutes of Health, National Center for Complementary and Integrative Health.

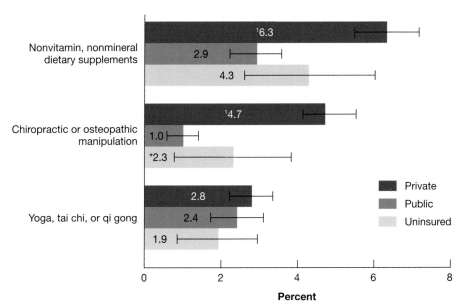

FIGURE 8.1 Age-adjusted percentages of children aged 4 to 17 years who used selected complementary health approaches during the past 12 months, by health insurance status: United States 2012. (Source: Black LI, Clarke TC, Barnes PM, Stussman BJ, Nahin RL. Use of complementary health approaches among children aged 4–17 years in the United States: National Health Interview Survey, 2007–2012. *Natl Health Stat Report.* 2015;(78):1–19. PMID: 25671583; PMCID: PMC4562218..

*Estimates are considered unreliable. Data have a relative standard error greater than 30% and less than or equal to 50% and should be used with caution.
[1]Significantly different from public and uninsured (*p* < .001).
NOTE: Estimates are based on household interviews of a sample of the civilian noninstitutionalized population.
SOURCE: CDC/INCHS. National Health Interview Survey. 2012.

CLINICIAN KNOWLEDGE ABOUT COMPLEMENTARY AND INTEGRATIVE MEDICINE

Clinicians should ask AYAs about their use of any form of complementary and integrative medicine, especially herbal products and supplements, at every health care visit. This is important information that allows AYAs and their clinician to partner and be transparent about the use of all therapies that a patient is taking or using. The clinician can use this conversation to help the AYAs learn about drug–herb interactions, and the safety and efficacy of the products they are taking or the interventions they are using. A nonjudgmental and knowledgeable approach goes far with the AYA patient and can be quite effective to illustrate that "natural" may not mean safe, and an endorsement on an internet site does not guarantee efficacy. Open communication between the clinician and patient and/or family leads to a more informed and trusted relationship, and allows for joint decision making.

An ethical and legal dilemma may present itself to the clinician when a patient wishes to utilize an integrative treatment where there may be a lack of sufficient evidence to support its use and a paucity of safety data.

Questions to consider include those described in a 2005 paper[7]:
1. Will effective care be utilized when the patient's condition is life-threatening?
2. Will using a treatment deflect from conventional treatment?
3. What is known about the safety and/or efficacy of the treatment?
4. Would this proposed therapy be acceptable to another clinician?
5. Does this treatment have some support in the medical literature?
6. Will this treatment interfere with any treatments the patient is currently taking?

HERBS/SUPPLEMENTS

Overview and Regulation

According to the American Botanical Council (ABC), adult consumers in the United States spent an estimated $9.602 billion on herbal dietary supplements in 2019, an 8.6% increase in total U.S. sales from the previous year.[8]

The Dietary Supplement Health and Education Act of 1994 defines herbal products as supplements because they are not tested according to the same scientific standards as conventional drugs. Packaging or marketing information does not need to be approved by the U.S. Food and Drug Administration (FDA) before a product reaches the market. Supplements cannot be marketed for the diagnosis, treatment, cure, or prevention of disease, despite evidence to the contrary. They can only describe how the "structure and function" of the human body is affected. No protection is offered against misleading or fraudulent claims.

Drug Interactions and Toxicity

Clinicians should be aware of potential herb/supplement–drug interactions.[9] Safety concerns include direct toxicities and contamination with active pharmaceutical agents.[10] Antiplatelet activity and interaction with the cytochrome P450 3A4 enzyme system are two significant effects noted in many herbs, in particular St. John's wort (SJW). For this reason, patients who suffer a trauma and visit an emergency room or those who are undergoing surgery, should be questioned about the use of herbal remedies. These AYAs should be counseled on the discontinuation of herbal remedies at least 2 weeks before surgery.[11]

A lack of quality control and regulation has resulted in contamination and misidentification of plant species. Herbal preparations may be contaminated with heavy metals or bacteria/fungal organisms while being manufactured or stored. One study, using the FDA's Adverse Event Reporting System on food and dietary supplements database between 2004 and 2015, reported severe medical events in those aged 0 to 25 years including death, disability, life-threatening events, hospitalization, emergency room visits, and/or intervention to prevent permanent disability.[12]

Dosing Issues and Active Compounds

Clinicians have become accustomed to using pharmaceutical products standardized with the same strength and high quality; this is not always the case with herbs/supplements. Because herbs/supplements represent complex entities, it is difficult to find one particular component representing the active agent. Patients should be counseled on the use of a clinically studied specific extract in an herb/supplement. Manufacturers may have their products tested for contamination and standard strength/quality, and the results of these assays are available online with the purchase of a membership with consumer lab (www.consumerlab.com). This company, through independent testing of products, assists clinicians identify health and nutritional products that are free from contamination and purely produced via quality and standard certification programs.

Long-Term Use

Long-term effects of herbs/supplements are not traditionally studied. For this reason, herbs/supplements should only be used on a limited basis until more data are available regarding long-term safety.

Use in Pregnancy and Lactation

Females contemplating pregnancy, currently pregnant, or nursing should not use herbs/supplements given the lack of evidence and safety studies.

Commonly Used Herbs/Supplements

Adolescents and young adults are likely to use herbs/supplements to treat a number of conditions, including eating disorders, obesity, polycystic ovary syndrome (PCOS), athletic performance enhancement, depression, anxiety, sleep disorders, and upper respiratory tract infections.

ST. JOHN'S WORT (HYPERICUM PERFORATUM)

Uses

St. John's wort has historically been used for depression.

Mechanism of Action

The two active ingredients are hypericin and hyperforin which inhibit the reuptake of serotonin, norepinephrine, and dopamine as well as neurotransmitters.

Clinical Studies

For patients with mild-to-moderate depression, SJW has equivalent efficacy and safety when compared to selective serotonin reuptake inhibitors (SSRIs).[13]

Adverse Effects

These include GI symptoms, dizziness, and confusion. Phototoxicity may occur with ingestion of high doses.

Herb–Drug Interactions

There is a significant interaction with cyclosporine, oral anticoagulants, oral contraceptives, and certain antiretroviral agents including indinavir due to SJW's ability to induce the cytochrome P450 3A4 enzyme system. The concomitant use of SJW with standard antidepressants is also contraindicated because of the risk of serotonin syndrome.

VALERIAN ROOT (VALERIANA OFFICIANALIS)

Uses

Valerian root is used for insomnia and as a sedative. It is also used for migraine headaches, fatigue, and intestinal cramps.

Mechanism of Action

Valerian root has sedative effects which may be due to effects on gamma aminobutyric acid (GABA) receptors.

Clinical Studies

In one meta-analysis of 60 studies looking at subjective sleep quality and anxiety reduction, valerian was found to be a safe and effective herb to promote sleep and prevent associated disorders.[14]

Adverse Effects

These include headache, excitability, uneasiness, and cardiac disturbances.

Herb–Drug Interactions

Care should be exercised when combining valerian root with other sedative agents and alcohol due to additive effects.

CHAMOMILE (MATRICARIA CHAMOMILLA)

Uses

Chamomile has been used for GI discomfort, peptic ulcer disease, pediatric colic, and mild anxiety.

Mechanism of Action

Chamomile may act via binding to central benzodiazepine receptors and has anti-inflammatory and antioxidant effects.

Clinical Studies

A recent meta-analysis showed a significant improvement in sleep quality after chamomile administration.[15]

Adverse Effects

Several cases of allergic reactions to chamomile have been reported; no significant toxicity has been reported.

Herb–Drug Interactions

No drug–herb interactions have been noted.

ELDERBERRY (SAMBUCUS)

Uses

Elderberry has been used for treating upper respiratory infections and fevers, and to help expectoration in bronchitis and asthma.

Mechanism of Action

Elderberry inhibits H1N1 influenza activities by **binding to H1N1 virions** and **blocking host cell recognition and entry**. Elderberry showed mild inhibitory effect at the early stages of the influenza virus cycle, with considerably stronger effect in the postinfection phase. It blocks viral glycoproteins and increases expression of interleukin 6, interleukin 8, and tumor necrosis factor (TNF).

Clinical Studies

Elderberry may not reduce the risk of developing upper respiratory infections but it may reduce the duration and severity of upper respiratory infections.[16]

Adverse Effects

Adverse effects include nausea, vomiting, stomach cramps, dizziness, and weakness.

Herb–Drug Interactions

Elderberry has no known severe, serious, or moderate interactions with other drugs.

ECHINACEA (E. ANGUSTIFOLIA, E. PALLIDA, E. PURPUREA)

Uses

Echinacea has been used for the treatment of upper respiratory infections, and as a topical analgesic for snake bites, stings, and burns. It has become popular as an immune booster.

Mechanism of Action

Echinacea protects the integrity of the hyaluronic acid matrix by stimulating the alternate complement pathway. It can promote nonspecific T-cell activation by binding to T cells and increasing interferon production. The polysaccharides arabinogalactan and echinacin are the active ingredients of *Echinacea* and therefore, may have immune-modulating effects on the body. Other ingredients include glycosides, alkaloids, alkylamides, polyacetylenes, and fatty acids which may inhibit viral replication, improve the motility of polymorphonuclear cells, and enhance phagocytosis.

Clinical Studies

One Cochrane review reported that *Echinacea* does not prevent or treat upper respiratory infections.[17] Patients with progressive systemic diseases such as multiple sclerosis, tuberculosis, systemic lupus erythematosus, autoimmune diseases, and human immunodeficiency virus (HIV) infection should not use *Echinacea* because of its possible immunomodulation.

Adverse Effects

These include skin rash, GI distress, and diarrhea.

Herb–Drug Interactions

Echinacea should not be used in patients on immunosuppressant medications.

 ## FEVERFEW (TANACETUM PARTHENIUM)

Uses

Feverfew is an herbal remedy for prevention and treatment of migraine headaches. It has also been used for upper respiratory infections, and depression.

Mechanism of Action

Feverfew may inhibit prostaglandin, thromboxane, and leukotriene synthesis. It also can reduce serotonin release from thrombocytes and polymorphonuclear leukocytes.

Clinical Studies

A prospective observational study demonstrated benefit from use of feverfew in combination with magnesium and coenzyme Q10 for prevention of migraine.[18]

Adverse Effects

Adverse effects include mouth ulcerations, contact dermatitis, dizziness, diarrhea, and heartburn.

Herb–Drug Interactions

Feverfew may interact with anticoagulants and antiplatelet agents due to its platelet aggregation inhibition.

 ## BUTTERBUR (PETASITES HYBRIDUS)

Uses

Butterbur has been used to treat migraine headaches, chronic cough, and urinary tract spasms.

Mechanism of Action

The active constituents of butterbur are the sesquiterpene compounds, petasin, and isopetasin. Butterbur is thought to have antispasmodic effects on smooth muscle and vascular walls and may have anti-inflammatory effects by inhibiting leukotriene synthesis.

Clinical Studies

Butterbur has been shown to be helpful in the pediatric populations as a prophylactic in decreasing migraine frequency.

Adverse Effects

Butterbur containing pyrrolizidine alkaloids is unsafe due to the hepatotoxicity of the alkaloids. Preparations that don't contain these alkaloids are considered safe.

Herb–Drug Interactions

Butterbur has no known severe, serious, or moderate interactions with other drugs.

 ## MELATONIN

Uses

Melatonin has been used for jet lag, insomnia, shift work disorder, circadian rhythm disorders in individuals who are visually impaired, and benzodiazepine and nicotine withdrawal.

Mechanism of Action

Melatonin appears to increase the binding of GABA to its receptors (Fig. 8.2).

Clinical Studies

Melatonin improves sleep in AYAs with attention deficit hyperactivity disorder, autism, and for individuals receiving cancer treatment.[19–21]

Adverse Effects

These include inhibition of ovulation, impair glucose utilization, and a decrease in prothrombin activity. Concomitant use of melatonin with alcohol, benzodiazepines, or other sedative drugs might cause additive sedation.

Herb–Drug Interactions

Melatonin has no known severe, serious, or moderate interactions with other drugs.

 ## INOSITOL

Uses

Inositol is used in those with metabolic syndrome and in those with PCOS.

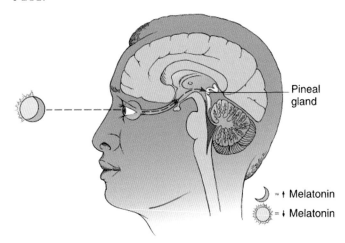

FIGURE 8.2 Melatonin (and subsequently serotonin) levels depend on exposure to sunlight. Melatonin induces sleep during dark hours and is suppressed by daylight. Dark months result in seasonal affective disorder for some people. (From Timby BK, Smith NE. *Introductory Medical-Surgical Nursing.* 12th ed. Lippincott Williams & Wilkins; 2017.)

Mechanism of Action

Inositol is an essential component of cell membrane phospholipids. It has weak lipotropic activity, and can shift fat out of liver and intestine cells. Inositol has a variety of stereoisomers, including myo-inositol (MI) and D-chiro-inositol (DCI). Myo-inositol is the most abundant form of cell membrane phospholipids in the central nervous system.

Clinical Studies

A recent meta-analysis assessed MI supplementation alone or in combination with DCI in females with PCOS. Nine randomized controlled trials involving 247 cases and 249 controls revealed significant decreases in fasting insulin and homeostasis model assessment index. A slight trend in reduction of testosterone concentration by MI was reported where androstenedione levels were unaffected. These results suggest the beneficial effect of MI in improving the metabolic profile of females with PCOS, concomitantly reducing their hyperandrogenism.[22]

Adverse Effects

It can interfere with the clotting cascade and can cause death in those with prolonged QT syndrome.

Herb–Drug Interactions

Inositol has no known severe, serious, or moderate interactions with other drugs.

 ACUPUNCTURE

Mechanism of Action

Originating in China more than 2,000 years ago, acupuncture is an ancient Chinese therapeutic treatment based on the premise that energy (*Qi*, Chi) flows through the body along channels known as meridians, connected by acupuncture points. The flow of *Qi* is manipulated by insertion of fine needles at acupuncture points along the involved meridians (Fig. 8.3). In acupuncture treatment, there is a segmental inhibition of pain impulses at the local site of needle stimulation through a disruption and inhibition of pain transmitting unmyelinated C fibers and sensory A delta fibers.

In assessing AYAs, an acupuncturist takes a history and then performs an examination, which includes the determination of the shape, color, and coating of the tongue and the force, flow, and character of the radial pulse. The specific treatment is based on the diagnosis and may include solid sterile needle placement, moxibustion (the practice of burning dried herbs over the acupuncture needles), acupressure, or cupping, a form of acupuncture where cups are placed on skin to create suction, which is believed to mobilize blood flow in order to promote healing.

Uses

Acupuncture is used in those with acute pain, substance use disorders, chronic back and neck pain, and headaches.

Clinical Studies

In one systematic review, acupuncture was superior to both artificial and no-acupuncture control for pain. Patients receiving acupuncture had less back and neck pain, osteoarthritis, and chronic headache. Evidence for efficacy of acupuncture has been noted in those with dental pain, postoperative pain, and nausea and vomiting associated with chemotherapy. Findings have shown a lower efficacy of acupuncture in those with migraine headaches, back pain, and dysmenorrhea.[23]

Battlefield acupuncture, a form of auricular acupuncture where a sequence of acupuncture needles are placed at up to five specific sites in one or both ears, has not been shown to be more effective

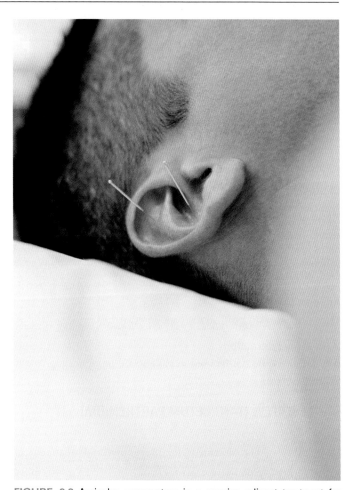

FIGURE 8.3 Auricular acupuncture is a growing adjunct treatment for chemical dependency. Practitioners place small needles under the skin of the outer ear to deliver an electrical impulse to the brain. Resulting relaxation may foster adherence to other substance abuse treatments and manage stress so that clients do not feel the need to engage in drinking or use of drugs. (From Videbeck SI. *Psychiatric-Mental Health Nursing.* 8th ed. Lippincott Williams & Wilkins; 2019.)

than placebo for pain intensity. However, more rigorous randomized controlled trials are needed to evaluate its efficacy in pain management.[24]

Adverse Effects

Adverse effects of acupuncture include pneumothorax, angina, septic sacroiliitis, epidural, and temporomandibular abscess.

 YOGA

Mechanism of Action

Yoga is widely known for helping to build strength and flexibility through a combination of meditation, controlled breathing, and stretches.

Uses

It is used for anxiety, hypertension, heart disease, back pain, and cancer.

Clinical Studies

Extensive research has explored yoga's potential value as an adjunct treatment for such health problems as anxiety, hypertension, heart disease, depression, low back pain, headaches, and cancer.[25] More studies are needed to evaluate the efficacy of this intervention.

Adverse Effects

None reported.

BIOFEEDBACK

Mechanism of Action

Biofeedback is a technique where the AYA, after being connected to electrical sensors, learns to control some of their body's functions, such as heart rate, temperature, muscle tension, and the breath. During a biofeedback session, the patient is taught to relax certain muscles, breathe in a different way and lower their heart rate to ultimately reduce pain and the effect of stress on their body. Adolescents and young adults learn to control their physiology through modification of electromyography, skin temperature, galvanic skin response or electrodermal response, respiratory rate, heart rate, heart rate variability, and neurofeedback.

Uses

It is used in those with chronic headaches, anxiety, and depression.

Clinical Studies

Studies have shown efficacy for migraine and chronic daily headache.[26,27]

Adverse Effects

None reported.

HYPNOSIS

Mechanism of Action

Clinical hypnosis is an effective mind–body tool that utilizes self-directed therapeutic suggestions to foster creativity and ingenuity and can facilitate the mind–body connection, leading to positive emotional and physical well-being.

Uses

It is used in those with chronic headaches, recurrent abdominal pain, anxiety, and depression.

Clinical Studies

Studies show promise in those with chronic headaches, recurrent abdominal pain, anxiety, depression, phobias, anger, family stressors, and sleep disorders.[28]

Adverse Effects

None reported.

MANUAL THERAPIES: CHIROPRACTIC, OSTEOPATHIC MANIPULATION, AND MASSAGE

Manual therapies include hands-on approaches, such as chiropractic medicine, osteopathic manipulative treatment (OMT), and massage therapy. The goal of manual therapies is to correct alignment, alleviate pain, and improve function to help support the body's innate ability to heal itself.

Mechanism of Action

Chiropractic Mechanism of Action

Chiropractic is based on the theory that all diseases could be traced to malpositioned bones in the spinal column called "subluxations," which lead to the entrapment of spinal nerves. Subluxations produce symptoms of disease because optimal functioning of tissues and organs is not allowed. Physical adjustment of the spine restores proper alignment of the spine by relieving nerve entrapments.

Osteopathic Manipulation Mechanism of Action

According to the American Osteopathic Association, with an advanced understanding of the interrelationships between the body's structure and function, and an understanding of how the body can be influenced by human's emotional or spiritual nature, the Doctors of Osteopathy (DO) use palpation and manipulation to provide patient-specific care that promotes health and treats disease.

Uses

Chiropractic and osteopathic manipulation is used for those with low back pain, cervical pain, headache, otitis media, dysmenorrhea, and carpal tunnel syndrome.

Clinical Studies

Positive studies exist for adults with low back pain[29] and for fibromyalgia.[30]

Adverse Effects

It is important for patients, families, parents/caregivers, and clinicians to be aware of the adverse effects of chiropractic manipulation in the AYA population. Chiropractic therapies have been associated with pain, cerebrovascular accidents, myelopathies, and radiculopathies after cervical manipulation and therefore caution is advised.[31] Adverse outcomes are most likely to occur when an improper manipulative method is used. Well-designed studies are needed to evaluate chiropractic care for select AYA conditions.

MASSAGE

Mechanism of Action

Massage therapy is thought to release muscle tension, remove toxic metabolites, and facilitate oxygen transport to cells and tissues. Massage promotes well-being through application of pressure to manipulate muscles, connective tissue, tendons, and ligaments to enhance relaxation and reduce pain. The most common form of massage therapy is traditional European or Swedish massage. The focus is to relax the muscles and improve circulation (Fig. 8.4). Another form of massage is the deep muscle or deep tissue technique commonly used in sports. Structural massage and movement integration, also called bodywork, utilizes deep tissue massage to correct posture problems and movement imbalances.

Uses

It is used in those with back pain, diabetes, eating disorders, cystic fibrosis, asthma, depression, atopic dermatitis, and juvenile rheumatoid arthritis.

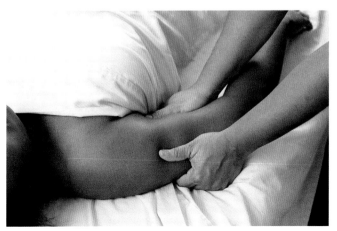

FIGURE 8.4 Wellness massage is a massage to decrease stress, promote relaxation, and support the body's natural restorative mechanisms.

TABLE 8.2

Talking with AYAs about Complementary and Integrative Medicine

Be open-minded. Most patients are reluctant to share information about their use of **complementary and integrative medicine** therapies because they are concerned that their clinicians will disapprove. By remaining open-minded, you can learn a lot about your patients' use of **complementary and integrative medicine.** These strategies will help foster open communication.

Ask the question. Ask every patient about his or her use of integrative therapies during routine history taking. One approach is simply to inquire, "Are you doing anything else for this condition?" It is an open-ended question that gives the patient the opportunity to tell you about his or her use of other clinicians or therapies. Another approach is to ask, "Are you taking any over-the-counter remedies such as vitamins/supplements or herbs?"

Do not dismiss any therapy as a placebo. If a patient tells you about a therapy that you are unaware of, make a note of it in the patient's record and schedule a follow-up visit after you have learned more—when you will be in a better position to negotiate the patient's care. If you determine the therapy might be harmful, you will have to ask the patient to stop using it. If it is not harmful and the patient feels better using it, you may want to consider incorporating the therapy into your care plan.

Discuss clinicians as well as therapies. Another way to help your patients negotiate the maze of integrative therapies is by stressing that they see appropriately trained and licensed clinicians. Know who to refer to in your area. Encourage your patients to ask integrative clinicians about their background and training and the treatment modalities they use. By doing so, your patients will be better equipped to make educated decisions about their health care.

Discuss complementary and integrative medicine therapies with your patients at every visit. Charting the details of their use will remind you to raise the issue. It may also help alert you to potential complications before they occur.

AYAs, adolescents and young adults.

Clinical Studies

There have been studies showing efficacy in those with back pain, diabetes, and juvenile rheumatoid arthritis. Less robust evidence is noted in those with atopic dermatitis, cystic fibrosis, depression, asthma, and eating disorders.[32]

Adverse Effects

None reported.

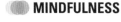 **MINDFULNESS**

Mechanism of Action

Jon Kabat-Zinn, the founder of Mindfulness-Based Stress Reduction (MBSR), defined mindfulness as "the awareness that emerges through paying attention on purpose, in the present moment, and nonjudgmentally to the unfolding of experience moment by moment." Mind–Body Medicine uses the ability of thoughts and emotions to shape physical health. Mind–body therapies can galvanize the relaxation response to reduce stress and improve overall well-being. The basic elements for eliciting the relaxation response include a nonjudging receptive awareness, a mental focus, such as repetition of the word, phrase, prayer, or image. A comfortable position and a quiet environment are helpful, but not essential. The relaxation response counters the harmful effects of stress and trauma responses.[33,34]

Mindfulness can easily be taught to AYAs. Online resources for families that explain mindfulness in developmentally appropriate ways are available.

Uses

Mindfulness is used for anxiety, insomnia, stress reduction, and chronic pain.

Clinical Studies

Mindfulness in combination with and without hypnosis, has been successfully combined for anxiety management and would benefit from additional study.[35-37]

Adverse Effects

None reported.

 SUMMARY

There are many complementary and integrative health care options available to AYAs and their families. Open, honest, and nonjudgmental discussions will enable AYAs to make informed choices.[38] Improved communication can be addressed by following the recommendations outlined in **Table 8.2.** Clinicians should inquire frequently and regularly about the use of complementary and integrative medicine in their AYA patients. Complementary and integrative approaches can be used safely and provide health benefits.

REFERENCES

1. McClafferty H. An overview of pediatric integrative medicine. *Pediatr Ann.* 2019;48(6):e216–e219. doi: 10.3928/19382359-20190515-04
2. Wang C, Preisser J, Chung Y, Li K. Complementary and alternative medicine use among children with mental health issues: results from the National Health Interview Survey. *BMC Complement Altern Med.* 2018;18(1):241. doi: 10.1186/s12906-018-2307-5. PMID: 30157825; PMCID: PMC6116551.
3. Black LI, Clarke TC, Barnes PM, et al. Use of complementary health approaches among children aged 4–17 years in the United States: National Health Interview Survey, 2007–2012. *Natl Health Stat Report.* 2015;(78):1–19.
4. Rhee TG, Evans RL, McAlpine DD, et al. Racial/ethnic differences in the use of complementary and integrative medicine in US adults with moderate mental distress. *J Prim Care Community Health.* 2017;8(2):43–54.
5. Elewonibi BR, BeLue R. Prevalence of complementary and alternative medicine in immigrants. *J Immigr Minor Health.* 2016;18(3):600–607. https://doi.org/10.1007/s10903-015-0210-4
6. National Center for Complementary and Integrative Health. *NCCIH Strategic Plan FY 2021–2025: Mapping the Pathway to Research on Whole Person Health.* National Center for Complementary and Integrative Health website accessed at https://nccih.nih.gov/about/nccih-strategic-plan-2021-2025 on 27 Jun 2022.
7. Cohen MH, Kemper KJ. Complementary therapies in pediatrics: a legal perspective. *Pediatrics* 2005;115(3):774–780. doi: 10.1542/peds.2004-1093
8. Smith T, May G, Eckl V, et al. US sales of herbal supplements increase by 8.6% in 2019. *HerbalGram.* 2020;127:54–69. Accessed August 31, 2020. http://cms.herbalgram.org/herbalgram/issue127/hg127-mktrpt-2019.html
9. Parvez MK, Rishi V. Herb-drug interactions and hepatotoxicity. *Curr Drug Metab.* 2019;20(4):275–282. doi: 10.2174/1389200220666190325141422
10. www.nccih.nih.gov/health/providers/digest/herb-drug-interactions-science accessed 27 Jun 2022.
11. Posadzki P, Watson LK, Ernst E. Adverse effects of herbal medicines: an overview of systematic reviews. *Clin Med.* 2013;13(1):7–12.
12. Or F, Kim Y, Simms J, Austin SB. Taking stock of dietary supplements' harmful effects on children, adolescents, and young adults. *J Adolesc Health.* 2019;65(4):455–461. doi: 10.1016/j.jadohealth.2019.03.005. Epub 2019 Jun 5. PMID: 31176525.
13. Ng QX, Venkatanarayanan N, Ho CYX. Clinical use of Hypericum perforatum (St John's wort) in depression: a meta-analysis. *J Affect Disord.* 2017;210:211–221. doi: 10.1016/j.jad.2016.12.048. Epub 2017 Jan 3.
14. Shinjyo N, Waddell G, Green J. Valerian root in treating sleep problems and associated disorders—a systematic review and meta-analysis. *J Evid Based Integr Med.* 2020;25:2515690X20967323. doi: 10.1177/2515690X20967323
15. Hieu TH, Dibas M, Surya Dila KA, et al. Therapeutic efficacy and safety of chamomile for state anxiety, generalized anxiety disorder, insomnia, and sleep quality: a systematic review and meta-analysis of randomized trials and quasi-randomized trials. *Phytother Res.* 2019;33(6):1604–1615. doi: 10.1002/ptr.6349. Epub 2019 Apr 21.
16. Wieland LS, Piechotta V, Feinberg T, et al. Elderberry for prevention and treatment of viral respiratory illnesses: a systematic review. *BMC Complement Med Ther.* 2021;21(1):112. doi: 10.1186/s12906-021-03283-5
17. Karsch-Völk M, Barrett B, Kiefer D, et al. Echinacea for preventing and treating the common cold. *Cochrane Database Syst Rev.* 2014;2(2):CD000530.
18. Guilbot A, Bangratz M, Ait Abdellah S, et al. A combination of coenzyme Q10, feverfew and magnesium for migraine prophylaxis: a prospective observational study. *BMC Complement Altern Med.* 2017;17(1):433. doi: 10.1186/s12906-017-1933-7
19. Maras A, Schroder CM, Malow BA, et al. Long-term efficacy and safety of pediatric prolonged-release melatonin for insomnia in children with autism spectrum disorder. *J Child Adolesc Psychopharmacol.* 2018;28(10):699–710. doi: 10.1089/cap.2018.0020. Epub 2018 Oct 11.
20. Esposito S, Laino D, D'Alonzo R, et al. Pediatric sleep disturbances and treatment with melatonin. *J Transl Med.* 2019;17(1):77. doi: 10.1186/s12967-019-1835-1
21. Andersen LPH, Gögenur I, Rosenberg J, et al. The safety of melatonin in humans. *Clin Drug Investig.* 2016;36(3):169–175. doi: 10.1007/s40261-015-0368-5
22. Unfer V, Facchinetti F, Orrù B, et al. Myo-inositol effects in women with PCOS: a meta-analysis of randomized controlled trials. *Endocr Connect.* 2017;6(8):647–658. doi: 10.1530/EC-17-0243

23. Nielsen A, Wieland LS. Cochrane reviews on acupuncture therapy for pain: a snapshot of the current evidence. *Explore (NY)*. 2019;15(6):434–439. doi:10.1016/j.explore.2019.08.009

24. Yang J, Ganesh R, Wu Q, et al. Battlefield acupuncture for adult pain: a systematic review and meta-analysis of randomized controlled trials. *Am J Chin Med*. 2021;49(1):25–40. doi: 10.1142/S0192415X21500026. Epub 2020 Dec 29.

25. Wieland LS, Skoetz N, Pilkington K, et al. Yoga treatment for chronic nonspecific low back pain. *Cochrane Database Syst Rev*. 2017;1(1):CD010671. doi:10.1002/14651858.CD010671.pub2

26. Blume HK, Brockman LN, Breuner CC. Biofeedback therapy for pediatric headache: factors associated with response. *Headache*. 2012;52(9):1377–1386.

27. Banerjee S, Argáez C. *Neurofeedback and Biofeedback for Mood and Anxiety Disorders: A Review of Clinical Effectiveness and Guidelines [Internet]*. Canadian Agency for Drugs and Technologies in Health; 2017.

28. Sawni A, Breuner CC. Clinical hypnosis, an effective mind-body modality for adolescents with behavioral and physical complaints. *Children (Basel)*. 2017;4(4):19.

29. Vining R, Long CR, Minkalis A, et al. Effects of chiropractic care on strength, balance, and endurance in active-duty U.S. military personnel with low back pain: a randomized controlled trial. *J Altern Complement Med*. 2020;26(7):592–601.

30. Schneider M, Vernon H, Ko G, et al. Chiropractic management of fibromyalgia syndrome: a systematic review of the literature. *J Manipulative Physiol Ther*. 2009;32(1):25–40.

31. Todd AJ, Carroll MT, Robinson A, et al. Adverse events due to chiropractic and other manual therapies for infants and children: a review of the literature. *J Manipulative Physiol Ther*. 2015;38(9):699–712. doi: 10.1016/j.jmpt.2014.09.008. Epub 2014 Oct 30.

32. Field T. Pediatric massage therapy research: a narrative review. *Children (Basel)*. 2019;6(6):78. doi:10.3390/children6060078

33. Ortiz R, Sibinga EM. The role of mindfulness in reducing the adverse effects of childhood stress and trauma. *Children (Basel)*. 2017;4(3):16. doi: 10.3390/children4030016

34. SECTION ON INTEGRATIVE MEDICINE. Mind-body therapies in children and youth. *Pediatrics*. 2016;138(3):e20161896. doi: 10.1542/peds.2016-1896. Epub 2016 Aug 22.

35. Jayawardena W, Erbe R, Lohrmann D, et al. Use of treatment and counseling services and mind-body techniques by students with emotional and behavioral difficulties. *J Sch Health*. 2017;87(2):133–141.

36. Kaiser P, Kohen DP, Brown ML, et al. Integrating pediatric hypnosis with complementary modalities: clinical perspectives on personalized treatment. *Children (Basel)*. 2018;5(8):108

37. Burnett-Zeigler I, McLeod D. Diversifying Mindfulness: Reflections from Our Journeys Applying Mindfulness-Based Interventions in the Black Community. *Journal of Integrative and Complementary Medicine*. 2022:110–113. http://doi.org/10.1089/jicm.2021.0440

38. Jou J, Johnson PJ. Nondisclosure of complementary and integrative medicine use to primary care physicians: findings from the 2012 National Health Interview Survey. *JAMA Intern Med*. 2016;176(4):545–546.

ADDITIONAL RESOURCES AND WEBSITES

Additional Resources and Websites for Clinicians:

Benson-Henry Institute—https://bensonhenryinstitute.org/

The Center for Mind-Body Medicine—www.cmbm.org/trainings

MAYO Clinic—Integrative medicine—Mayo Clinic

National Center for Complementary and Integrative Health—www.nccih.nih.gov/training/videolectures

Online updates on Biofeedback Applied Psychophysiology and Biofeedback—www.aapb.org/i4a/pages/index.cfm?pageid=3653

Rakel D. *Integrative Medicine*. 4th ed. Elsevier; 2017

The University of Minnesota—www.csh.umn.edu/education/online-modules-and-resources/learning-modules-healthcare-professionals

Additional Resources and Websites for Parents/Caregivers:

A Parent's Guide to Complementary and Integrative Medicine—Keep Kids Healthy—https://keepkidshealthy.com/2018/08/10/a-parents-guide-to-complementary-and-integrative-medicine/

National Center for Complementary and Integrative Health—https://www.nccih.nih.gov/

Whole Health—Home—TakeCare—https://takecare.org

Additional Resources and Websites for Adolescents and Young Adults:

Meditations—Benson-Henry Institute—https://bensonhenryinstitute.org/

National Center Complementary and Integrative Health info for teens -7 Things to Know About Mind and Body Practices for Children and Teens—https://www.nccih.nih.gov/health/tips/things-to-know-about-mind-and-body-practices-for-children-and-teens

Vo D. The Mindful Teen: Powerful Skills to Help You Handle Stress One Moment at a Time (The Instant Help Solutions Series)

CHAPTER

9

Technology and Social Media

Megan A. Moreno
Ellen M. Selkie

KEY WORDS

- Apps
- Cyberbullying
- Electronic health record (EHR)
- Internet
- Problematic internet use (PIU)
- Social media
- Technology
- Telehealth

 INTRODUCTION

Digital technology is omnipresent in an adolescent's and young adult's (AYA's) life as smartphones, tablets, and personal computers have proliferated in homes and schools. Rapid advancements in technology over the past decade have provided AYAs with numerous benefits, including expansive access to knowledge and far-reaching communication tools. Today's AYAs are "digital natives" who have grown up with access to computers and the internet from an early age. However, there are concomitant risks to technology use. This chapter provides an overview of technology with particular focus on social media use—the most popular form of internet use—including benefits and risks. The chapter concludes with discussion of opportunities to use these tools to improve health for AYAs.

SOCIAL MEDIA AND TECHNOLOGY USE RATES

Internet and social media use are now nearly universal among AYAs. Among young adults, a 2019 study found that 96% reported owning a smartphone, with rates up from 67% in 2012 and 56% in 2011.[1] In recent years, the digital divide in internet access between high and low socioeconomic groups has narrowed but still exists. Whereas 94% of higher-income households have a computer, only 73% of lower-income households have the same. Similarly, 89% of high-income teens have a smartphone compared with 74% of low-income teens.[2]

SOCIAL MEDIA

What Is Social Media?

The first iteration of the web was known as Web 1.0 and its purpose was to provide information to consumers. Technologic advancements led to Web 2.0, a new web that both provided information to consumers and empowered users to view, create, and share multimedia data with peers and the public. Web 2.0 led to what has been called social media, also called immersive or interactive media. Social media represent a set of Web 2.0 tools that are centered on interaction and sharing of content with others, although users may also consume content passively.

The idea of interacting and sharing content via media is a remarkable concept in the area of media studies. Traditional media, such as television, typically featured a corporation creating content that viewers consumed. Messages were unidirectional, easily represented by a single arrow pointing from the corporation to the consumer. In the world of social media, internet users became both creators and consumers of content. Messages now flow in all directions, from corporations to users, among users, and back to corporations through a seemingly endless array of potential paths. Thus, today's AYAs have increased capacity to interact with each other and the larger world using media, enhanced opportunities to explore and experiment via media, and an increased likelihood of being influenced or even harmed by media experiences.

The majority of AYAs report ownership of at least one social media account or profile.[2] Specific social media platforms vary in popularity among AYAs, but the top current platforms are listed below. With the exception of YouTube, all of these platforms allow for direct messaging between users in addition to specific functionalities unique to each platform.

- YouTube: Users can view and/or create video content and may comment on other users' videos. YouTube is often a primary source of news for AYAs.
- Snapchat: With this "ephemeral" app, users post photos or videos, either publicly or to selected individuals, that are automatically deleted in 24 hours.
- Instagram: Originally an image-based platform, Instagram now allows users to post photos and short videos (other users can comment), ephemeral posts in "stories," or longer form videos through the Instagram TV (IGTV) function. Instagram is owned by Facebook.
- TikTok: This short-form video platform allows users to post short videos with filters, text, and music. Other users can comment on these posts.
- Reddit: A platform valued for its anonymity, Reddit is a text-based website in which users write and comment on posts in a forum-style format. Popular comments/posts are "upvoted" or "downvoted" by the community, modulating their visibility.
- Facebook: One of the first social media sites, Facebook allows users to post photos, text, and videos to their personal "friend" network (which may extend to the friends of their friends). Facebook users can also form groups based on interests or geographic location. Despite public perception of the platform as one for older generations, many AYAs continue to maintain Facebook profiles to connect with family and friends.
- Twitter: Users can post short messages of up to 280 characters with or without photos or media.

The above list is not exhaustive—each year, sites change in popularity, new sites emerge, and older sites die out, leading to a constantly changing social media landscape. For example, in recent years, platforms have developed more functions to create ephemeral or anonymous content, but other, more permanent content also remains popular among youth.

How Social Media Sites Are Used

Adolescents report using technology to access social media for around 2 hours per day.[2] However, the ways in which this time is spent may vary and encompass both active and passive use. Active use represents activities such as content creation and posting, commenting on or otherwise engaging with (i.e., sharing, liking) others' posts, and conversing in direct messages or group chats. On the other hand, passive use includes scrolling through or viewing other users' content or news without responding or contributing.[3] Most AYAs' use of social media combines active and passive use.

Social media platforms offer different affordances, or characteristics, that allow users to express and share content in different ways. For some adolescent users, video or photographic content may be a way to share personal aspects of their lives. Memes (humorous images, videos, or text) are commonly shared widely as are quotes, song lyrics, and news stories. In summary, these sites offer many opportunities for self-expression, a means of peer communication and feedback, as well as connection to an online social network.

Influence of Social Media

Social media combines peer and media effects and thereby represents a powerful motivator of behavior whether by content created by individuals or simply found and shared with peers. It has been argued that social media may have greater influence than traditional media, as social media combines the power of interpersonal persuasion with the reach of mass media. Facebook, which has been described as "the most significant advance in persuasion since the radio was invented in the 1890s," initiated a new form of persuasion labeled "mass interpersonal persuasion." As such, a small number of content creators with large numbers of followers can earn money through advertisers in a manner similar to traditional celebrities. This has made full-time content creation a career aspiration for some youth.

Prior research has delineated four potential constructs, or paths of influence, of social media on AYAs[4] (Table 9.1): (1) *Connection*: Social media provides and enhances peer communication, networking, and connection; (2) *Comparison*: Social media allows comparison between peers to take place using tangible information such as photos, stated behaviors, and the ability to note peer comments; (3) *Identification*: Social media allows a profile owner to develop an online identity through a profile. Profile owners can then reflect and revise that identity via feedback from peers' comments and "likes," or by personal perusal through the social media profile. The ability to develop one's identity in real-time provides a unique multimedia view of the self; and, (4) *Immersive experience:* Social media combines text, images, videos, and other visual elements to create an immersive user experience.

Benefits of Social Media and Other Digital Technologies

There are many ways in which use of social media and technology benefits today's AYAs. Described below are key features of social media, particularly of social networking sites, that may provide unique benefits to this population.

Social Support and Social Capital

Virtual communities play an increasing role in the lives of today's youth. Previous work has described social connections via social media as similar in value to family connections,[5] and supported that social media may play an important role in the life course of AYAs' development of social connectedness.[6] Indeed, the majority of adolescents describe using social media to develop and sustain friendships. Epidemiologic studies over the years have repeatedly demonstrated that as the size of one's social network increases, physical and mental health improve. Online-only friends (i.e., those someone has never met in person) can oftentimes provide support to AYAs equivalent to that of offline friends. Such support has even been shown to attenuate suicidal ideation in the face of relational stress. Furthermore, online social media activity can increase social capital and strengthen offline friendships.[7] During the COVID-19 pandemic, these digital connections were especially important as in-person connections were more limited.

The varied social media sites available also allow AYAs to develop new arenas in which social support can be built and cultivated. Multiple studies have described social media as a desirable venue for help-seeking behaviors in mental health.[8] Aspects unique to social media (e.g., privacy from parents, anonymity, accessibility) allow AYAs the opportunity to explore relationships and social connections at their own pace. This can be particularly important for AYAs of marginalized identities including racial and ethnic minorities, sexual and gender minorities, and neurodivergent populations.[9]

Identity Development

Youth can use social media to manage their self-presentation or influence how others see them. Self-disclosure on social media, especially authentic expressions of self, can aid in identity clarification and evolution in response to feedback and new social media experiences.[10] Observing representation of individuals of different racial and ethnic identities can be helpful in shaping one's own racial and/or ethnic identity through social comparison.[11] While identity experimentation is less common on large-scale social media platforms such as Facebook and Instagram, smaller or "niche" social media platforms continue to be used by AYAs to explore and shape their identity. For those AYAs with interests outside the mainstream culture, social media provides an outlet to meet new people who share their interests through, for example, hobby and fandom communities. These online peer groups may provide AYAs with the support they need to develop and reinforce their identities.[12]

Education and Civic Engagement

There are several ways in which technology use can contribute to education. Youth in high school, technical school, and colleges/universities can use the internet to find information for reports, or augment classroom learning on specific topics. The internet can provide audio, video, or multimedia sources to complement traditional textbooks. Further, technology can be used as a means of communication between students as well as between students and teachers to discuss assignments and projects. During the COVID-19 pandemic, youth leveraged technology to advance their education through a myriad of ways, from seeking mental health resources for peers to learning how to fix their own bicycles.

Technology and social media can also contribute to AYAs' civic engagement. One feature of social media platforms such as Facebook is the ability to create groups and events, which can be private or publicly available to others. Many of the existing groups on Facebook are dedicated to political, religious, or community purposes. Other social media such as Twitter allow rapid and wide transmission of news and information. These platforms provide AYAs opportunities for exposure to new ideas and information, which can then lead to action through advocacy and/or political activism.[13]

Health Access and Illness Support

Social media allows AYAs to access health information for topics that may be stigmatized or embarrassing, such as sexual behavior or substance use. A key issue is to ensure that AYAs have knowledge of and access to sites that provide accurate and reliable information. To that end, numerous health organizations, such as Planned

TABLE 9.1

Areas of Influence Adapted from the Facebook Influence Model

Area of Influence	Cluster Topics within This Area	Example Items That Represent the Cluster
Connection	Connection to people	Allows people to constantly stay updated with other's lives Way to get to know acquaintances almost instantly Keep in touch with people you would not call or text
	Far-reaching	Ability to reach many people with one website Can reach anyone, young and old, rich and poor Bonding across cultures and distances
	Fast communication	Feel connected and in the loop constantly Puts everyone you know and what they are doing in one place Updates on people's lives faster than with a cell phone
	Business and promotion	Ability to plan influential events such as protests or sit-ins Statuses provide a way to blog instantly about events or political topics Every company uses it to promote business or provide deals
	Accessible and adaptable	Largest network in human history Easy to use and navigate Widely known and talked about
	Data and information	Huge database of information Compiled data from millions of individuals News feature
Identification	Identity expression	Freedom to express things and let them be heard Present the best side of yourself Show off accomplishments to everyone you are friends with on social media, not just close friends
	Influence on identity	Provides others with pictures that can influence perceptions Display aspects of yourself that you wouldn't share in offline life (sexuality, substance use) Wonder if you should be doing what you see everyone doing in pictures
Comparison	Curiosity about others	Can know what people are up to without asking them about it and without them knowing you know Creep culture/Stalking See who associates with whom through pictures and comments
	Social media establishing social norms	Reinforces beliefs or opinions by seeing that others hold same beliefs or opinions Can see what is popular by observation Can follow norms
Social media as an experience	Distractions	Procrastination Addictive Huge distraction
	Positive experiences	Social media content is referenced in daily life Provides entertainment at any time Status updates can promote a good mood
	Negative experiences	Changes the nature of communication from face-to-face to screen-to-screen People willing to sacrifice privacy Inspires competition in people

Moreno MA, Kota R, Schoohs S, et al. The Facebook influence model: a concept mapping approach. *Cyberpsychol Behav Soc Netw.* 2013;16(7):504–511.

Parenthood, maintain a social media presence. Many of these social media sites allow real-time interactions to answer questions or provide resources. Technology and social media also provide opportunities for AYAs with chronic illnesses, or their parents, to connect to groups to find support during challenging times or share stories with others. Social media has been described as a "mechanism of empowerment" for patients.[14] Some patients use technology or social media to interact with classmates, or even virtually attend classes, during prolonged hospital stays.

Risks of Social Media

While AYAs are rapid adopters of new technologies and may be particularly savvy in using online tools, the constantly evolving landscape of social media and frequent changes to design aspects of platforms can still create vulnerability. Many AYAs report moderating what they share online due to privacy concerns—for example, avoiding disclosure of personal information in profiles or to strangers.[15] Even so, information that is shared with online contacts an AYA "trusts" may have negative consequences if their relationships change. Furthermore, AYAs may not be aware of the large amounts of data that are collected by social media platforms and used for targeted advertising and other customized content.

Risks Related to Posted Content

Adolescence is frequently a time of behavioral experimentation, which, for some adolescents, includes experimentation with health-risk behaviors. As social media give adolescents the opportunity to post information about their personal lives, such as likes, dislikes, and activities, they also allow adolescents to display information about risky behaviors. Over a decade of research has found that many AYAs choose to represent health-risk behaviors including alcohol, substance use, sex, and other risks on social media.[16]

Future impact: Schools and employers. Displaying health-risk behavior information, such as information about sexual activity or substance use, on social media can make the information available in a globally public venue. Content displayed on social media can be copied, downloaded, or distributed by any profile viewer. Even ephemeral content, such as on Snapchat, can be shared via screenshot or external image capture. Therefore, all such information should be considered published, public, permanent, and persuasive. This information may then be accessed by people who the profile owner would prefer not view it, such as potential employers, teachers, or educational institutions. Though many AYAs understand these risks, some may remain unclear about or unmotivated to maintain security settings that protect their displayed content on social media.

Influencing others. Regardless of whether displayed content on social media is real, AYAs may respond to another's disclosures as if they were real and this in turn may influence intentions and behaviors. A previous study found that adolescents viewed displayed alcohol references on social media profiles as accurate and influential representations of alcohol use.[17] Content promoting eating disorders (e.g., pro-anorexia or "pro-ana" and pro-bulimia or "pro-mia") is also common on social media sites.

Sexting. The term "sexting" refers to sending, receiving, or forwarding sexually explicit messages or pictures using a cell phone, computer, or other digital devices. Across multiple studies, 14.8% of adolescents reported sending a sext and 27.4% reported receiving one. The prevalence of sexting increases with age, and the majority of sexting occurs using mobile devices.[18] Sexting is correlated with in-person sexual activity and has been associated with risky sexual behaviors (e.g., multiple sexual partners, lack of contraception) and psychosocial concerns,[19] although there is little longitudinal evidence to confirm or refute a causal relationship.

Sexting is increasingly conceptualized by adolescent development experts as normative behavior among AYAs. Exchanges of sexts between existing or prospective romantic and sexual partners are common and represent an extension of sexual behavior in the digital age. Still, sexting by AYAs can have unintended negative consequences such as embarrassment, regret, or being harassed as a result of sending a sext. The sext can also be distributed beyond the target recipient—studies have reported that 12% of adolescents have forwarded a sext to someone else without the consent of the original sexter.[18] There are also potential legal consequences, which can include prosecution under child pornography statutes, a potentially devastating consequence. As such, there have been calls for the criminal justice system in the United States to clarify the legality of these behaviors by establishing consistent, sexting-specific laws.

Cyberbullying. Cyberbullying is often defined as the deliberate use of technology including social media to attack or cause harm to another individual. It can include name-calling, spreading rumors, pretending to be someone else, sending unwanted pictures or texts, distributing pictures without consent, making threats, or asking someone to do something sexual. There are some unique aspects of the online environment that may increase the potential impact of cyberbullying incidents on victims. For instance, cyberbullying can occur at any time, not just when one is face-to-face. In addition, given the wide use of social media, cyberbullying has the potential to reach a large audience.

Among adolescents, cyberbullying is less common compared to traditional forms of bullying, and is commonly associated with other traditional bullying behaviors. Prevalence rates vary wildly, with studies estimating lifetime cyberbullying victimization rates from ~5% to 65% and perpetration rates from ~2% to 44%. Current data also suggest that up to 20% of college students have experienced cyberbullying. A key challenge in understanding the prevalence of cyberbullying is the varied definitions that have been used in research studies.[20] Multiple longitudinal studies have shown that both cyberbullying victimization and perpetration predict later substance use, depression, anxiety, self-harm, and suicidal ideation. Furthermore, both perpetration and victimization are associated with decreased academic achievement.[21]

Problematic Use and Multitasking

Problematic internet use (PIU) is a public health concern for AYAs that is defined as internet use that is risky, excessive, or impulsive in nature leading to adverse life consequences, including physical, emotional, social, or functional impairment.[22] Several studies in the United States and internationally suggest links between internet overuse and negative mental and physical health consequences.[23] Problematic digital media use has also included definitions and measurements designed to apply to more narrow types of use, such as video gaming (internet gaming disorder), compulsive cell phone use, and social media addiction.

Media multitasking is defined as using more than one media device or program concurrently. Media multitasking is an area in need of further study, as it is unclear what impact multitasking has on brain development during this critical time. It has been argued that the fragmentary nature of attention while multitasking may impact a teen's ability to sustain focus during tasks such as studying. Conversely, some have argued that in today's modern media society, multitasking is a necessary strategy to get work completed.

VIDEO GAMES AND ONLINE GAMING

Video games and gaming software are also frequently used by adolescents. Games can be played through consoles such as Playstation or Xbox, or they can be played on computers, tablets, or mobile phones. Many games offer players the opportunity to be creative by designing their own avatars or building structures within the game. Some games involve only the individual playing, while other games have social aspects in which players form teams to compete against each other or complete a task collectively. In these games, users can chat via text or voice. Several platforms such as YouTube and Twitch allow players to record or livestream themselves playing video games for others to observe.

TELEHEALTH

The Centers for Medicare and Medicaid Services (CMS) defines *telehealth* as the use of telecommunications and information technology to provide access to health assessment, diagnosis, intervention, consultation, supervision, and information across distance.[24] Telehealth includes health services and treatment delivered via telecommunications technology, such as phones, patient portals, and videoconferencing. Studies examining telehealth have found that delivering health services in this manner is feasible, acceptable, and has been effective across many different types of illnesses and conditions.[25] During the COVID-19 pandemic, there was a rapid expansion of telehealth as many clinicians adapted and integrated increased telehealth options to serve patients. While most literature to date has examined telehealth in the care of adult patients, a growing body of literature in adolescent health is demonstrating positive outcomes similar to those among adults.[26]

Advantages of telehealth for AYAs include convenience, particularly for adolescents who would need to travel a long distance to access health care. Further, less time traveling to health care appointments may mean less disruption of school and other activities. Additional potential advantages include lower costs of visits and increased comfort for teens engaging in care in a familiar setting such as their bedroom or living room. Clinicians must ensure high quality of care at all times, particularly given the limitations of telehealth without in-person interviews or physical examinations. Another key concern for adolescents is the capacity to provide confidential care through telehealth. For some adolescents, confidential care may be achieved by physically going to their own room during the visit, but for others who live in more constrained spaces, it may be more challenging. Another critical issue is ensuring equitable access to telehealth for all AYAs.

ELECTRONIC HEALTH RECORDS

While not a form of social media, electronic health records (EHRs) are digital medical records that can be shared electronically across clinicians. Many EHRs also offer patient portals that allow a patient, or a patient proxy, to communicate with the clinician and access personal health information. Thus, EHRs may share characteristics with social media in allowing AYAs increased opportunities to communicate, connect, and share information. Adolescents and young adults frequently go online to access health information, including information about sexually transmitted infections, nutrition, exercise, and sexuality. Given AYAs' comfort with seeking health information online, and high rates of internet access and use, this group is poised to uniquely benefit from increasing rates of EHR use.

Electronic health records are now a national expectation for hospitals in the United States. Further, the 21st Century Cures Act is intended to increase access, use, and exchange of electronic health information.[27] A study of parents of children and adolescents found that parents of younger children were more likely to utilize EHR portals compared to parents of adolescents.[28]

There are many potential benefits for AYAs having access to personal EHR portals. Studies have consistently shown health literacy benefits among adult patients who use online health portals, including obtaining prescription refills, asking nonurgent questions, and obtaining lab results. Further, studies in adult patients have shown improved clinician access, patient–clinician relationship, and continuity of care.

However, there are also barriers to access to EHR patient portals, particularly for adolescents. Many health care systems allow parents to have proxy access to their children's EHR during childhood. Often, access is blocked to both parents and patients when adolescents are between the ages of 13 and 17 due to concerns about confidentiality and consent.

Distinguishing standard medical information from protected or confidential adolescent health information remains a major challenge. At present, there is no widely available technology that can distinguish between confidential and standard medical record information. Addressing this concern may require creative solutions, such as allowing AYA patients to review their online medical information and sequester any information that can be legally protected as confidential; this could be done in the clinic setting or from a home computer.

Given the rise of EHRs and the potential benefits of improving health care access and engagement by AYAs, the Society for Adolescent Health and Medicine published a position paper[9] which advocated for EHR design, implementation, and use that address the needs of AYAs for access to health information and protection of confidentiality. Thus, EHR vendors need to develop systems that meet regulatory requirements and address the unique privacy needs of AYAs by building privacy settings into all aspects of their products. Further, health care systems implementing EHRs must provide training to all staff in techniques to protect confidential patient information as per national and state laws, as well as institutional policies.

APPS

The past few decades have seen growth in another area of digital media in the form of mobile applications, often referred to as apps. Apps are designed to be used across a number of consumer products including smartphones, tablets, and wearables. Apps represent many functionalities in digital media that overlap with other topics in this chapter, including social media, gaming, and health information access. A growing area of research focuses on using apps to improve adolescent health, including impacting health behaviors such as exercise or dietary intake, and providing mental health support. A critical tension in this area is between industry-developed apps which generally get to market quickly yet lack evidence, and research-developed apps which are often slower to reach the consumer marketplace.[30]

ROLE OF THE ADOLESCENT AND YOUNG ADULT CLINICIAN REGARDING DIGITAL TECHNOLOGY USE

Fortunately, there are strategies available for clinicians, educators, and parents to help AYAs avoid risks and amplify benefits associated with technology use. One approach is through focusing on three key concepts: balance, boundaries, and communication.[31]

Balance: The balance between online and offline time is a critical concept to discuss with AYAs. Spending time offline, including hanging out with friends and family, exercising, or spending time outside, is critical to AYA development. Further, achieving balance provides protection against risks such as PIU.

Boundaries: Boundaries refers to setting limits around what AYAs are willing to display about themselves online or on social media, as well as setting limits on where adolescents spend their time online. Discussing guidelines on what types of personal information are not appropriate to post on social media sites with teens can help prevent them from several online safety risks. These risks include being targets of bullying, unwanted solicitation, or embarrassment.

Communication: Just as with other core domains of adolescent health, parents should discuss social media and technology with their adolescents early and often. Establishing home rules for social media and technology use as soon as the child begins using these tools is an important way to promote healthy technology use from the beginning.

Adolescent and young adult clinicians can consider these core constructs in their efforts toward prevention, education, screening, and intervention. Specific strategies to consider include the following:

Prevention
- *Supervision and co-viewing*
  - Encourage parents to take an active role in supervising and providing guidance regarding technology use during the early adolescent years. Examples of this may include co-viewing of internet content with discussion of teachable moments or having parents follow their child's social media profiles.
  - Learning to engage in technology should involve a period of time in which sessions are supervised and guidance is offered, followed by a gradual progression to independent use once skills have been learned and demonstrated.
  - Co-viewing and co-playing with technology can foster enjoyment of technology and facilitate role modeling of appropriate technology use.
- *Balance*
  - There are many approaches to promoting balance with teens including setting a "media curfew" after which no technology is used, such as after 9 PM. This may involve, for example,

turning off the household Wi-Fi at a set time, or charging devices outside of an adolescent's bedroom.

- Some families establish "media-free times," such as family dinners, to provide time and space for families to interact without technologic interruptions. Such family communication may be beneficial for improving AYA mental health and mitigating negative impacts of cyberbullying.
- Young adults can consider engaging in media-free periods, such as a "screen-free week" or avoiding social media for a period of time to promote increased awareness of their offline environment. The amount of time spent on social media and other mobile applications can be self-monitored and even set to be limited (e.g., shutting down Twitter after 30 minutes of use) with a variety of mobile phone tools and apps.
- *Boundaries*
  - Among younger adolescents, it is important for families to discuss setting boundaries around what types of sites are appropriate for teens, as well as what actions to take if an adolescent stumbles onto a site with concerning content.
  - Shared decision making between adolescents and their parents about rules can increase trust. For example, if an adolescent is targeted by cyberbullying, the fear of having their device taken away may make them hesitant to tell an adult. If open, nonjudgmental communication has been established ahead of time, adolescents may feel safer in approaching parents in such a situation.
  - Promoting boundaries often involves helping AYAs see connections between their online and offline personas and audiences. One proposed guideline suggested by a teen is: "If what you're going to post is something you wouldn't want your grandmother to see, don't post it."
- *Media multitasking*
  - Encourage AYAs to avoid media multitasking, particularly when doing homework or academic tasks, as multitasking is associated with lower academic performance.
  - For high school students heading to college, clinicians can offer a timely reminder of the importance of avoiding media multitasking during study periods.
- *Communication*
  - Clinicians can encourage parents to regularly check in on an adolescent's social media presence and to revisit household rules as an adolescent gets older.
  - For the older adolescents or young adults living outside the home, parents can still play a role in prompting their child to take care in how much personal information they display online, and in maintaining a healthy balance of offline and online time.

Education

- Adolescent clinicians may consider working with schools or community groups to offer talks or educational sessions on these topics and to share resources. Concerns regarding social media and technology use by youth are shared among clinicians, educators, the legal and law enforcement community, other youth-oriented community groups, and even by youth themselves.

Screening

- *Balance*
  - Ask AYAs about their media and technology use, as well as how much time they spend each day without media.
  - Ask AYAs about what rules, if any, they or their family use to regulate or monitor media use.
- *Boundaries*
  - Ask AYAs about their privacy settings on social media sites, and how often they update or check these settings to ensure they are current.

- *Communication*
  - Ask AYAs about how often they discuss their social media and technology use with their parents/caregivers or other adults.
  - Ask AYAs if they have ever seen or been involved in anything that makes them feel unsafe online, and have them identify trusted adults in whom they can confide if safety concerns arise.
- *Problematic internet use*
  - Among AYAs who express concerns with overuse or overengagement with the internet, screening for PIU may be indicated. The Problematic and Risky Internet Use Screening Scale (PRIUSS-18) has been validated for use in AYAs.
  - A shorter scale, the PRIUSS-3 is a brief three-item scale that can be used in prescreening within clinical and school-based settings.[32]
- ***Ask patients directly about risk behaviors such as sexting***
  - As studies suggest that sexting is associated with offline sexual behaviors, screening for sexual health risks among teens who engage in sexting is indicated.
  - If AYAs are engaging in sexting, explore whether this behavior is consensual or if they feel pressured by partners to sext, as this may be a warning sign for intimate partner violence.
- ***Ask patients about experiences with online harassment or cyberbullying***
  - Since older AYAs may not consider cyberbullying a form of "bullying," consider using other terms such as online harassment or electronic harassment. For teens who have engaged as cyberbullies or victims, provide support and offer counseling as needed to address common consequences including negative self-esteem and depression. Involve parents, schools, and/or law enforcement if there are any concerns about safety.

Intervention

- One approach for prevention and intervention to promote healthy technology use is the Family Media Plan. This approach was developed by the American Academy of Pediatrics to align with their 2016 media policy statements. The tool is available online and free at this website: https://www.healthychildren.org/English/media/Pages/default.aspx, and does not collect personal information.
  - The Family Media Plan allows adolescents and their parents to co-develop a set of guidelines and rules for their media use. The tool provides a list of categories of rules, such as "media-free times" and "safety first," and a range of options to select within each category. Write-in rules and guidelines are also allowed. At the conclusion of the process, families can print out the list of rules and post it in the house for family members to follow.
  - The second part of the tool is a Media Time Calculator that allows adolescents to track how much time they spend each day on key activities, including sleep, meals, school, homework, physical activity, and socialization. Media time is then calculated in the context of these other activities, so that an individual can determine an appropriate amount of time to commit to media and technology use.
- ***Balance.*** Clinicians can help AYAs, particularly those struggling with balance or showing early signs of PIU, to develop media use plans or media-free times during the day. For some AYAs who have a more impaired relationship with the internet or technology, counseling may be indicated.
  - While there are currently no validated interventions for PIU, counseling may assist AYAs in developing strategies to reduce their use and cope with associated symptoms and signs such as social isolation or impulsivity.
- ***Boundaries.*** Encourage families to have scheduled check-ins with their adolescents to view social media profiles together.

This practice can ensure that security settings are up to date and that displayed information does not endanger the adolescents. Among young adults who live outside the home, this type of approach is less feasible, though clinicians can emphasize the impact that displayed personal information may have on the young adults' employment prospects.

SUMMARY

Technology and social media are integral parts of AYAs' lives. They offer AYAs a new world of opportunities but also create novel risks to their health and safety. Clinicians can apply a framework of balance, boundaries, and communication to counsel patients regarding their social media and technology use to maximize the benefits and minimize the risks of these novel tools. Electronic health records with patient portals offer many opportunities to engage and involve AYAs in their health care; however, barriers exist to providing confidential care in the EHR realm.

REFERENCES

1. Anderson M. Mobile technology and home broadband 2019. *Internet Technol*. 2019. https://www.pewresearch.org/internet/2019/06/13/mobile-technology-and-home-broadband-2019/
2. Rideout V, Robb MB. *The Common Sense Census: Media Use by Tweens and Teens, 2019*. Common Sense Media; 2019.
3. Orben A. Teenagers, screens and social media: a narrative review of reviews and key studies. *Soc Psychiatry Psychiatr Epidemiol*. 2020;55(4):407–414.
4. Moreno MA, Kota R, Schoohs S, et al. The facebook influence model: a concept mapping approach. *Cyberpsychol Behav Soc Netw*. 2013;16(7):504–511.
5. Geraee N, Eslami AA, Soltani R. The relationship between family social capital, social media use and life satisfaction in adolescents. *Health Promot Perspect*. 2019;9(4):307–313.
6. Wheatley D, Buglass SL. Social network engagement and subjective well-being: a life-course perspective. *Br J Sociol*. 2019;70(5):1971–1995.
7. Dredge R, Schreurs L. Social media use and offline interpersonal outcomes during youth: a systematic literature review. *Mass Commun Soc*. 2020;23(6):885–911.
8. Pretorius C, Chambers D, Coyle D. Young people's online help-seeking and mental health difficulties: systematic narrative review. *J Med Internet Res*. 2019;21(11):e13873.
9. Odgers CL, Schuller SM, Ito M. Screen time, social media use, and adolescent development. *Annu Rev Develop Psychol*. 2020;2:485–502.
10. Luo M, Hancock JT. Self-disclosure and social media: motivations, mechanisms and psychological well-being. *Curr Opin Psychol*. 2020;31:110–115.
11. Behm-Morawitz E. Media use and the development of racial and ethnic identities. In: Van den Bulck J, ed. *The International Encyclopedia of Media Psychology*. Wiley Blackwell-ICA; 2020.
12. Ito M, Martin C, Pfister RC, et al. *Affinity Online: How Connection and Shared Interest Fuel Learning*. New York University Press, 2018;256.
13. Middaugh E, Clark LS, Ballard PJ. Digital media, participatory politics, and positive youth development. *Pediatrics*. 2017;140(Suppl 2):S127–S131.
14. Shaw RJ, Johnson CM. Health information seeking and social media use on the internet among people with diabetes. *Online J Public Health Inform*. 2011;3(1):ojphi.v3i1.3561.
15. Third A, Bellerose D, De Oliveira JD, et al. *Young and Online: Children's Perspectives on Life in the Digital Age (The State of the World's Children 2017 Companion Report)*. Western Sydney University; 2017.
16. Reid Chassiakos YL, Radesky J, Christakis D, et al; Council on Communications and Media. Children and adolescents and digital media. *Pediatrics*. 2016;138(5):e20162593.
17. Moreno MA, Briner LR, Williams A, et al. Real use or "real cool": adolescents speak out about displayed alcohol references on social networking websites. *J Adolesc Health*. 2009;45(4):420–422.
18. Madigan S, Ly A, Rash CL, et al. Prevalence of multiple forms of sexting behavior among youth: a systematic review and meta-analysis. *JAMA Pediatr*. 2018;172(4):327–335.
19. Mori C, Temple JR, Browne D, et al. Association of sexting with sexual behaviors and mental health among adolescents: a systematic review and meta-analysis. *JAMA Pediatr*. 2019;173(8):770–779.
20. Kowalski RM, Limber SP, McCord A. A developmental approach to cyberbullying: prevalence and protective factors. *Aggression Violent Behav*. 2019;45:20–32.
21. Marciano L, Schulz PJ, Camerini AL. Cyberbullying perpetration and victimization in youth: a meta-analysis of longitudinal studies. *J Comput-Mediated Commun*. 2020;25(2):163–181.
22. Moreno MA, Jelenchick LA, Christakis DA. Problematic internet use among older adolescents: a conceptual framework. *Comput Human Behav*. 2013;29(4):1879–1887.
23. Moreno MA, Jelenchick L, Cox E, et al. Problematic internet use among US youth a systematic review. *Arch Pediatr Adolesc Med*. 2011;165(9):797–805.
24. Telemedicine. [cited June 27, 2022]. https://www.medicaid.gov/medicaid/benefits/telemedicine/index.html
25. Myers K, Nelson EL, Rabinowitz T, et al. American telemedicine association practice guidelines for telemental health with children and adolescents. *Telemedicine and e-Health*. 2017;23(10):779–804.
26. Gloff NE, LeNoue SR, Novins DK, et al. Telemental health for children and adolescents. *Int Rev Psychiatry*. 2015;27(6):513–524.
27. Carlson J, Goldstein R, Hoover K, et al. NASPAG/SAHM statement: the 21st century cures act and adolescent confidentiality. *J Adolesc Health*. 2021;68(2):426–428.
28. Thompson LA, Martinko T, Budd P, et al. Meaningful use of a confidential adolescent patient portal. *J Adolesc Health*. 2016;58(2):134–140.
29. Gray SH, Pasternak RH, Gooding HC, et al; Society for Adolescent Health and Medicine. Recommendations for electronic health record use for delivery of adolescent health care. *J Adolesc Health*. 2014;54(4):487–490.
30. Bry LJ, Chou T, Miguel E, et al. Consumer smartphone apps marketed for child and adolescent anxiety: a systematic review and content analysis. *Behav Ther*. 2018;49(2):249–261.
31. Moreno MA. *Sex, Drugs 'N Facebook: A Parent's Toolkit for Promoting Healthy Internet Use*. Hunter House, Inc; 2013.
32. Moreno MA, Arseniev-Koehler A, Selkie E, Development and testing of a 3-item screening tool for problematic internet use. *J Pediatr* 2016;176:167–172.e1.

ADDITIONAL RESOURCES AND WEBSITES

Additional Resources and Websites for Clinicians:
Affordances of social media review paper—https://pubmed.ncbi.nlm.nih.gov/30912754/
Cyberbullying—https://cyberbullying.org/Cyberbullying-Top-Ten-Tips-Health-Care-Providers.pdf
Family media use plan—https://www.healthychildren.org/English/media/Pages/default.aspx
Family media use plan intervention paper—https://pubmed.ncbi.nlm.nih.gov/33492346/
General review on media and adolescent development—https://www.annualreviews.org/doi/abs/10.1146/annurev-devpsych-121318-084815
I to M. *Hanging Out, Messing Around, and Geeking Out: Kids Living and Learning with New Media*. The MIT Press; 2013.

Additional Resources and Websites for Parents/Caregivers:
Breen G. *Kindness Wins: A Simple, No-Nonsense Guide to Teaching Our Kids How to Be Kind Online*. Booktrope; 2015.
Commonsense media—https://www.commonsensemedia.org/
Family media use plan—https://www.healthychildren.org/English/media/Pages/default.aspx
Family Online Safety Institute—https://www.fosi.org/good-digital-parenting-resource/social-media-guide
Livingstone S, Blum-Ross A. *Parenting for a Digital Future: How Hopes and Fears About Technology Shape Children's Lives*. Oxford University Press; 2020.

Additional Resources and Websites for Adolescents and Young Adults:
Born this way foundation—https://bornthisway.foundation/
Do Something (Activism)—https://www.dosomething.org/us
Teen Ink (Art)—https://www.teenink.com/ and @teen.ink on instagram
The Trevor Project (LGBTQ+ teens)—https://www.thetrevorproject.org/
Your life, your voice—https://www.yourlifeyourvoice.org/Pages/home.aspx

CHAPTER 10

Chronic Health Conditions in Adolescents and Young Adults

Susan M. Sawyer

KEY WORDS

- Adherence
- Chronic illness
- Contraception
- Disability
- Fertility
- Clinicians
- Parents
- Quality
- Sexual and reproductive health
- Special health care needs
- Transition to adult health care

INTRODUCTION

Adolescents and young adults (AYAs) with chronic health conditions face the same challenges as their healthy peers in their transition to adulthood in terms of individuation and autonomy, relationships with family and peers, education and employment, and sexuality. The usual developmental challenges experienced by healthy young people at this time are commonly amplified by the presence of a chronic health condition, while families, peers, schools, and the community may not provide the same opportunities for social and emotional learning. A major difference for AYAs with chronic health conditions is the level of health care that many of them require and their need to negotiate the complexities of the health care system over these years. Specific health conditions bring particular challenges, but the basis of this chapter is that AYAs face common issues as a result of the experiences they face growing up with a chronic health condition. These challenges benefit from common responses from families and health care systems, including patient- and family-centered care.

HOW ARE CHRONIC HEALTH CONDITIONS DEFINED?

Beyond diagnostic or systems definitions (e.g., asthma or chronic respiratory diseases), there is no single definition of a chronic health condition, even for its duration. Most definitions require some form of impairment, reflecting impacts on activities of daily living (e.g., needs help with mobility), increased use of health care (e.g., prescription medication, medical appointments), or special needs (e.g., special diets). Typically, a chronic health condition includes the following elements:

- It may have a complex etiology.
- There can be a lengthy period in which symptoms fluctuate in severity and functional impact.
- There is a prolonged course of illness in which other conditions or comorbidities may arise.
- There is associated impairment or disability.

Beyond medical or physical conditions (e.g., diabetes), chronic health conditions include behavioral disorders (e.g., sleep disorders), pain syndromes, developmental disorders (e.g., attention deficit hyperactivity disorder [ADHD]), and mental health disorders (e.g., anorexia nervosa, anxiety, substance use disorders) when associated with impairments or disability. In this regard, disability is viewed as an overarching term for impairments at the level of the body, the person, and the person in social situations, which result in limitation of activities or restrictions to full participation in age-appropriate activities.

Many conditions, illnesses, and disorders commonly co-occur. Thus, while the pain of a chronic regional pain syndrome most commonly follows acute injury, pain is also a feature of chronic medical conditions (e.g., cystic fibrosis) and physical disabilities (e.g., spastic cerebral palsy). There are also bidirectional impacts. Thus, mental health disorders are more commonly experienced in AYAs with chronic medical conditions, especially those with cognitive impacts, while AYAs with mental health disorders have higher rates of chronic medical conditions (e.g., obesity).

In the United States, children with special health care needs (CSHCNs) are defined as those who "have or who are at increased risk of having a physical, mental, emotional or other type of health condition requiring a type or amount of health and related services beyond that required by children generally."[1] The term equally applies to AYAs as it does to children.

Globally, the term noncommunicable diseases (NCDs) is increasingly used to group different categories of chronic health conditions, with a policy emphasis within adult medicine on the proportion that are preventable (e.g., type 2 diabetes). Initially, NCDs did not include mental health disorders or physical disabilities, although this is now changing.

Similarly used as a framework to group different chronic health conditions, rare (or orphan) diseases are conditions that are singularly uncommon. About half are genetically determined and unlike NCDs, most are not preventable or curable.

HOW PREVALENT ARE CHRONIC HEALTH CONDITIONS?

Over the past century, technical advances in medicine, surgery, and anesthesia as well as new models of care coordination have resulted in dramatic improvements in the survival of children with medical conditions that were once considered fatal in childhood, such as congenital heart disease, cystic fibrosis, and spina bifida. The majority of adolescents with such conditions now expect to survive into adulthood.[2]

Disease-specific surveys are able to describe the incidence and prevalence of individual conditions, and how this has changed over time. There has been a real increase in the *incidence* of certain conditions, such as type 1 diabetes, celiac disease, allergies and anaphylaxis, and chronic inflammatory bowel disease.[3–5] Other surveys demonstrate increasing prevalence in certain conditions over time, such as overweight and obesity with a resultant increase in hypercholesterolemia, hypertension, metabolic syndrome, and type 2 diabetes, especially in young adults.[6,7] In many parts of the world, successful treatment of human immunodeficiency virus (HIV) infection has resulted in HIV/acquired immunodeficiency syndrome now being largely considered to be a chronic health condition.

The extent of developmental, behavioral, and mental health disorders in AYAs is increasingly appreciated,[8–10] as are the biologic effects of puberty on disease onset and stability and health across the life course.[11,12] Varying by method of assessment, age, diagnosis, and region, about one in five adolescents has a mental health disorder,[10] and the 12-month prevalence of depression is around 10%.[9] While population patterns of mental health diagnoses change from childhood into adolescence and then again into young adulthood, the most common mental health disorders are anxiety and mood disorders (e.g., depression), behavioral and neurodevelopmental disorders (e.g., ADHD, conduct disorder), and substance use disorders.[10] Less common psychiatric disorders with substantial morbidity include anorexia nervosa. Within the same person, the diagnosis of mental health disorders commonly changes with age.[10] For example, an adolescent with type 1 diabetes is at greater risk than others of developing anxiety in later childhood, anorexia nervosa in adolescence, and bulimia nervosa in young adulthood.

Beyond true differences in the prevalence of specific conditions by ethnicity (e.g., sickle cell disease, celiac disease), the use of different definitions of chronic health conditions within different surveys yields inconsistent estimates. The difficulty in obtaining a picture of the incidence and prevalence of chronic health conditions in adolescence and young adulthood is further compounded by poor assessment across adolescence and young adulthood.[13,14] Many surveys span childhood and adolescence but often do not report adolescent data separately (e.g., 0 to 17 years) or use variable age ranges (e.g., 10 to 19, 10 to 17, 12 to 18) and age cuts (e.g., 10 to 14, 15 to 19 years; 12 to 14, 15 to 18 years; 10 to 13, 15 to 17 years) to report adolescent data. In the same way, assessing the prevalence of chronic health conditions in young adulthood can be challenging as age-cuts even more commonly fail to bring visibility to this age group (e.g., 14 to 65 years, 18 to 40 years, 18 to 65 years).[15] Even surveys of AYAs use different age ranges and age-cuts due to different definitions of when adolescence (and young adulthood) start and end. Globally, within the 10- to 24-year-old age range, the age cuts of 10 to 14 years, 15 to 19 years, and 20 to 24 years are increasingly used to differentiate age groups within the AYA population.[15]

Advocacy for AYAs with chronic health conditions has successfully influenced policy by focusing on a specific condition or group of similar conditions (e.g., mental health disorders, cancers). In this regard, disease-specific surveys can be very valuable in measuring the changing incidence or prevalence of a particular condition, the presence and type of unmet health care needs, access (or lack of access) to health insurance, and particular educational or employment challenges.

Beyond advocacy related to specific conditions, policies are best advanced by understanding common issues affecting AYAs with chronic health conditions. For example, policy to redress the consistently poorer outcomes in socioeconomically deprived AYAs with chronic health conditions are more powerfully served by surveys that measure outcomes and socioeconomic factors across different chronic health conditions.[13,14] Similarly, knowledge of the extent of comorbid physical, mental health and behavioral conditions has the potential to inform and improve models of health care delivery to AYAs.[16]

In the United States, the CSHCN Screener, a five-item, parent-reported screening survey, has been used to monitor prevalence of chronic health conditions in nationally representative studies by assessing: (1) the need or use of prescription medication; (2) above-routine use of medical, mental health, or educational services compared to other children of the same age; (3) activity limitations in day-to-day life compared to similar age children; (4) need or use of specialized therapies; and (5) need or use of treatment or counseling for an emotional, behavioral, or developmental condition or a condition that has or is expected to last at least 12 months.[13] Over time, studies show that around 15% to 20% of U.S. children have some form of special health care need.[13,14] Mental health disorders are significantly more common in adolescents with pre-existing physical conditions.[17] In some high-income countries, mental health disorders, behavioral disorders, and neurologic disabilities have become more prevalent than chronic medical conditions.[18]

In a New Zealand school-based population survey of 13- to 17-year-olds, 18% reported a chronic health condition.[19] Two-thirds (65%) reported no impact of the condition on their activities or socialization but over a quarter (27.5%) reported difficulties with everyday activities and nearly a 10th (7.6%) reported that their chronic health affected their ability to socialize with their peers.

In summary, there has been a doubling of the prevalence of any chronic health condition in children and adolescents over the past 40 years. As children mature into adolescents and then into young adulthood, chronic health conditions become more common, including mental health disorders.

INTERACTION OF ADOLESCENT DEVELOPMENT AND CHRONIC HEALTH CONDITIONS

A feature of chronic health conditions is the extent to which impacts change across the life course, reflecting disease biology, growth and cognitive development, as well as different expectations of peer relationships, educational participation, and employment. The two defining aspects of biologic development in adolescence and young adulthood are puberty and neurocognitive maturation which can have profound implications for AYAs with chronic health conditions.

The interaction of chronic health conditions with adolescent development is complex and bidirectional; the health condition may affect development and development may affect the condition. For example, some chronic health conditions, such as chronic renal failure, can cause pubertal delay, changing the timing and trajectory of peak height velocity. When extreme, these changes can result in stunting of adult height. For conditions such as asthma, the onset of puberty can reduce the severity of the disease, while the reverse is more typical in diabetes mellitus, with pubertal onset associated with poorer metabolic control. Regular monitoring of growth and its correlates is an important component of health care for all adolescents with chronic health conditions. For example, while the underlying neurologic disturbance of cerebral palsy is static, physical growth in adolescence and associated musculoskeletal impairments, pain, increased body mass, as well as fatigue variably contribute to changes in motor function and mobility in young adulthood.

During adolescence, the fundamental cognitive and problem-solving skills acquired in earlier childhood also undergo further development. Cognitive maturation results in greater capacity for insights around the significance of life-limiting conditions, such as cystic fibrosis, which may contribute to anxiety and depression. Growing capacity to maintain attention, greater working memory, and inhibitory control of emotions promotes the development of more goal-directed activities, which bring greater capacity for self-management of chronic health conditions. Importantly, future planning skills continue to develop well into the mid-20s, with implications for adherence to treatment. Social cognition, or the ability to make sense of the world through the processing of signals from others, accelerates from puberty and is central to interpersonal functioning, mental health and well-being, educational attainment, and future employment.[20] The effects of deficits in such cognitive skills, that can occur in a range of neurodevelopmental conditions, are commonly amplified in late childhood and adolescence. Fewer opportunities for peer engagement contribute to reduced opportunities for social and emotional learning, social confidence, and self-esteem, regardless of the cause (e.g., mobility limitations, parental overprotectiveness).

THE SOCIAL CONTEXT OF HEALTH-RELATED BEHAVIORS AND STATES

Social determinants of health have profound influence on health outcomes among AYAs, and this is also the case for those with chronic health conditions.[14] Structural determinants such as national economic wealth will influence the availability and quality of health services, health insurance, education (including inclusive education for those with cognitive and physical disabilities), and employment. These factors not only affect health outcomes during adolescence but have relevance for future health and life opportunities. More proximal determinants, also known as risk and protective factors, operate within the individual and their family, peers, school, and community.[21] A chronic health condition is a risk factor within the individual domain that, when compounded by risks within other domains (e.g., family dysfunction, bullying, unsupportive schooling, high rates of youth unemployment), can influence AYAs' engagement in health-related behaviors (e.g., tobacco use) and states (e.g., depression). For example, bullying increases the likelihood of a number of health-related behaviors and states, including substance misuse, unsafe sex, depression, antisocial and illegal activities, and dangerous driving.[21]

Given the importance of academic success for future employment, promoting school engagement by minimizing school absenteeism from illness and medical appointments is important. However, beyond academic achievement, schools are also important social environments for adolescents with chronic health conditions that promote peer connections, emotional control, and well-being.[22] Extracurricular activities with healthy peers can provide a pathway to friendships, while peer support groups for young people with chronic health conditions can help to normalize the differences they experience. Both are strategies to promote emotional well-being and continued engagement with schooling.

Many studies have explored the question of whether adolescents with chronic physical health conditions have a higher rate of mental health disorders. Most studies suggest that this group has a substantially elevated risk that is likely to be mediated by the same factors as observed among healthy young people, such as family connectedness.[14,17] Youth with certain conditions, such as physical and cognitive disabilities, appear to be at higher risk, which will be exacerbated by reduced opportunity for meaningful social relationships.

Some clinicians might assume that AYAs with chronic health conditions would be less likely than their healthy peers to engage in behaviors such as unsafe sex, or unsafe alcohol or drug use, especially when the chronic condition is severe. However, there is little evidence to support this notion, with some evidence suggesting that these AYAs may be at higher risk. Part of the explanation may be due to higher rates of depression, but it is also likely that biologic differences in cognitive processing (e.g., ADHD) result in a different appreciation of the risk associated with particular social situations. A simpler explanation may be the greater challenge to feel "normal" experienced by many AYAs with chronic health conditions, which may render them more sensitive to perceived peer norms in order to fit in socially.

What is apparent is that the risks of certain behaviors are greater for AYAs with particular chronic health conditions.[2] For example, while smoking is unhealthy for all young people, it is even more damaging for AYAs with diabetes due to its effect on microvascular and macrovascular disease. It is similarly riskier for young people with chronic lung or cardiac conditions. In the same way, heavy alcohol use is unsafe for all; however, alcohol can lower the seizure threshold for young people with epilepsy, and make blood glucose control more challenging in AYAs with diabetes.

QUALITY HEALTH SERVICES

The predominant orientation of children's health services is toward young children, the age group that was historically the major user of their facilities. Around the world, as the upper age of specialist pediatrics increases and the proportion of adolescents managed by pediatricians and specialist children's services grows, services and facilities need to become as oriented to adolescents as they historically have been to parents and families.[23] A strength of adult services is their focus on patient-centered care. However, many older AYAs are still learning to take responsibility for their health care, regardless of whether they live at home or not.[24] For different reasons, the notion of patient- and family-centered care is equally relevant in both child and adult settings, with its emphasis on respect, care coordination, appropriate provision of information, high-quality communication, patient involvement in decisions about care, and the ability of clinicians to listen to patient needs.

The World Health Organization describes adolescent-friendly health care as an approach to better orient the provision of health services to the needs of young people.[25] Also referred to as youth-friendly health care, this approach emerged out of concerns about the lack of developmentally appropriate primary health care for adolescents in low- and middle-income countries. The approach is equally relevant to AYAs in high-income countries and for specialist services.

The conceptual framework for adolescent-friendly health care in hospital settings is salient in advancing the concept of providing quality health care to young adults with chronic health conditions in various settings, including primary care.[26] As outlined in Figure 10.1, the provision of adolescent-friendly health care (a term synonymous with quality health care) is embedded in the notion of patient- and family-centered care, and implemented through a strong focus on providing a positive experience of care for the young person and evidence-based care to treat the underlying condition. Both depend on the other; that is, evidence-informed care or guideline-based care will not be

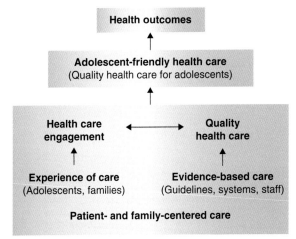

FIGURE 10.1 Conceptual framework of adolescent-friendly health care. (Reproduced with permission from Sawyer SM, Ambresin AE, Bennett KE, et al. A measurement framework for quality healthcare for adolescents in hospitals. *J Adolesc Health.* 2014;55(4):484–490.)

as effectively implemented unless AYAs are actively engaged in their health care, have a positive experience of care with the clinician and the health service, and have the opportunity for their families to be as engaged as they would like them to be. Engagement with care reflects both the quality of AYAs' experiences with individual staff as well as their wider experiences of the health service. This might include how welcome AYAs feel in attending a clinic or hospital, the age appropriateness of the physical spaces (e.g., waiting areas), the extent to which AYAs feel sufficiently involved in decisions about their health care, and the types of support services provided (e.g., educational and employment support). A critical element for AYAs with chronic health conditions is that active engagement by patients (and their families) is required to set expectations around self-management practices (e.g., adherence to treatment), as well as future engagement with health services (e.g., transition to adult health care).

THE ELEMENTS OF QUALITY HEALTH CARE FOR ADOLESCENTS AND YOUNG ADULTS WITH CHRONIC HEALTH CONDITIONS

There are myriad elements for clinicians to keep in mind in providing developmentally appropriate health care to AYAs with chronic health conditions, as portrayed in Figure 10.2. Putting this into practice can be simplified when the clinician *attends to the young person* with chronic health condition by applying the principles of AYA medicine, *works with the young person and their family* to promote the young person's growing capacity for self-management as they mature, and *understands health care delivery in the context of the health care system* in which they practice.

One of the key differences in working with AYAs with chronic health conditions is the need to balance the focus on the patient with that of the family. This balance varies with patient age, experience, and context. In addition, the balance is influenced by patient preference and cultural expectations. Parents of AYAs, especially those with chronic health conditions that were diagnosed during earlier childhood, commonly develop deeply trusting relationships with their child's clinicians. In these contexts, clinicians need to explicitly attend to developing a relationship with the AYA patient.

Parents continue to provide a high level of support to AYAs with chronic health conditions.[24] Ideally, parents can set appropriately high expectations for their children with chronic health conditions, and balance the care they provide while fostering their child's developing autonomy and independence. Supporting young people's emerging capacities is a critical role for parents of AYAs

with chronic health conditions. Parents are important in helping AYAs negotiate the health care system by accompanying their children to appointments, supervising treatments at home, supporting the actual transfer to adult health care, negotiating the complexity of health insurance, and clarifying what questions to explore with clinicians.[26] At times, however, parents may inadvertently foster dependency, reduce opportunities for social learning, and undermine young people's social confidence and resilience. This can include unintentionally undermining the potential learning to be gained within the health consultation itself.[27]

During adolescence, it is especially important that health care visits include time during which the clinician meets confidentially with the adolescent alone. There is no single "right" way to do this; some clinicians consult briefly with the adolescent and parent together, then spend the bulk of the consultation with the adolescent alone, before bringing the parent back into the consultation to sum up. In this context, it is critical that the notion of confidentiality is carefully reviewed with both the adolescent and the parent. Confidential consultations provide a respectful opportunity for clinicians to check the adolescent's understanding of their condition and its treatment (rather than assume that they know as much as their parents), and set expectations about their engagement in self-management, including adherence behaviors. Typically, as time goes on, the proportion of the consultation spent with the adolescent alone increases.

In adult-oriented settings, parents are not expected to be nearly as physically present within consultations, if at all. Yet, when complex or difficult decisions need to be made, many young adults wish for their parents, carers, or partners to be included within consultations, and commonly continue to rely on their parents for emotional support around managing their health. Many young adults with cognitive disabilities or prominent physical disabilities are much more reliant on their families for emotional and practical supports. Notwithstanding this, clinicians also need to primarily direct communication to the patient and not to their parents or carers, while also respectfully engaging them.

The following section briefly highlights three specific issues to consider when managing AYAs with chronic health conditions: adherence with treatment; sexual and reproductive health care; and transition to adult health care.

Adherence with Treatment

The majority of AYAs with chronic health conditions struggle to adhere to their treatment regimen. Adherence with medication is

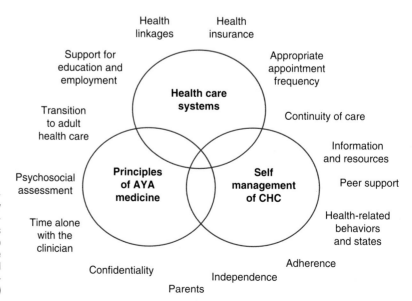

FIGURE 10.2 A Venn diagram that outlines the three major components for clinicians to attend to in providing adolescent-friendly health care for AYAs with chronic health conditions (CHC). Developmentally appropriate care is provided by applying the principles of AYA medicine, working with the young person and their family to promote the young person's capacity for self-management, in the context of the health care system in which they practice. (Modified from Kennedy A, Sawyer S. Transition from pediatric to adult services: are we getting it right? *Curr Opin Pediatr.* 2008;20(4):403–409.)

problematic at all ages, with only about half of all patients adhering to treatment recommendations. The responsibility lies with clinicians to routinely address adherence around all aspects of recommended treatment. The challenge for clinicians (and parents) is that, compared to adults, AYAs have not yet developed the same extent of goal-directed behaviors, remain less influenced by longer term fears of health complications, need greater assistance to develop treatment routines, and are more price-sensitive when having to pay for treatment.

There is no "right" age by which adolescents can be expected to no longer rely on their parents to support adherence-promoting behaviors. Indeed, parents continue to play a critical role for many years in supporting some AYAs with their medical treatments. The young adult years can be especially challenging in relation to poor adherence; parents are typically less influential at this time but the capacity of young adults to adhere does not magically improve on their 18th birthday. Rather, it continues to evolve across the 20s.

Given this, one responsibility for clinicians is to simplify treatment regimens wherever possible (e.g., twice-daily medication rather than three times daily). Attending to adherence behaviors at every consultation is another important role for clinicians. In the first instance, it is important to be clear about what treatment is recommended, why, and for how long. Consider the following principles:

* Be clear about the rationale for why every medication or treatment is prescribed.
* As adherence can differ for each medication or treatment, questions about adherence must be treatment specific.
* Make it easier for AYAs to be honest about poor adherence by asking questions that assume that adherence is poor rather than good.
* Respectfully engage with parents/caregivers to confirm AYA reports about their adherence behaviors.
* Acknowledge positive behaviors (and intentions). In doing so, seek clarification about why adherence is good for a particular medication/treatment at this time (i.e., has anything changed?).
* Identify barriers to adherence behaviors, including social barriers (e.g., dislike taking medication at school or at work).
* Be prepared to negotiate alternative approaches, especially if the effect of a drug holiday can be tested with an objective measure of health (e.g., "n-of-one" experiments).
* Explore with the young person about what they think might work for them (e.g., more or less support from parents, telephone alarms as reminders, adherence apps).
* Consider the contribution of mental health symptoms or disorders (e.g., depression) to poor adherence.
* When all else fails, be prepared to tolerate less than ideal adherence but with expectations that adherence will change with maturation, life experiences, and changing goals.

Sexual and Reproductive Health Care

Adolescents with chronic health conditions, including disabilities, become sexually active at a similar age to their healthy peers. For this group, the health risks of sexual activity may be exacerbated by the illness itself, the medications used to treat it, or by maladaptive emotional responses to illness. Many AYAs with chronic health conditions have concerns about their sexual attractiveness, the normalcy of their reproductive system and sexual response, fertility, safety of contraception use, and genetic aspects of their disease. In this context, it is concerning how little information AYAs receive from their clinicians about sexuality education that is specific to their chronic health condition.[28] The extent of sexual abuse and sexual assault, especially among AYAs with cognitive disability, is also concerning.

Some chronic health conditions are associated with infertility, either related to the disease itself or to its treatment. For example, males with cystic fibrosis are infertile, yet are still biologically able to father children using sperm aspiration and assisted reproductive techniques. In contrast, females with cystic fibrosis are fertile, and experience high rates of unplanned pregnancy. While there may be many explanations for this, the most obvious one is failure by health care services to appropriately discuss the importance of contraception for sexually active AYAs who do not desire pregnancy. Treatment of cancer variably affects fertility, hence the importance of timely fertility-preserving interventions.

Long-acting reversible contraceptives (LARCs) are the most effective form of contraception for healthy young AYA females. While there are many contraindications to individual contraceptive agents for young people with different chronic health conditions, LARCs are safer than oral contraceptive pill for many health conditions. For example, the combined oral contraceptive pill should be avoided in conditions with a thrombotic diathesis, in the context of severe liver disease, or in the presence of indwelling intravenous access. Discussions about fertility, contraception, and pregnancy risks for the mother and fetus (e.g., teratogenicity of medication) are important to have throughout adolescence into adulthood with young people as well as their parents, when appropriate.[28]

Given the risks of immunosuppression in AYAs with various conditions (e.g., transplantation), immunization with the human papillomavirus vaccine is an important element of preventive care for adolescent boys as well as girls.

Transition to Adult Health Care

Transition to adult health care refers to the planned movement of AYAs with chronic health conditions from child-oriented to adult-oriented health services.[29] As such, transition is a *process* that is initiated by child health services and continues well after the actual *event* of transfer to the adult service.

Historically, the notion of transition to adult health care related to specialist services. In the 1970s, 80s, and even the 90s, there were few adult specialist services interested in accepting the "survivors" of chronic illness in childhood and little planning by pediatric health services in developing closer linkages between pediatric and adult services. At that time, neither specialist pediatric nor adult services had much understanding of AYA development, and adolescents and their parents were poorly prepared to transfer to adult health care. In this context, it is not surprising that once AYAs transferred to adult care, negative experiences led to poor engagement with adult services and high rates of service "drop out" within the first year or so after transfer, sometimes with dire consequences for health outcomes.

Increasing attention is now paid to the needs of AYAs to better prepare AYAs and their families prior to transfer, and to better support their engagement in adult health care once they have transferred to adult services. Transition to adult health care is now appreciated to be as relevant for primary care as it is for specialist services. For those who transfer from specialist pediatric to adult specialist services, primary care can function to support the continuity of care across adolescence and young adulthood. A wider role for primary care is in supporting the large cohort of young people whose care is coordinated by primary care rather than specialist pediatric services, but for whom a change in orientation to more independently focused care is still required. At this time, many older AYAs move away from home for education or employment, which will commonly necessitate a shift in the primary care clinician as well as specialist services.

The critical aspect of transition to adult health care is that it is embedded in the knowledge that health care functions as a complex system that AYAs must negotiate to make it work for them. Some of the transition literature, especially from subspecialist areas, uses the term "transition to adult health care" synonymously with "quality health care" for AYAs or "developmentally appropriate health care." Indeed, there is much blurring in the literature of these various terms and themes. In Figure 10.2, transition to adult health care is described as an individual element which is of relevance to both the orientation of health care systems and the principles of AYA health care. Thus, supporting transition to adult health care is part of, but not synonymous with the totality of providing quality health care to AYAs with chronic health conditions.

Regardless of what we call it, there is room for improvement. For example, in the 2009 to 2010 survey of parents of 12- to 17-year-olds with special health care needs in the United States,[30] parents were asked how often their adolescent's clinicians encouraged their child to take responsibility for their health care needs, including taking medication, understanding their diagnosis, or following medical advice. While the majority were positive, 22% reported that this did not usually occur. More concerning was that only 40% of 12- to 17-year-olds met the standard to make an effective transition to adult health care. This was based on parents reporting that their children received anticipatory guidance on a number of key areas and that their clinicians usually or always encouraged them to take responsibility for their health. It was especially concerning that adolescents whose conditions more severely affected their daily activities were half as likely to achieve this objective as those whose conditions never affect their daily activities (26% vs. 52%). Children living in poverty were also half as likely as those in the highest-income bracket to receive transition services (25% vs. 52%).

The following points summarize some of the key elements of transition planning:

- Early planning helps prepare patients, families, and health care teams.
- Transition planning is an individualized, collaborative process between the adolescent and their family, and their various health care services including primary care.
- Tailored, written transition plans can help foster progressive development of disease-related knowledge and self-management skills. Transition plans can be used to set goals for adolescents and allow for regular review of progress by clinicians.
- While the timing of transfer to adult care might ideally be informed by patient readiness rather than age, in reality, planning around transfer to adult health care is done in the context of the age policies of specialist health services.
- It is better to transfer health care at a time of disease stability than in a crisis or period of instability.
- Structured transition programs that allow AYAs to meet with new clinicians before transfer increase clinic attendance within the adult health care system and increase patient satisfaction.
- Transition coordinators act as liaisons between pediatric and adult health care systems. They can promote continuity of care during the transition process by supporting patients and their families to navigate complex health care systems.

Within child-oriented services, many complex health conditions are managed by multidisciplinary teams. Such teams often have a strong focus on internal communication between team members, which can support the delivery of coordinated, accessible care, especially when facilitated by an electronic health record. Such teams have historically been less common within adult health care services. In their absence, many AYAs and their families, supported by their primary care clinician, end up developing their individual teams. Such teams can be equally effective in the longer term, although they risk being associated with delayed access to health care in the short term.

Some patient groups struggle to identify appropriate adult specialist services. This is particularly the case for AYAs with disabilities including those with complex physical disabilities, or developmental disorders such as intellectual disability, autism, and ADHD. Adolescents and young adults with mental health disorders may also struggle to identify appropriate services, especially in terms of ongoing care. Identifying an appropriate adult specialist clinician can also be difficult for those conditions that sit at the interface of specialist medical and mental health care within pediatric services, such as eating disorders. All too often, in the absence of adult specialist clinicians, the responsibility for care then lies with primary care professionals.

SUMMARY

Adolescents and young adults with chronic health conditions face the same challenges as otherwise healthy young people, with additional challenges due to the uncertainty and adversity created through living with a chronic health condition. A series of navigational capabilities are key to young people's ability to negotiate their changing relationships with families, peers (including intimate relationships), the education system and employment, and the health care system as they mature. These capabilities and assets are enriched by emotional intelligence, communication skills, and a positive mindset which underpin the determination, energy, and resilience that many AYAs with chronic health conditions need to achieve their current and future goals. These capabilities are shaped by day-to-day interactions, including interactions with clinicians.

REFERENCES

1. McPherson M, Arango P, Fox H, et al. A new definition of children with special health care needs. *Pediatrics.* 1998;102(1 Pt 1):137–140.
2. Sawyer SM, Drew S, Yeo MS, et al. Adolescents with a chronic condition: challenges living, challenges treating. *Lancet.* 2007;369(9571):1481–1489.
3. Vehik K, Dabelea D. The changing epidemiology of type 1 diabetes: why is it going through the roof? *Diabetes Metab Res Rev.* 2011;27(1):3–13.
4. Catassi C, Gatti S, Fasano A. The new epidemiology of celiac disease. *J Pediatr Gastroenterol Nutr.* 2014;59(Suppl 1):S7–S9.
5. Loh W, Tang MLK. The epidemiology of food allergy in the global context. *Int J Environ Res Public Health.* 2018;15(9):2043.
6. NCD Risk Factor Collaboration (NCD-RisC). Worldwide trends in body-mass index, underweight, overweight, and obesity from 1975 to 2016: a pooled analysis of 2416 population-based measurement studies in 128.9 million children, adolescents, and adults. *Lancet.* 2017;390(10113):2627–2642.
7. Dong Y, Jan C, Zou Z, et al. Effect of overweight and obesity on high blood pressure in Chinese children and adolescents. *Obesity.* 2019;27(9):1503–1512.
8. Collishaw S. Annual research review: secular trends in child and adolescent mental health. *J Child Psychol Psychiatry.* 2015;56(3):370–393.
9. Mojtabai R, Olfson M, Han B. National trends in the prevalence and treatment of depression in adolescents and young adults. *Pediatrics.* 2016;138(6):e20161878.
10. Costello EJ, He JP, Sampson NA, et al. Services for adolescents with psychiatric disorders: 12-month data from the National Comorbidity Survey–adolescent. *Psychiatr Serv.* 2014;65(3):359–366.
11. Patton GC, Viner R. Pubertal transitions in health. *Lancet.* 2007;369(9567):1130–1139.
12. Hochberg Z, Belsky J. Evo-devo of human adolescence: beyond disease models of early puberty. *BMC Med.* 2013;11(1):113.
13. Bethell CD, Blumberg SJ, Stein REK, et al. Taking stock of the CSHCN screener: a review of common questions and current reflections. *Acad Pediatr.* 2015;15(2):165–176.
14. Bethell CD, Newacheck PW, Fine A, et al. Optimizing health and health care systems for children with special health care needs using the life course perspective. *Matern Child Health J.* 2014;18(2):467–477.
15. Sawyer SM, Azzopardi PS, Wickremarathne D, et al. The age of adolescence. *Lancet Child Adolesc Health.* 2018;2(3):223–228.
16. Fazel M, Townsend A, Stewart H, et al. Integrated care to address child and adolescent health in the 21st century: a clinical review. *JCPP Advances.* 2021;1(4):e12045.
17. Bennett S, Shafran R, Coughtrey A, et al. Psychological interventions for mental health disorders in children with chronic physical illness: a systematic review. *Arch Dis Child.* 2015;100(4):308–316.
18. Halfon N, Houtrow A, Larson K, et al. The changing landscape of disability in childhood. *Future Child.* 2012;22(1):13–42.
19. Denny S, de Silva M, Fleming T, et al. The prevalence of chronic health conditions impacting on daily functioning and the association with emotional well-being among a national sample of high school students. *J Adolesc Health.* 2014;54(4):410–415.
20. Goddings AL, Burnett Heyes S, Bird G, et al. The relationship between puberty and social emotion processing. *Dev Sci.* 2012;15(6):801–811.
21. Sawyer SM, Afifi RA, Bearinger LH, et al. Adolescence: a foundation for future health. *Lancet.* 2012;379(9826):1630–1640.
22. Sawyer SM, Raniti M, Aston R. Making every school a health-promoting school. *Lancet Child Adolesc Health.* 2021;5(8):539–540.
23. Sawyer SM, McNeil R, Francis KL, et al. The age of paediatrics. *Lancet Child Adolesc Health.* 2019;3(11):822–830.
24. Beresford B, Stuttard L. Young adults as users of adult healthcare: experiences of young adult with complex or life-limiting conditions. *Clin Med.* 2014;14(4):404–408.
25. Ambresin AE, Bennett K, Patton GC, et al. Assessment of youth-friendly health care: a systematic review of indicators drawn from young people's perspectives. *J Adolesc Health.* 2013;52(6):670–681.
26. Sawyer SM, Ambresin AE, Bennett KE, et al. A measurement framework for quality healthcare for adolescents in hospitals. *J Adolesc Health.* 2014;55(4):484–490.

27. Duncan RE, Jekel M, O'Connell MA, et al. Balancing parental involvement with adolescent friendly health care in teenagers with diabetes: are we getting it right? *J Adolesc Health.* 2014;55(1):59–64.

28. Frayman K, Sawyer SM. Sexual and reproductive health in cystic fibrosis: a life-course perspective. *Lancet Respir Med.* 2015;3(1):70–86.

29. Society for Adolescent Health and Medicine. Transition to adulthood for youth with chronic conditions and special health care needs. *J Adolesc Health.* 2020;66(5):631–634.

30. U.S. Department of Health and Human Services, Health Resources and Services Administration, Maternal and Child Health Bureau. *The National Survey of Children with Special Health Care Needs Chartbook 2009–2010.* U.S. Department of Health and Human Services, 2013.

ADDITIONAL RESOURCES AND WEBSITES

Additional Resources and Websites for Clinicians:

Centers for Disease Control and Prevention—Healthy Schools—https://www.cdc.gov/healthyschools/chronicconditions.htm This website contains links to various resources that aim to promote the role of schools for health, with the knowledge that health is both an enabler and outcome of education. There are links to whole-school approaches, policies and approaches including for students with chronic health conditions (e.g., asthma, diabetes, epilepsy, food allergies, and poor oral health).

Got Transition—https://www.gottransition.org/ a U.S. federally funded resource center on health care transition that has links to a range of resources for health professionals, parents, and AYAs.

Meaningful Youth Engagement—https://pmnch.who.int/resources/publications/m/item/global-consensus-statement-on-meaningful-adolescent-and-youth-engagement This statement on the importance of meaningful youth engagement provides a policy context for greater engagement of AYAs in all matters that affect them, including health services. It was developed by the Partnership for Maternal, Newborn and Child Health.

World Health Organization—Health Promoting Schools—https://www.who.int/publications/i/item/9789240029392 This link is to the WHO website for access to Global Standards on Health Promoting Schools. There is also a link to a global guideline on School Health Services.

Additional Resources and Websites for Parents/Caregivers:

Got Transition—https://www.gottransition.org/parents-caregivers/ A U.S. federally funded resource center on health care transition that has links to a range of resources for health professionals, parents, and AYAs.

Raising Children Network—The direct link to chronic health conditions is https://raisingchildren.net.au/teens/mental-health-physical-health/chronic-conditions the Australian Parenting website. Funded by the Australian Government, the website provides evidence-based, practically oriented information to parents, including teenagers.

Society for Adolescent Health and Medicine—https://www.adolescenthealth.org/Resources/Resources-for-Adolescents-and-Parents.aspx The link below is to their parenting and adolescent resources site, which has a wide variety of links to different topics.

Additional Resources and Websites for Adolescents and Young Adults:

Got Transition—https://www.gottransition.org/youth-and-young-adults/ A U.S. federally funded resource center on health care transition that has links to a range of resources including a transition quiz.

Society for Adolescent Health and Medicine—https://www.adolescenthealth.org/Resources/Resources-for-Adolescents-and-Parents.aspx The link below is to their parenting and adolescent resources site, which has a wide variety of links to different topics.

CHAPTER 11

Palliative Care and End of Life in Adolescents and Young Adults

Chana B. Korenblum

Abby R. Rosenberg

KEY WORDS

- Adolescents and young adults
- End-of-life care
- Hospice
- Life-limiting illness
- Palliative care

INTRODUCTION

Given that adolescence and young adulthood are characterized by great biologic, psychological, and social changes, it follows that the experience of a serious illness during these years can have a profound impact.[1] Due to advances in medical care, youth with complex chronic diseases are living longer into adulthood than ever before, and many suffer from increasingly intractable symptoms.[2] This situation is deeply disruptive to achievement of developmental milestones related to emerging independence, identity, relationships, and career development, further amplifying distress.

Despite growing evidence of multiple benefits, supportive care for these conditions is often limited, and is often not offered until the end of life. Adolescents and young adults (AYAs) with these illnesses are thus left with a unique set of unmet needs. They tend to experience more complex, severe, and prolonged distress than younger children, or older adults with similar conditions.[3] They wish to be viewed as people, not defined by their underlying disease, and want to collect new life experiences, find meaning in life, and be remembered.[2] They generally prefer to be informed about their clinical status, to maintain control over their bodies, and to be respected in their decisions.[2] Ultimately, AYAs and their families must confront the possibility of dying at a time in life normally dedicated to establishing autonomy and planning for the future.

The provision of developmentally appropriate palliative care for AYAs is critical. This group often finds themselves between pediatric and adult health care systems,[1] with most institutions on both sides lacking in dedicated palliative care programming or resources.[4] Growing evidence supports early introduction of targeted palliative care interventions to help support AYAs and their families navigate the challenges of serious illnesses, regardless of prognosis.[2] In this chapter, a holistic approach to care for young people with life-limiting or life-threatening conditions will be presented.

DEFINITIONS

Palliative care has been defined by the World Health Organization (WHO) as:

"The active total care of patients whose disease is not responsive to curative treatment. Control of pain, of other symptoms, and of psychological, social, and spiritual problems is paramount. The goal of palliative care is achievement of the best quality of life for patients and their families."[5] More recently, the term has encompassed support of patients at any stage of a life-threatening illness, in contrast to a historical focus solely on the end-of-life period (Table 11.1).

As increasing numbers of children with life-limiting conditions (LLCs) survive into adolescence and early adulthood, the need for developmentally tailored palliative care services has grown in tandem. Estimating from available global data, the annual mortality rate for young people aged 15 to 24 years with LLCs is approximately 26.5 per 1,00,000, with cancer as the most common cause.[7]

An important consideration is the need for more intensive support during certain points along the disease trajectory, for example, in times of uncertainty and suffering.[8] Trajectories themselves will vary from young people who have lived with their condition since birth or early childhood and who may be expected to have a shortened lifespan, to those who may have led healthy lives until young adulthood when diagnosed with an incurable disease like cancer (Table 11.2). Flexibility, adaptability, and personalization are therefore key features of palliative care for young people. A multidisciplinary team approach can incorporate these features into

TABLE 11.1
What Is Palliative Care?[6]

Palliative care:
- provides relief from pain and other distressing symptoms
- affirms life and regards dying as a normal process
- intends neither to hasten nor to postpone death
- integrates the psychological, social, and spiritual aspects of patient care
- offers a support system to help patients live as actively as possible until death
- offers a support system to help families cope during patients' illnesses and in their own bereavement
- uses a team approach to address the needs of patients and families, including bereavement counseling, if indicated
- will enhance quality of life and may also positively influence the course of illness
- is applicable early in the course of illness, in conjunction with other therapies that are intended to prolong life, and includes those investigations needed to understand and manage distressing clinical complications
- requires a broad multidisciplinary approach that includes the family and makes use of available community resources; it can be successfully implemented even if resources are limited
- can be provided in tertiary care facilities, in community health centers, and even in homes

Adapted from World Health Organization. Definition of Palliative Care. http://www.who.int/cancer/palliative/definition/en/

TABLE 11.2
Types of Life-limiting Conditions in Young People[8]

1. Conditions for which curative treatment may be feasible and can fail (exclusions: young people in long-term remission or following successful curative treatment). Examples: cancer and irreversible organ failure of the heart, liver, or kidney
2. Conditions where there may be long periods of intensive treatment aimed at prolonging life and allowing participation in normal activities, and premature death is still possible or inevitable. Examples: cystic fibrosis, Duchene muscular dystrophy, and HIV/AIDS
3. Progressive conditions without curative treatment options, where treatment is exclusively palliative and may extend over many years. Examples: Batten disease, mucopolysaccharidosis, and Creutzfeldt–Jakob disease
4. Severe neurologic disability that may cause weakness and susceptibility to health complications. Deterioration may be unpredictable and not usually progressive. Examples: severe multiple disabilities following brain or spinal cord injuries and severe cerebral palsy

Adapted from the Joint Report on *Palliative Care for Young People.*

care, where AYAs and their families work in close partnership with skilled nurses, doctors, social workers, psychologists, and other allied clinicians in hospital, hospice, or at home.[2]

While some physical and psychological symptoms in AYAs with LLCs may overlap with those reported in younger children and older adults, how health care team members perceive and treat these symptoms may differ due to level of exposure to and comfort with this age group. Finally, the psychosocial needs of AYAs may be quite distinct, as described in more detail in the next section.

PSYCHOSOCIAL NEEDS OF ADOLESCENTS AND YOUNG ADULTS WITH LIFE-LIMITING CONDITIONS

Psychological Needs

The psychological needs of AYAs with LLCs are understandably complex, given the pronounced neurodevelopmental changes already characterized by this life stage. Identity formation in youth is based on a sense of immortality—an expectation of a future where anything is possible—a process shattered by a diagnosis of an LLC.[9] Adolescents and young adults are thus forced to take on a new identity and life perspective, experienced as multiple losses of their former self, control over their lives, and anticipated future achievements and relationships.[10] Younger AYAs may not have well-established plans, whereas older AYAs may grieve the inability to fulfill career or family planning goals, or worry about the welfare of their own children after they die.

Feelings can include loneliness, isolation, anger, frustration, depression from disruption of normal routines and connections, and fears about medical procedures, family members, and death itself. Adolescents and young adults with incurable cancer have significantly higher rates of anxiety and depression than younger children,[11] and around one in four meet criteria for post-traumatic stress disorder, and up to 90% report symptoms of post-traumatic stress.[12] Physical consequences of the disease and/or its treatment, especially those related to appearance and body image, can be demoralizing and may further lower self-esteem.[1] Opportunities to explore and experience sexuality and romantic relationships can be limited and development of professional identities and financial independence can also be significantly impacted.

Adolescents and young adults need a private space to express their thoughts and worries and to have these acknowledged and validated.[9] Creating and maintaining a sense of control where possible, including giving options, can be helpful, especially if medical nonadherence or an increase in risk-taking behaviors is noted.[1] Clinicians need to anticipate these issues in advance, and initiate

opportunities for frequent interdisciplinary assessments including screening for depression and anxiety.[9] Professional psychosocial support (from social workers, psychologists, creative arts therapists, child life specialists, youth workers, etc.) can be valuable to support adaptive coping.[4,10]

Social Needs

An LLC in adolescence or young adulthood has the potential to disrupt not only psychological development, but also the achievement of social milestones. At a time in life defined by individuation from parental figures, serious illness often forces a young person to depend on one or more primary caregivers for practical and emotional support, a dilemma placing significant stress on interactions with family members.[4] Family may inevitably become one of the main sources of social support and companionship, requiring both the young person and their parents to acknowledge the importance of the relationship, despite the drive for separation.[9]

Peer support is another developmentally oriented critical coping tool for AYAs. Continued connections with friends and participation in social events (e.g., school formals, graduation ceremonies) can be important.[13] Compared with the challenges of living with an LLC, however, goals and priorities of healthy peers may seem trifling or frivolous. Adolescents and young adults often describe the feeling of a life on pause, while their friends are moving ahead with their own life goals.[2] Facilitating connections with other AYAs with similar diagnoses can help combat the pervasive, profound sense of social isolation. One-on-one or facilitated group support by experienced professionals, where available, can also be impactful.

Access to web-based support programs and social networking sites can become key sources of social interaction, especially for patients with barriers to socializing outside of their homes.[4] Social media enables AYAs to update friends and family on their condition, providing a venue for patient engagement, and can increase access to health information and research study participation.[2] However, close guidance may be needed around coping with perceived perfection of others' images, protecting privacy, navigating exposure to misinformation, and avoiding financial exploitation.[14] Overall, health care team members, especially those with longstanding relationships with patients, can play an important role in helping AYAs enhance communication and strengthen social connections with family, partners, and peers.[15]

Spiritual and Cultural Needs

When faced with the possibility of an early death, a young person's need to find meaning and purpose can become more pronounced. Some AYAs may embrace or reject a spiritual system more fully, while maintaining hope is a common theme.[16] The palliative care team (see *Introduction of Palliative Care to Adolescents and Young Adults*) may offer spiritual support in an individualized way, including facilitating the expression of fears and doubts or exploring religious beliefs.[16]

Cultural humility is an approach that facilitates expression and exploration of an AYA's background, value system, life experience, and preferences, and how these elements of their identity intersect with clinical care.[17] Issues related to race/ethnicity, indigenous heritage, country of origin, sexual orientation, gender, education, and socioeconomic status are just some of the factors that can impact the illness experience, including at the end of life.[16] Clinicians should use a culturally humble lens to help ensure AYAs' wishes are thoughtfully considered.[16]

Needs of Close Others

The looming deterioration and death of a young family member, partner, or peer is typically an unfamiliar, unanticipated situation.[18] Despite playing a central caregiving role, most parents/caregivers will lack the knowledge and skills to care for their child and appreciate access to guidance and emotional support.[18] Primary carers experience high levels of psychological distress, as well as emotions such as fear, regret, and guilt both before and after the AYA's death.[10] Parents/caregivers can struggle with supporting their child's autonomy if it means contradicting their own views, and can grieve in anticipation of the loss of expected milestones, burdens which may go unnoticed. Regular, supportive parent/caregiver services from the time of diagnosis through bereavement can help alleviate this distress and prevent longer lasting mental health sequelae.[4,15]

Siblings, peers, and romantic partners may have similar psychosocial needs. They may be the closest person emotionally and developmentally to the AYA. Siblings worry also about their parents' coping and may feel displacement, deprivation, anger, injustice, loneliness, and vulnerability.[9] Opportunities to make final memories and say goodbye, to hear health information with the permission of the AYA, and to be involved in the palliative care process including funerals and memorials are important. These opportunities can help mitigate the potential negative impacts of the loss, including increased rates of anxiety, depression, and substance use.[2]

Needs of Clinicians

While medical care of AYAs can be extremely rewarding due to the privilege of witnessing resilience and growth in the face of adversity, it too can be emotionally burdensome, especially when witnessing a premature death.[1,18] Many clinicians may be young themselves and identify with the patient, or may be older and identify with the parent/caregiver. This identification creates an emotional proximity which may interfere with clinical decision making (see *Decision making and Advance Care Planning*).[1] Regular support and supervision, self-awareness, and maintenance of professional boundaries can help staff avoid responding to young people as peers or as their own child.[9]

Many clinicians do not feel comfortable caring for AYAs with complex chronic illnesses.[19] Reasons include lack of knowledge about age-appropriate care, fear of not knowing how to provide psychosocial support to young people, and needing to broach sensitive topics such as disability or end-of-life issues before rapport has been built. An approach that may deepen the relationship between the professional and the AYA involves the belief that positive outcomes can emerge from tragedy—helping the young person have a "good death."[8] Palliative care teams can also help relieve the care burden by bridging the knowledge gap with education about developmentally appropriate care for this age group.[1]

⬤ INTRODUCTION OF PALLIATIVE CARE TO ADOLESCENTS AND YOUNG ADULTS

How, When, Where, and by Whom

Early introduction of palliative care is a rapidly growing approach, to help patients and families adjust to their diagnosis and later face challenges that emerge as the disease progresses.[15] This care should be offered concurrently, alongside disease-targeted treatment, to normalize the importance of quality of life, emotional support, and symptom management throughout the illness course (Table 11.3).[4] Poor communication around symptoms and prognosis can lead to futile, invasive interventions that do not change the outcome in the end,[2] whereas early introduction of palliative care principles has been shown to decrease suffering, improve quality of life, and promote physical and emotional well-being.[20]

Negative associations with the term "palliative care" abound. Health care team members may have hesitations around initiating this type of discussion, including concerns that patients and families may think they are "giving up," may lose hope, or may become more distressed.[4] Adolescents and young adults and family members may want to avoid this conversation to protect each other from facing the reality of the illness trajectory, or for fear that

---

TABLE 11.3

Strategies for Introducing Palliative Care to AYAs[21]

When	**Introduce palliative care team members early to facilitate opening conversations to difficult and/or end-of-life concepts before disease/symptom-related "crises" or the cessation of active (curative) treatment.**
	Raise the possibility of palliative care at various time points in the treatment journey, including key transition points during care, when disease status changes, or where symptom burden may have increased.
Who	**Ensure the wider multidisciplinary team is confident and adequately skilled to support difficult and/or end-of-life conversations with AYAs.**
	Check understanding of current and/or end-of-life priorities and treatment goals with AYAs and families, while simultaneously focusing on their current and future quality of life.
	Check who they want to be involved in that conversation.
What/How	**Tailor the content of the conversation to the individual patient and family, and the unique context of the particular time point the conversation is being introduced.**
	Explore patient and family culture, values, and preferences.
	Provide honest and complete information regarding disease progression.
	Keep AYAs informed about their diagnosis, treatment, and prognosis even if treatment is ineffective or prognosis is poor (note: can be culturally dependent).
	Use structured advance care planning tools to scaffold conversations, and as a mechanism to facilitate communication.
	Address AYAs and/or families willingness and comfort with opening difficult and/or end-of-life conversations by acknowledging their concerns, while also gently outlining the ways in which such conversations may be helpful.
	Empower the AYA/family to determine how much they wish to delve into these topics at each given conversation opportunity.
	Be aware of concerns AYAs may have around involving/including family and loved ones (e.g., concerns about burdening family) and how the treating team can support them.
	Support the young person by maintaining quality of life, continuing and pursuing current activities, spending time in the environments they want to as far as possible, and exploring/identifying place of death preferences, as well as preference for how they may be remembered and/or their family/loved ones supported after their eventual death.

AYAs, adolescents and young adults.

Adapted from Sansom-Daly UM, Wakefield CE, Patterson P, et al. End-of-Life Communication Needs for Adolescents and Young Adults with Cancer: Recommendations for Research and Practice. *J Adolesc Young Adult Oncol.* 2020;9(2):157–165. doi: 10.1089/jayao.2019.0084. Epub 2019 Oct 29. PMID: 31660768; PMCID: PMC7360106.

it would lead to discontinuation of active treatment. The resulting "conspiracy of silence" can be a significant barrier to accessing appropriate comprehensive care,[4] and there is no evidence that the referral changes either hope or distress.[11] More comprehensive explanation of palliative care services to families and clinicians may change perceptions and increase uptake,[15] creating opportunities for tackling anticipated challenging symptoms, openly discussing advance care planning, and following the lead of AYAs and their families.[2]

Service Provision and Resources

To meet AYAs' current and anticipated palliative care needs, coordination of services is paramount. Where possible, a multidisciplinary palliative care team should be identified that connects with other professionals, and links hospital to community and home settings.[2] The palliative care team should have extra training in a holistic, biopsychosocial approach to the unique needs of AYAs, and should address access to services, prognostic communication, advance care planning, symptom assessment and management, and decision making.[2] Virtual connection to teams via phone or video conferencing may help break down geographical barriers, share expertise with patients and professionals in more remote areas, and enable patients to stay closer to home for longer periods.[4]

Adolescents and young adults should be informed about their options in terms of location of care, including home, hospital, and hospice where possible. Young people and their families should be able to visit a hospice beforehand and should have access to respite care if needed. The best outcome requires flexibility and choice, with the young person making decisions if they would like and are able, to ensure a good death in their preferred place.[2]

SYMPTOM MANAGEMENT

Symptom control is a cornerstone of palliative care in general and should be no different with AYAs. An individualized symptom assessment and management plan can occur alongside treatment of the underlying disease, and may have a holistic focus, including pharmacologic and nonpharmacologic interventions.[2] While a detailed management approach is beyond the scope of this chapter, some general principles can be used to guide the process.

A biopsychosocial lens can be very helpful when asking AYAs about their symptoms.[2] Types of physical symptoms will depend on the diagnosis and commonly include pain, fatigue, shortness of breath, decreased mobility, and poor appetite.[16] Low mood, anxiety, and disrupted sleep are typical psychological symptoms, which can in turn impact how AYAs experience pain and other physical symptoms. Distress related to social elements of loss, such as changes in relationships with friends and partners, can similarly influence a young person's perception of pain.[2]

The intensity of physical symptoms is often heightened in AYAs versus other age groups.[1] Adolescents and young adults may thus require higher medication doses and adjuvant medications, and may mistakenly be characterized as "drug-seeking."[1,15] A related concern shared by AYAs, families, and clinicians alike is that of medication abuse or misuse, in particular opioids. Reassurance should be given that the risk of addiction in the terminal phase of illness is extremely low, and symptom control during this phase is critical. Alternatively, AYAs may decline certain medications and endure distressing symptoms to exercise their autonomy, and avoid unwanted or uncomfortable side effects.

Other symptom management strategies used by AYAs may include the use of medical cannabis or herbal remedies. Where the evidence base is limited, efforts may be made in an open and nonjudgmental fashion to gather information about what patients are using and evaluate for potential interactions with other treatments. More research is needed to investigate the risks and benefits of medical cannabis and other nontraditional therapies for AYAs with LLCs.[13]

In summary, AYAs require comprehensive relief of physical and emotional suffering, and multidisciplinary modalities where available—including creative arts therapies, child life specialists, spiritual care practitioners, physical and occupational therapies, massage, meditation, and mindfulness—to create additional opportunities to exercise choice and control.[2]

DECISION MAKING AND ADVANCE CARE PLANNING

Assessing Readiness

Recognition of a young person's maturity level and amount of dependence on others is crucial when it comes to AYA care in general, and decision making in particular. Another consideration is that in many jurisdictions, parents or guardians may have a legal responsibility to make decisions, and in the process may withhold information from the AYA in an attempt to protect them from harm.[15] While many AYAs may lack life experience and fully formed executive functioning, most understand what is happening to them and prefer to be informed and involved in open, honest shared decision making. Not having this opportunity can feel frightening or disempowering, while allowing youth to participate helps maintain their autonomy in an uncontrollable situation, build trust with their parents/caregivers and care team, alleviate distress about uncertainty, and enable realistic priority setting.[15,17]

The degree of involvement in discussions may vary among AYAs, with some preferring distilled information and others deferring completely to their parents/caregivers. Finding a balance between the young person's autonomy and parents' rights to protect their children can be delicate.[17] Helpful points to cover from an early stage can include asking how much information they want to be told, who they would like to hear it from, and who they want with them (if anyone).[9] The Advance Care Planning Readiness Assessment is another way to check-in with an AYA regarding planning for end of life.[22] The measure consists of three yes/no questions relating to: (1) whether talking about what would happen if treatments were no longer effective would be helpful, (2) whether talking about medical care plans ahead of time would be upsetting, and (3) whether they would be comfortable writing down/discussing what would happen if treatments were no longer effective.

A set of core attributes has been described to promote successful communication with youth, including: (1) a systematic approach, with consistent time points for conversation and allowance of patient and family processing time; (2) direct, compassionate, nonjudgmental, concrete, and developmentally appropriate language; and (3) engagement of family, friends, and others who provide the patient with social support.[17] Participation by AYAs in these conversations can help parents/caregivers and health care team members make informed decisions, alleviate distress, avoid decisional regret, and respect the youth's values, beliefs, and preferences.[23] These conversations also impact how patients live their last days, how they die, and how their families and friends grieve.[17]

Tools

To help start the conversation, AYA-specific advance care planning documents such as Voicing My CHOiCES can be used to facilitate communication between AYAs and their families, friends, and health care team.[9] Voicing My CHOiCES is developmentally tailored to meet the specific needs of young people and addresses preferences such as how patients wish to be supported so they do not feel alone, who they would want to make their medical care decisions if they cannot make them on their own, what they wish their friends and family to know about them, and how they want to be remembered.[3] FAmily-CEntered Advance Care Planning (FACE) is another evidence-based tool, a guided conversation in three parts that puts the adolescent and their family at the center.[24]

Decision-making tools such as these are appreciated by AYAs, who tend to prefer that the medical team initiate these discussions.

Some examples of how to introduce tools to AYAs and families include the following[22]:

1. *While we are hopeful that your treatment will be effective against your disease, we have learned from other families like your own that not suggesting that you give some thought to some difficult issues early on is irresponsible of us. For example, it would be great if you would communicate with each other about who would be the person to make medical decisions for you if you became very ill and are not able to do so on your own.*

2. *Although we are hoping that this next treatment (medicine) will be helpful, many people your age have told us that they found it helpful to have a say about what they would want or not want if treatment doesn't go as expected. In fact, people your age helped create a guide so that they could put down on paper the things that are important to them.*

Conflict in Decision Making

Despite using a compassionate approach, assessing readiness, and providing tools to facilitate difficult conversations, disagreements between AYAs, parents/caregivers, family members, or clinicians may arise. A young person who is fully informed by their team about risks and benefits may choose to decline further treatment, potentially if it is in direct conflict with parents'/caregivers' preferences.[2] Some AYAs may lose or never achieve the complex cognitive processing required to analyze the consequences of a decision. Even where AYAs have the capacity, parents/caregivers and professionals may prefer not to include them in conversations, with the good intention of protecting them from emotional distress.[9] Some parents/caregivers may struggle to accept that their child is mature enough to make these choices, while others may feel such important decisions should only be made by adults. Some professionals or family members may want to uphold the AYA's "right to know everything" and others feel that the responsibility involved is too great.[9]

The role of the health care team is to support and share the burden of the decision with the AYA, while exploring families' hesitations and concerns in an open and nonjudgmental way.[2] Involving social workers, psychologists, palliative care clinicians, or bioethics consultants may help keep the best interests of the patient and family at the forefront. In the words of one expert group, "although gently and persistently involving the adolescent in most cases is ideal, this pathway is not always open or optimal; however, compassionate exploration of patient-, parent/caregiver-, and family-level values always is."[17]

⬤ TRANSITION TO THE ADULT HEALTH CARE SYSTEM

Many AYAs with LLCs may age out of pediatric care. The transition process is already complex for most teenagers with chronic illnesses and can become more so toward the end of life. Some pediatric centers may be able to continue caring for patients beyond the age of 18, especially for patients approaching death or for those with developmental considerations. For AYAs who have outgrown pediatric care, it can be difficult for patients, families, and professionals to "let go"—with a reluctance and fear to leave behind a relationship that sometimes spans years—and feel comfortable in an unfamiliar adult health care system.[25] This can be particularly hard for AYAs with rare conditions not often seen in the adult setting.

Evidence supporting a specific transition model for palliative care is sparse.[2] In some conditions, such as cystic fibrosis or congenital heart disease, transition may be more streamlined because a clearly identified adult service is on the receiving end.[25] Other conditions do not fit easily into a disease or system-specific category, and many young people may be seeing multiple specialists concurrently.

Pediatric and adult clinicians should proactively partner, where possible, to enhance the transition process and bridge the gap between two very disparate worlds.[26] Each system must adapt to and collaborate with the other; adult services need to better understand certain health conditions to provide more confident care and pediatric services need to better understand what the other side can offer to be able to manage expectations.[26] A focus on patient priorities—having knowledgeable clinicians providing coordinated care, promoting autonomy, and respecting values—will ensure that the transition process maximizes opportunities for young people with limited lives.[26]

⬤ END-OF-LIFE CARE

The care of AYAs at the end of life necessitates clear communication and review of preferences regarding the level of medical intervention, monitoring, goals, and place of death.[2] The minority of AYAs die where they want to, be that at home or in the hospital.[27] In addition, lack of communication may translate to unnecessary higher-intensity care. At the very end of life, nearly a quarter of AYAs will receive care in an intensive care unit or visit the emergency department for care needs.[27]

Decision making about location of care at the end of life should involve accommodating the wishes of young people and their families as much as possible, while considering practical limitations around service provision. A critical element may not necessarily be the place itself or whether the young person died in their preferred place, but rather if the youth and their family were given the information and choices about the possible options.[13]

Adolescents and young adults at end of life still find themselves caught in the middle, with most pediatric and adult hospices having limited experience caring for this age group. Some pediatric practitioners may be less comfortable managing higher AYA symptom needs than typically seen in younger children, and may end up providing hospice-level care if adult centers do not have the expertise either. Some countries have set up dedicated AYA hospices supporting young people with a variety of medical conditions.[13] In most cases, however, it will be essential for AYAs, their families, and clinicians to make links with specialized palliative care services where possible, which can provide developmentally tailored, high-quality end-of-life care.

⬤ BEREAVEMENT

When a young person dies, it is generally viewed as a disruption in the "normal" trajectory of a life course.[8] Children are meant to outlive parents and grandparents, making it more difficult to find meaning after such an event. Thus, the death of an AYA poses bereavement challenges distinct from those that follow the death of an older person. Responses will vary by culture and generation, but will have a profound impact on parents/caregivers, siblings, grandparents, partners, children, friends, and health care team members.[16] Although it is the same youth who has died, each person's reflections, emotions, and experiences will be very different.[8]

There may not be an expected or predictable pattern to the feelings, which can include shock despite a protracted illness, relief that the pain or suffering is over, guilt that more wasn't done to save the person or that they have died while others remain alive, failure that the person could not be protected from death, anger, helplessness, anxiety, numbness, yearning, and loneliness.[8] Bereaved parents, siblings, and peers are at higher risk of developing complicated grief,[16] a chronic, impairing reaction with more intense and prolonged symptoms.[28] Timely referral to psychological or psychiatric services by identifying risk factors (e.g., prior history of mental health or substance use issues) may be helpful in mitigating downstream consequences of untreated complicated grief.[2]

Connection to bereavement supports should be part of any AYA palliative care approach. Some parents/caregivers and siblings may benefit from specific group supports, while others may prefer one-on-one counseling.[2] Maintaining some form of contact with the treating care team may also be beneficial. Despite the magnitude of the loss, most parents are able to continue with everyday tasks, and over time, many report a sense of personal growth, becoming more expressive of feelings and feeling closer to surviving family members.[29]

SUMMARY

In this chapter, the impact of LLCs on youth and the people around them has been explored. An individualized, tailored approach that considers the intersection between illness and achieving developmental milestones is crucial to address comprehensively the unique physical, emotional, social, spiritual, and cultural needs of this population. For the clinician, the challenge is to follow the lead of the AYA to ensure that they are fully informed, respected, and supported in their choices.

Where possible, a multidisciplinary team with expertise should be involved to manage symptoms, plan for transition to adult care, prepare for end of life, and care for family and friends through bereavement. With appropriate support, a young person's sense of individuality, autonomy, value, and continuity can be cultivated and nurtured in order to embrace what the future may hold.[9] In the words of one expert, "although such deaths may never feel right, perhaps they can be made to feel less 'wrong'."[30]

REFERENCES

1. Clark JK, Fasciano K. Young adult palliative care: challenges and opportunities. *Am J Hosp Palliat Care*. 2015;32(1):101–111.
2. Chisholm J, Hough R, Soanes L, eds. *A Practical Approach to the Care of Adolescents and Young Adults With Cancer*. Springer International Publishing; 2018.
3. Donovan KA, Knight D, Quinn GP. Palliative care in adolescents and young adults with cancer. *Cancer Control*. 2015;22(4):475–479.
4. Pritchard S, Cuvelier G, Harlos M, et al. Palliative care in adolescents and young adults with cancer. *Cancer*. 2011;117(10 Suppl):2323–2328.
5. World Health Organization. *Cancer Pain Relief and Palliative Care*. Technical Report Series 804. WHO; 1990.
6. *Global Burden of disease study 2019 query tool website*. Accessed May 26, 2021. http://ghdx.healthdata.org/gbd-results-tool
7. Kelly D, Gibson F. *Cancer Care for Adolescents and Young Adults*. Blackwell Publishing Ltd.; 2008.
8. Hain R, Goldman A, Rapoport A, et al., eds. *Oxford Textbook of Palliative Care for Children*. Oxford University Press; 2021.
9. Ngwenya N, Kenten C, Jones L, et al. Experiences and preferences for end-of-life care for young adults with cancer and their informal carers: a narrative synthesis. *J Adolesc Young Adult Oncol*. 2017;6(2):200–212.
10. Bell CJ, Skiles J, Pradhan K, et al. End-of-life experiences in adolescents dying with cancer. *Support Care Cancer*. 2010;18(7):827–835.
11. Kazak AE, Alderfer M, Rourke MT, et al. Posttraumatic stress disorder (PTSD) and posttraumatic stress symptoms (PTSS) in families of adolescent childhood cancer survivors. *J Pediatr Psychol*. 2004;29(3):211–219.
12. Pinkerton R, Donovan L, Herbert A. Palliative care in adolescents and young adults with cancer-why do adolescents need special attention? *Cancer J*. 2018;24(6):336–341.
13. Gentile D, Markham MJ, Eaton T. Patients with cancer and social media: harness benefits, avoid drawbacks [published online ahead of print, 2018 Nov 1]. *J Oncol Pract*. 2018;JOP1800367.
14. Rosenberg AR, Wolfe J. Palliative care for adolescents and young adults with cancer. *Clin Oncol Adolesc Young Adults*. 2013;2013(3):41–48.
15. Upshaw NC, Roche A, Gleditsch K, et al. Palliative care considerations and practices for adolescents and young adults with cancer. *Pediatr Blood Cancer*. 2021;68(1):e28781.
16. Rosenberg AR, Wolfe J, Wiener L, et al. Ethics, emotions, and the skills of talking about progressing disease with terminally Ill adolescents: a review. *JAMA Pediatr*. 2016;170(12):1216–1223.
17. Kenten C, Ngwenya N, Gibson F, et al. Understanding care when cure is not likely for young adults who face cancer: a realist analysis of data from patients, families and healthcare professionals. *BMJ Open*. 2019;9(1):e024397.
18. McLaughlin SE, Machan J, Fournier P, et al. Transition of adolescents with chronic health conditions to adult primary care: factors associated with physician acceptance. *J Pediatr Rehabil Med*. 2014;7(1):63–70.
19. Levine DR, Mandrell BN, Sykes A, et al. Patients' and parents' needs, attitudes, and perceptions about early palliative care integration in pediatric oncology. *JAMA Oncol*. 2017;3(9):1214–1220.
20. Zadeh S, Pao M, Wiener L. Opening end-of-life discussions: how to introduce Voicing My CHOiCES™, an advance care planning guide for adolescents and young adults. *Palliat Support Care*. 2015;13(3):591–599.
21. Wiener L, Zadeh S, Wexler LH, et al. When silence is not golden: engaging adolescents and young adults in discussions around end-of-life care choices. *Pediatr Blood Cancer*. 2013;60(5):715–718.
22. Dallas RH, Kimmel A, Wilkins ML, et al. Acceptability of family-centered advanced care planning for adolescents with HIV. *Pediatrics*. 2016;138(6):e20161854.
23. Linebarger JS, Ajayi TA, Jones BL. Adolescents and young adults with life-threatening illness: special considerations, transitions in care, and the role of pediatric palliative care. *Pediatr Clin North Am*. 2014;61(4):785–796.
24. Chambers L. Stepping up: a guide to developing a good transition to adulthood for young people with life-limiting and life-threatening conditions. *Bristol: Together Short Lives*. 2015. https://www.togetherforshortlives.org.uk/app/uploads/2018/02/ProRes-Stepping-Up-Transition-Care-Pathway.pdf
25. Mack JW, Chen LH, Cannavale K, et al. End-of-life care intensity among adolescent and young adult patients with cancer in Kaiser Permanente Southern California. *JAMA Oncol*. 2015;1(5):592–600.
26. Shear MK, Simon N, Wall M, et al. Complicated grief and related bereavement issues for DSM-5. *Depress Anxiety*. 2011;28(2):103–117.
27. Callahan D. Death, mourning, and medical progress. *Perspect Biol Med*. 2009;52(1):103–115.
28. Kelly D. The challenge of caring for adolescents and young adults. *Int J Palliat Nurs*. 2013;19(5):211.
29. World Health Organization website. Accessed May 25, 2021. https://www.who.int/health-topics/palliative-care
30. Sansom-Daly UM, Wakefield CE, Patterson P, et al. End-of-life communication needs for adolescents and young adults with cancer: recommendations for research and practice. *J Adolesc Young Adult Oncol*. 2020;9(2):157–165.

ADDITIONAL RESOURCES AND WEBSITES

Additional Resources and Websites for Clinicians:
Goldstein NE, Morrison RS. *Evidence-Based Practice of Palliative Medicine*. Saunders; 2013. https://www.elsevier.com/books/evidence-based-practice-of-palliative-medicine/goldstein/978-1-4377-3796-7
Rosenberg AR, Wolfe J, Wiener L, et al. Ethics, emotions, and the skills of talking about progressing disease with terminally ill adolescents: a review. *JAMA Pediatr*. 2016;170(12):1216–1223. https://doi.org/10.1001/jamapediatrics.2016.2142
Sansom-Daly UM, Wakefield CE, Patterson P, et al. End-of-Life communication needs for adolescents and young adults with cancer: recommendations for research and practice. *J Adolesc Young Adult Oncol*. 2020;9(2):157–165. https://doi.org/10.1089/jayao.2019.0084
Voicing My CHOiCES advance care planning tool—https://store.fivewishes.org/ShopLocal/en/p/VC-MASTER-000/voicing-my-choices
Wiener L, Zadeh S, Wexler LH, et al. When silence is not golden: engaging adolescents and young adults in discussions around end-of-life care choices. *Pediatr Blood Cancer*. 2013;60(5):715–718. https://doi.org/10.1002/pbc.24490
Wolfe J, Hinds PS, Sourkes BM. *Textbook of Interdisciplinary Pediatric Palliative Care*. Elsevier/Saunders; 2011. https://www.elsevier.com/books/textbook-of-interdisciplinary-pediatric-palliative-care/wolfe/978-1-4377-0262-0
Zadeh S, Pao M, Wiener L. Opening end-of-life discussions: how to introduce Voicing My CHOiCES™, an advance care planning guide for adolescents and young adults. Palliat Support Care. 2015;13(3):591–599. https://doi.org/10.1017/S1478951514000054

Additional Resources and Websites for Parents/Caregivers:
Beecham J, Ortlip K. *Living with Dying: A Complete Guide for Caregivers*. Starcatcher Press; 2016. http://livingwithdying.com/
Courageous Parents Network—https://courageousparentsnetwork.org/
Grollman A. *Straight Talk about Death for Teenagers: How to Cope with Losing Someone You Love*. Beacon Press; 1993.
A Caregiver's Challenge: Living, Loving, and Letting Go.
Stickney D. *Water Bugs and Dragonflies: Explaining Death to Young Children*. The Pilgrim Press; 2004.
Voicing My CHOiCES advance care planning tool—https://store.fivewishes.org/ShopLocal/en/p/VC-MASTER-000/voicing-my-choices
Wolfelt AD. *Finding the Words: How to Talk with Children and Teens About Death, Suicide, Homicide, Funerals, Cremation, and Other End-of-Life Matters*. Companion Press; 2013.
Wolfelt AD. *Healing Your Grieving Heart: 100 Practical Ideas*. Companion Press; 2001.

Additional Resources and Websites for Adolescents and Young Adults:
Katz, A. *This Should Not Be Happening: Young Adults with Cancer*. Oncology Nursing Society; 2014. http://www.drannekatz.com/project/this-should-not-be-happening-young-adults-with-cancer/
Living Out Loud—https://livingoutloud.life/
Voicing My CHOiCES advance care planning tool—https://store.fivewishes.org/ShopLocal/en/p/VC-MASTER-000/voicing-my-choices

12

Quality Improvement Concepts in Adolescent and Young Adult Health

Alene Toulany
Jill S. Huppert

KEY WORDS
- Adolescent and young adult health
- Plan-do-study-act (PDSA) cycle
- Quality improvement
- Quality indicators

INTRODUCTION

The next generation of clinicians has two important roles as clinicians: providing care and improving care. Most health care training programs focus on helping physicians, nurses, and other clinicians learn how best to treat patients within a health system. Less emphasis has traditionally been placed on helping clinicians learn how to improve their practices or the system itself, as knowledge evolves. This chapter focuses on encouraging quality improvement (QI) knowledge and skills for clinicians engaged in adolescent and young adult (AYA) health care.

Quality in Health Care

Quality improvement has been a discipline in health care since at least the 1980s, but did not become widely recognized until the Institute of Medicine (IOM) in the United States released its report "To Err is Human" in 1999.[1] This report generated intense media attention with its disclosure that every year in the United States, between 44,000 and 98,000 patients die in-hospital from preventable medical errors, the equivalent of one jumbo jet crashing every day. It also sounded an alarm that there was a crisis in quality of care and started what we now know as the modern QI movement. In the past 15 to 20 years, there has been an explosion of awareness, studies, and literature on QI, with quality of care and accountability increasingly being demanded by patients, hospital boards, and the government.

What exactly does quality care mean? There are many definitions, however, this one captures most of the key elements: providing the right care, to the right patient, at the right time. In 2001, the IOM released its report "Crossing the Quality Chasm," which identifies six aims for a quality health care system.[2] These are considered to be the six domains of quality.
1. Safe: avoiding injuries to patients (e.g., medical errors)
2. Timely: reducing wait times and delays in receiving care
3. Efficient: avoiding waste (e.g., not repeating tests unnecessarily)
4. Effective: practicing evidence-based medicine
5. Equitable: providing high-quality care to all, regardless of demographics, geographical location, or socioeconomic status
6. Patient centered: ensuring that patient values guide clinical decisions

Some people think of QI as taking a problem that falls within one of these domains (e.g., access to care), identifying the gap (e.g., patients are waiting too long for procedure X), and then applying QI methods to close the gap. No discussion of QI is complete without a jumbo jet analogy. Airlines have used QI methods to achieve and maintain excellent safety records. The airline industry is definitely considered a very safe one, but falls short when other domains of quality are considered. For example, the airline industry is not that "equitable" (consider the first-class cabin), not that "client or patient centered" (consider typical airline food), and not that "timely" or "efficient" (consider long lines at customs and/or lost luggage).

Health care is not that different. Often, compromises are made in the QI work—improving one domain of quality may put another at risk. For example, shortening emergency department wait times may address issues of "timeliness" and "access," and even "safety" for that patient sitting in the waiting room waiting to be triaged who might have a life-threatening condition, however, this may put other elements of quality at risk. Many approaches to improving flow in the emergency department involve methods such as rotating patients in and out of stretchers or admitting patients to hallways, none of which are very "patient centered" and may not be equitable.

CLINICAL IMPORTANCE OF QUALITY IMPROVEMENT

There are many reasons why the clinician should care about QI, and why it is important to know how to effectively engage in QI activities in one's clinical practice. First, patients expect physicians to deliver the highest possible quality of care. Governments increasingly demand accountability from hospitals and physicians, to demonstrate that they are using health care dollars effectively and efficiently, and meeting accepted benchmarks of quality care. More and more, sustainable health care funding is tied to achieving standards of quality care (i.e., quality-based procedures/care). The media is also drawing attention to high-profile medical errors and lapses in care, so public awareness of quality issues is currently very high.

Unlike conducting clinical research, where any direct benefits to patients are far downstream and can take years to be realized, a QI project can have an immediate and direct impact on the day-to-day care provided to patients, which can be very rewarding. Increasingly, it is a professional expectation that all physicians engage in QI as part of their work. For example, many community hospitals now explicitly mandate that any new physicians have previous training or experience in QI. Hospitals look to clinicians to lead QI initiatives across their institutions. Quality improvement is also recognized as a valued academic activity, alongside education and research. There are many journals that publish QI studies (i.e., Pediatrics, British Medical Journal Quality Improvement Reports) but each has its own particular focus.

Finally, QI concepts have been incorporated throughout the physician competency frameworks[3] (e.g., Canadian Medical Education Directives for Specialists and the Accreditation Council for Graduate Medical Education) and curricula have been developed across the learning continuum.[4] In addition, after training, physicians are all required to engage in regular self-assessment of their clinical practice to earn maintenance of certification credits for continuing professional development. It is now a requirement of all practicing physicians in Canada and the United States to reflect on their practices and assess their clinical performance for the purpose of QI.

QUALITY IMPROVEMENT METHODS IN PRACTICE: IDENTIFYING AND PRIORITIZING QUALITY PROBLEMS

It is not hard to identify opportunities for improvement in one's clinical environment, but some ideas are better suited for a QI project than others. There are several key factors to consider when picking an appropriate target for a QI project. Initially, pick an issue that is important to patients, that is, something that occurs frequently enough and has high impact, in terms of improving the care received by the patients and/or cost savings. Next, choose something that one has some direct control over. For example, it might be difficult to try to improve the turnaround time on a lab test result, unless there is very strong buy-in and participation from stakeholders working in the lab, because most of the factors that would delay a test result are outside of one's control. Think about how feasible it will be to implement the project, in terms of possible organizational or logistical barriers, time, resources, and budget constraints. Also consider the possibility of unintended consequences. Improving care in one area may inadvertently cause problems in other areas. Finally, try to align the project with other QI activities in the organization to help accelerate progress.[5] This may allow one to tap into funding and resources to help the project along and gain the support of senior leaders who can help in dealing with obstacles that arise.

INSTITUTE FOR HEALTH CARE IMPROVEMENT MODEL FOR IMPROVEMENT

There are many different models for how to do a QI project, such as Lean and Six Sigma,[6,7] but the simplest and most commonly used is the Model for Improvement,[8] which is organized around three basic questions (Fig. 12.1):

1. What are we trying to accomplish?
2. How will we know that a change is an improvement?
3. What changes can result in improvement?

A basic principle is that not all change is improvement but that all improvement requires change.[9]

What Are We Trying to Accomplish?

The planning stage is the most important and time-consuming step in QI. Investing the time early on in really understanding the process and selecting the right intervention to target the problem will have much higher odds of success.

Defining an aim will help to focus the project and ensure that all team members are on the same page. An aim statement needs to be specific in defining what measure one is hoping to improve and setting a deadline by which to achieve it. When choosing a target for "how much," consider setting a stretch goal (an ambitious goal to aim for within a certain time), not something that can easily be achieved (like a 5% improvement). If time and work are going to be invested into a project, the aim should be to make

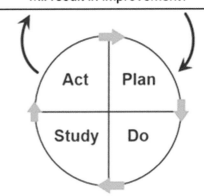

FIGURE 12.1 Model for improvement. (Used with permission from Langley GJ, Moen RD, Nolan KM, et al. *The Improvement Guide: A Practical Approach to Enhancing Organizational Performance.* 2nd ed. John Wiley and Sons; 2009.)

a significant improvement. While writing an aim statement may seem straightforward, in practice, it is hard to write an aim statement before actually starting a project. Some of the reasons are the measures have not been selected yet and one does not know how well they are currently performing, so it is hard to set a meaningful and realistic target for improvement. In addition, the causes of the quality problem are unclear at the outset and potential opportunities for improvement have not been realized. Previous interventions that have already been tried to close the quality gap may be unknown, as well as how successful or unsuccessful they were. It is very common to generate an aim statement at the beginning of a QI project, and then revise it after there is a better understanding of the quality problem (e.g., after doing a chart audit and root cause analysis, as will be explained later in the chapter).

A useful mnemonic that is often used to remind teams about the key elements of an effective aim statement is SMART. Be as **Specific** as possible and keep the project focused. When writing the aim statement, indicate clearly what measure will track success, and include a clear target for the amount of change wished to be seen in the measure. While "stretch" goals are desirable, set targets that are realistic and **Attainable**. It is helpful to look to the literature to see what other groups have been able to achieve using a similar intervention—that may help guide the team to determine what is possible. Otherwise, the target may be based on some preliminary pilot work that the group has done. More often than not, attempts are made to set a realistic target that is both achievable and meaningful. Finally, establish an aim that is targeting important process problems that are **Relevant** and that are likely to result in improved care.

How Will We Know That a Change Is an Improvement?

In order to know if a change has resulted in an improvement, a family of measures needs to be collected and studied including outcome, process, and balancing measures. Outcome measures are the clinically relevant outcomes to try to improve (e.g., mortality or major complication rate, adverse medication event rate). They are the measures that evaluate the effects of health care delivery on patients and populations. Process measures reflect the actions that makeup health care delivery. They could evaluate how well the steps or parts in the system are working, or how well the plan is being implemented. Process measures that specifically look at whether the intervention is being implemented as intended are often referred to as "measures of fidelity." In other words, is the intervention being implemented as expected and planned? If the change involves the use of a checklist to standardize a process, a measure of the fidelity of the intervention might evaluate whether the checklist is being used consistently. Balancing measures are used to ensure that the change does not result in any unintended or additional problems, for example, increased costs, decreased patient or staff satisfaction, or increased workload. As outcome measures are often far downstream, the project may be focused on improving process measures. Often significant improvements in process measures can be detected earlier than in outcome measures.

What Changes Can Result in Improvement?

Once the problems in the process have been identified, the next step is to pick appropriate solutions for them. It is important to articulate a theory that ties the proposed solution with the problem that it aims to solve. One must link the problem at hand to a theory, a change concept that is mapped to this theory, and then come up with some change ideas. A change concept is the general notion or approach to change whereas the change idea is the specific idea or intervention one might implement in their practice, to lead to an improvement. Some common change concepts include elimination of waste (remove unnecessary steps), error proofing (forcing functions, standardization, reminders), and managing time (reduce delays, wait times).

A classic example of the solution not matching the problem was the campaign to reduce antibiotic prescription for uncomplicated otitis media. Millions of dollars were spent on educating primary care physicians about not prescribing antibiotics, through mailings, conferences, or continuing medical education. Despite this, antibiotic prescription rates did not decrease because parents were still showing up demanding antibiotics for their children and refusing to leave their doctor's office until they had a prescription. If the theory is that clinician knowledge is the problem, then clinician education is the solution. But if patient knowledge is the issue, then the focus should be on patient education instead. In this case, a public health campaign, information pamphlets for parents, or posters in the waiting room may have been more effective interventions.

● STAKEHOLDER PARTICIPATION

Stakeholder input is very important. Stakeholders are anyone affected by a problem and anyone who will be involved with and/or affected by the change.[10] In order to identify the stakeholders, consider all the people who are affected by the QI project, have influence or power over the QI project, and/or have an interest in the QI project's successful (or unsuccessful) conclusion. This may include other physicians, interprofessional team members, patients, administrative staff, or other departments (e.g. diagnostic Imaging, lab). The reasons to identify and engage stakeholders are numerous. Stakeholders really understand the problem and can inform, build commitment, and promote successful implementation of the change.

By speaking with the stakeholders, one will get a sense of their reaction to the project. Stakeholders can generally be classified into four categories[11]:
1. Champions—constituting 10% of stakeholders, typically in a leadership position. They believe in the project, will help to remove barriers to success, and encourage others to help.
2. Helpers—another 10% of stakeholders. They share the team's goals and are willing to help operationalize the idea. These are great to recruit to the QI team.

3. Bystanders—the majority of people, about 60%. They are busy and have their own work to worry about. They won't oppose the project but won't help out either. However, if early results from the project are positive, they may come to believe in the value of the project and may convert to be helpers later on.
4. Resisters—20% of stakeholders. They actively disagree with the change idea and will try to prevent the project from succeeding. They may well have valid concerns and may be worried about consequences that have not been foreseen. Resisters need to be managed most carefully, as they can spread pessimism about the project and dissuade the support of others.

The approach taken with each stakeholder depends on how they are classified. Talk to the stakeholders and find out how they feel about the project. As all stakeholders will be affected to some degree, they should be kept informed of project developments, especially when the rolled out intervention will impact them. Helpers can be invited to join the QI team. Resisters are the trickiest to deal with. One may decide to proceed and work around them. But if left unchecked, they may undermine the project (directly, or by influencing others' opinions). If engaged, they may raise legitimate concerns, as well as possible solutions, to improve the odds of the project's success. The approach taken with resisters should be decided on a case-by-case basis.

Understanding Your Quality Improvement Problem Using Quality Improvement Tools

Quality problems need to be investigated thoroughly, and there are several tools to help. Fishbone diagrams (also called cause-and-effect diagram, Ishikawa diagram) are a simple but powerful tool for identifying possible variables influencing a problem.[12] An example Fishbone diagram shown in Figure 12.2 addresses the problem of long wait time for test results. Fishbone diagrams help to sort many possible causes for problem into useful categories. In this example, the team has used the patients, clinicians, equipment and organization categories, but not all problems will fit these categories and may have other facets. Also, this is a working document, with shorthand terms understandable to the team such as "FIFO" and "do-over." Ideally, the diagram is generated through a group brainstorming session, involving all the different participants or stakeholders in a process. A comprehensive understanding of the issue will result, if discussed as a group, rather than just by oneself or by only speaking with other physicians. Quality improvement almost always requires an interprofessional approach. Patients may also be engaged in this process.

A driver diagram is another tool used in QI to help better understand the quality problem at hand. Key driver diagrams depict the relationship between the project's aim, which was written in the beginning, the primary drivers that contribute directly to achieving the aim, and the changes or interventions that could cause the desired effects on the primary drivers. The diagram represents the team members' shared theories of "cause and effect" in the system—what changes will lead to the desired outcome. The diagram should be updated regularly as the team acquires new knowledge and experience. Figure 12.3 depicts an example driver diagram of a project aimed to increase the percentage of females with a sexually transmitted infection (STI) who are notified of their results within 7 days.[13] The problem identified was that teens treated in the emergency department were treated empirically and not consistently given their test results. The team identified four drivers and a set of possible changes for each driver that helped to focus their work.

One of the principles of QI is that even though one may think they understand the process, they really don't understand it until they go through a detailed process mapping exercise. Constructing a process map (also known as flowchart) helps to visually capture

Example: Cause and Effect Diagram

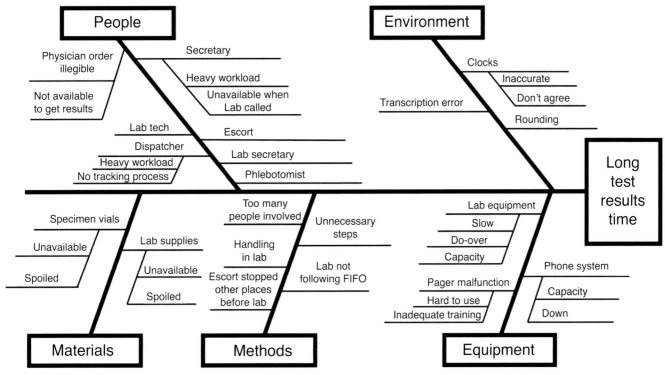

FIGURE 12.2 Example Fishbone diagram (also known as cause-and-effect diagram) of long wait times and test results. (Source: QI Essentials Toolkit: Cause and Effect Diagram. Institute for Healthcare Improvement, 2017. [Reprinted from www.IHI.org with permission of the Institute for Healthcare Improvement (IHI), ©2022.])

how various activities relate to one another in a health care process.[14,15] This map can be used to define an existing process or develop a new one.

Everyone makes assumptions about how things run in a hospital or clinic, but the reality is often quite different. The best way to draw an accurate process map is to physically go to where the process takes place, and follow it step by step from start to finish. It may be surprising to learn the number of steps and handoffs needed

to successfully complete the process, or to discover numerous and unnecessary delays in care. As with drawing the Fishbone diagram, one needs to speak to all the participants in the process to really understand what is going on. Once the process is mapped out, the rate-limiting or most problematic step will usually become clearer. In addition, variations in practice and opportunities to standardize procedures also become more apparent. The information gleaned from the process map will, therefore, help inform the target for

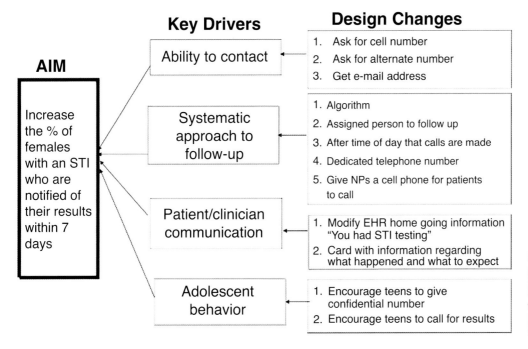

FIGURE 12.3 Example driver diagram. (Source: QI Essentials Toolkit: Driver Diagram. Institute for Healthcare Improvement, 2017. [Reprinted from www.IHI.org with permission of the Institute for Healthcare Improvement (IHI), ©2022.])

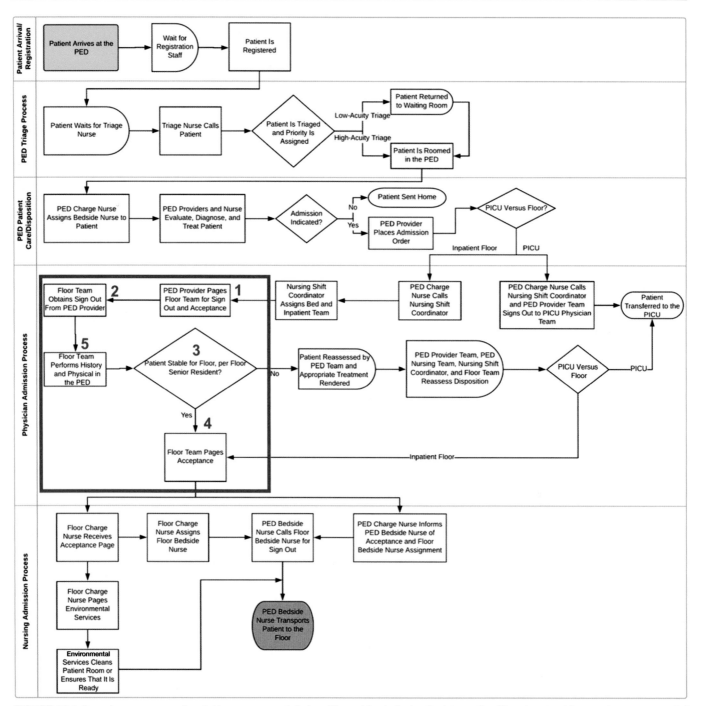

FIGURE 12.4 Example process map of pediatric emergency admissions. The *red box* indicates the intervention. The educational interventions recommended changing their workflow to the sequence indicated by the *red numbers* (steps 1–5).[16] (Source: QI Essentials Toolkit: Flow Chart. Institute for Healthcare Improvement, 2017. [Reprinted from www.IHI.org with permission of the Institute for Healthcare Improvement (IHI), ©2022.])

the QI intervention. A high-level process map or a very detailed one can be created. The level of detail depends on the process and quality problem that one is trying to understand. The process map needs to have sufficient detail to determine the best QI strategy to use. Figure 12.4 is an example process map of pediatric emergency admissions.[16] The team used the map to identify a bottleneck when the floor team was called to evaluate the patient, and focused their efforts there.

PLAN-DO-STUDY-ACT CYCLE

The systematic process of testing changes to see if one's ideas have improved their system is referred to as a "PDSA" or a

plan-do-study-act cycle.[17] Quality improvement consists of many of these cycles. There are four steps in PDSA cycle. Fundamentally, this is the standard scientific method in simpler terms. Set out with an aim, develop a hypothesis, test it in the real world and collect data, interpret the results, and potentially plan for another PDSA cycle based on what was learned during the first cycle.

Although P stands for Plan, this can be thought of as "Predict" where a hypothesis is formulated about a problem, then a bit of data is collected, analyzed, and interpreted, and conclusions drawn that allow the iteration of the next hypothesis. It is key to understand the importance of making predictions when doing PDSA work. Ask "what do you predict will happen when you introduce a change?" and then reflect on what happens, what resulted from the

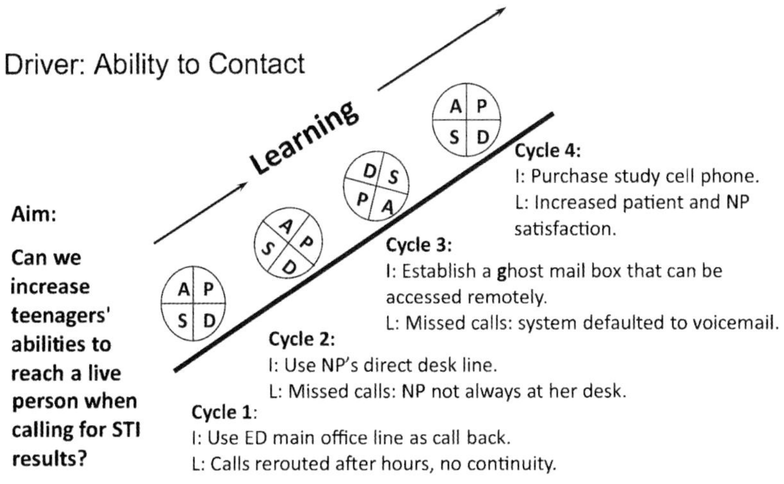

Driver: Ability to Contact
Learning
Aim:
Can we increase teenagers' abilities to reach a live person when calling for STI results?
A P S D
Cycle 4:
I: Purchase study cell phone.
L: Increased patient and NP satisfaction.
Cycle 3:
I: Establish a ghost mail box that can be accessed remotely.
L: Missed calls: system defaulted to voicemail.
Cycle 2:
I: Use NP's direct desk line.
L: Missed calls: NP not always at her desk.
Cycle 1:
I: Use ED main office line as call back.
L: Calls rerouted after hours, no continuity.

FIGURE 12.5 Learning from multiple PDSA cycles to increase ability to make voice-to-voice contact with adolescent females who have a positive STI test result. I, intervention; L, learning.[13] (Used with permission from Huppert JS, Reed JL, Munafo JK, et al. Improving notification of sexually transmitted infections: a quality improvement project and planned experiment. *Pediatrics*. 2012;130(2):e415–e422.)

change being tested, and decide on what was learned that can help advance the QI project.

Multiple cycles of these prediction–reflection loops are often required in QI projects, yet many do not take this approach in their QI work.[18] Many changes don't work out the first time they are tried, which is why QI projects will typically need to go through many PDSAs before they achieve their intended aim. A single PDSA cycle is not intended to lead to improvement; it tests a hypothesis and the results of the test help to strengthen the understanding of what does or does not work. It is the collective learning from multiple PDSAs that leads to a refined intervention and is more likely to lead to improvement. An example of the learning from the STI test result example is shown in Figure 12.5.[13]

While there are many benefits of doing PDSA cycles, few studies that mention doing PDSA actually demonstrate authentic application of this method. Plan-do-study-act is not just about going through the motions and saying "you are doing QI"—it is the key to success of the project. When going through authentic PDSA cycles, one will appreciate how each cycle increases confidence that the change will produce improvement because it allows the recognition of missing ingredients or necessary refinements that the intervention needs to be more successful. In addition, the process of implementing changes one PDSA cycle at a time is much more palatable for stakeholders in an organization that may have resisters to the change. For example, when an initiative is rolled out in one large swoop, some people can be taken aback by the rapid change. On the other hand, doing a small PDSA cycle and piloting a change at a small scale is generally not met with the same resistance.

DISPLAYING DATA

The second question in the Model for Improvement asks, "how will we know that a change is an improvement?" When a team wants to display their QI data to demonstrate whether the changes that they've introduced have resulted in an improvement, the most common tools to display data are that of a run chart or statistical process control (SPC) chart.[19] Figure 12.6 is an example SPC chart showing the percentage of charts with confidential number documented in the electronic health record (EHR) for females with STI testing.[13]

When one is new to QI, run charts are the easiest place to start. Run charts are a simple tool used to display data to determine if a system is demonstrating nonrandom patterns. The basic premise of these charts is to take data and display it over time rather than aggregate it. Aggregating data does not provide the full picture, and that run chart data can provide insight into what is happening with the improvement work.

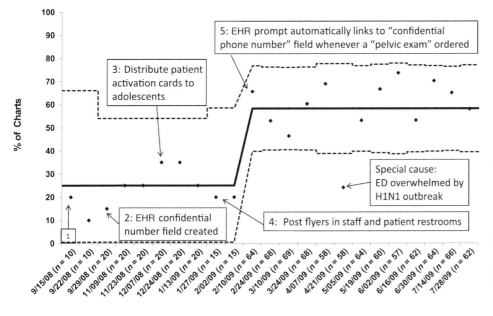

% of Charts
0
10
20
30
40
50
60
70
80
90
100
1
2: EHR confidential number field created
3: Distribute patient activation cards to adolescents.
4: Post flyers in staff and patient restrooms
5: EHR prompt automatically links to "confidential phone number" field whenever a "pelvic exam" ordered
Special cause: ED overwhelmed by H1N1 outbreak
9/15/08 (n = 10)
9/22/08 (n = 10)
9/29/08 (n = 20)
11/09/08 (n = 20)
11/23/08 (n = 20)
12/07/08 (n = 20)
12/24/08 (n = 20)
1/13/09 (n = 20)
1/27/09 (n = 15)
2/02/09 (n = 15)
2/10/09 (n = 64)
2/24/09 (n = 68)
3/10/09 (n = 69)
3/24/09 (n = 68)
4/07/09 (n = 58)
4/21/09 (n = 58)
5/05/09 (n = 64)
5/19/09 (n = 60)
6/02/09 (n = 57)
6/16/09 (n = 62)
6/30/09 (n = 64)
7/14/09 (n = 66)
7/28/09 (n = 62)

FIGURE 12.6 Example statistical process control chart showing percentage of charts with confidential number documented in the EHR for females with STI testing, over time. *n*, number of charts per interval. *Solid line*: mean percentage. *Dotted lines*: control limits. Initial intervention (box 1): Email ED staff reminders to collect confidential number whenever STI tests ordered. *Arrows* indicate subsequent interventions.[13] (Used with permission from Huppert JS, Reed JL, Munafo JK, et al. Improving notification of sexually transmitted infections: a quality improvement project and planned experiment. *Pediatrics*. 2012;130(2):e415–e422.)

Interpreting data on a run or control chart requires an understanding of variation to determine whether or not there is a "signal" or simply "noise." In QI, the typical variation that one might observe around a series of measurements is referred to as "common cause"—this is the random noise that one might observe. For example, if someone drove to work every day, they would arrive at work at slightly different times, sometimes a few minutes early, other times a few minutes late. This variation in arrival time is called common cause variation. In QI, data is plotted on a run chart to try to identify "special cause" variation—variation that is a result of more than just random chance—evidence that there is a "signal." Again, if someone is recording their arrival time to work (assuming they leave at the same time), maybe 1 day they arrive 15 minutes late because there was construction and they closed a lane on the road they take to work or maybe they consistently arrive 10 minutes earlier in the morning because in the summer, the traffic is lighter. Constructing a run chart using this outcome or process measures can help to display data over time to distinguish this "signal" from "noise."

There are several advantages of displaying QI data over time using a run chart. It makes performance visible and helps to make determinations about whether changes led to improvements and about the sustainability of QI efforts. Once special cause variation has occurred, the key is to determine why it occurred and what degree of confidence there is that the changes that were introduced actually led to the variation. In the example in Figure 12.6, one special cause was a QI intervention (intervention #5: change to the EHR), while another special cause was extraneous to the QI plan (an H1N1 outbreak).

KEY DIFFERENCES BETWEEN RESEARCH AND QUALITY IMPROVEMENT

Questions frequently arise about whether or not certain projects qualify as research or if they are considered QI. The confusion

---

TABLE 12.1

Adolescent-Focused Topics That Are Included in Well-Defined Quality Measures. Each Reference Provides Details on Definitions of the Outcomes, Numerators, Denominators, and Exclusions So That Local Results Can Be Compared with National Benchmarks

Source	Topic	Details
HEDIS	Adolescent well-care visits (AWC)[22]	Adolescents and young adults 12–21 y of age who had at least one comprehensive well-care visit with a primary care practitioner or an obstetrics and gynecology (OB/GYN) practitioner during the measurement year.
HEDIS	Metabolic monitoring for children and adolescents on antipsychotics (APM)[23]	Percentage of children and adolescents with ongoing antipsychotic medication use who had metabolic testing during the year.
HEDIS	Use of first-line psychosocial care for children and adolescents on antipsychotics (APP)[24]	Percentage of children and adolescents newly started on antipsychotic medications without a clinical indication who had documentation of psychosocial care as first-line treatment.
HEDIS	Nonrecommended cervical cancer screening in adolescent females (NCS)[25]	Adolescent females 16–20 y of age who were screened unnecessarily for cervical cancer.
HEDIS/ CMS	Weight assessment and counseling for nutrition and physical activity for children/adolescents (WCC)	Children and adolescents 3–17 y of age who had an outpatient visit with a primary care practitioner or OB/GYN during the measurement year and documentation of: • Body mass index (BMI) percentile • Counseling for nutrition • Counseling for physical activity
HEDIS/ CMS	Immunizations for adolescents (IMA)[26]	Adolescents 13 y of age who had one dose of meningococcal vaccine, one Tdap vaccine, and the complete human papillomavirus vaccine series by their 13th birthday.
HEDIS/ CMS	Medication management for people with asthma and asthma medication ratio	Adults and children 5–64 y old identified as having persistent asthma • Dispensed appropriate asthma medications that they remained on for at least 75% of their treatment period. • Ratio of controller medications to total asthma medications of ≥0.50 during the measurement year.
HEDIS/ CMS	Preventative care and screening: screening for clinical depression and follow-up plan[27]	The percentage of members ≥12 y old who were screened for clinical depression using a standardized instrument and, if screened positive, received follow-up care.
NQF	Adolescent assessment of preparation for transition (ADAPT) to adult-focused health care (NQF 2789)[28]	Patient survey completed by youth 16–17 y old with a chronic health condition. Measures • Counseling on transition self-management • Counseling on prescription medication • Transfer planning
NQF	Consumer assessment of Healthcare providers and systems hospital survey—child version (child HCAHPS) (NQF 2548)[29]	This 39-item survey asks parents of children under 18 y old about inpatient hospital experiences.
PQMP	Pediatric quality measures program[30]	The Agency for Healthcare Research and Quality (AHRQ) and CMS work together to improve children's health care quality across and within State and Federal health plans by establishing pediatric quality measures.

HEDIS, Healthcare Effectiveness Data and Information Set; CMS, Centers for Medicare and Medicaid Services; NQF, National Quality Forum; PQMP, Pediatric Quality Measures Program.

often stems from the many similarities: both involve a systematic investigation that is carefully designed to achieve reliable and valid results. While QI uses rigorous methodologies, the goals are different than research and, therefore, the design of a QI project will be different. In research, the aim is to prove a theory, generate new knowledge, and produce results that are generalizable. In QI, processes are analyzed in a local environment and try to improve care directly for patients. Quality improvement is not intended to be generalizable, but rather to generate local and specific results. If the project is successful, it may eventually disseminate the results and spread the improvements, but the scale is smaller and the benefits for patient care are immediate. In clinical research, randomization often occurs at the patient level and requires patient consent. Research also tries to control as many variables as possible, to test a hypothesis under ideal conditions. In QI, however, randomization often occurs at the system level and no consent is required when new and old processes are both considered standard of care. Variable conditions are also accepted as they are because that is the real-world context in which practice occurs. Another important distinction is that in research, generally, as many patients as possible are recruited to increase the power of a study. In QI, just enough data is needed to show that the processes are improving, and the changes are having the desired effect.

QUALITY IMPROVEMENT IN ADOLESCENT AND YOUNG ADULT HEALTH

There are some unique aspects of AYA health that may affect how to approach QI. Some institutions and colleagues might shy away from projects that seem too close to research because of issues with consent from minor patients and their guardians. Some conditions that might desperately need QI, such as reproductive health and mental health follow-up, will have to be carefully designed so that the new process does not inadvertently breach confidentiality. For example, an intervention to improve documentation of vaping might get printed onto an after-visit or discharge summary.

There are several areas that lend themselves well to QI: these topics have well-established evidence of benefits, but often inadequate implementation. One example is annual chlamydia screening for sexually experienced females under age 25. Despite decades of evidence and guidelines, the most recent estimate is that only about 52% of females received the recommended screening.[20] This kind of evidence to practice gap is a good place to start. "Do you know how your practice is doing on this measure? Our clinic thought we were above 90%, until we looked at our actual numbers."

If uncertain where to start, one could investigate how well they are performing on established quality and "pay for performance" measures. Center for Medicare and Medicaid Services (CMS) "pay for performance" is tied to several measures that apply to adolescent care.[21] The Healthcare Effectiveness Data and Information Set (HEDIS) is one of health care's most widely used performance improvement tools, and includes several benchmarks for quality in adolescent care (**Table 12.1**).

Another option for a QI project is to study any new processes that are implemented. For example, a health system required change in clinic scheduling procedures may impact access to care (third next available) or no-show rates. In addition, QI methods might help gather pilot qualitative or quantitative data before proposing a new research project. For example, stakeholder input may be needed on whether staff and patients would trust text messaging for test results.

There are often many clinicians, programs, and hospitals working on similar QI projects simultaneously. **Table 12.2** identifies some organizations that can be resources to help improve the health and quality of care of patients.

SUMMARY

At its core, QI is about providing the right care, to the right patient, at the right time. Unlike clinical research, where any direct benefits to patients are usually realized years later, QI projects have more immediate and direct impact on the front-line care provided to patients. The simplest and most commonly used model in QI

TABLE 12.2		
Glossary of Organizations That Support Quality and Practice Improvement in Health Care		
Abbreviation	**Name**	**Role**
NCQA	National Committee for Quality Assurance	Founded in 1990 as an independent nonprofit to improve quality and accountability in U.S. health care. NCQA oversees **HEDIS**.[31]
HEDIS	Healthcare Effectiveness Data and Information Set	Insurance plans voluntarily submit performance measures. HEDIS data help calculate national performance statistics and benchmarks, set accreditation standards, and allow the public to compare quality of care across health plans.
NQF	National Quality Forum[32]	Established in 1999, NQF is a private sector standard-setting organization whose efforts center on the evaluation and endorsement of standardized performance measures. Evidence-based approaches to improving care must meet rigorous criteria to be endorsed by NQF. Many government and private-sector organizations use NQF's endorsed measures to evaluate performance and share information with patients and families. NQF's measure search tool helps find measures that have been endorsed. Learn how others are defining outcomes, numerators, denominators, and exclusions.
IHI	Institute for Healthcare Improvement[17]	IHI began in the late 1980s as part of the National Demonstration Project on Quality Improvement in Health Care. Mission: Improve health and health care worldwide. IHI offers training and resources on the science of improvement to health systems and clinicians.
CMS	Centers for Medicare and Medicaid Services[33]	CMS uses quality measures in its quality improvement, public reporting, and pay-for-reporting programs for specific clinicians. The CMS Quality Measures Inventory lists each measure by program, reporting measure specifications including numerator, denominator, exclusion criteria, Meaningful Measures domain, measure type, and National Quality Forum (NQF) endorsement status.

is the Model for Improvement,[8] which is organized around three basic questions: (1) What are we trying to accomplish? (2) How will we know that a change is an improvement? (3) What changes can result in improvement? Before embarking on a QI project, it is critical that the identified problem is investigated thoroughly, and there are several helpful tools to consider including Fishbone diagrams, driver diagrams, and process mapping. Quality improvement consists of several systematic processes of testing change, referred to as "PDSA" or plan-do-study-act cycles.[17] Using these well-established QI tools and methods, the health and quality of care for AYAs may be improved and health system performance more easily compared across jurisdictions with national benchmarks and measures.

REFERENCES

1. Institute of Medicine, Committee on Quality of Health Care in America. In: Kohn LT, Corrigan JM, Donaldson MS, eds. *To Err Is Human: Building a Safer Health System*. National Academies Press (US); 2000.
2. Institute of Medicine, Committee on Quality of Health Care in America. *Crossing the Quality Chasm: A New Health System for the 21st Century*. National Academies Press (US); 2001.
3. Frank JR SL, Sherbino J, eds. *CanMEDS 2015 Physician Competency Framework*. Royal College of Physicians and Surgeons of Canada; 2015.
4. Massagli TL, Zumsteg JM, Osorio MB. Quality improvement education in residency training: a review. *Am J Phys Med Rehabil*. 2018;97(9):673–678.
5. Levy FH, Brilli RJ, First LR, et al. A new framework for quality partnerships in children's hospitals. *Pediatrics*. 2011;127(6):1147–1156.
6. Ahmed S, Manaf NHA, Islam R. Effects of lean six sigma application in healthcare services: a literature review. *Rev Environ Health*. 2013;28(4):189–194.
7. de Koning H, Verver JPS, van den Heuvel J, et al. Lean six sigma in healthcare. *J Healthc Qual*. 2006;28(2):4–11.
8. Langley GJ, Nolan TW, Norman CL, et al. *The Improvement Guide: A Practical Approach to Enhancing Organisational Performance* (2nd ed.). Jossey-Bass; 2009.
9. Berwick DM. A primer on leading the improvement of systems. *BMJ* (Clinical research ed.). 1996;312(7031):619–622.
10. Brugha R, Varvasovszky Z. Stakeholder analysis: a review. *Health Policy Plan*. 2000;15(3):239–246.
11. Beatty CA, Barker Scott BA. *Building Smart Teams: A Roadmap to High Performance*. Sage Publications; 2004.
12. Wong KC. Using an Ishikawa diagram as a tool to assist memory and retrieval of relevant medical cases from the medical literature. *J Med Case Rep*. 2011;5:120.
13. Huppert JS, Reed JL, Munafo JK, et al. Improving notification of sexually transmitted infections: a quality improvement project and planned experiment. *Pediatrics*. 2012;130(2):e415–e422.
14. McLaughlin N, Rodstein J, Burke MA, et al. Demystifying process mapping: a key step in neurosurgical quality improvement initiatives. *Neurosurgery*. 2014;75(2):99–109.
15. Holbrook A, Bowen JM, Patel H, et al. Process mapping evaluation of medication reconciliation in academic teaching hospitals: a critical step in quality improvement. *BMJ Open*. 2016;6(12):e013663.
16. Kouo T, Kleinman K, Fujii-Rios H, et al. A resident-led QI initiative to improve pediatric emergency department boarding times. *Pediatrics*. 2020;145(6):e20191477.
17. Institute for Healthcare Improvement. *How to improve*. Accessed March 30, 2021. http://www.ihi.org/resources/pages/howtoimprove/default.aspx
18. Taylor MJ, McNicholas C, Nicolay C, et al. Systematic review of the application of the plan-do-study-act method to improve quality in healthcare. *BMJ Qual Saf*. 2014;23(4):290–298.
19. Provost LMS. *The Healthcare Data Guide*. Jossey-Bass; 2011.
20. NCQA. *Chlamydia Screening in Women (CHL)*. https://www.ncqa.org/hedis/measures/chlamydia-screening-in-women/
21. Centers for Medicare & Medicaid Services. *Consensus Core Set: Pediatric Measures Version 1.0*. https://www.cms.gov/Medicare/Quality-Initiatives-Patient-Assessment-Instruments/QualityMeasures/Downloads/Pediatric-Measures.pdf
22. NCQA. *Child and Adolescent Well-Care Visits*. https://www.ncqa.org/hedis/measures/child-and-adolescent-well-care-visits/
23. NCQA. *Metabolic Monitoring for Children and Adolescents on Antipsychotics (APM)*. https://www.ncqa.org/hedis/measures/metabolic-monitoring-for-children-and-adolescents-on-antipsychotics/
24. NCQA. *Use of First-Line Psychosocial Care for Children and Adolescents on Antipsychotics (APP)*. https://www.ncqa.org/hedis/measures/use-of-first-line-psychosocial-care-for-children-and-adolescents-on-anti-psychotics/
25. NCQA. *Non-Recommended Cervical Cancer Screening in Adolescent Females (NCS)*. https://www.ncqa.org/hedis/measures/non-recommended-cervical-cancer-screening-in-adolescent-females/
26. NCQA. *Immunizations for Adolescents (IMA)*. https://www.ncqa.org/hedis/measures/immunizations-for-adolescents/
27. NCQA. *Depression Screening and Follow-Up for Adolescents and Adults (DSF)*. https://www.ncqa.org/hedis/measures/depression-screening-and-follow-up-for-adolescents-and-adults/
28. Sawicki GS, Garvey KC, Toomey SL, et al. Development and validation of the adolescent assessment of preparation for transition: a novel patient experience measure. *J Adolesc Health*. 2015;57(3):282–287.
29. Toomey SL, Zaslavsky AM, Elliott MN, et al. The development of a pediatric inpatient experience of care measure: child HCAHPS. *Pediatrics*. 2015;136(2):360–369.
30. AHRQ-CMS. *Pediatric Quality Measures Program (PQMP)*. https://www.ahrq.gov/pqmp/measures/all-pqmp-measures.html
31. Marjoua Y, Bozic KJ. Brief history of quality movement in US healthcare. *Curr Rev Musculoskelet Med*. 2012;5(4):265–273.
32. National Quality Forum. Measures. Reports & Tools. http://www.qualityforum.org/Measures_Reports_Tools/
33. Goodrich K, Garcia E, Conway PH. A history of and a vision for CMS quality measurement programs. *Jt Comm J Qual Patient Saf*. 2012;38(10):465–470.

🛜 ADDITIONAL RESOURCES AND WEBSITES

Additional Resources and Websites for Clinicians:
Basics of Quality Improvement. The American Academy of Family Physicians—https://www.aafp.org/family-physician/practice-and-career/managing-your-practice/quality-improvement-basics.html
Berwick DM. A primer on leading the improvement of systems. *BMJ* (Clinical research ed.). 1996;312(7031):619–622.
HEDIS Measures and Technical Resources. National Committee for Quality Assurance—https://www.ncqa.org/hedis/measures/
How to Improve. Institute for Healthcare Improvement—http://www.ihi.org/resources/pages/howtoimprove/default.aspx
Langley GJ, Nolan TW, Norman CL, et al. *The Improvement Guide: A Practical Approach to Enhancing Organizational Performance*. Jossey-Bass; 2009.
Measures, Reports and Tools. National Quality Forum—https://www.qualityforum.org/Measures_Reports_Tools.aspx
Additional Resources and Websites for Parents/Caregivers:
Brittain AW, Tevendale HD, Mueller T, et al. The teen access and quality initiative: improving adolescent reproductive health best practices in publicly funded health centers. *J Community Health*. 2020;45(3):615–625.
Committee on Adolescence. Achieving quality health services for adolescents. *Pediatrics*. 2016;138(2):e20161347. doi: 10.1542/peds.2016-1347
Involving Youth. Youth.Gov—https://youth.gov/youth-topics/involving-youth-positive-youth-development
Person- and Family-Centered Care Overview. Institute for Healthcare Improvement—http://www.ihi.org/Topics/PFCC/Pages/Overview.aspx
Person- and Family-Centered Care Resources. Institute for Healthcare Improvement—http://www.ihi.org/Topics/PFCC/Pages/Resources.aspx

CHAPTER 13

Research with and about Adolescents and Young Adults

Elissa R. Weitzman
Lauren E. Wisk

KEY WORDS

- Adolescence
- Data sources
- Ethics
- Measurement
- Participatory research
- Privacy and safety
- Research methods
- Youth engagement

INTRODUCTION

The second decade of the 21st century has seen a remarkable focus on adolescent and young adult (AYA) health, driven in part by recognition that a historically large portion of the world's population (approximately 40%) comprises persons between 10 and 24 years old.[1] Interest in adolescence and young adulthood is intense among scientists, clinicians, policymakers, and even writers as evident in the abundance of "young adult" novels and media characterizing the turbulence of this period. Changes in roles, relationships, responsibilities, and physiology are hallmarks of adolescence, a time when health-related attitudes and behaviors solidify, and youth turn from dependence on parents and caregivers toward autonomy and acute sensitivity to peer and social influences. Beliefs and behaviors that take shape in the second decade of life impact near and long-term health trajectories, with effects that reverberate throughout life and impact many aspects of society. It is no wonder that this group draws the attention of researchers seeking to answer questions about health and development, underlining the importance of understanding the opportunities, as well as constraints of research with and about AYAs.

Recognizing the importance of promoting research across the lifespan, in 2017, the National Institutes of Health (NIH) broadened its policies to promote research among children, a group that includes adolescents, and older adults, requiring researchers to explicitly justify the exclusion of any of these groups in relation to a study's scientific aims.[2] Not quite children or adults, AYAs occupy a special developmental status that requires sophistication and consideration in how they are approached and engaged in research. Many institutional review boards/research ethics boards (IRBs/REBs) desire input from an AYA expert, reflecting again on the unique issues that arise in research that pertains to this group. This chapter summarizes essential aspects of conducting health research with and about AYAs. Topics include ethical frameworks for ensuring human subject protections, the importance of collaborative and youth-engaged research, research designs and settings, measurement, and secondary data resources.

ETHICS AND OVERSIGHT

Federal policy for the protection of human subjects in the United States, known as the Common Rule as it applies across many U.S. federal agencies, allows research which involves children. Federal policies of European Union member states and other countries have developed their own guidelines and regulations.[3] Regulation 45 Code of Federal Regulations (CFR) part 46, subpart D of the Department of Health and Human Services Common Rule outlines the conditions under which children, including adolescents, may be involved in research (Table 13.1). Institutional review boards or similar ethics committees within an institution committed to providing oversight of human subjects, ultimately determine the appropriateness of research protocols involving adolescents and investigators should be familiar with the regulatory frameworks guiding IRB decisions. In the United States, many ethical guidelines and related regulations are different when the focus of research is on adolescents who are legal minors (<18 years of age) compared to those who are legal adults (≥18 years of age); research with minors often requires additional protections compared to research involving only adults.

Assent and developmental status. Increasingly, adolescents (youth, ≥12 years old) are considered able to decide for themselves whether to participate in research, although decisional capacity varies by child and is influenced by age, socioeconomic status/affluence, and level of health literacy.[4,5] Biologic age is the primary criterion for demarcating child from adult and persons younger than 18 years are legally considered children. Informed consent is a requirement for research with persons aged 18 years and older while *assent* is required from persons younger than 18 years,[6] but older than about 7 or 8 years when parents may typically be approached to provide proxy consent. The Common Rule 45 CFR 46.402(b) defines assent as: "… *a child's affirmative agreement to participate in research. Mere failure to object should not, absent affirmative agreement, be construed as assent.*" Active affirmation of willingness to participate in research is thus a condition for recruiting an adolescent.

Institutional review board oversight of research protocols involving children includes determining whether investigators are using appropriate strategies to ascertain the willingness of youth to participate in research. Institutional review boards are directed to provide approval of a research protocol that involves children based on the child's age, maturity, and psychological state. In the United States, Health and Human Services (HHS) guidance includes a high level of discretionary judgment on the part of IRBs: "*The IRB has the discretion to judge children's capacity to assent for all of the children to be involved in a proposed research activity, or on an individual basis.*"[6,7] Investigators should make sure to establish a framework for working with their IRB to ensure a thoughtful and

TABLE 13.1

Regulatory Conditions for Engaging Adolescents/Young Adults in Research in the United States

Health and Human Services Common Rule Regulation 45 CFR 46, subpart D

Regulation Part	Risk and Benefit	Conditions
45 CFR 46.404	Minimal risk to the children	• No greater than minimal risk to the children; *and* • Adequate provisions are made for soliciting the assent of the children and the permission of their parents or guardians, as set forth in HHS regulations at 45 CFR 46.408
45 CFR 46.405	Greater than minimal risk but prospect of direct benefit to participating child	• Risk justified by anticipated benefits to the subjects; • Relation of anticipated benefit to risk at least as favorable to subjects as that provided by available alternative approaches; *and* • Adequate provisions are made for soliciting assent of the children and permission of parents or guardians, per HHS regulations at 45 CFR 46.408.
45 CFR 46.406	Greater than minimal risk, no direct benefit to child, but likely to yield to generalizable knowledge about the subject's condition/disorder	• Risk represents a minor increase over minimal risk; • Intervention or procedure presents experiences to the child subjects that are reasonably commensurate with those inherent in their actual, or expected medical, dental, psychological, social, or educational situations; • The intervention or procedure is likely to yield generalizable knowledge about the subject's disorder or condition which is of vital importance for the understanding or amelioration of the disorder or condition; *and* • Adequate provisions are made for soliciting the assent of the children and the permission of their parents or guardians, as set forth in HHS regulations at 45 CFR 46.408.
45 CFR 46.407 **Secretary of HHS/designee approval and public review, beyond IRB**	Does not meet 45 CRF 46.404–406, but presents an opportunity to understand, prevent, or alleviate a serious problem affecting the health or welfare of children.	• Research presents a reasonable opportunity to further the understanding, prevention, or alleviation of a serious problem affecting the health or welfare of children; • Research will be conducted in accordance with sound ethical principles; *and* • Adequate provisions are made for soliciting the assent of children and the permission of their parents or guardians, as set forth in HHS regulations at 45 CFR 46.408.

CFR, Code of Federal Regulations; HHS, Department of Health and Human Services.

proactive process for reviewing and approving research involving adolescents and for providing them with developmentally appropriate information about the nature of a research protocol and its attendant risks, protections, and benefits.[6] Assent may be obtained with or without parent/guardian permission, depending on the study design and balance of risk and benefit. If assent is obtained without the permission of a parent/guardian, investigators must obtain a waiver from the IRB[7] under either 45 CFR 46.116(c) or (d) or where parental/guardian permission is not a reasonable requirement to protect the adolescent subject. Overall, investigators should consider that involving adolescents in research reflects a process and consideration of the complex factors that contribute to a considered understanding on the part of a young person to participate.

Privacy and Safety for the Adolescent Study Participant

In the United States, the Health Insurance Portability and Accountability Act of 1996 (HIPAA), Public Law 104–191, and its Privacy Rule, set the regulatory standards for the protection of privacy of personal health information[8] including for research purposes. For adults, these rules require patient authorization for disclosure of protected health information, yet for adolescents (under 18 years old), these rules allow expanded access to a youth's medical records by their parent/guardian with some exceptions, including additional regulations that vary by state.[9] In certain situations where youth disclose risks to their health and well-being, researchers have a duty to inform the participant's clinicians and parents/guardians and depending on the study protocol and circumstance, there may be a duty to report to child protective services. In advance of these situations, including a statement in the assent/consent process that explains this potential disclosure is warranted.

Adolescents' and young adults' willingness to share personal health information including electronic health information is generally high although willingness can vary for different types of information, research purposes, sociodemographic factors, and approaches to safeguarding privacy.[10,11] Privacy is a multidimensional construct that requires attention throughout all stages of research, from study design to implementation, analysis, reporting, and archiving of data. Privacy safeguards for research should be designed along the same dimensions that pertain to clinical care, namely those pertaining to the informational, psychological, social, and physical spaces that AYAs occupy.[12]

Informational privacy aligns with our understanding of confidentiality and is a dominant area of concern for research activities. Informational privacy is defined by a young person's right to control to whom, when, and under what conditions information collected for research is released and shared. Informational privacy is central to the management of research materials and an important condition for assent. Institutional review boards evaluate the adequacy of planned approaches for protecting the privacy of research information, including the growing number of studies that make use of digital information. Secondary use of data from digital devices and social media for research purposes may not be actively assented or even known. Privacy rules for these more novel data types are evolving and can be challenging to navigate, communicate, and enforce.[13] Social media data are often considered public and not covered by research protections. Where they are collected by private entities, research activities may be broadly defined and covered under unique terms. Breach of privacy and misuse of personal information from online sources is a particular concern for research with and about AYAs who are heavy users of digital systems and because regulatory controls are so weak. In the United

States, the Children's Online Privacy Protection Act (COPPA) of the U.S. Federal Trade Commission imposes limits on the information that websites can collect from children younger than age 13 and hinges on parental control over youth involvement. However, COPPA does not cover adolescents aged 13 to 17. Further, compliance with COPPA is largely voluntary and self-regulated,[14] leaving adolescents vulnerable to predatory use of their data including for research with few, if any, privacy protections. Similarly, privacy protections for children are afforded by the European Union's General Data Protection Regulation for children or "kids" (commonly referred to as the GDPR-K).[15] Under the GDPR-K, the age of consent for children is 16 years old, with variation by member states.

Adolescents and young adults are acutely sensitive to others' views of them underscoring the importance of **psychological privacy,** defined as protection from having one's attitudes, beliefs, and values disclosed to or judged by others. Accordingly, research interviews, assessment tools, and study protocols should reflect values for being curious, neutral, and nonjudgmental—features that may help establish rapport, promote collection of high-quality information, and protect the dignity and well-being of youth. Staff training and oversight is essential to maintaining the atmosphere of respect that undergirds psychological privacy. Fostering an ethos of respect is essential to interactions between staff and study participants and to interactions among research team members who review and discuss research materials. The latter is important inasmuch as judgments and opinions expressed among study staff may pervade and color research interactions with participants and even interpretation of study data.

Finally, research activities should be designed with care to protect **physical privacy** of AYAs. Physical privacy may involve ensuring that a young person can answer questions openly without risk of being observed or overheard. Research interviews may need to occur "out of earshot" and view of others, including telephone and computer-assisted interviews. Advance planning and use of screening questions can be helpful for identifying the adequacy of physical privacy. Asking AYAs whether they are "in a private space?" or "feel sufficiently private" at the start of an interview is a simple strategy for ascertaining the adequacy of physical privacy. Physical privacy is also important for biometric studies such as those that involve measuring height, weight, blood/fluids, and so on, as these experiences may be sensitive and experienced as embarrassing, stigmatizing, and even shaming for youth. If a physical examination is required for the research, sensitivity around performing sexual maturity ratings should also be acknowledged and communicated to AYAs at the time of study recruitment. Pretesting research operations, including in the spaces where interviews and observations are planned to occur, can help investigators identify threats to physical privacy—including the likelihood of intrusions and being visible or audible to others, with the goal being identification of problems and practical solutions. For example, use of a polarizing screen affixed to a computer tablet will block over-the-shoulder views of research information by a parent, guardian, clinician, or stranger, while folding room screens can provide a physical barrier around a scale in a hall or vestibule.

Informational and psychological privacy may all be infringed when recruiting AYAs to research via social media and exceptional care must be taken to outline protocols that offer privacy protections for use on these platforms which are attuned to these dimensions.[16,17]

Balancing Privacy and Safety

Concern for protecting privacy is balanced by concern for protecting a young person through relevant safety protocols. This balancing is necessarily complex as a young person's right to privacy can be abrogated if their safety is at risk, as may be the case if, for example, an adolescent discloses suicidality or victimization in the context of a research interview. Such a situation may require

protective intervention and intentional breach of confidentiality. Intentions regarding how safety risks will be responded to should be discussed when obtaining informed consent. Safety risks can also arise from breach of privacy and nonpermissioned sharing of personal health information as when study personnel are overheard discussing a research subject, or when study materials are not secured. Breach of privacy can result in adverse consequences to personal integrity (youth may feel betrayed, shamed, or exposed and subject to mistreatment/judgment); interpersonal relationships (sensitive information may be shared with friends or family contributing to tensions or difficult situations); and harms to educational or employment opportunity as when information about a chronic illness, psychological or behavioral health problem is shared that negatively impacts insurance eligibility or cost, education, or employment. Notably, safety protocols for collecting sensitive health information (i.e., reports of substance use and mental health status) from adolescents in clinical research have been shown to be highly acceptable to patients. In a recent study, investigators were able to consent >900 adolescents to reporting about sensitive behaviors after informing them that survey responses indicating potential risk for acute harm would be shared with a clinician, for safety follow-up. This protocol allowed for the research team to break confidentiality under consent in specific situations and was implemented without negative effects on adolescent engagement or clinical practice workflows.[18]

Certificate of Confidentiality

In the United States, federal certificates of confidentiality are also available to investigators to protect them from having to release sensitive information about AYAs collected as part of a research protocol, such as information about alcohol and other substance use or information about reproductive health and health care behaviors. Depending on the project and funders, Certificates of Confidentiality (COCs) will be required or optional. The NIH determines if the research should be protected by a COC if it meets one of the following requirements: (1) involves human subjects, defined by 45 CEF Part 46 (see above); requires (2) collection or use of biospecimens that are identifiable to the participant; (3) there is a risk that information and biospecimens can be used to identify the participant; or (4) research involves individual human genomic data.[19] More information about applying for COC can be found on the NIH Grants and Funding webpage.[20] Investigators should consider making use of these protections when planning research with and about AYAs.

ENGAGEMENT AND REPRESENTATION OF ADOLESCENTS AND YOUNG ADULTS IN RESEARCH

Adolescents and young adults are important partners as well as study participants in research about their health status and behaviors. AYAs may play key roles as partners and advisors in AYA-focused research. Building mechanisms within research projects for AYA engagement can increase a study's chances for success. Adolescent and young adult engagement can help to sharpen the implementation approach to best fit the experiences of AYAs, and help to ensure the relevance of research questions to the lives of AYAs who can also participate in the interpretation of findings. Youth and adult perspectives, priorities, and concerns are not the same. Therefore, creating opportunities for AYA involvement may bring the research enterprise closer to the target population, increasing the relevance of a study to the lives of the young person and smoothing the path for applying findings. Emerging evidence suggests that engaging young people in research through participatory models is also good for them—providing opportunities for them to develop leadership, confidence, a sense of self-worth and empowerment, and connection to and awareness of the world around them.[21]

Investigators are encouraged to identify opportunities to involve and partner with AYAs at every stage of the research cycle. While the benefits of engaging youth as stakeholders and partners in research are manifold, most studies do not employ participatory and youth-involved designs—by one count, fewer than 1% of over 400 studies published in 2019 about adolescents included adolescents in an advisory board capacity, one of the less intensive levels of youth research involvement.[22] Understanding the range of opportunities and modes of participation for involving AYAs in research may help investigators develop study designs and protocols that are youth-centered and youth-involving.

Models and frameworks for AYA engagement and representation in research are varied. However, it is helpful to consider a continuum of youth engagement options, holding aside unethical or coercive participation which should be guarded against through reviewing protocols and carefully considering disparities in power between adults/authorities and adolescents.[23] At a first level, studies may afford *no opportunities* for youth participation—all aspects of the study are determined by adult researchers and youth are only engaged as participants. At the next level, studies may involve AYAs in a *consultative* role. At this level, AYAs provide input and reactions to studies that adults initiate and manage. A next possible level of participation is *collaborative*, where studies are still initiated by adults, but AYAs have partnership opportunities and are afforded freedom to question, influence, or challenge how the research is undertaken and the results interpreted. Finally, the highest level of participatory research is where studies are *AYA-led* and adults take on the role of consultant, enabler, facilitator, and collaborator. For these studies, AYAs identify the problem or question driving research activities, and they manage and control the research process at every step of the research cycle.

In considering the range of opportunities for AYAs to participate in research, careful consideration of the many benefits to young people and to investigators for optimizing youth enfranchisement and involvement is recommended. In the best of all worlds, the goals of understanding young people and improving their well-being may be well served by enfranchising them through choice of consultative, collaborative, and even AYA-led research protocols. In all instances, investigators need to pay close attention to the complex power dynamics inherent in the differing roles and resources available to children and adults, developmental capacities, and the duty to protect young people from harm (i.e., in studies where political or social unrest may pose a danger to youth, or the topic of an investigation is a controversial topic that could in some settings pose a safety risk). Similarly, investigators should evaluate the terms of research involvement and whether they are fair and equitable. For example, in many instances, youth involvement through voluntary mechanisms can be developmentally enriching and educational. In some situations, voluntary participation could actually be coercive and abusive of the "AYA". Reviewing an organization's rules for youth participation is important when developing a research protocol that includes AYAs as part of the research team. The terms of involvement should provide for clearly communicated plans and agreements around compensation, and specify protections including trusted advisors or "third parties" to whom youth can turn if they have questions or complaints.

🔵 RESEARCH DESIGN AND METHODS

Outlined below is a brief exploration of the main study designs, considerations for data collection and analysis, and methodologic issues relevant to AYA populations. While the specific primary goal of research can vary dramatically, oftentimes investigators are interested in understanding the relationship between exposure to certain pre-existing or acquired characteristics or interventions and subsequent outcomes. In a best-case scenario, researchers are able to isolate the (causal) effects of an exposure on an outcome, by mitigating or minimizing the effects of bias (e.g., self-selection into various groups), chance (e.g., naturally occurring variation), and confounding (e.g., presence of phenomenon related to the exposure and outcome) that can obfuscate measurement of the exposure, outcome, and/or the relationship between them. Similarly, in the case of qualitative research, researchers may be interested in exploring similar topics including the subjective understanding of relationships among exposures and outcomes, and the meaning of these phenomena to study participants. In order to select the best study design (Table 13.2) to address a particular causal or associative question, researchers are often limited by practical considerations and must consider both what is feasible, as well as the potential trade-off from the aforementioned threats to validity from bias, chance, and confounding.

In addition to the main study designs outlined in the table, there are many variants of these approaches (e.g., case-cohort studies, ecologic studies) that have different strengths and limitations. The specific choice of which study design to use will depend on the research question being addressed, and on factors such as setting, timing, and available resources (see Additional Resources). Further, many studies are descriptive in nature, rather than analytical, where the goal is not to analyze the association between exposure and outcome but rather to describe features of a particular group. Because of the descriptive nature of the question being asked, many limitations related to timing of assessment do not necessarily apply but threats from selection into these samples are still common and have the greatest potential to undermine the validity of such studies.

Data Collection and Analysis

Once a researcher has selected their study design, they will turn their attention to determining data collection procedures (including selection of measurement/assessment tools). The data being collected might take multiple forms (e.g., laboratory values, biometric measurements, questionnaires) and come from multiple sources (e.g., medical records, in-person surveys), so careful design and coordination of data collection are essential. Researchers should begin by outlining the data elements that they want to collect and the proposed sources for each data element. Minimizing the number of sources will allow for a more straightforward set of data collection procedures. Moreover, clearly articulating data sources prior to beginning data collection will assist in finalizing a sufficiently detailed data collection plan to support development of a project manual of procedures, training plan, timeline, and approach to data quality checks—all of which are necessary for a smooth research project. As an example, simply stating that data will be extracted from a medical record is less concrete than specifying that data from the first outpatient evaluation and management visit in a calendar year will be extracted. Similar specificity regarding data elements is also warranted. Quantitative data can be measured on different scales that will lend themselves to different types of variables and analytic opportunities. As an example, a researcher may wish to capture body composition and could operationalize this as a continuous numeric element (e.g., measured weight in kg), discrete interval element (e.g., weight-for-age percentile based on growth charts), ordinal element (e.g., body mass index [BMI] categories [underweight, normal, overweight, obese]), or nominal/categorical element (e.g., living with or without obesity). Numeric elements are considered to include the highest level of "detail" and nominal elements the least. Investigators should keep in mind that post data collection, it is easier to redefine study data from a more to a less detailed element or definition (e.g., using measured weight to determine obesity) while the reverse (less to more detailed) is much harder.

Analog sources and approaches to data collection (e.g., paper-based forms) are often plagued by potential for errors that can result in data loss without great attention to details such as handwriting readability to paper storage practices to transcription of records into digital format for eventual analysis. Anticipatory planning may

TABLE 13.2

Research Designs and Adolescent and Young Adult Populations

Research Design	Major Strengths	Major Limitations	Considerations for Use With Adolescents and Young Adults
Experimental research is defined by exogenous/investigator-initiated intervention or exposure and subsequent follow-up to ascertain certain events (outcomes).	When experimental design involves careful randomization of individuals into groups with and without exposure to some exogenous factor, these studies are most likely to create the opportunity to identify causal relationships between the exposure and outcome under investigation.	Experimental designs are often the most resource intensive, including with respect to ethical oversight. Relatedly, because of strict but necessarily ethical guidance for the introduction of an intervention, experimental research is not always best suited for the study of naturally occurring phenomenon as exposures.	Because of the dynamic nature of adolescence/emerging adulthood, extra care is needed to partition out effects from outcomes changing naturally over time relative to changes caused by investigator-delivered interventions.
Cohort studies involve identification of groups of individuals based on certain defining/pre-existing features of that group, who are followed for a certain period of time, either prospectively or retrospectively, to ascertain outcomes.	A key advantage of cohort studies is the ability to establish a well-defined temporal relationship between exposure and outcome. These are also well suited when investigators wish to consider multiple exposures or outcomes simultaneously.	Like experimental research, cohort studies tend to be time and resource intensive, especially when studies involve prospective data collection or wish to investigate a rare outcome.	The longitudinal nature of many cohort studies requires researchers to consider how changing contexts or developmental milestones can impact phenomenon under investigation, as well as how measurements may need to be modified across developmental stages.
Case-control studies identify individuals for inclusion on the basis of outcome status (e.g., presence or absence of a disease) and involve ascertainment of prior exposure.	Optimizes speed of data collection (as the primary outcome of interest has occurred) and can thus represent an efficient study design, especially for rare outcomes.	Because ascertainment of exposure often relies on retrospective recall, these studies tend to be more subject to issues of recall bias.	The period of time in which a retrospective recall is considered accurate (e.g., in the last year vs. in the last 5 y) may be shorter for youth than for older adults.
Cross-sectional studies are those in which the exposure and outcome are simultaneously assessed.	These studies tend to be the most efficient in terms of time and cost for data collection. Cross-sectional studies can also provide useful preliminary data to inform subsequent studies utilizing more costly designs.	When exposure and outcome are assessed at the same point in time, these studies are not always able to establish that the exposure preceded the outcomes, which is a necessary precondition for establishing a causal relationship.	Cross-sectional studies often rely on sampling from specific settings (e.g., schools, clinics) in which youth differentially engage; attention to selection effects is especially warranted as a result.
Qualitative studies are those best suited for investigating: novel areas where structured questions are not yet developed; associations among health issues or subjective beliefs; refining prevention and intervention materials before they are field tested, or after they are used (to understand acceptability).	Qualitative studies can advance new thinking and research hypotheses; they are usefully applied at key junctures in a translational research cycle where insight can guide design of measures and programs, and in understanding outcomes, including participation, acceptability, and unintended consequences.	These studies do not produce generalizable information and are subject to selection bias; care is needed to protect against subjectivity. Suitable care is needed to protect the research relationship, privacy, confidentiality, and respect for person (study subject), given the personal nature of a research interview and observational protocol.	Youth, especially younger AYAs, may not always feel comfortable disclosing personal or sensitive information in interviews or focus groups without first building rapport with the interviewer and/or other interviewees. Especially for focus groups, characteristics of those interviewed together may impact what AYAs choose to disclose.

AYAs, Adolescents and Young Adults.

be especially important for smooth processing of data from analog sources. For research being conducted in low-resource settings or other situations where use of electronic tools is not feasible, these more traditional approaches may be necessary and will require additional attention to establishing and implementing standard operating procedures (SOPs) and best practices. When feasible, researchers can employ one of the multiple software options to help organize their data collection. Many of these options offer a range of functionalities from simply storing a collection of records in electronic form to more sophisticated survey design and administration tools.

Many free or low-cost software options exist. An important consideration when choosing data collecting and processing tools is the security and HIPAA compatibility of different platforms. As previously discussed, HIPAA sets the regulatory standards for the protection of personal health information and therefore its standards also govern choice of data collection and storage tools. Researchers should thus make sure that their processes involve systems that implement the necessary security procedures to safeguard access to participant data per HIPAA (or related) regulations.

Data quality control and assurance is an essential part of data collection procedures. Regardless of analog versus digital data collection, researchers need to develop SOPs that outline how, when, where, and by whom each data element will be collected and provide the necessary training for their research staff to implement such procedures systematically and consistently. In many cases, these plans may not need to be excessively complex but stronger SOPs will outline contingency protocols in addition to standard practices. Moreover, when working with AYA populations, it is often necessary to include a plan for addressing safety-related events in a research SOP.

Ensuring data quality also requires inspection and auditing of the data itself. Part of this process is best done *before* any real data are actually collected, by thoroughly testing the research procedures to ensure that they operate as intended and that the data outputs meet expectations for form and content. In the context of implementing a questionnaire, this is especially important when branching logic is used (i.e., receipt of one question is conditional on the response provided to a prior question) as unclear instructions (for paper surveys) or incorrect programming (for digital surveys) could create problems at the data management/analysis stages (best case) or render some data unusable (worst case). In studies that rely on data transcription or manual data entry, this process might also involve duplicate data entry (e.g., processing 20% of records twice) to evaluate the concordance between the original and facsimile records and correct any errors. Quality control processes should further be regularly implemented to identify any irregularities that arise during real-world data collection. When implemented early and often, these processes facilitate prompt identification and correction of any issues that arise and yield higher-quality data as a result.

For many investigators, the thought of **primary data collection** (generation or compilation of new data) can be extremely daunting. Fortunately, there is a wealth of pre-existing and publicly available data sources (**Table 13.3**) that can serve as a resource to answer research questions in AYA populations via **secondary data analyses**. Consideration of these datasets is encouraged, noting several key points about their use. First, many relevant publicly available datasets use complex sampling designs whereby the probability of selection into the study relies on participants' geographic location and other characteristics. For these types of samples, researchers should expect to use special statistical procedures to account for the unequal probabilities that persons are selected into study samples. Nearly all of the most popular programs for statistical analysis include procedures that account for complex sampling designs. Moreover, most of the studies and programs that support these datasets for public use also provide guidance, including detailed written guidance, on how to implement these statistical procedures with their data. Second, existing data are not free from complications. Even where samples were developed with the goal of population representativeness, bias can be introduced during the various stages of analysis depending on many common decisions that investigators must make (e.g., treatment of missing data or operationalization of race/ethnicity variables). Finally, while the large size of many of these datasets is seen as a considerable strength, for investigators who are interested in studying less common exposures, outcomes, or small subgroups of persons, analytic samples can quickly dwindle in size and challenge robust investigations. Combining multiple years of data is one way to mitigate this concern (which may require slight modifications to the adjustments for sampling design), but this strategy may not always be sufficient to generate sufficiently large samples or analytic precision; researchers should carefully evaluate the distribution of their unweighted sample to ensure that the data are adequate for the planned study purpose.

Selection of study design is an important early step in the research process, but is certainly not the only consideration when proactively addressing study validity for those who choose to pursue primary data collection. Across all study designs, attention to measurement of exposure(s), outcome(s), and covariates is critical to minimize many of the most common threats to validity. Even with the use of a secondary dataset, attention to how existing variables are reshaped or combined is warranted to optimize internal validity. While the following section outlines several of the most common measurement issues for research with AYAs, solutions to these measurement challenges require both prospective considerations in the design phase as well as ongoing attention when constructing and implementing an analytic strategy. For clinical and/or junior investigators with more limited technical experience, the importance of enlisting the help of statistical experts to assure that data analysis is appropriate and rigorous cannot be overstated.

Whether analyzing primary or secondary data, investigators may want to begin with a table describing the study sample in terms of key characteristics, which may also include a description of the primary exposure or outcome by each characteristic and appropriate statistical tests. "*A picture is worth a thousand words*" and researchers may also consider creative use of figures to describe key features of their sample. In general, the best tables are ones that are self-explanatory, well-organized, and consistent (e.g., in reporting decimal places) and the best figures are ones that are simple yet effective, with appropriate use of color/shapes/symbols, and accompanied by a descriptive legend. When it comes time to publish results, different academic journals will have their own unique formatting requirements that should be followed but well-designed tables and figures will be compatible across a range of journals.

For analytic research questions where the goal is to estimate the association between an exposure and outcome, researchers may wish to progress to the use of more advanced statistical models. Investigators should be guided by a clear research question and ideally, a well-considered **conceptual model** that outlines the structure or mechanism of the association under investigation, including confounders and other causal factors (i.e., mediators and moderators). Such a model, often depicted graphically, is informative for formulating an appropriate analytic (statistical) approach and can also help investigators to assess antecedent and consequent factors that may be targets for intervention. Linear and logistic regression are some of the most commonly used statistical techniques in medical research and are most useful for estimating the impact of exposure variables (also called independent variables or predictors) on continuous or binary outcome variables (also called dependent variables), respectively, with the ability to control for potential confounding factors. There are several other regression extensions that can be used for different types of outcomes (e.g., ordinal or Poisson regression) and the principles underlying regression inform many additional techniques that are used in other situations. For instance, in situations where investigators propose understanding a web of interrelated factors, path analysis or structural equation models may be helpful. In situations where analytic models are complicated by the presence of repeated measures over a period of time, or where observational units tend to be clustered together in a way that makes their data correlated to each other (e.g., adolescents clustered in schools), hierarchical models or generalized estimating equations can be used.

Regardless of planned analytic strategy, researchers ought to consider the wealth of statistical software available to assist in both data management and analysis. Selection of specific software is highly personal, often discipline or institution specific, and mostly irrelevant to the actual conduct of research since nearly all packages are capable of performing the most essential statistical procedures. In general, it is recommended to utilize a package with which the research team has prior experience and for which the institution and local experts (in biostatistics, epidemiology, or related fields) can offer support.

METHODOLOGIC ISSUES FOR RESEARCH WITH ADOLESCENTS AND YOUNG ADULTS

Adolescence and emerging adulthood constitute a sensitive and critical period of human development,[24–26] complicated by rapid and asynchronous physical, mental, emotional, and social changes.

TABLE 13.3

TABLE 13.3

Publicly Available Secondary Datasets Including Adolescents and Young Adults

Dataset	Description
Specific focus on adolescents/young adults	
Adolescent Brain & Cognitive Development (ABCD Study) https://abcdstudy.org/scientists/data-sharing/	The ABCD is a long-term study of brain development and child health in the United States. The primary goal is to determine how childhood experiences interact with each other and a child's changing biology to affect brain development and social, behavioral, academic, health, and other outcomes.
Growing Up Today Study (GUTS) http://nhs2survey.org/gutswordpress/	GUTS collects data annually from over 26,000 participants in order to evaluate the factors that influence health throughout the life cycle. Participants are children of the females who enrolled as participants in the second cohort of the Nurses' Health Study. Combined, the GUTS and the Nurses' Health Study can be considered a cross-generational study.
High School & Beyond (HSB) http://nces.ed.gov/surveys/hsb	HSB is a nationally representative, longitudinal study of 10th and 12th graders in 1980. It includes follow-up surveys conducted throughout the students' postsecondary years, surveys of teachers and parents of sampled students, and high school and postsecondary transcripts to enhance analysis.
Monitoring the Future (MTF) http://www.monitoringthefuture.org/	The MTF is a repeated series of surveys in which the same segments of the population (8th, 10th, and 12th graders; college students; and young adults) are presented with the same set of questions over a period of years to see how answers change over time. The purpose is to study changes in the beliefs, attitudes, and behavior of young people in the United States.
National Longitudinal Study of Adolescent to Adult Health (Add Health) www.cpc.unc.edu/projects/addhealth	Add Health is a longitudinal study of adolescents in grades 7–12 in the United States during the 1994–95 school year. This cohort has been followed into young adulthood with subsequent in-home interviews to collect social, environmental, behavioral, and biologic data with which to track the emergence of chronic disease as the cohort moves through their fourth decade of life.
Youth Risk Behavior Surveillance System (YRBSS) www.cdc.gov/healthyyouth/data/yrbs/	YRBSS was developed in 1990 to monitor priority health-risk behaviors that contribute markedly to the leading causes of death, disability, and social problems among youth in the United States. YRBSS surveys are conducted every 2 y, usually during the spring semester and include national, state, territorial, tribal government, and local school-based surveys of 9th through 12th grade students.
Cape Area Panel Study (CAPS) http://www.caps.uct.ac.za	CAPS began in 2002 and is a longitudinal study of the lives of youths and young adults in metropolitan Cape Town, South Africa. The study is split into four waves that interview about 4,800 randomly selected young people between ages 14–22 and reinterview them in different years between 2003 and 2006. The study's outcomes include schooling, employment, health, family formation, and intergenerational support systems.
Global School-based Student Health Survey (GSHS) https://www.who.int/ncds/surveillance/gshs/en/	GSHS was developed by the World Health Organization (WHO) in collaboration with United Nations' UNICEF, UNESCO, UNAIDS, and CDC; it is a school-based survey conducted primarily among students aged 13–17 y across the world.
World Health Organization (WHO) Adolescent Data https://www.who.int/data/maternal-newborn-child-adolescent-ageing/adolescent-data	The WHO curates an adolescent data portal that provides information on adolescents' demographics, mortality, morbidity, health risk factors, policies, and the health system's responsiveness to adolescent health needs. It also provides the access to adolescent health country profiles.
Inclusion of adolescents/young adults	
California Health Interview Survey (CHIS) http://healthpolicy.ucla.edu/chis/Pages/default.aspx	The California Health Interview Survey (CHIS) is the largest state health survey in the nation. It is an annual, random-dial telephone survey that asks questions on a wide range of health topics. CHIS provides representative data on all 58 counties in California and provides a detailed picture of the health and health care needs of California's large and diverse population.
Medical Expenditure Panel Survey (MEPS) https://meps.ahrq.gov/mepsweb/	MEPS, which began in 1996, is a set of large-scale surveys of families and individuals, their clinicians (doctors, hospitals, pharmacies, etc.), and employers across the United States. MEPS collects data on the specific health services that Americans use, how frequently they use them, the cost of these services, and how they are paid for, as well as data on the cost, scope, and breadth of health insurance held by and available to individuals. This is a panel survey that collects two calendar years of data on every member of participating families.
National Health and Nutrition Examination Survey (NHANES) https://www.cdc.gov/nchs/nhanes/	NHANES is a cross-sectional biannual study that combines interviews and physical examinations to obtain demographic, socioeconomic, dietary, and health-related (medical, dental, and physiologic and lab measurements) data on adults and children in the United States.

(continued)

TABLE 13.3

Publicly Available Secondary Datasets Including Adolescents and Young Adults (*Continued*)

Dataset	Description
National Health Interview Survey (NHIS) https://www.cdc.gov/nchs/nhis/	NHIS data are used to monitor trends in illness and disability and to track progress toward achieving national health objectives, including characterizing those with various health problems, determining barriers to accessing and using appropriate health care, and evaluating Federal health programs. This is a cross-sectional annual survey that collects health data (including behaviors and utilization) on every member of participating families, with additional data for one randomly selected adult and child.
National Immunization Surveys (NIS) https://www.cdc.gov/vaccines/imz-managers/nis/about.html	The NIS are a group of phone surveys used to monitor vaccination coverage among children 19–35 mo and teens 13–17 y, and flu vaccinations for children 6 mo–17 y. Data collection for the first survey began in April 1994 to check vaccination coverage after measles outbreaks in the early 1990s. The NIS provide current, population-based, state, and local area estimates of vaccination coverage among children and teens using a standard survey methodology. The surveys collect data through telephone interviews with parents or guardians in all 50 states, the District of Columbia, and some U.S. territories.
National Longitudinal Surveys (NLS) http://www.bls.gov/nls/	NLS are a set of surveys designed to gather information at multiple points in time on the labor market activities and other significant life events of males and females in the United States. NLS-Youth (NLSY) are a set survey of U.S. youth (NLSY97 respondents aged 12–17 when first interviewed in 1997), often interviewing youth annually to obtain information on a variety of topic, including labor market activity, education, and household composition.
National Survey of Children with Special Health Care Needs (NS-CSHCN) www.childhealthdata.org/learn/NS-CSHCN	The NS-CSHCN is a cross-sectional, MCHB-funded survey that has been conducted several times since 2001. It was designed to look at the health and functional status of children with special health care needs in the United States—their physical, emotional, and behavioral health, along with critical information on access to quality health care, care coordination of services, access to a medical home, transition services for youth, and the impact of chronic condition(s) on the child's family.
National Survey of Children's Health (NSCH) www.childhealthdata.org/learn/NSCH	The NSCH is a cross-sectional, MCHB-funded survey that has been conducted several times since 2003. It provides rich data on multiple, intersecting aspects of children's lives—including physical and mental health, access to quality health care, and the child's family, neighborhood, school, and social context.
National Survey of Family Growth (NSFG) http://www.cdc.gov/nchs/nsfg/	NSFG gathers information on family life, marriage and divorce, pregnancy, infertility, use of contraception, and general and reproductive health. The first NSFG surveys were conducted as 5 periodic Cycles from 1973 to 1995, with data on U.S. females 15–44 y of age; the 6th cycle beginning in 2002 included data on males. Starting in 2006, the NSFG began continuous interviewing across several years, with data released in waves.
National Survey on Drug Use and Health (NSDUH) https://nsduhweb.rti.org/respweb/homepage.cfm	NSDUH is an annual cross-sectional survey that provides national and state-level data on the use of tobacco, alcohol, illicit drugs (including nonmedical use of prescription drugs) and mental health among U.S. individuals aged 12 and older. Data is freely available via an application process.
Panel Study of Income Dynamics (PSID) https://psidonline.isr.umich.edu/	PSID is the longest running longitudinal household survey in the world; it began in 1968 with a nationally representative sample of over 18,000 individuals living in 5,000 families in the United States. Information on these individuals and their descendants has been collected continuously, including data covering employment, income, wealth, expenditures, health, marriage, childbearing, child development, philanthropy, education, and numerous other topics.
Kids' Inpatient Database (KID) https://www.hcup-us.ahrq.gov/kidoverview.jsp	The KID is the largest publicly available, all-payer pediatric inpatient care database in the United States; it has been produced every 3 y since 1997. Data include hospital inpatient stays and discharge data for patients younger than 21 y of age, and are structured like claims data, with ICD-9/10 codes, so can be used to look at health care utilization, access, charges, quality, and outcomes. Data are available for a fee.
Pediatric Health Information System (PHIS) www.childrenshospitals.org	PHIS is a comparative pediatric database, which includes clinical and resource utilization data for inpatient, ambulatory surgery, emergency department, and observation unit patient encounters for more than 45 children's hospitals. Data are available for a fee.
NCD Risk Factor Collaboration (NCD-RisC) https://ncdrisc.org/	NCD-RisC is a network of health scientists around the world that provides rigorous and timely data on major risk factors for noncommunicable diseases for all of the world's countries. The Collaboration currently has data from over 2,545 population-based surveys from 193 countries since 1957, with nearly 129 million participants whose risk factor levels have been measured.

This table is not a comprehensive list of all available datasets that could be used to study adolescent/young adult health, but rather a brief list of popular datasets that are well suited to address adolescent/young adult health research.

Measurement of these processes is inherently complicated by their dynamic nature and highlights the importance of the concept of time in AYA research. For instance, researchers interested in studying substance use in adolescents (either as an exposure or outcome) must consider that use behaviors can vary widely across age (e.g., middle vs. high school), period (e.g., final examinations vs. spring break), and cohorts (e.g., adolescents of the "Boomer" vs. "Millennial" generations).[27] It is important to understand that the phenomenon under investigation can vary across all these domains of time. Therefore, researchers must either construct a discrete and specific question/hypothesis with respect to time, selecting appropriate samples and measures accordingly, or utilize suitable statistical techniques that can capture dynamic processes across time. While a myriad of such statistical models exist, novice researchers or those with more limited analytic support may wish to employ the former option.

A related issue stems from issues with measurement validity across developmental periods. Because of dynamic changes, assessment tools or survey instruments may have different psychometric properties when administered to children versus adolescents versus adults. For example, the Patient Health Questionnaire (PHQ) is one of the most commonly used screening tools to identify symptoms of depression, but the "original" PHQ was developed and validated for use with adults. Modified versions of the PHQ have been developed and validated for use with adolescents,[28] while use of the original version may require modified scoring to improve predictive ability in younger populations. Similarly, decisions to use adolescent-reported measures versus parent-reported measures or the same tool administered in different settings can also influence the accuracy of tools and should be a consideration when constructing questionnaires. When planning research, investigators should assess the availability of measurement tools that have been validated with AYAs, to ensure they are using measures that matter to the young person and have demonstrable validity. The NIH has invested in the development of an expanding range of patient-reported outcome measures that are being validated with adolescent cohorts (i.e., youth aged 12 to 18 years). For example, the Patient-Reported Outcomes Measurement Information System (PROMIS) is developing pediatric item banks for youth self-report. Patient-Reported Outcomes Measurement Information System Pediatric measures offer tools for assessing dimensions of physical, social, and mental health of a young person using measures that are different from but are analogous to adult measures (i.e., measures that adults use to describe their health) and parent proxy measures (i.e., measures that parents/guardians complete on behalf of their child).[29] The PROMIS Pediatric measures have been validated with young people across a range of health conditions, are normed on child/adolescent populations, and have empirically defined cutpoints associated with youth health status and change. Similarly, selecting measures that correspond to the unique developmental periods of adolescence and young adulthood—such as those pertaining to health care transition and the growing autonomy and role changes of a young person—may be uniquely valuable for research with and about AYAs.

Perhaps the most common methodologic issue is that of missing data. Missing data can arise when by accident or intention, data elements are incompletely populated. Virtually all studies suffer from some level of missing data, which can complicate or undermine analyses, but this issue is often overlooked. Given that missing data is a near ubiquitous issue, investigators should always conduct a careful review of their data to understand the structure and extent of missingness, and select an approach for addressing it. The "best" case situations are those in which missingness is infrequent and data are **missing completely at random**. Here, the missingness is unrelated to the underlying value (data that would be present if not missing) and unrelated to other data elements. In such situations, most analyses can proceed using available data (i.e., complete case analysis) or with more straightforward imputation approaches (i.e., mean or mode imputation) with little threats to validity. Worse situations are those in which missingness is highly prevalent or data are **missing not at random**. Finding "structure" to missing data tends to be an especially common problem in research with AYAs where sensitive topics are often the focus of research and an AYA's decision to provide or refrain from sharing information is systematic. Here, investigators may opt to use more advanced techniques, such as multiple imputation or full information maximum likelihood methods in order to minimize bias and optimize usable information. Careful consideration is needed to guide use of more complex approaches to address missing data given these strategies are not free of certain assumptions for their use. Careful documentation and transparency in reporting data cleaning and analysis procedures are best practices.

In the case of longitudinal studies, attrition can be a major cause of missing data and can also introduce selection bias to an otherwise well-sampled study. Sample retention itself constitutes a considerable methodologic challenge that requires participant engagement to encourage continued participation as well as administrative investment for participant tracking and recontact (especially complicated when participants include a highly mobile group such as AYAs). Engaging with AYAs as research collaborators is one approach that may be particularly useful for longitudinal studies to ensure that retention efforts are effective.

Ultimately, when engaging in research on AYAs, or any other population, the ability of investigators to articulate clearly their procedures and honestly discuss potential limitations are key requirements for advancing methodologically rigorous, as well as thoughtful and informative research. Close, early collaboration with experts in study design and statistical methodologies is the best way to ensure rigor from study conceptualization through data collection, analysis, and reporting phases of research. These efforts can help safeguard against "fatal flaws" that can undermine the eventual conclusions of the study. Involvement and engagement of AYAs as stakeholders or outright collaborators can improve the acceptability of a research project and the acuity of insights gleaned from research, so that findings are meaningful to AYAs. Importantly, no study is perfect, but those that are ethically conducted, analyzed, and interpreted are fundamental for the translation of research into meaningful improvements to the lives of AYAs.

SUMMARY

Supporting the well-being of young people and through them, their families and communities, requires "measuring what matters" to young people, and with regard to the health issues they experience and the systems through which they move. Developing the field of AYA health and medicine requires investment in building the evidence base and a cadre of AYA health scientists. Effective research with and about AYAs is best done with an appreciation of the relevant ethical and regulatory frameworks governing this work, using approaches that seek to recognize and balance a youth protective stance with supports for autonomy and agency. Investigators should cultivate an understanding of these frameworks and wherever possible, strive to enfranchise youth within their study teams recognizing that doing so may benefit youth and the acuity and relevance of the research. A myriad of study designs are available to help investigators answer questions about AYA health and the efficacy of ameliorative programs, treatments, and policies. Careful review of a study's goals and questions in light of the abilities of a research design to deliver answers and insight is vital. Workshopping ideas with colleagues can help flag questions and concerns that investigators miss early in the development of a project, and improve the chances for a study's success. A rich array of analytic strategies, measures, and data systems exist from which to choose when developing a research project. Taking the time to work through these options and committing to planning, pretesting, and documenting decisions and procedures will pay dividends to the AYA health researcher and community. Statistical support can be essential even for the experienced investigators and nourishing collaborative relationships with other AYA health researchers and statisticians is enormously helpful.

REFERENCES

1. Patton GC, Sawyer SM, Santelli JS, et al. Our future: a Lancet commission on adolescent health and wellbeing. *Lancet.* 2016;387(10036):2423–2478. doi:10.1016/S0140-6736(16)00579-1
2. National Institutes of Health. Inclusion across the lifespan | grants.nih.gov. Accessed March 31, 2021. https://grants.nih.gov/policy/inclusion/lifespan.htm
3. Child participation in research. *European Union Agency for Fundamental Rights.* Published online 2014. Accessed March 31, 2021. https://fra.europa.eu/en/publication/2014/child-participation-research
4. Nelson LR, Stupiansky NW, Ott MA. The influence of age, health literacy, and affluence on adolescents' capacity to consent to research. *J Empir Res Hum Res Ethics.* 2016;11(2):115–121. doi:10.1177/1556264616636232
5. National Institutes of Health. *Guidelines for the Review of Inclusion on the Basis of Sex/Gender, Race, Ethnicity, and Age in Clinical Research Scientific Review Group (SRG) Responsibilities.* Accessed March 31, 2021. https://grants.nih.gov/grants/peer/guidelines_general/Review_Human_subjects_Inclusion.pdf
6. Field MJ, Behrman RE, Institute of Medicine (US) Committee on Clinical Research Involving Children, eds. *Ethical Conduct of Clinical Research Involving Children.* National Academies Press (US); 2004. doi: 10.17226/10958
7. U.S. Department of Health and Human Services. Research with Children–FAQs. Published online 2011:1–11. Accessed March 31, 2021. https://www.hhs.gov/ohrp/regulations-and-policy/guidance/faq/children-research/index.html
8. Summary of the HIPAA Privacy Rule | HHS.gov. Published 2013. Accessed March 31, 2021. https://www.hhs.gov/hipaa/for-professionals/privacy/laws-regulations/index.html
9. Guttmacher Institute. An overview of consent to reproductive health services by young people. *State Policies in Brief.* Published 2016. Accessed March 31, 2021. https://www.guttmacher.org/state-policy/explore/overview-minors-consent-law
10. Vaala SE, Lee JM, Hood KK, et al. Sharing and helping: predictors of adolescents' willingness to share diabetes personal health information with peers. *J Am Med Inform Assoc.* 2018;25(2):135–141. doi:10.1093/jamia/ocx051
11. Karampela M, Ouhbi S, Isomursu M. Connected health user willingness to share personal health data: questionnaire study. *J Med Internet Res.* 2019;21(11):e14537. doi:10.2196/14537
12. Britto MT, Tivorsak TL, Slap GB. Adolescents' needs for health care privacy. *Pediatrics.* 2010;126(6):e1469–e1476. doi:10.1542/peds.2010-0389
13. U.S. Department of Health and Human Services. *Examining Oversight of the Privacy & Security of Health Data Collected by Entities Not Regulated by HIPAA;* 2016. Accessed March 31, 2021. https://www.healthit.gov/sites/default/files/non-covered_entities_report_june_17_2016.pdf
14. Federal Trade Commission. Children's Privacy | Federal Trade Commission. Accessed March 31, 2021. https://www.ftc.gov/tips-advice/business-center/privacy-and-security/children%27s-privacy
15. Blackmer WS. EU general data protection regulation. *Am Fuel Petrochemical Manuf AFPM–Labor Relations/Human Resour Conf 2018.* 2018;2014(March 2014):45–62. https://journals.sagepub.com/doi/full/10.1177/1461444816686327
16. Hokke S, Hackworth NJ, Quin N, et al. Ethical issues in using the internet to engage participants in family and child research: a scoping review. *PLoS One.* 2018;13(9):e0204572. doi:10.1371/journal.pone.0204572
17. Gelinas L, Pierce R, Winkler S, et al. Using social media as a research recruitment tool: ethical issues and recommendations. *Am J Bioeth.* 2017;17(3):3–14. doi:10.1080/15265161.2016.1276644
18. Levy S, Tennermann N, Marin AC, et al. Safety protocols for adolescent substance use research in clinical settings. *J Adolesc Health.* Published online 2020. doi:10.1016/j.jadohealth.2020.07.030
19. Anderson EE, Corneli A. What is a certificate of confidentiality? *100 Questions (and Answers) About Research Ethics;* 2020:46–46. doi:10.4135/9781506348681.n25 https://methods.sagepub.com/book/100-questions-and-answers-about-research-ethics/i526.xml
20. National Institutes of Health. *Certificates of Confidentiality (CoC)—Human Subjects.* Accessed March 31, 2021. https://grants.nih.gov/policy/humansubjects/coc.htm
21. Anyon Y, Bender K, Kennedy H, et al. A systematic review of youth participatory action research (YPAR) in the United States: methodologies, youth outcomes, and future directions. *Heal Educ Behav.* 2018;45(6):865–878. doi:10.1177/1090198118769357
22. Sellars E, Pavarini G, Michelson D, et al. Young people's advisory groups in health research: scoping review and mapping of practices. *Arch Dis Child.* 2021;106:698–704. doi:10.1136/archdischild-2020-320452
23. Lansdown G, UNICEF Innocenti Research Centre. *Conceptual framework for measuring outcomes of adolescent participation.* Published 2018. Accessed March 31, 2021. https://www.unicef.org/media/59006/file
24. Ben-Shlomo Y, Mishra G, Kuh D. Life course epidemiology. In: Ahrens W, Pigeot I. (eds.) *Handbook of Epidemiology: Second Edition.* Vol. 57; 2014:1521–1549. Springer, New York, NY. https://doi.org/10.1007/978-0-387-09834-0_56
25. Fuhrmann D, Knoll LJ, Blakemore SJ. Adolescence as a sensitive period of brain development. *Trends Cogn Sci.* 2015;19(10):558–566. doi:10.1016/j.tics.2015.07.008
26. Blakemore SJ, Mills KL. Is adolescence a sensitive period for sociocultural processing? *Annu Rev Psychol.* 2014;65:187–207. doi:10.1146/annurev-psych-010213-115202
27. Gu J, Guo X, Veenstra G, et al. Adolescent marijuana use in the United States and structural breaks: an age-period-cohort analysis, 1991 to 2018. *Am J Epidemiol.* Published online December 16, 2020. doi:10.1093/aje/kwaa269
28. Richardson LP, Rockhill C, Russo JE, et al. Evaluation of the PHQ-2 as a brief screen for detecting major depression among adolescents. *Pediatrics.* 2010;125(5):e1097–e1103. doi:10.1542/peds.2009-2712
29. Intro to PROMIS—Health Measures http://www.healthmeasures.net/explore-measurement-systems/promis/intro-to-promis. Accessed March 31, 2021.

🛜 ADDITIONAL RESOURCES AND WEBSITES

Additional Resources and Websites for Clinicians:
The following resources provide additional guidance regarding adolescent health research, including sourcebooks about research methodologies.
About YouthRules! Accessed April 1, 2021. https://www.dol.gov/agencies/whd/youthrules
Involving young people in health research. Accessed April 1, 2021. https://wellcome.org/reports/involving-young-people-health-research#downloads-cb2d
Ozer EJ. Youth-Led Participatory Action Research. Developmental and Equity Perspectives. *Advances in Child Development and Behavior.* Vol. 50. Academic Press Inc.; 2016:189–207. https://pubmed.ncbi.nlm.nih.gov/26956074/
Szklo M, Javier N. *Epidemiology: Beyond the Basics.* 4th ed. Jones & Bartlett; 2019.
UNICEF Innocenti Research Centre. Conceptual framework for measuring outcomes of adolescent participation. Accessed March 31, 2021. https://www.unicef.org/media/59006/file
Young TK. *Population Health: Concepts and Methods.* Oxford University Press; 2004.

Additional Resources and Websites for Parents/Caregivers:
The following resources may be helpful for parents who seek to learn about protections and opportunities for adolescent health research.
Citizen Science for Health. Accessed April 1, 2021. https://www.citizenscienceforhealth.org/
Clinical Trials—U.S. National Library of Medicine. Accessed April 1, 2021. https://clinicaltrials.gov/
Institutional Review Boards Frequently Asked Questions—Guidance for Institutional Review Boards and Clinical Investigators. Accessed April 1, 2021. https://www.fda.gov/regulatory-information/search-fda-guidance-documents/institutional-review-boards-frequently-asked-questions
Research Match. Accessed April 1, 2021. https://www.researchmatch.org/
Research with Children FAQs. Accessed April 1, 2021. https://www.hhs.gov/ohrp/regulations-and-policy/guidance/faq/children-research/index.html
UNICEF Innocenti Research Centre. Conceptual framework for measuring outcomes of adolescent participation. Accessed March 31, 2021. https://www.unicef.org/media/59006/file

Additional Resources and Websites for Adolescents and Young Adults:
The following resources may be helpful for adolescents who seek to learn about and participate in health research, and understand some of the protections available to them as workers.
About YouthRules! Accessed April 1, 2021. https://www.dol.gov/agencies/whd/youthrules
Citizen Science for Health. Accessed April 1, 2021. https://www.citizenscienceforhealth.org/
Clinical Trials—U.S. National Library of Medicine. Accessed April 1, 2021. https://clinicaltrials.gov/
List of citizen science projects—Wikipedia. Accessed April 1, 2021. https://en.wikipedia.org/wiki/List_of_citizen_science_projects
Research Match. Accessed April 1, 2021. https://www.researchmatch.org/
Research with Children FAQs. Accessed April 1, 2021. https://www.hhs.gov/ohrp/regulations-and-policy/guidance/faq/children-research/index.html
UNICEF Innocenti Research Centre—Conceptual framework for measuring outcomes of adolescent participation. Accessed March 31, 2021. https://www.unicef.org/media/59006/file

PART II

Endocrine Disorders

CHAPTER 14

Abnormal Growth and Development

Toni Eimicke
Jonathan M. Swartz

KEY WORDS
- Constitutional delay of puberty
- Delayed puberty
- Growth
- Precocious puberty
- Puberty
- Short stature

INTRODUCTION

This chapter focuses on the adolescent whose growth and/or development falls outside the range of normal. These issues are usually of concern to adolescents and their families, and the clinician must have a clear understanding of how to evaluate and manage these problems. In evaluating growth during adolescence, it is necessary to assess whether a teen has reached puberty, whether puberty is proceeding normally, and whether the bony epiphyses are still open to permit further growth.

SHORT STATURE WITHOUT DELAYED PUBERTY

Adolescents who are progressing normally through puberty may present with concerns about short stature. Most of these teens have genetic or familial short stature, with other major categories including chronic disease, constitutional delay of growth and development, and endocrine diseases. Girls who are short may seek medical attention for this complaint when they have just reached menarche and worry that future growth in height will be limited. Boys may present as their pubertal growth spurt slows and they are still shorter than they had hoped. Most hormonal deficiencies, chronic diseases, and malabsorptive states that slow growth will also cause at least some delay in puberty or failure to progress normally through puberty; these are less likely causes for the short stature in teens who have normal puberty.

Definition of Short Stature

Adult height is strongly dictated by genetic factors; therefore, evaluation of short stature must be assessed considering the heights of family members. In general, 2 standard deviations (SDs) (2.3 percentile) below the mean height on a cross-sectional growth chart is used as the lower limit of normal.

Criteria for Evaluation: An adolescent should be considered for an evaluation of short stature if:

1. Linear growth rate is ≤4 cm/y during the years prior to the normal age for peak linear growth velocity.
2. No evidence of a peak linear growth velocity during puberty
3. Deceleration below an individual's established growth velocity occurs

4. The adolescent's height is more than 2 SDs below the mean (height below 2 SDs for age and sex within the population). Consideration should be given to carrying out a full evaluation, especially if growth pattern is inconsistent with family; at a minimum, a careful history and physical examination, screening laboratory tests, and observation of growth for 6 months are warranted.
5. The adolescent's height is more than 2 SDs below the calculated midparental height (see Chapter 2).

Differential Diagnosis

1. Familial short stature
2. Constitutional delay of growth and development
3. Chronic illness—can include diseases such as celiac disease, inflammatory bowel disease (IBD), severe asthma, cystic fibrosis, human immunodeficiency virus (HIV) infection, congestive heart failure, and renal failure, among others
4. Endocrine—can include hypothyroidism, isolated growth hormone (GH) deficiency, hypercortisolism, adrenal insufficiency, and poorly controlled diabetes mellitus
5. Congenital syndromes, including Down syndrome (trisomy 21), Turner syndrome (45,X), Noonan, Hurler, Silver–Russell syndrome, Laron syndrome (GH receptor gene mutations), short stature homeobox gene (SHOX) deficiency, and other skeletal dysplasias including chondrodysplasias
6. Intrauterine growth restriction or small for gestational age

Evaluation

History

1. Maternal pregnancy history—medical illnesses and medication use
2. Birth weight and length, and estimate of gestational age—important because premature infants with appropriate small weight tend to have a normal growth potential, whereas infants with intrauterine growth restriction who are inappropriately small for gestational age may not exhibit catch-up growth
3. Complete review of systems
   a. Renal—polyuria and polydipsia for hypothalamic and/or pituitary disorders
   b. Cardiac—peripheral edema, murmurs, and cyanosis
   c. Gastrointestinal—diarrhea, flatulence (malabsorption), vomiting, and/or abdominal pain
   d. Pulmonary—sleep apnea, asthma, or symptoms suggestive of cystic fibrosis
   e. Neurologic—headaches, visual field defects suggesting pituitary neoplasms
4. Growth history—review of symptoms and growth charts

5. Family history—final adult height, and patterns of growth and puberty in first- and second-degree relatives
6. Dietary history
7. Social history—psychosocial stressors[1]

Physical Examination

A complete physical examination is the next step in the evaluation and should include the following:
1. Height and weight (including past [whenever possible] and current growth measurements that are plotted on appropriate developmental charts for height, weight, and body mass index [BMI])
2. Arm span and upper-to-lower (U/L) body-segment ratio
3. Sexual maturity ratings (SMRs)—specifically breast and genital development, and not pubic hair only
4. A general physical examination, with special attention to the thyroid gland, visual fields assessment, neurologic examination, and stigmata of congenital syndromes

Laboratory/Radiologic Evaluation

The laboratory evaluation of short stature should include the following:
1. Routine laboratory screening: Complete blood cell (CBC) count with differential, erythrocyte sedimentation rate (ESR), chemistry profile including serum creatinine, insulin-like growth factor-1 (IGF-1), insulin-like growth factor binding protein 3 (IGFBP-3), and thyroid-stimulating hormone (TSH) and free thyroxine (free T_4). Screening for celiac disease with total immunoglobulin A (IgA) and anti-tissue transglutaminase (TTG) antibodies is also advised in asymptomatic children who are short.
2. Bone age: X-ray of the left hand and wrist for bone age (since the bone age can determine if there is more potential for growth and be used to estimate predicted final height).[2]
3. Midparental height calculation: It is also useful to obtain the parents' heights and calculate a midparental height (formula provided in Chapter 2). Although there are many genes involved in stature, and an offspring's height frequently varies considerably from midparental height, the midparental or target height can still give a good clue that the short stature is genetic.
4. Karyotype: A karyotype is useful when signs of Turner syndrome are present, as well as in any girl with unexplained short stature and otherwise normal labs. It can also be useful in boys with genital anomalies.
5. Referral to genetics can be considered if unexplained developmental delay and dysmorphic features are present in a patient with short stature.
6. Other tests: Other tests may be indicated depending on the history and physical examination and may include the following:
   a. Central imaging studies—cranial magnetic resonance imaging (MRI) with contrast
   b. Gastrointestinal studies
   c. Endocrine studies
      (1) Serum levels of IGF-1 and IGFBP-3 are often assessed when the growth pattern is concerning for GH deficiency. Insulin-like growth factor binding protein 3 can be useful in underweight or nutritionally deficient children who have low IGF-1 levels. Interpretation is often completed by pediatric endocrinologists in context of entire clinical picture.
      (2) Growth hormone stimulation testing is usually carried out by a pediatric endocrinologist using one of several protocols that involve two different agents (agents used include insulin, glucagon, arginine, L-dopa, or clonidine). Two agents are administered at different time points during the testing and a series of stimulated GH

levels are obtained and interpreted. In prepubertal adolescents, priming with sex steroids before stimulation testing should be considered for maximal GH release.

Suggestions for Diagnosis

1. Constitutional delay of puberty: Most short stature in adolescents is the result of either constitutional delay of puberty or familial short stature. Guidelines for diagnosis are outlined later in this chapter.
2. Genetic or familial short stature: Suggested by the following:
   a. Normal history and physical examination findings
   b. Family history of short stature
   c. Growth curve that generally parallels the third percentile
   d. Bone age that is appropriate for chronologic age (within 2 SDs)
3. Chronic illness: Chronic renal disease and Crohn disease are additional causes of short stature. These diseases are usually diagnosed by history, physical examination findings, or results of tests including, but not limited to, CBC, ESR, and chemistry studies.
4. Endocrine causes: Endocrine causes of short stature, such as hypothyroidism, GH deficiency, adrenal insufficiency, and adrenocortical excess, are less common. Hypothyroidism and adrenocortical excess can usually be detected by the patient's history, physical examination including a growth chart, or screening laboratory tests. Adolescents with classic GH deficiency can be difficult to differentiate from those with constitutional delay of puberty. This is particularly difficult during the time of expected peak linear growth velocity, when the growth of an adolescent with constitutional delay of puberty slows from the normal growth curve as other adolescents accelerate their growth velocities. Individuals with classic GH deficiency have normal body proportions. Additional features and findings may include a microphallus, child-like face, and/or history of hypoglycemia.

Treatment of Short Stature with Growth Hormone
Growth Hormone Deficiency

Patients with classic GH deficiency have marked benefit in statural outcome as the result of GH treatment. In addition, those with complete GH deficiency benefit from the metabolic effects of continuation of GH treatment after growth completion/epiphyseal fusion. These benefits include improvement of bone density, decreased fat mass, and improvement of muscle strength. These subjects should continue GH treatment at a markedly reduced dose, compared with that used for growth augmentation, throughout life.

Recombinant GH has been available since the 1980s. Patients with classical GH deficiency usually present with extreme short stature and slow growth (<4 cm/y) well before adolescence, although acquired GH deficiency, sometimes due to head trauma or tumors, may present in adolescence with slow growth and relatively delayed puberty.[3]

Other Conditions

Turner Syndrome Growth hormone has been used to increase height velocity and increase final adult height in patients who do not have true GH deficiency. Growth hormone is approved for use in patients with short stature due to Turner syndrome using a higher dose than is recommended for GH deficiency. Insulin-like growth factor-1, thyroid screens, and bone age x-rays are monitored during therapy, as well as close monitoring of linear growth using the growth chart for children with Turner syndrome (**Table 14.1**, Fig. 14.1). Patients with Turner syndrome should have baseline renal ultrasonography and periodic cardiac MRI and echocardiograms to screen for aortic root enlargement (Figs. 14.2 and 14.3). Aortic dissection is a rare but potentially fatal cause of severe chest pain in patients with Turner syndrome. Growth hormone treatment should ideally be

TABLE 14.1

General Health Screening Recommendations in Turner Syndrome

Screening/Evaluation	At Diagnosis	After Diagnosis (Child)	After Diagnosis (Adult)
Weight/BMI	Yes	Every visit	Every visit
Blood pressure	Yes	Every visit	Every visit
Thyroid function (TSH and free T_4)	Yes	Annually	Annually
Lipid panel			Annually if at least one cardiovascular risk factor[a]
Aminotransferase, GGT, and alkaline phosphatase		Annually after age 10 y	Annually
25-Hydroxyvitamin D		Every 2–3 y after age 9–11 y	Every 3–5 y
Celiac screen		Starting at age 2 y; then every 2 y	If symptomatic
Renal ultrasound	Yes		
Audiometric evaluation	Yes, at age 9–12 mo	Every 3 y	Every 5 y
Ophthalmologic evaluation	Yes, at age 12–18 mo		
Dental evaluation	Yes, if no prior care established		
Clinical assessment for congenital hip dysplasia	Yes, in newborns		
Skin examination	Yes	Annually	Annually
Bone mineral density			Every 5 y and when discontinuing estrogen
Skeletal assessment		Age 5–6 y and age 12–14 y	

[a]Cardiovascular risk factors: hypertension, overweight, tobacco, diabetes, and physical inactivity.
Adapted from Gravholt CH, Andersen NH, Conway GS, et al. Clinical practice guidelines for the care of girls and women with Turner syndrome: proceedings from the 2016 Cincinnati International Turner Syndrome Meeting. *Eur J Endocrinol.* 2017;177(3):G1–G70. doi: 10.1530/EJE-17-0430

initiated early in childhood when growth rate begins to fall off. Estrogen replacement is often delayed to age 12 to 14, to maximize height gain in patients with Turner syndrome. Growth hormone can also be used similarly in Noonan syndrome.

Intrauterine Growth Restriction and Other Indications Growth hormone is also approved by the U.S. Food and Drug Administration (FDA) for use in patients with short stature due to intrauterine growth restriction without catch-up growth, Prader–Willi syndrome, and chronic renal failure before transplantation. Growth hormone has also been approved for treatment of children and adolescents with idiopathic short stature who are more than 2.25 SDs below the mean in height and who are unlikely to catch up in height.[4] Patients who qualify for a trial of treatment with human GH for idiopathic short stature must have open epiphyses permitting further height gain. Patients with severe short stature who desire treatment with GH should be referred to a pediatric endocrinologist.

◼ DELAYED PUBERTY

Review of Normal Development

The pattern of normal puberty is discussed in detail in Chapter 2.

Definition and General Guidelines for Evaluating Puberty

In general, 2 SDs above and below the mean are used to define the range of normal variability. Chapter 2 is helpful in determining

guidelines for evaluation, and further guidelines are discussed subsequently.

Delayed development is defined by the absence of breast budding by age 13 in girls or the lack of testicular enlargement by age 14 in boys, both 2.5 SDs beyond the average age at onset of these changes. Alterations in the chronologic relationship of pubertal events are also common causes for evaluation. These include phallic enlargement in the absence of testicular enlargement in boys or the absence of menarche by age 16, or 4 years after the onset of breast development, in girls. If puberty is interrupted, there is a regression or failure to progress in the development of secondary sexual characteristics, accompanied by a slowing in growth rate. All these factors should be considered in the context of the adolescent's family history as it relates to growth and pubertal development, the adolescent's prior growth pattern, and the review of systems.

Differential Diagnosis

Delayed development occurs more commonly in boys than in girls. Most patients who present for an evaluation of slow growth and delayed development are high school–aged boys who are concerned about their short stature, as well as their lack of muscular and secondary sexual development, which may lead to worry about being at a disadvantage among their peers. Most of these boys have constitutionally delayed development; however, the clinical presentation of the patient with constitutional delay may be

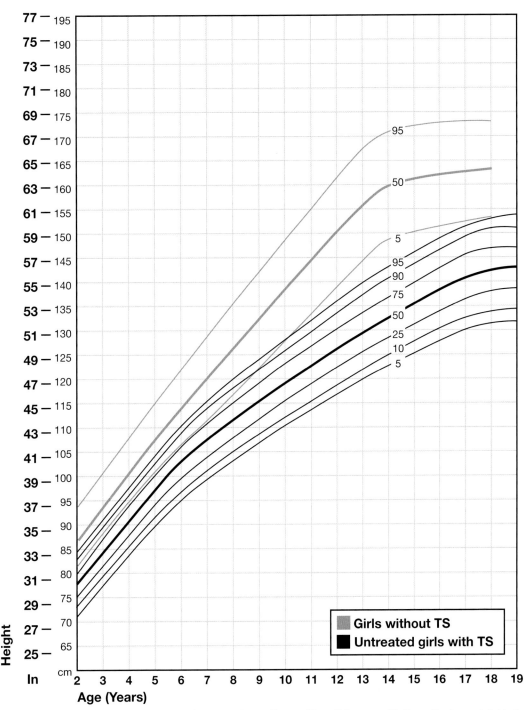

FIGURE 14.1 Growth chart for children with Turner syndrome. (Source: Rieser P, Davenport M. *Turner Syndrome: A Guide for Families.* Turner Syndrome Society of the United States; 2002. Data derived from Lyon et al.[7])

indistinguishable from that of the patient whose pubertal delay is the result of an organic lesion.

Constitutional Delay of Puberty

Adolescents with constitutional delay of puberty have often been slow growers throughout childhood. In the absence of sex steroids of puberty, growth may slow even further to <5 cm/y as these children reach an age when puberty would normally occur. Growth velocity increases into the normal range when these teens finally enter puberty. Adolescents with constitutional delay of puberty often have a family history of delayed growth and development in relatives. Teens with constitutional delay of puberty eventually

enter puberty on their own. Although they have a longer time to grow before their epiphyses close, they tend to have a less exuberant growth spurt than earlier developers.

Functional Causes of Delayed Puberty

Gonadotropin-releasing hormone (GnRH) secretion can be inhibited centrally by the following:

1. Inadequate nutrition, including eating disorders
2. Chronic disease including chronic heart disease, severe asthma, IBD, celiac disease, rheumatoid arthritis, chronic renal failure, renal tubular acidosis, sickle cell anemia, diabetes mellitus, systemic lupus erythematosus, cystic fibrosis, and infection with HIV

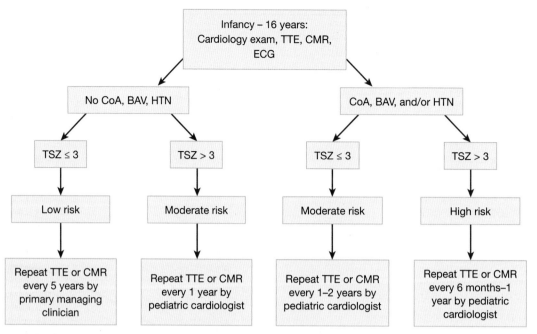

TTE, transthoracic echocardiography; CMR, cardiac magnetic resonance imaging; ECG, electrocardiogram; CoA, coarctation of aorta; BAV, bicuspid aortic valve; HTN, hypertension; TSZ, Turner syndrome specific Z-score of the aorta (see text for explanation).

FIGURE 14.2 Suggested cardiac monitoring protocol for patients with Turner syndrome from infancy to 16 years. (Source: Gravholt CH, Andersen NH, Conway GS, et al. Clinical practice guidelines for the care of girls and women with Turner syndrome: proceedings from the 2016 Cincinnati International Turner Syndrome Meeting. *Eur J Endocrinol.* 2017;177(3):G1–G70. doi: 10.1530/EJE-17-0430)

3. Severe environmental stress
4. Intensive athletic training
5. Severe hypothyroidism and excess cortisol states

Eating disorders associated with self-imposed restriction of caloric intake can delay or interrupt the progression of puberty. Anorexia nervosa most often develops in girls in early to middle adolescence, who have already entered puberty. Young adolescent boys or girls who are dieting because of fear of obesity may

present with the complaint of delayed development. Crohn disease or celiac disease may also present with delayed development and poor growth as the major symptoms. Since adolescence is normally a period of rapid growth and weight gain, failure to gain weight or small amounts of weight loss may be manifestations of significant nutritional insufficiency. Poor growth and delayed puberty are common in cystic fibrosis, thalassemia major, renal tubular acidosis, renal failure, cyanotic congenital heart disease, sickle

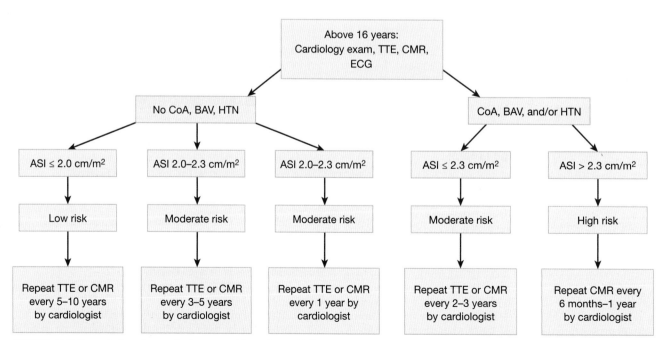

FIGURE 14.3 Suggested cardiac monitoring protocol for patients with Turner syndrome >16 years. (Source: Gravholt CH, Andersen NH, Conway GS, et al. Clinical practice guidelines for the care of girls and women with Turner syndrome: proceedings from the 2016 Cincinnati International Turner Syndrome Meeting. *Eur J Endocrinol.* 2017;177(3):G1–G70. doi: 10.1530/EJE-17-0430)

cell anemia, systemic lupus erythematosus, acquired immune deficiency syndrome, or very poorly controlled asthma or type 1 diabetes mellitus. Patients who are on stimulants such as methylphenidate for treatment of attention deficit hyperactivity disorder may have decreased appetite because of the medication and slower growth rates as a result of nutritional insufficiency.

Hypothyroidism may present in an adolescent with slowing of height velocity (height-dropping percentiles on the growth chart) whose weight is well preserved for height or who is mildly overweight, sometimes with delayed or interrupted pubertal development. The classic signs are often only present with severe hypothyroidism and include dull dry skin, decrease in pulse rate and blood pressure, constipation, and cold intolerance. A goiter is not always present. Autoimmune thyroiditis is the most common cause of hypothyroidism in teens. There may be a family history of hypothyroidism or autoimmune issues.

Cushing syndrome, whether due to endogenous glucocorticoid overproduction (rare) or chronic exposure to high doses of glucocorticoids for medical treatment, causes excessive weight gain, slowing of height velocity, and may interrupt or delay puberty. Conversely, if endogenous sex steroid production is also increased, it may present with precocious puberty without a growth spurt.

Hypothalamic Causes of Delayed or Absent Puberty

The ability of the hypothalamus to secrete GnRH may be damaged by the following:

1. Local tumors (germinomas, craniopharyngiomas, astrocytomas, or gliomas)
2. Infiltrative lesions such as central nervous system (CNS) leukemia or histiocytosis X
3. Central nervous system irradiation
4. Traumatic gliosis
5. Mass lesions such as brain abscesses or granulomas due to sarcoidosis or tuberculosis
6. Congenital defects in the ability to secrete GnRH (including isolated hypogonadotropic hypogonadism and Kallman syndrome). Studies have confirmed a large number of genes involved in cases of hypogonadotropic hypogonadism.
7. Congenital brain malformations associated with inability to secrete GnRH including optic nerve hypoplasia.

Pituitary Causes of Delayed Puberty

Puberty may not begin or may fail to proceed if the pituitary cannot respond to GnRH stimulation with luteinizing hormone (LH) and follicle-stimulating hormone (FSH) production. This may be due to the following:

1. Pituitary tumor
2. Selective impairment of gonadotrope function by hemochromatosis
3. Congenital hypopituitarism is usually diagnosed either in the neonatal period or with poor growth during childhood; causes include genetic defects that interfere with pituitary formation and empty sella syndrome.
4. Acquired hypopituitarism
5. Prolactinoma—excessive prolactin production by a pituitary adenoma (prolactinoma) or other tumors may interrupt or prevent puberty by interfering with gonadotropin production. Patients with prolactinomas most often present with secondary amenorrhea often with galactorrhea, but may present with stalled puberty. Headaches are sometimes present. Prolactinomas are more common in girls than boys, but can occur in both. Psychotropic drugs such as antipsychotics are a frequent cause of hyperprolactinemia.

Gonadal Failure

If the gonads are unable to respond to LH and FSH, puberty will not proceed.

The causes of gonadal failure with abnormal karyotype include the following:

1. Gonadal dysgenesis: The most common cause of gonadal failure is gonadal dysgenesis, which occurs in association with abnormalities of sex chromosomes. The gonads fail to develop and become rudimentary streaks. These patients are phenotypic females with normal immature female genitalia. The most common phenotype is Turner syndrome, which is caused by absence of part or all of a second sex chromosome. These patients are typically short with a final untreated height averaging 143 cm. Other identifying features of Turner syndrome are low-set ears, a webbed neck, widely spaced nipples, a trident hairline, an increased carrying angle of the lower arms, and short fourth and fifth fingers and toes. Renal abnormalities such as duplications and horseshoe kidney, and left-sided cardiovascular abnormalities such as bicuspid aortic valve, dilatation of the aortic root, and coarctation of the aorta are also associated with Turner syndrome. Half of these patients have 45,X karyotypes, whereas the rest have a mosaic form or have various X chromosome abnormalities or deletions.
2. Klinefelter syndrome: Males with Klinefelter syndrome (47,XXY) may present with poorly progressing puberty caused by partial gonadal failure (Fig. 14.4). Their testes can make some testosterone when driven by high levels of gonadotropins (LH and FSH) and they tend to have significantly impaired sperm production.[5] In the 47,XXY patient with pubertal development, the testes become small and firm because they become fibrotic. Gynecomastia and eunuchoid body habitus are often seen.

The causes of gonadal failure with normal karyotype include the following:

1. Acquired gonadal disorders
   a. Infection—viral or tubercular orchitis or oophoritis
   b. Trauma—bilateral testicular torsion resulting in anorchia is another cause of gonadal failure in males.
   c. Postsurgical removal
   d. Radiation, chemotherapy with agents such as cyclophosphamide
   e. Autoimmune oophoritis or orchitis (sometimes with multiple autoimmune endocrine abnormalities)
   f. Fragile X may present as secondary amenorrhea in females with ovarian failure.
   g. Cryptorchidism—the testes may fail to function, particularly if they remain intra-abdominal beyond infancy.
2. Congenital gonadal disorders
   a. Anorchism: In the "testicular regression syndrome," the testes are absent in a phenotypic male, presumably as a result of destruction in utero.
   b. Pure gonadal dysgenesis: This presents as absent puberty in patients with a normal karyotype (46,XX or 46,XY), normal stature, and a female phenotype.
   c. Enzyme defects in androgen and estrogen production: Enzymatic defects, such as 17α-hydroxylase or 20,22-desmolase deficiency, which render the gonad unable to produce estrogens or androgens, are other rare causes of primary gonadal failure.
   d. Gonadal failure is associated with other diseases such as congenital galactosemia in girls and ataxia telangiectasia.
3. Androgen-receptor defects
   a. Complete androgen insensitivity presents as a patient who is a phenotypic female with tall stature, normal breast development, and timing of puberty, but with absence of sexual hair and absence of menarche. The vagina ends in a blind pouch and there is no cervix or uterus. The karyotype is 46,XY, and testosterone levels are elevated.
   b. Partial androgen insensitivity (previously referred to as a variety of syndromes, including Reifenstein syndrome).

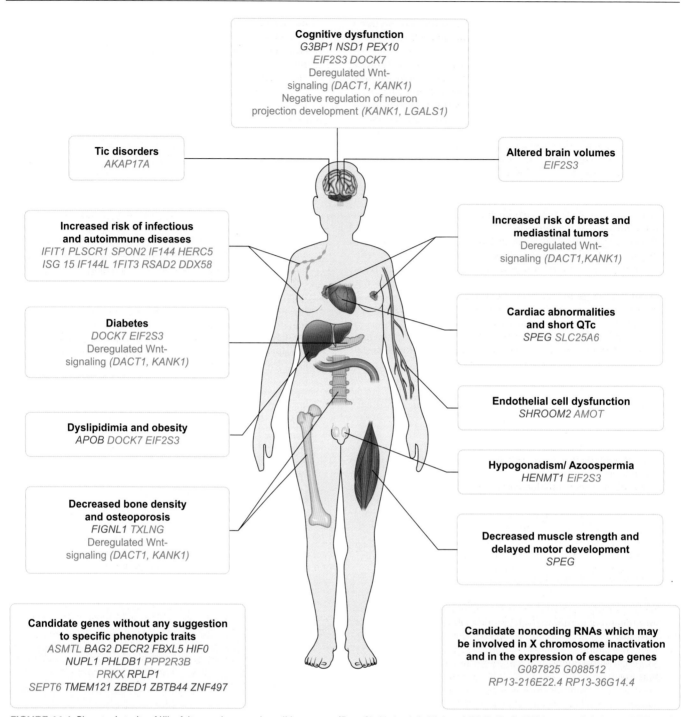

FIGURE 14.4 Phenytopic traits of Klinefelter syndrome and candidate genes. (From Skakkebaek A, Nielsen MM, Trolle C. DNA hypermethylation and differential gene expression associated with Klinefelter syndrome. *Sci Rep.* 2018;8(1):13740. doi:10.1038/s41598-018-31780-0)

Syndromes Associated with Pubertal Delay

There are several syndromes that are characterized by extreme obesity, short stature, and delayed puberty. These include the following:
1. Prader–Willi (extreme obesity, developmental delay, small hands and feet, and chromosome 15 deletion)
2. Bardet–Biedl syndrome (obesity, polydactyly, retinitis pigmentosa, genital hypoplasia, developmental delay)
3. Borjeson–Forseeman–Lehman (obesity, severe cognitive impairment, microcephaly, epilepsy, and skeletal anomalies)

Another congenital syndrome is congenital absence of the uterus and upper vagina (Mayer–Rokintansky–Kuster–Hauser syndrome). This is associated with normal puberty, but absent menses.

WORKUP OF DELAYED PUBERTY

Most adolescents with delayed maturation have constitutional delay of puberty. However, this diagnosis is made by excluding other causes of delayed puberty. A detailed history and physical examination will help focus and minimize the laboratory testing needed to evaluate an adolescent with delayed development.

History

1. Neonatal history: The neonatal history should include birth weight, history of previous maternal miscarriages, and congenital lymphedema (Turner syndrome). The past medical

history should focus on any history of chronic disease, congenital anomalies, previous surgery, radiation exposure, chemotherapy, or drug use.

2. Growth records: Past growth measurements that are plotted on appropriate growth charts for height, weight, and BMI are important in evaluating the adolescent with delayed puberty. The overall pattern of growth and changes in that pattern often lead to a diagnosis. The child whose delayed puberty is associated with a nutritional deficiency due to an eating disorder, IBD, celiac disease, or other chronic disease will show a greater decline in weight gain than in height and be underweight for height. In contrast, the child who has delayed puberty on the basis of an endocrinopathy such as acquired hypothyroidism or gonadal dysgenesis will have a greater slowing in height gain than in weight gain, and have weight well preserved for height, often being mildly overweight.

3. Review of systems: Special attention should be paid to weight changes, dieting, environmental stress, exercise and athletics, gastrointestinal symptoms, headache, neurologic symptoms (including abnormal peripheral vision and anosmia), and symptoms suggestive of thyroid disease.

4. Nutritional history and eating habits: This helps to assess the possibility of chronic malnutrition.

5. Family history: The family history should include the heights, timing of secondary sexual development and fertility of family members, and a history of endocrine disorders.

Physical Examination

A complete physical examination is indicated for the adolescent with delayed puberty, but the following areas are of particular importance:

1. Overall nutritional status and measurements of height, weight, and vital signs, including plotting of anthropometric data on growth curves.

2. Body measurements including the following:
   a. Arm span
   b. Upper-to-lower segment ratio: This can be measured by measuring symphysis pubis to floor for lower, subtracting lower from total height for upper. This measurement can be useful for patients who have either short extremities (short bone syndromes, congenital short stature syndromes) or long extremities (eunuchoid appearance).

3. Congenital anomalies, including midline facial defects.

4. Staging of sexual maturity: The patient should be examined for a delay in pubertal development as assessed by staging of breast and pubic hair in girls, and genitalia and pubic hair in boys (see Chapter 2). Pubic hair may be present, although the genitalia are prepubertal in a boy who had normal adrenarche, but lacks gonadal activation. Any evidence of heterosexual development, such as clitoromegaly or hirsutism in girls or gynecomastia in boys, should be noted.

5. Thyroid: Inspect for evidence of goiter. However, not all adolescents with hypothyroidism present with goiter.

6. Chest: Examine for evidence of chronic pulmonary disease.

7. Cardiac: Assess for evidence of congenital heart disease.

8. Abdomen: Check for abdominal distension as a sign of a malabsorptive disease and check for evidence of liver or spleen enlargement as a sign of a chronic systemic disorder.

9. Genital examination: The examination of the external genitalia in girls should focus on obvious congenital anomalies and an assessment of estrogen effect. Pale pink-gray vaginal mucosa with white secretion indicates the current presence of estrogen. A pelvic examination is not necessary as a part of the initial evaluation of a girl with delayed secondary sexual development, but an assessment of the depth of the vagina should be done, if possible, to rule out gynecologic congenital anomalies in a girl who has normal pubertal development

but delayed menarche. The examination should be carried out by a practitioner who is familiar with the techniques used for examining nonsexually active teenage girls.

10. Neurologic examination: Ophthalmoscopic examination and visual field assessment are done to look for abnormalities of the optic nerves and signs of intracranial hypertension.

Laboratory Tests

Laboratory evaluation should be focused according to the clinical impression. In the patient who is underweight for height, studies would include screening tests for chronic disease or malabsorptive states such as celiac disease.

Bone Age

The most useful initial examination in delayed puberty and slow growth is often a x-ray of the left hand and wrist for a bone age assessment. This information can be used to assess how much height growth potential remains in the patient with short stature and delayed development. A predicted adult height can be obtained using the Bayley–Pinneau tables in the Atlas of Skeletal Maturation by Greulich and Pyle.[6]

1. Constitutional delay of puberty: The patient with constitutional delay of puberty will usually have an equal delay of height age and bone age. Caution should be used in height estimates in patients with constitutional delay of puberty since bone age height predictions are less accurate in this group.

2. Delayed bone age: Patients with GH deficiency, hypothyroidism, and chronic disease usually have bone ages that are delayed several years behind their chronologic age.

3. Normal bone age: Typically seen with familial short stature. Bone age may also be used in conjunction with height age and chronologic age to give clues about a diagnosis as indicated below. Height age is determined by locating the corresponding age at which the patient's height would be equal to the 50th percentile.

Routine Laboratory Tests Initial laboratory studies to be considered in the adolescent with delayed puberty include a CBC count, ESR, or C-reactive protein (CRP) (useful as a screening test for chronic illness such as IBD), along with a comprehensive metabolic panel (CMP) including electrolytes, renal function, and liver function tests.

Screening for Celiac Disease or Inflammatory Bowel Disease Screening for celiac disease and IBD should include discussion of symptoms such as increased frequency of stooling, presence of blood in stool, urgency, and/or nighttime awakening to stool. Initial labs may include a TTG IgA along with a total IgA, as well as an ESR and/or CRP. If screening is positive, referral to a gastroenterologist is warranted for more extensive and confirmatory testing.

Central Imaging Studies If there is a suspicion of a CNS tumor, cranial MRI with contrast is the best way to evaluate the hypothalamus and pituitary. A computed tomography scan is a less sensitive alternative.

Hormonal Tests Hormonal tests to be considered include thyroid function tests (free T_4, TSH), prolactin, LH and FSH, dehydroepiandrosterone sulfate (DHEAS), testosterone or estradiol, and IGF-1 and IGFBP-3.

In the early stages (SMR 2) of puberty, breast budding and vaginal maturation in girls and penile and testicular enlargement in boys are more sensitive indicators of pubertal neuroendocrine–gonadal function than a single daytime measurement of gonadotropin (LH and FSH) levels, estradiol, or testosterone. Luteinizing hormone, FSH, and testosterone or estradiol may be in the prepubertal range on a daytime sample even though these hormones are actively being secreted at night. A first morning value to catch overnight activity is often more valuable in early puberty. Testosterone or estradiol levels may be valuable in following the patient whose puberty is not progressing normally by clinical assessment of growth and secondary sexual development.

Growth hormone is secreted primarily during sleep and in a pulsatile fashion, so random, daytime levels are commonly low. Insulin-like growth factor-1 and IGFBP-3 are used to assess GH sufficiency. Insulin-like growth factor-1 levels should be compared with normal ranges for SMR stage or bone age rather than chronologic age since the levels increase during puberty. Insulin-like growth factor-1 levels are low in patients with nutritional insufficiency. Patients with delayed puberty and slow growth often have temporarily decreased GH secretion simply due to pubertal delay, which increases to normal as puberty begins. If GH deficiency is suspected, the patient should be referred to a pediatric endocrinologist for GH stimulation testing. Patients with constitutional delay of puberty who are prepubertal may appear GH deficient on GH stimulation testing unless primed with estrogen before the test.

Luteinizing hormone and FSH determinations are only useful if they are consistent with puberty since these hormones are secreted primarily during sleep in the early phases of puberty. Early to mid-pubertal levels (SMR B2) are indistinguishable from prepubertal levels if not checked early in the morning using an ultrasensitive assay. Abnormally elevated LH and FSH levels (above upper limit of normal for the reference range given) are suggestive of primary gonadal failure. If LH and FSH levels are abnormally elevated, further laboratory evaluation would include blood karyotyping in search of a chromosomal abnormality such as 45,X. Patients with gonadal dysgenesis who have Y chromosomal material present should have their gonads removed surgically because of an increased risk for gonadoblastoma. If the chromosomes are normal in the patient with gonadal failure, antiadrenal (21-hydroxylase) and antithyroid antibodies (antithyroid peroxidase and antithyroglobulin) may be obtained to look for autoimmune issues associated with gonadal insufficiency. Screening for fragile X premutation should also be considered in the setting of unexplained ovarian insufficiency. Pelvic ultrasonography may be used to visualize the uterus and ovaries, but should be interpreted with caution since the prepubertal uterus is small and may be missed on ultrasonography. A vaginal ultrasonography is usually postponed until adulthood.

If the initial prolactin level is elevated, it should be repeated without a breast examination or other breast manipulation on the day of the testing, and ideally in a fasting state. Patients with significantly elevated prolactin levels should have a cranial MRI with contrast.

Neuroendocrine Pharmacologic Testing If there is a question of multiple pituitary hormone defects, the patient may be referred to an endocrinologist for pharmacologic and physiologic tests of neuroendocrine function.

Constitutional Delay of Puberty

The chief diagnostic challenge in the patient with pubertal delay is to distinguish between constitutional delay and true GnRH deficiency. About 90% to 95% of delayed puberty is constitutional delay of puberty. No single test reliably separates patients with constitutional delay from those with idiopathic hypogonadotropic hypogonadism.[7] This diagnosis is made by excluding the other causes, as discussed. However, using the guidelines in **Table 14.2**, one can confidently make a provisional diagnosis (**Table 14.2**).

Clues to Other Diagnoses

1. Gonadotropin deficiency
   a. Low serum FSH and LH levels, particularly if bone age is more than 13 years
   b. Low response to GnRH
   c. Abnormal central imaging study results

TABLE 14.2

Criteria for Provisional Diagnosis of Constitutional Delay of Puberty

Required Features

Detailed negative review of systems
Evidence of appropriate nutrition
Linear growth of at least 3.7 cm/y
Normal findings on physical examination, including genital anatomy, sense of smell, and U/L body-segment ratio
Normal CBC, sedimentation rate, normal thyroid function, and prepubertal levels of serum LH and FSH
Bone age delayed 1.5–4.0 y compared with chronologic age

Supportive Features

Family history of constitutional delay of puberty
Height between 3rd and 25th percentiles for chronologic age

U/L, upper-to-lower; CBC, complete blood cell; LH, luteinizing hormone; FSH, follicle-stimulating hormone.
From Barnes HV. Recognizing normal and abnormal growth and development during puberty. In: Moss AV, ed. *Pediatrics Update: Reviews for Physicians.* Elsevier–North Holland Publishing; 1979:103, with permission.

   d. History of neurologic symptoms, CNS infections, radiation, or disease
   e. Possible anosmia (Kallmann syndrome)
The presence of midline facial defects, anosmia, cryptorchidism, or microphallus strongly suggests idiopathic hypogonadotropic hypogonadism; however, the diagnosis cannot be firmly established until the patient reaches the age of 18 years and is still prepubertal. Genes for hypothalamic hypogonadism have been identified, as have some genes for familial pubertal delay.
2. Gonadal disorder
   a. History of gonadal radiation, surgery, infection, or trauma
   b. Significantly elevated FSH and LH
   c. Abnormal karyotype, such as 46,XY in a phenotypic girl
   d. Low upper/lower body-segment ratio
   e. Arm span may exceed height by >2 inches
   f. Significant gynecomastia in a boy
   g. Testes that are small for a given stage of puberty can be associated with 47,XXY (Klinefelter syndrome, see Fig. 14.4).
3. Turner syndrome: Excluding constitutional delay of puberty, one of the more common causes of maturation delay is Turner syndrome. The patient may have a 45,X karyotype, a mosaic karyotype such as 45,X/46,XX or ring or isochromosomes. Patients with Turner syndrome usually have some of the following characteristics:
   - Short stature
   - Streak gonads
   - Absent pubertal growth spurt
   - Poor development of secondary sexual characteristics, with less breast development than pubic hair development
   - Lymphedema
   - High arched palate
   - Strabismus
   - Hearing deficit due to chronic otitis
   - Cubitus valgus
   - Webbing of the neck
   - Low hairline
   - Shield-shaped chest
   - Coarctation of the aorta
   - Horseshoe kidneys
   - Short fourth metacarpal
   - Multiple pigmented nevi
   - Normal vagina, cervix, and uterus
   - Poor space-form perception

A karyotype is recommended in all girls with unexplained short stature, delayed puberty, webbed neck, lymphedema, or coarctation of the aorta.[8] Karyotype should also be considered for girls with a height below the fifth percentile and two or more features of Turner syndrome, such as high palate, nail dysplasia, short fourth metacarpal, and strabismus.

1. Chronic illness
   a. Abnormal findings on review of systems or physical examination
   b. Falling off height and weight curves at onset of disease
   c. Abnormal CBC count, sedimentation rate, or chemistry panel results

MANAGEMENT OF DELAYED PUBERTY

Once the presence of pubertal delay is established in a young person, an initial evaluation should be obtained, and it is reasonable to continue to closely monitor growth and development every 6 months for a year. If desired, it is also appropriate to refer to a pediatric endocrinologist for more specialized assessment. The young person should have interval measurements of growth, assessment of pubertal status by physical examination, and reassurance if progression of secondary sexual development is evident. There is no clinically available lab test that distinguishes constitutional delay from isolated hypogonadotropic hypogonadism, and close monitoring remains the best approach. After the first signs of testicular or breast enlargement are observed, follow-up at regular intervals is desirable to reassure the patient and parents that puberty is progressing. Since the testes begin to enlarge in males before increased testosterone production and increased growth velocity occur, support and guidance in dealing with the frustrations of delayed puberty are important, even after there is evidence that secondary sexual development has begun.

If the evaluation reveals primary gonadal insufficiency, cyclic estrogen and progestin therapy in girls or testosterone therapy in boys will be necessary. Adolescents with hypogonadotropic hypogonadism or hypopituitarism will also need estrogen or testosterone replacement, often with replacement of other hormones as well. Short courses of estrogen or testosterone are sometimes prescribed by pediatric endocrinologists to initiate development in constitutional delay of puberty.

Treatment for Females

In girls, there are several regimens for replacing estrogen and progesterone. If maximal preservation of linear growth is desired, estrogen is begun at a low dose, since height velocity is greater at low estrogen doses, and higher doses cause more rapid epiphyseal closure. The three phases of estrogen replacement are the following:

1. Induction of breast development and increase in height velocity in the patient with no secondary sexual development
2. Establishment of normal menses and increase in bone mineralization
3. Long-term maintenance of a normal estrogen state

Induction of Breast Development

In the first phase of pubertal induction for girls, estrogen replacement is administered at a low dose that is gradually increased every 6 to 12 months. The most common options include oral estrogens (micronized estradiol vs. conjugated estrogens) and transdermal estrogen (estradiol). Transdermal estrogens are preferred given increasing evidence of beneficial impacts on bone health and less alteration of clotting proteins (compared to oral preparations).[9] Injectable forms of estradiol can also be administered, but are less common. The induction of puberty with estrogen treatment is most appropriately managed by a pediatric endocrinologist. See **Table 14.3** for an estrogen dosing guideline.

TABLE 14.3

Recommended Estrogen Replacement Options for Feminization in Adolescent Turner Syndrome

Preparation	Pubertal Initiation Dose	Adult Dosing
Transdermal E2	3–7 mcg/d	25–100 mcg/d
Micronized 17β oral E2	0.25 mg/d	1–4 mg/d
Ethinyl estradiol	2 mcg/d	10–20 mcg/d
Depot E2	0.2 mg/mo	2 mg/mo

Adapted from Gravholt CH, Andersen NH, Conway GS, et al. Clinical practice guidelines for the care of girls and women with Turner syndrome: Proceedings from the 2016 Cincinnati International Turner Syndrome Meeting. *Eur J Endocrinol.* 2017;177(3):G1–G70. doi: 10.1530/EJE-17-0430

Induction of Menses

In the second phase of pubertal induction for females, menses are induced with an oral progestin (commonly micronized progesterone or medroxyprogesterone) that is administered monthly for 10 to 12 days. Progestin treatment is typically initiated either once breakthrough bleeding occurs or after 18 months to 2 years of estrogen treatment due to the risk of endometrial hyperplasia associated with prolonged unopposed estrogen.[10]

Long-Term Estrogen Replacement

In the third phase, a long-term approach is established and can either involve one of aforementioned forms of estrogen plus monthly progestin treatment given 10 to 12 days per month or replacement can be given as a combined estrogen–progestin preparation, orally or transdermally.

Oral estrogens pass first through the liver, which could increase side effects, including the hepatic synthesis of clotting proteins. Transdermal alternatives include estradiol patches (Vivelle Dot, Climara, Alora, and Estraderm), which are changed once or twice a week depending on the preparation. An oral progestin (medroxyprogesterone 10 mg or micronized progesterone 200 mg) is added for 10 to 12 days each month.

Many patients with delayed puberty have decreased bone density for age. The optimal dose of estrogen replacement for increasing bone density in adolescents remains to be established, but it is probably higher than in menopausal females. A bone density measurement by dual-energy x-ray absorptiometry (DXA) of the hip and spine at baseline and every 2 years is sometimes recommended in adolescents on estrogen or testosterone replacement. Bone density is compared with age-matched norms. The importance of appropriate calcium (1,300 mg/d for adolescents) intake by diet or supplements and at least 600 IU vitamin D to support bone calcification should be stressed at each visit. The timing of initiation of sex steroid therapy to achieve maximum height depends on the patient's chronologic and skeletal age and current height velocity.

Treatment for Boys

In boys with constitutional delay of puberty, 6-month courses of intramuscular (IM) testosterone enanthate or cypionate 50 mg monthly can be used to initiate secondary sexual development. Exposure to testosterone may speed the onset of the patient's own puberty. Since sex steroids cause fusion of epiphyses, care must be taken in the timing and monitoring of these therapies so that final height is not compromised. These patients should therefore be referred to an endocrinologist for treatment. The timing of such an intervention must take into account such complex issues as psychosocial stress, self-image, and school performance, which appear to be more affected by pubertal delay than by short stature alone.

Males with gonadal failure, hypopituitarism, or hypothalamic hypogonadism are maintained on long-term testosterone replacement using testosterone gel or IM testosterone replacement. They should receive adequate dietary calcium and vitamin D and should consider DXA scans for spinal and hip bone density measurements since they are at risk for a low bone mass. In both males and females whose delayed puberty is due to abnormalities in hypothalamic GnRH secretion that do not correct with time, fertility can be achieved using a small pump to deliver pulses of GnRH intravenously or subcutaneously for weeks or months. Some GnRH-deficient males will achieve spermatogenesis with human chorionic gonadotropin (hCG) alone or in combination with FSH. Ovulation can be induced by FSH and hCG in GnRH-deficient females.

Treatment of Specific Conditions

Hypothyroidism

Treatment is begun with levothyroxine (see Chapter 12). Thyroid function tests should be repeated in 6 weeks and the dose is adjusted to maintain the TSH concentration in the reference interval. Nonadherence with medication is often the underlying issue in teens whose TSH is elevated despite receiving unusually high doses of thyroid replacement. A 7-day pill package and adult supervision of doses may be helpful. Once the dose is established, thyroid tests are repeated at 6-month intervals. Catch-up growth is expected when thyroid hormone replacement is initiated, but patients who have been untreated for several years will lose some adult height.

Turner Syndrome and Gonadal Dysgenesis

Short stature associated with Turner syndrome can be treated with human growth hormone (hGH). The FDA and other worldwide regulatory agencies have approved the use of hGH for statural improvement in Turner syndrome. The hGH therapy should be ideally started before adolescent years, around age 4 to 6 or younger if indicated, and preferably before 12 to 13 years if the child is deemed an appropriate candidate for treatment. Indications for initiation of treatment include evidence of growth failure over 6 months without other identified treatable causes of poor growth.[11] The dose used is approximately double that used for subjects with classic GH deficiency. Data from the National Cooperative Growth Study from Genentech have shown GH to be effective in improving the final height of girls with Turner syndrome. Growth hormone treatment is most commonly managed by a pediatric endocrinology team. Estrogen replacement is usually initiated around age 12 to 13 (by age 14) unless the patient is predicted to be extremely short, in which case some delay of estrogen administration can be appropriate.

If there is a Y chromosome present on the karyotype to diagnose Turner syndrome, the patient will require gonadectomy. However, Y chromosomal material, rather than a full Y chromosome, may be present in girls who are virilized, either at birth or with puberty. These girls should have fluorescent in situ hybridization for the Y chromosome to ensure that no Y chromosomal material has been translocated. The presence of any Y material is an indication for gonadectomy, to prevent potential malignant neoplasias. Surgery should be followed by hormonal replacement therapy during and after puberty.

Chronic Illness

Treatment of pubertal delay caused by chronic illness necessitates treating the underlying disorder. For example, cystic fibrosis transmembrane conductance regulator (CFTR) potentiators in cystic fibrosis, gluten-free diet in celiac disease, corrective surgery for congenital heart disease, and hyperalimentation in IBD usually result in catch-up growth and maturity. Medications such as steroids or antimetabolites can inhibit growth. Catch-up growth can be observed after discontinuation of treatment with these drugs. In patients with chronic renal failure, there may be some growth after improved nutrition and hemodialysis or transplantation. However, many patients with chronic renal failure remain short. Growth hormone can be administered to subjects with chronic renal failure before transplantation to improve height, without causing deterioration of underlying renal function.

 PATIENT EDUCATION

Young adolescents are preoccupied with their physical appearance. Any variation from the normal timing of sexual development is a major source of embarrassment to them and evokes feelings of personal inadequacy. A review of a patient's progress on their individual pubertal growth and growth chart can help reassure them that growth is proceeding in a pattern that is appropriate. For patients who have a permanent defect in reproductive function, counseling and support from both the primary health clinician and medical specialist can be helpful in enabling the patient to establish a positive self-image of themself as a capable adult. Further counseling by a mental health professional may be necessary. Questions about fertility should be answered as they arise, with emphasis on the patient's ability to function normally as a marriage partner and parent of adopted children. With current technology, pregnancies are possible using in vitro fertilization with donor eggs and other assisted reproductive technologies in patients with ovarian insufficiency.

PRECOCIOUS PUBERTY

Definition

In boys, development before age 9 years is considered precocious. Early development in boys is rare. There are 10 times as many girls with precocious puberty as boys. There has been controversy over the definition of precocious puberty in North American girls, and more specifically the age at which a more extensive workup is warranted. In girls, the cutoff has traditionally been 8 years or 2.5 SDs below the average of breast development. There are practice variations in the extent of workup for girls between ages 6 and 7 years. Girls with central precocious puberty under age 6 years typically undergo MRI, but the yield in girls between ages 6 and 7 years has led to debate regarding the cost-effectiveness of this intervention given the relatively low rate of identifiable pathology.[12–13]

In addition, girls with precocious puberty with rapid progression or unusual progression of puberty, a predicted height below 150 cm or 2 SDs below target midparental height, those with neurologic symptoms, pubertal timing that is a significant outlier from family, or girls who are having psychological difficulty due to early puberty should be referred for further evaluation and consideration of possible suppression of puberty with GnRH analog therapy. Puberty is normally held back in humans during childhood by inhibitory connections to the hypothalamus, which suppress GnRH pulsations. If these inhibitory connections are damaged, GnRH pulse amplitude increases and central puberty ensues. There is often a family history of early puberty in girls with precocious puberty, and studies in recent years have begun to identify genes associated with precocious puberty including MKRN3, DLK1, KISS1, and KISS1R.

The vast majority of girls with central precocious puberty have idiopathic precocious puberty. Boys are much more likely to have a specific lesion causing their precocity.

Causes

Central causes of precocious puberty include the following:
1. Central nervous system tumors (optic gliomas, craniopharyngiomas, dysgerminomas, ependymoma)
2. Central nervous system malformations (hamartomas, arachnoid and suprasellar cysts, hydrocephalus, septo-optic dysplasia)
3. Infiltrative lesions (histiocytosis, granulomas, abscess)
4. Central nervous system damage (irradiation, trauma, meningitis, encephalitis)

Gonadotropin-independent causes of precocity in girls include the following:

1. Ovarian cysts, sometimes with McCune–Albright syndrome
2. Ovarian or adrenal estrogen-secreting tumors
3. Severe hypothyroidism
4. Exposure to exogenous estrogen

In boys, in addition to the central causes listed above, precocious puberty can be caused by androgen exposure, congenital adrenal hyperplasia, gonadal and adrenal tumors secreting androgens, hCG secreting tumors, and familial activating mutations of the LH receptor.

Incomplete Forms of Precocious Puberty

Premature Thelarche

Premature thelarche occurs often in female infants and toddlers. Self-limited breast budding, which is also transient, occurs in girls aged 6 and above. There is no sustained growth spurt or bone age advancement in these girls. Breast budding may appear and recede several times before sustained puberty ensues.

Premature Adrenarche

Benign premature adrenarche presents with underarm odor, and pubic and/or axillary hair development usually at ages 6 to 8 years. Bone age is often slightly advanced (1 year) and adrenal androgens are in the pubertal range. Premature adrenarche has been associated with an increased risk of developing ovarian hyperandrogenism (often known as polycystic ovary syndrome).[14] Patients with a history of intrauterine growth restriction followed by excessive weight gain and insulin resistance in childhood may present with premature adrenarche. They are also at increased risk for polycystic ovary syndrome and sometimes glucose intolerance as teens. Virilization in girls is rare and can be due to an androgen-secreting adrenal or ovarian tumor, topical androgen exposure, or congenital adrenal hyperplasia. Symptoms of virilization include deepening of the voice, clitoromegaly, or muscular development, along with rapid growth and bone age advancement. A thorough evaluation is required.

Evaluation of Precocious Puberty

History

History includes a review of family history of endocrine or pubertal disorders, timing of puberty in family members, use of estrogen- or androgen-containing gels by family members, and heights of family members. The patient's past history should be reviewed for evidence of predisposing medical conditions. The growth chart should be obtained.

Physical Examination

The physical examination includes careful measurement of height and weight, vital signs, examination of the skin for large irregular café au lait spots suggestive of McCune–Albright syndrome, examination of the fundi, assessment for thyroid enlargement, abdominal examination, and examination of SMR (measurement of breast or testicular and phallic dimensions, and pubic hair staging). The vaginal introitus can be examined for signs of estrogen effect on the labia minora and presence of leukorrhea in the frog-leg position. Internal examination is not necessary unless unexplained vaginal bleeding is present in which case an experienced observer can often visualize the vagina and cervix in the knee–chest position without instrumentation. In boys, the testicular examination should focus on any testicular asymmetry or masses, or phallic enlargement without testicular enlargement suggesting a source of androgens outside of the testes, such as congenital adrenal hyperplasia.

Laboratory Evaluation

A bone age x-ray of the left hand and wrist is useful. If the bone age is greater than 2 SD advanced, additional evaluation should be considered. A baseline prediction of adult height can be made using the average charts from the Bayley–Pinneau table at the back of the *Greulich and Pyle Atlas of Skeletal Maturation* (see Chapter 1 for details).

Laboratory evaluation might include an 8 am LH, FSH, estradiol, DHEAS, 17-hydroxyprogesterone (17-OH progesterone), and TSH in girls, and a testosterone and 8 am 17-OH progesterone and DHEAS, hCG, LH, and FSH in boys. The LH and FSH will be in the prepubertal range in the early stages of central puberty, with an LH level typically less than 0.1 to 0.3 I U/L depending on the assay. By the time breast or gonadal development is in SMR stage 3, LH and FSH are often in the pubertal range. To confirm central puberty, it is sometimes necessary to do a GnRH or GnRH analog stimulation test (GnRH itself is now unavailable) during which GnRH or GnRH analog is administered and LH, FSH, and estradiol/testosterone are assessed at 1, 2, and 3 hours. If estradiol is markedly elevated (more than 100 pg/mL) and LH and FSH are suppressed, an ovarian cyst or more rarely tumor is suspected. A pelvic ultrasonography can be done in girls if an ovarian cyst or tumor is thought to be the cause of the precocity. In boys, an hCG level should be checked to rule out an hCG-producing tumor that could be causing testosterone production. A cranial MRI with contrast should be done to rule out CNS lesion in all boys with central precocious puberty, in all girls younger than 6 years, and should be considered in girls between 6 and 8 years of age depending on the clinical history. An adrenocorticotropic hormone stimulation test may be needed if congenital adrenal hyperplasia is suspected as a cause of androgen excess.

Treatment of Precocious Puberty

If the evaluation has not revealed a specific treatable cause of precocious puberty and the child has central precocious puberty, GnRH analog treatment should be considered. Most girls in the 7- to 9-year range do not require treatment for suppression of puberty.[15] Many girls in this age range have a slow intermittent progression of their puberty and reach a final height that is not short. Often, parents are most worried about how they will handle menses in a grade school child, and can be reassured that menarche may not be imminent in most cases and that menses can be suppressed if necessary. Untreated girls should be followed up at 6-month to 1-year intervals. GnRH analog therapy can be administered for precocious puberty if indicated and comes in various formulations including 1-month, 3-month, and 6-month depot form, as well as a histrelin-acetate implant. Luteinizing hormone, FSH, and estradiol in girls or testosterone in boys can be obtained 1 to 2 hours after the depot leuprolide to document adequate suppression of puberty on therapy after 2 to 3 months of treatment. Partial suppression of puberty has been achieved in girls with gonadotropin-independent puberty (McCune–Albright syndrome) with aromatase inhibitors. Similar regimens with antiandrogens and aromatase inhibitors have been used in boys with familial LH-activating mutations.

SUMMARY

In order to identify abnormal growth and development, it is important to have a clear understanding of normal growth and development while also recognizing that an individual's adult height and timing of puberty are strongly influenced by genetic factors. The range of normal variability in growth is defined as 2 SDs above and below the mean. Concerns that would prompt evaluation of statural growth include linear growth rate <4 cm/y prior to average age of peak growth velocity, lack of appropriate growth acceleration during puberty, or unexpected deceleration of linear growth. A projected height more than 2 SDs below mean for age or more than 2 SDs below the midparental target height would also warrant an evaluation. The timing and tempo of pubertal development varies and is often dictated by genetic factors, though can also be affected by external influences such as poor health or environmental and social stressors. Delayed puberty is defined by absence of breast budding by 13 years in females or lack of testicular enlargement by 14 years in boys, both are 2.5 SDs beyond average age of onset. Precocious puberty is defined in boys as development before age 9 years and is uncommon and more concerning for pathology. The definition of precocious puberty in North American girls is less straightforward and traditionally has been defined as development before 8 years. There are practice variations around the evaluation of girls who develop between age 6 and 7 years and they may be less extensive than the evaluation of a girl who develops before the age of 6 years, which would include an MRI of the pituitary region. The treatment of linear growth concerns and abnormal pubertal development can be nuanced and complicated, hence often are best directed by pediatric endocrinologists.

REFERENCES

1. Muñoz-Hyoys A, Molina-Carballo A, Augustin-Morales M, et al. Psychosocial dwarfism: psychopathological aspects and putative neuroendocrine markers. *Psychiatry Res.* 2011;188(1):96–101. doi: 10.1016/j.psychres.2010.10.004
2. Gruelich WW, Pyle SI. *Atlas of Skeletal Development of the Hand and Wrist.* 2nd ed. Stanford University Press; 1959.
3. Grimberg A, DiVall SA, Polychronakos C, et al. Guidelines for growth hormone and insulin-like growth factor-1 treatment in children and adolescents: growth hormone deficiency, idiopathic short stature, and primary insulin-like growth factor-1 deficiency. *Horm Res Paediatr.* 2016;86(6):361–397. doi: 10.1159/000452150
4. Bell J, Parker, KL, Swinford RD, et al. Long term safety of recombinant human growth hormone in children. *J Clin Endocrinol Metab.* 2021;95(1):167–177.
5. Aksglaede L, Juul A. Testicular function and fertility in men with Klinefelter syndrome: a review. *Eur J Endocrinol.* 2013;168(4):R67–R76. doi:10.1530/EJE-12-0934
6. Bayley N, Pinneau SR. Tables for predicting adult height from skeletal age: revised for use with the Greulich–Pyle hand standards. *J Pediatr.* 1952;40(4):423–441. Accessed April 24, 2015. http://www.ncbi.nlm.nih.gov/pubmed/14918032
7. Harrington J, Palmert MR. Clinical review: distinguishing constitutional delay of growth and puberty from isolated hypogonadotropic hypogonadism: critical appraisal of available diagnostic tests. *J Clin Endocrinol Metab.* 2012;97(9):3056–3067. doi: 10.1210/jc.2012-1598
8. Apperley L, Das U, Ramakrishnana R, et al. Mode of clinical presentation and delayed diagnosis of Turner syndrome: a single centre UK study. *Int J Pediatr Endocrinol.* 2018;2018:4. doi: 10.1186/s13633-018-0058-1
9. Misra M, Katzman D, Miller KK, et al. Physiologic estrogen replacement increases bone density in adolescent girls with anorexia nervosa. *J Bone Miner Res.* 2011;26(10):2430–2438. doi: 10.1002/jbmr.447
10. Klein KO, Rosenfield RL, Santen RJ, et al. Estrogen replacement in Turner syndrome: literature review and practical considerations. *J Clin Endocrinol Metab.* 2018;103(5):1790–1803. doi: 10.1210/jc.2017-02183
11. Gravholt CH, Andersen NH, Conway, GS, et al. Clinical practice guidelines for the care of girls and women with Turner syndrome: proceeding from the 2016 Cincinnati International Turner Syndrome Meeting. *Eur J Endocrinol.* 2017;177(3):G1–G70. doi: 10.1530/EJE-17-0430
12. Cantas-Orsdemir S, Garb JL, Allen HF. Prevalence of cranial MRI findings in girls with central precocious puberty: a systematic review and meta-analysis. *J Pediatr Endocrinol Metab.* 2018;31(7):701–710. doi: 10.1515/jpem-2018-0052
13. Gohil A, Eugster EA. Delayed and precocious puberty: genetic underpinnings and treatments. *Endocrinol Metab Clin North Am.* 2020;49(4):741–757. doi: 10.1016/j.ecl.2020.08.002
14. Ibáñez L, Oberfield SE, Witchel S, et al. An international consortium update: pathophysiology, diagnosis, and treatment of polycystic ovarian syndrome in adolescence. *Horm Res Paediatr.* 2017;88(6):371–395.
15. Carel JC, Eugster EA, Rogol A, et al. Consensus statement on the use of gonadotropin-releasing hormone analogs in children. *Pediatrics.* 2009;123(4):e752–e762. doi:10.1542/peds.2008-1783

🛜 ADDITIONAL RESOURCES AND WEBSITES

Additional Resources and Websites for Clinicians:
https://academic.oup.com/jcem/article/89/7/3140/2844076
Clinical Resource Library | Pediatric Endocrine Society (pedsendo.org)
http://pedsendo.org/clinical-resource/consensus-on-use-of-gonadotropin-releasing-hormone-analogs-in-children-pediatrics-2009/
https://mk0pesendoklgy8upp97.kinstacdn.com/wp-content/uploads/2020/09/Child-with-suspected-short-stature-final.pdf

Additional Resources and Websites for Parents/Caregivers:
MAGIC Foundation—https://www.magicfoundation.org/
PES delayed puberty in boys handout—https://pedsendo.org/patient-resource/delayed-puberty-boys/
PES delayed puberty in girls handout—https://pedsendo.org/patient-resource/delayed-puberty-girls/
PES precocious puberty handout—https://pedsendo.org/patient-resource/precocious-puberty/
PES short stature handout—https://pedsendo.org/patient-resource/short-stature/
The Turner Syndrome Society of the United States—https://turnersyndromefoundation.org/

Additional Resources and Websites for Adolescents and Young Adults:
The Every Body Book: The LGBTQ+ Inclusive Guide for Kids about Sex, Gender, Bodies, and Families. By Rachel E Simon, Noah Grigni
https://kidshealth.org/en/teens/sexual-health/?WT.ac=t-nav-sexual-health
Short: Walking Tall When You're Not Tall at All. By John Schwartz—https://www.amazon.com/dp/B003H4I4HM/ref=cm_sw_r_em_api_glt_TJ429JBM39CGNRTWDJYF
The Turner Syndrome Society of the United States—https://turnersyndromefoundation.org/

15

Thyroid Function and Disease in Adolescents and Young Adults

Cecilia A. Larson

KEY WORDS

- Goiter
- Graves disease
- Hyperthyroidism
- Hypothyroidism
- Thyroid cancer
- Thyroid nodules
- Thyroid-stimulating hormone

INTRODUCTION

The thyroid is both affected by and contributes to diverse aspects of development, including physical and intellectual growth and sexual development. There are thyroid receptors throughout the body that mediate the effects of thyroid hormone, that is itself regulated by pituitary thyroid-stimulating hormone (TSH), which in turn is regulated by hypothalamic thyroid-releasing hormone (TRH). Disruption of the normal process of thyroid regulation affects thyroid function, causing either underactivity (hypothyroidism) or overactivity (hyperthyroidism) of the thyroid gland. In addition to disorders of thyroid function, adolescents and young adults (AYAs) are susceptible to structural disorders of the thyroid, including thyromegaly and nodular thyroid disease. Timely detection and treatment of thyroid disease during adolescence and early adulthood is essential for normal growth and development. This chapter discusses both functional and growth disorders of the thyroid, and presents an approach to detection, evaluation, and management of these disorders. The framework for recognition of thyroid disorders relies on an understanding of thyroid development, a complete medical history, physical examination, and laboratory and imaging evaluations.

THYROID MIGRATION, GROWTH, AND FUNCTION DURING DEVELOPMENT

- The thyroid gland forms during the first trimester of fetal development from the medial and lateral anlagen and follows a complex migratory path.
- Insufficient migration can lead to a lingual thyroid. Lingual thyroids may cause obstruction of the upper airway or develop thyroid cancer, but are not routinely removed if complications do not develop.
- Partial nonclosure of the migratory tract can lead to a thyroglossal duct cyst; thyroglossal duct cysts are usually benign and not of clinical significance unless infection of the cyst occurs, which may require surgical intervention.
- Postnatally and up to age 8 years, thyroid growth is similar and steady in males and females.

- During puberty, there is more than a fourfold increase in thyroid volume, which correlates not only with age and gender, but also with weight, height, body mass index (BMI), and pubertal stage.[1]
- By the end of puberty, the average weight of the female thyroid is 14.4 g, and for the male, it is 16.4 g.[2]
- Despite the significant increase in growth of the thyroid during puberty, levels of free thyroxine (fT_4) and TSH decrease from age 1 year to adulthood.
- There is an increase in thyroid disorders of both structure and function during puberty.

FOCUSED MEDICAL HISTORY

Medical conditions and genetic syndromes that are associated with an increased risk of thyroid functional disorders include the following:
- Trisomy 21
- Turner syndrome
- Klinefelter syndrome
- Autoimmune disorders (personal or family history)
  - Rheumatoid arthritis
  - Diabetes mellitus type 1
  - Celiac disease
  - Autoimmune polyglandular syndrome
  Iodine exposure increases risk of thyroid functional disorders.
- Computed tomography (CT) scan with iodinated contrast
- Kelp or seaweed supplements
- Amiodarone which contains iodine
  Medications that can affect thyroid function include the following:
- Lithium
- Valproate
- Amiodarone
- Interferon
- Thionamides
- Interleukin-2
- Tyrosine kinase inhibitors
- Dopamine
- Dobutamine
- Glucocorticoids
- Bexarotene
  Thyroid cancer risk is increased in specific syndromes and with positive family history of certain types of thyroid cancer:
- Cowden syndrome
- Bannayan–Riley–Ruvalcaba syndrome
- Gardner syndrome
- Multiple endocrine neoplasia (MEN) type 2
- Familial medullary thyroid cancer (MTC)

- Familial papillary thyroid cancer (PTC)
- Carney complex type 1

Ionizing radiation exposure increases risk of both functional (hypothyroidism) and structural disorders, increasing the risk of both benign nodule and cancer formation.

- Radiation treatment for childhood cancers
- Fallout from nuclear reactor accidents

The review of symptoms is especially relevant since thyroid hormone affects so many different tissues and organ systems. For a list of functional symptoms associated with thyroid activity, see **Table 15.1**.

Structural symptoms such as airway or esophageal obstruction and hoarseness are less common than functional symptoms, although structural signs such as an enlarged thyroid commonly lead to thyroid evaluation.

PHYSICAL EVALUATION OF THYROID STRUCTURE

- Inspection, palpation, and imaging by ultrasound, CT, or magnetic resonance imaging (MRI), all provide information about the physical aspects of the thyroid gland.
- Inspection (see Fig. 15.1) and palpation are best evaluated while the patient swallows, causing the thyroid to elevate. Ultrasound of the thyroid is the preferred imaging modality to assess thyroid gland structure. It allows for quantification of the size of the gland or a lesion, so it can be monitored and compared with a subsequent ultrasound. In addition, it can also identify features that aid in clarifying the diagnosis of thyroid enlargement.

TABLE 15.1
Clinical Effects of Thyroid Hormone

Clinical Effect	Hyperthyroidism	Hypothyroidism
Height velocity	Increased	Decreased
Weight	Decreased	Increased
Temperature	Increased in extreme cases	Decreased in extreme cases
Hair and skin	Oily and hair loss diffusely Pretibial myxedema[a]	Dry Myxedema generalized
Fingernails	Ridges	Brittle
Bowels	Increased frequency	Constipation
Cardiac	Increased heart rate Atrial fibrillation	Decreased heart rate
Menstruation	Lighter flow, irregular menses	Heavier flow, irregular menses
Skeleton	Bone loss Advanced bone age	Normal bone density Delayed bone age
Blood pressure	Systolic hypertension Increased mean arterial pressure	Diastolic hypertension
Eyes	Stare, lid lag, dry eye, exophthalmos[a]	Periorbital edema
Reflexes	Normal	Delayed relaxation
Cognition	Decreased school performance	Decreased school performance

[a]Associated specifically with Graves hyperthyroidism.

- While thyroid function and gland size and structure are sometimes related, it is important to recognize that hypo-, hyper-, and euthyroidism can exist in normal, small, enlarged (goitrous), or nodular thyroid glands. Thus, it is critical to assess both structure and function of the thyroid.
- Autoimmune thyroiditis
  - Diffuse heterogeneity is present; thyroid enlargement may or may not be present.
- Nodule(s)
  - Lower risk for cancer; nodule typically palpable
    - Hyperechoic peripheral vascularity
    - Spongiform appearance
    - Resembles puff or Napoleon pastry
    - Comet-tail shadowing
  - Increased risk for cancer
    - Hypoechoic
    - Microcalcifications
    - Central vascularity
    - Irregular margins
    - Incomplete halo
    - Nodule is taller than wide.
    - Significant growth of nodule

LABORATORY EVALUATION OF THYROID FUNCTION

Thyroid function is typically assessed by measuring blood tests associated with thyroid activity, and can aid in determining whether the signs and symptoms that the individual displays are indeed related to thyroid status. The most useful test is TSH, followed by fT_4. In selected situations, total triiodothyronine (T_3), reverse T_3 (rT_3), and thyroid antibody testing are necessary and helpful in establishing a diagnosis and/or monitoring response to therapy.

- Thyroid-stimulating hormone is the most sensitive assay of thyroid function in steady-state situations.
- When TSH is abnormal, and/or if a central (hypothalamic or pituitary) abnormality is suspected, fT_4 is also measured.
- Total T_3 is helpful when TSH is suppressed to identify and monitor response to antithyroid treatment in Graves disease.
- In inflammatory thyrotoxicosis due to release of preformed thyroid hormone, the ratio of T_4:T_3 is preserved (4:1).
- When acute illness is a factor, rT_3 levels can be measured. If rT_3 is elevated, this finding suggests that the changes observed in TSH, including early suppression followed by elevation, are associated with the acute illness and recovery phases. A "sick-euthyroid" pattern may also be reflected by a low total T_3, a pattern common in AYAs with eating disorders.
- The most specific thyroid antibody is thyroid-stimulating antibody (TSAb), which is typically measured in hyperthyroid patients to confirm Graves disease.
- Thyroid peroxidase (TPO) antibody is the most sensitive antibody to detect autoimmune thyroid disease and can be elevated in patients with either hypo- or hyperthyroidism. It is most helpful in subclinical hypothyroidism where fT_4 is normal, while there is a mild TSH elevation (i.e., <10 mIU/L). In this clinical setting, the presence of elevated TPO antibodies is associated with higher risk for overt hypothyroidism and can be an indication for thyroid hormone treatment.

RADIOLOGIC EVALUATION OF THYROID FUNCTION

The nuclear medicine thyroid scans allow the use of a small dose of a radioactive tracer whose thyroid and whole-body uptake can be imaged and quantified. There are three main uses of nuclear medicine studies for thyroid disorders:

1. Quantification of uptake in hyperthyroidism where increased uptake is consistent with Graves disease, while decreased

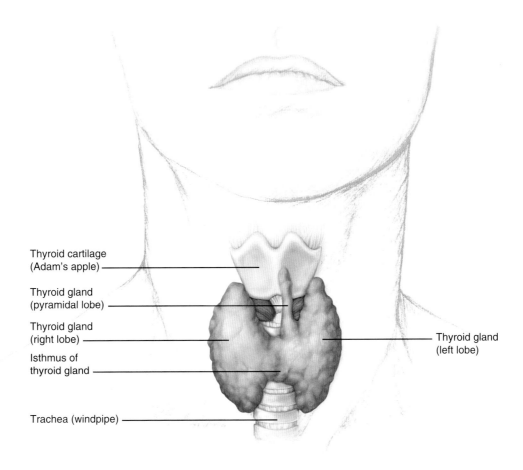

Thyroid cartilage
(Adam's apple)

Thyroid gland
(pyramidal lobe)

Thyroid gland
(right lobe)

Isthmus of
thyroid gland

Thyroid gland
(left lobe)

Trachea (windpipe)

FIGURE 15.1 Location of the thyroid. (Asset provided by Anatomical Chart Co.)

uptake suggests either exogenous thyroid ingestion or release of preformed thyroid hormone associated with inflammatory thyroiditis

2. Assessment of pattern of uptake to determine if a nodule is toxic or cold
   - Toxic nodule—nodule takes up tracer and suppresses the rest of the gland; fine-needle aspiration generally not necessary.
   - Cold nodule—nodule takes up less tracer than the rest of the gland; this requires further evaluation by fine-needle aspiration.
3. Determination if iodine-avid thyroid tissue exists after complete thyroidectomy for thyroid cancer

ROLE OF GENETIC TESTING IN THYROID DISEASE

Many genes have been identified that affect thyroid development and function, as well as the risk of thyroid cancer.
- The paired box gene (PAX-8), tissue transcription factor (TTF-2), and connexin genes are associated with abnormally located or absent thyroid glands in neonates.[3]
- Rearrangements in peroxisome proliferator-activated receptor gamma and PAX-8 genes are found in follicular thyroid cancers (FTCs).[4]
- Rearranged during transfection (RET) oncogene rearrangements are common in PTC in children.[5]
- Mutations in the v-raf murine sarcoma viral oncogene homolog B1 (BRAF) are common in adults with PTC.[6]
- Multiple endocrine neoplasia type 2 and familial medullary thyroid carcinoma syndromes are associated with RET oncogene mutations.

There are currently two specific situations where genetic testing has led to improved outcomes:
1. Screening at-risk individuals for the presence of specific RET mutations has helped identify and guide timing for prophylactic thyroidectomy, even prior to the development of MTC. Screening has improved outcome.[7]
2. In adults, fine-needle aspiration specimens with atypia of unknown significance for the presence of gene expression classifiers can be useful for identifying nodules associated with a high risk of cancer.[8]

It is likely that additional genetic testing will be developed to aid in risk stratification for individuals with nodules and for individuals with positive family history of thyroid cancer.

THYROID DISORDERS

Thyroid Structural Disorders
Thyromegaly
- Worldwide, the leading cause of an enlarged thyroid (goiter) is *iodine deficiency* leading to hypothyroidism with TSH-stimulated thyroid growth in an attempt to better capture the limited iodine in the diet.
- In *iodine-sufficient* areas such as the United States, the leading cause of an enlarged gland is inflammatory thyroiditis.
- Thyroid size is a function of gender, weight, BMI, and age. A simplified formula for estimation of normal size of the gland is $T = 1.48 + 0.054A$ where T is weight of the thyroid in grams and A is the age in months.[9]

- It is important to distinguish thyroid enlargement from other causes of neck swelling such as the following:
  - Neck fold fatty tissue
  - Increased strap muscle tissue
  - Lymph node or other glandular or soft tissue swelling

If it is not possible to discern the cause of the neck swelling, ultrasound of the neck can be helpful. The clinician should indicate the region of concern at the time of the ultrasound.

The serum TSH concentration is the pivotal test in determining what additional labs and imaging are necessary. When TSH is suppressed, the most common cause of thyromegaly is Graves disease with symmetric and diffuse gland hypertrophy, followed by nodular goiter, which usually causes asymmetric and irregular gland enlargement. The necessary additional testing is as follows:

- Free thyroxine
- Total T_3
- Thyroid-stimulating antibody
- Thyroid scan followed by ultrasound, if necessary

If TSH is normal or elevated, the additional labs and imaging needed are the following:

- Free thyroxine
- Thyroid peroxidase antibodies
- Thyroid ultrasound—this will show signs of inflammation, nodules, or cysts, and also quantify the gland dimensions.

Rarely, thyroid glands require surgery due to their size and location causing obstructive symptoms (e.g., dysphonia, hoarseness, difficulty swallowing or breathing, or cough). When obstructive symptoms exist, it may be helpful to get additional studies such as the following:

- Pulmonary function to assess for airway obstruction
- Swallowing study
- Direct laryngoscopy to look for vocal cord dysfunction

Thyroid Nodules

Thyroid nodules can be palpated in 1.8% of children between the ages of 11 and 18 years old. However, only 0.45% of these same individuals will have nodules 20 years later, indicating that many nodules spontaneously regress without intervention.[10] The concern about thyroid nodules is the potential for malignancy. While malignancy is rare (0.5% of all nodules), morbidity and mortality are increased in thyroid cancer that is detected late. Nodules that are associated with obstructive symptoms (e.g., hoarseness, or difficulty swallowing) are more likely to be cancerous.

After detecting a nodule, the next step is measurement of TSH. There is a correlation between TSH and risk of thyroid cancer; increases in TSH carry higher cancer risk, which may relate to the pathogenic role of TSH elevation in carcinogenesis. Furthermore, toxic thyroid nodules carry a low risk of thyroid cancer; thus, if TSH is suppressed, the thyroid should next be imaged by nuclear thyroid scanning with I-123. If the nodule concentrates iodine, it can be managed as a toxic thyroid nodule, but such nodules are rare in adolescence. If the TSH is suppressed and the nodule does not concentrate iodine, or if the TSH is elevated or normal, thyroid ultrasound is indicated. Nodules greater than 0.9 cm are generally biopsied, especially if other concerning ultrasound findings are present. Biopsy can be performed by fine-needle aspiration typically done with ultrasound guidance. There are numerous potential pathologic results detected by fine-needle aspiration, with varying positive predictive values for the presence of malignancy. The spectrum of results includes the following:

1. Nondiagnostic specimens with insufficient material for diagnosis
2. Benign, consistent with macrofollicular adenoma
3. Atypical cells of unknown significance
4. Consistent with follicular neoplasm
5. Suspicious for PTC
6. Suspicious for other malignancy
   i. Medullary thyroid cancer
   ii. Intrathyroidal lymphoma
   iii. Metastases from another primary tumor

It is important to prepare the patient and the family for this wide range of results prior to biopsy and to guide them through the next diagnostic and treatment steps based on the pathologic findings.

Thyroid Cancers

Differentiated thyroid cancers (PTC and FTC) and MTC should generally be treated initially with complete thyroidectomy by an experienced, high-volume thyroid surgeon. Long-term outcomes for these two categories differ. The survival rates for MTC at 15 and 30 years are 86% and 15%, respectively. At the same time points, the survival rates for PTC and FTC are 95% to 97% and 91% to 92%, respectively.[11]

Management of Differentiated Thyroid Cancer Ninety-five percent of thyroid cancer in adolescents is of the differentiated thyroid cancer type, of which the vast majority is PTC. Although there is a higher risk for multifocal disease and presence of extrathyroidal extension of tumor at diagnosis, prognosis for differentiated thyroid cancer survival is as good as or better than that of adults.

- Adolescents and young adults should undergo complete thyroidectomy.
- Use of radioiodine ablation can be reserved for those with the following high-risk features[12]:
  - Distant metastases
  - Vascular invasion
  - Gross extrathyroidal extension
  - Tumor size >1.0 to 2.0 cm
  - Tumor type: Tall cell, columnar cell, insular or poorly differentiated
- Follow-up consists of lifelong monitoring of the following:
  - Thyroid-stimulating hormone (aim to keep at the lower range of normal)
  - Thyroglobulin
  - Thyroglobulin antibodies
  - Neck exam and ultrasound
  - Iodine imaging when necessary

Management of Medullary Thyroid Cancer In individuals with a history of MTC, monitoring includes the following:

- Calcitonin
- Carcinoembryonic antigen
- Ultrasound follow-up

Thyroglobulin levels and iodine scanning/treatment are not indicated since the cell of origin for medullary thyroid cancer is the neuroendocrine C cell, which does not take up iodine or produce thyroglobulin. In kindreds with MTC, the RET gene is autosomal dominant with high penetrance and there is a strong genotype–phenotype correlation, such that there are age-specific guidelines for RET testing and, if necessary, prophylactic thyroidectomy.[7,13]

Functional Thyroid Disorders

The thyroid gland produces the two thyroid hormones T_4 and T_3 in a 4:1 ratio. The overabundance of T_4 (relative to T_3) serves as a reservoir of available thyroid hormone that can quickly be upregulated or downregulated, depending on the need for active thyroid hormone.

In addition to making thyroid hormones, the thyroid also produces thyroglobulin, which binds to the thyroid hormones within the thyroid follicles.

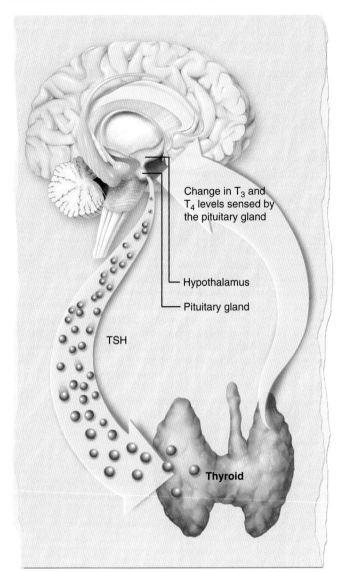

FIGURE 15.2 Feedback loop for thyroid hormone production. (Asset provided by Anatomical Chart Co.)

Peripherally, the thyroid hormones are principally bound to thyroid-binding globulin and albumin and other serum proteins made in the liver.

The thyroid gland is regulated by the hypothalamic and pituitary hormones, TRH and TSH, in a negative feedback loop system (Fig. 15.2). Excess amounts of thyroid hormone down-regulate production of TRH and TSH, which in turn leads to reduced production of the thyroid hormones, T_3 and T_4, as well as thyroglobulin.

Thyroid hormone T_4 contains four iodine molecules, and a deiodinase removes one iodine and converts T_4 to T_3. It is the free T_3 that binds to the thyroid receptor to mediate thyroid hormone effects.

The signs and symptoms of excess thyroid hormone (thyrotoxicosis) or underactivity (hypothyroidism) of the thyroid gland are manifested in the thyroid-responsive organs such as the skin, brain, heart, skeletal system, and intestinal and reproductive tracts (see Table 15.1).

Excess thyroid hormone can be either TSH or non-TSH mediated. In the case of TSH mediated, the TSH and thyroid hormones are both elevated, and this is due to central (secondary or tertiary) hyperthyroidism, an extremely rare entity usually associated with a pituitary tumor or hypothalamic lesion.

Most of the time, however, TSH is appropriately suppressed in response to elevated thyroid hormone levels. Elevated thyroid hormones can be due to release from preformed, stored thyroid hormone, or be due to *de novo* thyroid hormone production (hyperthyroidism).

Excess thyroid hormone levels occurring as a consequence of excessive release of already synthesized and stored T_4 and T_3 are characterized by the following:
- The ratio of T_4 to T_3 is 4:1.
- Thyroglobulin levels are not elevated.
- The duration of excess thyroid hormone levels is limited by the amount of preformed, stored thyroid hormone, and usually lasts a few weeks to a couple of months.
- The thyrotoxic phase can be followed by a late and sometimes permanent hypothyroidism.
- It occurs as a consequence of trauma to or inflammation of the thyroid.
  - Types of inflammatory thyrotoxicosis include the following:
    - Painful subacute thyroiditis
    - Postpartum thyroiditis
    - Painless sporadic thyroiditis

Hyperthyroidism

Hyperthyroidism is a specific subset of thyrotoxicosis where there is ongoing overproduction of thyroid hormone, which can be due to the following (in declining frequency in AYAs):
- Graves disease
- Excessive iodine load
- Autonomous nodular thyroid disease
- Inappropriate TSH overproduction by a pituitary tumor
- Overactive ectopic thyroid tissue (e.g., struma ovarii)

Graves Disease Graves disease is the most common cause of hyperthyroidism in AYAs. The prevalence of Graves disease in children is 1:5,000; however, between the ages of 15 and 25 years, there is a dramatic increase in Graves disease, especially in females. The female-to-male ratio in AYAs is approximately 5:1. Graves disease is an autoimmune disease caused by the production of TSAb, which are capable of directly stimulating thyroid tissue to overproduce thyroid hormones T_3 and T_4. There is lymphocytic infiltration of the thyroid and when glycosaminoglycans and lymphocytes accumulate in the orbital connective tissue and pretibial skin it can lead to exophthalmos (Fig. 15.3) and pretibial myxedema; both these clinical signs are pathognomonic for Graves disease. The other symptoms and signs of Graves disease are similar to that of other thyrotoxicoses (see Table 15.1).

The diagnosis of Graves disease can be made when the following clinical or laboratory findings are present:
- Pathognomonic clinical findings are present (thyrotoxicosis with pretibial myxedema and/or exophthalmos and/or thyroid bruit).

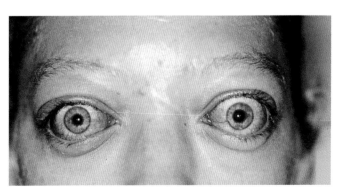

FIGURE 15.3 Patient with Graves ophthalmopathy. (From Penne RB. *Wills Eye Institute—Oculoplastics.* 2nd ed. Lippincott Williams & Wilkins; 2011.)

- Thyroid-stimulating antibodies are present
- Thyroid nuclear medicine scan demonstrating diffuse increased thyroid uptake in the context of a suppressed TSH

Initial treatment of Graves disease can include the use of a beta blocker (e.g., daily atenolol) to control adrenergic hyperthyroid symptoms (e.g., palpitations and tremors), as well as more specific antithyroid therapy, which can be used as a bridge to definitive therapy, or for 1 to 2 years in an attempt to achieve remission. Methimazole (MMI), an antithyroid therapy, decreases thyroid hormone production and is usually highly effective. However, some patients may develop adverse reactions, including severe skin allergy, hepatitis (much less common than with propylthiouracil [PTU] use), or rarely, agranulocytosis. Such side effects may limit the use of MMI. If a severe adverse reaction is suspected (rash, fever or sore throat, or right upper quadrant pain or jaundice), the MMI (or PTU) should be discontinued and definitive therapy with radioiodine or surgery is indicated.

Some experts recommend radioiodine ablation therapy routinely for Graves disease due to high rates of relapse (up to 50%) after antithyroid therapy is discontinued. Others favor a trial of antithyroid therapy before definitive (surgery or radioiodine ablation) therapy of Graves disease. There is consensus that definitive therapy is indicated when:

- Serious adverse response to antithyroid therapy occurs.
- Relapse after withdrawal of antithyroid medication occurs.
- Patient prefers individualized therapy based on availability (high-volume thyroid surgeon and/or radioiodine) and advantages/disadvantages of each type of treatment.
- Coexistence of concerning nodular thyroid disease, or severe Graves eye disease when thyroid surgery may be indicated.

When initiating antithyroid therapy, the dose is based on the following:

- Degree of thyroid overactivity and gland size
- In patients with a small goiter and a milder degree of hyperthyroid symptoms and slightly elevated fT_4 and total T_3 concentrations, a dose of 0.25 mg/kg/day MMI is used.
- A higher dose of MMI between 0.5 to 1.0 mg/kg/day is reserved for those with a large goiter and higher fT_4 and total T_3 levels.

Thyroid function tests are monitored every 4 to 6 weeks initially and dose is titrated in 0.25 mg/kg increments to achieve normal thyroid levels with dosage reduction beginning when fT_4 drops (even if TSH is still suppressed). Once TSH has stabilized and is normal, monitoring can be every 3 to 4 months.

Predictors of remission include the following:

- Smaller gland size
- Rapid restoration of euthyroidism (<3 months)
  - Low dose of antithyroid medication
- Higher BMI

Risk of relapse is greatest in the first year following discontinuation of antithyroid therapy, but can occur much later and lifelong thyroid function monitoring is indicated.

Autonomous nodule(s) that overproduce thyroid hormone independent of TSH are rare in younger patients and the risk for such nodules increases with age. Such nodules are usually >2 cm in size if they are producing sufficient thyroid hormone such that TSH is suppressed. Treatment of toxic nodules can include antithyroid medication, radioiodine, or surgery.

Hypothyroidism

The vast majority, >99%, of hypothyroidism occurs due to primary failure of the thyroid gland to make sufficient thyroid hormone. Abnormally located and partial thyroid glands are usually detected in the newborn period, mostly by mandatory heel stick newborn screening thyroid hormone levels. Hypothyroidism in the AYAs is usually acquired from underactivity of the thyroid gland. When the gland itself is unresponsive to the stimulatory signal TSH, it is termed primary hypothyroidism. However, sometimes, the regulatory signal is deficient, causing secondary (TSH) or tertiary (TRH) hypothyroidism. The common factor for all types of hypothyroidism is a reduced and falling level of thyroid hormone (fT_4). The symptoms and signs of primary hypothyroidism (see **Table 15.1**) are the same as seen in secondary and tertiary hypothyroidism.

Because thyroid receptors are located in virtually all tissues throughout the body, there is a constellation of symptoms and signs seen in hypothyroidism and these include the following:

- Decreased energy
- Sluggishness
- Constipation
- Dry skin and hair
- Decreased heart rate
- Decreased rate of linear growth despite increases in body weight
- In girls, there can be delayed, missed, or heavy menses

The signs and symptoms of hypothyroidism are nonspecific and can be easily attributed to other causes. Thyroid function evaluation by testing fT_4 and TSH levels is generally required to confirm or exclude the diagnosis of hypothyroidism.

In primary hypothyroidism, there is reduced fT4 and an elevated TSH. The majority of the time, thyroid antibodies (usually TPO and thyroglobulin antibodies) are also positive, as the usual pathogenesis of hypothyroidism is autoimmune-mediated thyroid failure or Hashimoto disease. Other causes of hypothyroidism include surgical resection of the gland, radioiodine ablation by I-131, or as an unintended consequence of ionizing radiation treatment for treatment of head and neck cancers.

- Regardless of cause, hypothyroidism is treated with T_4 (levothyroxine) replacement therapy.
- Triiodothyronine (liothyronine) is not necessary because the conversion of T_4 to T_3 still proceeds normally unless there is a selenium deficiency or other cause for deiodinase inactivity.
- The usual dose of T_4 is 2 to 4 mcg/kg in 10- to 15-year-olds and 1.6 mcg/kg in adulthood.[14]
- The dose of thyroid hormone is usually less than what is commonly needed for patients with congenital hypothyroidism.
- Dosing in primary hypothyroidism is titrated to normalize TSH and target TSH between 0.5 μL/mL and 3.0 μL/mL, which is usually associated with an fT_4 in the upper half of the normal range.
- Thyroid-stimulating hormone monitoring is typically 4 to 6 weeks after dosage adjustments. (Note: in secondary and tertiary hypothyroidism, the dose is based on achieving fT_4 levels in the upper half of normal without monitoring TSH.)
- Monitoring should be every 4 to 6 months in growing individuals, and yearly in those who have attained maximal height.
- Levels should be monitored if symptoms of hypo- or hyperthyroidism develop and if diseases involving the gastrointestinal tract such as celiac disease, gastric bypass, or diabetes-associated diarrhea develop and/or if medications that affect thyroid hormone requirements are added. In most cases, treatment is lifelong.

Nonthyroidal Illness

The thyroid axis has a complex response to both an acute illness and recovery from an acute illness.

- Acute illness (including sustained malnutrition)—there is a reduction in thyroid hormone production.
- Recovering from acute illness—there is a stage when the TSH is elevated to prompt restoration of normal thyroid levels.

If testing occurs during the recovery phase, it may appear to represent primary hypothyroidism (with elevation of TSH) but thyroid antibodies are typically negative, and if the patient improves clinically, the TSH and fT_4 typically normalize with time and without intervention.

Another feature of recovery from acute illness is that the rT_3 is usually elevated early in the process, and this can be measured when it is difficult to distinguish hypothyroidism from recovery from acute illness. Low T_3 levels in nonthyroidal illness predict worse clinical outcomes, and it is not clear whether T_4 and or T_3 treatment has an effect on outcome. Measurement of total T_3 levels can be especially helpful in the care of AYAs with eating disorders, as a low level of this hormone can indicate a more significant energy deficit.

PREGNANCY AND THYROID DISORDERS

While it is not routine to screen for thyroid disease in asymptomatic female AYAs who are (or are contemplating becoming) pregnant, the symptoms of thyroid disorders are nonspecific and common, so that, many reproductive-aged females undergo thyroid testing. While overt hypothyroidism in pregnancy is rare (elevated TSH >4.0 mIU/L or trimester-specific reference range and low fT_4), if it is found, it should be promptly treated at the usual 1.6 mcg/kg T_4 dose. Likewise, subclinical hypothyroidism should be treated (elevated TSH >4.0 mIU/L and normal fT_4) at 1 mcg/kg. There is still debate about treatment strategies when TSH is between 2.6 and 4 mIU/L, so experts usually individualize therapy based on pregnancy history, medical history, TPO status, and personal preference factors.[15]

Female AYAs with pre-existing hypothyroidism typically need a 30% to 40% increase in thyroid dose during pregnancy and can be instructed to increase their dose by two pills per week (e.g., continue one pill daily Monday to Friday and two pills on Saturday and Sunday) as soon as they know they are pregnant. Monthly monitoring allows appropriate adjustment of maternal thyroid dose with an aim of keeping the TSH <2.5 mIU/L.

In females with a history of Graves disease, there is a risk of hyperthyroidism in the fetus and newborn, even if the mother has had definitive treatment for the Graves disease and is on thyroid hormone replacement therapy. This occurs because the maternal TSAbs mediate the fetal effects—rapid fetal heart rate, poor growth, goiter, and exophthalmos. If the fetus shows signs of hyperthyroidism such as intrauterine growth retardation, tachycardia, and reduced amniotic fluid, the mother is typically treated with the antithyroid medication PTU that crosses the placenta and can treat the fetus. If only the fetus has hyperthyroidism and the mother is euthyroid or hypothyroid, the mother needs to be treated with thyroid hormone (to maintain/restore her euthyroidism) and antithyroid medication (for the fetus).

Radioactive iodine, even tracer doses, is not used during pregnancy or during breastfeeding, and ultrasound is the only imaging used during and shortly after pregnancy.

Postpartum thyroid disorders occur in 5% to 10% of U.S. pregnancies, and also may occur after pregnancy loss or termination. These thyroid issues can manifest any time during the first-year postpartum and can cause transient hyperthyroidism (which must be distinguished from newly detected Graves disease in the postpartum period) or hypothyroidism, which can be transient or permanent. Females who have had postpartum thyroid issues in prior pregnancies are at increased risk for recurrence of thyroid issues with subsequent pregnancies.

Thyroid nodules detected during pregnancy are evaluated in the same way as nodules detected in nonpregnant individuals with the exception that nuclear medicine thyroid scans are not obtained in pregnant females. Thyroid cancers detected during pregnancy can be surgically removed in the second trimester or after the pregnancy.

SUMMARY

Adolescents and young adults require timely detection and treatment of thyroid disease for normal growth and sexual and intellectual development, and during puberty, there is a fourfold increase in thyroid volume which is not associated with increased thyroid hormone levels, but with increased risk of structural and functional thyroid disorders during a developmental period when radiation sensitivity is also increased.

- Thyroid ultrasound is the most important imaging for thyroid structural disorders because it gives precise anatomic location and size information, as well as morphologic features of nodules that are predictive of cancer risk.
- Suspicious nodules require fine-needle aspiration biopsy.
- Management of differentiated thyroid cancers, which account for 95% of thyroid cancer in AYAs, includes complete thyroidectomy by an experienced high-volume thyroid surgeon, and radioiodine ablation only in instances where high-risk features are present.
- The cell of origin in MTC is the neuroendocrine C cell which makes calcitonin, which should be measured along with genetic testing for the RET oncogene for evaluation and ongoing monitoring.
- Thyroid-stimulating hormone is the most sensitive assay of thyroid function in the steady state, with suppressed levels generally indicating hyperthyroidism, normal levels indicating euthyroidism, and persistent high levels indicating hypothyroidism.
- Hyperthyroidism can be treated with surgery, radioiodine ablation, or antithyroid medication.
- Graves disease is the most common cause of hyperthyroidism in AYAs and is mediated by TSAbs which stimulate the thyroid gland to overproduce thyroid hormones.
- Hypothyroidism in most AYAs is caused by autoimmune Hashimoto disease which is associated with positive TPO and thyroglobulin antibody.
- The usual treatment dose of T_4 for hypothyroidism is 2 to 4 mcg/kg in 10- to 15-year-olds and 1.6 mcg/kg in adulthood with an aim to normalize the TSH.

REFERENCES

1. Fleury Y, Van Melle G, Woringer V, et al. Sex-dependent variations and timing of thyroid growth during puberty. *J Clin Endocrinol Metab*. 2001;86:750.
2. Pankow BG, Michalak J, McGee MK. Adult human thyroid weight. *Health Phys*. 1985;49:1097.
3. Polak M, Sura-Trueba S, Chauty A, et al. Molecular mechanisms of thyroid dysgenesis. *Horm Res*. 2004;62(suppl 3):14–21.
4. Foukakis T, Au AYM, Wallin G, et al. The Ras effector NORE1A is suppressed in follicular thyroid carcinomas with a PAX8-PPARgamma fusion. *J Clin Endocrinol Metab*. 2006;91:1143–1149.
5. Fenton CL, Lukes Y, Nicholson D, et al. The ret/PTC mutations are common in sporadic papillary thyroid carcinoma of children and young adults. *J Clin Endocrinol Metab*. 2000;85:1170–1175.
6. Penko K, Livezey J, Fenton C, et al. BRAF mutations are uncommon in papillary thyroid cancer of young patients. *Thyroid*. 2005;15:320–325.
7. Wells SA Jr, Asa SL, Waguespack SG, et al. Revised American Thyroid Association guidelines for the management of medullary thyroid carcinoma. *Thyroid*. 2015;25(6):567–610.
8. Alexander EK, Kennedy GC, Baloch ZW, et al. Preoperative diagnosis of benign thyroid nodules with indeterminate cytology. *N Engl J Med*. 2012;367(8):705.
9. Kay C, Abrahams S, McClain P. The weight of normal thyroid glands in children. *Arch Pathol*. 1966;82:349.
10. Rallison ML, Dobyns BM, Keating FR Jr, et al. Thyroid nodularity in children. *JAMA*. 1975;233(10):1069–1072.
11. Hogan AR, Zhuge Y, Perez EA, et al. Pediatric thyroid carcinoma: incidence and outcomes in 1753 patients. *J Surg Res*. 2009;156(1):167.
12. Haugen BR, Alexander EK, Bible KC, et al. 2015 American Thyroid Association management guidelines for adult patients with thyroid nodules and differentiated thyroid cancer: the American Thyroid Association Guidelines Task Force on thyroid nodules and differentiated thyroid cancer. *Thyroid*. 2016;26(1):1–133.
13. Romei C, Tacito A, Molinaro E, et al. Twenty years of lesson learning: how does the RET genetic screening test impact the clinical management of medullary thyroid cancer? [published online ahead of print December 2, 2014]. *Clin Endocrinol*. 2015;82(6):892–899. doi:10.1111/cen.12686
14. LaFranchi S. Thyroiditis and acquired hypothyroidism. *Pediatr Ann*. 1992;21:29.
15. Alexander EK, Pearce EN, Brent GA, et al. 2017 Guidelines of the American Thyroid Association for the diagnosis and management of thyroid disease during pregnancy and the postpartum. *Thyroid*. 2017:27:315.

📶 ADDITIONAL RESOURCES AND WEBSITES

Additional Resources and Websites for Clinicians:

American Association of Clinical Endocrinology—https://pro.aace.com/disease-state-resources/thyroid

American Thyroid Association—www.thyroid.org

Professional Version of the Merck Manual—https://www.merckmanuals.com/professional/SearchResults?query=Overview+of+the+Thyroid+Gland&icd9=MM101

Additional Resources and Websites for Parents/Caregivers:

American Thyroid Association—www.thyroid.org

Consumer Version of the Merck Manual—https://www.merckmanuals.com/home/hormonal-and-metabolic-disorders/thyroid-gland-disorders/overview-of-the-thyroid-gland

Additional Resources and Websites for Adolescents and Young Adults:

American Thyroid Association—www.Thyroid.org

https://www.yourhormones.info/glands/thyroid-gland/

https://www.endocrineweb.com/conditions/thyroid-nodules/thyroid-gland-controls-bodys-metabolism-how-it-works-symptoms-hyperthyroi

https://www.btf-thyroid.org/what-is-thyroid-disorder

CHAPTER 16

Diabetes Mellitus

Laura Kester Prakash
Tamara S. Hannon

KEY WORDS

- Diabetes complications
- Hyperglycemia
- Insulin
- Insulin resistance
- Patient-centered care
- Prediabetes
- Type 1 diabetes
- Type 2 diabetes

INTRODUCTION

Diabetes mellitus (diabetes) is a spectrum of metabolic diseases characterized by hyperglycemia resulting from defects in insulin secretion, insulin action, or both. Diabetes is a relatively common chronic disease, occurring in approximately 1 in 300 youth by 18 years old. The most common cause of diabetes in youth is type 1 diabetes, the etiology of which is usually autoimmune destruction of pancreatic β-cells. However, the prevalence of type 2 diabetes characterized by insulin resistance and β-cell dysfunction is increasing among adolescents and young adults (AYAs).

CLASSIFICATION AND ETIOLOGY

Classification of diabetes is based on the presumed etiology, rather than the mode of treatment (i.e., insulin vs. no insulin). Common types of diabetes include the following (see Table 16.1 for characteristics of type 1, type 2, maturity-onset diabetes of youth, and atypical forms):

1. Type 1 diabetes is the result of β-cell destruction leading to absolute insulin deficiency.
   a. Immune mediated (type 1A): Genetic risk for type 1 diabetes is linked to the class II HLA region where genes encoding HLA-DR, HLA-DQ, and HLA-DP molecules that present antigen epitopes to T cells are located.[1] Poorly defined environmental factors/exposures promote autoreactive T cells to recognize islet cell autoantigens and the inflammatory process leads to immune destruction and dysfunction of the β-cells. Adolescents and young adults at risk for or diagnosed with type 1 diabetes typically have one or more circulating islet-specific autoantibodies (insulin, glutamic acid decarboxylase 65, IA-2 antigen, zinc transporter 8).
   b. Nonimmune mediated (type 1B): The origin of the β-cell impairment is not known in cases of diabetes classified as type 1B, sometimes referred to as idiopathic type 1 diabetes or ketosis-prone atypical diabetes mellitus. Ketosis-prone atypical diabetes mellitus has been identified in approximately 10% of African Americans with youth-onset diabetes; it is also recognized among Asian populations.

2. Type 2 diabetes is a significant and increasing burden in AYAs.[2] The pathophysiology of type 2 diabetes includes insulin resistance generally associated with obesity, and progressive β-cell dysfunction resulting in relative insulin deficiency. Type 2 diabetes is more prevalent in adolescent girls than boys and disproportionately affects youth of racial–ethnic minority groups.

3. Genetic disorders associated with diabetes
   a. Maturity-onset diabetes of youth (MODY) is associated with monogenetic defects in β-cell function, impaired insulin secretion with minimal or no defects in insulin action, autosomal-dominant inheritance, and onset usually before the age of 25 years.[3] Maturity-onset diabetes of youth is rare (~1% of cases) and frequently misdiagnosed as type 1 or type 2 diabetes.
   b. Mitochondrial DNA: This very rare form of diabetes is characterized by specific genetic defect and is almost always associated with other symptoms—deafness, neurologic disorders, cardiac failure, renal failure, and myopathy. The mutations may be sporadic or maternally inherited. Various genetic defects of insulin action are known. These include type A insulin resistance, leprechaunism, Rabson–Mendenhall syndrome, lipoatrophic diabetes, and others.

4. Diseases of the exocrine pancreas leading to destruction of endocrine function
   a. Cystic fibrosis–related diabetes (CFRD) is associated with decreased pulmonary function, protein catabolism, and loss of weight. It results primarily from insulinopenia, although insulin resistance may be severe during steroid treatments for pulmonary inflammation. Early and adequate insulin treatment is associated with increased body weight and improved pulmonary function.[4]
   b. Others: Pancreatitis, trauma/pancreatectomy, neoplasia, hemochromatosis, fibrocalculous pancreatopathy.

5. Endocrinopathies including acromegaly, Cushing syndrome, hyperthyroidism, polycystic ovary syndrome, and pheochromocytoma

6. Drugs including glucocorticoids, atypical antipsychotics, pentamidine, protease inhibitors, thyroid hormone, diazoxide, and thiazides

7. Genetic syndromes associated with diabetes are Down syndrome, Klinefelter syndrome, Turner syndrome, Wolfram syndrome, Friedreich ataxia, Huntington chorea, Laurence–Moon syndrome, myotonic dystrophy, and Prader–Willi syndrome.

8. Gestational diabetes mellitus (GDM). The risk for subsequent development of diabetes is elevated; approximately

TABLE 16.1

Characteristics of Common Types of Diabetes

	Type 1	Type 2	Atypical	Maturity-Onset Diabetes of Youth or Monogenic Diabetes (MODY)
Age	Peaks at 5–9 y and midadolescence	Pubertal	Pubertal	Child, adolescent (usually < age 25)
Onset	Acute; severe	Insidious to severe	Acute; severe	Insidious or mild
Insulin secretion	Very low	Variable	Moderately low	Variable
Insulin sensitivity	Normal or decreased	Decreased	Normal	Normal
Insulin dependence	Permanent	None to progressive disease with insulin dependence	Variable	Usually no, until late
Racial/ethnic groups at increased risk	All (low in Asians)	African Americans, Hispanic Americans, Native Americans, Asian and Pacific Islanders	African American and Asian	All
Genetics	Polygenic	Polygenic	Presumed autosomal dominant	Autosomal dominant
Association: obesity	No	Strong	Variable	No
Acanthosis nigricans	No	Yes	No	No
Autoimmune etiology	Yes (small subset nonautoimmune)	No	No	No

Adapted from Rosenbloom AL, Joe JR, Young RS, et al. Emerging epidemic of type 2 diabetes in youth. *Diabetes Care.* 1999;22:345–354, with permission.

17% develop type 1 diabetes and 17% to 70% develop type 2 diabetes.

EPIDEMIOLOGY

1. Prevalence
   a. Type 1: The prevalence of type 1 diabetes varies by race/ethnicity and country, with the highest rates in areas most distant from the equator. The prevalence of type 1 diabetes in U.S. youth is approximately 1 in 300 by the age of 18 years. The incidence is increasing by 2% to 5% annually worldwide.[5]
   b. Type 2: There has been a steady worldwide increase in the prevalence of type 2 diabetes.[6,7] The vast majority of youth diagnosed with type 2 diabetes are pubertal.
      • Racial distribution: All races/ethnicities are affected. Persons of Hispanic, Black, Native American, and South Asian heritage are disproportionately affected.
      • Gender: Female preponderance in youth-onset type 2 diabetes
      • Family history: The majority of AYAs with type 2 diabetes have a family history of type 2 diabetes in a first- or second-degree relative. Also, an association with exposure to maternal undernutrition or overnutrition/gestational diabetes in utero.
      • Emergence of type 2 diabetes during puberty: Normal physiology of puberty is associated with relative insulin resistance. Insulin sensitivity decreases during puberty, around sexual maturity rating (SMR) stage 2, and is close to prepubertal levels by SMR 5. The degree of insulin resistance that is present during puberty is greatly impacted by obesity and lifestyle (diet, physical activity levels). Girls are more insulin resistant; this is only partially explained by higher body mass index (BMI).

DIAGNOSIS

Glycosylated hemoglobin or hemoglobin A1c (HbA1c), fasting plasma glucose (FPG), and the oral glucose tolerance test (OGTT) are approved measures for the diagnosis of diabetes (Table 16.2). The level of FPG and HbA1c has largely replaced the OGTT as it is cumbersome and costly, underutilized, and has poor repeated test reproducibility. HbA1c cut-point of 6.5% is not recommended as a single test for the diagnosis of diabetes, unless there is unequivocal evidence of hyperglycemia. Impaired fasting glucose (IFG) and impaired glucose tolerance (IGT) results are now considered to indicate prediabetes, but are not, of themselves, diagnostic of diabetes.[8]

TABLE 16.2

Criteria for the Diagnosis of Diabetes Mellitus; American Diabetes Association, 2020

1. Symptoms of diabetes plus casual plasma glucose concentration ≥200 mg/dL (11.1 mmol/L). Casual is defined as any time or day without regard to time since last meal.

   or

2. FPG ≥126 mg/dL (7.0 mmol/L). Fasting is defined as no caloric intake for at least 8 h.[a]

   or

3. HbA1c ≥6.5% (48 mmol/mol). The test should be performed in a laboratory using a method that is certified (National Glycohemoglobin Standardization Program [NGSP]) and standardized to the Diabetes Control and Complications Trial (DCCT) assay.[a]

4. 2-h PG ≥200 mg/dL (11.1 mmol/L) during an OGTT. The test should be performed as described by the World Health Organization.

[a]In the absence of unequivocal hyperglycemia, diagnosis requires two abnormal test results from the same sample or in two separate test samples.

OGTT, oral glucose tolerance test; FPG, fasting plasma glucose; PG, plasma glucose.

From The Expert Committee on the Diagnosis and Classification of Diabetes Mellitus. Report of the expert committee on the diagnosis and classification of diabetes mellitus. *Diabetes Care.* 2020;43(Suppl 1):S14–S31.

SCREENING

1. Type 1 diabetes: No universal screening is recommended.
2. Type 2 diabetes[8,9] (Fig. 16.1)
   a. Screen with HbA1c (or FPG) every other year, starting at 10 years or at the onset of puberty (if puberty occurs at a younger age).
   b. Screen
      - Overweight or obese patients (BMI at or above the 85th percentile for age and sex, those with weight for height at or above the 85th percentile, or weight of more than 120% of ideal for height weight) PLUS
      - Those who have any of the following risk factors:
         – Family history of type 2 diabetes in first- or second-degree relative
         – Race/ethnicity: Native American, African American, Hispanic, Asian/Pacific Islander
         – Signs of insulin resistance or conditions associated with insulin resistance, such as acanthosis nigricans, hypertension, dyslipidemia, polycystic ovary syndrome, exposure to gestational diabetes in utero, or history of intrauterine growth restriction

PREVENTION

- Type 1 diabetes—There is no effective prevention currently. However, advances have been made in the understanding of interventions to slow the autoimmune disease process.
- Type 2 diabetes—Screen at-risk individuals and recommend lifestyle modification (see Fig. 16.1).

EVALUATION AND TREATMENT

At initial presentation, the state of hydration and acid–base balance determine the need for fluids and insulin. It is important to determine the type of diabetes as soon as possible. Measurement of autoantibodies is useful if the etiology is unclear; for example, patients with a type 2 diabetes phenotype who may have both insulin deficiency due to type 1 diabetes and insulin resistance. Evidence of autoimmunity helps to guide therapy and is associated with a need for insulin. If type 1 diabetes is diagnosed, measurement of thyroid autoantibodies (thyroid peroxidase antibody) and thyroid function is indicated because of associated thyroiditis in 10% to 15% of patients. Type 2 diabetes usually, but not always, has an insidious presentation and is suggested by obesity, family history of type 2 diabetes in first- and/or second-degree relatives, acanthosis nigricans, and dyslipidemia. Normal weight and mild symptoms suggest early type 1 diabetes or MODY (in which case genetic testing should be pursued).

The goals of treatment of diabetes in AYAs are to achieve and maintain near-normal glycemic control (HbA1c <7%), identify and treat comorbid conditions (hypertension, dyslipidemia, depression/anxiety, sleep disorders), prevent and screen for long-term complications, and avoid unplanned pregnancy. Excellent glycemic control of type 1 diabetes is associated with substantially reduced incidence of complications and comorbidities, improved quality of life, and significant cost reduction.[10]

Unfortunately, glycemic control in AYAs with type 1 diabetes is generally suboptimal. Data from a U.S. type 1 diabetes registry indicate that mean HbA1c in 2016 to 2018 increased from 8.1% at the age of 5 years to 9.3% between ages 15 and 18, and then decreased to 8% by age 28. At that time, the American Diabetes Association (ADA) HbA1c goal of <7.5% was achieved by only 17%. Adolescents had a higher mean HbA1c in 2016 to 2018 than in 2010 to 2012.[11]

1. Education: In addition to the recommended information about diabetes, blood glucose (BG) testing, hypoglycemia, hyperglycemia and insulin administration, education and periodic education by a certified diabetes educator should include information about driving, smoking, alcohol use, use of contraception, and preconception counseling.
2. Meals, food, and nutrition: There is no standard ADA meal plan; rather, diet is adjusted for the individual to provide sufficient calories and nutrients to grow/maintain normal weight. Carbohydrate counting has replaced the meal-planning "exchange system" because it permits greater flexibility and offers the potential for adjusting the dose of rapid-acting insulin before each meal. Reducing the overall carbohydrate content by reducing concentrated sweets and processed foods while increasing vegetables and lean sources of protein can be beneficial to improve glycemic control and reduce insulin resistance.
3. Accessing glycemic control: The goal is to lower BG level, and resultant HbA1c to achieve maximum prevention of complications, taking into account patient safety and the ability to carry out the treatment regimen. Although normal levels of BG are the goal (70 to 120 mg/dL before meals and fasting), most patients (adults and adolescents) are not able to achieve consistently *normal* levels of HbA1c. Any lowering of HbA1c will reduce the risks of long-term complications.
   a. BG testing: Self-monitoring of BG has evolved to utilize continuous glucose monitoring (CGM), which is considered standard care. If not utilizing CGM, persons with type 1 diabetes should self-monitor glucose levels multiple times daily (up to 6 to 10 times/day), including premeal, prebedtime, and as needed for safety with exercise or driving. The recommended frequency of testing for type 2 diabetes is the same as type 1 diabetes if treatment includes insulin.
   b. HbA1c should be measured at each visit (generally quarterly). HbA1c values reflect the average BG over the previous 8 to 12 weeks, so BG records must also be examined to identify swings in BG that would not be evident in the percentage of glycated hemoglobin. Based on the Diabetes Control and Complications Trial, HbA1c values, the target HbA1c level is ≤7%.
4. Insulin: Humanized insulins (DNA origins) or insulin analogues in which one or more amino acids have been substituted on the α chain or β chain afford specific patterns of insulin release into the bloodstream. Rapid-acting preparations have a shorter duration of action; they may be given just before or at mealtime. Extended-acting analogs provide basal (background) insulin. Many different devices are available for insulin delivery (syringes, pens, pumps; see the "Internet Resources" section).
5. Treatment of patients who require insulin: Insulin therapy is always necessary for type 1 diabetes, those with insulin deficiency, and is recommended for patients with type 2 diabetes with poor glycemic control on oral and/or injectable antidiabetes regimens (HbA1c ≥8.5% to 9.0%). Insulin pump therapy with continuous subcutaneous infusion of insulin or multiple daily injections using basal and bolus insulin and carbohydrate counting is standard of care.

BASAL INSULIN DOSE

Basal insulin dose = ~40 to 50% of total daily dose (TDD). Adolescents typically require a TDD of approximately 0.7 to 1.2 unit/kg body weight/day as a starting point (40% to 50% basal and the rest as short-acting insulin boluses). Insulin dose requirements typically decrease in adulthood, after the physiologic insulin resistance associated with puberty decreases. At all ages, the actual insulin requirement depends on body habitus, insulin resistance, overall glycemic control, physical activity levels, nutritional status, diet, normal hormone fluctuations, and other factors.

BOLUS INSULIN DOSE = FOOD DOSE + CORRECTION DOSE

- Food dose to cover carbohydrates at meal or snack
   - One unit of short- or rapid-acting insulin will usually "cover" about 4 to 15 g of carbohydrate (carbohydrate

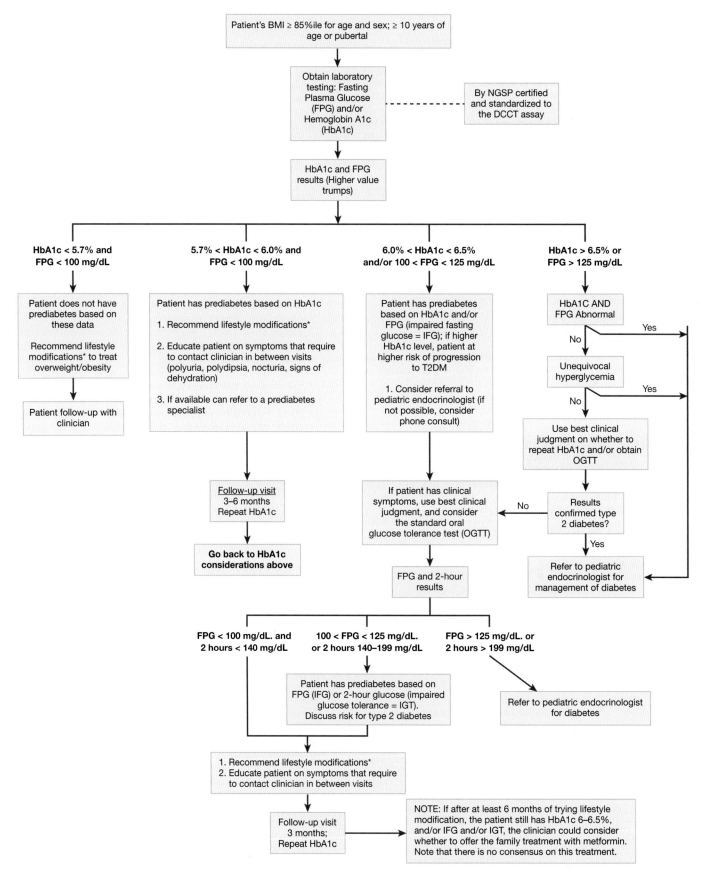

FIGURE 16.1 Diabetes screening algorithm. (From Magge SN, Silverstein J, Elder D, et al. Evaluation and treatment of prediabetes in youth. *J Pediatr.* 2020;219:11, used with permission.)

A <u>Lifestyle Modification Recommendations:</u>
1. Meet with a pediatric nutritionist for assessment and recommendations
2. At least 60 minutes of moderate-vigorous physical activity every day (can work up this gradually if deconditioned)
3. ≤2 hours screen time per day (includes TV, video games, computer use not related to school, tablets, texting, etc.)
4. Get enough sleep to promote optimal health. The AAP recommends children 6 to 12 years of age sleep 9 to 12 hours per 24 hours, and teenagers 13 to 18 years of age sleep 8 to 10 hours per 24 hours

<u>Diet Recommendation:</u>
Eliminate sugar-sweetened beverages
At least 5 servings of fruits and vegetables per day
Portion sizes (palm for meat, fist for everything else)

Set short-term goals and track progress

B <u>Oral Glucose Tolerance Test</u>
- Use 1.75 g/kg dextrose, 75 g max
- Done with 8–12 hours fasting
- Done before 10 AM
- Blood draws to occur at t = 0 and t = 120 minutes

C In situations in which an OGTT is not feasible, pediatric clinician can consider having family/patient check fasting and 2-hour postprandial blood sugars by home glucometer, with instructions to call clinician if blood sugars are falling within the diabetes range. Clinician can then refer to pediatric endocrinologist.

D <u>Criteria for the diagnosis of diabetes</u>
- FPG ≥126 mg/dL (7.0 mmol/L). Fasting is defined as no caloric intake for at least 8 hours.
                    OR
- 2-hour PG ≥200 mg/dL (11.1 mmol/L) during the OGTT. The test should be performed as described by the WHO, using glucose load containing the equivalent of 75 g anhydrous glucose dissolved in water.
                    OR
- A1C ≥6.5% (48 mmol/mol). The test should be performed in a laboratory using a method that is a method that is NGSP certified and standardized to the DCCT assay.
                    OR
- In a patient with classic symptoms of hyperglycemia or hyperglycemia crisis, a random glucose ≥200 mg/dL (11.1 mmol/L)

In the absence of unequivocal hyperglycemia, results should be confirmed by repeat testing.

E <u>Metformin Dosing</u>
- Gradually increase dose by 500-mg increments per week until patient achieves highest dose tolerated or 1,000 mg PO b.i.d. with food
- LFTs and CBC, ALT, AST, Creatinine Q6 mo
- Stop metformin if patient has macrocytic anemia and/or AST/ALT >2.5 x upper limit of normal. In the case of elevated liver enzymes, if stopping metformin is likely to result in suboptimal control, consider consultation with pediatric gastrointestinal/liver specialist.

FIGURE 16.1 (*Continued*)

to insulin ratio of 4 to 15) meaning that 1 unit of rapid-acting insulin will be required for each 4 to 15 g of carbohydrate consumed. This varies according to BMI, type of foods eaten, and degree of insulin resistance.

- Food dose = grams of carbohydrate consumed/carbohydrate to insulin ratio
- Correction dose: The correction dose of insulin is added to the food dose when the premeal BG is above target range and is administered before that meal. The correction dose may also be used to correct for hyperglycemia at other times of the day independent of meals.
  - The rule of 1,800 may be used to estimate more closely the initial "insulin sensitivity factor" (the estimated point drop in BG per unit of rapid-acting insulin) used for the corrective dose:
    - The sensitivity factor = 1,800/TDD = the approximate BG drop per unit of insulin administered. For example, a sensitivity factor of 30 implies that 1 unit of insulin will drop the BG 30 mg/dL when given as a correction dose.
  - Correction dose = (measured BG − target BG)/insulin sensitivity factor
6. Treatment of type 2 diabetes and MODY: Treatment should be based on the known pathophysiology—insulin resistance, hepatic overproduction of glucose, and relative insulin deficiency.
   a. Acute management of newly diagnosed symptomatic patients: Individuals who are ketotic and those with significant hyperglycemia at diagnosis (BG >250 mg/dL) will require initially insulin therapy to reduce BG levels. Several studies of adults and adolescents have demonstrated that intensive treatment with insulin results in improved glycemic control 1 year later. Metformin therapy is generally begun when the patient is no longer ketotic. Insulin can be slowly withdrawn over the subsequent weeks as glycemic control is achieved.
   b. Patients with insidious onset and milder hyperglycemia (HbA1c ≤8.5%) can be initially managed with metformin, recommendations for dietary modification, and education to increase physical activity.

Nutrition: Management of nutritional intake is a crucial component of diabetes treatment. Avoidance of foods with added sugar, as well as sugary beverages, and limiting fat to <35% of total energy intake (<10% saturated fat) is recommended to reduce the risk of development of cardiovascular and fatty liver disease. Medical nutritional therapy should be individualized, and patient-centered goal setting should be pursued to decrease portion sizes of processed foods, increase consumption of vegetables, and decrease carbohydrate consumption to amounts recommended for meeting nutritional and growth requirements. Limiting the amount of carbohydrate takes into account the inherently abnormal insulin secretory pattern and reduces insulin requirements. The effect of carbohydrate restriction (as part of total caloric reduction) may be seen within 4 days, with a reduction in postprandial BG. It is generally recommended that carbohydrates from vegetables, fruit, dairy, legumes, and whole grains provide 45% to 50% of total daily energy intake; this may require a reduction in carbohydrate intake from highly processed foods from baseline, but provides recommended nutrients for normal growth and development during adolescence. Neither the International Society for Pediatric and Adolescent Diabetes (ISPAD) nor the ADA has endorsed very–low-carbohydrate diets or further carbohydrate restriction for AYAs.

Physical activity: Routine physical activity will increase insulin sensitivity independent of weight changes. In addition, it improves endothelial function, lipid profile, and psychological health in youth with type 1 and type 2 diabetes. Currently, both aerobic (walking, jogging, running, cycling, and swimming) as well as anaerobic (resistance/strength training) physical activity is recommended. A minimum of 60 minutes (cumulative) of moderate to vigorously intense aerobic physical activity is recommended per day and at least 20 to 30 minutes of vigorous muscle and bone strengthening should be encouraged 3 days per week via strength/anaerobic training. This may be a challenge for less active youth, in which case a patient-centered goal should be identified with a plan of increasing to the recommended goal over time as tolerated. Purposeful walking is an ideal option for an introductory activity for the sedentary patient. Patients treated with insulin have variability in their glucose response to different types of physical activity and these considerations should be incorporated into specific recommendations for type and duration of experience.

Medications: Medications currently approved for treatment of type 2 diabetes in children and adolescents are metformin, insulin, and liraglutide, a glucagon-like peptide-1 (GLP-1) analog. Although more medications are U.S. Food and Drug Administration approved for adults, these medications are also first-line for young adults.

- Insulin is required initially for patients who present with metabolic derangement (ketosis or HbA1c ≥9.0%) and may be weaned and discontinued as glycemic control improves. More than 50% of adolescents with type 2 diabetes require insulin therapy to control hyperglycemia despite treatment with other agents.
- Metformin is the first-line therapy for patients presenting without ketosis or severe hyperglycemia (HbA1c ≥9%). Treatment with metformin improves insulin resistance, decreases hepatic glucose production, and often improves lipid profiles. The initial response to metformin may include decreased appetite and food intake with transient weight loss. Side effects are primarily gastrointestinal: increased frequency of bowel movements, gas, bloating, diarrhea, nausea, and rarely vomiting. Although metformin is generally tolerated by AYAs, when side effects occur, they generally, but do not always, improve over time. Side effects may be minimized or reduced by starting at a low dose and increasing the dose over a few weeks. Hypoglycemia does not occur with metformin treatment alone, and lactic acidosis, a potentially serious condition associated with the predecessor biguanide (phenformin), is also exceedingly rare with the only available agent in this class, *metformin.* Discontinue and ensure adequate hydration prior to contrast studies that may impair renal function and with dehydration or critical illness.
- Liraglutide is an injectable, FDA-approved GLP-1 analog for use in adolescents with type 2 diabetes. The GLP-1 analogs function as incretins and increase glucose-dependent insulin secretion while delaying gastric emptying and decreasing appetite. Side effects include gastrointestinal discomfort, nausea, and rarely vomiting. Use of these agents is often associated with modest weight loss, which is beneficial. For this reason, liraglutide is increasingly utilized prior to insulin when treatment with metformin has not resulted in achievement of glycemic control.

COMPLICATIONS, ASSOCIATED CONDITIONS, AND FOLLOW-UP CARE

The ADA "Standards of Medical Care in Diabetes," updated annually, provides components of diabetes care, treatment goals, and up-to-date resources for clinicians.[12] Position and Consensus Statements focusing on youth with diabetes are also available.[13–16]

1. Autoimmune disorders (type 1 diabetes only): Approximately 10% to 15% of patients with type 1 diabetes develop autoimmune thyroiditis. Initial antithyroid antibody levels do not predict subsequent involvement. Annual thyroid studies to detect hypothyroidism are recommended; thyroid-stimulating hormone is generally sufficient. Other autoimmune diseases affecting the adrenal, pituitary, ovary, or parathyroid are uncommon.

2. Microvascular complications: Microvascular complications are directly correlated with the level of glycemic control and duration of diabetes, and are exacerbated by hypertension.
   a. Retinopathy: Yearly dilated funduscopic examination.
   b. Nephropathy: Annual screening for urinary albumin. The level of random urinary microalbumin: creatinine ratio is highly correlated with timed specimens. Meticulous attention to blood pressure is important (both systolic and diastolic); attempt to maintain BP ≤130/80 mm Hg. Angiotensin-converting enzyme (ACE) inhibitors or angiotensin receptor antagonists and improved control represent the treatments for persistent microalbuminuria because they have been shown to delay the progression of nephropathy.
   c. Neuropathy occurs but is rarely symptomatic during adolescence. Examination of the feet for pulses, sensation, deep tendon reflexes, hygiene, calluses, and evidence of infection is indicated. The Semmes–Weinstein monofilament test for sensation is a rapid, sensitive screening test for distal sensory neuropathy. Symptomatic autonomic neuropathy (heart rate invariability and/or postural hypotension) and gastroparesis (postprandial nausea or vomiting, postprandial hypoglycemia, and diarrhea or constipation) occur rarely in this age group.
3. Macrovascular complications: Diabetes-associated accelerated cardiovascular disease may not be preventable with improved glycemic control, although the risk is decreased with tight control of hypertension and hyperlipidemia.[10]
4. Dyslipidemia: Dyslipidemia is common in type 2 diabetes and poorly controlled type 1 diabetes. It increases the risk for cardiovascular disease two- to fourfold and reflects various degrees of insulin resistance, obesity, diet, and poor glycemic control. The typical pattern is elevated triglycerides and decreased HDL-C. Although all hypoglycemic agents used in AYAs tend to lower triglycerides and LDL-C, if LDL-C levels of less than 100 mg/dL have not been attained with better glycemic control and dietary recommendations, treatment with lipid-lowering medications is indicated. New-generation "statin" drugs are generally preferred. Yearly measurement of fasting lipid profiles is recommended among those with previously abnormal profiles or ongoing poor glycemic control. Measurement every 5 years is sufficient if initial LDL-C is <100 mg/dL.
5. Hypertension: Hypertension even with mild elevations (>130/80 mm Hg) is associated with an increased risk of microvascular complications. The appearance often coincides with the onset of persistent microalbuminuria. Angiotensin-converting enzyme inhibitors/receptor antagonists are the drugs of choice.
6. Gluten sensitivity: Gluten sensitivity is estimated to be present in 5% of individuals with type 1 diabetes. The benefit of universal screening of all individuals with type 1 diabetes is not well established. Evaluate with Ig-A antiendomysial or Ig-A antitissue transglutamase antibodies (accompanied by measurement of IgA, as well) if symptoms are suggestive of malabsorption or unexplained postprandial hypoglycemia.
7. Eating disorders: Disordered eating can occur in patients with any form of diabetes. It can present in a variety of forms, including dietary restriction, self-induced vomiting, binge eating, and/or underdosing/omitting insulin usage. Eating disorders may be present in up to 30% of females and 20% of males with type 1 diabetes and lead to elevated HbA1c levels and acute and chronic complications, including an increased risk of retinopathy, kidney disease, and nerve damage.[17] The presence of an eating disorder in a patient with diabetes, increases the mortality rate of the patient to 14.5, which exceeds the standard mortality rate for either type 1 diabetes (4.06) or an eating disorder (8.86) alone.[18] As for all adolescents, it is important to screen for concerns with body image issues and the desire to gain or lose weight.

8. Hypoglycemia: Severe hypoglycemia is common with intensified regimens targeting euglycemia. An episode of severe hypoglycemia increases the risk for additional hypoglycemia because it is associated with a reduced magnitude of autonomic and neuroglycopenic symptoms, counterregulatory hormone responses, and cognitive dysfunction during subsequent hypoglycemia. These return to normal with strict avoidance of hypoglycemia. Patients at risk for hypoglycemia and the people with whom they spend significant time should be well versed in signs, symptoms, and treatment for hypoglycemia.
9. Alcohol use: Alcohol use is not recommended for minor adolescents, including those with diabetes. For those who do drink, provide education about its potential to cause hypoglycemia. Alcohol inhibits gluconeogenesis and interferes with the counterregulatory responses to insulin-induced hypoglycemia. It also impairs judgment. Severe hypoglycemia may result many hours after as little as 2 ounces of alcohol is consumed, particularly on an empty stomach. Anticipatory guidance should include moderation, eating additional carbohydrates at the time of alcohol consumption, avoiding alcohol use while driving, and informing others they are with both of their diabetes, and hypoglycemia recognition and management.

SPECIAL CONSIDERATIONS FOR PATIENT-CENTERED CARE WITH ADOLESCENTS AND YOUNG ADULTS

Self-management of diabetes is burdensome for patients and families. Consideration should be given to developing patient-centered, evidence-based practices at the individual, family, community, and systems levels to improve health outcomes.[19]

1. Together, identify reasons for poor glycemic control and develop strategies for remediation. Consider the Pediatric Self-Management Model for self-management behaviors, as there are numerous modifiable (treatments, lifestyle and habits, clinic visits, monitoring) and nonmodifiable (cognitive differences, resources, severity of disease) influences on self-care behaviors. Serious psychopathology (including eating disorders) and recurrent diabetic ketoacidosis (DKA) are indications for referral.
2. Identify one reasonable and measurable target behavior for action (number of BG tests, recording carbohydrates at a specific meal, self-insulin adjustment based on BG or carbohydrate intake). It is important to focus on desired behavior that can be controlled rather than outcome that cannot be.
3. Identify short-term reinforcers relevant to the AYA. Reinforcers can include the discussion of fewer symptoms (hypoglycemia or nocturia), improved physical performance, more flexibility in timing and content of meals, as well as the allocation of rewards from parents, and greater independence.
4. Establish a realistic time frame for accomplishments, based on the behavior and goal, using a SMART (specific, measurable, achievable/actionable, relevant, time-based) goal framework. Remember HbA1c levels reflect average blood sugar level over 8 to 12 weeks, so even a small reduction is significant.
5. Adolescents and young adults may benefit from more frequent visits with their clinician with shorter time intervals between visits to access implementation and sustainability of developed plan, as well as barriers to implementation and sustainability. More frequent visits offer more opportunities for reassessing goals and progress.
6. Examine the extent of parental support and monitoring; more support and monitoring by parents of adolescents is associated with increased BG testing and lower HbA1c. Also assess additional supports that may be beneficial in diabetes management.

7. Group coping-skill training improves long-term glycemic control and quality of life.
8. All youth with diabetes should be referred for consultation with a pediatric endocrinologist.

TRANSITION TO ADULT CARE

Transition from adolescence into young adulthood can be a time of overwhelming change with an exponentially increasing responsibility. For patients with diabetes, this can add additional accountability to their growing independence creating a potentially high-risk period for their diabetes management. Multiple factors can contribute to the outcomes during this period, including change in dynamic of clinic visits and the hurdles of engaging with new adult clinicians, potential challenges with insurance coverage, changes in routine with new schools and/or jobs, as well as new exposures to substances such as alcohol. New stressors have the potential to compound existing psychological challenges, including diabetes distress. This is particularly concerning considering the realization that glycemic control is least controlled in adolescents with diabetes. Current recommendations for the ADA to improve transition for adolescents include[20]:

1. Increasing collaboration between pediatric clinicians, patient, and family to develop a transition plan at least 1 year prior to transition.
2. Graduated increase in patient responsibility of their independent diabetes management, which includes glucose self-management, scheduling appointments, monitoring and refilling diabetes supply, knowing how and when to contact clinicians with questions or concerns.
3. Educating the patient regarding differences between pediatric and adult care of diabetes in the medical setting.
4. The pediatric/adolescent clinician should provide new adult clinician with written summary of active problem list (including mental health concerns), medications, diabetes self-assessment skills, glycemic control history, and diabetes comorbidities.
5. Patients should be provided with contact information/options for adult care adult care clinicians to initiate care appointment within 3 to 4 months following last pediatric clinician. Additional information should be provided on what to do if this transition is not successful and they become lost to follow-up.
6. Individualized and developmentally appropriate plans should be created to ensure patient is best equipped to adhere to their diabetes care considering all transition-related factors. This may include additional re-education as needed.
7. Existing comorbidities should be addressed and controlled as much as possible prior to transition, including eating disorders, mental health concerns, and micro- or macrovascular complications. For those comorbidities that are not controlled, a plan should be discussed with the patient and family, incorporating the new clinician, if possible, to ensure a smooth transition of these care needs.

SUMMARY

Diabetes is a relatively common chronic disease that is increasing in prevalence in AYAs across the globe. Regardless of the etiology of diabetes, chronic hyperglycemia is associated with long-term microvascular (retinopathy, nephropathy, and neuropathy) and accelerated macrovascular (coronary artery disease and stroke) complications. A chronic disease model of care to maintain routine medical and mental health checks, as well as continued counseling for prevention of acute and secondary complications of diabetes is important for all AYAs with diabetes. As adolescents prepare to transition to adult-based care, shared-decision making and increasing autonomy with self-care are increasingly important.

REFERENCES

1. Ilonen J, Lempainen J, Veijola R. The heterogeneous pathogenesis of type 1 diabetes mellitus. *Nat Rev Endocrinol.* 2019;11:635.
2. Nadeau KJ, Anderson BJ, Berg EG, et al. Youth-onset type 2 diabetes consensus report: current status, challenges, and priorities. *Diabetes Care.* 2016;39:1635.
3. Anık A, Çatlı G, Abacı A, et al. Maturity-onset diabetes of the young (MODY): an update. *J Pediatr Endocrinol Metab.* 2015;28:251.
4. Granados A, Chan CL, Ode KL, et al. Cystic fibrosis related diabetes: pathophysiology, screening and diagnosis. *J Cyst Fibros.* 2019;18:S3.
5. Maahs DM, West NA, Lawrence JM, et al. Epidemiology of type 1 diabetes. *Endocrinol Metab Clin North Am.* 2010;39:481.
6. Dabelea D, Mayer-Davis EJ, Saydah S, et al. Prevalence of type 1 and type 2 diabetes among children and adolescents from 2001 to 2009. *JAMA.* 2014;311:1778.
7. Lascar N, Brown J, Pattison H, et al. Type 2 diabetes in adolescents and young adults. *Lancet Diabetes Endocrinol.* 2018;6:69.
8. Magge SN, Silverstein J, Elder D, et al. Evaluation and treatment of prediabetes in youth. *J Pediatr.* 2020;219:11.
9. Styne DM, Arslanian SA, Connor EL, et al. Pediatric obesity-assessment, treatment, and prevention: an endocrine society clinical practice guideline. *J Clin Endocrinol Metab.* 2017;102:709.
10. Nathan DM; DCCT/EDIC Research Group. The diabetes control and complications trial/epidemiology of diabetes interventions and complications study at 30 years: overview. *Diabetes Care.* 2014;37:9.
11. Foster NC, Beck RW, Miller KM, et al. State of type 1 diabetes management and outcomes from the T1D exchange in 2016–2018. *Diabetes Technol Ther.* 2019;21:66.
12. American Diabetes Association. Standards of medical care in diabetes-2021. *Diabetes Care.* 2021;44(Suppl 1):S4.
13. American Diabetes Association. 13. Children and Adolescents: standards of medical care in diabetes-2021. *Diabetes Care.* 2021;44:S180.
14. Cameron FJ, Garvey K, Hood KK, et al. ISPAD Clinical Practice Consensus Guidelines 2018: diabetes in adolescence. *Pediatr Diabetes.* 2018;19(Suppl 27):250.
15. Chiang JL, Maahs DM, Garvey KC, et al. Type 1 diabetes in children and adolescents: a position statement by the American Diabetes Association. *Diabetes Care.* 2018;41:2026.
16. Zietler P, Arslanian S, Fu Junfen, et al. ISPAD Clinical Practice consensus Guidelines 2018: type 2 diabetes mellitus in youth. *Pediatr Diabetes.* 2018;19(Suppl 27):28.
17. Doyle EA, Quinn SM, Ambrosino JM, et al. Disordered eating behaviors in emerging adults with type 1 diabetes: a common problem for both men and women. *J Pediatr Health Care.* 2017;31:327.
18. Nielsen S, Emborg C, Mølbak AG. Mortality in concurrent type 1 diabetes and anorexia nervosa. *Diabetes Care.* 2002;25:309.
19. Modi AC, Pai AL, Hommel KA, et al. Pediatric self-management: a framework for research, practice, and policy. *Pediatrics.* 2012;129:e473.
20. Peters A, Laffel L, the American Diabetes Association Transitions Working Group. Diabetes care for emerging adults: recommendations for transition from pediatric to adult diabetes care systems: a position statement of the American Diabetes Association, with representation by the American College of Osteopathic Family Physicians, the American Academy of Pediatrics, the American Association of Clinical Endocrinologists, the American Osteopathic Association, the Centers for Disease Control and Prevention, Children with Diabetes, The Endocrine Society, the International Society for Pediatric and Adolescent Diabetes, Juvenile Diabetes Research Foundation International, the National Diabetes Education Program, and the Pediatric Endocrine Society (formerly Lawson Wilkins Pediatric Endocrine Society). *Diabetes Care.* 2011;34:2477.

ADDITIONAL RESOURCES AND WEBSITES

Additional Resources and Websites for Clinicians:
American Diabetes Association—http://www.diabetes.org
Association of Certified Diabetes Educators—http://www.aadnet.org/
Children with Diabetes—http://www.childrenwithdiabetes.com
International Society for Pediatric and Adolescent Diabetes—https://www.ispad.org
Juvenile Diabetes Research Foundation—http://www.jdrf.org

Additional Resources and Websites for Parents/Caregivers:
AboutKidsHealth—https://www.aboutkidshealth.ca/Article?contentid=2509&language=English
AboutKidsHealth—https://www.aboutkidshealth.ca/Search/Pages/AKHResults.aspx?k=diabetes&language=English
Association of Certified Diabetes Educators—http://www.aadnet.org
Children with Diabetes—http://www.childrenwithdiabetes.com
Juvenile Diabetes Research Foundation—https://www.jdrf.ca/type-1-diabetes-and-covid-19-going-back-to-school/?gclid=EAIaIQobChMI89nOyoOf8gIVdSs4Ch2viAALEAAYASAAEgIshPD_BwE
Patient-focused online publication and organization—https://diatribe.org

Additional Resources and Websites for Adolescents and Young Adults:
Diabetes Canada—https://www.diabetes.ca/managing-my-diabetes/kids,-teens—diabetes/teens—diabetes
FRED—https://www.diabetes-children.ca/en/type-1-diabetes/type-1-diabetes/?gclid=EAIaIQobChMIg5j_uP2e8gIVamtvBB3RSAMnEAAYASAAEgI_sfD_BwE
Juvenile Diabetes Research Foundation—https://www.jdrf.org/t1d-resources/newly-diagnosed/teens/-Juvenile
Patient-focused online publication and organization—https://diatribe.org

PART III

Cardiovascular and Pulmonary Disorders

CHAPTER 17

Cardiovascular Health and Cholesterol Disorders

Holly C. Gooding
Jacob C. Hartz

KEY WORDS

- Atherosclerosis
- Cardiovascular disease
- Cholesterol
- Dyslipidemia
- Familial hypercholesterolemia
- Ideal cardiovascular health
- Prevention
- Risk assessment

INTRODUCTION

In 2010, the American Heart Association (AHA) set as its 2020 Impact Goal the improvement of cardiovascular health of all Americans by 20% over the next decade, a goal they reaffirmed in 2020 with a further commitment to equitably increase healthy life expectancy worldwide.[1] In setting these strategic goals, the AHA defined the new construct of *ideal cardiovascular health*. Cardiovascular health is comprised of seven individual metrics that, when present together at ideal levels, are associated with lower cardiovascular disease (CVD) and total mortality and increased years lived free of CVD.[2] By scoring each metric as poor (0), intermediate (1), or ideal (2) using specific definitions for adults 20 years of age and older and for children and adolescents, clinicians and researchers can calculate a comprehensive cardiovascular health score ranging from 0 to 14 (Table 17.1).

This chapter will review the concept of cardiovascular health and its role in the prevention of CVD. The chapter will focus on the role of cholesterol levels, one of the seven cardiovascular health metrics, in the pathophysiology of atherosclerosis. Screening for abnormal cholesterol levels in childhood and adolescence is a cornerstone of the 2011 National Heart Lung Blood Institute (NHLBI) Expert Panel on Integrated Guidelines for Cardiovascular Health and Risk Reduction in Children and Adolescents.[3] Identification of specific lipid disorders and their treatment are also discussed. Readers are referred to the individual chapters for each of the other six metrics that comprise cardiovascular health: nutrition (Chapter 6), diabetes (Chapter 16), blood pressure (Chapter 20), physical activity (Chapter 23), body mass index (BMI) (Chapter 37), and tobacco exposure (Chapter 70).

CARDIOVASCULAR HEALTH

Numerous studies from populations around the world have confirmed the benefit of achieving ideal cardiovascular health in childhood and retaining it into middle age. A 2016 meta-analysis of nine prospective cohort studies including 12,828 middle aged and older adults from China, Korea, the United Kingdom, and the United States found that having greater than or equal to 5 ideal cardiovascular health metrics or a total cardiovascular health score of greater than 10 out of a possible 14 was associated with lower risk of all-cause mortality (relative risk [RR] 0.55; 95% confidence interval [CI] 0.37 to 0.80), cardiovascular mortality (RR 0.25; 95% CI 0.10 to 0.63), CVD (RR 0.20; 95% CI 0.11 to 0.37), and stroke (RR 0.31; 95% CI 0.25 to 0.38).[2] In addition, the Coronary Artery Risk Development in Young Adults (CARDIA) study found that having a high cardiovascular health score of 12 or greater at ages 18 to 30 years was associated with a significantly lower risk of CVD events (adjusted hazard ratio [aHR] 0.14; 95% CI 0.09 to 0.22) and CVD mortality (aHR 0.07; 95% CI 0.03 to 0.19) over 32 years of follow-up.[4] Importantly, the population attributable fraction for CVD mortality was 0.81 (95% CI 0.55 to 0.92) in this study, meaning that 81% of the variation in early CVD death before the age of 65 was explained by having less than ideal cardiovascular health in young adulthood.

Studies from childhood cohorts confirm the benefit of having ideal cardiovascular health even at younger ages. In a pooled analysis of data from five pediatric cohorts from the United States and Finland following 9,388 participants from 8 years of age up to 55 years of age, maintaining ideal cardiovascular health throughout the study was associated with less carotid intima media thickness in middle age, a marker of atherosclerosis.[5] Notably, 25% of participants in these cohorts already had less than ideal cardiovascular health in childhood, and trajectory analysis identified late adolescence as a common period of cardiovascular health loss.

Together these studies highlight the importance of a life course approach to achieving and maintaining cardiovascular health (Figure 17.1). Prenatal and perinatal factors affect cardiovascular health at birth. Children born preterm, small or large for gestational age, and exposed in utero to hypertension, preeclampsia, or gestational diabetes, are at higher risk for poor cardiovascular health.[6] Early feeding, sleep, and activity patterns are important for reversing some of this risk and promoting cardiovascular health.[7] Adolescence represents a particularly critical inflection point for cardiovascular health given both the biologic changes of puberty and the psychosocial development that characterize this life stage.[8] The transition to young adulthood is another critical window, as adolescents and young adults (AYAs) establish health behavior patterns and often become parents, solidifying patterns for the generations to come.[9]

Unfortunately, the prevalence of ideal cardiovascular health is generally low. In population health surveys from the National Health and Nutrition Examination Surveys, only 13% of American adults and 47% of American adolescents meet at least five of the seven ideal cardiovascular health metrics.[10] For adolescents, the prevalence is lowest for ideal dietary patterns (essentially 0%) and ideal physical activity levels (25.4%) and highest for ideal (non)-smoking (95.7%), ideal blood pressure (89.1%), and ideal fasting

TABLE 17.1

American Heart Association Definitions of Ideal Cardiovascular Health for Children and Adolescents Under 20 Years of Age and Adults 20 Years of Age and Older[10]

Metric	Level of Cardiovascular Health for Each Metric		
	Poor	Intermediate	Ideal
Tobacco Smoking			
Children and adolescents 12–19 y	Tried during the prior 30 d	Not applicable	Never tried; never smoked a whole cigarette
Adults 20 y and older	Current smoking	Former, quit less than 12 mo ago	Never or quit greater than 12 mo ago
Physical Activity			
Children and Adolescents 12–19 y	None	>0 and <60 min of moderate or vigorous every day	≥60 min of moderate or vigorous every day
Adults 20 y and older	None	1–149 min/wk moderate intensity or 1–74 min/wk vigorous intensity	≥150 min/wk moderate intensity or ≥75 min/wk vigorous intensity
Healthy Diet Pattern, number of components from AHA diet score[a]			
Children and Adolescents 5–19 y	<2	2–3	4–5
Adults 20 y and older	<2	2–3	4–5
Body Mass Index			
Children and Adolescents 2–19 y	>95th percentile for age/sex	85th–95th percentile for age/sex	<85th percentile for age/sex
Adults 20 y and older	≥30 kg/m²	25–29.9 kg/m²	<25 kg/m²
Total Cholesterol, mg/dL			
Children and Adolescents 6–19 y	≥200	170–199	<170
Adults 20 y and older	≥240	200–239 or treated to goal	<200 without need for medication
Blood Pressure			
Children and Adolescents 8–19 y	>95th percentile for age/sex/height	90–95th percentile or SBP ≥120 mm Hg or DBP ≥80 mm Hg	<90th percentile for age/sex/height
Adults 20 y and older	SBP ≥140 or DBP ≥90 mmHg	SBP 120–139 or DBP 80–89 mm Hg or treated to goal	SBP <120 and DBP <80 mm Hg without need for medication
Fasting Plasma Glucose, mg/dL			
Children and Adolescents 12–19 y	≥126	100–125 or treated to goal	<100 without need for medication
Adults 20 y and older	≥126	100–125 or treated to goal	<100 without need for medication

AHA, American Heart Association; SBP, systolic blood pressure; DBP, diastolic blood pressure.

[a]Ideal diet is defined by the number of categories met: (1) at least 4.5 cups per day of fruits and vegetables, (2) at least two 3.5-ounce servings a week of fish, (3) less than 1,500 mg a day of sodium, (4) fewer than 36 ounces a week of sugar sweetened beverages, (5) at least three 1-ounce servings a day of whole grains, scaled to a 2,000 kcal/d dietary intake for children.

glucose (86.2%). The prevalences of ideal cholesterol levels (77.2%) and ideal BMI (63.4%) are moderate for adolescents. Each of the metrics, with the exception of diet and physical activity, are more likely to be at ideal levels in adolescents compared to adults (Figure 17.2), again highlighting the importance of the transition to adulthood for the loss or preservation of ideal cardiovascular health.

ATHEROSCLEROSIS

Atherosclerosis, the pathophysiologic process underlying CVD, begins when the endothelial cells lining the inner surface of arteries attract white blood cells through expression of adhesion molecules

(Figure 17.3).[11] Once inside the tunica intima of the arterial wall, monocyte-derived macrophages engulf lipoprotein particles and become foam cells. These foam cells are eventually covered with a fibrous cap, known as an atheroma, consisting of extracellular matrix molecules produced from smooth muscle cells within the vessel wall. The atheroma slowly accumulates more lipids and cellular debris and develops a necrotic core. Large atheromas, also known as atherosclerotic plaques, can cause physical stenosis, which gradually limits blood flow and causes tissue ischemia. They can also rupture and release proinflammatory molecules from the lipid core, leading abruptly to thrombosis and blockage of blood flow. Pieces of the atherosclerotic plaque can also break off or

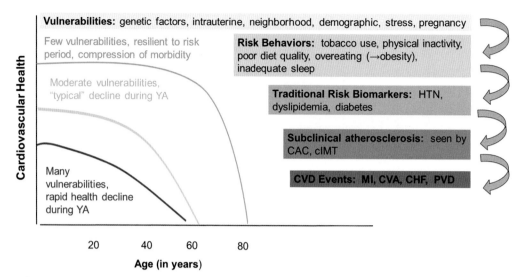

FIGURE 17.1 Causes of variation in trajectories of cardiovascular health. The three cases illustrated in the figure vary from having a low early vulnerability burden that allows CVH to develop maximally (*green curve*) to having a high vulnerability burden that constrains the development of CVH (*red curve*). The comparison of the *green* and *yellow curves* illustrates that the clinical impact of such a rapid loss of CVH varies depending upon its timing in the life course. CAC, coronary artery calcium; CHF, congestive heart failure; CIMT, carotid intima media thickness; CVA, cerebral vascular accident; CVD, cardiovascular disease; CVH, cardiovascular health; HTN, hypertension; MI, myocardial infarction; PVD, peripheral vascular disease; YA, young adulthood. (*Source:* Gooding HC, Gidding SS, Moran AE, et al. Challenges and opportunities for the prevention and treatment of cardiovascular disease among young adults: report From a National Heart, Lung, and Blood Institute Working Group. *J Am Heart Assoc.* 2020;9(19). doi:10.1161/JAHA.120.016115)

embolize and cause ischemia by lodging in smaller blood vessels further down the vascular tree.

Each of the components of ideal cardiovascular health contributes to the process of maintaining a healthy vasculature or conversely, to atherosclerosis if absent. Inflammation is key to the initial formation of foam cells and progression to atheromas.[11]

Smoking, obesity, and diabetes promote inflammation while physical activity and a diet rich in antioxidants can reduce inflammation. Hypertension increases tension in the arterial wall leading to proliferation of smooth muscle cells and oxidative stress, further fueling the formation of atheromas. Cholesterol-containing low-density lipoprotein (LDL) particles form the basis of the lipid core.

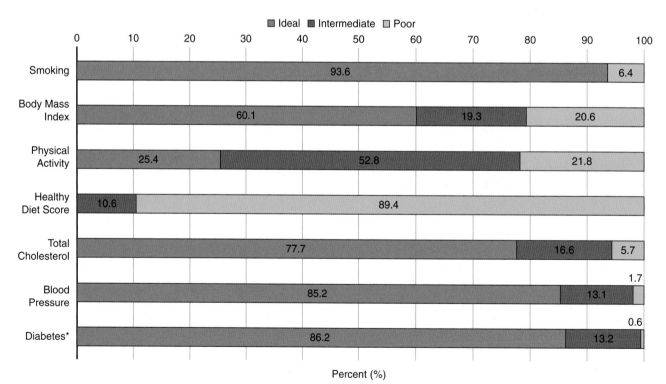

FIGURE 17.2 Prevalence of adolescents ages 12 to 19 years and adults ages 20 years and older in the National Health and Nutrition Examination Survey meeting the American Heart Association Definitions of Poor, Intermediate, and Ideal Cardiovascular Health for each of the seven metrics.[10] BMI, body mass index; CVH, cardiovascular health. (*Source:* National Center for Health Statistics, NHANES, 2015 to 2016 (healthy diet score, 2013 to 2014) as reported in "Heart Disease and Stroke Statistics—2020 Update" from the American Heart Association.)

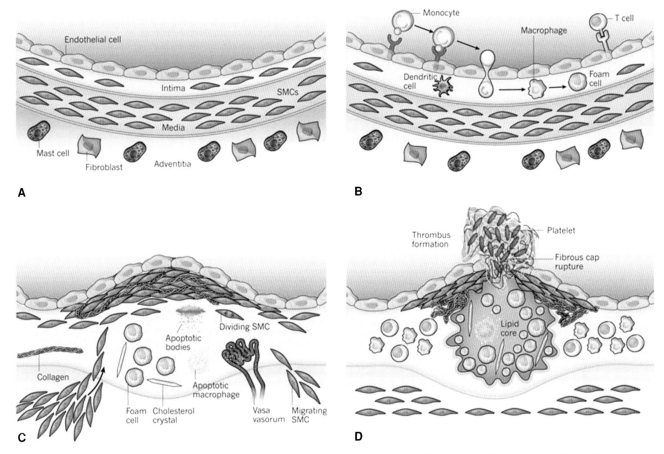

FIGURE 17.3 Development of atherosclerotic lesions. **A:** The normal artery contains three layers. The inner layer, the tunica intima, is lined by a monolayer of endothelial cells that is in contact with blood overlying a basement membrane. The middle layer, or tunica media, contains smooth muscle cells (SMCs) embedded in a complex extracellular matrix. The adventitia, the outer layer of arteries, contains mast cells, nerve endings, and microvessels. **B:** The initial steps of atherosclerosis include adhesion of blood leukocytes to the activated endothelial monolayer, directed migration of the bound leukocytes into the intima, maturation of monocytes (the most numerous of the leukocytes recruited) into macrophages, and their uptake of lipid, yielding foam cells. **C:** Lesion progression involves the migration of SMCs from the media to the intima and the heightened synthesis of extracellular matrix macromolecules such as collagen, elastin, and proteoglycans. Extracellular lipid derived from dead and dying cells can accumulate in the central region of a plaque, often denoted the lipid or necrotic core. **D:** Thrombosis, the ultimate complication of atherosclerosis, often complicates a physical disruption of the atherosclerotic plaque. (*Source:* Libby P, Ridker PM, Hansson GK. Progress and challenges in translating the biology of atherosclerosis. *Nature*. Published online 2011. doi:10.1038/nature10146)

In contrast, cholesterol-poor high-density lipoprotein (HDL) particles can remove cholesterol particles and take them back to the blood stream.

There is definitive evidence that atherosclerosis begins in childhood and progresses during the AYA years. Autopsy studies dating back to the early 1900s have found fatty streaks, the earliest precursors to atherosclerosis, in children.[12] Some of the clearest evidence comes from the Pathobiological Determinants of Atherosclerosis in Youth (PDAY) study which collected arteries, blood, tissue, and clinical data from 15- through 34-year-olds who died of accidents, homicides, or suicides in the 1980s.[12] The prevalence of fatty streaks and raised atherosclerotic lesions increased with age and was higher in males compared to females. The extent of atherosclerosis was greater in those with higher non-HDL cholesterol, hypertension, hyperglycemia, and smoking, and was inversely associated with HDL-cholesterol. Obesity was associated with greater atherosclerosis in males only.[12] Importantly, fatty streaks and raised lesions were seen even in those with normal lipid profiles, although non-HDL cholesterol was the greatest risk factor beyond age and showed a linear relationship with advanced atherosclerotic lesions starting at levels as low as 130 mg/dL. This is consistent with recent epidemiologic studies demonstrating that non-HDL cholesterol in childhood is a stronger predictor of coronary artery calcium than lipid levels measured later in life.[13]

LIPID PHYSIOLOGY AND LIPID DISORDERS

The lipids found in humans include sterols (primarily cholesterol) and fatty acids. While dyslipidemia is associated with an increased risk of CVD, lipids are an important component of a number of physiologic processes. For instance, cholesterol plays a role in the fluidity of cell membranes, steroid hormones, and bile acids, while fatty acids are the primary energy store for humans, are a constituent of phospholipids, and play a role in cell signaling.

As lipids are hydrophobic, they need to be carried in the circulation packaged as lipoproteins. Lipoproteins are composed of cholesterol (free cholesterol and cholesterol esters), triglycerides, and apolipoproteins (Figure 17.4). Lipoproteins can be differentiated based on their content of triglycerides and cholesterol; size and density; electrophoretic properties; and composition of apolipoproteins. They can be categorized as chylomicrons (and chylomicron remnants), very low density lipoproteins (VLDL), intermediate density lipoproteins (IDL), LDL, and HDL. The key to the physiology of the lipoprotein particle lies in its composition of apolipoproteins. The apolipoproteins provide structure, act as ligands

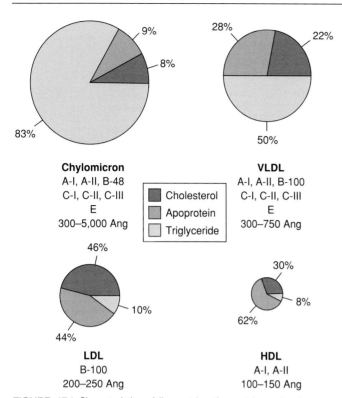

Chylomicron
A-I, A-II, B-48
C-I, C-II, C-III
E
300–5,000 Ang

VLDL
A-I, A-II, B-100
C-I, C-II, C-III
E
300–750 Ang

Cholesterol
Apoprotein
Triglyceride

LDL
B-100
200–250 Ang

HDL
A-I, A-II
100–150 Ang

FIGURE 17.4 Characteristics of lipoproteins. Apoproteins and volume are detailed below each lipoprotein. Ang, angstroms; VLDL, very low–density lipoprotein; LDL, low-density lipoprotein; HDL, high-density lipoprotein. (Adapted from Hardoff D, Jacobson MS. Hyperlipidemia. *Adolesc Med State Arts Rev.* 1992;3:475.)

for receptors, and activate enzymes necessary for lipid metabolism (Figure 17.4).

The production of these lipoproteins requires sterols and fatty acids derived from the diet or produced endogenously, primarily in the liver. The dietary sterols are composed of both cholesterol (75%) and plant sterols (25%) and enter the enterocyte via the Niemann–Pick C1-Like 1 protein. Cholesterol is then converted to cholesterol ester by acyl-coenzyme A [acyl-CoA] cholesterol acyltransferase in the enterocyte, which traps the cholesterol ester within the cell. Plant sterols (also called phytosterols), though, are not retained within the enterocyte, but are excreted back to the intestinal lumen through adenosine triphosphate binding cassette subfamilies G5 and G8 (ABCG5 and ABCG8). Although plant sterols competitively inhibit the absorption of cholesterol, and theoretically may have positive health benefits, defects in ABCG5 and ABCG8 lead to excessive absorption of plant sterols, a condition known as sitosterolemia. Sitosterolemia is associated with hemolytic anemia, xanthomas, and joint discomfort. However, its role in the development of CVD is less clear.

Free fatty acids are absorbed from the intestinal lumen into the enterocyte through a different mechanism that remains poorly understood. Once absorbed, free fatty acids and cholesterol esters combine with apolipoproteins to form chylomicrons. One important step in this process is the transfer of fatty acids to the primary structural protein of chylomicrons, Apolipoprotein B (Apo B), by microsomal triglyceride transport protein (MTP). Mutations in MTP lead to abetalipoproteinemia, in which chylomicrons are not formed correctly and accumulate in the enterocytes. Symptoms include severe hypocholesterolemia, steatorrhea, insufficient absorption of fat-soluble vitamins, failure to thrive, acanthocytosis, and retinitis pigmentosa. Lomitapide (Juxtapid) is an MTP inhibitor that dramatically reduces the production of chylomicrons as well as VLDL through its actions in the liver, but leads to significant

fat malabsorption and hepatic steatosis. It is currently approved for patients with homozygous familial hypercholesterolemia (FH), but its use is limited by its adverse effects.

A process similar to the formation of chylomicrons occurs in the endogenous production of VLDL in the liver. One significant difference between VLDL and chylomicrons is that the Apo B produced in the liver is Apo B100, whereas the Apo B isoform incorporated in chylomicrons is Apo B48. Apo B48 is not recognized by the LDL receptor, preventing premature uptake of chylomicron contents. Once the chylomicron and VLDL enter the circulation, they are quickly cleared as they deliver triglycerides to muscle and adipose tissue. Lipoprotein lipase is responsible for hydrolyzing the triglycerides in the chylomicron and VLDL. Importantly, insulin is critical for lipoprotein lipase function. Hence, insulin resistance is associated with inadequate lipoprotein lipase activity and the clinical finding of hypertriglyceridemia. Further, defects in any component of the lipoprotein lipase [LPL] apparatus, such as GPIHBP1, Apo CII, or Apo A-V will cause hypertriglyceridemia. Evinacumab, an Angiopoietin-Like 3 (ANGPTL3) inhibitor, lowers triglycerides and also dramatically reduces LDL cholesterol, although the mechanism behind the latter effect is unclear.

As chylomicrons lose triglycerides, they are called chylomicron remnants; as VLDL loses triglycerides, it becomes IDL and eventually LDL. As LDL is the most ubiquitous lipoprotein, the efficiency of its removal from the circulation is critical to the risk of CVD. LDL is primarily removed by the liver through LDL receptors, the number and function of which are genetically determined. Defects in the number or function of LDL receptors are the most common cause of FH. As the number of functional LDL receptors is inherited, changes to a patient's diet and physical activity level will have only modest effects on LDL cholesterol values. It should be noted that LDL has no known physiologic role and its value can approach zero without known harm.

While in the circulation, chylomicron remnants gain apolipoprotein E [Apo E], the ligand for the LDL receptor, and are removed from the blood stream. However, if Apo E is defective, chylomicron remnants are cleared less efficiently, leading to familial dysbetalipoproteinemia, which involves increases in both cholesterol and triglyceride levels.

Dyslipidemia is a general term referring to the occurrence of one or more abnormal values on a standard clinical lipid profile (Table 17.2). Typically, this includes an elevated triglyceride level (hypertriglyceridemia), a low HDL cholesterol level (hypoalphalipoproteinemia), or an elevated LDL cholesterol (hyperbetalipoproteinemia). In clinical practice, the most common lipid disorders are hypertriglyceridemia in the setting of insulin resistance and an elevated LDL cholesterol secondary to FH. Familial hypercholesterolemia is the most common disease inherited in an autosomal dominant fashion and affects approximately 1 in 250 people. It is most often caused by defects in the LDL receptor, but can also be a result of gain-of-function mutations in the *PCSK9* gene or in the *APOB* gene that drives Apo B production. Without treatment, FH increases the risk of CVD by as much as 20-fold.

Identification of patients with FH is often difficult as the family history has been shown to be unreliable and the disease is asymptomatic, except among the most severely affected, who may have xanthomas. While genetic testing and a number of validated criteria can be used to formally diagnose FH, they rarely influence clinical decisions as treatment is based on LDL cholesterol values. Currently, patients with FH typically are classified as either having heterozygous or homozygous FH, but may be better classified based on the phenotypic severity of the disease. Patients with homozygous FH, which occurs in about 1 in 1 million individuals, have severely elevated LDL cholesterol levels, often above 800 mg/dL. A majority of patients with homozygous FH have mutations in both alleles of the LDL receptor, but also may have one mutation in the LDL receptor and an additional mutation in *APOB* or *PCSK9*. Unlike

TABLE 17.2

Classification of Lipid Disorders

Disease	Causes/Variants	Lipids	Notes
Familial hypercholesterolemia	1) LDL receptor defect 2) *APOB* defect (Familial Defective Apo B-100) 3) PCSK9 4) LDLRAP1 (autosomal recessive hypercholesterolemia)	↑↑ LDL-C	Heterozygous familial hypercholesterolemia is the most common autosomal dominant inherited disease (~1/250 people). Defects in the LDL receptor are most common. Patients with homozygous FH have LDL-C that is often above 800 mg/dL.
Familial chylomicronemia syndrome	1) LPL deficiency 2) APO-CII deficiency (co-factor for LPL) 3) LMF1 4) APO-A5 5) GP1HBP1 (Structural support protein for LPL)	↑↑ TG	Severely elevated TG levels, often >1,000 mg/dL, but varies widely. Primary treatment goal is lowering TG to reduce risk of triglyceride-induced pancreatitis.
Lysosomal acid lipase deficiency (Wolman disease) and CESD	Defect in *LIPA* gene	↑ TG ↓ HDL-C	Wolman disease is a more severe phenotype and presents in infancy with cholestasis, liver disease, failure to thrive, malabsorption, and adrenal insufficiency. CESD presents later with liver disease and dyslipidemia.
Familial dysbetalipoproteinemia	Apo E-2 defect	↑ TC −/↓ LDL-C ↑↑ TG ↓ HDL-C	Diagnosis is made when the triglyceride to Apo B ratio is <10.
Familial hypertriglyceridemia	Polygenic with ↑ VLDL production	↑↑ TG	Often associated with other comorbidities, particularly insulin resistance.
Sitosterolemia	ABCG5/ABCG8	↑ LDL	Hemolytic anemia and joint pain. Often responds poorly to statins, but well to diet modification. Patients may present with xanthomas with LDL-C levels lower than would be expected.
Cerebrotendinous xanthomatosis	Defect in 27-hydroxylase (CYP27A1)	↓ HDL-C ↑ LDL-C	Primarily a neurologic disease secondary to cholesterol and cholestanol in the brain. Symptoms begin in the second decade of life, with a diagnosis made in the third or fourth decade of life. Additional symptoms include, elevated cholestanol levels, increased bile alcohols in urine, jaundice, early atherosclerotic events, cataracts, chronic diarrhea, and osteoporosis. LDL-C levels are lower than would be expected in the presence of xanthomas.

LDL, low-density lipoprotein; HDL, high-density lipoprotein; Apo, apolipoprotein; FH, familial hypercholesterolemia; PCSK9, proprotein convertase subtilisin/kexin type 9; LDLRAP1, low-density lipoprotein receptor adaptor protein-1; TG, triglyceride; CESD, cholesteryl ester storage disease; LMF1, lipase maturation factor-1; GP1HBP1, glycosylphosphatidylinositol-anchored high-density lipoprotein-binding protein1; TC, total cholesterol.

those with heterozygous FH, patients with homozygous FH often present in childhood with xanthomas or a family history of severe hypercholesteremia. Unfortunately, if missed, patients may present in early adolescence with signs and symptoms of coronary ischemia. Patients with homozygous FH also are unlikely to respond to conventional medical therapy and must be treated with weekly or biweekly LDL apheresis, despite being on multiple lipid-lowering medications.

Clinically, clinicians most often make clinical decisions based on lipid panels that report the cholesterol content of the various lipoproteins. The goal of risk reduction is to reduce the presence of Apo B particles, and the LDL cholesterol value is simply a surrogate marker of the prevalence of Apo B in the circulation. This can lead to discordance in which there is a high level of Apo B particles circulating, but LDL cholesterol appears to be normal or only slightly elevated. This is most likely to occur in the setting of hypertriglyceridemia. In these cases, the Apo B level will help clarify the individual's CVD risk, which will be misrepresented by the LDL cholesterol and non-HDL cholesterol levels.

CARDIOVASCULAR RISK SCREENING

In 2011, the NHLBI Expert Panel on Integrated Guidelines for Cardiovascular Health and Risk Reduction in Children and Adolescents,[3] endorsed by the American Academy of Pediatrics (AAP), recommended comprehensive cardiovascular screening for all children beginning in infancy. A developmentally appropriate approach to each of the seven cardiovascular health factors, plus an assessment of family history of early CVD, was recommended for patients at birth to 12 months and ages 1 to 4, 5 to 9, 9 to 11, 12 to 17, and 18 to 21 years.

In adolescence (ages 12 to 17 years) and early young adulthood (ages 18 to 21 years), clinicians should:

- Update **family history** at each nonurgent health encounter, inquiring about early CVD (males ≤55 years, females ≤65 years) in parents, grandparents, aunts, and uncles.
- Assess **tobacco exposure**, reinforce a strong antismoking message, and provide smoking cessation assistance or referral as needed (see Chapter 70).
- Obtain a **dietary history** and review healthy dietary patterns, providing counseling as needed (see Chapter 6).

- Obtain a **physical activity** history and recommend ≥1 hour per day of moderate to vigorous physical activity and less than 2 hours per day of screen/sedentary time for adolescents and ≥150 minutes of physical activity for young adults (see Chapter 23).
- Chart **height/weight/ BMI**, intensify diet and activity counseling for those with a BMI in the overweight category, and address obesity per established algorithms (see Chapter 37)
- Check **blood pressure** annually, work-up and manage elevated blood pressure per current AAP guidelines (as updated in 2017, see Chapter 20).
- Measure fasting plasma **glucose**, hemoglobin A1C, or 2-hour plasma glucose during a 75-g oral glucose tolerance test in those with overweight or obesity and one or more risk factors per American Diabetes Association guidelines (as updated in 2000, see Chapter 16).
- Obtain a **universal lipid screen** with nonfasting non-HDL-C or fasting lipid profile in preadolescence at ages 9 to 11 years and again at ages 17 to 21 years; obtain a fasting lipid profile at ages 12 to 16 years if members of the family are newly identified with early CVD events, a parent has dyslipidemia or total cholesterol ≥240 mg/dL, or the adolescent has diabetes, hypertension, overweight/obesity, smokes cigarettes, or has another condition associated with elevated CVD risk (see **Table 17.3**).

These guidelines are consistent with the 2016 AHA Statement on CVH Promotion in Children[14] and the 2018 American College of Cardiology (ACC)/AHA Guideline on the Management of Blood Cholesterol.[15] The 2019 AHA Statement on Cardiovascular Risk Reduction in High-Risk Pediatric Patients[16] makes further recommendations for those children and adolescents with accelerated CVD risk due to multiple concurrent CVD risk factors or other comorbidities (see **Table 17.3**).

The 2011 NHLBI recommendation of universal lipid screening at ages 9 to 11 and 17 to 21 was met with some controversy.[17] Critics remain concerned about the safety of statins in children, the harms of diagnosing children with lipid disorders other than FH for which evidence-based treatment beyond lifestyle changes has not been established, and the cost effectiveness of screening and treatment relative to population health measures to promote better diet and physical activity for all. Proponents point to the ability of universal screening to identify more children with genetic FH than the previously recommended family history–based screening, the safety of statins in short term trials in adolescents, and strong epidemiologic data connecting lifetime exposure to elevated cholesterol to CVD events. Notably, in 2016 the U.S. Preventive Services Task Force reaffirmed their 2007 "I" statement on cholesterol screening in children and adolescents, concluding that there was insufficient evidence to recommend for or against screening before the age of 20 years.[18] While they acknowledged the prevalence of FH is estimated at 1 in 250 to 500 adolescents, they were unable to identify studies demonstrating the benefit of early detection and treatment on adult mortality (nor did they identify clear evidence of harms of screening).

This controversy, as well as the complexity of the 2011 NHLBI Guidelines, has likely contributed to the low uptake of universal lipid screening by pediatricians. Only 42.4% of pediatricians surveyed by the AAP in 2014 reported usually or always screening healthy 17- to 21-year-olds for elevated cholesterol.[19] More than half (54%) were not familiar with the 2011 NHLBI Guidelines, and 23% felt cholesterol screening was a low priority. Pediatricians endorsed heart healthy lifestyle counseling for all children and adolescents but noted many barriers, including lack of access to healthy foods and exercise opportunities for patients, and also noted a lack of pediatric lipid specialists for referral if screening identified problems. Only 21% felt comfortable prescribing a statin to older teens and young adults.

Results from the initial cholesterol screen should be categorized as acceptable, borderline, or high (**Table 17.4**). The cholesterol screening algorithm in the 2011 NHLBI Guidelines recommends 2 fasting lipid profiles to confirm the diagnosis of high LDL cholesterol ≥130 mg/dL or high triglycerides ≥130 mg/dL in adolescents. Those with extremely elevated levels (i.e., LDL-C ≥250 mg/dL or triglycerides ≥500 mg/dL) should be referred to a pediatric lipid specialist. All others should have an evaluation for other CVD risk factors and risk conditions (see **Table 17.3**) as well as secondary causes (**Table 17.5**) followed by a 6-month trial of intensive health behavior changes. This should include a diet with only 25% to 30% of calories from fat, ≤7% from saturated fat, ~10% from monounsaturated fat, and <200 mg/d of cholesterol while avoiding trans fats as much as possible. Ideally, these recommendations should be made during consultation with a registered dietician.

Pharmacologic therapy is recommended for all AYAs with a persistently elevated LDL cholesterol ≥190 mg/dL as this is consistent with the FH phenotype.[3,15] The 2011 NHLBI Guidelines also recommend treatment for those with LDL cholesterol ≥160 mg/dL to 189 mg/dL and: (a) 1 high-level risk factor, or (b) ≥2 moderate-level risk factors (see **Table 17.3**); or LDL cholesterol ranging from 130 mg/dL to 159 mg/dL and (a) 2 or more high-level risk factors or (b) 1 high-level risk factor plus 2 or more moderate-level risk factors (see **Table 17.3**). The 2018 ACC/AHA Guidelines recommend shared decision-making regarding statins for AYAs with LDL cholesterol from ≥160 mg/dL to 189 mg/dL, as this may represent the FH phenotype and elevated lifetime risk for CVD.

Estimates from the National Health and Nutrition Examination Surveys indicate abnormal cholesterol affects 1 in 5 children and adolescents,[20] although only 0.4% have very high levels of elevated LDL cholesterol ≥190 mg/dL. Many more have less elevated levels of total cholesterol (7.4%) or low HDL cholesterol (13.4%) levels, for which diet and exercise changes are recommended. Not surprisingly, the 2011 NHLBI Guidelines recommend pharmacologic treatment for an estimated 483,500 more young adults ages 17 to 21 years compared to the 2018 ACC/AHA Guidelines given their more explicit consideration of other CVD risk factors.[21]

TREATMENT OF LIPID DISORDERS

As noted earlier, health behavior changes remain the cornerstone of treatment as they have a number of benefits beyond reducing CVD risk. However, recommendations in the current guidelines in children, adolescents, and adults are based on epidemiologic data and very few prospective, controlled trials. As a result, there has been a shift from recommendations on specific amounts of saturated fat, cholesterol, and salt obtained in the diet, to broader recommendations in the 2019 ACC/AHA Guideline on the Primary Prevention of Cardiovascular Disease.[22] These guidelines recommend that the diet be largely composed of fruits and vegetables; include whole grains compared to refined grains; and that fats predominantly be monounsaturated and polyunsaturated rather than saturated fat. The 2019 ACC/AHA Guideline on the Primary Prevention of Cardiovascular Disease recommends the complete elimination of *trans*-fats and notes the contribution of sugar-sweetened beverages to excess caloric intake.

The Diet Intervention Study in Children[23] was a randomized controlled trial designed to assess the safety and efficacy of a reduced-fat dietary intervention among prepubertal children with elevated LDL cholesterol. The intervention group received counseling to reduce saturated fat in their diet. Although the changes in LDL cholesterol were neither clinically nor statistically different between the two groups at the last visit, there also were no adverse effects of the low-fat diet.

Pharmacologic Agents

Statins

Statins are the first-line treatment for reducing Apo B levels (**Table 17.6**). Statins inhibit the enzyme HMG-CoA reductase, the

TABLE 17.3

Definitions of Children and Adolescents At-Risk, At-Moderate-Risk, and At-High-Risk for Cardiovascular Disease According to the American Heart Association[16]

Category	Condition	Screening Interval	Level to Consider Pharmacotherapy (mg/dL)	Goal Level (mg/dL)
High risk	• Type 1 diabetes mellitus • Type 2 diabetes mellitus • End-stage renal disease • Kawasaki disease with persistent aneurysms ($Z_{max} \geq 2.5$) • Solid-organ transplant vasculopathy • Childhood cancer survivor (or stem cell recipient) *Or* • Moderate risk *plus* ≥2 at-risk factors	Annually	LDL-C ≥130 or Non-HDL-C ≥145	LDL-C <100 Non-HDL-C <130
Moderate risk	• Severe obesity (BMI ≥1.2 × 95th percentile) • Heterozygous familial hypercholesterolemia • Hypertension • Aortic coarctation • Aortic stenosis • Elevated Lipoprotein(a) • Chronic kidney disease not requiring dialysis • Childhood cancer survivor or received chest radiation *Or* • ≥3 at-risk factors	Every 2 y	LDL-C ≥160 or Non-HDL-C ≥190	LDL-C <130
At risk	• Obesity (BMI ≥95th percentile) • Insulin resistance with comorbidities (NAFLD, PCOS) • White-coat hypertension • Cardiomyopathy • Pulmonary hypertension • Chronic inflammatory conditions • Previous coronary artery translocation for anomalous coronary artery or transposition of the great arteries • Childhood cancer (cardiotoxic chemotherapy only) • Kawasaki disease with regressed aneurysms	Every 3 y	LDL-C ≥160 or Non-HDL-C ≥190	LDL-C <130

LDL, low-density lipoprotein; HDL, high-density lipoprotein; BMI, body mass index; NAFLD, nonalcoholic fatty liver disease; PCOS, polycystic ovary syndrome.

TABLE 17.4

Acceptable, Borderline, and Abnormal Plasma Lipid, Lipoprotein, and Apolipoprotein Concentrations in Adolescents

	Acceptable (mg/dL)	Borderline (mg/dL)	High (mg/dL)[a]
Total cholesterol	<170	170–199	>200
LDL cholesterol	<110	110–129	>130
Non-HDL cholesterol	<120	120–144	>145
Apolipoprotein B	<90	90–109	>110
Triglycerides (10–19 y)	<90	90–129	>130
HDL cholesterol	>45	40–45	<40
Apolipoprotein A-1	>120	115–120	<115

[a]Low cut points for HDL and apolipoprotein A-1 represent approximately the 10th percentile. Cut points for high and borderline represent approximately the 95th and 75th percentiles, respectively.
LDL, low-density lipoprotein; HDL, high-density lipoprotein.
Values for plasma lipid and lipoprotein levels are from the NCEP Expert Panel on Cholesterol Levels in Children. Non-HDL cholesterol values from the Bogalusa Heart Study are equivalent to the NCEP Pediatric Panel cut points for LDL cholesterol. Values for plasma apolipoprotein B and apolipoprotein A-1 are from the National Health and Nutrition Examination Survey III.
Adapted from Expert Panel on Integrated Guidelines for Cardiovascular Health and Risk Reduction in Children and Adolescents; National Heart, Lung, and Blood Institute. Expert panel on integrated guidelines for cardiovascular health and risk reduction in children and adolescents: summary report. *Pediatrics.* 2011;128(suppl 5):S213–S256.

rate-limiting factor in cholesterol synthesis, thus decreasing intracellular cholesterol levels. This in turn increases the clearance of LDL cholesterol by increasing the number of LDL receptors. As a class, statins are generally interchangeable, with the major differences being in potency and interactions with other medications. Depending on the statin and its dose, statins decrease LDL cholesterol by 25% to 45%. As a rule of thumb, doubling the dose of a statin will decrease LDL cholesterol by an additional six percent from the baseline change. Statins also lower triglycerides by 15% to 30%. There is growing evidence to support the role of statins in primary prevention, particularly in patients with FH. The table describes indications for starting statins based on the 2019 recommendations.

Adverse effects are commonly attributed to statins, but there is little data to support statins' role in causing these effects. The most common adverse effect in adults is myalgias. While a proportion of patients will not be able to tolerate statins, there was no significant difference in the rate of reported myalgias compared to nonusers or discontinuation of statins in a report by the AHA.[24] In studies of AYAs, myalgias are infrequently reported. The more serious potential complication is a risk of rhabdomyolysis, which is exceedingly rare. It is not clear that routine measurements of creatine kinase levels are needed after statin initiation or that they can be used to prevent rhabdomyolysis with dose adjustments. A second common concern is liver injury. Although statins primarily act in the liver, clinically relevant liver injury is rare, although mild elevations in liver transaminases are common. It is reasonable to obtain liver transaminase levels prior to, and following, initiation of a statin. Serial measurements are most likely unnecessary.

TABLE 17.5

Secondary Causes of Dyslipidemia in Adolescents and Young Adults

Exogenous	• Alcohol (especially binge drinking) • Medications (corticosteroids, isotretinoin, oral contraceptives containing estrogen, HIV antiretroviral agents)
Endocrine/Metabolic	• Hypothyroidism • Diabetes (type 1 and 2) • Pregnancy • Polycystic ovary syndrome • Anorexia nervosa • Congenital metabolic conditions (Glycogen Storage disease, Gaucher disease, Tay–Sachs, Niemann–Pick disease)
Other Conditions	• Renal diseases (chronic kidney disease, hemolytic uremic syndrome, nephrotic syndrome) • Liver diseases (cholestatic conditions, cirrhosis) • Inflammatory diseases (systemic lupus erythematosus, juvenile rheumatoid arthritis, Kawasaki disease) • Solid-organ transplant recipient • Childhood cancer survivor
Infections	• Acute viral/bacterial infection • Human immunodeficiency virus (HIV) infection • Acute hepatitis

The risk of developing diabetes mellitus also is of concern and there is likely a small, increased risk.[25] Despite this risk, patients who develop diabetes mellitus after starting a statin generally continue treatment based on the significant benefits of statins in patients with diabetes mellitus. Female patients of reproductive age should be counseled that statins are potentially teratogenic and that they should either not take statins or use appropriate methods of birth control. In addition to these concerns, nonspecific symptoms such as fatigue, headaches, and gastrointestinal discomfort have been reported. In general, statins are remarkably well tolerated by AYAs.

There appears to be no effect on growth and development with statin initiation before or during puberty. Further, there appears to be no impact on cognition. These can be explained by the fact that LDL does not participate in the delivery of cholesterol for hormone synthesis, nor does it cross the blood–brain barrier. Further, as demonstrated in landmark studies in adults, extremely low LDL cholesterol levels (<50 mg/dL) are well tolerated.[26] When considering starting a statin in adolescents, it should be noted that there does not appear to be a dose-related increase in adverse effects nor do adverse effects increase with length of time on the medication.

Statins interact with a number of commonly prescribed medications. The most frequent interactions occur through metabolism by OATP1B1, which is an enzyme that transports statins and other medications into the cell. The most commonly prescribed medications that inhibit OATP1B1 are clarithromycin, ritonavir, indinavir, saquinavir, and cyclosporine. These all lead to increased statin concentrations. Fluvastatin has been recommended in patients prescribed immunosuppression because it appears to be the least dependent on OATP1B1. A number of statins also are metabolized by the CYP3A4 enzymes. Atorvastatin, lovastatin, and simvastatin are most dependent on the CYP3A4 enzymes. Fluvastatin is

TABLE 17.6

Common Pharmacologic Agents Used in the Treatment of Lipid Disorders

Medication Class	Proposed Mechanisms of Action	Expected Effects	Notes
Statins	Inhibits HMG-CoA, which is the rate-limiting step of cholesterol synthesis	↓↓ LDL-C ↓ TG ↑ HDL-C	Effects depend on potency and dose of statin. Higher doses of rosuvastatin and atorvastatin are most effective.
Ezetimibe	Inhibits cholesterol absorption at Niemann–Pick C1-like 1 Inhibits reabsorption of cholesterol in bile salts	↓ LDL-C –/↓ TG –/↑ HDL-C	Rare adverse effects Most commonly used in combination with a statin Effective in treatment of sitosterolemia
Fibrates	↑ LPL activity ↓ TG production ↓ peroxisome proliferator-activated receptor gamma	↓ LDL-C ↓↓ TG ↑ HDL-C	Typically restricted to treating severe hypertriglyceridemia as role in CVD reduction is limited. Gemfibrozil should not be used with a statin. Typically contraindicated in renal and liver failure
PCSK9 inhibitors	Inhibits PCSK9, thereby increasing availability of LDL receptors	↓↓ LDL-C ↓ TG ↑ HDL-C ↓ Lp(a)	Primarily used as adjunct to statins or in patients with statin intolerance
Omega-3 fatty acid supplements	Inhibits synthesis of fatty acids by blocking the transcription factor, sterol regulatory element binding protein-1	↓↓ TG	Vascepa (Icosapent ethyl) is the purified form of EPA. Lovaza is a concentrated form of EPA and DHA. Over-the-counter supplements vary in Docosahexaenoic acid (DHA) and EPA content and are not regulated by the FDA.
Bempedoic acid	Inhibits adenosine triphosphate citrate lyase	↓ LDL – TG ↓ HDL	Primarily used as adjunct to statins or in patients with statin intolerance

LDL, low-density lipoprotein; HDL, high-density lipoprotein; EPA, eicosapentaenoic acid; FDA, Food and Drug Administration.

metabolized primarily by CYP2C9 and CYP2C8, while pitavastatin and rosuvastatin are primarily metabolized through other pathways. Typically, these interactions cause no clinical adverse effects in AYAs, but should be discussed with a clinician at the time of medication initiation in case dose adjustments or temporary discontinuation of the statin are needed.

Ezetimibe

In patients who resist taking a statin, have a contraindication to statins, or have not reached goal LDL cholesterol, ezetimibe is often recommended. Although initial trials showed mixed results regarding the efficacy of ezetimibe, the publication of the IMPROVE-IT study not only changed the perception of ezetimibe, but also gave increased credence to the "LDL hypothesis."[27] The mechanisms of action of ezetimibe are not entirely clear, but it likely interferes with cholesterol absorption at the intestinal brush border through the Niemann–Pick C1-Like 1 protein and with the reabsorption of cholesterol in bile salts. When added to a statin, ezetimibe is expected to reduce LDL cholesterol by approximately 20% and triglycerides by 5% to 11%, and increase HDL cholesterol by 3% to 5%. Although adverse effects such as hepatotoxicity and myalgias have been reported, adverse reactions are rare.

Proprotein Convertase Subtilisin/Kexin Type 9 (PCSK9) Inhibitors

Over the past two decades, the emergence of PCSK9 inhibitors has helped change the approach to the management of patients with elevated LDL cholesterol. PCSK9 is an intracellular enzyme that acts to recycle LDL receptors after they are internalized. By inhibiting PCSK9, these agents prevent the intracellular destruction of the LDL receptor, thereby increasing their availability to return to the cell surface. PCSK9 inhibitors can lower LDL cholesterol by up to 70% when used as monotherapy and by an additional 60% for patients already taking a statin. PCSK9 inhibitors can reduce triglycerides up to 31% and HDL cholesterol as much as 9%. Unlike statins, PCSK9 inhibitors may reduce lipoprotein(a) by up to 36%, whereas statins may lead to a modest increase in lipoprotein(a) levels. Despite the remarkable lowering of LDL cholesterol, alirocumab and evolocumab have only been shown to reduce CVD events, not overall mortality.[28]

PCSK9 inhibitors are well tolerated. In adults, this is particularly important as they can be an alternative treatment option for those who cannot tolerate statins or are not at goal despite maximally tolerated statin therapy. However, as adolescents typically tolerate statins without issue, PCSK9 inhibitors are rarely used. The most common adverse effect is injection site reaction, with other adverse effects no more common than among patients receiving placebo.

Omega-3 Polyunsaturated Fatty Acids

As discussed previously, the addition of polyunsaturated fats to the diet has a small, but statistically significant impact on CVD risk. The use of one class of polyunsaturated fatty acid, omega-3 polyunsaturated fatty acids, has gained particular interest. Omega-3 fatty acids can be purchased as "fish oil" in which it is found in combination with omega-6 fatty acids and omega-9 fatty acids. Although the formulation and dose ultimately determine the effects of omega-3 fatty acid supplements on the lipid profile, high doses (4 g/d) decrease triglycerides by 30% to 45%, while increasing LDL cholesterol by 20% to 30% and increasing HDL cholesterol by 10% to 15%.

Icosapent ethyl (Vascepa), which is the purified form of the omega-3 fatty acid, eicosapentaenoic acid (EPA), was shown in the Reduction of Cardiovascular Events with Icosapent Ethyl–Intervention Trial (REDUCE-IT)[29] to reduce the risk of the CVD events by approximately 25%. However, the Long-Term Outcomes Study to Assess Statin Residual Risk with Epanova in High Cardiovascular Risk Patients with Hypertriglyceridemia (STRENGTH)[30] was recently halted because of futility. The results of the STRENGTH trial along with concerns about the placebo used in REDUCE-IT have raised concerns about the benefits of purified omega-3 supplements in preventing CVD. In addition, omega-3 supplements have significant adverse effects, including bad taste, belching, bleeding risk, and an increased risk of atrial fibrillation.

Bile Acid Sequestrants

Once the lipid-lowering medication of choice, bile acid sequestrants have largely been replaced by other agents based on their lower efficacy and poor tolerability. Historically, the three most common bile acid sequestrants were cholestyramine, colesevelam, and colestipol. These medications block reabsorption of bile salts leading to cholesterol excretion in the feces. LDL cholesterol lowering is dose dependent, but ranges from 15% to 30%. The adverse effects are related to the bile acid sequestrants being suspended in a solution. Most patients will discontinue bile acid sequestrants because of nausea, flatulence, and constipation. There are systemic concerns such as coagulopathies, poor absorption of iron, calcium, and water-soluble vitamins, but these are rare.

Fibrates

Fibrates are primarily used to treat hypertriglyceridemia and have little-to-no role in the treatment of elevated LDL cholesterol. The mechanism of action of fibrates likely includes increasing lipoprotein lipase activity, decreasing endogenous triglyceride production, and inhibiting peroxisome proliferator-activated receptor gamma. Fibrates are generally well tolerated, but may lead to gastrointestinal discomfort (e.g., diarrhea and gallstones), myalgias, and increased appetite. Fibrates also are generally contraindicated in patients with liver or kidney disease. However, when used to reduce severely elevated triglyceride levels, this risk should be weighed against the risk of triglyceride-induced pancreatitis. While gemfibrozil should not be used in combination with a statin because of an increased risk of myalgias, fenofibrate can be used.

Niacin

Niacin (Vitamin B3, nicotinic acid) also affects the lipid profile, primarily by lowering the triglyceride level. Niacin reduces triglyceride levels by up to 40%, possibly through inhibition of diacylglycerol acyltransferase 2, the final step in triglyceride synthesis. It also reduces LDL cholesterol by 20%, possibly through decreased VLDL production, and increases HDL cholesterol by 30% through unclear mechanisms. However, several trials have failed to show additional benefit when niacin was added to a baseline statin. In addition, adverse effects have generally limited its utility. Several of the most important include flushing, inhibition of platelet function, gout, clinically important decreases in insulin sensitivity, and liver injury.

Additional Agents

While statins and ezetimibe remain the most commonly used medications to treat dyslipidemia in adolescents, newer medications provide options for adolescents who have not sufficiently reduced their LDL cholesterol or have refractory hypertriglyceridemia due to monogenic causes. Bempedoic acid is an alternative for patients who cannot tolerate a statin. It blocks production of cholesterol by inhibiting adenosine triphosphate citrate lyase, which is distal to the site of action of statins. While bempedoic acid monotherapy is not as effective at lowering LDL cholesterol as statin monotherapy, adverse muscle effects are thought to be less frequent since its active metabolite is present only in the liver. When bempedoic acid is added to ezetimibe, nearly a 50% reduction in LDL cholesterol can be seen. When added to a statin, LDL cholesterol is reduced by an additional 26%. Bempedoic acid has no effect on triglycerides and may decrease HDL cholesterol slightly. Whether bempedoic acid reduces CVD events as much as statins do is yet to be determined, but it is a promising oral medication for a select group of patients, particularly those who are not eligible for PCSK9 inhibitors or statins.

Lomitapide is approved only for patients with homozygous FH. By inhibiting microsomal transfer protein, VLDL and chylomicrons are not appropriately assembled, and are not secreted. Although as much as a 50% reduction in LDL cholesterol has been observed in small trials, the accumulation of lipids within hepatocytes and enterocytes leads to significant adverse effects, particularly fatty liver disease and intolerable gastrointestinal symptoms. Although the gastrointestinal adverse effects can be mitigated with a low-fat diet, adherence to this diet is difficult for many patients. Mipomersen also inhibits the production of functional Apo B, but is an antisense oligonucleotide that inhibits Apo B messenger ribonucleic acid. It reduces LDL cholesterol by 25% to 40%, but has similar adverse effects as lomitapide, which has limited its use.

Evinacumab was approved in the United States in 2021 for patients with homozygous FH. Evinacumab significantly lowers both LDL cholesterol and triglycerides by interfering with angiopoietin-like protein 3, although the role of angiopoietin-like protein 3 in LDL cholesterol and triglyceride metabolism is not well understood. In clinical trials, evinacumab lowered triglycerides and LDL cholesterol by up to 60% in patients with homozygous FH.

SUMMARY

Cardiovascular health is essential to the population's health. Adolescence and young adulthood represent a critical time in the life course for the promotion of cardiovascular health and the prevention of CVD. Clinicians caring for this age group should assess cardiovascular health metrics, including cholesterol levels, and appropriately classify and treat any identified lipid disorders to ensure the future health of their patients. Studies of the most effective methods of predicting accelerated CVD risk for AYAs, and of communicating this risk in a way that leads to sustained behavior change, are ongoing.

REFERENCES

1. Angell SY, Mcconnell MV, Anderson CAM, et al. The American Heart Association 2030 impact goal: a presidential advisory from the American Heart Association. *Circulation.* 2020;141(9):e120–e138. doi:10.1161/CIR.0000000000000758
2. Fang N, Jiang M, Fan Y. Ideal cardiovascular health metrics and risk of cardiovascular disease or mortality: a meta-analysis. *Int J Cardiol.* 2016;214:279–283. doi:10.1016/j.ijcard.2016.03.210
3. Expert Panel on Integrated Guidelines for Cardiovascular Health and Risk Reduction in Children and Adolescents, National Heart, Lung, and Blood Institute. Expert Panel on Integrated Guidelines for Cardiovascular Health and Risk Reduction in Children and Adolescents: summary report. *Pediatrics.* 2011;128(Suppl 1):S1–S44. doi:10.1542/peds.2009-2107A
4. Perak AM, Ning H, Khan SS, et al. Associations of late adolescent or young adult cardiovascular health with premature cardiovascular disease and mortality. *J Am Coll Cardiol.* 2020;76(23):2695–2707. doi:10.1016/j.jacc.2020.10.002
5. Allen NB, Krefman AE, Labarthe D, et al. Cardiovascular health trajectories from childhood through middle age and their association with subclinical atherosclerosis. *JAMA Cardiol.* 2020;5(5):557–566. doi:10.1001/jamacardio.2020.0140
6. Barker DJP. Developmental origins of chronic disease. *Public Health.* 2012;126(3):185–189. doi:10.1016/j.puhe.2011.11.014
7. Gillman MW. Primordial prevention of cardiovascular disease. *Circulation.* 2015;131(7):599–601. doi:10.1161/CIRCULATIONAHA.115.014849
8. Daniels SR, Pratt CA, Hollister EB, et al. Promoting cardiovascular health in early childhood and transitions in childhood through adolescence: a workshop report. *J Pediatr.* 2019;209:240–251.e1. doi:10.1016/j.jpeds.2019.01.042
9. Gooding HC, Gidding SS, Moran AE, et al. Challenges and opportunities for the prevention and treatment of cardiovascular disease among young adults: report from a National Heart, Lung, and Blood Institute working group. *J Am Heart Assoc.* 2020;9(19):e016115. doi:10.1161/JAHA.120.016115
10. Virani SS, Alonso A, Benjamin EJ, et al. Heart disease and stroke statistics—2020 update: a report from the American Heart Association. *Circulation.* 2020;141(9):e139–e596. doi:10.1161/CIR.0000000000000757
11. Libby P, Ridker PM, Hansson GK. Progress and challenges in translating the biology of atherosclerosis. *Nature.* 2011;473(7347):317–325. doi:10.1038/nature10146
12. McGill HC Jr, McMahan CA, Gidding SS. Preventing heart disease in the 21st century: implications of the Pathobiological Determinants of Atherosclerosis in Youth (PDAY) study. *Circulation.* 2008;117(9):1216–1227. doi:117/9/1216 [pii]10.1161/CIRCULATIONAHA.107.717033
13. Armstrong MK, Fraser BJ, Hartiala O, et al. Association of non–high-density lipoprotein cholesterol measured in adolescence, young adulthood, and mid-adulthood with coronary artery calcification measured in mid-adulthood. *JAMA Cardiol.* 2021;6(6):661–668. doi:10.1001/jamacardio.2020.7238
14. Steinberger J, Daniels SR, Hagberg N, et al. Cardiovascular health promotion in children: challenges and opportunities for 2020 and beyond. *Circulation.* 2016;134(12):e236–255. doi:10.1161/CIR.0000000000000441
15. Grundy SM, Stone NJ; Guideline Writing Committee for the 2018 Cholesterol Guidelines. 2018 cholesterol clinical practice guidelines: Synopsis of the 2018 American Heart Association/American College of Cardiology/Multisociety Cholesterol guideline. *Ann Intern Med.* 2019;170(11):779–783. doi:10.7326/M19-0365
16. De Ferranti SD, Steinberger J, Ameduri R, et al. Cardiovascular risk reduction in high-risk pediatric patients: A scientific statement from the American Heart Association. *Circulation.* 2019;139(13):e603–e634. doi:10.1161/CIR.0000000000000618
17. Gillman MW, Daniels SR. Is universal pediatric lipid screening justified? *JAMA.* 2012;307(3):259–260. doi:10.1001/jama.2011.2012
18. U.S. Preventive Services Task Force, Bibbins-Domingo K, Grossman DC, et al. Screening for lipid disorders in children and adolescents: US Preventive Services Task Force Recommendation Statement. *JAMA.* 2016;316(6):625–633. doi:10.1001/jama.2016.9852.
19. De Ferranti SD, Rodday AM, Parsons SK, et al. Cholesterol screening and treatment practices and preferences: a survey of United States pediatricians. *J Pediatr.* 2017;185:99–105.e2. doi:10.1016/j.jpeds.2016.12.078
20. Nguyen D, Kit B, Carroll M. Abnormal cholesterol among children and adolescents in the United States, 2011–2014. *NCHS Data Brief.* 2015;(228):1–8.
21. Gooding HC, Rodday AM, Wong JB, et al. Application of pediatric and adult guidelines for treatment of lipid levels among US adolescents transitioning to young adulthood. *JAMA Pediatr.* 2015;169(6):569–574. doi:10.1001/jamapediatrics.2015.0168
22. Arnett DK, Blumenthal RS, Albert MA, et al. 2019 ACC/AHA guideline on the primary prevention of cardiovascular disease: a report of the American College of Cardiology/American Heart Association Task Force on clinical practice guidelines. *Circulation.* 2019;140(11):e596–e646. doi:10.1161/CIR.0000000000000678
23. Van Horn L, Obarzanek E, Barton BA, et al. A summary of results of the Dietary Intervention Study in Children (DISC): lessons learned. *Prog Cardiovasc Nurs.* 2003;18(1):28–41. doi:10.1111/j.0889-7204.2003.01007.x
24. Newman CB, Preiss D, Tobert JA, et al. Statin safety and associated adverse events: a scientific statement from the American Heart Association. *Arterioscler Thromb Vasc Biol.* 2019;39(2):E38–E81. doi:10.1161/ATV.0000000000000073
25. Mach F, Ray KK, Wiklund O, et al. Adverse effects of statin therapy: perception vs. the evidence – focus on glucose homeostasis, cognitive, renal and hepatic function, haemorrhagic stroke and cataract. *Eur Heart J.* 2018;39(27):2526–2539. doi:10.1093/eurheartj/ehy182
26. Ridker PM, Danielson E, Fonseca FAH, et al. Rosuvastatin to prevent vascular events in men and women with elevated C-reactive protein. *N Engl J Med.* 2008;359(21):2195–2207. doi:10.1056/NEJMoa0807646
27. Cannon CP, Blazing MA, Giugliano RP, et al. Ezetimibe added to statin therapy after acute coronary syndromes. *N Engl J Med.* 2015;372(25):2387–2397. doi:10.1056/NEJMoa1410489
28. Kolber MR, Nickonchuk T, Turgeon R. Do PCSK9 inhibitors reduce cardiovascular events? *Can Fam Physician.* 2018;64(9):669.
29. Bhatt DL, Steg PG, Miller M, et al. Cardiovascular risk reduction with icosapent ethyl for hypertriglyceridemia. *N Engl J Med.* 2019;380(1):11–22. doi:10.1056/NEJMoa1812792
30. Nicholls SJ, Lincoff AM, Garcia M, et al. Effect of high-doseomega-3 fatty acids vs corn oil on major adverse cardiovascular events in patients at high cardiovascular risk: The STRENGTH randomized clinical trial. *JAMA.* 2020;324(22):2268–2280. doi:10.1001/jama.2020.22258

ADDITIONAL RESOURCES AND WEBSITES

Additional Resources and Websites for Clinicians:
American Heart Association Professional Heart Daily—https://professional.heart.org/en
Familial Hypercholesterolemia Foundation—https://thefhfoundation.org/

Additional Resources and Websites for Parents/Caregivers:
American Heart Association—https://www.heart.org/en/healthy-living
Familial Hypercholesterolemia Foundation—https://thefhfoundation.org/

Additional Resources and Websites for Adolescents and Young Adults:
Center for Young Men's Health—https://youngmenshealthsite.org/guides/heart-disease/
Center for Young Women's Health—https://youngwomenshealth.org/2019/11/21/heart-disease/
Teens Health—https://kidshealth.org/en/teens/cholesterol.html

CHAPTER 18

Syncope, Vertigo, and Sudden Cardiac Arrest

Amy Desrochers DiVasta
Mark E. Alexander

KEY WORDS

- Fainting
- Hypertrophic cardiomyopathy
- Long QT syndrome
- Palpitations
- Preparticipation examination
- Sudden cardiac arrest
- Supraventricular tachycardia
- Syncope
- Vertigo

 ## INTRODUCTION

Cardiac symptoms in adolescents and young adults (AYAs) are very common; true cardiac disease is not. Syncope is a frequent complaint, often raising concerns of future sudden cardiac arrest (SCA).[1] The clinician's critical task is to distinguish between benign and worrisome syncope. The epidemiology almost always favors innocent causes.

SYNCOPE

Etiology

Syncope is a sudden, transient loss of consciousness (TLOC) and postural tone, lasting several seconds to a minute, followed by spontaneous recovery. Syncope is common, particularly among adolescent females 13 to 18 years old,[1,2] and the prevalence may be increasing.[3] Any condition that leads to decreased cerebral perfusion may cause syncope.

Classification

The three major categories of syncope are: (1) neurocardiogenic (vasovagal/reflex, postural orthostatic tachycardia); (2) cardiovascular (structural, arrhythmogenic); and (3) noncardiovascular (epileptic, psychogenic). Syncope of unknown origin (i.e., *simple syncope*) and neurocardiogenic syncope account for 85% to 90% of events.[4,5] In these cases, ineffective cerebral blood flow, resulting from inadequate cardiac output, leads to loss of consciousness. Only 1% to 5% of patients with syncope have significant cardiac disease. Seizures or psychiatric causes account for only a small minority of episodes. Broadly, these events are classified as episodes of TLOC. Focusing on TLOC that is less than 2 to 3 minutes clarifies the focus to events that could be syncope. Longer periods of apparent LOC, by definition, are not syncope and require alternative explanations.

History and Physical Examination

A detailed history (including family history) and thorough physical examination are typically sufficient to make an accurate diagnosis. Key elements of the history include:
1. Onset and frequency of episodes

2. Surrounding circumstances, such as exercise, posture, or other precipitating factors
3. Prodromal symptoms, including dizziness, diaphoresis, nausea, pallor, palpitations, chest pain, or dyspnea
4. Complete or incomplete loss of consciousness, duration, and time to recovery
5. Abnormal movements, incontinence, or injuries
6. Previous medical history and medication use
7. Family history of sudden death (particularly if <40 years old), similar episodes, or early onset of heart disease

"Warning signs" that suggest a more worrisome etiology include syncope during exercise, syncope in a supine position, family history of sudden death, personal history of cardiac disease, or an event precipitated by a loud noise, intense emotion, or fright.[6] Mid-exertional syncope, where the collapse occurs during short bursts of exercise (i.e., climbing a rope, swimming a 100-meter race, sprinting in basketball or soccer) is particularly worrisome. Nearly half of mid-exertional syncope events have a specific cardiac cause.[7]

The physical examination should include a neurologic assessment and a dynamic cardiac examination to evaluate for a pathologic murmur. Examining the patient supine, immediately upon standing, and then during and following a squat gives the opportunity to induce murmurs of mitral valve prolapse and hypertrophic cardiomyopathy (HCM), and informs the examiner about their immediate response to orthostatic stress. Close attention also should be paid to nutritional factors and emotional health during syncope evaluations given their importance throughout adolescence.

Table 18.1 presents a differential diagnosis for a syncopal event. Common etiologies are discussed below.

Neurocardiogenic Syncope

Neurocardiogenic syncope (i.e., *vasovagal syncope*) is the most common form of syncope.
1. Duration: Few seconds to minutes
2. Onset: Gradual, typically with a prodrome
3. Etiology: Precipitating factors (fear, anxiety, pain, hunger, overcrowding, fatigue, injections, sight of blood, prolonged upright posture) are usually identifiable.
4. Prodromal symptoms: Nausea, dizziness, visual spots or dimming, feelings of apprehension, pallor, yawning, diaphoresis, and feelings of warmth
5. Syncopal event: Brief loss of consciousness with gradual loss of muscle tone
6. Syncopal seizures: Rarely, a brief period of opisthotonus will occur following syncope.
7. Recovery: Rapid (<1 minute to consciousness), though residual fatigue, malaise, weakness, nausea, and headache are common.

TABLE 18.1

Differential Diagnosis of a Syncopal Event

	Typical/Vasovagal	Cardiac	Atypical/Conversion	Vertigo
Position	Upright	Supine or upright	Either	Change in position
Prodrome	Frequent	None	Variable	Rare
Duration	<1 min	<1 min	Minutes	Brief, may cluster
Color	Pale	May be normal	Flushed/normal	Normal
Visual symptoms	Gradual dimming	Abrupt dimming	Variable	Room spinning
Exercise	Postexertional or no relationship	Peak exercise	Variable	Uncommon
Palpitations	Hard	Rapid, precedes faints	Variable	Uncommon
Injury/incontinence	Rare	Moderately frequent	Rare	Rare
Frequency	Isolated or episodic	Isolated or episodic	Often very frequent	Episodic
School disability	Rare	Rare	Frequent	Rare
Family history	Possibly "fainting" but otherwise negative	Often positive		Rare
ECG	Normal or nonspecific PR <220 ms QTc <460 ms Right atrial enlargement Borderline LVH	T-wave inversion QTc >480 ms WPW QRS >120 ms, bundle branch block	Normal or nonspecific	Normal or nonspecific
Comments	Borderline ECG findings likely nonspecific though consultation appropriate	Often established cardiac diagnosis	Typical event as a trigger	

ECG, electrocardiogram; WPW, Wolff–Parkinson–White; LVH, left ventricular hypertrophy.

8. Pathophysiology: Neurally mediated syncope results from a combination of inappropriate peripheral vasodilation and cardiac slowing, resulting in a transient period of inadequate cerebral (and other organ) blood flow. This physiology is mediated by several normal reflexes. Fainting restores cerebral blood flow and permits those reflexes to return to normal.

9. Specific situational syncope syndromes, including needle phobia, hair-grooming syncope, stretch syncope, micturition syncope, and post-tussive syncope, require minimal investigation.

10. There is likely some decline in the preponderance of neurocardiogenic syncope and a small increase in the frequency of "adult" causes of syncope as AYAs age into their mid to late 20s. This shift in disease frequency is subtle, but may influence diagnostic approaches.

Diagnostic Evaluation of Neurocardiogenic Syncope

Adolescents and young adults with a true syncopal event should undergo a thorough history, physical examination, and electrocardiogram (ECG).[8] A normal diagnostic screen (reassuring history, benign examination, and normal ECG) is generally sufficient to exclude cardiac disease. Additional testing is needed only if further concerns for cardiac or neurologic disease remain.[9] Unnecessary testing may inappropriately elevate patient care costs.[10]

1. Routine laboratory investigation, electroencephalogram (EEG), and intracranial imaging are not needed.

2. Echocardiogram has very low yield for routine evaluation; it should be utilized to evaluate exertional syncope or syncope with other high-risk features. There will be a 5% to 10% incidence of incidental, unrelated findings.[8]

3. Exercise testing is required if syncopal episodes occur during exercise.

4. Tilt table testing: Specificity is poor (35% to 100%) and sensitivity is variable (75% to 85%); 40% of healthy AYAs have a positive tilt test. Head-up tilt testing has fallen out of favor because of these poor test characteristics. While there continue to be groups that strongly advocate for tilt table testing, the authors and most North American pediatric cardiologists have dramatically limited their use of this test.

5. Ambulatory ECG monitoring can be useful for correlating symptoms and rhythm. The choice of monitoring (Holter monitor, external loop recorder, implantable loop recorder) requires consideration of symptom frequency, severity, and need for more precise data. Implantable loop records are very effective at correlating symptoms and rhythm.[11] Recently, 3-, 7-, and 14-day patch recorders permit extended monitoring using a single lead. These devices are increasingly used as an intermediate step in evaluating frequent syncope.

6. When situational triggers are identified, either behavioral or medical therapies aimed at those triggers are appropriate. Common examples include syncope triggered by dysmenorrhea/abdominal pain or events following phlebotomy.

Management of Neurocardiogenic Syncope

Management includes (1) reassurance; (2) hydration and caffeine/alcohol avoidance; (3) recognition of prodromal symptoms and implementation of preventative techniques, including supine positioning or increasing postural tone (isometric contractions of the extremities, folding the arms, or crossing the legs); (4) upright, weight-bearing exercise; and (5) pharmacotherapy for refractory cases that do not respond to supportive therapy (Table 18.2). Generally, a 12-month symptom-free interval is considered a reasonable duration of treatment, after which a trial off of any medications is warranted.

TABLE 18.2

Pharmacologic Treatment Options for Neurocardiogenic Syncope

Drug	Dose	Proposed Mechanism of Action	Side Effects	Quality of Data
Fludrocortisone	0.1–0.2 mg/d	↑ Renal Na⁺ absorption	Bloating or edema	
		↑ Circulating blood volume	Hypokalemia	+
			Hypertension	
Midodrine	5–10 mg q4h	α-Agonist	Piloerection	
	Maximum four doses/d	↑ Peripheral vascular resistance	Scalp pruritus	
			Hypertension	++
			Urinary retention	
			Difficult adherence to treatment	
β-Blockers		Blocks excess sympathetic response (paradoxical effect)	Fatigue	
Atenolol	25–50 mg daily		Depression	±
Metoprolol	25–50 mg b.i.d.			
SSRIs		↑ Extracellular serotonin leads to downregulation of receptor density	Headache	
Fluoxetine	20 mg daily		Insomnia	±
Sertraline	50 mg daily		GI effects	

+, moderate data to support efficacy; ++, strong data to support efficacy; ±, mixed data to support efficacy; SSRIs, selective serotonin reuptake inhibitors; GI, gastrointestinal.

Postural Orthostatic Tachycardia Syndrome

Postural orthostatic tachycardia syndrome (POTS) is a heterogeneous disorder of autonomic regulation. Characterized by a marked pulse change (>40 bpm) or excessive tachycardia (>120 bpm) when the patient moves from a supine to upright position, patients often report fatigue, dizziness, and exercise intolerance with upright position. Adolescents and young adults have enough ability to increase their heart rate in response to position change that there is typically little or no blood pressure change. POTS is likely a result of both ineffective vascular constriction with standing (hence an appropriate tachycardia) and an exaggerated sympathetic response. This physiology is created in normal subjects with spaceflight or even modest periods of bed rest. Chronic fatigue syndrome and POTS overlap considerably.[12] Treatment includes fluids and vasoconstrictors for symptom relief.[13] β-Blockers are also commonly used. The heterogeneity of management practices reflects the variable physiology and symptomatology of POTS, inconsistencies in the diagnostic approaches used by clinicians, and the lack of clear "best practices" in managing the condition. Though often difficult to implement, slowly progressive physical reconditioning may be the most important therapy.[14]

Orthostatic Hypotension

Orthostatic hypotension (systolic blood pressure decrease >20 mm Hg or diastolic blood pressure decrease >10 mm Hg with upright posture typically without sinus tachycardia) is less common in AYAs. Etiologies of orthostatic hypotension include pregnancy, malnutrition, volume depletion, medication side effects, and neurologic disorders. There can be both immediate forms (within seconds of standing) and delayed orthostatic hypotension that is apparent by several minutes after standing. For many AYAs, compensatory sinus tachycardia mitigates this physiology resulting in classification as POTS.

Cardiovascular Syncope

Cardiovascular syncope is an acute collapse with few premonitory symptoms, often in association with exercise or exertion. It occurs secondary to arrhythmia, obstructed left ventricular (LV) filling, obstructed LV outflow, or ineffective myocardial contraction (Table 18.3). When this event persists for more than a minute or so, it represents an SCA. Cardiac syncope should be suspected in patients with a personal history of significant cardiac disease and when any of the "warning signs" are present

TABLE 18.3

Differential Diagnosis of Cardiac Syncope

Structural/Functional	Electrical	Acquired
HCM	LQTS (inherited or secondary)	Commotio cordis
Dilated cardiomyopathy		Drugs (cocaine, stimulants, inhalants)
Coronary artery anomalies	Brugada syndrome	
Arrhythmogenic cardiomyopathy	WPW syndrome	
	Short QT syndrome	Atherosclerotic coronary artery disease
Aortic stenosis	Heart block (congenital or acquired)	
Aortic dissection/Marfan syndrome		Myocarditis
Pulmonary hypertension	Catecholaminergic polymorphic ventricular tachycardia	Postoperative congenital heart disease
Pulmonic stenosis		
Tetralogy of Fallot		Fontan surgery
Transposition of the great arteries		
Hypoplastic left heart syndrome		
Coarctation of the aorta		

HCM, hypertrophic cardiomyopathy; LQTS, long QT syndrome; WPW, Wolff–Parkinson–White.

TABLE 18.4	
"Warning Signs" of Syncope That May Be due to Cardiovascular Causes	
Historical Signs	**Examination/ECG Signs**
While in supine position	Abnormal cardiac rhythm
During exertion	Hypertension
Precipitated by noise, strong emotion, stress	Pathologic murmur or click
Lack of prodromal symptoms	Abnormal QTc interval
Family history of sudden death or heart failure in relative age <40	Heart block

ECG, electrocardiogram.

(Table 18.4). Important historical details include prior episodes, exercise intolerance, exertional chest discomfort, and a family history of premature coronary artery disease, sudden death, syncope, or hypertension.[15] Many patients with cardiac syncope will have previously recognized cardiac conditions; the clinician should seek urgent cardiology input for these patients.

Clues to cardiac disease on examination include hypertension, abnormal cardiac rhythm, heart murmur, or features suggestive of Marfan syndrome.[16] However, the majority of patients with new cardiac etiologies (and those at risk of SCA) will have a completely normal physical examination. The ECG is a convenient screening tool, but is often normal. Echocardiography that includes adequate visualization of the coronary arteries is essential. Exercise electrocardiography is useful in patients with exertional chest discomfort, syncope, exercise intolerance, or worrisome palpitations. Patients should be referred to a cardiologist if cardiac disease is suspected. Strenuous activities, including sports and driving, should be restricted until cardiology evaluation is completed.

Palpitations, Arrhythmias, and Wolff–Parkinson–White Syndrome

Palpitations can result from sustained or nonsustained arrhythmias or from symptomatic sinus tachycardia. The typical history for supraventricular tachycardia (SVT) is an abrupt onset of palpitations, often during a rapid position change such as standing up after tying a shoe or a sudden jump. These palpitations are sensed as being quite rapid, may be associated with dizziness and lightheadedness at onset, and can last for minutes to hours. When palpitations persist and are present during the medical evaluation, the diagnosis is readily apparent. When palpitations self-terminate, the classic history is that they stop abruptly, though in practice this history is often unclear. Sustained SVT usually results from either an accessory pathway or atrioventricular node reentry.

Supraventricular tachycardia is bothersome but not life-threatening unless the patient has Wolff–Parkinson–White (WPW) syndrome, an arrhythmia identified by the typical delta wave on resting ECG (Figure 18.1). Most patients who are diagnosed with WPW syndrome warrant referral for possible catheter ablation.[17]

Isolated atrial and ventricular premature beats can produce a sense of skipped heart beats, but usually these beats are asymptomatic and recognized only during physical examination. Infrequent, isolated ectopy is a variant of normal, and may not require more evaluation than an examination and ECG. More frequent or sustained ectopy warrants further evaluation.

An ECG is a good first step in the evaluation of palpitations.[18] A normal ECG early in the evaluation permits triaging of any further cardiac evaluation. In the absence of associated cardiac symptoms or family history of cardiomyopathy, an AYA with infrequent, self-limited palpitations, a normal ECG, and reasonable access to medical care can be managed via an expectant approach. For more worrisome cases, further investigation may be needed. Different ambulatory monitoring techniques each have advantages and limitations and should be selected based on the frequency and duration of symptoms. Traditional Holter monitors and longer-term patch monitors (Zio and Bardy among others) permit 1 to 14 days of continuous recordings. Smartphone-enabled recorders or implantable long-term event monitors are required for correlating symptoms to possible arrhythmia if symptoms occur less frequently.

Noncardiovascular Syncope

Hyperventilation frequently causes dizziness, but true syncope is rare. The history may include details of peripheral tingling and anxiety that may be reproduced in the office. Metabolic disturbances such as hypoglycemia or anemia can also lead to syncope.

Psychogenic or pseudosyncope is typically characterized by a gradual slump to the floor, without injury, anxiety, or vital sign instability. The history is often difficult to characterize, and the frequency of the episodes may cluster and increase over time. A detailed history can help distinguish between typical syncope, epilepsy, and psychogenic events.[19] A history of more than 50 spells, a sense that consciousness waxes and wanes, and five or more hospitalizations are each associated with psychogenic nonepileptic events. This diagnosis, like functional neurologic disorder, requires

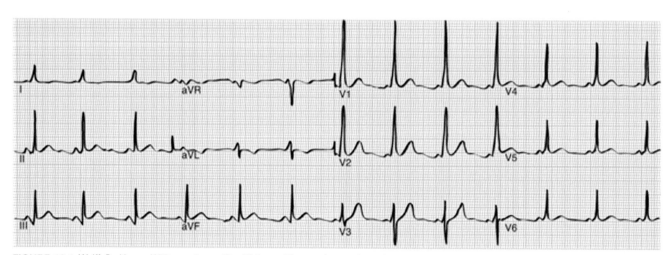

FIGURE 18.1 Wolff–Parkinson–White syndrome. The PR interval is very short and prominent delta waves are present. Delta waves are easily seen in the precordial leads but are less prominent in the frontal plane (I, II, III, avR, avL, avF). This suggests the common left-sided location of the accessory pathway. The pre-excitation and abnormal ventricular activation results in prominent anterior (V1, V2) voltages and somewhat wider QRS than normal for age. Right-sided and septal pathways are typically more obvious. (From Perpetua EM; Keegan Consulting, LLC. *Cardiac Nursing*. 7th ed. Lippincott Williams & Wilkins; 2020.)

thorough clinical evaluation, a high degree of clinical suspicion for atypical etiologies, and thoughtful assessment strategies to effectively correlate events and physiology.

Rare etiologies include subclavian steal syndrome and cerebral occlusive disease. Migraine sufferers can have syncope, vertigo, or dizziness preceding or accompanying their headaches.

VERTIGO

Vertigo is a sensation of rotary movement/spinning, rather than dizziness. Causes of true vertigo (Table 18.5) may be either peripheral (accompanied by tinnitus and/or hearing loss) or central (accompanied by ataxia or other motor signs).

History

The history can distinguish vertigo from syncope and seizures, and may also reveal a specific etiology for the vertigo. In most cases, the diagnosis is established through history and negative physical examination findings.

1. Descriptions of the episode and any previous attacks
2. Circumstances preceding the attack
3. Precipitating factors
4. Alleviating factors: recumbence, food, fresh air, and sudden movements

Physical Examination

General physical examination with special emphasis on the following:

1. Neurologic examination:
   Evidence of cranial nerve deficits, particularly III, IV, VI, VII, and VIII; funduscopic examination
   Focal motor deficits
   Tendon reflexes: focal loss, asymmetry, and hyperreflexia
   Cerebellar function: Truncal or appendicular ataxia
   Nystagmus with straight gaze: Horizontal nystagmus suggests a peripheral etiology, whereas vertical and diagonal nystagmus suggest a central etiology.
   Sensory abnormalities: Peripheral sensory loss suggests neuropathy
   Asymmetry of skin color or temperature suggestive of autonomic neuropathy
2. Special examination maneuver for vertigo:
   a. The Dix–Hallpike maneuver or Nylen–Bárány test: This maneuver may be the most helpful test to perform on patients with vertigo. It has a positive predictive value of 83% and a negative predictive value of 52% for the diagnosis of benign positional vertigo. Have the patient sit at the edge of a table. Holding on to their head, have them abruptly lie back as you place their head 45 degrees below the table and at a 45-degree angle to one side. Repeat the test with the

head at a 45-degree angle to the opposite side. Elicitation of nystagmus indicates a "positive" test result, suggesting benign positional vertigo.

For sustained vertigo or vertigo that seems positional in origin, referral to a neurologist or otolaryngologist is advisable for further evaluation and testing. An otolaryngologist should promptly evaluate patients with abrupt onset of vertigo and auditory symptoms. Treatment of vertigo is difficult. Short-term therapy for vertigo and vomiting may include antihistamines such as meclizine, antiemetics, or mild sedatives.

SUDDEN CARDIAC ARREST IN ADOLESCENTS AND YOUNG ADULTS

Sudden cardiac arrest accounts for only about 10% of the overall sudden death rate in the AYA population, with an incidence of 1 to 2/100,000 patient-years.[20] Hypertrophic cardiomyopathy is the most common cause of SCA in the United States among patients 15 to 35 years old. Competitive athletes are likely at minimally higher risk for SCA than their sedentary peers or recreational athletes.[21] Most SCA occurs at rest or even during sleep.[22]

Etiologies of Sudden Unexpected Cardiac Death in Adolescents and Young Adults

Structural anomalies, electrical abnormalities, sequelae of congenital heart disease, and acquired conditions can all lead to SCA, and mirror the etiologies of cardiac syncope (see Table 18.4). Many of these conditions may be familial.[20] Any patient with a suspected cardiac condition should be referred to a cardiologist for a full evaluation and determination of appropriate athletic and recreational limitations. Despite large case-control studies that do not show a link between stimulant use and cardiac events, therapy for attention deficit hyperactivity disorder may be delayed because of concerns about these risks. Screening in that cohort is essentially identical to population-based screening. Common SCA etiologies are reviewed below.

Hypertrophic Cardiomyopathy (See Chapter 19)[23,24]

Long QT Syndrome

1. Definition: Long QT syndrome (LQTS) is a disorder of delayed ventricular repolarization, leading to risk for arrhythmias (torsades de pointes, ventricular fibrillation), syncope, seizure, and SCA. Patients may be asymptomatic.
2. Familial LQTS: Estimated frequency 1/2,000. While traditionally described as both an autosomal recessive (Jervell and Lange-Nielsen syndrome) and autosomal dominant disease (Romano–Ward), modern genetic investigations have demonstrated more than a dozen important ion channels that contribute to the final phenotype.[25] The majority are disorders of potassium channels (KCNQ1 and KCNH2) or sodium channels (SCN5A). With this understanding, familial LQTS represents a spectrum from homozygous and compound heterozygous disease that can include mutations that are latent in the parent.
3. Acquired LQTS: May be related to an underlying disease state or secondary to medication effects (Table 18.6).
4. Diagnosis: Begins with an ECG, but requires careful patient-specific and family investigation. Acute illnesses, several medications, and neurally mediated syncope may transiently prolong the QT. Long QT syndrome is rare when QTc <450 ms, and frequently confirmed when QTc >480 to 500 ms. The diagnosis is most challenging for QTc values between 450 and 480 ms.
5. Treatment: To decrease the mortality rate, all patients should be referred to a cardiologist for discussion of treatment, which includes:
   a. Avoidance of medications known to prolong the QT interval (http://crediblemeds.org) and emotional stressors or vigorous activities that may precipitate a syncopal episode.

TABLE 18.5

Etiologies of Vertigo

Peripheral	Central
Vestibular neuritis (acute labyrinthitis)	Tumors of the brainstem and cerebellum
Benign positional vertigo	Demyelinating diseases
Ototoxic drugs	Vasculitis
Acoustic neuromas	Cerebral infarctions
Ménière disease	Infections of the nervous system
Perilymphatic fistulas	Postinfectious inflammatory demyelination
Otitis media	Basilar migraine
Motion sickness	Brain injury due to head trauma
Ear obstruction	

TABLE 18.6

Conditions/Medications Associated with QT Interval Prolongation

Conditions	Medications
Electrolyte abnormality[a]	Antiarrhythmic drugs
Recent syncope	Tricyclic antidepressants
Coronary artery disease	Azole antifungals
Myocarditis	Macrolide antibiotics
Alcoholism	Arsenic
Eating disorders	Diuretics (via electrolyte changes)
Liquid protein diets	Antipsychotics
Hypothyroidism	Fluoroquinolones
Cerebrovascular accident	Methadone
Encephalitis	Antimalarials
Traumatic brain injury	Trazodone
Subarachnoid hemorrhage	
Diabetic ketoacidosis	

[a]Electrolyte abnormality: hypokalemia, hypocalcemia, hypomagnesemia.
For a frequently updated list, please visit crediblemeds.org

b. Restriction from competitive athletics and prudent changes in recreational activities.[26] This practice is evolving and requires detailed discussion and shared decision making.

c. Cascade screening beginning with an ECG should be obtained in first-degree relatives of patients diagnosed with LQTS.

d. β-Blockers: The initial treatment of choice, β-blockers, decrease cardiac events, but do not change the QT interval nor provide absolute protection against SCA. Medication compliance is essential; life-threatening arrhythmia can occur if the medication is suddenly discontinued.

e. Implantable cardioverter-defibrillators are being used less frequently for most LQTS, but remain important for those with a history of cardiac arrest or recurrent syncope.

f. Left cervical sympathectomy is a thoracoscopic procedure that offers significant benefit in selected patients.

Other Ion Channel Defect Disorders

Brugada syndrome is a distinctive mutation of the cardiac sodium channel gene that leads to dynamic right ventricular conduction delays; patients often present with syncope or cardiac arrest.[27] Other ion channel defects include catecholaminergic polymorphic ventricular tachycardia and a short QT syndrome. Catecholaminergic polymorphic ventricular tachycardia is notable for having normal resting ECGs and sometimes requiring vigorous exercise to elicit the typical bidirectional ventricular tachycardia or rapid atrial tachycardia that permits clinical diagnosis.

Sudden Cardiac Arrest and Genetic Screening

Increasingly, familial heart diseases are being recognized due to both better care of those with the disorders and increased recognition of less severely affected family members. Obtaining details regarding heart disease in first-degree relatives (parents, siblings) allows for better informed care of AYAs. An affected family member will more frequently have a genetic diagnosis, because precise genetic testing is now technically feasible in 50% to 80% of families. Genetic testing also allows for relatively prompt identification of unaffected family members. For those families without a clear genetic marker, regular follow-up is warranted to track the potential phenotype. Given the significant costs and sometimes ambiguous results of current genetic testing, referral for cardiology consultation is a more efficient approach for AYAs with a family history of these disorders but no signs/symptoms and no familial genetic marker.[28]

Prevention: To Screen or Not to Screen?

Universal cardiac screening programs targeting either high school athletes or all adolescents remain controversial.[29] The epidemiology of SCA is relatively clear. Most developed countries report approximately 1 to 2 deaths per 100,000 patient-years, which corresponds to 1 to 2 high school students per year in most states. When SCA occurs in athletes, it results in significant local press coverage and appropriately heightened concern and anxiety among families.[30]

The risk of SCA appears elevated in athletes compared to other AYAs. Among athletes, SCA is most prevalent in Black basketball players, and is less common in both females and in athletes competing in other sports.[31] In many schools, more than 70% of students participate in sports at the level that requires a signed "clearance." The rarity of SCA and the large numbers of youth participating in athletics create challenging questions about where to focus screening efforts. Universal screening efforts in other countries have had mixed results. The success of screening in Italy has been challenged by multiple contradictory experiences. Those observations, combined with the need to potentially screen three to five million students per year, have informed current U.S. recommendations against using routine ECGs for primary care or school-based screening.

Several small to moderate efforts have incorporated ECGs into systematic screening. When ECG screening is performed, approximately 4% to 8% of the ECGs are abnormal. Recent efforts focused on reducing the number of false positives have decreased the referral rate to <3%.[32] The scale of these efforts has been insufficient to provide accurate estimates for discovering HCM or LQTS. In one demonstration project in Texas that used ECGs and immediate performance of a limited echocardiogram, 19% of those with potentially critical diagnoses never returned to follow-up or therapy.[33]

While the ECG can identify some heart disease, it is a marginal screening test for previously unrecognized heart disease in AYAs. Specificity is quite poor given the rarity of the relevant diseases and the number of borderline ECGs that occur. HCM, the most common cause of SCA for AYAs, will usually result in an abnormal ECG. However, the second most common cause of athletic SCA is anomalous coronary arteries. These patients will have a normal ECG and examination; diagnosis can be difficult, even with echocardiogram. Arrhythmias contributing to SCA (WPW, LQTS) will also typically have an abnormal ECG.

While the ECG itself is inexpensive, the downstream evaluation of possible findings is substantial. This results in significant cost associated with ECG screening, which is a drawback to universal screening. There is also a concern that universal screening may create unnecessary barriers to youth participation in athletics and other physical activities. Thus, universal screening could have the unintended consequence of contributing to morbidity and mortality from obesity, diabetes, and hypertension in adulthood. In contrast, supporters of universal screening maintain that utilizing both ECGs and echocardiograms can substantially reduce the false-positive rate. Supporters argue that these studies can be performed at very high volume, with high quality, and at minimal cost.

Primary care and adolescent medicine clinicians can reduce morbidity and mortality by preventing heat injury, increasing the availability of school-based automated external defibrillators, and assuring that there are emergency action plans in place.[34] In addition, given the frequency of premonitory symptoms in youth with subsequent SCA, prompt investigation of patients with syncope, palpitations, and similar symptoms remains important. In contrast to universal screening, those youth with a significant family history, abnormal examination, or symptoms (palpitations, chest pain, or syncope) should be referred for further evaluation.

⬤ SUMMARY

Syncope, vertigo, and SCA are complex and varied clinical issues that can impact AYAs. Clinicians can elucidate important clinical details and distinguish among a broad range of possible problems through a structured and thoughtful approach that includes thorough history taking, careful physical assessment, and judicious use of testing modalities.

REFERENCES

1. Kenny RA, Bhangu J, King-Kallimanis BL. Epidemiology of syncope/collapse in younger and older Western patient populations. *Prog Cardiovasc Dis.* 2013;55(4): 357–363.
2. Anderson JB, Czosek RJ, Cnota J, et al. Pediatric syncope: National Hospital Ambulatory Medical Care survey results. *J Emerg Med.* 2012;43(4):575–583.
3. Roston TM, Tran DT, Sanatani S, et al. A population-based study of syncope in the young. *Can J Cardiol.* 2018;34(2):195–201.
4. Shen WK, Sheldon RS, Benditt DG, et al. 2017 ACC/AHA/HRS guideline for the evaluation and management of patients with syncope: executive summary: a report of the American College of Cardiology/American Heart Association Task Force on Clinical Practice Guidelines and the Heart Rhythm Society. *J Am Coll Cardiol.* 2017;70(5):620–663.
5. Zavala R, Metais B, Tuckfield L, et al. Pediatric syncope: a systematic review. *Pediatr Emerg Care.* 2020;36(9):442–445.
6. Dalal A, Czosek RJ, Kovach J, et al. Clinical presentation of pediatric patients at risk for sudden cardiac arrest. *J Pediatr.* 2016;177:191–196.
7. Miyake CY, Motonaga KS, Fischer-Colbrie ME, et al. Risk of cardiac disease and observations on lack of potential predictors by clinical history among children presenting for cardiac evaluation of mid-exertional syncope. *Cardiol Young.* 2016;26(5):894–900.
8. Paris Y, Toro-Salazar OH, Gauthier NS, et al. Regional implementation of a pediatric cardiology syncope algorithm using standardized clinical assessment and management plans (SCAMPS) methodology. *J Am Heart Assoc.* 2016;5(2):e002931.
9. Shanahan KH, Monuteaux MC, Brunson D, et al. Long-term effects of an evidence-based guideline for emergency management of pediatric syncope. *Pediatr Qual Saf.* 2020;5(6):e361.
10. Redd C, Thomas C, Willis M, et al. Cost of unnecessary testing in the evaluation of pediatric syncope. *Pediatr Cardiol.* 2017;38(6):1115–1122.
11. Bezzerides VJ, Walsh A, Martuscello M, et al. The real-world utility of the LINQ implantable loop recorder in pediatric and adult congenital heart patients. *JACC Clin Electrophysiol.* 2019;5(2):245–251.
12. Kizilbash SJ, Ahrens SP, Bruce BK, et al. Adolescent fatigue, POTS, and recovery: a guide for clinicians. *Curr Probl Pediatr Adolesc Health Care.* 2014;44(5):108–133.
13. Chen G, Du J, Jin H, et al. Postural tachycardia syndrome in children and adolescents: pathophysiology and clinical management. *Front Pediatr.* 2020;8:474.
14. Shibata S, Fu Q, Bivens TB, et al. Short-term exercise training improves the cardiovascular response to exercise in the postural orthostatic tachycardia syndrome. *J Physiol.* 2012;590(15):3495–3505.
15. Drezner JA, Fudge J, Harmon KG, et al. Warning symptoms and family history in children and young adults with sudden cardiac arrest. *J Am Board Fam Med.* 2012;25(4):408–415.
16. Schunk PC, Ruttan T. Pediatric syncope: high-risk conditions and reasonable approach. *Emerg Med Clin North Am.* 2018;36(2):305–321.
17. Pappone C, Vicedomini G, Manguso F, et al. Wolff-Parkinson-White syndrome in the era of catheter ablation: insights from a registry study of 2169 patients. *Circulation.* 2014;130(10):811–819.
18. Sedaghat-Yazdi F, Koenig PR. The teenager with palpitations. *Pediatr Clin North Am.* 2014;61(1):63–79.
19. Reuber M, Chen M, Jamnadas-Khoda J, et al. Value of patient-reported symptoms in the diagnosis of transient loss of consciousness. *Neurology.* 2016;87(6):625–633.
20. Bagnall RD, Singer ES, Tfelt-Hansen J. Sudden cardiac death in the young. *Hear Lung Circ.* 2020;29(4):498–504.
21. Asif IM, Rao AL, Drezner JA. Sudden cardiac death in young athletes: what is the role of screening? *Curr Opin Cardiol.* 2013;28(1):55–62.
22. Tsuda T, Fitzgerald KK, Temple J. Sudden cardiac death in children and young adults without structural heart disease: a comprehensive review. *Rev Cardiovasc Med.* 2020;21(2):205–216..
23. Elliott PM, Anastasakis A, Borger MA, et al. 2014 ESC guidelines on diagnosis and management of hypertrophic cardiomyopathy: the task force for the diagnosis and management of hypertrophic cardiomyopathy of the European Society of Cardiology (ESC). *Eur Heart J.* 2014;35(39):2733–2779.
24. Miron A, Lafreniere-Roula M, Steve Fan CP, et al. A validated model for sudden cardiac death risk prediction in pediatric hypertrophic cardiomyopathy. *Circulation.* 2020;142(3):217–229.
25. Wallace E, Howard L, Liu M, et al. Long QT syndrome: genetics and future perspective. *Pediatr Cardiol.* 2019;40(7):1419–1430.
26. Chambers KD, Ladouceur VB, Alexander ME, et al. Cardiac events during competitive, recreational, and daily activities in children and adolescents with long QT syndrome. *J Am Heart Assoc.* 2017;6(9):e005445.
27. Dechert BE, LaPage MJ, Cohen MI. Suspicion and persistence: a case of pediatric brugada syndrome. *Pediatrics.* 2019;144(1):e20183296.
28. Ackerman M, Atkins DL, Triedman JK. Sudden cardiac death in the young. *Circulation* 2016;133(10):1006–1026.
29. Lehman PJ, Carl RL. The preparticipation physical evaluation. *Pediatr Ann.* 2017;46(3):e85–e92.
30. Dubin AM. Screening ECGs for young competitive athletes: it is complicated. *Curr Opin Pediatr.* 2015;27(5):604–608.
31. Harmon KG, Drezner JA, Wilson MG, et al. Incidence of sudden cardiac death in athletes: a state-of-the-art review. *Heart.* 2014;100(16):1227–1234.
32. Drezner JA, Ackerman MJ, Anderson J, et al. Electrocardiographic interpretation in athletes: the "Seattle Criteria." *Br J Sports Med.* 2013;47(3):122–124.
33. Zeltser I, Cannon B, Silvana L, et al. Lessons learned from preparticipation cardiovascular screening in a state funded program. *Am J Cardiol.* 2012;110(6): 902–908.
34. DeFroda SF, McDonald C, Myers C, et al. Sudden cardiac death in the adolescent athlete: history, diagnosis, and prevention. *Am J Med.* 2019;132(12): 1374–1380.

ADDITIONAL RESOURCES AND WEBSITES

Additional Resources and Websites for Clinicians:
Adult-Oriented Clinical Review of POTS—https://onlinelibrary.wiley.com/doi/full/10.1111/joim.12852
An Approach to Pediatric ECGs—https://www.youtube.com/watch?v=jVqRUkVqC5o
Guide to Patient Education for AYA with POTS—https://onlinelibrary.wiley.com/doi/abs/10.1111/pace.13571
Pediatric Syncope Systematic Review—https://www.ncbi.nlm.nih.gov/pmc/articles/PMC7469873/

Additional Resources and Websites for Parents/Caregivers:
Explanation of sudden cardiac death—https://www.healthychildren.org/English/health-issues/injuries-emergencies/sports-injuries/Pages/Sudden-Cardiac-Death.aspx
Listing of medications that prolong the QT interval—www.crediblemeds.org
Syncope resource from the American Heart Association—https://www.heart.org/en/health-topics/arrhythmia/symptoms-diagnosis–monitoring-of-arrhythmia/syncope-fainting

CHAPTER 19

Heart Murmurs, Congenital Heart Disease, and Acquired Heart Disease

Amy Desrochers DiVasta
Suellen Moli Yin
Mark E. Alexander

KEY WORDS

- Congenital heart disease
- Connective tissue disorder
- Endocarditis
- Hypertrophic cardiomyopathy
- Mitral valve prolapse
- Murmur
- Pericarditis

 INTRODUCTION

Cardiac murmurs occur in at least 50% of all normal children and often persist into adolescence and young adulthood. Murmurs are the most frequent reason for referral to a cardiologist. The vast majority are considered to be "innocent" or "physiologic" in origin. In most patients with a cardiac murmur, a careful history and physical examination establish the diagnosis and/or guide further referral and evaluation.

HISTORY

Murmurs first heard during childhood or adolescence are more likely to be innocent murmurs. However, complaints of fatigue, decreased exercise tolerance, exertional chest pain, or palpitations are suggestive of pathologic heart disease.[1] Any adolescent or young adult (AYA) with syncope or near-syncope during exercise should undergo cardiac evaluation (Chapter 18). A thorough family history should be obtained, paying particular attention to any history of sudden death or structural cardiac abnormalities in first-degree relatives.

PHYSICAL EXAMINATION

A careful, stepwise examination is crucial, including performance of a dynamic cardiac examination (sitting, supine, and squatting or with the Valsalva maneuver). In higher resource environments, most patients with any concern for cardiac structural disease will have an echocardiogram. In lower resource environments or more geographically isolated locations in which echocardiograms may not be easily obtained, a careful examination can help confirm whether additional testing is truly needed. Key examination components include:

1. General appearance, including assessment of growth and maturation
2. Pulses in upper and lower extremities
3. Blood pressures in both arms and a leg with an appropriately sized blood pressure cuff
4. Palpation:
   a. A thrill, heave, or lift over the precordium or suprasternal notch is usually pathologic.
   b. Increased intensity and/or lateral displacement (away from the midclavicular line) of the point of maximal impulse suggests left ventricular (LV) enlargement.
5. Auscultation (see individual diagnoses for details):
   a. First heart sound (S_1): S_1 is produced by closure of the mitral and then the tricuspid valve and is best heard at the cardiac apex. Splitting of S_1 can be a normal finding. However, auscultation of another sound close to S_1 is usually either a fourth heart sound (S_4) or an ejection click.
   b. Second heart sound (S_2): The first component (aortic valve closure, A_2) and the second component (pulmonary valve closure, P_2) of S_2 should be of equal intensity. Normally, there is respiratory variation or physiologic splitting of the S_2, with widening of the separation with inspiration and narrowing or disappearance of the split with exhalation. Wide, fixed splitting suggests right ventricular (RV) volume overload such as that seen with an atrial septal defect (ASD). A single S_2 is also abnormal.
   c. Third heart sound (S_3): S_3 may be a normal finding in AYAs, and is more prominent in hyperdynamic states.
   d. Fourth heart sound (S_4): S_4 may be normal in older adults, but is almost always pathologic in AYAs. Practically, the distinctions can be challenging and are influenced by heart rate and clinical context.
   e. Clicks: Sharp, high-frequency sounds that are important clues to organic disease.
   f. Murmurs: Assess murmur characteristics, including timing, loudness, length, tonal quality, and location. All diastolic murmurs, except venous hums, should be considered pathologic.

DIAGNOSTIC CLUES SUGGESTIVE OF INNOCENT (NORMAL) MURMURS

1. History: Asymptomatic with no family history of cardiac disease
2. Physical examination: Normal, other than the presence of the murmur
3. Timing of murmur: Early systolic; almost never diastolic or holosystolic
4. Intensity: Usually grade 1 to 3/6, and often changing with position (louder in supine position and quieter with sitting or standing)
5. Quality: Vibratory with no clicks. There is physiologic splitting of S_2
6. Location: May vary, but frequently at lower or upper left sternal border (LSB), without extensive radiation

TYPES OF INNOCENT (NORMAL) MURMURS

Still's Murmur

- A grade 1/6 to 3/6 low-to-medium–pitched midsystolic murmur with a vibratory or musical quality best heard at lower LSB. The murmur decreases with sitting or standing.
- Still's murmur can be differentiated from the murmur of hypertrophic cardiomyopathy (HCM) because the Still's murmur decreases with standing, and is less harsh than a murmur associated with a ventricular septal defect (VSD).

Pulmonary Flow Murmur

- A grade 1/6 to 3/6 short crescendo–decrescendo midsystolic murmur best heard at the upper LSB, between the second and third left intercostal spaces. The murmur is decreased by inspiration and sitting. It is often heard in the setting of tachycardia due to fever, anxiety, or exertion.
- A pulmonary flow murmur is differentiated from valvular pulmonary stenosis by the absence of a click and from an ASD because S_2 splits normally.

Cervical Venous Hum

- A medium-pitched, soft, blowing continuous murmur heard best above the sternal end of the clavicle, at the base of the neck.
- The murmur is increased by rotating the head away from the side of the murmur. The murmur is decreased by jugular venous compression or assuming a supine position—unique for a normal murmur.

Supraclavicular (Carotid) Bruit

- A short, high-pitched early systolic murmur, usually grade 2/6, heard best above the clavicles with radiation to the neck while the AYA is sitting. The murmur is decreased by hyperextending the shoulders (bringing the elbows behind the back).

DIAGNOSTIC CLUES SUGGESTIVE OF PATHOLOGIC MURMURS

1. History: Growth failure, decreased exercise tolerance, exertional syncope or near-syncope, exertional chest pain
2. Physical examination: Clubbing, cyanosis, decreased or delayed femoral pulses, apical heave, palpable thrill, tachypnea, inappropriate tachycardia
3. Murmur: Diastolic, holosystolic, loud or harsh, extensive radiation, increases with standing, associated with a thrill, abnormal S_2 (Table 19.1)

MURMURS ASSOCIATED WITH STRUCTURAL HEART DISEASE

Mildly symptomatic congenital heart disease may not be recognized until adolescence, particularly in underserved populations (Table 19.2).

Atrial Septal Defect

1. Physical examination: Signs and symptoms depend on the size of the shunt.
   a. Hyperdynamic precordium with RV lift with sizable shunt; no thrill
   b. Widely split and fixed S_2
   c. Pulmonary flow murmur: Grade 2/6 to 3/6 systolic ejection murmur at upper LSB
   d. Mid-diastolic rumble at lower LSB
2. Further evaluation
   a. Electrocardiogram (ECG): Right-axis deviation, RV conduction delay (rSR′ pattern), right atrial enlargement, or RV hypertrophy

TABLE 19.1

Types of Pathologic Murmurs

Murmur Type	Characteristics	Common Defects
Systolic ejection	Crescendo–decrescendo Begins after S_1; ends before S_2 Best heard with diaphragm	Aortic stenosis Pulmonary stenosis Coarctation of the aorta ASD
Holosystolic	Begins with and obscures S_1 Ends at S_2 Heard at LSB or apex	VSD Mitral regurgitation
Early diastolic	Decrescendo Begins immediately after S_2 High–medium pitch	Aortic insufficiency Pulmonary insufficiency
Mid-diastolic	Low pitch Rumble Best heard with bell	ASD VSD Mitral stenosis
Continuous	Extend up to and through S_2 Continue through all/part of diastole Best heard with diaphragm	PDA

ASD, atrial septal defect; LSB, left sternal border; VSD, ventricular septal defect; PDA, patent ductus arteriosus.

   b. Chest x-ray: Mild to moderate cardiomegaly with increased pulmonary vascularity
   c. Echocardiogram: Diagnostic with visualization of location and size of defect
   d. Cardiac magnetic resonance imaging (MRI) allows excellent imaging of the atrial septum and RV volume.
3. Management: Both surgical closure and transcatheter device closure are safe, effective, and popular management choices.

Ventricular Septal Defect

1. Physical examination: Shunt volume determines findings.
   a. With increasing shunt size, the precordium becomes increasingly hyperdynamic. A thrill may be present with either a large or small shunt.
   b. S_2 is normal with small shunts and accentuated with larger shunts. An S_3 may be present. A loud P_2 (suggesting pulmonary hypertension) is a worrisome finding.
   c. Grade 2/6 to 3/6 holosystolic murmur at lower LSB
   d. Mid-diastolic rumble at the apex with large shunts
2. Further evaluation
   a. ECG: Normal in small defects; LV hypertrophy with large defects
   b. Chest x-ray: Normal in small defects; cardiomegaly with increased pulmonary vascularity in large defects
   c. Echocardiogram: Provides anatomical detail of location and size of defect; color Doppler permits visualization of very small defects
3. Management: Depends on RV pressure and may require catheterization to make appropriate therapeutic decisions. Prophylaxis for infective endocarditis (IE) is no longer recommended for VSD.

Patent Ductus Arteriosus

1. Physical examination: Shunt volume determines findings.
   a. Normal precordium with small shunt; hyperdynamic with a thrill with large shunt
   b. Grade 2/6 to 4/6 continuous murmur at upper LSB
   c. Wide pulse pressure and bounding pulses with large shunt

TABLE 19.2

Clues to Specific Cardiac Diseases

Diagnosis	Auscultation	Other Findings	Chest X-ray	ECG
Patent ductus arteriosus	Continuous murmur LUSB and subclavicular area	Wide pulse pressure Bounding pulses	Prominent pulmonary artery	Normal LAE/LVH
ASD	Fixed, widely split S_2 Systolic ejection murmur at LUSB Mid-diastolic rumble at LLSB	RV lift	Prominent RV outflow	Incomplete RBBB (rSR' pattern)
Pulmonary stenosis	Systolic ejection click (mild PS) P_2 delayed and soft SEM at LUSB	RV lift Thrill at LUSB	Prominent RV outflow Poststenotic dilation	RVH RAE
Aortic stenosis	Early systolic murmur RUSB, transmitted to neck Systolic ejection click (mild AS) Soft A_2	LV lift Decreased pulses	LVE	LVH
Mitral regurgitation	Holosystolic murmur with radiation to axilla; soft S_1	LV lift	Large LA and LV	Bifid P waves Left-axis deviation
MVP	Midsystolic click; mid- or late systolic murmur			Abnormal T waves Arrhythmias
Hypertrophic cardiomyopathy	Midsystolic murmur at LLSB, increased with standing and decreased with Valsalva maneuver	Rapid carotid upstroke	±LVE ±LAE	LVH ±Q waves
VSD	High-pitched, harsh holosystolic murmur at LLSB	Thrill at LLSB	Normal	Normal (if small VSD)
Pulmonary hypertension	Loud P_2 No murmur or regurgitant murmur at LLSB	Clubbing	Variable	RAE RVH
Coarctation of aorta	Continuous/systolic precordial murmur Systolic ejection click from bicuspid aortic valve	SBP lower in legs than arms Decreased/delayed femoral pulses	Rib notching Increased pulmonary markings	LVH

ECG, electrocardiogram; LUSB, left upper sternal border; LAE, left atrial enlargement; LVH, left ventricular hypertrophy; LLSB, left lower sternal border; RV, right ventricular; RBBB, right bundle-branch block; PS, pulmonic stenosis; RVH, right ventricular hypertrophy; RAE, right atrial enlargement; SEM, systolic ejection murmur; RUSB, right upper sternal border; AS, aortic stenosis; LV, left ventricular; LA, left atrium; LVE, left ventricular enlargement; VSD, ventricular septal defect.

2. Further evaluation
   a. ECG: Often normal; LV hypertrophy seen if left-to-right shunting is significant
   b. Chest x-ray: Cardiomegaly and increased pulmonary vascularity with large shunt
   c. Echocardiogram: Visualization with two-dimensional and color Doppler imaging
3. Management: Cardiac catheterization is rarely required for diagnosis but is commonly done for coil or device occlusion.

Valvular Pulmonary Stenosis

1. Physical examination: Severity of obstruction determines findings.
   a. RV lift with systolic thrill at upper LSB in more severe forms
   b. Systolic ejection click at upper LSB, which is louder with expiration (more difficult to hear with severe stenosis)
   c. S_2 normal or widely split, depending on severity of stenosis

d. Grade 2 to 4/6 harsh systolic ejection murmur at upper LSB; may radiate to the lung fields and back.
2. Further evaluation
   a. ECG: Normal, with progression to RV hypertrophy (upright T wave in lead V1) as stenosis increases
   b. Chest x-ray: Prominent pulmonary artery segment with normal vascularity
   c. Echocardiogram: Permits evaluation of valve morphology
   d. Cardiac catheterization is rarely required for diagnosis.
3. Management: Treatment of choice is balloon pulmonary valvuloplasty.

Valvular Aortic Stenosis

1. Physical examination: Severity of obstruction determines findings.
   a. Prominent apical impulse and systolic thrill (at upper RSB or suprasternal notch)
   b. Intensity of S_1 may be diminished due to poor ventricular compliance.

c. Systolic ejection click at lower LSB/apex that radiates to aortic area at upper RSB; no respiratory variation

d. Grade 2 to 4/6 long, harsh systolic crescendo–decrescendo ejection murmur at upper RSB

e. High-frequency early diastolic decrescendo murmur of aortic regurgitation

f. Careful assessment for features of associated Turner or Williams syndrome

2. Further evaluation

a. ECG: May be normal or indicate LV hypertrophy, with strain pattern (ST-segment depression and T-wave inversion in left precordium) indicating severe stenosis.

b. Chest x-ray: Normal heart size with prominent ascending aorta

c. Echocardiogram: Permits evaluation of valve morphology and determination of level of stenosis; 70% to 85% of stenotic valves are bicuspid.

d. Cardiac catheterization is rarely required for diagnosis.

3. Management: In select cases, aortic balloon valvuloplasty may be an initial palliative procedure.

Hypertrophic Cardiomyopathy (Fig. 19.1)

1. Definition: This cardiac muscle disorder leading to myocardial hypertrophy is usually genetic. For the HCM typical sarcomeric mutations, the prevalence is 1 in 500 in the general population. There are rarer forms associated with other genetic disorders (such as Noonan syndrome) and the potential for HCM with neither a clear genetic finding nor a family history. Idiopathic HCM is more frequently diagnosed in older adults.

2. Natural history: Genetically and phenotypically heterogeneous. Most patients are asymptomatic. If symptoms develop, usual complaints include exertional chest pain, exercise intolerance, shortness of breath, and syncope.

3. Physical examination

a. Associated features of skeletal myopathy such as peripheral weakness and myopathic facies are usually previously recognized.

b. Normal to hyperdynamic precordium with increased LV impulse, dynamic thrill

c. Auscultation may be normal. Dynamic examination demonstrates systolic ejection murmur at the lower LSB with *increasing* intensity in the standing position and *decreasing* intensity with squatting or Valsalva maneuver.

d. Dynamic murmur of mitral insufficiency or LV outflow obstruction

4. Further evaluation

a. ECG: Normal in some cases; LV and/or septal hypertrophy, ST-T wave changes, and atrial enlargement may be seen.

b. Echocardiogram: Essentially diagnostic, with excessive LV wall thickness, impaired ventricular filling, variable degrees of LV outflow tract obstruction, left atrial enlargement, and variable systolic anterior motion of the mitral valve. May require differentiation from athletic heart.

c. Cardiac MRI: Specific attention to delayed enhancement on cardiac MRI has become an early part of staging HCM.

d. Exercise testing: May be beneficial to evaluate the dynamic structure of their outflow tract obstruction, evaluate blood pressure responses to exercise, and quantify exercise performance. Hypertrophic cardiomyopathy represents the cardiovascular disease with the highest frequency of serious events during pediatric exercise testing,[2] so some practices will appropriately defer that testing.

5. Management: Management of HCM is highly individualized, but may include use of an implantable defibrillator, surgical

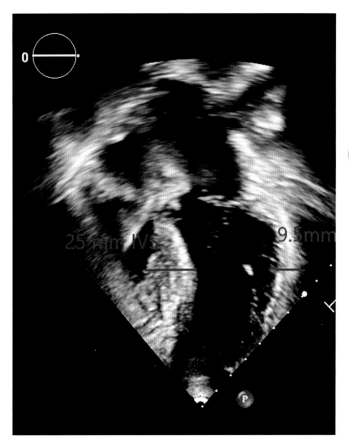

FIGURE 19.1 Hypertrophic cardiomyopathy. Apical echo image on a 14-year-old girl who was effectively resuscitated from an out-of-hospital arrest after which was diagnosed with hypertrophic cardiomyopathy. This demonstrates marked asymmetry with a 25-mm interventricular septum (IVS, Z score 15) with a sigmoid shape, no resting left ventricular outflow tract obstruction, and a normal size lateral wall measuring 9.5 mm. Genetic evaluation demonstrated a heterozygous myosin heavy chain mutation. She was the index case in the family. Her younger sister and her asymptomatic father had nearly identical echocardiograms and the same genetic findings.

or catheter treatment, or drug therapy.[3] The AYA is restricted from competitive sports.[4] Prophylaxis for IE is no longer recommended. The European Society of Cardiology HCM risk calculator is normed for Europeans who are 16 years or older. However, it is used by many to help estimate risk and assist in decisions regarding implantable cardiac defibrillators.[5] There are now more robust pediatric data that note that neither increased septal thickness nor increased outflow tract gradients are associated with increased risk in younger patients.[6] Given the nature of the management choices, HCM management increasingly relies on a shared decision-making model. Primary care clinicians can play a critical role in assuring that families are referred for cascade screening of affected siblings (and parents), and reinforcing the genetic risks for children.

Mitral Valve Prolapse

Mitral valve prolapse (MVP) is a heterogeneous disorder, with a wide spectrum of pathologic, clinical, and echocardiographic manifestations. The modern understanding of MVP identifies the mitral valve involvement as either part of global connective tissue abnormalities—such as Marfan syndrome, Ehlers–Danlos syndrome (EDS), or osteogenesis imperfecta—or as an isolated finding. Mitral valve prolapse has also been found to be more common in malnourished AYAs with anorexia nervosa. Weight loss decreases the size of the

LV muscle mass, but the valvular connective tissue does not change in size. This mismatch leads to a large, redundant valve and MVP. Most AYA patients with MVP have an excellent prognosis. Those with other connective tissue diseases are at increased risk for the development of mitral regurgitation, IE, cerebral embolism, life-threatening arrhythmia, and sudden death. This important distinction helps the clinician to alleviate unnecessary anxiety and to avoid activity limitations or antibiotic prophylaxis in otherwise healthy young people.

The prevalence of MVP in the general population is estimated at 2% to 3%, with equal gender distribution.[7] Although the diagnosis of MVP is common, clinically important MVP occurs infrequently.[8] Mitral valve prolapse may be diagnosed at any age. Like HCM, the frequency of MVP and symptomatic MVP increases as adolescents age into adulthood; therefore, symptoms are more likely among older AYAs.

Many cardiac symptoms (including chest pain, palpitations, exercise intolerance, and syncope) that were historically attributed to the presence of MVP are no more common than in the general population and are unrelated to MVP.[8]

Malignant MVP (or arrhythmic MVP), is a rare but serious form of MVP with more ventricular arrhythmia and specific features on echocardiogram. This is typically identified as patients move out of the AYA age range, but can be seen in AYAs. Surveillance for malignant MVP and for development of significant mitral insufficiency both motivate episodic cardiac evaluation in patients with MVP, particularly those who have new symptoms or changes in their examination.[9]

1. Physical examination: (a) Dynamic mid-to-late systolic click that moves later into systole with supine position or squatting and earlier into systole with standing or the Valsalva maneuver; (b) high-pitched, late systolic murmur, heard best at the apex of the heart; some AYA patients have no click and only a late systolic murmur; (c) associated physical abnormalities including scoliosis, pectus excavatum, decreased anteroposterior diameter, and stigmata of associated connective tissue disorders.
2. Further evaluation: (a) ECG is normal; (b) chest x-ray is normal; (c) ambulatory ECGs (Holter or event monitoring) may be indicated to evaluate for arrhythmia if the AYA has palpitations that disrupt activities of daily living or cause severe symptoms (syncope, dizziness); (d) echocardiogram allows visualization of the mitral valve, assessment for mitral regurgitation, and confirmation of the diagnosis of MVP. Mild bowing of a mitral leaflet, a normal variant, should not be misdiagnosed as frank prolapse.
3. Management: (a) Asymptomatic AYAs without mitral regurgitation need reassurance but do not need activity restriction, antibiotic prophylaxis, or follow-up echocardiography; (b) adolescents and young adults with mitral insufficiency, ventricular arrhythmias, history of cardiac syncope, or family history of premature sudden death may require activity restriction and careful consideration of athletic choices[10]; (c) Routine prophylaxis for IE is no longer recommended for MVP; (d) β-Blocking agents may be indicated for either symptomatic relief or to target a specific arrhythmia; there is no evidence that β-blockade decreases the already low risk of sudden death[8]; (e) mitral regurgitation is generally well tolerated during pregnancy and delivery[11]; (f) first-degree relatives of patients with substantial MVP should be considered for evaluation and echocardiogram because of the high prevalence of the diagnosis within families.
4. Complications: Complications of MVP are rare unless significant disease is present; however, (a) arrhythmias are the most frequent complication, including premature ventricular contractions, supraventricular tachyarrhythmia, ventricular tachycardia, and bradyarrhythmia; (b) there is increased risk of IE in patients with MVP and mitral regurgitation; (c) progressive mitral regurgitation can occur, but is rare in otherwise healthy AYAs; (d) there is very low risk of sudden cardiac death, but the incidence is still greater than that in the general population, likely due to ventricular arrhythmia; and (e) there remains a controversial risk of stroke.

Mitral Valve Regurgitation

1. Physical examination: Findings depend on severity of regurgitation. (a) Normal to hyperdynamic precordium; (b) grade 2/6 to 4/6 high-frequency holosystolic apical murmur; may radiate toward the base (upper LSB); (c) low-frequency apical mid-diastolic rumble with severe regurgitation.
2. Further evaluation: (a) ECG: Bifid P wave of left atrial enlargement if regurgitation is chronic and severe; (b) chest x-ray is normal or shows cardiomegaly; (c) echocardiogram demonstrates the cause of valve abnormality and severity of regurgitation.
3. Management: (a) Adolescent and young adult patients no longer require IE prophylaxis; (b) adolescents and young adults are followed to determine the need for afterload reducing agents or for surgery.

SYSTEMIC CONNECTIVE TISSUE DISEASE AND THE HEART

Marfan Syndrome

Marfan syndrome is an autosomal dominant global connective tissue disorder with specific ocular, musculoskeletal, and cardiac involvement (Fig. 19.2). Cardiac management of MVP in patients with Marfan syndrome is based upon aortic root dilation. β-Blockers are used as prophylaxis to try to slow dilation, which may progress rapidly during pregnancy.[12] Adolescents and young adults with Marfan syndrome are generally restricted from high intensity and collision sports.[13]

Ehlers–Danlos Syndromes

Ehlers–Danlos syndromes are a range of connective tissue disorders characterized by abnormalities in collagen and musculoskeletal involvement (Fig. 19.3). Mitral valve prolapse is relatively common in the classic subtype of EDS. Aortic root dilation is less severe and less frequent than in Marfan syndrome. Patients with EDS may experience palpitations, presyncope, and syncope associated with autonomic dysregulation and the neurally mediated hypotension accompanying postural orthostatic tachycardia.[14]

Fragile X Syndrome

This alteration in the *FMR1* gene is associated with intellectual disability, joint laxity, and some incidence of aortic root dilation and MVP. The cardiac involvement may not be apparent until adolescence. Periodic cardiac screening may be warranted.

ACQUIRED INFECTIOUS AND INFLAMMATORY HEART DISEASE

Bacterial Endocarditis: Recognition and Prophylaxis

Adolescents and young adults with significant valvular heart disease, unrepaired or residual VSD, prosthetic valves, and many other forms of congenital heart disease are at increased risk of acute or subacute IE. Infective endocarditis can be a devastating infection resulting in stroke or acute valve failure, and may require extended therapy. Given that many of these infections are the result of oral flora, the most important protective maneuvers are maintaining good oral hygiene and recognizing the potential for infection. Routine use of antibiotics prior to dental cleaning does not reliably prevent either acute or subacute IE, and may interfere with regular care. Current recommendations from the American Heart Association significantly reduce the indications for antibiotic prophylaxis of IE (Tables 19.3 to 19.6).[15] This shift in preventative strategy does not eliminate the need to be vigilant about potential IE. Appropriate testing with blood cultures and consultation for persistent unexplained fever in the at-risk patient remain the keys to recognize these infections.[16]

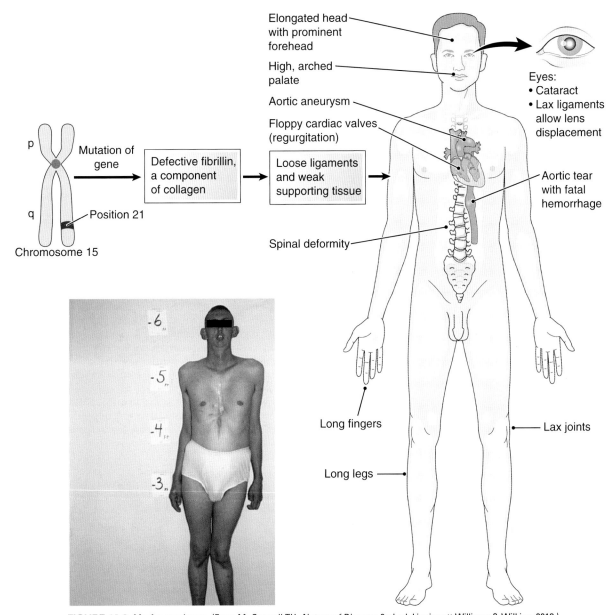

FIGURE 19.2 Marfan syndrome. (From McConnell TH. *Nature of Disease.* 2nd ed. Lippincott Williams & Wilkins; 2013.)

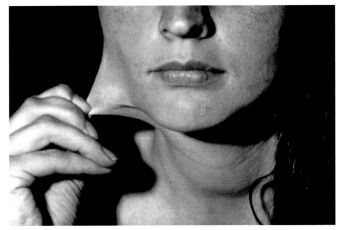

FIGURE 19.3 Ehlers–Danlos syndrome. (Courtesy of V. Voigtländer, Klinikum Ludwigshafen.)

Inflammatory Heart Disease

Lyme Carditis

Lyme disease is an epidemic infection in many areas caused by the tick-borne spirochete *Borrelia burgdorferi.* Cardiac involvement occurs during the early disseminated phase concurrent with potential neurologic manifestations. The carditis ranges from asymptomatic first-degree block to advanced heart block to a fulminant myocarditis with hemodynamic collapse. An ECG is not warranted for localized Lyme disease with only a target lesion or for late Lyme arthritis. With early disseminated disease (such as facial palsy or meningitis), an ECG allows for rapid triage. PR intervals >220 ms should raise suspicion for some cardiac involvement. PR intervals >300 ms are associated with progression to more advanced heart block; these patients should have inpatient monitoring while intravenous therapy is initiated.

Myopericarditis

Viral or idiopathic myopericarditis is a spectrum of diseases ranging from relatively benign inflammation localized to the pericardium

TABLE 19.3
Cardiac Conditions Associated with Endocarditis

Endocarditis Prophylaxis Recommended	Endocarditis Prophylaxis Not Recommended

Prosthetic cardiac valve
Previous infectious endocarditis
Congenital heart disease (CHD)[a]
  Unrepaired cyanotic CHD, including palliative shunts and conduits
  Completely repaired congenital heart defect with prosthetic material or device, whether placed by surgery or by catheter intervention, during the first 6 mos after the procedure[b]
  Repaired CHD with residual defects at the site or adjacent to the site of a prosthetic patch or prosthetic device (which inhibits endothelialization)
Cardiac transplantation recipients who develop cardiac valvulopathy
	Innocent murmurs
	Mitral valve prolapse
	Hypertrophic cardiomyopathy

[a]Antibiotic prophylaxis is no longer recommended for forms of congenital heart disease other than those described above.
[b]Prophylaxis is recommended because endothelialization of prosthetic material occurs within 6 mo after the procedure.
Adapted from Wilson W, Taubert KA, Gewitz M, et al. Prevention of infective endocarditis: guidelines from the American Heart Association. *Circulation.* 2007;115:1.

TABLE 19.4
Summary of Major Changes in 2007 American Heart Association's Guidelines on Prevention of Infective Endocarditis

Bacteremia resulting from daily activities is much more likely to cause infective endocarditis (IE) than bacteremia associated with a dental procedure

Only an extremely small number of cases of IE might be prevented by antibiotic prophylaxis even if prophylaxis is 100% effective

Antibiotic prophylaxis is not recommended based solely on an increased lifetime risk of acquisition of IE

IE prophylaxis is recommended only to those with conditions listed in Table 19.3

Antibiotic prophylaxis is no longer recommended for any other form of CHD, except for the conditions listed in Table 19.3

Antibiotic prophylaxis is recommended only for patients with underlying cardiac conditions associated with the highest risk of adverse outcome from IE (Table 19.3) when undergoing any dental procedures that involve manipulation of gingival tissues or the periapical region of teeth or perforation of oral mucosa

Antibiotic prophylaxis is recommended only for patients with underlying cardiac conditions associated with the highest risk of adverse outcome from IE (Table 19.3) when undergoing procedures on the respiratory tract or infected skin, skin structures, or musculoskeletal tissues

Antibiotic prophylaxis solely to prevent IE is not recommended for genitourinary or gastrointestinal tract procedures

The writing group reaffirms the procedures noted in the 1997 prophylaxis guidelines for which endocarditis prophylaxis is not recommended and extends this to other common procedures, including ear and body piercing, tattooing, and vaginal delivery and hysterectomy

Adapted from Wilson W, Taubert KA, Gewitz M, et al. Prevention of infective endocarditis: guidelines from the American Heart Association. *Circulation.* 2007;115:1.

TABLE 19.5
Dental Procedures and Recommendations for Endocarditis Prophylaxis (for Patients in Table 19.3)

Prophylaxis Is Recommended for:	Prophylaxis *Is Not* Recommended for:
• Manipulation of gingival tissue • Manipulation of the periapical region of teeth • Perforation of the oral mucosa	• Routine anesthetic injection through noninfected tissue • Dental x-rays • Placement of removable prosthodontic or orthodontic appliances • Adjustment of orthodontic appliances • Placement of orthodontic brackets • Shedding of deciduous teeth • Bleeding from trauma to lips or oral mucosa

to catastrophic involvement with large effusions, arrhythmias, or hemodynamic collapse. Myopericarditis can be occult and nearly asymptomatic or present as acute and quickly life-threatening "fulminant" myocarditis. When chest pain is a presenting symptom, the pain is usually more severe and lasts longer than "typical" musculoskeletal pain. Electrocardiogram typically demonstrates diffuse ST-T wave changes. Cardiac auscultation frequently reveals abnormalities including tachycardia, arrhythmia, or pericardial rubs. Serum troponin levels are usually elevated. Urgent cardiology consultation is warranted when significant chest pain is associated with any suggestion of syncope, arrhythmia, or hemodynamic instability.

TABLE 19.6
Regimens for Dental Procedures

Situation	Agent	Regimen: Single Dose 30–60 min Before Procedure	
		Adults	Children
Oral	Amoxicillin	2 g	50 mg/kg
Unable to take oral medication	Ampicillin OR Cefazolin OR Ceftriaxone	2 g IM or IV 1 g IM or IV	50 mg/kg IM or IV 50 mg/kg IM or IV
Allergic to penicillins or ampicillin—oral	Cephalexin[a,b] OR Clindamycin OR Azithromycin OR Clarithromycin	2 g 600 mg 500 mg	50 mg/kg 20 mg/kg 15 mg/kg
Allergic to penicillins or ampicillin and unable to take oral medication	Cefazolin OR Ceftriaxone[b] OR Clindamycin	1 g IM or IV 600 mg IM or IV	50 mg/kg IM or IV 20 mg/kg IM or IV

[a]Or other first- or second-generation oral cephalosporin in equivalent adult or pediatric dosage.
[b]Cephalosporins should not be used in an individual with a history of anaphylaxis, angioedema, or urticaria with penicillins or ampicillin.
IM, intramuscular; IV, intravenous.

There is evidence that severe COVID-19 illness or multisystem inflammatory syndrome in children (MIS-C) and adults (MIS-A) can result in myocarditis and myocardial dysfunction. Patients with less severe symptoms also have risk of developing myopericarditis, although it is much less common. Early small observational studies indicated that up to 78% of nonhospitalized patients had findings indicative of myocardial inflammation after resolution of acute COVID-19 symptoms,[17] but more recent reports of a large number of young adult athletes indicate that the true prevalence of myocarditis may be as low as 0.5% to 3%.[18] The clinical significance of this diagnosis of subclinical myocarditis remains unknown.

As there is a known association between myocarditis and sudden cardiac arrest in athletes, a number of guidelines have been developed for cardiovascular risk screening prior to return to exercise after COVID-19.[19] These range from guidelines recommending extensive testing (including cardiac MRI, troponin level, echocardiogram, and ECG) for higher-level competitive athletes to more targeted approaches requiring only examination or ECG initially, with additional testing if clinically indicated for younger athletes.[19,20] Current expert consensus holds that the risk of myocarditis (and therefore sudden cardiac arrest) is increased for those who: (1) have more systemic inflammation during acute COVID-19 illness; (2) are older and participate in more intense sports; (3) have cardiac symptoms such as chest pain, exertional dyspnea, palpitations, or syncope; or (4) have abnormal initial screening test results (ECG, echocardiogram, or troponin level).[20] These guidelines and practices will continue to evolve as more knowledge is gained regarding the risk factors and prevalence of post–COVID-19 myocarditis, especially with increasing vaccination rates and the emergence of COVID-19 variants. Multisystem inflammatory syndrome in children and overall severe pediatric disease are exceptionally rare in fully vaccinated children, as is the case in adults.

Vaccine-related myocarditis from mRNA vaccines has now been well recognized with a maximum estimated incidence of ~1/14,000 in adolescent males. This complication presents within 7 days of vaccination, typically within 2 to 3 days, and more frequently after the second dose. These AYAs present with combinations of chest pain, shortness of breath, fever, and headache. Laboratory evaluation will show an elevated troponin level and ECGs are frequently abnormal with ST-segment changes. Over 80% of patients have normal ventricular function on echocardiogram, and the others have mild dysfunction. The hospital course is typically benign.[21]

GENERAL CONSIDERATIONS IN THE EVALUATION OF HEART LESIONS

By adolescence and young adulthood, most patients with significant congenital heart disease have been previously identified. New disease is most likely to be diagnosed in underserved populations, or as a result of an acquired process (e.g., acute myocarditis, acquired cardiomyopathy). Slowly progressive valvular disease (e.g., bicommissural aortic valve disease, MVP, and mitral insufficiency) may first become apparent during adolescence. The identification of arrhythmias and complex ion channel disorders also increases during later adolescence and young adulthood.

A careful history and examination should allow differentiation of normal from pathologic murmurs. Electrocardiograms and chest x-rays do not add to the accuracy of diagnosis. Echocardiography adds little to the diagnosis of a "normal" murmur. The cost-effective choice between referring to a pediatric cardiologist (which often includes an echocardiogram) and directly obtaining an echocardiogram depends on the relative cost of the test, the accessibility of consultation, and the skill of the individual practitioner in identifying pathologic murmurs.[22] If the murmur is deemed innocent, the clinician should emphasize that the heart is normal. This helps prevent healthy AYAs from being labeled with cardiac diagnoses, and reduces needless patient, parental, and clinician anxiety.

CONGENITAL HEART DISEASE IN ADOLESCENTS AND YOUNG ADULTS

Because of advances in surgical and medical management, many types of congenital heart disease have very low early and late mortality rates. As a result, an increasing number of youth with congenital heart disease survive to adulthood.[23] Over a million Americans currently have a history of repaired or palliated heart disease.

For all but the most serious disorders, adolescence is often a period of medical quiescence. Youth feel well, and are coping with the usual tasks of adolescence with little to remind them of their need for medical care. However, though the quantitative risks vary substantially, many of these repairs carry long-term risks of arrhythmias, myocardial failure, and valve dysfunction (Table 19.7).

Even without progression of hemodynamic or "cardiac" concerns, a history of neonatal and childhood cardiac surgery is associated with a nearly dose-dependent decline in health-related well-being.[24] The more complex the operation, the more operations they need, the more follow-up that they need (and get), and the worse their health-related quality of life. Somewhat paradoxically, patients systematically report that they have good exercise performance and feel well; thus, very specific questioning about daily activities and well-being is a critical part of understanding their true cardiac status. For most complicated defects, peak exercise capacity is clearly decreased, while submaximal exercise capacity is relatively preserved.[25] Accurate assessment of expected and actual exercise capacity may help in choosing appropriate recreational and vocational activities.[26]

For the primary care clinician, the most critical tasks are to ensure routine health maintenance including immunizations, counseling regarding risk-taking behaviors, reproductive health issues, and effective transition to adulthood, while also facilitating continued specialized cardiac care.[27,28] Children with significant heart disease are often lost to follow-up toward the end of elementary school and again during the transition to adulthood. Even in a publicly funded health system, over a quarter had lapsed follow-up by age 12, with over 50% having minimal follow-up by age 22.[29] The medical home is an ideal place to evaluate and optimize school and social function for patients with established heart disease. Deficits in cognitive testing at the start of school have been associated with each of the following: a history of cardiac bypass, complex cardiac repair, or long stays in the intensive care unit.[30] The impact of these deficits on school performance during adolescence is not yet known. A history of prior cardiac surgery is almost always a reasonable indication for further testing and development of an Individualized Educational Program when there are concerns. Many congenital heart programs can facilitate that evaluation.

There are also guidelines for participation in competitive and recreational athletic activities for youth with known heart disease.[31–34] These guidelines provide a reasonable starting point for discussing athletic participation and can help the clinician to determine when specialty consultation may be needed prior to clearance for participation in athletic endeavors.

Transition to Adult Care for Youth with Congenital Heart Disease

Specialized care during the transition to adulthood may take a variety of forms, and is influenced by the severity of the underlying disease, the locally available resources, and clinician or patient/family preference. Some youth may remain with the cardiologist who cared for them during childhood, while others may transition to an adult cardiologist or to a specialized adult congenital center (if available).[35,36]

TABLE 19.7

Common Forms of Congenital Heart Disease and Potential Issues in Adolescence

	Common Issues	Rare Concerns
Simple CHD		
Repaired ASD		Atrial tachycardia Heart block
Repaired VSD	Residual VSD Right bundle branch block	Arrhythmias
Mild pulmonary stenosis		
Moderate complexity CHD		
Tetralogy of Fallot	Pulmonary insufficiency Atrial tachycardia RV dysfunction	Ventricular tachycardia LV dysfunction
Ebstein anomaly	Arrhythmias Exercise intolerance	Cyanosis
Aortic valve disease	Widely variable	
Aortic coarctation	Additional aortic/ mitral valve disease Hypertension	
Arterial switch for d-transposition	Neoaortic valve disease Mild coronary insufficiency Branch pulmonary artery stenosis	
AV canal defects	Arrhythmias Mitral insufficiency	
High complexity CHD		
Complex tetralogy of Fallot	Conduit obstruction Branch pulmonary artery stenosis	
Single ventricular- Fontan	Sinus node dysfunction Exercise intolerance Arrhythmias Fluid retention	Protein-losing enteropathy Ventricular failure
Truncus arteriosus	Conduit obstruction Truncal valve dysfunction	
Atrial switch for d-TGA	Arrhythmias Systemic RV failure	

CHD, congenital heart disease; ASD, atrial septal defect; VSD, ventricular septal defect; AV, arterioventricular; d-TGA, dextro-transposition of the great arteries; RV, right ventricle; LV, left ventricle.

Congenital heart disease in the young adult can be broadly categorized by the ability of the initial intervention to cure or palliate the disease, the number of initial interventions, and the expected need for future interventions. The American College of Cardiology/American Heart Association 2018 Consensus paper regarding the

adult with congenital heart disease provides a useful framework.[37] Three classifications from simple to complex congenital disease are used:

- **Simple congenital heart disease** includes such lesions as mild valvar pulmonary stenosis and repaired ASD or VSD. These "nearly normal" patients will require little to no activity restriction, no endocarditis prophylaxis, and infrequent follow-up. Most can be cared for in the general medical community.
- The young adult with **congenital heart disease of moderate complexity** often feels well but has significant risk of requiring additional interventions. Tetralogy of Fallot and aortic coarctation are two examples where the residual disease may be slowly progressive or occult. Also included in this category is the patient with moderate but asymptomatic valve disease who may require future intervention. These young adults should be seen periodically at regional adult congenital heart centers.
- The young adult with **congenital heart disease of great complexity**—characterized by repairs involving conduits, functional single ventricle physiology, and/or pulmonary hypertension—requires regular, often intensive, support from specialized adult congenital heart disease centers.

Clinicians caring for youth with congenital heart disease should guide patients and families in preparing for transition to adulthood during early and middle adolescence. The goal is to facilitate a planned, purposeful transition to adult-oriented care for youth and families rather than an abrupt transfer to adult care during a time of crisis.[35] Pregnancy (and prepregnancy planning) is an example of one of many times during the transition to adulthood that specialized resources for youth and families will be needed.[38]

● SUMMARY

Cardiac murmurs are common among AYAs, and a detailed history and thorough physical examination are typically sufficient to differentiate between physiologic and pathologic causes. Targeted testing and collaboration with a cardiologist can help establish a diagnosis and treatment plan when congenital or acquired heart disease is suspected. Importantly, most congenital heart disease will have already been identified prior to adolescence and young adulthood. Assuring appropriate life-long follow-up for AYAs with repaired congenital heart disease is critical. Finally, it is important to keep in mind that there are significant forms of inherited heart disease where AYAs can either be the index case or develop the phenotype.

REFERENCES

1. Sumski CA, Goot BH. Evaluating chest pain and heart murmurs in pediatric and adolescent patients. *Pediatr Clin North Am.* 2020;67(5):783–799.
2. Barry OM, Gauvreau K, Rhodes J, et al. Incidence and predictors of clinically important and dangerous arrhythmias during exercise tests in pediatric and congenital heart disease patients. *JACC Clin Electrophysiol.* 2018;4(10):1319–1327.
3. Maron BJ. Clinical course and management of hypertrophic cardiomyopathy. *N Engl J Med.* 2018;379(7):655–668.
4. Maron BJ, Levine BD, Washington RL, et al. Eligibility and disqualification recommendations for competitive athletes with cardiovascular abnormalities: task force 2: preparticipation screening for cardiovascular disease in competitive athletes: a scientific statement from the American Heart Association and American College of Cardiology. *Circulation.* 2015;132(22):e267–e272.
5. Elliott PM, Anastasakis A, Borger MA, et al. 2014 ESC guidelines on diagnosis and management of hypertrophic cardiomyopathy: the task force for the diagnosis and management of hypertrophic cardiomyopathy of the European Society of Cardiology (ESC). *Eur Heart J.* 2014;35(39):2733–2779.
6. Miron A, Lafreniere-Roula M, Steve Fan CP, et al. A validated model for sudden cardiac death risk prediction in pediatric hypertrophic cardiomyopathy. *Circulation.* 2020;142(3):217–229.
7. Guy TS, Hill AC. Mitral valve prolapse. *Annu Rev Med.* 2012;63:277–292.
8. Althunayyan A, Petersen SE, Lloyd G, et al. Mitral valve prolapse. *Expert Rev Cardiovasc Ther.* 2019;17(1):43–51.
9. Muthukumar L, Jahangir A, Jan MF, et al. Association between malignant mitral valve prolapse and sudden cardiac death: a review. *JAMA Cardiol.* 2020;5(9):1053–1061.
10. Caselli S, Mango F, Clark J, et al. Prevalence and clinical outcome of athletes with mitral valve prolapse. *Circulation.* 2018;137(19):2080–2082.

11. Lerman TT, Weintraub AY, Sheiner E. Pregnancy outcomes in women with mitral valve prolapse and mitral valve regurgitation. *Arch Gynecol Obstet*. 2013;288(2):287–291.

12. Koo HK, Lawrence KA, Musini VM. Beta-blockers for preventing aortic dissection in Marfan syndrome. *Cochrane Database Syst Rev*. 2017;11(11):CD011103.

13. Braverman AC, Harris KM, Kovacs RJ, et al. Eligibility and disqualification recommendations for competitive athletes with cardiovascular abnormalities: Task Force 7: aortic diseases, including Marfan syndrome: a scientific statement from the American Heart Association and American College of Cardiology. *Circulation*. 2015;132(22):e303–e309.

14. Hakim A, O'Callaghan C, De Wandele I, et al. Cardiovascular autonomic dysfunction in Ehlers–Danlos syndrome—Hypermobile type. *Am J Med Genet C Semin Med Genet*. 2017;175(1):168–174.

15. Wilson W, Taubert KA, Gewitz M, et al. Prevention of infective endocarditis: guidelines from the American Heart Association: a guideline from the American Heart Association Rheumatic Fever, Endocarditis and Kawasaki Disease Committee, Council on Cardiovascular Disease in the Young, and the Council on Cardiovascular Disease in the Young, and the Council on Clinical Cardiology, Council on Cardiovascular Surgery and Anesthesia, and the Quality of Care and Outcomes Research Interdisciplinary Working Group. *J Am Dent Assoc*. 2007;138(6):739–745, 747–760.

16. Baltimore RS, Gewitz M, Baddour LM, et al. Infective endocarditis in childhood: 2015 update: a scientific statement from the American Heart Association. *Circulation*. 2015;132(15):1487–1515.

17. Puntmann VO, Carerj ML, Wieters I, et al. Outcomes of cardiovascular magnetic resonance imaging in patients recently recovered from coronavirus disease 2019 (COVID-19). *JAMA Cardiol*. 2020;5(11):1265–1273.

18. Daniels CJ, Rajpal S, Greenshields JT, et al. Prevalence of clinical and subclinical myocarditis in competitive athletes with recent SARS-CoV-2 infection: results From the Big Ten COVID-19 Cardiac Registry. *JAMA Cardiol*. 2021;6(9):1078–1087.

19. Wilson MG, Hull JH, Rogers J, et al. Cardiorespiratory considerations for return-to-play in elite athletes after COVID-19 infection: a practical guide for sport and exercise medicine physicians. *Br J Sports Med*. 2020;54(19):1157–1161.

20. American Academy of Pediatrics. COVID-19 Interim Guidance: Return to Sports and Physical Activity. https://www.aap.org/en/pages/2019-novel-coronavirus-covid-19-infections/clinical-guidance/covid-19-interim-guidance-return-to-sports/#:~:text=The%20AAP%20recommends%20that%20decisions,COVID%2D19%20can%20be%20decreased.

21. Truong DT, Dionne A, Muniz JC, et al. Clinically suspected myocarditis temporally related to COVID-19 vaccination in adolescents and young adults: suspected myocarditis after COVID-19 vaccination. *Circulation*. 2022;145(5):345–356.

22. Danford DA. Cost-effectiveness of echocardiography for evaluation of children with murmurs. *Echocardiography*. 1995;12(2):153–162.

23. Best KE, Rankin J. Long-term survival of individuals born with congenital heart disease: a systematic review and meta-analysis. *J Am Heart Assoc*. 2016;5(6):e002846.

24. Mellion K, Uzark K, Cassedy A, et al. Health-related quality of life outcomes in children and adolescents with congenital heart disease. *J Pediatr*. 2014;164(4):781–788.e1.

25. Mueller GC, Stark V, Steiner K, et al. Impact of age and gender on cardiac pathology in children and adolescents with Marfan syndrome. *Pediatr Cardiol*. 2013;34(4):991–998.

26. Kempny A, Dimopoulos K, Uebing A, et al. Reference values for exercise limitations among adults with congenital heart disease. Relation to activities of daily life–single centre experience and review of published data. *Eur Heart J*. 2012;33(11):1386–1396.

27. Haberer K, Silversides CK. Congenital heart disease and women's health across the life span: focus on reproductive issues. *Can J Cardiol*. 2019;35(12):1652–1663.

28. Gupta P. Caring for a teen with congenital heart disease. *Pediatr Clin North Am*. 2014;61(1):207–228.

29. Mackie AS, Rempel GR, Rankin KN, et al. Risk factors for loss to follow-up among children and young adults with congenital heart disease. *Cardiol Young*. 2012;22(3):307–315.

30. McGrath E, Wypij D, Rappaport LA, et al. Prediction of IQ and achievement at age 8 years from neurodevelopmental status at age 1 year in children with D-transposition of the great arteries. *Pediatrics*. 2004;114(5):e572–e576.

31. Van Hare GF, Ackerman MJ, Evangelista JAK, et al. Eligibility and disqualification recommendations for competitive athletes with cardiovascular abnormalities: task force 4: congenital heart disease: a scientific statement from the American Heart Association and American College of Cardiology. *Circulation*. 2015;132(22):e281–e291.

32. Maron BJ, Zipes DP, Kovacs RJ. Eligibility and disqualification recommendations for competitive athletes with cardiovascular abnormalities: preamble, principles, and general considerations: a scientific statement from the American Heart Association and American College of Cardiology. *Circulation*. 2015;132(22):e256–e261.

33. Selamet Tierney ES. The benefit of exercise in children with congenital heart disease. *Curr Opin Pediatr*. 2020;32(5):626–632.

34. Dean PN, Battle RW. Congenital heart disease and the athlete: what we know and what we do not know. *Cardiol Clin*. 2016;34(4):579–589.

35. Talluto C. Establishing a successful transition care plan for the adolescent with congenital heart disease. *Curr Opin Cardiol*. 2018;33(1):73–77.

36. Moceri P, Goossens E, Hascoet S, et al. From adolescents to adults with congenital heart disease: the role of transition. *Eur J Pediatr*. 2015;174(7):847–854.

37. Stout KK, Daniels CJ, Aboulhosn JA, et al. 2018 AHA/ACC guideline for the management of adults with congenital heart disease: executive summary: a report of the American College of Cardiology/American Heart Association Task Force on clinical practice guidelines. *Circulation*. 2019;139(14):e637–e697.

38. Abarbanell G, Tepper NK, Farr SL. Safety of contraceptive use among women with congenital heart disease: a systematic review. *Congenit Heart Dis*. 2019;14(3):331–340.

📶 ADDITIONAL RESOURCES AND WEBSITES

Additional Resources and Websites for Clinicians:

Guidelines for Prevention of Infectious Endocarditis—http://circ.ahajournals.org/content/116/15/1736.full.pdf

Additional Resources and Websites for Parents/Caregivers:

Adult Congenital Heart Association: A patient/physician partnership with engaged joint physician/patient leadership and educational events—https://www.achaheart.org/

Family Support Groups: There are a number of disease-specific family support groups that have clinical advisors to support participants and assure accurate content. In addition, camps for children and adolescents with congenital heart disease offer opportunities for children to play and share experiences with each other—Littlehearts.org; Mendedlittlehearts.org; https://www.sistersbyheart.org/

Fontan Outcomes Network: A family-driven group that is part of the national pediatric cardiology quality improvement collaborative—https://www.fontanoutcomesnetwork.org/

Infective Endocarditis Wallet Card—http://www.heart.org/HEARTORG/Conditions/More/ToolsForYourHeartHealth/Infective-Bacterial-Endocarditis-Wallet-Card_UCM_311659_Article.jsp

Sudden Arrhythmic Death Syndromes Foundation: Focused on families with inherited arrhythmia syndromes and those with survivors or victim of sudden cardiac arrest—https://www.sads.org/

Transplant Families: Parent founded and focused on the patient/family experience of all pediatric solid organ transplant—https://www.transplantfamilies.org/

CHAPTER 20

Systemic Hypertension

Matthew B. Rivara
Joseph T. Flynn

KEY WORDS

- Blood pressure
- Exercise
- Guideline
- Heart
- Kidney
- Left ventricular hypertrophy
- Obesity
- Sodium

 INTRODUCTION

Hypertension is one of the most common chronic diseases in adults, affecting about 45% of adults of all ages and 22% of younger adults 18 to 39 years of age.[1,2] In children <18 years of age, however, hypertension is much less common, with most screening studies demonstrating a 3% to 4% prevalence of persistent hypertension. Some studies have reported a higher prevalence of up to 5% in adolescents living with obesity, reflecting an impact of the obesity epidemic similar to that seen in adults.[3,4] Other recent analyses have demonstrated an increase in prevalence of hypertension in children and adolescents ≤18 years of age, again likely because of the obesity epidemic.[5] Furthermore, due to changes in the pediatric normative blood pressure (BP) data published in 2017, there has been an increase in the percentage of adolescents who would be classified as hypertensive.[6] In those ≥18 years of age, however, when accounting for changes in threshold definitions of hypertension based on clinical practice guidelines (CPG), the prevalence of hypertension has remained relatively stable over time.[3]

Most adolescents and adults with hypertension have primary hypertension—that is, no identifiable underlying cause can be found for their BP elevation. Since most hypertensive adolescents and young adults (AYAs) ≤39 years of age are asymptomatic, particularly those with primary hypertension, it is imperative to measure BP whenever an AYA is seen for health care in order to detect hypertension and institute appropriate measures to reduce future cardiovascular risk.

 DEFINITION OF HYPERTENSION

The cardiovascular end points used to define hypertension in adults (e.g., myocardial infarction, stroke) do not occur in children and adolescents. Therefore, the definition of hypertension in those <13 years of age is a statistical one derived from analysis of a large database of BPs obtained from healthy children.[7] The 2017 American Academy of Pediatrics (AAP) Clinical Practice Guideline on High Blood Pressure in Children and Adolescents revised this approach for adolescents ≥13 years of age, and adopted the same BP cut-points as used in the revised American Heart Association/American College of Cardiology (AHA/ACC) adult guideline, also

published in 2017.[8] This was done deliberately to align the adult and pediatric guidelines, recognizing that adolescent hypertension is similar in many respects to adult hypertension, and that such alignment would facilitate transition of care from adolescence to adulthood.

For AYAs ≥13 years, any systolic BP (SBP) reading ≥130 or diastolic BP (DBP) reading ≥80 mm Hg is considered hypertensive, regardless of age or gender. Individuals with BP values of this magnitude when based on an average of 2 or more readings on two or more occasions are considered to have hypertension.[8] Of note, the threshold BP of 130/80 for defining hypertension in AYAs was established in the pediatric and adult hypertension CPGs mentioned above, with prior guidelines having used a higher threshold of ≥140/90 for adults, and percentile-based definitions for adolescents <18 years old. As in adolescents, use of the new definition has resulted in an increase in the prevalence of hypertension among young adults and in the intensity of antihypertensive medication treatment for many young adults taking BP lowering medications.[9]

Observational studies evaluating the prognostic value of the new definition of hypertension among young adults have shown that young adults diagnosed with hypertension have a higher risk of developing adverse cardiovascular events later in life compared to young adults with normal BP.[10] Analyses of the impact of the revised pediatric guidelines have demonstrated a stronger link between BP and other intermediate markers of cardiovascular risk such as metabolic syndrome and left ventricular hypertrophy (LVH), as well as better prediction of adult hypertension.[6,11]

Elevated BP

Common to both the pediatric (<18 years of age) and adult BP classification schemes is the concept of "elevated BP," referring to BPs between the normal and hypertensive ranges. This term is meant to serve as an alert to patients and clinicians to the potential for future development of hypertension and of the need to make lifestyle changes that might prevent this from occurring. The same BP value of 120 to 129/<80 mm Hg is used in both adolescents and adults to designate elevated BP.

Staging

Also common to both the pediatric and adult BP classification schemes is the concept of "staging" the severity of hypertension. The staging system helps to determine how rapidly a hypertensive patient should be evaluated and when antihypertensive drug therapy should be initiated. The currently accepted staging systems for hypertension in children and in AYAs are compared in **Table 20.1**.[7,8]

TABLE 20.1

Classification of BP in Children and AYAs

BP Classification	Children 1–<13 y of Age[a]	AYAs ≥13 y of Age[b]
Normal	SBP and DBP <90th percentile	SBP <120 mm Hg and DBP <80 mm Hg
Elevated BP	SBP or DBP 90–95th percentile; or if BP is >120/80 even if <90th percentile	SBP 120–129 mm Hg and DBP <80 mm Hg
Stage 1 hypertension	SBP or DBP ≥95th to 99th percentile plus 5 mm Hg	SBP 130–139 mm Hg or DBP 80–89 mm Hg
Stage 2 hypertension	SBP or DBP >99th percentile plus 5 mm Hg	SBP ≥140 mm Hg or DBP ≥90 mm Hg

[a]Adapted from Flynn JT, Kaelber DC, Baker-Smith CM, et al. Clinical Practice Guideline for screening and management of high blood pressure in children and adolescents. *Pediatrics.* 2017;140(3):e20171904.
[b]Adapted from Whelton PK, Carey RM, Aronow WS, et al. 2017. ACC/AHA/AAPA/ABC/ACPM/ AGS/APhA/ASH/ASPC/NMA/PCNA Guideline for the prevention, detection, evaluation, and management of high blood pressure in adults: a report of the American College of Cardiology/ American Heart Association Task Force on Clinical Practice Guidelines. *J Am Coll Cardiol.* 2018;71(19):2199–2269.
AYAs, adolescents and young adults; BP, blood pressure; DBP, diastolic blood pressure; SBP, systolic blood pressure.

FACTORS THAT INFLUENCE BP

Height and Weight

Height, given its importance as a surrogate marker of growth and maturation in childhood, has been incorporated into the normative BP percentiles used in children and adolescents since the 1996 "Working Group" report published by the National High BP Education Program, and is still part of the definition of normal and abnormal BP for adolescents <13 years old.[7] Weight is also an important factor in determining BP, as it has a positive association with BP. Increased body mass index (BMI) is also one of the most important influences on BP in adults ≥18 years old.[3]

Age

Blood pressure increases with age in a nonlinear manner through adolescence; this is likely related to growth. Beyond adolescence, BP, especially SBP, continues to increase in a significant percentage of individuals as the result of genetic and environmental factors, as well as age-associated vascular changes.

Sodium and Other Dietary Constituents

Numerous studies have done little to settle the controversy concerning the relationship of sodium intake to BP. For individuals with normal BP, dietary sodium restriction does not appear to lead to a clinically meaningful change in SBP or DBP.[12] However, in adults (including young adults) with hypertension, sodium restriction does appear to lower SBP and DBP to a modest degree, and this effect is amplified in certain salt-sensitive individuals.[13] There are fewer studies of the association of salt intake on BP s in children and adolescents, and those that have been done have shown only a modest association.

Other studies have found a link between potassium intake and both elevated and low BP, although the preponderance of evidence appears to show a protective effect of increased potassium intake.[14] In contrast, efforts to correlate calcium and other divalent cations with BP have been equivocal. Similarly, suggested correlations between BP and vitamins A, C, and E remain to be proved. Falkner et al.[15] noted that dietary modification of certain nutrients when instituted at an early age could contribute to the prevention of hypertension in urban minority adolescents at risk for hypertension.

Stress and Adverse Childhood Experiences

Both physical and mental stressors evoke changes in BP. Indeed, the degree of change has been thought by some to be useful in predicting later-life hypertension. Early studies have demonstrated that hypertensive adolescents had significantly greater increases in heart rate, SBP, and DBP during mental stress (performance of difficult arithmetic problems) than normotensive adolescents, an effect that may be mediated by impaired renal sodium handling.[16] In adults, including young adults, high perceived stress over time has been shown to contribute to the development of hypertension and other cardiovascular diseases, suggesting that stress may have lifelong adverse cardiovascular effects.[17] Studies of meditation and other stress-reduction interventions have unfortunately not shown a significant impact on BP in individuals with hypertension. Thus it is currently uncertain whether stress is a modifiable risk factor for hypertension outcomes.

Recent studies have identified a link between adverse childhood experiences and the development of hypertension and other cardiovascular risk factors. Adverse childhood experiences include such events as loss of a parent, physical/sexual abuse, and emotional neglect. Analysis of data on self-reported adverse childhood experiences from the Behavioral Risk Factor Surveillance System have demonstrated that experiencing even one such event is associated with an increased risk of hypertension, dyslipidemia, and diabetes, with the risk increasing in a dose-response fashion as the number of such events experienced increases. Potential mechanisms are under study, but may include such factors as alterations in immunity/inflammation, and/or vasoactive factors. Identifying and addressing these has been identified as another important aspect of primordial prevention.[18]

Race/Ethnicity

Over the past two decades, it has been increasingly recognized that race is primarily a social construct that does not accurately represent genetic ancestry, and is a poor proxy for human biologic variation. There are increasing calls to abandon its use in clinical medicine in favor of more precise analytics and tools that better capture risk of disease and response to treatments. Racial and ethnic differences in disease prevalence are often more likely due to structural and social determinants of health rather than representations of true biologic differences. In the case of hypertension prevalence, there are substantial racial and ethnic disparities for adults ≥18 years of age, with non-Hispanic Blacks having the highest rates of hypertension.[1] Additionally, survey data have shown that for individuals <18 years of age, recent increases in hypertension prevalence have been more pronounced among Black and Mexican American youth than in non-Hispanic Whites, suggesting that such racial and ethnic disparities are present at all ages.[19]

There has been much debate regarding whether there might be a pathophysiologic basis of these observations, including hypotheses focused on differences between Blacks and individuals of other racial backgrounds in plasma renin activity and sodium reabsorption in the kidney.[20] Such hypotheses at least partially underlie current recommendations to incorporate race in the selection of an initial antihypertensive agent in adults with hypertension (no such recommendation exists for pediatric patients). We believe that all antihypertensive medication options should be considered for all patients, irrespective of perceived or self-identified race or ethnicity, with therapy adjusted based on medication response and occurrence of side effects.

Genetics

Both familial aggregation BP studies and twin studies indicate a strong positive correlation between hereditary influences and BP measurements. Family history has been shown to be an important determinant of overall cardiovascular risk.[21] It is estimated that about one-third of variations in BP among individuals are heritable, most likely from several genes.[22] Additionally, several single-gene defects have been described, which account for hypertension in a small number of patients, especially those with a family history of severe, early-onset hypertension.[23]

Birth Weight and Other Perinatal Factors

The "fetal origins" hypothesis maintains that low birth weight is a risk factor for the subsequent development of primary hypertension in adulthood.[24] This hypothesis stems from findings of large population studies that demonstrate an inverse correlation between birth weight and adult BP.[25] One proposed explanation for this effect is deficient maternal nutrition, possibly leading to development of a reduced number of nephrons in utero. Studies suggest that maternal smoking during pregnancy and bottle-feeding of newborns may also lead to hypertension later in life.[26,27] Other epidemiologic studies have found that adult BP is more closely related to early childhood growth than to birth weight.[28]

 ETIOLOGY

At least 80% to 90% of adolescents with hypertension have no known cause for their disorder and are labeled as having primary or essential hypertension. As in younger children, kidney diseases are the most common secondary cause in adolescents. Primary hypertension in adolescents is frequently characterized by isolated SBP elevation, whereas DBP elevation is more likely to be present in secondary hypertension.[7] Obesity and a positive family history of hypertension are also common in adolescents with primary hypertension.

Primary or essential hypertension accounts for 90% to 95% of all cases of hypertension in adults ≥18 years of age.[29] Unfortunately, there are no data available on specific etiologies of hypertension in young adults 18 to 25 years of age compared to other age groups. A high index of suspicion in the clinician caring for hypertensive young adults is therefore needed for detection of cases of secondary hypertension.

 DIAGNOSIS

Blood Pressure Measurement

There are several important points regarding measurement of BP that should be considered in patients of any age. They are as follows:

1. Pediatric and adult guidelines differ regarding the recommended technique for BP measurement. The 2017 AAP CPG recommends auscultation for BP measurement in youth, primarily because currently available normative BP values are based upon auscultation. The 2017 ACC/AHA guideline, however, recommends the use of automated, oscillometric devices.[7,8]
2. Proper cuff bladder size is critical regardless of technique. The length of the cuff bladder should be at least 80% of the mid-arm circumference. For practical purposes, use the largest cuff that fits the arm while leaving the antecubital fossa free for auscultation. Given the obesity epidemic, many AYAs will require large adult or even thigh-sized cuffs because of increased arm circumferences.
3. Blood pressure measurements should be taken while the patient is seated with feet on the floor, back supported, and the arm at heart level. The arm (preferably the right) used for the measurement should be recorded in the chart. Ideally,

the patient should have rested for several minutes and should not have smoked or ingested caffeine in the 30 minutes before measurement.
4. For apprehensive patients, BP measurements obtained outside of the office setting may provide insight as to the existence of "white coat" hypertension (WCH). In adults, home BP measurement has been shown to be an appropriate method of assessing potential WCH. A lack of validated devices and normative values precludes the use of home BP in children and adolescents. Ambulatory BP monitoring (ABPM), in which BP measurements are obtained over a 24-hour period with an automated device, is considered the optimal technique for diagnosing WCH, and can be performed in all AYAs.[30]

Confirmation of Hypertension Diagnosis

In adolescents <18 years of age, three BP determinations on different days must show a high (≥95th percentile) SBP or DBP or both before a diagnosis of hypertension is made. This is because BP in this age group has been shown to be quite labile, leading to the possibility of overdiagnosis if only one or two BP readings are relied upon.[7] As stated above, assessment for WCH, ideally with ABPM, is now recommended by the 2017 AAP CPG.[7] Studies suggest that WCH may actually be a prelude to sustained hypertension, and others have shown that adolescents with WCH have early evidence of target-organ damage.[31] Further, one recent study has shown that BP profiles in adolescents are not stable over time, implying that repeated ABPM may be appropriate in some patients.[32]

Confirmation of hypertension in adults requires documentation of elevated BP (≥130/80) on just two occasions.[8] Twenty-four-hour ABPM or home measurement of BP is now recommended in adults to confirm the diagnosis of hypertension and for titration of BP-lowering medications. Additionally, home BP monitoring or ABPM are recommended to evaluate for possible WCH and masked hypertension phenotypes.[8]

Diagnostic Evaluation

Once the diagnosis of hypertension is made, a diagnostic evaluation and management plan can be initiated. The diagnostic evaluation must be tailored to the individual, taking into account age, sex, family history, and level of hypertension. For example, a 12-year-old female with a past medical history of recurrent urinary tract infections, no family history of hypertension, and a BP of 150/115 mm Hg would be a candidate for an aggressive evaluation for secondary causes (particularly kidney disease, specifically reflux nephropathy). In contrast, invasive studies to identify a secondary cause are unlikely to be helpful in a 21-year-old male with obesity, a family history of hypertension, and a BP of 150/78 mm Hg.

1. History: A detailed history should assess for possible secondary causes, target-organ damage, and other cardiovascular risk factors. Ask about (1) symptoms of urinary tract infections or renal disease; (2) birth/perinatal history; (3) family history of hypertension or other cardiovascular disease; (4) physical activity, dietary patterns, and other lifestyle habits; and (5) alcohol, tobacco, and substance use. Substances that may elevate BP are listed in Table 20.2, and historical clues suggestive of secondary hypertension are in Table 20.3.
2. Physical examination: A thorough examination is also an essential part of the diagnostic evaluation. The examination should evaluate for evidence of a secondary cause or end-organ damage and include the following:
   a. Height, weight, and calculated BMI
   b. BP in both arms and a lower extremity
   c. Femoral pulses
   d. Neck: Carotid bruits or an enlarged thyroid gland
   e. Fundi: Arteriolar narrowing, arteriovenous nicking, hemorrhages, exudates
   f. Abdomen: Bruits, hepatosplenomegaly, flank masses

TABLE 20.2
Substances That May Elevate BP

Prescription Medications	Nonprescription Medications	Others
Calcineurin inhibitors (cyclosporine, tacrolimus)	Caffeine	Cocaine
Dexedrine[a]	Ephedrine	Ethanol
Erythropoietin	Nonsteroidal anti-inflammatory drugs[a]	Heavy metals (lead, mercury)
Glucocorticoids	Pseudoephedrine	3,4-Methylenedioxy-methamphetamine ("Ecstasy")
Methylphenidate[a]		Tobacco
Oral contraceptives		Herbal preparations (*Ephedra, Glycyrrhiza*)
Phenylpropanolamine		
Pseudoephedrine		
Tricyclic antidepressants[a]		

[a]These cause elevated blood pressure relatively infrequently compared with the other agents in the table.

g. Heart: Rate, precordial heave, clicks, murmurs, arrhythmias
h. Extremities: Pulses, edema
i. Nervous system
j. Skin: Striae, acanthosis nigricans, café-au-lait spots, neurofibromas

3. Physical examination findings suggestive of secondary causes of hypertension are listed in Table 20.3. In addition, the clinician should remember that severe hypertension in AYAs who are not obese suggests a secondary cause, particularly kidney disease. Acute onset should prompt evaluation for acute renal disease.
4. Laboratory testing: Basic/screening studies should be performed in all patients with confirmed BP elevation. Specific testing is indicated when secondary hypertension is suspected or for those with stage 2 hypertension. Clinical practice guidelines for adults suggest screening for secondary causes of hypertension in individuals with drug-resistant (≥3 drugs), abrupt onset, age <30 years, unprovoked or minimally provoked hypokalemia, and in individuals with severe target-organ damage.[8]
   a. *Screening tests*—should be done in all patients:
      • Electrolytes, blood urea nitrogen, and creatinine
      • Urinalysis, with attention to the presence of hematuria and/or albuminuria (urine cultures should be obtained if history or urinalysis suggest infection)
      • Lipid profile (initial test does not have to be fasting)
      • Fasting glucose or hemoglobin A1c (hemoglobin A1C is preferred in children and adolescents <18 years) to screen for impaired glucose tolerance/hyperinsulinemia.
   b. *Specific laboratory tests* should be directed by findings on history and physical examination, or from the screening test results. Examples include (1) antinuclear antibody test and erythrocyte sedimentation rate in a hypertensive female adolescent with a malar rash, and (2) plasma renin activity and aldosterone if there is hypokalemia and metabolic alkalosis.
   c. *Advanced testing* should only be done when secondary causes of hypertension are suspected. For example, obtain plasma metanephrines if pheochromocytoma is suspected or a 24-hour urine collection for protein if there is persistent proteinuria.
   d. *Imaging studies* are indicated only in specific circumstances. Kidney ultrasound should be obtained for all adolescents <18 years with stage 2 hypertension, or for those with stage 1 hypertension and an abnormal urinalysis.[7] Routine kidney imaging is not currently recommended for

TABLE 20.3
History and Physical Examination Findings Suggestive of Secondary Causes of Hypertension

Present in History	Suggests
Known UTI/UTI symptoms	Reflux nephropathy
Joint pains, rash, fever	Vasculitis, SLE
Acute onset of gross hematuria	Glomerulonephritis, renal thrombosis
Renal trauma	Renal infarction, RAS
Abdominal radiation	Radiation nephritis, RAS
Renal transplant	Transplant RAS
Precocious puberty	Adrenal disorder
Muscle cramping, constipation	Hyperaldosteronism
Excessive sweating, headache, pallor, and/or flushing	Pheochromocytoma
Known illicit drug use	Drug-induced HTN
Present on Examination	**Suggests**
BP >140/100 mm Hg at any age	Secondary hypertension
Leg BP < arm BP	Aortic coarctation
Poor growth, pallor	Chronic renal disease
Turner syndrome	Aortic coarctation
Café-au-lait spots	Renal artery stenosis
Delayed leg pulses	Aortic coarctation
Precocious puberty	Adrenal disorder
Bruits over upper abdomen	Renal artery stenosis
Edema	Renal disease
Excessive pigmentation	Adrenal disorder
Striae in a male	Hypercortisolism

BP, blood pressure; HTN, hypertension; RAS, renal artery stenosis; SLE, systemic lupus erythematosus; UTI, urinary tract infection.

evaluation of hypertensive patients ≥18 years of age. Chest x-ray should only be obtained if the cardiac examination is abnormal. More advanced imaging studies such as nuclear-medicine scans or angiography are only useful in a small percentage of hypertensive AYA patients and should only be obtained under the direction of a hypertension specialist.

THERAPY

Prevention

Optimally, measures to prevent or minimize the effects of hypertension should be applied to all patients at risk for developing hypertension. The difficulty lies in identifying those at risk and deciding what measures to apply. Though prevention studies for AYAs with long-term follow-up are lacking, a reasonable starting point is to consider patients with the characteristics listed below as being at risk. They should be counseled about nonpharmacologic approaches to maintain lower BP and should be periodically monitored:

1. Elevated BP (BP ≥120 to 129/80 mm Hg)
2. BMI >85th percentile, particularly if parents are living with obesity
3. Hyperlipidemia or a family history of the disorder, particularly if there is a family history of coronary artery disease or stroke
4. Two or more family members with treated hypertension

Nonpharmacologic Interventions

Weight loss, aerobic exercise, and dietary modifications have all been shown to successfully reduce BP in hypertensive patients of all ages. These interventions should be part of the treatment plan for all AYAs with hypertension:

1. Weight reduction: Excess body weight is correlated closely with increased BP. Weight reduction reduces BP in a large proportion of hypertensive individuals who are >10% above ideal weight.
2. Dietary changes: Moderate sodium restriction in hypertensive individuals has been shown to reduce SBP, on average, by 4.9 mm Hg and DBP by 2.6 mm Hg. The so-called "DASH (Dietary Approaches to Stop Hypertension) diet," which is lower in sodium and higher in potassium and calcium content, has been demonstrated to be of benefit in hypertensive adults and adolescents.[33]
3. Exercise: Regular aerobic physical activity, adequate to achieve at least a moderate level of physical fitness, may be beneficial for both prevention and treatment of hypertension. Consistent activity (≥30 minutes/session, 4 to 5 days/week) can reduce SBP in hypertensive patients by approximately 10 mm Hg.
4. Other lifestyle changes: Smoking cessation and avoidance of alcohol excess, misuse of medications, and drugs (e.g., cocaine, amphetamines) are also important considerations. Cigarette smoking increases BP and is a major risk factor for cardiovascular disease. Excessive alcohol intake can raise BP and cause resistance to antihypertensive therapy.

Pharmacologic Treatment—Adolescents ≤18 Years

1. Antihypertensive medications are definitely indicated for patients with[7]:
   a. Symptoms of hypertension
   b. Stage 2 hypertension without a modifiable problem such as obesity
   c. Evidence of hypertensive end-organ damage
   d. Type 1 or type 2 diabetes
   e. Secondary hypertension
2. If none of these indications are present, drug treatment can be withheld. The lifestyle modifications discussed earlier should be recommended. If BP remains elevated after a reasonable trial of these measures (usually 6 to 12 months), then medication should be prescribed.
3. It is now recommended to obtain an echocardiogram at the time of initiation of antihypertensive medications to assess for LVH and left ventricular dysfunction.
4. Once-daily medications should be used if possible to improve adherence for what may be a lifelong but asymptomatic problem.
5. Explicit education should be provided about hypertension and the reasons for therapy using language the adolescent understands.
6. Adolescents should generally be responsible for taking their own medications, but parents should be encouraged to help adolescents maintain adherence.
7. Antihypertensive agents should be chosen to obtain the maximum benefit and minimize side effects. The ideal hypertensive agent would.
   a. Lower BP in almost all hypertensive individuals
   b. Address specific pathogenic mechanisms
   c. Be associated with few biochemical changes

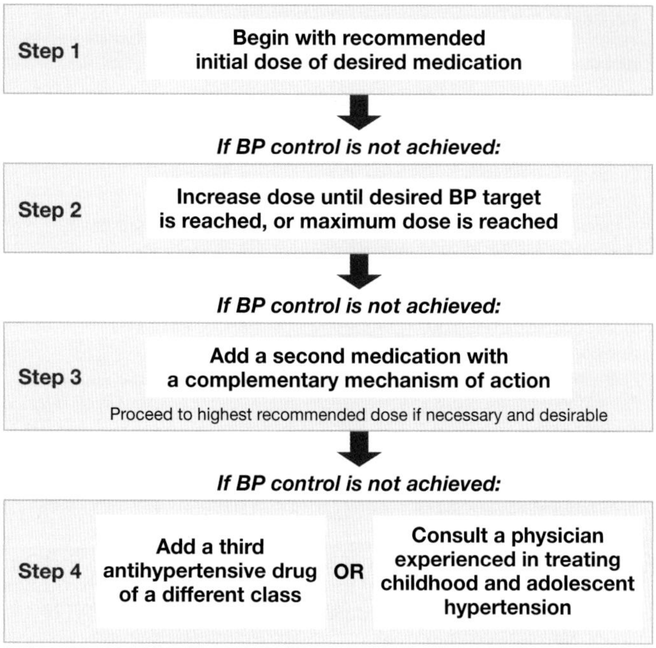

FIGURE 20.1 Stepped-care approach to antihypertensive therapy in adolescents <18 years of age. BP, blood pressure.

Step 1: Begin with recommended initial dose of desired medication

If BP control is not achieved:

Step 2: Increase dose until desired BP target is reached, or maximum dose is reached

If BP control is not achieved:

Step 3: Add a second medication with a complementary mechanism of action
Proceed to highest recommended dose if necessary and desirable

If BP control is not achieved:

Step 4: Add a third antihypertensive drug of a different class **OR** Consult a physician experienced in treating childhood and adolescent hypertension

   d. Be associated with few or no adverse effects
   e. Be dosed once or, at most, twice daily
   f. Be inexpensive
   Unfortunately, the ideal antihypertensive agent does not exist. The AAP has stated that first-line agents may include thiazide diuretics, long-acting calcium channel blockers, angiotensin-converting enzyme inhibitors, or angiotensin receptor blockers (ARBs).[7] Comprehensive reviews have been published that may help guide the clinician in selecting from among these agents.
8. As illustrated in Figure 20.1, a stepped-care approach is usually followed when prescribing antihypertensive agents in patients <18 years. In this approach, a monotherapy drug regimen is superimposed on nonpharmacologic therapy as initial treatment.[7]
9. Suggested initial and maximum doses of various antihypertensive agents for patients <18 years are given in Table 20.4. Many have pediatric-specific Food and Drug Administration (FDA)-approved labeling as a result of recent trials in children and adolescents.
10. For adolescents <18 years with either primary or secondary hypertension, target BP should be <130/80; for those with chronic kidney disease, target BP should be 24-hour mean arterial pressure <50th percentile on ABPM.[7]
11. Laboratory monitoring should be performed as appropriate if an agent with potential metabolic side-effects is prescribed. Either home or repeat ABPM may be used to assess BP control; annual ABPM should be obtained in hypertensive adolescents with chronic kidney disease.[7]
12. After an extended course of drug therapy and sustained BP control, a gradual reduction in or withdrawal of medication can be attempted with close observation and continuation of nonpharmacologic therapy.

Pharmacologic Treatment—Young Adults ≥18 Years

1. Drug therapy is generally initiated in all adults for SBP ≥140 mm Hg and/or DBP ≥90 mm Hg, and in adults with an estimated 10-year atherosclerotic cardiovascular risk of ≥10% and SBP ≥130 mm Hg or DBP ≥80 mm Hg.[8] This is based on epidemiologic evidence of reduction in stroke, myocardial infarction, and other cardiovascular disease with effective antihypertensive treatment.

TABLE 20.4

Antihypertensive Agents for Use in Chronic Treatment of Hypertension in Adolescents <18 Years Old[a]

Class	Drug	Starting Dose	Interval	Maximum Dose[b]
Angiotensin-converting enzyme inhibitors	Benazepril	0.2 mg/kg/d up to 10 mg/d	q.d.	0.6 mg/kg/d up to 40 mg/d
	Enalapril	0.08 mg/kg/d	q.d.	0.6 mg/kg/d up to 40 mg/d
	Fosinopril	0.1 mg/kg/d up to 10 mg/d	q.d.	0.6 mg/kg/d up to 40 mg/d
	Lisinopril	0.07 mg/kg/d up to 5 mg/d	q.d.	0.61 mg/kg/d up to 40 mg/d
	Quinapril	5–10 mg/d	q.d.	80 mg/d
	Ramipril	2.5 mg/d	q.d.	20 mg/d
Angiotensin receptor blockers	Candesartan	4 mg/d	q.d.	32 mg q.d.
	Losartan	0.75 mg/kg/d up to 50 mg/d	q.d.–b.i.d.	1.44 mg/kg/d up to 100 mg/d
	Olmesartan	20–35 kg: 10 mg/d ≥35 kg: 20 mg/d	q.d.	20–35 kg: 20 mg/d ≥35 kg: 40 mg/d
	Valsartan	6–17 y: 1.3 mg/kg/d up to 40 mg/d	q.d.	6–17 y: 2.7 mg/kg/d up to 160 mg/d
Calcium channel blockers	Amlodipine	0.10 mg/kg/d	q.d.	0.6 mg/kg/d up to 10 mg/d
	Felodipine	2.5 mg/d	q.d.	10 mg/d
	Isradipine	0.05–0.15 mg/kg/dose	t.i.d.–q.i.d.	0.8 mg/kg/d up to 20 mg/d
	Extended-release nifedipine	0.25–0.5 mg/kg/d	q.d.–b.i.d.	3 mg/kg/d up to 120 mg/d
Diuretics	Chlorthalidone	0.3 mg/kg/d	q.d.	2 mg/kg/d up to 50 mg/d
	HCTZ	1 mg/kg/d	b.i.d.	3 mg/kg/d up to 50 mg/d
	Spironolactone	1 mg/kg/d	q.d.–b.i.d.	3.3 mg/kg/d up to 100 mg/d
	Triamterene	1–2 mg/kg/d	b.i.d.	3–4 mg/kg/d up to 300 mg/d
Peripheral α-antagonists	Doxazosin	1 mg/d	q.d.	4 mg/d
	Prazosin	0.05–0.1 mg/kg/d	t.i.d.	0.5 mg/kg/d
	Terazosin	1 mg/d	q.d.	20 mg/d
Vasodilators	Hydralazine	0.25 mg/kg/dose	t.i.d.–q.i.d.	7.5 mg/kg/d up to 200 mg/d
	Minoxidil	0.1–0.2 mg/kg/d	b.i.d.–t.i.d.	1 mg/kg/d up to 50 mg/d

[a]Consult comprehensive reviews or other references for specific side effects.
[b]The maximum recommended adult dose should never be exceeded. Note that for some drugs, the maximum adult dose may be higher than what is listed in this table.
b.i.d., twice daily; HCTZ, hydrochlorothiazide; q.d., once daily; q.i.d., four times daily; t.i.d., three times daily.

a. Several months of nonpharmacologic measures can be implemented before drug therapy is begun in patients with stage 1 hypertension.

b. Patients with stage 2 hypertension, secondary hypertension, diabetes, or underlying kidney disease warrant immediate initiation of drug therapy.

2. The general comments made above about the ideal antihypertensive agent for adolescents apply also to young adult patients.

3. In adults, the most recent CPG from the ACC and AHA recommends choosing from several classes of antihypertensive medications. In general, the initial antihypertensive agent should be a thiazide-type diuretic, an ACE inhibitor or ARB, or a calcium channel blocker. For adults with chronic kidney disease, an ACE inhibitor or ARB is preferred.[8] Beta blockers are not first-line therapy for hypertension, except in patients with atherosclerotic cardiovascular disease or heart failure.

4. If a diuretic, ACE inhibitor, or ARB is started, serum creatinine and serum potassium should be monitored approximately 2 weeks after initiation of therapy. Irrespective of antihypertensive agent choice, all patients started on drug therapy should be followed closely for BP response and therapy intensified or changed to achieve the goal BP.

5. Combination preparations are acceptable as first-line therapy, particularly for patients with stage 2 hypertension, and may improve both adherence and the ability to reach treatment goals.

6. Similar to the stepped-care approach illustrated in Figure 20.1, medication doses should be titrated to achieve goal BP, and additional medications added as needed if BP control cannot be achieved with the initial regimen chosen.

7. As with adolescents, the goal BP for young adults taking anti-hypertensive medication is <130/80.

8. Withdrawal of antihypertensive medications after a period of drug treatment may be attempted if the patient is motivated to continue lifestyle changes.

Pharmacologic Treatment—Special Populations

1. Females who take oral contraceptives: Most females who take oral contraceptives have small increases in SBP and DBP but usually within the reference range. Hormonal contraceptives, mainly those that contain estrogen, can increase angiotensinogen in some individuals, with resultant increases in angiotensin II and BP. Many of the studies of BP and oral contraceptive agents involved higher doses of both estrogen and progesterone than are used currently. If concurrent treatment with an oral contraceptive and antihypertensive medication is needed, consideration should be given to using a low-estrogen or progestin-only contraceptive.

2. Adolescents with asthma: Beta-blocking medications can worsen bronchoconstriction and are therefore relatively contraindicated for patients with asthma and hypertension. Cardioselective β_1 receptor selective agents such as metoprolol or bisoprolol may be tried, especially in those with mild asthma.

3. Diabetes: The diagnosis of hypertension or even elevated BP in an AYA with either type 1 or type 2 diabetes is an indication to initiate antihypertensive drug therapy. ACE inhibitors or ARBs should be used as the initial agent in patients with diabetes and hypertension because of their potential benefit in slowing or preventing diabetic nephropathy.

4. Pregnancy: Hypertension in pregnant females is a risk factor for both complications of pregnancy such as preeclampsia, and future hypertension in offspring. Additionally, only a small number of antihypertensive agents are known to be safe during pregnancy. Given this, hypertension during pregnancy should be managed with the guidance of an obstetrician.

⬤ HYPERTENSIVE EMERGENCIES

Rarely, an AYA will have signs of encephalopathy or heart failure at presentation and be found to have extraordinarily high BP, at levels well above stage 2 hypertension. This constitutes a true emergency and may have life-threatening target-organ effects unless efforts to lower the BP are begun at once. Assistance from an expert in hypertension should be sought. Meanwhile, the patient should be hospitalized and an intravenous line placed. Usually, a continuous infusion of either nicardipine or labetalol should be started at a low dose and then titrated as needed to slowly reduce the BP. The initial reduction should be no more than 25% of the planned reduction over the first 8 hours in order to prevent cerebral, cardiac, or kidney ischemia from overly rapid BP reduction.[34] Blood pressure can then be lowered further over the next 24 to 48 hours. When adequate BP control has been achieved, oral antihypertensive agents can be gradually introduced and the intravenous agents discontinued. A thorough evaluation to determine the cause of the hypertension must be made once the patient's condition has been stabilized.

⬤ SUMMARY

Recent updates to adult and pediatric CPGs on hypertension have led to significant alignment regarding the detection, evaluation, and management of hypertension in AYAs. Most notably, the diagnostic thresholds for normal and high BP are identical starting at age 13, which should facilitate identifying AYAs with high BP. The approaches to evaluation and therapy are also similar, albeit with some differences regarding initiation of antihypertensive medications and specifically recommended medications. Many data gaps remain, especially regarding the outcomes of hypertension in this age group. However, there is general agreement that attention to high BP in AYAs is of paramount importance in reducing the long-term burden of cardiovascular disease.

REFERENCES

1. Ostechega Y, Fryar CD, Nwankwo T, et al. *Hypertension Prevalence Among Adults Aged 18 and Over: United States, 2017–2018*. National Center for Health Statistics; 2020.
2. Dorans KS, Mills KT, Liu Y, et al. Trends in Prevalence and control of hypertension according to the 2017 American College of Cardiology/American Heart Association (ACC/AHA) guideline. *J Am Heart Assoc.* 2018;7(11):e008888.
3. Egan BM, Li J, Hutchison FN, et al. Hypertension in the United States, 1999 to 2012: progress toward Healthy People 2020 goals. *Circulation.* 2014;130(19):1692–1699.
4. Flynn J. The changing face of pediatric hypertension in the era of the childhood obesity epidemic. *Pediatr Nephrol.* 2013;28(7):1059–1066.
5. Hardy ST, Sakhuja S, Jaeger BC, et al. Trends in blood pressure and hypertension among US children and adolescents, 1999–2018. *JAMA Netw Open.* 2021;4(4):e213917.
6. Blanchette E, Flynn JT. Implications of the 2017 AAP clinical practice guidelines for management of hypertension in children and adolescents: a review. *Curr Hypertens Rep.* 2019;21(5):35.
7. Flynn JT, Kaelber DC, Baker-Smith CM, et al. Clinical Practice Guideline for screening and management of high blood pressure in children and adolescents. *Pediatrics.* 2017;140(3):e20171904.
8. Whelton PK, Carey RM, Aronow WS, et al. 2017 ACC/AHA/AAPA/ABC/ACPM/AGS/APhA/ASH/ASPC/NMA/PCNA Guideline for the prevention, detection, evaluation, and management of high blood pressure in adults: Executive Summary: A Report of the American College of Cardiology/American Heart Association Task Force on Clinical Practice Guidelines. *J Am Coll Cardiol.* 2018;71(19):2199–2269.
9. Muntner P, Carey RM, Gidding S, et al. Potential US population impact of the 2017 ACC/AHA high blood pressure guideline. *Circulation.* 2018;137(2):109–118.
10. Yano Y, Reis JP, Colangelo LA, et al. Association of blood pressure classification in young adults using the 2017 American college of cardiology/American heart association blood pressure guideline with cardiovascular events later in life. *JAMA.* 2018;320(17):1774–1782.
11. Du T, Fernandez C, Barshop R, et al. 2017 Pediatric hypertension guidelines improve prediction of adult cardiovascular outcomes. *Hypertension.* 2019;73(6):1217–1223.
12. Graudal NA, Hubeck-Graudal T, Jurgens G. Effects of low sodium diet versus high sodium diet on blood pressure, renin, aldosterone, catecholamines, cholesterol, and triglyceride. *Cochrane Database Syst Rev.* 2011;(11):CD004022.
13. Juraschek SP, Miller ER, Weaver CM, et al. Effects of sodium reduction and the DASH diet in relation to baseline blood pressure. *J Am Coll Cardiol.* 2017;70(23):2841–2848.
14. Aaron KJ, Sanders PW. Role of dietary salt and potassium intake in cardiovascular health and disease: a review of the evidence. *Mayo Clin Proc.* 2013;88(9):987–995.
15. Falkner B, Sherif K, Michel S, et al. Dietary nutrients and blood pressure in urban minority adolescents at risk for hypertension. *Arch Pediatr Adolesc Med.* 2000;154(9):918–922.
16. Harshfield GA, Dong Y, Kapuku GK, et al. Stress-induced sodium retention and hypertension: a review and hypothesis. *Curr Hypertens Rep.* 2009;11(1):29–34.
17. Spruill TM, Butler MJ, Thomas SJ, et al. Association between high perceived stress over time and incident hypertension in black adults: findings from the Jackson heart study. *J Am Heart Assoc.* 2019;8(21):e012139.
18. Godoy LC, Frankfurter C, Cooper M, et al. Association of adverse childhood experiences with cardiovascular disease later in life: a review. *JAMA Cardiol.* 2021;6(2):228–235.
19. Din-Dzietham R, Liu Y, Bielo M-V, et al. High blood pressure trends in children and adolescents in national surveys, 1963 to 2002. *Circulation.* 2007;116(11):1488–1496.
20. Spence JD, Rayner BL. Hypertension in blacks: individualized therapy based on renin/aldosterone phenotyping. *Hypertension.* 2018;72(2):263–269.
21. Giussani M, Antolini L, Brambilla P, et al. Cardiovascular risk assessment in children: role of physical activity, family history and parental smoking on BMI and blood pressure. *J Hypertens.* 2013;31(5):983–992.
22. Colhoun H. Confirmation needed for genes for hypertension. *Lancet.* 1999;353(9160):1200–1201.
23. Lifton RP, Gharavi AG, Geller DS. Molecular mechanisms of human hypertension. *Cell.* 2001;104(4):545–556.
24. Lurbe E, Ingelfinger J. Developmental and early life origins of cardiometabolic risk factors. *Hypertension.* 2021;77(2):308–318.
25. Zureik M, Bonithon-Kopp C, Lecomte E, et al. Weights at birth and in early infancy, systolic pressure, and left ventricular structure in subjects aged 8 to 24 years. *Hypertension.* 1996;27(3 Pt 1):339–345.
26. Beratis NG, Panagoulias D, Varvarigou A. Increased blood pressure in neonates and infants whose mothers smoked during pregnancy. *J Pediatr.* 1996;128(6):806–812.
27. Singhal A, Cole TJ, Lucas A. Early nutrition in preterm infants and later blood pressure: two cohorts after randomised trials. *Lancet.* 2001;357(9254):413–419.
28. Edvardsson VO, Steinthorsdottir SD, Eliasdottir SB, et al. Birth weight and childhood blood pressure. *Curr Hypertens Rep.* 2012;14(6):596–602.
29. Carretero OA, Oparil S. Essential hypertension. Part I: definition and etiology. *Circulation.* 2000;101(3):329–335.
30. Flynn JT, Urbina EM. Pediatric ambulatory blood pressure monitoring: indications and interpretations. *J Clin Hypertens (Greenwich).* 2012;14(6):372–382.
31. Conen D, Aeschbacher S, Thijs L, et al. Age-specific differences between conventional and ambulatory daytime blood pressure values. *Hypertension.* 2014;64(5):1073–1079.

32. Hanevold CD, Miyashita Y, Faino AV, et al. Changes in ambulatory blood pressure phenotype over time in children and adolescents with elevated blood pressures. *J Pediatr.* 2020;216:37–43.e2.

33. Ferguson MA, Flynn JT. Rational use of antihypertensive medications in children. *Pediatr Nephrol.* 2014;29(6):979–988.

34. Sarafidis PA, Georgianos PI, Malindretos P, et al. Pharmacological management of hypertensive emergencies and urgencies: focus on newer agents. *Expert Opin Investig Drugs.* 2012;21(8):1089–1106.

📶 ADDITIONAL RESOURCES AND WEBSITES

Additional Resources and Websites for Clinicians:

American College of Cardiology selection of tables and figures from 2017 Clinical Practice Guideline for the Prevention, Detection, Evaluation, and Management of High Blood Pressure in Adults—https://www.acc.org/~/media/Non-Clinical/Files-PDFs-Excel-MS-Word-etc/Guidelines/2017/Guidelines_Made_Simple_2017_HBP.pdf

American Heart Association Hypertension Guideline Toolkit—http://aha-clinical-review.ascendeventmedia.com/books/aha-high-blood-pressure-toolkit/

Muntner P, Shimbo D, Carey RM, et al. Measurement of blood pressure in humans: a scientific statement from the American Heart Association. *Hypertension.* 2019;73:e35–e66—https://www.ahajournals.org/doi/full/10.1161/HYP.0000000000000087

PediaLink: Blood Pressure Measurement in Children (Video)—A video tutorial highlighting suggested steps for accurately collecting blood pressure measurement in children—https://www.youtube.com/watch?v=JLzkNBpqwi0

Screening and Management of High Blood Pressure in Children and Adolescents Guideline Overview – Highlights the key action statements and recommendations from the AAP's guideline on high blood pressure in children and adolescents—https://www.aap.org/en-us/_layouts/15/WopiFrame.aspx?sourcedoc=/en-us/Documents/Screening%20and%20Management%20of%20High%20Blood%20Pressure%20in%20Children%20and%20Adolescents.pptx&action=default

Additional Resources and Websites for Parents/Caregivers and Adolescents and Young Adults:

CDC website for high blood pressure—https://www.cdc.gov/bloodpressure/index.htm

International Pediatric Hypertension Association—http://www.iphapediatrichypertension.org/

National Heart, Lung and Blood Institute: High Blood Pressure—https://www.nhlbi.nih.gov/health-topics/high-blood-pressure

National Institutes of Health information page on the DASH Eating Plan—https://www.nhlbi.nih.gov/health-topics/dash-eating-plan

Screening & Treating Kids for High Blood Pressure: AAP Report Explained—https://www.healthychildren.org/English/health-issues/conditions/heart/Pages/High-Blood-Pressure-in-Children.aspx

Seattle Children's Hospital—Pediatric Hypertension Questions and Answers—https://www.seattlechildrens.org/clinics/pediatric-hypertension/qa/

CHAPTER 21

Pulmonary Problems

Lori L. Vanscoy
Peter J. Mogayzel Jr

KEY WORDS

- Asthma
- Cystic fibrosis
- E-cigarette or vaping product use associated lung injury
- Pectus excavatum
- Primary ciliary dyskinesia
- Vocal cord dysfunction

 INTRODUCTION

Respiratory complaints are quite common among adolescents and young adults (AYAs). While the majority of pulmonary symptoms in the AYA population are benign, some will be indicative of underlying pulmonary disease. The individual with a chronic pulmonary condition diagnosed earlier in childhood may experience exacerbations, lung function decline, or the appearance of disease complications during adolescence or early adulthood. For other individuals, the initial presenting symptoms of respiratory disease may first occur during this period. This chapter reviews the most common respiratory diseases affecting AYAs as well as less common pulmonary conditions that can lead to significant morbidity and mortality if unrecognized and untreated. Asthma, exercise-induced bronchospasm, and pectus excavatum are common respiratory disorders in the AYA population. Exercise-induced laryngeal obstruction (EILO) and habit cough are also encountered with significant regularity, with symptoms that can mimic those of asthma, leading to misdiagnosis. Disorders of mucociliary clearance, including cystic fibrosis (CF) and primary ciliary dyskinesia (PCD), are less common but can result in significant morbidity, especially in the second and third decades of life. Finally, electronic cigarette (e-cigarette) use, which is gaining popularity among AYAs presents significant risks to lung health. This chapter reviews the clinical characteristics, diagnosis, and treatment strategies for each of these entities to empower the AYA clinician to identify and treat these respiratory conditions when encountered.

ASTHMA

Asthma is a chronic airways disease characterized by recurrent variable airflow limitation leading to episodes of cough, chest tightness, and wheezing. It affects approximately 10% of AYAs in the United States, or approximately 5 million individuals.[1] Risk factors for asthma include a family history of asthma, presence of other atopic disease, personal or secondhand smoke exposure, and obesity.[2] Premature delivery, particularly <30 weeks gestation, is also associated with increased risk of asthma in adolescence and adulthood.[3] The symptoms of asthma include dry cough, chest tightness or pain, shortness of breath with exertion, and wheezing. Cough is often worse at night or in the early morning and may disrupt sleep. Asthma triggers vary among individuals and include viral illness, environmental allergen exposure, exercise, cold air or weather changes, personal or secondhand smoke exposure, air pollutants, strong smells, and stress.

The clinical history is critical to making the diagnosis and should include symptom history, response to short acting beta-agonists, presence of other atopic features, and family history. Physical examination is often normal in people with asthma, but characteristic findings can include chest hyperinflation and diffuse polyphonic wheezing. Wheezing may be absent in the individual suffering a severe asthma exacerbation due to extreme airflow limitation, although other signs of respiratory distress would be expected. Other findings of atopic disease, such as "allergic shiners," edema and pallor of the nasal mucosa, nasal polyps, and eczema are frequently present. There is no single definitive diagnostic test for asthma, though documentation of expiratory airflow limitation and assessment of bronchodilator response is strongly recommended to support an asthma diagnosis. Ideally this measurement should be performed prior to beginning controller therapy, which is anticipated to improve lung function and reduce the airflow variability characteristic of asthma. Spirometry provides the most robust assessment of airflow limitation and may be available in the primary care setting. Spirometry graphically represents lung function with the flow-volume loop, with expiratory and inspiratory flow (y-axis) plotted versus volume (x-axis). Characteristic spirometry findings of airflow obstruction include reduced forced expiratory volume in 1 second (FEV1) and reduced ratio of FEV1 to forced vital capacity (FEV1/FVC). These abnormalities are visualized by a concave or "scooped" appearance of the expiratory limb of the flow–volume loop. Following bronchodilator administration, improvement of ≥12% in the FEV1 indicates airway reactivity. If spirometry is not readily available, twice daily peak expiratory flow (PEF) measurements may be obtained over a 1- to 2-week period to determine airflow variability. Daily diurnal variability in PEF is calculated using the following equation: ([day's highest PEF − day's lowest PEF]/[mean of the day's highest and lowest PEF]). A weekly average of PEF diurnal variability exceeding 10% is consistent with asthma.[4]

Bronchial provocation testing, allergy testing, and fractional concentration of exhaled nitric oxide (FeNO) may help to support the diagnosis of asthma,[4] but all are nonspecific. Bronchial provocation testing typically uses inhaled methacholine or exercise to induce airflow limitation. Bronchial provocation testing can induce airflow limitation with disorders other than asthma, so this study may be the most useful for exclusion of asthma when the test is normal. Bronchial provocation testing is frequently requested prior to entry into military service for AYAs with a remote history of asthma. Cardiopulmonary exercise testing, using a treadmill or stationary bike, can be helpful in determining if exercised-induced dyspnea is due to asthma. Skin prick testing or measurement of serum allergen-specific immunoglobulin E (IgE) can identify allergic sensitization, supporting a diagnosis of allergic asthma. Elevated

FeNO is associated with eosinophilic airway inflammation, a feature of allergic asthma. However, increased FeNO is observed in disorders other than asthma, such as allergic rhinitis and eczema, and is not elevated in neutrophilic asthma. Additionally, FeNO values can be impacted by a variety of factors including viral illness, bronchoconstriction, smoking, and use of e-cigarettes, so the utility of FeNO for asthma diagnosis is not clearly defined.

Assessment of symptom control and risk for future exacerbations guides asthma management decisions.[4] Symptom control can be determined from the frequency of daytime and nighttime symptoms, frequency of short-acting beta agonist (SABA) use for symptom relief, and activity limitation. Asthma symptoms occurring more than twice per week during the day, SABA use for symptoms more than twice weekly, presence of any nighttime awakenings due

to asthma, and activity limitation due to asthma indicate suboptimal asthma control. In addition to poor asthma control, risk factors for future exacerbations include a history of exacerbations in the previous year, frequent SABA use, poor adherence (which includes incorrect use of inhaler devices), comorbidities such as obesity and food allergy, smoke exposure, adverse socioeconomic circumstances, psychosocial problems, and low lung function.[4]

All individuals with asthma should have rescue medication for episodic symptomatic relief, while those with poor asthma control require daily controller therapy. Stepwise management strategies are well detailed in national and international guidelines (Figs. 21.1 and 21.2),[4,5] which differ slightly in their preferred treatment recommendations. A notable recent addition to asthma treatment strategies is the use of single maintenance and

AGES 12+ YEARS: STEPWISE APPROACH FOR MANAGEMENT OF ASTHMA

Treatment	Intermittent Asthma — STEP 1	Management of Persistent Asthma in Individuals Ages 12+ Years				
		STEP 2	STEP 3	STEP 4	STEP 5	STEP 6[c]
Preferred	PRN SABA	Daily low-dose ICS and PRN SABA or PRN concomitant ICS and SABA▲	Daily and PRN combination low-dose ICS-formoterol▲	Daily and PRN combination medium-dose ICS-formoterol▲	Daily medium-high dose ICS-LABA + LAMA and PRN SABA▲	Daily high-dose ICS-LABA + oral systemic corticosteroids + PRN SABA
Alternative		Daily LTRA[a] and PRN SABA or Cromolyn,[a] or nedocromil,[a] or zileuton,[a] or theophylline,[a] and PRN SABA	Daily medium-dose ICS and PRN SABA or Daily low-dose ICS-LABA, or daily low-dose ICS + LAMA,▲ or daily low-dose ICS + LTRA,[a] and PRN SABA or Daily low-dose ICS + theophylline[a] or zileuton,[a] and PRN SABA	Daily medium-dose ICS-LABA or daily medium-dose ICS + LAMA, and PRN SABA▲ or Daily medium-dose ICS + LTRA,[a] or daily medium-dose ICS + theophylline,[a] or daily medium-dose ICS + zileuton,[a] and PRN SABA	Daily medium-high dose ICS-LABA or daily high-dose ICS + LTRA,[a] and PRN SABA	
		Steps 2-4: Conditionally recommend the use of subcutaneous immunotherapy as an adjunct treatment to standard pharmacotherapy in individuals ≥ 5 years of age whose asthma is controlled at the initiation, build up, and maintenance phases of immunotherapy▲			Consider adding Asthma Biologics (e.g., anti-IgE, anti-IL5, anti-IL5R, anti-IL4/IL13)[b]	

Assess Control

- First check adherence, inhaler technique, environmental factors,▲ and comorbid conditions.
- **Step up** if needed; reassess in 2-6 weeks
- **Step down** if possible (if asthma is well controlled for at least 3 consecutive months)

Consult with asthma specialist if Step 4 or higher is required. Consider consultation at Step 3.

Control assessment is a key element of asthma care. This involves both impairment and risk. Use of objective measures, self-reported control, and health care utilization are complementary and should be employed on an ongoing basis, depending on the individual's clinical situation.

Abbreviations: ICS, inhaled corticosteroid; LABA, long-acting beta₂-agonist; LAMA, long-acting muscarinic antagonist; LTRA, leukotriene receptor antagonist; SABA, inhaled short-acting beta₂-agonist

[a]Cromolyn, nedocromil, LTRAs including zileuton and montelukast, and theophylline were not considered for this update, and/or have limited availability for use in the United States, and/or have an increased risk of adverse consequences and need for monitoring that make their use less desirable. The FDA issued a Boxed Warning for montelukast in March 2020.

[b]The AHRQ systematic reviews that informed this report did not include studies that examined the role of asthma biologics (e.g., anti-IgE, anti-IL5, anti-IL5R, anti-IL4/IL13). Thus, this report does not contain specific recommendations for the use of biologics in asthma in Steps 5 and 6.

[c]Data on the use of LAMA therapy in individuals with severe persistent asthma (Step 6) were not included in the AHRQ systematic review and thus no recommendation is made.

FIGURE 21.1 Treatment management approach from 2020 Focused Updates to the Asthma Management Guidelines of the National Heart Lung Blood Institute. (NIH Publication No. 20-HL-8142. December 2020.)

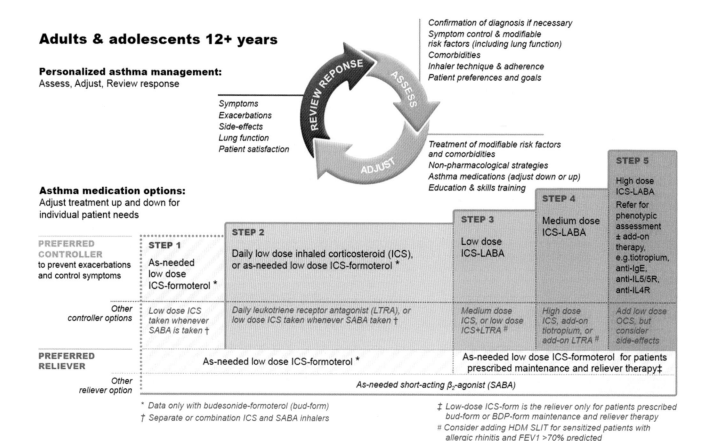

FIGURE 21.2 Personalized management for adults and adolescents to control symptoms and minimize future risk. (©2020 *Global Initiative for Asthma*, reprinted with permission. Available from www.ginasthma.org)

reliever therapy (SMART), in which a single-combination inhaler containing an inhaled corticosteroid (ICS) (budesonide) and the long-acting beta agonist (LABA) formoterol is used both as daily maintenance therapy and as rescue medication. The SMART treatment strategy is associated with a decrease in asthma exacerbations requiring systemic corticosteroids, emergency department visits, and hospitalizations.[6] The Global Initiative for Asthma (GINA) no longer recommends use of SABA alone for AYAs with mild asthma, instead recommending intermittent use of ICS-formoterol as the quick relief medication of choice.[4] In contrast, the National Heart Lung and Blood Institute Asthma Management Program prefers SABAs as the rescue medication in mild asthma.[5] Both programs prefer the SMART treatment strategy beginning with Step 3 management.[4,5] For those whose asthma cannot be controlled with ICS/LABAs and management of comorbidities and environmental triggers, novel biologic therapies can be of significant benefit and are being utilized with increasing frequency in the AYA population.

Interval assessment is critical to asthma management, with treatment intensified until symptom control is achieved and then decreased as tolerated to minimize side effects while maintaining adequate symptom control. Before stepping up therapy for AYAs with suboptimal asthma control, a careful assessment of medication adherence, environmental triggers, and comorbidities should be conducted. Poor asthma medication adherence is extremely common. However, selecting medications that are taken once rather than twice daily and that do not require spacer use (such as dry powder inhalers) may help to mitigate this barrier to achieving good asthma control in the AYA population. Initial treatment choice within each medication class is frequently dependent upon the individual's insurance coverage. There are a myriad of available ICS and ICS/LABA combination medications. Most of these maintenance medications

are dosed twice daily, but a few are available for once daily use. Once daily options include the ICS fluticasone furoate (approved for patients ≥5 years of age) and the ICS/LABA, fluticasone furoate-vilanterol trifenatate (approved for patients ≥18 years).

Asthma exacerbations represent acute or subacute worsening of symptoms and lung function and can be triggered by viral illness, allergen exposures, environmental factors, season or weather changes, and poor adherence to controller therapy. Anyone experiencing an exacerbation should receive treatment with an inhaled reliever medication. This may be a SABA or, for those using the SMART protocol, an increase in frequency of ICS-formoterol use up to a maximum total daily dose of 72 mcg of formoterol (equivalent to 16 puffs of budesonide/formoterol combination inhaler), though such high usage was rarely necessary in clinical trials.[4] Increased controller therapy during exacerbations should be considered for those using only a SABA as their reliever. A short course of an oral corticosteroid should be added (typically 40 to 60 mg/d for 5 to 7 days) for patients who fail to improve with reliever therapy after 2 to 3 days, who deteriorate rapidly or whose PEF is <60% of their personal best, or who have a history of sudden severe exacerbations. A steroid taper is unnecessary for a course of systemic steroids that is <2 weeks duration. Patients should be empowered to manage asthma in the outpatient setting by providing sufficient education regarding proper technique and indications for inhaled medication use, avoidance strategies for common triggers, and interventions to be employed during exacerbations. Some patients benefit from regular monitoring of PEF in the home setting, though for the majority, symptom monitoring is equally effective. Each patient should have a written asthma action plan that clearly details his or her individualized comprehensive asthma treatment recommendations (see the GINA Patient Guide in ancillary online resources for AYAs).

RESPIRATORY DISORDERS TRIGGERED BY EXERCISE

Shortness of breath is a common respiratory concern of the adolescent, and can occur in individuals with no prior respiratory problems. Exercise-induced bronchoconstriction (EIB) and EILO should be considered in the differential diagnosis for these AYAs.

Exercise-Induced Bronchoconstriction

Exercise-induced bronchospasm is limitation of airflow triggered by exercise, resulting in symptoms of chest tightness, shortness of breath, and wheezing. The pathophysiology of EIB is related to dehydration of the airways during periods of increased ventilation, creating a hyperosmotic environment that triggers mast-cell degranulation with release of leukotrienes, histamine, tryptase, and prostaglandins that induce bronchoconstriction and airway inflammation.[7] Treatment of EIB consists of premedication with SABAs 15 minutes before strenuous exercise and SABA use for symptomatic relief following exercise. Alternatively, combination ICS-formoterol medications can also be used 15 minutes prior to exercise. Frequent use of SABAs can be associated with development of tolerance, making the medication less effective over time.[7] Individuals with recurrent EIB symptoms and frequent SABA use should be evaluated for poorly controlled persistent asthma and treated with daily controller therapy if appropriate. Leukotriene receptor antagonists (LTRAs) used daily or intermittently may help to prevent EIB. However, LTRAs carry a black box warning due to concerns about increased risk of neuropsychiatric events, including suicidal thoughts and actions,[8] so should be used with caution only in individuals not responding to other treatment options. Finally, AYAs with EIB should be encouraged to allow sufficient warm-up time prior to exercise, which can be very helpful in preventing EIB symptoms.

Exercise-Induced Laryngeal Obstruction

Exercise-induced laryngeal obstruction is the partial or complete closure of the laryngeal inlet during exercise, resulting in exertional dyspnea. Vocal cord dysfunction (VCD) has also been used to describe this condition, but EILO is more appropriate because the airflow obstruction can occur at the level of the glottis or vocal folds, at the supraglottis, or at both locations. Exercise-induced laryngeal obstruction is almost as common as asthma, with an estimated prevalence of 5% to 7% in AYAs,[9] and appears to have a strong female predominance ranging from 61% to 100% in several case series.[9] Symptoms of EILO include shortness of breath and noisy breathing with exertion that resolve quickly with rest. The noisy breathing is frequently described by the patient and observer as wheezing, but is actually inspiratory stridor, which is often audible to the individual. Syncope is not a typical feature of EILO, and if present, should prompt an evaluation to rule out cardiac pathology. Interestingly, literature suggests that there is a behavioral phenotype associated with EILO that is characterized by perfectionism or underlying anxiety.[10] Exercise-induced laryngeal obstruction often occurs in competitive athletes, especially as the level of intensity of the sport increases. Asthma and EILO can coexist, and it is important to consider EILO for the individual whose exercise-related symptoms are not responding to asthma therapy.

The preferred diagnostic test for EILO is continuous laryngoscopy during exercise (CLE) to directly visualize and characterize upper airway obstruction with exertion.[10] In centers not equipped to perform CLE, an alternative approach is to perform flexible fiberoptic laryngoscopy following exercise that has provoked symptoms. This latter approach may fail to identify upper airway obstruction, because many individuals experience quick resolution of symptoms upon stopping exercise. Treatment of EILO consists of education about the disorder, reassurance that EILO is not life-threatening, and referral to speech–language pathology for rescue breathing techniques.[11] Treatment of comorbid conditions, including asthma, gastroesophageal reflux, sinus disease, and anxiety may also be indicated.

HABIT COUGH (TIC COUGH OR SOMATIC COUGH SYNDROME)

Cough is another common respiratory complaint of AYAs. A characteristic feature of most chronic pulmonary conditions, cough is part of the body's natural defense system serving to mobilize mucus from the lower airways to expel foreign particles such as dust, pollen, or infectious organisms from the lungs. Cough is an appropriate response to viral illness, environmental allergies, air pollution, and aspiration. However, a cough persisting for more than a month is deemed chronic, and often leads the affected individual to seek medical care.

Evaluation of the individual with chronic cough should include a thorough history to define the circumstances of cough onset; quality and timing of cough; presence of any associated symptoms such as fever, rhinitis, wheezing, chest pain, weight loss, and hemoptysis; treatments that have been attempted to date including antibiotics, antihistamines, short-acting bronchodilators, and inhaled or systemic steroids; and results of any diagnostic testing such as viral antigen panels or chest imaging. Prior history of asthma or wheezing should be elicited. A thorough physical examination should be conducted, with findings of fever, hypoxemia, weight loss, focal abnormalities on lung auscultation, or digital clubbing alerting the clinician to potential underlying infection or chronic pulmonary disease. Pulse oximetry should be performed as part of the evaluation and chest imaging should be obtained for any individual with hypoxemia or focal abnormalities on pulmonary exam. When the physical examination is normal and review of systems is unremarkable, the diagnosis of habit cough should be considered.

Habit cough often has a clear trigger, such as a viral illness, asthma exacerbation, or flare of environmental allergies. However, the cough persists even after resolution of the inciting event. Features of habit cough are quite characteristic. The hallmark of habit cough is the disappearance of the cough with distraction and during sleep, though the young person often will report difficulty falling asleep because of cough. The individual with habit cough is usually able to anticipate the onset of cough and feels relief after coughing. Cough quality is classically loud, brassy, or barking, but can also have a repetitive throat clearing nature. The cough can be severe, leading to post-tussive emesis, and is very troublesome to the family and to the school environment. In fact, the individual with habit cough may have been excluded from school because of the disruptive nature of the cough and concerns about infectious risks to his or her classmates.

Habit cough is a clinical diagnosis. Recognizing habit cough can spare the affected individual unnecessary diagnostic testing and inappropriate treatment with asthma medications and antibiotics. In communicating the diagnosis to the patient and parent/caregiver, it is important to stress that this cough is not volitional despite its habitual nature. Treatment of habit cough requires empowering the affected individual to break the cough cycle. Suggestion therapy is a treatment strategy that can employ distraction and reinforcement to delay cough onset for longer and longer intervals until the cough eventually extinguishes. Suggestion therapy has been well described by Hurvitz and Weinberger,[12] and can lead to resolution of even long-standing habit cough in a single brief treatment session, as illustrated at www.habitcough.com.

PECTUS EXACAVATUM

Pectus excavatum is the most common chest wall abnormality, with incidence estimated between 1 and 8 per 1,000.[13] Male AYAs are affected more frequently than female AYAs. Pectus excavatum is a depression of the anterior chest wall with dorsal deviation of the sternum and costal cartilage. Though typically an isolated defect, pectus excavatum can be associated with

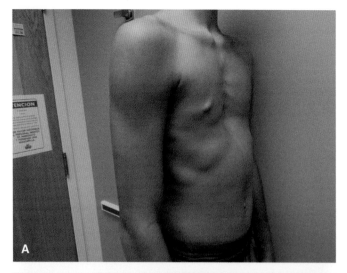

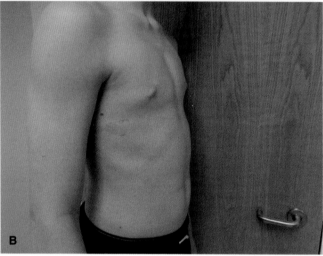

FIGURE 21.3 Pectus excavatum before (**A**) and after (**B**) Nuss procedure. (Photos courtesy of the Pediatric Nuss Center at the Children's Hospital of the King's Daughter's in Norfolk, VA.)

underlying syndromes—particularly Marfan, Noonan, and Turner syndromes.[13] Pectus excavatum is usually first recognized in childhood and becomes more apparent during the rapid skeletal growth of puberty. Symptoms associated with pectus excavatum include chest pain, shortness of breath, exercise intolerance, and fatigue. Cosmetic appearance can also be of significant concern to individuals with a prominent chest wall deformity.

The majority of those with pectus excavatum do not have parenchymal lung or airways disease, and their poor exercise tolerance is often multifactorial. Abnormal chest wall mechanics in individuals with pectus excavatum may limit their ability to generate increased tidal volumes during exercise. Pectus excavatum deformity may also lead to right ventricular (RV) compression impeding RV filling during exercise.

Pectus excavatum is identified by visual inspection of the chest (Fig. 21.3). Serial caliper measurement of the distance from the deepest sternal depression to the top of the rib cage can track progression of the deformity over time. The severity of pectus excavatum is defined by the Haller index, which is the ratio of the transverse chest diameter to the narrowest anterioposterior diameter, calculated from chest computed tomography (CT).[14] A Haller index of 2.5 is normal, with higher values indicating more significant deformity. Additional diagnostic evaluation should include echocardiogram to identify heart anomalies such as mitral valve

prolapse and right atrial or RV compression. Pulmonary function testing may identify a restrictive defect and cardiopulmonary exercise testing can assess for exercise limitation and dyspnea, which may help to inform treatment decisions.

Treatment of pectus excavatum is usually surgical. The primary indications for pectus excavatum repair are related to the degree of perceived impairment related to the deformity. Patients with pectus excavatum who are experiencing exercise limitation or chest pain, or who are experiencing body image concerns or anxiety related to their chest wall deformity should be referred for surgical evaluation, with the diagnostic work-up above being directed by or in consultation with the surgical team. Clinically, patients often experience significant improvement in exercise-related symptoms following pectus excavatum repair, even if baseline pulmonary function testing and echocardiograms are normal. In a large series of 1,270 patients followed at the Children's Hospital of the King's Daughters in Norfolk, VA from 1985 to 2018, 95% reported improvement in exercise tolerance following pectus excavatum repair.[15] Repair also typically results in significant cosmetic improvement, which can have important psychological benefits. The most common surgical repair is the minimally invasive Nuss procedure, in which a steel or titanium bar is placed beneath the sternum and remains in place for 2 years or more until desired sternal shape is achieved.[14] Optimal timing for the Nuss procedure is toward the end of the pubertal growth spurt, usually between 10 and 15 years of age with preference toward older ages. An alternative surgical option is the open Ravitch procedure, which may be considered for individuals with more complex deformities or for those with recurrent deformities. Timing of repair is important in achieving desired outcomes, so adolescents with pectus excavatum who experience exercise limitation or pain should be referred promptly for surgical evaluation.

For individuals with mild deformities or for those who desire nonoperative management, the vacuum bell can be used. This device applies suction to the anterior chest wall to elevate the sternum, modifying chest wall shape over time. The device is used for up to several hours each day for a period of months to years. The vacuum bell can achieve modest improvements in pectus excavatum deformities, with the most noted benefits for younger children, for milder baseline deformities, and for those with higher daily device use and duration of use.[16,17] Because of the quite significant commitment required to achieve good results with the vacuum bell, this treatment option is best reserved for the highly motivated individual.

DISORDERS OF MUCOCILIARY CLEARANCE

Cystic fibrosis and PCD are genetic disorders that result in impaired mucociliary clearance, leading to chronic productive cough, recurrent bronchitis, and development of bronchiectasis. In CF, the underlying pulmonary pathophysiology results from defective chloride transport at the epithelial cell surface, resulting in dehydration of the airway-surface liquid and mucus. In contrast, individuals with PCD have abnormal ciliary structure, motion, or reduced numbers of cilia lining the airway. Both CF and PCD predispose to chronic bacterial infection of the airways. The most prevalent microorganism in the CF airway until midadolescence is *Staphylococcus aureus*, with *Pseudomonas aeruginosa* becoming the predominant airway pathogen in adults with CF.[18] The PCD airway is typically infected with respiratory organisms such as *Streptococcus pneumoniae* or *Haemophilus influenzae*. However, infections with the same organisms identified in CF airways can be present. Pulmonary manifestations of CF and PCD are similar, but other clinical features may help to distinguish between the two entities (**Table 21.1**).

Cystic Fibrosis

Cystic fibrosis is a multisystem, autosomal recessive genetic disorder characterized by progressive obstructive lung disease, exocrine pancreatic insufficiency, abnormal sweat-chloride concentration,

TABLE 21.1

Clinical Manifestations of Cystic Fibrosis and Primary Ciliary Dyskinesia by Organ System

Organ System	Cystic Fibrosis	Primary Ciliary Dyskinesia
Ear, Nose, and Throat	Pansinusitis, Nasal polyps	Chronic or recurrent otitis media with effusion, conductive hearing loss, chronic rhinorrhea, sinusitis, nasal polyps
Cardiac	No clinical manifestations	>50% have situs inversus or situs ambiguus, 12% heterotaxy
Gastrointestinal	Exocrine pancreatic insufficiency (90%), loose or malodorous stools, constipation, delayed gastric emptying, rectal prolapse, liver disease, distal intestinal obstruction syndrome (DIOS), meconium plugging or ileus in newborn	Situs inversus in approximately half of individuals
Skin	Elevated sweat chloride concentration	No skin manifestations
Endocrine	CF-related diabetes (often presenting in adolescence)	No related endocrine manifestations
Reproductive	Male infertility due to congenital bilateral absence of the vas deferens	Reduced fertility in both males and females

CF, cystic fibrosis.

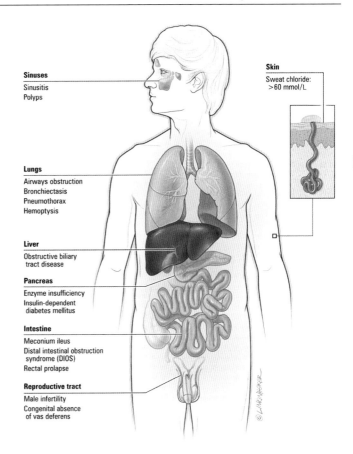

Sinuses
Sinusitis
Polyps

Lungs
Airways obstruction
Bronchiectasis
Pneumothorax
Hemoptysis

Liver
Obstructive biliary tract disease

Pancreas
Enzyme insufficiency
Insulin-dependent diabetes mellitus

Intestine
Meconium ileus
Distal intestinal obstruction syndrome (DIOS)
Rectal prolapse

Reproductive tract
Male infertility
Congenital absence of vas deferens

Skin
Sweat chloride: >60 mmol/L

FIGURE 21.4 Manifestations of cystic fibrosis by organ system. (Reprinted with permission of the author, Michael Linkinhoker, Link Studio.)

and male infertility (Fig. 21.4). Cystic fibrosis occurs most frequently in individuals of European descent, but affects all ethnicities. Approximately 56% of the 35,000 individuals with CF in the United States are 18 years of age or older, with median predicted survival of 23.3 years in 2020.[18] Once a disease of childhood, survival has steadily increased as therapeutics improve; the average life expectancy of an individual with CF in the United States in 2020 was 50.0 years and is anticipated to continue to climb.[18] Cystic fibrosis is caused by mutations in the CF transmembrane conductance regulator (CFTR) gene, which encodes the CFTR protein, an ion channel that regulates chloride and bicarbonate transport. To date, more than 2,000 variants in the *CFTR* gene have been identified, of which at least 360 are CF-causing and 48 are of varying clinical significance.[19] Information about specific mutations can be found at www.CFTR2.org.

Pulmonary complications account for the majority of morbidity and mortality in individuals with CF. Respiratory symptoms include: chronic cough, sputum production, and hemoptysis. Wheezing can occur, but is not a hallmark of the disease. Cough and dyspnea develop as obstructive lung disease progresses. Gastrointestinal symptoms of CF are related to malabsorption, primarily of fat, and include abdominal pain, loose or malodorous stools, and constipation. Other complications that become more common in adolescence and young adulthood include CF-related diabetes, liver disease, and distal intestinal obstruction syndrome (DIOS). Classic physical examination findings in CF include nasal polyposis, chest hyperinflation (barrel chest), crackles on pulmonary auscultation, and clubbing of the distal phalanges of the fingers and toes. However, many adolescents diagnosed in infancy, and receiving appropriate CF therapy, will have an entirely normal physical examination.

The majority of AYAs with CF are diagnosed in infancy by newborn screening, which has been routinely conducted in all states in the United States since 2010. However, any individual with a suggestive clinical history should undergo sweat chloride testing. Sweat chloride ≥60 mmol/L is diagnostic of CF, while individuals with a sweat chloride <30 mmol/L are unlikely to have the disease. Indeterminate values between 30 and 59 mmol/L require additional diagnostic testing. Cystic fibrosis transmembrane conductance regulator genetic analysis is also a critical component of the CF evaluation and should be conducted for all individuals with sweat chloride ≥30 mmol/L and for those with sweat chloride <30 mmol/L who have a suspicious clinical history.[20]

Traditionally, CF treatments have been focused on ameliorating the symptoms of the disease. Symptom-targeted pulmonary therapies include: airway clearance to mobilize thick, tenacious sputum; inhaled mucus-modulating agents (hypertonic saline, dornase alfa, and mannitol) to thin abnormal airway secretions; inhaled antibiotics specifically for eradication of newly acquired or suppression of chronic *P. aeruginosa* infection; and oral or intravenous antibiotics to treat periodic exacerbations of lung disease. Nutritional support consists of pancreatic enzyme replacement therapy (PERT) for those who have exocrine pancreatic insufficiency along with fat-soluble vitamin and salt supplementation. Individuals with CF-related diabetes mellitus are treated with insulin. CF transmembrane conductance regulator (CFTR) modulators are mutation-specific medications that target the defective CFTR protein to restore chloride channel function at the cell-surface. Approximately 90% of AYAs with CF are eligible for CFTR modulator therapy; treatment with CFTR modulators for individuals with qualifying variants has resulted in remarkable improvements in lung function, reduced frequency of pulmonary exacerbations, reductions in sweat chloride concentrations, and improved weight gain.[21-23] It is anticipated that the AYA population with CF will become healthier over time as CFTR modulator therapies become available for the youngest children.

Primary Ciliary Dyskinesia

Primary ciliary dyskinesia is a genetic disorder leading to immobile or hypomobile cilia affecting approximately 1 in 10,000-15,000 individuals.[24] Mutations of more than 40 different genes encoding for the proteins comprising the cilia ultrastructure, most of which are inherited in an autosomal recessive fashion, have been reported to cause PCD.[24] The hallmark of the PCD clinical phenotype is daily wet cough and chronic rhinitis, which typically begin in early infancy. Organ laterality defects occur in over 50% of people with PCD.[25] Approximately, 80% of individuals with PCD have a history of neonatal respiratory distress despite full-term delivery.[24]

Diagnosis of PCD relies on multiple modalities, some of which are available only at specialized care centers. Exhaled nasal nitric oxide concentration in individuals with PCD is low, typically 10 times less than in healthy individuals. However, low nasal nitric oxide concentrations can also occur with tobacco smoking, nasal obstruction, and CF. E-cigarette use may also impact exhaled nasal nitric oxide measurements, though the effects are not well characterized. Electron microscopy evaluation of cilia biopsies from the carina or inferior nasal turbinate may demonstrate abnormalities of the cilia ultrastructure, though cases of PCD with normal cilia ultrastructure have been reported. High-speed video microscopy analysis (HSVMA) of live samples, obtained by nasal brushing, can assess ciliary beat frequency and pattern. Finally, genetic testing for variants associated with PCD can now identify 65% to 70% of people with the disease.[24]

There is no cure for PCD and large clinical trials of therapies have not been conducted because of the rarity of the disease; therefore, treatment recommendations are largely extrapolated from CF care. Airway clearance is the mainstay of therapy and aerobic exercise, which may assist in mucous clearance, is encouraged. As in CF, liberal use of oral or intravenous antibiotics directed toward the individual's known airway pathogens for episodic increases in respiratory symptoms is recommended.

⬤ E-CIGARETTE OR VAPING PRODUCT USE-ASSOCIATED LUNG INJURY

Electronic cigarettes are popular among adolescents, with 19.6% of high school students and 4.7% of middle school students (totaling approximately 3.6 million youth) reporting current e-cigarette use in the 2020 National Youth Tobacco Survey. Among high school current e-cigarette users, 38.9% report frequent and 22.5% report daily e-cigarette use.[26] Among young adults aged 18 to 24 years in 2019, 9.3% reported using e-cigarettes and more than half of these individuals (56.0%) reported never having smoked combustible cigarettes.[27] While e-cigarette devices are frequently marketed as a safer alternative to traditional combustible tobacco and even incorporated into tobacco cessation programs, there is accumulating evidence for harm. The most alarming clinical entity is e-cigarette or vaping product use associated lung injury (EVALI), which was initially described in 2019, following several reported clusters of acute pulmonary illness in young adults who used e-cigarettes. As of February 18, 2020, 2807 hospitalizations and 68 deaths due to EVALI had been reported to the Centers for Disease Control, with cases from all 50 states, the District of Columbia, Puerto Rico, and the U.S. Virgin Islands.[28] Electronic-cigarette or vaping product use-associated lung injury is defined as acute lung injury occurring within 90 days of e-cigarette use, with radiographic abnormalities, and exclusion of alternative diagnoses. Investigation of the outbreaks has linked most, but not all, EVALI cases to vaping of

tetrahydrocannabinol (THC)-containing products. In one study of 51 patients with EVALI from 16 states, vitamin E acetate, commonly used as a diluent for THC-vaping products, was recovered from bronchoalveolar lavage (BAL) fluid in 48 patients with EVALI, but from none of the matched controls, implicating vitamin E acetate as one potential factor in EVALI pathophysiology.[29]

Symptoms of EVALI include shortness of breath, chest pain, cough, and rarely hemoptysis. The majority of patients with EVALI report gastrointestinal symptoms, including nausea, vomiting, abdominal pain, and occasionally diarrhea. Constitutional symptoms of fever, fatigue, malaise, and weight loss may also occur.[30] On physical examination, patients with EVALI can be ill-appearing with tachypnea, tachycardia, and hypoxemia but typically have clear breath sounds on pulmonary auscultation. Characteristic laboratory findings include markedly elevated erythrocyte sedimentation rate, elevated C-reactive protein, and mild leukocytosis with neutrophil predominance. Mild hyponatremia and mild transaminitis have also been reported.[31] Chest radiography or CT demonstrate a variety of imaging patterns, but most EVALI cases have consolidations and ground glass opacities (Fig. 21.5), often with lower lobe predominance and subpleural sparing.[32] Bronchoalveolar lavage findings are nonspecific and include predominance of macrophages and neutrophils; most have lipid-laden macrophages. Though EVALI is considered a diagnosis of exclusion, suspicion for it should be high in a previously healthy adolescent or young adult with characteristic clinical presentation and a history of recent e-cigarette use, particularly for those who vape THC products. Additional diagnostic testing should be directed toward identifying alternative diagnoses, such as

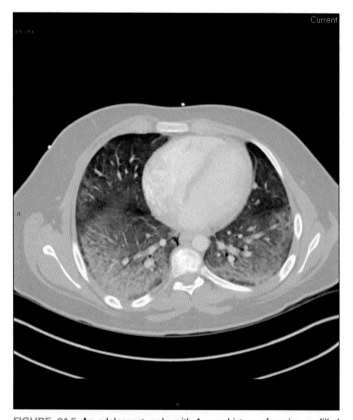

FIGURE 21.5 An adolescent male with 1-year history of vaping prefilled counterfeit THC-cartridges. He presented with pleuritic chest pain, progressive dyspnea, and hypoxia to the mid-80s. Chest CT scan demonstrated basilar-predominant ground-glass opacities with septal thickening and pneumomediastinum. (Reprinted with permission of the American Thoracic Society. Copyright © 2022 American Thoracic Society. All rights reserved. Cite: MA Lu, NA Jabre, and PJ Mogayzel, Jr./2020/Vaping-related Lung Injury in an Adolescent/AJRCCM/Volume 201, Number 4/481-482. The American Journal of Respiratory and Critical Care Medicine is an official journal of the American Thoracic Society.)

infection in immunocompromised individuals or pulmonary hemorrhage in the patient suspected of having systemic autoimmune disease based on other clinical features.

Treatment of EVALI is largely supportive, with respiratory needs ranging from supplemental oxygen to intubation and mechanical ventilation. Patients with EVALI are often empirically treated with antibiotics for community-acquired pneumonia, but this is necessary only for those with likely or confirmed concomitant infection. Systemic corticosteroids appear to be beneficial, leading to rapid improvement in symptoms in one series of adolescent patients with EVALI.[33] Finally, sustained cessation of e-cigarette use is critical to successful treatment of EVALI; referral to nicotine or substance cessation programs, as appropriate, is strongly recommended (see Chapters 70 and 71 for additional information). The long-term sequelae of EVALI and of chronic e-cigarette use are unknown at this time and remain active areas of investigation.

SUMMARY

Respiratory complaints are common among the AYA population. Careful review of symptoms and past medical history is critical to distinguish benign, self-limited conditions from more serious underlying pulmonary disease, to guide further diagnostic evaluation, and to inform treatment decisions. Asthma is the most common disorder encountered in primary care and has quite typical clinical features and well-prescribed diagnostic and therapeutic recommendations. Disorders that mimic asthma can be discerned from characteristic clinical features, such as inspiratory stridor with exertion (EILO) and absence of nighttime cough (habit cough). A chronically productive cough should alert the clinician to potential disorders of mucociliary clearance. All AYA clinicians should be alert to potential e-cigarette use as a trigger or cause of pulmonary symptoms in this population. Familiarity with the conditions discussed in this chapter will enable clinicians to successfully identify and treat the most common pulmonary disorders encountered in clinical practice and to optimize the respiratory health of the AYA population.

REFERENCES

1. Centers for Disease Control and Prevention. Accessed March 24, 2021. www.cdc.gov/asthma/most_recent_national_asthma_data.htm
2. American Lung Association Asthma Risk Factors. Accessed July 7, 2021. https://www.lung.org/lung-health-diseases/lung-disease-lookup/asthma/asthma-symptoms-causes-risk-factors/asthma-risk-factors
3. Been JV, Lugtenberg MJ, Smets E, et al. Preterm birth and childhood wheezing disorders: a systematic review and meta-analysis. *PLoS Med.* 2014;11(1):e1001596.
4. Global Initiative for Asthma. *Global Strategy for Asthma Management and Prevention, 2020.* Accessed March 25, 2021. www.ginasthma.org
5. Expert Panel Working Group of the National Heart, Lung, and Blood Institute (NHLBI) administered and coordinated National Asthma Education and Prevention Program Coordinating Committee (NAEPPCC). Cloutier MM, Baptist AP, Blake KV, et al. Focused updates to the asthma management guidelines: A report from the National Asthma Education and Prevention Program Coordinating Committee Expert Panel Working Group. *J Allergy Clin Immunol.* 2020;146(6):1217–1270. doi:10.1016/j.jaci.2020.10.003. Erratum in: *J Allergy Clin Immunol.* 2021;147(4):1528–1530. PMID: 33280709; PMCID: PMC7924476.
6. Sobieraj DM, Weeda ER, Nguyen E, et al. Association of inhaled corticosteroids and long-acting beta-agonists as controller and quick relief therapy with exacerbations and symptom control in persistent asthma: a systematic review and meta-analysis. *JAMA.* 2018;319(14):1485–1496.
7. Weiler JM, Brannan JD, Randolph CC, et al. Exercise-induced bronchoconstriction update-2016. *J Allergy Clin Immunol.* 2016;138(5):1292–1295.
8. U.S. Food & Drug Administration. *FDA requires Boxed Warning about serious mental health side effects for asthma and allergy drug montelukast (Singulair); advises restricting use for allergic rhinitis.* Accessed March 25, 2021. www.fda.gov/drugs/drug-safety-and-availability/fda-requires-boxed-warning-about-serious-mental-health-side-effects-asthma-and-allergy-drug
9. Nordang L, Norlander K, Walsted ES. Exercise-induced laryngeal obstruction—An overview. *Immunol Allergy Clin North Am.* 2018;38(2):271–280.
10. Olin JT. Exercise-induced laryngeal obstruction: When pediatric exertional dyspnea does not respond to bronchodilators. *Front Pediatr.* 2019;7:52.
11. Shaffer M, Litts JK, Nauman E, et al. Speech-language pathology as a primary treatment for exercise-induced laryngeal obstruction. *Immunol Allergy Clin North Am.* 2018;38(2):293–302.
12. Hurvitz M, Weinberger M. Functional respiratory disorders in children. *Pediatr Clin North Am.* 2021;68(1):223–237.
13. Cobben JM, Oostra RJ, Van Dijk FS. Pectus excavatum and carinatum. *Eur J Med Genet.* 2014;57(8):414–417.
14. Abdullah F, Harris J. Pectus excavatum: more than a matter of aesthetics. *Pediatr Ann.* 2016;45(11):e403–e406.
15. Obermeyer RJ, Cohen NS, Jaroszewski DE. The physiologic impact of pectus excavatum repair. *Semin Pediatr Surg.* 2018;27(3):127–132.
16. Obermeyer RJ, Cohen NS, Kelly RE Jr, et al. Nonoperative management of pectus excavatum with vacuum bell therapy: a single center study. *J Pediatr Surg.* 2018;53(6):1221–1225.
17. St-Louis E, Miao J, Emil S, et al. Vacuum bell treatment of pectus excavatum: an early North American experience. *J Pediatr Surg.* 2019;54(1):194–199.
18. Cystic Fibrosis Foundation Patient Registry 2020 Annual Data Report, Bethesda, Maryland.
19. Clinical and Functional Translation of CFTR. Accessed March 17, 2021. http://www.cftr2.org
20. Farrell PM, White TB, Ren CL, et al. Diagnosis of cystic fibrosis: consensus guidelines from the cystic fibrosis foundation. *J Pediatr.* 2017;181S:S4–S15.
21. Ramsey BW, Davies J, McElvaney NG, et al. A CFTR potentiator in patients with cystic fibrosis and the G551D mutation. *N Engl J Med.* 2011;365(18):1663–1672.
22. Middleton PG, Mall MA, Drevinek P, et al. Elexacaftor-tezacaftor-ivacaftor for cystic fibrosis with a single Phe508del Allele. *N Engl J Med.* 2019;381(19):1809–1819.
23. Heijerman HGM, McKone EF, Downey DG, et al. Efficacy and safety of the elexacaftor plus tezacaftor plus ivacaftor combination regimen in people with cystic fibrosis homozygous for the F508del mutation: a double-blind, randomized, phase 3 trial. *Lancet.* 2019;394(10212):1940–1948.
24. Lucas JS, Davis SD, Omran H, et al. Primary ciliary dyskinesia in the genomics age. *Lancet Respir Med.* 2020;8(2):202–216.
25. Shapiro AJ, Davis SD, Ferkol T, et al. Laterality defects other than situs inversus totalis in primary ciliary dyskinesia: insights into situs ambiguus and heterotaxy. *Chest.* 2014;146:1176–1186.
26. Wang TW, Neff LJ, Park-Lee E, et al. E-cigarette use among middle and high school students—United States, 2020. *MMWR Morb Mortal Wkly Rep.* 2020;69:1310–1312.
27. Tobacco Product Use Among Adults—United States, 2019. Accessed July 23, 2021. https://www.cdc.gov/mmwr/volumes/69/wr/mm6946a4.htm?s_cid=mm6946a4_w
28. Outbreak of Lung Injury Associated with the Use of E-Cigarette, or Vaping, Products. Accessed March 23, 2021. cdc.gov/tobacco/basic_information/e-cigarettes/severe-lung-disease.html.
29. Blount BC, Karwowski MP, Shields PG, et al. Vitamin E acetate in bronchoalveolar-lavage fluid associated with EVALI. *N Engl J Med.* 2020;382(8):697–705.
30. Aberegg SK, Maddock SD, Blagev DP, et al. Diagnosis of EVALI: general approach and the role of bronchoscopy. *Chest.* 2020;158(2):820–827.
31. Layden JE, Ghinai I, Pray I, et al. Pulmonary illness related to E-cigarette use in Illinois and Wisconsin—final report. *N Engl J Med.* 2020;382(10):903–916.
32. Henry TS, Kanne JP, Kligerman SJ. Imaging of vaping-associated lung disease. *N Engl J Med.* 2019;381(15):1486–1487.
33. Rao DR, Maple KL, Dettori A, et al. Clinical features of E-cigarette, or vaping, product use-associated lung injury in teenagers. *Pediatrics.* 2020;146(1):e20194104.

ADDITIONAL RESOURCES AND WEBSITES

Additional Resources and Websites for Clinicians:
Asthma:
https://ginasthma.org/reports/
https://ginasthma.org/asthma-education-videos/
https://www.nhlbi.nih.gov/health-topics/asthma-management-guidelines-2020-updates
Cystic fibrosis:
https://www.cff.org/
https://www.cff.org/Care/Clinical-Care-Guidelines/
E-cigarettes and vaping:
https://www.cdc.gov/tobacco/basic_information/e-cigarettes/index.htm
Primary ciliary dyskinesia:
https://www.nhlbi.nih.gov/health-topics/primary-ciliary-dyskinesia

Additional Resources and Websites for Parents/Caregivers:
Asthma:
https://www.cdc.gov/asthma/parents.html
Cystic fibrosis:
https://www.cff.org/
E-cigarettes and vaping:
https://www.cdc.gov/tobacco/basic_information/e-cigarettes/Quick-Facts-on-the-Risks-of-E-cigarettes-for-Kids-Teens-and-Young-Adults.html
https://downloads.aap.org/RCE/ENDShandout_Parents.pdf
https://www.healthychildren.org/English/health-issues/conditions/tobacco/Pages/Facts-For-Parents-About-E-Cigarettes-Electronic-Nicotine-Delivery-Systems.aspx
Habit cough:
www.habitcough.com
Pectus excavatum:
https://youtu.be/T-E5eSraulY

Additional Resources and Websites for Adolescents and Young Adults:
Asthma:
https://ginasthma.org/wp-content/uploads/2021/05/GINA-Patient-Guide-2021-copy.pdf
https://www.thoracic.org/patients/patient-resources/resources/asthma.pdf
https://www.thoracic.org/patients/patient-resources/resources/asthma-and-exercise.pdf
https://www.thoracic.org/patients/patient-resources/resources/asthma-treatment.pdf
Cystic fibrosis:
https://www.cff.org/
https://www.cff.org/Life-With-CF/Daily-Life/
E-cigarette use (how to quit):
https://teen.smokefree.gov/quit-vaping
Vocal cord dysfunction:
https://www.thoracic.org/patients/patient-resources/resources/vocal-cord-dysfunction.pdf

PART IV

Musculoskeletal Problems and Sport Medicine

CHAPTER 22

Common Musculoskeletal Problems

Ashley Rowatt Karpinos
Keith J. Loud

KEY WORDS

- Ankle
- Core
- Growth plates
- Hip
- Knee
- Musculoskeletal care
- Shoulder
- Spine
- Stress fractures

INTRODUCTION

Musculoskeletal problems, including injuries and pain, are among the most common reasons for adolescents and young adults (AYAs) to seek medical attention, regardless of their activity level. Appropriate management of these concerns can facilitate healthy participation in physical activity and earn the confidence of the patient.

Most common conditions can be managed adequately in the medical home without referral to a specialist since they improve with supportive care and conservative treatments. When clinicians need assistance with diagnosis and management, or when musculoskeletal conditions are not improving as expected with initial care, the patient should be referred to a sports medicine or orthopedic specialist with expertise in these conditions.

This chapter outlines a general approach to musculoskeletal concerns, including important elements of the history and physical examination, triage and initial management, indications for imaging and referral, and principles of treatment and rehabilitation. Conditions commonly seen in AYAs affecting the ankle, knee, hip, shoulder, and spine[1] are reviewed with a focus on care that can be provided in the medical home. Common musculoskeletal conditions by body part are listed in Table 22.1. With a focused history and physical examination, the clinicians should be able to prioritize likely diagnoses and develop initial management plans.

GENERAL PRINCIPLES OF MUSCULOSKELETAL INJURY CARE

Elements of Musculoskeletal History

Evaluation of a musculoskeletal concern begins with a thorough history, which should include the following:

- Anatomic location of symptoms (ask patient to point with one finger to localize)
- Injury mechanism or inciting factors
- Onset and timing of pain
- Presence of swelling or popping
- Perception of joint instability or locking
- Natural course of symptoms since onset
- Alleviating factors (ice, rest, bracing, medications)
- Provoking factors (certain positions, movements)
- Baseline physical activities and intensity prior to symptoms and subsequent changes

Obtaining the history of musculoskeletal concerns may lead to conversations with AYA patients about activities that are important to them and give the clinicians insight into risk-taking behaviors that contribute to some injuries.

Elements of Musculoskeletal Physical Examination

Using a standard approach to the physical examination focusing on the anatomic area of concern can facilitate effective evaluation. The important elements of a musculoskeletal physical examination are explained in Table 22.2. Findings on the musculoskeletal examination may lead the clinician to consider the presence of systemic disorders (e.g., pectus excavatum or carinatum [Marfan syndrome], joint hypermobility and/or hyperextensible skin [Ehler–Danlos], café-au-lait spots and/or axillary freckling [neurofibromatosis], and high arches of the feet and hammer-toes [spinal dysraphism or peripheral neuropathy]).

General Indications for Imaging in Musculoskeletal Evaluations

In general, plain x-rays are necessary for any of the following circumstances:

1. Significant pain with systemic signs (pain with fever or pain that awakens a patient from sleep)
2. Any new pain with a history of cancer

X-rays should be considered for any of the following circumstances:

1. Acute injury with history or examination suggestive of fracture (i.e., pain, swelling, instability)
2. Unexplained or persistent complaints

Advanced imaging, such as magnetic resonance imaging (MRI), ultrasound, or computed tomography (CT) scan are not commonly indicated for the initial evaluation of musculoskeletal concerns and should usually be reserved for evaluation of specific conditions by musculoskeletal specialists.

General Indications for Referral to a Musculoskeletal Specialist for Patients with Acute Trauma of an Extremity

When in doubt about diagnosis and management, the clinicians should recommend rest from provoking activities and refer to a musculoskeletal specialist. Regardless of the injury site,

TABLE 22.1

Common Musculoskeletal Injuries in Adolescents and Young Adults by Body Part

Body Part	Acute Injuries	Insidious/Overuse Injuries
Head/neck	Cervical muscle strain ("whiplash") Cervical root and brachial plexus neurapraxia ("stinger") Cervical spine fractures Concussion Cranial fractures	Cervical muscle strain (chronic)
Spine	Vertebral fracture Vertebral ligament injury	Lumbar spondylolysis/spondylolisthesis Lumbar spondylosis Muscular strain Scheuermann disease (vertebral endplates)
Chest	Rib fracture Chest wall contusion	Rib stress fracture
Shoulder	Acromioclavicular joint sprain Fracture Instability (subluxation/dislocation) Labral tear	Bicep tendonitis Multidirectional glenohumeral instability Proximal humeral epiphysiolysis (Little League shoulder) Rotator cuff strain Scapular dyskinesis Subacromial bursitis/impingement syndrome
Elbow	Fracture (radial head vs. supracondylar)	Medial epicondyle apophysitis (Little League elbow) Ulnar collateral ligament (UCL) sprain Lateral epicondylitis (tennis elbow) Medial epicondylitis Ulnar neuropathy of the elbow
Wrist/hand	Fracture Joint sprain	Carpal tunnel syndrome De Quervain tenosynovitis Extensor tendonitis Flexor tendonitis Triangular fibrocartilage complex tear
Hip	Fracture (avulsion vs. other) Muscle strain Sacroiliac sprain	Greater trochanteric bursitis Iliac crest apophysitis Iliotibial (IT) band syndrome Femoroacetabular impingement (FAI) Pelvic/femoral stress fracture Slipped capital femoral epiphysis (SCFE) Snapping hip syndrome/iliopsoas tendinopathy
Knee	Anterior cruciate ligament (ACL)/posterior cruciate 　ligament (PCL) rupture Bone bruise Fracture Medial collateral ligament (MCL)/lateral collateral 　ligament (LCL) sprain Meniscus tear Patellar instability (dislocation, subluxation)	Iliotibial (IT) band syndrome Osteochondritis dissecans (OCD) Patellofemoral pain (PFP) Patellar tendonitis Pes anserinus bursitis Tibial tubercle apophysitis (Osgood–Schlatter)
Foot/ankle/leg	Fracture Ligament sprain	Calcaneal apophysitis Medial tibial stress syndrome (shin splints) Stress fracture (tibia, metatarsal) Plantar fasciitis

immediate consultation should be considered for any of the following criteria:

1. Obvious deformity
2. Acute locking (joint cannot be moved actively or passively past a certain point)
3. Inability of patient to actively move joint in a specific plane of motion (e.g., inability to extend knee)
4. Penetrating wound of major joint, muscle, or tendon
5. Neurologic deficit or vascular compromise
6. Joint instability perceived by the patient or elicited on examination
7. Bony crepitus

General Concepts in Treatment and Rehabilitation of Injuries

The prevention of long-term sequelae of injury depends on complete rehabilitation, characterized by full, pain-free range of motion (ROM) and normal strength, endurance, and proprioception.

TABLE 22.2

Approach to a Standard Musculoskeletal Physical Examination

Inspection	• Look for swelling, bruising, or deformity • Assess baseline level of comfort • Observe for alterations to general movements
Palpation	• Touch the anatomic structures at the source of the pain and nearby to determine the primary anatomical location of symptoms • Look for specific tenderness at commonly injured and important areas relevant to the specific anatomical area of concern (e.g., base of the 5th metatarsal in lateral ankle injury) • Ensure adequate vascular perfusion of affected areas
Range of motion (ROM)	• Ask the patient to perform active ROM of the affected and nearby joints in each plane of motion • Perform passive ROM with attention to asymmetry
Strength	• Offer manual resistance to the patient moving the joint in each plane of motion with attention to significantly decreased strength and asymmetry that may indicate muscle or tendon rupture or nerve injury
Special testing (joint-specific)	• Each anatomical area has specific musculoskeletal examination maneuvers that help with diagnosis, such as the Lachman test for a torn anterior cruciate ligament of the knee • Test reflexes and sensation if there is concern for neurologic injury • Test functions such as balance, walking, running, or throwing

There are four phases of rehabilitation:

1. Limit further injury and control pain and swelling.
2. Improve strength and ROM of injured structures.
3. Achieve near-normal strength, ROM, endurance, and proprioception of injured structures.
4. Return to exercise or sport without symptoms.

Since AYAs progress through these phases at different rates, clinicians should avoid predicting definite time frames for return to participation. Referral to a rehabilitation specialist, such as a physical therapist or certified athletic trainer, is often necessary to guide the patient through rehabilitation phases 2 through 4. Some schools have certified athletic trainers, which can improve access and affordability.

Phase 1: Limit Further Injury and Control Pain and Swelling

The initial treatment of many musculoskeletal conditions focuses on limiting injury and controlling pain and swelling. The mnemonic PRICE is a useful way to recall the general principles of phase 1 (Table 22.3). Uninjured structures should be exercised to maintain fitness and psychological health. Athletes may be able to perform stretching, core exercises, or cross-training of unaffected areas.

Phase 2: Improve Strength and Range of Motion of Injured Structures

Specific exercises should be done within a pain-free ROM. Isometric exercises can be started on the first day if there is little pain-free ROM and the patient is able to contract the muscles. Recommend relative rest, avoiding activities that cause pain while continuing activities that do not cause pain or result in recurrence of symptoms within 24 hours. Nonsteroidal anti-inflammatory drugs (NSAIDs) may be used to interrupt the cycle of pain, muscle spasm, inflexibility, weakness, and decreased endurance. However, NSAIDs should not be used to mask pain and allow premature return to play. Ice is a good analgesic and reduces swelling. Adolescents and young adults should maintain general fitness, as described for phase 1.

Phase 3: Achieve Near-Normal Strength, Range of Motion, Endurance, and Proprioception of Injured Structures

Exercise that does not cause recurrence of symptoms can be gradually increased. Healing is characterized by minimal discomfort or laxity with provocative testing, normal ROM, no point tenderness to palpation, no pain with stretching, and progressively less pain with activities of daily living.

Phase 4: Return to Exercise or Sport without Symptoms

Functional rehabilitation should be sport-specific, practicing components at a decreased level and advancing gradually to full-force exertion. Premature return to sports is likely to result in further injury or another injury. Successful rehabilitation minimizes the risk of reinjury and returns the injured structures to baseline ROM, strength, endurance, and proprioception.

TABLE 22.3

The Mnemonic PRICE (Protection, Rest, Ice, Compression, Elevation)

P • Protection	• The affected structure must be protected, using appliances (e.g., soft wrap, splint, crutches, walking boot, sling) as necessary to achieve pain relief • If the patient is unable to walk without a limp, some form of protection is needed • Re-evaluate frequently to avoid extended use of crutches or bracing without indication
R • Rest	• Resting the affected structures limits further injury and facilitates healing • Protective appliances can help • Advise avoidance of activities that cause pain
I • Ice	• Anti-inflammatory treatments can reduce pain and swelling • Cryotherapy, such as ice, can be applied for 20 min at a time, 3–4 times a day for the first few days • Nonsteroidal anti-inflammatory drugs, if prescribed, should be dosed regularly (rather than "as needed") to achieve therapeutic steady-state levels, but limited to 5–10 d
C • Compression	• Compression, such as with a soft wrap, brace, or compressive sleeve can provide comfort and help reduce swelling • Ensure compressions are allowing routine blood flow through vascular structures involved
E • Elevation	• Elevating affected structures helps reduce swelling which can facilitate return of function

In the clinician's office, safe return to participation in physical activities can be advocated when the patient demonstrates:

1. No residual deformities or edema in the injured body part. An exception to this rule is the ankle, which may demonstrate persistent soft tissue swelling (not effusion) after functional restoration has been achieved.
2. Full and equal ROM compared to the uninjured, paired joint
3. At least 90% muscle strength compared to the uninjured, paired extremity
4. No pain at rest or with activity

GROWTH PLATE DISORDERS

Younger AYAs are susceptible to injury at growth plates until skeletal maturity has been reached. Growth plates include physes (ossification centers near the end of a long bone) and apophyses (ossification centers at the attachment of a major tendon or ligament group). Growth plates close at various times over the course of several years depending on anatomic location and pubertal development. While growth plates are open, they are typically weaker than surrounding tissues and prone to acute injuries, such as Salter–Harris fractures (see Ankle Fractures), and chronic injuries, such as humeral epiphysiolysis, or "Little League Shoulder."

Chronic stress and repetitive motions can also lead to injury at apophyses, called "apophysitis." These injuries can lead to focal pain in younger adolescents. A common example is tibial tubercle apophysitis (Osgood–Schlatter disease), a chronic apophyseal injury at the tibial tubercle apophysis causing anterior knee pain (described later in the chapter). Similarly, calcaneal apophysitis (Sever disease) is a cause of heel pain especially common in physically active 9- to 15-year-olds. Medial epicondyle apophysitis ("Little League Elbow") is a cause of elbow pain in younger adolescents who pitch or throw repetitively. Apophysitis may not be detected on x-ray. Apophyses can also be injured acutely with a sudden forceful pull of a tendon at the apophysis. In these cases, x-rays may show displacement of the apophysis and clinicians should refer to a musculoskeletal specialist.

THE ANKLE

Acute ankle injuries, including sprains and fractures, are common in physically active and inactive AYAs.

History of Ankle Symptoms

Adolescents and young adults can generally demonstrate the mechanism that caused an ankle injury. While lateral ankle injuries resulting from ankle inversion (turning the ankle in, with the sole facing medially) are most common, injuries resulting from ankle eversion can be more serious.

Physical Examination of the Ankle

1. Inspect for visible abnormalities, asymmetry, swelling, and bruising.
2. Palpate for bony tenderness.
3. Assess active and passive ROM in plantarflexion, dorsiflexion, inversion, and eversion. Evaluate discomfort with passive ROM.
4. Test strength in plantarflexion, dorsiflexion, inversion, and eversion.
5. Perform special testing of the ankle which includes anterior drawer and talar tilt to assess ligament laxity. Check for vascular integrity. Assess for pain-free weight-bearing with normal gait and if present, then assess heel-and-toe walking. If the AYA is ambulating without a limp, assess core strength and single-leg balance.

Imaging of the Ankle

The Ottawa ankle rules (Fig. 22.1) are a well-validated set of clinical decision rules used to determine the need for an ankle x-ray.[2] A standard ankle x-ray series includes an anteroposterior (AP), lateral, and mortise view. A standard foot x-ray series includes AP, lateral, and oblique. Foot and ankle x-rays should be obtained weight-bearing.

Treatment of the Ankle

Most ankle injuries in AYAs can be treated nonoperatively by the clinicians based on the specific diagnosis.

Ankle Sprain

Definition and Etiology

A sprain is an injury to a ligament that occurs when a force stretches a ligament through a greater ROM than normal without causing a fracture of a nearby bone. The most common ankle sprain is an injury to the anterior talofibular ligament after ankle inversion. In more severe lateral ankle sprains, the calcaneal fibular ligament and posterior talofibular ligament can also be injured (Fig. 22.2).

Epidemiology

Among AYAs, ankle sprains are more common in males aged 15 to 19 years. Half of all ankle sprains occur during athletic activity, most commonly during indoor/court sports.[3]

Clinical Manifestation

1. History
   a. Ankle inversion or eversion while walking, stepping off a curb, or running
   b. Immediate pain, with some ability to bear weight
2. Physical Examination
   a. Lateral ankle swelling and bruising may persist for several weeks. Bruising may migrate during recovery.
   b. Tenderness with palpation of the injured ligament(s) and possibly at the attachment to the associated bone
   c. Decreased ROM and pain with passive ROM of the injured ligament
   d. Decreased strength due to pain
   e. Laxity of the sprained ligament may be present in acute or remote ankle sprain. Most patients with ankle sprains can bear weight but may have a limp.

Diagnosis

The diagnosis of an ankle sprain can be made clinically based on history and physical examination. X-rays may be needed to exclude ankle fracture as per Ottawa ankle rules.

Treatment

An initial goal of the acute treatment of an ankle sprain is to limit disability while promoting decrease in pain and swelling and recovery of ROM, strength, and proprioception. Mainstays of initial treatment are the following:

1. Relative rest from activities, ice, compression, and elevation
2. Braces: Initially, compression and stability can be provided by an air-stirrup–type ankle brace, which should be used for many acute sprains not complicated by fracture. Within a few weeks, the AYA can transition into a more functional soft stirrup or lace-up ankle stabilizing brace. These ankle braces provide stability to inversion and eversion, allowing for active dorsiflexion and plantarflexion during weight-bearing gait, which is a key to successful rehabilitation.
3. Crutches: Crutches are rarely needed in ankle sprains. If crutches are needed for significant pain with weight-bearing, the patient should be instructed in partial weight-bearing techniques and advised to discontinue use of crutches as soon as tolerated.

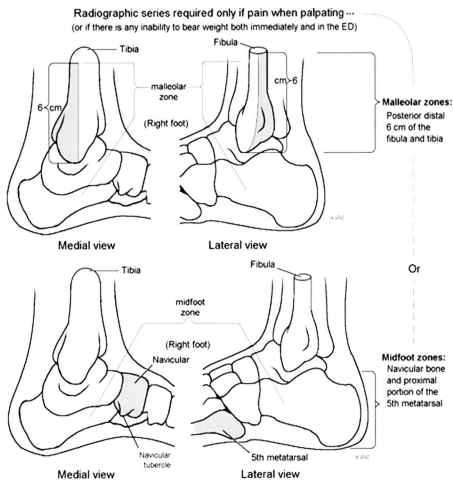

FIGURE 22.1 Ottawa ankle rules for suspected fracture. (From Chila A; American Osteopathic Association. *Foundations of Osteopathic Medicine.* 3rd ed. Lippincott Williams & Wilkins; 2010.)

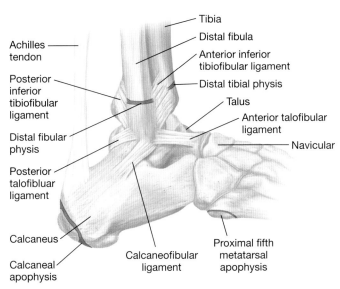

FIGURE 22.2 Lateral ankle anatomy includes the anterior talofibular ligament (ATFL), calcaneal fibular ligament (CFL), and posterior talofibular ligament (PTFL) can be injured in lateral ankle sprains. If the physis of the distal fibula (growth plate) is open, it can be injured in younger adolescents during ankle inversion injuries.

Rehabilitation of ankle sprains should start on the first day of evaluation with active ROM exercises such as spelling the alphabet with the toes and stretching the calf muscles. Many patients will benefit from referral to a rehabilitation specialist for guidance through the process of rehabilitation and complete return to prior function.

Prognosis

Adolescents and young adults can typically return to normal activities 2 to 6 weeks after an ankle sprain, depending on the severity of injury. Adolescents and young adults who experience one ankle sprain are likely to have a recurrent ankle sprain. The stirrup or lace-up-type ankle brace should be worn in competition sports for 6 months after the injury to help prevent recurrent ankle sprains. Guiding the AYA through a full recovery and rehabilitation program after an ankle sprain promotes return of optimal strength, balance, and function to prevent future injuries. Some athletes with chronic ankle sprains and ligament laxity develop chronic pain from ankle impingement syndrome.

Ankle Fractures

Fractures can occur in isolation or with ankle sprains. The most common sites of ankle fracture are the distal fibula, base of the fifth metatarsal, talus, and tibia. A small avulsion fracture at the tip of the distal fibula or tibia may be treated identically to a common ankle sprain. However, if the fracture is at a different anatomic location, refer to a specialist for further management. If there is bony tenderness without fracture on imaging, immobilize for 1 week with weight-bearing as tolerated, then re-evaluate.

If there is bony tenderness at a physis in an adolescent with open growth plates, assume that a fracture is present even if the x-ray is normal. Before an adolescent has reached skeletal maturity, physes (growth plates) are open. Under force, an open growth plate may be weaker than a ligament. In an inversion injury, a younger adolescent may sustain an injury to the physis of the distal fibula, such as in a Salter–Harris fracture (see Fig. 22.2). An older AYA is more likely to sprain a lateral ankle ligament. The history, physical examination, and x-rays, if indicated, can differentiate these injuries, although a type I Salter-Harris injury is indistinguishable from ligament sprain on x-ray. Fortunately, the treatment of both injuries is similar.

THE KNEE

Knee injuries and pain syndromes are among the most common chief complaints in AYAs. Knee anatomy is shown in Figure 22.3.

History of Knee Symptoms

1. Atraumatic Knee Pain With Physical Activities
   a. Chronic pain: Patellofemoral pain (PFP) and Osgood–Schlatter disease are common causes. In general, if the patient does not give a history of the knee giving out or locking, sharp pain, effusion, the sensation of something loose in the knee, or the sensation that something tore with an initial injury, then the injury will likely heal with conservative nonsurgical management.
   b. Acute pain: Acute knee pain without an injury suggests osteochondritis dissecans (OCD), pathologic fracture, infection, arthritis, or referred pain from the hip. Unless the examination provides a diagnosis, any adolescent with acute knee pain without a history of trauma should have an x-ray of the knee. If the knee x-rays are normal, evaluate and obtain x-rays of the hip to rule out hip disorders such as slipped capital femoral epiphysis (SCFE) manifesting as knee pain.
2. Traumatic Knee Pain
   a. Knee injury during weight-bearing, cutting, or pivoting while running, or an unplanned fall can cause internal derangement including ligamentous, meniscal tears, patellar instability (dislocation or subluxation), fracture, and bone bruising. A patient who injures the knee while cutting or pivoting without contact by another player has a high likelihood of having an anterior cruciate ligament (ACL) tear or patellar instability. After an ACL injury, patients frequently report a "pop" and a sensation of knee instability.
   b. A valgus knee injury: A valgus motion is a common mechanism for injury of the medial collateral ligament (MCL), and possibly the ACL or meniscus.

Physical Examination of the Knee

1. Inspect for superficial swelling, discoloration, effusion, or deformity. Reduced bulk and tone of the quadriceps may indicate a serious or chronic internal knee injury.
2. Palpate for knee effusion. The presence or absence of a knee effusion is important in determining an initial differential diagnosis. An acute knee effusion within 24 hours of a knee injury is a hemarthrosis and suggests a specific set of acute traumatic knee injuries (Table 22.4). Palpate anatomic landmarks including the patella, patellar tendon, tibial tubercle, medial and lateral joint lines, MCL, lateral collateral ligament (LCL), iliotibial (IT) band, pes anserinus, and head of the fibula.
3. Observe active ROM in knee extension and flexion. Note that a knee effusion limits extremes of knee extension and flexion. Use passive ROM to evaluate quadriceps and hamstring flexibility.
4. Evaluate strength in resisted knee flexion and extension.
5. Special testing for ligamentous laxity includes Lachman and pivot shift to evaluate the ACL, posterior drawer, and sag sign to evaluate the posterior cruciate ligament (PCL), valgus stress to evaluate the MCL, varus stress to evaluate the LCL, and McMurray test to evaluate meniscus tears. Assess core strength first with a single leg stance and, if stable, then with a single leg squat.

Imaging of the Knee

The Ottawa knee rule is a validated clinical decision rule[4] which suggests an x-ray is indicated after an acute knee injury if any one of the following criteria is present:
1. Inability to bear weight
2. Fibular head tenderness

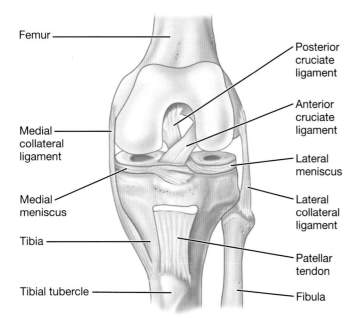

FIGURE 22.3 Right knee joint (anterior view). (From Anderson MK, Barnum M. *Foundations of Athletic Training*. 7th ed. Lippincott Williams & Wilkins; 2021.)

TABLE 22.4

Knee Conditions in Adolescents and Young Adults with and without Effusion

	Traumatic Injuries	Atraumatic Knee Pain
Knee effusion present	ACL/PCL rupture Bone bruise Fracture Meniscus tear (effusion may not be visible initially) Patellar or knee dislocation	Early osteoarthritis (postsurgical) Reactive arthritis Joint infection (including gonococcal, Lyme) Osteochondritis dissecans (OCD) Systemic juvenile idiopathic arthritis
No knee effusion	MCL/LCL sprain or rupture	Iliotibial (IT) band syndrome Patellofemoral pain (PFP) Patellar tendonitis Pes anserinus bursitis Tibial tubercle apophysitis (Osgood–Schlatter)

MCL, medial collateral ligament; LCL, lateral collateral ligament; ACL, anterior cruciate ligament; PCL, posterior cruciate ligament.

3. Isolated tenderness of the patella
4. Inability to flex the knee beyond 90 degrees

Common conditions such as PFP, Osgood–Schlatter, and iliotibial (IT) band syndrome do not require x-rays to establish a diagnosis. Adolescents and young adults presenting with knee effusion should have x-rays as part of the initial evaluation. When knee x-rays are indicated, a standard x-ray series includes bilateral AP and unilateral sunrise and lateral of the affected side, with bilateral sunrise views if concerned for patellar instability or a unilateral tunnel view if effusion and suspecting OCD or ACL tear. Knee x-rays should be obtained weight-bearing when able. Magnetic resonance imaging evaluation is not routinely indicated in the acute or chronically injured knee. However, if a clinician strongly suspects an acute ACL rupture, MRI can be considered while awaiting referral for definitive management.

Treatment of the Knee

Chronic knee pain is treated according to the specific cause. The following approach guides the treatment of acute traumatic knee injuries.

1. Use the history, physical examination, and imaging, if indicated, to establish a working diagnosis.
2. Protect the knee with a hinged knee brace. Allow the patient to bear weight if they can ambulate without pain or a limp with the knee protection. Prescribe crutches if the patient cannot bear weight without pain or there is suspicion of fracture. Knee immobilizers are rarely indicated and can lead to decreased strength and ROM. Only use a knee immobilizer in a patellar fracture or dislocation and refer urgently to a specialist.
3. Relative rest includes avoiding activities that cause knee pain or could exacerbate the injury. In an acute traumatic knee injury, recommend avoidance of all running, jumping, cutting, and pivoting initially. In the absence of fracture or knee dislocation, the patient may walk.
4. Recommend ice and analgesics as needed.
5. Compression, such as with an elastic wrap, should be used for swelling.
6. Instruct patients to elevate the leg by propping up the foot or lower leg with the knee in extension, not using a pillow under a bent knee, which can lead to decreased ROM. Recommend the patient start isometric quadriceps contractions or supine straight leg lifts in the first few days if possible. This can help prevent the rapid quadriceps atrophy that delays recovery.
7. Refer to a musculoskeletal specialist for definitive evaluation and management.

Patellofemoral Pain

Definition

Patellofemoral pain syndrome, also known as "runner's knee," is the most common cause of anterior knee pain among AYAs, with a prevalence of about 10% to 25%.[5] Patellofemoral pain syndrome is more common in females.

Etiology

Patellofemoral pain originates from the patellofemoral joint, the articulation of the patella with the trochlear groove of the femur. The condition may result from abnormal biomechanical forces that occur across the patella due to muscle imbalances or hypermobility.

Clinical Manifestations

Pain from PFP occurs around or behind the patella and is worsened by at least one activity that loads the patellofemoral joint during weight-bearing on a flexed knee, such as running, jumping, squatting, and going up or down stairs. The following clinical manifestations are common in PFP:

1. History
   a. Insidious onset of atraumatic achy anterior knee pain. The patient may grip the front of the knee and patella with the whole hand when describing the pain.
   b. Pain is worse with activities such as running, jumping, squatting, and stairs.
   c. Theatre sign: Pain is worse after prolonged sitting with the knee in flexion.
   d. Pain is chronic or recurrent, and patients may present with several months or years of pain.
   e. Sharp pain may cause sensation of buckling, especially on stairs, but knees do not actually give way.
2. Physical Examination
   a. Inspection of the patient with PFP is usually normal.
   b. Palpation of the patellar edges or facets results in tenderness.
   c. ROM and strength are usually normal.
   d. Squatting may cause pain.
   e. The dynamic patellar compression test, grind sign or Clarke sign, is performed by compressing the superior aspect of the patella between thumb and index finger as the patient actively tightens the quadriceps in 10 degrees of flexion. Pain or apprehension suggests PFP. Direct compression of the patella against the femur with the knee flexed may also elicit pain.

Diagnosis

The diagnosis of PFP is usually made by a compatible history and physical examination. The differential diagnosis includes patellar tendinopathy, medial plica syndrome, patellar instability, patellofemoral cartilage defects, or early osteoarthritis. X-rays are rarely needed and are only indicated to exclude other conditions if the diagnosis is not certain.

Treatment

1. Most patients respond well to nonoperative management. Use the principles of PRICE (**Table 22.3**) to help with symptom management. Nonsteroidal anti-inflammatory drugs may offer temporary relief.
2. The most important treatment for PFP is physical therapy for muscle strengthening. Due to the chronic and recurrent nature of symptoms, most patients benefit from a formal physical therapy referral where they can learn specific stretching and strengthening exercises with a focus on quadriceps, hamstrings, and core muscles. Once patients learn their therapy program, they can be moved to a home program.
3. A graduated running program can be started after symptoms are controlled and strength is improving. Ice may be helpful immediately after exercise.
4. A knee sleeve with a cutout for the patella may be helpful to the patient for some activities.
5. Kinesiotaping may provide short-term pain relief and is not harmful.[6]

Prognosis

The prognosis for PFP is good, especially initially with focused treatments. The symptoms can be recalcitrant or recur, thus, it is important for AYAs to learn the specific stretching and strengthening exercises early and maintain these long-term in order to participate in the activities they enjoy most. Sometimes PFP causes long-term modification of activities, such as decreased running and/or a transition to lower impact sports such as swimming.

Osgood–Schlatter Disease

Definition and Etiology

Osgood–Schlatter disease, or tibial tubercle apophysitis, is inflammation and stress at the tibial tubercle apophysis. It is characterized by discomfort at the tibial tubercle in a skeletally immature patient. With puberty, the developing quadriceps muscle mass places the small tibial tubercle ossification center under great traction stress from the patellar tendon during running and jumping activities. Osgood–Schlatter is most common in physically active males aged 11 to 15 years, during the period of rapid linear growth.

Clinical Manifestations

1. History
   a. Pain focally at the tibial tubercle
   b. Pain aggravated by activity and relieved by rest
   c. Recent history of growth spurt, high levels of running and jumping, or overall increase in activity level
   d. Unilateral involvement is more common than bilateral involvement.
   e. Duration is usually several months but can last longer.
2. Physical Examination
   a. Point tenderness at the tibial tubercle
   b. Mild swelling at the tibial tubercle
   c. Normal knee joint with full ROM

Diagnosis

X-rays are not essential for diagnosis and are generally done only to eliminate the possibility of other processes and evaluate skeletal maturity. The x-ray may reveal soft tissue swelling anterior to the tibial tubercle and in an older AYA, a nonossified fragment of the tibial tubercle may be seen.

Treatment

As Osgood–Schlatter is also an anterior knee pain syndrome, many of the same principles of treatment for PFP apply. Additional considerations include the following:

1. Careful explanation of the condition and expected duration, noting that symptoms can persist until skeletal maturity.
2. If symptoms are mild, the patient may continue in the chosen sport. If symptoms are more severe, limit running and jumping activities for 2 to 4 weeks, or until pain improves.
3. If symptoms are severe or fail to respond to restriction of activity, immobilization with a knee immobilizer for a few weeks is effective. Immobilization should also be strongly considered when the patient has difficulty actively bringing the knee to full extension.
4. Knee pads should be used for activities in which kneeling or direct knee contact might occur.
5. Surgery is rarely indicated. If the patient continues to have symptoms after skeletal maturity and x-rays reveal a persistent unfused fragment, surgical excision often provides relief.

Prognosis

The symptoms of Osgood–Schlatter abate when the tibial tubercle apophysis matures and fuses with the tibia. While the prognosis is excellent, AYAs should be informed that the process might recur with increases in physical activity before skeletal maturity. After bony maturation is completed a prominent tubercle may always be visible. Some patients may still have difficulty kneeling on the prominent tubercle, even into adulthood.

Osteochondritis Dissecans

Osteochondritis dissecans is an important idiopathic condition of focal avascular necrosis in which bone and overlying articular cartilage separate from the medial femoral condyle, or less commonly, from the lateral femoral condyle. The peak incidence is in the preadolescent age-group. The clinical course and treatment vary according to the age at onset, with children and young adolescents having a better prognosis than older adolescents and adults. Insidious onset of intermittent, nonspecific knee pain that

does not respond to PFP treatment should raise suspicion for OCD, especially if associated with intermittent effusion or a sensation of knee locking. Diagnosis of OCD requires specific radiographic views (e.g., "tunnel" or "notch") and should prompt referral to a musculoskeletal specialist.

THE HIP

Adolescents and young adults may use the term hip pain to describe an array of concerns originating from the femoroacetabular joint, thighs, buttocks, low back, and pelvis. The large muscle masses in this area and the proximity to the lower abdomen and genitourinary systems necessitates an expanded differential diagnosis beyond musculoskeletal concerns. Hip pain that originates from the femoroacetabular joint most commonly presents as anterior groin pain and includes some of the more serious causes of hip pain in AYAs, including femoroacetabular impingement (FAI), labral tears, SCFE, and femoral stress fracture.

History of Hip Symptoms

Begin by asking the patient to point to the specific area of greatest pain, trying to differentiate anterior, lateral, or posterior hip area symptoms, which can guide the remainder of the history. It is important to elicit the duration, acuity, and character of the pain, as well as exacerbating and relieving activities.

Physical Examination of the Hip

1. Inspect for swelling, bruising, or deformity at rest.
2. Palpate for areas of maximal tenderness, including at the anterior groin and laterally at the greater trochanter.
3. Test passive ROM in flexion, extension, internal rotation, and external rotation.
4. Perform strength testing of flexion, extension, abduction, and adduction.
5. Special tests of the hip include flexion abduction external rotation (FABER), which suggests iliopsoas pathology or sacroiliac dysfunction, and flexion adduction internal rotation (FADIR), which suggests FAI, labral tear, or femoral stress fracture. The single leg hop test, hopping a few times on one leg, is a nonspecific test that may be used to elicit and localize bony pain, as in a stress fracture.

Imaging of the Hip

X-rays of the hips and pelvis should be obtained sparingly in AYAs, given their child-bearing potential and the risks associated with radiation. When needed, initial imaging with an AP of the pelvis and frog-leg lateral (which provides a lateral view of both femoral necks) or cross-table lateral (which provides a lateral view of one hip) is sufficient.

Treatment of the Hip

The treatment of most hip conditions is based on rehabilitation with physical therapy. Due to the complexity of hip injuries and the risk of morbidity in inadequately treated hip conditions, clinicians should refer to a rehabilitation and/or musculoskeletal specialist for management of hip conditions that are severe or not improving.

Femoroacetabular Impingement and Labral Tears

Femoroacetabular impingement results from abnormal contact between the femoral head and the rim of the acetabulum. Impingement of the bony structures can cause pain and predispose to tears of the labrum, a ring of flexible cartilage around the rim of the acetabulum that deepens the socket. Both circumstances can occur in adolescents but are more common in young adults. AYAs present with pain in the anterior groin, usually worse with activities. On examination, they may have decreased ROM and pain with FADIR. X-rays can confirm the anatomic changes that predispose to FAI but are not required to initiate treatment. The mainstay of treatment for FAI is physical therapy. Refer to a musculoskeletal specialist if AYAs do not improve with this treatment.

Slipped Capital Femoral Epiphysis

Definition

Slipped capital femoral epiphysis is a true orthopedic surgical emergency and must be recognized by clinicians caring for adolescents. In SCFE, the anatomic relationship between the femoral head and neck is altered secondary to a disruption at the level of the physis. A "stable" slip progresses slowly with insidious onset of pain. An "unstable" slip present acutely with inability to bear weight and is a surgical emergency.

Etiology

The femoral head slips posteriorly, inferiorly, and medially on the femoral metaphysis. This occurs through the hypertrophic cell layer of the epiphysis that widens during the accelerated growth of puberty. Obesity may alter the mechanics, increasing the vector of shear force acting at the physis, in addition to the increased forces caused by excess body weight itself. Most cases of SCFE are unrelated to an endocrine disorder, although hypopituitarism, hypogonadism, and hypothyroidism, are associated with an increased risk for bilateral slips. Endocrine abnormalities should be considered in patients with SCFE at the extremes of the adolescent age-group (before age 9 or after age 16).

Epidemiology

The prevalence of SCFE is two to four times higher in males than in females. Symptoms usually occur shortly before or during the period of accelerated growth (10 to 13 years in girls, 12 to 15 years in boys). Nearly 90% occur in patients affected by overweight or obese.

Clinical Manifestations

1. History
   a. Pain is localized to the anterior hip or groin in most patients, although pain may occur in the thigh or knee, referred from the obturator nerve.
   b. Some patients present with a painless limp.
2. Physical Examination
   a. On inspection, the affected leg is often held in slight external rotation and abduction at rest and in slight external rotation with ambulation.
   b. Range of motion is decreased in internal rotation, adduction, and flexion.
   c. A limp is present in 50% of patients, although an adolescent with an unstable slip typically refuses to bear weight due to pain.

Diagnosis

The condition should be considered in any adolescent with hip or knee pain or a limp. X-rays of the pelvis are necessary. In a normal AP x-ray of the hip, a line drawn on the superior edge of the femoral neck intersects the epiphysis; in a slip, the epiphysis falls below this line (Fig. 22.4). This is sometimes referred to as the "ice cream" (femoral head) falling off the "cone" (the femoral neck). Early and more subtle slips are more clearly seen on frog-leg lateral views. In suspected early cases that have normal x-rays, MRI may be helpful, demonstrating edema around the physis on T2-weighted images.

Treatment

1. Patients with SCFE should be made non–weight-bearing, either on crutches or in a wheelchair immediately in the primary care office.
2. Urgent orthopedic referral for surgery should occur to prevent progression.

Prognosis

Avascular necrosis and early hip osteoarthritis can be complications of SCFE. Avascular necrosis occurs more commonly after unstable slips. Premature degenerative joint disease is a frequent late development in many patients with severe, chronic slips, after fixation in situ, and can present in late adolescence and young adulthood.

THE SHOULDER

The glenohumeral joint, commonly referred to as the shoulder joint, is the most injured shoulder structure. However, shoulder injuries may also include problems at the acromioclavicular (AC) joint, the scapula, or proximal humerus. Acute rotator cuff tears that require surgery are rare in AYAs and more common in older adults. In evaluating shoulder concerns in AYAs, clinicians should also consider referred pain from the neck or abdomen.

History of Shoulder Symptoms

The history should focus on the location of discomfort, acuity of onset, duration of symptoms, sensation of instability or movement, popping, radiating patterns, as well as previous treatments. It is important to assess for the dominant hand and ask about repetitive and overhead activities.

Physical Examination of the Shoulder

1. Inspect for swelling, bruising, and deformity at rest. The history should focus on the location of discomfort, acuity of onset, duration of symptoms, sensation of instability or movement,

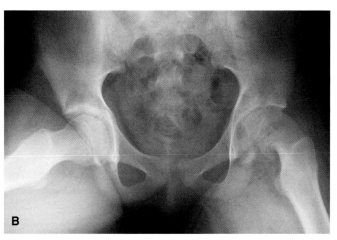

FIGURE 22.4 **A:** In the normal hip on the right, a line drawn on the superior femoral neck intersects the proximal femoral epiphysis. In the hip on the left with a slipped epiphysis, the epiphysis lies completely below a line drawn on the superior femoral neck. **B:** This is better visualized on the frog-lateral views.

popping, radiating patterns, as well as previous treatments. It is important to assess for the dominant hand and ask about repetitive and overhead activities.

2. Palpate for areas of maximal tenderness, including at the sternoclavicular joint, clavicle, AC joint, head of the humerus, and scapula.

3. Evaluate active ROM of the neck to observe for reproduction of shoulder pain. Test active and passive ROM in forward elevation, abduction, and internal and external rotation, noting asymmetry.

4. Perform strength testing for (1) the rotator cuff muscles with abduction and resisted flexion in the scapular plane (supraspinatus), (2) external rotation (infraspinatus and teres minor), and (3) internal rotation (subscapularis).

5. Special tests of the shoulder include the "empty can" test for impingement symptoms and dynamic labral shear test for labral tears. Posterior observation of scapular symmetry and winging after forward elevation indicates scapular dyskinesis, a common underlying cause of shoulder symptoms (Fig. 22.5).

Imaging of the Shoulder

X-rays of the shoulder are not commonly needed in initial assessment of most shoulder symptoms. X-rays are indicated to evaluate for fracture and widening of the physis of the proximal humerus in humeral epiphysiolysis. When indicated, x-rays should include an AP view, axillary, and scapular Y-view. Magnetic resonance imaging with specific protocols is needed to evaluate for labral tears or rotator cuff tears and can be performed by specialists if indicated.

Treatment of the Shoulder

Most shoulder concerns in AYAs can be successfully treated with several weeks of physical therapy. Activities such as sitting with poor posture, typing, and reading can lead to shoulder symptoms that are treated effectively with specific strengthening exercises. Adolescents and young adults with shoulder symptoms that are

not improving with conservative treatments or that are preventing participation in preferred activities should be referred to a musculoskeletal specialist.

Acute Shoulder Injuries

Acromioclavicular Joint Sprain

Acromioclavicular joint sprain, a disruption of the AC ligament, is a common acute shoulder injury in AYAs. The primary mechanism of injury is falling directly onto the lateral shoulder with the arm in adduction at the side, or a direct lateral blow. Patients present with focal pain and tenderness to palpation localized to the AC joint, as well as pain with forward elevation, abduction, and rotator cuff testing. X-rays are used to assess widening at the AC joint and to rule out clavicle fracture. Initial treatment with PRICE (Table 22.3) is helpful. Most patients will require a sling for initial protection and rest, but the sling can usually be discontinued as soon as pain improves. Focused physical therapy will usually lead to recovery of full strength and ROM, which are required before returning to activities.

Shoulder Dislocation

Acute glenohumeral joint dislocations occur in traumatic shoulder injuries due to the relatively shallow articulation of the glenoid or "socket" with the humeral head or "ball" and the wide ROM available at this joint. Anterior dislocations are most common. If the humeral head moves out of the glenoid and does not spontaneously reduce, the athlete will have extreme pain and loss of ROM that usually results in emergent presentation. A humeral head dislocation can be reduced acutely by a knowledgeable care professional. X-rays confirm positioning and evaluate for fracture. Acute shoulder dislocations can result in acute labral tears. These patients should be referred to a specialist for evaluation and management, which can include physical therapy or surgery.

In glenohumeral subluxations, the humeral head moves out of the glenoid socket only briefly and then spontaneously returns. A patient may present in the office with shoulder pain and report a "pop" or sensation of movement. On examination, they usually have nearly full strength and ROM. These patients can be treated with a brief sling for comfort and physical therapy.

Chronic Shoulder Injuries

Chronic Shoulder Instability with Glenoid Labrum Injuries

In contrast to acute traumatic shoulder dislocations, some AYAs have chronic shoulder instability, which includes recurrent shoulder subluxations as well as excess motion or laxity at the glenohumeral joint. Patients may give a history of known injuries or may present with chronic atraumatic shoulder pain. Chronic shoulder instability is common in athletes in overhead sports, such as volleyball, swimming, baseball, softball, and in AYAs with general ligamentous laxity. Shoulder instability results in movement of the humeral head at the glenoid and can lead to chronic tearing of the labrum. Laxity and signs of labral tearing can be appreciated on physical examination. Most patients with chronic shoulder instability are treated successfully with physical therapy.

Shoulder Impingement Syndrome

Shoulder impingement syndrome is a cause of shoulder pain in overhead athletes and AYAs who have repetitive shoulder movements. Impingement syndrome is a general term that includes a constellation of anatomic conditions, including chronic shoulder instability, muscle imbalances, or bony protrusions, that result in narrowing of the subacromial space. Narrowing of the subacromial space can lead to inflammation of the contained structures including the rotator cuff tendons and subacromial bursa, which results in pain. Initially, patients have pain when their shoulder is raised in overhead positions. However, the pain can progress to occur

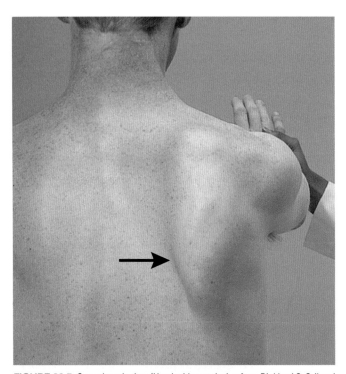

FIGURE 22.5 Scapular winging. (Used with permission from Bickley LS, Szilagyi PG, Hoffman RM, et al. *Bates' Guide to Physical Examination and History Taking.* 13th ed. 2020.)

with everyday activities or at rest. Physical examination maneuvers including the "empty can" test elicit pain. In the empty can maneuver, the AYA's arm is elevated to 90 degrees and the elbow is extended. The AYA rotates the shoulder causing the thumb to point down (as though emptying a can). The examiner stabilizes the shoulder while applying downward force to the arm. The test is positive if the AYA experiences pain or has weakness when trying to resist the examiner's downward force. Initial symptoms can be improved with rest from overhead activities, ice, and anti-inflammatories. Identifying the contributing causes is essential to successful rehabilitation. Most patients improve with physical therapy.

Weak Scapular Stabilizing Muscles

The scapular stabilizing muscles are a group of muscles that attach to the scapula and provide support at the scapulothoracic articulation. It is common for these muscles to become weak through general disuse in everyday activities, such as hunching forward over a device, or even in physically active athletes who do not focus on strengthening these muscles. A stable scapula provides a base from which the upper extremity gains a range of pain-free motions. Weak scapular stabilizing muscles are an underlying contributor to many common causes of shoulder pain and injury. Weak scapular muscles may cause scapular winging on physical examination (see Fig. 22.5). The scapular stabilizers can be strengthened with specific upper back exercises. Adolescents and young adults can learn these strengthening exercises through a course of physical therapy and continue to use these exercises throughout their lifetime. For overhead athletes in sports, routine scapular stabilizer strengthening is important for prevention of injury.

Humeral Epiphysiolysis

Humeral epiphysiolysis, or Little League Shoulder results from microtrauma to the physis at the proximal humerus in skeletally immature athletes. Chronic stress from a repetitive activity, such as throwing, can lead to widening or separation at the physis with resulting pain, weakness, and disability. This is common in younger adolescent boys who have open growth plates and are participating in frequent and competitive throwing sports. In older AYAs in whom growth plates at the proximal humerus are closed, other soft tissue structures are more likely to be injured. The diagnosis is suggested by pain in the proximal humerus and confirmed by x-rays. The treatment is rest from throwing and physical therapy. Patients should be referred to work with a therapist who is knowledgeable in throwing mechanics and specific rehabilitation progressions.

THE SPINE

Several abnormalities of the spine, including scoliosis and kyphosis, present during adolescence and young adulthood. Differentiating the causes requires a systematic approach to the history, physical examination, and appropriate utilization of x-rays.

History of Spine Symptoms

The history of spine symptoms should include inquiry about the duration and quality of discomfort, presence of observed deformity, and exacerbating and relieving positions. It is important to assess for associated fever, loss of bowel or bladder functioning, bilateral lower extremity paresthesia or weakness, and history of cancer which may be indicative of an urgent or malignant cause of spine symptoms.

Physical Examination of the Spine

1. Observe from the front, side, and behind for spine deformity and shoulder asymmetry. Observe for leg-length discrepancy by placing fingers on the iliac crests.
2. Palpate each spinous process, the paraspinous musculature, the iliac crests, and sacroiliac articulations to evaluate for the

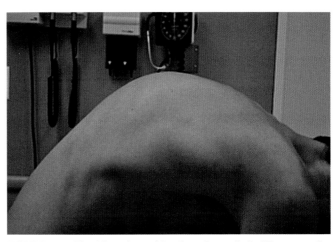

FIGURE 22.6 The Adams forward bend test for scoliosis. When assessing for an abnormal spinal curve, look for a prominent rib cage (rib hump), asymmetrical thoracic spine, and asymmetrical waistline. (From *Lippincott's Nursing Advisor 2009*. Lippincott Williams & Wilkins; 2009.)

location of discomfort. Prone positioning during the examination may help with relaxation and identification of structures.
3. Assess ROM in forward flexion, extension, right and left lateral flexion, and rotation while the patient is standing.
4. Perform lower extremity strength testing while the patient is seated.
5. Special tests of the spine include the Adams forward bend test, in which the patient bends forward at the waist with feet shoulder-width apart and hands palm-to-palm in the midline. Prominences along the spine on one or both sides at different levels suggest scoliosis (Fig. 22.6). Other specific tests include straight leg and crossed leg raise to evaluate for discogenic back pain, lumbar spine extension standing on a single leg to evaluate for pars interarticularis pain, and specific reflex and sensory examination.

Imaging of the Spine

Most AYAs who present with back pain do not require imaging. However, AYAs with a history of spine trauma, severe midline pain, neurologic changes, or spinal deformity, need x-rays. The initial spinal series should include an AP and lateral of the cervical, thoracic, or lumbar spine. Oblique images may be needed to evaluate for spondylosis. A scoliosis series should be obtained for obvious spinal deformity. Magnetic resonance imaging is not needed in initial evaluation of most spine syndromes but can confirm disc pathology, nerve root involvement, and tumors.

Treatment of the Spine

Most causes of spine pain can be treated with directed physical therapy and modification of activities and positioning. Some spinal conditions can be treated with focused injections and bracing, while others require surgical treatments. Correctly diagnosing and treating spine pain in young patients can help improve quality of life and activity levels.

Spondylolysis/Spondylolisthesis
Definition

1. Spondylolysis represents a stress fracture through the pars interarticularis of the vertebra (Fig. 22.7A), most commonly at L5. Spondylolysis occurs primarily in adolescents.
   a. Spondylolisthesis occurs when one vertebral body is anteriorly positioned relative to the one below (Fig. 22.7B). Isthmic spondylolisthesis develops in many cases of bilateral spondylolysis as the fractures free the vertebral body from

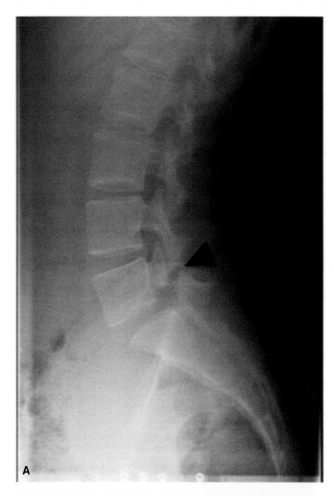

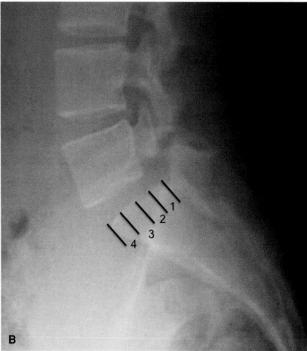

FIGURE 22.7 **A:** Spondylolysis (*arrow*) seen on a lateral lumbar x-ray as a lucency in the pars interarticularis of L5. **B:** Spondylolisthesis (same patient). The amount of slip is graded based on how far anteriorly the superior vertebral body has moved on the inferior one. This patient has Grade 1 spondylolisthesis (0% to 25%). Further progression is classified as Grade 2 (26% to 50%), Grade 3 (51% to 75%), and Grade 4 (76% to 100%).

the stabilization that normally occurs posteriorly. Progression typically occurs prior to skeletal maturity, but patients may develop occult spondylolysis and progression to spondylolisthesis that does not present until young adulthood.

Etiology

Increased stress on the pars interarticularis due to repetitive back extension such as in ballet, gymnastics, figure skating, and playing on the offensive or defensive lines in American football (in which collisions with the opposing line occur repeatedly) may contribute to development of spondylolysis or spondylolisthesis. Biomechanical factors such as increased lordosis in the lumbar spine, tight hamstrings, and/or Scheuermann kyphosis may contribute to excess stress and progression of these conditions.

Clinical Manifestations

1. History
   a. Insidious onset of focal low back pain with activity that becomes more pervasive without treatment
2. Physical Examination
   a. Loss of lumbar lordosis
   b. Pain with lumbar hyperextension in standing position ("Stork test") (**Table 22.5**)
   c. Pain with palpation of the midline lumbar spine
   d. Radicular signs are rare.

Diagnosis

Initial x-rays can identify an obvious fracture, evidence of spondylolisthesis, or other diagnoses (destructive lesions, congenital vertebral anomalies). Additional evaluation may include x-rays with oblique views, bone scan, CT, or MRI.

Treatment

The goals of treatment are resolution of symptoms and decreasing risk of progression of spondylolysis to spondylolisthesis. These patients should be referred to a specialist.

Prognosis

Unilateral spondylolysis can heal with conservative treatments. If pain improves, repeat imaging is not required. However, patients with spondylolisthesis require referral to a specialist for routine x-rays to monitor the grade of slip (Fig. 22.8B).

Discogenic Back Pain

Definition

Discogenic back pain refers to back pain originating from an injury or change in the vertebral discs, most commonly of the lumbar spine. Disc injuries are more common in older populations but can present in AYAs. In athletes and physically active AYAs, disc injuries are less common than spondylolysis.

TABLE 22.5			
Clinical Findings of Causes of Low Back Pain			
	Spondylolysis	**Discogenic**	**Nonspecific/ Muscular**
Pain at rest	+/–	+	+/–
Pain with activity	+	+	+/–
Pain on forward bending	–	+	+/–
Pain on backward bending	+	–	+/–
Radiating pain	– (rarely +)	+	–

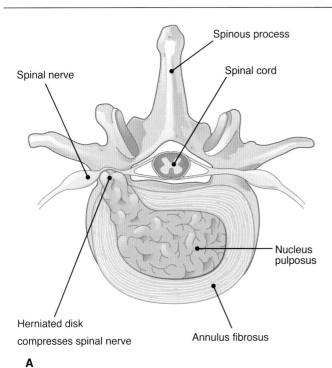

Spinous process

Spinal nerve

Spinal cord

Nucleus pulposus

Herniated disk compresses spinal nerve

Annulus fibrosus

A

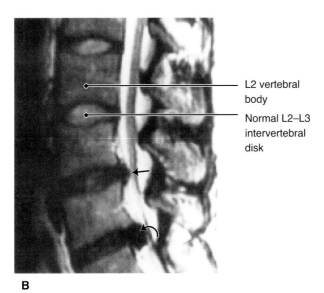

L2 vertebral body

Normal L2–L3 intervertebral disk

B

FIGURE 22.8 Herniated disk. **A:** The central mass of the disk protrudes into the spinal canal, putting pressure on the spinal nerve. **B:** MRI of the lumbar spine, sagittal section, showing herniated disks at multiple levels. There is a bulging L3–L4 disk (*straight arrow*) and an extruded L4–L5 lumbar disk (*curved arrow*). (From Cohen BJ, DePetris A. *Medical Terminology.* 7th ed. Lippincott Williams & Wilkins; 2013.)

Etiology

The most common disc change is herniation of the nucleus pulposus (Fig. 22.8). A resulting mass effect in the neural foramina causes radicular symptoms over the distribution of the nerve root exiting below the level of involvement (e.g., L5-S1 disc herniation typically results in symptoms involving the distribution of S1).

Clinical Manifestations

1. History
   a. Acute or insidious onset of low back pain, which can be quite bothersome and prompt a change in daily activities.
   b. Pain radiating unilaterally in a radicular pattern suggests involvement of a nerve root (**Table 22.5**).

   c. Bilateral radicular pain or neurologic symptoms are not consistent with discogenic back pain and should prompt aggressive evaluation of the central nervous system (CNS).
2. Physical Examination
   a. Decreased ROM and pain with forward flexion
   b. Focal pain at the midline and/or paraspinous muscles of the low back
   c. Positive straight-leg raise or crossed leg raise indicates a nerve rot may be involved.
   d. In acute or severe cases, gait may be antalgic.

Diagnosis

Clinical history and examination are usually sufficient for diagnosis. X-rays are usually negative but can help rule out fracture. Magnetic resonance imaging is rarely indicated in the primary care setting or in initial evaluations. Magnetic resonance imaging is indicated for patients with bilateral lower extremity findings, neurologic deficits, or failure to respond to the initial 6 weeks of conservative treatments.

Treatment

1. Nonsteroidal anti-inflammatory drugs and sometimes muscle relaxants are used to treat pain. Narcotic analgesics should be avoided.
2. Physical therapy is essential to address mechanics and postural awareness.
3. Patients who do not improve with physical therapy or have persistent radicular pain should be referred to a spine specialist to consider injections.
4. Patients not responsive to physical therapy and injection may be candidates for microdiscectomy.

Prognosis

Most patients with discogenic back pain improve symptomatically with conservative treatments. However, the anatomic changes, such as the presence of a disc herniation, do not necessarily resolve. Adolescents and young adults who experience discogenic back pain may have recurrent episodes of back pain in their lifetime. Effectively managing back pain is important to promote physical activities since staying physically active helps back pain. These patients can benefit from early and clear education on the condition, incorporation of back and core exercises into routine physical activity, modification of daily motions to support spine health (such as squatting rather than flexing the lumbar spine to lift, sitting with proper posture), and avoiding certain activities, such as Olympic lifting and axial loading.

Nonspecific Low Back Pain

Definition

Nonspecific low back pain, also termed "mechanical" or "muscular" low back pain refers to low back pain in which a specific underlying etiology is not apparent. Nonspecific low back pain is the most common cause of back pain in adolescents.[7]

Etiology

Although specific spinal pathology is not present, most patients have symptoms that suggest a muscular component and relationship to altered mechanics. Psychosocial factors such as feeling chronically fatigued and being in an emotionally abusive relationship have also been associated with back pain.

Clinical Manifestations

1. History
   a. General discomfort across the low back
   b. Pain is usually insidious in onset, although occasionally an acute strain can cause more abrupt onset of symptoms.
   c. Pain worsens with inactivity, although intermittent activity may worsen pain (see **Table 22.5**).

2. Physical Examination
   a. Mild decrease in ROM and discomfort with ROM testing
   b. General tenderness diffusely or variably across the low back, predominantly in the paraspinous muscles
   c. Movement may be slow, but not as limited as in acute discogenic back pain.

Diagnosis

The diagnosis of nonspecific low back pain can be made with a compatible history and physical examination. Imaging is not indicated in initial evaluation.

Treatment

1. Physical therapy should focus on postural awareness, spinal mobility, core and back strengthening, and hamstring and hip flexor stretching.
2. Acetaminophen and NSAIDs can be used temporarily. Narcotic analgesics are not indicated.

Prognosis

The prognosis for improvement of symptoms with conservative treatment is good. However, as with discogenic back pain, symptoms can be recurrent. Patients benefit from education and continuing back health management programs to prevent exacerbations and persistent symptoms. Some patients with chronic low back pain may benefit from cognitive behavioral therapy.

Scoliosis

Definition

Scoliosis is an abnormal lateral curvature of the vertebral column of >10 degrees in the coronal plane as measured by the Cobb angle on a full-length posteroanterior x-ray. Adolescent idiopathic scoliosis (AIS) occurs in patients over 10 years old and is the most common form of scoliosis. Scoliosis may involve the thoracic spine, lumbar spine, or both. Spinal curves <10 degrees are more appropriately called "spinal asymmetry" and represent variations in postural alignment that frequently resolve, whereas true scoliosis does not resolve and will remain present throughout adulthood.

Congenital scoliosis involves vertebral body malformations and defects of segmentation, such as hemivertebrae and/or bars. Congenital scoliosis is often diagnosed incidentally on x-rays performed for other reasons. Congenital scoliotic curves often progress during child and adolescent growth and require annual monitoring by a spine specialist.[8]

Etiology

The cause of AIS is likely multifactorial. Genetics seems to play a role as the risk of scoliosis is higher in first-degree relatives. Suspected causative factors include muscle, connective tissue, and bone disorders, as well as minor abnormalities of the CNS and hormone expression.

Epidemiology

Adolescent idiopathic scoliosis occurs in 2% of adolescents with similar rates in males and females. Scoliosis curve onset prior to 10 years old is considered "early-onset" scoliosis and carries a high risk of progression. A history of early-onset scoliosis in an adolescent presenting with spinal or lower extremity complaints warrants attention because of higher rates of underlying conditions such as CNS diseases, genetic syndromes, or neuromuscular disorders. The clinician should consider additional consultation and/or spine MRI.

Clinical Manifestations

1. History
   a. Scoliosis does not typically cause pain, though some patients present with a muscular discomfort.

2. Adolescents and young adults or their parents may notice shoulder or waist asymmetry or a spinal curve and ask for evaluation. However, some AYAs are not aware of any spinal curve.
3. Physical Examination
   a. The Adams forward-bend test is used to evaluate spinal asymmetry (see Fig. 22.7).
   b. If an inclinometer is used in the office to quantify axial rotation of the trunk during the Adams forward bend test, a rotation of 5 to 7 degrees warrants x-rays or referral to a spine specialist if imaging is not available.[9]
   c. Right-sided thoracic and left lumbar curves are the most common. Left-sided thoracic curves are atypical and carry a higher association with CNS malformations, requiring referral to a spine specialist.
   d. If scoliosis is identified, perform a thorough physical examination to look for neurologic or connective-tissue disorders.

Diagnosis

Scoliosis is suspected based on physical examination and confirmed by x-rays demonstrating a lateral spine curvature of over 10 degrees.

Treatment

1. The goal of treatment is to prevent progression of the scoliosis curve to avoid the onset of symptoms or need for surgery. Most young adolescents with scoliosis will require clinical and radiographic monitoring. If the spinal curve is not progressive over time and the adolescent is asymptomatic, no treatment is needed. After skeletal maturity, curve progression is rare. Thus, most young adults with scoliosis do not require any radiographic monitoring or treatment.
2. If AYAs have muscular back discomfort associated with their curve, physical therapy is an effective treatment.
3. If scoliosis curves have a Cobb angle greater than 20 degrees on x-rays or are progressive in a young adolescent, refer to a spine specialist for evaluation and treatment.
4. For skeletally immature adolescents aged 10 to 15 years with scoliosis and a Cobb angle of 20 to 40 degrees, spine bracing using a rigid thoracic lumbar sacral orthosis brace can slow the progression to the surgery threshold.[10] Bracing is most effective if the adolescent wears the brace for at least 13 hours each day.[10] Adolescents can remove the brace for physical activities. Bracing is discontinued when the adolescent reaches skeletal maturity or progresses to require surgery.
5. Surgery to fuse the spine is indicated for adolescents with a Cobb angle of 50 degrees or greater.

Prognosis

The risk of scoliosis curve progression is higher among those with younger age at onset, more skeletal immaturity, and higher magnitude curves. Curve progression after skeletal maturity is rare for curves <50 degrees. The majority of AYAs with AIS will not be clinically impacted by scoliosis.

Scheuermann Kyphosis

Scheuermann kyphosis is a structural deformity in the sagittal plane of the thoracic spine that can cause back pain. Scheuermann kyphosis must be differentiated from poor posture, in which the kyphotic curve is flexible and resolves once the patient lies down. Scheuermann kyphosis appears as a more severe angulation and the kyphosis persists in the supine position. Lateral spine x-rays demonstrate anterior wedging of at least three thoracic vertebrae. Scheuermann kyphosis, like scoliosis, typically progresses during skeletal growth, requiring regular radiographic monitoring. Adolescents and young adults with kyphosis should be referred to a spine specialist. Physical therapy is the mainstay of treatment.

STRESS FRACTURES

Definition/Etiology

Stress fractures occur when the repetitive forces or impact loading on a bone exceed available bone strength and health, rather than a single traumatic force causing an acute fracture. Stress fractures most commonly occur in the tibia and metatarsals, but are also found in the tarsal bones, femur, and pelvis. Spondylolysis of the spine is a type of stress fracture. Femoral and pelvic stress fractures can occur in AYAs who participate in endurance weight-bearing sports, such as running, or have energy or nutritional deficiencies. A heightened awareness for these injuries in exercising AYAs with eating disorders should prompt aggressive attention to any focal lower extremity bony discomfort.

Epidemiology

Stress fractures are a concern in athletes who participate in high-impact endurance activities, such as cross-country running[11,12] as well as in basic training for AYA military recruits. Stress fractures are more common in AYAs with a prior history of stress fracture and in females. Adolescents and young adults with decreased bone health from eating disorders or relative energy deficit, amenorrhea or oligomenorrhea, or other low estrogen states are at higher risk.[13–15]

Clinical Manifestations

1. History
   a. Insidious onset of aching discomfort without an injury, though the pain may worsen acutely over a few days.
   b. A gradual increase in pain with symptoms progressing from discomfort during/after activity to discomfort with walking or at rest
   c. When severe, a dull aching pain at rest, such as laying down at night
   d. A history of increased activity or prolonged activity in a state of relative energy deficiency, including in disordered eating
2. Physical Examination
   a. Pain may occur with direct bony palpation of the involved anatomic area, although pain is sometimes diffuse and difficult to localize at the pelvis and femur.
   b. Pain with ROM or strength testing may be present.
   c. Focal pain elicited with a single leg hop test can localize the area of concern and is used to monitor clinical improvement over time.

Diagnosis

The diagnosis of a stress fracture can be made clinically. The role of imaging is to rule out other insidious bony conditions, confirm anatomic location, grade severity, and evaluate healing. Within the first month of pain from a stress fracture, x-rays may be normal because no bony healing callous is yet apparent. If early imaging is necessary to confirm a stress fracture, noncontrast MRI should be considered.

Treatment

1. The primary treatment of stress fractures is rest of the involved anatomic structure from impact loading to provide time for healing. If lower extremity, the patient must limit running, jumping, and high-impact activities. Many stress fractures can be treated with time and rest alone.
2. If pain is present with weight-bearing or the patient has a limp, the patient should use crutches or a walking boot until they can walk without pain.
3. If the patient has adequate nutrition and energy availability and is able to ambulate without pain, they can be advised to cross-train in nonimpact activities that do not cause discomfort.

4. Concurrent with treatment for stress fracture, the clinician should address possible risk factors associated with stress fracture: nutritional energy deficiencies, training changes, low bone density, oligomenorrhea/amenorrhea.
5. Often, successful treatment of stress fractures in energy deficiency requires involvement of a multidisciplinary team including physician, athletic trainer or physical therapist, dietitian, and sometimes therapist or psychiatrist.

Prognosis

The prognosis of most stress fractures is good as these injuries heal with rest, time, and attention to risk factors. However, the healing process can take several weeks or months, especially among AYAs with underlying risk factors, and injuries can be recurrent.

High-risk stress fractures are a subset of stress fractures that are at risk for progression to complete fracture, prolonged recovery, or nonunion, including those in the femoral neck (tension side), patella, anterior tibia, talus, tarsal navicular, proximal fifth metatarsal, great toe sesamoids, and medial malleolus.[16] Adolescents and young adults with high-risk stress fractures should be treated with crutches initially and referred to a specialist who can guide AYAs through the healing process.

THE CORE

The core refers to a diverse group of centrally located muscles that provide stabilization of the extremities (Table 22.6). Strengthening core muscles requires intentional exercise and is important for both injury prevention and rehabilitation. Relative deficiencies in core muscle strength can contribute to movement patterns responsible for more distal injuries and overuse pains. Common core strengthening exercises are listed in Table 22.6.

SUMMARY

Many AYAs seek medical care within the medical home for musculoskeletal injuries and pain. Clinicians who care for AYAs can develop a standard approach to the history and physical examination for

TABLE 22.6

The Core: Muscle Groups That Contribute to Core Stabilization and Common Core Strengthening Exercises

Muscle Groups That Contribute to Core Stabilization	Core Strengthening Exercises
Abdominal muscles	Curl-up (abdominal crunch)
External obliques	Dead bug (supine alternating hand to knee)
Internal obliques	Pelvic tilt
Rectus abdominis	Plank
Transversus abdominis	Plank clam shell
Back muscles	Prone hip extension
Erector spinae	Prone superman (hip and shoulder extension)
Hip muscles	Prone swimmer (alternating hip and shoulder extension)
Gluteus minimums	Quadrupled alternating arms
Gluteus medius	Quadrupled alternating legs
Tensor fascia latae	Quadrupled alternating arms and legs (bird dog)
	Side plank
	Side-lying clam shell
	Side-lying hip abduction
	Sit-up
	Supine hip bridge
	Supine single-leg hip bridge

evaluation of these concerns. Many musculoskeletal conditions are treated with conservative measures. However, if AYAs are not improving as expected with initial treatments, or if the diagnosis is uncertain, they should be referred to a sports medicine or orthopedic specialist. It is important to ensure AYAs with musculoskeletal concerns have proper rehabilitation and return to prior functional status to facilitate participation in physical activities that are often a source of physical, emotional, and social well-being.

⬤ ACKNOWLEDGMENT

The authors wish to acknowledge Blaise A. Nemeth for his contributions to previous versions of this chapter.

REFERENCES

1. Patel DR, Yamasaki A, Brown K. Epidemiology of sports-related musculoskeletal injuries in young athletes in United States. *Transl Pediatr.* 2017;6(3):160–166.
2. Tiemstra JD. Update on acute ankle sprains. *Am Fam Physician.* 2012;85(12):1170–1176.
3. Doherty C, Delahunt E, Caulfield B, et al. The incidence and prevalence of ankle sprain injury: a systematic review and meta-analysis of prospective epidemiological studies. *Sports Med.* 2014;44(1):123–140.
4. Gould SJ, Cardone DA, Munyak J, et al. Sideline coverage: when to get radiographs? A review of clinical decision tools. *Sports Health.* 2014;6(3):274–278.
5. Crossley KM, Stefanik JJ, Selfe J, et al. 2016 Patellofemoral pain consensus statement from the 4th International Patellofemoral Pain Research Retreat, Manchester. Part 1: terminology, definitions, clinical examination, natural history, patellofemoral osteoarthritis and patient-reported outcome measures. *Br J Sports Med.* 2016;50(14):839–843.
6. Gaitonde DY, Ericksen A, Robbins RC. Patellofemoral pain syndrome. *Am Fam Physician.* 2019;99(2):88–94.
7. Yang S, Werner BC, Singla A, et al. Low back pain in adolescents: a 1-year analysis of eventual diagnoses. *J Pediatr Orthop.* 2017;37(5):344.
8. Hresko MT. Clinical practice. Idiopathic scoliosis in adolescents. *N Engl J Med.* 2013;368(9):834–841.
9. Labelle H, Richards SB, De Kleuver M, et al. Screening for adolescent idiopathic scoliosis: an information statement by the Scoliosis Research Society International Task Force. *Scoliosis.* 2013;8(1):17.
10. Weinstein SL, Dolan LA, Wright JG, et al. Effects of bracing in adolescents with idiopathic scoliosis. *N Engl J Med.* 2013;369(16):1512–1521.
11. Changstrom, BG, Brou L, Khodaee M. Epidemiology of stress fracture injuries among US high school athletes, 2005–2006 through 2012–2013. *Am J Sports Med.* 2015;43(1):26–33.
12. Rizzone KH, Ackerman KE, Roos KG, et al. The epidemiology of stress fractures in collegiate student-athletes, 2004–2005 through 2013–2014 academic years. *J Athl Train.* 2017;52(10):966–975.
13. Joy E, De Souza MJ, Nattiv A, et al. 2014 Female Athlete Triad coalition consensus statement on treatment and return to play of the female athlete triad: 1st international conference held in San Francisco, California, May 2012 and 2nd international conference held in Indianapolis, Indiana, May 2013. *Br J Sports Med.* 2014;48(4):289.
14. Mountjoy M, Sundgot-Borgen J, Burke L, et al. The IOC consensus statement: beyond the Female Athlete Triad–Relative Energy Deficiency in Sport (RED-S). *Br J Sports Med.* 2014;48:491–497.
15. Tenforde AS. Carlson JL, Chang A, et al. Association of the Female Athlete Triad risk assessment stratification to the development of bone stress injuries in collegiate athletes. *Am J Sports Med.* 2017;45(2):302–310.
16. McInnis KC, Ramey LN. High-risk stress fractures: diagnosis and management. *PM R.* 2016;8(3 Suppl):S113–S1124.

🛜 ADDITIONAL RESOURCES AND WEBSITES

Additional Resources and Websites for Clinicians:
Care of the Young Athlete, 2nd Edition—an encyclopedic reference of conditions common to athletes focused on children and adolescents, published jointly by the American Academy of Pediatrics (AAP) and American Academy of Orthopedic Surgeons (AAOS).
Essentials of Musculoskeletal Care, 5th Edition—a comprehensive, practical guide to the diagnosis and treatment of orthopedic problems encountered in primary care practice, published by the AAOS.
The 5-Minute Sports Medicine Consult Premium, 3rd Edition—quick reference for diagnosis and treatment of common musculoskeletal conditions in alphabetical order, with optional online access, with optional online access.
Orthobullets.com—an orthopedic learning and collaboration community for physicians—https://www.orthobullets.com/
Pediatric Orthopaedics and Sports Injuries, 2nd Edition—a quick reference guide of common pediatric orthopedic conditions and injuries, published by the AAP.
Sports Medicine in the Pediatric Office, by Jordan Metzl—a case-based text and DVD that demonstrates hands-on examination techniques.
The Sports Medicine Patient Advisor, by Pierre Rouzier—a thorough compilation of patient education materials including handouts with rehabilitative exercises for specific conditions.

Additional Resources and Websites for Parents/Caregivers:
The AAP Parenting Website—safety information for all ages, including for athletes and specific sports—https://www.healthychildren.org/English/Pages/default.aspx
Centers for Disease Control and Prevention. Child Safety and Injury Prevention—Sports Safety—https://www.cdc.gov/safechild/sports_injuries/index.html
OrthoInfo—American Academy of Orthopaedic Surgeons resources for patients to manage bone and joint health—https://orthoinfo.org
The Sports Medicine Patient Advisor, by Pierre Rouzier—a thorough compilation of patient education materials including handouts with rehabilitative exercises for specific conditions—http://www.sportsmedpress.com/
Stop Sports Injuries—resources to find a musculoskeletal specialist—https://www.stopsportsinjuries.org/STOP/Find_a_Specialist.aspx

Additional Resources and Websites for Adolescents and Young Adults:
The AAP Parenting Website—safety information for all ages, including for athletes and specific sports—https://www.healthychildren.org/English/Pages/default.aspx
Centers for Disease Control and Prevention. Child Safety and Injury Prevention—Sports Safety—https://www.cdc.gov/safechild/sports_injuries/index.html
OrthoInfo—American Academy of Orthopaedic Surgeons resources for patients to manage bone and joint health—https://orthoinfo.org/
Stop Sports Injuries—https://www.stopsportsinjuries.org/
TeenHealth—Sport Safety Tips—https://kidshealth.org/en/teens/#teenquiz

Guidelines for Promoting Physical Activity and Sports Participation

Ashley Rowatt Karpinos
Ashlee LaFontaine Enzinger

KEY WORDS

- Athletics
- Exercise prescription
- Injury prevention
- Medical eligibility
- Overuse injury
- Physical activity
- Preparticipation physical evaluation
- Safety
- Sports participation

INTRODUCTION

Physical activity (PA) and sports participation play an important role in the health and well-being of adolescents and young adults (AYAs). In the United States, it is estimated that up to $117 billion of health care costs and 10% of early deaths per year are related to inactivity.[1] Recent youth surveys show that adolescent participation in PA is at a record low. Up to 15% of youth report not being active for at least 1 hour on any day the prior week and only about a quarter are meeting current exercise recommendations.[2,3] This is concerning considering that activity levels tend to decline as age increases and nations reporting the lowest levels of PA have the highest rates of individuals affected by overweight and obesity.[1]

Creating positive activity-related habits at a young age provides numerous physical, cognitive, and psychosocial health benefits through adulthood.[1,3] Clinicians have an important role in encouraging healthy PA while minimizing the associated risks. This includes screening for activity deficiency, identifying barriers to participation, performing a thorough evaluation prior to sports clearance, and providing individualized injury prevention and PA recommendations. A primary goal of clinicians should be promoting PA to meet the objectives set forth by the U.S. government's Healthy People 2030 initiative.[4]

PHYSICAL ACTIVITY AND SPORTS

Physical activity is defined as any movement that requires energy. Exercise is usually a planned set of movements to reach a certain physical fitness (PF). Sport is some amount of PA or exercise that follows a set of rules, is competition based, and performed by an individual or a team. Sport includes PA used as training toward a specific goal or skill set. Physical fitness is the ability to perform exercise without extreme fatigue and with enough energy left to perform daily activities. As PA increases, PF and its health benefits increase. Physical fitness includes five main components:
- Cardiorespiratory fitness—activity for long periods of time (endurance or aerobic power)
- Musculoskeletal fitness—muscle strength, endurance (includes bone health and strength)

- Flexibility—range of motion (ROM) of joints or groups of joints
- Balance—maintaining equilibrium while stationary or moving
- Speed of movement—agility or ability to move the body quickly

Physical activity can be described by different degrees of intensity—light, moderate, or vigorous—depending on the level of energy expended, as measured by a metabolic equivalent of task (MET). For example, 1 MET would be the energy used while sitting at rest. Sedentary activity is waking activity using less than 1.5 MET while sitting or reclining (e.g., screen time). Light activity is nonsedentary activity less than 3 MET, such as walking, cooking, or household chores. Moderate activity is 3 to 6 MET, such as brisk walking or yard work, and should increase breathing, sweating, and heart rate (HR). Vigorous activity is 6 MET or more, such as running, stairs, or biking, and significantly increases breathing, HR, and sweating.[1] Most exercise recommendations target levels of moderate to vigorous physical activity (MVPA).

EPIDEMIOLOGY OF PHYSICAL ACTIVITY AND SPORTS PARTICIPATION

Among AYAs, the lowest rates of participation can be found in adolescent girls, youth with special health care needs, historically marginalized populations, and those with low socioeconomic status. Activity decreases in these groups with increasing age.[2,3] The 2019 Youth Risk Behavior Survey of U.S. high school students reported only 23% being active at daily recommended activity levels. Just under 50% reported muscle strengthening at least 3 days per week and 16% met the current aerobic and strengthening guidelines. About one in four report doing physical education (PE) 5 days per school week, and a little over half played on at least one sports team. These self-reported levels fall short of the 2020 Healthy People Goals for PA, which are set each decade to promote better population health, fitness, and quality of life. From 2011 to 2019, overall levels of aerobic and strengthening activity in adolescents had a significant linear decline with no change in PE (except for a decrease among females) or sports participation.[3]

The 2017 U.S. Bureau of Labor Statistics reports only about 18% of people age 15 and older being active on any given day. Of those being active, walking (30%) was the most popular, followed by lifting weights (9.1%), using cardiovascular equipment (9.1%), and running (8.6%). Adolescents and young adults aged 15 to 24 years were more likely to participate in team sports than individual activities. Males were more likely to engage in sports like football, basketball, soccer, and golf whereas females were more likely to do yoga or aerobic activities.[5] Interestingly, many adolescents may overreport their level of activity, with some studies using objective measurements of PA finding that only 8% meet current recommendations for daily exercise.[1,2]

TABLE 23.1

Recommendations for Physical Activity[1]

	Ages 6–17 y	Adults 18 y or Older
Aerobic[a]	60 min/d MVPA	150 min/wk moderate or 75 min/wk vigorous or equal combo
Muscle/Bone strengthening[b]	3 d/wk	2 d/wk
Additional benefits	Fun, appropriate for skill level/age, variety of body movements	>300 min/wk moderate or 150 min/wk vigorous

MVPA, moderate to vigorous physical activity.
[a]Done in one session or bouts of 8–10 min spread during the day or week.
[b]Can be incorporated into aerobic activity.

RECOMMENDATIONS FOR PHYSICAL ACTIVITY

Current PA recommendations in the United States were set by the 2018 Physical Activity Guidelines and are supported by the American Academy of Pediatrics (AAP), American Academy of Family Medicine (AAFP), American Medical Society for Sports Medicine (AMSSM), American College of Sports Medicine (ACSM), American Orthopedic Society for Sports Medicine (AOSSM), American Osteopathic Academy of Sports Medicine (AOASM), and the U.S. Centers for Disease Control and Prevention (CDC).[1] These recommendations highlight aerobic activity levels (Table 23.1).

Resistance Training and Flexibility

Strength training starts with no-load or body weight resistance exercises focusing on all major muscle groups and increases gradually once proper technique is learned. It is ideal to perform 8 to 15 repetitions in 2 to 3 sets, or to the point it is difficult to do another repetition, known as muscle fatigue.[1,2] Using lighter weights at higher repetitions increases muscle endurance. Using heavier weights with lower repetitions increases strength. Proper lifting technique is characterized by a slow, continuous speed through a full muscle ROM. It is important to use well-maintained equipment, appropriate protective devices, a reasonable starting weight, and supervision by a qualified professional. Recently, the AAP changed its position on one-repetition maximum (1RM) lifting in adolescents, to include that 1RM has been shown to be a safe and effective method of assessing strength and guiding training programs if done with proper technique monitored closely by a qualified professional.[6,7]

Flexibility exercises are also an important part of training. Although there are insufficient data to recommend for or against routine stretching, it can be of help for some AYAs dealing with prior injury or musculoskeletal issues (e.g., Osgood–Schlatter Disease). Flexibility is attained through smooth, slow stretching of all major joints or musculotendinous areas, holding positions for at least 20 to 30 seconds at a time. Stretching can count toward daily activity goals and be included in warm-up and cool-down periods that protect against injury.[1]

Additional Types of Activity

Recent studies show that high-intensity interval training (HIIT) may provide similar or greater cardiovascular benefit than MVPA and can be encouraged in certain populations as an alternative activity. High-intensity interval training includes short bursts of maximal training effort alternating with lower-intensity periods of recovery. This type of training can increase insulin sensitivity, decrease blood pressure (BP), and improve body composition in adults. High-intensity interval training provides greater cardiovascular benefits

for individuals living with overweight, obesity, or at risk for type 2 diabetes or cardiovascular disease than for healthy adults with normal weight.[1] However, it should be used with caution in those with underlying medical conditions and level of intensity should be increased gradually.

Electronic active gaming has become an increasingly popular means of activity with the development of interactive video games. Although active gaming can include short periods of MVPA, it primarily involves light activity. Electronic active gaming should not replace regular PA as it is not known if gaming can help individuals reach activity goals or provide health benefits. Adolescents and young adults spend, on average, more than 7 hours per day (or 55% of waking time) sedentary or using screens. It is still important to limit total screen time, including gaming, to less than 2 hours per day in favor of regular exercise, sports participation, social interactions, structured daily routines, and adequate sleep.[1,2]

CLINICIANS' ROLES IN PROMOTING PHYSICAL ACTIVITY

Obesity is a global health crisis with rates increasing over the past few decades as activity levels have decreased.[2] One in five adolescents live with obesity and/or prediabetes, which increases the risk of developing type 2 diabetes and cardiovascular disease.[3] In AYAs, inactivity is a predictor of poor health as well as future alcohol and drug use. In adults, inactivity is associated with increased cardiovascular disease, cancer, diabetes, and all-cause mortality. Regular exercise is central to improving overall health and preventing disease.[1,2]

Benefits of Physical Activity

Moderate to vigorous PA, including aerobic and strength training, has numerous health benefits:

- Decreased cardiometabolic risk factors with lower rates of early death, hypertension, stroke, heart disease, type 2 diabetes, and cancer
- Improved cardiovascular (aerobic) and muscular fitness, with increased muscle mass and strength, decreased body fat, and improved bone density
- Improved balance with decreased risk for falls or injury in the young and old
- Improved psychosocial and neurocognitive health: better focus and memory in students; improved energy, sleep, and quality of life; increased ability to plan, organize, and initiate tasks; better control of emotions and mental health; and decreased rates of fatigue, smoking, anxiety, and depression[1,2,8]

Studies show that youth living with obesity who exercise regularly have better glucose control, insulin sensitivity, and cardiorespiratory fitness. Many studies also show a positive effect on learning that may be dose dependent with academic performance improving as activity levels increase.[2] Benefits of PA can build within days to weeks of being physically active. Even one episode of MPVA can improve health. The largest gains occur in those who are inactive and become even insufficiently active, with more positive effects as activity increases. If levels reach at least 150 minutes per week, all-cause mortality can decrease as much as 33% compared to those who are inactive. These benefits are widespread despite age, sex, race, ethnicity, or current weight.[1]

Barriers and Predictors of Participation

Adolescence and young adulthood are important life transition periods with possible barriers to PA. Barriers may include increased workloads and decreased time, opportunities, energy, or motivation. However, there are no data to support that PA has negative effects on schoolwork. Other barriers include the baseline high levels of inactive or insufficiently active AYAs and the lack of knowledge of the PA guidelines by some clinicians. Typical AYAs are more likely to participate in diverse activities that are interesting to them, less competitive, and enjoyed with friends. The strongest predictors for participating in and maintaining PA include favorable attitudes toward exercise or sports, awareness of benefits, individual motivation, good body image, perceived competence in the activity, accessibility, enjoyment, and influence from friends, family, and PE teachers.[2,4] An understanding of motivators and barriers may be helpful for clinicians as they make recommendations to AYAs.

Puberty and Bone Maturation

Because of musculoskeletal changes that occur during puberty, adolescent athletes warrant special attention. Rapid increases in height and weight amplify injury risk in contact and collision sports (e.g., concussion) due to increased force of impact from higher speed and body mass (Table 23.2). Flexibility is relatively decreased in puberty, as bone grows faster than soft tissues. Decreased flexibility coupled with increases in muscle mass and strength may lead to bony avulsions or stress injuries of the comparatively weak growing bone and growth plates. Once athletes reach skeletal maturity, tendon or ligamentous injuries (e.g., anterior cruciate ligament [ACL] tears) become more common than the bone injuries seen in younger adolescents.

How to Promote Safe Activity

Since the greatest risk of injury or cardiac event occurs with sudden increases in activity level or intensity, AYAs who do not

TABLE 23.2

Sports Classified by Contact Level

Collision	Hitting or colliding with people or objects purposefully; usually using great force	Boxing[a], diving, gymnastics, ice hockey[b] (mens), lacrosse (mens), rodeo, roller derby, rugby, tackle football[c], water polo, wrestling
Contact	Contact occurs with people or objects; not purposeful and generally with less force than collision sports	Basketball, downhill skiing, field hockey, ice hockey (womens), lacrosse (womens), martial arts[d], snowboarding, soccer, ultimate frisbee
Limited contact	Unintended or infrequent contact; usually has rules to prevent contact	Baseball, bicycling, cross-country, fencing, flag/touch football, floor hockey, handball, horseback, martial arts[d], racquetball, skating, softball, volleyball
Noncontact	Rare or unexpected contact; usually rules do not allow any contact	Archery, badminton, bowling, dance, golf, jump rope, powerlifting/bodybuilding[e], riflery, running, sailing, swimming, tennis, track and field

Adapted from Council on Sports Medicine and Fitness. Medical conditions affecting sports participation. *Pediatrics.* 2008;121:841–848. Please see article for expanded list of sports.
[a]AAP opposes boxing for children and AYAs due to the risk of head and face injuries.
[b]AAP recommends limiting body checking in hockey for players aged 15 and under to reduce injuries. Body checking not allowed in women's hockey or women's lacrosse.
[c]AAP has no specific recommended age for tackling but emphasizes focus on proper technique and following rules.
[d]Martial arts has multiple forms, including judo, jujitsu, tae kwon do; some are contact and others are limited contact.
[e]AAP recommends limiting powerlifting and bodybuilding until adolescent sexual maturity rating 5.

exercise should begin with a low-moderate intensity, low impact, and low collision activity (e.g., walking on synthetic track, golf). Adolescents and young adults with concerns about PA should be encouraged to start by increasing general movement throughout the day. Any amount of PA is better than none and can still provide health gains.[1] Three 10-minute periods of exercise daily can provide similar benefits to a single, continuous 30-minute session.[8] A lifestyle approach promoting common activities such as dancing, yard work, stairs instead of the elevator, or parking further away from locations can increase activity safely among previously inactive AYAs. The activity should be fun and not feel like a burden or chore. The goal should be intensity that is at least moderate (able to talk but not sing) or vigorous (only able to say a few words before needing to take a breath or stop talking) and should include a variety of exercise types.[1] Counsel AYAs to increase activity gradually, always warm-up and cool-down, stretch frequently, allow proper recovery times, listen to their bodies, avoid exercise when ill, and seek medical evaluation if they have concerns. Starting with reasonable and attainable goals helps build confidence, supports long-term adherence, and protects from injury.[8] For AYAs working to increase PA, limit increases to 10% per week and recommend 1 to 2 days of rest between strengthening sessions. Exercise should be gradually increased in the following order (maximize each step before going to the next)[6,8]:
1. Frequency of activity (days/week)
2. Time of activity (duration of exercise sessions)
3. Intensity of activity (from low-moderate intensity) to meet desired goals

Practical Guidance for Clinicians

Developing healthy habits at a young age leads to better outcomes as an adult. Early, diverse, and positive PA experiences increase the likelihood that AYAs will adopt and maintain a healthy lifestyle. A thorough explanation of PA benefits may foster the AYA's interest. Studies in adults show that PA counseling by a clinician who uses an exercise referral system (such as an exercise prescription) can increase rates of activity for up to 12 months. Physical therapy, athletic trainers, exercise specialists, physiatrists, sports medicine physicians, recreational departments, PE teachers, electronic applications, or free online fitness videos may be helpful in sustaining PA among AYAs. Simply encouraging adolescents to actively participate in PE at school can meet up to 40% of their daily PA goal.[3] Including family members in counseling also increases positive attitudes toward PA. Parents can help by role modeling and providing financial or transportation support.

WRITING AN EXERCISE PRESCRIPTION

An exercise prescription creates an individualized and specific exercise routine that is safe for the patient based on their activity preference, current fitness level, and health goals. Exercise prescriptions can improve a patient's physical literacy and help them to feel confident and competent with PA, which improves initiation of and adherence to activity. Like a medication prescription (that includes dose, frequency, and duration), exercise prescriptions are a type of treatment safer than most medications and written using a comparable structure known as the FITT principle.[8] Written prescriptions for exercise should include recommendations for:
  Frequency—times per week
  Intensity—light, moderate, or vigorous
  Time—minutes per day
  Type—aerobic (walking, running), strengthening (weights), flexibility (yoga), varied (sport)
Studies show that patients are more likely to comply with activity recommendations if a prescription is written and/or if provided by a clinician who is physically fit themselves.[2,6,8]

Establishing a Baseline of Physical Activity

Clinicians should document time spent both in sedentary and PA behaviors and use the Physical Activity Guidelines[1] to classify their patients by current activity level:

- Inactive—no PA beyond the basic movements of daily life
- Insufficiently active—some MVPA per day but less than daily recommendations
- Active—meets daily target activity levels
- Highly active—exceeding the target range for daily activity

The ACSM Exercise is Medicine (EIM) initiative encourages all clinicians to document self-reported physical activity as a vital sign (PAVS) at every visit. In adult studies, integration of PAVS data into the electronic health record has led to improvement in weights in patients living with obesity, hemoglobin A1c in patients with diabetes, and PA-related counseling by clinicians.[2,8] Physical activity as a vital sign is defined as the number of days/week engaged in MVPA × time (minutes/day) = total minutes/week of MVPA.

Motivational Interviewing

Self-efficacy is vital to changing sedentary behaviors and creating positive PA changes over time. Motivational interviewing facilitates this process by determining the AYA's receptiveness to change, identifying barriers, and creating collaborative behavioral change strategies and goals. A precontemplative person who is not exercising or intending to exercise should have an assessment and documentation of barriers to PA. In addition, nonjudgmental support and education about the health benefits of PA should be provided. A contemplative or infrequently exercising AYA should be assessed for barriers to PA, receive counseling about realistic goals, and receive guidance in developing an initial exercise plan. An approach that encourages the AYA to maximize personal strengths can aid behavior changes. Adolescents and young adults in the action stage who are meeting goals should receive positive feedback and recognition for being self-motivated, which helps maintain PA levels.[6,8]

Creating an Action Plan for Physical Activity

1. Perform a thorough history and physical or use a recent Preparticipation physical evaluation (PPE) to identify safety risks and contraindications to immediate PA, such as exercise-related cardiac symptoms that may require further work-up or specialty evaluation (see the Preparticipation Physical Evaluation section).
2. Determine the preferred activity or exercise type (crucial to PA confidence and adherence).
3. Negotiate and agree on a PA action plan. Write the exercise prescription using the FITT principle (see Writing an Exercise Prescription). The prescription should be written to begin the initial activity at an acceptable minimum frequency and include suggestions for safe incremental increases. An exercise session includes[6,8]:
   - Warm-up period of lower intensity for 5 to 10 minutes. Helps to warm muscles, increase flexibility, and gradually increase HR and circulation.
   - Cardiorespiratory period of 20 to 60 minutes. Can include a nonaerobic activity, such as strengthening. There is little cardiovascular benefit after 30 minutes of aerobic activity and the risk for adverse events increases. Consider smaller, cumulative increments.
   - Cool-down period of lower intensity for 5 to 10 minutes. Helps gradually decrease HR and BP back to resting values and can include muscle strengthening or stretching.

Reaching Physical Activity Goals

An exercise prescription should include attainable metrics written with consideration of the AYA's short-term (e.g., initiating PA, increasing amount, involving others) and long-term (e.g., better

cardiovascular health, body image, or sports participation) goals.[8] Plan to review short-term goals at each visit with adjustments as necessary to meet long-term objectives. An insufficiently active person should increase MVPA slowly in small and fun ways to meet goals. Adolescents and young adults actively meeting goals can obtain additional health benefits from increasing activities safely. Adolescents and young adults exceeding daily activity recommendations should vary their exercise to decrease risk of injury. Activities can be diversified while maintaining fitness levels.[1,6] Some may prefer to exercise alone, especially initially. However, AYAs are more likely to sustain PA if they have a partner or external advocate. Establishing a support system, such as including parents in discussions, or encouraging small activity changes over time that progressively includes friends or family members can help AYAs reach and maintain goals.[2]

Evaluating Physical Activity Goals

Frequent reassessment ensures a safe progression to meet goals and allows for further guidance or referral if needed. There are three phases of exercise progression[6]:

1. Initial (4 to 6 weeks)—body acclimates to activity
2. Improvement (4 to 6 months)—increase in activity until desired level or health goal
3. Maintenance (> 6 months)—goals met, no increase necessary, vary PA and avoid burnout (see Sport Specialization)

At subsequent visits, clinicians should monitor the effects of activity. This may include changes in weight, BP, and mood, as well as an assessment for injuries.[1] Assess whether an individual is following the prescription safely and meeting goals. Use self-reported methods, which can overestimate actual levels, and/or objective measures (e.g., activity logs, pedometers, electronic applications, or other fitness trackers).[2] Give a new FITT-based exercise prescription at each visit geared toward reaching all goals. Adolescents and young adults are more likely to be successful and adhere to an exercise prescription when clinicians make reasonable suggestions to increase activity that fits into the context of current lifestyle and health status. Resources to aid clinicians include the *ACSM Guidelines for Exercise Prescription*. The EIM *Healthcare Provider's Action Guide*, free on the EIM website (www.exerciseismedicine. org), includes a step-by-step process to develop action plans with example prescriptions and patient and clinician handouts.

PREPARTICIPATION PHYSICAL EVALUATION

The Preparticipation Physical Evaluation (PPE), 5th Edition, or *The Monograph*,[9] is a collaboration of leading medical societies and is the definitive guide for clinicians who evaluate AYAs before training or competition. *The Monograph* is an essential tool for promoting the health and safety of athletes. Since the second edition in 1997, it includes the American Heart Association (AHA) and American College of Cardiology (ACC) recommendations concerning cardiovascular screening.[10] State laws determine which clinicians can legally perform the PPE, but any clinician who performs the PPE should be competent in screening athletes. While activity can be safely recommended for almost all AYAs, the PPE guides formal medical evaluation before PA.

Goals and Context of the Preparticipation Physical Evaluation

The goals of the PPE according to *The Monograph*[9] are to:

1. Screen for life-threatening or disabling conditions.
2. Screen for conditions that lead to injury or illness.
3. Establish adolescents without a primary care provider (PCP) or medical home into the health care system.
4. Assess general physical and mental health.
5. Promote discussions about general health and lifestyle concerns.

The AAP recommends an annual, comprehensive preventive health visit during adolescence. The PPE should be incorporated into this visit and conducted by the AYA's PCP within an established medical home. A group-based private station setup (several AYAs rotate through private stations receiving portions of the physical examination at each station) is a less desirable but acceptable alternative, especially when AYAs have no medical home or there are barriers to receiving medical care. Mass screenings in large rooms such as gymnasiums are not appropriate.

There is no evidence to guide the frequency of the PPE specifically, and state and organizational recommendations differ. The PPE is commonly incorporated annually at a preventive health visit as a periodic athlete health evaluation. There are many other essential components of a thorough preventive health evaluation that are not included in the PPE (see Chapter 5).

The Preparticipation Physical Evaluation History

The history detects about 75% of the medical and orthopedic conditions that are identified during PPEs. *The Monograph's* PPE History Form is shown in Figure 23.1. For adolescents younger than 18 years, the athlete and parent should complete the history form together. The clinician should confirm key written responses verbally.

The AHA/ACC recommended history for cardiovascular screening[10,11] is incorporated in the PPE history questions:
1. Family history of unexpected or unexplained death before age 35
2. Family history of a genetic heart problem
3. Family history of pacemaker or implanted defibrillator before age 35
4. Personal history of heart condition (murmur, hypertension)
5. Personal history of prior cardiac testing (e.g., electrocardiogram (ECG) or echocardiography)
6. Personal history of seizure
7. Personal history of syncope, near syncope, palpitations, excessive or progressive shortness of breath, or chest pain or discomfort, particularly with exertion

The remainder of the history should assess for:
1. Previous exclusion from sports for any reason
   Medical conditions (past and current) including recent illnesses (e.g., COVID-19, See section on Coronavirus Disease 2019 below), concussion and head injuries, sickle cell trait, missing organs (e.g., spleen, testicle, kidney)
2. Past and current musculoskeletal injuries
3. Past surgical history
4. Medications and supplements
5. Allergies
6. Symptoms of asthma, bronchospasm, hernia, skin conditions (e.g., herpes simplex virus [HSV] or methicillin-resistant *Staphylococcus aureus*), transient neurologic conditions, heat illness, or vision problems
7. Menstrual history in females
8. A history of weight concerns, rapid changes in body weight, dieting or food restrictions, and eating disorders
9. Anxiety and depression (Patient Health Questionnaire- 4 [PHQ-4] is a brief screening tool)

Positive responses to the screening history should prompt more in-depth evaluation. Though the goal of the history is to identify all conditions that confer unacceptable risk to participation, it is impossible to ensure PA participation without any risk even with a thorough history.

The Preparticipation Physical Evaluation Physical Examination

The PPE requires a directed physical examination to identify medical problems or deficits that could worsen an athlete's performance or health. *The Monograph's* PPE Physical Examination Form is shown in Figure 23.2.

Many conditions that significantly impact participation in sports, such as congenital heart disease and hemophilia, are identified in the preadolescent age-group and are not subtle. However, subtle presentations of congenital defects or acquired diseases may be initially detected during the physical examination. The most common abnormalities detected in the examination are abnormal visual acuity, high BP, and prior musculoskeletal injuries or deficits that have not been fully rehabilitated.

The physical examination should include assessment of the following:
1. Height, weight, and body mass index (BMI): Low BMI should prompt consideration of energy deficiency and eating disorders. High BMI should prompt discussion of the increased risk of heat illness.
2. Blood pressure and pulse: BP should be taken with a properly sized cuff while resting in a seated position and not talking (see Elevated Blood Pressure). Asymptomatic bradycardia in the 40- to 50-beats per minute range occurs commonly in the highly conditioned athlete and does not need an evaluation if asymptomatic.[12] However, bradycardia (with and without symptoms) may also be an indicator of energy deficiency and should prompt the clinician to evaluate for disordered eating and eating disorders.
3. Visual acuity and pupil equality: Adolescents and young adults with corrected visual acuity worse than 20/20 should be referred for evaluation. If corrected vision is worse than 20/40 in one eye, eye protection is encouraged (Table 23.3). It is important to document the presence of baseline anisocoria or other ocular defects before any closed head injury occurs.
4. Skin: Infections that are highly contagious (e.g., varicella, impetigo, HSV) should be identified. Athletes should not return to sports in which skin-to-skin contact is possible until they are determined to be noninfectious (see Table 23.3).
5. Teeth and mouth: Retrognathia is a stigmata of Marfan syndrome.
6. Cardiac examination includes AHA/ACC recommendations[10,11]:
   a. Perform precordial auscultation in supine and standing positions (or with Valsalva) to identify heart murmurs consistent with dynamic left ventricular outflow obstruction. Evaluate for the presence of murmurs, clicks, or rubs (see Chapter 19). Benign murmurs are characteristically low-intensity systolic murmurs that decrease in intensity from supine to standing. In contrast, if a murmur is present from hypertrophic cardiomyopathy (HCM), it is a harsh systolic ejection murmur that increases in intensity when the patient moves from squatting to standing position or with Valsalva.
   b. Assess femoral artery or lower extremity pulses to evaluate for aortic coarctation.
   c. Recognize the physical stigmata of Marfan syndrome including: hypermobility of the wrist or thumb (or both), pectus carinatum or excavatum, hindfoot deformity, facial features, skin striae, increased arm span to height ratio and reduced upper segment to lower segment ratio, or a murmur associated with mitral valve prolapse. The diagnosis relies on a set of defined criteria centered on the cardinal features of aortic root dilation and ectopic lens with family history and genetic evaluation.[9]
7. Abdomen: Adolescents and young adults with organomegaly should be withheld from collision/contact or limited-contact sports until definitive evaluation and individual assessment for clearance has been completed.
8. Genitalia: Routine examination is no longer recommended as part of the PPE unless there is a concerning history. Symptomatic hernias must be evaluated further prior to play. An undescended testicle is not a contraindication to contact sports; however, the athlete should wear a protective cup to protect

---

This form should be placed into the athlete's medical file and should **not** be shared with schools or sports organizations.

■ PREPARTICIPATION PHYSICAL EVALUATION

HISTORY FORM

Note: Complete and sign this form (with your parents if younger than 18) before your appointment.

Name: _____   Date of birth: _____

Date of examination: _____   Sport(s): _____

Sex assigned at birth (F, M, or intersex): _____   How do you identify your gender? (F, M, or other): _____

List past and current medical conditions. _____
_____

Have you ever had surgery? If yes, list all past surgical procedures. _____
_____

Medicines and supplements: List all current prescriptions, over-the-counter medicines, and supplements (herbal and nutritional).
_____
_____

Do you have any allergies? If yes, please list all your allergies (ie, medicines, pollens, food, stinging insects).
_____
_____

Patient Health Questionnaire Version 4 (PHQ-4)

Over the last 2 weeks, how often have you been bothered by any of the following problems? (Circle response.)

	Not at all	Several days	Over half the days	Nearly every day
Feeling nervous, anxious, or on edge	0	1	2	3
Not being able to stop or control worrying	0	1	2	3
Little interest or pleasure in doing things	0	1	2	3
Feeling down, depressed, or hopeless	0	1	2	3

(A sum of ≥3 is considered positive on either subscale [questions 1 and 2, or questions 3 and 4] for screening purposes.)

GENERAL QUESTIONS (Explain "Yes" answers at the end of this form. Circle questions if you don't know the answer.)	Yes	No
1. Do you have any concerns that you would like to discuss with your provider?		
2. Has a provider ever denied or restricted your participation in sports for any reason?		
3. Do you have any ongoing medical issues or recent illness?		
HEART HEALTH QUESTIONS ABOUT YOU	**Yes**	**No**
4. Have you ever passed out or nearly passed out during or after exercise?		
5. Have you ever had discomfort, pain, tightness, or pressure in your chest during exercise?		
6. Does your heart ever race, flutter in your chest, or skip beats (irregular beats) during exercise?		
7. Has a doctor ever told you that you have any heart problems?		
8. Has a doctor ever requested a test for your heart? For example, electrocardiography (ECG) or echocardiography.		

HEART HEALTH QUESTIONS ABOUT YOU (CONTINUED)	Yes	No
9. Do you get light-headed or feel shorter of breath than your friends during exercise?		
10. Have you ever had a seizure?		
HEART HEALTH QUESTIONS ABOUT YOUR FAMILY	**Yes**	**No**
11. Has any family member or relative died of heart problems or had an unexpected or unexplained sudden death before age 35 years (including drowning or unexplained car crash)?		
12. Does anyone in your family have a genetic heart problem such as hypertrophic cardiomyopathy (HCM), Marfan syndrome, arrhythmogenic right ventricular cardiomyopathy (ARVC), long QT syndrome (LQTS), short QT syndrome (SQTS), Brugada syndrome, or catecholaminergic polymorphic ventricular tachycardia (CPVT)?		
13. Has anyone in your family had a pacemaker or an implanted defibrillator before age 35?		

FIGURE 23.1 PPE History Form. (Used with permission from O'Connor FG. *ACSM's Sports Medicine: A Comprehensive Review.* Wolters Kluwer; 2012.)

BONE AND JOINT QUESTIONS	Yes	No
14. Have you ever had a stress fracture or an injury to a bone, muscle, ligament, joint, or tendon that caused you to miss a practice or game?		
15. Do you have a bone, muscle, ligament, or joint injury that bothers you?		

MEDICAL QUESTIONS	Yes	No
16. Do you cough, wheeze, or have difficulty breathing during or after exercise?		
17. Are you missing a kidney, an eye, a testicle (males), your spleen, or any other organ?		
18. Do you have groin or testicle pain or a painful bulge or hernia in the groin area?		
19. Do you have any recurring skin rashes or rashes that come and go, including herpes or methicillin-resistant *Staphylococcus aureus* (MRSA)?		
20. Have you had a concussion or head injury that caused confusion, a prolonged headache, or memory problems?		
21. Have you ever had numbness, had tingling, had weakness in your arms or legs, or been unable to move your arms or legs after being hit or falling?		
22. Have you ever become ill while exercising in the heat?		
23. Do you or does someone in your family have sickle cell trait or disease?		
24. Have you ever had or do you have any problems with your eyes or vision?		

MEDICAL QUESTIONS (*CONTINUED*)	Yes	No
25. Do you worry about your weight?		
26. Are you trying to or has anyone recommended that you gain or lose weight?		
27. Are you on a special diet or do you avoid certain types of foods or food groups?		
28. Have you ever had an eating disorder?		

FEMALES ONLY	Yes	No
29. Have you ever had a menstrual period?		
30. How old were you when you had your first menstrual period?		
31. When was your most recent menstrual period?		
32. How many periods have you had in the past 12 months?		

Explain "Yes" answers here.

_____

_____

_____

_____

_____

_____

_____

_____

_____

_____

_____

_____

I hereby state that, to the best of my knowledge, my answers to the questions on this form are complete and correct.

Signature of athlete: _____

Signature of parent or guardian: _____

Date: _____

© 2019 American Academy of Family Physicians, American Academy of Pediatrics, American College of Sports Medicine, American Medical Society for Sports Medicine, American Orthopaedic Society for Sports Medicine, and American Osteopathic Academy of Sports Medicine. Permission is granted to reprint for noncommercial, educational purposes with acknowledgment.

FIGURE 23.1 (*Continued*)

the other, descended testis. An evaluation for the undescended testis is necessary.

9. Sexual maturation rating: Sexual maturity rating is part of the adolescent physical examination but does not affect PA eligibility.

10. Musculoskeletal screening: General screening includes muscle and joint inspection, palpation, ROM, strength, and joint-specific special testing (see Chapter 22, Table 22.2). A more in-depth examination of the specific body parts, which can be found in *The Monograph* along with illustrations, should be performed if concerns arise from the history or screening examination.[9]

If the physical examination is abnormal, common conditions (listed in parentheses) should be considered:

a. Body symmetry:
   • Dressed in clothing for inspection of the body (such as shorts and a shirt), ask the AYA to stand with arms at the sides. Look for a head that is tilted or turned to side (cervical spine injury, muscle spasm), asymmetry of shoulder heights (trapezius spasm, neck or shoulder injury, scoliosis), enlarged acromioclavicular (AC) joint (prior AC joint sprain or "shoulder separation"), asymmetrical iliac crest heights (scoliosis, leg-length difference, back spasm), knee effusion (knee injury; see Chapter 22, Table 22.4), prominent tibial tuberosity (Osgood–Schlatter disease), or ankle swelling (ankle sprain not rehabilitated). Any swollen joint without prior injury or trauma should be evaluated for other etiology, such as overuse, inflammatory, neoplastic, or infectious conditions.
   • Ask the athlete to contract ("tighten") the quadriceps muscles and look for atrophy of the vastus medialis (any knee or lower extremity injury in which the athlete chronically avoids normal use of that leg).

b. Neck screening: This is especially important in players with a previous history of neck injury or brachial plexopathy (referred to as *stingers* or *burners*).
   • Have the athlete perform cervical flexion (look at the floor), extension (look at the ceiling), lateral rotation

This form should be placed into the athlete's medical file and should **not** be shared with schools or sports organizations.

■ PREPARTICIPATION PHYSICAL EVALUATION

PHYSICAL EXAMINATION FORM

Name: _____   Date of birth: _____

PHYSICIAN REMINDERS

1. Consider additional questions on more-sensitive issues.
   - Do you feel stressed out or under a lot of pressure?
   - Do you ever feel sad, hopeless, depressed, or anxious?
   - Do you feel safe at your home or residence?
   - Have you ever tried cigarettes, e-cigarettes, chewing tobacco, snuff, or dip?
   - During the past 30 days, did you use chewing tobacco, snuff, or dip?
   - Do you drink alcohol or use any other drugs?
   - Have you ever taken anabolic steroids or used any other performance-enhancing supplement?
   - Have you ever taken any supplements to help you gain or lose weight or improve your performance?
   - Do you wear a seat belt, use a helmet, and use condoms?
2. Consider reviewing questions on cardiovascular symptoms (Q4–Q13 of History Form).

EXAMINATION			
Height:	Weight:		
BP: / (/) Pulse:	Vision: R 20/ L 20/ Corrected: ☐ Y ☐ N		

MEDICAL	NORMAL	ABNORMAL FINDINGS
Appearance • Marfan stigmata (kyphoscoliosis, high-arched palate, pectus excavatum, arachnodactyly, hyperlaxity, myopia, mitral valve prolapse [MVP], and aortic insufficiency)		
Eyes, ears, nose, and throat • Pupils equal • Hearing		
Lymph nodes		
Heart[a] • Murmurs (auscultation standing, auscultation supine, and ± Valsalva maneuver)		
Lungs		
Abdomen		
Skin • Herpes simplex virus (HSV), lesions suggestive of methicillin-resistant *Staphylococcus aureus* (MRSA), or tinea corporis		
Neurological		

MUSCULOSKELETAL	NORMAL	ABNORMAL FINDINGS
Neck		
Back		
Shoulder and arm		
Elbow and forearm		
Wrist, hand, and fingers		
Hip and thigh		
Knee		
Leg and ankle		
Foot and toes		
Functional • Double-leg squat test, single-leg squat test, and box drop or step drop test		

[a] Consider electrocardiography (ECG), echocardiography, referral to a cardiologist for abnormal cardiac history or examination findings, or a combination of those.

Name of health care professional (print or type): _____   Date: _____

Address: _____   Phone: _____

Signature of health care professional: _____, MD, DO, NP, or PA

© 2019 American Academy of Family Physicians, American Academy of Pediatrics, American College of Sports Medicine, American Medical Society for Sports Medicine, American Orthopaedic Society for Sports Medicine, and American Osteopathic Academy of Sports Medicine. Permission is granted to reprint for noncommercial, educational purposes with acknowledgment.

FIGURE 23.2 PPE Physical Examination Form. (Used with permission from O'Connor FG. *ACSM's Sports Medicine: A Comprehensive Review.* Wolters Kluwer; 2012.)

TABLE 23.3

Medical Conditions and Sports Participation

Condition	May Participate
Atlantoaxial instability (instability of the joint between cervical vertebrae 1 and 2) Explanation: See Athletes with a Disability and Special Health Care Needs.	Qualified yes
Bleeding disorder Explanation: Athlete needs evaluation.	Qualified yes
Cardiovascular disease[a] Myocarditis Explanation: Carditis may result in sudden cardiac arrest with exertion. See section on Coronavirus Disease 2019 below (COVID-19).	No
Hypertension Explanation: See Elevated Blood Pressure.	Qualified yes
Congenital heart disease Explanation: Consultation with a cardiologist is recommended.	Qualified yes
Dysrhythmia Explanation: Consultation with a cardiologist is advised.	Qualified yes
Heart murmur Explanation: If the murmur is innocent (does not indicate heart disease), full participation is permitted. Otherwise, athlete needs evaluation.	Qualified yes
Structural/Acquired heart disease Hypertrophic cardiomyopathy Coronary artery anomalies Arrhythmogenic right ventricular cardiomyopathy Acute rheumatic fever with carditis Ehlers–Danlos syndrome, vascular form Marfan syndrome Mitral valve prolapse Anthracycline use Explanation: Consultation with a cardiologist is recommended. Most of these conditions carry a significant risk of sudden cardiac arrest associated with intense physical exercise. Hypertrophic cardiomyopathy requires thorough and repeated evaluations because disease may change manifestations during later adolescence. Marfan syndrome with an aortic aneurysm can also cause sudden death during intense physical exercise. An athlete who has received chemotherapy with anthracyclines may be at increased risk of cardiac problems because of the cardiotoxic effects of the medications, and resistance training in this population should be approached with caution; strength training that avoids isometric contractions may be permitted.	Qualified no
Vasculitis/Vascular disease Kawasaki disease (coronary artery vasculitis) Pulmonary hypertension Explanation: Consultation with a cardiologist is recommended.	Qualified yes
Cerebral palsy Explanation: Athlete needs evaluation to assess functional capacity to perform sports-specific activity.	Qualified yes
Diabetes mellitus Explanation: All sports can be played with proper attention and appropriate adjustments to diet (particularly carbohydrate intake), blood glucose concentrations, hydration, and insulin therapy. Blood glucose concentrations should be monitored before exercise, every 30 min during continuous exercise, 15 min after completion of exercise, and at bedtime.	Yes
Diarrhea, infectious Explanation: Unless symptoms are mild and athlete is fully hydrated, no participation is permitted, because diarrhea may increase risk of dehydration and heat illness (see Fever).	Qualified no
Eating disorders Explanation: Athlete with an eating disorder needs medical and psychiatric assessment before participation. See section on Eating Disorders and Energy Deficiency below.	Qualified yes

(*continued*)

TABLE 23.3

Medical Conditions and Sports Participation (*Continued*)

Condition	May Participate
Eyes One functional eye (best-corrected visual acuity worse than 20/40 in the poorer-seeing eye) Loss of an eye Detached retina or family history of retinal detachment at young age High myopia Connective tissue disorder, such as Marfan or Stickler syndrome Previous intraocular eye surgery or serious eye injury Explanation: An athlete who has lost an eye and/or who has only one functional eye would suffer significant disability if the functional eye was seriously injured. Specifically, boxing and full-contact martial arts are not recommended for these athletes, because eye protection is impractical and/or not permitted. Some athletes who previously underwent intraocular eye surgery or had a serious eye injury may have increased injury risk because of weakened eye tissue. Availability of eye guards approved by the American Society for Testing and Materials and other protective equipment may allow participation in most sports, but this must be judged on an individual basis.	Qualified yes
Conjunctivitis, infectious Explanation: Athlete with active infectious conjunctivitis should be excluded from swimming.	Qualified no
Fever Explanation: Elevated core temperature may be indicative of a pathologic medical condition (infection or disease) that is often manifest by increased resting metabolism and heart rate. Accordingly, during athlete's usual exercise regimen, the presence of fever can result in greater heat storage, decreased heat tolerance, increased risk of heat illness, increased cardiopulmonary effort, reduced maximal exercise capacity, and increased risk of hypotension because of altered vascular tone and dehydration. On rare occasions, fever may accompany myocarditis or other conditions that make usual exercise dangerous.	No
Gastrointestinal conditions Malabsorption syndromes (celiac disease or cystic fibrosis) Explanation: Athlete needs individual assessment for general malnutrition or specific deficits resulting in coagulation or other defects; with appropriate treatment, these deficits can be treated adequately to permit normal activities. Short-bowel syndrome or other disorders requiring specialized nutritional support, including parenteral or enteral nutrition Explanation: Athlete needs individual assessment for collision, contact, or limited-contact sports. Presence of central or peripheral, indwelling, venous catheter may require special considerations for activities and emergency preparedness for unexpected trauma to the device(s).	Qualified yes
Heat illness, history of Explanation: Because of the likelihood of recurrence, athlete needs individual assessment to determine the presence of predisposing conditions and behaviors. Develop a prevention strategy that includes sufficient acclimatization (to the environment and to exercise intensity and duration), conditioning, hydration, and salt intake, as well as other effective measures to improve heat tolerance and to reduce heat injury risk (i.e., protective equipment and uniform configurations).	Qualified yes
Hepatitis (viral) Explanation: See Blood-Borne Pathogens and Sports Participation below.	Yes
HIV infection Explanation: If viral load is detectable, then athletes should be advised to avoid high-contact sports such as wrestling and boxing. See Blood-Borne Pathogens and Sports Participation below.	Yes
Kidney, absence of one Explanation: Athlete needs individual assessment for contact, collision, and limited-contact sports. Protective equipment may reduce risk of injury to the remaining kidney sufficiently to allow participation in most sports, providing such equipment remains in place during activity.	Qualified yes
Liver, enlarged Explanation: If the liver is acutely enlarged, then participation should be avoided because of risk of rupture. If the liver is chronically enlarged, then individual assessment is needed before collision, contact, or limited-contact sports are played. Patients with chronic liver disease may have changes in liver function that affect stamina, mental status, coagulation, or nutritional status.	Qualified yes
Malignant neoplasm Explanation: Athlete needs individual assessment.	Qualified yes
Musculoskeletal disorders Explanation: Athlete needs individual assessment (see Chapter 22).	Qualified yes

TABLE 23.3

Medical Conditions and Sports Participation (*Continued*)

Condition	May Participate
Neurologic disorders History of serious head or spine trauma or abnormality, including craniotomy, epidural bleeding, subdural hematoma, intracerebral hemorrhage, second-impact syndrome, vascular malformation, and neck fracture Explanation: Athlete needs individual assessment for collision, contact, or limited-contact sports.	Qualified yes
History of concussion Explanation: Athlete needs individual assessment. See Sport-Related Concussion.	Qualified yes
Myopathies Explanation: Athlete needs individual assessment.	Qualified yes
Recurrent headaches Explanation: Athlete needs individual assessment.	Yes
Recurrent plexopathy (burner or stinger) and cervical cord neuropraxia with persistent defects Explanation: Athlete needs individual assessment for collision, contact, or limited-contact sports; regaining normal strength is important benchmark for return to play.	Qualified yes
Seizure disorder, well controlled Explanation: Risk of seizure during participation is minimal.	Yes
Seizure disorder, poorly controlled Explanation: Athlete needs individual assessment for collision, contact, or limited-contact sports. The following noncontact sports should be avoided: archery, riflery, swimming, weightlifting, power lifting, strength training, and sports involving heights. In these sports, occurrence of a seizure during activity may pose a risk to self or others.	Qualified yes
Obesity Explanation: Because of the increased risk of heat illness and cardiovascular strain, athlete with obesity particularly needs careful acclimatization (to the environment and to exercise intensity and duration), sufficient hydration, and potential activity and recovery modifications during competition and training.	Yes
Organ transplant recipient (and those taking immunosuppressive medications) Explanation: Athlete needs individual assessment for contact, collision, and limited-contact sports. In addition to potential risk of infections, some medications (e.g., prednisone) may increase tendency for bruising.	Qualified yes
Ovary, absence of one Explanation: Risk of severe injury to remaining ovary is minimal.	Yes
Pregnancy/Postpartum Explanation: See Physical Activity during Pregnancy.	Qualified yes
Respiratory conditions Pulmonary compromise, including cystic fibrosis Explanation: Athlete needs individual assessment but, generally, all sports may be played if oxygenation remains satisfactory during graded exercise test. Athletes with cystic fibrosis need acclimatization and good hydration to reduce risk of heat illness.	Qualified yes
Asthma Explanation: With proper medication and education, only athletes with severe asthma need to modify their participation. For those using inhalers, recommend having a written action plan and using a peak flowmeter daily. Athletes with asthma may encounter risks when scuba diving.	Yes
Acute upper respiratory infection Explanation: Upper respiratory obstruction may affect pulmonary function. Athlete needs individual assessment for all except mild disease (see Fever).	Qualified yes
Rheumatologic diseases Juvenile rheumatoid arthritis Explanation: Athletes with systemic or polyarticular juvenile rheumatoid arthritis and history of cervical spine involvement need x-rays of vertebrae C1 and C2 to assess risk of spinal cord injury. Athletes with systemic or HLA-B27-associated arthritis require cardiovascular assessment for possible cardiac complications during exercise. For those with micrognathia (open bite and exposed teeth), mouth guards are helpful. If uveitis is present, risk of eye damage from trauma is increased; ophthalmologic assessment is recommended. If visually impaired, guidelines for functionally one-eyed athletes should be followed.	Qualified yes

(*continued*)

TABLE 23.3

Medical Conditions and Sports Participation (*Continued*)

Condition	May Participate
Juvenile dermatomyositis, idiopathic myositis Systemic lupus erythematosus Raynaud phenomenon Explanation: Athlete with juvenile dermatomyositis or systemic lupus erythematosus with cardiac involvement requires cardiology assessment before participation. Athletes receiving systemic corticosteroid therapy are at higher risk of osteoporotic fractures and avascular necrosis, which should be assessed before clearance; those receiving immunosuppressive medications are at higher risk of serious infection. Sports activities should be avoided when myositis is active. Rhabdomyolysis during intensive exercise may cause renal injury in athletes with idiopathic myositis and other myopathies. Because of photosensitivity with juvenile dermatomyositis and systemic lupus erythematosus, sun protection is necessary during outdoor activities. With Raynaud phenomenon, exposure to the cold presents risk to hands and feet.	
Sickle cell disease Explanation: Athlete needs individual assessment. In general, if illness status permits, all sports may be played; however, any sport or activity that entails overexertion, overheating, dehydration, or chilling should be avoided. Participation at high altitude, especially when not acclimatized, also poses risk of sickle cell crisis. **Sickle cell trait** Explanation: Athletes with sickle cell trait generally do not have increased risk of sudden death or other medical problems during athletic participation under normal environmental conditions. However, when high exertional activity is performed under extreme conditions of heat and humidity or increased altitude, such catastrophic complications have occurred rarely. Athletes with sickle cell trait, like all athletes, should be progressively acclimatized to the environment and to the intensity and duration of activities, and should be sufficiently hydrated to reduce the risk of exertional heat illness and/or rhabdomyolysis. According to National Institutes of Health management guidelines, sickle cell trait is not a contraindication to participation in competitive athletics, and there is no requirement for screening before participation (outside certain organizations, such as the NCAA).	Qualified yes
Skin infections, including herpes simplex, molluscum contagiosum, verrucae (warts), staphylococcal, and streptococcal infections (furuncles [boils], carbuncles, impetigo, methicillin-resistant *Staphylococcus aureus* [cellulitis and/or abscesses]), scabies, and tinea Explanation: During contagious periods, participation in gymnastics or cheerleading with mats, martial arts, wrestling, or other collision, contact, or limited-contact sports is not allowed.	Qualified yes
Spleen, enlarged Explanation: If the spleen is acutely enlarged, then participation should be avoided because of risk of rupture. If the spleen is chronically enlarged, then individual assessment is needed before collision, contact, or limited-contact sports are played. See Mononucleosis.	Qualified yes
Testicle, undescended or absence of one Explanation: Certain sports may require a protective cup.	Yes

Adapted from Council on Sports Medicine and Fitness. Medical conditions affecting sports participation. *Pediatrics.* 2008;121:841–848.
NCAA, National Collegiate Athletic Association.
[a]Cardiovascular-specific considerations in the eligibility and disqualification of competitive athletes with cardiovascular abnormalities from the AHA/ACC are periodically updated.[15]

(look over the left and then over the right shoulder), and lateral flexion (put right ear on right shoulder, then left ear on left shoulder). Look for limited or asymmetric motion with these maneuvers (neck injury, congenital cervical abnormalities). Any athlete with limitation of ROM, weakness, or pain on neck examination should undergo further evaluation before engaging in sports.

c. Shoulder screening:
- Have the athlete raise the arms from the side and touch the hands above the head, keeping elbows extended (full abduction). Look for asymmetric shoulder elevation before arms reach 90 degrees (shoulder weakness, brachial plexopathy, impingement syndrome, shoulder instability) or inability to raise arms to full abduction position (shoulder weakness, brachial plexopathy, impingement, or apprehension from subluxation or dislocation).
- Have the athlete hold the arms in front of the body (forward flexion) and then to the side (90 degrees abduction); examiner should push the hands down. Look for asymmetric atrophy or fasciculations of anterior and middle deltoid muscles and pain and/or weakness (may be indicative of a variety of shoulder problems).

- Have the athlete put hands behind the head (maximal external rotation/abduction). Look for the inability to get hands behind the head (i.e., lack of external rotation of shoulder) or apprehension or inability to pull the elbows, symmetrically, posterior to the shoulder (anterior subluxation or dislocation). An athlete with limitation of ROM should be evaluated further before clearance is granted for participation.

d. Elbow and hand screening:
- Have the athlete extend and flex elbows with arms at 90 degrees abduction. Look for asymmetric elbow motion (prior dislocation or fracture, osteochondritis dissecans).
- With arms at sides and elbows flexed 90 degrees, have the athlete pronate and supinate forearms. Look for asymmetry (residual of forearm fractures, Little League elbow, osteochondritis dissecans of elbow). The cause of limited motion should be established before cleared for participation, especially in throwing sports.
- In the same position, have the athlete spread fingers and then make a fist. Look for lack of finger flexion, swollen joints, or finger deformity (residuals of sprains, fractures). Hand injuries should be evaluated and recommendations for sports participation should be based on the severity

of the injury and the specific sport. An athlete with evidence of prior fracture or tendon rupture complication should have further assessment before participation.

e. Back and leg screening:
- Have the athlete stand facing away from the examiner. Look for asymmetry of waist (scoliosis, leg-length difference) or increased lordosis (spondylolysis, tight hip flexors, weak hamstrings). Idiopathic scoliosis is not usually a contraindication for participation unless the angle is severe (i.e., Cobb angle >45 degrees).
- Have the athlete bend forward at waist/hips (lumbar flexion). Look for twisting or deviation of the side (paraspinous muscle spasm), asymmetric prominence of rib cage (scoliosis, Fig. 22.6), or inability to reverse lumbar lordosis (spondylolysis, muscle spasm caused by chronic inflammatory conditions such as ankylosing spondylitis).
- Have the athlete stand straight and rise onto toes. Look for asymmetry of heel elevation (calf weakness, restricted ankle motion from injury) or asymmetry of calf (atrophy from incompletely rehabilitated injury, neurologic condition).
- Have the athlete rise onto heels. Look for asymmetry of elevation of forefoot or toes (weakness of ankle dorsiflexors, limitation of ankle motion from ankle injury). If asymmetry on toe or heel raising is detected, further evaluation and treatment are indicated before the athlete is cleared for full sports participation.

f. Hip and knee screening:
- Have the athlete slowly assume a painless squatting position (buttocks on heels). If the athlete cannot do this, further evaluation is indicated.
- Ask the athlete to take four steps forward in this squatting position ("duck walk"), then turn 180 degrees in this squatting position and take four more steps. Look for asymmetric heel height off ground (limited ankle motion or Achilles tendon tightness from tendonitis or injury), asymmetric knee flexion, difference in heel-to-buttock height from the rear view, or inability to get down as far on one side as on the other (knee effusion, torn meniscus, quadriceps tightness, patellofemoral pain, Osgood–Schlatter disease). Pain at any point in the range of knee flexion should be evaluated for cause and rehabilitated before allowing return to participation without restrictions.

g. Ankle screening:
- Have the athlete hop five times as high as possible on each foot. Inability to complete this suggests an undiagnosed or unrehabilitated lower leg, ankle, or foot injury. The ankle should be evaluated and fully rehabilitated before full participation is allowed.

h. Core screening:
- Have the athlete stand on each leg individually and observe from behind for asymmetric drop in posterior superior iliac spine (weak core muscles).
- Have the athlete perform a single leg squat and look for instability or valgus knee positioning (weak core muscles, see Table 22.6, see Anterior Cruciate Ligament Injury Prevention).

Diagnostic Tests and Laboratory Evaluation

1. Hemoglobin and ferritin—Hemoglobin is recommended for athletes at risk of anemia. Ferritin can be helpful to assess iron stores (see Iron Deficiency and Anemia).
2. Electrocardiogram (ECG)—Not universally recommended for routine screening alone. Can be used if clinicians and health care systems determine benefit outweighs harm (see Sudden Cardiac Arrest).[13]
3. Vitamin D—Not routinely recommended unless at high risk for vitamin D deficiency (see Calcium and Vitamin D).

4. Sickle cell trait—Not routinely recommended unless athlete participating in National Collegiate Athletic Association (NCAA). Screening for Sickle cell trait is required by the NCAA due to a legal settlement though there are no data to support routine screening after the newborn period. Evaluation is included in newborn screening in all states.
5. Urinalysis—Not routinely recommended in asymptomatic athletes.

Determining Medical Eligibility for Physical Activity

The goal of the PPE is promotion of safe PA for all AYAs. After evaluation, the patient should be given one of the following recommendations documented on the PPE Medical Eligibility Form[9]:
1. Medically eligible for all sports without restriction
2. Medically eligible for all sports without restriction with recommendations for further evaluation or treatment of a certain condition(s)
3. Medically eligible for certain sports
4. Not medically eligible pending further evaluation
5. Not medically eligible for any sport

Recommendations for athletic participation are made according to available expert panel or evidence-based guidelines for participation with known medical conditions. The AAP guidelines on medical conditions affecting sports participation are detailed in **Table 23.3**. Detailed cardiovascular-specific considerations in the eligibility and disqualification of competitive athletes with cardiovascular abnormalities from the AHA/ACC are periodically updated.[11] These are guidelines and each AYA should be evaluated individually.

Only current myocarditis (See section on Coronavirus Disease 2019 below) and fever (within 24 hours) are specific reasons for strict immediate exclusion from all PA (see **Table 23.3**). However, many conditions may require temporary restriction for further evaluation or treatment. Clinicians should be comfortable recommending that athletes are not medically eligible pending further evaluation, regardless of how excited or concerned an AYA may be for immediate participation. Subspecialty evaluation is often indicated. If considering a recommendation that an AYA is not medically eligible for any sport, relevant specialty consultation is highly recommended.

Conditions leading to complete exclusion from sports are rare and the goal is to help all AYAs engage safely in physical activities. When AYAs are not medically eligible for a particular sport, alternative PAs should be offered. Assistive devices and accommodations should be explored (see Athletes with a Disability and Special Health Care Needs). When AYAs have medical considerations that require restrictions or qualifications to participate, these recommendations, including the risks and benefits of continued participation, should be discussed clearly with the athlete and, when indicated, the guardians. With a signed medical release, communication with the relevant organization or coach may be helpful. Athletes should be monitored for the physical and emotional effects of not being allowed to participate in the desired activities.[9]

Medical–Legal Issues in Exclusion from Sports Participation

A team physician and institution have the legal ability to restrict an AYA from participating in athletics if the decision is individualized, reasonably made, and based on competent medical evidence.[9] Athletes and their parents may seek to participate in a sport against medical advice, citing the Americans with Disabilities Act of 1990 or section 504(a) of the Rehabilitation Act of 1973, which prohibits discrimination against an athlete who is disabled if that person has the capabilities and skills required to play a competitive sport. All clinicians may not evaluate risk identically. However, courts have supported the decision of physicians, if the decision is based on sound medical judgment.[9]

Medical eligibility and athletic participation recommendations should be clearly documented and defensible using evidence-based or expert opinion guidelines and specialty consultation when needed.[9] The Monograph's Medical Eligibility Form[9] includes a specific statement that the athlete does not have any apparent clinical contraindications to participation as recommended. However, if conditions arise after the athlete has been cleared for participation, the physician may rescind the medical eligibility until the problem is resolved.[9] It may be helpful to include in communications that while reasonable medical standards indicate the AYA may participate, the AYA (and/or guardian) should consider the individual risks and benefits of participation and understand that a determination of medical eligibility is not a guarantee against future medical problems or adverse outcomes. Performing the PPE in the context of the medical home and established relationships often facilitates these communications.

Effectiveness of the Preparticipation Physical Evaluation

The PPE was not developed as an evidence-based process. More long-term studies are needed to assess the true efficacy of PPEs and the most beneficial way to apply them to the AYA population. For now, they can play an important role in the (1) routine and comprehensive health care of AYAs and (2) promotion of safe PA.

COMMON CONSIDERATIONS IN PHYSICAL ACTIVITY EVALUATION

Eating Disorders and Energy Deficiency

The PPE includes tools to screen for eating disorders and energy deficiency states. Athletes are at high risk to develop eating disorders and should receive appropriate treatment[9] (see Chapter 38). Some AYAs do not meet criteria for a diagnosed eating disorder but have energy deficiency states. The term Female Athlete Triad is a historical term that describes the negative effect of energy deficiency, with and without associated eating disorders, on bone health and menstrual function.[14] It is important for clinicians to recognize the physiologic changes of energy deficiency before the clinical outcomes of osteoporosis and functional hypothalamic amenorrhea are apparent. Relative energy deficiency in sport (RED-S)[15] is the newer term to describe the range of possible pathophysiologic effects that are seen in energy deficiency with PA, including impairments in menstrual function (oligomenorrhea, amenorrhea), bone health (stress fractures), metabolic rate, immunity, protein synthesis, and cardiovascular health (**Table 23.4**). Similar physiologic changes can occur in males and females with low energy availability.[15] Energy deficiency can also have negative effects on training and performance (**Table 23.4**).

Given the high levels of energy expenditure by some athletes, energy deficiency states can occur intentionally or unintentionally. Energy availability of 45 kilocalories per kilogram of fat-free mass (kcal/kg FFM) per day is optimal for health and a minimum of 30 kcal/kg FFM per day is needed to support normal menstrual cycles, bone health, and metabolism.[14,15] Thus, meticulous attention to energy balance and nutrition including total caloric requirements, macronutrients (carbohydrates, fats, proteins) and micronutrients (vitamins and minerals) is an important aspect of care for many athletes. However, it can be difficult for athletes to access the specific dietary resources needed to support high levels of PA. Many athletes only access dietary resources when pathophysiologic consequences of energy deficiency become apparent, such as through repeated stress fractures, secondary amenorrhea, or weight loss.

The PPE provides opportunities to evaluate energy deficiency and health consequences. Body mass index can be low or preserved in these states, and clinical assessment of other historical

TABLE 23.4

Potential Health and Performance Consequences of Relative Energy Deficiency in Sport (RED-S)

Potential Health Consequences from RED-S	Potential Performance Consequences from RED-S
Menstrual function	Decreased endurance performance
Bone health	Increased injury risk
Endocrine	Decreased training response
Metabolic	Impaired judgment
Hematologic	Decreased coordination
Growth/Development	Decreased concentration
Psychological[a]	Irritability
Cardiovascular	Depression
Gastrointestinal	Decreased glycogen stores
Immunologic	Decreased muscle strength

Adapted from Mountjoy M, Sundgot-Borgen J, Burke L, et al. The IOC consensus statement: beyond the female athlete triad–relative energy deficiency in sport (RED-S). Br J Sports Med. 2014;48(7):491–497.
RED-S, relative energy deficiency in sport.
[a]Psychological consequences can precede or result from RED-S.

elements, such as menstrual function, nutritional patterns, and stress fractures may aid in identifying athletes with low energy availability. Cumulative risk assessment and return to play guidelines can help determine PA participation levels. The RED-S Clinical Assessment Tool and the Female Athlete Triad Cumulative Risk Assessment are tools that may help clinicians evaluate risk and make return to play recommendations for athletes with energy deficiency.[14,16] Safe Exercise at Every Stage (www.safeexerciseateverystage.com) offers tools for guiding exercise during eating-disorder treatment.

The first-line treatment for energy deficiency is nutrition therapy to restore energy balance. Combined oral contraceptives are not recommended as a first-line therapy because they have not been shown to protect or improve bone health. Additionally, exogenous estrogen often results in return of menses which may be falsely interpreted by athletes as an indicator of menstrual health and energy availability. Transdermal estrogen has been shown to increase bone mineral density in adolescents with anorexia nervosa, although it does not result in complete catch-up of bone mineral density. Athletes who require contraception should be counseled in order to make an informed decision about the most appropriate method based on their individual circumstances (see Chapter 46). To improve bone health, energy and micronutrient intake should be optimized.[14,15]

A multidisciplinary team is helpful in the treatment of energy deficiency states in athletes and may include a primary care physician, team physician, dietitian, therapist, psychiatrist, athletic trainer, as well as family members and coaches. Treatment contracts can help athletes and treatment teams define shared expectations for treatment plans.[16] Clinicians can educate all athletes and families on the importance of optimal nutrition for health and athletic performance.

Cardiovascular Considerations in Exercise
Sudden Cardiac Arrest

A goal of the PPE is to identify cardiovascular conditions that predispose AYAs to sudden cardiac arrest (SCA). Exercise is a trigger for SCA. The estimated prevalence of sudden cardiac death (SCD) is 1.25 cases per 100,000 high school student athletes per year and 2 per 100,000 college student athletes per year.[9] The common causes for SCA in AYA athletes include HCM, myocarditis, coronary artery anomalies, arrhythmogenic right ventricular cardiomyopathy, dilated cardiomyopathy, long QT syndrome, Wolff–Parkinson–White syndrome, and aortic dissection. Atherosclerotic coronary artery disease is a cause of SCA starting at about age 20. Additionally, athletes may experience SCA without structural causes, in which case arrhythmias are the likely cause.

Careful attention to the personal and family history is essential during the PPE. The physical examination should include cardiac auscultation while the AYA is supine and standing (or with Valsalva maneuver), observation for stigmata of Marfan syndrome, and palpation of femoral pulses. An ECG can be used for screening if clinicians and health care systems determine the benefits outweigh the harms.[13] When screening ECG is used in trained athletes, specific guidelines for interpretation should be referenced.[12] Detailed recommendations for the eligibility and disqualification of competitive athletes with cardiovascular abnormalities are available through a series of specific task force recommendations.[11] Clinicians should consult this resource and specialists as needed to determine athletic eligibility for AYAs with cardiovascular conditions. Sporting organizations should have automatic external defibrillators (AEDs) and individuals trained in cardiopulmonary resuscitation (CPR) immediately available as these are the life-saving interventions needed to treat SCA.

Elevated Blood Pressure

Although clinicians may assume that athletes who regularly engage in aerobic activities have optimal cardiovascular health, high BP is the most common cardiovascular abnormality encountered at the PPE.

Physical activity is an effective nonpharmacologic treatment for elevated BP. Over time, routine aerobic activity lowers resting systolic and diastolic BP. Acutely, aerobic activity raises systolic BP while diastolic BP decreases or remains unchanged.

The definitions of normal BP and hypertension are listed in Table 23.5. Athletes with any abnormal BPs should receive further evaluation, monitoring, and treatment (see Chapter 20). Athletes with stage 2 hypertension or with end-organ damage should not be allowed to compete in competitive sports or high-static activities (e.g., weightlifting) until BP has been adequately evaluated and treated.[17]

When BP lowering medications are needed, angiotensin-converting enzyme inhibitors (ACE inhibitors) and angiotensin II receptor blockers (ARBs) are preferred in athletes who have no risk of pregnancy. Otherwise, calcium channel blockers can be used due to their neutral effects on training. Beta-blockers and diuretics should be avoided due to negative effects on cardiac output in training and because they may be banned in certain sports or organizations.

Micronutrients, Supplements, and Fluids

With attention to proper nutrition and fluid consumption, most athletes who are eating a well-balanced diet of sufficient calories should not require supplements. Athletes should pay particular attention to adequate intake of protein, iron, calcium, and vitamin D.[18] If recommended daily requirements cannot be met in the diet alone, supplementation may be needed (Table 23.6).

TABLE 23.5

Blood Pressure Categories in Adolescents and Adults

Blood Pressure Category	Adolescents >12 y Old and Adults
Normal	SBP <120 mm Hg and DBP <80 mm Hg
Elevated	SBP 120–129 mm Hg and DBP <80 mm Hg
Stage 1 hypertension	SBP 130–139 mm Hg or DBP 80–89 mm Hg
Stage 2 hypertension	SBP ≥140 mm Hg or DBP ≥90 mm Hg

SBP, systolic blood pressure; DBP, diastolic blood pressure.

TABLE 23.6

Daily Recommended Intake of Protein and Micronutrients in Athletes

Recommended Daily Intake	Children 9–18 y	Adults (19–50 y)
Protein	About 6-ounce equivalents of protein foods	Normal activity level: 0.8 g/kg[a] Endurance sports: 1.2–1.4 g/kg Strength and resistance sports: 1.6–1.7 g/kg
Iron	15 mg 12 mg	18–22 mg (females) 8 mg (males)
Calcium	1,300 mg	1,000 mg
Vitamin D	15 mcg (600 IU)	15 mcg (600 IU)

Recommendations are from American College of Sports Medicine, American Academy of Pediatrics, and U.S. Department of Agriculture, and U.S. Department of Health and Human Services.
[a]g/kg/day—grams of protein intake per kilogram of AYA body weight per day.
IU, international units; mg, milligram; mcg, microgram.

Iron Deficiency and Anemia

Iron deficiency is the most common nutritional deficiency in athletes, particularly in females with heavy menstrual cycles. Iron deficiency anemia can lead to decreased performance; therefore, treatment is recommended. In athletes with iron deficiency without anemia (normal hemoglobin and low ferritin), iron supplementation may improve measures of physical performance.[19] Thus, many athletes and coaches request assessment of anemia and iron status. It is reasonable to screen at-risk athletes for anemia and iron deficiency and recommend treatments to normalize iron stores to a minimum ferritin level of at least 30 to 50 ng/mL. Increasing dietary intake of iron is optimal and AYAs should be recommended to eat a diet high in iron (see Table 23.6). If supplements are used, oral supplementation every other day may be sufficient.

Calcium and Vitamin D

Calcium and vitamin D are important for musculoskeletal health. Adolescence is a critical period for increasing lifelong bone mineral density as peak bone mass is achieved in the early twenties. Accrual of skeletal calcium and optimal bone health during adolescence is important in the prevention of bone stress injuries, low bone mineral density, and osteoporosis. Calcium is best obtained through sufficient dietary intake (see Table 23.6); but in athletes with dietary intolerances or low intake, supplements may be needed. Vitamin D can be more difficult to obtain in the diet. Adolescents and young adults with malabsorption, obesity, bone stress injuries, or high dermatologic melanin may be at risk for vitamin D deficiency. When vitamin D levels are inadequate, supplements are indicated. Oral vitamin D supplementation is preferable to encouraging AYAs to seek more sunlight exposure. While ultraviolet (UV) rays from sunlight can activate vitamin D, UV exposure also increases the risk of skin cancer.

Supplements

Supplement use among athletes is common and knowledgeable clinicians can help guide AYAs in appropriate use. For the majority of athletes who can consume routine balanced meals, all nutrient requirements can be met through food. However, protein supplements (in recommended amounts) can be used safely in athletes with high training demands who are unable to consume adequate protein in their diet. Some caffeine can be used safely in training and competition for older AYAs, with careful attention to hydration and amounts allowed by specific sporting organizations. Energy drinks are not recommended.[20]

Some AYAs are interested in using supplements to enhance strength or performance. It is important that athletes be aware that most supplements are not approved by the Food and Drug Administration (FDA) and may contain unwanted substances. Resources such as National Sanitation Foundation International Certified for Sport®, ConsumerLab, and United States Pharmacopeia Verification can assist in determining more reliable sources for supplements, like protein and vitamins, when recommended. Taking banned substances, such as anabolic steroids, can have many negative health consequences. Additionally, some commonly prescribed medications, such as diuretics, are banned by many sports organizations. Clinicians should seek updated information on banned substances for athletes in specific organizations and advise athletes on substance use risks.

Fluids

Adolescents and young adults should maintain a status of euhydration with normal electrolytes before, during, and after exercise. Adolescents are more prone to dehydration than adults. Athletes should consume adequate fluids to slake thirst throughout the day. There is no benefit to hyperhydration for exercise, and this practice can lead to problems such as hyponatremia. The use of sports drinks can help with glucose and electrolyte balance but are usually not needed in shorter-duration exercise. Clinicians can advise AYA athletes that one gulp is typically equivalent to one ounce (oz) of fluids:

1. Before exercise—2 to 4 hours prior to exercise, consume 12 to 20 oz (5 to 10 mL/kg body weight) of water.
2. During exercise–consume 4 oz of water every 20 minutes. The goal is to replace fluids and electrolytes lost in sweat, so exact needs depend on sweat rates. For intense exercise over 1-hour duration, sports drinks may be needed.
3. After exercise—for most AYAs, recommend 8 to 20 oz of fluid after exercise. If athletes have at least 12 hours between training sessions, they can likely recover to a state of euhydration by drinking noncaffeinated beverages (water or milk) to thirst. If athletes are training intensely or multiple times daily, they need to actively consume hydrating beverages at a rate of 20 oz fluid per pound of weight lost. Intravenous fluids are rarely needed.

Mental Health Considerations

Athletes and physically active AYAs experience similar mental health conditions as their peers. While PA typically provides many positive mental health benefits, clinicians should recognize what aspects of sports participation may be contributing to mental health disorders. Some unique aspects of sports participation that may affect mental health include performance stress, body concerns (including sociocultural and sport-specific pressure to change body weight, shape, and/or appearance), overtraining and burnout, transition out of competitive sports, and injuries. Undiagnosed or untreated mental health issues can lead to unsafe behavior such as extremes of activity (overly sedentary or overtraining), poor adherence to treatment plans, unmonitored supplement or illegal substance use, or unhealthy weight control measures. In addition, the experience of a sport-related injury can unmask or trigger mental health disorders.[21] Screening for depression, anxiety, and eating disorders is part of the PPE. Treatment of mental health conditions for physically active AYAs is similar to that of the general population (see Chapter 74).

Sport-Related Concussion

Sport-related concussion is a traumatic brain injury induced by biomechanical forces from an athletic activity and are common in AYAs. Athletes should be screened for past concussions and counseled about the risks of concussion from athletic activities and concussion prevention and recognition. For most AYAs, sport-related concussion symptoms usually resolve within 2 weeks; however, younger athletes are at higher risk for prolonged symptoms.[22] Adolescents and young adults with sport-related concussion need to be followed by knowledgeable clinicians for guidance on rest, exercise, rehabilitation, return to educational activities, and return to sport. These AYAs can be cared for by knowledgeable clinicians within the medical home using clinical tools[22] or referred to medical specialists familiar with the care of sport-related concussion (see Chapter 24).

Attention Deficit Hyperactivity Disorder

Many AYAs with attention deficit hyperactivity disorder (ADHD) participate in a variety of PAs and exercise can have positive effects on ADHD symptoms.[23] If AYAs require treatment with stimulants, clinicians should pay careful attention to cardiovascular effects, weight maintenance, and temperature regulation. Medications may increase core temperature or delay a sense of fatigue and cause athletes to be more susceptible to heat illness. Adolescents and young adults with ADHD should undergo the standard preparticipation cardiovascular evaluation. Clinicians should counsel AYAs with ADHD about signs of medication side effects that may be enhanced by PA and monitor therapy regularly.

Some athletes may perceive that their athletic performance is enhanced with the use of stimulants. Care should be taken to ensure accurate diagnosis and management of ADHD in all AYAs. Clinicians caring for athletes with ADHD should be aware of potential regulations in ADHD management among sport governing bodies. For example, stimulants are banned by the World Anti-Doping Agency (WADA) and the International Olympic Committee (IOC). However, stimulants are permitted by the NCAA when athletes and clinicians are following specific guidelines for evaluation and management of ADHD. Stimulants are not specifically regulated in most youth sports.

Mononucleosis

Mononucleosis, or "mono," caused by Ebstein–Barr virus (EBV) or cytomegalovirus (CMV), commonly results in splenomegaly, which increases the risk for splenic rupture. Though splenic rupture is rare, it is a medical emergency. Splenic rupture can occur spontaneously, though the risk may be increased with a sudden increase in portal venous pressure such as with a Valsalva maneuver, PA, and direct trauma. About 74% of splenic rupture occurs in the first 21 days and 91% occurs within the first 31 days.[24] Consensus guidelines currently recommend individuals with mononucleosis avoid all PA for at least 3 weeks; however, restricting all PA for 31 days is a more conservative approach. To restart PA after mononucleosis, AYAs should be assessed for clinical improvement and absence of palpable splenomegaly before gradually restarting exercise. Given the risks associated with PA in undiagnosed mononucleosis, physically active AYAs and athletes with clinical syndromes suggestive of mono should be withheld from exercise until the diagnosis can be confirmed. Given the decreased sensitivity of the heterophile antibody "monospot" test during the first week of illness, viral titers can be helpful in the early diagnosis of athletes (see Chapter 33).

Blood-Borne Pathogens and Sports Participation

Human immunodeficiency virus (HIV), hepatitis B virus (HBV), and hepatitis C virus (HCV) are the blood-borne pathogens most relevant to PA. Exercise is beneficial to the health of AYAs living with HIV, HBC, and HCV.[25] Therefore, AYAs who are infected with blood-borne pathogens, including HIV, should not be restricted from routine participation. The risk of transmission during athletics is extremely low. There are no documented cases of HIV or HCV transmission during sports participation. There are reports of HBV transmission during physical activity, likely due to contact with open wounds from the carrier.

Universal screening for blood-borne pathogens is not specifically recommended before PA. All AYAs should be screened according to existing health guidelines for the general population. All individuals with open wounds should cover the wound properly with a sturdy occlusive dressing for the duration of PA. Prevention of infection should focus on immunization against HBV, universal precautions for care of bleeding injuries in athletics, and reduction of nonathletic associated risky behaviors in AYAs.

Coronavirus Disease 2019 (COVID-19)

The novel virus SARS-CoV-2 that emerged in late 2019 causing a global pandemic required clinicians to rapidly consider a new aspect of promoting safety and health in physical activities. Adolescents and young adults need to be advised on optimal measures to prevent viral transmission and infection during PAs. The safety of participation in group PAs depends on AYA's underlying medical conditions, local virus activity, and implementation of control measures, such as vaccination, physical distancing, masking, and ventilation.

The cardiac effects of infection by SARS-CoV-2, like other viruses, include viral myocarditis, which is a risk for SCA among exercising AYAs. As the global scientific community learns more about the important considerations of SARS-CoV-2 in PA, recommendations are updated regarding safety in sports participation during a pandemic, screening for coronavirus disease 2019 (COVID-19) during the PPE, evaluating AYAs for potential cardiovascular effects after COVID-19, and guidance for gradual return to exercise after COVID-19. Clinicians should be aware of current recommendations and practices for AYAs seeking advice on physical activities during each phase of the COVID-19 pandemic and after viral infections.

PROMOTING PHYSICAL ACTIVITY IN ALL POPULATIONS

Physical activity provides mental and physical health benefits. Promoting participation among AYAs can help develop healthy activity patterns and habits for a lifetime. Thus, informed policies can promote inclusion for all AYAs in structured PA opportunities regardless of gender, intellectual abilities, physical abilities, pregnancy status, and other considerations, except for rare medical exclusions.

Female Athlete

The institution of Title IX of the Educational Amendments Act of 1972, which requires that males and females in educational programs receiving federal aid have equitable opportunities to participate in sports, has led to higher rates of athletic participation among females. Females now account for almost half of high school and college athletes. Females should be encouraged to participate in PAs throughout all phases of the menstrual cycle. Clinicians should pay careful attention to evaluation of females' risk for ACL injury, concussion, joint dislocations, anemia, energy availability, and nutritional status.

Transgender/Nonbinary Athletes

Transgender and nonbinary (TNB) AYAs should be encouraged to participate in PAs given the physical and mental health benefits of exercise for all individuals. Sporting organizations are encouraged to actively promote inclusive and supportive environments for all AYAs to participate, regardless of their gender identity. Many elite level organizations have policies to help guide competition for TNB athletes receiving gender-affirming care.[9] However, in the United States, many youth, community, and high school organizations do not have established policies for these athletes. Clinicians may need to advocate for AYAs with all gender identities to be included fairly in PAs and sports.

Athletes with a Disability and Special Health Care Needs

Adolescents and young adults with physical and cognitive impairments should be encouraged to participate safely in physical activities for the mental, social, and physical health benefits that many AYAs experience. For athletes with certain disabilities, being physically active can also have unique health benefits. For example, rates of pressure ulcers, infections, and hospitalizations are lower for athletes with paraplegia when compared to inactive peers with paraplegia.[26]

Through the PPE, clinicians can provide specific guidance on safe activities and assess the need for accommodations. Clinicians should use the standard PPE Athletes with Disabilities Form: Supplement to the Athlete History.[9] The physical examination should include careful attention to ocular, cardiovascular, neurologic, dermatologic, and musculoskeletal function. Consultation with a physical therapist, physiatrist, or primary specialist may be needed.

A common consideration is atlantoaxial instability (AAI), which is more prevalent in Down syndrome (see **Table 23.3**). Though usually asymptomatic, athletes with symptomatic AAI need lateral cervical spine x-rays in flexion and extension to measure changes in the atlantodens interval and should be restricted from sports with excessive neck motion or impact. Some organizations, such as the Special Olympics, require that all athletes with Down syndrome competing in certain sports have a screening x-ray series for asymptomatic AAI. The PPE may not be able to be completed in a single office visit and AYAs with a disability or special health care need may require further specialty evaluation or rehabilitation before participation.[9]

Physical Activity during Pregnancy

Exercise during pregnancy can offer health benefits including decreased rates of gestational diabetes mellitus, preterm birth, and lower birth weight, as well as increased rates of vaginal delivery and shorter postpartum recovery times.[27] Exercise during the postpartum period can help to prevent depression.[27] Females who routinely engaged in vigorous-intensity aerobic activity or were physically active before pregnancy can safely continue those activities during uncomplicated pregnancies. Females who were not physically active before pregnancy should receive guidance about initiating and advancing PA.

Females should engage in at least 150 minutes of moderate-intensity aerobic activity spread throughout the week during pregnancy and the postpartum period.[1] High-risk PAs, such as scuba diving, alpine skiing, water skiing, and pole vaulting should be avoided in pregnancy. Organizations such as the NCAA, recommend an ethic of caring and inclusion for pregnant athletes. Females with pregnancy complications should receive individualized PA recommendations from their obstetric clinician.

INJURY PREVENTION

Sports Injury Epidemiology

In the United States, the most common activity associated with injury is general exercise.[28] The most common exercise-related injuries are musculoskeletal and occur in about 1/1,000 hours of walking and less than 4/1,000 hours of running.[1] Females tend to have more lower extremity (e.g., ACL, patellofemoral) and spine (e.g., spondylolysis) injuries. Males tend to injure upper extremities (e.g., Little League shoulder [overuse injury caused by stress to the humerus]). In 2015, there were 50 youth sport-related deaths. The most common medical cause of death was SCA, and the most common injury-related cause of death was brain trauma. The sport with the highest injury rate of 4.08 per 1,000 athlete exposures is American-style football.[28] Overall, the injury rate in all high school sports is relatively low at 2.32 injuries per 1,000 athlete exposures.[28]

Risk of injury or reinjury is highest among AYAs with (1) less PA and lower baseline activity levels, (2) sudden increases in activity level or intensity, and (3) a history of prior injury.[1,28] Risk increases as activity intensity, frequency, duration, training level, and contact level increase. Age, current fitness level, and experience play an important role in injury risk. Whereas AYAs can safely increase activity in small amounts every 1 to 2 weeks, older adults may need 2 to 4 weeks. Less fit people or those with prior injuries also require a slower rate of increase.[28] Due to the risk of head injuries, the AAP recommends against youth participating in boxing.

Sports Specialization

Sport specialization refers to intense training in a single sport to the exclusion of other athletic activities. A societal shift from attention to participation and fun in youth sports to a focus on early sporting success has led to a trend of more young adolescents specializing in sports. It is estimated that about one in five youth athletes specialize in a single sport by age 12 to 14 years.[29] Early sport specialization (before age 14 to 15 years) does not appear to be beneficial for achieving elite athletic status in most team sports, and those who participate in multiple sports through mid-adolescence are successful in a variety of sports. Early sport specialization may be beneficial for athletic success in a few individual sports with repetitive skills where peak performance occurs before puberty, such as figure skating and gymnastics.[29]

For most adolescents, sport specialization should be delayed until after puberty, into late adolescence. Clinicians should encourage young adolescents to participate in a variety of athletic activities they enjoy, rotating different sports throughout the year. Adolescents should not participate in multiple sports during the same season, or for multiple teams (school and community-based teams) concurrently. This approach may help prevent burnout, overuse injuries, and facilitate enjoyment of daily PAs as a component of lifetime wellness.

Burnout

Adolescents and young adults can experience burnout from sports participation as a result of chronic stress during activities, and burnout may lead to sport discontinuation.[30] Youth sport experiences should focus on healthy psychological development, physical development, targeted skill development, and appropriate training loads. The relationship between sport specialization and burnout is an area of active research. If youth do experience burnout from competitive sports, they should be encouraged to explore new PAs for the mental and physical health benefits.

Overuse Injuries

Repetitive activities and high training loads are risk factors for overuse injury. Overuse injuries are more common than traumatic injuries. Adolescents are at particular risk for overuse injuries during the period of maximal growth velocity. Sport specialization may be a risk factor for injury risk independent of training load.[29] Overuse injuries may cause some AYAs to discontinue athletic participation before adulthood. Along with prevention strategies, highly active AYAs who participate in vigorous PA more than 1 hour per day most days of the week should be encouraged to take one day of rest and recovery each week with several weeks of rest intermittently throughout the year.

Athletes participating in endurance sports and sports with repetitive motions should be counseled about overuse injury prevention. For example, overhead athletes (those who use upper arm and shoulder in an arc overhead such as pitching, volleyball, tennis etc.) and swimmers who are prone to shoulder injuries should be advised to engage in scapular strengthening exercises routinely (see Chapter 22). Some sports, such as youth running and baseball, have developed guidelines to reduce overuse injuries. While youth

baseball has formal guidelines for daily and weekly limits on pitch counts to reduce injury rates, athletes, families, and coaches do not always adhere to these guidelines. Though softball pitching is associated with injury risk, no guidelines for softball pitch counts have been developed. More evidence and education are needed to help prevent overuse injuries in AYAs.

Anterior Cruciate Ligament Injury Prevention

One of the most successful injury prevention initiatives is the development of proprioceptive and neuromuscular strengthening programs that decrease the risk of ACL rupture. Injuries to the ACL are more common in females and may be related to increased landing with valgus knee positioning and lack of hamstring activation. Prevention programs can decrease ACL injuries substantially and are among the most well-studied injury prevention initiatives for acute athletic injuries.

Anterior cruciate ligament injury prevention programs consist of proprioceptive and neuromuscular training, plyometrics, agility drills, functional balance, and core strengthening exercises (see Chapter 22) that should be integrated into exercise sessions by athletes and teams routinely. Several different ACL injury prevention programs have been developed and are recommended by the AAP to be used by coaches, teams, and athletes. Clinicians should advise athletes on the benefits of ACL injury prevention programs.

Equipment

Clinicians should encourage the use of recommended sport-specific safety equipment. Well-conditioned helmets decrease the risk of traumatic head injuries, though not concussions, in many sports. Eye protection and mouthguards decrease the risk of ophthalmologic and oral trauma, respectively. Shin, knee, wrist, and shoulder pads can decrease injury severity in blunt traumas. Chest wall protectors and safety balls help decrease the risk of SCA from chest wall blows (commotio cordis) in baseball and softball. Athletic cups are specifically recommended for athletes with a single testicle.

Guidelines and Rules

Adolescents and young adults should follow established conditioning guidelines and sport-specific rules. For example, athletes should gradually increase exercise in warmer environments for heat acclimatization to help prevent heat illness. Athletes should start exercise sessions with proper energy stores, stay well-hydrated throughout exercise (see Fluids), and follow ACL injury prevention programs (see Anterior Cruciate Ligament Injury Prevention). Adolescents and young adults should rest if they are nearing exhaustion or experiencing exertional cardiopulmonary symptoms. Coaches and athletes should be familiar with rules of specific sports and proper technique to help prevent injury. For example, American-style football athletes should follow recommendations for proper tackling (such as avoiding spear tackling) to help prevent spine and spinal cord injuries. Soccer athletes should avoid heading the ball until they acquire the strength and coordination to master proper technique.

Athletic Organizations and Facilities

Clinicians can help local athletic organizations and schools develop policies to enhance safety in youth sports. For example, AEDs should be available in locations where AYAs engage in PA. Community members and leaders should be encouraged to seek certification in CPR and first-aid training. Facilities should be well-maintained with proper ventilation, sanitation, lighting, and be located away from traffic, electrical, and water hazards. Organizations should establish informed weather policies (e.g., lightening, heat, and humidity) and promote a culture of healthy engagement in activities with awareness for signs of exhaustion, concussion, and athlete distress. Clinicians, AYAs, coaches, athletic trainers, and families can work together to promote patterns of safe PA with lasting health benefits.

SUMMARY

Adolescence and young adulthood are critical periods for developing behavioral patterns and making lifestyle choices that affect health in adulthood. A primary goal for clinicians is to encourage habits that optimize health and decrease risk for future morbidity and mortality. A PPE helps to identify issues that may need evaluation prior to sports participation. However, studies show that PA can be safe for everyone and the benefits generally outweigh the risks.[1] Adolescents and young adult who engage in more daily PAs, routine exercise, or sports are generally happier, have higher quality of life, and have decreased rates of obesity, chronic disease, and premature death. Current minimum activity recommendations are 60 minutes daily for adolescents and 150 minutes weekly for adults. Beginning with reasonable and realistic recommendations utilizing an exercise prescription, clinicians can aid AYAs to successfully initiate activity to reach and maintain health and exercise goals. Physical activity is one of the safest and single most important treatments a clinician can promote to improve the overall health of a person at any age and through any medical consideration.

ACKNOWLEDGMENT

The authors wish to acknowledge Keith J. Loud for his contributions to previous versions of this chapter.

REFERENCES

1. 2018 Physical Activity Guidelines Advisory Committee. *2018 Physical Activity Guidelines Advisory Committee Scientific Report*. U.S. Department of Health and Human Services; 2018.
2. Lobelo F, Muth ND, Hanson S; Council on sports medicine and fitness; section on obesity. Physical activity assessment and counseling in pediatric clinical settings. *Pediatrics*. 2020;145(3):e20193992.
3. Merlo CL, Jones SE, Michael SL, et al. Dietary and physical activity behaviors among high school students—youth risk behavior survey, United States, 2019. *MMWR Suppl*. 2020;69(Suppl-1):64–76.
4. U.S. Department of Health and Human Services, Office of Disease Prevention and Health Promotion. *Healthy People 2030*. Accessed January 22, 2021. https://health.gov/healthypeople
5. Woods R; US Bureau of Labor Statistics. *Sport and exercise*, 2017. Accessed April 1, 2021. https://www.bls.gov/spotlight/2017/sports-and-exercise/home.htm
6. Gauer RL, O'Connor FG; United States Army Center for Health Promotion and Preventive Medicine. *How to write an exercise prescription*. Accessed February 1, 2021. https://www.move.va.gov/Move/docs/Resources/CHPPM_How_To_Write_And_Exercise_Prescription.pdf
7. Stricker PR, Faigenbaum AD, McCambridge TM. AAP council on sports medicine and fitness. Resistance training for children and adolescents. *Pediatrics*. 2020;145(6):e20201011.
8. Riebe D, Ehrman JK, Liguori G, et al. eds. *ACSM's Guidelines for Exercise Testing and Prescription*. 10th ed. Wolters Kluwer/Lippincott Williams & Wilkins Health, 2018.
9. Bernhardt DT, Roberts WO, eds. *PPE Preparticipation Physical Evaluation*. 5th ed. American Academy of Pediatrics, 2019.
10. Maron BJ, Friedman RA, Kligfield P, et al. Assessment of the 12-lead ECG as a screening test for detection of cardiovascular disease in healthy general populations of young people (12-25 years of age): a scientific statement from the American Heart Association and the American College of Cardiology. *Circulation*. 2014;130(15):1303–1334.
11. Maron BJ, Levine BD, Washington RL, et al. Eligibility and disqualification recommendations for competitive athletes with cardiovascular abnormalities: task force 2: preparticipation screening for cardiovascular disease in competitive athletes: a scientific statement from the American Heart Association and American College of Cardiology. *Circulation*. 2015;132(22):e267–e272.
12. Drezner JA, Sharma S, Baggish A, et al. International criteria for electrocardiographic interpretation in athletes: consensus statement. *Br J Sports Med*. 2017;51(9):704–731.
13. Drezner JA, O'Connor FG, Harmon KG, et al. AMSSM position statement on cardiovascular preparticipation screening in athletes: current evidence, knowledge gaps, recommendations, and future directions. *Clin J Sport Med*. 2016;26(5):347–361.
14. Joy EA, Nattiv A. Clearance and return to play for the female athlete triad: clinical guidelines, clinical judgment, and evolving evidence. *Current Sports Med Reports*. 2017;16(6):382–385.
15. Mountjoy M, Sundgot-Borgen JK, Burke LM, et al. IOC consensus statement on relative energy deficiency in sport (RED-S): 2018 update. *Br J Sports Med*. 2018;52(11):687–697.
16. Mountjoy M, Sundgot-Borgen J, Burke L, et al. RED-S CAT. Relative energy deficiency in sport (RED-S) clinical assessment tool (CAT). *Br J Sports Med*. 2015;49(7):421–423.
17. Baker-Smith CM, Pietris N, Jinadu L. Recommendations for exercise and screening for safe athletic participation in hypertensive youth. *Pediatr Nephrol*. 2020;35(5):743–752.
18. Thomas DT, Erdman KA, Burke LM. American College of Sports Medicine Joint Position Statement. Nutrition and athletic performance. *Med Sci Sports Exerc*. 2016;48(3):543–568. Erratum in: Med Sci Sports Exerc. 2017;49(1):222.
19. Rubeor A, Goojha C, Manning J, et al. Does iron supplementation improve performance in iron-deficient nonanemic athletes? *Sports Health*. 2018;10(5):400–405.
20. Committee on Nutrition and the Council on Sports Medicine and Fitness. Sports drinks and energy drinks for children and adolescents: are they appropriate? *Pediatrics*. 2011;127(6):1182–1189.
21. Chang C, Putukian M, Aerni G, et al. Mental health issues and psychological factors in athletes: detection, management, effect on performance, and prevention: American Medical Society for Sports Medicine position statement. *Clin J Sport Med*. 2020;30(2):e61–e87.
22. Harmon KG, Clugston JR, Dec K, et al. American Medical Society for Sports Medicine position statement on concussion in sport. *Clin J Sport Med*. 2019;29(2):87–100.
23. Pujalte GGA, Maynard JR, Thurston MJ, et al. Considerations in the care of athletes with attention deficit hyperactivity disorder. *Clin J Sport Med*. 2019;29(3):245–256.
24. Sylvester JE, Buchanan BK, Paradise SL, et al. Association of splenic rupture and infectious mononucleosis: a retrospective analysis and review of return-to-play recommendations. *Sports Health*. 2019;11(6):543–549.
25. McGrew C, MacCallum DS, Narducci D, et al. AMSSM position statement update: blood-borne pathogens in the context of sports participation. *Clin J Sport Med*. 2020;30(4):283–290.
26. Lape EC, Katz JN, Losina E, et al. Participant-reported benefits of involvement in an adaptive sports program: a qualitative study. *PM&R*. 2018;10(5):507–515.
27. Physical activity and exercise during pregnancy and the postpartum period: ACOG committee opinion, number 804. *Obstet Gynecol*. 2020;135(4):e178–e188.
28. Patel DR, Yamasaki A, Brown K. Epidemiology of sports-related musculoskeletal injuries in young athletes in United States. *Transl Pediatr*. 2017;6(3):160–166.
29. Kliethermes SA, Marshall S, LaBella CT, et al. Defining a research agenda for youth sport specialization in the United States: the AMSSM youth early sport specialization summit. *Clin J Sport Med*. 2021;31(2):103–112.
30. DiFiori JP, Benjamin HJ, Brenner J, et al. Overuse injuries and burnout in youth sports. *Clin J Sport Med*. 2014;24(1):3–20.

ADDITIONAL RESOURCES AND WEBSITES

Additional Resources and Websites for Clinicians:
American College of Sports Medicine—Physical activity guidelines—https://www.acsm.org/read-research/trending-topics-resource-pages/physical-activity-guidelines
American Medical Society for Sports Medicine—Position statements from the professional organization for nonsurgical sports medicine physicians—https://www.amssm.org/Publications.php
Exercise Is Medicine—Resources from American College of Sports Medicine for physical activity assessment and promotion—https://www.exerciseismedicine.org
Healthy People 2030—U.S. Department of Health and Human Services, including evidence-based resources for physical activity—https://health.gov/healthypeople/objectives-and-data/browse-objectives/physical-activity/evidence-based-resources
National Center for Catastrophic Sports Injury Research—http://nccsir.unc.edu
Physical Activity Guidelines for Americans, 2nd Edition. U.S. Department of Health and Human Services—https://health.gov/sites/default/files/2019-09/Physical_Activity_Guidelines_2nd_edition.pdf
Preparticipation Physical Evaluation Monograph, 5th edition—Monograph available for purchase and PPE forms available to download for free—https://www.aap.org/en-us/advocacy-and-policy/aap-health-initiatives/Pages/PPE.aspx
Relative energy Deficiency in Sport (RED-S) Clinical Assessment Tool (CAT)—https://bjsm.bmj.com/content/bjsports/49/7/421.full.pdf
Safe Exercise at Every Stage (SEES)—Clinical guideline for managing and incorporating exercise into eating disorder treatment—https://www.safeexerciseateverystage.com/
Sport Concussion Assessment Tool, 5th Edition (SCAT5)—https://bjsm.bmj.com/content/bjsports/early/2017/04/26/bjsports-2017-097506SCAT5.full.pdf

Additional Resources and Websites for Parents/Caregivers:
Centers for Disease Control and Prevention. Child Safety and Injury Prevention—Sports safety—https://www.cdc.gov/safechild/sports_injuries/index.html
Centers for Disease Control and Prevention. HEADS Up—Concussion resources for Parents—https://www.cdc.gov/headsup/index.html
The Female and Male Athlete Triad Coalition—Education about nutrition and energy needs for athletes—https://www.femaleandmaleathletetriad.org/athletes/what-is-the-triad/
HealthyChildren.org—The AAP parenting website—https://www.healthychildren.org/English/Pages/default.aspx
Healthy People 2030—U.S. Department of Health and Human Services data to support population health—https://health.gov/healthypeople
Let's Move—Action plan for activities to do every day to improve health—https://letsmove.obamawhitehouse.archives.gov
National association for Physical Literary—Resources for promoting physical activity in communities—http://naplusa.org/

Project Adam—Programs to enhance community and school preparedness for SCA management—https://www.projectadam.com/

Stop Sports Injuries—Youth sports injury prevention—https://www.stopsportsinjuries.org/

U.S. Department of Health and Human Services. Move Your Way® Campaign—Tips and tools for families to get more active—health.gov/our-work/nutrition-physical-activity/physical-activity-guidelines

Additional Resources and Websites for Adolescents and Young Adults:

Centers for Disease Control and Prevention. HEADS Up—Concussion resources for Athletes—https://www.cdc.gov/headsup/index.html

The Female and Male Athlete Triad Coalition—Education about nutrition and energy needs for athletes—https://www.femaleandmaleathletetriad.org/athletes/what-is-the-triad/

HealthyChildren.org—The AAP parenting website—https://www.healthychildren.org/English/Pages/default.aspx

Let's Move—Action plan for activities to do every day to improve health—https://letsmove.obamawhitehouse.archives.gov/

NCAA Sport Science Institute—Health & safety guidance in collegiate sports—https://www.ncaa.org/sport-science-institute

OrthoInfo—American Academy of Orthopaedic Surgeons' safe exercise tips—https://orthoinfo.aaos.org/en/staying-healthy/safe-exercise/

SportsMedToday.com—Comprehensive sports medicine resource for athletes, coaches, and parents from American Medical Society for Sports Medicine—https://www.sportsmedtoday.com/

Stop Sports Injuries—Youth sports injury prevention—https://www.stopsportsinjuries.org/

U.S. Department of Health and Human Services. Move Your Way® Campaign—Tips and tools for families to get more active—https://health.gov/our-work/nutrition-physical-activity/physical-activity-guidelines

CHAPTER 24

Concussion

Michael A. Beasley
Cynthia J. Stein
William P. Meehan III

KEY WORDS

- Chronic traumatic encephalopathy (CTE)
- Management
- Mild traumatic brain injury (TBI)
- Return-to-learn
- Return-to-play
- Second impact syndrome
- Sport-related concussion (SRC)

INTRODUCTION

Sport-related concussion (SRC) has become a leading focus of concern, research, and advanced clinical care in pediatric and adolescent and young adult (AYA) athletes. Most commonly occurring with direct trauma to the head, concussion may follow any injury to the body that results in a rapid rotational force to the head, or whiplash-type injury. Symptoms following SRC vary widely in severity and duration and may include somatic, vestibular, cognitive, sleep, and emotional domains. These symptoms typically develop soon after injury and for most athletes resolve within days or weeks. Longer recovery periods are seen which are probably influenced by increased awareness and anxiety surrounding the injury. The foundation of concussion management has historically been physical and cognitive rest, though growing literature supports progressive activity early after injury as symptoms allow. For those with prolonged recovery, symptom-guided therapies and a multidisciplinary approach may be helpful. Concussion remains a clinical diagnosis and advances in imaging, neurocognitive testing, and assessment are needed to improve diagnosis, treatment, and prevention of injury.

DEFINITION

To date, there is no universally accepted definition for the diagnosis of concussion. The most recent definition of concussion as outlined in the 5th International Conference Consensus Statement is as follows[1,2]:

Sport-related concussion is a traumatic brain injury induced by biomechanical forces. Several common features that may be utilized in clinically defining the nature of a concussive head injury include the following:
- Sport-related concussion may be caused either by a direct blow to the head or any part of the body where force is transmitted to the head.
- Sport-related concussion typically results in the rapid onset of short-lived impairment of neurologic function that resolves spontaneously. However, in some cases, signs and symptoms evolve over a number of minutes to hours.
- Sport-related concussion may result in neuropathologic changes, but the acute clinical signs and symptoms largely reflect a functional disturbance rather than a structural injury and, as such, no abnormality is seen on standard neuroimaging studies.
- Sport-related concussion results in a range of clinical signs and symptoms that may or may not involve loss of consciousness (LOC).
- Resolution of symptoms typically follow a sequential course, and in some cases symptoms may be prolonged.

The clinical signs and symptoms cannot be explained by drug, alcohol, or medication use, other injuries (such as cervical injuries, peripheral vestibular dysfunction, etc.) or other comorbidities (e.g., psychological factors or coexisting medical conditions).

Though dozens of grading scales based on symptom severity or LOC have been published, none have been scientifically validated. It is currently recommended that all classification or severity scales be abandoned and replaced by individualized assessment for clinical resolution.

PATHOPHYSIOLOGY

Sport-related concussion is primarily a functional rather than gross, structural injury. While the pathophysiology of concussion is incompletely understood, animal studies suggest a "complex cascade of ionic, metabolic, and pathophysiologic events."[3] One proposed model includes a stretch injury to neuronal cell membranes and axons altering cellular makeup, neurotransmitter release, and mitochondrial dysfunction, that ultimately results in increased reactive oxygen species production and glucose utilization to address ion imbalances.[3] Increased glucose metabolism coincides with a reduction in cerebral blood flow which may be protective in nature, but ultimately creates an energy crisis that may last up to 4 weeks after injury.[4,5]

EPIDEMIOLOGY

The reported incidence of concussion has greatly increased over the last 20 years, likely due to increased awareness of SRC.[6] Accurate tracking of SRC diagnoses is complicated by varied definitions and diagnostic criteria, lack of surveillance systems, underreporting by athletes, and varied points of entry into the medical system.[5] Currently, the majority (75%) of SRCs in 5- to 17-year-olds are diagnosed initially through their primary care provider.[7]

Epidemiologic studies of SRC most frequently track organized sport-related injuries per athlete exposures (AEs).[5] Sport-related concussion incidence data illustrates that:

- the incidence in males is highest in American football, lacrosse, ice hockey, and wrestling.
- the incidence in females is highest in soccer, lacrosse, field hockey, and basketball.
- in sports played by similar rules for both sexes (soccer, basketball), female athletes appear to have a higher risk of SRC than male athletes.
- the incidence appears higher in collegiate than high school athletes.
- SRC occurs more frequently in competition than in practice: threefold higher in tackle football competition than practice; sevenfold higher in male lacrosse and soccer competition than practice; and fivefold higher in female lacrosse, soccer, and basketball competition than practice.[8]

It is not fully understood why female athletes appear to be at higher risk for SRC. Proposed reasons for the differences include intrinsic factors such as limited head and neck stabilization or influence of hormones, as well as extrinsic factors such as willingness to report injuries and symptoms.[5] Recent data however, indicate no statistical difference in time to full return-to-play (RTP) between sexes across comparable sports at the collegiate level.[9]

DIAGNOSIS

Definitive diagnosis of concussion can be difficult and sometimes controversial due to variability of signs and symptoms, lack of standardized objective criteria or diagnostic testing, reliance on self-reporting of symptoms, and overlap of symptoms with other common conditions.

- Headache is the most commonly reported symptom, both acutely and chronically.
- Dizziness, difficulty concentrating, confusion, and fatigue are all frequent complaints.[5]
- Loss of consciousness is not required for diagnosis, occurring in fewer than 5% of SRC.[5]
- Oculomotor and vestibular dysfunction are increasingly recognized after SRC.[10]

Postconcussion symptom checklists are helpful for initial evaluation of number and severity of symptoms at diagnosis and for monitoring recovery (Table 24.1).

On-Field Assessment

"When in doubt, sit them out," has become a universally accepted call to immediately remove from play any athlete suspected of having sustained a concussion. Athletes who suffer an SRC may be more likely to suffer additional head and musculoskeletal injuries, and are likely at increased risk for cerebral edema and poor outcomes, a phenomenon known as second-impact syndrome (SIS).[11] Acute evaluation, particularly in the setting of LOC, should begin with assessment of the "ABCs": airway, breathing, and circulation. The mechanism that leads to concussion can also lead to structural head and cervical spine injuries. If cervical spine injury cannot be ruled out, the athlete should be immobilized and transferred to an advanced emergency center immediately. After emergent cervical or neurologic injury has been addressed or ruled out, the athlete should be evaluated further for concussion off the field.

Sideline Assessment

Many sideline assessment tools have been developed to assist clinicians in the initial evaluation for SRC.[12] The sport concussion assessment tool (SCAT) is one of the most frequently used sideline assessments. The sport concussion assessment tool 5 (SCAT5), represents the most recent revision of the tool[13]: The SCAT5 is designed for athletes age 13 years or older and the Child SCAT5

is for athletes 5 to 12 years old. The SCAT5 consists of individually validated components including the Maddocks memory assessment questions, Glasgow Coma Scale, a cervical spine assessment, the postconcussion symptom scale, cognitive screening, and a balance assessment with the modified Balance Error Scoring System (mBESS). While the SCAT5 and similar tools facilitate a standardized and comprehensive evaluation, they are not designed as a stand-alone method to exclude or confirm the diagnosis of concussion and should be used by clinicians trained in assessing and managing SRC.[13] Additional tools are being developed in an attempt to improve SRC detection but available evidence is still insufficient to recommend their use for sideline SRC screening.[12]

Concussion signs and symptoms may evolve over time, and repeated assessments of athletes suspected of SRC are recommended. Any athlete demonstrating worsening symptoms, deteriorating level of consciousness, weakness into extremities, repeated emesis, or seizure activity should be referred to an emergency department.

Clinic Assessment

Assessments which occur in the hours or days following the injury should focus on confirming the concussion diagnosis and ruling out additional neurologic and/or musculoskeletal concerns. Confirmation of SRC as a diagnosis typically requires a clear mechanism of injury, a constellation of symptoms and timeline consistent with SRC, and the elimination of alternative etiologies of symptoms.[3] Designed specifically for sideline SRC screening, the effectiveness of the SCAT decreases 3 to 5 days after injury, and symptoms may resolve prior to in-office examination.[3,13] For athletes with ongoing symptoms, the postconcussion symptom scale is beneficial for monitoring recovery.[2] As cervical injury can co-occur with SRC, a complete cervical exam should be completed to rule out additional skeletal injury and evaluate for an additional source of persistent headaches. Clinicians should screen for pre-existing conditions, including mood, headache, and learning disorders so that symptoms present prior to the SRC are not mistakenly attributed to the new injury.[2]

Growing evidence supports the use of the vestibular/oculomotor screening (VOMS) tool in assessing athletes as a sensitive indicator of symptoms directly from SRC or associated peripheral vestibular conditions.[14] With symptom provocation, the VOMS tool may assist in identifying SRC as well those patients most likely to benefit from additional vestibular/oculomotor therapy.[2,14]

Advanced Diagnostics

Neuroimaging

Conventional neuroimaging such as computed tomography (CT) and magnetic resonance imaging (MRI) may help rule out structural injury (e.g., skull fractures, intracranial bleeding), but does not establish or exclude the diagnosis of concussion. With worsening symptoms or lack of improvement, MRI is the preferred neuroimaging modality as it is superior to CT in identifying cerebral contusion and white matter injury.[5] Though the primary use of MRI in patients with SRC is to assess for structural abnormalities, only 0.5% of patients with SRC with persistent symptoms will have imaging findings attributable to injury; over 14% will have unrelated structural abnormalities with the majority being benign.[15] Further research is needed before routine clinical use is recommended.[3,5]

Biologic Fluid Biomarkers

Investigation in the use of biomarkers in blood, saliva, and cerebrospinal fluid is ongoing. Currently, however, there are no evidence-based recommendations for the use of any biologic fluid biomarkers in concussion diagnosis, management, or clearance for return to sport.

Neurocognitive Testing

The use of computerized neurocognitive tests in SRC evaluation has increased dramatically at all levels of sport, from youth leagues to professional organizations, because it allows for standardized,

TABLE 24.1

Postconcussion Symptom Scale

Symptoms	No Symptoms	Mild		Moderate		Severe	
Headache	0	1	2	3	4	5	6
Pressure in head	0	1	2	3	4	5	6
Neck pain	0	1	2	3	4	5	6
Nausea or vomiting	0	1	2	3	4	5	6
Dizziness	0	1	2	3	4	5	6
Blurred vision	0	1	2	3	4	5	6
Balance problems	0	1	2	3	4	5	6
Sensitivity to light	0	1	2	3	4	5	6
Sensitivity to noise	0	1	2	3	4	5	6
Feeling slowed down	0	1	2	3	4	5	6
Feeling "in a fog"	0	1	2	3	4	5	6
"Don't feel right"	0	1	2	3	4	5	6
Difficulty concentrating	0	1	2	3	4	5	6
Difficulty remembering	0	1	2	3	4	5	6
Fatigue/low energy	0	1	2	3	4	5	6
Confusion	0	1	2	3	4	5	6
Drowsiness	0	1	2	3	4	5	6
More emotional	0	1	2	3	4	5	6
Irritability	0	1	2	3	4	5	6
Sadness	0	1	2	3	4	5	6
Nervous or anxious	0	1	2	3	4	5	6
Trouble falling asleep	0	1	2	3	4	5	6

The symptom checklist should be completed by the athlete in a resting state. Number of symptoms and total symptom score can be tracked at each visit to monitor progress.

objective, rapid, and uniform testing that can be monitored over time. Though potentially helpful as part of a comprehensive concussion evaluation, these tests have potential limitations and should be interpreted by a neuropsychologist or clinician with specialized training in test interpretation and neurologic principles of SRC treatment and management. Factors unrelated to SRC including sleep, co-occurring conditions (e.g., attention deficit hyperactivity disorder), effort and focus during testing, testing environment, and previous exposure to testing, all have the potential to affect baseline and postinjury scores.[2,5]

MANAGEMENT

Initial management of concussion consists of protection from reinjury, brief physical and cognitive rest, and education of the athlete and family on expectations. Initial removal from play and protection from recurrent injury can have significant impact on overall concussion recovery. Athletes who continue to play after injury

may be more likely to have more severe symptoms, worse neurocognitive scores, and a higher likelihood for prolonged recovery.[16] Once protected, treatment of concussion focuses on symptom management, including headache relief, sleep management, and appropriate rest. While prior recommendations stressed cognitive and physical rest until symptom resolution, there is growing evidence that extended rest in the setting of improving symptoms may in fact prolong recovery. Brief cognitive rest and return to academics as symptoms allow, may not worsen outcome and reduces academic setback and social isolation.[17] Similarly, there is growing support for early reintroduction of light exercise as symptoms allow, rather than complete rest until symptom resolution.[18] This "subthreshold" early exercise may have improved effects on the athlete's mood, sleep, and overall symptom profile and possibly hasten recovery.[19]

The majority (80% to 90%) of concussions among AYAs resolve within 2 weeks,[20] with younger athletes possibly taking longer, but typically becoming symptom free by 4 weeks.[21] The number and

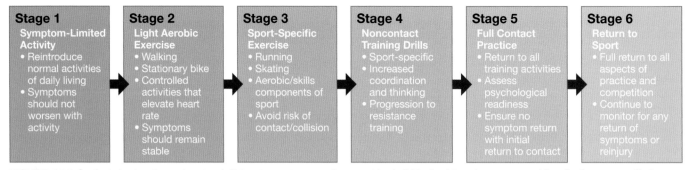

FIGURE 24.1 Graduated return-to-sport protocol. Return-to-sport progressions must be individualized based on extent and length of symptoms. Each stage requires a minimum of 24 hours before progressing, with a consideration for longer times at each stage in prolonged recovery. Return to previous step with worsening symptoms. (Adapted from Harmon KG, Clugston JR, Dec K, et al. American Medical Society for sports medicine position statement on concussion in sport. *Br J Sports Med.* 2019;53(4):213–225.)

severity of initial symptoms are the most consistent predictor of prolonged recovery.[3] Pre-existing depression or anxiety may also be associated with prolonged symptoms.[22] Postconcussion syndrome (PCS) describes persistence of concussion symptoms beyond the normal course of recovery; however, no consensus definition exists. Postconcussion syndrome is increasingly being referred to as persistent postconcussive symptoms (PPCS), a collection of nonspecific symptoms, rather than a specific pathophysiology, and includes the possibility of confounding or coexisting factors rather than ongoing concussion physiology.[2]

Return-to-Play

Some degree of formalized RTP is supported by all major consensus statements, practice guidelines, and laws in all 50 U.S. states and the District of Columbia. These laws typically have three major components: (1) education for coaches, athletes, and families; (2) removal from play with any suspicion of concussion and restriction from return the same day if confirmed; and (3) requirement of written medical clearance for RTP by a clinician with training in diagnosing and managing SRC.[2,3,5] Once symptoms have resolved, a graduated RTP protocol should be used to progressively test the athlete with advancing activity (Fig. 24.1). Each RTP stage requires a minimum of 24 hours, with progression to the next stage if the athlete remains symptom free. Longer symptom-free waiting periods between stages may be prudent in younger patients or those with more prolonged recovery. In addition, mounting evidence suggests that progressive noncontact exercise as tolerated prior to full symptom resolution is unlikely to be harmful and may be beneficial.

Return to Academics

After a concussion, some athletes have difficulty returning to school. Cognitive difficulties, including trouble with memory and decreased focus and concentration, may be magnified by symptoms including headaches, fatigue, and sleep disturbance. While the school setting and associated bright lights and noisy environment may worsen symptoms, use of remote learning with increased screen time can worsen headaches and visual symptoms.[23] It is important to reassure athletes, families, and schools that while academics may worsen symptoms, this does not represent new brain injury, and students with minimal or resolved symptoms can return to normal academics as soon as tolerated. Students with more significant symptoms may require academic accommodations and a guided, progressive return-to-learn protocol (Fig. 24.2). Those requiring prolonged academic restrictions may benefit from a more formalized return strategy such as an individualized education plan (IEP) or 504 plan (a U.S. federally recognized plan in public schooling systems designed to accommodate students with disabilities).[24] The American Academy of Pediatrics Councils on

Sports Medicine and Fitness and School Health have developed recommendations for return to learning.[24] Additionally, the Centers for Disease Control and Prevention provides free online resources for students, parents, school officials, and managing clinicians.

Pharmacologic Therapy

There is no medication available to treat the underlying pathophysiology of concussion; medication use is directed at alleviating symptoms. Initially, patients should be managed solely with physical and cognitive rest as symptoms require. For those who suffer severe or prolonged symptoms, medication for headaches, sleep disturbance, dizziness, and cognitive function may be considered.[5,24] Acetaminophen and nonsteroidal anti-inflammatories are frequently used for head pain, though chronic use may be associated with rebound/overuse headaches.[5] Use of medications such as melatonin for sleep dysfunction, tricyclic antidepressants for prolonged headaches, amantadine for cognitive difficulties, and methylphenidate for focus and concentration difficulties have been reported by primary care providers and specialists.[5,24] These medications should be administered by clinicians experienced in concussion management and reserved for AYAs with prolonged recovery, whose symptoms are significantly negatively impacting their quality of life. Any patient being considered for RTP should be symptom-free while off medications that may have been used to treat concussion-related symptoms.[9]

Targeted Therapies

Athletes with more severe or prolonged symptoms may require a symptom-limited guided exercise protocol.[3] Cervical injuries may contribute to headaches, neck pain, and activity intolerance; identification and treatment of cervicalgia through physical therapy may hasten recovery.[4] Similarly, treating athletes struggling with vestibular and oculomotor symptoms with guided vestibular therapy may increase tolerance of exercise and academics, possibly improving outcomes in prolonged recovery.[3] Anxiety, depression, and other mood disturbances may occur after SRC resulting from symptoms of the injury, exacerbation of the underlying disturbance, or adjustment reaction to imposed limitations following the injury. Standard therapies aimed at these symptoms may benefit patients, especially those with prolonged recovery.[1,9]

⬤ COMPLICATIONS AND CHRONIC EFFECTS

There is growing concern that sustaining multiple concussions may have cumulative effects. Evidence suggests that repeated concussions may be associated with acute and chronic changes, including cognitive impairment, dementia, mood disorders, and memory difficulties. Though evidence on long-term sequelae from recurrent concussions is inconsistent and actively debated, the potential risk

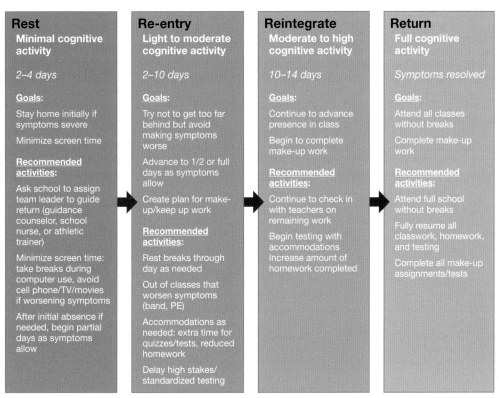

Rest **Minimal cognitive activity**	Re-entry **Light to moderate cognitive activity**	Reintegrate **Moderate to high cognitive activity**	Return **Full cognitive activity**
2–4 days	*2–10 days*	*10–14 days*	*Symptoms resolved*
Goals: Stay home initially if symptoms severe Minimize screen time	**Goals:** Try not to get too far behind but avoid making symptoms worse Advance to 1/2 or full days as symptoms allow Create plan for make-up/keep up work	**Goals:** Continue to advance presence in class Begin to complete make-up work	**Goals:** Attend all classes without breaks Complete make-up work
Recommended activities: Ask school to assign team leader to guide return (guidance counselor, school nurse, or athletic trainer) Minimize screen time: take breaks during computer use, avoid cell phone/TV/movies if worsening symptoms After initial absence if needed, begin partial days as symptoms allow	**Recommended activities:** Rest breaks through day as needed Out of classes that worsen symptoms (band, PE) Accommodations as needed: extra time for quizzes/tests, reduced homework Delay high stakes/standardized testing	**Recommended activities:** Continue to check in with teachers on remaining work Begin testing with accommodations Increase amount of homework completed	**Recommended activities:** Attend full school without breaks Fully resume all classwork, homework, and testing Complete all make-up assignments/tests

FIGURE 24.2 Academic recovery guidelines. Academic reintegration must be individualized based on symptoms and tolerance of the athlete. While increasing academic work may worsen symptoms, it does not create new brain injury, thus students may skip steps and return to academics as soon as symptom allow. (Adapted from Boston Children's Hospital Concussion Clinic, Academic Recovery Guidelines After Concussion.)

of these complications should be made clear to athletes who have suffered multiple concussions as they consider return to sport.[1,3]

Second-Impact Syndrome

Second-impact syndrome typically refers to a catastrophic injury involving an athlete who, while still suffering symptoms from an initial concussion, receives a secondary injury to the head. Second-impact syndrome remains rare and variably defined.[9,25] Most definitions include consecutive concussive events leading to cerebral edema and catastrophic brain injury. This definition distinguishes SIS from malignant cerebral edema resulting from a single injury.[25] While SIS is poorly understood, the potential for severe consequences following reinjury remains a primary impetus to restrict athletes from returning to contact or collision risk until they are entirely asymptomatic.

Mental Health and Wellness

Sport participation with regular exercise is an effective intervention in the prevention and reduction of depression.[26] Though studies have suggested football players with prior concussions are more likely to suffer depression, former high school football players showed lower risk of depression than nonathletes late into adulthood.[27] Research is needed to understand the mental health risks and benefits of sports participation and concussion.

Chronic Traumatic Encephalopathy

Chronic traumatic encephalopathy (CTE) is a distinct tauopathy and associated degenerative brain changes studied primarily in retired contact and collision athletes, linked to recurrent head trauma. The Berlin consensus statement includes a systematic review of possible long-term effects of SRC, including CTE and other neuropathologies.[28] Though there is no method for diagnosing CTE in living individuals, clinicians who care for patients with concussion must be aware of and be able to discuss the developing

knowledge surrounding CTE. A clear cause-and-effect relationship between CTE and prior SRC or participation in contact sports has yet to be established.[2,28]

Disqualification and Retirement from Sport

There are no current evidence-based guidelines for clinicians to recommend disqualification or retirement from sport, nor is there an accepted number of concussions prohibiting further participation.[3,5] Retirement or disqualification of the athlete must be individualized because of variability in symptoms, recovery time, exposure risk, and acceptance of risk by the patient or family. Persistent behavioral changes, mood disorders, and neurologic deficits may all have direct and indirect relation to injuries. Shared decision making between the athlete, family, and an expert in SRC is recommended for any retirement or disqualification discussion.[3,5]

⬤ PREVENTION

Advanced personal protection, rule changes, and legislation have all been proposed as potential methods of preventing SRCs and their sequelae. Although critical in prevention of structural injuries, there is no compelling evidence that protective equipment in the form of helmets, headgear, or mouth guards prevents SRCs.[5] Moreover, there are concerns that the use of protective equipment may provide a false sense of protection, leading to an increase in dangerous behavior.[10] Strengthening the neck and shoulder musculature has been proposed as a possible preventative measure. Evidence suggests that poor neck strength is a predictor of concussion, whereas increase in neck strength reduces SRC risk.[29] Rule changes to minimize high-risk situations in sport may reduce concussion rates.[2,5] Raising the age of introduction of checking/tackling, training in contact techniques, and limiting contact in practices all have potential to decrease frequency of head contact, potentially decreasing incidence of SRC.[2]

SUMMARY

Sport-related concussions are common in AYA athletes. While most athletes recover quickly and without complication, there is an increasing awareness and focus on persistent postconcussive symptoms. Any athlete suspected of having a concussion should be removed from play immediately and be evaluated by an experienced medical professional before RTP is allowed. The foundation of concussion management is conservative, with brief initial physical and cognitive rest, followed by progressive return to activities as symptoms allow. In prolonged recovery, a variety of advanced treatment options are available. Research is ongoing to improve the prevention, diagnosis, and treatment of concussion and to increase awareness of possible long-term sequelae.

REFERENCES

1. McCrory P, Feddermann-Demont N, Dvořák J, et al. What is the definition of sports-related concussion: a systematic review. *Br J Sports Med.* 2017;51(11):877–887.
2. McCrory P, Meeuwisse W, Dvorak J, et al. Consensus statement on concussion in sport--the 5th international conference on concussion in sport held in Berlin, October 2016. *Br J Sports Med.* 2017;51(11):838–847
3. Harmon KG, Clugston JR, Dec K, et al. American Medical Society for Sports Medicine position statement on concussion in sport. *Br J Sports Med.* 2019;53(4):213–225.
4. Meier TB, Bellgowan PSF, Singh R, et al. Recovery of cerebral blood flow following sports-related concussion. *JAMA Neurol.* 2015;72(5):530–538.
5. Halstead ME, Walter KD, Moffatt K, et al. Sport-related concussion in children and adolescents. *Pediatrics.* 2018;142(6):e20183074.
6. Colvin JD, Thurm C, Pate BM, et al. Diagnosis and acute management of patients with concussion at children's hospitals. *Arch Dis Child.* 2013;98(12):934–938.
7. Arbogast KB, Curry AE, Pfeiffer MR, et al. Point of health care entry for youth with concussion within a large pediatric care network. *JAMA Pediatr.* 2016; 170(7):e160294.
8. O'Connor KL, Baker MM, Dalton SL, et al. Epidemiology of sport-related concussions in high school athletes: National Athletic Treatment, Injury and Outcomes Network (NATION), 2011–2012 through 2013–2014. *J Athl Train.* 2017;52(3): 175–185.
9. Master CL, Katz BP, Arbogast KB, et al. Differences in sport-related concussion for female and male athletes in comparable collegiate sports: a study from the NCAA-DoD Concussion Assessment, Research and Education (CARE) Consortium. *Br J Sports Med.* 2021;55(24):1387–1394.
10. Master CL, Scheiman M, Gallaway M, et al. Vision diagnoses are common after concussion in adolescents. *Clin Pediatr.* 2016;55(3):260–267.
11. Broglio SP, Cantu RC, Gioia GA, et al. National Athletic Trainers' Association position statement: management of sport concussion. *J Athl Train.* 2014;49(2): 245–265.
12. Patricios J, Fuller GW, Ellenbogen R, et al. What are the critical elements of sideline screening that can be used to establish the diagnosis of concussion? A systematic review. *Br J Sports Med.* 2017;51(11):888–894.
13. Echemendia RJ, Meeuwisse W, McCrory P, et al. The sport concussion assessment tool 5th Edition (SCAT5): background and rationale. *Br J Sports Med.* 2017; 51(11):848–850.
14. Mucha A, Collins MW, Elbin RJ, et al. A brief vestibular/ocular motor screening (VOMS) assessment to evaluate concussions: preliminary findings. *Am J Sports Med.* 2014;42(10):2479—2486.
15. Bonow RH, Friedman SD, Perez FA, et al. Prevalence of abnormal magnetic resonance imaging findings in children with persistent symptoms after pediatric sports-related concussion. *J Neurotrauma.* 2017;34(19):2706–2712.
16. Elbin RJ, Sufrinko A, Schatz P, et al. Removal from play after concussion and recovery time. *Pediatrics.* 2016;138(3):e20160910.
17. Brown NJ, Mannix RC, O'Brien MJ, et al. Effect of cognitive activity level on duration of post-concussion symptoms. *Pediatrics.* 2014;133(2):e299–e304.
18. Howell DR, Mannix RC, Quinn B, et al. Physical activity level and symptom duration are not associated after concussion. *Am J Sports Med.* 2016;44(4): 1040–1046.
19. Mychasiuk R, Hehar H, Ma I, et al. Reducing the time interval between concussion and voluntary exercise restores motor impairment, short-term memory, and alterations to gene expression. *Eur J Neurosci.* 2016;44(7):2407–2417.
20. McCrea M, Guskiewicz K, Randolph C, et al. Incidence, clinical course, and predictors of prolonged recovery time following sport-related concussion in high school and college athletes. *J Int Neuropsychol Soc.* 2013;19(1):22–33.
21. Zemek R, Barrowman N, Freedman SB, et al. Clinical risk score for persistent postconcussion symptoms among children with acute concussion in the ED. *JAMA.* 2016;315(10):1014–1025.
22. Iverson GL, Gardner AJ, Terry DP, et al. Predictors of clinical recovery from concussion: a systematic review. *Br J Sports Med.* 2017;51(12):941–948.
23. Halstead ME, McAvoy K, Devore CD, et al. Returning to learning following a concussion. *Pediatrics.* 2013;132(5):948–957.
24. Kinnaman KA, Mannix RC, Comstock RD, et al. Management strategies and medication use for treating paediatric patients with concussions. *Acta Paediatr.* 2013;102(9):e424–e428.
25. Stovitz SD, Weseman JD, Hooks MC, et al. What definition is used to describe second impact syndrome in sports? A systematic and critical review. *Curr Sports Med Rep.* 2017;16(1):50–55.
26. Cooney GM, Dwan K, Greig CA, et al. Exercise for depression. *Cochrane Database Syst Rev.* 2013;(9):CD004366..
27. Deshpande SK, Hasegawa RB, Rabinowitz AR, et al. Association of playing high school football with cognition and mental health later in life. *JAMA Neurol.* 2017;74(8):909–918.
28. Manley G, Gardner AJ, Schneider KJ, et al. A systematic review of potential long-term effects of sport-related concussion. *Br J Sports Med.* 2017;51(12):969–977.
29. Collins CL, Fletcher EN, Fields SK, et al. Neck strength: a protective factor reducing risk for concussion in high school sports. *J Prim Prev.* 2014;35(5):309–319.

ADDITIONAL RESOURCES AND WEBSITES

Additional Resources and Websites for Clinicians:

Bloom J, Blount JG. Sideline evaluation of concussion. Last updated November 16, 2020. https://www.uptodate.com/contents/sideline-evaluation-of-concussion

Centers for Disease Control and Prevention. Heads up to healthcare providers. https://www.cdc.gov/headsup/providers/index.html

Evans RW, Whitlow CT. Acute mild traumatic brain injury (concussion) in adults. Last updated March 17, 2021. https://www.uptodate.com/contents/acute-mild-traumatic-brain-injury-concussion-in-adults

Halstead ME, Walter KD, Moffatt K, et al. Sport-related concussion in children and adolescents. *Pediatrics.* 2018; 142(6):e20183074.

Harmon KG, Clugston JR, Dec K, et al. American Medical Society for Sports Medicine position statement on concussion in sport. *Br J Sports Med.* 2019;53(4):213–225.

Meehan WP III. *Concussions.* Greenwood/ABC-CLIO, LCC, 2017.

Meehan WP III, O'Brien MJ. Concussion in children and adolescents: management. Last updated September 14, 2020. https://www.uptodate.com/contents/concussion-in-children-and-adolescents-management

McCrory P, Meeuwisse W, Dvorak J, et al. Consensus statement on concussion in sport–the 5th international conference on concussion in sport held in Berlin, October 2016. *Br J Sports Med.* 2017;51(11):838–847.

Printable forms of both the SCAT5 (https://bjsm.bmj.com/content/51/11/851) and Child-SCAT5 (https://bjsm.bmj.com/content/51/11/862)

Additional Resources and Websites for Parents/Caregivers:

Centers for Disease Control and Prevention (CDC). Heads up to parents. https://www.cdc.gov/headsup/parents/index.html

International Concussion Society. Concussion 101 or parents. https://www.concussion.org/news/concussion-101-for-parents/

Meehan WP III. *Kids, Sports, and Concussion: a Guide for Coaches and Parents.* 2nd ed. Praeger; 2018.

MomsTeam. Youth Sports Concussion Safety Center. https://www.momsteam.com/

Nationwide Children's Hospital. A parent's guide to concussions. https://www.nationwidechildrens.org/specialties/concussion-clinic/concussion-toolkit/a-parents-guide-to-concussions

Torres AR. Concussions: what parents need to know. Last updated November 30, 2020. https://www.healthychildren.org/English/health-issues/injuries-emergencies/sports-injuries/Pages/Concussions.aspx

Additional Resources and Websites for Adolescents and Young Adults:

Centers for Disease Control and Prevention (CDC). Heads up for athletes: a fact sheet for high school athletes. Revised January 2019. ttps://www.cdc.gov/headsup/pdfs/highschoolsports/athletes_fact_sheet-508.pdf

Centers for Disease Control and Prevention (CDC). Heads up for athletes:a fact sheet for middle school athletes. Revised January 2019. https://www.cdc.gov/headsup/pdfs/highschoolsports/middleschool_athletes_fact_sheet-a.pdf

Centers for Disease Control and Prevention (CDC). Heads up for athletes: concussion information sheet. Revised January 2019. https://www.cdc.gov/headsup/pdfs/youthsports/Parent_Athlete_Info_Sheet-a.pdf

National Collegiate Athletic Association (NCAA), Sports Science Institute (SSI). Concussion safety: what student-athletes need to know. Last updated Summer 2020. https://ncaaorg.s3.amazonaws.com/ssi/concussion/SSI_ConcussionFactSheet_StudentAthletes.pdf

National Collegiate Athletic Association (NCAA), Sports Science Institute (SSI). Concussion safety video for student-athletes. https://youtu.be/cXOLhtEwySw

PART

V

Skin Disorders

CHAPTER 25

Acne

Lindsay C. Strowd
Daniel P. Krowchuk

KEY WORDS
- Acne
- Acne vulgaris

INTRODUCTION

Acne vulgaris is the most common skin disease, it affects at least 85% of adolescents and young adults (AYAs). Although sometimes dismissed as trivial, acne may cause emotional distress and physical scarring. For these reasons, clinicians caring for AYAs should be familiar with the pathogenesis, clinical manifestations, and options for management of acne.[1]

ETIOLOGY

Acne is a disease of pilosebaceous units, composed of a follicle, sebaceous gland, and vellus hair. These structures are concentrated on the face, chest, and back, explaining the occurrence of acne in these areas. Several factors contribute to the pathophysiology of acne:

1. Androgens and sebum production: At adrenarche, rising levels of dehydroepiandrosterone sulfate (DHEA-S), likely after conversion to testosterone and 5-α-dihydrotestosterone, cause sebaceous glands to enlarge and produce more sebum. Increased sebum production contributes to obstruction within follicles and correlates with acne severity.
2. Bacteria and the innate immune response: *Cutibacterium acnes* is an anaerobic gram-positive rod that colonizes pilosebaceous follicles following increases in sebum production. *C. acnes* elaborates lipases that can damage the follicle wall and releases several chemotactic factors and proinflammatory mediators.
3. Abnormal keratinization: Epithelial cells lining the follicle proliferate more rapidly and become more cohesive. The result is a collection of cells and sebum that leads to the development of the primary acne lesion, the microcomedo.[1] As obstruction increases, the follicle may rupture with spread of its contents into surrounding tissues, an event that contributes to inflammation.

CLINICAL MANIFESTATIONS

Acne Lesions

1. Obstructive lesions (comedones): Obstruction within follicles initially is microscopic (i.e., microcomedones) but ultimately becomes apparent as open and closed comedones. Open comedones (blackheads) have a dilated follicular orifice and a

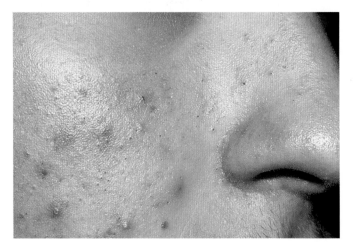

FIGURE 25.1 This patient has moderate mixed (inflammatory and comedonal) acne. He has inflammatory papules and pustules, erythematous macules (resolving inflammatory lesions), and open comedones. (From Jensen S. *Nursing Health Assessment.* 3rd ed. Lippincott Williams & Wilkins; 2018.)

black color (thought to be due to oxidized melanin, altered transmission of light through epithelial cells, or the presence of certain lipids in sebum) (Fig. 25.1). Closed comedones (whiteheads) are small (1 mm in diameter) white to skin-colored papules (Fig. 25.2).

2. Inflammatory lesions: Rupture of obstructed follicles leads to the formation of erythematous papules (<5 mm in diameter),

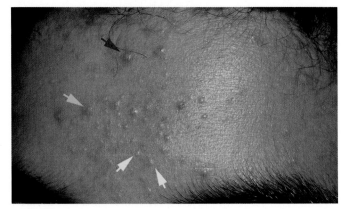

FIGURE 25.2 This patient has moderate mixed acne (inflammatory and comedonal) with closed comedones (*yellow arrows*), papules (*green arrow*), and pustules (*blue arrow*).

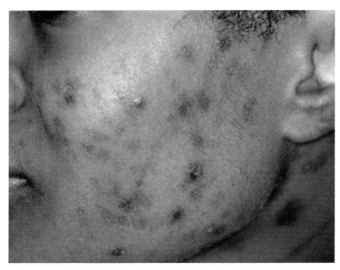

FIGURE 25.3 In persons with skin of color, resolving inflammatory lesions may produce hyperpigmented macules. (From Lugo-Somolinos A, McKinley-Grant L, Goldsmith LA, et al. *Essential Dermatology in pigmented skin.* Lippincott Williams & Wilkins; 2011.)

pustules, and nodules (>5 mm in diameter) (see Fig. 25.1). As inflammatory lesions resolve, they often leave erythematous (see Fig. 25.1), violaceous, or hyperpigmented macules (Fig. 25.3) that may persist for as long as a year. Patients often mistake these lesions for scars. Some patients develop cysts, compressible nodules that lack overlying inflammation.

3. Scars: Scarring is most likely to occur in those who have large inflammatory lesions (i.e., nodules). On the face, scars appear as small pits (Fig. 25.4), while on the trunk they are hypopigmented macules. Occasionally, patients develop hypertrophic scars (i.e., keloids).

Acne Variants

1. Pomade acne: Caused by physical obstruction of follicles, most often from inadvertent application of hairstyling products (e.g., pomades, greases) to facial skin. Comedones are concentrated on the forehead near the scalp and in the temporal fossae.

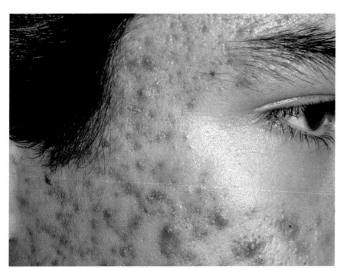

FIGURE 25.4 Acne scars on the face appear as small pits as seen here in the temporal fossa. Based on the presence of scars and numerous inflammatory lesions, this patient has severe acne. (From Burkhart C, Morrell D, Goldsmith LA, et al. *Essential Pediatric Dermatology.* Lippincott Williams & Wilkins; 2009.)

2. Acne conglobata: A severe form of acne in which cysts, abscesses, and draining sinuses develop on the face, chest, or back (e-Fig. 25.1). Extensive scarring and keloid formation are common.

3. Acne fulminans: This severe acne variant is characterized by the abrupt onset of painful nodules and cysts that become hemorrhagic and ultimately suppurate. Ulcers form and heal slowly, often leaving extensive scarring. Fever, chills, weight loss, myalgias, or arthritis may be present. Patients may have leukocytosis, anemia, elevated inflammatory markers and transaminases, and periosteal reaction suggestive of osteomyelitis.

4. Gram-negative folliculitis: Infection with gram-negative bacteria that complicates long-term oral antibiotic treatment of acne. The organisms most often responsible include *Escherichia coli, Enterobacter* spp, *Serratia marcescens,* and *Klebsiella* spp. Patients exhibit inflammatory papules and pustules concentrated around the nose.

5. Steroid acne: Patients who have Cushing syndrome or who are being treated with systemic corticosteroids may develop an eruption composed of monomorphous erythematous papules or pustules located on the face, upper trunk, and arms.

EVALUATION

Elements of the history that may be helpful are presented in **Table 25.1.** At a minimum, the physical examination should include the face, chest, and back. To aid in assessing the effect of treatment, one can document the approximate number and types of acne lesions present on the face (forehead, each cheek, and chin), chest, and back. Including photographs in an electronic health record is especially helpful.

An assessment of acne severity serves to inform the development of a treatment plan. The method presented here focuses on the face, but involvement of the trunk should be considered.[1]

1. Mild acne: A minority of the face is involved; a few papules and pustules are present, but there are no nodules or scars.

2. Moderate acne: Approximately one-half of the face is involved; papules and pustules are more numerous, but nodules are few (see Fig. 25.1).

3. Severe acne: The majority of the face is involved; papules and pustules are numerous, and there are several nodules; scarring may be present (see Fig. 25.4).

Although androgens play an important role in acne, most patients have normal hormone concentrations. As a result, measuring concentrations of DHEA-S, free testosterone, and 17-hydroxy-progesterone should be reserved for young women who have acne and other evidence of androgen excess (e.g., oligo- or amenorrhea, hirsutism, female-pattern alopecia, clitoromegaly).

DIFFERENTIAL DIAGNOSIS

Some conditions that mimic acne and differentiating features are presented below. In each of these disorders, comedones are absent.

1. Keratosis pilaris (KP): Small skin-colored papules located on the cheeks. A keratin plug emanating from the follicular orifice may be seen or palpated (differentiating the lesions from those of acne) (e-Fig. 25.2). Keratosis pilaris often also affects the upper outer arms, thighs, and buttocks, which are areas not involved by acne.

2. Periorificial dermatitis: May arise de novo or occur in AYAs using potent topical or inhaled corticosteroids. It is characterized by erythematous papules, pustules, and scaling concentrated around the mouth, nose, or eyes. Unlike in acne, lesions are not present on the forehead or cheeks (e-Fig. 25.3).

3. Rosacea: Erythematous papules, pustules, and scaling involve the central face. Flushing and telangiectasias are present and distinguish it from acne (e-Fig. 25.4).

TABLE 25.1

Key Elements of the History

Questions for All Patients	Rationale
When did your acne begin?	Early- or late-onset acne may indicate the presence of androgen excess.
What medications have you tried and how did they work for you?	If the patient has used a medication you're planning to prescribe, was it effective? If not, was it ineffective due to improper use or the occurrence of adverse effects?
Are you taking other medications?	Are there potential drug interactions? Could the medication be exacerbating acne (as might occur with depot medroxyprogesterone acetate, oral corticosteroids, lithium, diphenylhydantoin, phenobarbital, or isoniazid)?
Do you have "sensitive" skin or eczema?	Individuals who have sensitive skin or atopic dermatitis may be less likely to tolerate medications that are irritating or drying (e.g., topical retinoids).
What skin or hair care products do you use?	Occlusive preparations placed on the skin may physically obstruct follicles and worsen acne. Advise the use of products that are labeled "nonacnegenic," "noncomedogenic," or "won't block pores." Hair greases used for hairstyling may obstruct follicles if inadvertently applied to facial skin.
Are there other factors that may worsen acne?	Pressure applied by athletic gear (especially pads or chin straps) or tight clothing may worsen acne.
Questions for Young Women	**Rationale**
Are you having menstrual periods and, if so, how often?	Oligo- or amenorrhea may suggest androgen excess as might occur in polycystic ovary syndrome or late-onset congenital adrenal hyperplasia. Premenstrual acne flares may occur.
Are you using birth control? If so, what form?	Progestin-containing long-acting reversible contraceptives may worsen acne. Combined oral contraceptives (even those without a specific FDA indication for acne) may improve acne.

4. *Pityrosporum* folliculitis: Folliculitis caused by *Pityrosporum ovale* results in pruritic erythematous papules and pustules on the back, chest, and shoulders. In contrast to acne, the face is spared (e-Fig. 25.5). A potassium hydroxide preparation performed on a pustule roof may reveal spores and short hyphae.
5. Facial angiofibromas (adenoma sebaceum): Erythematous papules or nodules that are fixed in location (unlike acne lesions) and involve the nasolabial folds, nose, and medial cheeks (e-Fig. 25.6). Lesions typically appear in childhood, earlier than would be anticipated for acne.

MANAGEMENT

Managing acne requires an understanding of the pathophysiology of the disease, its degrees of severity, and the mechanisms of action and adverse effects of various treatments. Evidence-based guidelines for acne management exist,[2–4] but treatment should be individualized, taking into consideration the patient's perception of the severity of their disease, past experiences with medications, and the ability to consistently adhere to a therapeutic plan. Suggested treatment plans for mild, moderate, and severe disease are presented in **Tables 25.2** to **25.4**, respectively. Ideally, plans should be as simple as possible and employ medications that target various disease mechanisms.

Patient Education

The key components of patient education are outlined below. During the initial visit (and at return visits if needed), one should attempt to:
1. Dispel myths
   a. Acne is not caused by dirt, and frequent washing will not be beneficial. In fact, washing too often or using harsh cleansers or applying toners (designed to remove oil, cosmetics, and dirt) may irritate the skin and limit one's ability to

tolerate topical medications.[2] Advise washing the face twice daily with a mild nonsoap cleanser (e.g., a synthetic detergent such as Cetaphil or Dove bar, or a lipid-free cleanser such as Cetaphil, CeraVe, or Aquanil).
   b. The role of diet in causing or worsening acne is an issue of ongoing debate. Studies have suggested associations between acne and both a high glycemic load diet and the intake of milk.[1,2] At present, however, there is insufficient evidence to support dietary manipulation as an adjunct to acne management.[1–4]
2. Educate about the disease and its management.
   a. Describe the causes of acne as it relates to increased oil production and overgrowth of skin bacteria.
   b. Discuss the role of aggravating factors such as pressure applied by helmet chin straps or other athletic gear,

TABLE 25.2

Options for Managing Mild Acne

Face
- Inflammatory or mixed
  - BPO once daily ± topical retinoid
  - Alternatives if available (once daily):
    - BPO/antibiotic fixed-dose combination product
    - BPO/topical retinoid fixed-dose combination product
    - Topical antibiotic/topical retinoid fixed-dose combination product
- Comedonal
  - Topical retinoid (as single agent) or topical retinoid–containing fixed-dose combination product once daily

Chest and back
- Inflammatory or mixed: BPO wash once daily in shower
- Comedonal: Salicylic acid wash once daily in shower

If no improvement, proceed to Table 25.3.
BPO, benzoyl peroxide.

TABLE 25.3
Options for Managing Moderate Acne

Only the face is involved
- Topical retinoid at bedtime
  - Individual product (like tretinoin cream 0.025% or adapalene cream 0.1%) **OR**
  - Fixed-dose combination product (like BPO/adapalene or clindamycin/tretinoin)
- Topical antimicrobial each morning
  - BPO (if topical retinoid alone prescribed), **OR**
  - BPO/topical antibiotic fixed-dose combination product (if topical retinoid alone prescribed)

Face and chest or back involved
- Topical retinoid at bedtime to the face (as above), **AND**
- Oral antibiotic (like doxycycline, minocycline, or sarecycline)
- Consider adding BPO wash once daily in the shower to the chest and back

If no improvement, proceed to Table 25.4 or refer to a dermatologist.
BPO, benzoyl peroxide.

application of occlusive substances to the skin (such as hair greases or thick emollients), and occupational exposure to oils or greases.

c. Advise the use of skin care products (moisturizers, cosmetics, sunscreens) that are labeled "nonacnegenic," "noncomedogenic," or "won't block pores."

d. Discuss expectations for therapy and advise the patient that:
- Eight weeks or longer may be required to see improvement once treatment has begun. This is critically important to mention as many patients expect results within days, and lack of perceived efficacy may be a reason for premature treatment cessation.
- Currently available medications (with the possible exception of oral isotretinoin) are not curative. As a result, most patients require sustained therapy to control the disease.
- The goal of treatment is to reduce the number and severity of lesions and prevent scarring. Although many patients desire skin that is free of acne, for many this is not possible.
- Advise against picking at or "popping" acne lesions. Doing so can prolong the healing process, lead to secondary infection, or cause scarring.
- Provide guidance about using medications and prepare the patient for possible adverse effects. Topical agents should be applied as a thin coat to all acne-prone areas, not only to lesions. When the entire face is to be treated, dispense an amount the size of a pea onto a fingertip (some products employ a pump to dispense an appropriate amount). Touch the medication to each side of the forehead, each cheek, and the chin. Use the fingertips

TABLE 25.4
Options for Managing Severe Acne

Consider referral to a dermatologist, OR maximize the treatment plan
- Topical retinoid at bedtime to the face: If a low-potency agent was prescribed previously, consider increasing the potency (e.g., tretinoin microgel 0.04% or 0.1%)
- Oral antibiotic (like doxycycline, minocycline, or sarecycline)
- Add BPO once daily to the face (if not being used as part of a fixed-dose combination product)
- For females, consider a combined oral contraceptive

If no improvement, consider isotretinoin therapy, which usually involves referral to a dermatologist.
BPO, benzoyl peroxide.

to spread the medication, covering the entire face while avoiding the angles of the mouth, eyes, and alar folds (areas prone to irritation).

Topical Medications
Benzoyl Peroxide
1. Mechanism of action: Primarily bactericidal and somewhat comedolytic.
2. Dosing:
   a. Benzoyl peroxide (BPO) is considered by the U.S. Food and Drug Administration (FDA) to be generally safe and effective. Therefore, it is available without a prescription in concentrations ranging from 2.5% to 10% in a variety of vehicles (gels, creams, lotions, washes, and soaps). Some prescription forms remain, but they are often more expensive and may not be covered by insurance.
   b. For the face, consider using a gel in a 5% concentration applied once daily (gels are more effective than other vehicles). Increasing the concentration to 10% does not greatly enhance the therapeutic effect but increases the likelihood of drying and irritation.
   c. For the chest and back, consider a 10% wash that can be used once daily in the shower. Washes are convenient for treating large areas, although their efficacy is less than that of products applied to the skin and left on for several hours.
3. Adverse effects:
   a. Redness, drying, and peeling: Can be moderated by applying a moisturizer, decreasing the concentration of BPO, changing the vehicle (e.g., if the patient is using a gel, consider prescribing one that is water based or changing to a cream or lotion), or decreasing frequency of use to every other day.
   b. Bleaching: Benzoyl peroxide bleaches fabrics (including clothing, wash cloths, towels, pillowcases) and hair.
   c. Contact dermatitis: Uncommon occurrence that produces a pruritic eruption composed of erythema, small papules, or vesicles.

Topical Antibiotics
1. Mechanism of action: Reduce concentrations of *C. acnes*, inflammatory mediators, and possibly free fatty acids. As a result, these agents are useful in the management of mild to moderate inflammatory facial acne.
2. Dosing: Most products are used twice daily. However, if used in conjunction with another topical agent (e.g., a retinoid at bedtime), they may be applied once daily (in the morning).
   a. Single agents: Clindamycin, erythromycin, and sodium sulfacetamide (with or without sulfur). Using a topical antibiotic as monotherapy is discouraged because of the potential for the development of antibiotic resistance.[2,3] For this reason, consider adding BPO in the form of a fixed-dose combination product (below) or as a separate agent.
   b. Fixed-dose combination products: Products that combine a topical antibiotic and BPO have greater efficacy than either of the individual components; the inclusion of BPO reduces the likelihood of antibiotic resistance. Fixed-dose combination products are convenient and likely increase adherence. Cost may be a significant disadvantage. Available products include BPO 5%/erythromycin 3%, BPO 5%/clindamycin 1%, and BPO 2.5%/clindamycin 1%.
3. Adverse effects: As single agents, topical antibiotics are well tolerated. When combined with BPO, the adverse effects discussed previously may occur.

Topical Retinoids
1. Mechanism of action: Normalize keratinization within follicles, thereby reducing obstruction and the risk of follicular

TABLE 25.5

Topical Retinoids

Product	Vehicle/Concentration
Single agents	
• Tretinoin (generic, Retin-A [and other brands])[a]	• Cream: 0.025%, 0.05%, 0.1% • Gel: 0.01%, 0.025% • Lotion: 0.05% • Microgel: 0.04%, 0.06%, 0.08%, 0.1%
• Adapalene (generic and Differin)[b]	• Cream: 0.1% • Gel: 0.1%, 0.3% • Lotion: 0.1%
• Tazarotene (Tazorac, Avage)	• Cream: 0.05%, 0.1% • Gel: 0.05%, 0.1% • Lotion: 0.045% • Foam: 0.1%
Fixed-dose combinations	
• Adapalene/benzoyl peroxide (Epiduo)	• Gel: adapalene 0.1%/benzoyl peroxide 2.5%, adapalene 0.3%/benzoyl peroxide 2.5%
• Tretinoin/clindamycin (Ziana, Veltin)	• Gel: tretinoin 0.025%/clindamycin 1%

[a]Tretinoin (but not adapalene) may be inactivated by benzoyl peroxide. Therefore, the two agents should not be applied simultaneously.
[b]Adapalene gel 0.1% is available without a prescription.

rupture, and enhancing the penetration of other topical medications. They also have anti-inflammatory properties.
2. Dosing: Available as single agents or in fixed-dose combination products (Table 25.5). Factors to consider in selecting an agent include the following:
   a. Determine if your patient would benefit from a single agent (retinoid alone) or a fixed-dose combination product based on the following:
      • Cost: Is the fixed-dose combination product on the patient's medication formulary, and, if not, can they access and use a drug savings card or other discount mechanism?
      • Severity of inflammatory acne: Will topical BPO or clindamycin (the agents contained in fixed-drug combination products) be sufficient to control the inflammatory component of acne? Will BPO be beneficial to manage bacterial antibiotic resistance?
   b. If a retinoid-only product is desired, select a low-potency agent (such as tretinoin cream 0.025% or adapalene cream 0.1%) to reduce the likelihood of adverse effects. If the patient advises you that they have dry or sensitive skin, use a cream vehicle; if they have oily skin, consider a gel (such as tretinoin microgel 0.04% or adapalene 0.1%).
   c. With any topical retinoid, begin by applying it every second or third night and progress to nightly application as tolerated over 2 to 3 weeks.
3. Adverse effects:
   a. Dryness, redness, and peeling are most common. In addition to the strategies described previously, to prevent drying, advise the regular use of a noncomedogenic emollient, especially during cold weather months. Using a product that contains a sunscreen will protect against retinoid-induced photosensitivity. Temporary worsening of acne may occur 2 to 3 weeks after beginning a topical retinoid.

   b. Hyperpigmentation: In persons of color, retinoid-induced inflammation may cause hypo- or hyperpigmentation. This is an important reason to begin treatment with a low-potency agent, gradually increase application frequency, and use an emollient.
   c. Teratogenicity: Because tretinoin is structurally similar to isotretinoin, concern exists about potential teratogenicity. However, there have been no reports of malformations occurring in infants exposed to tretinoin in utero.[1] Nevertheless, tretinoin and adapalene should be avoided during pregnancy and are classified category C (risk to the fetus cannot be ruled out). Tazarotene, in contrast, is category X (contraindicated in pregnancy) due to teratogenicity concerns. This issue should be discussed if the drug is to be prescribed for a woman of childbearing potential.

Azelaic Acid (20%)
1. Mechanism of action: Antibacterial and comedolytic. As a result, it is most useful in the management of mild to moderate facial acne in those who cannot tolerate a topical retinoid.
2. Dosing: Applied twice daily
3. Adverse effects: Generally well tolerated but some patients experience pruritus, stinging, or erythema

Dapsone
1. Mechanism of action: A topical sulfone antibiotic that has anti-inflammatory activity. More effective in females with acne than in adolescents.
2. Dosing: Applied twice daily. Available as a gel.
3. Adverse effects: Using BPO products with dapsone gel may cause temporary (lasting as long as several weeks) orange-brown skin discoloration. Glucose-6-phosphate dehydrogenase testing is not required.[3]

Salicylic Acid
1. Mechanism of action: Promotes desquamation from follicles. May be beneficial for those who have comedonal acne but are unable to tolerate a topical retinoid.
2. Dosing: Applied once or twice daily. Available without a prescription as washes, scrubs, or pads.
3. Adverse effects: Drying, irritation

Oral Medications
Antibiotics
Oral antibiotics have greater efficacy than topical formulations and, for this reason, are used to treat more severe or extensive (i.e., chest and back) inflammatory acne. They should be used in conjunction with BPO (to reduce the likelihood of antibiotic resistance) and a topical retinoid. To avoid the development of antibiotic cross-resistance, avoid the simultaneous use of different oral and topical antibiotics. Once the inflammatory component of the disease has been controlled and an appropriate topical treatment program is in place, discontinue the oral antibiotic (ideally in 3 to 4 months, although some patients require more prolonged treatment).[3] Doxycycline, minocycline, or sarecycline often are preferred because they may be taken once daily, have better penetration into follicles, and have a lower prevalence of bacterial resistance.[2-6]
1. Doxycycline: Often a first choice.
   a. Dosing: 50 to 100 mg once or twice daily (or subantimicrobial-dose doxycycline containing 20 mg twice daily).
      • To avoid gastrointestinal upset and pill esophagitis, take with food and a large glass of water.
      • To prevent staining of dental enamel, use only in those >8 years of age.
      • To prevent photosensitivity, advise the use of a noncomedogenic broad-spectrum sunscreen (one with ultraviolet A and B protection).

b. Adverse effects (most common): Gastrointestinal upset, pill esophagitis, photosensitivity, vulvovaginal candidiasis, and headaches (including those caused by idiopathic intracranial hypertension). The risk of idiopathic intracranial hypertension is greatly increased when doxycycline is used in conjunction with oral isotretinoin so this should be avoided.

2. Minocycline: May be a first choice for severe acne or a second choice if doxycycline is ineffective.
   a. Dosing: 50 to 100 mg once or twice daily
      • To prevent gastrointestinal upset, take with food.
      • To prevent staining of dental enamel, use only in those >8 years of age.
   b. Adverse effects: Vertigo, dizziness, hyperpigmentation, and headaches (including those caused by idiopathic intracranial hypertension). Uncommon but important autoimmune adverse effects include drug hypersensitivity syndrome, lupus-like syndrome, hepatitis, and other hypersensitivity reactions.[3]

3. Sarecycline: A newer oral tetracycline that is more expensive than doxycycline or minocycline. Dosing is weight based and adverse effects are similar to those of doxycycline.[6]

4. Other antibiotics: A number of other antibiotics have been used to treat acne including trimethoprim-sulfamethoxazole, erythromycin, azithromycin, amoxicillin, and cephalexin.[3]

Hormonal Therapy

1. Combined oral contraceptives (COCs) improve acne by increasing sex hormone–binding globulin and suppressing ovarian androgen production. Although four COCs have an FDA indication for the treatment of acne (Ortho Tri-Cyclen, Estrostep, Yaz, Beyaz), others likely are beneficial.[1,2] Combined oral contraceptives typically are not viewed as monotherapy for acne but as adjuncts to standard treatment in those who have resistant disease. The use of COCs and their possible adverse effects are discussed in Chapter 48. Of note, existing evidence does not support interactions between COCs and non-rifampin antibiotics.[7]

2. Spironolactone has antiandrogenic properties and is used by some (off label) to treat female adolescents and young adults who have recalcitrant severe acne and signs of androgen excess.[3,4]

Isotretinoin

Indicated for the treatment of severe, scarring acne recalcitrant to standard treatment. However, it is also used to treat moderate acne that is refractory to oral antibiotics or that relapses rapidly after their discontinuation.[3] Those wishing to prescribe isotretinoin must register with iPLEDGE, a risk management system intended to prevent fetal exposure to the drug (https://www.ipledgeprogram.com). Recognizing that the vast majority of patients receive isotretinoin from a dermatologist, this section is intended to inform clinicians about the drug and possible adverse effects.

1. Mechanism of action: Vitamin A derivative that reduces sebum production, normalizes follicular keratinization, decreases *C. acnes* colonization.

2. Dosing: Often begun at 0.5 mg/kg/d and increased 1 month later to 1.0 mg/kg/d; treatment is continued for 16 to 20 weeks.[1,3] Most patients experience sustained clearing of acne after discontinuation of the medication. All patients are required to visit their prescriber every 30 days to receive medication counseling and obtain their next prescription.

3. Adverse effects: The most important of these include the following:
   a. Teratogenicity: Isotretinoin use during pregnancy is contraindicated due to the increased risk of spontaneous abortion and fetal malformations.[3] iPLEDGE requires that young women use two forms of effective contraception beginning 1 month before and extending to 1 month after the completion of treatment. Two negative pregnancy tests are required prior to receiving the initial prescription, and pregnancy tests are conducted monthly during treatment. Male patients are not required to use contraception while on isotretinoin but must pledge not to share their medication with anyone else, especially female patients.
   b. Dermatologic: The most common adverse effect is cheilitis (erythema, fissuring, and peeling of the lips). Drying of nasal mucosae may lead to epistaxis. Dry skin and dry eyes (that may result in contact lens intolerance) are common.
   c. Musculoskeletal: Myalgias are common, and hyperostoses (bone spurs and calcification of tendons and ligaments) may occur, especially in those receiving therapy lasting longer than 6 months.[2] Premature epiphyseal closure occurs rarely.[2,3]
   d. Gastrointestinal: Elevation of transaminases, triglycerides, and cholesterol may occur and regular monitoring is performed. Reversal of these abnormal results generally occurs despite continued therapy. Concern has been raised about an association between isotretinoin use and the development of inflammatory bowel disease (IBD), although several well-designed studies have found no increased risk.[3,8]
   e. Neuropsychiatric: A possible association between isotretinoin use and depression and suicidal ideation remains an issue of some concern. For most patients, successful acne treatment improves depressive symptoms and quality of life.[3] In addition, many studies, including a large meta-analysis, indicate no association with depression; suicide rates are lower among those receiving isotretinoin than would be expected among the general population.[3,4,9] However, there are well-documented cases in which depressive symptoms appeared after beginning isotretinoin, resolved when the drug was withdrawn, and returned with rechallenge.[10] In view of this and the possibility that idiosyncratic reactions might occur, those caring for persons receiving isotretinoin should remain alert for the development of symptoms of depression and suicidality.

● TREATMENT FOLLOW-UP

Except for those being treated with isotretinoin, patients should return 3 to 4 months after beginning treatment. However, they should be encouraged to contact their clinician sooner with questions or concerns about medication use or adverse effects. At the return visit, one can assess adherence, adverse effects, and the effect of treatment. Based on this information, the treatment plan can be maintained or revised.

● SUMMARY

Acne vulgaris is a common skin disease among AYAs. The pathogenesis is multifactorial, involving androgens and sebum production, bacteria and the innate immune response, and abnormal keratinization. Management tips include:

a. Clinical counseling is essential to treatment success and should include education about the disease, its causes, common myths, routine skin care, possible aggravating factors, appropriate use of medications, and anticipated outcomes.

b. For all but the mildest forms of acne, treatment regimens should address more than one component of disease pathophysiology (i.e., using BPO to address *C. acnes* and a topical retinoid to address follicular obstruction).

c. A topical retinoid is essential to the management of moderate or severe acne, regardless of the lesion types observed.

d. Topical or oral antibiotics should not be used as monotherapy due to the risk of bacterial resistance.

REFERENCES

1. Krowchuk DP, Gelmetti C, Lucky AW. Acne. In: Schachner LA, Hansen RC, eds. *Pediatric Dermatology*. 4th ed. Mosby-Elsevier; 2011:827–850.
2. Eichenfield LF, Krakowski AC, Piggott C, et al. Evidence-based recommendations for the diagnosis and treatment of pediatric acne. *Pediatrics*. 2013;131(Suppl 3):S163–S186.
3. Zaenglein AL, Pathy AL, Schlosser BJ, et al. Guidelines of care for the management of acne vulgaris. *J Am Acad Dermatol*. 2016;74(5):945–973.
4. Mwanthi M, Zaenglein AL. Update in the management of acne in adolescence. *Curr Opin Pediatr*. 2018;30(4):492–498.
5. Thiboutot DM, Dréno B, Abanmi A, et al. Practical management of acne for clinicians: an international consensus from the Global Alliance to Improve Outcomes in Acne. *J Am Acad Dermatol*. 2018;78(2 Suppl 1):S1–S23.e1.
6. Sarecycline (Seysara) – another oral tetracycline for acne. *Med Lett Drugs Ther*. 2019;61(1568):43–44.
7. Simmons KB, Haddad LB, Nanda K, et al. Drug interactions between non-rifampin antibiotics and hormonal contraception: a systematic review. *Am J Obstet Gynecol*. 2018;218(1):88–97.e14.
8. Etminan M, Bird ST, Delaney JA, et al. Isotretinoin and risk for inflammatory bowel disease: a nested case-control study and meta-analysis of published and unpublished data. *JAMA Dermatol*. 2013;149(2):216–220.
9. Huang YC, Cheng YC. Isotretinoin treatment for acne and risk of depression: a systematic review and meta-analysis. *J Am Acad Dermatol*. 2017;76(6):1068–1076.e9.
10. Prevost N, English JC. Isotretinoin: update on controversial issues. *J Pediatr Adolesc Gynecol*. 2013;26(5):290–293.

ADDITIONAL RESOURCES AND WEBSITES

Additional Resources and Websites for Clinicians:

Ashton R, Weinstein M. Acne vulgaris in the pediatric patient. *Pediatr Rev*. 2019;40(11):577–589.

Eichenfield LF, Krakowski AC, Piggott C, et al. Evidence-based recommendations for the diagnosis and treatment of pediatric acne. *Pediatrics*. 2013;131(Suppl 3): S163–S186.

Sambhi RD, Kalaichandran R, Tan J. Critical analysis of features and quality of applications for clinical management of acne. *Dermatol Online J*. 2019;25(10):13030. This study identified 358 Apple and 256 Google apps dealing with acne; 12 and 13, respectively, dealt with clinical management. All were considered by the authors to be of variable quality and lacked features essential for effective disease management.

Zaenglein AL. Acne vulgaris. *N Eng J Med*. 2018;379:1343–1352.

Additional Resources and Websites for Parents/Caregivers and Adolescents and Young Adults:

Acne Resource Center: Website of the American Academy of Dermatology—Accessed April 21, 2020. https://www.aad.org/public/diseases/acne

Manufacturer websites: Manufacturers of brand-name products have websites that provide information about acne, offer discount cards, or offer apps to track the progress of one's treatment. Use any search engine using the product name.

CHAPTER 26

Miscellaneous Skin Conditions

Lindsay C. Strowd
Daniel P. Krowchuk

KEY WORDS

- Alopecia
- Dermatitis
- Drug eruptions
- Fungal infections
- Hypersensitivity reactions
- Papulosquamous diseases

 INTRODUCTION

The identification and management of skin disorders is an important component of adolescent and young adult (AYA) health care. According to the National Ambulatory Medical Care Survey, a dermatologic diagnosis was made in 17.8% of AYA primary care visits.[1] This chapter reviews the identification and management of skin diseases that affect AYAs, addressing the conditions most likely to be encountered by clinicians. For additional information, readers should consult a standard dermatology text or atlas. Of note, infestations (scabies and pediculosis) and molluscum contagiosum are discussed in Chapter 67.

 DERMATITIS

The term dermatitis (or eczema) refers to inflammation of the epidermis and superficial dermis. Common forms of dermatitis that affect AYAs include atopic, allergic contact, and seborrheic.

Atopic Dermatitis

Atopic dermatitis (AD) is a chronic disease that is the result of multiple factors, including genetics, epidermal barrier dysfunction, immune dysregulation, and immune response to *Staphylococcus aureus*. Among the more than 20% of children who develop AD, most have a resolution of symptoms by adolescence or adulthood. However, 10% to 30% do not and a smaller number experience the onset of disease as an adult.[2]

Clinical Manifestations

1. In AYAs, AD is characterized by erythematous patches located in flexural areas, such as the antecubital and popliteal fossae, superimposed on a background of xerotic skin. The face (including the eyelids), neck, and hands also may be involved (Fig. 26.1). A variant of dermatitis is dyshidrotic eczema in which intensely pruritic vesicles involve the lateral aspects of the digits or palms (e-Fig. 26.1). In persons of color, AD lesions are less erythematous and may be papular and lichenified (thickened). In addition, there may be areas of hypo- or hyperpigmentation.

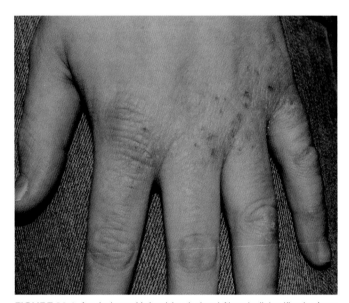

FIGURE 26.1 Atopic dermatitis involving the hand. Note the lichenification (over the metacarpophalangeal joint of the index finger) and small crusted erosions.

2. Individuals who have AD also commonly exhibit:
   a. Xerosis
   b. Hyperlinear palms
   c. Keratosis pilaris: Keratotic papules centered around follicles; typically located on the upper outer arms, thighs, and face (e-Fig. 26.2)
   d. Dennie–Morgan lines: Prominent skin folds located beneath the eyes
   e. Ichthyosis vulgaris: Polygonal scales located on the anterior and lateral legs
   f. Lichenification: Thickening of the skin with accentuated skin creases (due to chronic scratching)
   g. Pityriasis alba: Hypopigmented macules often located on the face; the borders are not sharply demarcated, rather there is a gradual transition from normal to abnormal color (e-Fig. 26.3)

Complications

Individuals who have AD are often colonized with *S. aureus*, likely because of increased bacterial adherence and a decrease in cutaneous antimicrobial peptides. In addition, defects in antimicrobial peptide production and T-cell function increase susceptibility to viral infections, including molluscum contagiosum, warts, and eczema herpeticum.

Treatment

1. Daily measures
   a. Avoid irritants: Use fragrance-free skin-care products; a nonsoap cleanser for bathing (e.g., a synthetic detergent like Cetaphil or fragrance-free Dove bar or a lipid-free cleanser like Cetaphil, CeraVe, or Aquanil); an additive-free laundry detergent (e.g., All Free Clear, Tide Free, and others); avoid dryer sheets and fabric softeners; choose cotton clothing over synthetic fabrics and wool.
   b. Hydrate the skin: Apply generous amounts of a fragrance-free emollient immediately after a bath or shower. Lotions work well for many individuals but preservatives in some products may cause stinging. Creams or ointments are more effective emollients, although they may leave a greasy feel that some individuals find unpleasant. Applying products immediately after bathing allows for enhanced percutaneous absorption and can help minimize the greasy feeling. Using a cool mist room humidifier can also help, particularly in low-humidity climates and seasons.
2. Management of exacerbations
   a. Topical corticosteroid: Apply twice daily if needed. Ointments offer greater efficacy and tolerability; however, as with emollients, some patients prefer creams because ointments have a greasy feel. Prescribe a sufficient amount of product. Approximately 3 g is required to cover an entire adult arm once.
      • Face: Use a low-potency preparation (e.g., hydrocortisone 1% or 2.5%).
      • Extremities or trunk: Use a mid-potency agent (e.g., triamcinolone acetonide 0.1% or fluocinolone acetonide 0.025%). For resistant or lichenified areas or when treating the hands, a higher-potency agent (e.g., fluocinonide 0.05% or mometasone furoate ointment 0.1%) may be needed. These agents should be used with caution since prolonged application may cause skin atrophy.
   b. Topical calcineurin inhibitors (e.g., tacrolimus [Protopic] and pimecrolimus [Elidel])
      • Most useful for the management of AD in areas where potent corticosteroids cannot be used due to concerns about skin atrophy (e.g., the face, groin, axillae) or in areas of resistant disease (where they are often used in conjunction with topical corticosteroids [e.g., a topical corticosteroid is applied in the morning and the topical calcineurin inhibitor in the evening]).
      • Tacrolimus is indicated for the treatment of moderate-to-severe AD (the 0.03% concentration is approved for those 2 to 15 years of age and the 0.1% concentration for those ≥16 years of age); pimecrolimus is indicated for the treatment of mild-to-moderate AD in those ≥2 years of age.
   c. Topical phosphodiesterase inhibitor (e.g., crisaborole [Eucrisa])
      • Similar to topical calcineurin inhibitors, crisaborole 2% ointment will not cause skin atrophy. Crisaborole is approved for treatment of mild-to-moderate AD for those aged 3 months and older.
   d. Antihistamine: A first-generation (sedating) antihistamine, like diphenhydramine or hydroxyzine, may be used at bedtime to provide relief from pruritus.
   e. Antibiotic: If signs of secondary bacterial infection are present (e.g., oozing, crusting), an antistaphylococcal antibiotic may be administered orally for 7 to 10 days. For those who have severe or resistant AD, consider attempting to reduce *S. aureus* colonization by recommending (1) twice-weekly bleach baths (1/4 cup of household bleach in a half-full bathtub) or sodium hypochlorite cleanser and (2) intranasal mupirocin twice daily for 5 days.

3. Recalcitrant disease: For patients who have an inadequate response to topical therapy, consultation with a dermatologist is indicated to modify the program or consider systemic therapy. Options include the following:
   a. Dupilumab (Dupixent)
      • Dupilumab is an interleukin-4 (IL-4) receptor antagonist that blocks both IL-4 and IL-13, two cytokines that are important in the pathogenesis of AD. Dupilumab is approved by the U.S. Food and Drug Administration (FDA) for use in those ≥6 years with moderate-to-severe AD.[3]
      • The drug is delivered by a subcutaneous injection that is self-administered every 14 to 28 days. In clinical trials, dupilumab significantly decreased AD severity and improved itch in most patients.
      • Dupilumab is considered relatively safe and does not require ongoing laboratory monitoring.
   b. Cyclosporine: Oral cyclosporine is FDA-approved for use in severe refractory AD in adults, but in some cases is used off-label for treatment of severe AD in younger patients. Due to concerns about potential nephrotoxicity, it is used for very short periods of time as a bridge to other systemic therapy.
   c. Other agents: Methotrexate, azathioprine, and mycophenolate have been used off-label to treat refractory AD. All have potentially serious side effects and require ongoing laboratory monitoring.
   d. Corticosteroids: Avoid using oral corticosteroids to treat AD. Frequently, patients experience a rebound exacerbation of AD after cessation.

Allergic Contact Dermatitis

Allergic contact dermatitis (ACD) occurs when an antigen penetrates the epidermis and sensitizes T lymphocytes. Within 12 to 24 hours of re-exposure to the antigen, an eruption appears at the site of contact. Often the offending agent can be identified based on the appearance of lesions and their distribution. In a minority of cases, dermatologic referral for patch testing may be necessary.

1. **Plant** (e.g., poison ivy, oak, or sumac)
   a. Clinical manifestations: Allergic contact dermatitis due to plants results in an acute dermatitis with erythematous papules, vesicles, or bullae. Lesions are present on exposed areas (e.g., face, extremities) and may be arranged in a linear distribution (at the site of contact with resin emanating from a damaged plant) (Fig. 26.2). If the exposure is indirect (e.g., hugging a dog that has run through poison ivy),

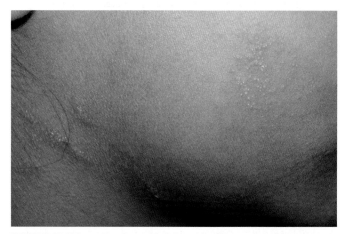

FIGURE 26.2 In contact dermatitis due to poison ivy, small erythematous papules are present, often in a linear arrangement as seen on the neck and the angle of the mandible.

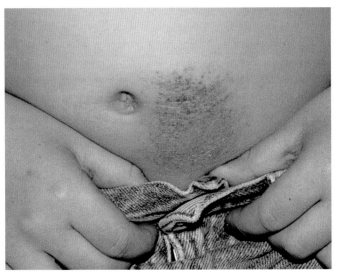

FIGURE 26.3 Contact dermatitis due to nickel in a clothing snap. There is an erythematous patch near the umbilicus. (From Goodheart HP. *Goodheart's Photoguide of Common Skin Disorders*. 4th ed. Lippincott Williams & Wilkins; 2015.)

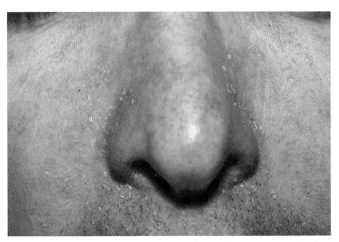

FIGURE 26.4 In adolescents and young adults, seborrheic dermatitis often involves the nasolabial folds with erythema and scaling. (From Goodheart HP. *Goodheart's Photoguide of Common Skin Disorders*. 4th ed. Lippincott Williams & Wilkins; 2015.)

a linear distribution of lesions is unlikely and one may see fine erythematous papules, not vesicles.

  b. Treatment: If the eruption is mild and limited in extent (e.g., <10% to 15% of the body surface), therapy may include a mid-potency topical corticosteroid (e.g., triamcinolone acetonide 0.1%), a topical nonsensitizing anesthetic (e.g., pramoxine), and an oral first-generation antihistamine. When the eruption is extensive, severe, or involves critical areas (e.g., face, perineum), systemic corticosteroid therapy (e.g., prednisone orally for 12 to 21 days in a tapering dose) is indicated.

2. **Metal**: Nickel is the most common contact allergen worldwide.[4] Nickel allergy produces a chronic dermatitis characterized by minimal erythema, scaling, and thickening of the skin. Commonly affected sites include the lobules of the ears (earrings), area below the umbilicus (belt buckle or clothing snap), umbilicus (piercing jewelry), neck (necklace), or wrist (bracelet or watch) (Fig. 26.3). Treatment is with an appropriate topical corticosteroid and nickel avoidance. Patients may be advised to:

  a. Choose low or no nickel jewelry and eyeglass frames (i.e., items made of surgical-grade stainless steel, 18-karat yellow gold, platinum, titanium, or sterling silver).

  b. Purchase clothing with snaps, buttons, and fasteners that are plastic or metal that is plastic coated or painted.

  c. Wear watchbands made of plastic, leather, or cloth.

3. **Preservatives, fragrances**: These products cause erythema and tiny papules. Commonly affected sites include the face or eyelids (cosmetics), axillae (deodorant), or neck (perfume). Treatment is avoidance of the offending agent (once identified) and the application of an appropriate topical corticosteroid.

Seborrheic Dermatitis

Seborrheic dermatitis is a chronic and relapsing inflammatory disorder that occurs in areas with numerous sebaceous glands. It affects 1% to 3% of adults and is especially common in AYAs in whom sebaceous glands are most active.[5] Although the cause is not clearly understood, it may involve an inflammatory response to the yeasts of the genus *Malassezia* (formerly *Pityrosporum*).

Clinical Manifestations

Typical findings are scaling of the scalp (i.e., dandruff), or scaling and erythema of the eyebrows, eyelids, glabella, nasolabial or retroauricular creases, beard or sideburn areas, or ear canals (Fig. 26.4).

Treatment

1. Scalp: Advise the use of an antiseborrheic shampoo containing pyrithione zinc (e.g., Head and Shoulders, DHS Zinc, and others), selenium sulfide (e.g., Selsun, Exsel, and others), or ketoconazole (e.g., Nizoral). If facial skin is involved, allow some of the shampoo to contact these areas and then rinse (this is a useful adjunct to the topical therapies discussed below). If signs of inflammation are present (e.g., erythema or erosions), a topical corticosteroid solution (e.g., fluocinolone acetonide 0.1%) may be applied at bedtime if needed.

2. Skin: Control can be achieved using a low-potency topical corticosteroid (e.g., hydrocortisone 1%) and/or an agent active against yeast (e.g., clotrimazole, miconazole nitrate, or ketoconazole) applied twice daily if needed.

⬤ FUNGAL INFECTIONS

Tinea Versicolor

Tinea (pityriasis) versicolor is a common superficial infection caused by yeasts of the genus *Malassezia* (formerly *Pityrosporum*). Sebum-rich environments appear to support lipophilic *Malassezia* spp. Although these organisms are part of the normal skin flora, hot and humid weather, sweating, and use of oils on the skin may trigger a change from the yeast form to the hyphal form, resulting in the appearance of rash.

Clinical Manifestations

Most patients have no symptoms but some report pruritus. The eruption is composed of well-defined round macules that may coalesce into large patches; scale may be present. Although lesions may be hypo- or hyperpigmented, most often, in more deeply pigmented individuals, they are hypopigmented (Fig. 26.5). The trunk is the primary site of involvement, but the proximal extremities and sides of the neck also may be affected. Tinea versicolor is usually diagnosed clinically. If uncertainty exists, a potassium hydroxide preparation performed on the scale from a lesion will demonstrate short hyphae and spores (i.e., "spaghetti and meatballs") and a Wood's lamp examination will reveal a yellow-gold fluorescence from affected areas.

Differential Diagnosis

Eruptions that may be concentrated on the trunk and mimic tinea versicolor include the following:

1. Pityriasis rosea (PR): Lesions are thin, erythematous, oval plaques (not macules) with long axes oriented parallel to lines of skin stress.

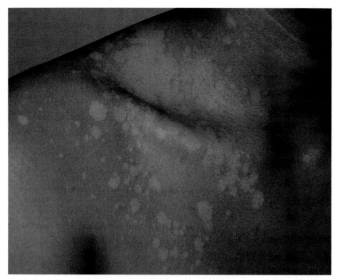

FIGURE 26.5 In this example of tinea versicolor, there are numerous round hypopigmented macules. In the supraclavicular area, macules have coalesced to form a hypopigmented patch.

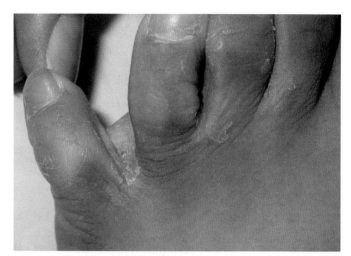

FIGURE 26.6 In the most common form of tinea pedis, scaling and maceration are present in the interdigital spaces.

2. Vitiligo: Lesions are depigmented (not hypopigmented) and lack scale.
3. Secondary syphilis: The eruption is composed of erythematous to violaceous to red-brown scaling papules. Lesions are widespread (not limited to the trunk) and often involve the palms and soles. Affected individuals have systemic symptoms, including fever, malaise, and lymphadenopathy.
4. Confluent and reticulated papillomatosis of Gougerot and Carteaud: This uncommon disorder is often confused with tinea versicolor. Reticulated areas of hyperpigmentation that are hyperkeratotic (and, therefore, have a rough texture) are present on the central chest or back. Well-defined round or oval macules are not seen (e-Fig. 26.4).

Treatment

Several options exist for treatment. Because recurrence is common, monthly prophylaxis for 3 months is recommended following any of the treatments below. One option is a single 8- to 12-hour application of selenium sulfide. It is important to counsel patients that even with effective treatment, several months will be required for normalization of pigmentation.
1. Topical agents
   a. Selenium sulfide lotion 1% (available without a prescription) or 2.5% (requires prescription): Apply a thin coat to affected and adjacent areas for 10 minutes then shower. Repeat daily for 1 week.
   b. Ketoconazole shampoo: Apply for 5 minutes once daily for 1 to 3 days.
   c. Terbinafine spray: Apply twice daily for 2 to 3 weeks.
   d. Imidazole creams (e.g., clotrimazole, miconazole nitrate, ketoconazole, and others): Effective for localized infection (not practical for treatment of large areas).
2. Oral agents: Usually reserved for resistant infections or patients who cannot tolerate or effectively use a topical agent. Off-label options include the following:
   a. Itraconazole: 400 mg once or 200 mg/day for 7 days
   b. Fluconazole: 400 mg once or 300 mg once repeated in 1 week

Tinea Pedis (Athlete's Foot)

Tinea pedis is the most prevalent dermatophyte infection in AYAs.

Clinical Manifestations

1. Interdigital form (caused by *Trichophyton [T.] rubrum* or *Epidermophyton [E.] floccosum*): Pruritus, fissuring, scaling, and maceration between the toes (Fig. 26.6)
2. Moccasin form (caused by *T. rubrum*): Widespread scaling that involves much or all of the sole and sides of the foot
3. Inflammatory form (caused by *T. mentagrophytes*): Vesicles or bullae located on the instep of the foot (Fig. 26.7).

Differential Diagnosis

Several disorders involve the feet and may mimic tinea pedis. In each case, a potassium hydroxide preparation or fungal culture would be negative.
1. Contact dermatitis due to shoes: Involves the dorsum of the feet, not the interdigital spaces or plantar surfaces.
2. Juvenile plantar dermatosis: Typically occurs in older children and less often in adolescents. Causes erythema, dryness, lichenification, and fissuring primarily of the plantar surfaces of the forefeet.
3. Psoriasis: Causes erythema and thick (not fine) scale of the feet. Individuals often have lesions of psoriasis elsewhere.

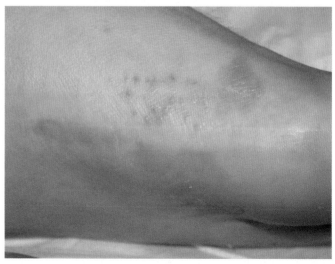

FIGURE 26.7 The inflammatory form of tinea pedis produces papules and vesicles near the instep of the foot.

Treatment

For most infections, a fungistatic topical imidazole (e.g., miconazole nitrate, clotrimazole, econazole, etc.) applied twice daily until clearing occurs (typically 2 to 4 weeks) is effective. If this treatment fails, consider a topical agent that is fungicidal (e.g., terbinafine, naftifine). For widespread or resistant infection, an oral agent (e.g., griseofulvin, terbinafine, itraconazole, or fluconazole) may be required. If there is concomitant nail involvement (i.e., onychomycosis), oral terbinafine or itraconazole will be necessary.

Onychomycosis

The terms onychomycosis (nail infection by any fungus) and tinea unguium (infection by fungi called dermatophytes) are often used interchangeably. Most fungal nail infections are caused by dermatophytes (usually *T. rubrum*, *T. mentagrophytes*, and *E. floccosum*). The prevalence of onychomycosis in the United States is estimated to be 2% to 14%. Infection is uncommon before puberty and highest in those >60 years of age.[6]

Clinical Manifestations

Two forms of infection are recognized.

1. Subungual onychomycosis: The most prevalent form of infection that causes thickening of the nail and a yellow discoloration distally or laterally (the result of separation of the nail from the underlying nail bed) (Fig. 26.8)
2. Superficial white onychomycosis: Produces a white discoloration of the surface of the nail with powdery scale

Differential Diagnosis

The clinical features of the disorders listed below often permit their differentiation from onychomycosis. However, if uncertainty exists, a fungal culture of a nail scraping or clipping can be helpful.

1. Candidiasis: Uncommon in adolescents and usually involves the fingernails. Causes a chronic paronychia characterized by erythema and swelling of the proximal nail fold, loss of the cuticle, and nail dystrophy (that lacks yellow discoloration).
2. Psoriasis: Usually causes pitting of the nails; lesions of psoriasis are present elsewhere.
3. Pachyonychia congenita: Results in thickening and discoloration of the nails that may be difficult to differentiate clinically from onychomycosis. The condition usually has its onset in early childhood but may be delayed until adolescence.
4. Lichen planus: Causes longitudinal ridging or splitting of nails. Typical skin lesions (purple polygonal papules and plaques) are present elsewhere.

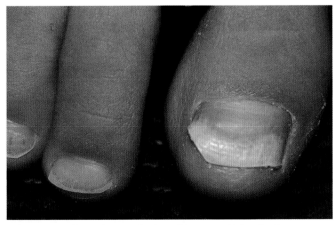

FIGURE 26.8 In onychomycosis, the nail becomes thick and yellow.

Treatment

Superficial white onychomycosis may respond to topical antifungal therapy. However, subungual onychomycosis requires one of the oral therapies listed below for adults.[7] One should consider potential drug interactions, adverse effects, and the need for laboratory monitoring.

1. Terbinafine 250 mg daily for 12 weeks (preferred due to higher cure rate and lower likelihood of adverse effects)
2. Itraconazole 200 mg daily for 12 weeks
3. Fluconazole is preferred by some but is not FDA-approved for the treatment of onychomycosis.

Cure rates with oral therapy are as high as 70%; however, recurrences are common. To reduce the chance of recurrence, advise patients to dry carefully after bathing or showering and to apply an absorbent powder containing an antifungal agent (e.g., tolnaftate [e.g., Tinactin and others], or miconazole nitrate [e.g., Micatin, Desenex, Zeasorb AF, Lotrimin AF, and others]).

Tinea Cruris

Tinea cruris represents infection of the inguinal folds with the dermatophytes *T. mentagrophytes* or *E. floccosum*. It affects males more often than females and is uncommon before puberty.

Clinical Manifestations

Appears as a well-demarcated erythematous patch involving the proximal thigh and crural fold (may be unilateral or bilateral). The border of the lesion is elevated and scaling and is typically more erythematous than the center. The scrotum and penis are spared (Fig. 26.9).

Differential Diagnosis

Clinical examination is usually sufficient for diagnosis. If uncertainty exists, a potassium hydroxide preparation or fungal culture can be helpful. These would be negative in uncomplicated intertrigo and erythrasma and would demonstrate pseudohyphae and spores in candidiasis.

1. Candidiasis: Bright red patch in the crural fold that also involves the scrotum and penis; satellite papules may be present.
2. Intertrigo: Maceration resulting from rubbing of moist skin surfaces creates a superficial erosion that is not as well defined as tinea cruris and lacks border elevation.
3. Erythrasma: Superficial infection caused by *Corynebacterium minutissimum* that produces erythematous to brown patches

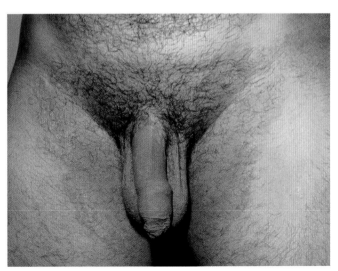

FIGURE 26.9 Tinea cruris is characterized by an erythematous patch that involves the proximal thigh and crural fold. Involvement may be bilateral as shown here or unilateral. (From Craft N, Taylor E, Tumeh PC, et al. *VisualDx: Essential Adult Dermatology.* Lippincott Williams & Wilkins; 2010.)

in intertriginous areas (groin, axillae, gluteal cleft). Scale may be present, but the borders of lesions are not elevated. Wood's lamp examination reveals a "coral-red" color fluorescence.

Treatment

Apply a topical imidazole cream twice daily as described in the section on tinea pedis. Tinea cruris may be a recurrent problem. Counsel patients to dry carefully after bathing or showering, avoid tight-fitting or occlusive clothing, and apply a talc-free absorbent powder to reduce moisture and friction.

VIRAL INFECTIONS

Warts

Warts are epidermal growths caused by various types of human papillomavirus (HPV). Human papillomavirus types are often related to the clinical presentation; for example, types 1, 2, and 4 cause common warts on the hands and plantar warts, while types 2 and 10 cause flat warts. Warts are spread by direct contact, auto-inoculation, or fomites (like showers or pool decking in the case of plantar warts).

Clinical Manifestations

1. Common warts: Skin-colored, often dome-shaped papules with a rough (i.e., verrucous) surface (e-Fig. 26.5). Occasionally, they exhibit a finger-shaped (i.e., filiform) appearance. Black specks that represent thrombosed capillaries may be seen on the surface of the wart.
2. Plantar warts: Skin-colored papules, nodules, or plaques that have a rough surface that are located on the plantar surface of the foot (e-Fig. 26.6). Because of the pressure exerted by walking, plantar warts are less elevated than common warts.
3. Flat warts: Skin-colored or pink, small (1 to 3 mm), smooth, flat-topped papules often located on the face or legs (e-Fig. 26.7).
4. Anogenital warts: Condylomata acuminata are skin-colored papules or plaques that involve the genitalia or perianal region (see Chapter 66).

Treatment

Warts often regress spontaneously and, therefore, observation without intervention is reasonable. However, many patients find the lesions unsightly and will request treatment. Several therapeutic options exist but those most commonly employed are salicylic acid and cryotherapy (which have comparable efficacy).[8] Patients should be counseled that HPV may remain in the skin after successful treatment and, as a result, recurrence is possible.

1. Salicylic acid: Application of salicylic acid 17% liquid (available without a prescription) is a safe and effective first-line treatment, especially for common and plantar warts. Depending on the size of the wart, several weeks to 3 months may be required for resolution. A typical treatment plan is as follows:
   a. In the evening, shower, bathe, or otherwise moisten the wart and then dry with a towel.
   b. Rub the wart with an emery board or nail file (to debride the wart).
   c. Apply salicylic acid to the wart and allow it to dry. To avoid irritation, avoid applying salicylic acid to normal skin.
   d. Occlude the wart with tape.
   e. In the morning, remove the tape (which facilitates debridement).
   f. Repeat the above steps daily.
2. Cryotherapy: Destruction of a wart by freezing is effective but painful. Although several cryogens are available for in-office or home use, liquid nitrogen is most effective due to its lower temperature. The goal of treatment is to create a blister within the epidermis.

   a. Liquid nitrogen is applied using a spray device or a cotton-tipped applicator reinforced with additional cotton (to hold liquid nitrogen).
   b. It is applied until the wart and a 1-mm rim of normal skin turn white (typically 10 to 15 seconds).
   c. When the wart thaws, a second treatment may be performed.
   d. Counsel the patient that a blister may form and provide wound-care instructions.
   e. If no blister forms or if wart tissue remains after a blister heals, begin salicylic acid treatment as described above.
   f. Repeat cryotherapy in 4 weeks if necessary.
3. Cimetidine: Oral cimetidine has immunomodulatory effects, enhancing T-cell function and cytokine production. Although data are conflicting, it may be of benefit, particularly in those who have numerous or resistant warts. A typical dose for AYAs is 400 mg twice daily for 6 to 8 weeks. Cimetidine is not FDA-approved for the treatment of warts. If it is used, some recommend concomitant salicylic acid treatment as described previously.
4. Tretinoin: Topical tretinoin has been used off-label to treat flat warts. The mechanism of action is not fully understood but it may be the result of the inflammatory response created in the skin. Tretinoin is applied to lesions nightly as tolerated.
5. Other treatment options include (a) intralesional injection of skin test antigens (e.g., *Candida*, *Trichophyton*); measles, mumps, and rubella vaccine; or bleomycin; or (b) the application of squaric acid. None of these are FDA-approved for the treatment of warts. Referral for laser treatment or electrodesiccation and curettage may be considered for recalcitrant warts.

BACTERIAL INFECTIONS

Crusted (Nonbullous) Impetigo

Crusted impetigo is an infection with *S. aureus* that produces erosions with a "honey-colored" crust often located near the nares. The differential diagnosis includes nummular eczema (often located on the extremities or trunk) or herpes simplex virus infection (typically produces clustered vesicles on an erythematous base). If infection is localized, a topical agent (e.g., mupirocin, retapamulin) may be used. For widespread or multifocal infection, an oral agent active against *S. aureus* is indicated.

Bullous Impetigo

Bullous impetigo is an infection with specific phage types of *S. aureus* that elaborate an epidermolytic toxin. The toxin damages intercellular adherence resulting in the formation of fragile bullae that easily rupture leaving round, crusted erosions. The differential diagnosis includes thermal burns, insect bite reactions, or immunobullous diseases. Treatment with an oral antistaphylococcal agent is indicated.

Folliculitis

Folliculitis represents inflammation centered around follicles. The most common form is caused by *S. aureus*. Hot tub folliculitis is caused by *Pseudomonas aeruginosa* acquired from hot tubs, swimming pools, or water parks.

Clinical Manifestations

Follicular-centered pustules with surrounding erythema (Fig. 26.10). Common sites of involvement are the thighs or buttocks, or areas exposed to pressure or friction applied by clothing. In those who have hot tub folliculitis, lesions are often concentrated in areas covered by bathing garments.

Treatment

Treatment options for staphylococcal folliculitis are presented below. Hot tub folliculitis requires no specific therapy as lesions

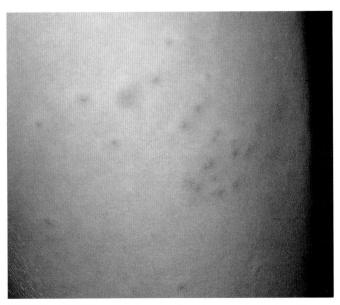

FIGURE 26.10 Follicular-centered erythematous papules and pustules are observed in folliculitis. This patient acquired infection from a hot tub.

resolve spontaneously over several days. Occasional patients experience a complication (e.g., conjunctivitis, otitis externa, cystitis) that requires appropriate antibiotic therapy.

1. Localized disease: Topical antibiotic (e.g., clindamycin, mupirocin, retapamulin)
2. Widespread disease: Oral antistaphylococcal antibiotic for 7 to 10 days
3. Prevention
    a. Use an antibacterial cleanser containing chlorhexidine (avoid ear canals) or sodium hypochlorite daily.
    b. Avoid tight-fitting clothing.
    c. If folliculitis is linked to shaving, change razor blades frequently and use an antibacterial cleanser after shaving.
    d. If the above strategies fail, consider twice-weekly bleach baths (1/4 cup of household bleach in a half-full bathtub) and/or intranasal mupirocin twice daily for 5 days.

PAPULOSQUAMOUS DISEASES

These diseases are characterized by elevated lesions (papulo) that have scale (squamous). The two most common papulosquamous diseases affecting AYAs are pityriasis rosea (PR) and psoriasis.

Pityriasis Rosea

Pityriasis rosea is a condition of unknown cause that may be the result of a viral infection. Pityriasis rosea occurs most often in AYAs.

Clinical Manifestations

1. Patients are usually well, although a minority experience a brief prodrome of malaise, headache, lymphadenopathy, or pharyngitis 1 to 2 weeks before the onset of the rash.
2. In 50% to 80% of patients, the rash begins with a herald patch, a scaling round or oval patch measuring 2 to 10 cm in diameter. The herald patch is usually located on the trunk, but may appear elsewhere.
3. Two to 21 days after the appearance of the herald patch, a generalized eruption begins that may be associated with pruritus. The generalized eruption involves thin, scaly oval plaques; the scale is located on the trailing edge of the lesions (i.e., toward the center of lesions). This is unlike the scale of tinea corporis that is located at the leading edge of lesions (i.e., peripherally). Lesions are distributed symmetrically on the trunk with relative

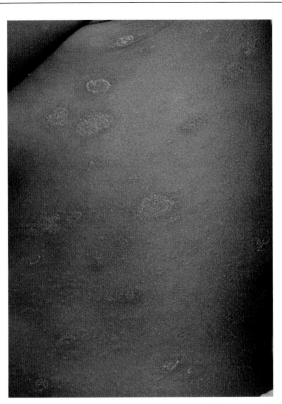

FIGURE 26.11 In this example of pityriasis rosea, there are oval scaling thin plaques on the lateral trunk. The long axes of lesions are arranged parallel to lines of skin stress.

sparing of the face and extremities (Fig. 26.11). The long axes of lesions are arranged parallel to lines of skin stress, so that on the back, the arrangement of lesions suggests the appearance of the branches of a fir tree. In persons with skin of color, lesions may be papular and distributed "inversely" (i.e., concentrated on the extremities or in the groin with relative sparing of the trunk).

Differential Diagnosis

1. Tinea corporis or nummular eczema: May mimic the herald patch of PR. A lesion of nummular eczema usually exhibits crust not scale.
2. Viral exanthems or morbilliform drug eruptions: Lesions do not have scale or the unique orientation of those of PR.
3. Secondary syphilis: Unlike patients who have PR, those who have secondary syphilis are ill with fever and lymphadenopathy and often have lesions on the palms or soles.

Treatment

There is no specific treatment; resolution typically occurs in 6 to 8 weeks (range 2 to 12 weeks). Pruritus may be managed with a topical corticosteroid, an emollient containing menthol or phenol (agents that act as counterirritants distracting the body from the sensation of pruritus), or an oral first-generation antihistamine (sedating). Judicious sun exposure may reduce pruritus or cause the eruption to resolve more rapidly.

Psoriasis

Psoriasis is an immune-mediated inflammatory skin disorder that affects an estimated 2% of the population.[9] In approximately one-third of patients, the disease first appears during childhood or adolescence.

Clinical Manifestations

The lesions of psoriasis are well-defined erythematous papules and plaques that possess a thick, adherent scale. If scale is removed,

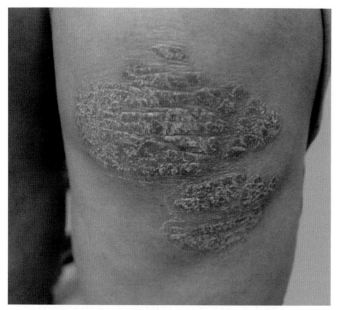

FIGURE 26.12 The lesions of psoriasis are erythematous scaling papules and plaques. Lesions are often located on the extensor surfaces of the extremities. (From Werner R. *Massage Therapist's Guide to Pathology.* 5th ed. Lippincott Williams & Wilkins; 2012.)

punctate areas of bleeding appear (Auspitz sign). The eyebrows, ears, extensor surfaces of the elbows and knees, umbilicus, and gluteal cleft are commonly affected (Fig. 26.12). Lesions may appear at sites of trauma (the Koebner phenomenon), likely explaining involvement of the extensor elbows and knees. Many individuals have scalp disease with erythema and scale. Pitting, yellowing, or thickening of the nails occurs in a minority of patients. Although psoriasis may be associated with an oligoarthritis involving the metacarpophalangeal or proximal interphalangeal joints or axial skeleton, this occurs rarely in AYAs.

Treatment

Typical topical treatment options are listed below. They are most useful for those who have a limited number and extent of lesions. Patients who have more widespread disease or those who fail to respond to topical treatment should be referred to a dermatologist for consideration of other topical or systemic agents.

1. Topical corticosteroid: For lesions on the trunk or extremities, a mid-potency agent like triamcinolone acetonide 0.1% may be applied twice daily. Those who fail to respond (or whose lesions are thick) may require a higher-potency product (like fluocinonide 0.05% [class 2]). However, when using potent preparations, caution should be exercised to avoid prolonged application that might result in skin atrophy. One way to avoid this is to apply the medication twice a day for 2 weeks and then twice daily Saturday and Sunday (beginning about a week later). This "pulsed" treatment maintains the steroid effect but reduces the likelihood of skin atrophy. Scalp involvement requires a solution (like fluocinolone acetonide oil 0.01% [class 6] or clobetasol propionate 0.05% [class 1]) or foam (like clobetasol propionate 0.05%).

2. Topical calcipotriene 0.005%: For those who do not respond adequately to a topical corticosteroid, calcipotriene may be valuable. It is a vitamin D_3 analog that normalizes epidermal proliferation. It is used in conjunction with a topical corticosteroid (each drug applied once daily). Although expensive, the most convenient formulation contains a class 1 corticosteroid combined with calcipotriene; it is applied once daily as needed.

3. Other treatments: Although effective, tars and anthralin are cosmetically displeasing and are generally considered second-line therapies. Tazarotene is a topical retinoid occasionally used in conjunction with a topical corticosteroid. A shampoo containing salicylic acid or tar can help remove thick scale from the scalp.

HYPERSENSITIVITY REACTIONS

Urticaria

Urticaria is a form of cutaneous hypersensitivity reaction in which there is vasodilation (causing erythema) and fluid leak from vessels (causing swelling). The lifetime prevalence of the disorder is 20%.[10] Urticaria may be separated into acute (lasting <6 weeks) and chronic (lasting ≥6 weeks) forms. Acute urticaria may have a number of triggers, most commonly infection (e.g., viral, streptococcal, parasitic), foods (e.g., shellfish, peanuts, eggs, strawberries), medications (e.g., antibiotics [e.g., penicillin, sulfonamides], nonsteroidal anti-inflammatory agents, others [e.g., barbiturates, codeine]), or insect stings.

Clinical Manifestations

The lesions are wheals (hives) and can take many shapes, including rings, arcs, plaques, or papules (Fig. 26.13). Individual lesions are evanescent, typically lasting less than 3 hours and never longer than 24 hours.

Differential Diagnosis

Disorders that may mimic urticaria include the following:

1. Erythema multiforme (EM): Lesions are fixed in location (not evanescent); have a uniform morphology (not multiple lesion shapes); exhibit a central duskiness, vesicle, or crust; and favor the extremities with relative sparing of the trunk.

2. Urticarial vasculitis: Lesions last longer than 24 hours and have central duskiness or purpura.

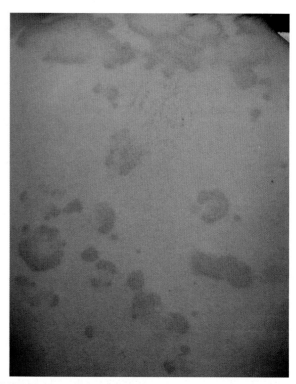

FIGURE 26.13 In urticaria, lesions take many shapes. In this patient there are erythematous papules, circles, incomplete circles, and plaques with polycyclic borders.

3. Serum sickness-like eruption: Lesions are large, often purple rings or plaques associated with periarticular swelling; fever and arthralgias are often present.

Evaluation

Evaluation for a precipitating factor should be dictated by the history and physical examination.

Treatment

1. Treat or remove any identified precipitant and avoid the use of nonsteroidal anti-inflammatory agents that may exacerbate urticaria.
2. H1-antihistamines are first-line therapy. Although a first-generation agent (e.g., diphenhydramine or hydroxyzine) is often used, sedation may be a problem. As a result, it may be prudent to begin therapy with a second-generation (e.g., loratadine, cetirizine) or third-generation (e.g., desloratadine, fexofenadine, levocetirizine) agent. If a response is not achieved, a first-generation antihistamine could be added at bedtime or the dose of the second- or third-generation drug increased (some advocate increasing the dose to two to four times that recommended).[10] Once lesions have resolved, treatment may be continued for several additional days and then discontinued.
3. Oral corticosteroids are second-line therapies generally reserved for severe disease. It is not uncommon for patients to experience a reappearance of lesions when corticosteroids are withdrawn.
4. Most episodes of urticaria resolve in about 2 weeks. If the condition persists or is recurrent, or if accompanied by an episode of anaphylaxis, allergy consultation is indicated.

Erythema Multiforme

Erythema multiforme represents a cutaneous hypersensitivity reaction that occurs most commonly in young adults. Traditionally, it is separated into two forms, EM minor and EM major. For convenience, both entities will be discussed here.

1. **Erythema multiforme (formerly called EM minor)**
   a. *Clinical manifestations:* Most cases (90%) are caused by infections, especially herpes simplex virus (a history of herpes labialis is reported by 50% of patients with EM). Prodromal symptoms are absent, and the rash begins as erythematous papules that have a predilection for acral surfaces, including the palms, soles, and face, with relative sparing of the trunk. Lesions remain fixed in location for up to 2 to 3 weeks before resolving. Over several days, a central violaceous discoloration or, occasionally, a vesicle or crust develops (Fig. 26.14). One-half of those who have EM have oral erosions that are few in number.
   b. *Treatment:* Erythema multiforme is self-limited, resolving in 2 to 3 weeks. No specific therapy is indicated. If EM is recurrent and thought to be the result of herpes simplex virus infection, consider daily oral antiviral prophylaxis.
2. **Stevens–Johnson syndrome (SJS) (formerly called EM major) and toxic epidermal necrolysis (TEN):** Stevens–Johnson syndrome and TEN represent more severe and potentially life-threatening hypersensitivity reactions to drugs (e.g., antibiotics [trimethoprim-sulfamethoxazole], anticonvulsants [lamotrigine, carbamazepine, phenytoin, phenobarbital], nonsteroidal anti-inflammatory agents) or, less commonly, infectious agents (e.g., *Mycoplasma pneumoniae*). Stevens–Johnson syndrome and TEN may represent the same disease process, differing only in extent of cutaneous involvement. The annual incidence of SJS and TEN worldwide is 1.2 to 6 and 0.4 to 1.9 per million people, respectively.[11]

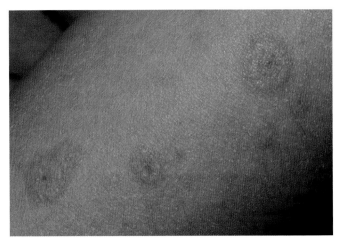

FIGURE 26.14 In erythema multiforme, target lesions are observed. These are erythematous papules that develop a central violaceous discoloration, vesicle, or crust.

   a. *Clinical manifestations:* Stevens–Johnson syndrome/TEN typically begins 6 days to 2 weeks after initiating a drug.[4]
      • Patients experience prodromal symptoms, including fever, sore throat, rhinitis, cough, headache, vomiting, or diarrhea.
      • Within 14 days, erythematous or purpuric macules and patches appear on the trunk and extremities. Blisters form rapidly and rupture leaving large areas of denuded skin (e-Fig. 26.8). In SJS, there is epidermal loss of <10% of the body surface, while TEN is diagnosed when patients lose >30% of the epidermal surface; those with involvement of 10% to 30% are said to have SJS/TEN overlap. In SJS and TEN, target lesions are absent or few in number.
      • Mucosal involvement is prominent with hemorrhagic crusting of the lips (e-Fig. 26.9), oral ulcers, and purulent conjunctivitis. The trachea, bronchi, and gastrointestinal tract may be involved.
   b. *Treatment:* Early discontinuation of the offending drug is essential. The use of systemic corticosteroids is controversial. Intravenous immunoglobulin may be beneficial. Immunosuppressants or biologic agents occasionally are used but the evidence regarding their efficacy is limited. Supportive care (with careful attention to skin, eye, and fluid and electrolyte status) in a burn unit or intensive care unit is imperative. Monitoring for secondary bacterial infection is important since sepsis leading to multiorgan failure is the leading cause of death.[12]
   c. *Prognosis:* The mortality rate of SJS is 1% to 5%, and that of TEN is 25% to 30%.[12] Long-term complications involve the eye (impaired tear production and drainage, aberrant lashes), skin (altered pigmentation), and nails (dystrophy).

Erythema Nodosum

Erythema nodosum (EN) is a hypersensitivity reaction that results in inflammation of fat (panniculitis). Precipitants include infection (e.g., *Streptococcus pyogenes* [the most common infectious cause], tuberculosis, Epstein–Barr virus, *Yersinia enterocolitica*, histoplasmosis, coccidioidomycosis, leptospirosis), medications (e.g., estrogen in oral contraceptives, sulfonamides), inflammatory bowel disease, or collagen vascular disease. However, in most cases, no precipitating factor is identified.

Clinical Manifestations

Patients develop tender erythematous nodules that are typically located on the extensor surfaces of both legs. Over several days,

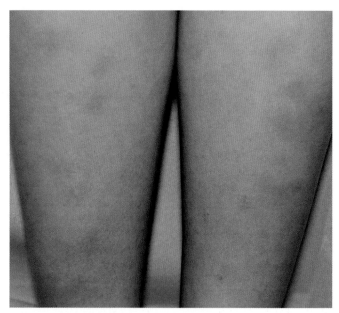

FIGURE 26.15 Erythema nodosum is characterized by violaceous nodules often located on the extensor surfaces of the legs.

the nodules evolve from red to brown-red or purple and later to yellow-green (Fig. 26.15).

Evaluation

The evaluation is guided by the findings on history and physical examination. In patients who have no known precipitants and appear healthy, some recommend limited screening studies, including measurement of antistreptolysin-O and/or anti-DNase B titers, complete blood count, serum calcium, stool hemoccult testing, chest x-ray and screening for tuberculosis (purified protein derivative [PPD] skin test or interferon gamma receptor assay).

Treatment

If identified, a precipitating factor should be treated or removed. Erythema nodosum generally resolves within several days to a few weeks. First-line treatment includes a nonsteroidal anti-inflammatory agent and relative rest. For those who fail to respond, consultation with a dermatologist is appropriate to consider treatment with saturated solution of potassium iodide, colchicine, or prednisone.

Drug Eruptions

Drug eruptions represent a distinct form of hypersensitivity reaction. The major forms are discussed below (urticarial drug eruptions, SJS, and TEN were addressed previously).

1. **Exanthematous (morbilliform):** The most common form of drug eruption is one that mimics the appearance of a viral exanthem. Erythematous macules that may become slightly elevated begin on the trunk and spread to the face and extremities. The eruption appears 7 to 14 days after beginning a medication but may occur earlier if there has been prior drug exposure. Aminopenicillins, cephalosporins, sulfonamides, and anticonvulsants are most often responsible. Treatment involves removing the offending drug and administering an antihistamine. If the suspected drug is essential and no alternative exists, some advocate continuing the agent despite the eruption ("treating through"). In such cases, the eruption usually resolves but occasional patients experience worsening.

2. **Drug-induced hypersensitivity syndrome** (DIHS, also known as drug reaction with eosinophilia and systemic symptoms [DRESS]): Drug-induced hypersensitivity syndrome is a severe reaction that likely results from defects in the metabolism of certain drugs. The agents most commonly implicated are anticonvulsants (e.g., phenobarbital, phenytoin, carbamazepine, and lamotrigine), antibiotics (e.g., sulfonamides, minocycline), and allopurinol. Drug-induced hypersensitivity syndrome begins 2 to 6 weeks after initiating a drug. Patients develop fever and erythematous macules and papules (i.e., a morbilliform eruption); facial edema is often present. Hepatitis (possibly fulminant), pneumonitis, myocarditis, and nephritis may occur. Early withdrawal of the suspected drug is essential; systemic corticosteroids are employed in severe cases.

3. **Fixed drug eruption:** This unique eruption is characterized by an erythematous or dusky oval patch or plaque that occurs at the same body location each time the offending drug is administered (usually within 24 hours of restarting the agent). Lesions may blister and heal with hyperpigmentation (e-Fig. 26.10). Common sites of involvement are the distal extremities and the penis. Many drugs may cause a fixed drug eruption, including antibiotics (e.g., sulfonamides, tetracyclines), anticonvulsants (e.g., barbiturates, carbamazepine), and nonsteroidal anti-inflammatory agents.

4. **Photosensitivity eruptions:** May be classified as phototoxic or photoallergic.
   a. Phototoxic reactions: Occur when ultraviolet (UV) light (typically UVA) activates a drug. Phototoxic eruptions are mediated by nonimmunologic mechanisms (e.g., free radical damage to cells). Clinically, an exaggerated sunburn-like erythema appears 2 to 6 hours after exposure. Drugs commonly responsible include tetracyclines (doxycycline and other tetracyclines), nonsteroidal anti-inflammatory agents, sulfonamides, fluoroquinolones, phenothiazines, and diuretics (e.g., furosemide, thiazide, hydrochlorothiazide).
   b. Photoallergic: Photoallergy is an uncommon disorder that is thought to be the result of delayed hypersensitivity. Once sensitized, within 24 hours of re-exposure to the drug, an eczematous eruption (e.g., papules and vesicles) appears on sun-exposed areas. Extension of the rash to protected areas may occur. Sunscreens, particularly those containing benzophenones, are usually responsible.

● OTHER CONDITIONS

Hair Loss

Hair loss without associated scarring of the scalp may be separated into generalized and localized forms. The most common causes of hair loss are discussed below.

1. Generalized hair loss
   a. Telogen effluvium: Normally, approximately 90% of hairs are in a growing (anagen) state and 10% in a resting (telogen) state; 50 to 100 are lost each day. A stressful event such as a significant febrile illness, delivering an infant, or being born may shift the majority of hairs to a telogen state. Two to 4 months following the event, resting hairs are lost and replaced by growing hairs. Since hair regrowth occurs spontaneously, no treatment is necessary. Other causes of telogen effluvium include endocrine diseases (e.g., hypothyroidism, hypopituitarism) and medications (e.g., certain anticonvulsants, isotretinoin, cimetidine, terbinafine). Discontinuing an oral contraceptive also may be responsible.[13]
   b. Androgenetic alopecia (AGA): In males, AGA is believed to result from the effects of androgens on genetically susceptible hair follicles. Under the influence of dihydrotestosterone, genes are activated that reduce the length of the hair growth cycle and size of the follicles. As a result, shorter and finer hairs are produced. The role of androgens

in females is less clear. In males, AGA usually begins in the 20s or 30s but may have its onset earlier (the prevalence in boys 15 to 17 years has been estimated to be 14%).[13] It is characterized by temporal and eventually frontal hairline recession. An estimated 3% of females aged 20 to 29 years develop AGA.[13] They experience diffuse hair loss that is most noticeable at the vertex. For females who have marked temporal recession or other signs of androgen excess, hormonal evaluation is indicated. The initial treatment of AGA in males is minoxidil 5% topically or finasteride orally; in females, minoxidil 2% topically or spironolactone orally may be employed.

2. Localized hair loss
   a. Alopecia areata: Alopecia areata is an autoimmune disorder that results in one or more round or oval patches of complete hair loss; scaling and inflammation of the scalp are absent. At the periphery of lesions, one may see exclamation point hairs, short hairs that are broader distally than proximally. A minority of patients experience loss of all scalp hair (alopecia totalis) or body hair (alopecia universalis). For those who have one or two small patches of hair loss, no intervention is an option since there is a high rate of spontaneous remission within 1 year. Initial treatment generally involves a potent topical corticosteroid (like clobetasol foam) or intradermal corticosteroid injections performed every 4 to 6 weeks. One regimen for topical therapy is to apply the steroid at bedtime five consecutive nights followed by two nights without treatment (to avoid cutaneous atrophy). Minoxidil is often used in conjunction with a corticosteroid, especially if some hair regrowth is observed. If involvement is extensive, consultation with a dermatologist is indicated. The National Alopecia Areata Foundation is a source of support and resources for patients and families (www.naaf.org).
   b. Traction alopecia: Thinning of the hair may result from constant, excessive traction as might result from tight braiding or ponytails. The hair loss is incomplete, symmetrically distributed, and located at sites where the hair is parted. Reducing traction on the hair generally results in regrowth.
   c. Trichotillomania (TTM) (hair-pulling disorder): Repetitive twirling, twisting, rubbing, or pulling of hair may cause it to break, a disorder termed TTM. The American Psychiatric Association's *Diagnostic and Statistical Manual of Mental Disorders*, 5th edition categorizes TTM among the obsessive-compulsive and related disorders and provides specific criteria for this diagnosis.[14] Affected individuals often feel anxious or tense before pulling their hair and relief afterward. Most often the scalp is involved, and affected individuals have well-defined patches of relative alopecia; within the patches are hairs of differing lengths. Scaling is absent but petechiae or erosions may be present, particularly if hair is pulled. Other sites of involvement include the eyebrows, eyelashes, or extremities. For those with significant disease, consultation with a mental health clinician may be helpful to consider cognitive behavioral therapy (e.g., relaxation training or habit reversal therapy). No FDA-approved medications exist for the treatment of TTM. Selective serotonin reuptake inhibitors are frequently prescribed, but no studies have demonstrated their efficacy.[15]

Acanthosis Nigricans

Most often, acanthosis nigricans (AN) occurs in association with obesity and reflects insulin resistance. Acanthosis nigricans also may occur in certain syndromes (e.g., the HAIR-AN syndrome [*hyperandrognemia, insulin resistance, acanthosis nigricans*]) and

in older adults may be associated with malignancy (in such cases, AN is of abrupt onset and widespread).

Clinical Manifestations

Acanthosis nigricans is a hyperpigmented "velvety" thickening of the skin typically observed at the nape and sides of the neck and in the axillae.

Treatment

If weight reduction can be achieved, the appearance of AN will improve. A topical retinoid applied daily or a keratolytic (like ammonium lactate or urea) applied twice daily may benefit some individuals.

Hidradenitis Suppurativa

Hidradenitis suppurativa is a chronic inflammatory disease of apocrine glands. It begins during the second or third decade of life and occurs more commonly in females. The prevalence is often stated to be 1%, although one study suggests that it may be as low as 0.053%.[16]

Clinical Manifestations

Involvement of the axillae or groin is typical; patients develop recurrent, tender nodules that rupture and drain. Over time, sinus tracts or hypertrophic scars may form (e-Fig. 26.11).

Treatment

Initial treatment includes long-term oral antibiotic therapy (with doxycycline or minocycline), twice-daily application of a topical antibiotic (like clindamycin), and regular use of an antibacterial soap (e.g., one containing chlorhexidine or sodium hypochlorite). For those who have severe recalcitrant disease, surgical excision of the affected areas may be curative.

Hyperhidrosis

Hyperhidrosis, excessive sweating, affects up to 3% of the U.S. population.[17] It may be primary (idiopathic) or secondary (resulting from an underlying disorder or medication). Primary hyperhidrosis typically has its onset in adolescence or young adulthood.[17]

Clinical Manifestations

Most often, primary hyperhidrosis involves the axillae, palms, and soles. Severe forms can adversely impact quality of life, compromising social or occupational activities.

Treatment

For axillary hyperhidrosis, one can recommend an over-the-counter antiperspirant containing aluminum chloride. If this fails, consider one of the following strategies:

1. Recommend a product containing a higher concentration of aluminum chloride (like Certain Dri [12%]) or prescribe a product containing aluminum chloride hexahydrate (like Xerac AC [6.25%] or Drysol [20%]). Ideally, these are applied at bedtime under occlusion with plastic wrap. If sweating is controlled (requires several days), occlusion can be discontinued, and the frequency of application decreased (to every few days as needed).
2. The newest FDA-approved topical product for hyperhidrosis is towelettes containing glycopyrronium (Qbrexa). They can be used in children aged 9 and older for axillary involvement.
3. For some individuals, tap-water iontophoresis may be beneficial. Devices are available to treat the underarms, hands, and feet. Information may be obtained at www.drionic.com.
4. An oral anticholinergic like glycopyrrolate is often effective but may cause dry mouth, dry eyes, or bladder or bowel dysfunction.
5. For those with recalcitrant axillary hyperhidrosis, intradermal injection of botulinum toxin or treatment with a device that

employs electromagnetic energy may be useful. In those who have severe or widespread symptoms, thoracic sympathectomy may be considered.

Sun Exposure

Sun exposure is linked to the development of skin cancer and skin aging (i.e., wrinkling and laxity of the skin, mottled pigmentation, blackheads). Most skin cancers are nonmelanoma skin cancers (NMSCs, e.g., basal cell carcinoma and squamous cell carcinoma) that are associated with cumulative lifetime sun exposure. Approximately 3 million individuals in the United States develop an NMSC each year and the incidence is rising, including among those <40 years of age. Rates of malignant melanoma also have been increasing. It was estimated that in 2020, 100,350 persons in the United States would be diagnosed with malignant melanoma and 6,850 would die of this disease.[18] Among new cases, 0.4% are diagnosed in those <20 years of age and 5.1% in those 20 to 34 years of age.[19] Malignant melanoma is associated with intermittent intense UV exposure. Of note, both NMSC and malignant melanoma have been linked to tanning bed use; young age of use and UV dose appear to be important risk factors. Essential recommendations for sun protection for those at risk include the following:

- Use a broad-spectrum sunscreen (one that provides UVA and UVB protection). The sun protection factor (SPF) is primarily a measure of UVB protection; it is the ratio of the minimum dose of UV radiation needed to produce sunburn in sunscreen-protected skin to that of unprotected skin. In principle, therefore, application of an SPF 8 product would protect against sunburn eight times longer than using no sunscreen.[20] In the United States, there is no rating system for UV-A protection.
  - Apply the sunscreen liberally—using too little will reduce the effective SPF. To provide a margin of error if too little is applied, choose a product with an SPF of 30 or more.
  - Reapply the sunscreen frequently if sweating or swimming. All sunscreen labels now state the length of time the sunscreen is considered active on the skin, typically either 40 or 80 minutes.
  - Consider an alcohol-free product (to prevent stinging of the eyes) and one that is labeled "nonacnegenic," "noncomedogenic," or "won't block pores" (to avoid worsening acne).
- Wear sun-protective clothing (like a hat with a brim or shirts having a UV protective factor).
- Wear sunglasses that provide UV protection (labeled as blocking 100% of the full UV spectrum).
- Avoid tanning beds—consider sunless tanning products that can be applied at home or in a tanning facility.

Vitiligo

Vitiligo represents an acquired loss of pigment. It is likely an autoimmune phenomenon that occurs in genetically predisposed individuals. In the United States and Europe, the prevalence is approximately 1%.[21]

Clinical Manifestations

Lesions are well-defined macules or patches that are depigmented. Vitiligo may be separated into two forms: generalized (i.e., lesions are symmetrically distributed on the extremities, trunk, face, and neck) and segmental (i.e., involves only one area of the body and does not cross the midline). Occasionally, vitiligo is associated with other autoimmune disorders, including thyroiditis, adrenal insufficiency, pernicious anemia, and gonadal dysfunction. Many experts recommend the performance of thyroid function studies and antithyroid antibodies, with other testing only if indicated based on symptoms or signs.

Differential Diagnosis

The complete loss of pigment in vitiligo distinguishes it from other disorders characterized by a reduction in pigment (i.e., hypopigmentation), including tinea versicolor, pityriasis alba and other forms of postinflammatory hypopigmentation, and nevus depigmentosus. In addition, the lesions of tinea versicolor and pityriasis alba often have scale, and the lesions of pityriasis alba have indistinct borders.

Treatment

The treatment of localized vitiligo is with a potent topical corticosteroid or a calcineurin inhibitor (the latter is especially useful in the treatment of facial lesions where the use of a potent topical corticosteroid may cause skin atrophy). Often the two drugs are used in combination (e.g., the calcineurin inhibitor is applied twice daily Monday to Friday and the corticosteroid twice daily Saturday and Sunday [to reduce the possibility of steroid-induced atrophy]). For those who have extensive disease, referral to a dermatologist is prudent (for consideration of UV light or laser therapy). Information and support can be found at the following sites: American Vitiligo Research Foundation (www.avrf.org) and Vitiligo Support International (www.vitiligosupport.org).

Body Modifications

Tattoos and piercings are common among AYAs.[22] In a Harris Poll published in 2016, 29% of all adults and 47% of millennials (aged 18 to 35 years) reported having one or more tattoos. Although most of those surveyed viewed their tattoo(s) positively, 23% reported some regret.[23] Among college students, one survey found that 51% had at least one body piercing.[22]

a. Almost all states have laws that affect one or more aspects of body modification. For example, at least 45 states have laws prohibiting minors from obtaining tattoos. Thirty-eight states prohibit piercing and tattooing of minors without parental permission.[24]
b. Although the rate of complications associated with tattooing or piercing is not known, it is likely quite low, especially if procedures are performed by a professional. The most important of these complications are discussed below.

Complications of Tattooing

Infections Infection may occur if inappropriate hygiene practices are employed (e.g., the artist fails to wear gloves, fails to disinfect the skin, or uses contaminated needles or ink). The most common forms are local infections like folliculitis or abscess due to *Staphylococcus aureus* (including methicillin-resistant *S. aureus*) or cellulitis caused by *Streptococcus pyogenes*. Management is with an appropriate topical or oral antibiotic depending on the severity of infection. Systemic infection occurs rarely, although severe infections such as infective endocarditis, spinal abscess, and gangrene occurring following tattooing have been reported. Nontuberculous mycobacterial (NTB) infection, characterized by the appearance of papules, nodules, or abscesses within the tattoo, has been reported following the use of contaminated ink. If NTB infection is suspected, consultations with a dermatologist (for diagnostic biopsy) and an infectious diseases specialist (regarding treatment) are appropriate. Bloodborne pathogens, including hepatitis B, hepatitis C, and human immunodeficiency virus, may be transmitted during tattoo placement but the likelihood is low when the procedure is done in a licensed establishment.

Inflammatory Reactions Localized erythema and edema are common in the days following tattoo placement. However, the appearance of an eruption within an established tattoo suggests an inflammatory response to tattoo pigment(s). These eruptions may be eczematous (pruritic erythematous patches), lichenoid (flat-topped papules), or granulomatous (nodules). Often these reactions can be managed with the application of a potent topical corticosteroid. However, failure to respond should prompt consultation with a dermatologist. In addition, there have been rare reports of cutaneous vasculitis and skin cancer (arising within tattoo pigmentation) occurring in tattoo recipients.

Tattoo Removal

For those desiring tattoo removal, picosecond and Q-switched lasers are first-line treatments. The laser type and wavelength selected are determined by the tattoo's colors and the patient's skin type. Those considering removal should be counseled that laser removal is costly, multiple treatments are required, ink removal may be incomplete, and there may be permanent changes in skin pigmentation and texture.

Complications of Piercing

Infection Minor local bacterial infection (i.e., cellulitis, abscess formation) is the most common complication of piercing. In many cases, this can be prevented by appropriate wound care. Rarely, systemic infection may occur, including bacteremia, infective endocarditis, meningitis, and toxic shock syndrome. Some unique complications related to specific piercing sites include the following:

a. Chondritis due to *Pseudomonas* sp. infection may complicate piercings of ear cartilage.
b. Oral piercings may be complicated by glossitis and abscess formation that may involve anaerobic bacteria. Rarely, Ludwig angina, Lemierre syndrome, cerebellar abscess, and tetanus have been reported.
c. Genital piercings may become infected with gram-negative enteric bacteria like *Escherichia coli*.

Sensitivity to Materials Used in Piercing Jewelry Body piercing jewelry may be composed of stainless steel, gold, niobium, titanium, or alloys. Gold is often combined with nickel or other metals. Owing to the high prevalence of nickel sensitivity, it should be avoided. Niobium, titanium, and surgical stainless steel rarely produce an allergic response, although not all surgical stainless steel is nickel free.

Scarring Any trauma to the skin can result in scarring, but piercings are particularly susceptible to keloid scar formation. Particularly high-risk piercing sites include the ear lobe, ear cartilage, and nasal cartilage. Keloids can occur in any skin type, although they are more common in patients with darker skin types. There also appears to be some element of genetic predilection for keloid formation; if a patient has a personal or family history of keloid scarring, they should be counseled about the risk of this occurring with any new piercing. Although recent research has improved our understanding of the pathogenesis of scar formation and offered some novel treatment options, the treatment of keloids remains a challenge.

SUMMARY

The identification and management of skin disorders are important as nearly one in five visits by AYAs may be associated with a dermatologic diagnosis. This chapter has reviewed the disorders most likely to be encountered by clinicians, including forms of dermatitis, skin infections, hypersensitivity disorders, hair loss, consequences of sun exposure and photoprotection, and body modification.

REFERENCES

1. National Ambulatory Medical Care Survey. Accessed October 7, 2013. http://www.cdc.gov/nchs/ahcd.htm
2. Eichenfield LF, Tom WL, Chamlin SL, et al. Guidelines of care for the management of atopic dermatitis: section 1. Diagnosis and assessment of atopic dermatitis. *J Am Acad Dermatol.* 2014;70(2):338–351.
3. Gooderham MJ, Hong HCH, Eshtiaghi P, et al. Dupilumab: a review of its use in the treatment of atopic dermatitis. *J Am Acad Dermatol.* 2018; 78(3 Suppl 1):S28–S36.
4. Silverberg NB, Pelletier JL, Jacob SE, et al; Section on Dermatology, Section on Allergy and Immunology. Nickel allergic contact dermatitis: identification, treatment, and prevention. *Pediatrics.* 2020;145:e20200628.
5. Dessinioti C, Katsambas A. Seborrheic dermatitis: etiology, risk factors, and treatments: facts and controversies. *Clin Dermatol.* 2013;31(4):343–351.
6. Lipner SR, Scher RK. Onychomycosis: clinical overview and diagnosis. *J Am Acad Dermatol.* 2019;80(4):835–851.
7. Lipner SR, Scher RK. Onychomycosis. Treatment and prevention. *J Am Acad Dermatol.* 2019;80(4):853–867.
8. Kwok CS, Gibbs S, Bennett C, et al. Topical treatments for cutaneous warts. *Cochrane Database Syst Rev* 2012;(9):CD001781.
9. Boehncke WH, Schön MP. Psoriasis. *Lancet.* 2015;386(9997):983–994.
10. Schaefer P. Acute and chronic urticaria: evaluation and treatment. *Am Fam Physician* 2017;95(11):717–724.
11. Schwartz RA, McDonough PH, Lee BW. Toxic epidermal necrolysis, Part I: introduction, history, classification, clinical features, systemic manifestations, etiology, and immunogenesis. *J Am Acad Dermatol.* 2013;69(2):173.e1–e13.
12. Schwartz RA, McDonough PH, Lee BW. Toxic epidermal necrolysis, Part II: prognosis, sequelae, diagnosis, differential diagnosis, prevention, and treatment. *J Am Acad Dermatol.* 2013;69(2):187.e1–e16.
13. Tackett BN, Hrismalos EN. Alopecia in adolescents. *Adolesc Med State Art Rev.* 2011;22(1):16–34.
14. American Psychiatric Association. *Diagnostic and Statistical Manual of Mental Disorders.* 5th ed. American Psychiatric Association; 2013.
15. Rothbart R, Amos T, Siegfried N, et al. Pharmacotherapy for trichotillomania. *Cochrane Database Syst Rev* 2013;(11):CD007662.
16. Cosmatos I, Matcho A, Weinstein R, et al. Analysis of patient claims data to determine the prevalence of hidradenitis suppurativa in the United States. *J Am Acad Dermatol* 2013;68(3):412–419.
17. McConaghy JR, Fosselman D. Hyperhidrosis: management options. *Am Fam Physician* 2018;97(11):729–734.
18. Skin Cancer Foundation. Accessed May 13, 2020. https://skincancer.org/skin-cancer-information/skin-cancer-facts/
19. National Cancer Institute Surveillance, Epidemiology, and End Results Program. Accessed May 13, 2020. https://seer.cancer.gov/statfacts/html/melan.html
20. Sambandan DR, Ratner D. Sunscreens: an overview and update. *J Am Acad Dermatol.* 2011;64(4):748–758.
21. Ezzedine K, Eleftheriadou V, Whitten M, et al. Vitiligo. *Lancet.* 2015;386(9988):74–84.
22. Breuner CC, Levine DA; Committee on Adolescence. Adolescent and young adult tattooing, piercing, and scarification. *Pediatrics.* 2017;140(4):320171962.
23. Shannon-Missal L. *Tattoo takeover: three in ten Americans have a tattoo, and most don't stop at one. Harris Poll No. 12.* 2016. Accessed July 19, 2020. https://theharrispoll.com/tattoos-can-take-any-number-of-forms-from-animals-to-quotes-to-cryptic-symbols-and-appear-in-all-sorts-of-spots-on-our-bodies-some-visible-in-everyday-life-tableothers-not-so-much-but-one-thi/
24. National Conference of State Legislatures. *Tattooing and body piercing. State laws, statutes, and regulations.* 2019. https://www.ncsl.org/research/health/tattooing-and-body-piercing.aspx

ADDITIONAL RESOURCES AND WEBSITES

Additional Resources and Websites for Clinicians:

Atopic Dermatitis
Yang EJ, Sekhon S, Sanchez IM, et al. Recent developments in atopic dermatitis. *Pediatrics.* 2018;142:e20181102.

Hair Loss
Henkel ED, Jaquez SD, Diaz LZ. Pediatric trichotillomania: review of management. *Pediatr Dermatol.* 2019;36:803–807.
Strazzulla LC, Wang EHC, AvilaL, et al. Alopecia areata: an appraisal of new treatment approaches and overview of current therapies. *J Am Acad Dermatol.* 2018;78:15–24.
Strazzulla LC, Wang EHC, Avila L, et al. Alopecia areata: disease characteristics, clinical evaluation, and new perspectives on pathogenesis. *J Am Acad Dermatol.* 2018;78:1–12.

Hyperhidrosis
Nawrocki S, Cha J. The etiology, diagnosis and management of hyperhidrosis: a comprehensive review. Etiology and clinical work-up. *J Am Acad Dermatol.* 2019;81:657–666.
Nawrocki S, Cha J. The etiology, diagnosis and management of hyperhidrosis: a comprehensive review. Therapeutic options. *J Am Acad Dermatol.* 2019;81:669–680.

Sunscreens
Mancuso JB, Maruthi R, Wang SQ, et al. Sunscreens: an update. *Am J Clin Dermatol.* 2017;18:643–650.

Urticaria
Antia C, Baquerizo K, Korman A, et al. Urticaria: a comprehensive review. Epidemiology, diagnosis, and work-up. *J Am Acad Dermatol.* 2018;79:599–614.
Antia C, Baquerizo K, Korman A, et al. Urticaria: a comprehensive review: treatment of chronic urticaria, special populations, and disease outcomes. *J Am Acad Dermatol.* 2018;79:617–633.

Additional Resources and Websites for Parents/Caregivers and Adolescents and Young Adults:
American Academy of Dermatology (https://www.aad.org/public): Information on diseases and conditions.
Society for Pediatric Dermatology (https://pedsderm.net/for-patients-families/): Patient information handouts, patient videos, and links to patient organizations.

PART VI

Neurologic and Sleep Disorders

CHAPTER 27

Epilepsy

Shilpa B. Reddy
Emma G. Carter

KEY WORDS

- Anti-seizure medication (ASM)
- Epilepsy
- Females with epilepsy
- People with epilepsy (PWE)
- Seizures
- Seizure precautions
- Sudden unexpected death in epilepsy (SUDEP)

INTRODUCTION

About one in 26 people in the United States will develop epilepsy in their lifetime, making epilepsy the fourth most common neurologic disorder in this country. About 50 million people worldwide are diagnosed with epilepsy.[1,2] Epilepsy has a bimodal age distribution with the most common age groups being young children and older adults. Among children and adolescents age 17 years and younger in the United States, approximately 0.6% or 470,000 children have active epilepsy.[1] If people with epilepsy (PWE) are accurately diagnosed and treated, up to 70%, could have seizure-free lives.[2] Recognition of seizure activity, accurate seizure classification, and appropriate determination of the etiology of seizures are vital in providing optimal treatment for the individual person with epilepsy. In addition, the field of epilepsy has been advanced by new electroencephalography (EEG) modalities, neurodiagnostic imaging, neurogenetic testing, and both medical and surgical treatment options.

In treating adolescents and young adults (AYAs) with epilepsy, important considerations include contraception and pregnancy, seizure precautions specific for this age group, seizure detection devices, methods to improve medication adherence, comorbidities such as mental-health diagnoses, and sudden unexpected death in epilepsy (SUDEP). Epilepsy awareness has improved over the years with the growth of the internet and social media. However, stigma and discrimination are significant problems for many PWE and their families, especially outside of the United States. Seizure and epilepsy education remain highly relevant and a worldwide public health priority for patients, clinicians, and communities.

DEFINITIONS

The International League Against Epilepsy (ILAE) defines an epileptic seizure as a transient occurrence of signs and/or symptoms due to abnormal excessive synchronous neuronal activity in the brain.[3] Seizures are then further distinguished into two groups: unprovoked seizures and acute symptomatic seizures. Unprovoked seizures are seizures occurring without a potentially responsible clinical condition or occurring in a timeframe beyond the estimated interval for the occurrence of acute symptomatic seizures.[3] Acute symptomatic seizures are seizures occurring in close temporal relationship with an acute central nervous system (CNS) insult.[4] This insult may be secondary to inflammatory, structural, toxic, or metabolic etiologies.[4]

The definition of epilepsy was redefined in 2014 from having two unprovoked seizures greater than 24 hours apart to one of the following[3]:

1. At least two unprovoked seizures occurring more than 24 hours apart
2. One unprovoked seizure and a probability of further seizures similar to the general recurrence risk (at least 60%) after two unprovoked seizures occurring over the next 10 years (i.e., in some cases a diagnosis of epilepsy can be made after only one seizure if the known risk of having another seizure is high)
3. Diagnosis of an epilepsy syndrome

The general recurrence risk is considered high in patients with a remote insult, such as traumatic brain injury (TBI), with seizure activity occurring more than 1 month after the TBI or a single seizure with a structural or remote symptomatic etiology and an abnormal EEG.[3]

Other important epilepsy terms include status epilepticus and seizure clusters.[5] Status epilepticus is defined as a condition resulting from either the failure of the mechanisms responsible for terminating a seizure or from the initiation of mechanisms that lead to prolonged seizures.[5] The duration of a seizure deemed "continuous seizure activity" (5 minutes), and the seizure duration associated with long-term consequences (30 minutes) are derived from animal models and clinical research of generalized tonic–clonic status epilepticus.[5] Unlike status epilepticus, seizure clusters are not well-defined and there is no agreed upon definition.[6] Several definitions have been proposed including ≥ three seizures within 24 hours; ≥ two seizures within 24 hours; or ≥ two seizures in 6 hours.[6] Despite the lack of a consensus definition, seizure clusters are predominantly seen in patients that have refractory epilepsy. They often require benzodiazepine rescue medication to abort these clusters, which prevents long-term consequences and limits the need for additional medical care in the hospital setting.[6]

EPIDEMIOLOGY

Epilepsy affects individuals worldwide without association with specific gender, race, ethnicity, socioeconomic status, or geographic location. Epilepsy has been described for thousands of years with the earliest known references to PWE occurring in 4000 BC.[1] It is estimated that 50 million people worldwide have epilepsy and approximately 2.4 million people are newly diagnosed each year.[2] In developing countries, the median prevalence is 1% to 1.5% while

TABLE 27.1

Classification of Seizure Types, The International League Against Epilepsy 2017

Seizure Type	Description	Clinical Features
Focal aware seizures	Focal onset seizures with retained awareness of self and environment	Motor: automatisms, atonic, clonic, epileptic spasms, hyperkinetic, myoclonic, tonic Nonmotor: autonomic, behavior arrest, cognitive, emotional, sensory
Focal impaired awareness seizures	Focal onset seizures with impaired awareness of self and environment	
Generalized onset seizures	Generalized onset seizures (all have impaired awareness)	Motor: tonic–clonic, clonic, tonic, myoclonic, myoclonic–tonic–clonic, myoclonic–atonic, atonic, epileptic spasms Nonmotor (i.e., absence): typical, atypical, myoclonic, eyelid myoclonia
Unknown onset seizures	Inability to classify seizure type based on clinical and/or electrographic features	May involve clinical features that overlap or uncertain clinical history

in developed countries the prevalence is lower (0.4% to 1%).[1,2] There is a higher incidence of new cases in low- to middle-income countries, which is thought to be attributable to disparities in medical access and quality of medical care as well as endemic diseases such as neurocysticercosis.[1]

Common risk factors for epilepsy include a history of febrile seizures, stroke or vascular malformation, CNS tumor, congenital brain malformation, cerebral palsy, autism spectrum disorder, or a family history of seizures, developmental delay, genetic disorders, or neurocutaneous syndromes.[1,7] Risk factors for epilepsy should always be reviewed when there is clinical suspicion for seizures.

THE INTERNATIONAL LEAGUE AGAINST EPILEPSY CLASSIFICATIONS

The ILAE 2017 classification of seizure types are intended to provide simple and logical terminology that may be communicated among clinicians worldwide.[8,9] Within this classification system (Table 27.1), there are basic and expanded versions.

ETIOLOGY

Acute symptomatic seizures occur in close temporal proximity to a metabolic, infectious, structural, or toxic insult and represent approximately 40% of all seizures.[4] Acute symptomatic seizures are thought to be provoked, and some etiologies are treatable and reversible. Other etiologies such as structural lesions carry a high risk of recurrent seizures, and therefore, may warrant maintenance antiseizure medication (ASM), at least in the short term. Table 27.2 lists common etiologies for acute symptomatic seizures.

Etiologies for epilepsy may be subdivided into structural, genetic, immune, metabolic, or unknown as seen in Table 27.3.[4] Some diagnoses may fit into more than one category (i.e., tuberous sclerosis has an underlying genetic etiology associated with tubers, which are structural epileptogenic lesions). Lennox–Gastaut syndrome (LGS) is defined as an epileptic encephalopathy characterized by multiple seizure types, cognitive impairment, and EEG with specific epileptiform and background abnormalities.[8,10] The diagnosis of LGS is not reflective of a particular etiology of epilepsy, and any of the etiologies listed may meet criteria for LGS depending on severity and clinical course.

DIFFERENTIAL DIAGNOSIS FOR PAROXYSMAL EVENTS

Several psychiatric, neurologic, and other medical conditions have symptoms that can mimic seizures. Because management of these symptoms will differ from seizure management, a detailed

TABLE 27.2

Etiologies of Acute Symptomatic Seizures

Metabolic	Toxins	CNS Infections	Structural
Hyponatremia	Alcohol withdrawal	Bacterial	Traumatic brain injury (TBI)
Hypomagnesemia	Alcohol intoxication	Viral (most common HSV-1)	Ischemic stroke
Hypocalcemia	Cocaine	Fungal	Hemorrhagic stroke
Hypoglycemia	Stimulant overdose		Diffuse anoxic injury
Hyperglycemia	Meperidine		Posterior reversible encephalopathy syndrome (PRES)
	Methaqualone		Cerebral venous thrombosis
	Hallucinogens		Eclampsia
	Phencyclidine (PCP)		
	Barbiturate withdrawal		
	Benzodiazepine withdrawal		
	Carbon monoxide poisoning		

HSV-1, Herpes simplex virus-1.

TABLE 27.3

Common Etiologies of Epilepsy

Structural	Genetic	Metabolic	Immune
CNS tumor	SCN1A mutation	GLUT-1 deficiency	Rasmussen encephalitis
Encephalomalacia	Autosomal Dominant Frontal Lobe	Pyridoxine-dependent epilepsy	Anti-NMDA receptor encephalitis
Mesial temporal lobe epilepsy	Epilepsy (CHRNA4, CHRNA2, or	Porphyria	Leucine-rich glioma-inactivated 1
(MTLE) with hippocampal	CHRNB2 mutations)	Aminoacidopathy	(LGI1) antibody encephalitis
sclerosis	Neurofibromatosis type I		
Hypothalamic hamartoma	Progressive myoclonic epilepsies:		
Sturge–Weber syndrome	• Lafora body disease		
Malformations of cortical	• Unverricht–Lundborg disease		
development:	• Neuronal ceroid lipofuscinoses		
• Lissencephaly	• Myoclonic epilepsy with ragged		
• Polymicrogyria	red fibers		
• Focal cortical dysplasia	Tuberous sclerosis complex		
• Hemimegalencephaly	Juvenile myoclonic epilepsy		
	Juvenile absence epilepsy		
	Generalized epilepsy with eyelid		
	myoclonia		

CNS, central nervous system; CHRNA, cholinergic receptor nicotinic alpha; CHRNB, cholinergic receptor nicotinic beta; NMDA, N-methyl-D-aspartate.

history and physical examination and an EEG of appropriate duration should be obtained to confirm the diagnosis of seizures/epilepsy. The event history should elicit preceding symptoms, evolution, stereotyped nature (i.e., does every episode look the same), duration, triggers, responsiveness, awareness, post-event symptoms, and frequency. With the ubiquity of cell phones, obtaining a video of a typical event may help narrow the differential diagnosis and tailor the evaluation, preventing unnecessary testing.[11] The most common nonepileptic diagnoses are functional neurologic disorder which includes psychogenic pseudosyncope (apparent loss of consciousness without associated EEG changes seen in syncope) and psychogenic nonepileptic events (see Table 27.4 for semiologic differences that help distinguish these events from bilateral tonic–clonic seizures). Other common diagnoses to consider are syncope, postural orthostatic tachycardia syndrome, migraine, panic attack, catatonia, transient ischemia attack, stroke, postsyncopal convulsion, movement disorders (i.e., tic disorder, chorea, paroxysmal dyskinesia, nonepileptic myoclonus, dystonia, tremor), and sleep disorders (i.e., cataplexy, benign sleep myoclonus, parasomnias, confusional arousals, restless leg syndrome, sleepwalking, REM behavior sleep disorder).

🔵 DIAGNOSTIC EVALUATION

Diagnostic evaluation of an AYA with a first-time seizure should be deferred until the AYA is medically stable and seizure activity has stopped. Initial diagnostic evaluation should focus on identifying acute provoking factors, especially potentially treatable or reversible etiologies (see above). In addition to a detailed history and physical examination, the evaluation should include basic metabolic panel to rule out electrolyte disturbance, urine drug screen for intentional or accidental intoxication, and complete blood count to screen for infection.[12,13] Depending on presence of focal seizure semiology and/or neurologic deficits and altered mental status, further work-up with lumbar puncture to evaluate for meningitis or encephalitis and head computed tomography (CT) to rule out gross structural abnormalities (i.e., intracranial hemorrhage, neoplasm) may be warranted.[12,13]

In the setting of a first-time unprovoked seizure, the next steps in evaluation help stratify risk of seizure recurrence and in turn, guide decisions about starting maintenance ASM.[12,13] Factors that suggest an increased risk of recurrent seizures include nocturnal seizure, abnormal neurologic examination, significantly abnormal head imaging, and epileptiform abnormalities on EEG.[12,13] The absolute risk of seizure recurrence after one unprovoked seizure in the AYA population is not precisely known. Separately analyzed data in patients <18 years old estimate the overall risk of recurrence is less than 50% while the risk of recurrence for patients >18 years old is greater than 50%.

If seizure semiology and/or EEG indicates focal epilepsy, a brain magnetic resonance imaging (MRI) should be obtained to evaluate for potential structural etiology (see Management of Epilepsy). If brain MRI is unremarkable (nonlesional focal epilepsy), additional imaging studies should be obtained to help localize the epileptogenic zone, in preparation for potential epilepsy surgery[14] (Table 27.5).

If the evaluation does not reveal a structural etiology for either generalized or focal epilepsy, or, if structural abnormalities are

TABLE 27.4

Distinguishing Features between Bilateral Tonic–Clonic Seizure and Convulsive Psychogenic Nonepileptic Events (PNEE)

Symptoms	Bilateral Tonic–Clonic Seizure	Convulsive PNEE
Tongue biting	Lateral	Tip
Incontinence	May be present	May be present
Shaking	Rhythmic, synchronous, sustained	Nonrhythmic, asynchronous, intermittent
Responsiveness	Unresponsive	Responsive to noxious stimuli
Pelvic thrusting	Not present	May be present
Forced eye closure	Not present	May be present
Postevent breathing pattern	Sonorous	Hyperventilation

TABLE 27.5

Summary of Tools in Seizure Onset Localization

Tool	Strengths	Limitations
Scalp EEG	Ability to localize to a lobe or lateralize	May not be accurate localization or lateralization
MRI	Identify lesion	May be negative even with (microscopic) lesion
PET	Identify dysfunction	Dysfunction is nonspecific
Ictal SPECT	Identifies networks of ictal activation	May not identify onset Results dependent on observer identifying seizure onset and injecting rapidly
MEG	Resection of tight MEG dipoles associated with high rates of seizure freedom	May be negative
SEEG	Identifies seizure onset and network	Identification of seizure onset dependent on where electrodes are placed Invasive Expensive High failure rates in MRI-negative cases

PET, positron emission tomography; SPECT, single photon emission computed tomography; MEG, magnetoencephalography; SEEG, stereoelectroencephalography; MRI, magnetic resonance imaging; EEG, electroencephalography.

commonly associated with specific gene mutations (i.e., tubers with tuberous sclerosis complex, cortical malformations with mechanistic target of rapamycin pathway mutations, lissencephaly) a genetic epilepsy panel may be sent, which contains >300 genes associated with epilepsy.[15] If no pathogenic variants are seen on a genetic epilepsy panel, referral to a genetics clinic for consideration of whole exome sequencing may be helpful, particularly if there are comorbidities and/or family history of epilepsy.

MANAGEMENT OF EPILEPSY

There are three broad categories in the treatment of epilepsy: medication, surgical intervention, and dietary therapy. Management should be individualized to each patient based on epilepsy classification, potential benefit, and potential adverse effects. The following sections explore specific treatment options within each category.

Medications

Medications for the treatment of seizures in AYAs are listed in Table 27.6. Initiation of ASM in this population requires careful consideration of side effects and potential interactions with contraception and other medications.[16–18]

Surgical Options

Intractable epilepsy (also known as drug-resistant epilepsy) is defined as persistent seizures after failing maximum doses of at least two ASMs (administered consecutively or concurrently) appropriate for a patient's specific type of epilepsy.[19] Approximately one-third of PWE will meet the definition of intractable epilepsy

and warrant timely referral to a comprehensive epilepsy center to explore nonmedication treatment options, such as surgery or diet therapy.[19] If surgical intervention is pursued, realistic expectations about seizure and quality of life outcomes should be discussed with patient and family. Expectations will vary based on degree of independence, comorbidities, number of ASMs, epilepsy syndrome, and baseline frequency of seizures.

For patients with intractable focal epilepsy confirmed by semiology and ictal EEG findings (seizure with EEG onset in one region or hemisphere of the brain), a brain MRI should be obtained to evaluate for a potential structural etiology. Symptomatic lesional focal epilepsy patients have improved seizure-free outcomes after resection compared to nonlesional focal epilepsy.[19,20] In patients with nonlesional focal epilepsy, additional testing after brain MRI may be needed to localize and/or lateralize seizure onset (see Diagnostic Evaluation). In some multidisciplinary epilepsy programs, invasive stereo-EEG (SEEG) or subdural grid electrodes may be utilized to localize the epileptogenic zone further.[19] In cases where SEEG or subdural grid elucidates more than one seizure foci or in cases where resection of the seizure focus would lead to long-term neurologic deficits (i.e., involving eloquent cortex), patients may be considered for responsive neurostimulation (RNS). This device, approved by the U.S. Food and Drug Administration (FDA) for adults with intractable focal epilepsy, continuously monitors intracranial EEG data using proprietary algorithms that detect seizure activity.[21] Once detected, RNS rapidly responds with high frequency neurostimulation designed to disrupt seizure propagation.[21]

Hemispherectomy is a surgical procedure creating functional or anatomical disconnection between the two cerebral hemispheres.[22] This procedure should be considered in AYAs with intractable symptomatic focal epilepsy secondary to a large structural lesion and/or injury involving a majority of one hemisphere (i.e., remote perinatal stroke or TBI with subsequent encephalomalacia, Rasmussen encephalitis, Sturge–Weber syndrome). In children, hemispherectomy is associated with high seizure-free rates (up to 80%) and low risk of worsening baseline neurologic function.[22] The limited data for hemispherectomy in patients older than 16 years also demonstrate similar long-term seizure-free rates and stable functional outcomes.[22]

A vagal nerve stimulator (VNS) may be a treatment option for patients with intractable generalized epilepsy or focal epilepsy that is not amenable to or has failed surgical interventions.[21] This battery-powered device has leads that are placed in the carotid sheath around the left vagus nerve and connected to a subcutaneous programmable pacemaker in the left upper chest.[21] The VNS device can acutely reduce seizure duration with device activation and may reduce seizure frequency and duration, providing a chronic progressive-prophylactic effect.[23] In addition to RNS and VNS, the newest neuromodulation device uses deep brain stimulation (DBS), which was FDA approved in 2018 for the treatment of intractable focal epilepsy for adults.[21]

Corpus callosotomy may be a palliative surgical option for AYAs with symptomatic generalized epilepsy.[24] This procedure involves either partial or complete disruption of the white matter connections between the two cerebral hemispheres, preventing bihemispheric and generalized seizure propagation and in turn, clinical manifestation of seizure activity.[24] The procedure has demonstrated high rates of efficacy in atonic seizures.

Dietary Therapy

For AYAs with intractable epilepsy that are not amenable to, or failed prior surgical epilepsy treatments, dietary therapies may be considered. There are four main dietary therapies used as adjunctive seizure treatment: classic ketogenic diet (KD), modified Atkin diet (MAD), low glycemic index treatment (LGIT), and medium-chain triglyceride ketogenic diet (MCTKD). Although the

TABLE 27.6

Antiseizure Medications

Medication	Seizure Type or Epilepsy Syndrome	Potential Side Effects	Special Considerations
Levetiracetam	Broad spectrum	Mood and behavior changes	Similar mechanism of action as brivaracetam
Brivaracetam	Broad spectrum	Sedation	Similar mechanism of action as levetiracetam, lower risk of mood and behavior side effects
Zonisamide	Broad spectrum	Decreased appetite/weight loss, kidney stones, oligohydrosis	Similar mechanism of action as topiramate
Topiramate	Broad spectrum, LGS	Decreased appetite/weight loss, kidney stones, oligohydrosis, cognitive slowing, teratogenicity	Similar mechanism of action as zonisamide, decreased effectiveness of estrogen-containing birth control (>200 mg/d)
Lamotrigine	Broad spectrum, LGS	Stevens–Johnson rash, insomnia	May exacerbate myoclonic seizures, follow levels closely with estrogen-containing birth control and during pregnancy.
Valproic acid	Broad spectrum, absence, LGS	Teratogenicity, weight gain, acne, hair loss, dose-dependent thrombocytopenia, elevated liver enzymes, PCOS	Enzyme inhibitors thus adjust dose with concurrent lamotrigine or rufinamide.
Oxcarbazepine	Focal	Dizziness, blurry vision, hyponatremia	May exacerbate generalized seizures, risk of withdrawal seizures with abrupt discontinuation, decreased effectiveness of estrogen-containing birth control (>1,200 mg/d).
Carbamazepine	Focal	Dizziness, blurry vision	May exacerbate generalized seizures, risk of withdrawal seizures with abrupt discontinuation, autoinduction, enzyme inducer thus follow levels closely and use cautiously with other ASMs and medication classes.
Eslicarbazepine	Focal	Dizziness, blurry vision	Similar mechanism of action to oxcarbazepine and carbamazepine with a longer half-life
Lacosamide	FDA approved for focal and primary generalized tonic–clonic seizures	Dizziness, blurry vision	Avoid with other sodium channel drugs and medications that can prolong PR interval.
Ethosuximide	Absence	Abdominal pain, nausea and vomiting, agranulocytosis, elevated liver enzymes	—
Rufinamide	Atonic, LGS	Prolonged QT syndrome	Adjust dose with concurrent valproic acid use.
Perampanel	Broad spectrum	Mood changes	—
Vigabatrin	Infantile spasms and refractory focal	Irreversible peripheral vision loss, nonspecific MRI changes	May exacerbate myoclonic seizures.
Clobazam	LGS	Sedation	Similar mechanism of action to clonazepam
Clonazepam	Broad spectrum	Sedation	Tachyphylaxis with long-term use
Felbamate	LGS	Aplastic anemia, liver failure, weight loss	—
Cenobamate	FDA approved for focal but no contraindications for generalized	Sedation, dizziness	—
Phenytoin	Focal, status epilepticus	Hirsutism, gingival hyperplasia, cerebellar atrophy, osteoporosis, teratogenicity	May exacerbate myoclonic and generalized seizures
Phenobarbital	Broad spectrum, status epilepticus	Sedation, adverse neurodevelopmental outcomes, teratogenicity	Risk of withdrawal seizures with abrupt discontinuation
Gabapentin	Focal	Sedation	May exacerbate myoclonic and generalized seizures, similar mechanism of action to pregabalin.
Pregabalin	Focal	Sedation	May exacerbate myoclonic and generalized seizures, similar mechanism of action to gabapentin.
Cannabidiol	LGS, Dravet syndrome	Elevated liver enzymes, diarrhea	May increase clobazam metabolite.
Fenfluramine	Dravet syndrome	Decreased appetite/weight loss	Baseline ECHO, use caution with concurrent SSRI, may increase clobazam metabolite

LGS, Lennox–Gastaut syndrome; ECHO, echocardiogram; SSRI, selective serotonin reuptake inhibitor; ASM, antiseizure medication; MRI, magnetic resonance imaging; FDA, U.S. Food and Drug Administration.

mechanism of action for seizure control is not fully understood, each of these dietary therapies aim to use ketones as an energy source for the brain instead of glucose.[25] Adolescents and young adults that feed by mouth and/or per tube may be eligible for all dietary therapies, but all patients should work closely with a dietitian trained in these diets. Patients can theoretically be on KD and other dietary therapies indefinitely, but it is important to re-evaluate efficacy and safety with a ketogenic dietitian and epileptologist at least every 2 years.

The KD uses a low carbohydrate to high fat ratio while the MAD limits the total carbohydrate intake.[26] Studies of KD and MAD in patients <18 years old with intractable epilepsy have demonstrated 50% reduction in seizures in 50% to 60% of patients.[25] However, there is limited evidence for any dietary therapy in patients >18 years old. Moreover, AYAs (both typically developing and those with intellectual disability) who take food by mouth are likely to face challenges adhering to one of these restrictive diets.

CONSIDERATIONS FOR FEMALES WITH EPILEPSY

Prepregnancy counseling and contraception are especially important topics to discuss with AYA females with epilepsy because many ASMs interact with hormonal contraception and may have teratogenic effects. These topics should ideally be discussed before the AYA patient becomes sexually active and reviewed at interval visits. Other important topics of discussion for AYA females with epilepsy include folic acid supplementation, ASM adjustments during pregnancy, polycystic ovarian syndrome (PCOS), bone health, and catamenial epilepsy.

Contraception

When counseling AYAs about contraception, clinicians should be aware that: (1) certain ASMs induce hepatic enzymes that can reduce effectiveness of hormonal contraception and (2) estrogen-containing contraception can alter the effectiveness of certain ASMs.[26] Antiseizure medications that induce hepatic enzymes and that may result in failure of some hormonal birth control include phenobarbital, phenytoin, carbamazepine, and higher doses of oxcarbazepine and topiramate.[26] Progesterone or copper intrauterine devices and depot medroxyprogesterone acetate (DMPA) injections are highly effective and are the preferred form of birth control for AYA females taking these ASMs. Clinicians may consider giving DMPA injections more frequently (i.e., every 10 weeks instead of every 12 weeks). Combination or progestin-only oral contraceptive pills (OCPs), transdermal patches, vaginal rings, or progestin implants should not be used for contraception by AYAs taking these ASMs. Antiseizure medications that do not induce hepatic enzymes and that may be safely used with all types of hormonal contraception include: ethosuximide, valproate, gabapentin, pregabalin, clonazepam, levetiracetam, tiagabine, zonisamide, vigabatrin, lacosamide, and ezogabine.[26] Estrogen increases glucuronidation in the liver and may increase metabolism of lamotrigine and oxcarbazepine by approximately 50%.[26] Adjustments in the dosages of lamotrigine or oxcarbazepine may be needed to prevent breakthrough seizures when OCPs containing estradiol are prescribed to AYAs taking these ASMs. The teratogenicity of ASMs is a particular concern when treating female AYAs. There are several ASM and pregnancy registries which report the prevalence of congenital malformations with ASMs, including the International Registry of Antiepileptic Drugs and Pregnancy, North American Antiepileptic Drugs and Pregnancy Registry, and UK Epilepsy and Pregnancy Register.[26] Reported rate ranges of congenital malformation associated with ASMs include carbamazepine (2.6% to 5.5%), lamotrigine (2.0% to 2.9%), levetiracetam (0.7% to 2.8%), oxcarbazepine (2.2% to 3.0%), phenobarbital (5.5% to 6.5%), phenytoin (2.9% to 6.4%), topiramate (3.9% to 4.3%), and valproate (6.7% to 10.3%).[26]

Pregnancy

Adult females with epilepsy have been shown to have 50% higher rates of infertility than the general population. This is thought to be attributable to other neuroendocrine disorders or the effects of some ASMs on fertility.[26] When planning for pregnancy, AYAs need preconceptual counseling reviewing seizure burden, potential pregnancy complications. optimizing ASM regimen and addressing the need for ASM monitoring, and folic acid supplementation. Once pregnant, females with epilepsy typically have improved seizure control or may remain seizure free due to the increased levels of progesterone and its anticonvulsant effects.[26] The absorption, distribution, metabolism, and excretion of some ASMs may be affected by physiologic changes that occur during pregnancy. Lamotrigine, levetiracetam, topiramate, zonisamide, and oxcarbazepine levels may be lower in pregnancy and may require frequent monitoring (i.e., 1 to 2 baseline levels prior to pregnancy, obtain level once pregnant, and then check level every month during pregnancy) along with periodic dose adjustments based on changes in the levels and seizure burden.[26]

Breastfeeding

The current standard of care is to counsel females who are taking ASMs that breastfeeding is safe.[26] For unclear reasons, females with epilepsy are significantly less likely to breastfeed than those without epilepsy. For those who plan to breastfeed, clinician should counsel that lipid soluble ASMs may transfer into breast milk, but the amount is typically low and does not produce side effects.[26] Ethosuximide, zonisamide, lamotrigine, benzodiazepines, and barbiturates are associated with elevated ASM levels in the breast milk and have potential side effects, such as sedation and irritability.[26] Despite the low risk of short-term effects, the use of ASMs in females who are breastfeeding has been shown to have no adverse effects on development in several prospective studies.[26]

Polycystic Ovarian Syndrome

Polycystic ovarian syndrome is caused by an imbalance of reproductive hormones and associated with several symptoms including dysmenorrhea, irregular menstrual cycles, hirsutism, acne, hair loss or thinning hair, weight gain, infertility, and skin tags and darkening of the skin.[26] The general prevalence of PCOS is 5% to 10% in AYAs between age 15 to mid-40s. Adolescents and young adults taking valproate are at an even higher risk of developing PCOS.[26] Valproate should usually be avoided in AYAs with epilepsy given that it is associated with an increased risk of PCOS and because of the risk of teratogenicity.

Bone Health

Adolescents and young adults with epilepsy have lower bone mineral density than healthy controls of the same age and is attributable to ASM exposure.[26] Cerebral palsy and conditions that limit mobility may further lower bone mineral density.[26] While there are no official screening recommendations in AYAs with epilepsy, clinicians should be aware that vitamin D levels may be lower in patients taking phenobarbital, phenytoin, carbamazepine, and oxcarbazepine as these ASMs can interfere with vitamin D metabolism.[26] Dual energy x-ray absorptiometry scans are the most sensitive assessment of bone mineral density, but no specific guidelines for whom to screen and how frequently to do so exist for AYAs taking ASMs.[26] Likewise, there is no clear consensus on the dosing of vitamin D for AYAs who take ASMs who have low bone density.[26]

Catamenial Epilepsy

Catamenial epilepsy is defined as a variation in seizure frequency during the menstrual cycle and is typically characterized by an increase in seizure burden around menstruation.[26] The timing of the increase in seizure burden is variable with some AYAs having an increase in seizures during menstruation and others experiencing increases in seizure activity immediately before or after menses, or mid cycle.[26] While the etiology is not precisely known, research suggests that decreased progesterone levels may be the cause. Progesterone is metabolized to the active metabolite, allopregnanolone, which is thought to have anticonvulsant properties via postsynaptic inhibitory Gamma Amino Butyric Acid (GABA)-A receptors. In contrast, estrogen is thought to have proconvulsant properties via excitatory effects on glutamate receptors.[26] However, there is no conclusive evidence that combination OCPs increase seizure activity. Studies using progesterone supplements have been difficult to interpret given the variable timing of increased seizure burden in relation to the menstrual cycle.[26] A few studies with mostly small sample sizes have shown seizure reduction with medroxyprogesterone acetate or other progesterone supplements.[26] More research is needed in AYAs with catamenial epilepsy to determine optimal treatment regimens.

EPILEPSY COMORBIDITIES

There are several neuropsychiatric diagnoses that occur at higher rates in AYAs with epilepsy compared to the general population. Mood disorders are the most common psychiatric comorbidity, occurring in up to 50% in all PWE, thus AYAs with epilepsy should be screened frequently for depression and anxiety and treated as appropriate.[14] In addition to mental-health counseling, pharmacologic treatment of depression and anxiety may be warranted.[14] In AYAs with epilepsy, medications that decrease seizure threshold should be avoided, including bupropion, clomipramine, and maprotiline. Other medications should be used cautiously for the same reason, including tricyclic antidepressants and lithium.[14] Selective serotonin reuptake inhibitors, specifically citalopram, have the lowest risk of decreasing seizure threshold and have relatively fewer interactions with ASMs.[14] It is important to counsel AYAs that all ASMs carry an FDA warning about increased risk of suicidal thoughts and behavior.[16] In addition, it is important for clinicians to be aware that levetiracetam and perampanel are associated with relatively higher rates of mood and behavior disturbances.[16]

Learning disorders are also frequently seen in PWE, with approximately 50% of children with epilepsy having some degree of learning difficulty (compared to 15% of the general population).[14] In addition, PWE are more likely to be diagnosed with the inattentive type of attention deficit hyperactivity disorder (ADHD). In patients with ADHD, treatment with stimulants has a theoretical risk of decreasing seizure threshold, but stimulant use is not contraindicated in PWE.[14]

Sleep disorders, behavior issues, movement disorders (depending on etiology of epilepsy), and headaches are also frequently seen in AYAs with epilepsy.[14] Addressing sleep disorders may lead to improved seizure control by optimizing sleep duration and quality.

LIVING WITH EPILEPSY

Seizure Precautions

Adolescents and young adults with epilepsy should take precautions in certain environments and activities that place them at higher risk of injury if they were to have a seizure. For most AYAs, independence plays a key role in identity formation and mental health. Clinicians and parents/caregivers should help the AYA to balance independent activities and safety. **Table 27.7** lists general seizure precautions for AYAs. Clinicians should advise AYAs to avoid baths, because drowning in a bathtub is the most common cause of accidental death in PWE.[14,27] Although driving laws vary by state, the ILAE recommends no driving for at least 3 months after stopping ASMs.[4] Adolescents and young adults should also be aware of potential seizure triggers, such as alcohol use, sleep deprivation, and flashing lights (for those

TABLE 27.7
General Seizure Precautions
Wear medic alert bracelet that has "epilepsy" listed as diagnosis.
Download "in case of emergency" app on cell phone (*emergency information saves as lock screen image so first responder only needs to power up phone to access).*
Use caution with breakable dishes.
Use caution with hot food and liquids.
Avoid baths *(take showers with rubber mat).*
Avoid using a stove when possible.
Move bed away from walls and tables.
Pad edges of tables.
Avoid sleeping on lofted bed.
Avoid using power tools.
No babysitting
Keep hallways and rooms clear of items that can be tripped over *(cords, toys, etc.).*

with photosensitive epilepsy). Medication adherence should also be encouraged and monitored because missed doses of ASMs is one of the most common causes for status epilepticus.[14]

Adolescents and young adults with epilepsy should be encouraged to stay active, as exercise is good for both physical and mental health and is not a common trigger for seizures. Note that patients with incompletely controlled absence epilepsy may be at risk for hyperventilation-induced absence seizures, thus should be cautious about strenuous exercise that causes shortness of breath. Recreational precautions for AYAs with seizures are listed in **Table 27.8**.

Sudden Unexpected Death in Epilepsy

Sudden unexpected death in epilepsy is rare, occurring in approximately 1 in 1,000 PWE per year,[27] though rates for the AYA population is unknown. The pathophysiology of SUDEP is not completely understood but there are several factors associated with higher risk of SUDEP, such as frequent bilateral tonic–clonic seizures, nocturnal

TABLE 27.8
Recreational Seizure Precautions
Always use helmets and other protective gear on bike, scooter, all-terrain vehicles, etc.
Always wear a life jacket and have adult swim buddy in open water.
Avoid automatic exercise machines such as treadmill, elliptical, etc.
Use caution and always wear appropriate protective gear in contact sports such as football, rugby, hockey.
Use harness on ski lifts.
Avoid risk recreational activities such as scuba diving, rock climbing, hang gliding, shooting guns, backcountry skiing.

seizures, duration of epilepsy, ASM polytherapy, and male gender.[27] Similarly, improved seizure control is associated with reduced risk of SUDEP. Adolescents and young adults with epilepsy should be encouraged to avoid seizure triggers, improve medication adherence with pillbox or cell phone reminders, and communicate regularly with clinicians about seizures and seizure management. Interventions such as direct or indirect supervision during sleep, seizure detection devices, and bed alarms have limited evidence to support their use for SUDEP prevention.[27] However, as AYAs transition to more independent living, the use of an FDA-approved seizure detection watch can help reduce parent/caregiver and patient anxiety. These devices are designed to detect changes in heart rate, temperature, sweat, and motion that usually accompany bilateral tonic–clonic seizures then send an alert to designated parent's/caregiver's cell phone.[27] As awareness and research continue to expand, there is hope for more evidence-based strategies to prevent SUDEP.

Seizure Action Plan

All AYAs with epilepsy attending school, living in care facilities, holding jobs, and participating in recreational activities should have a detailed Seizure Action Plan they can share with appropriate supervisors. A template for a Seizure Action Plan is available from the Epilepsy Foundation (https://epilepsy.com). Supervisors should be aware of steps to provide first aid for a seizure which are detailed in Table 27.9.[14]

Employment

For AYAs with epilepsy looking for a job, the Americans with Disabilities Act (ADA) states that "private employers with 15 or more employees cannot discriminate against an employee that can do the essential function of the job with reasonable accommodations."[14] Also, under the ADA, employers cannot ask whether a person has epilepsy and applicants do not have to disclose if they have epilepsy or are taking prescription medications.[14] However, an AYA with epilepsy will need to disclose if they need accommodations (i.e., scheduled breaks to take medication, time off for doctor's appointments, avoidance of heights). For safety reasons, AYAs are encouraged to disclose their Seizure Action Plan with coworkers and supervisors.[14]

● SUMMARY

Approximately half of children with epilepsy require seizure management into adulthood, making AYAs with epilepsy a relatively prevalent population with unique health care needs. After epilepsy

is diagnosed, management must be tailored based on gender, etiology, comorbidities, and individual quality of life goals. Patients and parents/caregivers should be counseled about common seizure triggers and potential limitations as AYAs seek more independence. Families of AYAs with epilepsy may face additional emotional and medical challenges during the transition from pediatric to adult epilepsy programs, which may be improved by early discussions and support from clinicians.

REFERENCES

1. Singh A, Trevick S. The epidemiology of global epilepsy. *Neurol Clin.* 2016;34(4):837–847.
2. World Health Organization website. https://www.who.int/news-room/fact-sheets/detail/epilepsy. Accessed November 2, 2020.
3. Fisher RS, Acevedo C, Arzimanoglou A, et al. ILAE official report: a practical clinical definition of epilepsy. *Epilepsia.* 2014;55(4):475–482.
4. Falco-Walter JJ, Scheffer IE, Fisher RS. The new definition and classification of seizures and epilepsy. *Epilepsy Res.* 2018;139:73–79.
5. Trinka E, Cock H, Hesdorffer D, et al. A definition and classification of status epilepticus–report of the ILAE task force on classification of status epilepticus. *Epilepsia.* 2015;56(10):1515–1523.
6. Jafarpour S, Hirsch LJ, Gaínza-Lein M, et al. Seizure cluster: definition, prevalence, consequences, and management. *Seizure.* 2019;68:9–15.
7. Beghi E, Giussani G, Sander JW. The natural history and prognosis of epilepsy. *Epileptic Disord.* 2015;17(3):243–253.
8. Pack AM. Epilepsy overview and revised classification of seizures and epilepsies. *Continuum.* 2019;25(2):306–321.
9. Fisher RS, Cross JH, D'Souza C, et al. Instruction manual for the ILAE 2017 operational classification of seizure types. *Epilepsia.* 2017;58(4):531–542.
10. Pearl PL. Epilepsy syndromes in childhood. *Continuum.* 2018;24:186–209.
11. Piña-Garza JEJ, James KC, eds. *Fenichel's Clinical Pediatric Neurology: A Signs and Symptoms Approach.* 8th ed. Elsevier; 2019.
12. Gavvala JR, Schuele SU. New-onset seizure in adults and adolescents: a review. *JAMA.* 2016;316(24):2657–2668.
13. American Academic of Neurology website. https://www.aan.com/policy-and-guidelines. Accessed March 15, 2021.
14. Epilepsy Foundation website. https://www.epilepsy.com. Accessed March 13, 2021.
15. Weber YG, Biskup S, Helbig KL, et al. The role of genetic testing in epilepsy diagnosis and management. *Expert Rev Mol Diagn.* 2017;17(8):739–750.
16. Abou-Khalil BW. Update on antiepileptic drugs 2019. *Continuum.* 2019;25(2):508–536.
17. Lagae L, Sullivan J, Knupp K, et al. Fenfluramine hydrochloride for the treatment of seizures in Dravet syndrome: a randomised, double-blind, placebo-controlled trial. *Lancet.* 2019;394(10216):2243–2254.
18. Lattanzi S, Trinka E, Zaccara G, et al. Adjunctive cenobamate for focal-onset seizures in adults: a systematic review and meta-analysis. *CNS Drugs.* 2020;34(11):1105–1120.
19. Ryvlin P, Cross JH, Rheims S. Epilepsy surgery in children and adults. *Lancet Neurol.* 2014;13(11):1114–1126.
20. West S, Nevitt SJ, Cotton J, et al. Surgery for epilepsy. *Cochrane Database Syst Rev.* 2019;6(6):CD010541.
21. Benbadis SR, Geller E, Ryvlin P, et al. Putting it all together: options for intractable epilepsy: an updated algorithm on the use of epilepsy surgery and neurostimulation. *Epilepsy Behav.* 2018;88S:33–38.
22. McGovern RA, ANV Moosa, Jehi L, et al. Hemispherectomy in adults and adolescents: seizure and functional outcomes in 47 patients. *Epilepsia.* 2019;60(12):2416–2427.
23. Pérez-Carbonell L, Faulkner H, Higgins S, et al. Vagus nerve stimulation for drug-resistant epilepsy. *Pract Neurol.* 2020;20(3):189–198.
24. Chan AY, Rolston JD, Lee B, et al. Rates and predictors of seizure outcome after corpus callosotomy for drug-resistant epilepsy: a meta-analysis. *J Neurosurg.* 2018;1:1–10.
25. Martin-McGill KJ, Bresnahan R, Levy RG, et al. Ketogenic diets for drug-resistant epilepsy. *Cochrane Database Syst Rev.* 2020;6:CD001903.
26. Stephen LJ, Harden C, Tomson T, et al. Management of epilepsy in women. *Lancet Neurol.* 2019;18(5):481–491.
27. Maguire MJ, Jackson CF, Marson AG, et al. Treatments for the prevention of Sudden Unexpected Death in Epilepsy (SUDEP). *Cochrane Database Syst Rev.* 2020;2(4):CD011792.

ADDITIONAL RESOURCES AND WEBSITES

Additional Resources and Websites for Clinicians:
Centers for Disease Control and Prevention: Epilepsy First Aid website—https://www.cdc.gov/epilepsy/about/first-aid.htm
Empatica website—https://www.empatica.com/embrace2
Epilepsy Foundation: Find an Epilepsy Center website—https://www.epilepsy.com/connect/find-epilepsy-specialist/find-epilepsy-center
Epilepsy Foundation website—https://www.epilepsy.com
Wyllie, E, eds. *Wyllie's Treatment of Epilepsy: Principles and Practice.* 6th ed. Wolters Kluwer; 2015.

Additional Resources and Websites for Parents/Caregivers:
Centers for Disease Control and Prevention: Managing Epilepsy Parent Toolkit website—https://www.cdc.gov/epilepsy/toolkit/resource_guide.htm
Epilepsy Foundation Facebook website—https://www.facebook.com/EpilepsyFoundationofAmerica
Epilepsy Foundation Instagram website—https://www.instagram.com/epilepsyfdn

TABLE 27.9

First Aid for Seizure

Try to stay calm.
Ease person to the floor and roll onto side.
Loosen anything around their neck (i.e., tie, scarf).
Cushion head.
Do not put anything or take anything out of person's mouth.
Clear area around person from furniture or other objects that may cause injury.
Administer (nonoral) emergency seizure medication if seizure lasts more than 5 min and call 911.
When person regains consciousness, talk in gentle voice, and stay until person is awake and oriented enough to return to usual activities.

Epilepsy Foundation Twitter website—https://twitter.com/EpilepsyFdn

Epilepsy Foundation: Your Local Epilepsy Foundation website—https://www.epilepsy.com/affiliates

Kobau R. Nearly one in five adults with active epilepsy lives alone based on findings from the 2010 and 2013 US National Health Interview Surveys. US Centers for Disease Control and Prevention, Epilepsy Program. Epilepsy Behav. 2015;51:259–260.

Parent to Parent USA website—https://www.p2pusa.org/about

Social Security Administration: Disability Evaluation Under Social Security website—https://www.ssa.gov/disability/professionals/bluebook/11.00-Neurological-Adult.htm

Additional Resources and Websites for Adolescents and Young Adults:

Epilepsy Foundation: Driving Laws website—https://www.epilepsy.com/driving-laws

Epilepsy Foundation Instagram website—https://www.instagram.com/epilepsyfdn

Epilepsy Foundation: Living with Epilepsy website—https://www.epilepsy.com/living-epilepsy/epilepsy-foundation-my-seizure-diary

Epilepsy Foundation: Managing your Epilepsy website—https://www.epilepsy.com/learn/managing-your-epilepsy/what-managing-epilepsy-well-network/texting-4-control

Epilepsy Foundation Twitter website—https://twitter.com/EpilepsyFdn

Epilepsy Foundation: Your Local Epilepsy Foundation website—https://www.epilepsy.com/affiliates

U.S. Equal Employment Opportunity Commission website—https://www.eeoc.gov/laws/guidance/epilepsy-workplace-and-ada

Headaches

Christopher B. Oakley

KEY WORDS

- Acute treatment
- Cluster headache
- Headache
- Migraine headache
- New daily persistent headache
- Posttraumatic headache
- Primary headache
- Prophylactic treatment
- Secondary headache
- Tension-type headache

INTRODUCTION

Headache is one of the most common problems that is encountered in the care of adolescents and young adults (AYAs) and is the most common neurologic sign or symptom seen in this population. While most headaches are not indicative of a concerning underlying process, certain situations and presentations warrant further evaluation. Even headaches that have a benign etiology may lead to significant disruption and diminished quality of life for AYAs. For these reasons, it is imperative that AYAs presenting with headaches receive a thorough, detailed history and physical examination. Imaging, laboratory evaluation, ancillary testing, and referrals should be used as necessary to narrow the differential diagnosis. Once a diagnosis has been made, a multitiered treatment approach should be employed. A systematic approach to the evaluation and management of headaches will help to minimize the disruption that headache symptoms have on the lives of AYAs and their families.

EPIDEMIOLOGY

Headaches are common among AYAs. Over half of all adolescents report experiencing a headache and by young adulthood, over 80% report experiencing headaches of some type.[1,2] The incidence of migraine headaches, among the most common and disabling headache types, increases with age affecting about one in three young adults.[3] The prevalence of chronic headaches, including chronic migraine, also increases with age, reaching almost 10% by young adulthood.[4] The incidence of headaches is higher among female AYAs, particular after puberty. Postpubertal AYA females are nearly twice as likely to develop headaches, and specifically migraines, as males.[2,3] Genetic and hormonal differences are thought to account for the differences between females and males, particularly with primary headaches such as migraine. Approximately 80% to 90% of AYAs with headaches and nearly two-thirds of AYAs with migraine have a first-degree relative with headache. At least four specific genetic markers have been linked to migraines and more than 20 others have been proposed.[5] In population studies, migraine and severe/frequent headache is highest among White and Native Americans, with slightly lower prevalence among Black and Hispanic Americans, and significantly lower prevalence among Asian Americans. The reasons for differences in prevalence are not clear, but likely reflect differences in symptom reporting, health care access, and treatment.[6]

HEADACHE CLASSIFICATION AND TYPES

Headaches have been described for thousands of years, but a formal diagnostic system and criteria were not established until the 1980s. The first International Classification of Headache Disorders (ICHD-1) was published in 1988 with the most recent edition, ICHD-3, published in 2018. The ICHD divides headaches into three broad categories: (1) primary headaches or headaches without an identified specific etiology, (2) secondary headaches or headaches with a specific identified etiology, and (3) cranial neuralgias, central and primary facial pain, and other headaches. This third category is heterogeneous and includes headaches that do not meet criteria for primary or secondary headaches.[7]

Most headaches among AYAs fall under the classification of primary headaches, including migraines, tension-type headache (TTH), cluster headaches, as well as a specific chronic daily headache known as new daily persistent headache (NDPH). The list of secondary headaches is nearly limitless given that any headache caused by a specific underlying etiology is included in this broad category. Some of the more commonly encountered secondary headaches include posttraumatic headache, medication overuse headache (MOH), and idiopathic intracranial hypertension (IIH). Additionally, headaches associated with intracranial structural abnormalities (e.g., cerebral venous sinus thrombosis [CVST], mass or tumor, Chiari malformation, hydrocephalus), substance use, or comorbid medical conditions are also examples of secondary headaches. Cranial neuralgias, facial pain, and other headaches will not be discussed as they are uncommon among AYAs.

Most primary and secondary headaches, have an episodic form and a chronic form. In general, the chronic form is distinguished from the episodic form by being present more than half the days of the month for at least three consecutive months—this distinction is generally applicable, though episodic and chronic forms of certain headache types are distinguished differently.[7] Table 28.1 lists characteristics that help distinguish primary from secondary headaches.

COMMON PRIMARY HEADACHES

Migraine

Migraine is among the most problematic headache types seen in AYAs because it is common and can be disabling. There are two main types of migraines—those with a preceding warning sign, also

TABLE 28.1

Historical Features Distinguishing Primary and Secondary Headaches

Historical Features	Primary Headache	Secondary Headache
Presentation	Chronic, >6 mo	Acute, <6 mo
Pattern	Recurrent or daily	Progressive
Location	Frontal, lateral >posterior	Posterior >frontal, lateral
Quality	Throbbing, pressure	Pressure, ache
Time of day	Anytime	Early morning (4–7 AM)
Frequency/duration	Varies: hours–days	Constant
Nausea/vomiting	Nausea >> vomiting	Vomiting
Visual aura/diplopia	Aura	Diplopia
Photo/phonophobia	+++	−

monosodium glutamate [MSG]-containing foods, processed meats and cheeses)[9]
• Symptoms improvement by quiet, dark, rest, and/or sleep

An understanding of aura is critical to delineating specific types of migraines. Aura is a symptom, typically sensory in nature, which precedes a migraine headache. Aura typically builds over a few minutes and then may last about an hour before dissipating. The migraine headache typically begins as the aura is resolving or after the aura has resolved. Visual changes, either positive or negative, are the most common aura. The second most common aura is sensory changes, typically described as paresthesias. Other aura symptoms occur less commonly and include language and speech disturbances, mental status changes, vertigo, and motor weakness.

Migraine with Brainstem Aura (Previously Known as Basilar Migraine)

Migraine with brainstem aura is a specific type of migraine with aura that is commonly seen in AYAs, particularly females. This subset accounts for up to 20% of migraines in AYAs. It accounts for a smaller proportion of migraines in adults, possibly due to a relative lack of subclassification, beyond migraine with aura, in the adult population.[8] At least two of the following aura symptoms must be present to make the diagnosis: vertigo, ataxia not from sensory deficit, dysarthria, tinnitus, hypacusis, diplopia, and/or decreased level of consciousness. Importantly, the presence of motor weakness excludes the diagnosis of migraine with brainstem aura. There is a purported connection between migraine with brainstem aura and hemiplegic migraine as both subtypes are often seen within families and there is an overlap in genetic markers for both (See section on Hemiplegic Migraine).[7,11]

Hemiplegic Migraine

Though relatively uncommon, hemiplegic migraine is a concerning migraine type, particularly because its presentation mimics a stroke. It is important to make the diagnosis and treat appropriately and aggressively to limit these headaches and to avoid unnecessary and potentially harmful evaluation and treatment of stroke such as the administration of tissue plasminogen activator (tPA). The aura of hemiplegic migraine must consist of fully reversible motor weakness and may include other more typical aura

known as an aura, and those without an aura. Migraine without aura (previously known as the common migraine) accounts for about 75% of all migraine headaches and migraine with aura (previously known as the classic migraine) accounts for the remaining 25%.[8] Migraine with aura is subdivided further into specific migraine with aura subtypes. Table 28.2 lists the ICHD-3 diagnostic criteria for migraine with and without aura. Adolescents and young adults with migraine will often report these common historical features:
• Family history of migraines
• Childhood history of migraine precursors such as motion sickness, abdominal migraine, cyclic vomiting syndrome, benign paroxysmal vertigo of childhood, or infantile colic[10]
• Migraine triggers such as puberty and/or pregnancy (likely attributable to hormone changes), stress, or diet (e.g., caffeine, alcohol,

TABLE 28.2

Criteria for Migraine Headaches: International Classification of Headache Disorders-3[9]

Migraine without Aura (Common Migraine)

A. At least five attacks fulfilling criteria B–D
B. Headache attacks last 4–72 h (untreated or unsuccessfully treated).[b]
C. Must have two of the following:
  1. Unilateral location[c]
  2. Pulsating quality
  3. Moderate to severe pain intensity
  4. Aggravation by or causing avoidance of routine physical activity
D. At least one of the following
  1. Nausea and/or vomiting
  2. Photophobia and phonophobia
E. Not better accounted for by another ICHD-3 diagnosis

Migraine with Aura (Classic Migraine)[a]

A. At least two attacks fulfilling criteria B and C
B. One or more of the fully reversible aura symptoms
  1. Visual[d]
  2. Sensory[e]
  3. Speech and/or language
  4. Motor
  5. Brainstem
  6. Retinal
C. At least three of the following six characteristics
  1. At least one aura symptom spreads gradually over 5+ min.
  2. Two or more aura symptoms occur in succession.
  3. Each aura symptom lasts 5–60 min.
  4. At least one aura symptom is unilateral.
  5. At least one aura symptom is positive.
  6. Aura is accompanied, or followed within 60 min, by headache.[f]
D. Not better accounted for by another ICHD-3 diagnosis

ICHD-3, International Classification of Headache Disorders-3.
[a]These criteria are for migraine with aura in general. Specific subtypes of migraine with aura may have varying criteria.
[b]In patients <18 years old, attacks may last 2–72 hours.
[c]In patients <18 years old, pain is more often bilateral.
[d,e]Visual aura is most common aura, accounting for over 90% of migraine with aura patients; sensory aura is second most common.
[f]While the headache is typically migraine in nature, it does not always have to meet the full criteria for migraine without aura to qualify. Headache typically follows the aura but aura may linger into the headache or even present after the headache has commenced.

symptoms. Hemiplegic migraine has several genetic familial sub-types including type 1 (CACNA1A), type 2 (ATP1A2), and type 3 (SCN1A). Other loci have been suggested, but are yet to gain their own specific subtype.[7]

Migraines and Menses

Hormonal milieu and migraines are so intertwined that many AYAs with migraine report a connection to their menstrual cycles, usu-ally in one of two ways: (1) pure *menstrual migraines*, character-ized by migraines that occur only a few days before or after the first day of the menstrual cycle, and (2) *menstrual-related migraines* characterized by migraines that occur around the start of the cycle but that may also be present at other times during the menstrual cycle. In both cases, the pattern should be present over several cycles in close proximity.[7] Hormone management, usually in the form of low estrogen–containing pills or patches or non-estrogen–containing options, may be helpful in the management and even prevention of these specific types of migraines.[12]

Tension-Type Headache

Tension-type headache is the most common type of headache seen in all populations, including AYAs. Up to 80% of young adults have reported having some degree of TTH. Though common, it is unusual for patients to seek medical attention for TTH as they tend to be mild to moderate and do not generally lead to disability or dysfunction. Tension-type headaches are typically described as a generalized, band-like pressure pain that lasts between 30 minutes to 1 week. Additionally, scalp tenderness may be present but is not required.[7,13] In some individuals, TTH can be difficult to distinguish from migraines. One key differentiator between the two is that TTH can occur with isolated photo- or phonophobia, whereas both photo- and phonophobia are required to meet the particular associ-ated symptom classification of migraine (see **Table 28.2**). Another potential differentiator is that TTH should not have associated gastrointestinal (GI) symptoms, whereas the presence of nausea and/or vomiting are among the symptoms used for the diagnosis of migraine.

Cluster Headache

Cluster headache is the third most common primary headache type, but remains a relatively uncommon headache among AYAs. Still, cluster headaches may present in late adolescents and early adulthood.[14] Cluster headaches are often mistaken for migraine because the presentation of both headaches have overlapping char-acteristics. Unlike migraines, cluster headaches are more preva-lent in AYA males than females. The ICHD-3 criteria for cluster headache is a severe, unilateral pain around the eye and temple area that lasts between 15 minutes and 3 hours. Cluster headaches are the most notable of the broader category of primary headache called trigeminal autonomic cephalalgias (TACs). Trigeminal auto-nomic cephalalgias are differentiated from other headaches by the presence of at least one notable ipsilateral parasympathetic auto-nomic feature (conjunctival injection and/or lacrimation, nasal congestion and/or rhinorrhea, eyelid edema, forehead/facial sweat-ing, miosis and/or ptosis) and/or a marked sense of agitation or restlessness.[7] These headaches can occur up to several times a day in the most severe cases. It is important to recognize cluster headaches and treat aggressively as they can be disabling. Cluster headaches have the unfortunate moniker of "the suicide headache" due to their severity.

New Daily Persistent Headache

Each of the previously noted primary headache types may occur episodically or chronically. New daily persistent headache differs from the former categories in that there is only a chronic version. By definition, NDPH is a primary headache disorder that pres-ents from the onset as a persistent, daily headache. To make the

diagnosis, headache onset should be clearly recalled with the head-ache becoming constant and unremitting within the first day and then lasting for a minimum of 3 months.[7] Unlike most other pri-mary headaches, a medical evaluation is typically recommended given the abrupt onset and constancy of the headache. While no specific recommendations exist for the medical evaluation, it is not uncommon for patients to have imaging of the head and laboratory tests (including complete blood count, complete metabolic panel, thyroid studies, inflammatory markers, and screening for auto-immune or infectious diseases) to look for a possible underlying etiology. Once diagnosed, the expectations for symptom manage-ment of NDPH are often different than for other headache types. Given the refractory nature of NDPH, the treatment goal is often to minimize the associated disability and dysfunction rather than to achieve headache cessation.[15]

COMMON SECONDARY HEADACHES

While most headaches in AYAs are primary headaches, second-ary headaches also occur. Secondary headaches are those with an identifiable underlying etiology. When an adolescent or young adult presents with new-onset headaches, the challenge for clinicians is to determine if the headache is the onset of a primary headache disorder or a more insidious process warranting evaluation. The list of secondary headaches is expansive, but among the more seri-ous life-threating types are central nervous system infection, intra-cranial mass/lesion, intracranial bleed, CVST, and stroke. Because these headaches herald potentially life-threating conditions, clini-cians should be aware of "Red Flag" characteristics in clinical pre-sentation and examination findings (see Headache Clinic Visit and Evaluation). **Table 28.1** lists distinguishing features of primary and secondary headaches and **Table 28.3** lists "Red Flags" that should prompt the clinician to consider referral to an emergency depart-ment, neurologist, and/or headache specialist for urgent evalua-tion. In addition, clinicians should also be aware that headaches can be a presenting sign for mental health concerns among AYAs.[16]

Posttraumatic Headache

Posttraumatic headache, or headache attributed to trauma or injury to the head and/or neck, includes all headaches that occur, typically within 1 week, of a head or neck injury, including con-cussion. When the headaches persist for more than 3 months, the headache is classified as chronic posttraumatic headache.[7] These are among the most common types of secondary headaches seen in AYAs. Headaches are typically one of the first symptoms to present following a head injury and one of the last symptoms to resolve.[17]

Headaches Related to Substances, Including Medications

Headaches can occur because of the use of both illegal and legal substances, including medications. In the AYA population, these headaches typically arise from a lack of understanding regarding how to treat headaches or from experimentation with medication

---

TABLE 28.3
"Red Flags" in the Evaluation of Headaches[17–19]

- Explosive new-onset, marked changes in headaches, or worst headache of life
- Early morning or overnight headache, especially with associated signs/symptoms concerning for increased intracranial pressure such as vomiting
- Rapid and/or steady progression of headaches
- Worsening with straining, bearing down, or position change
- Presence of other concomitant neurologic concerns such as seizure
- Mood, mental status, school or work performance change
- Abnormal neurologic and/or fundoscopic examination

or substances. Medication overuse headache (previously called rebound headache) occurs as a result of overuse of over-the-counter treatments as well as prescription treatments. The features and ICHD-3 diagnostic criteria for MOH include the following:[7]

- Headaches ≥15 days/month in a patient with pre-existing headaches
- >3 months of overuse of a medication that is taken for acute symptomatic relief of headaches
- Headaches are not better explained by another ICHD-3 diagnosis

When considering MOH, the following frequencies constitute overuse: Ergotamine or triptans ≥10 days/month; NSAIDs or acetaminophen ≥15 days/month.[7]

Treatment for MOH is challenging because it typically involves removing the offending agent. Because of this, AYAs will often experience worsening headache symptoms before improvement. It is important that AYAs know how to appropriately use the acute or rescue medications for their discrete headaches to both facilitate successful treatment and reduce the likelihood that they will fall back into an MOH.[20]

Other prescription drugs, illicit drugs, and alcohol use and/or withdrawal can also lead to headaches in AYAs. Drugs that are frequently associated with the development of headaches include alcohol, cocaine, marijuana, ecstasy, steroids, and stimulants. Additionally, opioids and barbiturates can be overused but these are not recommended and should not be used in the treatment of headaches.[7]

Idiopathic Intracranial Hypertension

Previously called pseudotumor cerebri, IIH is a type of secondary headache attributed to elevated cerebrospinal fluid (CSF) pressure without an underlying identifiable reason. Criteria for elevated CSF pressures per ICHD-3 is 250 mm H_2O in adults (≥18 years) and 280 mm H_2O in adolescents, but typically CSF pressure is over 300 mm H_2O. When IIH is suspected, adolescent or young adult should have an evaluation to exclude an intracranial process (tumor, CSF obstruction and hydrocephalus, CVST). In addition, adolescent or young adult should have full ophthalmology evaluation (including formal visual field testing) to establish the urgency for treatment because IIH can lead to irreversible visual loss. Lumbar puncture (LP) is both diagnostic and therapeutic. Lowering the CSF pressure to a normal level via LP can lead to resolution of symptoms, including headaches. Common IIH presentation and features include the following:[7,21]

- Common in AYA females of childbearing age
- Overweight and obesity are risk factors.
- History and physical examination findings include optic nerve edema (papilledema once increased CSF pressure confirmed), visual field and blind spot changes, cranial nerve VI palsy, reported pulsatile tinnitus
- May be related to the following medications: oral contraceptives, tetracyclines, vitamin A and D, retinoids, steroid withdrawal, immunosuppressants, thyroxine

Headache Related to Cerebral Venous Sinus Thrombosis

Similar to IIH, headaches related to CVST are often characterized by dull, generalized pain that may be accompanied by signs of increased intracranial pressure such as vomiting. Headaches related to CVST are more common in AYA females of childbearing age. While strokes related to CVST are atypical, 75% occur in young women.[18] Bleeding disorders, coagulopathies, oral contraceptives, and other hormone treatments are known risk factors for CVST.[7,18]

🔵 HEADACHE CLINIC VISIT AND EVALUATION

When evaluating an adolescent or young adult with headaches, the history and physical examination are critical in determining the diagnosis, the need for further evaluation, and the treatment of choice. The history should include the following:[17,22]

- Headache description: onset including any possible contributing events/circumstances, frequency, pattern over time, different types of headaches, timing of headache within the day/week/year, prodrome or aura, location, quality and intensity of pain, associated symptoms (especially photo- and phonophobia, nausea, vomiting), and any recent change in headache pattern or characteristics
- Triggers, alleviating factors including medications, symptoms between attacks, treatments tried (both preventative and acute)
- "Red Flags"—see **Table 28.3**
- Possible exacerbating lifestyle factors (sleep, hydration, diet, activity, stress)
- Mood and psychiatric screen
- Past medical history (especially neurologic, psychiatric, substance use, and head injury/trauma), other current medical or mental health concerns, and family history (especially headache)

The history should also seek to differentiate primary from secondary headaches (see **Table 28.1**).

The physical examination should include the following:[17]

- Vital signs, including orthostatic blood pressure measurements when indicated
- General examination—with particular focus on the head, eyes, ears, nose, and throat; cardiac; respiratory; GI; musculoskeletal; skin
- Complete neurologic examination with particular focus on mental status, eye movements, pronator drift or other subtle signs of asymmetric weakness, gait, balance and coordination or other signs of ataxia, and reflexes
- Fundoscopic examination

The history and physical examination should lead to a diagnosis or at least narrow the differential diagnosis. Additional evaluation is warranted when there is concern for a secondary headache. It should also be considered in the diagnosis of some primary headache, namely NDPH and those primary headaches in which symptoms are worsening and/or refractory despite appropriate treatment.

The evaluation of headache can be separated into 4 categories: (1) imaging, (2) laboratory, (3) ancillary neurologic testing, and (4) referral to an emergency department (ED) or specialist.[17,23]

1. Imaging—obtained when concerned for secondary headache, acute onset, or marked change in headache pattern. Magnetic resonance imaging (MRI) provides better detail, especially of the posterior fossa but computed tomography (CT) should be obtained in an acute situation or when MRI is unavailable. Contrast-enhanced imaging is helpful when infection or inflammatory conditions are in the differential diagnosis.
2. Laboratory studies—generally not considered part of a headache evaluation unless general medical or metabolic concerns are being considered. Laboratory evaluation may be needed with certain medications.
3. Ancillary neurologic testing—is not usually indicated in the evaluation of headache, though LP and examination of CSF may be needed to evaluate for suspected infection, inflammatory process, or pressure-related headache. Electroencephalogram and electromyography are not usually indicated for evaluation of headache.
4. Referral–a patient with an acute severe headache, abnormal examination (especially neurologic), or other "Red Flags" (Table 28.3) should be referred to the ED for acute evaluation and care. Referral to a specialist in neurology or headache medicine is indicated when the adolescent or young adult's headache is refractory to management or beyond the clinician's scope of care.

🔵 HEADACHE TREATMENT

The treatment of headaches begins with a trusting relationship between adolescent or young adult and their clinician. An explanation of the headache diagnosis and reassurance (when appropriate) are foundational and may substantially reduce worry by adolescent or young adult and/or their family. When headache treatment is needed, a multitiered approach should be recommended. A discussion of the expectations of headache management is important because there are no known cures for headaches. The goal of treatment should be to reduce the frequency of headaches as much as possible and to make headache management simple and effective. The use of a headache diary may be helpful for tracking treatment effectiveness and progress. Diary entries should include headache frequency, use of abortive/acute/rescue interventions, and any disability attributed to the headache. While treatment duration is not well established, it should continue for some time once good control is achieved to try to prevent relapse or recurrence.[24]

The Multitiered Approach

1. Lifestyle modifications (what the patient can control)
2. Nonpharmacologic therapies, including nutraceuticals (any substance that is derived from a food source that provides medical or health benefits)
3. Pharmacologic interventions (prophylactic and abortive)
4. Other/special considerations

Lifestyle Modifications

The way in which a person lives can contribute to the development of headaches and can also contribute to the improvement of headaches. Five key areas for focus in improving headaches are sleep, hydration, diet, exercise or activity, and stress management.[22]

- Sleep—good sleep hygiene including sleep routine, minimizing electronics before bed, and adequate sleep (8 hours/night for adolescents and 7 to 8 hours/night for young adults) (See Chapter 29)
- Hydration and diet—adequate nutrition and hydration throughout the day is crucial for maintaining brain energy and metabolism and helping to reduce headaches. Water is the best form of hydration but other noncaffeinated drinks (juice, milk, etc.) are good hydration options. Adequate hydration can be judged by setting a certain volume or by monitoring the frequency/volume/color of urine. Adequate nutrition includes eating three well-balanced meals, as well as snacks as needed, daily. Maintaining a healthy weight is important because obesity has also been linked to headaches.[19] Alcohol and excessive caffeine may worsen or provoke headaches and certain foods may trigger headaches such as migraines (see online additional resources).[9]
- Exercise/activity—daily cardiovascular exercise for 20 to 30 minutes should be recommended. When the adolescent or young adult is too busy for daily cardiovascular exercise, recommend that they start exercising 3 to 5 days weekly initially.
- Stress management—stress can be a potent contributor to headache onset, frequency, and intensity. Stress management, including counseling, can be helpful in improving headaches that are stress-induced.

Nonpharmacologic Therapies

The second tier of headache management includes nonpharmacologic therapies that may be useful for prevention and for acute intervention. Mind–body therapies such as cognitive behavioral therapy, pain counseling/therapy, biofeedback, physical therapy (multiple modalities), and acupuncture have been shown to improve and prevent headaches.[17,25] Additionally, nutraceuticals such as melatonin, magnesium, vitamin B2, coenzyme Q10 have been shown in some studies to be effective as prophylactic treatment for various types of headaches and in certain situations may have a role in acute interventions.[25] Nutraceuticals for headache management have not been approved by the U.S. Food and Drug Administration (FDA) and are not regulated, therefore they should be used cautiously.

In addition, some of these therapies can be expensive, and access to experienced clinicians may be limited. The other challenge when considering complementary and alternative therapies is that they may not be covered by insurance.

Pharmacology—Prophylactic and Acute/Rescue

Table 28.4 lists medication options for acute management and prevention of common headache types seen in AYAs. Prophylactic (also called preventative) medications should be considered when adolescent or young adult is having dysfunction or disability related to their headache burden. It is important for adolescent or young adult to know that prophylactic medications (1) are not curative; (2) can take several months to titrate and reach full potential; (3) will need to be continued for at least 6 months beyond the time when good headache control is achieved; and (4) should not be discontinued suddenly. In addition, AYAs should know that there are several medications and classifications and finding a medication that works for an individual may take time and several trials. Finally, chronic and refractory headaches may require more than one medication for effective treatment.

Acute (also called rescue) medications may be used with or without preventive medications. The medication options for acute treatment may be wide-ranging, depending on the type of headache. Headaches are typically best treated as early in the headache as possible, at the correct dose, utilizing the right combination of medications. The adolescent or young adult should be aware to use medications as prescribed or recommended to avoid developing headaches attributable to medication overuse.

Hormone Therapy

Headaches that are associated with the menstrual cycle may be improved with hormone therapy such as estrogen–progestin contraceptives to reduce the fluctuations in estrogen and progestin associated with the menstrual cycle. Adolescents and young adults with menstrual or menstrual-related migraine without aura may consider the use of combined estrogen–progesterone contraception to reduce headaches, although headaches are not always improved with these therapies. When combined estrogen–progesterone contraceptions are considered for headache management, low (≤35-mcg ethinyl-estradiol [EE]) or very low (≤20-mcg EE) estrogen options are often recommended as these tend to be better for headache management. Minimizing the number of cycles using continuous or extended dosing of combined estrogen–progesterone contraception or vaginal rings can be beneficial by reducing the estrogen fluctuations which may trigger headache. While nonestrogen options provide contraception and are considered the safest with respect to stroke risk, they may not be as beneficial for headache management.[12,30]

The use of combined estrogen–progesterone contraception in AYAs with migraine with aura remains controversial. Several organizations, including the World Health Organization, have considered migraines with aura to be an absolute contraindication to the use of combined hormonal contraception.[30] To date, however, there are limited data on the risk of stroke with combined estrogen–progesterone contraception and there are no good quality studies on the risk associated with using low-dose estrogen. At present, the data suggest that the absolute risk for developing stroke is low in females with migraine with aura using combined estrogen–progesterone contraception[30] As such, the International Headache Society Task Force does not indicate that migraine with aura is an absolute contraindication for combined estrogen–progesterone contraception. They suggest that decisions regarding contraceptive choice in females with migraine with aura should be considered on an individual basis with careful assessment of risks and benefits, including the assessment of risk factors for stroke or cardiovascular disease (i.e., tobacco use, dyslipidemia, family history of arterial disease age <45 years, obesity, diabetes, known vascular disease).[31] For instance, it may be necessary to consider estrogen-containing contraceptives for the treatment of endometriosis or polycystic ovary syndrome. In addition, AYAs with migraine with aura should also consider contraceptive options that confer no-risk for stroke including progestin-only contraceptives, subdermal implant, depot-medroxyprogesterone, and copper or levonorgestrel-releasing intrauterine devices.[12,30]

TABLE 28.4

Common Acute and Prophylactic Therapies for Managing Headaches[13,15–17,18,20,26–30]

Headache Type	Therapies Used for Acute Episodes	Therapies Used for Prophylaxis
Migraine	• Nonsteroidal anti-inflammatory drugs (NSAIDs) • Triptans (almotriptan, eletriptan, frovatriptan, naratriptan, rizatriptan, sumatriptan, zolmitriptan, lasmiditan[a]) • *Gepants*[b] (rimegepant and ubrogepant) • Antiemtics (antidopaminergic agents [prochlorperazine and metoclopramide] and odansetron can be used; often works better paired with NSAIDs, triptan, and/or gepant) • Dihydroergotamine (DHE) (intravenous or intranasal) **Emergency Department/Inpatient management** • NSAIDs, antiemetic, fluids are typical first line • Other therapies (i.e., valproic acid, magnesium, steroids) utilized as necessary	• Antiepileptics (topiramate, valproic acid, zonisamide commonly used; gabapentin and levetiracetam may be helpful) • Antihypertensives (beta blockers [propranolol, atenolol, metoprolol, nadolol], angiotensin receptor blockers (candesartan). Calcium channel blockers (less commonly used because of conflicting evidence of efficacy, however verapamil is still recommended for hemiplegic migraine) • Antidepressants (tricyclic antidepressants and serotonin–norepinephrine reuptake inhibitors; selective serotonin reuptake inhibitors may be beneficial) • Antihistamines (cyproheptadine) • CGRP monoclonal antibodies[c] (three subcutaneous monthly agents [galcanezumab, erenumab, fremanezumab] and one quarterly IV agent [eptinezumab] available) • Gepants[b] (rimegepant, atogepant)
Cluster	• Triptans (especially subcutaneous sumatriptan) • High-flow oxygen • Steroid burst • Nerve blocks (occipital and sphenopalatine ganglion [SPG])	• Verapamil • Indomethacin • High-dose melatonin • High-dose galcanezumab
Tension-type headache (TTH)	• NSAIDs	• Often not warranted • Amitriptyline and topiramate often first line when needed but could consider other prophylactic options noted above.
New daily persistent headache	• Similar to migraine and TTH, depending on headache presentation/characteristics • Be careful to avoid medication overuse.	• Similar to migraine and TTH depending on headache presentation/characteristics
Posttraumatic headache	• NSAIDs • Nerve blocks	• Amitriptyline often first line but can use other options similar to migraine and TTH, depending on headache presentation/characteristics.
Special Circumstances		
Menstrual related	• NSAIDs • Triptans (often used as a small burst with daily use for 3–5 days correlating to timing of the menstrually related headache/migraine)	• Consider hormone therapy for headaches without aura.
Pregnancy	• Consider referral. • Nerve blocks • Medications should be used cautiously.	• Consider referral • Serial nerve blocks • Medications should be used cautiously.

[a]Triptan (5HT1B and 5HT1D) like acute medication that is 5HT1F agonist; can be considered in patients with certain contraindications to triptans such as cardiac or vascular concerns due to binding a nonvascular receptor.
[b]New class designed specifically for headache/migraine as a small-molecule CGRP blockers with options available for both acute and prophylaxis. Need to try and fail two to three standard treatments before approval is likely.
[c]New class designed specifically for headache/migraine prevention. Need to try and fail two to three standard treatments before approval is likely.

Adolescents and young adults with migraine with aura should be offered counseling about the variety of contraceptive options. It may be best to consider a collaborative approach that includes specialists in headache medicine, adolescent medicine, and/or a gynecology. The headache specialist should ask the adolescent or young adult to describe their migraines and aura including: (1) new auras or associated symptoms develop, (2) changes to their auras or migraine headaches, and/or (3) prolonged auras or symptoms that develop. These changes may lead the headache specialist to recommend changing or stopping the combined hormone therapy.[30]

Other Procedures

In addition, procedures such as nerve blocks, trigger point injections, and onabotulinumtoxinA (Botox) may be helpful in the management of headaches, but are usually performed by specialists in headache management.[27,28]

 SUMMARY

Headaches are common among AYAs and can lead to marked dysfunction and disability, especially if the headaches are not appropriately diagnosed and treated. While most headaches are primary in nature, comprehensive history and physical examination are critical to identify those headaches that are secondary to an underlying condition. Fortunately, the history and physical examination will be sufficient to diagnose a primary headache in most cases. Adolescents and young adults with primary headaches are likely to benefit from reassurance and conservative headache management. For AYAs who require treatment beyond lifestyle modification and reduction of triggers, a multitiered approach, including pharmacologic intervention or even more specialized approaches or options should be considered.

REFERENCES

1. Linet MS, Stewart WF, Celentano DD, et al. An epidemiologic study of headache among adolescents and young adults. *JAMA*. 1989;261(15):2211–2216.
2. Abu-Arafeh I, Razak S, Sivaraman B, et al. Prevalence of headache and migraine in children and adolescents: a systematic review of population-based studies. *Dev Med Child Neurol*. 2010;52(12):1088–1097.
3. Stewart WF, Wood C, Reed ML, et al. Cumulative lifetime migraine incidence in women and men. *Cephalalgia*. 2008;28(11):1170–1178.
4. Buse DC, Manack AN, Fanning KM, et al. Chronic migraine prevalence, disability, and sociodemographic factors: results from the American Migraine Prevalence and Prevention Study. *Headache*. 2012;52(10):1456–1470.
5. Bron C, Sutherland HG, Griffiths LR. Exploring the hereditary nature of migraine. *Neuropsychiatr Dis Treat*. 2021;17:1183–1194.
6. Stewart WF, Lipton RB, Liberman J. Variation in migraine prevalence by race. *Neurology*. 1996;47(1):52–59.
7. Headache Classification Committee of the International Headache Society. The International Classification of Headache Disorders, 3rd edition. *Cephalalgia*. 2018;38:1–211.
8. Lewis DW. Pediatric migraine. *Neurol Clin*. 2009;27(2):481–501.
9. Yamanaka G, Morichi S, Suzuki S, et al. A review on the triggers of pediatric migraine with the aim of improving headache education. *J Clin Med*. 2020;9(11):3717.
10. Gelfand AA. Episodic syndromes that may be associated with migraine: A.K.A. "the childhood periodic syndromes." *Headache*. 2015;55(10):1358–1364.
11. National Center for Advancing Translational Sciences. Genetic and Rare Diseases Information Center. Information on migraine with brainstem aura. Available at: https://rarediseases.info.nih.gov/diseases/5896/migraine-with-brainstem-aura#ref_8347). Accessed August 9, 2022.
12. Mathew PG, Dun EC, Luo JJ. A cyclic pain: the pathophysiology and treatment of menstrual migraine. *Obstet Gynecol Sur*. 2013;68(2):130–140.
13. Pacheva I, Milanov I, Ivanov I, et al. Evaluation of diagnostic and prognostic value of clinical characteristics of migraine and tension type headache included in the diagnostic criteria for children and adolescents in International Classification of Headache Disorders—second edition. *Int J Clin Prac*. 2012;66(12):1168–1177.
14. Lambru G, Matharu M. Management of trigeminal autonomic cephalalgias in children and adolescents. *Curr Pain Headache Rep*. 2013;17(4):323.
15. Olesen J, Yamani N. New daily persistent headache: a systematic review of an enigmatic disorder. *J Headache Pain*. 2019;20(1):80.
16. Dindo LN, Recober A, Haddad R, et al. Comorbidity of migraine, major depressive disorder, and generalized anxiety disorder in adolescents and young adults. *Int J Behav Med*. 2017;24(4):528–534.
17. Kelly M, Strelzik J, Langdon R, et al. Pediatric headache: overview. *Curr Opin Pediatr*. 2018;30(6):748–754.
18. Paner A, Jay WM, Nand S, et al. Cerebral vein and dural venous sinus thrombosis: risk factors, prognosis and treatment—a modern approach. *Neuroophthalmology*. 2009;33(5):237–247.
19. Verrotti A, Di Fonzo A, Penta L, et al. Obesity and headache/migraine: the importance of weight reduction through lifestyle modifications. *Biomed Res Int*. 2014;2014:420858.
20. Chiang CC, Schwedt TJ, Wang SJ, et al. Treatment of medication-overuse headache: a systematic review. *Cephalalgia*. 2016;36(4):371–386.
21. Mollan SP, Davies B, Silver NC, et al. Idiopathic intracranial hypertension: consensus guidelines on management. *J Neurol Neurosurg Psychiatry*. 2018;89(10):1088–1100.
22. Merison K, Jacobs H. Diagnosis and treatment of childhood migraine. *Curr Treat Options Neurol*. 2016;18(11):48.
23. Lewis DW, Ashwal S, Dahl G, et al. Practice parameter: evaluation of children and adolescents with recurrent headaches: report of the Quality Standards Subcommittee of the American Academy of Neurology and the Practice Committee of the Child Neurology Society. *Neurology*. 2002;59(4):490–498.
24. Oskoui M, Pringsheim T, Billinghurst L, et al. Practice guideline update summary: pharmacologic treatment for pediatric migraine prevention: report of the guideline development, dissemination, and implementation subcommittee of the American Academy of Neurology and the American Headache Society. *Neurology*. 2019;93(11):500–509.
25. Powers SW, Kashikar-Zuck SM, Allen JR, et al. Cognitive behavioral therapy plus amitriptyline for chronic migraine in children and adolescents: a randomized clinical trial. *JAMA*. 2013;310(24):2622–2630.
26. Barmherzig R, Rajapakse T. Nutraceuticals and behavioral therapy for headache. *Curr Neurol Neurosci Rep*. 2021;21(7):33.
27. Gerwin R. Treatment of chronic migraine headache with onabotulinumtoxinA. *Curr Pain Headache Rep*. 2011;15(5):336–338.
28. Szperka CL, Gelfand AA, Hershey AD. Patterns of use of peripheral nerve blocks and trigger point injections for pediatric headache: results of a survey of the American Headache Society Pediatric and Adolescent Section. *Headache*. 2016;56(10):1597–1607.
29. Robbins MS. Diagnosis and management of headache: a review. *JAMA*. 2021;325(18):1874–1885.
30. Sacco S, Merki-Feld GS, Ægidius KL, et al. Hormonal contraceptives and risk of ischemic stroke in women with migraine: a consensus statement from the European Headache Federation (EHF) and the European Society of Contraception and Reproductive Health (ESC). *J Headache Pain*. 2017;18(1):108.
31. Bousser MG, Conard J, Kittner S, et al. Recommendations on the risk of ischaemic stroke associated with use of combined oral contraceptives and hormone replacement therapy in women with migraine. The International Headache Society Task Force on combined oral contraceptives & hormone replacement therapy. *Cephalalgia*. 2000;20(3):155–156.

🛜 ADDITIONAL RESOURCES AND WEBSITES

Additional Resources and Websites for Clinicians:
American Academy of Neurology Practice Guidelines—https://www.aan.com/Guidelines/home/ByTopic?topicId=16Neurology (aan.com)
American Headache Society—https://americanheadachesociety.org/resources/
The International Classification of Headache Disorders 3rd edition—https://ichd-3.org/
Loder EW, Buse DC, Golub JR. Headache and combination estrogen-progestin oral contraceptives: integrating evidence, guidelines, and clinical practice. *Headache*. 2005;45(3):224–231.
MacGregor EA. Migraine, menopause and hormone replacement therapy. *Post Reprod Health*. 2018;24(1):11–18. https://americanmigrainefoundation.org/resource-library/oral-contraceptives-and-migraine/
Szperka CL, VanderPluym J, Orr SL, et al. Recommendations on the use of anti-CGRP monoclonal antibodies in children and adolescents. *Headache*. 2018;58(10):1658–1669. doi:10.1111/head.13414

Additional Resources and Websites for Parents/Caregivers:
Advocating for Your Child with Migraine | AMF—americanmigrainefoundation.org
Creating A Routine for Children with Migraine | AMF—americanmigrainefoundation.org
The Harm of Migraine Stereotypes in Media—americanmigrainefoundation.org
Identifying and Removing Dietary Triggers in Children | AMF—americanmigrainefoundation.org
Migraine in Children | American Migraine Foundation
Migraine Prevention 101: What It Is, When To Use It and Why—americanmigrainefoundation.org
Pediatric Migraine Action Plan | American Migraine Foundation
Pediatric Migraine Content Hub | American Migraine Foundation
7 Tips to Help Children With Migraine At School | AMF—https://americanmigrainefoundation.org/resource-library/7-tips-to-help-children-with-migraine-have-a-successful-school-year/

Additional Resources and Websites for Adolescents and Young Adults:
How To Cancel Plans When You Need Self-Care | AMF—americanmigrainefoundation.org
Identifying and Removing Dietary Triggers in Children | AMF—americanmigrainefoundation.org
Patient Guides | American Migraine Foundation
Pediatric Migraine Action Plan | American Migraine Foundation
Pediatric Migraine Content Hub | American Migraine Foundation
7 Tips to Help Children With Migraine At School | AMF—americanmigrainefoundation.org
Transitioning to Adult Migraine Care Webinar Recap—https://americanmigrainefoundation.org/resource-library/transitioning-webinar-recap/

CHAPTER 29

Sleep Disorders

Gabrielle Rigney
Shelly K. Weiss

KEY WORDS

- Apnea
- Excessive sleepiness
- Insomnia
- Parasomnias
- Prevention
- Screening
- Sleep
- Sleep disorders
- Sleep habits
- Treatment

INTRODUCTION

Sleep is one of our basic needs. It is important for our physical, intellectual, and emotional health. Lack of sleep makes us tired and irritable, decreases short-term memory, and can result in decreased productivity at work and/or school, as well as sleep-related accidents. Sleep disturbances are common in adolescents and young adults (AYAs). Many young people acknowledge difficulties with sleep (often not obtaining adequate sleep) when specifically asked, although it may not be their chief complaint.

Given the variation in classification systems (*Diagnostic and Statistical Manual of Mental Disorders-5, International Classification of Diseases-10, International Classification of Sleep Disorders-3*), rather than taking a purely diagnostic approach, this chapter focuses on common sleep problems experienced by AYAs, as they may be addressed by clinicians working in non–sleep specialty settings. These include sleep deprivation and excessive daytime sleepiness and the various sleep-related behaviors and disorders that are associated with them (e.g., insomnia, delayed sleep phase syndrome, sleep-disordered breathing [SDB] including obstructive sleep apnea [OSA] and narcolepsy). Although less common in adolescence and young adulthood than in childhood, we also briefly describe parasomnias—undesirable physical (motor or autonomic) phenomena that occur exclusively or predominantly during sleep.

As in younger children and older adults, sleep disturbances in AYAs are multifactorial in etiology. They may arise from physiologic and physical processes and symptoms (e.g., changes in chronobiology, difficulties in the transition from sleep to wakefulness, hormonal changes throughout the menstrual cycle, pain, gastrointestinal reflux); symptoms related to mental health issues (e.g., anxiety, depression, stressors, and trauma); environmental and lifestyle factors (e.g., use of technology before bedtime and through the night, busy academic, social, or work schedules); parenting demands; and substance use (e.g., stimulants, barbiturates, or use of caffeine, nicotine, alcohol, hallucinogens, cannabinoids, or other nonprescription substances).

SLEEP PHYSIOLOGY

Sleep is divided into rapid eye movement (REM) sleep and nonrapid eye movement (NREM) sleep. Studies of sleep physiology are carried out using polysomnography, which usually includes electroencephalogram (EEG), electrooculogram, electromyogram, and measures of respiratory function such as airflow, oxygen saturation, and end-tidal PCO_2 levels.

Rapid Eye Movement Sleep

Rapid eye movement sleep occupies about 25% of sleep time in AYAs and is characterized by a high autonomic arousal state including increased cardiovascular and respiratory activity, very low voluntary muscle tone, and rapid synchronous nonpatterned eye movements. The EEG pattern shows a low-voltage variable frequency resembling the awake state. Most dreams occur during REM sleep.

Nonrapid Eye Movement Sleep

Nonrapid eye movement sleep occupies 70% to 80% of sleep time in AYAs and is divided into three stages:

1. N1: Very light or transitional sleep, characterized on EEG by less than 50% alpha rhythm, and low-amplitude mixed-frequency activity
2. N2: Medium-deep sleep, characterized on EEG by the presence of sleep spindles, K-complexes, occupies about 50% of sleep.
3. N3: Progressively deeper sleep, characterized on EEG by a general slowing of frequency and an increase in amplitude (delta waves). Muscular and cardiovascular activities are decreased and little dreaming occurs.

SLEEP PATTERN AND CHANGES DURING ADOLESCENCE AND YOUNG ADULTHOOD

Normal sleep usually consists of a brief period of N1 and N2, followed by a lengthier interval of N3 (slow-wave sleep). After approximately 70 to 100 minutes of NREM sleep, a 10- to 25-minute REM period occurs. This cycle is repeated four to six times throughout the night. The REM periods usually increase by 5 to 30 minutes each cycle, increasing the amount of REM sleep occurring in the second half of the night. The percentage of slow-wave sleep decreases and N2 increases between infancy and adolescence, a pattern that continues into adulthood.[1]

Another documented change in sleep, emerging in adolescence, is a delay in the circadian rhythm timing system.[2] With progressive pubertal development (documented by increasing sexual maturity ratings), there is a tendency toward a lengthening of the internal day and greater eveningness (a preference for later bedtimes and rise times). This tendency persists into young adulthood, before beginning to shift back to earlier bed and rise times in the early 20s.[2] Combined with lifestyle factors that further reinforce later bedtimes (e.g., social activities, electronic media use) and require early rising (e.g., academic and vocational schedules), sleep duration in AYAs is often truncated and insufficient. Although most adolescents require 8 to 10 hours of sleep per night,[3] evidence from worldwide data shows that millions of adolescents are sleeping for less than 8 hours, particularly on school nights.[4] Similarly, although young adults require approximately 7 to 9 hours of sleep,[3] the average sleep durations for these individuals are likely substantially less,[5] particularly when weeknight (vs. weekend) sleep is considered. Only 35% of 18- to 29-year-olds report getting 8 or more hours of sleep on weeknights, whereas 60% report this amount of sleep on weekends.[6] A common reason reported by almost half of the adult population for insufficient sleep is that they do not have enough time for sleep.[7] It should be noted that attempts to catch up on sleep during the weekend are counterproductive, contributing to irregular sleep schedules and making sufficient weekday sleep more difficult to achieve.

COMMON SLEEP DISTURBANCES AND DISORDERS

Sleep Deprivation and Excessive Daytime Sleepiness Due to Insufficient Sleep

Excessive daytime sleepiness is common among AYAs. In a recent report of the American College Health Association (2019), 19.7% of college undergraduates endorsed that daytime sleepiness is a big or very big problem.[7] In the same publication, it was noted that 12.7% of undergraduate college students reported that they had no days in the past week where they had enough sleep to feel rested, and a further 32.1% reported that they only had enough sleep in 1 to 2 days of the past week. Although excessive daytime sleepiness may be caused by any factor that disrupts sleep (e.g., OSA) or can be a symptom of narcolepsy, the most common cause of excessive daytime sleepiness is related to insufficient sleep ("inadequate sleep"). Inadequate sleep may be due to poor sleep practices or late bedtimes. Demanding schedules that include academics, employment, and extracurricular activities, combined with circadian delays and early weekday wake times, can leave insufficient time for sleep. Electronic devices and social media, commonly used by AYAs, may further disrupt sleep during the night.[8] In addition, young adults who are parents face additional sleep disruption associated with caring for young children who may themselves have difficulty sleeping.[9] This chronic sleep deprivation can cause complaints of fatigue or difficulty staying awake during school or work, adversely affecting performance. Mood, physical health, and safety may be compromised, with drowsy driving presenting a notable risk to the 16- to 25-year-old driver.[10] There are a wide variety of medications prescribed for AYAs (both for mental or physical health disorders) that can interfere with sleep, leading to insomnia or excessive daytime sleepiness. Compensatory behaviors, such as stimulant use, napping, sleeping in on weekends, poor food choices (e.g., excessive caffeinated foods or beverages), and reductions in activity, can be iatrogenic, maintaining inadequate sleep and precipitating other sleep disturbances (e.g., insomnia, phase delays, SDB/apnea).

Insomnia

Insomnia is characterized by dissatisfaction about sleep quality or duration. Subjective complaints include difficulty falling asleep at bedtime, waking up at night and having difficulty going back to sleep, waking up too early in the morning with an inability to return to sleep, or a complaint of nonrestorative sleep. The nocturnal difficulties lead to daytime symptoms including fatigue, decreased energy and/or problems with cognitive functions, and mood disturbance.[11-13] Adolescents and young adults most typically have insomnia that manifests as difficulties initiating sleep at bedtime or returning to sleep during the night following a typical period of arousal. Mechanisms underlying insomnia include maladaptive sleep-related cognitions (e.g., concerns about the effects of not getting enough sleep, doubt about one's own ability to change sleep patterns) and behaviors (e.g., leaving inadequate time to relax and unwind before attempting to initiate sleep; use of technology before bed; using the bed and bedroom for activities other than sleep, thereby reducing the association between sleep and bed). Stress, anxiety, mood disorders, and substance use disorder may all be bidirectionally associated with insomnia, and a growing body of literature suggests that insomnia predicts the development of psychological disorders over time.[14] Other less common causes of insomnia include physical illnesses associated with pain or discomfort, increased time in bed, or significant disruptions to sleep and daytime routines.

Medications, such as selective serotonin reuptake inhibitors, stimulants, sympathomimetics, and corticosteroids, may also precipitate or perpetuate symptoms of insomnia. Patients should be questioned specifically about the use of cannabis, either for insomnia or other purposes. Cannabis is known to be used widely (an illicit substance in some U.S. states, with legalization in Canada and other countries) for both recreational and increasingly medicinal and therapeutic purposes. Although AYAs may be using cannabis for insomnia, there is a lack of literature to support this use. A recent literature review (2019) of clinical studies examining the effects on subjective and objective measures of sleep, suggests that cannabinoids may have favorable impact on sleep disturbance. It was concluded that the evidence suggests that "the administration of tetrahydrocannabinol (THC) and THC-derivatives alone, or in combination with cannabidiol may improve self-reported sleep."[15] However, this critical review reported that the vast majority of the studies investigated sleep as a secondary outcome, and there is to date, a lack of placebo-controlled trials examining the use of cannabinoids specifically for treatment of sleep disorders. These studies are needed to investigate the potential benefits, or harms (e.g., side effects) of the use of cannabinoids for sleep disorders.[15]

Delayed Sleep Phase

A delayed sleep phase syndrome (DSPS) is a circadian phase disorder in which the timing of sleep is delayed. Adolescents and young adults are particularly prone to this problem because of their busy evening schedules and an intrinsic biologic preference for a later bedtime. When allowed to sleep for a normal length of time (e.g., weekends, vacations), the delayed sleep onset time will result in delayed waking time. Upon awakening, the individual will be refreshed. However, given the demands of early school and work start times, most individuals with DSPS will not be able to achieve sufficient sleep. They will have difficulty arising, experience daytime sleepiness, and be at risk for the myriad negative outcomes associated with inadequate sleep. When asked to fall asleep at a normal bedtime, well before physiologically ready, they will be at increased risk of engaging in the maladaptive cognitions and behaviors associated with insomnia (described above). Difficulties with academic and occupational functioning, conflict with parents or significant others, and compensatory behaviors may further increase risk of developing comorbid insomnia or other disorders. Based in part on normative data, Auger and Crowley[16] have proposed a weekday bedtime later than 12 AM as a potential indicator of DSPS in adolescents over age 14 years. Using a similar approach, Robillard et al.[17] have used a 1:30 AM or later sleep onset time and a 10:00 AM or later waking time as indicators of sleep phase delay in young adults, aged 19 to 24 years. It is important to note that these times are guidelines only.

Sleep-Disordered Breathing/Obstructive Sleep Apnea

The main cause of SDB is OSA syndrome. This is the presence of complete or partial obstruction of the upper airway during sleep and is associated with the following history: frequent snoring (>3 nights/week), labored breathing during sleep, gasps/snorting noises, observer episodes of apnea, daytime sleepiness, and/or daytime neurobehavioral abnormalities plus others.[18] Sleep-disordered breathing/obstructive sleep apnea, either alone or in combination with other sleep disturbances, places AYAs at significant risk of inadequate sleep and its negative correlates including, but not limited to, excessive daytime sleepiness.[19]

Narcolepsy

Narcolepsy is a chronic neurologic disorder characterized by two major abnormalities—excessive and overwhelming daytime sleepiness and intrusion of REM sleep phenomenon into wakefulness. The age at onset is usually between 10 and 25 years; however, the diagnosis is often delayed.[20] The first and primary manifestation of narcolepsy is excessive daytime sleepiness. The disorder is characterized by four classic symptoms: sleep attacks, cataplexy, sleep paralysis, and hypnagogic (wakefulness to sleep) and hypnopompic (sleep to wakefulness) hallucinations.

Sleep Attacks

Sleep attacks are intrusive and debilitating periods of sleep during the day that may last anywhere from a few seconds to 30 minutes. These periods are often precipitated by sedentary, monotonous activity, and are more frequent after meals and later in the day. Sleepiness is transiently relieved after short naps, but will gradually increase again within the 2 to 3 hours following the nap.

Cataplexy

Cataplexy refers to abrupt, brief periods (seconds to minutes), bilateral loss or reduction of postural muscle tone while conscious, precipitated by intense emotions (e.g., anger, fright, surprise, excitement, or laughter). This is the most valuable symptom in the diagnosis of narcolepsy.

Sleep Paralysis

Sleep paralysis refers to the temporary loss of muscle tone occurring with the onset of sleep or upon awakening. This can be experienced by 8% of adults who do not have narcolepsy.[21]

Hypnagogic Hallucinations

Hypnagogic hallucinations occur with the onset of sleep, while hypnopompic hallucinations occur upon awakening; hallucinations can be visual, auditory, tactile, or kinetic (with sensation of movement).

People without narcolepsy may have occasional sleep paralysis and/or hypnagogic hallucinations. In addition, people with narcolepsy may have automatic activity during periods of altered consciousness. Sleep attacks occur in 100% of individuals with narcolepsy, sleep attacks and cataplexy occur in 70%, sleep paralysis occurs in 50%, and hallucinations occur in 25%. Approximately 10% of individuals will experience all four classic symptoms.

Narcolepsy is a complex disorder caused by the loss of hypocretin (orexin)-producing neurons in the hypothalamus region of the brain.[22] The close association between narcolepsy–cataplexy and the human leukocyte antigen allele DQB1*0602 suggests an autoimmune etiology. There has been interest in the association of narcolepsy with H1N1 influenza and vaccinations. A recent systematic review determined that this association is only related to one vaccine (Pandemrix R) and not to the infection, and is interpreted with caution due to possible bias in the available literature.[23] Narcolepsy is diagnosed by clinical history and documentation of objective findings using both overnight polysomnography and daytime multiple sleep latency test (MSLT) and supported by genetic evaluation. The overnight polysomnography will exclude other sleep disorders, such as sleep apnea. The MSLT is a useful investigation in the diagnosis of narcolepsy. It will show a shortened time to sleep onset (sleep latency) and early onset of REM sleep.

Parasomnias

Parasomnias are undesirable phenomena that occur exclusively or predominantly during sleep. In general, the prevalence of parasomnias decreases with age.[24] Compared to the disturbances and disorders described above, the parasomnias described next, in and of themselves, are less frequently targeted for clinical intervention. Intervention is recommended when the parasomnia is severe enough to cause distress or dysfunction (e.g., nightmares significantly disrupt sleep or precipitate insomnia) or the individual is at risk of injury or harm (e.g., sleepwalking resulting in falls or leaving the house). Parasomnias may also be addressed during the course of intervention in an associated mental health disorder (e.g., anxiety- or trauma-related disorders). In this section, we focus on the more common parasomnias: nightmares, sleepwalking, and sleep terrors.

Nightmares

Nightmares occur during REM sleep, usually occurring in the last one-third to one-half of the sleep episode. They are the most common type of REM-related parasomnia (Table 29.1), with frequent nightmares affecting approximately 5% of the population and are more common in children than adults. Onset is usually before age 10 years; later onset is more suggestive of psychological causes, such as anxiety, distress, and trauma. Drug withdrawal, particularly from benzodiazepines, barbiturates, or alcohol, can also lead to nightmares. Nightmare content is often reflective of developmental milestones and stages, with AYAs expressing more social, academic, occupational, and safety-related concerns.[24] Nightmares may contribute to insomnia by increasing anxiety and therefore sleep onset latency (which is the time it takes to fall asleep after lights are turned off at bedtime).

Sleepwalking and Sleep Terrors

Sleepwalking (somnambulism) and sleep terrors (paver nocturnus) are disorders of impaired and partial arousal from deep slow-wave sleep. Both conditions occur in the first third of the sleep episode, during the rapid transition from N3 (slow-wave sleep) to lighter stages (N1/N2) of sleep. They are infrequently seen beyond adolescence. Characterized by a low level of awareness, clumsiness, a blank expression, and indifference to the environment, sleepwalking episodes usually last from 1 to 30 minutes. Sleep terrors, which are easily confused with, but distinct from nightmares (Table 29.1),

TABLE 29.1
Characteristics of Sleep Terrors versus Nightmares

Characteristic	Sleep Terrors	Nightmares
Vocalization	Intense	Limited
Timing	In first 1/3 of night	Usually in second half of night
Autonomic activity	Marked increase	Slight increase
Arousal	Difficult	Easy
Motility	Marked	Limited
Recall	Minimal	Vivid
Sleep stage	NREM sleep	REM sleep

NREM, nonrapid eye movement; REM, rapid eye movement.

are characterized by the outward expression of intense anxiety, fear, and vocalizations in the form of screams, moans, or gasps. Autonomic features include tachycardia, tachypnea, and sweating. As with sleepwalking, the individual experiencing a sleep terror appears to be relatively nonresponsive to the external environment or efforts to arouse him or her. Upon awakening, there is usually no recall of the experience. Psychological disturbances are thought to be a more likely cause of sleep terrors or sleepwalking if the onset is after age 12 years, the condition has persisted for several years, there is a negative family history, and there is maladaptive daytime behavior.

Sleep Disturbance due to the COVID-19 Pandemic

The COVID-19 pandemic has had a profound impact on the daily routines of AYAs, including changes to sleep behavior. COVID-19 has been found to impact AYAs' sleep, both positively and negatively based on research published to date. Bedtimes and waketimes were found to shift later during the pandemic, leading to an increase in sleep duration.[25-27] These changes in sleep behavior have been found to be particularly beneficial for adolescents, as the delayed bedtime and waketime are more aligned with adolescent physiologic sleep needs. Throughout the pandemic, many adolescents benefitted from sleeping the required 8 hours on school nights that was previously not attained. These changes also resulted in less daytime sleepiness being reported.[25,26] In contrast, young adults reported an increase in sleep difficulties associated with sleep onset difficulties, night awakenings, and nightmares during the COVID-19 lockdown.[26] Other behaviors such as greater screen time and increased family stress compared to before COVID-19 have also been hypothesized to contribute to changes in sleep behavior. It is recommended that clinicians working with AYAs throughout the pandemic assess and monitor sleep behavior. The lessons learned from COVID-19 and its impact on sleep will be important in preparing for improvements in sleep health for AYAs during other unexpected challenges.

PREVENTION, IDENTIFICATION, AND TREATMENT

Although specific disturbances and disorders require unique assessments and interventions, comorbidity among disorders, shared risk and maintenance factors, and overlap in intervention strategies permit a staged approach to prevention, identification, and treatment. This approach may be particularly helpful in non–sleep specialty settings.

Prevention and Screening

Like diet and exercise, conversations about the promotion of healthy sleep habits should start early. Ideally, these conversations would be part of universal preventative health measures occurring across multiple systems and settings (e.g., home, school, media, clinicians' offices) and start early in children's lives. As independence and autonomy increase into adolescence and young adulthood, so can the individual's responsibility for maintaining healthy sleep habits. Some degree of monitoring by parents, while in the family home, and clinicians can be helpful. Although the transition out of the family home and into independent, peer, or romantic shared living arrangements can be a time when healthy sleep habits are vulnerable to disruption, a solid sleep foundation may help young adults maintain, or at least return to, healthier patterns following this transitional period.

In addition to fostering healthy sleep, preventive counseling and screening can preclude the development of certain sleep disorders that are secondary to poor sleep habits. Prevention should include sleep education, monitoring of sleep and sleep habits, and building motivation to engage in healthy sleep behaviors. The ABCs of SLEEPING,[28] designed to organize sleep hygiene recommendations, can be used to structure screening and counseling efforts (**Table 29.2**).

TABLE 29.2

The ABCs of Sleeping

The ABCs of SLEEPING[28] can be used to screen for and target sleep hygiene-related difficulties:

- **A**ge-appropriate **B**edtimes and waketimes with **C**onsistency: Ensure enough time for sleep, maintain regular sleep and rise times.
- **S**chedules and routines: Reduce presleep arousal ("unwind" before bed), work with circadian rhythms.
- **L**ocation: Minimize disturbances, reinforce associations between the bedroom and sleep.
- No **E**lectronics in the bedroom or before bed.
- **E**xercise and diet: Increase daytime activity, especially outdoors; reduce alcohol, energy drinks, caffeine, etc.
- **P**ositivity and relaxation: Address stress, anxiety, worries during the day; focus on relaxation, calm before bed.
- **I**ndependence when falling asleep: Avoid becoming dependent on external stimuli (e.g., television, radio) to initiate sleep.
- **N**eeds met during the day: Make time for socialization and entertainment earlier in the day rather than at night.
- All of the above equals **G**reat sleep.

To learn more about this tool, see "Additional Resources" (online ancillary content).

Other helpful screening and educational resources for teenagers include the BEARS (Bedtimes, Excessive sleepiness, Awakenings, Restlessness, and Snoring)[29] screener, which provides a broad method of querying for many of the sleep disturbances described in this chapter and the sleep-smart tips for teens (which are also applicable to young adults) from the National Sleep Foundation (www.sleepfoundation.org). For young adults, the Pittsburgh Sleep Quality Index is a prominent screening tool used worldwide.[30]

History Taking, Sleep Diary, and Physical Examination

History

Following positive screening, the presenting sleep complaint(s) should be described and a history of other sleep problems in the individual and family should be explored. Information collected should include age at onset, timing during sleep, and the duration, frequency, and intermittent or continuous nature of the complaint. Daytime symptoms and effects should also be queried, including sleepiness, fatigue, and energy levels, mood and anxiety, cognitive difficulties (e.g., attention, memory, learning), and occupational and academic functioning. Symptoms of SDB/OSA should be elicited, if possible, from a parent, sibling, roommate, or partner. Compensatory behaviors (e.g., napping, substance use) and any treatment previously tried (description, length of trial, and result) should also be assessed. An academic and psychosocial history may further elucidate daytime factors that can be both consequences of, and contributors to, sleep disturbances. Corroborative history from parent(s) may be useful to determine if the perception of the complaint differs between people in the family. Thacher[5] provides an interesting discussion of the role of parents in diagnosing and treating sleep problems in young adults. If there is a bed partner or roommate, the significant other may also be asked to provide information. This can be particularly helpful for parasomnias, restlessness, and SDB.

Sleep History Tool

If not previously assessed using a tool like the ABCs of SLEEPING,[28] a description of the bedroom environment; bedtime (weekdays and weekends) and bedtime routines (what is done before sleep); sleep onset location; and the presence of light, noise, television, computer, or other electronics in bedroom should be requested, as should a description of sleep generally (i.e., time to fall asleep, amount of sleep, regularity of sleep and wake schedules). Additional information about what occurs after sleep onset (e.g., frequency, timing, and duration of arousals; behavior during arousals; presence of amnesia for event; response to intervention at the time of arousal) can assist with the differential diagnoses of sleep disturbances such as difficulty returning to sleep related to insomnia, nightmares, sleep terrors, and other parasomnias.

Sleep Diary

A 1- to 2-week sleep diary, listing bedtimes, nighttime symptoms, time on awakening, daytime fatigue or sleepiness, and daytime naps, can be a very helpful tool in evaluating a sleep disturbance. Other assessment tools can include questionnaires and objective measures, such as home videos of nocturnal behaviors (e.g., for parasomnias) and actigraphy (a device that resembles a wristwatch and is a computerized motion detector that measures activity as a proxy for sleep and waking). Medical, psychiatric, and surgical history (including history of tonsillectomy and adenoidectomy) should also be collected or considered, including prescription and over-the-counter medications, herbal products, dietary supplements, weight-loss products, performance-enhancing substances, stimulants, as well as alcohol, cannabis, and other nonprescription drugs.

Sleep Wearables

Consumer sleep-tracking devices commonly known as "wearables," include popular devices such as FitBit and Garmin, which are widely used worldwide. Wearables use an accelerometer to measure movement and translate these into sleep/wake data. These devices are typically worn on the wrist and used for tracking physical activity. However, around 25% of wearable users have also used their device to track their sleep behavior.[31] A recent study tested the performance of the latest consumer devices alongside validated objective measures of sleep (i.e., actigraphy and polysomnography), and found that most wearable devices perform well in detecting sleep and at detecting wake. FitBit devices were found to be better at sleep tracking than Garmin devices. It's important to note that sleep wearables are not able to effectively identify sleep stages and are likely to demonstrate more accurate results on nights where the consumer has slept well.[31]

Physical Examination

Depending on the particular sleep complaint, clinicians may also wish to conduct a targeted physical examination. For example, a physical examination related to SBD/OSA may reveal evidence of tonsillar hypertrophy, adenoidal facies, micrognathia/retrognathia, high-arched palate, failure to thrive, hypertension, and growth abnormalities (either underweight or overweight).[18] It is important to note, however, that even if OSA is present, there may be no abnormalities seen on physical examination.

Referral for Further Assessment

A referral for further assessment should be made in certain circumstances. It is often of benefit to refer to a sleep consultant about the need for a sleep study (overnight polysomnography), rather than ordering a sleep study right away. Sleep studies are used to evaluate a variety of conditions including SDB, some parasomnias, and disorders of hypersomnolence (combined with a daytime MSLT), but are often not necessary in the evaluation of other sleep disorders (e.g., insomnia).

Treatment

A staged approach to treatment is outlined below. The treatment of all sleep disorders is beyond the scope of this chapter. The following strategies are foundational and will apply across most disturbances and disorders when there is an element of behavioral insomnia or inadequate sleep duration:

1. Identify sleep hygiene factors using data provided during screening and history taking, which may be contributing to or maintaining sleep disturbances (e.g., insufficient time for sleep, use of electronics in bedroom, variable sleep schedules).

2. Identify and encourage sleep-promoting behaviors (e.g., regular exercise; regularizing bedtime and wake time, including on weekends; reducing use of substances such as caffeine, alcohol, nicotine, and illicit substances; practicing wind-down routines; increasing exposure to bright natural light in the morning, darkness at night).

3. Provide (or refer for) counseling related to existing situational stressors.

4. Use motivational interviewing (MI) techniques to assist with treatment planning and engagement. Although treatment will result in improved sleep and additional benefits, the changes required (e.g., earlier bedtimes, turning off electronics) will come at a cost (e.g., loss of social opportunities). Motivational interviewing can prevent these costs from becoming treatment barriers.

5. Provide instruction or resources to facilitate the use of relaxation techniques. Once these strategies are in place, more disorder-specific treatments can be applied, focusing on the more unique causes and characteristics of each disorder. These strategies are described in the Additional Resources.

Sleep Disorder Clinics

For severe sleep disorders or diagnostic dilemmas, referral to a sleep disorder clinic or sleep consultant can be helpful. The National Sleep Foundation keeps an updated state-wise list of accredited sleep disorder centers (www.sleepfoundation.org). In addition, clinics in the United States accredited by the American Academy of Sleep Medicine (listed by state) are available at www.aasmnet.org. Clinics in Canada (listed by province) are available on the website of the Canadian Sleep Society at www.css-scs.ca.

SUMMARY

Sleep plays a critical role in healthy development, and understanding what sleep is, how it is regulated, and how sleep physiology is unique for AYAs is important to inform both assessment and treatment of sleep problems. Throughout adolescence and young adulthood, there are a range of biopsychosocial factors that interact and contribute to the etiology of sleep problems. A staged approach to prevention, identification, and treatment of sleep problems is recommended, which includes starting early with primary prevention and screening for sleep problems in AYAs. The use of tools such as a sleep diary or wearable devices is also recommended to obtain a history of the sleep complaint. Where necessary, referral for further assessment (e.g., at a sleep disorder clinic) is recommended.

REFERENCES

1. Ohayon MM, Carskadon MA, Guilleminault C, et al. Meta-analysis of quantitative sleep parameters from childhood to old age in healthy individuals: developing normative sleep values across the human lifespan. *Sleep*. 2004;27:1255–1273.
2. Crowley SJ, Wolfson AR, Tarokh L, et al. An update on adolescent sleep: new evidence informing the perfect storm model. *J Adolesc*. 2018;67:55–65.
3. Hirshkowitz M, Whiton K, Albert SM, et al. National Sleep Foundation's sleep time duration recommendations: methodology and results summary. *Sleep Health*. 2015;1(1):40–43.
4. Gradisar M, Gardner G, Dohnt H. Recent worldwide sleep patterns and problems during adolescence: a review and meta-analysis of age, region, and sleep. *Sleep Med*. 2011;12(2):110–118.
5. Thacher PV. Late adolescence and emerging adulthood: a new lens for sleep professionals. In: Wolfson AR, Montgomery-Downs HE, eds. *The Oxford Handbook of Infant, Child, and Adolescent Sleep and Behavior*. Oxford University Press; 2013:586–602.
6. National Sleep Foundation 2002 Sleep in America Poll Task Force. 2002 "Sleep in America Poll." 2002. Available at http://sleepfoundation.org/sites/default/files/2002SleepInAmericaPoll.pdf
7. American College Health Association. *National College Health Assessment II, Reference Group Data Report Undergraduate Students Spring 2019*. Hanover, MD: American College Health Association; 2019.
8. Hale L, Kirschen GW, LeBourgeois MK, et al. Youth screen media habits and sleep: sleep-friendly screen behavior recommendations for clinicians, educators, and parents. *Child Adolesc Psychiatr Clin N Am*. 2018;27(2):229–245.
9. Stremler R. Postpartum sleep: impact of infant sleep on parents. In: Wolfson AR, Montgomery-Downs HE, eds. *The Oxford Handbook of Infant, Child, and Adolescent Sleep and Behavior*. Oxford University Press; 2013:58–69.

10. Higgins JS, Michael J, Austin R, et al. Asleep at the wheel—the road to addressing drowsy driving. *Sleep.* 2017;40(2).

11. Morin C. Insomnia rounds (non-peer reviewed). 2012. Available at https://css-scs.ca/insomnia-rounds/

12. American Psychiatric Association. *Diagnostic and Statistical Manual of Mental Disorders.* 5th ed. American Psychiatric Publishing; 2013.

13. American Academy of Sleep Medicine. *International Classification of Sleep Disorders: Diagnostic & Coding Manual.* 3rd ed. American Academy of Sleep Medicine; 2013.

14. Harvey AG, Alfano CA, Clarke G. Mood disorders. In: Wolfson AR, Montgomery-Downs HE, eds. *The Oxford Handbook of Infant, Child, and Adolescent Sleep and Behavior.* Oxford University Press; 2013:515–531.

15. Kuhathasan N, Dufort A, MacKillop J, et al. The use of cannabinoids for sleep: a critical review on clinical trials. *Exp Clin Psychopharmacol.* 2019;27(4):383.

16. Auger RR, Crowley SJ. Circadian timing: delayed sleep phase disorder. In: Wolfson AR, Montgomery-Downs HE, eds. *The Oxford Handbook of Infant, Child, and Adolescent Sleep and Behavior.* Oxford University Press; 2013:327–346.

17. Robillard R, Naismith SL, Rogers NL, et al. Delayed sleep phase in young people with unipolar or bipolar affective disorders. *J Affect Disord.* 2013;145(2):260–263.

18. Marcus CL, Brooks LJ, Draper KA, et al. Diagnosis and management of childhood obstructive sleep apnea syndrome. *Pediatrics.* 2012;130:576–584.

19. Archbold KH. Pediatric sleep apnea and adherence to positive airway pressure (PAP) therapy. In: Wolfson AR, Montgomery-Downs HE, eds. *The Oxford Handbook of Infant, Child, and Adolescents Sleep and Behavior.* Oxford University Press; 2013:362–369.

20. Morse AM. Narcolepsy in children and adults: a guide to improved recognition, diagnosis and management. *Med Sci (Basel).* 2019;7(12):106.

21. Sharpless BA. A clinician's guide to recurrent isolated sleep paralysis. *Neuropsychiatr Dis Treat.* 2016;12:1761.

22. Singh AK, Mahlios J, Mignot E. Genetic association, seasonal infections and autoimmune basis of narcolepsy. *J Autoimmun.* 2013;43:26–31.

23. Sarakanen TO, Alakuijala APE, Dauvilliers YA, et al. Incidence of narcolepsy after H1N1 influenza and vaccinations: systematic review and meta-analysis. *Sleep Med Rev.* 2018;38:177–186.

24. Ivanenko A, Larson K. Nighttime distractions: fears, nightmares, and parasomnias. In: Wolfson AR, Montgomery-Downs HE, eds. *The Oxford Handbook of Infant, Child, and Adolescent Sleep and Behavior.* Oxford University Press; 2013:347–361.

25. Becker SP, Dvorsky MR, Breaux R, et al. Prospective examination of adolescent sleep patterns and behaviors before and during COVID-19. *Sleep.* 2021;44(8):zsab054.

26. Socarras LR, Potvin J, Forest G. COVID-19 and sleep patterns in adolescents and young adults. *Sleep Med.* 2021;83:26–33.

27. Bruni O, Malorgio E, Doria M, et al. Changes in sleep patterns and disturbances in children and adolescents in Italy during the Covid-19 outbreak. *Sleep Med.* 2022;91:166–174.

28. Howlett M, Jemcov A, Adams A, et al. ABCs of SLEEPING tool: improving access to care for pediatric insomnia. *Clin Pract Pediatr Psychol.* 2020;8(1):1.

29. Owens JA, Dalzell V. Use of the "BEARS" sleep screening tool in a pediatric residents' continuity clinic: a pilot study. *Sleep Med.* 2005;6:63–69.

30. Buysse DJ, Reynolds CF III, Monk TH, et al. The Pittsburgh Sleep Quality Index: a new instrument for psychiatric practice and research. *Psychiatry Res.* 1989;28(2):193–213.

31. Chinoy ED, Cuellar JA, Huwa KE, et al. Performance of seven consumer sleep-tracking devices compared with polysomnography. *Sleep.* 2021;44(5):zsaa291.

📶 ADDITIONAL RESOURCES AND WEBSITES

Additional Resources and Websites for Clinicians:
American Academy of Sleep Medicine—www.aasm.org
Canadian Sleep Society—www.css-scs.ca
International Pediatric Sleep Association—www.pedsleep.org
National Sleep Foundation—www.sleepfoundation.org
Pediatric Sleep Problems: A Clinician's Guide to Behavioural Interventions. Meltzer LJ, McLaughlin Crabtree V. American Psychological Association. 2019—https://doi.org/10.1037/14645-000
World Sleep Society—www.worldsleepsociety.org

Additional Resources and Websites for Parents/Caregivers:
American Academy of Sleep Medicine—www.aasm.org
Canadian Sleep Society—www.css-scs.ca
National Sleep Foundation—www.sleepfoundation.org
Snooze… or Lose! 10 "No War" Ways to Improve Your Teen's Sleep Habits. Emsellem HA. Joseph Henry Press. 2006
World Sleep Society—www.worldsleepsociety.org

Additional Resources and Websites for Adolescents and Young Adults:
The Awesome Power of Sleep: How Sleep Super-Charges Your Teenage Brain. Morgan N. Walker Books Ltd. 2021
Goodnight Mind for Teens. Carney CE. Instant Help Books, 2020
The Insomnia Workbook for Teens: Skills to Help You Stop Stressing and Start Sleeping Better. Tompkins MA, Thompson MA. Instant Help Books, 2018
National Sleep Foundation—www.sleepfoundation.org
Sensible Sleep—www.sensiblesleep.com

PART VII

Genitourinary Disorders

CHAPTER 30

Renal and Genitourinary Tract Infections in Adolescents and Young Adults

Lawrence J. D'Angelo
Shamir Tuchman

KEY WORDS

- Cystitis
- Drug resistance
- Dysuria
- Epididymitis
- Extended spectrum beta lactamase (ESBL)
- Prostatitis
- Pyelonephritis
- Urinary tract infection (UTI)

 INTRODUCTION

Genitourinary tract infections are common in adolescents and young adults (AYAs). All of these infections share a common pathogenesis of colonization of the vaginal introitus (in females) or urethral meatus (males and females) by bacterial or other flora followed by ascension via the urethra into the bladder. If the infection is contained by host factors or medical intervention to the bladder, then patients have what is now designated as an uncomplicated urinary tract infection (UTI). Such infections are usually described as urethritis, cystitis, or asymptomatic bacteriuria. Further extension can lead to less commonly diagnosed but more complicated infections such as pyelonephritis in both males and females and epididymitis and prostatitis in males. Spread of these infections is often accompanied by malaise, fever, chills, flank pain, costovertebral angle tenderness, and testicular, pelvic, or perineal pain, particularly in males with epididymitis or prostatitis. This progression of symptoms is the most reliable and consistent way to define a specific infection as either uncomplicated or complicated.

This chapter will review the epidemiology, diagnosis, and treatment of the most common infections seen in AYAs. Challenges in diagnosis and in treatment of the expanding number of resistant organisms now causing UTIs will also be discussed.

UNCOMPLICATED INFECTIONS

Cystitis

Epidemiology

1. Over the course of a lifetime, UTIs occur three to five times more commonly in females than in males. For adolescents, this difference may be as great as 50-fold.
2. One in three female AYAs will have at least one episode of acute cystitis during adolescence or young adulthood.[1] An even higher annual incidence of lower UTI was demonstrated in a cohort of sexually active female university students: 0.7 infections/person-year.[2] One infection appears to predispose an

individual to more, with 24% of young women having at least one recurrence within 6 months and up to 50% of those with one recurrence experiencing a second recurrence in this same time period.[3]

3. Risk factors for infection
   a. Female AYAs: Female AYAs are at greater risk than male AYAs because of a short urethra, which has close proximity to vaginal and rectal microorganisms. Other risk factors for UTIs include the following (although many of these risk factors are not well substantiated in the literature):
      - Coitus and coital behaviors (diaphragm use, coital frequency, use of spermicide-coated condoms, and having a new sexual partner)
      - Pregnancy
      - Previous UTIs
      - Nonsecretor of ABO blood group antigens (secondary to differential binding of bacteria to vaginal epithelial cells)[4]
      - Catheterization or instrumentation of the urethra[5]
      - Anatomical or functional abnormalities (e.g., urethral stenosis, neurogenic bladder, and nephrolithiasis)
      - Obesity[6]
      - Having a first-degree relative with a history of UTIs[7]
   b. Male AYAs: Because UTIs in general and cystitis in particular are so much less frequent in male AYAs, risk factors and pathophysiology are less well understood. In nonsexually active male AYAs, bladder and renal infections are more likely to result from structural or functional abnormalities of the perineum and/or urinary tract. Additional factors may include the following:
      - Blood group B or AB nonsecretor; P1 blood group phenotype
      - Insertive anal intercourse[8]
      - Sexual partner with vaginal colonization by uropathogens
      - Uncircumcised[9]

Microbiology and Resistance

Females The most common organism causing acute cystitis is *Escherichia coli* (75% to 90%).[10] Internationally, *Staphylococcus saprophyticus* may play a major role in such infections in AYAs,[11] but it now appears that in the United States, other gram-negative organisms cause most of the remainder of the infections. Organisms such as *Klebsiella* species, *Pseudomonas aeruginosa*, *Enterobacter* and *Proteus* species, *Staphylococcus aureus*, *Streptococcus faecalis*, and *Serratia marcescens* may play a greater role in recurrent or chronic, rather than in acute, infections. Gram-positive organisms such as *Staphylococcus saprophyticus*, enterococci, and group B streptococcus are less frequent chronic infection pathogens; recent studies have shown that in females with symptoms suggestive of UTI, positive midstream cultures for the latter two organisms have a very low positive predictive value when compared to catheterized specimens,[12] implying that these are likely colonizers of the external periurethral area.

Males Approximately three-fourths of UTIs in male AYAs are due to gram-negative bacilli, but *E. coli* infections are not nearly as common as in females. Gram-positive organisms, particularly enterococci and coagulase-negative staphylococci, account for approximately one-fifth of infections. Sexually transmitted pathogens such as *Trichomonas vaginalis, Neisseria gonorrhoeae, Chlamydia trachomatis, Mycoplasma hominis,* and *Gardnerella vaginalis* can cause urethral, epididymal, and prostatic infections that can be confused with UTIs in AYAs.[13] Furthermore, *M. genitalium* has been shown to cause nongonococcal urethritis (NGU) in males, with the highest prevalence in males who are *C. trachomatis* negative.

Resistance

Rates of resistance in urinary tract pathogens have continued to increase in the past decade.[14] This has been documented primarily in complicated infections, but has also been noted in uncomplicated cystitis in both AYA males and females.[15] The most worrisome of these resistance mutations have been "extended spectrum beta lactamase (ESBL) producing *Enterobacteriaceae*" which are more likely to be detected in hospitalized patients. These organisms are major contributors to the growing resistance to fluoroquinolones.

Risk factors for the presence of resistant organisms as the cause of uncomplicated or complicated UTIs include the following[16]:
• Prior antibiotic use in the past 60 to 90 days
• Inpatient stay at a health care facility in the past 120 days
• Recent travel to parts of the world with high rates of multiresistant organisms
• Prior history of an infection caused by a multiresistant organism

Symptoms and Signs

Females In females, the most common symptoms of UTIs are dysuria, frequency, hesitancy, suprapubic pain or pressure, overt pyuria, and hematuria. These symptoms are often difficult to localize. For example, dysuria can be related to infections in the bladder, urethra, vulva, or vagina. The location and timing of the dysuria are occasionally helpful. Dysuria associated with cystitis or urethritis is often described as internal pain and is usually worse when a patient initiates micturition. External pain or "terminal pain" (at the end of micturition) is more often associated with other conditions such as a vulvar inflammation, upper genital tract infection, or a herpes simplex infection.

Table 30.1 lists the pathogens, incidence of pyuria and hematuria, urine culture findings, and signs and symptoms of acute dysuria in females.

Males Apart from the preceding symptoms, male patients may also have symptoms associated with infections in the prostate (penile, perineal, or rectal pain), epididymis (scrotal discomfort or tender epididymis), or testicles (testicular pain and swelling).

Differential Diagnosis of Acute Dysuria

The most common complaint arousing suspicion of a UTI is dysuria. However, dysuria may be a symptom of infection elsewhere in the urinary or genital tract, particularly in AYAs.[17] The differential diagnosis of dysuria includes the following:

Female Adolescents and Young Adults
1. Acute vaginitis and possible associated Skene glands infection secondary to sexually transmitted pathogens
2. Vulvovaginitis
3. Local dermatitis from chemicals and other agents such as soaps, contraceptive agents and foams, and feminine hygiene products
4. Subclinical pyelonephritis: Some with only dysuria have a complicated UTI. These infections may be more difficult to eradicate. There are no reliable and simple methods to distinguish them from uncomplicated UTIs if upper tract or systemic symptoms are not present.
5. Acute urethral syndrome: Symptomatic females with pyuria but no growth of urinary pathogens on culture are likely infected with one or more sexually transmitted pathogens and should be evaluated for these.[18]

Males The differential diagnosis of cystitis and dysuria includes the following:
1. Urethritis (secondary to sexually transmitted organisms, including *N. gonorrhoeae, C. trachomatis, T. vaginalis, M. genitalium,* and others)
2. Prostatitis/epididymitis/orchitis
3. Irritation from agents such as lubricants or spermicides
4. Trauma (usually associated with masturbation)

Diagnosis

1. History
   a. In young women, it is important to elicit symptoms suggestive of vulvovaginitis, such as an abnormal vaginal discharge or vaginal itching; with a vaginal infection, symptoms of frequency and urgency are less common. In young men, a history of sexual exposure, type of sexual activity, past urinary tract problems, or penile trauma is important.
   b. Similarly, in female AYAs, it is helpful to know if the patient uses any medications or potential irritants such as douches, intravaginal feminine hygiene products, strong soaps, bubble

TABLE 30.1						
Differential Diagnosis of Acute Dysuria in Females						
Condition	**Pathogen**	**Pyuria**	**Hematuria**	**Bacteriuria**	**Urine Culture**[a]	**Signs and Symptoms**
Cystitis	*E. coli, S. saprophyticus, Proteus, Klebsiella* sp	Usually	Sometimes	Usually	$10^2->10^5$	Acute onset, severe symptoms, dysuria, frequency, urgency, suprapubic or low back pain, suprapubic tenderness, internal dysuria
Urethritis	*C. trachomatis, N. gonorrhoeae, M. genitalium, herpes simplex virus*	Usually	Rarely	Rarely	$<10^2$	Gradual onset, mild symptoms, vaginal discharge or bleeding, lower abdominal pain, new sexual partner, cervical or vaginal lesions on examination
Vaginitis	*Candida* sp, *T. vaginalis*	Rarely	Rarely	Rarely	$<10^2$	Vaginal discharge or odor, pruritus, dyspareunia, external dysuria, no frequency or urgency; vulvovaginitis on examination

[a]Colony forming units (CFU)/mL.

baths, or intravaginal contraceptive products that could cause a local dermatitis. In male AYAs, a history of mechanical irritation including frequent masturbation is important.

c. For both male and female AYAs, inquiring about specific sexual practices is important.

d. Determining whether there are signs of a complicated infection of the upper genitourinary tract is important. Fever and flank pain suggest acute pyelonephritis. Other important historical factors predisposing to complicated infections include underlying urinary tract abnormalities, diabetes mellitus, UTIs in childhood, three or more previous UTIs, or complicated infections like acute pyelonephritis in the past.

2. Physical examination

a. In both sexes, an examination of the abdomen and flank for tenderness should be performed.

b. In female AYAs, an external genital or pelvic examination should be considered if the patient is sexually active or if there is history of a vaginal discharge.

c. In male AYAs, examination should include inspection and palpation of the genitals to check for urethral discharge, meatal erythema, inflammation of the glans penis, penile lesions, an enlarged or tender epididymis or testis, or inguinal lymphadenopathy. A rectal examination is necessary if a diagnosis of prostatitis is under consideration.

3. Laboratory studies[19]

a. Nonculture examination of urine

   • Both direct examination of *uncentrifuged* urine or Gram stain of a similar specimen are insensitive diagnostic tests unless the culture has a bacteria colony count of at least 10^5 organisms/mL. Similarly, microscopic detection of pyuria on unspun urine necessitates counting cells in a hemocytometer (with ≥ 8 cells/mm^3 correlating with positive urine cultures) and is rarely performed. Examination of centrifuged urine sediment, while possible, is not reliably standardized and may be positive with any cause of pyuria.

   • Several other chemical tests that use nitrate glucose oxidase or catalase to detect the presence of nitrites are commonly used diagnostic tests. Available by "dipstick," they are unfortunately dependent on the conversion of nitrate to nitrite, which is usually only associated with infections caused by members of the Enterobacteriaceae family including *E. coli*. When the infection is caused by other organisms such as *S. saprophyticus* or *Enterococcus*, this test is most often negative.

   • Chemical testing for the presence of leukocyte esterase has limitations as well, although it may be conveniently combined on a dipstick for testing for urinary nitrites. When combined, these tests still have relatively low sensitivity but high predictive value if both are positive. If nonculture testing is utilized, urine should be examined within 2 hours of collection.

b. Urine culture

   • Urine cultures (UC) are not a routine part of the evaluation of every patient with symptoms consistent with an uncomplicated UTI. For older AYAs who are able to provide a reliable history, urine culture is not typically obtained before starting antibiotic therapy. For prepubertal girls and younger adolescents who may have difficulty characterizing their symptoms—especially if this is likely their first UTI—culture should be considered. They are, however, necessary for those individuals who have recurrent or complicated infections (pyelonephritis) or in those who have failed initial treatment. Older criteria of a colony count of >100,000 CFU/mL of a typical urinary pathogen have been replaced by colony counts as low as $\geq 10^2$ CFU/mL or more commonly a count of 10^4 in a voided midstream specimen. However, while true for Enterobacteriaceae, this technique of sampling and diagnostic standard does not apply if other bacterial species (such as *enterococci* or group B strep) are isolated.[12]

4. Other tests

a. Females: Prepubertal girls or those with three infections within 1 to 2 years should receive a more complete urinary tract evaluation, which may include urine culture, a renal ultrasound, and a voiding cystourethrogram. In postpubertal female AYAs with uncomplicated cystitis, evaluation after recurrent episodes other than urine culture is unlikely to reveal significant abnormalities that would change either therapy or prognosis.

b. Males: Although some authorities recommend a full investigation after the first infection, this is probably of greater importance in the young child or infant. In AYAs, there is less evidence for such studies unless there is a suspected renal abnormality or if there is no response to therapy.

Recurrent Infections in Female Adolescents and Young Adults

Approximately 20% to 25% of young women will have recurrent UTIs, defined as two infections in 6 months or three in 1 year.[20] Most of these female AYAs do not have anatomical or functional abnormalities of the urinary tract. However, female patients with a relapse of symptoms within 2 weeks of completion of therapy should have their urine cultured, be treated with the selected antibiotic regimen for at least 7 days, and should have careful follow-up including a "test-of-cure" culture. Similarly, females with recurrent cystitis within 3 months of the original infection should have a urine culture so that antibiotic therapy can be targeted to the causative organism. Repeated infections which are not related to coitus, associated with persistent hematuria or renal insufficiency or result in more complicated infections such as pyelonephritis, should result in an evaluation for an occult source of infection or urologic abnormality.

Evidence-based techniques for preventing recurrent infections include stopping intravaginal feminine hygiene and intravaginal contraceptive use, postcoital voiding, increased fluid intake (>3 L daily), daily or every other day antimicrobial prophylaxis, postcoital antibiotic prophylaxis, and symptom-directed patient-initiated treatment.[21] More controversial and still unsubstantiated approaches include daily lactobacilli product administration, methenamine salts, d-mannose products, ascorbic acid treatment, cranberry products, and a vaginal "vaccine" made of heat-killed uropathogenic bacteria.[21]

ASYMPTOMATIC BACTERIURIA

The prevalence of asymptomatic bacteriuria (reproducible growth of $>10^5$ CFU/mL) ranges from approximately 1% to 7%. There is a tendency toward spontaneous cure. However, young women with this condition are at increased risk of an overt UTI (8% in the week after documented bacteria in the urine),[22] and, in individuals whose infection begins in childhood, there is a suggestion that their infection can lead to renal impairment. Asymptomatic bacteriuria during pregnancy is a risk factor for the development of acute pyelonephritis, for lower fetal birth weight, and for a higher incidence of prematurity. Treatment is mainly indicated for individuals who are (1) pregnant; (2) male; (3) have a renal tract abnormality or are immunocompromised (diabetes, sickle cell disease, HIV infection, etc.); or (4) young women with a history of UTI recurrence and concomitant pyuria.[23] Treatment should be with appropriate antibiotics selected based on culture and subsequent sensitivities.

COMPLICATED INFECTIONS

Complicated infections are those which have signs and symptoms that suggest spread beyond the bladder. These include the following:
- Fever
- Systemic symptoms (chills, nausea and vomiting, malaise, myalgias, etc.)
- Flank or back pain
- Costovertebral angle tenderness
- Pelvic or perineal pain

The presence of these signs and symptoms may suggest infections that require a more careful selection of antibiotics and more intentional follow-up.

Pyelonephritis
Etiology

The most common complicated UTI is pyelonephritis, an infection of the renal pelvis and medulla. Risk factors for pyelonephritis are similar to those for uncomplicated UTIs (with the strongest factors being recent intercourse, a new sexual partner, and spermicide use), but also include diabetes and a maternal history of a complicated UTI.[24] Most infections occur from bacterial ascent through the urethra and bladder to the ureters and the kidneys.

The microbiology of pyelonephritis is like that of uncomplicated infections. However, because patients with pyelonephritis are more likely to have had previous infections, resistant organisms are more likely to be cultured.

Diagnosis

The clinical manifestations may include the signs and symptoms listed above. Laboratory findings usually include one or more of the following: elevated leukocyte count, erythrocyte sedimentation rate and/or C-reactive protein, urinalysis revealing leukocytes and bacterial and cellular casts, and a positive urine culture result.

The range of symptoms varies from mild to those suggesting septicemia (high fever, organ dysfunction, shock, and renal insufficiency). Like uncomplicated infections, most cases of acute pyelonephritis in young women are caused by E. coli (>80%). Pyuria and gram-negative bacteria are usually present on examination of the urine. Urine culture specimens should always be obtained even if antibiotics have recently been initiated. Blood cultures should also be obtained from those whose diagnosis is uncertain, from immunosuppressed patients, from those in whom a hematogenous source is suspected, or from those who are ill enough to be hospitalized. If fever and flank pain persist after 72 hours of treatment, cultures should be repeated, and ultrasonography or computed tomography should be considered to evaluate for obstruction or the presence of an abscess. Additional indications for imaging studies include recurrent pyelonephritis and persistent hematuria.[25] Indications for hospitalization include persistently high fever, pregnancy, persistent vomiting, suspected sepsis, uncertain diagnosis, and coincident urinary tract obstruction. Other relative indications include anatomical urinary tract abnormalities, immunocompromised status, and inadequate access to follow-up care.

Epididymitis/Prostatitis
Etiology

Epididymitis and prostatitis are inflammatory reactions of the male "upper" sexual/urinary tract. Epididymitis is the considerably more common of the two, but both are relatively infrequent and when they do occur in this age-group, they are usually secondary to sexually transmitted infections such as N. gonorrhoeae or C. trachomatis. Coliform bacteria, S. saprophyticus, M. hominis, U. urealyticum, and T. vaginalis have also been implicated as causative agents. Retrograde spread of pathogens is the usual mechanism of infection.[26]

Risk factors for both infections include sexual activity, strenuous physical activity, and prolonged periods of sitting such as that associated with long trips or sedentary jobs. Anatomical factors such as posterior urethral valves or urethral or meatal stenosis can also be a predisposing factor.

Diagnosis

Epididymitis usually presents with acute to subacute scrotal pain. Pain can affect one or both testes. Symptoms of lower UTI may be present (dysuria, frequency, hematuria) as can systemic symptoms such as fever, nausea, and vomiting.

If epididymitis is suspected, nucleic acid antibody testing for N. gonorrhoeae and C. trachomatis should be initiated from either a urethral swab or urine. Urine dipsticks positive for leukocyte esterase or nitrates help to support the diagnosis in combination with clinical signs and symptoms. Physical findings may include scrotal swelling, tenderness of the epididymis, and associated tenderness of the testicle.

When testicular pain is the main presenting symptom and physical examination cannot distinguish between epididymal and testicular tenderness, the differential diagnosis must include testicular torsion. Immediate urologic consultation should be requested in addition to obtaining a scrotal ultrasound with blood flow studies to assess perfusion and anatomy (see Chapter 59).

In prostatitis, symptoms and signs usually include penile/scrotal, suprapubic, perineal, groin, or back pain or pain that occurs during ejaculation. There may also be frequency, dysuria, and hesitation as well as systemic symptoms such as chills, fever, and malaise. Other symptoms may include hematospermia and hematuria. Physical examination usually reveals tenderness on rectal examination when the prostate is palpated.

In either condition, urinalysis may reveal bacteriuria or pyuria and urine cultures may be positive. However, absence of these laboratory findings does not eliminate either diagnosis if history and/or physical examination suggest infection.

TREATMENT OF UNCOMPLICATED AND COMPLICATED URINARY TRACT INFECTIONS

In the face of a significant increase in the number of urinary pathogens demonstrating resistance to antibiotics historically used to treat UTIs, such as trimethoprim-sulfamethoxazole, ampicillin and amoxicillin, and some quinolones,[27] the guidelines for treating acute uncomplicated UTIs have been updated. This growing resistance to medications necessitates that local resistance patterns be consulted before prescribing any antibiotic for treatment of UTIs. Trimethoprim-sulfamethoxazole should only be used if the local resistance rates of uropathogens do not exceed 20%. Ampicillin or amoxicillin should never be used as empirical treatment of UTIs; they should only be used if culture results show that the isolated bacteria are sensitive to these agents.[28] Table 30.2 summarizes the current recommendations for treating both lower and upper tract infections.

Oral antibiotic treatment remains appropriate for patients with pyelonephritis with mild to moderate illness and no associated nausea or vomiting (Table 30.2). Any of these regimens may be initiated with an initial one-time dose of an intravenous (IV) or intramuscular (IM) agent such as 1 g of ceftriaxone, ertapenem 1 g IV or IM, or 5 mg/kg of gentamicin IV or IM, depending on local community resistance patterns.

Patients with severe illness, those who are unable to tolerate oral regimens, or those with significant underlying health issues (patients with pregnancy, diabetes, sickle cell disease, or immunodeficiency) should be admitted to the hospital and treated with one of the IV regimens listed in Table 30.2.[29]

Patients with recurrent infections who elect either postcoital or daily prophylaxis should follow one of the regimens listed in Table 30.2, as determined by their urine culture and sensitivity results.

TABLE 30.2

Treatment of Genitourinary Tract Infections in AYAs

Oral treatment options for uncomplicated urinary tract infections (UTIs)/cystitis[a]
- Nitrofurantoin monohydrate/macrocrystals (100 mg every 12 hours [h] for 5 days [d])
- Trimethoprim-sulfamethoxazole (160/800 mg every 12 h for 3 d)
- Cefpodoxime proxetil (200 mg every 12 h for 3–7 d)

Intramuscular treatment option for uncomplicated UTIs/cystitis[a]
- Fosfomycin (3 g intramuscular [IM] in single dose)

In older adolescents (older than 16 y), the following oral treatment options are also acceptable if there is low risk of community resistance to quinolones (<10%)[a]
- Ciprofloxacin (250 mg every 12 h for 3 d)
- Ofloxacin (200 mg every 12 h for 3 d)
- Levofloxacin (500 mg once daily for 3 d)

In pregnancy, a 7-d regimen of the following is preferred
- Nitrofurantoin (100 mg orally every 12 h for 5 d)

Oral treatment options for postcoital or continuous prophylaxis to prevent recurrent infections in high-risk patients with asymptomatic bacteriuria, or those with recurrent infections
- Trimethoprim (100 mg postcoital or daily)
- Trimethoprim-sulfamethoxazole (40/200 mg postcoital or daily)
- Nitrofurantoin (50–100 mg postcoital or daily)
- Norfloxacin (200 mg postcoital or daily)

Complicated UTIs/pyelonephritis—outpatient regimens
All of the outpatient regimens listed below should be initiated with a one-time dose of one of the following parenteral medications:
- Ceftriaxone (1 g intravenous (IV) or IM)
- Ertapenem (1 g IV or IM)
- Gentamicin (5 mg/kg IV or IM)

Oral outpatient therapy for complicated UTIs/pyelonephritis
- Trimethoprim-sulfamethoxazole (160/800 mg every 12 h for 7–10 d)
- Cefpodoxime proxetil (200 mg every 12 h for 10–14 d)
- Cefdinir (300 mg every 12 h for 10–14 d)
- Cefadroxil (1 g every 12 h for 10–14 d)

In older adolescents (older than 16 y), if there is low risk of community resistance to quinolones (<10%), the following are also acceptable:
- Ciprofloxacin (500 mg every 12 h for 7–10 d)
- Levofloxacin (750 mg once daily for 5–7 d)

Intravenous inpatient therapy for complicated UTIs/pyelonephritis
- Ceftriaxone (1 g every 12–24 h)
- Piperacillin/tazobactam (4.5 g every 6 h)
- Ciprofloxacin (400 mg every 12 h) (if there is <10% community resistance to quinolones)
- Imipenem/cilastatin (500 mg every 6 h) (if there is risk of an ESBL organism)
Add the following if enterococcus is suspected
- Vancomycin 15 to 20 mg/kg every 8–12 h
These regimens should be maintained for 48–72 h or until the patient is afebrile and able to tolerate one of the oral medication regimens listed above. They should then complete 14 total days of antibiotic therapy.

Epididymitis
For acute epididymitis most likely caused by chlamydia or gonorrhea:
- Ceftriaxone (500 mg IM in a single dose)
PLUS
- Doxycycline (100 mg PO b.i.d. for 10–14 d)
Likely enteric organism or sexually transmitted organism (history of insertive anal intercourse)
- Ceftriaxone (500 mg IM in a single dose)
PLUS
- Levofloxacin (500 mg orally once daily for 10 d)

Prostatitis
Patients with symptoms of prostatitis at risk for or with laboratory evidence of (e.g., gram-negative intracellular diplococci on Gram stain of a specimen obtained via urethral swab) *N. gonorrhoeae* or *C. trachomatis* should be treated with:
- Ceftriaxone (500 mg IM in a single dose)
PLUS
- Doxycycline (100 mg PO b.i.d. for 10–14 d)
For acute prostatitis not likely due to *N. gonorrhoeae* or *C. trachomatis*:
- Levofloxacin (500 mg orally q.d. for 28–42 d) or
- Trimethoprim-sulfamethoxazole (160/800 mg every 12 h for 28–42 d)

[a]Patients with potentially complicating problems (diabetes, sickle cell disease, etc., a history of a recent previous UTI, or symptoms for >1 wk) use a 7-d regimen of the above medications.
AYAs, adolescents and young adults; ESBL, extended spectrum beta lactamase.

In epididymitis and prostatitis, treatment should be empirically initiated if either diagnosis is strongly considered, in accordance with the regimens listed in Table 30.2. Although antibiotics have good penetration into an acutely inflamed prostate gland or epididymis, epididymitis should be treated for 10 to 14 days while prostatitis should ideally be treated for 14 to 28 days.

THE FUTURE OF PREVENTION AND TREATMENT OF URINARY TRACT INFECTIONS

Organisms causing both complicated and uncomplicated UTIs have continued to show increasing resistance to many antibiotics. This has contributed to both the spread and severity of these infections. While concern has been focused on ESBLs and the resistance they confer toward cephalosporins, many carbapenems and extended spectrum penicillins, other plasmid-derived resistance mutations have contributed to limiting the usefulness of aminoglycosides, sulfonamides, and quinolones. However, new treatment strategies are emerging.[30] New antimicrobials resistant to inactivation by ESBLs are under development and are being paired with new classes of beta-lactamase inhibitors.

At the same time, vaccines targeting bacterial adhesion, bacterial toxins and proteases, and bacterial siderophore systems may soon play a major role in preventing infections. Similarly, "small molecules" targeting ureases and bacterial adhesion may limit the colonization that is the forerunner of most infections. These may ultimately replace the only marginally successful behavioral alterations that have been tried for years with mixed success.

SUMMARY

Urinary tract infections represent a continued source of morbidity in AYAs. Despite a significant number of behavioral interventions to prevent infections, they continue to occur with a predictable incidence. While most uncomplicated infections remain easily treatable, growing resistance to antibiotics makes potentially simple infections complicated and complicated infections potentially life-threatening. Luckily, new antibiotics, enhanced behavioral interventions, possible vaccines, and other methods to inhibit bacterial colonization will hopefully reduce the occurrence and severity of these infections.

REFERENCES

1. Foxman B. Urinary tract infection syndromes: occurrence, recurrence, bacteriology, risk factors, and disease burden. *Infect Dis Clin North Am.* 2014;28(1):1–13.
2. Hooton TM, Scholes D, Hughes JP, et al. A prospective study of risk factors for symptomatic urinary tract infection in young women. *N Engl J Med.* 1996;335(7):468–474.
3. Foxman B, Gillespie B, Koopman J, et al. Risk factors for second urinary tract infection among college women. *Am J Epidemiol.* 2000;151(12):1194–1205.
4. Sakallioglu O, Sakallioglu AE. The effect of ABO-Rh blood group determinants on urinary tract infections. *Int Urol Nephrol.* 2007;39(2):577–579.
5. Shuman EK, Chenoweth CE. Urinary catheter-associated infections. *Infect Dis Clin North Am.* 2018;32(4):885–897.
6. Semins MJ, Shore AD, Makary MA, et al. The impact of obesity on urinary tract infection risk. *Urology.* 2012;79(2):266–269.
7. Scholes D, Hawn TR, Roberts PL, et al. Family history and risk of recurrent cystitis and pyelonephritis in women. *J Urol.* 2010;184(2):564–569.
8. Breyer BN, Vittinghoff E, Van Den Eeden SK, et al. Effect of sexually transmitted infections, lifetime sexual partner count, and recreational drug use on lower urinary tract symptoms in men who have sex with men. *Urology.* 2012;79(1):188–193.
9. Morris BJ, Wiswell TE. Circumcision and lifetime risk of urinary tract infection: a systematic review and meta-analysis. *J Urol.* 2013;189(6):2118–2124.
10. Flores-Mireles AL, Walker JN, Caparon M, et al. Urinary tract infections: epidemiology, mechanisms of infection and treatment options. *Nat Rev Microbiol.* 2015;13(5):269–284.
11. Lo DS, Shieh HH, Barreira ER, et al. High frequency of Staphylococcus saprophyticus urinary tract infections among female adolescents. *Pediatr Infect Dis J.* 2015;34(9):1023–1025.
12. Hooton TM, Roberts PL, Cox ME, et al. Voided midstream urine culture and acute cystitis in premenopausal women. *N Engl J Med.* 2013;369:1883–1891.
13. den Heijer CDJ, van Dongen MCJM, Donker GA, et al. Diagnostic approach to urinary tract infections in male general practice patients: a national surveillance study. *Br J Gen Pract.* 2012;62(604):e780–e786.
14. Walker E, Lyman A, Gupta K, et al. Clinical management of an increasing threat: outpatient urinary tract infections due to multidrug-resistant uropathogens. *Clin Infect Dis.* 2016;63(7):960–965.
15. Brosh-Nissimov T, Navon-Venezia S, Keller N, et al. Risk analysis of antimicrobial resistance in outpatient urinary tract infections of young healthy adults. *J Antimicrob Chemother.* 2019;74(2):499–502.
16. Larramendy S, Deglaire V, Dusollier P, et al. Risk factors of extended-spectrum beta-lactamases-producing Escherichia coli community acquired urinary tract infections: A systematic review. *Infect Drug Resist.* 2020;13:3945–3955.
17. Huppert JS, Biro F, Lan D, et al. Urinary symptoms in adolescent females: STI or UTI? *J Adolesc Health.* 2007;40(5):418–424.
18. Tomas ME, Getman D, Donskey CJ, et al. Overdiagnosis of urinary tract infection and underdiagnosis of sexually transmitted infection in adult women presenting to an emergency department. *J Clin Microbiol.* 2015;53(8):2686–2692.
19. Chu CM, Lowder JL. Diagnosis and treatment of urinary tract infections across age groups. *Am J Obstet Gynecol.* 2018;219(1):40–51.
20. Gupta K, Trautner BW. Diagnosis and management of recurrent urinary tract infections in non-pregnant women. *BMJ.* 2013;346:f3140.
21. Geerlings SE, Beerepoot MAJ, Prins JM. Prevention of recurrent urinary tract infections in women: antimicrobial and nonantimicrobial strategies. *Infect Dis Clin North Am.* 2014;28(1):135–147.
22. Cai T, Mazzoli S, Mondaini N, et al. The role of asymptomatic bacteriuria in young women with recurrent urinary tract infections: to treat or not to treat? *Clin Infect Dis.* 2012;55:771–777.
23. Nicolle LE, Gupta K, Bradley SF, et al. Clinical practice guideline for the management of asymptomatic bacteriuria: 2019 update by the Infectious Diseases Society of America. *Clin Infect Dis.* 2019;68(10):1611–1615.
24. Scholes D, Hooton TM, Roberts PL, et al. Risk factors associated with acute pyelonephritis in healthy women. *Ann Intern Med.* 2005;142(1):20–27.
25. American College of Radiology. *ACR appropriateness criteria® radiation dose assessment introduction.* Accessed October 14, 2021. https://www.acr.org/-/media/ACR/Files/AppropriatenessCriteria/RadiationDoseAssessmentIntro.pdf
26. Banyra O, Shulyak A. Acute epididymo-orchitis: staging and treatment. *Cent European J Urol.* 2012;65(3):139–143.
27. Swami SK, Liesinger JT, Shah N, et al. Incidence of antibiotic-resistant Escherichia coli bacteriuria according to age and location of onset: a population-based study from Olmsted County, Minnesota. *Mayo Clin Proc.* 2012;87(8):753–759.
28. Gupta K, Bhadelia N. Management of urinary tract infections from multidrug-resistant organisms. *Infect Dis Clin North Am.* 2014;28(1):49–59.
29. Bader MS, Loeb M, Leto D, et al. Treatment of urinary tract infections in the era of antimicrobial resistance and new antimicrobial agents. *Postgrad Med.* 2020;132(3):234–250.
30. Flores-Mireles AL, Walker JN, Caparon M, et al. Urinary tract infections: epidemiology, mechanisms of infection and treatment options. *Nat Rev Microbiol.* 2015;13(5):269–284.

ADDITIONAL RESOURCES AND WEBSITES

Additional Resources and Websites for Clinicians:
https://emedicine.medscape.com/article/1958794-overview?src=ppc_google_rlsa-traf_mscp_emed-hdle-cohort_md_us
https://www.uptodate.com/contents/acute-complicated-urinary-tract-infection-including-pyelonephritis-in-adults?search=urinary%20tract%20infection%20adult&source=search_result&selectedTitle=1~150&usage_type=default&display_rank=1
https://www.uptodate.com/contents/acute-simple-cystitis-in-women?search=urinary%20tract%20infection%20adult&source=search_result&selectedTitle=4~150&usage_type=default&display_rank=2#H899949262
https://www.niddk.nih.gov/health-information/urologic-diseases/bladder-infection-uti-in-adults

Additional Resources and Websites for Parents/Caregivers:
https://www.webmd.com/women/guide/avoid-uti
https://www.womenshealth.gov/a-z-topics/urinary-tract-infections
https://youngwomenshealth.org/parents/
https://www.everydayhealth.com/urinary-tract-infections/resources/
https://www.acog.org/womens-health/faqs/urinary-tract-infections

Additional Resources and Websites for Adolescents and Young Adults:
https://youngwomenshealth.org/2013/01/02/uti/
https://youngmenshealthsite.org/guides/urinary-tract-infection/
https://www.healthlinkbc.ca/illnesses-conditions/infectious-diseases/complicated-urinary-tract-infections
https://kidshealth.org/en/teens/uti.html
https://10faq.com/health/urinary-tract-infection-symptoms/
https://www.healthline.com/health/UTI after sex

CHAPTER 31

Enuresis in Adolescents and Young Adults

Joana Dos Santos
Martin A. Koyle

KEY WORDS

- Adolescents and Young Adults
- Bedwetting
- Daytime incontinence
- Enuresis
- Monosymptomatic enuresis
- Nocturnal enuresis
- Nonmonosymptomatic enuresis
- Primary enuresis
- Secondary enuresis
- Teenagers

INTRODUCTION

Enuresis, or bedwetting, affects up to 20% of 6-year-olds, and its prevalence progressively decreases by approximately 15% per year.[1-3] Although reported in 0.2% to 4.5% of adolescents and young adults (AYAs),[1-5] enuresis is very likely underreported, especially in older patients, due to associated social stigmata, negative impact on self-esteem, and resultant significant psychosocial burden. The more severe and the longer pediatric enuresis takes to resolve, the more likely it will persist into adulthood.[5,6] This condition is more common in boys (ratio of 2:1) and in the presence of a positive family history in first-degree relatives.[1-4] Enuresis in AYAs is more often associated with daytime incontinence and/or lower urinary tract symptoms (LUTS). Therefore, before addressing bedwetting, it is important to identify and treat underlying contributing factors such as voiding dysfunction, obstructive sleep apnea (OSA), neurogenic conditions, obesity, neurodevelopmental problems, and concomitant psychiatric disorders in order to increase the chance of treatment success and avoid frustration. In addition, AYAs with conditions affecting renal concentration such as sickle cell anemia, diabetes mellitus, and diabetes insipidus, and those taking certain psychotropic medications are more prone to enuresis.[5,6] Research and evidence-based treatments for bedwetting in AYAs are limited; however, similar to pediatric primary enuresis, the use of the bedwetting alarm remains the first-line treatment for AYAs. Finally, the combination of desmopressin and anticholinergics, and neurostimulation modalities such as transcutaneous electrical neurostimulation and sacral neurostimulation are potential alternative therapies for refractory enuresis in this population.[7-9]

DEFINITIONS

Terminology of lower urinary tract dysfunction has historically been confusing and not standardized until recently. However, it is crucial for the clinician to be aware of different types of enuresis and specific nomenclature of LUTS to accurately diagnose and treat bedwetting and reduce confusion among clinicians.

The International Children's Continence Society (ICCS) has standardized bedwetting terminology for children and adolescents[10]:

Incontinence: Refers to the involuntary leakage of urine.

Enuresis: Episodes of intermittent urinary incontinence that occur during sleep beyond 5 years of age, when most children are expected to achieve bladder control. The presence of intermittent incontinence both while the child is awake and during sleep must be named daytime incontinence and enuresis, respectively.

Monosymptomatic enuresis (ME): Enuresis occurring in AYAs without other LUTS and no history of bladder dysfunction. Teens with ME present with bedwetting only, but no daytime accidents or other urinary symptoms.

Nonmonosymptomatic enuresis (NME): Enuresis associated with other LUTS, including daytime incontinence, increased or decreased urinary frequency, urgency, dysuria, straining, hesitancy, or a weak or intermittent urinary stream. Nonmonosymptomatic enuresis is more common than ME in AYAs.[2-5] Hence, it is essential to identify and treat bladder dysfunction before addressing enuresis. This will increase the likelihood of treatment success and avoid frustration.

Primary enuresis: When dryness during sleep has never been achieved for a period longer than 6 months.

Secondary enuresis: Bedwetting that occurs in AYAs who have been previously dry for longer than 6 months. It is essential to rule out organic causes such as urinary tract infection (UTI), constipation, conditions associated with renal concentration impairment (i.e., sickle cell anemia, diabetes insipidus, and diabetes mellitus), use of medications that increase the risk of enuresis (i.e., risperidone and clozapine) and neurogenic bladder. Secondary enuresis may also occur during or following stressful life events for AYAs. However, more commonly, the exact cause remains unknown. Both primary and secondary enuresis can be either monosymptomatic or nonmonosymptomatic.

Daytime incontinence: Incontinence while the individual is awake during the day. Among AYAs who experience enuresis, 18% to 55% also have significant daytime symptoms.[1,2,5] Female AYAs often have more daytime symptoms than male AYAs and these symptoms may be associated with bladder and bowel dysfunction (BBD) and UTIs. Rarely, late presentation of posterior urethral valves (PUV) and Hinman syndrome (severe nonneurogenic neurogenic bladder) present with LUTS, persistent daytime incontinence, and/or enuresis.

Bedwetting in AYAs is more commonly NME and will require specialty care.[1] For instance, BBD is a common, but underdiagnosed condition in AYAs with NME, that describes a constellation of LUTS associated with functional constipation. Enuresis is often present in AYAs with BBD.[10] In the absence of red flags that warrant immediate referral, the clinician is encouraged to initiate investigations and appropriate treatment of underlying conditions. In addition to limiting fluids before bed, initial conservative management with timed voiding and constipation treatment is recommended for at least 3 to 6 months for all AYAs with enuresis and BBD. While limiting fluids before bedtime is important, increased fluid intake during the day is essential to support timed voiding (promote bladder cycling) and decrease evening thirst. Given the severe psychosocial burden of this condition, a referral to the urologist is warranted without delay if no improvement is seen within this time frame. In this chapter, we focus on the etiology, diagnosis, and management of primary ME, which can usually be managed by the general practitioner and adolescent medicine specialist.

ETIOLOGY

The pathophysiology of primary monosymptomatic enuresis (PME) is complex and multifactorial, involving genetic factors, central nervous system abnormalities (delayed maturation of neuronal pathways responsible for sleep arousal), increased nocturnal urinary production, and bladder dysfunction.[9,11,12]

Genetics

Approximately 50% of children with PME will have one parent with previous PME and 70% of affected children have a first-degree relative with a similar history.[1,3,12,13] The pattern of inheritance of ME is most frequently autosomal dominant with high penetrance. However, somatic, and environmental factors are known to play remarkable epigenetic modulatory effects.[13] A recent study reported a significant association of specific loci on chromosomes 6 and 13 with enuresis. More importantly, potential risk genes mapped in this study have known roles in sleep patterns, urine production, and bladder function. Therefore, those genes could represent potential drug targets for therapy in the future.[11]

Central Nervous System Abnormalities

Sleep arousal disorder: Children, adolescents, and adults with all types of enuresis are deep sleepers.[1–3,6,10,13–17] Typically, bladder filling and detrusor contractions elicit strong arousal stimuli; however, in AYAs with enuresis, sleep arousal is reduced and they cannot wake up to a full bladder. Enuresis occurs in all sleep stages, but especially during nonrapid eye movement sleep.[13] Delayed maturation of brain arousal mechanisms during sleep is a known major contributor to the pathogenesis of enuresis. These findings are supported by recent functional magnetic resonance imaging studies demonstrating microstructure changes in areas associated with central micturition control such as the thalamus, medial frontal gyrus, anterior cingulate cortex, and insula.[14,15]

Nocturnal Polyuria

Excessive overnight urinary production, named nocturnal polyuria, occurs in a subset of AYAs with enuresis[1–4] and is defined as overnight urinary output greater than 130% of expected bladder capacity (EBC) for age.[10] The EBC for age is commonly calculated using the Koff formula: EBC (mL) = (age [years] +2) × 30 for ages 2 to 12, and 400 to 600 mL in adults.[16] Decreased overnight secretion of antidiuretic hormone (ADH) has been reported in previous case-control studies, leading to an excessive production of dilute urine during sleep.[12] Once nocturnal polyuria is identified with a volume voiding diary, conditions that are commonly associated with increased diuresis overnight such as OSA, diabetes insipidus, metabolic diseases (i.e., type 1 and type 2 diabetes mellitus), and those affecting renal concentration (i.e., hemoglobinopathies, tubulopathies) must be considered.

Bladder Dysfunction

Decreased bladder capacity and nocturnal detrusor overactivity have been described in children and AYAs with ME and are attributed to a lack of inhibition of the micturition reflex during sleep.[13] In addition to the microstructural brain abnormalities described above, delayed maturation of the pontine micturition center, which is responsible for bladder control, has been reported.[13,18] Furthermore, AYAs with NME often present with associated voiding dysfunction (i.e., BBD, overactive bladder [OAB], dysfunctional voiding).[4,6,9,10,12,13]

PSYCHOSOCIAL BURDEN

Significant psychosocial burden is well described in AYAs with enuresis.[1–6,20] They commonly report stigmatization, negative self-image, poor school performance, peer relationship issues, family stress, and social isolation, especially when enuresis is associated with daytime incontinence.[20] In addition, these AYAs more frequently present with depressive symptoms, and are at higher risk of domestic violence.[21] High prevalence of NME has been reported in AYAs with anorexia nervosa, attention deficit hyperactivity disorder, and other behavioral disorders, and is often refractory to treatment when co-occurring with these conditions.[22,23] Clinicians should be aware that AYAs with enuresis may require psychological support, and treatment of associated comorbidities is essential to achieve dryness.

DIAGNOSIS AND EVALUATION OF ENURESIS IN ADOLESCENTS AND YOUNG ADULTS

A thorough history, physical examination, 2- to 7-day voiding diary (including voided volumes), and urinalysis (Table 31.1) are the mainstays of enuresis diagnosis. Further investigations and treatment will be guided by the specific type of enuresis. For instance, a teenager with NME and OAB will have a history of urgency, possibly daytime incontinence, increased urinary frequency, and small voided volumes (less than the EBC) on voiding diary. This clinical presentation with normal urinalysis is usually sufficient to confirm the diagnosis of OAB, without the need for urodynamic studies. Significant organic causes are infrequent with ME. The prevalence of organic or psychological causes is higher in secondary enuresis and/or NME.

TREATMENT

Treatment for enuresis in AYAs should be based on information gathered from history, voiding diary, physical examination, and urinalysis and directed to specific causes. Likewise, the AYA's and family's level of motivation to treat enuresis must be considered. It is important to emphasize that enuresis is a common condition not under voluntary control and that punishment is not only ineffective but worsens the psychosocial burden of bedwetting.

Lifestyle Changes

Lifestyle changes should be the first step to treat both ME and NME.[1–4] All AYAs with enuresis should try to limit fluids before bed. It is important that they reach the recommended daily fluid intake of 2 to 2.5 liters daily, so that they do not feel thirsty by the end of the day. Dehydration would lead to higher fluid intake in the evening, making enuresis challenging to treat. Clinicians should recommend that AYAs drink 80% of their recommended daily fluid intake by 4 PM, with only 20% after that, and, whenever possible, no fluids 2 hours before bed (except when practicing sports in the evening, or in small amounts needed for any evening medications). In addition, timed voiding every 2 hours during the day (and immediately before bed), and the treatment of constipation are initially recommended, especially for AYAs with NME.[24] In such patients, daytime symptoms must be addressed prior to treating the bedwetting to increase the chance of achieving dryness and to avoid frustration with treatment failure.

TABLE 31.1

Diagnosis and Evaluation of Enuresis in AYAs: History, Physical Examination, Laboratory and Other Tests

	History	Voiding Diary	Physical Examination	Laboratory and Further Tests
Enuresis quantification	Number of wet nights per week/ month Most consecutive dry nights Period of dryness >6 mo Age of toilet training Nocturia	Number of voids per day, last void before bedtime Volume of voids Weight of overnight pull-ups Daily and evening fluid intake, drinking habits	Often completely normal	UA: All AYAs with enuresis[10]: check for glucose, protein, white blood cells, and specific gravity screen for UTI, DM, DI Hematuria: Urethral stricture, meatal stenosis Urine culture: If UA suggests UTI
NME	Intermittent daytime incontinence Frequency, urgency, hesitancy, dysuria, holding maneuvers Interrupted stream, weak stream, and straining UTIs Constipation/ Straining during evacuation Encopresis, blood in stools	Type of stools (BSC) Frequency of bowel movements	Abdomen: Palpable masses, stools	Uroflowmetry[a]: Not routinely needed. Ultrasound with pre- and postvoid residual[b]: Not routinely needed
Red flags for organic disease	Polydipsia, increased appetite, weight loss (DM, DI) CNS trauma, headache, vomiting, seizures, visual changes Gait changes, lower limb weakness, numbness (spinal tumors, transverse myelitis, neuromuscular disorders) Continuous daytime incontinence (girls with ectopic ureter)	High voided volumes Nocturnal polyuria	Check BP GU: Urethral meatus location, stenosis Watch urine stream: Forceful, narrow, dribbling, straining Back exam: Midline defects, gluteal fold abnormalities, hair tufts Neurologic exam: Gait, lower limb motor and sensory, deep tendon reflexes, perineal sensation, rectal sphincter tone Perianal and perineal excoriations and vulvovaginitis are concerning for sexual abuse and warrant further evaluation. However, a normal exam does not rule out abuse	
Family history	Enuresis in relatives Voiding dysfunction, "small bladders" Sleep disorders, difficulty arousing from sleep OSA, snoring			
Social adjustment to enuresis	Family member responsible for changing sheets and laundry Prior treatments and results Level of motivation to treat enuresis Psychological review of family, peers, school			

[a]Uroflowmetry is a noninvasive urodynamic study that evaluates the urinary flow rate and postvoid residual, usually ordered by the urologist, in certain cases of NME (OAB, dysfunctional voiding, neurogenic bladder, urethral stricture/meatal stenosis).

[b]Except if urethral obstruction or neurogenic bladder is suspected. In that case, refer to the urologist and consider spine MRI to look for spinal cord abnormalities.

AYAs, adolescents and young adults; BP, Blood pressure; BSC, Bristol Stool Chart; DI, Diabetes insipidus; DM, Diabetes mellitus; GU, Genitourinary exam; OSA, Obstructive sleep apnea; UA, Urinalysis; UTI, Urinary tract infection; NME, nonmonosymptomatic enuresis; CNS, central nervous system.

Specific Treatments

Bedwetting alarms: The bedwetting alarm is generally considered first-line treatment for children and AYAs with primary or ME, who did not respond to lifestyle changes and wet the bed at least twice per week.[1–4,10] However, when nocturnal polyuria is present, treatment with desmopressin (DDAVP) should be considered as first line. A recent Cochrane review including four trials (127 children, mostly 5 to 16) showed that alarms may decrease the number of wet nights per week at treatment completion compared to controls or no treatment.[25] Long-term cure rates with the bedwetting alarm are approximately 70% to 80%, higher than any medication used to treat enuresis.[1–3,25,26–28] Desmopressin has similar efficacy, but higher relapse rates.[27] Bedwetting alarms are conditioning systems connected through wire or Bluetooth to moisture sensors in the youth's underwear that work by setting off a loud sound and/or vibratory signal when patients start to wet themselves. The primary goal of the alarm is to condition the young person's brain to recognize when the bladder is full, so that they should now wake up and go to the toilet. Initially, the teenager wakes up after the fact, but the hope is that over time, the full bladder triggers arousal from sleep. Newer alarms feel lighter and patients describe them as comfortable. Some brands offer recording apps and a convenient extra wireless receiver (one to be carried by the patient and the second for the parent's/caregivers' bedroom). The disadvantages of bedwetting alarms are that they are time consuming and that family members must be equally invested in waking up the teenager, at least initially. In addition, wearing alarms are not a discrete choice and can be challenging for AYAs who share the bedroom with others at home or at college/university. Adherence to alarm treatment is often low among AYAs.[1,26,27] Bedwetting alarms are often covered by private health insurance with prescription; prices vary from 40 to 160 U.S. dollars. The ICCS recommends the alarm treatment for 8 to 12 weeks,[10] but if no improvement is seen after 6 weeks of wearing the device nightly, success with the alarm is unlikely. The alarm treatment can be stopped after at least 14 consecutive dry nights.[1–4,10,12,13] If the enuresis relapses, use of the bedwetting alarm can be successfully reinitiated, possibly due to the conditioning achieved with previous use. The most common cause of failure is the teenager's inability to wake up to the alarm. It is essential to set expectations beforehand, and tell patients and families that AYAs with enuresis are deep sleepers, and as such, family support is paramount. Enuretic AYAs often need to be awakened by a family member when the alarm goes off during the first few weeks of treatment. To help facilitate arousal, each time the AYA is awakened by the parent, they should be given a new password and instructed to remember it. In the morning, the AYA should try to remember the password from the previous evening (similarly to how one person is more likely to wake up to a 3 AM alarm when this individual knows that they need to catch an early flight). Other causes of alarm failure are not trying the alarm for a sufficient period of time or lack of motivation leading to noncompliance with any treatments (i.e., lifestyle changes, alarm, and/or medication).

Medications

Medications are as effective as the bedwetting alarm for the short-term resolution of enuresis.[26] Higher success rates have been reported with medications than lifestyle changes to treat enuretic patients over the long term.[27] The choice of medication should target the cause of the enuresis. For instance, the primary goal of nocturnal polyuria treatment should be to decrease overnight urinary production; therefore, DDAVP should be used as first-line treatment. More frequently, the intermittent use of DDAVP is indicated as needed for adolescents with primary ME during camp, sleepovers, and trips. On the other hand, a patient with NME and OAB who fails conservative management, should be treated with anticholinergic medications.[24,27] Drugs used to treat enuresis include the following:

Desmopressin: Synthetic analogue of the ADH that increases water reabsorption and urine concentration in the distal tubules, ultimately reducing overnight urine production. Studies have reported 70% success rates with DDAVP in patients with nocturnal polyuria[1]; however, relapses are relatively common after it is stopped.[1–4,27] Desmopressin is available as tablets (200 to 400 mcg) and sublingual melts (120 to 360 mcg). The advantages of the melts are rapid onset of action and that fluids are not needed to swallow tablets. Desmopressin nasal spray is no longer available due to risk

of overdose. Desmopressin should be taken 1 hour before bedtime. The adolescent or young adult must be instructed not to drink fluids from 1 hour prior to until 8 hours after taking DDAVP to prevent severe hyponatremia and seizures. In addition to dilutional hyponatremia, rare reported side effects are abdominal pain, nausea, headaches, nasal congestion, rhinitis, nosebleeds, and sore throat.[8–12] These symptoms usually improve with dose reduction. The dose should be increased by one tablet or melt per day until dryness is achieved to a maximum of 400 mcg (tablets) or 360 mcg (melts) daily. The response to DDAVP should be reassessed 2 weeks after starting the medication. If there is at least a partial response, then treat for 3 months. In that case, it is important to check electrolytes, especially serum osmolality and sodium. In cases of intermittent use of DDAVP, the patient should try the medication at least 1 week prior to the planned event to titrate their optimal dose.

Anticholinergics: Anticholinergics act by decreasing uninhibited contractions and relaxing the detrusor muscle, ultimately increasing bladder capacity. These drugs are recommended for NME, to treat OAB, in the context of associated daytime incontinence and small bladder capacity, or as second-line treatment in combination with the bedwetting alarm and/or DDAVP in cases of refractory ME (Fig. 31.1).[24,27,29] Previous studies have reported higher efficacy and quicker improvement of ME with the combination of DDAVP and an anticholinergic than with DDAVP alone.[29] Five to 10 mg immediate-release oxybutynin is a good option to be taken 1 hour prior to bed in addition to DDAVP for AYAs who failed initial treatment with the alarm and/or DDAVP alone. Adolescents with OAB and associated daytime incontinence may benefit from extended-release oxybutynin, available in 5, 10, and 15 mg tablets (usual dose 10 mg, maximum 15 mg daily) or immediate-release 5 mg, orally, two to three times daily. Common side effects of anticholinergics are dry mouth, skin flushing, headache, nausea, drowsiness, constipation, and urinary retention. Likewise, solifenacin is a newer extended-release anticholinergic used to treat OAB that specifically targets M3 bladder receptors, thereby causing fewer side effects such as dry mouth and constipation.[29] Other anticholinergic drugs used to treat OAB are tolterodine and fesoterodine. Prior to initiating treatment with anticholinergics, it is important to document good bladder emptying by measuring the postvoid residual on ultrasound or uroflowmetry.

Mirabegron: Mirabegron is a selective agonist of the β3 adrenergic receptor, found in the bladder wall used to treat OAB; it acts by relaxing the detrusor muscle with a similar role in the management of NME and OAB. Mirabegron may be especially useful for patients with NME and OAB who also have constipation or for AYAs experiencing side effects with anticholinergic medications.[30]

Imipramine: Imipramine is a tricyclic antidepressant with anticholinergic effects that works by decreasing detrusor contractility and enhancing bladder capacity; its use for the treatment of enuresis has not been well investigated in AYAs. Studies assessing the use of tricyclic antidepressants in children with enuresis have shown complete resolution in 20% while taking treatment; similar relapse rates have been shown in both the treatment and placebo groups (approximately 99%) once treatment is discontinued.[28] A recent Cochrane systematic review showed that, compared to placebo, imipramine is effective at decreasing the number of wet nights per week during treatment (four trials, 347 children, mostly 5 to 16), but most children relapsed once treatment is discontinued. However, there was some evidence that tricyclics in combination with anticholinergics may be more effective than tricyclics alone in the long term. After treatment, 45% of children on imipramine and oxybutynin were still wetting the bed versus 83% taking only imipramine (one trial, 36 children).[28] Tricyclics should be recommended with caution as third-line treatment for refractory cases due to the potential severe side effects including cardiac arrhythmias, hypotension, central nervous system depression, liver

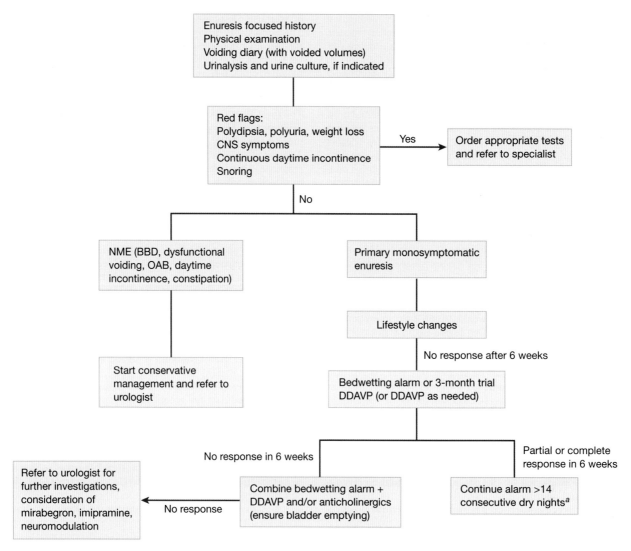

FIGURE 31.1 Proposed algorithm for the management of enuresis in adolescents and young adults. CNS, central nervous system; NME, nonmono-symptomatic enuresis; BBD, bladder and bowel dysfunction; OAB, overactive bladder; DDAVP, desmopressin. (Details regarding key features of history and physical exam and recommended tests are provided in Table 31.1)

toxicity, interaction with other drugs, and the risk of intoxication by accidental overdose.

Neuromodulation

Transcutaneous electrical neurostimulation (TENS) and sacral neurostimulation (SNS) are neuromodulation modalities that have been reported as safe and efficacious for the treatment of refractory cases of primary ME and NME.[9,31,32] While neuromodulation appears beneficial in children and younger adolescents, data in older adolescents and young adults (YA) are lacking at the moment. Both modalities provide electrical stimulation to sacral nerves responsible for bladder control. Transcutaneous electrical neurostimulation is a noninvasive procedure in which a device provides electrical stimulation to the lower back through four leads connected to adhesive pads that are attached to the skin at the level of sacral spinal nerves 2–4 (S2–S4). Treatment is typically recommended for 8 to 12 weeks. Frequency of treatment ranges from weekly to daily. Duration of stimulation also varies, from 20 minutes up to 1 hour daily. The physiotherapist works with each patient to achieve the optimal intensity and frequency of stimuli. The TENS machine can be purchased by the patient or rented from a physiotherapy clinic.

Sacral neurostimulation therapy involves a minor surgical procedure for placement of a wire lead into the S3 foramen and along the S3, with subcutaneous implantation of a stimulator to provide continuous, low-intensity electrical stimulation of the nerve. A meta-analysis including 292 individuals from seven nonheterogeneous randomized controlled trials (RCT) showed a significant reduction in the number of wet nights per week in pediatric patients with PME treated with either TENS or SNS.[9] No serious adverse effects were noted related to neurostimulation. In another RCT, none of the children with PME experienced complete remission of enuresis with TENS.[32] Because TENS is noninvasive, relatively inexpensive, and easy to implement, one may consider it a first alternative before trying the implantable device. Adolescents and young adults who did not respond to either lifestyle changes or bedwetting alarm, and/or who failed a combination of medications should be referred to the urologist for consideration of further investigations and/or neuromodulation options.

● SUMMARY

Primary monosymptomatic enuresis is associated with social stigma and low self-esteem in AYAs; therefore, it is important to identify and treat this condition as soon as possible to minimize the significant psychosocial burden in these individuals. Enuresis in AYAs is more often associated with daytime incontinence and/or LUTS. Hence, before addressing bedwetting, it is important to identify and treat underlying contributing factors such as voiding dysfunction, OSA, neurogenic conditions, obesity, neurodevelopmental problems, and concomitant psychiatric disorders. The bedwetting alarm is the first-line treatment for AYAs with enuresis. Finally, the combination of desmopressin and anticholinergics, and neuromodulation modalities such as transcutaneous electrical neurostimulation and sacral neurostimulation are potential alternative therapies for refractory enuresis in this population.

REFERENCES

1. Vande Walle J, Rittig S, Bauer S, et al. Practical consensus guidelines for the management of enuresis. *Eur J Pediatr.* 2012;171(6):971–983.
2. Robson WLM. Clinical practice. Evaluation and management of enuresis. *N Engl J Med.* 2009;360(14):1429–1436.
3. Bayne AP, Skoog SJ. Nocturnal enuresis: an approach to assessment and treatment. *Pediatr Rev.* 2014;35(8):327–335.
4. Bogaert G, Stein R, Undre S, et al. Practical recommendations of the EAU-ESPU guidelines committee for monosymptomatic enuresis-Bedwetting. *Neurourol Urodyn.* 2020;39(2):489–497.
5. Baek M, Park K, Lee HE, et al. A nationwide epidemiological study of nocturnal enuresis in Korean adolescents and adults: population based cross sectional study. *J Korean Med Sci.* 2013;28(7):1065–1070.
6. Yeung CK, Sreedhar B, Sihoe JDY, et al. Differences in characteristics of nocturnal enuresis between children and adolescents: a critical appraisal from a large epidemiological study. *BJU Int.* 2006;97(5):1069–1073.
7. Chua ME, Silangcruz JMA, Chang SJ, et al. Immediate 1-month efficacy of desmopressin and anticholinergic combination therapy versus desmopressin monotherapy in the treatment of pediatric enuresis: a meta-analysis. *J Pediatr Urol.* 2016;12(3):156.e1–156.e9.
8. Deshpande AV, Caldwell PHY, Sureshkumar P. Drugs for nocturnal enuresis in children (other than desmopressin and tricyclics). *Cochrane Database Syst Rev.* 2012;12(12):CD002238.
9. Chua ME, Fernandez N, Ming JM, et al. Neurostimulation therapy for pediatric primary enuresis: a meta-analysis. *Urology.* 2017;106:183–187.
10. Austin PF, Bauer SB, Bower W, et al. The standardization of terminology of lower urinary tract function in children and adolescents: update report from the standardization committee of the International Children's Continence Society. *Neurourol Urodyn.* 2016;35(4):471–481.
11. Jørgensen CS, Horsdal HT, Rajagopal VM, et al. Identification of genetic loci associated with nocturnal enuresis: a genome-wide association study. *Lancet Child Adolesc Health.* 2021;5(3):201–209. Epub 2021 Jan 15. doi: 10.1016/S2352-4642(20)30350-3
12. Caldwell PHY, Deshpande AV, Von Gontard A. Management of nocturnal enuresis. *BMJ.* 2013;347:f6259.
13. Kuwertz-Bröking E, von Gontard A. Clinical management of nocturnal enuresis. *Pediatr Nephrol.* 2018;33(7):1145–1154.
14. Lei D, Ma J, Du X, et al. Spontaneous brain activity changes in children with primary monosymptomatic nocturnal enuresis: a resting-state fMRI study. *Neurourol Urodyn.* 2012;31(1):99–104.
15. Lei D, Ma J, Shen X, et al. Changes in the brain microstructure of children with primary monosymptomatic nocturnal enuresis: a diffusion tensor imaging study. *PLoS One.* 2012;7(2):e31023.
16. Guerra LA, Keays MA, Purser MJ, et al. Pediatric cystogram: are we considering age-adjusted bladder capacity? *Can Urol Assoc J.* 2018;12(12):378–381.
17. Song QX, Wang L, Cheng X, et al. The clinical features and predictive factors of nocturnal enuresis in adult men. *BJU Int.* 2020;126(4):472–480.
18. Sinha R, Raut S. Management of nocturnal enuresis–myths and facts. *World J Nephrol.* 2016;5(4):328–338.
19. Grzeda MT, Heron J, von Gontard A, et al. Effects of urinary incontinence on psychosocial outcomes in adolescence. *Eur Child Adolesc Psychiatry.* 2017;26(6):649–658.
20. Sá CA, Gusmão Paiva AC, de Menezes MCLB, et al. Increased risk of physical punishment among enuretic children with family history of enuresis. *J Urol.* 2016;195(4 Pt 2):1227–1230.
21. Kanbur N, Pinhas L, Lorenzo A, et al. Nocturnal enuresis in adolescents with anorexia nervosa: prevalence, potential causes, and pathophysiology. *Int J Eat Disord.* 2011;44(4):349–355.
22. Von Gontard A, Equit M. Comorbidity of ADHD and incontinence in children. *Eur Child Adolesc Psychiatry.* 2015;24(2):127–140.
23. Im YJ, Lee JK, Park K. Time course of treatment for primary enuresis with overactive bladder. *Int Neurourol J.* 2018;22(2):107–113.
24. Caldwell PHY, Nankivell G, Sureshkumar P. Simple behavioral interventions for nocturnal enuresis in children. *Cochrane Database Syst Rev.* 2013;19(7):CD003637.
25. Caldwell PH, Codarini M, Stewart F, et al. Alarm interventions for nocturnal enuresis in children. *Cochrane Database Syst Rev.* 2020;5(5):CD002911.
26. Song P, Huang C, Wang Y, et al. Comparison of desmopressin, alarm, desmopressin plus alarm, and desmopressin plus anticholinergic agents in the management of paediatric monosymptomatic nocturnal enuresis: a network meta-analysis. *BJU Int.* 2019;123(3):388–400.
27. Park SJ, Park JM, Pai KS, et al. Desmopressin alone versus desmopressin plus an anticholinergic in the first-line treatment of primary monosymptomatic nocturnal enuresis: a multicenter study. *Pediatr Nephrol.* 2014;29(7):1195–1200.
28. Caldwell PHY, Sureshkumar P, Wong WCF. Tricyclic and related drugs for nocturnal enuresis in children. *Cochrane Database Syst Rev.* 2016;2016(1):CD002117.
29. Hsu FC, Weeks CE, Selph SS, et al. Updating the evidence on drugs to treat overactive bladder: a systematic review. *Int Urogynecol J.* 2019;30(10):1603–1617.
30. Allison SJ, Gibson W. Mirabegron, alone and in combination, in the treatment of overactive bladder: real-world evidence and experience. *Ther Adv Urol.* 2018;10(12):411–419.
31. Khedr EM, Elbeh KA, Baky AA, et al. A double-blind randomized clinical trial on the efficacy of magnetic sacral root stimulation for the treatment of monosymptomatic nocturnal enuresis. *Restor Neurol Neurosci.* 2015;33(4):435–445.
32. Jørgensen CS, Kamperis K, Borch L, et al. Transcutaneous electrical nerve stimulation in children with monosymptomatic nocturnal enuresis: a randomized, double-blind, placebo controlled study. *J Urol.* 2017;198(3):687–693.

🛜 ADDITIONAL RESOURCES AND WEBSITES

Additional Resources and Websites for Clinicians:

Bogaert G, Stein R, Undre S, et al. Practical recommendations for monosymptomatic enuresis-Bedwetting. Neurourol Urodyn. 2020;39(2):489–497.

Guidelines for evaluation from the European Association of Urology—https://uroweb.org/guideline/paediatric-urology/

Robson WLM. Clinical practice: evaluation and management of enuresis. N Engl J Med. 2009;360(14):1429–1436.

Vande Walle J, Rittig S, Bauer S, et al. Practical consensus guidelines for the management of enuresis. Eur J Pediatr. 2012;171(6):971–983.

Additional Resources and Websites for Parents/Caregivers:

American Academy of Pediatrics—https://www.healthychildren.org/English/health-issues/conditions/genitourinary-tract/Pages/Nocturnal-Enuresis-in-Teens.aspx

National Kidney Foundation—https://www.kidney.org/patients/bw/BWparents

Additional Resources and Websites for Adolescents and Young Adults:

American Academy of Pediatrics—https://www.healthychildren.org/English/health-issues/conditions/genitourinary-tract/Pages/Nocturnal-Enuresis-in-Teens.aspx

Continence Foundation of Australia—https://www.continence.org.au/information-incontinence-english/bedwetting-in-teenagers-and-young-adults

National Kidney Foundation: Questions Kids Ask—https://www.kidney.org/patients/bw/BW_faq

National Kidney Foundation—https://www.kidney.org/patients/bw/BWyoungadults

Nemours Children's Health/AboutKidsHealth—https://kidshealth.org/en/parents/about.html#caturinary

VII

CHAPTER 32

Asymptomatic Proteinuria and Hematuria

Shamir Tuchman
Lawrence J. D'Angelo

KEY WORDS

- Dipstick
- Fixed
- Glomerular
- Hematuria
- Nephrotic
- Proteinuria
- Postural
- Transient

INTRODUCTION

Proteinuria and hematuria represent two of the most common abnormalities encountered when testing the urine of adolescents and young adults (AYAs). The degree to which these findings represent a clinically meaningful sign of underlying kidney disease depends on a systematic and thorough investigation into the potential causes. A thorough history, physical examination, and microscopic examination of the urine sediment often facilitate identification of the potential cause of hematuria and/or proteinuria in many cases and may save the patient from unnecessary testing and evaluation. At other times, the investigation may identify significant underlying kidney disease requiring treatment to stop or slow the progression. This chapter is organized to provide a systematic approach to the evaluation and diagnosis of conditions presenting with isolated proteinuria, hematuria, or both. The approach is rooted in the understanding of the pathophysiology and prognosis of benign and nonbenign causes of each. This chapter will focus on the pathophysiology of different types of proteinuria, present a diagnostic approach to systematically identify potential causes, and describe clinical diagnoses that present with proteinuria as one, if not the only, clinical sign. This chapter also provides a description of the pathophysiology underlying the occurrence of hematuria, a diagnostic approach for evaluating hematuria, and a review of the diagnoses leading to hematuria encountered in AYAs.

ASYMPTOMATIC PROTEINURIA

Asymptomatic proteinuria is defined as increased urinary protein not associated with hematuria, hypertension, or other symptoms of renal insufficiency. Proteinuria is a common finding in the urine of AYAs; however, it is most often transient and therefore benign. However, persistent asymptomatic proteinuria may be an early marker of kidney disease. Routine urinary screening for proteinuria in AYAs is not recommended by the American Academy of Pediatrics or the U.S. Preventive Services Task Force, nor is it cost effective.[1] This is because although approximately 5% of AYAs will have proteinuria on routine urinalysis, a much smaller proportion will have persistent proteinuria with repeated testing.[2]

Nonetheless, routine urinalyses are commonly performed in otherwise healthy AYAs despite these recommendations. Screening *is* recommended in AYAs with conditions associated with an increased risk of chronic kidney disease (CKD). Therefore, the challenge for the clinician is to establish the significance of an isolated finding of proteinuria and identify the few individuals who require a more extensive evaluation.

Pathophysiology

Indexed to body surface area, normal urine protein excretion in AYAs is less than 100 mg/m²/day (approximately 4 mg/m²/hour). Levels of proteinuria up to 250 mg/day may be normal in AYAs with a larger body size, consistent with the adult value of <250 mg/day as an absolute threshold. Nephrotic range proteinuria is defined as protein excretion of ≥2,000 mg/day. Proteinuria detected on a screening urine dipstick may be quantified in two ways: (1) via a 24-hour urine collection (a cumbersome approach prone to over- or undercollection); or (2) by obtaining a spot urine protein-to-creatinine (Up/c) ratio (mg protein per mg creatinine). The latter provides a good approximation of the 24-hour excretion of protein in grams per day. A spot Up/c correlates well with the 24-hour urine protein excretion in idiopathic causes of proteinuria and to a lesser extent in systemic disorders such as systemic lupus erythematosus.[3,4] The "second voided urine" is the most ideal specimen for this approach.

Proteinuria may occur as the result of four different mechanisms (Table 32.1), including the following:

1. Increased permeability of the glomerular filtration membrane for mid– to high–molecular-weight proteins. Larger and more negatively charged plasma proteins (e.g., albumin) are not appreciably filtered. However, proteinuria can occur when the permeability of the membrane changes secondary to processes that include inflammation and immune-mediated injury.

2. Changes in tubular reabsorption of low–molecular-weight (LMW) proteins. Due to their smaller size, LMW proteins (<25,000 Daltons) are freely filtered at the glomerulus and almost completely reabsorbed in the proximal tubule. Any condition, whether acquired or congenital, that causes proximal tubular dysfunction can lead to LMW proteinuria.

3. Increased circulation of plasma proteins (e.g., overflow proteinuria). Adolescents and young adults with rhabdomyolysis may develop proteinuria due to the excessive production of myoglobin and other substances released from muscle, which may overwhelm the glomerular filtration membrane and alter glomerular permeability.

4. Functional proteinuria (e.g., fever, exercise, congestive heart failure) and orthostatic proteinuria due to changes in glomerular pressure and filtration.

TABLE 32.1
Categories of Proteinuria

Category	Example
Factitious proteinuria	Highly concentrated urine (elevated urine specific gravity) Gross hematuria Contamination with antiseptic (chlorhexidine or benzalkonium) High urine pH Radiographic contrast media (affects specific gravity) High levels of cephalosporin/penicillin analogs Sulfonamide metabolites
Transient proteinuria	Benign positional proteinuria Transient proteinuria associated with exercise, stress, fever Urinary tract infection

Fixed proteinuria	Glomerular
	  Hyperfiltration
	    Diabetic nephropathy
	    Renal dysplasia, hypoplasia
	    Reflux nephropathy
	    Focal segmental glomerulosclerosis
	  Primary glomerulopathies
	    Minimal change disease
	    Focal segmental glomerulosclerosis
	    Membranous nephropathy
	    Nail–patella syndrome
	  Systemic disease(s)
	    Systemic lupus erythematosus
	    Fabry disease
	  Tubulopathies (low–molecular-weight proteinuria)
	    Acquired
	      Nephrotoxic medications (antibiotics, nonsteroidal anti-inflammatory drugs)
	      Heavy metal poisonings (lead, mercury)
	    Inherited/genetic
	      Dent disease
	      Wilson disease
	      Genetic disorders associated with Fanconi syndrome

Overflow proteinuria	Monoclonal gammopathies (multiple myeloma) Myoglobinuria (rhabdomyolysis)

Epidemiology

Up to 5% of healthy AYAs may have proteinuria and/or microscopic hematuria detected on a random screening urine sample.[5] The prevalence falls significantly with repeated testing, so a diagnosis of persistent proteinuria should be based on three separate abnormal urine specimens. In a urine screening study of adolescents up to 15 years of age, the prevalence of persistent urinary abnormalities was 0.71%.[5]

Causes of Asymptomatic Proteinuria

The causes of asymptomatic proteinuria range from those that are known to be benign to those associated with significant kidney disease. Significant kidney disease is often suggested by higher amounts of proteinuria and the presence of associated findings like hypertension, hematuria, and/or elevated creatinine. Causes of asymptomatic proteinuria include the following:

Transient Proteinuria

Low-level proteinuria (<500 mg/m^2/day) may occur in the setting of recent exercise, stress, fever, dehydration, and urinary tract infection. Transient proteinuria has been reported in up to 6% of AYAs.[6] It is not associated with long-term renal morbidity. By definition, the proteinuria will resolve on repeat testing when the underlying cause is no longer present.

Postural Proteinuria (Orthostatic or Benign Positional Proteinuria)

Postural proteinuria is a condition in which low- to moderate-level proteinuria develops in the standing or upright position and disappears in the recumbent position. It is found in up to 20% of school-aged children, occurring more commonly in the second decade of life. Postural proteinuria is slightly more common in male AYAs and is one of the most common causes of proteinuria in this age group.[7] It often resolves by the end of young adulthood and is rarely associated with long-term kidney disease. The diagnosis of postural proteinuria is confirmed when a random urine dipstick is positive for protein and a first morning urine specimen is negative to trace for proteinuria. Patients with postural proteinuria may have up to 1,000 mg of protein in a 24-hour sample. Although almost always a benign condition, postural proteinuria can rarely become fixed proteinuria signaling the presence of true kidney disease; therefore, AYAs with postural proteinuria should have first morning urinalyses checked at regular visits (i.e., health maintenance visits) to evaluate for the emergence of fixed proteinuria.

Fixed Isolated Proteinuria

Persistent, nonorthostatic proteinuria that occurs in the absence of microscopic or gross hematuria may be due to glomerular and nonglomerular causes.

Glomerular Causes

Hyperfiltration Renal Injury An important risk factor for progressive CKD, hyperfiltration occurs when adaptation to nonreversible kidney injury leads to excessive filtration through remaining functioning nephrons to maintain the glomerular filtration rate (GFR). Over time, the hyperfiltration results in irreversible damage to these nephrons. This mechanism is important in diabetic and reflux nephropathies and renal dysplasia.

Glomerulopathies Isolated fixed proteinuria may be due to primary glomerular diseases. An important example of this is focal segmental glomerulosclerosis (FSGS), which can occur as a primary or secondary disease. Primary FSGS can be further subdivided into idiopathic disease or familial (monogenetic) forms.[8] Focal segmental glomerulosclerosis may present with a spectrum of diseases ranging from asymptomatic moderate-level (500 to 2,000 mg/day) proteinuria to symptomatic disease with frank nephrosis. It carries a worrisome long-term prognosis with a significant proportion of patients progressing to end-stage renal disease (ESRD). Glomerulopathies that classically present with nephrosis such as minimal change nephrotic syndrome (MCNS) or membranous nephropathy are rarely asymptomatic.

Systemic Disease Proteinuria manifesting as albuminuria may be a renal manifestation of systemic disorders. Kidney involvement occurs in about two-thirds of patients with systemic lupus erythematosus (SLE).[9] In those with isolated low-level proteinuria, this may be a sign of mild glomerular disease. However, in patients with nephrotic range proteinuria, this likely represents membranous disease. There is growing evidence that onset of SLE during adolescence and young adulthood is associated with more severe kidney disease at presentation.[10]

Monogenetic Disorders There are a group of rare genetic disorders associated with the occurrence of moderate- to nephrotic-range proteinuria that present in adolescence. One example is

Fabry disease, which is associated with low- to moderate-level proteinuria in addition to other diverse manifestations of the disease.

Tubular Causes

Tubulointerstitial kidney disease: Freely filtered LMW proteins are exclusively reabsorbed in the proximal tubule. As such, diseases causing generalized proximal tubular dysfunction may lead to low- to moderate-grade LMW proteinuria called renal Fanconi syndrome. Fanconi syndrome may manifest secondary to (1) monogenetic disorders such as cystinosis, tyrosinemia, Wilson disease, Dent disease, or other inborn errors of metabolism or (2) an acquired condition due to a reaction to penicillamine, aminoglycosides, heavy metals (mercury or lead), tenofovir, or other medications.

Overflow Causes

Conditions causing overflow proteinuria include myoglobinuria, hemoglobinuria, and multiple myeloma. These conditions are associated with overproduction of LMW proteins that can either overwhelm the resorptive capacity of the proximal tubule or cause damage to the filtration membrane or renal tubules directly. Myoglobinuria and hemoglobinuria are usually transient and multiple myeloma is rare.

Diagnostic Approach

History and Physical Examination

A detailed history and physical examination focused on specific elements will aid the practitioner in narrowing the differential diagnosis and in ordering appropriately targeted laboratory and imaging tests. Important aspects of the history to be elicited by the practitioner include the occurrence of the following:

- Recent illness or fever
- Decreased urine output
- "Frothy" and/or concentrated urine
- Recent weight gain
- Tighter fitting clothing
- Early morning edema noted in the face and around the eyes (e.g., periorbital edema)
- Joint pain and/or rash

The physical examination should focus on the presence of the following:

- Hypo- or hypertension
- Increased measured weight relative to a recent documented weight (if known)
- Edema (periorbital, facial, vaginal/penile, lower extremity)
- Abdominal distention/ascites
- Rash

Laboratory Testing

The urine dipstick test is the most common qualitative test for protein in the urine. Urine should be tested as soon after voiding as possible. Urine dipsticks contain tetrabromophenol blue, which undergoes a colorimetric reaction in the presence of proteins with abundant amino acid groups (most commonly, albumin). The result is different shades of color corresponding to the concentration of the reacting proteins. The qualitative urine dipstick does not detect the presence of globulins, Bence Jones proteins, or LMW proteins.

When the urine dipstick test is positive for protein (1+ to 4+), the following diagnostic approach may be used to isolate the etiology.

1. Rule out a false-positive test—a false-positive test is more likely when any of these conditions are present: Alkaline urine (pH >7.5), high urine specific gravity (≥1.025), exposure to iodinated contrast, or use of chlorhexidine antiseptic. If any are present, send the urine for a Up/c ratio to confirm the presence of true proteinuria.
2. If the Up/c ratio in the random urine specimen is elevated above 0.2 mg protein/mg creatinine, repeat a Up/c ratio on a

first morning urine specimen within 1 to 2 weeks to confirm the presence of persistent, nonorthostatic (e.g., fixed) proteinuria.

3. If the proteinuria is persistent and fixed, obtain a renal function panel (serum creatinine, sodium, potassium, chloride, bicarbonate, and phosphorus) to evaluate for abnormalities associated with underlying kidney disease.
4. If proteinuria is persistent and fixed, obtain a kidney ultrasound to evaluate for structural kidney disease.
5. If a kidney ultrasound fails to reveal structural disease, obtain tests to help diagnose systemic illness such as SLE as suggested by history and physical examination.
6. If the Up/c ratio is >2 mg protein/mg creatinine (a value typically indicating nephrotic range proteinuria), obtain a serum albumin and total cholesterol to confirm the presence of hypoalbuminemia and hypercholesterolemia, consistent with nephrotic syndrome.
7. If signs of renal tubulopathy such as glucosuria, acidosis, and/or hypophosphatemia are present, obtain a urinary retinol-binding protein (a marker of LMW proteinuria).
8. Consider a kidney biopsy. While indications for performing a kidney biopsy in asymptomatic proteinuria are not standardized, most nephrologists recommend obtaining a kidney biopsy in asymptomatic AYAs with persistent, fixed proteinuria exceeding 1,000 mg/day (e.g., Up/c ratio ≥1.0). In general, the prognosis for asymptomatic orthostatic or persistent proteinuria of <500 mg/day is good[11] and the yield of finding significant disease on kidney biopsy is low. In patients with abnormal kidney function and/or hypertension, lower levels of proteinuria should prompt consideration of kidney biopsy.

In AYAs with nephrotic range proteinuria, the decision to proceed with a kidney biopsy prior to a trial of corticosteroids hinges on the prebiopsy probability of diagnosing FSGS versus MCNS. Focal segmental glomerulosclerosis is likely to be resistant to treatment with corticosteroids. International data show the prevalence of FSGS on renal biopsy in pediatric and adult patients to be between 7% and 19%.[12] Focal segmental glomerulosclerosis is also more likely to be the cause of nephrotic syndrome in Black AYAs. The genetic underpinnings for this occurrence are now being elucidated with associations with apolipoprotein L1(ApoL1) gene variants being reported in large studies.[13] Therefore, a kidney biopsy should be considered early in the evaluation of fixed and persistent proteinuria in AYAs or younger Black adolescents.

Prognosis

In general, isolated low-grade proteinuria (<500 mg/m^2/day) is not associated with severe glomerular pathology. For proteinuria associated with clinical symptoms or other urinary/laboratory findings, the prognosis depends on the underlying pathology. Even low-level microalbuminuria is a risk factor for renal complications in youth with hypertension, glomerulopathies associated with hematuria, and diabetes mellitus.[14]

HEMATURIA

Hematuria may be gross (e.g., macroscopic) when blood in the urine is visible to the naked eye and microscopic when it is not. Microscopic hematuria is defined as the presence of red blood cells (RBCs) in the urine. Screening for hematuria can be done with conventional urine dipsticks. The urine dipstick is able to detect one to five RBCs per high-power field in urine, making this test very sensitive (>90%). Similarly, a negative urine dipstick test effectively excludes hematuria with a specificity approaching 99%. False-negative results for hematuria are rare but may occur in the presence of oxalates, urine pH <5.1, or ascorbic acid (vitamin C). False-positive results may occur in the presence of hemoglobin, myoglobin, or semen.[15] Hemoglobinuria may develop from lysis of RBCs in the urine or from hemoglobin filtered due to intravascular hemolysis. As a result, true hematuria can only be confirmed by visualization of the presence of whole RBCs in spun urine sediment.

Epidemiology

In AYAs, the prevalence of microscopic hematuria is approximately 5%.[16] On a repeat urinalysis, the prevalence decreases to 1%.

Pathophysiology

Hematuria (either gross or microscopic) may be of glomerular or nonglomerular origin. Symptoms, laboratory tests, and direct urine microscopy often help the clinician determine the cause. Glomerular hematuria may be due to active glomerular inflammation (e.g., glomerulonephritis) or inherited abnormalities of the glomerular filtration membrane. The finding on urine microscopy of dysmorphic RBCs with or without RBC casts is consistent with glomerular hematuria. Red blood cell casts form when RBCs are allowed to pass through the glomerulus and become obstructed in the tubular lumen, creating a mold of the lumen that is eventually flushed into the bladder. Glomerular hematuria is often accompanied by proteinuria, hypertension, and/or abnormal renal function.

When hematuria is nonglomerular, the presence of symptoms may suggest the source of bleeding. Processes that cause distention of the renal capsule or irritation of the uroepithelium (lining of the urinary collecting system) may cause back, flank, abdominal, or pelvic pain depending on the site of irritation. In addition to pain, lower urinary tract bleeding may be suggested by the presence of dysuria, nausea, urinary frequency and/or urgency, or the presence of clots in the urine. In contrast, bleeding within the renal parenchyma may be asymptomatic.

Differential Diagnosis

A systematic approach to evaluating hematuria includes determining whether the bleeding is glomerular or nonglomerular in origin. If glomerular hematuria is thought to be present, the differential diagnosis may include both primary structural abnormalities and acquired inflammatory/immunologic diseases. **Table 32.2** summarizes the most commonly encountered diagnoses.

Diagnostic Approach

History and Physical Examination

A detailed history and physical examination focused on specific elements will aid the practitioner in narrowing the differential diagnosis and in ordering appropriately targeted laboratory and imaging tests. Important aspects of the history to be elicited by the practitioner include the following:

- Illnesses with the presence of fever, sore throat, and/or rash occurring concurrently or within 5 to 21 days prior to the onset of hematuria
- Urinary symptoms of enuresis, dysuria, urgency, and/or frequency
- Recent trauma (even mild) to the abdomen, flank, or back
- Diarrheal illness, with or without bloody stools, starting 5 to 10 days prior to onset of gross hematuria
- Abdominal, flank, and/or back pain
- Gross hematuria occurring throughout the urinary stream versus at the end of urination
- Joint pain and/or rash
- Recent or current menses (assigned female at birth)
- Family history of hearing loss, CKD, early stroke, kidney stones, and/or vision loss

The physical examination should focus on the following:
- Hypertension
- Pallor
- Edema (periorbital)
- Palpable retroperitoneal masses
- Costovertebral tenderness to palpation

TABLE 32.2

Causes of Hematuria

Category	Example
Glomerular hematuria	
• Primary glomerulopathies:	Alport syndrome Thin basement membrane disease (TBMD)
• Acquired glomerulopathies	
Hypocomplementemic glomerulonephritis	Postinfectious glomerulonephritis (PIGN) C3 glomerulopathy Lupus nephritis Glomerulonephritis associated with chronic bacteremia Typical or atypical hemolytic uremic syndrome (HUS)
Normocomplementemic glomerulonephritis	IgA nephropathy Henoch–Schönlein purpura (HSP) nephritis Mesangioproliferative glomerulonephritis Pauci-immune glomerulonephritis Antiglomerular basement membrane disease (anti-GBM)
Nonglomerular hematuria	
• Structural parenchymal disease	
Cystic renal disease	Isolated renal cysts Autosomal-dominant polycystic kidney disease (ADPKD) Cystic renal disease in tuberous sclerosis (TS)
Noncystic renal disease	Medullary-sponge kidney with nephrocalcinosis/nephrolithiasis
• Renal parenchymal tumors	Renal cell carcinoma Renal medullary carcinoma (especially sickle cell disease/trait) Renal angiomyolipomas in TS
• Renal tubular hematuria	Acute papillary necrosis (sickle cell, diabetes, excessive analgesic use) Sickle cell trait–associated hematuria
• Renal trauma	Contusion, lacerations, disruption (increased risk in enlarged kidneys)
• Vascular disease	Malignant hypertension Arteriovenous malformations Renal arterial thrombi/renal vein thrombosis
• Urothelial bleeding	
Structural/functional	Ureteropelvic junction (UPJ) obstruction Urethrorrhagia (predominantly males) Athlete's (runner's) hematuria Loin pain hematuria syndrome
Inflammatory/ infectious	Acute cystitis/pyelonephritis BK virus–associated nephropathy (immunocompromised) Urethritis Prostatitis Schistosomiasis
Irritative	Nephrolithiasis Hypercalciuria Bladder tumors Hemorrhagic cystitis (cyclophosphamide exposure)
Coagulopathic (rare presentation)	Thrombocytopenia Congenital (hemophilia) or acquired (medication related) coagulation defects

C3, complement component 3; IgA, immunoglobulin A.

• Rash including the presence of petechiae and/or purpura
• Joint swelling

The initial approach to the adolescent or young adult with gross hematuria is summarized below:

1. Ensure that the urine is not being discolored by other pigments by microscopic examination for RBCs. Centrifugation of urine often offers an early clue to the presence of pigments in the urine as the supernatant will remain discolored after centrifugation.[17] Causes of pigmenturia may be endogenous (porphyrinuria, hemoglobinuria, myoglobinuria) or exogenous (foods and drugs).

2. Confirm that the hematuria originates from the kidneys or urinary tract. False hematuria can be caused by vaginal bleeding or factitious hematuria.

3. If a glomerular source of hematuria is confirmed (by the presence of dysmorphic RBCs and/or RBC casts), obtain a renal function panel to assess the GFR and electrolytes, as well as serum complement levels (C3 and C4) to narrow the differential diagnosis. If C3 is low, obtain additional laboratory testing to assess for further evidence of prior streptococcal infection or the presence of collagen vascular disease (e.g., antideoxyribonuclease B antibody, antistreptolysin O antibody, anti–double-stranded deoxyribonucleic acid antibody). If C3 is normal, consider anticytoplasmic neutrophil antibody (ANCA) associated vasculitis.

4. If possible, obtain urinalyses from parents and siblings to screen for a familial glomerulopathy.

5. In cases of coexisting proteinuria, a Up/c ratio and serum albumin will determine whether a nephritic/nephrotic syndrome is present.

6. If nonglomerular hematuria is present, further evaluation of potential etiologies is directed by the history, symptoms, associated comorbid conditions, and findings on microscopy. This includes a urine culture for suspected urinary tract infection.

7. Renal ultrasound is of limited diagnostic utility when a glomerular origin is suspected. Patients with active glomerulonephritis may have increased cortical echogenicity labeled as "medical renal disease." In contrast, a renal ultrasound should be obtained in the evaluation of nonglomerular gross hematuria to identify renal/bladder tumors, renal cysts, renal calculi, or hydronephrosis. Additional imaging, such as computed tomography, should be reserved for evaluating renal trauma, nephrolithiasis, or to further delineate renal lesions seen on ultrasound.

8. In nonglomerular hematuria without an identified cause, a urine calcium-to-creatinine ratio (mg Ca/dL divided by mg creatinine/dL) should be obtained to evaluate for hypercalciuria (defined as a ratio ≥0.22). Hypercalciuria is one of the most common risk factors for the development of kidney stones.[18] It is also the most common metabolic abnormality identified in AYAs with kidney stones, being present in up to 47% of patients.[19]

9. In AYAs with African ancestry who present with gross hematuria of unclear etiology, consider screening for the presence of sickle cell trait with hemoglobin electrophoresis.

10. A kidney biopsy is usually not indicated for AYAs with asymptomatic hematuria. It may be indicated when suspected glomerular hematuria occurs with hypertension, abnormal GFR, and/or proteinuria >1,000 mg/day, as these signs/symptoms are suggestive of more severe glomerular disease.

Specific Conditions Presenting with Gross or Microscopic Hematuria in Adolescents and Young Adults

Marathon Runner's (Athlete's) Hematuria

Gross or microscopic hematuria is associated with many forms of vigorous exercise.[20] The typical history is one of normal urine prior to exercise and hematuria on the first specimen voided after exercise. This may last 24 to 48 hours, possibly in association with dysuria and suprapubic discomfort. The hematuria may be caused by a decrease in renal plasma flow, local bladder trauma, or leakage of blood from spiral vessels in the adventitia of minor calyces. The prognosis is benign.

Loin Pain Hematuria Syndrome

This rare, poorly understood condition is characterized by recurrent bouts of gross or microscopic hematuria associated with unilateral or bilateral flank/abdominal pain. The pain may radiate to the pelvis and groin and can be severe and chronic. Examination of the urine reveals what appears to be glomerular hematuria with dysmorphic RBCs and/or RBC casts.[21] Loin pain hematuria syndrome occurs primarily in females (70% of patients diagnosed). Blood pressure and renal function are normal. The associated pain may be difficult to control, requiring consultation with specialists in pain medicine. The underlying pathogenesis has not been fully elucidated but structural abnormalities of the glomerular basement membrane have been noted in a kidney biopsy study.[21]

IgA Nephropathy (Berger Disease)

Immunoglobulin A (IgA) nephropathy is a relatively common cause of gross hematuria of glomerular origin in AYAs. Eighty percent of patients are diagnosed between 16 and 35 years of age. In North America, the male-to-female ratio is 2:1. IgA nephropathy occurs more commonly in Asian and White youth.[22] The disease is commonly characterized by recurrent bouts of hematuria (usually gross) occurring shortly after infections. Urinary protein excretion varies from normal to nephrotic range. The decision to proceed with kidney biopsy often hinges on the level of proteinuria. Renal function is usually normal at presentation, but up to 30% of individuals will progress to ESRD within 10 years of diagnosis.[22] Poor prognostic signs include hypertension, renal insufficiency, and persistent proteinuria (protein excretion >1 g/day).[23] The diagnosis can only be made by kidney biopsy. Henoch–Schönlein purpura can cause glomerular lesions that are indistinguishable from IgA nephropathy on histology.

Hereditary Nephritis (Alport Syndrome)

Alport syndrome can be inherited as an X-linked (typically), autosomal-dominant, or autosomal-recessive condition. It is caused by mutations in the alpha-5 chain of type IV collagen, which explains both its renal and extrarenal manifestations. Alport syndrome is usually more severe in male AYAs and may present with a spectrum of clinical disease. It leads to ESRD in most young men by the third to fourth decades of life.[24] In addition to hematuria, up to 90% of male AYAs have associated sensorineural hearing loss.[24] Ocular manifestations, including corneal opacities, anterior lenticonus, cataract, and retinal abnormalities, occur commonly in Alport syndrome. Often diagnostic for the presence of disease, ocular manifestations of Alport syndrome are present in up to 70% to 80% of adult males and a lower proportion of females.[25]

Thin Basement Membrane Disease

Thin basement membrane disease (TBMD) is characterized by glomerular hematuria (usually presenting with gross hematuria) and normal renal function. It is inherited as an autosomal-dominant disease due to mutations in either the alpha-3 or alpha-4 chains of type IV collagen. Kidney biopsy reveals diffuse thinning of the glomerular basement membrane. Thin basement membrane disease affects approximately 1% of the population.[26] It is now known to lead to progressive CKD in a minority of patients, necessitating regular screening for the development of proteinuria, hypertension, and abnormal GFR.

⬤ SUMMARY

The diagnoses leading to hematuria and/or proteinuria in AYAs are varied in both etiology, pathophysiology, and the prognosis for long-term preservation of kidney function. The challenge for the practitioner remains to systematically evaluate for potential causes and appropriately refer patients for further nephrology care when necessary. Early diagnosis and treatment for diseases associated with deterioration in renal function are important to slow or potentially halt the progression of disease. A careful history, physical examination, and targeted use of lab testing and imaging modalities can often significantly narrow the differential diagnosis in AYAs with hematuria and/or proteinuria.

ACKNOWLEDGMENT

This chapter was written by Dr. Shamir Tuchman in his private capacity. The content provided in this chapter does not represent the views of nor is endorsed by the U.S. Government or the Food and Drug Administration.

REFERENCES

1. Sekhar DL, Wang L, Hollenbeak CS, et al. A cost-effectiveness analysis of screening urine dipsticks in well-child care. *Pediatrics.* 2010;125(4):660–663.
2. Arslan Z, Koyun M, Erengin H, et al. Orthostatic proteinuria: an overestimated phenomenon? *Pediatr Nephrol.* 2020;35(10):1935–1940.
3. Medina-Rosas J, Yap KS, Anderson M, et al. Utility of urinary protein-creatinine ratio and protein content in a 24-hour urine collection in systemic lupus erythematosus: a systematic review and meta-analysis. *Arthritis Care Res.* 2016;68(9):1310–1319.
4. Montero N, Soler MJ, Pascual MJ, et al. Correlation between the protein/creatinine ratio in spot urine and 24-hour urine protein. *Nefrologia.* 2012;32(4):494–501.
5. Parakh P, Bhatta NK, Mishra OP, et al. Urinary screening for detection of renal abnormalities in asymptomatic school children. *Nephrourol Mon.* 2012;4(3):551–555.
6. Trihono PP, Wulandari N, Supriyatno B. Asymptomatic proteinuria in Indonesian adolescent students. *Saudi J Kidney Dis Transpl.* 2019;30(3):694–700.
7. Brandt JR, Jacobs A, Raissy HH, et al. Orthostatic proteinuria and the spectrum of diurnal variability of urinary protein excretion in healthy children. *Pediatr Nephrol.* 2010;25(6):1131–1137.
8. Fogo AB. Causes and pathogenesis of focal segmental glomerulosclerosis. *Nat Rev Nephrol.* 2015;11(2):76–87.
9. Barsalou J, Levy DM, Silverman ED. An update on childhood-onset systemic lupus erythematosus. *Curr Opin Rheumatol.* 2013;25(5):616–622.
10. Amaral B, Murphy G, Ioannou Y, et al. A comparison of the outcome of adolescent and adult-onset systemic lupus erythematosus. *Rheumatology.* 2014;53(6):1130–1135.
11. Baskin AM, Freedman LR, Davie JS, et al. Proteinuria in Yale students and 30-year mortality experience. *J Urol.* 1972;108(4):617–618.
12. O'Shaughnessy MM, Hogan SL, Thompson BD, et al. Glomerular disease frequencies by race, sex and region: results from the International Kidney Biopsy Survey. *Nephrol Dial Transplant.* 2018;33(4):661–669.
13. Genovese G, Friedman DJ, Ross MD, et al. Association of trypanolytic ApoL1 variants with kidney disease in African Americans. *Science.* 2010;329(5993):841–845.
14. Bjornstad P, Cherney DZ, Maahs DM, et al. Diabetic kidney disease in adolescents with type 2 diabetes: new insights and potential therapies. *Curr Diab Rep.* 2016;16(2):11.
15. Cyriac J, Holden K, Tullus K. How to use... urine dipsticks. *Arch Dis Child Educ Pract Ed.* 2017;102(3):148–154.
16. Ferris M, Hogan SL, Chin H, et al. Obesity, albuminuria, and urinalysis findings in US young adults from the Add Health Wave III study. *Clin J Am Soc Nephrol.* 2007;2(6):1207–1214.
17. Viteri B, Reid-Adam J. Hematuria and proteinuria in children. *Pediatr Rev.* 2018;39(12):573–587.
18. Issler N, Dufek S, Kleta R, et al. Epidemiology of paediatric renal stone disease: a 22-year single centre experience in the UK. *BMC Nephrol.* 2017;18(1):136.
19. Spivacow FR, Del Valle EE, Boailchuk JA, et al. Metabolic risk factors in children with kidney stone disease: an update. *Pediatr Nephrol.* 2020;35(11):2107–2112.
20. Van Biervliet S, Van Biervliet JP, Watteyne K, et al. Pseudonephritis is associated with high urinary osmolality and high specific gravity in adolescent soccer players. *Pediatr Exerc Sci.* 2013;25(3):360–369.
21. Urits I, Li N, Berger AA, et al. Treatment and management of loin pain hematuria syndrome. *Curr Pain Headache Rep.* 2021;25(1):6.
22. Hogg RJ. Idiopathic immunoglobulin A nephropathy in children and adolescents. *Pediatr Nephrol.* 2010;25(5):823–829.
23. Coppo R. Clinical and histological risk factors for progression of IgA nephropathy: an update in children, young and adult patients. *J Nephrol.* 2017;30(3):339–346.
24. Nozu K, Nakanishi K, Abe Y, et al. A review of clinical characteristics and genetic backgrounds in Alport syndrome. *Clin Exp Nephrol.* 2019;23(2):158–168.
25. Savige J, Sheth S, Leys A, et al. Ocular features in Alport syndrome: pathogenesis and clinical significance. *Clin J Am Soc Nephrol.* 2015;10(4):703–709.
26. Matthaiou A, Poulli T, Deltas C. Prevalence of clinical, pathological and molecular features of glomerular basement membrane nephropathy caused by COL4A3 or COL4A4 mutations: a systematic review. *Clin Kidney J.* 2020;13(6):1025–1036.

ADDITIONAL RESOURCES AND WEBSITES

Additional Resources and Websites for Clinicians:
American Urological Association—Diagnosis, Evaluation, and Follow-up of Asymptomatic Microhematuria (AMH) in Adults—https://www.auanet.org/x262.xml
Bignall ONR, Dixon BP. Management of hematuria in children. Curr Treat Options Pediatr. 2018;4(3):333–349. https://www.ncbi.nlm.nih.gov/pmc/articles/PMC6097192/
Ingold CJ, Bhatt H. *Orthostatic Proteinuria.* StatPearls Publishing; 2022. https://www.ncbi.nlm.nih.gov/books/NBK562308/
Kallash M, Rheault MN. Approach to persistent microscopic hematuria in children. Kidney. 360 2020;1(9):1014–1020. https://kidney360.asnjournals.org/content/1/9/1014
Leung AKC, Wong AHC, Barg SSN. Proteinuria in children: evaluation and differential diagnosis. Am Fam Physician. 2017;95(4):248–254. https://www.aafp.org/afp/2017/0215/p248.html
Samal L, Linder JA. The primary care perspective on routine urine dipstick screening to identify patients with albuminuria. CJASN. 2013;8(1):131–135. https://cjasn.asnjournals.org/content/8/1/131
Thomas B, Lerma EV. Proteinuria. *Medscape* (updated December 2021). https://emedicine.medscape.com/article/238158-overview

Additional Resources and Websites for Parents/Caregivers:
National Institute of Diabetes and Digestive and Kidney Diseases (NIDDK): IgA Nephropathy—https://www.niddk.nih.gov/health-information/kidney-disease/iga-nephropathy
National Kidney Foundation (NKF) Website: Hematuria in Children—https://www.kidney.org/atoz/content/hematuria
NephCure Proteinuria Resource Center—https://nephcure.org/livingwithkidneydisease/proteinuria-resource-center/
UpToDate: Patient education: Blood in the urine (hematuria) in children (Beyond the Basics)—https://www.uptodate.com/contents/blood-in-the-urine-hematuria-in-children-beyond-the-basics
UpToDate: Patient education: Protein in the urine (proteinuria) (Beyond the Basics)—https://www.uptodate.com/contents/protein-in-the-urine-proteinuria-beyond-the-basics

Additional Resources and Websites for Adolescents and Young Adults:
DaVita Kidney Care: Proteinuria—https://www.davita.com/education/kidney-disease/risk-factors/proteinuria
National Kidney Foundation (NKF) Website: Kidney Health Testing: Albumin-to-creatinine ratio—https://www.kidney.org/atoz/content/know-your-kidney-numbers-two-simple-tests
National Kidney Foundation (NKF) Website: Kidney Health Testing: Focal Segmental Glomerulosclerosis (FSGS)—https://www.kidney.org/atoz/content/focal
National Kidney Foundation (NKF) Website: What you should know about albuminuria (proteinuria)—https://www.kidney.org/atoz/content/proteinuriawyska
National Kidney Foundation (NKF) Website: Urinalysis and Kidney Disease: What You Need to Know—https://www.kidney.org/sites/default/files/11-10-1815_HBE_PatBro_Urinalysis_v6.pdf

PART VIII

Infectious Diseases

Infectious Mononucleosis

Catherine Miller
Terrill Bravender

KEY WORDS

- Epstein–Barr virus
- Hepatosplenomegaly
- Heterophile antibodies
- Infectious mononucleosis
- Lymphadenopathy
- Lymphocytosis

INTRODUCTION

Infectious mononucleosis (IM) was initially clinically described in the 1880s and first named by Sprunt and Evans in 1920.[1] Infectious mononucleosis most commonly presents in adolescents and young adults (AYAs) and is characterized by sore throat, fever, cervical lymphadenitis, and fatigue. Though this clinical picture can be associated with other viruses, over 90% of cases of IM are caused by Epstein–Barr virus (EBV).[2,3] Epstein–Barr virus is a herpes virus which establishes a lifelong latent infection. In this chapter, we will focus on IM caused by primary EBV infection.

Usually, IM is an acute, self-limited, and benign lymphoproliferative disease but symptoms can persist for months. Classic clinical symptoms along with atypical lymphocytosis suggest the diagnosis of IM, and rapid serologic testing for heterophile antibodies or EBV-specific antibodies confirm the diagnosis.[4] Severe complications such as airway compromise, splenic rupture, or fulminant EBV infection are rare.[5] The host immune system plays a key role in shaping the clinical manifestations of EBV infection and immunocompromised hosts are at higher risk of EBV-associated severe lymphoproliferative conditions. Epstein–Barr virus is also associated with the development of lymphoid and epithelial cancers.[1] Currently, there is neither an EBV vaccine nor definitive treatment beyond symptomatic care for IM.[6–8]

Etiology and Pathophysiology

Epstein–Barr virus is a fragile, enveloped DNA herpes virus and humans are the only known reservoir. Like all herpes viruses, acquisition leads to lifelong infection after the acute viral replication has been contained.[9] The virus is viable in saliva for a few hours outside of the host.[3] Transmission occurs primarily through exposure to oropharyngeal secretions (hence, its reputation as "the kissing disease").[2] Other described routes of transmission include transplantation or blood transfusion.[10] Epstein–Barr virus initially infects oral epithelial cells and B lymphocytes. Infection then spreads throughout the lymphoreticular system with rapid viral replication both in the oral cavity and periphery. There is a polyclonal B-cell proliferation, a significant T-cell response, and activation of natural killer (NK) cells.[11] The atypical white blood cells (WBCs), also called Downey cells, that are frequently seen on peripheral blood smears are mainly CD8 cytotoxic T cells.[9]

The immune response accounts for many of the clinical manifestations of IM such as lymphadenopathy and hepatosplenomegaly. For 3 to 4 months following acute infection, the number of infected cells decreases, but some infected memory B and T cells continue to circulate in the blood and oropharyngeal lymphoid tissue indefinitely.[11] Intermittently, the virus reactivates in the lymphoid tissues and this leads to lifelong unpredictable oral shedding of the virus in asymptomatic individuals.[11] Tight immune control is maintained over these latent and reactivation phases in immunocompetent hosts and a single episode of IM confers lifelong immunity.[11]

Epidemiology

Over 90% of adults worldwide have serologic evidence of past EBV infection.[2] The highest rates of IM are in the 15- to 24-year-old age group, with about 6 to 8 cases/1,000 persons per year.[4] Infectious mononucleosis is particularly common among AYAs living in close proximity to one another, such as in schools or the military.[3,5]

Age

Prior to age 10 years, most primary EBV infections are asymptomatic or result in mild illness not recognized as an EBV infection.[9] However, symptomatic EBV infections are more common in AYAs; 30% to 50% of AYAs who contract EBV will develop the symptoms of IM.[5] In developed countries, children seem to be acquiring primary EBV infection at a later age.[10] This trend may lead to a greater proportion of AYAs being susceptible to IM.[10]

Gender

There are no gender differences in prevalence.[3]

Sociodemographic Factors

Primary EBV infections occur at a younger age among persons living in overcrowded households and from lower versus higher socioeconomic backgrounds.[12]

Season

There is no seasonal variation in IM incidence.[5]

Clinical Manifestations

In those who develop IM, there is a long incubation period of 30 to 50 days after which there may be a 3- to 5-day prodrome of malaise, fatigue, headaches, anorexia, and myalgias.[3] The traditional triad of IM includes pharyngitis, lymphadenopathy, and fever.[9] A striking aspect of IM is the long duration of acute illness, with symptoms typically lasting 2 to 3 weeks, and occasionally lasting months.[8,10,13] Early on in IM, the WBC count will show a lymphocytosis with atypical immature lymphocytes.[4] Antibody response demonstrated by the presence of heterophile or EBV-specific antibodies are other key hematologic findings in IM.[4]

Signs and Symptoms

Signs and symptoms are summarized in Table 33.1. The sore throat can be severe and is associated with an exudative pharyngitis and palatal petechiae in up to 50% of individuals.[5] Adenopathy is usually symmetrical and significant. Anterior cervical lymphadenopathy is present in almost all patients, but this does not help in differentiating IM from other viral infections.[2] Posterior cervical, axillary, and inguinal lymphadenopathy are more specific for IM.[4] Fatigue is often the symptom with longest duration.[9] Liver involvement is considered part of the acute illness instead of a complication. Abnormal liver function tests are seen in 80% of patients and the liver involvement is subclinical in 90% to 95% of patients with IM.[9] Approximately 3% to 15% of individuals develop a rash that may take on several different appearances—morbilliform, macular, scarlatiniform, urticarial, petechial, or erythema multiforme.[14] The typical distribution involves the trunk and spares the extremities, and emergence is usually in the first days of illness resolving in 1 to 6 days.[15] Classic teaching about a high incidence of skin rashes (80% to 100%) in patients with IM who were treated with antibiotics has been called into question by more recent studies showing a much lower incidence of 15% to 33%.[14–16] Although the exact mechanism for the development of this antibiotic-associated rash is unknown, it appears that there may be two populations: one who have a transient EBV-associated loss of tolerance to a drug and a second group who develop a true and persistent delayed-type drug hypersensitivity.[14]

Complications

Complications of IM are summarized in Table 33.2. Overall, the complication rate of IM is approximately 1% to 2%.[10] Complications

TABLE 33.1

Signs and Symptoms of Infectious Mononucleosis[2,9,13,14]

Signs and Symptoms	Prevalence (%)
Cervical lymphadenopathy	76–95
Sore throat	>90
Fatigue	66–90
Headache	47–75
Fever	42–70
Upper respiratory symptoms (congestion and cough)	48–64
Decreased appetite	44–50
Myalgias	41–50
Abdominal pain	8–40
Splenomegaly	33
Hepatomegaly	25
Nausea and vomiting	<20
Periorbital and eyelid edema	10
Rash	3–15
Jaundice	<5

TABLE 33.2

Potential Complications of Infectious Mononucleosis[1–3,10]

Neurologic
Facial or peripheral nerve palsies
Meningoencephalitis
Aseptic meningitis
Optic neuritis
Transverse myelitis
Guillain–Barré syndrome
Acute psychosis
Perceptual distortions "Alice in Wonderland" syndrome

Hematologic
Splenic rupture
Coagulopathy
Aplastic anemia
Hemolytic anemia
Eosinophilia
Profound thrombocytopenia
Hemophagocytic lymphohistiocytosis

Cardiac
Pericarditis
Myocarditis
Electrocardiogram changes (nonspecific ST and T-wave abnormalities)

Pulmonary
Airway obstruction
Pneumonitis
Pleural effusions
Pulmonary hemorrhage

Gastrointestinal
Pancreatitis
Hepatitis with liver necrosis
Malabsorption
Acalculous cholecystitis

Dermatologic
Rash (may be cold induced)
Erythema multiforme

Renal
Glomerulonephritis
Nephrotic syndrome
Mild hematuria or proteinuria

Ophthalmologic
Conjunctivitis
Episcleritis
Uveitis

Other
Bullous myringitis
Orchitis
Genital ulcerations
Parotitis
Monoarticular arthritis

can be due to damage from the body's immune response or from tissue-invasive viral infection.[9] Occasionally, patients will present with a major complication as their presenting manifestation of the disease.[17]

Specific Complications

Splenic Rupture In IM, the spleen often increases to three to four times the normal size.[18] Splenic rupture, which can be fatal, is seen in approximately 0.1% to 0.5% of cases of IM.[5] At least half of

CHAPTER 33 • Infectious Mononucleosis   **321**

the cases are spontaneous without any history of trauma or unusual physical exertion. Typically, there is abrupt abdominal pain in the left upper quadrant that radiates to the top of the left shoulder. This is followed by generalized abdominal pain, pleuritic chest pain, and signs and symptoms of hypovolemia. However, the onset may be insidious.[18] Splenic rupture risk is highest in the first 3 weeks of illness and approximately half of cases occur during the peak of the acute illness.[5] All patients with IM should be considered at risk for splenic rupture and given information regarding the clinical warning signs for rupture, because clinical severity, laboratory results, and physical examination are not reliable predictors of risk.[18]

Airway Obstruction Airway obstruction is an uncommon but life-threatening complication of IM related to massive lymphoid hyperplasia and mucosal edema. It is more common in younger children and adolescents and may present with drooling, stridor, and difficulty breathing.[1,5] Supportive measures can include corticosteroids to reduce the edema and hypertrophy of the lymphoid tissue, close hospital observation, elevating the head of the bed, and supplemental oxygen.[19] In more severe cases, intubation, tracheostomy, or acute tonsillectomy may be indicated.[19]

Chronic Active Epstein–Barr Virus Infection Most patients with EBV-associated IM develop lifelong immunity. Rarely, individuals may develop active EBV disease with a chronic persistent course. These patients are unable to control the EBV infection and have very high levels of EBV in the blood and markedly high titers of EBV antibodies.[11] Chronic active EBV disease (CAEBV) is characterized by severe illness lasting >3 months, persistently elevated blood levels of EBV, and infiltration of tissues by EBV-positive lymphocytes. Chronic active EBV disease is more commonly seen in Asia and South and Central America.[20] Hematopoietic stem cell transplantation is currently the only proven effective treatment for CAEBV.[20]

Laboratory Evaluation

Antibody Testing

The standard rapid test for IM is the presence of heterophile antibodies. These immunoglobulin M (IgM) antibodies are induced during the immune upregulation in acute EBV infection and cross-react with unrelated antigens, typically, horse, sheep, or bovine erythrocytes.[10] These rapid test kits have sensitivities of 81% to 95% and specificities of 98% to 100% when compared to EBV-specific serologies, however, sensitivity is lower during the first week of infection and in younger children.[21] Heterophile antibodies can persist for a year or more and so are not always diagnostic of an acute infection.[10]

If the heterophile test is negative and IM is suspected, specific EBV antibody tests can be done. The EBV viral capsid antigen

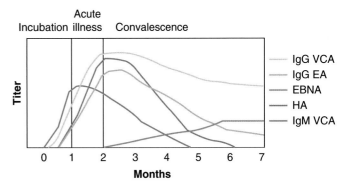

Antibody response to acute infection with EBV. VCA, virus capsid antigen; HA, heterophil antibody; EA, early antigen; EBNA, EBV nuclear antigen.

FIGURE 33.1 The evolution of antibodies to various EBV antigens in patients with IM is shown in the figure. IgM and IgG antibody responses to EBV capsid antigen develop during the acute phase, as does an IgG response to EBV EA in most cases. The IgG response lasts for life, but the IgM response is transient and is shortest in very young children. Antibody response to nuclear antigen lasts for life and is typically quite late in onset. (Source: Henle W, Henle G. Seroepidemiology of the virus. In: Epstein M, Achong B eds. *The Epstein-Barr Virus.* Springer-Verlag; 1979:61–79; and Tomkinson B, Sullivan J. Epstein-Barr virus infection and mononucleosis. In: Gorbach S, Bartlett J, Blacklow N eds. *Infectious Diseases.* WB Saunders; 1991:1348–1356.)

(VCA) IgM, which peaks early in the acute illness and persists for 1 to 3 months before disappearing, is the most specific and valuable serologic test for confirming the diagnosis of acute IM.[1] Immunoglobulin G (IgG) VCA antibodies peak later during the acute illness, and then usually persist life-long. Therefore, detection of VCA IgG alone will not distinguish between an acute and a remote infection.[1] Antibodies to early antigen (EA) are also detectable in most patients during the acute phase of IM. These EBV EA antibodies usually persist for 1 to 2 months but can persist at low titers for many years and high titers can be found in immunocompromised patients with high EBV replication.[1] Finally, about 2 to 3 months after symptom onset, antibodies against EBV nuclear antigen (EBNA) develop and persist indefinitely.[9] Figure 33.1 shows the characteristic EBV antibody responses to various EBV antigens. Table 33.3 shows the pattern of serologic results in various EBV stages.

Complete Blood Count

The WBC differential is a useful addition to the history and physical examination, as it can be abnormal early in the illness before rapid antibody-based tests yield positive results. Increases in the total percentage of WBCs that are lymphocytes (>50%) and percentage of atypical lymphocytes (at least 10%) significantly increase the likelihood of IM.[4] The total WBC count is often elevated in the

TABLE 33.3

Patterns of EBV Serology

Types of Infection	Heterophile Antibody	VCA-IgG	VCA-IgM	Early Antigen D-EA	R-EA	EBNA
Susceptible (nonimmune)	−	−	−	−	−	−
Acute primary infection	+	++	+	+	−	−
Remote past infection	−	+	−	−	−	+
Reactivated infection	+/−	+++	−	+	++	+/−

D-EA, diffuse early antigen; EBNA, Epstein–Barr nuclear antigen; Ig, immunoglobulin; R-EA, restricted early antigen; VCA, viral capsid antigen.

range of 10,000 to 20,000/mm³. Other common hematologic abnormalities include a mild granulocytopenia and thrombocytopenia in 25% to 50% of people.[1]

Hepatic Transaminases

Transaminase levels are elevated in 80% of individuals, peaking during the second or third week of symptoms.[2] Mild hepatitis is so common that entirely normal hepatic transaminases should lead the clinician to consider a diagnosis other than EBV infection.[9]

Epstein–Barr Viral Detection

Serum-based EBV DNA nucleic acid amplification tests have been developed, and the magnitude of the viral load has been correlated with severity of illness. However, EBV viral load tests are not readily available for clinical use, and the primary use of these tests has been in immunocompromised patients at risk for EBV-associated malignancy.[10]

Differential Diagnosis

In addition to other causes of EBV-negative mononucleosis such as cytomegalovirus, toxoplasmosis, rubella, adenovirus, and acute human immunodeficiency virus (HIV) infection, the differential diagnosis includes group A β-hemolytic streptococcal pharyngitis, nonspecific viral tonsillitis, mycoplasma pneumonia, Vincent angina (necrotizing ulcerative gingivitis), diphtheria, viral hepatitis, Lemierre syndrome due to *Fusobacterium necrophorum*, and lymphoproliferative disorders or acute leukemia.[4,22]

Diagnosis

The diagnosis is based on the following considerations:

Clinical Symptoms

Infectious mononucleosis should be suspected in an AYA with fatigue, fever, splenomegaly, adenopathy, and pharyngitis.

Abnormal White Blood Cell Count

Patients will usually have the following:
a. Relative lymphocytosis >50%
b. Absolute lymphocytosis >4,000/mm³
c. Relative atypical lymphocytosis >10%

Positive Serology

Almost all AYAs with IM have positive heterophile antibodies. If a patient continues to be symptomatic and heterophile antibodies are negative, antibody titers for EBV (including VCA and EBNA) should be evaluated.

Other Tests

While testing for group A β-hemolytic streptococcal pharyngitis may be indicated, a positive test does not exclude the possibility of IM.

Management

Most patients with IM will require only supportive symptomatic care.

Symptomatic Care

a. Rest: Recommend adjusting daily activities and resting as needed during the acute phase of illness. Make AYAs and their parents aware that the acute symptoms usually resolve over 2 weeks, although the associated fatigue may persist for 4 weeks, or sometimes longer. Many patients require up to 2 months for full recovery. About 10% of patients with IM report persistent fatigue 6 months after the onset of symptoms.[9,10]
b. Fever and pain control: Nonsteroidal anti-inflammatory agents or acetaminophen can be used regularly for fever and pain. The severity of throat pain can interfere with sleep and oral

intake, so adding anesthetic throat lozenges or gargles can be helpful.[9] Aspirin should be avoided because there is a rare association between EBV and Reye syndrome.
c. Fluids and nutrition: Attention to hydration and adequate nutrition is important, especially in the febrile stage of illness. Patients with severe pharyngitis may benefit from supplemental liquid nutrition.

Antimicrobials

In the absence of a bacterial co-infection, antibiotics should not be used.[3] The effectiveness of using antiviral agents is uncertain and studies to date provide only low-quality evidence.[7] Although antiviral agents may suppress viral shedding and reduce duration of lymphadenopathy, they do not impact the clinical course of IM.[7]

Corticosteroids

Corticosteroids are not indicated as studies have not shown clinical effectiveness and there are insufficient data on short- and long-term consequences.[8] The use of prednisone (20 to 60 mg daily, tapered over 1 to 2 weeks) is indicated only in patients with significant pharyngeal edema causing respiratory compromise or with immune-mediated hematologic complications.[1,3]

Vaccine Development

No licensed EBV vaccine is available, though research into a vaccine to prevent EBV infection and EBV-associated diseases has been ongoing for several decades.[6] Most of the vaccination studies have focused on glycoprotein 350 (gp350), the major EBV envelope protein. A candidate vaccine did decrease the incidence of IM but did not protect against EBV infection in a phase II clinical trial.[6,10]

Recommendations Regarding Physical Activity

Adolescents and young adults with IM should refrain from vigorous physical activity for at least 1 month after the onset of symptoms due to risk of splenic rupture. The likelihood of splenic rupture decreases over time, and 90% of splenic ruptures occur within 31 days of onset of illness.[17] Decisions about returning to play should be made on a case-by-case basis. Radiologic imaging of the spleen is not recommended. There is significant variability in splenic size, and such assessments have not been shown to predict splenic rupture risk.[23] It may take 3 to 6 months after IM recovery for athletes to regain their previous levels of physical fitness.[3]

Epstein–Barr Virus–Associated Conditions

Despite some clinical similarities, there is little evidence that EBV causes chronic fatigue syndrome, and a positive IgG test for EBV does not imply a causal relationship.[1,3]

Because of EBV's ability to alter cellular gene transcription combined with latent infection in B lymphocytes and epithelial cells, EBV is associated with a variety of lymphoid and epithelial cancers including nasopharyngeal carcinoma, leiomyosarcoma, and Burkitt and Hodgkin lymphoma.[24] In addition, development of IM (as opposed to asymptomatic primary EBV infection) has been linked to an increased risk for the development of Hodgkin lymphoma and multiple sclerosis.[25,26]

In the rare genetic disorder, X-linked lymphoproliferative syndrome, affected males are unable to control EBV infection and the majority will die after development of fulminant EBV IM.[5] Rarely, host T-cell infection with EBV may be associated with hemophagocytic syndrome, resulting in severe pancytopenia and hepatitis.[3]

Epstein–Barr virus is also a key factor in many cases of post-transplant lymphoproliferative disorder.[10] Post-transplant lymphoproliferative disorder is characterized by abnormal proliferation of lymphoid immune cells in immunosuppressed solid or hematopoietic transplant recipients with impaired immune surveillance.[10]

 SUMMARY

Infectious mononucleosis is caused by EBV, which is transmitted primarily through exposure to oropharyngeal secretions, and has a long incubation period of 30 to 50 days. Acute infection is characterized by pharyngitis, lymphadenopathy, fever, fatigue, and hepatosplenomegaly, along with a lymphocytosis with atypical immature lymphocytes. Symptoms typically last for 2 to 3 weeks, but fatigue can linger for months. Almost all AYAs with IM will have a positive rapid heterophile antibody test. If it is very early in the illness and the heterophile antibodies are negative, EBV-specific antibody titers for VCA IgM and EBNA should be evaluated. Severe complications such as splenic rupture and airway obstruction occur in less than 2% of cases. Symptomatic care includes rest, refraining from vigorous physical activity for 1 month, fever and pain control, and attention to hydration and nutrition. Antibiotics should not be used unless there is a bacterial coinfection and corticosteroids are only used if pharyngeal edema causes respiratory compromise or there is an immune-mediated hematologic complication.

REFERENCES

1. Jenson HB. Epstein-Barr virus. *Pediatr Rev.* 2011;32(9):375–384.
2. Dunmire SK, Hogquist KA, Balfour HH. Infectious mononucleosis. *Curr Top Microbiol Immunol.* 2015;390(Pt 1):211–240.
3. Kimberlin DW, Long SS, Brady MT, et al. *Red Book 2018 Report of the Committee on Infectious Diseases.* 31st ed. American Academy of Pediatrics; 2018.
4. Ebell MH, Call M, Shinholser J, et al. Does this patient have infectious mononucleosis?: the rational clinical examination systematic review. *JAMA.* 2016;315(14):1502–1509.
5. Womack J, Jimenez M. Common questions about infectious mononucleosis. *Am Fam Physician.* 2015;91(6):372–376.
6. van Zyl DG, Mautner J, Delecluse HJ. Progress in EBV vaccines. *Front Oncol.* 2019;9:104.
7. De Paor M, O'Brien K, Fahey T, et al. Antiviral agents for infectious mononucleosis (glandular fever). *Cochrane Database Syst Rev.* 2016;12(12):CD011487.
8. Rezk E, Nofal YH, Hamzeh A, et al. Steroids for symptom control in infectious mononucleosis. *Cochrane Database Syst Rev.* 2015;2015(11):CD004402.
9. Odumade OA, Hogquist KA, Balfour HH Jr. Progress and problems in understanding and managing primary Epstein-Barr virus infections. *Clin Microbiol Rev.* 2011;24(1):193–209.
10. Dunmire SK, Verghese PS, Balfour HH Jr. Primary Epstein-Barr virus infection. *J Clin Virol.* 2018;102:84–92.
11. Tangye SG, Palendira U, Edwards ESJ. Human immunity against EBV-lessons from the clinic. *J Exp Med.* 2017;214(2):269–283.
12. Gares V, Panico L, Castagne R, et al. The role of the early social environment on Epstein Barr virus infection: a prospective observational design using the Millennium Cohort Study. *Epidemiol Infect.* 2017;145(16):3405–3412.
13. Balfour HH Jr, Odumade OA, Schmeling DO, et al. Behavioral, virologic, and immunologic factors associated with acquisition and severity of primary Epstein-Barr virus infection in university students. *J Infect Dis.* 2013;207(1):80–88.
14. Thompson DF, Ramos CL. Antibiotic-induced rash in patients with infectious mononucleosis. *Ann Pharmacother.* 2017;51(2):154–162.
15. Chovel-Sella A, Ben Tov A, Lahav E, et al. Incidence of rash after amoxicillin treatment in children with infectious mononucleosis. *Pediatrics.* 2013;131(5):e1424–e1427.
16. Hocqueloux L, Guinard J, Buret J, et al. Do penicillins really increase the frequency of a rash when given during Epstein-Barr Virus primary infection? *Clin Infect Dis.* 2013;57(11):1661–1662.
17. Sylvester JE, Buchanan BK, Paradise SL, et al. Association of splenic rupture and infectious mononucleosis: a retrospective analysis and review of return-to-play recommendations. *Sports Health.* 2019;11(6):543–549.
18. Bartlett A, Williams R, Hilton M. Splenic rupture in infectious mononucleosis: a systematic review of published case reports. *Injury.* 2016;47(3):531–538.
19. Lloyd AM, Reilly BK. Infectious mononucleosis and upper airway obstruction: intracapsular tonsillectomy and adenoidectomy with microdebrider for prompt relief. *Ear Nose Throat J.* 2021;100(10_suppl):958S–960S.
20. Kimura H, Cohen JI. Chronic active Epstein-Barr virus disease. *Front Immunol.* 2017;8:1867.
21. Marshall-Andon T, Heinz P. How to use... the Monospot and other heterophile antibody tests. *Arch Dis Child Educ Pract Ed.* 2017;102(4):188–1893.
22. Holm K, Svensson PJ, Rasmussen M. Invasive Fusobacterium necrophorum infections and Lemierre's syndrome: the role of thrombophilia and EBV. *Eur J Clin Microbiol Infect Dis.* 2015;34(11):2199–2207.
23. Ceraulo AS, Bytomski JR. Infectious mononucleosis management in athletes. *Clin Sports Med.* 2019;38(4):555–561.
24. Cohen JI, Dropulic L, Hsu AP, et al. Association of GATA2 deficiency with severe primary Epstein-Barr virus (EBV) infection and EBV-associated cancers. *Clin Infect Dis.* 2016;63(1):41–47.
25. Endriz J, Ho PP, Steinman L. Time correlation between mononucleosis and initial symptoms of MS. *Neurol Neuroimmunol Neuroinflamm.* 2017;4(3):e308.
26. Hedström AK, Huang J, Michel A, et al. High levels of Epstein-Barr virus nuclear antigen-1-specific antibodies and infectious mononucleosis act both independently and synergistically to increase multiple sclerosis risk. *Front Neurol.* 2020;10:1368.

⟨⟨ ADDITIONAL RESOURCES AND WEBSITES

Additional Resources and Websites for Clinicians:

Ceraulo AS, Bytomski JR. Infectious mononucleosis management in athletes. *Clin Sports Med.* 2019;38(4):555–561.

De Paor M, O'Brien K, Fahey T, Smith SM. Antiviral agents for infectious mononucleosis (glandular fever). *Cochrane Database Syst Rev.* 2016;12:CD011487.

Ebell MH, Call M, Shinholser J, et al. Does this patient have infectious mononucleosis?: the rational clinical examination systematic review. *JAMA.* 2016;315(14):1502–1509.

https://www.cdc.gov/epstein-barr/hcp.html

Rezk E, Nofal YH, Hamzeh A, et al. Steroids for symptom control in infectious mononucleosis. *Cochrane Database Syst Rev.* 2015(11):CD004402.

Womack J, Jimenez M. Common questions about infectious mononucleosis. *Am Fam Physician.* 2015;91(6):372–376.

Additional Resources and Websites for Parents/Caregivers:

JAMA Patient Pages: Ebell MH. Infectious mononucleosis. *JAMA.* 2016;315(14):1532. doi:10.1001/jama.2016.2474

https://kidshealth.org/en/parents/mono.html
https://my.clevelandclinic.org/health/diseases/13974-mononucleosis
https://www.cdc.gov/epstein-barr/about-mono.html
https://www.healthychildren.org/English/health-issues/conditions/infections/Pages/Mononucleosis.aspx

Additional Resources and Websites for Adolescents and Young Adults:

https://newsnetwork.mayoclinic.org/discussion/infectious-diseases-a-z-when-a-kiss-is-more-than-a-kiss/
https://youngmenshealthsite.org/guides/mono/
https://youngwomenshealth.org/2013/10/08/mononucleosis/
https://www.mayoclinic.org/diseases-conditions/mononucleosis/expert-answers/mononucleosis/faq-20058444
https://www.mayoclinic.org/diseases-conditions/mononucleosis/expert-answers/mononucleosis/faq-20058564

CHAPTER 34

Infectious Respiratory Illnesses

Terrill Bravender
Alison C. Tribble

KEY WORDS
- Coronavirus
- COVID-19
- Influenza
- *Mycoplasma pneumoniae*
- Pertussis
- Pneumonia
- SARS-CoV-2
- Vaccines

INTRODUCTION

Infectious respiratory illnesses are common reasons for adolescents and young adults (AYAs) to seek medical care. While the majority of such illnesses are minor and self-limited, some infections may be severe or even life threatening, particularly in those with comorbid health conditions. This chapter focuses on two bacterial (*Mycoplasma pneumoniae* and pertussis) and two viral (influenza and SARS-CoV-2) illnesses that frequently affect the AYA population.

MYCOPLASMA AND COMMUNITY-ACQUIRED PNEUMONIA

Community-acquired pneumonia (CAP) is the most common infectious cause of death in the world. Although the majority of these deaths are in the elderly, CAP is a serious cause of illness in children, resulting in more than 150,000 hospitalizations each year in the United States. However, in the absence of severe asthma or cardiac disease, AYAs are unlikely to develop severe illness: in a recent review of CAP hospitalizations, infants and young children had a CAP hospitalization rate of 62.2/10,000 whereas AYAs had a rate of 4.2/10,000.[1]

The diagnosis of CAP is often straight forward: (1) evidence of infection such as fever and/or leukocytosis, (2) lower respiratory-tract signs and symptoms such as cough, sputum production, chest pain, or abnormal chest examination, and (3) an infiltrate on chest x-ray. Widespread vaccination of the pediatric population with conjugate pneumococcal vaccine has significantly reduced the rates of pneumococcal pneumonia whereas atypical bacteria, like *M. pneumoniae,* continue to be a prominent cause of CAP in the AYA population. Clinicians should consider this, as well as clinical presentation, as they choose antibiotic coverage for CAP.[2] This section will focus on *Mycoplasma pneumoniae*, a common cause of pneumonia in adolescents that may be asymptomatic but is often associated with pharyngitis, tracheobronchitis, and otitis media.

Etiology and Pathophysiology

Mycoplasma spp are about the same size as large viruses (~150 to 250 nm). They are prokaryotes that do not have cell walls. Instead, they are bound by cell membranes containing sterols. Because they lack cell walls, they are resistant to β-lactam antibiotics but are sensitive to antibiotics that interfere with protein synthesis, such as macrolides and tetracyclines.

By means of attachment proteins, *M. pneumoniae* adhere to ciliated and nonciliated respiratory epithelium, causing cellular damage to the trachea, bronchi, and bronchioles. The organism also causes ciliostasis, which may lead to prolonged cough. Transmission to the respiratory tract is through aerosolized inhalation. There is a high rate of transmission to family members and other close contacts, with an incubation period of 3 to 4 weeks. Many of the nonpulmonary findings are related to the immune response to infection.

Epidemiology

Laboratory testing for *M. pneumoniae* is more common now that it is included on most respiratory pathogen panels, but there is no routine surveillance program in the United States so prevalence data are scarce. Infection is endemic in many areas and may result in cyclical epidemic outbreaks every few years. Localized outbreaks often occur in schools, military bases, summer camps, college dormitories, and prisons. *M. pneumoniae* is likely responsible for 4% to 8% of CAP but may rise to 40% during outbreaks and as high as 70% in closed populations.[3]

Clinical Manifestations

Symptoms are often insidious in onset, heralded by malaise, headache, and low-grade fever. Cough develops after 3 to 5 days. Though initially nonproductive, cough may progress to production of frothy white sputum. Sputum production is not as copious as in typical bacterial pneumonia. The cough may become paroxysmal and occasionally chest pain and hemoptysis occur. In patients with no prior history of asthma, dyspnea is uncommon. Patients may also have nasal congestion and rhinorrhea.

Individuals do not usually appear very ill, and physical findings are often minimal. When present, individuals may have mild pharyngitis, conjunctivitis, or lymphadenopathy. Bilateral bullous myringitis is suggestive of mycoplasma infection, but this is rare, and the previously reported association has been questioned.[4] Chest examination is usually benign. If pneumonia is present, there may be isolated crackles or areas of wheezing over one or both of the lower lobes. Signs of pleural effusion are occasionally present.

Complications

Nonrespiratory infections and complications may occur 1 to 21 days after initial respiratory symptoms, related either to invasive *M. pneumoniae* or cross-reacting antibodies. Reported complications include almost every organ system, including the development of arthralgias and arthritis, *M. pneumoniae*-induced rash and mucositis (MIRM), hemolytic anemia, Guillain–Barré syndrome, conjunctivitis, and uveitis. The community-acquired respiratory distress syndrome (CARDS) toxin has recently been identified and exhibits some sequence homology with pertussis toxin (PT).[3]

Laboratory Evaluation

Traditionally, cold agglutinins have been used for bedside diagnosis; however, polymerase chain reaction (PCR) testing on nasal wash, nasopharyngeal, or pharyngeal swab affords the most utility. Serology may be helpful in the evaluation of more severely ill patients, but acute and convalescent titers are required. The white blood count (WBC) is usually normal. Radiographic findings may appear worse than the clinical observations. Chest x-ray often has a peribronchial interstitial pattern, frequently in the lower lobes. Hilar adenopathy and pleural effusions may also be seen.

Differential Diagnosis

The differential diagnosis includes streptococcal pneumonia, viral pneumonia (such as adenovirus, parainfluenza, and influenza), *Chlamydophila pneumoniae*, and *Legionella* pneumonia. In at-risk individuals, one should also consider tuberculosis, Q fever (*Coxiella*), rickettsial infections, and fungal infections.

Diagnosis

The diagnosis of *Mycoplasma* infections is usually based on clinical suspicion. In rare instances, a more precise diagnosis may be required (see laboratory evaluation described earlier).

Management

Although most infections with *M. pneumoniae* are self-limited and resolve without treatment, antibiotic therapy has been shown to decrease the length and severity of illness in AYAs. Macrolides are the preferred agent, although there have been increasing reports of macrolide-resistant *M. pneumoniae* since the early 2000s, particularly in Asia. Between 70% and 85% of isolates in China are macrolide resistant, as are 10% to 12% in North America.[5] If symptoms persist and there is concern about resistance, the use of doxycycline or levofloxacin should be considered. Acceptable oral regimens include:

a. Azithromycin: 500 mg on day 1, then 250 mg daily on days 2 through 5
b. Clarithromycin: 500 mg twice a day for 7 days
c. Erythromycin: 500 mg four times a day for 7 days
d. Doxycycline: 100 mg twice a day for 7 days
e. Levofloxacin 500 mg daily for 7 days

PERTUSSIS

Pertussis, meaning "intense cough," is frequently unrecognized and underdiagnosed in AYAs. The term *pertussis* is more appropriate than "whooping cough," because many patients, particularly AYAs, do not "whoop." Pertussis infection continues to cause fatal illness in vulnerable neonates and incompletely immunized infants. Adolescents and young adults are a major source of infection for these vulnerable populations.

Etiology

Bordetella spp are small Gram-negative coccobacilli. *Bordetella pertussis* is the sole cause of epidemic pertussis, and the usual cause of sporadic pertussis. Only *B. pertussis* produces PT, which plays a major role in the virulence of the infection. *B. parapertussis* may occasionally cause pertussis, but accounts for fewer than 5% of *Bordetella* isolates in the United States.

Transmission is through close contact with respiratory secretions. Intrafamilial spread is common in both immunized and unimmunized individuals. The incubation period is usually 5 to 10 days but may be as long as 21 days. Pertussis is primarily a mucosal disease; although the organism may invade alveolar macrophages, there is no bacteremic phase of the illness.

Epidemiology

Despite widespread vaccination, epidemiologic modeling suggests that there are approximately 24 million annual cases of pertussis worldwide, resulting in about 160,000 deaths. More than 90% of cases are in parts of the world where vaccination rates remain very low. The incidence of pertussis demonstrates a cyclic pattern, with peaks occurring every 2 to 5 years; this was true in the prevaccine era as well as today. Before widespread vaccine use, pertussis was the leading cause of death due to infectious disease in children under 14 years old. Routine childhood vaccination led to a significant decrease in disease burden, and the rate of pertussis infection reached its lowest level in 1976. Since then, rates of infection have increased significantly, even in highly immunized populations. There have been several epidemic outbreaks in the United States, but even the interepidemic rates have not returned to the low levels of 1976. The number of reported cases in the United States increased from 4,570 in 1990, to 25,827 cases in 2004, prior to the introduction of the adolescent pertussis booster vaccine in 2005. Reported cases then declined, but have since risen again, skyrocketing to 48,277 in 2012. Most recently in 2019, 15,662 cases were reported.[6] Most of the recent increase in pertussis illness has been attributed to disease in AYAs, who now account for half of all cases in the United States. The increased infection burden is thought to be a combination of waning immunity, vaccine refusal, and improved recognition and diagnosis of the illness. In AYAs with a cough illness lasting more than 3 weeks, up to one-third are caused by *B. pertussis* infection.[7]

Clinical Manifestations

The clinical severity of pertussis varies widely and may be influenced by age, immunization history, degree of exposure, past antibiotic administration, and concomitant infections. Classic pertussis is divided into three stages:

Catarrhal: This begins after the incubation period with nasal congestion and rhinorrhea, sometimes accompanied by low-grade fever, sneezing, and watery eyes. Patients are most contagious in this stage, but the symptoms are indistinguishable from a routine upper respiratory-tract infection. These symptoms begin to wane after 1 to 2 weeks, as the paroxysmal stage begins.

Paroxysmal: The onset of cough marks the beginning of the paroxysmal stage. Initially dry and intermittent, the cough progresses to the paroxysms that are characteristic of pertussis. An otherwise well-appearing patient may have episodic coughing fits with choking, gasping, and feelings of strangulation and suffocation. A forceful inspiratory gasp sounding like a "whoop" is most frequently seen in young infants. Posttussive emesis is common. At its peak, these episodes may occur hourly.

Convalescent: During this stage, the number, severity, and duration of the coughing paroxysms diminish.

The duration of classic pertussis is 6 to 10 weeks. Adolescents and young adults, particularly those who have been immunized, are unlikely to show distinct stages of illness. Adolescents and young adults may complain only of coughing episodes, without fever or congestion, but the illness often leads to days or weeks of interrupted sleep and time away from school. The physical examination between coughing episodes may be completely normal.

Pertussis is most contagious from approximately 1 to 2 weeks before the onset of cough and for 2 to 3 weeks after coughing begins. Complications are primarily seen in infants and young children and include seizures, pneumonia, apnea, encephalopathy, and death. Adolescents and young adults rarely develop serious complications, but secondary bacterial pneumonia and adult-respiratory distress syndrome have been reported.

Laboratory Evaluation

Complete blood count: Profound leukocytosis with WBC counts from 15,000 to as high as 100,000/mm^3 due to an absolute lymphocytosis may be seen, particularly in the catarrhal phase, most commonly in infants and young children.

Nucleic acid amplification tests (NAATs): PCR assays are the most commonly used laboratory method for detecting pertussis. They are rapid, accurate, and are most sensitive within the first 3 weeks of cough. Sensitivity is decreased following 5 days of antibiotics and in immunized individuals but is still better than culture.

Culture: The incubation period is 10 to 14 days, so culture rarely guides treatment decisions. False-negative cultures may occur after the second week of illness, if antibiotics have been administered, or if specimens are not collected and transported properly.

Serology: IgG antibodies to PT may be used in AYAs whose immunity has waned. Serologic testing may be difficult to interpret, particularly in adolescents and young adults who have been immunized in the past year. Acute and convalescent samples are no longer used clinically because of the high number of immunized individuals and their typical presentation late in the course of illness.

Differential Diagnosis

The differential diagnosis includes adenoviral infection, mycoplasma pneumonia, chlamydia pneumonia, and influenza.

Diagnosis

Based on recommendations developed at the 2011 Global Pertussis Initiative Conference, pertussis should be suspected in patients over 10 years old who present with paroxysms of cough without fever plus one of the following: whoop, apnea, sweating episodes between paroxysms, posttussive emesis, or worsening symptoms at night.[8]

When clinical suspicion warrants, confirmatory testing should be performed. Specimens for PCR testing must be obtained from the posterior nasopharynx and not the anterior nasopharynx or throat. Alternatively, nasopharyngeal aspiration with saline may yield better diagnostic results, but is not always practical in the clinical setting. The proper test is based on symptom duration:

1. Cough <2 weeks: PCR
2. Cough for 2 to 4 weeks: PCR and serology
3. Cough >4 weeks: serology

Management

All cases of suspected or confirmed pertussis should receive appropriate antibiotic therapy. Treatment provided in the catarrhal stage may provide some clinical benefit; thereafter, the benefit is primarily to decrease the spread of infection. Any of the following oral antibiotics may be used, with azithromycin being the preferred agent:

1. Azithromycin 500 mg on day 1 and 250 mg on days 2 to 5
2. Clarithromycin 500 mg twice daily for 7 days
3. Erythromycin 500 mg 4 times daily for 7 to 14 days
4. Trimethoprim-sulfamethoxazole one double-strength tablet twice daily for 14 days may be used for those who are unable to tolerate macrolides.

Symptomatic treatment of cough with various agents, including corticosteroids, inhaled beta agonists, montelukast, and antihistamines have minimal impact and are not recommended.[9]

Control Measures

1. Treatment with a full course of antibiotics is indicated for all household contacts of an infected patient within 3 weeks of symptom onset in the index patient regardless of immunization status. Other high-risk contacts may be treated as well. The dose and duration of prophylactic antibiotics are the same as used for treatment. Prompt antibiotic administration can limit secondary transmission. Since pertussis immunity is not absolute, even those with subclinical disease may be able to transmit the illness to others. Treatment is particularly important for those who have close contact with infants or young children.
2. Close contacts who are unimmunized or underimmunized should have immunization initiated or continued as soon as possible.
3. Contacts of the infected individual should be monitored for symptoms for 21 days after the most recent contact.
4. Students with pertussis should be excluded from school. Individuals are considered noninfectious after 5 days of antibiotic therapy and may return to school then. If unable to take antibiotics, individuals are considered infectious for 21 days after the onset of cough.

Immunization

Universal pertussis immunization is recommended for children starting at 2 months of age and has been widely used in combination with diphtheria and tetanus toxoids (diphtheria, tetanus, pertussis [DTP]) since the 1940s. Less reactogenic acellular pertussis vaccines (DTaP), containing purified inactivated components of the *B. pertussis* organism, are highly effective and have replaced the use of the whole cell vaccine in the United States.

Natural and vaccine-induced immunity to pertussis wanes over time, leaving adolescents and adults susceptible to infection. Two acellular pertussis vaccines are licensed for use in adolescents (Tdap). Adolescents (age 11 to 18 years) who have completed the recommended childhood DTaP series should receive a Tdap booster, preferably at their 11- or 12-year annual visit. Females should receive a dose of Tdap during each pregnancy between 27- and 36-weeks gestation regardless of previous receipt of Tdap.[10]

● INFLUENZA

Influenza is an acute respiratory illness that is highly contagious, affects all age groups, and has caused epidemics for hundreds of years. Although most influenza infections in AYAs are self-limited, those with chronic illnesses such as asthma or cardiac disease may develop a serious life-threatening infection. Additionally, AYAs often serve as the reservoir for influenza, and those who are unvaccinated may be responsible for infecting high-risk individuals such as infants.[11]

Etiology

Influenza viruses are orthomyxoviruses that are enveloped with two important surface glycoproteins: hemagglutinin (HA) and neuraminidase (NA). Influenza viruses are classified as A, B, or C. Influenza A and B viruses are responsible for seasonal epidemics, whereas C virus is responsible for mild, common-cold–like illnesses. Influenza A viruses are further categorized into subtypes based on HA and NA. Since 1977, there have been two predominant circulating subtypes, influenza A (H1N1) and influenza A (H3N2). Influenza B is not subtyped. Influenza A and B are indistinguishable clinically, but influenza A (H3N2) viruses are generally associated with the most severe epidemics.

Influenza viruses are negative-sense RNA viruses that contain eight separate gene segments. During virus replication, point mutations in the gene segments can lead to minor antigenic virus variants. Minor antigenic changes occur frequently and lead to yearly epidemics of influenza illness. Transmission is person to person through respiratory droplets or by direct contact with articles recently contaminated by nasopharyngeal secretions. The incubation period is only 1 to 4 days and a single infected person may transmit the virus to a large number of susceptible individuals. Individuals are most infectious during the 24 hours before and through the peak of symptoms. Viral shedding continues for approximately 7 days after the onset of symptoms. Seasonal epidemics typically occur during the winter. Local outbreaks can peak within 2 weeks of onset and last 4 to 8 weeks.

Epidemiology

Although influenza may be sporadically identified through the year, epidemics typically occur annually during the winter months. Influenza A generally occurs annually, whereas influenza B recurs every 3 or 4 years. Local epidemics are maintained by high-infection rates in young children. During these outbreaks, infection rates may be as high as 40% for school-aged and preschool children, as opposed to infection rates in young adults of 10% to 20%. For most adolescents, influenza results in nothing more than a "bad cold;" however, it is a cause of morbidity, particularly among young children and those with underlying medical conditions. The severity of outbreaks varies widely depending on influenza variants and vaccine uptake and effectiveness. For the past 4 years, hospitalization rates have ranged from 42 to 74 hospitalizations per 100,000 population for those ages 0 to 4 years, 10 to 20 for those 5 to 17 years, and 17 to 33 for those 18 to 49 years.[12] Hospitalization rates for those with high-risk conditions such as asthma or heart disease may be as high as 200 per 100,000 population. The impact of the mitigation responses for the COVID-19 pandemic resulted in a dramatic decrease in influenza activity for the 2020 to 2021 season, with a 61% decrease in testing specimens and a 98% reduction in the number positive specimens in the United States. Similar decreases in influenza activity have been reported internationally.[13]

Clinical Manifestations

Patients typically develop sudden onset fever and chills associated with a nonproductive cough, myalgias, sore throat, malaise, and headache. The fever, often as high as 40°C, peaks within 24 hours of the onset of symptoms, and may last 5 days. The dry, hacking cough may persist for 1 week after other symptoms have resolved. Nausea, vomiting, and diarrhea, seen in younger children, are infrequent in AYAs. Patients appear unwell, with injected conjunctiva, hyperemic mucous membranes, and clear rhinorrhea.

Complications

Influenza has been associated with primary viral pneumonia, secondary bacterial pneumonia, encephalitis, encephalopathy, Guillain–Barré syndrome, Reye syndrome, myocarditis, and myositis.

Laboratory Evaluation

During influenza season, particularly during a known influenza outbreak, diagnostic testing using a nasopharyngeal swab or wash should be considered in any patient with acute febrile respiratory symptoms if the test results will influence clinical management, and should be obtained in patients being admitted to the hospital. Rapid NAATs provide results in 10 to 30 minutes but do not distinguish influenza A subtypes which may be detected by molecular assays such as reverse transcription-polymerase chain reaction (RT-PCR).

Differential Diagnosis

The differential diagnosis includes bacterial infections such as streptococcal pneumonia, chlamydial pneumonia, and mycoplasma pneumonia, as well viral infections such as adenovirus, parainfluenza, respiratory syncytial virus, and rhinovirus.

Diagnosis

Even during peak influenza activity, the clinical diagnosis of influenza can be difficult because many other circulating respiratory viruses cause similar symptoms. During episodes of peak disease activity, it is impractical to test every patient with signs and symptoms of influenza. Therefore, the diagnosis is often made based on the clinical presentation informed by the prior probability of influenza based on local rates of influenza activity. There are few data examining the validity of the clinical diagnosis of influenza in adolescents. The reported positive predictive value of the clinical diagnosis in adults varies widely from 18% to 87%, compared to laboratory-confirmed influenza. During a seasonal outbreak, the diagnosis should be considered in any adolescent or young adult with sudden onset of fever and dry, nonproductive cough.

Management

Most AYAs who contract influenza will require supportive care only. Ibuprofen or acetaminophen may be used for fever, headache, and myalgia. Patients should be advised not to use aspirin because of the potential for the development of Reye syndrome. Antiviral medications should be prescribed for patients with underlying illness (regardless of timing) and otherwise healthy patients who present for treatment within 48 hours of the onset of symptoms. These medications have been shown to decrease the time to symptom resolution by 1 to 2 days and to decrease viral shedding. Due to resistance, amantadine and rimantadine are no longer recommended. Neuraminidase inhibitors that block the release of virions from infected cells continue to be effective. Two are currently available, one oral and one an inhaled powder: (1) oseltamivir, 75 mg by mouth twice daily for 5 days and (2) zanamivir two inhalations (5 mg each inhalation) twice daily for 5 days. Zanamivir may induce bronchospasm and should not be used in individuals with asthma or other respiratory disease. Baloxavir is a selective inhibitor of influenza cap-dependent endonuclease and is approved for ages 12 years and up who weigh ≥40 kg. For those 40 to 80 kg, the dose is 40 mg once, orally, and for those 40 to 80 kg, the dose is 80 mg once, orally.[14]

Immunization

Annual universal immunization is strongly recommended.[14] Multiple influenza inactivated vaccines are available in quadrivalent and trivalent formulations. All quadrivalent vaccines contain influenza A(H1N1), Influenza A(H3N2), B/Victoria, and B/Yamagata components. Trivalent vaccines do not include the B/Yamagata component. All inactivated egg-based vaccines are licensed for children 6 months and older. There is one cell-culture–based vaccine licensed for children 4 years and older, one recombinant vaccine licensed for those 18 years and older, and a high-dose vaccine licensed only for those 65 years and older. Finally, a live attenuated quadrivalent vaccine (LAIV4) is administered using an intranasal sprayer. Use of LAIV4 should be restricted to healthy adolescents only and should not be administered to those with high-risk medical conditions. In those with a history of severe egg allergy, vaccination should be administered in an inpatient or outpatient setting under the supervision of a clinician able to manage severe allergic conditions. When vaccine supply is limited, priority should be given to individuals who are immunosuppressed or those with underlying chronic disease such as asthma, diabetes, hemoglobinopathies, and renal dysfunction. Additionally, all clinicians and individuals who plan to be pregnant during the influenza season should make special efforts to be vaccinated.

CORONAVIRUS DISEASE 2019 (COVID-19)

Coronavirus disease 2019 (COVID-19) is a clinical syndrome caused by severe acute respiratory syndrome coronavirus 2 (SARS-CoV-2). While endemic mild coronavirus infections have been described since the 1960s, the first serious outbreak occurred in China in 2002, when severe acute respiratory syndrome (SARS) was first described and found to be due to a novel coronavirus variant, SARS-CoV. An additional coronavirus variant emerged in

Saudi Arabia in 2012, the Middle East respiratory syndrome coronavirus (MERS-CoV). The extent of these outbreaks was minimal, due to the limited transmissibility of SARS-CoV and lack of human-to-human transmission of MERS-CoV, which is transmitted from dromedary camels to humans. In December 2019, an outbreak of viral pneumonia was identified in Wuhan, China, and was quickly identified as a novel coronavirus, SARS-CoV-2. In February 2020, the World Health Organization designated the clinical disease as COVID-19. Since initial identification of the COVID-19, the impact on populations has waxed and waned in relation to the implementation of pandemic precautions such as social distancing and masking, the background rates of immunization, and the emergence of viral variants. The most impactful viral variants to date have been delta (B.1.617.2) which was first identified in India in late 2020 and omicron (B.1.1.529) first identified in South Africa in late 2021. Both variants are more transmissible than the original alpha SARS-CoV-2 variant. Delta resulted in more severe disease than alpha, whereas omicron resulted in less severe disease in most affected individuals. By early 2022, almost one million people in the United States and more than six million people worldwide had died due to COVID-19.[15]

Fortunately, most children and AYAs with COVID-19 tend to have minimal symptoms. Detected infection in children was initially much lower than in adults, but rates of infection in children and AYAs have increased with subsequent variants and as precautions have decreased. University students and others living in communal environments are likely to have a high prevalence of infection if pre-existing immunity is low and minimal precautions are in place, but most will have asymptomatic infections or symptoms similar to the common cold. Adolescents and young adults may serve as a reservoir of infection fostering community spread, and a few may develop severe complications.

Etiology and Pathophysiology

Coronaviruses are large, enveloped, single-stranded RNA viruses that typically cause mild upper respiratory symptoms in immunocompetent hosts. Animal reservoirs include dogs, cats, cattle, pigs, and bats. Coronaviruses are so named due to the presences of surface spike proteins giving them the appearance of the sun's corona. Early in SARS-CoV-2 infection, these spike proteins bind to angiotensin-converting enzyme 2 (ACE2) receptors in nasal, bronchial, and alveolar epithelial cells.[16] Because of the involvement of ACE2 receptors, there was concern that upregulation of these receptors (such as in patients being treated with ACE inhibitors) might lead to greater susceptibility to severe complications, but this has not been borne out in outcomes research.[17]

Like other coronaviruses, SARS-CoV-2 is transmitted via respiratory droplets during face-to-face exposure. However, unlike most other coronaviruses, SARS-CoV-2 has also been found to be transmitted at longer distances via inhalation of fine droplets and aerosol particles.[18] Still, risk of exposure is greatest within 3 to 6 feet of an infectious source, particularly with sustained exposure (typically >15 minutes). Inadequate ventilation or increased exhalation of infectious particles, such as with physical exertion or raised voices, also increases risk of exposure. In the health care setting, aerosolizing procedures such as high-flow oxygen administration, suctioning, and nebulizer treatments may be high risk, emphasizing the importance of appropriate personal-protective equipment use by clinicians. Surface transmission, which was a concern in the early days of the pandemic, is an insignificant contributor to transmission. Host viral load peaks around the time of symptom onset, with viral shedding beginning about 2 days prior.

Clinical Manifestations

The clinical spectrum of infection ranges from asymptomatic to deadly. The incubation period with earlier variants was 4 to 5 days but is as short as 3 days with the omicron variant. Typical symptoms include fever, cough, sore throat, fatigue, and myalgia. Anosmia and/or ageusia is reported by at least half of symptomatic patients, more commonly in females than males. These sensory impairments may precede onset of respiratory symptoms, and persist for greater than 4 weeks in about 10% of those affected.[19] While the vast majority of children have minimal symptoms, almost one-third of hospitalized children with SARS-CoV-2 infection require ICU admissions or invasive mechanical ventilation. In a large, multicenter study, obesity, diabetes mellitus, feeding-tube dependence, and developmental delay emerged as risk factors for severe COVID-19 among children 2 to 17 years.[20] Still, risks for AYAs remain lower than adults who are at greater risk for complications if they are elderly, or have obesity, type 2 diabetes, cardiovascular disease, or chronic lung disease.

Complications

Although uncommon, some AYAs may develop acute, severe complications similar to adults. These complications often start as respiratory distress during the second week of illness, and case reports have included pneumonia, acute respiratory failure, acute respiratory distress syndrome, and acute kidney injury.[21] An uncommon complication seen in children is the Kawasaki-disease–like clinical syndrome called multisystem inflammatory syndrome in children (MIS-C)[22] (**Table 34.1**). In a study comparing severe acute COVID-19 to MIS-C, children ages 6 to 12 were more likely to have MIS-C whereas those ages 13 to 20 and with underlying medical conditions were more likely to have severe acute COVID-19.[23] Another poorly understood potential complication is what has been termed "long COVID" or "persistent post-COVID syndrome." Symptoms may include vascular fibrosis, impairment of cardiac and pulmonary function, chronic fatigue, and depression.[24]

Differential Diagnosis

COVID-19 should be suspected in any AYA with fever, cough, shortness of breath, myalgias, sore throat, loss of smell or taste, headache, or with a known exposure. Aside from anosmia and ageusia, these symptoms are nonspecific, and the differential diagnosis is extremely broad and should be informed by community prevalence of SARS-CoV-2, influenza, and other viral illnesses.

TABLE 34.1

Case Definition for Multisystem Inflammatory Syndrome in Children (MIS-C). Consider MIS-C in Any Pediatric Death with Evidence of SARS-CoV-2 Infection[22]

Age <21 y

Fever ≥38.0 °C for ≥24 h or a report of subjective fever for ≥24 h

Laboratory evidence of inflammation (including, but not limited to an elevated C-reactive protein, erythrocyte sedimentation rate, fibrinogen, procalcitonin, d-dimer, ferritin, lactic acid dehydrogenase [LDH], or interleukin 6 [IL-6], elevated neutrophils, reduced lymphocytes, and low albumin)

Clinically severe illness requiring hospitalization

Multisystem (>2) organ involvement (cardiac, renal, respiratory, hematologic, gastrointestinal, dermatologic, or neurological)

Positive for current or recent SARS-CoV-2 infection or exposure to a suspected or confirmed COVID-19 case within the 4 wk prior to onset of symptoms

No alternative plausible diagnosis

Diagnosis

In a pandemic setting, testing of AYAs with symptoms concerning for COVID-19, even if mild, or of those who have recently been exposed, is critical to interrupting SARS-CoV-2 transmission and reducing community burden of disease. Available tests to detect infection include antigen and NAATs. Nucleic acid amplification tests are highly sensitive and specific, and may be performed on nasal, nasopharyngeal, oropharyngeal, sputum, and saliva samples. These tests typically have turnaround times of 1 to 3 days; rapid NAAT platforms are also available, albeit with slightly lower sensitivity.[25] Antigen testing of nasal or nasopharyngeal specimens allows for rapid point-of-care testing, but sensitivity is inferior to NAATs. Antigen testing performs better in symptomatic individuals; for example, one platform was 80% sensitive in those with symptoms compared to 41% in those without.[26] Serology for SARS-CoV-2 is available but is less useful for detecting acute infection, as antibodies are not detected until 1 to 2 weeks after symptom onset.[27] However, antibody testing has been useful in detecting past infection, and in particular, for identifying MIS-C. The utility of serology may wane as community exposure and vaccination expand, although the long-term persistence of SARS-CoV-2 antibody is unknown.

Management

Adolescents and young adults with symptoms concerning for COVID-19 should undergo testing and isolate while awaiting test results. Quarantine and isolation recommendations continue to evolve, and clinicians and patients should consult local and national public heath guidance for up-to-date recommendations. The majority of AYAs will require only symptomatic care, and treatment with over-the-counter antipyretic and anti-inflammatory medications as appropriate. For AYAs with COVID-19 who are at high risk of progression to severe disease, targeted therapeutic options have become available. Monoclonal antibodies given to outpatients early in disease are effective in reducing hospitalization and death and have been granted emergency use authorization (EUA) by the U.S. Food and Drug Administration (FDA); however, as SARS-CoV-2 variants have evolved, efficacy of individual antibody preparations has waned. With the emergence of the omicron subvariant, BA.2, only bebtelovimab is expected to retain efficacy. Remdesivir is an FDA-approved intravenous antiviral for adults and pediatric patients ≥12 years and ≥40 kg who are hospitalized with COVID-19, but it has also shown efficacy when given in shorter courses to high-risk outpatients.[28] Additionally, two oral antivirals are available under EUA for outpatients at high risk of progression to severe COVID-19 with symptoms ≤5 days: Paxlovid (nirmatrelvir and ritonavir) for those ≥12 years and ≥40 kg and molnupiravir for those ≥18 years. Paxlovid has efficacy similar to monoclonal antibodies for preventing severe outcomes, but significant drug–drug interactions may limit its use. Molnupiravir lacks such interactions but is less effective and contraindicated in pregnancy. Given the evolving nature of SARS-CoV-2 variants and therapeutic options, clinicians should routinely seek updated information from infectious diseases experts and national health authorities (https://www.covid19treatmentguidelines.nih.gov/).

Even though AYAs rarely experience severe COVID-19, the mental health, educational, employment, and social consequences of the pandemic have been significant. In order to limit viral spread, schools and colleges have shifted to online learning, limiting educational activities and isolating AYAs from peers and other developmentally critical activities. This isolation combined with the limited availability of employment opportunities has created financial hardships and stress resulting in increased rates of mental-health concerns.[29] The effects of the pandemic may persist for years. Adolescents and young adults entering the workforce are seeking employment during the most severe economic contraction since the great depression and the economic impact on these youth may persist throughout their working careers.

Immunization

Vaccine development progressed in record time following the identification of SARS-CoV-2, with numerous candidates using a variety of platforms. Two vaccines utilizing a novel messenger RNA (mRNA) platform, manufactured by Moderna and Pfizer-BioNTech, were the first to receive EUA in the United States in December 2020. These vaccines deliver mRNA encoding the viral spike protein to cells by encasing it in a lipid nanoparticle coating, and initial studies demonstrated 94% to 95% efficacy for prevention of symptomatic COVID-19, including severe disease.[30,31] Authorization was expanded down to 12 years of age in May 2021, and a lower dose of the Pfizer-BioNTech vaccine was authorized for children 5 to 11 years in October 2021. Both vaccines are now FDA approved for 16 years (Pfizer-BioNTech) or 18 years (Moderna) and older. The initial series requires administration of two doses, 3 to 4 weeks apart, with an additional dose indicated for immunocompromised patients. A third single-dose vaccine produced by Johnson & Johnson, which uses a modified adenovirus as a vector for DNA encoding the viral spike protein, was shown to be 66% effective against symptomatic COVID-19, with high efficacy against hospitalization and death.[32] Emergency use authorization for this vaccine was granted by the United States in February 2021. As the pandemic progressed, booster vaccines began to be recommended in late 2021, and the timing of and the populations benefiting from subsequent boosters remains in development.

In addition to vaccination, a long-acting monoclonal antibody product, EVUSHELD (tixagevimab copackaged with cilgavimab), was authorized in December 2021, as pre-exposure prophylaxis for the highest risk immunocompromised patients not expected to have a reliable response to vaccination. In initial trials, EVUSHELD offered significant protection from symptomatic COVID-19 for 6 months,[33] though efficacy may evolve as new variants emerge.

 ## SUMMARY

While most infectious respiratory illnesses in AYAs are self-limited, determining the etiology of the infection is important, particularly with regard to *M. pneumoniae*, pertussis, influenza and SARS-CoV-2, to guide treatment and implement infection control measures. When available, vaccination plays an important role in limiting disease spread and should be strongly encouraged.

REFERENCES

1. Jain S, Williams DJ, Arnold SR, et al. Community-acquired pneumonia requiring hospitalization among U.S. children. *N Engl J Med*. 2015;372(9):835–845.
2. Bradley JS, Byington CL, Shah SS, et al. The management of community-acquired pneumonia in infants and children older than 3 months of age: clinical practice guidelines by the Pediatric Infectious Diseases Society and the Infectious Diseases Society of America. *Clin Infect Dis*. 2011;53(7):e25–e76.
3. Waites KB, Xiao L, Liu Y, et al. Mycoplasma pneumoniae from the respiratory tract and beyond. *Clin Micorbiol Rev*. 2017;30(3):747–809.
4. Mellick LB, Verma N. The mycoplasma pneumoniae and bullous myringitis myth. *Pediatr Emerg Care*. 2010;26(12):966–968.
5. Ho J, Ip M. Antibiotic-resistant community-acquired bacterial pneumonia. *Infect Dis Clin North Am*. 2019;33(4):1087–1103.
6. Centers for Disease Control and Prevention. *2019 Provisional Pertussis Surveillance Report*. 2020. https://www.cdc.gov/pertussis/downloads/pertuss-surv-report-2019-508.pdf Accessed March 5, 2021.
7. Kilgore PE, Salim AM, Zervos MJ, et al. Pertussis: microbiology, disease, treatment, and prevention. *Clin Micobiol Rev*. 2016;29(3):449–486.
8. Cherry JD, Tan T, Wirsing von König C-H, et al. Clinical definitions of pertussis: summary of a global pertussis initiative roundtable meeting, February 2011. *Clin Infect Dis*. 2012;54(12):1756–1764.
9. Wang K, Bettiol S, Thompson MJ, et al. Symptomatic treatment of the cough in whooping cough. *Cochrane Database Syst Rev*. 2014;(9):CD003257.
10. Liang JL, Tiwari T, Moro P, et al. Prevention of pertussis, tetanus, and diphtheria with vaccine in the United States: recommendations of the Advisory Committee on Immunization Practices (ACIP). *MMWR Recomm Rep*. 2018;67(2):1–44.
11. Dharan NJ, Sokolow LZ, Cheng P-Y, et al. Child, household, and caregiver characteristics associated with hospitalization for influenza among children 6–59 months of age: an emerging infections program study. *Pediatr Infect Dis J*. 2014;33(6):e141–e150.
12. Xu X, Blanton L, Elal AIA, et al. Update: influenza activity in the United States during the 2018–2019 season and composition of the 2019–20 influenza vaccine. *MMWR Morb Mortal Wkly Rep*. 2019;68(24):544–551.

13. Olson SJ, Azziz-Baumgartner E, Budd AP, et al. Decreased influenza activity during the COVID-19 pandemic—United States, Australia, Chile, and South Africa, 2020. *MMWR Morb Mortal Wkly Rep.* 2020;69(37):1305–1309.

14. American Academy of Pediatrics Committee on Infectious Diseases. Recommendations for prevention and control of influenza in children, 2020–2021. *Pediatrics.* 2020;146(4):e2020024588.

15. Johns Hopkins Coronavirus Resource Center, https://coronavirus.jhu.edu/, Accessed March 30, 2022.

16. Wiersinga WJ, Rhodes A, Cheng AC, et al. Pathophysiology, transmission, diagnosis, and treatment of coronavirus disease 2019 (COVID-19). *JAMA.* 2020;324(8):782–793.

17. Armstrong K, Soltoff A, Rieu-Werden M, et al. Use of angiotensin converting enzyme inhibitors and angiotensin receptor blockers associated with lower risk of COVID-19 in household contacts. *PLOS One.* 2021;16(3):e0247548.

18. Centers for Disease Control and Prevention. *Scientific Brief: SARS-CoV-2 Transmission.* 2021. https://www.cdc.gov/coronavirus/2019-ncov/science/science-briefs/sars-cov-2-transmission.html?CDC_AA_refVal=https%3A%2F%2Fwww.cdc.gov%2Fcoronavirus%2F2019-ncov%2Fscience%2Fscience-briefs%2Fscientific-brief-sars-cov-2.html. Accessed April 3, 2022.

19. Mastrangelo A, Bonato M, Cinque P. Smell and taste disorders in COVID-19: from pathogenesis to clinical features and outcomes. *Neurosci Lett.* 2021;748:135694.

20. Woodruff RC, Campbell AP, Taylor CA, et al. Risk factors for severe COVID-19 in children. *Pediatrics.* 2021;e2021053418. doi: 10.1542/peds.2021-053418.

21. Rankin DA, Ralj R, Howard LM, et al. Epidemiologic trends and characteristics of SARS-CoV-2 infections among children in the United States. *Curr Opin Pediatr.* 2021;33(1):114–121.

22. Centers for Disease Control and Prevention. *Information for Healthcare Providers about Multisystem Inflammatory Syndrome in Children (MIS-C), Case Definition for MIS-C.* 2020. https://www.cdc.gov/mis-c/hcp/ Accessed March 5, 2021.

23. Feldstein LR, Tenforde MW, Friedman KG, et al. Characteristics and outcomes of US children and adolescents with multisystem inflammatory syndrome in children (MIS-C) compared with severe acute COVID-19. *JAMA.* 2021;325(11):1074–1087.

24. Oronsky B, Larson C, Hammond TC, et al. A review of persistent post-COVID syndrome (PPCS). *Clin Rev Allergy Immunol.* 2021;1–9.

25. Centers for Disease Control and Prevention. *Overview of Testing for SARS-CoV-2 (COVID-19).* 2021. https://www.cdc.gov/coronavirus/2019-ncov/hcp/testing-overview.html Accessed March 21, 2021.

26. Pray IW, Ford L, Cole D, et al. Performance of an antigen-based test for asymptomatic and symptomatic SARS-CoV-2 testing at two university campuses–wisconsin, September–October 2020. *MMWR Morb Mortal Wkly Rep.* 2021;69(5152):1642–1647.

27. Long Q-X, Liu B-Z, Deng H-J, et al. Antibody responses to SARS-CoV-2 in patients with COVID-19. *Nat Med.* 2020;26(6):845–848.

28. Gottlieb RL, Vaca CE, Paredes R, et al. Early remdesivir to prevent progression to severe covid-19 in outpatients. *N Engl J Med.* 2022;386(4):305–315.

29. Jones HE, Manze M, Ngo V, et al. The impact of the COVID-19 pandemic on college students' health and financial stability in New York city: findings from a population-based sample of City University of New York (CUNY) students. *J Urban Health.* 2021;98(2):187–196.

30. Polack FP, Thomas SJ, Kitchin N, et al. Safety and efficacy of the BNT162b2 mRNA Covid-19 vaccine. *N Engl J Med.* 2020;383(27):2603–2615.

31. Baden LR, El Sahly HM, Essink B, et al. Efficacy and safety of the mRNA-1273 SARS-CoV-2 vaccine. *N Engl J Med.* 2021;384(5):403–416.

32. Oliver SE, Gargano JW, Scobie H, et al. The advisory committee on immunization practices' interim recommendation for use of janssen COVID-19 vaccine—United States, February 2021. *MMWR Morb Mortal Wkly Rep.* 2021;70(9):329–332.

33. Tixagevimab and Cilgavimab (Evusheld) for pre-exposure prophylaxis of COVID-19. *JAMA.* 2022;327(4):384–385.

ADDITIONAL RESOURCES AND WEBSITES

Additional Resources and Websites for Clinicians:

American Academy of Pediatrics, Red Book Online—https://redbook.solutions.aap.org/

Centers for Disease Control and Prevention, Healthcare Workers: Information on COVID-19—https://www.cdc.gov/coronavirus/2019-ncov/hcp/index.html

Centers for Disease Control and Prevention, Mycoplasma pneumoniae Infections, For Clinicians and Laboratories—https://www.cdc.gov/pneumonia/atypical/mycoplasma/hcp/index.html

Centers for Disease Control and Prevention, Pertussis (Whooping Cough) Information for Healthcare Professionals—https://www.cdc.gov/pertussis/materials/hcp.html

Centers for Disease Control and Prevention, Seasonal Influenza Information for Health Professionals—https://www.cdc.gov/flu/professionals/index.htm

Johns Hopkins University Coronavirus Resource Center—https://coronavirus.jhu.edu/

Additional Resources and Websites for Parents/Caregivers:

American Academy of Pediatrics, healthychildren.org COVID-19—https://www.healthychildren.org/English/health-issues/conditions/COVID-19/Pages/default.aspx

Centers for Disease Control and Prevention, COVID-19, Information for parents and caregivers about COVID-19 in children and teens—https://www.cdc.gov/coronavirus/2019-ncov/daily-life-coping/children/symptoms.html

Centers for Disease Control and Prevention, COVID-19 Parental Resources Kit—Adolescence—https://www.cdc.gov/coronavirus/2019-ncov/daily-life-coping/parental-resource-kit/adolescence.html

Society for Adolescent Health and Medicine, COVID-19: Resources for Parents and Teens—https://www.adolescenthealth.org/COVID-19/COVID-19-Resources-for-Parents-and-Teens.aspx

United States, Department of Health and Human Services, Combat COVID—https://combatcovid.hhs.gov/

United States National Library of Medicine, Medline Plus: Pneumonia—https://medlineplus.gov/pneumonia.html

United States National Library of Medicine, Medline Plus: Whooping Cough—https://medlineplus.gov/whoopingcough.html

Additional Resources and Websites for Adolescents and Young Adults:

American College Health Association, Resources, Influenza—https://www.acha.org/ACHA/Resources/Topics/Flu.aspx

The Government of Canada: COVID-19 Resources for Youth, Students, and Young Adults—https://www.canada.ca/en/public-health/services/diseases/coronavirus-disease-covid-19/resources-youth-students.html

The Jed Foundation, COVID-19 Resource Guide for Students, Teens, & Young Adults—https://www.jedfoundation.org/covid-19-resource-guide-for-students-teens-young-adults/

Society for Adolescent Health and Medicine, COVID-19: Resources for Parents and Teens—https://www.adolescenthealth.org/COVID-19/COVID-19-Resources-for-Parents-and-Teens.aspx

University of Michigan Department of Psychiatry, Coping with the COVID-19 Pandemic as a College Student—https://medicine.umich.edu/dept/psychiatry/michigan-psychiatry-resources-covid-19/adults-specific-resources/coping-covid-19-pandemic-college-student

CHAPTER 35

Viral Hepatitis

Mary E. Romano
Anita K. Pai

KEY WORDS
- Hepatitis A
- Hepatitis B
- Hepatitis C
- Hepatitis vaccine
- Viral hepatitis

INTRODUCTION

Hepatitis refers to inflammation of the liver due to infectious or noninfectious causes. Infectious causes include hepatitis A, B, C, D, and E, Epstein–Barr virus, and cytomegalovirus. This chapter will discuss hepatitis A, B, C, D, and E.

HEPATITIS A

Hepatitis A virus (HAV) is a nonenveloped, small, single-stranded ribonucleic acid (RNA) virus in the *Picornaviridae* family. Only one serotype has been identified.

Epidemiology

Implementation of HAV vaccination decreased the incidence of HAV, but there was an 850% increased incidence from 2014 to 2018. This was attributed to community outbreaks among those experiencing homelessness and using illicit drugs.[1] More than half of HAV cases now occur in persons 30 to 49 years of age. When risk factors were reported, 50% reported intravenous (IV) drug use. Food-borne epidemics have occurred related to sewage-polluted waters, poor hygiene by fruit handlers, and contamination during food preparation. Outbreaks are monitored by the U.S. Centers for Disease Control (CDC), U.S. Food and Drug Administration (FDA), and U.S. Department of Health and Human Services (see Additional Resources).

Clinical Course

Hepatitis A replicates in the liver, is excreted in bile, and is shed in the stool, where it is the most highly concentrated. Transmission occurs via the fecal–oral route, contaminated food or water, sexual contact, and illicit drug use. Hepatitis A can be transmitted through close personal contact in group settings. It has an incubation period of 28 days with a range of 15 to 50 days.[1] Viral shedding and peak infectivity are highest 2 weeks before symptoms begin until 1 week after symptom onset. Infected children shed the virus longer than adults. Children <6 years are typically asymptomatic, have prolonged stool shedding of virus, and often go undiagnosed, making them an important infection source.[1]

Symptoms vary by age and patients may have a prodrome of malaise, vomiting, anorexia, or abdominal pain before the abrupt onset of fever, vomiting, abdominal pain, jaundice, or pruritus.

Adolescents and young adults (AYAs) are more likely to be symptomatic with jaundice, occurring in 70% of infected individuals.[2] Approximately 80% of adults will have severe hepatitis.[2] Clinical infection does not last longer than 2 months although 10% to 15% of symptomatic persons have prolonged or relapsing disease for up to 6 months.[2]

Chronic infection does not occur. Most infected individuals will recover with no permanent damage and it is rarely fatal among older people and/or those with underlying liver disease.[2] Extrahepatic complications include pancreatitis, pericarditis, thrombocytopenia, autoimmune hemolytic anemia, vasculitis, nephrotic syndrome, and Guillain–Barré syndrome. Relapsing HAV can occur, with a second episode of cholestatic hepatitis within 6 to 10 weeks of the first episode.

Viral Antigens and Antibodies

Acute HAV is defined by the presence of immunoglobulin M (IgM) antibody to HAV (IgM anti-HAV).[3] Figure 35.1 details the course of HAV serology.[1] Detection of IgM anti-HAV is >95% sensitive and specific for HAV and can be detected 5 to 10 days from exposure and shortly after vaccination. It remains positive for up to 6 months.[3] Immunoglobulin G (IgG) antibody to HAV (IgG anti-HAV) is present at the onset of disease and remains detectable. It is also present after vaccination. IgG confers lifelong immunity.

Treatment

Acute infection usually clears spontaneously and does not require therapy. Supportive care is recommended. There are no dietary restrictions, but patients should avoid alcohol. Patients should be monitored for signs of acute liver failure and if these develop, they should be transferred to a liver transplant center.

Prevention and Prophylaxis

The virus can survive outside of the body. Heating food and liquids to temperatures of 85 °C for at least 1 minute kills the virus.[1] Adequate hand hygiene, water sanitation, and food hygiene are essential to preventing infection. Travelers to endemic areas should be vaccinated and counseled about preventative measures. Hepatitis A vaccine and human serum immunoglobulin (HSIG) are available for prophylaxis.

Hepatitis A Vaccine

Vaccination is recommended for pre- and postexposure prophylaxis. Vaccination is recommended for all children and adolescents 12 months to 18 years, people at increased risk for HAV infection, people at increased risk for severe disease from HAV infection, and at risk/unvaccinated persons during outbreaks.[4] Table 35.1 outlines specific risk factors.

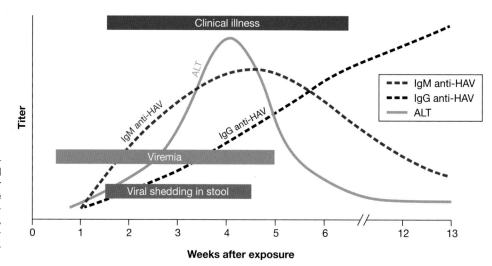

FIGURE 35.1 Immunologic course of hepatitis A virus infection with associated clinical and laboratory findings. Viremia occurs prior to onset of clinical symptoms. A carrier state does not occur and IgG antibodies are persistent and protective following infection. HAV, hepatitis A virus; anti-HAV, antibodies to hepatitis A virus; ALT, alanine aminotransferase. (Adapted from www.cdc.gov/hepatitis)

There are two single-antigen vaccines, HAVRIX (GlaxoSmithKline) and VAQTA (Merck), and one combination vaccine, Twinrix (GlaxoSmithKline), licensed for use in the United States. Single-antigen vaccines are available in pediatric and adult formulations for those ≥12 months. Twinrix, a combination HAV and HBV vaccine, is for use in persons ≥18 years. Dosing of all vaccines is 0.5 mL in persons ≤18 years and 1 mL for persons ≥19 years.

Single-antigen vaccines are given on a 2-dose schedule with a minimum interval of 6 months and a maximum interval of 12 months. If the series is interrupted/delayed, it does not need to be restarted. If the second dose is given in less than 6 months, it is invalid and needs to be repeated 6 months after the early second dose was given. Twinrix is given in a 3-dose series over 6 months.[4]

Efficacy An adequate/protective response to vaccination is defined as IgG anti-HAV levels of ≥10 mIU/mL. Levels of antibodies following vaccination are 10- to 100-fold lower than those seen with infection.[5] Adolescents and young adults have a good response to the vaccine with 97% of persons achieving appropriate antibody levels 1 month after the first dose and 100% within 1 month of the second dose.[4]

The exact duration of antibody protection after vaccination is unknown. In several studies, anti-HAV has been shown to remain ≥10 mIU/mL for at least 20 years in most adults vaccinated as

both children and adults. There is evidence of waning immunity beyond 20 years, although response to booster dosing indicates immune memory and ongoing protection. Individuals demonstrating decreased antibody response 1 month postvaccination include persons with immunocompromising conditions, human immunodeficiency virus (HIV) positive persons with low CD4 counts, and liver transplant recipients.[4]

Pre/Postvaccination Testing Prevaccination testing is only recommended in populations where there are high rates of HAV infection.[4] Postvaccination testing is not recommended except in individuals at risk for poor/inadequate response.[4]

There are limited data on revaccination, but it should be considered in persons who did not mount an adequate response following vaccination.[4] Revaccinated patients should be rechecked 1 month after vaccination. There is no evidence to support repeating the series again and those who fail to mount an adequate response with revaccination should be considered susceptible to HAV.

Human Serum Immunoglobulin

Human serum immunoglobulin protects against HAV (and measles, mumps and rubella) via the passive transfer of antibodies. GamaSTAN is the only FDA-approved HSIG available.[4] It is given intramuscularly and can be used for pre- or postexposure prophylaxis. Live virus vaccines can interact with HSIG and should be given at least 2 weeks prior or 6 months after HSIG administration.

Hepatitis A Virus Pre-exposure Prophylaxis If HSIG is used for travel pre-exposure prophylaxis, the dose is 0.1 mL/kg for 1 month of travel and 0.2 mL/kg for ≥2 months of travel. If extended travel is expected, HSIG should be given every 2 months for the duration of travel. Vaccination should also be given to unvaccinated individuals ≥6 months at a separate injection site. If vaccine series cannot be completed prior to travel/exposure, a single-antigen vaccine will induce an adequate response in most individuals within 2 weeks. A booster should be given 6 to 18 months following this dose.[4]

Hepatitis A Virus Postexposure Prophylaxis (PEP) Vaccination is recommended as soon as possible after exposure in unvaccinated persons ≥12 months. Infection risk is greatest with household contacts and sexual exposure. Household transmission rates are higher for infected children than for AYAs. Unvaccinated individuals should complete the series, but it is not required for PEP. Human serum immunoglobulin should also be given at a separate injection site (0.1 mL/kg) in high-risk individuals.[4] Efficacy of PEP has only been proven if given within 2 weeks of exposure.

TABLE 35.1

Populations at Increased Risk of Hepatitis A Infection

- **Populations at increased risk for HAV infection**
  - International travelers
  - Men who have sex with men
  - People who use drugs (injection or noninjection) and all those who use illegal drugs
  - People with occupational risk for exposure
  - People who anticipate close personal contact with an international adoptee
  - People experiencing homelessness
  - People living in group settings for those with developmental disabilities
  - People who are incarcerated

- **Populations at increased risk for severe disease from HAV infection**
  - People with chronic liver disease
  - People with human immunodeficiency virus infection
  - People ≥40 y of age
  - Pregnant females at risk for HAV infection or severe outcome from HAV infection

Considerations in Pregnancy

Vertical transmission of HAV is rare but has been reported. Preterm labor has been reported in >60% of females with infection during pregnancy. There is no risk to the infant from breastfeeding.[5] The CDC recommends vaccinating any pregnant woman who is identified to be at risk for HAV infection or who has risk of a serious outcome from infection.[4]

 HEPATITIS B

Hepatitis B virus (HBV) is a deoxyribonucleic acid (DNA) virus in the *Hepadnaviridae* family and includes genotypes A through J.

Epidemiology

Hepatitis B virus is transmitted through percutaneous or mucosal exposure to infected bodily fluids and/or blood. Exposure can occur through perinatal exposure, sexual contact, contaminated needles, or close personal contact with an infected individual. Among adults with HBV, about 50% report no risk factors for HBV infection.[6] Among those with risk factors, IV drug use and multiple sex partners are most commonly reported.[6]

Hepatitis B virus rates are low in children and adolescents. More than half of all acute infections occur in persons 30 to 49 years.[1] Prevalence has decreased in the United States, attributable to vaccination and a national strategy to eliminate infection.

The U.S. Preventive Services Task Force (USPSTF) recommends screening all at-risk AYAs including those that are HIV positive, have a household contact or sexual partner with HBV, engage in behaviors that would put them at risk, were born in countries with HBV prevalence >2%, or unvaccinated U.S.-born persons whose parents were born in regions of high prevalence.[7]

Clinical Course

Acute infection can vary from subclinical hepatitis to acute liver failure. Hepatitis B virus has an incubation period of 90 days with a range of 60 to 150 days. In symptomatic individuals, prodromal symptoms last about 10 days prior to onset of jaundice and may include a serum-sickness–like syndrome with fever, rash, and arthralgia. Jaundice lasts 1 to 3 weeks although malaise and fatigue may last up to 6 months.

Most children <10 years with HBV are asymptomatic. Perinatal acquisition is almost always asymptomatic. In contrast, up to 50% of those >10 years will have symptomatic infection.[2] Infection can also be associated with extrahepatic manifestations including rash, arthritis/arthralgias, cryoglobulinemia, thrombocytopenia, glomerulonephritis, Gianotti–Crosti syndrome (papular acrodermatitis), and polyarteritis nodosa.[2]

Progression to chronic HBV is most likely to occur in those with perinatal infection and occurs in 5% of persons who are infected as adults. Most individuals with chronic HBV are asymptomatic but still able to transmit infection. Approximately 15% to 25% of persons with chronic HBV will develop chronic liver disease including liver cancer. This is related to age of infection: 25% of people who become chronically infected during childhood and 15% of those who become chronically infected during adulthood die prematurely from cirrhosis or liver cancer.[2]

Viral Antigens and Antibodies

Acute HBV is diagnosed with the presence of hepatitis B surface antigen (HBsAg) *and* IgM antibody to HBV core antigen (IgM anti-HBc).[3] Figure 35.2A details the course of HBV serology in an acute infection. Table 35.2 outlines the interpretation of serologic test results.

Hepatitis B surface antigen can be detected 1 to 9 weeks after exposure and often precedes clinical symptoms. Hepatitis B virus DNA is a marker of infectivity and may be detectable before HBsAg

TABLE 35.2

Serologic Interpretation of Laboratory Screening for HBV

Serologic Test Results	HBsAg	Total anti-HBc	IgM Anti-HBc	Anti-HBs
Detected following vaccination or for 3–6 mo following receipt of HBIG	−	−	−	+
False positive (susceptible)				
Past infection (resolved)	−	+	−	−
"Low-level" chronic infection (unlikely to be infectious)				
Chronic infection	+	+	−	−
Past infection, with recovery, immunity to new infection	−	+	−	+
Acute infection	−	+	+	−
Early acute infection or recent vaccination	+	−	−	−
Never infected	−	−	−	−

HBsAg, HBV surface antigen; anti-HBc, antibody to HBV core antigen; anti-HBs, antibody to HBV surface antigen.
Adapted from www.cdc.gov/hepatitis

in acute infection. Following recovery from acute HBV, HBsAg, and HBV DNA wane over 4 to 6 months. Resolution of HBsAg is followed by detection of antibody to hepatitis B surface antigen (anti-HBs), a marker of immunity to HBV. There may be a "window period" in acute HBV, during which neither HBsAg nor anti-HBs is detectable. IgM antibody to HBV core antigen, a marker of acute HBV infection, may be the only detectable marker of infection during the "window period."[3,8]

The presence of HBsAg for >6 months indicates chronic infection. Figure 35.2B details the course of HBV serology in chronic infection.[3,8] Antibodies to hepatitis B core antigen (total anti-HBc), persists indefinitely as a marker of past infection.[3] Hepatitis B e-antigen (HBeAg) is another marker of HBV infectivity and active HBV replication. Seroconversion of HBeAg to anti-HBe heralds a period of remission and lower viral load.[3,8] Chronic HBV has distinct phases marked by varying rates of HBV replication and disease activity as is shown in Figure 35.2C. Monitoring DNA levels helps to determine the phase of infection and timing of therapy. Patients may transition between and/or may not go through all phases.[8]

Treatment

Infected patients should be counseled on how to minimize transmission. See Table 35.3 for specific recommendations.

Symptomatic Acute Hepatitis B Infection

Most immunocompetent adults with acute infection do not require therapy as >95% will spontaneously recover. Patients with severe infection progressing toward liver failure should be evaluated for transplantation and oral antiviral therapy may be indicated. Therapy should be continued until HBsAg is cleared or continue indefinitely if transplant occurs.[8]

Chronic Hepatitis B Infection

Treatment decisions are determined by phase of infection, genotype, existing comorbidities, and prior exposure or resistance to

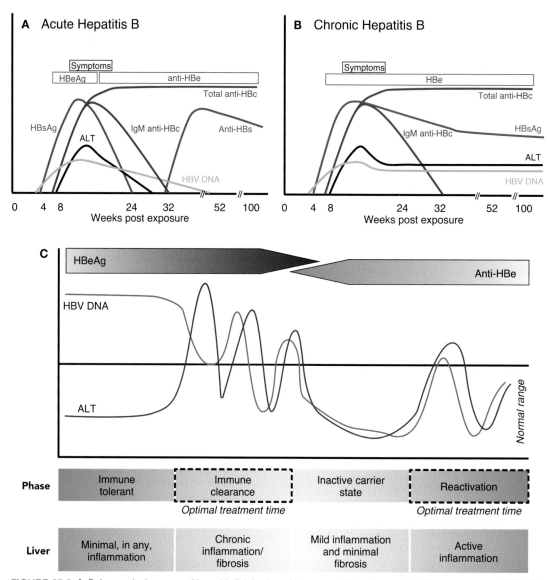

FIGURE 35.2 A, B: Immunologic course of hepatitis B infection with recovery. There is resolution/disappearance of HBV DNA, HBsAg, and HBeAg. **C:** Phases of chronic hepatitis B infection as determined by biochemical, virologic, and histologic activity of disease. HBV, hepatitis B virus; HBsAg, HBV surface antigen; anti-HBc, antibody to HBV core antigen; anti-HBs, antibody to HBV surface antigen; anti-HBe, antibody to HBV e-antigen; ALT, alanine aminotransferase. (A, B: Used with permission from Knipe DM. *Fields Virology.* 6th ed. Wolters Kluwer; 2013.)

HBV medications.[8] For those with inactive disease, annual testing to determine the presence of HBsAg is recommended.[8] The optimal timing of therapy is in the immune-active or reactivation phase with the goal being suppression of HBV DNA. Treatment decisions are also based on the presence of cirrhosis, HBeAg, degree of the aspartate transaminase (AST)/alanine transaminase (ALT) elevation, and HBV DNA levels.

Coinfection with hepatitis C (HCV), hepatitis D (HDV), or HIV will affect treatment. Patients who become immunocompromised may have a change in disease status necessitating a change in treatment. The American Association for the Study of Liver Diseases (AASLD) has developed guidance for HBsAg-positive recipients of liver transplants and HBV management in nonliver solid organ transplant recipients. In these patients, close monitoring of disease status is necessary.[8]

Prevention and Prophylaxis

Vaccination and HBV immunoglobulin (HBIG) are available for prophylaxis.

TABLE 35.3

Recommendations for Reducing Hepatitis B Transmission

People who are HBsAg POSITIVE should
- Have household and sexual contacts vaccinated
- Use barrier protection during sex if partner is unvaccinated or not immune
- Avoid sharing toothbrushes or razors
- Avoid sharing needles and glucose monitors
- Cover open cuts, scratches, sores
- Clean blood/bodily fluid with bleach solution
- Avoid donating blood, organs, or sperm

People who are HBsAG POSITIVE
- Can participate in all activities including contact sports
- Should not be excluded from daycare or school and should not be isolated from other children/peers
- Can share food and utensils and kiss others

HBsAg, HBV surface antigen; anti-HBc, antibody to HBV core antigen; anti-HBs, antibody to HBV surface antigen.

TABLE 35.4

Populations at Increased Risk of Hepatitis B Infection

- **Sexual Exposure**
  - People with partners who are HBsAg positive
  - People having >1 sex partner in the past 6 mo
  - People with a sexually transmitted infection
  - Men who have sex with men
- **Percutaneous or mucosal exposure to blood**
  - People who currently or have ever used intravenous drugs
  - Household contacts of individuals who are HBsAg positive
  - People living or working in a facility for the developmentally disabled
  - Health care workers with occupational exposure risk
  - People receiving hemodialysis
  - People with diabetes
- **Other people at risk for HBV infection**
  - Travelers to countries with HBsAg prevalence of ≥2%
  - People with hepatitis C virus infection
  - People with chronic liver disease
  - People with HIV infection
  - People who are incarcerated

Hepatitis B Vaccine

Vaccination is recommended for infants, children, and adolescents <19 years, persons at risk from exposure, other persons at risk for HBV infection, patients with chronic liver disease, and all persons seeking protection from infection. Table 35.4 outlines specific risk factors.

There are three single-antigen vaccines (Energix-B, Recombivax HB, and Heplisav-B) and two combination vaccines (PEDIARIX and TWINRIX). Heplisav-B is approved for persons ≥18 years, PEDIARIX for children between 6 weeks and 7 years, and TWINRIX for those ≥18 years. Vaccines are safe in pregnancy. Adverse reactions include soreness at the injection site, low-grade fever, myalgia, arthralgia, headache, and malaise.[6]

For AYAs, the vaccine schedule includes three intramuscular injections of a single-antigen vaccine given at 0, 1, and 6 months. There are alternate schedules approved with certain vaccines and/or specific patient populations. Immunocompromised persons should receive larger and/or additional doses. If the series is interrupted after the first dose, the second dose should be administered as soon as possible with the second and third doses separated by at least 8 weeks. If the vaccine series is interrupted after the second dose, the third dose should be administered as soon as possible.[6]

Efficacy A protective antibody response is seen in 95% of infants, children, and adolescents and 90% of adults ≤40 years following vaccination. All persons with anti-HBsAg levels >10 IU/mL following vaccination are considered to have mounted an adequate response. Risk factors for an inadequate response include older age, smoking, obesity, male sex, substance use, obesity, renal failure, diabetes, or any immunocompromising condition/medication that results in immunosuppression.[6]

All persons with initial antibody levels >10 IU/mL remain protected despite declining antibody levels which occurs in all persons postvaccination. Persons vaccinated at >1 year of age are more likely to have protective antibody levels 18 years postvaccination (74%) as compared to those who were vaccinated at <1 year of age (16%).[6]

Pre/Postvaccination Testing Adults at risk for infection should have complete serologic testing prior to vaccine administration. The vaccine can be administered without results as there is no risk in giving the vaccine to someone with unknown HBV status.[1]

Postvaccination testing should be done at 1 to 6 months and is recommended when immune status will direct clinical management. Testing is recommended in AYAs with ongoing occupational-exposure risk, on hemodialysis, with HIV or other immunocompromising conditions or those with sexual partner(s) with chronic HBV.[1]

Revaccination is recommended in certain populations.[6] Adolescents and young adults with ongoing occupational exposure should receive a booster dose and if levels remain inadequate, they should be revaccinated. Persons receiving hemodialysis should have antibody levels checked annually and a booster dose given if levels fall. Recommendations for other immunocompromised persons have not yet been determined. There is no maximum number of booster doses recommended and it is not recommended to repeat the series more than twice. Persons who do not have adequate antibody levels after revaccination should be considered at risk for HBV infection.

Hepatitis B Immunoglobulin

Hepatitis B immunoglobulin provides passive protection against HBV and is indicated after exposure in susceptible persons including infants born to HBsAg-positive mothers, unimmunized/partially immunized individuals, known vaccine nonresponders, sexual contacts of person with acute infection, and parenteral exposure to HBsAg-positive blood. HepaGam B and Nabi-HB are licensed for use in the United States. Vaccination is recommended at the same time at a separate injection site.[6]

Hepatitis B Postexposure Prophylaxis Postexposure prophylaxis should be given within 7 days for percutaneous/mucosal exposure and 14 days for sexual exposure.[6] Wounds and mucous membranes that have been in contact with bodily fluids should be thoroughly flushed with water and washed with soap. The application of caustic agents or antiseptics into open wounds is not recommended.[6]

In those with occupational exposure, prophylaxis with HBIG and/or HBV vaccine is indicated as soon as possible depending on vaccination status of the clinician and HBV positivity of exposure.[6] See Table 35.5 for specific recommendations.

Fully vaccinated individuals with nonoccupational exposure to blood or bodily fluids should receive booster dose when the source of exposure is known to be positive and postvaccination testing was not done in the exposed individual. Unvaccinated or partially vaccinated persons should receive HBIG and HBV vaccine simultaneously at separate injection sites. Partially vaccinated individuals need to complete the series. Treatment should not be delayed if results of serologic testing are pending.[6]

Considerations in Pregnancy

Perinatal mother-to-child transmission (MTCT) of HBV contributes to a significant portion of chronic HBV worldwide. The CDC recommends universal screening of all pregnant females early in pregnancy. Females with acute clinical hepatitis or high-risk behaviors and females without prenatal screening should be tested at delivery.[6]

Females who are HBsAg-positive should be screened for HBV DNA. Maternal antiviral therapy is recommended if viral load is >200,000 IU/mL.[6] The highest risk of MTCT is with a high viral load, even when the infant is treated. The AASLD recommends treatment at 28 to 32 weeks. Treatment is typically stopped at birth or 3 months after. Breastfeeding is not contraindicated as medications are only minimally excreted in breast milk, but there is insufficient long-term safety data and this should be discussed with the mother.[8]

The CDC has guidelines for the testing and treatment of infants born to HbsAg-positive mothers or when status is unknown.

TABLE 35.5					

Postexposure Prophylaxis for Health Care Workers after Occupational Hepatitis B Exposure

	Postexposure Testing		Postexposure Prophylaxis		
HCW Status	**Source Patient (HBsAg)**	**HCW Testing (anti-HBs)**	**HBIG**	**Vaccination**	**Postvaccination Serologic Testing**
Documented responder after complete series			No action needed		
Documented nonresponder after two complete series	Positive/unknown	—[a]	HBIG × 2 separated by 1 mo	—	N/A
	Negative		No action needed		
Response unknown after complete series	Positive/unknown	<10 mIU/mL	HBIG × 1	Initiate revaccination	Yes
	Negative	<10 mIU/mL	None	Initiate revaccination	Yes
	Any result	≥10 mIU/mL	No action needed		
Unvaccinated/incompletely vaccinated or vaccine refusers	Positive/unknown	—	HBIG × 1	Complete vaccination	Yes
	Negative	—	None	Complete vaccination	Yes

anti-HBs, antibody to hepatitis B surface antigen; HBIG, hepatitis B immunoglobulin; HBsAg, hepatitis B surface antigen; HCW, health care worker; N/A, not applicable.
[a]Not indicated.
Adapted from www.cdc.gov/hepatitis

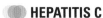

HEPATITIS C

Hepatitis C is an RNA virus in the *Flaviviridae* family. There are six major genotypes. In the United States, about 70% of cases are caused by genotype 1, 20% by genotype 2, 10% by genotype 3, and 1% by other genotypes.

Epidemiology

Hepatitis C is a blood-borne pathogen. In children, the primary route of transmission is maternal–fetal.[1] Screening procedures have eliminated HCV infection from blood products. Factors associated with an increased risk of infection in AYAs include IV drug use, intranasal illicit drug use, men who have sex with men, long-term hemodialysis, occupational needle/mucosal exposure in health care workers or public safety workers, HIV infection, and history of incarceration.[9] Coinfection with HIV/HCV increases the risk of HCV sexual transmission to uninfected partners.[9]

Rates of acute infection have increased significantly over the last 10 years with the largest increases occurring in adults 20 to 39 years with a history of IV drug use[1] The increase is due to increased IV drug use and surveillance.[4] There is a biphasic pattern of acute infection with a peak at 19 to 29 and 45 to 65 years. Rates increased in both genders, but are higher in males. Rates are greater in American Indians/Alaskan Natives and non-Hispanic Whites.

More than 50% of people who become infected with HCV will develop chronic HCV, making it the most common blood-borne infection.[1] Although prevalence rates are currently highest in adults born between 1945 and 1965, given the large increase in young adults, this is expected to shift.

The AASLD and the Infectious Diseases Society of America (IDSA) recommend one-time screening for all patients >18 years. Screening should be offered to patients younger than 18 years with behaviors that increase infection risk.[9]

Clinical Course

Identification of acute HCV can be difficult as patients may be asymptomatic or have nonspecific symptoms. Jaundice occurs in <25% of patients.[9] HCV has an incubation period of 2 to 23 weeks with a range of 2 to 26 weeks. Acute liver failure from acute HCV is uncommon.

Chronic disease develops in >50% of persons and is usually asymptomatic, though it can cause chronic fatigue and depression.[2] Liver disease usually progresses more slowly in children and adolescents but can be unpredictable. Although uncommon, chronic HCV can progress to cirrhosis and/or hepatocellular carcinoma (HCC). Children and adolescents with co-occurring conditions (nonalcoholic fatty liver disease, HIV or HBV coinfection, autoimmune hepatitis) need monitoring for disease progression. Extrahepatic manifestations of chronic HCV include diabetes mellitus, glomerulonephritis, essential mixed cryoglobulinemia, porphyria cutanea tarda, and non-Hodgkin lymphoma.[2]

Cirrhosis will develop over 5 to 20 years in 5% to 25% of persons with chronic HCV. Once cirrhosis has developed, there is a 1% to 4% annual risk for developing HCC. Risk factors for progression to cirrhosis include male gender, age >50 years, alcohol use, coinfection with HBV or HIV, nonalcoholic fatty liver disease, or immunosuppressive therapy.[2]

Viral Antigens and Antibodies

Hepatitis C is diagnosed in the presence of HCV RNA or viral antigen. Antibodies to HCV (anti-HCV) must also be present. Antibody testing cannot differentiate between acute, chronic, or resolved infection.[3] Figure 35.3 outlines the course of HCV serology.

Liver enzymes may be elevated during acute HCV. The presence of HCV RNA indicates viremia and occurs as early as 1 to 2 weeks after exposure. Anti-HCV is detectable in 40% of patients by 10 to 11 weeks, in 80% of patients by 15 weeks, and in nearly 100% of patients at 6 months. If HCV resolves, HCV RNA is no longer detectable. Anti-HCV may remain positive for life, but does not confer immunity. Anti-HCV may not be detected in immunocompromised patients or persons receiving dialysis. Patients with autoimmune disease may have a false-positive anti-HCV.[3]

Chronic HCV is defined as the persistence of anti-HCV and HCV RNA. Patients with detectable antibodies but negative RNA levels are not currently infected. If there is a known exposure, repeat

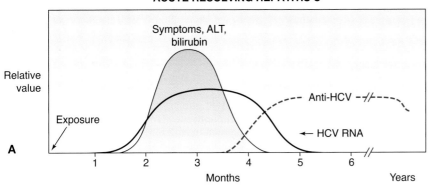

ACUTE RESOLVING HEPATITIS C

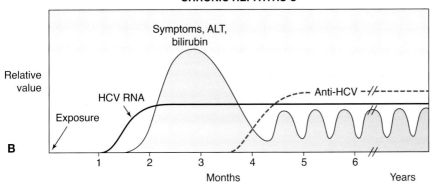

CHRONIC HEPATITIS C

FIGURE 35.3 Immunologic course of hepatitis C infection with associated clinical and laboratory findings. **A:** Acute resolving HCV. **B:** Chronic HCV. HCV, hepatitis C virus; anti-HCV, antibodies to HCV; ALT, alanine aminotransferase. (Used with permission from Ganti L. *Step-Up to USMLE Step 2 CK.* 5th ed. Wolters Kluwer; 2019.)

testing can be done after 6 months. Table 35.6 outlines the interpretation of serologic test results for HCV infection.

Treatment

Patients with HCV should be counseled on how to minimize transmission. Recommendations are similar to those for HBV as outlined in Table 35.3. Individuals should be encouraged to reduce risk-taking behaviors such as illicit drug use and reusing needles. Universal precautions include cleaning surfaces using a dilution of one part bleach to nine parts water.

Children and adolescents may face stigmatization in their schools or communities. Parents/caregivers should be counseled that HCV is not transmitted by casual contact and AYAs should be allowed to participate in school, sports, and other activities without restriction. Abstinence from alcohol should be encouraged. Hepatitis B and HAV vaccinations are recommended and pneumococcal vaccination is recommended in patients with cirrhosis. Hepatotoxic

TABLE 35.6
Sequence and Serologic Interpretation of Laboratory Screening for HCV

	Anti-HCV	HCV RNA
Never Infected/Susceptible[a]	NEGATIVE	NEGATIVE
Past/Resolved Infection[a]	POSITIVE	NEGATIVE
Current HCV Infection	POSITIVE	POSITIVE
False Positive	POSITIVE	NEGATIVE

HCV, hepatitis C; anti-HCV, antibodies to HCV; RNA, ribonucleic acid.
[a]If known exposure in the prior 6 months additional follow-up testing recommended.
Adapted from www.cdc.gov/hepatitis

medications or herbal therapies should be used with caution. Therapeutic doses of acetaminophen are permitted. Transplantation is not contraindicated in chronic HCV.[10]

Acute Hepatitis C

New recommendations from the AASLD–IDSA guidance panel call for the immediate treatment of acute HCV infection. Spontaneous resolution can occur and typically does so in 6 months. Serial negative HCV tests should be documented to ensure resolution. Patients who clear the infection do not require antiviral therapy but are not immune to reinfection.[11]

The same regimen is used for treatment of acute and chronic infection although shorter treatment courses for acute infection are being studied. Monitoring liver enzymes and international normalized ratio (INR) every 2 weeks is recommended. Patients with acute HCV can be managed in an outpatient setting unless symptoms require additional support. Although liver failure is rare (<1%), patients should be monitored and those with signs of liver failure should be referred to a transplant center.[11]

Chronic Hepatitis C

The goal of therapy is to achieve a sustained virologic response (SVR) and reduce risk of developing cirrhosis and HCC. Consultation with a hepatologist is recommended for treatment. The AASLD–IDSA updates treatment recommendations at https://www.hcvguidelines.org/. Treatment considerations include HCV genotype, tolerability and toxicity, optimal efficacy of different medications, and length of treatment. Other clinical considerations include the presence or absence of cirrhosis, prior treatment experience, co-occurring infections/conditions, and medication interactions.[12]

Pegylated-interferon-α (IFN) and ribavirin were previously the only therapeutic options, but direct-acting antivirals (DAAs) are now the mainstays of treatment.[4,13] Direct-acting antivirals target specific HCV proteins and disrupt viral replication. They are classified by their target proteins and mechanism of action (e.g., protease inhibitors, polymerase inhibitors). Most treatment regimens use a combination of DAAs. Sustained virologic response rate of >95% is achieved after 8 to 24 weeks of DAA therapy.[11]

Direct-acting antivirals are recommended for patients ≥3 years with certain DAAs approved for use in AYAs younger than 18 years.[11] It is important to take a thorough medication history that includes herbal therapies prior to initiating therapy because DAAs have significant medication interactions. Information about medication interactions can be found at the AASLD–IDSA website, package inserts for the individual medications, and at the online database of the University of Liverpool (https://www.hep-druginter-actions.org/).

Co-occurring conditions can affect the treatment of HCV. When HCV and HIV are present, the treatment of one virus can affect the other. In addition, medications used for the treatment of the viruses can interact. Information to guide treatment can be found at https://clinicalinfo.hiv.gov/en/guidelines. Specific treatment recommendations and modification should also be considered in those with renal disease, liver transplant recipients, or transplant recipients from an HCV-positive donor. The AASLD–IDSA website is a good source for recommendations in these situations.[11]

Monitoring during Hepatitis C Treatment Prior to treatment, patients should have testing for: HCV genotype, viral load, HIV, HBV, and an evaluation for autoimmune hepatitis. A liver biopsy may be indicated to further evaluate liver disease and degree of fibrosis. Patients should be monitored for adherence and adverse treatment effects including serial assessments of complete blood count, INR, hepatic function panel, and glomerular filtration rate. Viral load should be checked at the end of treatment and at 12 weeks to confirm SVR. Patients with advanced fibrosis and cirrhosis should be screened every 6 months for HCC with alpha-fetoprotein and ultrasound.[12]

Prevention and Prophylaxis

There is no prophylaxis for HCV. It is recommended that HCV testing be integrated into substance use treatment, needle service, and acute detoxification programs.

If exposure occurs, antibody and RNA testing should be completed within 48 hours. If negative, repeat testing should be done at 6 months. Treatment is recommended for patients who are RNA positive. For those with workplace exposure, there is a 0.2% risk for infection among those exposed to HCV-antibody–positive blood through needle stick or sharp injuries. There have been almost no cases of HCV acquisition through other workplace exposures.[1] Those with ongoing exposure should have testing as indicated and should be counseled on how to reduce transmission risk.

Considerations in Pregnancy

The CDC recommends that all pregnant females be screened during pregnancy unless HCV prevalence is <0.1%. Pregnant females with known risk factors should be tested with every pregnancy even in an area of low prevalence. Risk of transmission is estimated at 4% to 8% per pregnancy.[2]

Transmission can occur during pregnancy or childbirth and there are no options for prophylaxis. Risk of MTCT is higher if the mother has a high-viral load or is coinfected with HIV. Breastfeeding is not contraindicated unless the mother has cracked/bleeding nipples. Pregnant females with cirrhosis are at increased risk for adverse maternal and perinatal outcomes and should be managed by a maternal–fetal medicine obstetrician. Onset of jaundice and pruritus in pregnant patients with HCV should raise concern for intrahepatic cholestasis of pregnancy. Levels of HCV RNA can fluctuate with pregnancy and viral load should be reassessed after delivery.[13,14]

HEPATITIS D

A member of the *Deltaviridae* family, HDV is only transmitted in the presence of HBV. It is an RNA virus and requires a host enzyme for replication. There are eight genotypes; genotype 1 is most common in North America.

Epidemiology

Hepatitis D is transmitted primarily through blood and sexual contact. Patients with immunity to HBV, are not susceptible to HDV infection. It is uncommon in children, but can be acquired by AYAs with pre-existing HBV infection. Risk factors include IV drug use and high-risk sexual behaviors. The risk from contaminated blood products has been reduced due to improved screening techniques.[1] HDV can be contracted with HBV (coinfection) or can occur in the presence of chronic HBV (superinfection). Superinfection can result in rapid progression of pre-existing HBV infection.[2]

The risk of HDV is highest among persons living in or traveling to areas with high HDV prevalence—Eastern/Southern Europe, the Middle East, West/Central Africa, East Asia, and the Amazon Basin. It is uncommon in North America.[2]

Clinical Course

Coinfection and superinfection have an incubation period of 3 to 7 weeks. The clinical course with coinfection is variable. In most cases, it is self-limiting and improves with resolution of HBV. Less than 5% of coinfected individuals develop chronic infection. However, acute liver failure is more common with coinfection than in patients with acute HBV alone.[2] Liver enzymes have a biphasic pattern, rising with HBV replication and then with the emergence of HDV.

Acute hepatitis with superinfection can be more severe. Superinfection accelerates the progression of chronic HBV in 70% to 90% of people and >80% of persons will develop chronic HDV infection. Progression to cirrhosis occurs almost 10 years earlier in those with superinfection. Chronic HBV/HDV infection is associated with more rapid disease progression. Liver failure occurs within 5 to 10 years in 70% to 80% and 1 to 2 years in 15% of persons.[2]

Viral Antigens and Antibodies

There is no FDA-approved assay for HDV antigen, which is detectable 1 week after exposure. Ribonucleic acid quantitative polymerase chain reaction (PCR) is another marker of HDV infection. There are commercially available RNA assays that are not yet FDA approved. Hepatitis D antibody testing is needed to define infection status. Anti-HDV IgM antibodies are detectable 1 to 3 weeks from exposure and indicate acute infection or disease activity in chronic HDV infection. Anti-HDV IgG rises a few weeks after the primary infection and remains positive in patients with chronic infection. There are commercially available tests for HDV antibodies, but they are not FDA approved.[3]

Patients with coinfection have markers to HBV and HDV. Total antibodies to HDV are detected in 85% of infections. As HBV infection resolves, HDV antibodies will decline to undetectable levels. This coincides with an increase in anti-HBs antibodies. The presence of total anti-HBc and anti-HBs antibodies following coinfection indicates immunity to future infection with HBV and HDV. Anti-HDV antibodies persist indefinitely in those with superinfection.[3]

Treatment

See hepatitis B above.

Prevention and Prophylaxis

Prevention of HBV will prevent HDV. Persons with exposure to HBV and HDV should be treated the same as those exposed to HBV alone. Vaccination against HBV is protective against HDV.

Considerations in Pregnancy

There are no considerations for HDV during pregnancy.

 HEPATITIS E

Hepatitis E virus is an RNA virus in the *Hepeviridae* family. There are four genotypes. Types 1 and 2 are only found in humans. Types 3 and 4 are found in humans, pigs, and other animal species.

Epidemiology

Hepatitis E is more common in developing countries where it is primarily transmitted through the fecal–oral route. It is largely the result of environmental sanitation and contaminated water. Animals serve as reservoir for HEV and infection occurs from the ingestion of uncooked/undercooked meat.[15] Hepatitis E and HAV are the main causes of acute hepatitis worldwide. Hepatitis E is endemic in Asia, Africa, Mexico, and the Middle East.[15] There have been significant increases in HEV outbreaks in Europe during the last 10 years. These are due to sporadic outbreaks caused by environmental or food-borne infections.

Clinical Course

The incubation periods for HEV is 40 days with a range of 15 to 60 days. The clinical course of HEV is similar to HAV, with asymptomatic shedding of virus 1 week prior and 30 days after onset of jaundice/clinical symptoms.[2] Most patients are asymptomatic and/or have a self-limited course. In developing countries, symptomatic infection occurs most often in persons 15 to 44 years of age.[2] Overall mortality rates are low with a case fatality of about 1% in outbreaks. Severe illness and mortality are higher in pregnant persons and individuals with underlying chronic liver disease. In pregnant females, the case fatality rate has been reported as high as 25%, especially if the infection occurs during the third trimester.[14]

Chronic HEV does not occur in healthy persons but can occur in immunocompromised patients.[15] In 6% to 8% of patients, HEV infection is associated with extrahepatic manifestations, most commonly renal (membranous glomerulonephritis and membranoproliferative glomerulonephritis) and neurologic (Guillain–Barré syndrome, meningoencephalitis, and peripheral neuropathy).

Viral Antigens and Antibodies

Hepatitis E virus RNA can be detected 3 weeks after exposure and 1 week prior to the onset of symptoms. Viremia lasts for 2 weeks.[3] Liver enzyme elevation occurs 4 to 5 weeks after exposure and persists for 3 to 13 weeks. Detection in stool occurs 1 week prior and 1 week after symptoms, but may be detected longer in some people.

Hepatitis E antibodies are detectable 3 weeks after exposure. Hepatitis E IgG persists but IgM declines in convalescence and is negative by 13 weeks. Serologic testing is recommended when other causes of hepatitis have been ruled out or if travel has occurred to an endemic region.[3] Immunoassays for anti-HEV antibodies are commercially available but not FDA approved. Nucleic acid tests for HEV RNA also exist but are not commercially available.[3]

Treatment

Acute infection does not require therapy. Treatment may be indicated for patients who progress to acute liver failure and have decompensation of prior liver disease. Ribavirin may be used to reduce the viral load.

Prevention and Prophylaxis

Sanitation and access to clean drinking water can prevent infection. Travelers to endemic areas can reduce risk by avoiding ingestion of unpurified water or uncooked pork and venison. Boiling and chlorination of water can inactivate HEV. There is no vaccine available in the United States.[2]

Considerations in Pregnancy

Hepatitis E infection in pregnancy results in a higher rate of fulminant hepatitis and death. This is thought to be due to the effect of hormonal changes on the immune system—specifically deregulation of the progesterone receptor signaling pathway.[5] Maternal mortality is higher in the Middle East and Asia as compared to Europe and the United States. Vertical transmission may occur with a higher risk of stillborn birth and neonatal death with infection in the third trimester. Breastfeeding with acute infection is not recommended.[5] Ribavirin cannot be used due to its teratogenic effect.

 SUMMARY

Hepatitis A through E are a group of viruses that cause liver inflammation. Hepatitis A and E typically spread through contaminated food and water and cause acute, short-term infections. Hepatitis B, C, and D spread through contact with infected blood and/or contact with bodily fluids and can cause acute or chronic infections. Despite improvements in screening, vaccinations, pre/postexposure prophylaxis, and treatment options, there have been increases in rates of viral infection, mostly attributable to increases in IV drug use.

ACKNOWLEDGMENTS

The authors wish to acknowledge Praveen S. Goday and Lynette Gillis for contributions to previous versions of this chapter.

REFERENCES

1. Centers for Disease Control and Prevention. *Viral hepatitis surveillance—United States, 2018.* Published July 2020. Accessed February 2, 2021. https://www.cdc.gov/hepatitis/statistics/SurveillanceRpts.htm
2. Division of Viral Hepatitis, National Center for HIV/AIDS, Viral Hepatitis, STD, and TB Prevention. *Viral hepatitis.* Updated July 2020. Accessed March 5, 2021. https://www.cdc.gov/hepatitis
3. Centers for Disease Control and Prevention. *Viral hepatitis serology training.* Updated November 15, 2015. Accessed February 18, 2021. https://www.cdc.gov/hepatitis/resources/professionals/training/serology/training.htm
4. Nelson NP, Weng MK, Hofmeister MG, et al. Prevention of hepatitis A virus infection in the United States: Recommendations of the Advisory Committee on Immunization Practices, 2020. *MMWR Recomm Rep.* 2020;69(5):1–38.
5. Seto MTY, Cheung KW, Hung IFN. Management of viral hepatitis A, C, D and E in pregnancy. *Best Pract Res Clin Obstet and Gynaecol.* 2020;68:44–53.
6. Schillie S, Vellozzi C, Reingold A, et al. Prevention of hepatitis B virus infection in the United States: Recommendations of the Advisory Committee on Immunization Practices. *MMWR Recomm Rep.* 2018;67(1):1–31.
7. U.S. Preventive Services Task Force. Screening for hepatitis B virus infection in adolescents and adults: U.S. Preventive Services Task Force Recommendation Statement. *JAMA.* 2020;324(23):2415–2422.
8. Terrault NA, Lok ASF, McMahon BJ, et al. Update on prevention, diagnosis, and treatment of chronic hepatitis B: AASLD 2018 Hepatitis B guidance. *Hepatology.* 2018;64(4):1560–1599.
9. Ghany MG, Morgan TR, AASLD-IDSA Hepatitis C Guidance Panel. Hepatitis C guidance 2019 update: American Association for the Study of Liver Diseases–Infectious Diseases Society of America recommendations for testing, managing, and treating hepatitis C virus infection. *Hepatology.* 2020;71(2):686–721.
10. Owens DK, Davidson KW, Krist AH, et al; U.S. Preventive Services Task Force. Screening for hepatitis C virus infection in adolescents and adults: US Preventive Services Task Force Recommendation Statement. *JAMA.* 2020;323(10):970–975.
11. American Association for the Study of Liver Disease (AASLD) and Infectious Diseases Society of America (IDSA). *HCV guidance: recommendations for testing, managing, and treating hepatitis C.* Accessed March 23 2021. http://www.hcvguidelines.org
12. Heimbach JK, Kulik LM, Finn RS, et al. AASLD guidelines for the treatment of hepatocellular carcinoma. *Hepatology.* 2018;67(1):358–380.
13. Chappell CA, Krans EE, Bunge K, et al. A phase 1 study of ledipasvir/sofosbuvir in pregnant women with hepatitis C virus [abstract 87]. Conference on retroviruses and opportunistic infections, Seattle, WA; 2019.
14. Yattoo GN. Treatment of chronic hepatitis C with ledipasvir/sofosbuvir combination during pregnancy [Abstract]. *Hepatol Int.* 2018;12(Suppl. 2):S292–S293.
15. Hartard C, Gantzer C, Bronowicki J-P, et al. Emerging hepatitis E virus compared with hepatitis A virus: a new sanitary challenge. *Rev Med Virol.* 2019;29(6):e2078.

VIII

ADDITIONAL RESOURCES AND WEBSITES

Additional Resources and Websites for Clinicians:

Information from the American Association on the Study of Liver Disease and Infectious Disease Society of American on the management of Hepatitis C—http://www.hcvguidelines.org

Information from the CDC for providers on hepatitis diagnosis and treatment—http://www.cdc.gov/hepatitis/

Medication Interactions:

Potential drug interactions for medications used to treat hepatitis—https://www.hep-druginteractions.org

Potential drug interactions for medications used to treat hepatitis and HIV—www.aidsinfo.nih.gov/guidelines

Outbreaks and Surveillance:

Real-time notices of recalls and alerts from the U.S. Department of Agriculture (USDA) and U.S. Food and Drug Administration (FDA)—https://www.foodsafety.gov/recalls-and-outbreaks

Recalls and public health alerts put out the U.S. Federal Safety and Inspection Services—https://www.fsis.usda.gov/recalls#

This page provides links to public health alerts, consumer advisories, and other safety information related to food and dietary supplement products—https://www.fda.gov/food/recalls-outbreaks-emergencies/alerts-advisories-safety-information

Additional Resources for and Websites for Parents/Caregivers and Adolescents and Young Adults:

Patient information about hepatitis from the liver foundation—http://www.liverfoundation.org/abouttheliver/info/

Patient information about hepatitis from the National Foundation for infectious disease—https://www.nfid.org/?s=hepatitis Patient information about hepatitis—http://kidshealth.org/teen/sexual_health/stds/hepatitis.html

Patient information about hepatitis—http://kidshealth.org/parent/infections/bacterial_viral/hepatitis.html

Patient information from the CDC on hepatitis—http://www.cdc.gov/hepatitis/

36

Human Immunodeficiency Virus Infections and Acquired Immunodeficiency Syndrome

Jonathan D. Warus
Marvin E. Belzer

KEY WORDS

- Acquired immunodeficiency syndrome (AIDS)
- Antiretroviral therapy (ART)
- Exposure
- Human immunodeficiency virus (HIV)
- Postexposure prophylaxis (PEP)
- Pre-exposure prophylaxis (PrEP)
- Prevention
- Testing
- Transmission
- Treatment

INTRODUCTION

During the 40 years since the human immunodeficiency virus (HIV) epidemic began, there have been significant scientific advancements in the identification, detection, and treatment of HIV infection. As of November 2020, over 37.9 million people worldwide were living with HIV, the virus responsible for the advanced immunocompromised condition known as acquired immunodeficiency syndrome (AIDS). The number of people living with HIV continues to rise with the combined effects of improving therapies and high rates of new infections, particularly among adolescents and young adults (AYAs). While advances in antiretroviral therapy (ART) can allow most youth to live healthy lives with simple once-a-day regimens, existing challenges for clinicians involve identifying youth living with HIV, engaging them in care, and assisting them with long-term adherence to medications.

In the past 15 years, the HIV field has been further revolutionized by advancements in HIV prevention strategies including the recognition of treatment as prevention (TasP), nonoccupational use of postexposure prophylaxis (PEP), and the rollout of pre-exposure prophylaxis (PrEP). Utilizing these highly effective HIV prevention methods, the 2019 *Ending the HIV Epidemic (EHE): A Plan for America* aims to end the HIV epidemic in the United States by 2030.[1] As with challenges in HIV care, challenges also exist in the implementation and utilization of prevention strategies, and continued innovative research is needed to engage youth in HIV prevention.

ETIOLOGY, PATHOGENESIS, AND NATURAL HISTORY

Human immunodeficiency virus is a single-stranded RNA retrovirus that infects and leads to the destruction of CD4+ T lymphocytes and can result in severe immune deficiency over time. Human immunodeficiency virus-1 is the cause of most cases of AIDS in the world. Human immunodeficiency virus-2, a retrovirus related to HIV-1, is found primarily in Central Africa and generally has a slower progression (20 years vs. 5 to 10 years with HIV-1) but a similar spectrum of disease.

Acute HIV infection presents as a mononucleosis-like illness in many but not all patients, 2 to 6 weeks after infection. The illness typically lasts 1 to 2 weeks and causes nonspecific constitutional symptoms as well as myalgias, lymphadenopathy, and sore throat (Table 36.1). Without a high index of suspicion, the diagnosis often may not be recognized by clinicians.

While the phase of illness following acute infection is one of clinical latency, it is clear that viral production is steady at an estimated 10 billion virions daily. During this time, T-cell production and destruction remain precariously balanced.

A slow but steady depletion of CD4+ T cells occurs in all but a small percentage of untreated patients, who are referred to as long-term nonprogressors. Without treatment, the average rate of decline of CD4+ T cells is about $50/mm^3$/year and most patients develop AIDS (severe immune deficiency) over a period of 8 to 10 years. Approximately 10% of those with a new HIV infection will rapidly progress to an AIDS diagnosis within 4 years. Numerous studies indicate that ART can suppress the viral load to undetectable levels in most patients. Viral suppression is associated with a steady immune reconstitution in most patients. Even patients with severe depletion of their immune system can often return to excellent health after successful treatment.

Adolescents and young adults diagnosed relatively early in the course of HIV infection, who successfully initiate ART, should have a near-normal lifespan when medication adherence is supported and other health risks, such as substance use, are minimized.[2]

TABLE 36.1
Clinical Manifestations of Acute HIV-1 Infection

Features	Overall % ($n = 378$)
Fever	75
Fatigue	68
Myalgia	49
Skin rash	48
Headache	45
Pharyngitis	40
Cervical adenopathy	39
Arthralgia	30
Night sweats	28
Diarrhea	27

HIV, human immunodeficiency virus.
Adapted from Daar ES, Pilcher CD, Hecht FM. Clinical presentation and diagnosis of primary HIV-1 infection. *Curr Opin HIV AIDS.* 2008;3(1):10–15.

There is growing evidence that chronic HIV infection elicits systemic inflammation that accelerates risk for cardiovascular illness. Even with effective antiretroviral treatment, individuals living with HIV have higher cardiovascular risk and cardiovascular disease has emerged as an important cause of death in this population.[3]

Another area of emerging research is neurocognitive function in AYAs living with HIV. In one study, 67% of 220 youth diagnosed with HIV (mean age 21 years) naive to ART, demonstrated HIV-associated neurocognitive disorders on neuropsychological testing.[4] There were high rates of impairment in learning and memory as well as executive functioning that clearly impact clinicians' approaches to patient management. In multivariable models, these impairments were associated with some markers of HIV (e.g., CD4 cell counts) but also with other factors such as high-risk alcohol use and psychiatric distress.

 ## EPIDEMIOLOGY

Prevalence

At the end of 2018, the Centers for Disease Control and Prevention (CDC) estimated that 1,173,900 persons aged 13 and older were living with HIV infection in the United States. Of these individuals, it is estimated that 161,800 (13.8%) were living with undiagnosed HIV.[5]

Incidence

From 2014 through 2018, the number of new HIV infections in the United States remained stable, at approximately 36,000 new cases each year. In 2018, one in five new infections occurred in AYAs aged 13 to 24.[5]

Age

Adolescents and young adults are particularly impacted by HIV. In 2018, the CDC reported an estimated 7,600 new HIV infections in youth aged 13 to 24. Although young people in this age group represented 16% of the U.S. population in 2018, they accounted for 21% of all new HIV diagnoses made that year. Those 13 to 24 years old are also the age group with the largest percentage of undiagnosed HIV infections, with 44.9% of those living with HIV being unaware of the infection.[5]

Ethnicity

Communities of color continue to be disproportionately impacted by HIV infection. Among those in the United States aged 13 to 24, 41% of new infections occurred in Black youth and 26% in Latino youth in 2018.[5]

Gender

At the end of 2018, 78% of adolescents and adults aged 13 years or over living with HIV were assigned male at birth and 22% were assigned female. It is important to note that while transgender individuals are at high risk for HIV, data for these communities are lacking due to the absence of uniform data collection approaches.[5]

Global Epidemiology

As of 2019, the Joint United Nations Programme on HIV/AIDS (UNAIDS) estimated that 38.0 million individuals were living with HIV worldwide (with 20.7 million of these individuals residing within Eastern and Southern Africa) and the global prevalence of HIV in youth 15 to 24 years of age was 3.4 million. In 2019, there were approximately 1.7 million new HIV infections globally with 28% of these occurring in those 15 to 24 years of age.[6,7]

 ## TRANSMISSION

Human immunodeficiency virus can be transmitted only by the exchange of body fluids. Blood, semen, vaginal secretions, and breast milk are the only fluids documented to be associated with the transmission of HIV infection. Although HIV is found in saliva, tears, urine, and sweat, no case has been documented that implicates these fluids as agents of infection.

Transmission Routes

Table 36.2 shows the common routes of transmission for those diagnosed with HIV based on assigned sex at birth. Most new cases in individuals assigned male at birth occur in men who have sex with men (MSM), while the majority of new infections among those assigned female at birth are transmitted through heterosexual contact and injection drug use. Young men who have sex with men

TABLE 36.2

Diagnoses of HIV Infection among Male and Female Adolescents and Young Adults, by Age Group and Transmission Category, 2018–United States and Six Dependent Areas

Transmission Category	Males				Females			
	13–19 y		20–24 y		13–19 y		20–24 y	
	No.	%	No.	%	No.	%	No.	%
Male-to-male sexual contact	1,356	92.9	4,928	91.8	—	—	—	—
Injection drug use (IDU)	16	1.1	91	1.7	23	8.7	99	13.8
Male-to-male sexual contact and IDU	33	2.3	180	3.4	—	—	—	—
Heterosexual contact[a]	41	2.8	169	3.2	227	86.4	609	85.1
Other[b]	13	0.9	2	0.0	13	4.9	7	1.0
Total[c]	1,459	100	5,370	100	263	100	715	100

[a]Heterosexual contact with a person known to have, or to be at high risk for, HIV infection.
[b]Includes hemophilia, blood transfusion, perinatal exposure, and risk factor not reported or not identified.
[c]Because column totals for numbers were calculated independently of the values for the subpopulations, the values in each column may not sum to the column total.
HIV, human immunodeficiency virus.
Adapted from Centers for Disease Control and Prevention. National Center for HIV/AIDS, Viral Hepatitis, STD, and TB Prevention. Division of HIV/AIDS Prevention. *HIV Surveillance–Adolescents and Young Adults.* Slide set. Accessed March 22, 2021. http://www.cdc.gov/hiv/pdf/library/slidesets/cdc-hiv-surveillance-adolescents-young-adults-2018.pdf

(YMSM), especially Black and Latino YMSM, are at particularly high risk for HIV infection.[5]

Injection Drug Use

Human immunodeficiency virus is easily transmitted by needle sharing. Because of the unreliability and frequent lack of acceptance of needle bleaching and the frequent lack of acceptance or inaccessibility of substance use treatment, almost all public health organizations support needle exchange programs. In these programs, those who use injection drugs can exchange used needles for clean ones while at the same time gaining access to condoms, bleach, and referral resources. Many programs across the United States have shown that neither injection drug use prevalence in the community, nor the frequency of use among individuals, increases when needle exchange is available. In fact, HIV and other blood-borne disease transmissions (e.g., hepatitis) are markedly reduced with the availability of needle exchange programs.[8]

Sex

Sexual transmission of HIV is thought to have a hierarchy of relative risks based upon factors such as tissue involved, lubrication, friction, and potential for increased bodily fluid exchange. Receptive anal intercourse without condoms carries the highest risk, followed by insertive anal intercourse and vaginal intercourse. Oral sex is categorized as carrying lower risk but has been shown to result in HIV transmission. Studies have demonstrated that proper and consistent use of latex condoms or dental dams can markedly reduce the risk for HIV transmission during sex.[9]

Vertical Transmission

Universal opt-out HIV screening of pregnant females, antiretroviral treatment and prophylaxis, use of cesarean delivery when appropriate, and avoidance of breastfeeding have greatly reduced perinatal HIV transmission in the United States. With early diagnosis, appropriate treatment, and avoidance of breastfeeding, transmission risk is reduced to 2% or less. For those with an undetectable viral load during the entire pregnancy, the risk of vertical transmission is likely zero.[10]

⬤ HUMAN IMMUNODEFICIENCY VIRUS TESTING AND COUNSELING

The primary goal of HIV testing is to determine if an individual is or is not living with an HIV infection, with subsequent linkage to appropriate health care and supportive services for treatment or prevention, as needed. Early diagnosis and entry into care are critical steps in addressing the HIV epidemic, yet many individuals living with HIV, especially youth, remain unaware of the infection. For those without a current HIV infection who are at risk, testing is a gateway to further HIV prevention services. The importance of HIV testing cannot be overstated. Factors to keep in mind when approaching HIV testing in youth include consent and confidentiality, screening recommendations, types of HIV testing, and appropriate counseling.

Consent and Confidentiality

Clinicians must balance the protection of AYAs' rights against the amount of information needed to deliver proper care. Laws governing an individual's ability to consent for HIV testing and receive confidential care vary within the United States and from country to country. Current U.S. regulations are described here:

Individuals older than 18 years who are competent: The CDC recommends that patients in all health care settings receive HIV testing as part of routine primary medical care. Separate informed consent (from the general medical consent) is not needed, and prevention counseling should not be a prerequisite for HIV diagnostic testing or as part of HIV screening programs.

Individuals between 12 and 17 years: Laws vary widely from state to state. According to the Guttmacher Institute, all 50 states and the District of Columbia allow minors to consent to sexually transmitted infection (STI) services, although some states specify a minimum age (generally 12 or 14 years, but 16 years in South Carolina) one must reach before they can provide consent. Thirty-two states explicitly include HIV testing and treatment as part of STI services for which minors can consent.[11] Many states allow (but do not require) clinicians to notify a minor's parents that their child is seeking STI services.

Individuals younger than 12 years and incompetent adolescents: For these individuals, a third party (parent or legal guardian) authorizes testing. However, this authorization may be restricted by state laws.

An increasing number of states have statutes governing HIV testing. Without such a statute, general laws regarding minors apply. It is not clear whether HIV testing would fall under the category of consent for STI services in states that do not declare HIV to be an STI. Clinicians worldwide need to be familiar with local laws regarding the following:

1. Consent for testing: Who can consent? What is the required informed consent? Are pretest and posttest counseling available?
2. Who can receive the results of these tests and under what circumstances?
3. Where will test results be recorded?
4. What can be written in the chart regarding testing and test results?

To Whom Should Human Immunodeficiency Virus Testing Be Offered?

In 2006, the CDC modified its recommendations to advise that HIV testing be routine for all sexually active adolescents and adults between the ages of 13 and 64 years whenever they access health care. Youth should be advised that they will be tested and given the option to decline. All pregnant individuals should be screened for HIV at least once early during each pregnancy.[12] Following initial testing, persons at high risk should be screened at minimum once annually and be offered additional prevention methods such as PEP and PrEP. Clinicians in the United States can access more information regarding state-specific laws at http://www.cdc.gov/hiv/policies/law/states/index.html. Clinicians practicing outside of the United States should be familiar with local laws governing HIV testing and prevention.

The following groups are at high risk and should have repeat testing at least annually:

1. Men who have sex with men regardless of sexual orientation (note that many youth in this group may not self-identify as gay or bisexual).
2. Transgender individuals who have sex with cisgender men.
3. Youth who share needles (e.g., steroid injections and recreational drugs).
4. Youth with partners from the above three groups.
5. Youth who have had intercourse or shared needles with persons living with HIV.
6. Youth with other STIs.
7. Sexually active youth from economically disadvantaged areas or areas of known high seroprevalence.
8. Youth with multiple sexual partners.

Who Should Have Human Immunodeficiency Virus Testing Deferred?

Expert opinion suggests testing be deferred in the following situations:

1. Youth with severe mental illness who cannot provide consent for testing.
2. Youth with acute intoxication or experiencing drug withdrawal.

3. Youth experiencing suicidality and those who indicate that they would seriously consider suicide if given a diagnosis of HIV.

Youth-Specific Testing

Testing can occur in a number of settings. Many testing sites now have counselors (including peer health educators) who are specifically trained to work with AYAs and may therefore be perceived as youth friendly. Counselors should have specialized training to address identified risks and knowledge of effective interventions and resources for youth. Often, these sites are co-located where other services or activities are available for youth (e.g., homeless shelters, free clinics, schools, recreational centers, mobile testing vans). Youth-specific testing should be recommended whenever possible as it can be an effective component of prevention education. In particular, testing that is targeted to subpopulations of youth highly impacted by HIV can support goals outlined in *Ending the HIV Epidemic*. However, this youth-friendly approach should not deter from offering routine testing in all clinical settings, which is a strategy critical to identification of the 45% of youth living with HIV who are unaware of their status.

Human Immunodeficiency Virus Tests

The technology for HIV testing continues to evolve at a rapid pace, with the development of tests that are easier to perform, provide quicker results, and allow for earlier detection of HIV from the time of infection. Available assays rely on various methods, including detection of (1) HIV antibodies, (2) the viral p24 antigen, and (3) viral nucleic acid (ribonucleic acid [RNA]). See Table 36.3 for various available HIV testing methods, the target of detection, and the estimated window from infection to a positive test result.

Rapid Human Immunodeficiency Virus Testing

Rapid HIV tests (most provide results in as little as 1 to 20 minutes) are now available with sensitivities and specificities exceeding 99%, providing a critical opportunity for counseling and linkage to care and prevention while eliminating the need for return visits. This allows for rapid, low-cost screening in high-volume settings such as emergency departments and in mobile populations such

---

TABLE 36.3

HIV Diagnostic Testing Windows

Testing Method	Target of Detection	Estimated Window From Infection to Positive Result, Days
First-generation EIA	IgG antibody	35–45
Second-generation EIA	IgG antibody	25–35
Third-generation EIA	IgG and IgM antibody	20–30
Fourth-generation EIA	IgG and IgM antibody + p24 antigen	15–20
Western blot	IgG and IgM antibody	Indeterminate: 35–50
		Positive: 45–60
Viral load (cutoff 50 copies/mL)	HIV RNA	10–15
Viral load, ultrasensitive (cutoff 1–5 copies/mL)	HIV RNA	5

EIA, enzyme-linked immunoassay; IgG, immunoglobulin G; IgM, immunoglobulin M; HIV, human immunodeficiency virus; RNA, ribonucleic acid.

---

as those experiencing homelessness. For these reasons, rapid tests have become the screening test of choice in the United States and many parts of the world. Further, it has been shown that youth accept and prefer point-of-care testing over traditional tests.[13] Since 2002, the U.S. Food and Drug Administration (FDA) has approved a number of rapid HIV tests for use on serum, whole blood (fingerstick samples), and oral secretions. The CDC website (http://www.cdc.gov/hiv/testing/laboratorytests.html) has extensive information on the use of rapid HIV testing, including specific recommendations for clinicians regarding the Clinical Laboratory Improvement Amendments Program, counseling, and quality assurance guidelines. Rapid HIV tests report results as positive, negative, or indeterminate.

Antibody (First/Second/Third-Generation) Tests

All positive enzyme immunoassay (EIA) test results must be followed by confirmatory testing; a negative test result does not need to be confirmed. New testing algorithms have been adopted in many organizations that include the use of a second rapid test kit (different than initial) to confirm positive test results during the same visit. If a second rapid HIV test is used for confirmation, the patient is given a presumptive positive result and connected to services for further diagnostic evaluation (e.g., viral load). While Western blot may be used for confirmation, this practice has been largely replaced by viral load testing for HIV RNA through polymerase chain reaction (PCR). Use of a two-test rapid HIV testing algorithm rather than traditional confirmatory testing with a Western blot may improve linkage to care in some settings.[14]

Viral p24 Antigen (Fourth-Generation) Tests

Newer fourth-generation HIV tests have the advantage of detecting the viral p24 antigen as well as HIV antibodies. Combination antibody–antigen tests may allow HIV detection during acute infection before HIV antibodies are formed, effectively shortening the window period. These tests can be used for screening and are particularly helpful for use in acute settings such as delivery rooms and occupational exposures.

Viral Nucleic Acid (Viral Load) Tests

Viral nucleic acid tests remain the test of choice for detection of early or acute HIV infection. Polymerase chain reaction–based tests are frequently used to detect HIV RNA. Time to positivity is determined by the sensitivity of the individual test, and ultrasensitive assays are now capable of detecting very low levels of viremia as early as 5 days following infection.

Pretest Counseling

Prior to performing an HIV test, youth should be given the opportunity to review written and/or oral information regarding HIV infection, routine screening recommendations, and an explanation regarding the meaning of positive and negative testing results. The patient should have the opportunity to ask any questions prior to testing. It should also be made clear that an individual can decline HIV testing without consequences and this will not affect their ability to access future care or services.

Posttest Counseling

Negative Test Result

For some clinicians, when giving a patient a negative HIV testing result, there is no further discussion other than the result itself and sometimes recommendations for subsequent rescreening. Rather than ending the conversation at this point, clinicians should strive to engage all patients with a negative HIV test in a discussion regarding their individual risk for HIV and whether they could benefit from and/or desire further HIV prevention services (see the section on HIV Prevention).

Positive Test Result

Posttest counseling should be given in-person and should include the following:

1. Provide the results of the test: This should be done in a direct manner at the beginning of the posttest session. If a screening antibody test was reactive and a two-test rapid HIV testing algorithm is not standard care, then a fourth-generation (antibody/antigen) test or viral load is ordered. It is imperative to explain that while the screening test was positive, a definitive diagnosis cannot be made until confirmatory results return.

2. Allow the adolescent or young adult time to express feelings and reactions: It is important to recognize that the emotions and thoughts experienced by those receiving a new diagnosis of HIV vary widely. Validate the individual's experience and avoid minimizing any distress they may be feeling, while also providing education regarding the advances in medical treatment discussed during the pretest session to offer hope and support.

3. Assess the adolescent's or young adult's understanding of the result: This is best assessed by asking the adolescent or young adult directly what the test result means to them. The youth should be supported in identifying behavior change goals to reduce their risk of transmitting the virus to others. Adolescents and young adults should also understand that although the virus is probably present for life, a positive test does not mean one has AIDS. Youth with a new diagnosis of HIV should be advised as follows:

   a. Do not donate blood, semen, or body organs.

   b. Inform clinicians and dentists of HIV status.

   c. Encourage biologic children, sexual partners, and needle contacts to seek evaluation and testing (many counties in the United States and other countries have anonymous partner notification programs).

   d. Early in the course of HIV, there is increased risk of passing the virus to sexual partners. There are ways to prevent this from happening including abstinence, condoms, and prevention methods for partners such as PrEP.

   e. Over time, with appropriate, adequate, and consistent HIV treatment, the risk of passing the virus to sexual partners can be fully prevented.

   f. No evidence exists that HIV is transmitted to family household members or to close contacts by routes other than sexual intercourse, exposure to blood, and perinatal transmission.

   g. Household items (e.g., glasses, forks, dishes) may be shared by those living with HIV and other household members. Personal hygiene items (i.e., razors and toothbrushes) should not be shared.

   h. Bathroom facilities may be used by all household members.

4. Refer the patient to an HIV specialist, preferentially one who is experienced in working with AYAs. Ideally, the clinic will have an interdisciplinary team that includes a clinician, social worker, nurse, and other parents/caregivers to provide medical care and psychosocial support. It is highly advisable to get multiple contact methods (phone, email, Facebook, other social media, etc.) from the patient so that they can be reached in subsequent weeks to ensure they have been linked to care.

HUMAN IMMUNODEFICIENCY VIRUS PREVENTION

The HIV prevention paradigm has shifted significantly in recent years. Primary prevention efforts to reduce the HIV risk of those without HIV have expanded beyond behavioral interventions to include biomedical interventions such as PrEP, public health strategies like HIV counseling and testing, and structural interventions that address community partnerships and collaboration, including increasing access to condoms, dental dams, and needle exchange programs. The White House and other public health leaders have increasingly emphasized secondary prevention (reducing transmission risk from persons living with HIV) through "Treatment as Prevention." Globally, it is estimated that only one in three youth 15 to 24 years of age demonstrates accurate knowledge to prevent HIV infections.[7]

Primary Biomedical Prevention

If a patient completes HIV screening with a negative testing result, the next step for the clinician is to determine if the patient has had any potential exposure to HIV in the past 72 hours. If so, the patient may benefit from PEP. If there has been no exposure during this timeframe, the clinician should then have a discussion with the patient about their ongoing risk for HIV infection to determine if the patient could benefit from PrEP. Most clinicians are familiar with this type of approach when it comes to pregnancy testing and determinations about the use of emergency contraception and birth control. Postexposure prophylaxis is often described as the "emergency contraception" for HIV with PrEP being described as the "birth control" for HIV. Practitioners should become familiar with local minor consent laws related to these services when caring for those under 18 years of age.

Postexposure Prophylaxis

Postexposure prophylaxis was first recommended for occupational exposures to HIV (e.g., for needlesticks) and has since been expanded to include nonoccupational exposures such as through sexual activity, injection drug use, and other exposures to blood, genital secretions, or other potentially infectious body fluids (sometimes known as nPEP if the exposure is nonoccupational). If a patient (1) does not have a known HIV infection, (2) has either a negative rapid HIV test or pending HIV lab test, and (3) has had a substantial potential exposure to HIV in the past 72 hours, they can complete a 28-day course of medication that can provide up to an 81% reduction in the risk of acquiring HIV from the exposure. Postexposure prophylaxis is considered to be an emergency medical intervention and should be started as soon as possible after the exposure for optimal effectiveness. Once the patient is past the 72-hour window after the possible exposure, the benefits of PEP may not outweigh the risks of the medication.

Postexposure prophylaxis can be provided by any prescribing practitioner. When starting PEP, it is recommended to obtain a blood HIV test (rapid or lab testing), serum creatinine, liver function tests, screening for hepatitis B and C, syphilis, gonorrhea and chlamydia (site specific based on exposures), and a pregnancy test with emergency contraception if applicable. Postexposure prophylaxis should be started even if testing results are still pending due to the time sensitivity of the intervention.

According to the CDC guidelines, the recommended medication regimen for those ≥13 years of age with no known renal disease is a 28-day course of tenofovir disoproxil fumarate (TDF) 300 mg and emtricitabine 200 mg (packaged together in one pill) once daily *with either* dolutegravir 50 mg once daily *or* raltegravir 400 mg twice daily. Although these are the regimens approved by the FDA, it is important to note that adherence to the full course of medication is essential for optimal efficacy of PEP and there will likely never be head-to-head controlled trials of different PEP regimens. Acknowledging the difficulty with adhering to more complex regimens and in an attempt to optimize PEP adherence, many practitioners utilize one-pill-per-day options (three antiretroviral medications in one pill) as off-label PEP regimens.

Repeat testing is recommended upon completion of PEP and again 3 months after the potential HIV exposure. Upon completion of the PEP regimen, patients with ongoing risk for HIV infection can immediately transition to PrEP for ongoing protection against HIV. The CDC has comprehensive PEP guidelines for practitioners and expert consultation is also available through the National HIV/AIDS Clinician's Consultation Center PEPline at 1-888-448-4911.[15]

Pre-exposure Prophylaxis

Pre-exposure prophylaxis is an HIV prevention method that uses consistent doses of antiretroviral medications in those not living with HIV to reduce the risk of HIV from potential future exposures. In individuals not living with HIV, taking PrEP regularly every day reduces the risk of acquiring HIV by up to 99% for sexual exposures and by more than 70% for injection drug use. Pre-exposure prophylaxis was originally approved by the FDA in 2012 for use by those 18 years and older. In 2018, the FDA extended this approval to any individual weighing at least 35 kg. Pre-exposure prophylaxis can be provided by any prescribing practitioner after checking for any medication interactions with the recommended regimen. If a patient (1) does not have a known HIV infection, (2) has either a negative rapid HIV test or pending HIV lab test, (3) has not had a substantial potential exposure to HIV in the past 72 hours, and (4) is determined to have ongoing risk for HIV infection, they can likely benefit from PrEP. Pre-exposure prophylaxis only provides protection against HIV; patients should be counseled that it does not protect against other STIs or pregnancy. Consequently, PrEP should be combined with counseling about other risk reduction methods, including discussions about condom use, STI screening, and pregnancy prevention. The CDC has extensive PrEP guidelines for practitioners and expert consultation is also available through the National HIV/AIDS Clinician's Consultation Center PrEPline at 1-855-448-7737.[16]

Oral Pre-exposure Prophylaxis Oral regimens for use as PrEP each consist of a single pill per day containing two antiretroviral medications. For both regimens, side effects tend to be mild and most resolve after the first month. Tenofovir disoproxil fumarate 300 mg + emtricitabine 200 mg in a fixed-dose combination can be used in all patients; typical side effects include headache, nausea or abdominal pain, and rarely weight loss. Although long-term data are lacking, there is concern about adverse effects on bone density and renal function. Tenofovir alafenamide (TAF) 25 mg + emtricitabine 200 mg in a fixed-dose combination can be used in all patients *excluding those with ongoing exposures in vaginal/frontal tissue* due to lack of data in this population at the current time. Typical side effects include diarrhea and weight gain. Theoretically, there is a lower risk for adverse effects on bone or renal function with TAF compared to the other medication regimen, but again, long-term data are lacking.

When starting oral PrEP, it is recommended to obtain blood work including a baseline HIV test (rapid or lab testing), serum creatinine, and screening for hepatitis B and C, and syphilis. Pregnancy screening is recommended with possible contraception and/or emergency contraception, if applicable. Other screening including gonorrhea and chlamydia should be done and will be site specific and based on exposures. Pre-exposure prophylaxis can be started even if testing results are still pending and if there is low concern for comorbid conditions; PrEP can be discontinued if any concerns arise from the results. If taken daily, oral PrEP typically becomes fully effective after 7 days in rectal tissue and after 20 days in all other tissues.[16]

While oral PrEP is currently only FDA-approved as a daily pill, there is another possible dosing option available. Event-driven PrEP (ED-PrEP), also known as "on-demand" or "2-1-1" PrEP, is an alternative oral dosing option endorsed by the World Health Organization (WHO) for use only by MSM due to lack of data in other populations. Event-driven PrEP consists of taking two PrEP doses of the TDF formulation at the same time 2 to 24 hours prior to sex and then one dose at both 24 and 48 hours after sex (if ongoing sexual encounters, daily doses are taken until 48 hours after the last encounter). While this regimen may be appropriate for some patients with infrequent potential exposures to HIV, it may be difficult for many youth to anticipate upcoming sexual activity and to adhere to an irregular dosing schedule.[17]

Injectable Pre-exposure Prophylaxis In late 2021, the FDA announced the approval of the first injectable medication option for PrEP for all individuals weighing at least 35 kg. Cabotegravir 600 mg is injected by a clinician into the gluteal muscle at 0, 1, and 3 months, with subsequent injections every 2 months. Preliminary data show that this method may be superior to daily pill regimens for HIV prevention, likely due to its improved adherence. Typical side effects include local injection site reactions, headache, fever, fatigue, back pain, myalgias, or rash. Injection site reactions can be treated proactively with over-the-counter pain medication as needed for 1 to 2 days and a warm compress to the site for 15 to 20 minutes upon arriving home. For patients who are worried about side effects or have significant anxiety around using a long-acting medication, clinicians may do an optional 4-week oral cabotegravir trial of 30 mg daily.

When starting injectable PrEP, it is recommended to obtain a blood HIV-1 RNA test within 1 week prior to initiation. If clinicians wish to provide the first injection at the first visit, an additional rapid combined antigen/antibody test can be performed prior to the injection as the RNA results will not be immediately available. Additional testing includes syphilis, gonorrhea and chlamydia (site specific based on exposure), and pregnancy test with possible contraception and/or emergency contraception (if applicable). Based on clinical trial data, it is *not* recommended to check creatinine, lipid panels, hepatitis, or liver function testing when starting cabotegravir injections. Unlike oral PrEP, there are currently no data available to estimate the time to maximal protection from HIV when starting on injectable PrEP.[16]

Pre-exposure Prophylaxis Lab Monitoring For patients taking oral PrEP, it is recommended that blood HIV screening (rapid or lab testing) be performed every 3 months to ensure that HIV infection has not occurred. For those on injectable PrEP, HIV-1 RNA lab testing is recommended every 2 months at each injection appointment. Given that the medications used for PrEP are not adequate for HIV treatment, there is concern that over extended periods of time, HIV may acquire resistance to the medications in PrEP if infection is not detected. Patients on PrEP who later have a positive HIV test result should be linked to HIV care that incorporates viral resistance testing. Other follow-up testing for those on oral PrEP include repeat serum creatinine every 6 to 12 months (not needed in those on injectable PrEP). All patients taking PrEP should be offered repeat STI and pregnancy screening as indicated and as often as every 3 to 4 months.

While oral medications used for PrEP are shorter acting and protection will wane within 7 to 10 days after stopping daily oral dosing, injectable PrEP is longer acting and has a "tail period" of detectable medication levels after discontinuation. There is some concern that during this period, medication levels will fall below protective levels, but may still be sufficient to select for HIV strains with resistance mutations in those with ongoing HIV exposures, making HIV treatment more complex. It is recommended that those who are discontinuing injectable PrEP who have ongoing risk of HIV receive education about this "tail period." Further, these individuals should be offered oral PrEP within 8 weeks of the last cabotegravir injection, receive education about PEP if needed, and continue follow-up visits with HIV-1 RNA testing every 3 months for the next year.[16]

Pre-exposure Prophylaxis Utilization in Adolescents and Young Adults Although PrEP is known to be highly effective and medically simple to administer, many studies have shown that this method of HIV prevention remains widely underutilized, especially in the AYA populations. A 2018 survey of YMSM (13 to 17 years of age) revealed that 54.8% had heard of PrEP, but 56.1% of these individuals did not know how to access PrEP and only 2.5% reporting they had ever used PrEP.[18] Many other barriers to PrEP access have been identified for youth, including lack of knowledge, low perceived risk of HIV infection, cost/insurance, medical mistrust, racism, and PrEP- and HIV-related stigma. Many PrEP clinics have incorporated PrEP "navigators" to provide peer health education and assistance in navigating these barriers and the medical system to enhance PrEP uptake and adherence. In addition, mobile health (mHealth) interventions are currently in development and testing to assist with PrEP uptake and adherence in youth at risk for HIV infection.

Secondary Biomedical Prevention

Treatment as Prevention

Adolescents and young adults with a new diagnosis of HIV should be referred to an AYA HIV specialist as soon as possible for linkage to treatment, including the baseline laboratory assessment. Research has shown that early initiation of ART and adherence to treatment not only delays disease progression for the individual but can also prevent transmission of the virus to sexual partners. This method of secondary HIV prevention has been designated as TasP. The Prevention Access Campaign launched the public health slogan *Undetectable = Untransmittable (U = U)* in 2016 in response to three large studies showing that there was zero transmission of HIV from those living with HIV who were virally suppressed to their sexual partners.[19] The CDC officially recognized in 2017 that those who are living with HIV, take ART, and achieve an undetectable viral load for at least 6 months, have *zero risk* of transmitting the virus to their sexual partners.[20]

Behavioral Prevention

In order to optimize primary and secondary biomedical prevention of HIV, communities and clinicians must also strive to educate all AYAs regarding HIV prevention and promote behavioral change through risk reduction counseling.

Human Immunodeficiency Virus Prevention Education

Adolescents and young adults frequently receive general HIV education in school settings. More targeted approaches with high-risk populations like YMSM, transgender females, or females of color are best employed utilizing evidence-based interventions that are strongly connected to HIV and STI screening, such as those published by the CDC (https://www.cdc.gov/hiv/effective-interventions/index.html).

Appropriate educational intervention goals for AYAs include the following:

1. Reducing misinformation about and prejudice against individuals living with HIV
2. Helping to reduce behavior associated with HIV risk, including recommendations to decrease unprotected sexual activity, numbers of sexual partners, and substance use
3. Supporting AYAs who choose abstinence
4. Increasing use of condoms and other barrier methods by AYAs who are sexually active
5. Encouraging young people and their sexual partners to have regular HIV and STI screening with treatment of STIs as needed
6. Referral and/or linkage to behavioral and biomedical interventions (e.g., PEP and PrEP) as appropriate

Human immunodeficiency virus prevention education should be conducted through schools, religious organizations, youth organizations, medical facilities, and meetings with parents. Media (e.g., internet, social media, television) are powerful methods to impart information that may change AYAs' attitudes. Outreach to youth where they congregate can be an especially effective method of reaching certain populations with elevated risk for HIV, such as youth experiencing homelessness, involved in gang activity, or not enrolled in school. Involving peers in the education process can also be helpful. It is important to offer HIV/AIDS education in a language and format that the adolescent or young adult can understand. The information must be simple, accurate, and direct.

Risk Reduction Counseling

In order to optimize the strategies of primary and secondary biomedical prevention of HIV, clinicians must also be able to promote behavioral change for those at risk for HIV. Risk reduction counseling creates a patient-centered dialogue that acknowledges the patient's feelings, attitudes, beliefs, and values while attempting to increase patient knowledge, skills, and self-efficacy. By asking the patient to reflect upon existing behaviors (number of partners, sexual practices, condom use patterns, STI/HIV testing, substance use, pregnancy prevention, etc.), the clinician can then ask the patient to identify any behaviors they would like to change and facilitate the development of ideas regarding behaviors that may reduce the risk of HIV. Clinicians should strive to balance their own public health duties to end the HIV epidemic with patient autonomy, creating an open and affirming, sex-positive environment where youth feel comfortable expressing their questions, concerns, and desires to foster healthy sexuality.[21]

MANAGEMENT OF HUMAN IMMUNODEFICIENCY VIRUS INFECTION IN ADOLESCENTS AND YOUNG ADULTS

Initial Assessment

History and Physical Examination

The history and physical examination should evaluate the following:

1. Prior exposure to infections that have the potential to reactivate, including tuberculosis (TB), syphilis, herpes genitalis, herpes zoster, and cytomegalovirus (CMV) infections.
2. Number of children, their ages, and their health status.
3. Injection drug use history and history of alcohol and other substance use.
4. Sexual history, past history of STIs.
5. History of mental health problems such as anxiety, depression, and suicidality.
6. Prior immunizations.
7. A review of systems, focusing particularly on the following:
   a. Systemic: Anorexia, weight loss, fevers, night sweats.
   b. Skin: Pruritus, rashes, pigmented lesions.
   c. Lymphatic: Increased size or number of lymph nodes.
   d. Eyes, ears, nose, and throat: Change in vision, sinus congestion.
   e. Cardiopulmonary: Cough, dyspnea.
   f. Gastrointestinal: Dysphagia, abdominal pain, and diarrhea.
   g. Musculoskeletal: Myalgias, arthralgias.
   h. Neurologic: Memory loss, neuralgias, motor weakness, and headache.
   i. Genitourinary: Bumps, ulcers, dysuria, or discharge.
8. Careful measurement of weight, height, body mass index, and vital signs.
9. Careful physical examination assessing the following:
   a. Skin: Seborrhea, folliculitis, Kaposi sarcoma (KS) lesions, psoriasis, tinea, herpetic lesions, genital lesions, and molluscum contagiosum.
   b. Eye: Visual acuity and fields, cotton-wool spots, and hemorrhagic exudates on fundoscopic examination.
   c. Mouth: Periodontal disease (gingivitis), oral hairy leukoplakia (white plaques along lateral aspect of tongue), thrush, oral ulcers, and KS lesions.
   d. Lymphatic: Asymmetrical, tender, enlarged nodes, particularly posterior cervical, axillary, and epitrochlear nodes.
   e. Cardiopulmonary: Rales, murmurs (AYAs who inject drugs).
   f. Gastrointestinal: Hepatosplenomegaly.
   g. Genitourinary: Herpetic lesions, warts, penile discharge, cervical discharge, or vaginal discharge.

h. Anal: Perianal ulcers, fissures, and condyloma.
i. Neurologic: Focal findings, altered mental status.

Laboratory Evaluation

Initial assessment should include the following (usually acquired by the HIV specialist):
1. Complete blood count (anemia, leukopenia, or thrombocytopenia).
2. Chemistry panel (hypergammaglobulinemia, hypoalbuminemia, hypocholesterolemia, elevated liver enzymes, or decreased renal function).
3. Urinalysis.
4. CD4+ T-cell count and percentage.
5. Viral load (HIV RNA PCR).
6. HIV-resistance testing.
7. Tuberculosis screening with either interferon-gamma release assays (IGRA, preferred method)or purified protein derivative skin test (PPD, also acceptable).
8. Serology for hepatitis A, B, and C, toxoplasmosis, and varicella if previous infection or immunization status is not known.
9. Tests for syphilis, gonorrhea, and chlamydia infections if sexually experienced.
10. Papanicolaou test (Pap smear) in those with a cervix who have ever been sexually active for 1 year, regardless of age

Vaccinations

For more detailed information, refer to the Advisory Committee on Immunization Practices (ACIP) general recommendations on immunization (https://www.cdc.gov/vaccines/adults/rec-vac/health-conditions/hiv.html).[22]
1. Hepatitis A: Recommended for all previously unvaccinated individuals at risk for infection.
2. Hepatitis B: Recommended for all patients without evidence of hepatitis B immunity or chronic infection. Retrospective studies demonstrate that many AYAs living with HIV do not develop antibodies to hepatitis B after three immunizations. Clinicians can consider a fourth immunization or repeating the series after the patient begins ART.
3. Human papillomavirus (HPV): Recommended for all those living with HIV through the age of 26 years if they did not receive or complete the series (older patients up to 45 years may also benefit). Given the high HPV burden in those living with HIV, vaccination has the potential to be very beneficial.
4. Influenza: While intranasal vaccination is contraindicated, the inactivated vaccine should be offered annually.
5. Measles, mumps, rubella (MMR): Measles, mumps, rubella vaccination is generally considered safe in most patients with HIV but is contraindicated in individuals with severe immunosuppression (defined as CD4+ count below 200 cells/µL or CD4+ less than or equal to 15%).
6. Meningococcal vaccination: Individuals living with HIV are likely at increased risk for meningococcal disease. Their response rates to the vaccine may be suboptimal, however, and ACIP recommends a two-dose primary series with quadrivalent vaccine (given at least 8 weeks apart) for adolescents living with HIV receiving their first vaccine between the ages of 11 and 18 years. Meningococcal B vaccine may also be offered to those 16 to 23 years of age (preferably at the ages of 16 to 18 years).
7. Tetanus, diphtheria, and acellular pertussis (Tdap): Human immunodeficiency virus is not a contraindication to Tdap vaccination; follow general AYA vaccination schedules.
8. Pneumococcal: If neither pneumococcal conjugate vaccine (PCV13) nor pneumococcal polysaccharide vaccine (PPSV23) has been received previously, administer one dose of PCV13 as soon as possible after diagnosis and one dose of PPSV23 8

weeks later. If PCV13 has been received previously, administer one dose of PPSV23 at least 8 weeks after the most recent dose of PCV13. A single revaccination of PPSV23 5 years after the first dose is recommended for individuals living with HIV.
9. Polio: Patients requiring primary or booster immunizations should only receive the inactivated form.
10. Varicella (chickenpox): The ACIP recommends varicella vaccination for all patients living with HIV who lack varicella antibody as long as the patient's CD4+ count is >200 cells/µL at the time of vaccination.
11. SARS-CoV-2: Vaccination recommendations are evolving but vaccination against SARS-CoV-2 including administration of booster doses is strongly recommended.

Follow-Up

1. Patients should have their medical and psychosocial needs assessed at least every 3 to 6 months by an HIV specialist. Many patients on ART should be seen monthly as psychosocial and adherence issues frequently arise. These appointments should focus on identifying signs and symptoms of disease progression, assessing coping skills, and reinforcing secondary prevention education. The primary care clinician can provide much of this interval care with a focus on psychosocial issues, STI screening up to every 3 months, and updating immunizations and TB screening. A Venereal Disease Research Laboratory (VDRL) or a rapid plasma reagin (RPR) test for syphilis should be conducted yearly. These tests should be conducted more frequently for YMSM in high-prevalence regions.
2. Pap smear in those with a cervix and sexually active for 1 year. Then, annually for 3 consecutive years and, if normal, once every 3 years. While there are no specific guidelines on obtaining anal Pap smears in MSM, some clinicians screen annually.
3. Regular discussion of sexual risk reduction and family planning
4. Discussion of disclosure of HIV status including options for partner notification
5. Discussion of nutrition, exercise, disease progression, medication options, and potential clinical trials. Integrase inhibitors (dolutegravir and bictegravir) and TAF containing antiretrovirals have been associated with weight gain requiring monitoring for obesity and appropriate guidance.
6. Regular evaluation of mental health status
7. Ongoing referral and linkage to identified resources (e.g., housing, transportation, employment, education)

Manifestations of Human Immunodeficiency Virus Infection

Early manifestations of HIV are listed in Table 36.4.

Opportunistic diseases, including infections and neoplasms, typically occur after immune suppression reaches a certain level. Table 36.5 lists some common diseases and the corresponding CD4+ T-cell count associated with these illnesses.

TABLE 36.4

Early Clinical Manifestations of HIV Infection

Unexplained weight loss	Pruritic papular eruptions
Fatigue and malaise	Xerosis
Chronic lymphadenopathy	Recurrent tinea infections
Leukopenia	Severe molluscum contagiosum
Isolated thrombocytopenia	Seborrheic dermatitis
Oral hairy leukoplakia	Exacerbations of psoriasis

HIV, human immunodeficiency virus.

TABLE 36.5
Opportunistic Diseases

CD4+ T-cell Count (per mm³)	Condition
200–500	Thrush Kaposi sarcoma (KS) Tuberculosis reactivation Herpes zoster Bacterial sinusitis/pneumonia Herpes simplex
100–200	*Pneumocystis carinii* pneumonia All of the above
50–100	Systemic fungal infections Primary tuberculosis Cryptosporidiosis Cerebral toxoplasmosis Progressive multifocal leukoencephalopathy Peripheral neuropathy Cervical carcinoma
0–50	Cytomegalovirus disease Disseminated MAC Non-Hodgkin lymphoma Central nervous system lymphoma AIDS dementia complex

AIDS, acquired immunodeficiency syndrome; MAC, *Mycobacterium avium* complex.
From Phari JP, Murphy RL. *Contemporary Diagnosis and Management of HIV/AIDS Infections.* Handbooks in Health Care; 1999 with permission.

The management of conditions associated with HIV is beyond the scope of this chapter and is frequently left to HIV specialists. Updated treatment information is available on several websites listed at the end of this chapter.

Management of Sexually Transmitted Infections

1. Uncomplicated chlamydia, gonorrhea, trichomonas, and syphilis are treated in the same manner as in AYAs without HIV.
2. Pelvic inflammatory disease can be more difficult to treat in those living with HIV, especially in those with significant immune dysfunction (low CD4+ T-cell count). In general, the CDC treatment guidelines (http://www.cdc.gov/STD/treatment/) are followed but the threshold for hospitalization for administration of IV antibiotics is lowered.
3. Cervical dysplasia has been shown to be very prevalent in those living with HIV, who are at significantly higher risk for invasive cervical cancer than those not living with HIV. High-risk serotypes such as HPV-16 seem to be more common, and spontaneous regression appears to be less common. Abnormal Pap smears in those living with HIV should be managed following recommendations for the general population. Whenever possible, refer adolescents with HIV and abnormal Pap smear results to clinicians with HIV experience.

Management of Family Planning
Risk of Mother–Child Transmission

The CDC guidance indicates that HIV transmission to partners or to a fetus will not occur in individuals with an undetectable viral load (maintained for at least 6 months prior to sex/conception). However, because adherence to HIV treatment can vary, sexual partners should still be offered appropriate guidance including access to PrEP.[23]

Contraception

As with any AYA, it is important to discuss birth control with youth living with HIV. Unintended pregnancies can disrupt an already complex situation for youth living with HIV. As condom use frequently drops when youth use effective contraception, contraceptive counseling in these youth is complicated by the competing desires of preventing transmission of HIV to sexual partners (using condoms) and preventing unintended pregnancy (usually with a more effective method such as long-acting reversible contraceptives [LARC]). Condom use to prevent HIV/STI transmission is highly recommended for AYAs using all methods of contraception, including LARC; however, with HIV transmission eliminated in youth with undetectable viral loads, the personal decisions made with partners can be complex.

Medication interactions between contraceptives and ART are important to consider. Contraceptives utilizing estrogen may be less effective in patients using medications that increase estrogen metabolism, such as protease inhibitors (including antiretroviral boosting medications such as norvir), specific nonnucleoside reverse transcription inhibitors (efavirenz and nevirapine), and the combination ART pill elvitegravir/cobicistat/emtricitabine/TDF. For youth at high risk for pregnancy, the use of estrogen-containing contraception may be better paired with ART regimens that do not include these medications. Long-acting reversible contraceptives (implantable and intrauterine devices) are effective options in those living with HIV and offer the additional benefits of avoiding medication interactions with estrogen and not increasing pill burden. There is evidence that dolutegravir is associated with a three-fold increase in neural tube defects (data not is not yet available for a similar compound bictegravir). These are currently the preferred choices for ART due to their potency, durability, and tolerance. Consultation with an HIV specialist is advised in patients at high risk for pregnancy.

Sports Participation

Youth living with HIV have no restrictions on athletic activity and should be encouraged to maintain fitness similar to youth without HIV. If bleeding occurs, universal precautions are advised. Youth living with HIV with detectable viral loads should avoid activities like boxing where close contact and frequent bleeding might occur.

Evaluation of Specific Syndromes

The clinician's index of suspicion for opportunistic infections (OIs) should correlate with the state of the patient's immune system, best approximated by the CD4+ T-cell count. Clinicians should have a low threshold for seeking consultation with an HIV or infectious disease specialist for patients experiencing severe or persistent symptoms.

Pulmonary (Cough or Shortness of Breath)

1. If the CD4+ T-cell count is 200/μL or less or the percentage of CD4+ T cells is 14% or less, Pneumocystis pneumonia (PCP) should be considered. Workup for PCP should include chest x-ray (CXR) and pulse oximetry, induced sputum, and bronchoscopy.
2. In patients with a CD4+ T-cell count higher than 200/μL and a percentage higher than 14%, it is unlikely to be PCP. Evaluate for bronchitis, sinusitis, TB, and viral or bacterial pneumonia and consider CXR and sinus films. Sinus problems are frequent and often severe in individuals with HIV, especially those with advanced immune deficiency.

Fever

1. Diagnostic evaluation for those with severe immunosuppression (CD4+ T-cell count <200/μL) and without specific organ system signs or symptoms should include workup for PCP, *Mycobacterium avium* complex (MAC), and CMV.

VIII

a. Chest x-ray: Interstitial infiltrates are consistent with PCP or infection with MAC or CMV; focal infiltrates are consistent with TB or bacterial pneumonia

b. Labs: Anemia and elevated alkaline phosphatase are common with MAC; elevated lactate dehydrogenase is common in PCP.

c. Blood cultures or PCR for bacteria, virus (CMV), fungus, and acid-fast bacillus

d. Consider serum cryptococcal antigen.

If fever persists and above tests are inconclusive, consider the following:

e. Lumbar puncture: May detect cryptococcal infection.

f. Bone marrow biopsy: May identify disseminated MAC, CMV, or fungus.

g. Ophthalmology consultation: May detect evidence of CMV.

h. Sinus films

i. Body computed tomography (CT): May detect lymphoma.

2. In patients with mild immunosuppression (CD4+ T-cell count 200 to 500/μL), look for common illnesses (viral or bacterial) and consider TB, sinusitis, and pneumonia.

3. In patients with minimal immune suppression (CD4+ T-cell count >500/μL), avoid costly workups unless conservative evaluation fails to uncover a source.

Diarrhea

Always assess whether symptoms could be medication related.

1. In patients with severe immunodeficiency (CD4+ T-cell count <200/μL):

a. If diarrhea is mild, consider empiric treatment with diphenoxylate or loperamide.

b. If diarrhea is severe, check stool for ova and parasites and enteric pathogens including *Cryptosporidium*, *Cyclospora*, and *Isospora*.

c. If these tests are inconclusive, consider colonoscopy looking for CMV, MAC, *Microsporidia*, and *Isospora*.

2. In patients without severe immunodeficiency, diarrhea is usually self-limited, and costly evaluations should be avoided. Consider evaluation for parasites, *Clostridium difficile*, and bacteria if the patient is sexually active, is experiencing homelessness, or has traveled abroad recently.

Neurologic (New or Worsening Headaches, Seizures, Focal Neurologic Symptoms or Signs)

In patients with severe immunodeficiency (CD4+ T-cell count <200/μL):

1. Emergency CT or magnetic resonance imaging (MRI) of head: Multiple enhancing ring lesions are usually indicative of toxoplasmosis; primary central nervous system lymphoma is also common.

2. Lumbar puncture for cell count, protein, glucose, cryptococcal antigen, Gram stain, bacterial and fungal cultures, routine acid-fast bacillus, and VDRL

Dysphagia

In patients with severe immunodeficiency (CD4+ T-cell count <200/μL), if oral thrush is present, consider empiric treatment for *Candida* with fluconazole. In the absence of oral thrush or if empiric treatment fails, consider endoscopy to look for fungus, CMV, and herpes simplex virus.

Prophylaxis

Prophylaxis is one of the most important ways that patients with severe immunosuppression can maintain their health. Severe immunosuppression is now rare. The CDC publishes updated guidelines for primary prophylaxis that can be found on their website (http://aidsinfo.nih.gov/guidelines).

Tuberculosis

Initiate prophylaxis in AYAs with a positive PPD (>5 mm) or who have a positive IGRA without evidence of active TB and with no prior history of treatment for active or latent TB. Treat AYAs who are close contacts of a person with infectious TB, regardless of screening result. More information is available on the CDC website. Current guidelines now recommend the use of rifamycins which interact with many antiretrovirals. It is advised to consult these frequently changing guidelines or to consult with an HIV specialist when youth require prophylaxis for TB (https://www.cdc.gov/tb/topic/treatment/ltbi.htm).

Antiretroviral Therapy

Research has shown that early initiation of ART and adherence to treatment not only delays disease progression for the individual but can also prevent transmission of the virus to sexual partners (see section on TasP above).[24] Globally as of 2020, it is estimated that 73% of individuals living with HIV have access to ART with the highest rates (83%) in Western/Central Europe and North America and the lowest rates (43%) in the Middle East and Northern Africa.[25] The CDC regularly updates guidelines on the use of antiretrovirals for adolescents and adults (http://aidsinfo.nih.gov/guidelines) and should be consulted with the assistance of an HIV specialist in determining how a patient should be treated with ART. It should be noted that monthly injectable antiretrovirals (cabotegravir and rilpivirine) were approved in 2021. Although a full discussion of the use of antiretrovirals is beyond the scope of this chapter, some basic principles pertaining to youth are important.

Initiating Antiretroviral Therapy

1. All persons living with HIV should be offered ART.

2. Consideration of "quick start" (initiating ART at the first visit) should be discussed. Rapid referral to an HIV specialist is preferred.

3. Initial choices may be impacted by the desire for pregnancy or in those at high risk for pregnancy interested in contraception.

The patient's ability to adhere to the medication regimen must be considered. Research has indicated that physicians are notoriously poor at predicting how likely a patient is to take medication. Table 36.6 reviews some basic concepts about AYAs and adherence to ART. Predictors of poor adherence include psychosocial difficulties such as poor support, mental health concerns, substance use, and homelessness. Factors such as patients' trust in their clinicians or concerns that taking medication might inadvertently disclose their HIV status to family, friends, roommates, or coworkers must be considered. Also critical are medication-inherent factors such as the number of pills, the frequency of dosing, the size or taste of pills, potential side effects (many youth fear rashes that might disclose their HIV status), and food and timing requirements. Forgetting, not feeling like taking medication, and not wanting to be reminded of HIV infection were the most common barriers reported by participants in one sample of nearly 500 adolescents living with perinatally and behaviorally acquired HIV.[26]

Injectable cabotegravir–rilpivirine given monthly is now a treatment option for youth not wanting to take pills. Each medication is injected separately once a month with a primary side effect of local injection site pain. To screen for medication allergy, it is currently recommended to take the oral form of these medications for 1 month prior to initiating the first injections.

In general, one should try to keep regimens as simple and tolerable as possible. Because studies have demonstrated that AYAs' adherence to ART is often poor, it is important to choose regimens that avoid HIV resistance (integrase inhibitors or boosted protease inhibitors). Close monitoring for nonadherence by multiple clinicians including psychosocial support staff is critical and frequent follow-up appointments are needed for many patients. The use of pill boxes, cell phone alarms, and mobile applications can help youth stay organized, although these methods have yet to be studied in randomized trials. Youth nonadherent to HIV medications may benefit from daily text message reminders (CDC evidence-based intervention), frequent phone-based support, and cognitive behavioral therapy. Alternative interventions are under investigation.[27,28]

In summary, viral load suppression with ART in adolescents living with HIV not only impacts the individual's disease progression but also reduces HIV transmission in the population. Medication has been demonstrated in many cases to produce immune reconstitution in even the most damaged immune systems as long as the virus is sensitive to the medication and the patient has not developed a terminal or untreatable complication. Initiation and selection of a treatment regimen should occur only after a thoughtful conversation between the patient and clinician with expertise

TABLE 36.6
Barriers to Adherence

Barriers for the general population	1. Complexity of the medical regimen 2. Lack of social support 3. Adverse effects of treatment 4. Distrust of health care clinicians 5. Lack of understanding about the medication 6. Difficulty coming to terms with a life-threatening illness

Additional barriers for adolescents	Developmental capacities of adolescence can create barriers to adherence
	1. Early adolescence
	  a. Concrete, not yet abstract, thinking (undeveloped problem-solving skills)
	  b. Preoccupation with self and questions about pubertal changes
	2. Middle adolescence
	  a. Need for acceptance from peers (desire not to appear different)
	  b. Present orientation (decreased ability to plan for future doses and grasp future implications of disease)
	  c. Busy, unstructured lives (difficulty remembering to take pills)
	3. Late adolescence
	  a. Establishment of independence (the need to challenge authority figures and restructure regimens)
	  b. Feelings of immortality (disbelief that HIV can hurt them)

Additional barriers for adolescents living with HIV	1. For most, fear of disclosure of their HIV status to family and friends 2. For many, lack of adult or peer support to reinforce their adherence 3. For youth establishing independence, the conflict between needing to challenge authority figures and needing to depend on adult clinicians for support in taking ART 4. For asymptomatic adolescents, difficulty accepting the implications of a serious illness while they still feel well 5. For some who still think concretely, difficulty grasping the concept that there is a connection between strict adherence to ART and prevention of disease progression 6. For youth experiencing homelessness, lack of refrigeration or a place to store medicines and lack of a daily routine

ART, antiretroviral therapy; HIV, human immunodeficiency virus.

in HIV care, after taking into consideration the patient's ability to adhere and numerous psychosocial factors. Helping patients prepare for ART and maintain treatment once begun is a challenging task best undertaken by an interdisciplinary team.

SUMMARY

Recommendations for Clinicians
Primary care practitioners should:
1. Be aware of the disproportionate burden of HIV infection in youth, especially in high-risk populations such as YMSM, transgender youth, and AYAs of color.
2. Obtain thorough sexual histories from all patients and counsel regularly on risk reduction behaviors.
3. Understand HIV testing and counseling.
4. For all patients with a negative HIV screen, determine if the patient may benefit from postexposure prophylaxis (PEP, if potential exposure in the past 72 hours) and/or pre-exposure prophylaxis (PrEP, if at ongoing risk of HIV).
5. For all patients with a positive HIV screen, perform confirmatory testing and, if indicated, link to an HIV care specialist as soon as possible.
6. Comanage individuals living with HIV with their HIV specialists.
7. Initiate the evaluation of common symptoms such as fever, cough, headache, and diarrhea in those living with HIV.
8. Be familiar with community resources available for AYAs in need of more intensive HIV prevention or treatment interventions.

ACKNOWLEDGMENT

The authors wish to acknowledge Lisa K. Simons, MD for her contributions to previous versions of this chapter.

REFERENCES

1. Office of Infectious Disease and HIV/AIDS Policy, HHS. *What is ending the HIV epidemic in the U.S.* Accessed March 22, 2021. https://www.hiv.gov/federal-response/ending-the-hiv-epidemic/overview
2. Samji H, Cescon A, Hogg RS, et al. Closing the gap: increases in life expectancy among treated HIV-infected individuals in the United States and Canada. *PLoS One.* 2013;8(12):e81355.
3. So-Armah K, Benjamin LA, Bloomfield GS, et al. HIV and cardiovascular disease. *Lancet HIV.* 2020;7(4):e279–e293.
4. Nichols SL, Bethel J, Garvie PA et al. Neurocognitive functioning in antiretroviral therapy-naïve youth with behaviorally acquired human immunodeficiency virus. *J Adolesc Health.* 2013;53(6):763–771.
5. Centers for Disease Control and Prevention. Estimated HIV incidence and prevalence in the United States, 2014–2018. *HIV Surveillance Supplemental Report.* 2020;25(1). Published May 2020. Accessed March 22, 2021. http://www.cdc.gov/hiv/library/reports/hiv-surveillance.html
6. Joint United Nations Programme on HIV/AIDS (UNAIDS). *UNAIDS Data 2020.* Published July 2020. Accessed September 27, 2021. https://www.unaids.org/en/resources/documents/2020/unaids-data
7. Joint United Nations Programme on HIV/AIDS (UNAIDS). *Young people and HIV.* Published May 2021. Accessed September 27, 2021. https://www.unaids.org/en/resources/documents/2021/young-people-and-hiv
8. Javed Z, Burk K, Facente S, et al. *Syringe Services Programs: A Technical Package of Effective Strategies and Approaches for Planning, Design, and Implementation.* US Department of Health and Human Services, National Center for HIV/AIDS, Viral Hepatitis, STD and TB Prevention, Centers for Disease Control and Prevention; 2020. Published 2020. Accessed August 1, 2021. https://www.cdc.gov/ssp/docs/SSP-Technical-Package.pdf
9. Centers for Disease Control and Prevention. *Condoms and STDs: Fact Sheet for Public Health Personnel.* Accessed July 23, 2022. https://www.cdc.gov/condomeffectiveness/docs/Condoms_and_STDS.pdf
10. Centers for Disease Control and Prevention. *HIV and pregnant women, infants, and children.* Accessed March 22, 2021. https://www.cdc.gov/hiv/group/gender/pregnantwomen/index.html
11. Guttmacher Institute. *State laws and policies: minors' access to STI services.* Accessed March 22, 2021. https://www.guttmacher.org/state-policy/explore/minors-access-sti-services#
12. Branson BM, Handsfield HH, Lampe MA, et al; Centers for Disease Control and Prevention. Revised recommendations for HIV testing of adults, adolescents, and pregnant women in health-care settings. *MMWR Recomm Rep.* 2006;55(RR-14):1–17.
13. Turner SD, Anderson K, Slater M, et al. Rapid point-of-care HIV testing in youth: a systematic review. *J Adolesc Health.* 2013;53(6):683–691.
14. Martin EG, Salaru G, Paul SM, et al. Use of a rapid HIV testing algorithm to improve linkage to care. *J Clin Virol.* 2011;52(1):S11–S15.

VIII

15. Centers for Disease Control and Prevention, Department of Health & Human Services. *Updated guidelines for antiretroviral postexposure prophylaxis after sexual, injection drug use, or other nonoccupational exposure to HIV–United States, 2016.* Published 2016. Accessed March 28, 2021. https://www.cdc.gov/hiv/pdf/programresources/cdc-hiv-npep-guidelines.pdf

16. Centers for Disease Control and Prevention, Department of Health & Human Services. *Preexposure prophylaxis for the prevention of HIV infection in the United States–2021 update. A clinical practice guideline.* Published 2021. Accessed March 17, 2022. https://www.cdc.gov/hiv/pdf/risk/prep/cdc-hiv-prep-guidelines-2021.pdf

17. World Health Organization. *What's the 2+1+1? Event-driven oral pre-exposure prophylaxis to prevent HIV for men who have sex with men: update to WHO's recommendation on oral PrEP. Geneva;2019(WHO/CDS/HIV/19.8).* Published 2019. Accessed March 28, 2021. https://www.who.int/publications-detail-redirect/what-s-the-2-1-1-event-driven-oral-pre-exposure-prophylaxis-to-prevent-hiv-for-men-who-have-sex-with-men

18. Macapagal K, Kraus A, Korpak AK, et al. PrEP Awareness, uptake, barriers, and correlates among adolescents assigned male at birth who have sex with males in the U.S. *Arch Sex Behav.* 2020;49(1):113–124.

19. U=U taking off in 2017. *Lancet.* 2017;4(11):e475. doi: https://doi.org/10.1016/S2352-3018(17)30183-2

20. Centers for Disease Control and Prevention. *Dear Colleague Letter: September 27, 2017—National Gay Men's HIV/AIDS Awareness Day.* Published 2017. Accessed March 28, 2021. https://www.cdc.gov/nchhstp/dear_colleague/2017/dcl-092717-National-Gay-Mens-HIV-AIDS-Awareness-Day.html

21. National Network of STD/HIV Prevention Training Centers Curriculum Committee. *Behavioral counseling for STD/HIV risk reduction.* Published 2011. Accessed March 28, 2021. https://www.stdhivtraining.org/resource.php?id=19&ret=clinical_resources

22. National Center for Immunization and Respiratory Diseases. General recommendations on immunization—recommendations of the Advisory Committee on Immunization Practices (ACIP). *MMWR Recomm Rep.* 2011;60(2):1–64.

23. Centers for Disease Control and Prevention. *Recommendations for use of antiretroviral drugs in pregnant HIV-1-infected women for maternal health and interventions to reduce perinatal HIV transmission in the United States.* Published 2020. Accessed March 29, 2021. https://clinicalinfo.hiv.gov/sites/default/files/guidelines/documents/Perinatal_GL_2020.pdf

24. Cohen MS, Chen YQ, McCauley M, et al. Prevention of HIV-1 infection with early antiretroviral therapy. *N Engl J Med.* 2011;365(6):493–505.

25. Joint United Nations Programme on HIV/AIDS (UNAIDS). *Global HIV & AIDS statistics–Fact Sheet.* Published 2021. Accessed October 18, 2021. https://www.unaids.org/en/resources/fact-sheet

26. MacDonell K, Naar-King S, Huszti H, et al. Barriers to medication adherence in behaviorally and perinatally infected youth living with HIV. *AIDS Behav.* 2013;17(1):86–93.

27. Alcon S, Ahmed B, Sloane D, et al. Interventions to improve medication adherence in adolescents with HIV: a systematic review and meta-analysis. *J Investig Med.* 2020;68(7):1217–1222.

28. Garofalo R, Kuhns LM, Hotton A, et al. A randomized controlled trial of personalized text message reminders to promote medication adherence among HIV-positive adolescents and young adults. *AIDS Behav.* 2016;20(5):1049–1059.

🛜 ADDITIONAL RESOURCES AND WEBSITES

Additional Resources and Websites for Clinicians:

AIDS Education & Training Center: Clinical Consultation Hotlines—https://aidsetc.org/consultation. Telephone 1-800-933-3413 (HIV management). Additional clinical consultation hotlines located on the website related to PEP, PrEP, etc.

Avert: Global Information and Education on HIV and AIDS—https://www.avert.org/professionals/hiv-around-world

CDC, HRSA, NIH, et al.: Recommendations for HIV Prevention with Adults and Adolescents with HIV in the United States, 2014 (amended 2016)—https://stacks.cdc.gov/view/cdc/44064

CDC: Preventing Needlesticks and Sharps Injuries—http://www.cdc.gov/niosh/topics/bbp/sharps.html. CDC website about bloodborne infectious diseases and preventing needlesticks and sharps injuries.

CDC: Preventing New HIV Infections—https://www.cdc.gov/hiv/guidelines/preventing.html. Guidelines and implementation resources about prevention strategies and services.

CDC: Revised Recommendations for HIV Testing of Adults, Adolescents, and Pregnant Women in Health-Care Settings—https://www.cdc.gov/mmwr/preview/mmwrhtml/rr5514a1.htm

HIV information: Clinical Guidelines Portal—https://clinicalinfo.hiv.gov/en/guidelines. Links to CDC guidelines for antiretroviral treatment, management of opportunistic infections, preexposure prophylaxis (PrEP), occupational and nonoccupational postexposure prophylaxis (PEP), etc.

University of California San Francisco (UCSF): HIV InSite—http://hivinsite.ucsf.edu/. Up-to-date HIV information for providers and patients.

UCSF National Clinician Consultation Center: HIV/AIDS Guidelines—https://nccc.ucsf.edu/clinical-resources/hiv-aids-resources/hiv-aids-guidelines/. Up-to-date U.S. Public Health Service guidelines for HIV treatment, prevention, and bloodborne pathogen exposure.

UCSF National Clinician Consultation Center: PEPline—https://nccc.ucsf.edu/clinician-consultation/pep-post-exposure-prophylaxis/. Telephone 1-888-448-4911.

UCSF National Clinician Consultation Center: PrEPline—https://nccc.ucsf.edu/clinician-consultation/prep-pre-exposure-prophylaxis/. Telephone 1-855-448-7737 (1-855-HIV-PREP).

UNAIDS: AIDSinfo—https://aidsinfo.unaids.org/. Global data on HIV epidemiology and response.

United States Preventive Services Task Force Recommendation Statement: Preexposure Prophylaxis for the Prevention of HIV Infection—https://www.uspreventiveservicestaskforce.org/uspstf/document/RecommendationStatementFinal/prevention-of-human-immunodeficiency-virus-hiv-infection-pre-exposure-prophylaxis

World Health Organization: HIV/AIDS—https://www.who.int/health-topics/hiv-aids/. Worldwide resources and data related to HIV.

Additional Resources and Websites for Parents/Caregivers:

Nemours Kids Health—https://kidshealth.org/en/parents/hiv.html. Basic information for parents on HIV and AIDS.

Positive Peers—https://positivepeers.org/the-plus-side/blog/resources-parents-kids-living-hiv-2/. Resources for parents of children living with HIV.

Positive Peers—https://positivepeers.org/the-plus-side/blog/friend-family-member-tells-theyre-living-hiv/

University of Delaware—https://www.udel.edu/academics/colleges/canr/cooperative-extension/fact-sheets/hiv-aids-what-parents-need-to-know/HIV/AIDS: What Parents Need to Know.

Additional Resources and Websites for Adolescents and Young Adults:

Advocates for Youth—https://www.advocatesforyouth.org/issue/hiv/. Resources on youth HIV prevention, destigmatization, and care, as well as fact sheets on other health topics.

The Body—https://www.thebody.com/. HIV education site for patients.

CDC: HIV Basics—https://www.cdc.gov/hiv/basics/index.html. CDC website with many general resources and information about HIV, transmission, testing, prevention, etc.

CDC: National AIDS Hotline. Telephone 1-800-342-2437 or 1-800-344-7432 (Spanish) or 1-800-243-7889 (for hearing-impaired). Service for the public to ask questions about HIV/AIDS and can provide referrals to state and local resources.

CDC: PEP (Postexposure Prophylaxis)—https://www.cdc.gov/hiv/basics/pep.html. CDC website with basic information about postexposure prophylaxis.

CDC: PrEP (Preexposure Prophylaxis)—https://www.cdc.gov/hiv/basics/prep.html. CDC website with basic information about preexposure prophylaxis.

NAM AIDSmap: About HIV—https://www.aidsmap.com/about-hiv. Many general resources and robust information about HIV, testing, treatment, prevention, contraception, etc.

National Center for Youth Law—https://youthlaw.org/. Comprehensive resources and guidance related to supporting youth and the public agencies that serve them.

PART IX

Conditions Affecting Nutrition and Weight

CHAPTER 37

Obesity

Kristin M. W. Stackpole
Nancy Crimmins
Stavra A. Xanthakos

KEY WORDS

- Bariatric surgery
- Obesity
- Overweight
- Severe obesity

INTRODUCTION

Over the past 50 years, the prevalence of obesity has risen dramatically throughout the world in all age groups.[1] Overweight and obesity are major risk factors for cardiovascular disease, the leading global cause of death, and increase risk of additional diseases associated with decreased quality of life and premature death, including diabetes, fatty liver disease, certain cancers, adverse psychologic effects, and musculoskeletal disorders.[1] Clinicians who care for adolescents and young adults (AYAs) will encounter a substantial number of affected young people. As such, clinicians need to be prepared to diagnose accurately overweight and obesity and its related health problems and to implement prevention and treatment strategies for this age group.

DEFINITION OF OBESITY IN ADOLESCENTS AND YOUNG ADULTS

Body mass index (BMI) (kg/m²) is the most recommended tool to screen for excess adiposity in all ages. In adults (≥18 years old), overweight is defined as a BMI of ≥25 kg/m² and obesity (class I) as a BMI of ≥30 kg/m². Severe obesity in adults is further categorized as class II if BMI ≥35 kg/m² and class III if ≥40 kg/m². Due to growth during childhood, age- and gender-specific BMI percentile distributions are used to define overweight and obesity in children and adolescents <18 years of age, using either the Centers for Disease Control and Prevention (CDC) (www.cdc.gov/growthcharts/) or World Health Organization (WHO) growth charts (www.who.int/toolkits/child-growth-standards/standards/body-mass-index-for-age-bmi-for-age). Overweight in those <18 years of age is defined as a BMI of ≥85th percentile for age and gender or ≥25 kg/m² (whichever is lower), while obesity (class I) is defined as a BMI threshold of ≥95th percentile for age and gender or BMI of >30 kg/m² (whichever is lower).[2] Severe pediatric obesity is based on the percent of the 95th percentile for BMI, with class II obesity defined as a BMI of ≥120% of the 95th percentile BMI or ≥35 kg/m² (whichever is lower), and class III as a BMI of ≥140% of the 95th percentile BMI or ≥40 kg/m² (whichever is lower).[2,3]

While BMI remains the most widely recommended screening tool for overweight and obesity, it has some limitations.[4] A high BMI may reflect a larger fat-free mass in very athletic AYAs with high muscle mass. There are also racial and ethnic differences in percentages of body fat at the same BMI, with Mexican American and South Asian children having higher percentages of percent body fat and non-Hispanic Black children having lower percentages of body fat for the same BMI. Although skinfold thickness, waist circumference, dual-energy x-ray absorptiometry, and bioelectrical impedance analysis are also used to measure excess adiposity, these methods are not currently recommended as first–line screening methods for obesity, as they require specific training and/or equipment to perform accurately and consistently.[4]

EPIDEMIOLOGY OF OBESITY IN ADOLESCENTS AND YOUNG ADULTS

Data from national health surveys performed between 1976 and 2018 show that the prevalence of obesity in 12- to 19-year-olds in the United States has quadrupled from 1976–1980 to the present 2017–2018 survey[5] (Table 37.1). During this period, obesity rates rose from 5.0% to 21.2% in 12 to 19 years old.[5] The prevalence of obesity among individuals age 20 to 39 is even higher at 40.0%.[6] Additionally, disparities in obesity rates remain among ethnic and racial groups, with Hispanic and non-Hispanic Black youth having the highest prevalence, followed closely by non-Hispanic White youth, while non-Hispanic Asian youth have the lowest rates.[5]

During the same period, severe obesity in AYAs has risen to an estimated 6.1% of 12 to 19 years old and 9.2% of those ≥20 years of age in 2017 to 2018.[5,6] This trajectory may portend a substantial rise in premature mortality in the next generation of adults, given the steep increase in cardiovascular risk factors in youth with severe obesity, and greater likelihood to remain severely obese as adults.[3] Severe obesity at age 18 years was associated with a significant increased risk of premature death in adulthood, with a hazard ratio for all-cause mortality of 2.46 (95% confidence interval [CI], 1.91, 3.16), relative to normal weight at age 18 years.[7]

PATHOGENESIS OF OBESITY

Environmental and Behavioral Risk Factors

Major societal changes over the past century have contributed to the current epidemic of obesity. Many of these factors intersect and include:

1. Improvements in food production and government subsidies resulting in greater availability of cheaper, energy-dense, yet nutrient-poor foods that are high in sugar, refined carbohydrates, and/or saturated fat. These highly processed food products are often intensely appealing to natural human taste preferences for sweet, salty, and fatty foods.

TABLE 37.1

Obesity Prevalence in Adolescents Aged 12 to 19 Years (U.S. National Health and Nutrition Examination Surveys)

	All % (standard error)	Boys % (standard error)	Girls % (standard error)
1976–1980	5.0 (0.5)	4.8 (0.5)	5.3 (0.8)
1988–1994	10.5 (0.9)	11.3 (1.3)	9.7 (1.1)
1999–2000	14.8 (0.9)	14.8 (1.3)	14.8 (1.0)
2001–2002	16.7 (1.1)	17.6 (1.3)	15.7 (1.9)
2003–2004	17.4 (1.7)	18.2 (1.9)	16.4 (2.3)
2005–2006	17.8 (1.8)	18.2 (2.4)	17.3 (2.1)
2007–2008	18.1 (1.7)	19.3 (2.2)	16.8 (2.0)
2009–2010	18.4 (1.3)	19.6 (2.3)	17.1 (1.3)
2011–2012	20.5 (1.7)	20.3 (2.4)	20.7 (2.0)
2013–2014	20.6 (2.1)	19.8 (2.2)	21.4 (3.2)
2015–2016	20.6 (2.0)	20.2 (2.6)	20.9 (2.0)
2017–2018	21.2 (1.3)	22.5 (1.3)	19.9 (2.2)

Adapted from data presented in Fryar CD, Carroll MD, Afful J. Prevalence of overweight, obesity, and severe obesity among children and adolescents aged 2–19 years: United States, 1963–1965 through 2017–2018. *NCHS Health E-Stats.* 2020.

2. Changing cultural preferences contributing to a decrease in home-based meal preparation using more nutritious whole foods, in favor of greater reliance on commercially prepared foods
3. Greater food insecurity, in part due to reduced access to nutritious whole foods and increased reliance on highly processed, calorically dense yet nutrition-deficient food[8]
4. Concurrent technologic advances that have dramatically reduced energy expenditure in both work and leisure-time activities
5. Both lack of sleep and disturbances in the circadian cycle are associated with an increase in BMI through a variety of physiologic changes, including increased ghrelin levels and appetite,[9] decreased insulin sensitivity, and increased risk of diabetes.[10]
6. Endocrine disrupting chemical exposures have increased in the environment worldwide, with several classes of ubiquitous and pervasive chemicals linked to rises in metabolic diseases and obesity.[11]

Genetic Risk Factors

Weight is a heritable trait. The concordance of fat mass in monozygotic twins ranges from 70% to 90% compared to 35% to 45% in dizygotic twins. While mutations in several genes have been implicated in monogenic obesity, the genetic risk related to more common obesity likely reflects the contribution of multiple genetic susceptibility loci.[12]

1. Monogenic mutations: While relatively uncommon, clinical testing is now available for over 50 monogenic mutations which can lead to hyperphagia and obesity. The most common is an autosomal dominant mutation in the melanocortin-4 receptor (MC4R) that alters leptin–melanocortin signaling and reduces satiety. The prevalence of MC4R mutations in children with obesity ranges from 0.5% to 5.8%, with clinical onset of obesity by age 2 years.[13] Development is completely normal and there are no syndromic features. Mutations in

leptin or its receptor, LEP and LEPR, can also lead to early-onset obesity, as well as hyperphagia, delayed puberty, and immune dysfunction. Although true leptin deficiency is rare, mutations in LEPR have been reported in 3% of individuals with early-onset obesity and hyperphagia.[14] Although monogenic mutations in other genes in the leptin-signaling pathway are uncommon, setmelanotide, an MC4R receptor agonist, is now U.S. Food and Drug Administration (FDA) approved for mutations in leptin receptor, pro-opiomelanocortin (POMC), and proprotein convertase subtilisin/kexin type 1 (PCSK1).[15] Mutations in single-minded homolog 1 (SIM1), brain-derived neurotrophic factor (BDNF), and tropomyosin-related kinase B (TRKB) can also lead to early, severe obesity, but currently lack targeted therapies.[12]
2. Genetic syndromes associated with obesity: Prader–Willi, Bardet–Biedl, and Alstrom syndromes are associated with hyperphagia, obesity, and distinct phenotypic associations. Adolescents and young adults with developmental delay, dysmorphic features, or organ dysfunction should be referred to a genetics specialist for evaluation to rule out syndromic obesity.
3. Epigenetic mechanisms: Multiple environmental factors can drive changes in gene expression without altering the DNA sequence and further amplify obesity risk, including diet, physical activity, endocrine disruptors, glycemic load, and stress.[16]

Hormonal Abnormalities

Hormonal causes of obesity should be suspected in cases of poor linear growth and/or symptoms of endocrine disease. Thyroid disease rarely causes significant weight gain unless severe thyroid hormone deficiency exists. Mild elevation of thyroid-stimulating hormone with normal free thyroxine (T4), consistent with subclinical hypothyroidism, is common in patients with obesity and does not require L-thyroxine hormone replacement. Growth hormone (GH) deficiency should be suspected if insulin-like growth factor (IGF-1) and IGF-binding protein-3 levels are low, and can be confirmed with GH-stimulation testing. Cushing syndrome is very uncommon in adolescents, but first signs include weight gain accompanied by growth arrest. Subsequently, the classic signs and symptoms develop, including central obesity, thick striae, acne, facial flushing, virilization, and psychologic disturbances. Diagnosis of Cushing syndrome is difficult as no single test confirms the diagnosis and interpreting results require input from an endocrinologist. Furthermore, it must be determined if the cause of excess cortisol is adrenocorticotropic hormone (ACTH)-dependent (pituitary adenoma or ectopic production of ACTH such as by carcinoid tumor) or ACTH-independent (adrenal overproduction). Damage to the hypothalamus or tumors affecting it can also lead to insatiable appetite and to the rapid development of severe obesity.[17]

Medications

Certain medications can promote excess and rapid weight gain by increasing appetite, while others may cause fatigue or drowsiness, limiting one's motivation and ability to be physically active. Reviewing the medications that a patient is currently taking to determine if any are linked to weight gain is essential in the initial evaluation. Table 37.2 lists medications associated with weight-gain and potential alternative weight neutral or weight-loss promoting agents.[18–20]

HEALTH EFFECTS AND MEDICAL EVALUATION OF OBESITY

Complications due to obesity include a wide number of problems previously considered "adult" conditions (Fig. 37.1). The comorbidities associated with obesity may be related to the mass effect of increased weight or adiposopathy, a derangement in adipocytes and the secondary endocrine and immune responses. Because obesity affects a wide range of organ systems, AYAs with obesity should

TABLE 37.2
Weight-Gain Promoting Medications and Alternative Treatment

Weight Gain Promoting	Weight Neutral	Weight-Loss Promoting
Antidepressants		
Tricyclic antidepressants (amitriptyline, nortriptyline, imipramine, doxepin), trazadone, monoamine oxidase inhibitors, mirtazapine, SSRIs (selective serotonin reuptake inhibitors: paroxetine, citalopram, escitalopram)	Selective serotonin reuptake inhibitors (fluoxetine, sertraline)	Bupropion
Atypical Antipsychotics		
Aripiprazole (less weight gain), clozapine, olanzapine, quetiapine, risperidone	Ziprasidone	
Mood Stabilizers		
Lithium	Ziprasidone, lamotrigine	Topiramate
Antiepileptics		
Carbamazepine, oxcarbazepine, gabapentin, valproic acid		Topiramate, zonisamide
Attention Deficit Hyperactivity Disorder Medications		
		Methylphenidate, amphetamine, dextroamphetamine, lisdexamfetamine
Antihypertensives		
Alpha-adrenergic blockers (terazosin) Beta-adrenergic blockers (atenolol, metoprolol, nadolol, propranolol)	Angiotensin-converting enzyme (ACE) inhibitors, angiotensin receptor blockers, third-generation beta-adrenergic blockers (carvedilol, nebivolol), thiazides, calcium channel blockers	
Antihistamines		
Benadyl, hydroxyzine, cetirizine, fexofenadine	Loratidine	
Contraceptives		
Medroxyprogesterone	Nonhormonal contraception Oral contraceptive pills	
Systemic Glucocorticoids (for Chronic Inflammatory or Autoimmune Disease)		
Prednisone, methyl prednisone	Nonsteroidal immunosuppressive and anti-inflammatory agents	
Diabetes Medications		
Insulin, sulfonylureas, thiazolidinediones, meglitinides	Dipeptidyl peptidase-4 inhibitors	Metformin, amylin analog (pramlintide), exenatide. Glucagon-like peptide (GLP-1) agonist (liraglutide), sodium-glucose cotransporter-2 (SGLT-2) inhibitors (canagliflozin, dapagliflozin)

Note: not all medications listed have been approved by the U.S. Food and Drug Administration for people younger than 18 years.

undergo a thorough review of systems and comprehensive medical evaluation (Table 37.3).

The onset of puberty can also affect the risk of metabolic disease. A transient state of insulin resistance develops during puberty and peaks at sexual maturity rating 3 in both sexes. The exact mechanisms are not known, but likely due to the concurrent spike in GH secretion. Glucose tolerance is usually maintained by an increase in insulin production from β-cells in the pancreas. However, the pubertal increase in insulin resistance can cause metabolic disease

to manifest in peripubertal children with obesity, due to baseline insulin resistance and genetic predisposition to disease. Obesity can in turn impact the timing and characteristics of puberty. Adolescents with obesity tend to be taller than expected for genetic potential and advanced skeletal maturation is common. Females with obesity may undergo earlier sexual maturation, possibly due to higher levels of leptin, an adipokine that indicates adequate fat mass for reproduction and is thought to be permissive for pubarche. Conversion of adrenal androgens to estrogens in adipose tissue may also play a

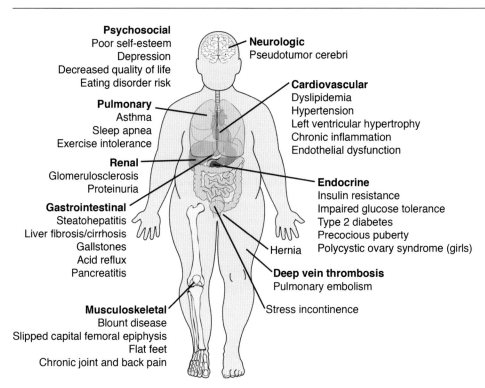

Psychosocial
Poor self-esteem
Depression
Decreased quality of life
Eating disorder risk

Neurologic
Pseudotumor cerebri

Pulmonary
Asthma
Sleep apnea
Exercise intolerance

Cardiovascular
Dyslipidemia
Hypertension
Left ventricular hypertrophy
Chronic inflammation
Endothelial dysfunction

Renal
Glomerulosclerosis
Proteinuria

Endocrine
Insulin resistance
Impaired glucose tolerance
Type 2 diabetes
Precocious puberty
Polycystic ovary syndrome (girls)

Gastrointestinal
Steatohepatitis
Liver fibrosis/cirrhosis
Gallstones
Acid reflux
Pancreatitis

Hernia

Deep vein thrombosis
Pulmonary embolism

Stress incontinence

Musculoskeletal
Blount disease
Slipped capital femoral epiphysis
Flat feet
Chronic joint and back pain

FIGURE 37.1 Health risks of obesity in adolescents and young adults (AYAs). (Adapted from Figure 1 in Xanthakos, SA, Daniels SR, Inge TH. Bariatric surgery in adolescents: an update. *Adolesc Med Clin.* 2006;17(3):589–612.)

role. Despite earlier sexual maturation, obese females often exhibit menstrual irregularities. Obesity and insulin resistance are risk factors for polycystic ovary syndrome (PCOS) (see Chapter 54), characterized by chronic anovulation and hyperandrogenism. However, obesity can also suppress gonadotropins independent of hyperandrogenism, with blunting of luteinizing hormone during sleep.

TREATMENT OF ADOLESCENTS AND YOUNG ADULTS WITH OBESITY

Avoiding Bias in the Treatment of Obesity

A pervasive, societal-wide stigma exists against obesity, and clinicians can be equally susceptible to this bias.[21] Biased assumptions that patients with obesity lack willpower, are "lazy" or "undisciplined" can lead to clinicians exhibiting less respect and empathy, which can hamper bilateral and patient-centered communication. For adolescents and their families, additional manifestations of bias can include assumptions of poor parenting ability, greater risk of bullying from peers, negative pressure or criticism from family members, or even lower expectations from educators.

When assessing AYAs with overweight and obesity, maintain open body language, use "people-first" language, and make sure the patient is feeling heard. Open-ended questions and motivational interviewing techniques are critical to partner with the patient and family to identify key factors playing into excess weight gain and to optimize treatment. Simplifying an assessment to "too many calories in" and "too little activity" and/or handing down a standard plan is unlikely to succeed. Focus on creating healthy behaviors and limiting obesity-related morbidity instead of defining success as normalization of BMI. Finally, the office space should include furniture that is sturdy without arms and tables that can accommodate large weights. Scales should be located in a private area and ideally provide an accurate weight up to 1,000 lb.

Prevention of Obesity in Adolescents and Young Adults

Prevention is the best cure for obesity. It is important to review BMI status and growth charts (for those <18 years) at clinic visits. Anticipatory guidance to promote a healthy-weight status for AYAs includes the following[22,23]:

1. Encourage healthy nutritional practices, particularly in early puberty when there is programmed propensity to increase fat cells (see Dietary Interventions below).
2. Identify unhealthy eating attitudes and harmful eating behaviors including restrictive dieting, overeating, and binging, all of which are associated with overweight.
3. Encourage regular physical activity and participation in age-appropriate household chores, family, and extracurricular activities.
4. Limit extended sedentary periods, including limiting nonacademic screen time (television viewing, video games, and other computer-based pastimes) to less than 2 h/d.
5. Encourage a healthy sleep schedule with adequate duration aligned with natural diurnal rhythms, with diurnal natural light exposure and limited artificial light around bedtime.
6. Counsel to avoid alcohol intake and substance use.

Treatment in the Primary Care Setting

Once overweight or obesity is present, the mainstay and initial course of action remains multifaceted behavioral interventions.[22,23] Surveying the patient to determine the outcome of past attempts is critical to avoid repeating unsuccessful recommendations and to identify and mitigate barriers to success.

1. Dietary interventions:
   - Avoid consumption of sugar-sweetened beverages and juice.
   - Increase intake of whole fruits and vegetables with a goal of ≥5 servings a day.
   - Eat regular meals, including breakfast, and avoid "grazing" throughout the day, especially between meals and at night.
   - Limit fast food to no more than once a week.
   - Encourage higher fiber foods and sufficient protein intake.
   - If feasible, involve a registered dietitian with expertise in weight management to help patients identify specific dietary risk factors and tailor an individualized and balanced dietary plan. A variety of dietary interventions, including both carbohydrate-modified and portion-controlled diets, can be effective in reducing BMI and body fat. The optimal dietary plan is therefore the one that the patient is most likely to follow. However, very low–calorie diets and intermittent

TABLE 37.3

Medical Evaluation of Obesity

History
- Family history of obesity, cardiovascular disease, hyperlipidemia, hypertension, type 2 diabetes, thyroid disease, nonalcoholic fatty liver disease, obstructive sleep apnea (OSA), polycystic ovarian syndrome
- Age of onset of obesity, triggers for weight gain (e.g., illness, injury, family stress, depression, medication usage), and past weight-loss efforts
- Diet history including diet recall (quality and quantity of food and drink consumed), frequency of restaurant food, family-eating patterns, unhealthy eating attitudes, dieting, binge eating, purging, and food insecurity
- Sedentary and physical activity history, including screen time, and barriers to physical activity (unsafe neighborhood, joint pain, asthma)
- Sleep schedule, timing of sleep, signs of OSA
- Current medications, particularly any that are weight promoting
- Screen for depression, anxiety, poor self-esteem/body image
- Full review of systems: headaches, exercise intolerance, snoring, daytime sleeping, abdominal pain, joint/hip pain, urinary frequency, polydipsia, polyuria, bowel changes, rashes, hirsutism, irregular menses or amenorrhea

Physical Examination
- Plot weight, height, body mass index (BMI) on CDC growth curves for those 18 and younger. Short stature, growth failure, or relative short stature (shorter than expected potential) may indicate endocrine cause.
- Measure blood pressure with an appropriately sized cuff.
- Pubertal staging: Asses for early puberty in girls (breast development before age 8). Delayed puberty in females suggests possibility of endocrine disorder.
- Skin, hair, and extremities:
  - Acanthosis nigricans suggests insulin resistance.
  - Striae that are thick, violet in color, and located on the abdomen, buttocks, and thighs are suggestive of Cushing syndrome.
  - Hirsutism is suggestive of polycystic ovary syndrome.
  - Polydactyly may indicate Bardet–Biedl syndrome.
- Papilledema suggests pseudotumor cerebri.
- Thyromegaly suggests hypothyroidism.
- Orthopedic abnormalities particularly involving lower extremities

Laboratory Tests and Diagnostic Evaluations
- Basic screening: Thyroid-stimulating hormone, fasting blood glucose, hemoglobin A1C, fasting lipid profile, and liver function tests
- For type 2 diabetes evaluation: fasting plasma glucose (FPG) 100–125 mg/dL represents impaired fasting glucose and FPG ≥126 mg/dL or above represents diabetes. Alternatively,
  - 2-h glucose tolerance test: Impaired glucose tolerance = glucose ≥140 mg/dL at 2 h and diabetes = glucose ≥200 mg/dL. Patient should be in usual state of health and not taking oral steroids or medications that can affect blood glucose for longer than 2 wks.
  - A casual glucose >200 mg/dL plus polyuria, polydipsia, and weight loss
- For diagnosis of polycystic ovarian syndrome: (1) clinical or biochemical evidence of androgen excess including acne, hirsutism, elevated testosterone or free testosterone; and (2) oligomenorrhea. Luteinizing hormone:follicle-stimulating hormone ratio of >2.0 supportive but not diagnostic alone. A 17-hydroxyprogesterone and dehydroepiandrosterone sulfate level can rule out late-onset congenital adrenal hyperplasia and adrenal tumors, respectively.
- If symptoms of OSA, a polysomnography study
- Request x-rays if concern for slipped capital femoral epiphysis or tibia vara (Blount disease)
- Consider echocardiogram for exercise intolerance, hypertension, OSA, or severe obesity.

fasting are currently not recommended for adolescents, given the lack of robust evidence of safety and efficacy.
2. Exercise and activity recommendations:
   - Engage in at least 1 hour of daily moderate to vigorous activity and in strength exercises at least twice a week.
   - Reduce sedentary activity to less than 2 hours of nonacademic screen time and avoid extended sedentary time.

- Because activity changes alone rarely lead to significant weight loss, patients must also be counseled to make dietary changes to be successful.
3. Psychosocial support:
   - Educate family members on how to create a healthy home environment and to model good habits. Family-based behavioral weight-loss treatments are generally more effective in younger children than adolescents.[22]
   - Screen for depression, anxiety, low self-esteem, and substance use which could impair motivation and the ability to implement and sustain lifestyle changes. Refer for psychological counseling if psychological problems or adverse family dynamics manifest.[22]
4. Sleep recommendations:
   - Evaluate the duration and quality of sleep and encourage sleep hygiene as discussed under Prevention above.

TERTIARY INTERVENTIONS WHEN LIFESTYLE AND DIETARY COUNSELING FAIL

Comprehensive Weight Management Programs

Multidisciplinary interventions are recommended for patients with progressive or severe weight gain despite lifestyle counseling. These programs involve more frequent visits, with psychologic support, physician supervision, and intensive dietitian and exercise support. However, such programs are resource intensive and may not always be covered by third-party payers. Access may also be limited by geography, as youth-focused programs are often located at larger medical centers. Further, the higher frequency of visits can conflict with employment or school commitments or be prohibitive if distance or transportation issues exist.

Medications

Adjunctive weight-loss medications may be attempted when intensive lifestyle modifications have failed or if significant obesity-related comorbidities exist. Table 37.4 lists FDA-approved medications for *long-term* use for weight loss in adults: orlistat (Xenical, Alli), phentermine combined with topiramate (Qsymia), naltrexone combined with bupropion (Contrave), and liraglutide (Saxenda). Only orlistat and liraglutide are FDA-approved for weight loss in patients 12 to 18 years old. Orlistat prevents the absorption of dietary fat by inhibiting gastrointestinal lipases and produced modest weight loss in clinical trials in adolescents (−2.61-kg placebo-subtracted weight loss after 1 year).[24] Side effects can include stomach pain, gas, diarrhea, and leakage of oily stool. Liraglutide is a glucagon-like peptide 1(GLP-1) receptor agonist which increases satiety and decreases gastric emptying. In children with obesity receiving lifestyle therapy, liraglutide reduced BMI nearly 5 kg/m² more than placebo.[25] The primary side effects were nausea, diarrhea, and vomiting.

Metformin is often used to treat impaired glucose tolerance or diabetes in AYAs. Although not FDA-approved for weight loss, use of metformin was associated with modestly reduced BMI in adolescents with obesity compared to placebo, while other studies suggest it may temper weight gain caused by atypical antipsychotic use in youth.[26]

For those 18 years and older, a once-daily, controlled-release combination of phentermine/topiramate was associated with a mean 9% reduction in weight over 2 years compared to placebo, and is generally well tolerated.[27] Because of the potential for significant birth defects (cleft lip/palate) primarily with first trimester fetal exposure, AYA females of reproductive potential should have effective contraception and pregnancy monitoring. The combination drug naltrexone and bupropion is associated with a 4.6% placebo-subtracted weight loss after 1 year of treatment.[28] Nausea, constipation, and headaches are among the most common side effects. A comparison of adults achieving at least 5% or 10% weight loss in clinical trials of the four FDA-approved weight-loss medications is shown in Figure 37.2.

TABLE 37.4

U.S. Food and Drug Weight-Loss Medications Approved for Long-Term Use[18,25]

Medication	Dose	Adverse Effects (AE)/ Contraindications (C)	Comments	FDA Approved
Orlistat • Pancreatic lipase inhibitor, blocks approximately 30% of fat absorption, may improve LDL cholesterol	• Start with 120 mg daily. May increase up to 120 mg t.i.d.	AE: flatulence, diarrhea, bloating, fat-soluble vitamin deficiency, increased urinary oxalate C: cholestasis, chronic malabsorption syndrome	• Recommend taking multivitamin. • Monitor fat-soluble vitamins.	≥12 y
Phentermine + Topiramate • Sympathomimetic amine, reduces hunger and possibly increases energy expenditure. • Enhances GABA (gamma-aminobutyric acid) receptor activity, inhibits carbonic anhydrase, reduces cravings.	• Start with 3.75 mg/23 mg × 14 d, then increase to 7.5 mg/46 mg, may slowly increase up to 15 mg/92 mg.	AE: dry mouth, restless, insomnia, palpitations, paresthesias, dysgeusia, cognitive impairment, depression C: active cardiovascular disease, uncontrolled hypertension, seizures, cardiac arrhythmias, hyperthyroidism, glaucoma, kidney stones, pregnancy, if taking MAOI (monoamine oxidase inhibitor), suicidal ideation	• Scheduled IV controlled substance (phentermine) • Counsel on use of birth control due to increased risk of cleft lip and palate • Pregnancy test to start	≥18 y
Naltrexone + Bupropion • Dopamine and norepinephrine reuptake inhibitor and opioid receptor antagonist, prevents autoinhibition of pro-opiomelanocortin (POMC) by β-endorphin, helps with excessive hunger and cravings.	• Week 1: 1 tablet (8 mg/ 90 mg) once daily • Week 2: 1 tablet twice daily • Week 3: 2 tablets in morning, 1 tablet in evening • Week 4: 2 tablet twice a day (for maximum daily dose of 32 mg/360 mg)	AE: insomnia, anxiety, headache, diarrhea, nausea, vomiting, dizziness, neuropsychiatric reactions including suicidal thoughts C: generalized anxiety disorder, seizures, uncontrolled hypertension, bulimia, cardiac arrhythmia, liver failure, cirrhosis, opioid use	• Avoid opioid use. • High fat diet increases bioavailability (avoid high fat diet). • Avoid in bipolar disorder.	≥18 y
Liraglutide • GLP-1 (glucagon-like peptide 1) receptor agonist, increases satiety, decreases gastric emptying.	• Start with 0.6 mg subcutaneous injection once daily and titrate each week up to 3.0 mg.	AE: nausea, vomiting, diarrhea, constipation, headaches; rarely: pancreatitis, gallbladder disease, renal impairment, suicidal thoughts, may cause hypoglycemia in diabetic patient on additional medication which causes hypoglycemia C: medullary thyroid cancer, MEN type II, history of pancreatitis	• Not recommended in severe renal or hepatic impairment	≥12 y with weight >60 kg and baseline body mass index (BMI) equivalent to ≥30 kg/m²

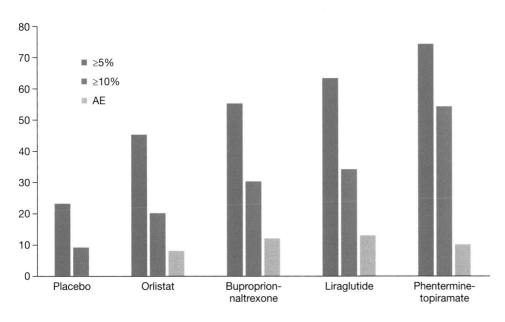

FIGURE 37.2 Proportion of adults with at least 5% or 10% weight loss at 12 months for FDA-approved drugs versus placebo. In clinical trials for weight-loss drugs approved for long-term use, adults achieving at least 5% weight loss at 12 months are depicted by *blue bars*, and those achieving at least 10% are depicted by *orange bars*. Adults who discontinued treatment due to adverse events (AE) are depicted in *gray bars*. (Adapted from eTable 4: Estimated Absolute Rate of Outcomes with Intervention, Khera R, Murad MH, Chandar AK, et al. Association of pharmacological treatment for obesity with weight loss and adverse events: a systematic review and meta-analysis. *JAMA*. 2016;315(22):2424–2434. doi:10.1001/jama.2016.7602)

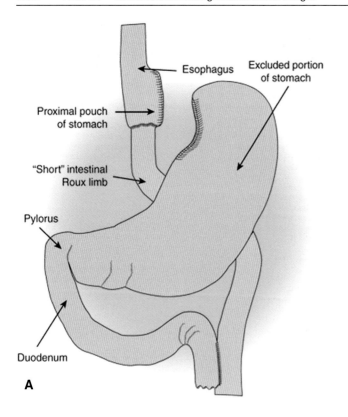

A

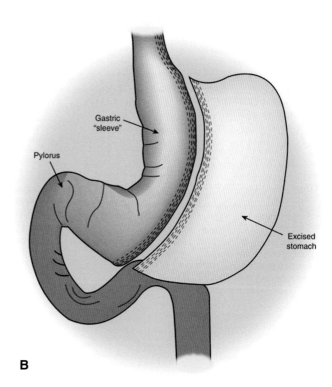

B

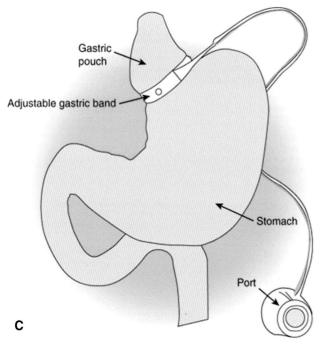

C

FIGURE 37.3 Types of weight-loss surgeries performed in adolescents and young adults (AYAs). **A:** Roux-en-Y gastric bypass (RYGB) creates a small gastric pouch by stapling off the body of the stomach. A Roux limb of jejunum is anastomosed to the gastric pouch, while the excluded stomach and bypassed duodenum are connected distally to the jejunum. **B:** The sleeve gastrectomy (SG) is created by stapling off and removing the body of the stomach, leaving a narrow gastric "sleeve" that remains in continuity with the bowel. **C:** Adjustable gastric band (AGB) is an inflatable silicone band placed around the neck of the stomach, which slows and decreases food consumption. A catheter connects the band to a subcutaneous port so that the band can be inflated or deflated by injecting or removing saline. (From Nettina SM. *Lippincott Manual of Nursing Practice.* 10th ed. Lippincott Williams & Wilkins; 2013.)

Phentermine is a sympathomimetic amine approved for *short-term* (up to 12 weeks) weight loss in adults. Phentermine is drug enforcement administration schedule IV stimulant agent and should not be used in patients with anxiety, overactive thyroid, glaucoma, uncontrolled hypertension, heart disease, seizures, drug abuse, pregnancy, or within 14 days of monoamine oxidase inhibitors (MAOIs).[18]

Bariatric Surgery

Bariatric surgery is currently the most effective treatment for achieving sustained weight loss in AYAs with severe obesity.

Current criteria for bariatric surgery in AYAs include a BMI ≥120% of the 95th percentile or 35 kg/m² (whichever is lower) for those with severe comorbidities (type 2 diabetes, pseudotumor cerebri, severe nonalcoholic steatohepatitis, or obstructive sleep apnea), or a BMI ≥140% of the 95th percentile or 40 kg/m² with or without comorbid conditions.[29] Absolute contraindications for surgery include inability to understand or provide informed assent/consent for the procedure, active psychiatric illness, problematic substance use, a medical cause for obesity that can be treated (i.e., Cushing syndrome) or planned pregnancy within 12 months of surgery.

Bariatric surgery techniques most frequently used in AYAs include the Roux-en-Y gastric bypass (RYGB) (Fig. 37.3A) and the sleeve gastrectomy (SG) (Fig. 37.3B). In the United States, the adjustable gastric band (AGB) (Fig. 37.3C) was never approved for use in adolescents, but was approved in several other countries. The use of AGB has steeply declined (peaking around 2008–2009), due in part to risk of device-related complications as well as suboptimal weight-loss outcomes.[30] At present, SG is the most common procedure in both AYA (≥70% of cases), due to comparable weight loss but lower operative risk compared to RYGB.[30] Although SG has lower nutritional risk than RYGB, both can result in chronic micronutrient deficiencies, especially iron and vitamin B12.[31] Lifelong supplementation and nutritional monitoring are critical after any type of bariatric procedure.

Recently, endoscopic bariatric procedures (intragastric balloons, endoscopic SG) have emerged as less invasive weight-loss procedures for adults, often as a bridge to traditional bariatric surgery.[32] Data on long-term safety and efficacy are currently insufficient to recommend use in adolescents.

● SUMMARY

Obesity remains a significant problem for AYA in the United States. Comprehensive screening for health complications is recommended. Lifestyle and dietary counseling in the primary care setting remains the first-line treatment for most patients, but if these measures fail, more intensive lifestyle interventions, adjunctive medications, and bariatric surgery may be considered.

REFERENCES

1. World Health Organization. Obesity and overweight. Accessed April 12, 2021. https://www.who.int/news-room/fact-sheets/detail/obesity-and-overweight.
2. Skinner AC, Ravanbakht SN, Skelton JA, et al. Prevalence of obesity and severe obesity in US children, 1999–2016. *Pediatrics.* 2018;141(3):e20173459.
3. Kelly AS, Barlow SE, Rao G, et al. Severe obesity in children and adolescents: identification, associated health risks, and treatment approaches: a scientific statement from the American Heart Association. *Circulation.* 2013;128(15):1689–1712.
4. Adab P, Pallan M, Whincup PH. Is BMI the best measure of obesity? *BMJ.* 2018; 360:k1274.
5. Fryar CD, Carroll MD, Afful J. Prevalence of overweight, obesity, and severe obesity among children and adolescents aged 2–19 years: United States, 1963–1965 through 2017–2018. *NCHS Health E-Stats.* 2020.
6. Hales CM, Carroll MD, Fryar CD, et al. Prevalence of obesity and severe obesity among adults: United States, 2017–2018. *NCHS Data Brief.* 2020;360:1–8.
7. Ma J, Flanders WD, Ward EM, et al. Body mass index in young adulthood and premature death: analyses of the US National Health Interview Survey linked mortality files. *Am J Epidemiol.* 2011;174(8):934–944.
8. Tester JM, Rosas LG, Leung CW. Food insecurity and pediatric obesity: a double whammy in the era of COVID-19. *Curr Obes Rep.* 2020;9(4):442–450.
9. Qian J, Morris CJ, Caputo R, et al. Ghrelin is impacted by the endogenous circadian system and by circadian misalignment in humans. *Int J Obes (Lond).* 2019;43(8):1644–1649.
10. Lee SWH, Ng KY, Chin WK. The impact of sleep amount and sleep quality on glycemic control in type 2 diabetes: a systematic review and meta-analysis. *Sleep Med Rev.* 2017;31:91–101.
11. Heindel JJ, Newbold R, Schug TT. Endocrine disruptors and obesity. *Nat Rev Endocrinol.* 2015;11(11):653–661.
12. Goodarzi MO. Genetics of obesity: what genetic association studies have taught us about the biology of obesity and its complications. *Lancet Diabetes Endocrinol.* 2018;6(3):223–236.
13. Valette M, Bellisle F, Carette C, et al. Eating behaviour in obese patients with melanocortin-4 receptor mutations: a literature review. *Int J Obes (Lond).* 2013;37(8): 1027–1035.
14. Farooqi IS, Wangensteen T, Collins S, et al. Clinical and molecular genetic spectrum of congenital deficiency of the leptin receptor. *N Engl J Med.* 2007;356(3):237–247.
15. Clement K, van den Akker E, Argente J, et al. Efficacy and safety of setmelanotide, an MC4R agonist, in individuals with severe obesity due to LEPR or POMC deficiency: single-arm, open-label, multicentre, phase 3 trials. *Lancet Diabetes Endocrinol.* 2020;8(12):960–970.
16. Rohde K, Keller M, la Cour Poulsen L, et al. Genetics and epigenetics in obesity. *Metabolism.* 2019;92:37–50.
17. Rosenfeld A, Arrington D, Miller J, et al. A review of childhood and adolescent craniopharyngiomas with particular attention to hypothalamic obesity. *Pediatr Neurol.* 2014;50(1):4–10.
18. Apovian CM, Aronne LJ, Bessesen DH, et al. Pharmacological management of obesity: an Endocrine Society Clinical Practice Guideline. *J Clin Endocrinol Metab.* 2015;100(2):342–362.
19. Saunders KH, Shukla AP, Igel LI, et al. Pharmacotherapy for obesity. *Endocrinol Metab Clin North Am.* 2016;45(3):521–538.
20. Tsai AG, Wadden TA. In the clinic: obesity. *Ann Intern Med.* 2013;159(5):ITC3-1-ITC3-15; quiz ITC3-16.
21. Phelan SM, Burgess DJ, Yeazel MW, et al. Impact of weight bias and stigma on quality of care and outcomes for patients with obesity. *Obes Rev.* 2015;16(4):319–326.
22. Cardel MI, Atkinson MA, Taveras EM, et al. Obesity treatment among adolescents: a review of current evidence and future directions. *JAMA Pediatr* 2020;174(6): 609–617.
23. Styne DM, Arslanian SA, Connor EL, et al. Pediatric obesity-assessment, treatment, and prevention: an Endocrine Society Clinical Practice Guideline. *J Clin Endocrinol Metab.* 2017;102(3):709–757.
24. Singhal V, Sella AC, Malhotra S. Pharmacotherapy in pediatric obesity: current evidence and landscape. *Curr Opin Endocrinol Diabetes Obes.* 2021;28(1):55–63.
25. Kelly AS, Auerbach P, Barrientos-Perez M, et al. A randomized, controlled trial of liraglutide for adolescents with obesity. *N Engl J Med.* 2020;382(22):2117–2128.
26. Kendall D, Vail A, Amin R, et al. Metformin in obese children and adolescents: the MOCA trial. *J Clin Endocrinol Metab.* 2013;98(1):322–329.
27. Smith SM, Meyer M, Trinkley KE. Phentermine/topiramate for the treatment of obesity. *Ann Pharmacother.* 2013;47(3):340–349.
28. Yanovski SZ, Yanovski JA. Naltrexone extended-release plus bupropion extended-release for treatment of obesity. *JAMA.* 2015;313(12):1213–1214.
29. Pratt JSA, Browne A, Browne NT, et al. ASMBS pediatric metabolic and bariatric surgery guidelines, 2018. *Surg Obes Relat Dis.* 2018;14(7):882–901.
30. Griggs CL, Perez NP Jr, Goldstone RN, et al. National trends in the use of metabolic and bariatric surgery among pediatric patients with severe obesity. *JAMA Pediatr.* 2018;172(12):1191–1192.
31. Xanthakos SA, Khoury JC, Inge TH, et al. Nutritional risks in adolescents after bariatric surgery. *Clin Gastroenterol Hepatol.* 2020;18(5):1070–1081.e5.
32. Sullivan S, Edmundowicz SA, Thompson CC. Endoscopic bariatric and metabolic therapies: new and emerging technologies. *Gastroenterology.* 2017;152(7): 1791–1801.

🛜 ADDITIONAL RESOURCES AND WEBSITES

Additional Resources and Websites for Clinicians:

Child & Teen Healthy Weight and Obesity | DNPAO | CDC—The CDC's Division of Nutrition, Physical Activity, and Obesity's collection of resources provides parents and caregivers, clinicians, and partners with tools and information to help children and teens maintain a healthy weight and prevent obesity.

USDA MyPlate—https://www.myplate.gov/—Includes free educational as well as print materials, available as downloadable PDFs.

Dietary Guidelines for Americans—https://www.dietaryguidelines.gov/—The Dietary Guidelines for Americans provides advice on what to eat and drink to meet nutrient needs, promote health, and prevent disease. It is developed and written for a professional audience, including policymakers, clinicians, nutrition educators, and Federal nutrition program operators.

Centers for Disease Control and Prevention Overweight and Obesity—https://www.cdc.gov/obesity/index.html—Up-to-date statistics on the epidemiology of overweight and obesity in the United States, and strategies for management.

Additional Resources and Websites for Parents/Caregivers:

Child & Teen Healthy Weight and Obesity | DNPAO | CDC—The CDC's Division of Nutrition, Physical Activity, and Obesity' has multiple resources for parents and caregivers, to help children and teens maintain a healthy weight and prevent obesity.

USDA MyPlate—https://www.myplate.gov/—Includes educational resources, recipes, and tracking tools for families and individuals. From the U.S. Department of Agriculture. Some resources available in Spanish.

EatFresh.org—https://eatfresh.org—is a project of the California Department of Social Services SNAP-Ed program and is a great resource for anyone who wants to improve their health. Available in multiple languages.

have a plant—https://fruitsandveggies.org—This resource offers simple ways to add more fruits and veggies to your day, expert advice, nutrition and storage information, shopping lists, healthy menus and recipes, kid-friendly recipes and healthy tips, as well as ways to save money using fruits and veggies.

Centers for Disease Control and Prevention Physical Activity Basics—https://www.cdc.gov/physicalactivity/basics/index.htm—Up-to-date information on physical activity guidelines and tips to become more active for adults and children.

Additional Resources and Websites for Adolescents and Young Adults:

Start Simple with MyPlate | MyPlate. https://www.myplate.gov/life-stages/teens Use the Start Simple with MyPlate app to pick simple daily food goals, see real-time progress and earn badges along the way.

Teens | MyPlate (https://www.myplate.gov/life-stages/teens) A section of the MyPlate.gov website that was designed for tweens and teens, by the U.S. Department of Agriculture. Some resources available in Spanish.

CHAPTER 38

Feeding and Eating Disorders

Debra K. Katzman
Neville H. Golden

CHAPTER

KEY WORDS

- Anorexia nervosa
- Atypical anorexia nervosa
- Avoidant restrictive food-intake disorder
- Binge-eating disorder
- Bulimia nervosa
- Family-based treatment
- Interdisciplinary
- Medical complications

INTRODUCTION

The focus of this chapter is on feeding and eating disorders in adolescents and young adults (AYAs). Feeding and Eating Disorders in the *Diagnostic and Statistical Manual of Mental Disorders, 5th edition* (DSM-5) include diagnostic classifications that represent disturbances in feeding and eating throughout the lifespan.[1] The diagnostic classifications in this section include (1) anorexia nervosa (AN); (2) bulimia nervosa (BN); (3) binge-eating disorder (BED); (4) avoidant restrictive food intake disorder (ARFID); (5) pica; (6) rumination disorder; (7) other specified feeding or eating disorder (OSFED) including atypical anorexia nervosa (AAN); and (8) unspecified feeding or eating disorder (USFED). This chapter focuses on feeding and eating disorders most commonly seen in AYAs: AN, BN, AAN, BED, and ARFID. These feeding and eating disorders are mental illnesses characterized by weight control behaviors and eating attitudes and behaviors that commonly result in medical complications. Individuals with feeding and eating disorders benefit from prompt diagnosis and aggressive interdisciplinary, developmentally appropriate treatment.

ANOREXIA NERVOSA

The core features of AN include significantly low weight, fear of gaining weight, and a disturbance in the way body weight, shape, or size is experienced. There are two subtypes: the restricting type, AN-R (those who control their weight through dieting, fasting, or exercising) and a binge-eating/purging subtype, AN-B/P (those who purge to control weight and/or routinely binge eat) (**Table 38.1**).[1]

Etiology

The etiology of AN is multifactorial with biologic, psychological, and sociocultural factors all contributing to the development of the disorder. Over the last decade, research has focused on the contributions of genetics to the biologic vulnerability, the personality type associated with AN, and the potential role of neurotransmitters in the etiology of the disorder.

There is a familial predisposition to eating disorders, with female relatives most often affected. There is a higher rate of AN

TABLE 38.1

DSM-5 Diagnostic Criteria for Anorexia Nervosa[1]

A. Restriction of energy intake relative to requirements, leading to a significantly low body weight in the context of age, sex, development trajectory, and physical health. Significantly low weight is defined as a weight that is less than minimally normal or, for children and adolescents, less than that minimally expected.

B. Intense fear of gaining weight or of becoming fat, or persistent behavior that interferes with weight gain, even though at a significantly low weight.

C. Disturbance in the way in which one's body weight or shape is experienced, undue influence of body weight or shape on self-evaluation, or persistent lack of recognition of the seriousness of the current low body weight.

Restricting type: During the last 3 mo, the individual has not engaged in recurrent episodes of binge-eating or purging behavior (i.e., self-induced vomiting or the misuse of laxatives, diuretics, or enemas). This subtype describes presentations in which weight loss is accomplished primarily through dieting, fasting, and/or excessive exercise.

Binge-eating/purging type: During the last 3 mo, the individual has engaged in recurrent episodes of binge-eating or purging behavior (i.e., self-induced vomiting or the misuse of laxatives, diuretics, or enemas).

---

among identical twins compared to fraternal twins. In addition, relatives of individuals with an eating disorder are at higher risk of developing an eating disorder. These findings suggest that genetic factors may predispose some people to eating disorders. To date, no single gene or combination of genes has been identified. Genome-wide association studies have identified a locus on chromosome 12 in AN. This locus is also associated with type 1 diabetes and other autoimmune diseases.[2]

Researchers have discovered disturbances in several different neurotransmitters including serotonin, norepinephrine, and dopamine in those with AN. There is evidence that starvation, binging, and excessive exercise can lead to changes in neurotransmitters and conversely, there is evidence that neurotransmitter abnormalities can lead to these behaviors. The role of disturbances in transmission of serotonin, a neurotransmitter known to play a role in modulating appetite, obsessional behavior, and impulsivity, has received particular interest.

Weight concerns and societal emphasis on thinness are pervasive in westernized societies and adolescent females tend to be more vulnerable to these influences. The slim body ideal is thought to be the key contributor to the gender differences seen in both AN and BN. In a biologically predisposed individual, feelings of ineffectiveness and loss of control during adolescence, compounded by societal pressures to be thin, can lead to dieting to obtain a sense of control. Dieting itself, leads to further preoccupation with shape and weight, perpetuating the cycle. Many of the behaviors, physical signs, and symptoms seen in AN can be attributed to malnutrition.

Epidemiology

1. Prevalence and incidence:
   a. Lifetime prevalence is 5.7% for females and 1.2% for males.[3]
   b. Incidence rates are highest in 15- to 19-year-old females.
   c. College students: 5.2% (6.2% females and 3.4% males) have a body mass index (BMI) <18.5 kg/m²; 1.4% of undergraduates state that an eating disorder disrupted their academics; 34.7% state that they are very or slightly overweight; and 52% state they are trying to lose weight.[4]
2. Age:
   a. Commonly begins during adolescence; >90% of individuals with eating disorders are diagnosed <25 years.
   b. Peak age at onset is mid-adolescence (13 to 15 years) with a range between 10 and 25 years.
   c. Increasing prevalence in children and younger adolescents
3. Gender:
   a. 85% to 90% of AYAs are females.
   b. 1/6 adolescents <14 years with AN are boys.[5]
4. Comorbidity:
   a. May coexist with other psychiatric disorders (e.g., anxiety disorders, depression, obsessive-compulsive disorder [OCD], and substance use disorders).
   b. May coexist with medical conditions (e.g., diabetes mellitus, cystic fibrosis, celiac disease, and inflammatory bowel disease [IBD]).

Risk Factors[6]

1. Age and gender:
   a. Adolescence
   b. Female
2. Early childhood eating problems:
   a. Picky eating, digestive, and early eating-related problems
   b. Struggles concerning meals
3. Weight concerns/negative body image/dieting:
   a. Adolescent females who diet are more likely to develop an eating disorder than females who do not diet.
4. Perinatal events:
   a. Prematurity, small for gestational age
   b. Females with a history of AN may also be at increased risk for adverse perinatal events.
5. Personality traits:
   a. Perfectionism
   b. Anxiety
   c. Low self-esteem
   d. Harm avoidance
   e. Obsessionality
6. Early puberty
7. Chronic illness
8. Physical and sexual abuse:
   a. Sexually abused individuals have the same or slightly higher incidence of AN as those not abused.
9. Family history/family psychopathology:
   a. Elevated rates of psychiatric disorders (anxiety disorders and mood disorders) in first-degree relatives of patients with AN
10. Competitive athletics:
    a. Participation in sports that place a high emphasis on body weight and appearance (e.g., ballet, gymnastics, and wrestling)

Clinical Manifestations

Behaviors

1. Dieting: May follow comments about body weight, shape, or size
2. Preoccupation with shape and weight
3. Distorted body image: Results in continued weight loss, leading to a state of emaciation
4. Unusual eating attitudes and behaviors:
   a. Denial of hunger
   b. Consumes low-calorie and/or low-fat foods
   c. Avoids previously enjoyed foods
   d. Eats the same foods at the same time each day
   e. Breaks food into small portions, hides food, or secretly throws food away
   f. May consume large amounts of water or diet sodas with caffeine to satisfy hunger or cause diuresis
   g. Enjoys reading cookbooks, collecting recipes, watching cooking shows, and cooking for others, although will not eat
5. Increased physical activity:
   a. May stand constantly, move arms and legs, run up and down stairs, jog, do floor exercises or calisthenics in an effort to expend energy
   b. Physical activity is obligatory and is often secretive or hidden.
   c. As weight loss continues, activity level often increases.
   d. Maintains rigid exercise regimen, despite fatigue, illness, or injury
6. Purging behaviors: May include vomiting, use of diuretics, fasting, excessive exercise, or herbal remedies or complementary and alternative medicines (CAM)
7. Frequent weighing:
   a. Weighing oneself daily or multiple times a day
   b. Weight on the scale determines how the individual feels about him/herself.
8. Wears baggy or layered clothing: Conceals weight loss or to keep warm
9. Poor self-esteem
10. Isolation:
    a. Withdrawal from friends and family
    b. Avoids social situations associated with food
11. Inflexibility: Difficulties with "set-shifting" (ability to flexibly shift a cognitive response) that may result in a strong sense of "right and wrong"
12. Irritability and mood changes:
    a. Starvation can cause mood changes.
    b. Comorbid mental illness can contribute to mood disturbance.

Signs and Symptoms

Signs and symptoms may be minimal but can include the following:
1. Signs:
   a. Weight loss:
      • Restriction of energy intake leading to a significantly low body weight in the context of age, sex growth, and developmental trajectory and physical health
      • Any significant or unexpected weight loss or failure to make expected weight gain during a period of growth is cause for concern.
      • Physical signs of malnutrition including loss of subcutaneous tissue, temporal, proximal muscle and gluteal wasting, loss of muscle mass, and prominence of bony protuberances.
   b. Amenorrhea or irregular menses in individuals assigned female sex at birth:
      • Amenorrhea is no longer a criterion for the diagnosis of AN, but 20% to 30% develop amenorrhea before significant weight loss; 50% develop it at the same time as the weight loss; and 25% develop it following weight loss.

c. Pubertal delay: AN can delay the onset or progression of puberty.

d. Growth: Impaired linear growth can occur if onset of AN happens before growth is complete. Examine the growth chart to determine whether the patient has crossed growth percentiles.

e. Skin and body hair:
   - Dry skin with hyperkeratotic areas
   - Yellow or orange discoloration, most noticeable on the palms and soles
   - Pitting and ridging of the nails
   - Lanugo hair—fine downy hair commonly seen on the back, stomach, or face
   - Hair loss or thinning

f. Recurrent fractures

g. Hypothermia: oral body temperature may be 35 °C or lower

h. Bradycardia: one of the most common cardiac arrhythmias

i. Hypotension: hypotension associated with significant postural changes

j. Acrocyanosis

k. Edema, usually dependent

l. Systolic murmur that may be associated with mitral valve prolapse

2. Symptoms:
   a. Cold intolerance
   b. Postural dizziness and fainting
   c. Early satiety, abdominal bloating, discomfort, and pain
   d. Constipation
   e. Fatigue, muscle weakness, and cramps
   f. Poor concentration
   g. Loss of libido

Laboratory Features

1. Hematologic:
   a. Leukopenia: may be a relative lymphocytosis
   b. Anemia: not common, usually a late finding
   c. Thrombocytopenia
   d. Decreased erythrocyte sedimentation rate (ESR); if elevated, consider other diagnoses.

2. Chemistry:
   a. Hypokalemia: hypokalemia with an increased serum bicarbonate level may indicate frequent vomiting or use of diuretics, whereas nonanion gap acidosis is common with laxative abuse. Caloric restriction alone does not usually cause hypokalemia.
   b. Hyponatremia: secondary to excess water intake, inappropriate secretion of vasopressin (the syndrome of inappropriate antidiuresis), or impaired renal sodium reabsorption
   c. Hypophosphatemia: at presentation or after initiation of refeeding
   d. Hypomagnesemia
   e. Hypocalcemia
   f. Increased blood urea nitrogen (BUN)
   g. Elevated serum transaminases (40% of patients)
   h. Increased cholesterol
   i. Increased serum carotene level (15% to 40% of patients)

3. Endocrine:
   a. Thyroid: Thyroid hormone disturbances represent adaptation to starvation, do not require thyroid hormone replacement, and will reverse with nutritional rehabilitation
      - Low Triiodothyronine (T3), representing increased conversion of thyroxine (T4) to reverse T3
      - T4: usually normal or slightly low
      - Thyrotropin (TSH) usually normal
   b. Growth hormone (GH):
      - Decreased insulin-like growth factor 1 (IGF-1) levels
      - Growth hormone levels normal or elevated, consistent with relative GH resistance

c. Prolactin: Usually normal

d. Gonadotropins:
   - Hypogonadotropic hypogonadism with low basal levels of luteinizing hormone (LH) and follicle-stimulating hormone (FSH)
   - Twenty-four-hour LH secretory pattern: Prepubertal with low LH levels and no spikes or occasional nocturnal spikes
   - Blunted response of FSH and LH to gonadotropin-releasing hormone (GnRH) stimulation

e. Sex steroids:
   - Estradiol: Low in females (<30 pg/mL)
   - Testosterone: Low in males

f. Cortisol:
   - Basal levels normal or slightly high
   - Decreased response of adrenocorticotropic hormone (ACTH) to corticotropin-releasing hormone
   - Normal cortisol response to ACTH stimulation

4. Cardiac:
   a. Electrocardiogram (ECG): Bradycardia, low-voltage changes, prolonged QTc interval, T-wave inversions, and occasional ST-segment depression
   b. Echocardiogram: Decreased cardiac size and left ventricular wall thickness, pericardial effusion and increased prevalence of mitral valve prolapse

5. Gastrointestinal (GI):
   a. Upper GI tract series: Usually normal findings; with occasional decreased gastric motility. May demonstrate features of the superior mesenteric artery syndrome
   b. Barium enema: Normal findings

6. Renal and metabolic:
   a. Decreased glomerular filtration rate
   b. Elevated BUN concentration
   c. Decreased maximum concentration ability (nephrogenic diabetes insipidus)
   d. Metabolic alkalosis
   e. Alkaline urine

7. Low bone mineral density (BMD):
   a. Both males and females with AN have low BMD and are at increased fracture risk.[7]
   b. Oral estrogen–progesterone combination pills have not been proven to be effective in increasing BMD.
   c. Bisphosphonates (alendronate and risedronate) have shown no significant effect on spine BMD in adolescents but a positive effect in adults.
   d. 17β-estradiol transdermal patch in older girls with AN (bone age ≥15 years) showed increased spine and hip BMD; complete catch-up did not occur.[8]
   e. Current recommendations for low BMD in AN include sustainable weight restoration through optimizing nutritional intake, resumption of spontaneous menses, and optimal calcium (1,300 mg/day of elemental calcium) and vitamin D (600 to 1,000 IU units/day) intake.[9] Despite intervention, BMD may not return to normal.
   f. In individuals assigned female sex at birth, measurement of baseline BMD with dual-energy x-ray absorptiometry (DXA) is recommended after 6 or more months of amenorrhea. There is no clear guidance available for males.[10]

Medical Complications

Table 38.2 outlines the medical complications seen in AYAs with AN.

Diagnosis and Differential Diagnosis

The diagnosis of AN should be suspected in AYAs with unexplained weight loss and food avoidance.

1. Medical conditions:
   a. Inflammatory bowel disease
   b. Malabsorption—cystic fibrosis, celiac disease

TABLE 38.2

Medical Complications of Eating Disorders

System	Anorexia Nervosa	Bulimia Nervosa	ARFID
Fluid and electrolytes	• Dehydration, elevated BUN/creatinine • Hypokalemia • Hyponatremia • Hypochloremic alkalosis • Hypophosphatemia • Hypomagnesemia • Hypoglycemia • Ketonuria • Edema	• Dehydration, elevated BUN/creatinine • Hypokalemia (from vomiting or from laxative or diuretic use) • Hypophosphatemia (especially when bingeing occurs after a prolonged period of dietary restriction) • Hypochloremic alkalosis • Hypomagnesemia • Edema	• Dehydration, elevated BUN/creatinine • Hypokalemia • Hyponatremia • Hypochloremic alkalosis • Hypophosphatemia • Hypomagnesemia • Hypoglycemia
Head, eyes, ears, nose and throat	• Dry, cracked lips and tongue	• Dry lips and tongue • Subconjunctival hemorrhages • Palatal scratches • Erosion of dental enamel • Dental caries	• Dry, cracked lips and tongue
Cardiovascular	• Bradycardia • Orthostatic blood pressure or heart rate changes • Cardiac arrhythmias • Electrocardiographic abnormalities (prolonged QTc interval, low voltage, T-wave abnormalities) • Reduced myocardial contractility • Mitral valve prolapse • Pericardial effusion • Congestive heart failure	• Dizziness • Orthostatic blood pressure or heart rate changes • Cardiac arrhythmias • Ipecac cardiomyopathy	• Bradycardia • Orthostatic blood pressure or heart rate changes • Cardiac arrhythmias • Electrocardiographic abnormalities (prolonged QTc interval, low voltage, T-wave abnormalities)
Gastrointestinal	• Delayed gastric emptying • Constipation • Elevated transaminases • Superior mesenteric artery syndrome • Rectal prolapse • Gallstones	• Parotid swelling • Esophagitis • Mallory–Weiss tears • Rupture of the esophagus or stomach • Acute pancreatitis • Paralytic ileus secondary to laxative abuse • Cathartic colon • Barrett esophagus	• Delayed gastric emptying • Constipation
Pulmonary		• Aspiration pneumonia • Pneumomediastinum	
Renal	• Elevated BUN/creatinine • Decreased glomerular filtration rate • Renal calculi • Edema • Renal concentrating defect • Enuresis (most commonly nocturnal)	• Elevated BUN/creatinine • Edema (after withdrawal of laxatives)	• Elevated BUN/creatinine
Endocrine	• Primary or secondary amenorrhea • Pubertal delay • Growth delay and short stature • Low T3 syndrome • Hypercortisolism • Partial diabetes insipidus	• Irregular menses	• Primary or secondary amenorrhea • Pubertal delay • Growth delay and short stature
Hematologic	• Anemia • Leukopenia • Thrombocytopenia • Low ESR		• Iron deficiency anemia
Musculoskeletal	• Muscle wasting and generalized muscle weakness • Reduced BMD • Increased fracture risk	• Fatigue, muscle weakness and cramps • Reduced BMD (if previously at a low weight or amenorrheic)	• Muscle wasting and generalized muscle weakness • Reduced BMD

IX

(continued)

TABLE 38.2

Medical Complications of Eating Disorders (*Continued*)

System	Anorexia Nervosa	Bulimia Nervosa	ARFID
Dermatologic	• Acrocyanosis • Dry, yellow skin (hypercarotenemia) • Lanugo • Brittle nails • Thin, dry hair • Hair loss	• Calluses on the dorsum of hand—(Russell sign)	• Cutaneous manifestation of nutritional deficiencies
Neurologic	• Syncope • Seizures • Peripheral neuropathies • Structural brain changes (enlarged lateral ventricles and deficits in both gray and white matter volumes) • Decreased concentration, memory, and thinking ability	• Syncope • Seizures	

BUN, blood urea nitrogen; BMD, bone mineral density; ESR, erythrocyte sedimentation rate.

c. Endocrine conditions—hyperthyroidism, Addison disease, diabetes mellitus
d. Collagen vascular disease
e. Central nervous system (CNS) lesions—hypothalamic or pituitary tumors
f. Malignancies
g. Chronic infections—tuberculosis, human immunodeficiency virus
h. Immunodeficiency
2. Psychiatric conditions:
a. ARFID
b. Mood disorders
c. Anxiety disorders
d. Somatization disorder
e. Substance abuse disorder
f. Psychosis

Evaluation

History

Helpful questions regarding eating, weight-control behavior, and other issues include:
1. Why has individual and/or family come for assessment?
2. How does the patient feel about their appearance?
3. Is the patient trying to change their appearance?
4. Any change in weight? If yes, what methods were used?
5. How much does the patient want to weigh?
6. Does the patient binge? Describe a "binge"? Frequency of binges?
7. What methods of purging are used (vomiting, laxative abuse, diuretics, ipecac, diet pills, excessive exercise, or CAM)?
8. Highest and lowest weight and when?
9. Feeling that one's body affects their mood?
10. Is there a part of the patient's body that the patient is uncomfortable with and why?
11. Does the disordered eating interfere with the individual's life? How much time does the patient spend preparing food, exercising, and weighing themself?
12. How much does the patient worry about eating or their weight?
13. Previous treatment, including hospitalizations? Where? What type and for how long?
14. Exercise history? Type, amount, and frequency?
15. Twenty-four-hour dietary recall?
16. In females, menstrual history including age of menarche, last normal menstrual period, frequency of menses, changes in menses, medications including hormonal contraceptives? In males, loss of early morning erections and diminished libido?
17. Family medical and psychiatric history (family members with an eating disorder, mental illness, or substance abuse disorder)?
18. Prior or current history of sexual, physical, or emotional abuse?
19. Family's understanding of patient's eating problem? What have parent(s)/caregiver/family members done to support the individual?

Instruments

Several instruments have been developed to aid in the diagnosis of eating disorders and the differentiation of AN from BN. These include the following:
1. *Eating Attitudes Test (EAT-26)*[11]: This validated screening test is a 26-item self-report questionnaire that examines attitudes and behaviors regarding food, weight, and body image in AYAs. A score >21 is suggestive of an eating disorder and warrants further evaluation.
2. *Eating Disorders Examination Questionnaire (EDE-Q)*: The EDE-Q[12] is a 28-item self-report questionnaire that assesses the range and severity of eating disorder features: restraint, eating concerns, weight, and shape concerns.
3. *Kids Eating Disorders Survey (KEDS)*: The KEDS[13] is a 14-item self-report instrument requiring a second-grade reading level. It includes a three-point scale and eight figure drawings for assessing body shape concerns. Normal values are available.

Nutritional Assessment

1. Twenty-four-hour dietary recall:
a. Types of foods and beverages
b. Portion sizes
c. Specific foods or food groups that are intentionally avoided (e.g., fats, carbohydrates, or protein)
d. Excessive amount of fluid intake including caffeinated products (coffee, tea, or soda) to reduce hunger and alter body weight
2. Diet products or CAM
3. Dietary calcium intake:
a. Adolescents require 1,300 mg of elemental calcium/day. Each 8-oz glass of milk, one 1.5-oz serving of cheese or one yogurt contains approximately 300-mg calcium.[9]
b. May require oral supplementation
4. Anthropometric measurements: height, weight, BMI, and skinfold measures

Physical Examination

1. Measure weight and height, calculate BMI, and plot on growth charts:
   a. Weight—measure in hospital gown after patient has emptied their bladder
   b. Calculate BMI = weight (kg)/height (m^2)
   c. Calculate percentage median BMI = patient's BMI/median BMI for age and sex × 100
   d. Obtain previous growth charts—may indicate falling off percentiles for weight, height, or BMI
2. Sexual maturity rating (SMR): assure that puberty is proceeding in a normal manner
3. Focus on signs of malnutrition described above

Recommended Laboratory Tests

1. Complete blood cell, platelet count, and ESR
2. Serum chemistry including BUN, creatinine, electrolytes (including calcium, phosphate, magnesium, and phosphorus) and liver function tests
3. Serum albumin level
4. T3, T4, and TSH levels
5. Females: LH, FSH, estradiol, and prolactin level if amenorrheic

Boys: LH, testosterone (free and total)
1. Electrocardiogram
2. Bone mineral density:
   a. Females: amenorrhea for >6 months
   b. Males: no definitive recommendations

Optional laboratory tests include:
1. Upper GI tract series and small bowel series
2. Barium enema
3. Celiac screen
4. Stool calprotectin (if IBD suspected)
5. Computed tomography or magnetic resonance imaging (MRI) of the head

Treatment

1. Team approach: Treatment is best conducted by an interdisciplinary team of individuals who are skilled and knowledgeable in working with AYAs with eating disorders.[14] The treatment team typically consists of a physician, therapist, and nutritionist. Excellent communication among team members is paramount.
2. Diagnosis: Early diagnosis and intervention is important.
3. Medical and nutritional intervention: Goals include nutritional rehabilitation, weight restoration, and reversal of the acute medical complications.
4. Psychological intervention: Research supports that family-based treatment (FBT) is an effective first-line outpatient treatment for adolescents with AN.[15] Family-based treatment is based on the importance of empowering parents/caregivers as the principal resource in weight restoration and effectively changing the eating disorder behaviors. Coexisting mental illness such as an anxiety disorder or depression should also be considered in making treatment recommendations.
5. Pharmacologic treatment: Evidence for the role of medications in the management of AN is limited and there are no U.S Food and Drug Administration (FDA)-approved medications for treatment of this disorder. Initial interest in the use of the selective serotonin reuptake inhibitors (SSRIs) has not been supported by randomized-controlled trials in underweight adults with AN or in relapse prevention after weight restoration. A recent randomized-controlled trial in adults with AN found a modest effect of olanzapine on weight gain but no significant benefit for psychological symptoms.[16] A placebo-controlled pilot study in AYAs with AN demonstrated no significant effect of olanzapine on weight gain or psychological symptoms.[17]

Despite the lack of proven efficacy, psychotropic medications are frequently prescribed for AYAs with eating disorders, usually for psychiatric comorbidity.[18] The most common medications prescribed are SSRIs such as fluoxetine, sertraline, paroxetine, fluvoxamine, and citalopram. These medications are also useful in treating comorbid depression or OCD. The FDA requires a "black box" warning on the label to warn of an increased risk of suicidal ideation and behavior in AYAs being treated with these medications. Finally, caution should be taken prescribing any medication that could prolong the QTc interval, which can be prolonged in underweight patients.

6. Treatment setting:
   a. Inpatient, outpatient, partial hospitalization, or residential settings. Most AYAs with AN can be treated as outpatients.
   b. Factors supporting hospitalization are outlined in **Table 38.3**.[14]
   c. Goals of hospitalization include weight gain and medical stabilization.
   d. Nutritional rehabilitation:
      • Essential for underweight or those who are medically compromised
      • Weight restoration via oral route, whenever possible
      • Short-term nasogastric feeding may be necessary
      • A recent study showed that higher calorie refeeding (starting at 2,000 kcal/day with increases by 200 kcals/d) restored medical stability earlier with shorter length of stay and no adverse safety events compared to lower calorie feedings (starting at 1,400 kcals/d and advancing by 200 kcal every other day).[19] Clinical remission rates at 1 year were similar in both groups with no increased rates of rehospitalization in the higher calorie group.[20]
      • Inpatient weight gain of 1 to 2 kg a week is optimal.

TABLE 38.3

Factors Supporting Hospitalization in an Adolescent with an Eating Disorder

One or more of the following justify hospitalization:

1. Severe malnutrition (weight ≤75% average body weight for age, sex, and height)
2. Dehydration
3. Electrolyte disturbances (e.g., hypokalemia, hyponatremia, hypophosphatemia)
4. Cardiac dysrhythmia
5. Physiologic instability
   Severe bradycardia (heart rate <50 beats/min daytime; <45 beats/min at night)
   Hypotension (<90/45 mm Hg)
   Hypothermia (body temperature <96 °F)
   Orthostatic changes in pulse or blood pressure (a drop of >20 mm Hg systolic BP or >10 mm Hg diastolic BP, a pulse increase of >30 bpm in adults and > 40 bpm in adolescents aged 12–19 y)[a]
6. Arrested growth and development
7. Failure of outpatient treatment
8. Acute food refusal
9. Uncontrollable binging and purging
10. Acute medical complications of malnutrition (e.g., syncope, seizures, cardiac failure, pancreatitis)
11. Acute psychiatric emergencies (e.g., suicidal ideation, acute psychosis)
12. Comorbid diagnosis that interferes with the treatment of the eating disorder (e.g., severe depression, obsessive–compulsive disorder, severe family dysfunction)

[a]More recent definitions of orthostatic intolerance in adolescents aged 12 to 19 years suggest that pulse differences up to 40 bpm may be normal.[22] At present, however, there is no definitive evidence on pulse differences in AYAs with eating disorders and expert consensus on the applicability of the evidence in healthy AYAs to patients with eating disorders requires further study.

Adapted with permission from Golden NH, Katzman DK, Sawyer SM, et al. Position Paper of the Society for Adolescent Health and Medicine: medical management of restrictive eating disorders in adolescents and young adults, 2015.[14]

- Refeeding syndrome—a constellation of cardiac, hematologic, and neurologic symptoms is associated with refeeding a malnourished AYA.
- Most serious feature of refeeding is sudden unexpected death associated with hypophosphatemia and cardiac arrhythmias.
- Refeeding hypophosphatemia is associated with the degree of malnutrition on admission, but not rate of refeeding.[21]

Some medical complications may not be completely reversible (growth retardation, reduced bone mass, and structural brain changes) with nutritional rehabilitation.

Outcome

Numerous studies have been conducted on the outcome of AYAs with AN with wide variability in the results due to differences in the definitions of recovered cases, length of follow-up, and type of data collected. The prognosis for AYAs with AN is better than that for adults, due in part to the shorter duration of symptoms. Between 40% and 70% of adolescents with AN recover, 20% to 30% improve but continue to have persistent symptoms, and 20% develop a chronic form of the illness.[6] Adolescents with AN can fully recover, but the time to recover may take many years. Findings pertaining to recovery include:

1. Weight restoration: 40% to 63% of adolescents achieve a weight >90% median BMI (mBMI) at 1-year follow-up.[23]
2. Menses: 68% of adolescents with AN followed for 1 year and 95% of those followed for 2 years were menstruating at follow-up.
3. Eating difficulties:
   a. Eating difficulties take longer to resolve.
   b. 1/3 of patients were eating normally at follow-up and 1/2 were still purposefully avoiding high-calorie foods.
4. Psychological disturbances:
   a. Psychological recovery lags behind weight restoration.
   b. Psychiatric comorbidity common in follow-up.
   c. Lifetime incidence of depression occurs in 50% to 68%; anxiety disorders (especially OCD and social anxiety disorder) in 30% to 65%; substance abuse in 12% to 21%; and comorbid personality disorders in 20% to 80%.
   d. Good or satisfactory psychosocial functioning ranged from 22% to 73%.
   e. 1/3 of patients with AN "cross over" to BN at some time in their illness.
5. Psychosocial: Most patients were engaged in full-time employment, with good work attendance.
6. Mortality:
   a. Mortality rates are among the highest of all psychiatric disorders.
      - Approximately 5.6% of patients with AN die per decade of illness.[6]
      - Weighted mortality rate of 5.86 deaths per 1000 person years.[24]
   b. Causes of death are suicide and the medical complications of starvation.
   c. Greatest risk for mortality occurs in the first 10 years of follow-up.
7. Factors associated with a good prognosis:
   a. Short duration of illness
   b. Early identification and intervention
   c. Early onset (<14 years old)
   d. No associated comorbid psychological diagnoses
   e. No binging and purging
   f. Supportive family
8. Factors associated with a poor prognosis:
   a. Longer duration of illness
   b. Binging and purging
   c. Comorbid mental illness (mood disorders, substance abuse)
   d. Lower body weight at presentation

Anorexia nervosa appears to have lower recovery rates than BN.

ATYPICAL ANOREXIA NERVOSA

Atypical anorexia nervosa is an eating disorder where AYAs present with all the criteria for AN except that, despite significant weight loss, their weight remains in the normal or above normal range. Many AYAs with AAN have a history of being overweight and frequently go unrecognized because weight loss is usually perceived as beneficial. As a result, AYAs with AAN often present for treatment after a longer duration of illness. Because AAN is classified under the category of "Other Specified Feeding and Eating Disorders," many clinicians perceive AAN to be less severe than AN. However, even though their body weight may be in the normal or above normal range, AYAs with AAN can have severe medical complications similar to those seen in AYAs with AN including bradycardia, orthostasis, electrolyte disturbances, hypothalamic–pituitary–gonadal axis suppression and low BMD. In addition, AYAs with AAN have higher distress related to eating and body image than those with AN.

The patient's prior growth trajectory can help guide the determination of a treatment goal weight (TGW). In females with AAN, resumption of menses can be used as one objective indicator of return to biologic health. One study found that some weight gain was necessary for resumption of menses in adolescents with AAN, and that these patients need to be at a higher mBMI percentage than those with AN to resume menses.[25] However, patients with AAN may not necessarily need to be restored to their premorbid highest weight to resume menses.

BULIMIA NERVOSA

Bulimia nervosa is an eating disorder characterized by recurrent binge eating accompanied by inappropriate compensatory behaviors including self-induced vomiting, laxative abuse, enemas, diuretics, excessive exercise, prolonged fasting, abuse of stimulants (including methylphenidate, cocaine, over-the-counter "natural" supplements, caffeine), and underdosing of insulin (for those with diabetes mellitus) to control weight or to purge calories consumed during binge eating. These behaviors must occur, on average, at least once a week for 3 months (Table 38.4).[1]

Epidemiology

1. Prevalence:
   a. Up to 15% of healthy individuals report binge eating or purging behaviors. The numbers are even higher for college students with 23% of college females and 14% of college males reporting binging at least once each week.
   b. Lifetime prevalence of BN in young females living in western industrialized countries is estimated to be 1% to 4%.

TABLE 38.4

DSM-5 Diagnostic Criteria for Bulimia Nervosa[1]

A. Recurrent episodes of binge eating. An episode of binge eating is characterized by both of the following:
   1. Eating, in a discrete period of time (e.g., within any 2-h period), an amount of food that is definitely larger than what most individuals would eat in a similar period of time under similar circumstances
   2. A sense of lack of control overeating during the episode (e.g., a feeling that one cannot stop eating or control what or how much one is eating)
B. Recurrent inappropriate compensatory behaviors in order to prevent weight gain, such as self-induced vomiting; misuse of laxatives, diuretics, or other medications; fasting; or excessive exercise
C. The binge eating and inappropriate compensatory behaviors both occur, on average, at least once a week for 3 mo.
D. Self-evaluation is unduly influenced by body shape and weight.
E. The disturbance does not occur exclusively during episodes of anorexia nervosa

2. Age:
   a. Onset during late adolescence or early adulthood
   b. Average age of onset 16 to 17 years
   c. Rare in those <14 years old
3. Gender:
   a. 3:1 female-to-male ratio[26]
   b. Recently, increased prevalence in males, particularly those who participate in sports with weight categories/restrictions (e.g., wrestlers)
4. Comorbidity:
   a. 80% of patients with BN report a lifetime prevalence of another psychiatric condition.
   b. Major comorbid conditions are mood disorders (50% to 80%), anxiety disorders (13% to 65%), personality disorders (20% to 80%), and substance abuse disorders (25%).[6]
   c. Patients tend to be more impulsive than those with AN.
   d. May engage in shoplifting, stealing, self-destructive acts, and sexual acting out.

Risk Factors

1. Age and gender:
   a. More likely to develop during adolescence.
   b. Females affected more than males.
2. Early childhood eating and health problems:
   a. Childhood eating problems (pica, early digestive problems, and weight reduction efforts)
3. Weight concerns, negative body image, and dieting
4. Personality traits:
   a. Negative affect, impulsivity, stressful life events, and family conflict
5. Early puberty/early menarche
6. Family history:
   a. Increased risk of developing BN if a family member has an eating disorder; concordance rates are higher for monozygotic than for dizygotic twins and range from 27% to 83%
   b. Susceptibility locus for BN has been identified on chromosome 10p.
7. Childhood sexual abuse

Clinical Manifestations

Behaviors

1. Binging and purging:
   a. Binging:
      • Rapid consumption of a large amount of high calorie food (as high as 3,000 to 5,000 kcal) in a short period of time (usually less than 2 hours)
      • Self-perceived loss of control overeating
      • Triggers—negative mood, interpersonal stress, hunger due to dietary restriction, and negative feelings related to body image. Typically occur in afternoon after skipping breakfast or lunch, or late in the evening.
   b. Purging (specific behaviors outlined above)
   c. Binge–Purge cycles:
      • After a binge, feelings of guilt and shame together with fear of weight gain result in purging.
      • Purging may have a calming effect and relieve guilt after a binge episode leading to recurrent cycles of binging and purging to help manage feelings of depression and anxiety.
      • Binging and purging are usually done secretly.
      • Patients distressed by abnormal eating behaviors.
         Initially, the binge–purge activity may be infrequent, but with time, it may increase to daily or even several times a day. Some individuals with BN will purge even after ingesting normal or small amounts of any food that might be considered high in calories or fat. Therefore,

over time, what began as a diet or weight-control measure turns into a means of mood regulation with the binging and purging behaviors becoming a source of coping.
2. Evidence of purging:
   a. Frequent trips to the bathroom, particularly after eating
   b. Signs and/or smells of vomit or packages of laxatives or diuretics
3. Evidence of binge eating:
   a. Disappearance of food or the presence of empty wrappers and containers indicating the consumption of large amounts of food.
   b. Stealing, hoarding, hiding food, or eating in secret
4. Frequently weighing
5. Preoccupation with food
6. Overly concerned with food, body weight, shape, and size
7. Self-evaluation is unduly influenced by body shape and weight.

Signs and Symptoms

1. Signs:
   a. Body weight is usually normal or above normal.
   b. Marked weight fluctuations
   c. Skin changes: Calluses on the dorsum of the hand secondary to abrasions from the central incisors when the fingers are used to induce vomiting (Russell sign)
   d. Enlargement of the parotid glands; usually bilateral and painless
   e. Perimolysis (dental enamel erosion): Usually occurs in the lingual, palatal, and posterior occlusal surfaces of the teeth.
   f. Edema
2. Symptoms:
   a. Weakness and fatigue
   b. Headaches
   c. Abdominal fullness and bloating
   d. Nausea
   e. Normal or irregular menses
   f. Muscle cramps
   g. Chest pain and heartburn
   h. Easy bruising (from hypokalemia/platelet dysfunction)
   i. Bloody diarrhea (in those who abuse laxatives)

Medical Complications

See Table 38.2 which outlines the medical complications seen in AYAs with BN.

Diagnosis and Differential Diagnosis

1. Medical conditions:
   a. Chronic cholecystitis
   b. Cholelithiasis
   c. Peptic ulcer disease
   d. Gastroesophageal reflux disease
   e. Superior mesenteric artery syndrome
   f. Malignancies (including CNS tumors)
   g. Infections—acute bacterial and viral GI infections, parasitic infections, and hepatitis
   h. Pregnancy
   i. Oral contraceptives: nausea can be a side effect of oral contraceptives/hormone replacement therapy
   j. Cannabinoid hyperemesis syndrome
   k. Medications—some have side effects that include nausea and vomiting, or food cravings.
2. Psychiatric conditions:
   a. AN-binge/purge subtype
   b. BED
   c. Major depressive disorder, with atypical features
   d. Borderline personality disorder

Evaluation

Evaluation includes a complete history and physical examination. Laboratory screening includes:
1. CBC and platelets
2. BUN and creatinine, electrolytes, glucose, calcium, phosphorus, magnesium
3. Serum amylase
4. ECG with rhythm strip
5. Urinalysis—specific gravity, ketones or protein

Treatment

The treatment requires an interdisciplinary team approach. The first step is to make a diagnosis and address the eating disorder as soon as possible. The principles of treatment include the following:
1. Medical and nutritional intervention: The goals include careful medical monitoring and the correction of any medical complication, in particular electrolyte abnormalities. A structured meal plan including three regular meals a day will reduce the physiologic drive to binge. Individuals should be encouraged and supported to avoid foods that trigger a binge (e.g., ice cream or baked goods). Moderate exercise can also be helpful. Patients should have routine dental care and consultation should be sought for those with dental damage secondary to vomiting.
2. Psychological intervention: In adults, cognitive-behavioral therapy (CBT) is the first-line therapy for BN. Treatment with CBT reduces binge eating and purging in 30% to 50% of patients and improves attitudes about body shape and weight. Cognitive-behavioral therapy focuses on strategies to cope with the emotional triggers that lead to binge eating and purging and addresses ways to modify abnormal attitudes to eating, body shape, and weight. In adolescents with BN, 39% of those treated with FBT were no longer binging or purging after 18 weeks compared with 18% receiving supportive psychotherapy. There was no significant difference in these two treatment groups at 1-year follow-up.[27]
3. Pharmacologic treatment: Multiple studies have demonstrated a positive effect of a number of different antidepressants for treating BN. Fluoxetine is the only FDA-approved medication for the treatment of adults with BN and is most effective at a dose of 60 mg daily.[6] Treatment with fluoxetine results in a decrease in binge eating and purging episodes in 55% to 65% of subjects. A combination of antidepressant medication and CBT appears to be superior to either modality alone. An SSRI (e.g., high dose fluoxetine) can be prescribed either initially or if there is minimal or no response after 6 weeks of psychotherapy.
4. Treatment settings: The treatment settings for AYAs with BN are similar to those outlined for AN. Most AYAs with BN can be treated as outpatients.

Outcome

Most individuals with BN recover over time with recovery rates ranging from 35% to 75% at 5 years of follow-up. Bulimia nervosa tends to be a chronic relapsing condition and approximately one third of patients relapse in 1 to 2 years. Comorbidity is frequent but mortality is low. Adolescents with BN are at increased risk for suicidal behaviors including suicidal ideation (5.93%), suicide attempts (6.56%), and multiple suicide attempts (5.64%). These rates are higher than what has been reported in adolescents with other eating disorders.[28]

Full recovery in BN is higher than in AN. A favorable outcome has been associated with a younger age at presentation, shorter duration of illness, absence of laxative abuse, close social connections, and a good therapeutic response within the first month of treatment.[26]

TABLE 38.5

DSM-5 Diagnostic Criteria for Binge-Eating Disorder[1]

A. Recurrent episodes of binge eating. An episode of binge eating is characterized by both of the following:
   1. Eating, in a discrete period of time (e.g., within any 2-h period), an amount of food that is definitely larger than what most people would eat in a similar period of time under similar circumstances
   2. A sense of lack of control overeating during the episode (e.g., a feeling that one cannot stop eating or control what or how much one is eating)
B. The binge-eating episodes are associated with three (or more) of the following:
   1. Eating much more rapidly than normal
   2. Eating until feeling uncomfortably full
   3. Eating large amounts of food when not feeling physically hungry
   4. Eating alone because of feeling embarrassed by how much one is eating
   5. Feeling disgusted with oneself, depressed, or very guilty afterward
C. Marked distress regarding binge eating is present
D. The binge eating occurs, on average, at least once a week for 3 mo.
E. The binge eating is not associated with the recurrent use of inappropriate compensatory behavior as in bulimia nervosa and does not occur exclusively during the course of bulimia nervosa or anorexia nervosa.

BINGE-EATING DISORDER

Binge-eating disorder became formally recognized as an eating disorder in the DSM-5 (Table 38.5).[1] Binge-eating disorder is characterized by recurrent and persistent binge-eating that occurs at least weekly, for more than 3 months, and is not associated with recurrent inappropriate compensatory behaviors. Adolescents and young adults with BED may eat rapidly, eat irrespective of hunger or satiety, eat alone because of embarrassment, and experience negative feelings after a binge.

Most studies report prevalence rates between 1% and 3%, with about twice as many females reporting binge eating compared to males; however, BED has the highest prevalence of any eating disorder in males.[29] Binge-eating disorder typically begins in adolescence or young adulthood and is as common among females from racial or ethnic minority groups as for White females. The disorder is more prevalent among those in weight-loss treatment than in the general population.

Although BED is not well studied, identified risk factors include dieting, negative affect, overvaluation of weight, eating in the absence of hunger, loss of control eating in childhood, and childhood obesity. Males are more likely to present with overexercise and steroid use.

Binge-eating disorder is associated with increased medical morbidity and mortality and increased health care utilization. Anxiety and depression are common comorbidities. Self-harm, suicidal ideation, substance abuse, and other impulsive or risk-taking behaviors are also seen but less so in younger adolescents. Mood lability and emotional dysregulation are common features.

The majority of AYAs with BED can be treated as outpatients. Hospitalization or day treatment should be considered for medical management, treatment resistance, suicide risk, or severe self-harm. Preliminary evidence for the treatment of BED suggests that interpersonal psychotherapy, CBT, and dialectical behavior therapy may show some efficacy. Internet or app-based interventions may also be helpful and more acceptable than in-person. Topiramate and sertraline have been found to be useful for adults with BED; these medications have not been studied in adolescents. Although the course for BED is comparable to that of BN, remission rates are higher for BED. Adolescents and young adults with BED tend not to "cross over" to other eating disorders. BED is associated with obesity in later life.

TABLE 38.6

DSM-5 Diagnostic Criteria for Avoidant Restrictive Food Intake Disorder[1]

A. An eating or feeding disturbance (e.g., apparent lack of interest in eating or food; avoidance based on the sensory characteristics of food; concern about aversive consequences of eating) as manifested by persistent failure to meet appropriate nutritional and/or energy needs associated with one (or more) of the following:
  1. Significant weight loss (or failure to achieve expected weight gain or faltering growth in children)
  2. Significant nutritional deficiency
  3. Dependence on enteral feeding or oral nutritional supplements
  4. Marked interference with psychosocial functioning
B. The disturbance is not better explained by lack of available food or by an associated culturally sanctioned practice.
C. The eating disturbance does not occur exclusively during the course of anorexia nervosa or bulimia nervosa, and there is no evidence of a disturbance in the way in which one's body weight or shape is experienced.
D. The eating disturbance is not attributable to a concurrent medical condition or not better explained by another mental disorder. When the eating disturbance occurs in the context of another condition or disorder, the severity of the eating disturbance exceeds what is routinely associated with the condition or disorder and warrants additional clinical attention.

AVOIDANT RESTRICTIVE FOOD INTAKE DISORDER

Avoidant restrictive food intake disorder is a disturbance in eating or feeding as exhibited by persistent failure to meet appropriate nutritional and/or energy needs leading to significant clinical consequences, such as weight loss, failure to achieve expected weight gain, or faltering growth in children; nutritional deficiency; dependence on enteral feeding or oral nutritional supplements; or marked interference with psychosocial functioning (**Table 38.6**).[1] Unlike AYAs with AN, those with ARFID do not have weight or shape concerns.

Epidemiology

Recent studies suggest that the incidence of ARFID among clinical populations ranges from 1.5% to 64%.[30] Avoidant restrictive food intake disorder is more common among males compared to those with AN or BN. Adolescents with ARFID have a low body weight, but not as low as that found in adolescents with AN. In addition, adolescents with ARFID are younger than those with other EDs, and have a longer duration of illness compared with children and adolescents with AN and BN. Common psychiatric comorbidities among AYAs with ARFID include anxiety disorders, autism spectrum disorder, and attention deficit hyperactivity disorder.[31]

Clinical Presentation

The literature suggests that ARFID includes a broad range of clinical presentations. The DSM-5 provides three examples of commonly seen clinical presentations: avoidance of food based on sensory characteristics, low appetite or disinterest in food, and fear of negative consequences of eating. These clinical presentations are intended as examples only. However, recent research suggests that ARFID is a heterogeneous diagnosis with three distinct clinical subtypes.

Medical Complications

Avoidant restrcitive food intake disorder can lead to severe medical consequences of malnutrition (see **Table 38.2**). Given the heterogeneity of ARFID, the medical complications may vary based on the clinical presentation.[32]

Evaluation

The evaluation of AYAs with ARFID is similar to AYAs with AN (see above) and should include a careful history of the AYA's eating behaviors: low appetite, disinterest, dislike, fear of specific foods, avoidance of particular textures, colors, tastes, or smells or a fear of negative consequences of eating such as choking or vomiting. It is important to ask about attitudes toward body weight, shape, or size; this will help distinguish ARFID from other eating disorders, in particular AN. Screening blood work and physical exam is similar to that outlined above for AYAs with AN.

Screening Instruments

  1. Eating Disturbances in Youth Questionnaire (EDY-Q) is a 12-item self-report measure designed to detect early-onset eating disturbances in 8- to 13-year-olds.
  2. Nine Item ARFID Screen (NIAS) is a brief multidimensional instrument to measure ARFID-associated eating behaviors.[33] The NIAS is validated for parent report about kids as young as 7 years old.

Diagnostic Instruments

  1. Pica, ARFID, and Rumination Disorder Interview (PARDI) is a multi-informant, semistructured interview designed to assess the global presence and severity of ARFID. The instrument has good internal consistency across all subscales and moderate interrater reliability.[34]
  2. Eating Disorder Examination-ARFID module (EDE-ARFID) is both a diagnostic instrument and a tool used to gather clinical information relating to ARFID psychopathology.

Treatment

Current treatment recommendations include a multimodal approach, characterized by interdisciplinary team that considers a wide range of interventions. The recommended treatment includes medical monitoring, and nutritional and psychological interventions. The first step in treatment is focused on increasing the amount or variety of food consumed by challenging the underlying driver of food avoidance or restriction. There is no evidence-based psychological treatment suitable for all forms of ARFID at this time. Evaluation of the efficacy of psychological treatments for ARFID—particularly, family-based, and cognitive-behavioral approaches, specifically cognitive-behavioral therapy for ARFID (CBT-AR) for AYAs is ongoing.[35]

MALES AND EATING DISORDERS

Eating disorders in males are reported to be underdiagnosed and misunderstood.[36] In contrast to females, body dissatisfaction and disordered eating in males is more related to muscularity and leanness than thinness. Males with eating disorders are often preoccupied with being too small and want to be bigger and lean. Existing diagnostic criteria and screening tools focus on thinness so clinicians may be missing large numbers of males with eating disorders.

Epidemiology

  1. Approximately 10% of AYAs suffering from eating disorders are male (10:1 female to male ratio).
  2. In community samples of youth under 13 years of age, the female to male ratio is 6:1.[5,37]
  3. Although eating disorders affect a higher proportion of males who identify as gay or bisexual, the majority of males with eating disorders are heterosexual.

Clinical Presentation

  1. Males with eating disorders often present for treatment late in the course of illness. One study found that at presentation, over half of the males met criteria for hospital admission.[38]

2. Males may engage in behaviors that include increasing exercise for the purpose of gaining muscle, increasing dietary protein intake to gain muscle mass, cycling between bulking and cutting activities, and using performance enhancing substances, both legal (e.g., creatine) and illegal (e.g., anabolic steroids).

3. In general, many of the medical complications in males are similar to those in females.

Medical Management

Medical management for males is similar to that for females with eating disorders, however, the following issues are specifically relevant to males:

1. Refeeding protocols: Caloric requirements for males with AN should be higher than for females because of larger size and increased muscle mass in males.

2. Determination of TGW: Unlike females where resumption of menses can be used as an objective measure of return to biologic health and inform decisions about TGW, there is no such indicator in males. Data are lacking on testosterone cut-offs to guide decisions about TGW.

3. There is no guidance on when to order baseline BMD measurements by DXA or how to monitor bone health in males with eating disorders.

RELATIVE ENERGY DEFICIENCY IN SPORT

Relative energy deficiency in sport (RED-S) is the result of energy deficiency relative to the balance between dietary energy intake and energy expenditure required for a young person's health and sporting activities.[39] Health consequences of this low-energy condition can alter many physiologic systems including, but not limited to, metabolic rate, menstrual function, bone health, immunity, growth and development, GI, cardiovascular, and psychological health. Relative energy deficiency in sport was formerly called the "Female Athlete Triad" (disordered eating, menstrual disturbance, low bone density), but has been adapted to include both females and males.

Early diagnosis of RED-S is imperative to prevent acute and long-term health consequences. Therefore, screening for RED-S in high-risk populations should be undertaken as part of the annual health examination. Clinicians should have a high index of suspicion among athletes, especially those who present with disordered eating or eating disorders, weight loss, poor growth and development, menstrual dysfunction, recurrent injuries, decreased performance, or mood changes. Screening should focus on evaluating an AYA's eating attitudes and behaviors; hormonal and metabolic function; body weight that is appropriate for one's age, sex, and height; and musculoskeletal system.

Risk Factors

1. Athletes in sports that have an emphasis on appearance, weight category sports, and endurance
2. Menstrual irregularities including amenorrhea
3. Stress fractures
4. Low body mass
5. Substantial weight loss
6. Dietary restriction, prolonged fasting
7. Pressure to lose weight and/or frequent weight cycling
8. Reduced growth/development
9. Recurrent illnesses
10. Iron deficiency anemia
11. Decreased BMD
12. Critical comments about eating or weight from others
13. Depression/mood changes
14. Self-induced vomiting
15. Laxatives, diuretics, or diet pills use for the purpose of losing weight or maintaining a thin physique
16. Early start of sport-specific training
17. Overtraining
18. Recurrent and nonhealing injuries
19. Family history of an eating disorder

Physical Signs

The following findings on physical examination would prompt further evaluation:

1. Height, weight (increased or decreased or no change when a change is expected)
2. Orthostatic hypotension
3. Lack of progression of expected SMRs
4. Lanugo hair
5. Hypercarotenemia
6. Parotid swelling
7. Russell sign
8. Musculoskeletal injuries or assessment (stress fractures, low BMD)

Treatment

The treatment of RED-S should include an interdisciplinary team of health professionals who understand the condition and the demands of the athlete's sport. The treatment team should work closely with the AYA, their family, and coach to return to optimal health. Treatment should focus on correcting the discrepancy between energy intake and energy expenditure. Intake of nutrients and other vitamins should be optimized for age and sex.[10] Assessment and possible treatment of comorbid mental health disorders may require psychotherapy and psychopharmacotherapy.

SUMMARY

The most common feeding and eating disorders seen in AYAs include AN, BN, AAN, BED, and ARFID. These disorders are highly prevalent and are associated with significant medical and psychological consequences. Early identification and aggressive evidence-based treatments will help prevent long-term morbidity and mortality in this population.

REFERENCES

1. American Psychiatric Association. *Diagnostic and Statistical Manual of Mental Disorders*, 5th ed. American Psychiatric Association; 2013.
2. Duncan L, Yilmaz Z, Gaspar H, et al. Significant locus and metabolic genetic correlations revealed in genome-wide association study of anorexia nervosa. *Am J Psychiatry*. 2017;174(9):850–858.
3. Smink FRE, Van Hoeken D, Oldehinkel AJ, et al. Prevalence and severity of DSM-5 eating disorders in a community cohort of adolescents. *Int J Eat Disord*. 2014;47(6):610–619.
4. American College Health Association. *National College Health Assessment II: Reference Group Undergraduates Executive Summary*. Hanover, MD, 2013.
5. Pinhas L, Morris A, Crosby RD, et al. Incidence and age-specific presentation of restrictive eating disorders in children: a Canadian Pediatric Surveillance Program study. *Arch Pediatr Adolesc Med*. 2011;165(10):895–899.
6. Walsh BT AE, Becker AE, Bulik CM, et al. Defining eating disorders. In Evans DL, Foa EB, Gur RE, et al., eds. Treating and Preventing Adolescent Mental Health Disorders: What We Know and What We Don't Know. 2nd ed. Oxford University Press; The Annenberg Foundation Trust at Sunnylands, and the Annenberg Public Policy Center of the University of Pennsylvania, 2017:289–313.
7. Misra M, Golden NH, Katzman DK. State of the art systematic review of bone disease in anorexia nervosa. *Int J Eat Disord*. 2016;49(3):276–292.
8. Misra M, Katzman DK, Miller KK, et al. Physiologic estrogen replacement increases bone density in adolescent girls with anorexia nervosa. *J Bone Miner Res*. 2011;26(10):2430–2438.
9. Golden NH, Abrams SA; Committee on Nutrition. Optimizing bone health in children and adolescents. *Pediatrics*. 2014;134(4):e1229–1243. doi: 10.1542/peds.2014-2173. PMID: 25266429.
10. Gordon RJ, Gordon CM. Adolescents and bone health. *Clin Obstet Gynecol*. 2020;63(3):504–511.
11. Garner DM, Garfinkel PE. The eating attitudes test: an index of the symptoms of anorexia nervosa. *Psychol Med*. 1979;9(2):273–279.
12. Fairburn CG, Beglin SJ. Eating disorder Examination Questionnaire (EDE-Q 6.0). In Fairburn CG, ed. *Cognitive Behavior Therapy and Eating Disorders*. Guilford Press; 2008.
13. Childress AC, Brewerton TD, Hodges EL, et al. The Kids' Eating Disorders Survey (KEDS): a study of middle school students. *J Am Acad Child Adolesc Psychiatry*. 1993;32(4):843–850.

14. Society for Adolescent Health and Medicine; Golden NH, Katzman DK, et al. Position paper of the Society for Adolescent Health and Medicine: medical management of restrictive eating disorders in adolescents and young adults. *J Adolesc Health*. 2015;56(1):121–125.

15. Lock J, Le Grange D, Agras WS, et al. Randomized clinical trial comparing family-based treatment with adolescent-focused individual therapy for adolescents with anorexia nervosa. *Arch Gen Psychiatry*. 2010;67(10):1025–1032.

16. Attia E, Steinglass JE, Walsh BT, et al. Olanzapine versus placebo in adult outpatients with anorexia nervosa: a randomized clinical trial. *Am J Psychiatry*. 2019;176(6):449–456.

17. Kafantaris V, Leigh E, Hertz S, et al. A placebo-controlled pilot study of adjunctive olanzapine for adolescents with anorexia nervosa. *J Child Adolesc Psychopharmacol*. 2011;21(3):207–212.

18. Monge MC, Forman SF, McKenzie NM, et al. Use of psychopharmacologic medications in adolescents with restrictive eating disorders: analysis of data from the National Eating Disorder Quality Improvement Collaborative. *J Adolesc Health*. 2015;57(1):66–72.

19. Garber AK, Cheng J, Accurso EC, et al. Short-term outcomes of the study of refeeding to optimize inpatient gains for patients with anorexia nervosa: a multicenter randomized clinical trial. *JAMA Pediatr*. 2021;175(1):19–27.

20. Golden NH, Cheng J, Kapphahn CJ, et al. Higher-calorie refeeding in anorexia nervosa: 1-year outcomes from a randomized controlled trial. *Pediatrics*. 2021;147(4):e2020037135.

21. Society for Adolescent Health and Medicine. Refeeding hypophosphatemia in hospitalized adolescents with anorexia nervosa. *J Adolesc Health*. 2014;55: 455–457.

22. Raj SR, Guzman JC, Harvey P, et al. Canadian Cardiovascular Society position statement on postural orthostatic tachycardia syndrome (POTS) and related disorders of chronic orthostatic intolerance. *Can J Cardiol*. 2020;36(3):357–372.

23. Forman SF, Grodin LF, Graham DA, et al. An eleven site national quality improvement evaluation of adolescent medicine-based eating disorder programs: predictors of weight outcomes at one year and risk adjustment analyses. *J Adolesc Health*. 2011;49(6):594–600.

24. Arcelus J, Mitchell AJ, Wales J, et al. Mortality rates in patients with anorexia nervosa and other eating disorders, a meta-analysis of 36 studies. *Arch Gen Psychiatry*. 2011;68(7):724–731.

25. Seetharaman S, Golden NH, Halpern-Felsher B, et al. Effect of a prior history of overweight on return of menses in adolescents with eating disorders. *J Adolesc Health*. 2017;60(4):469–471.

26. Castillo M, Weiselberg E. Bulimia nervosa/purging disorder. *Curr Probl Pediatr Adolesc Health Care*. 2017;47(4):85–94.

27. Le Grange D, Crosby RD, Rathouz PJ, et al. A randomized controlled comparison of family-based treatment and supportive psychotherapy for adolescent bulimia nervosa. *Arch Gen Psychiatry*. 2007;64(9):1049–1056.

28. Crow SJ, Swanson SA, Le Grange D, et al. Suicidal behavior in adolescents and adults with bulimia nervosa. *Compr Psychiatry*. 2014;55(7):1534–1539.

29. Bohon C. Binge eating disorder in children and adolescents. *Child Adolesc Psychiatr Clin N Am*. 2019;28(4):549–555.

30. Bourne L, Bryant-Waugh R, Cook J, et al. Avoidant/restrictive food intake disorder: a systematic scoping review of the current literature. *Psychiatry Res*. 2020;288:112961.

31. Norris ML, Spettigue W, Hammond NG, et al. Building evidence for the use of descriptive subtypes in youth with avoidant restrictive food intake disorder. *Int J Eat Disord*. 2018;51(2):170–173.

32. Norris ML, Robinson A, Obeid N, et al. Exploring avoidant/restrictive food intake disorder in eating disordered patients: a descriptive study. *Int J Eat Disord*. 2014;47(5):495–499.

33. Zickgraf HF, Ellis JM. Initial validation of the Nine Item Avoidant/Restrictive Food Intake disorder screen (NIAS): a measure of three restrictive eating patterns. *Appetite*. 2018;123:32–42.

34. Bryant-Waugh R, Micali N, Cooke L, et al. Development of the Pica, ARFID, and Rumination Disorder Interview, a multi-informant, semistructured interview of feeding disorders across the lifespan: a pilot study for ages 10–22. *Int J Eat Disord*. 2019;52(4):378–387.

35. Thomas JJ, Wons OB, Eddy KT. Cognitive-behavioral treatment of avoidant/restrictive food intake disorder. *Curr Opin Psychiatry*. 2018;31(6):425–430.

36. Nagata JM, Ganson KT, Murray SB. Eating disorders in adolescent boys and young men: an update. *Curr Opin Pediatr*. 2020;32(4):476–481.

37. Nicholls DE, Lynn R, Viner RM. Childhood eating disorders: British national surveillance study. *Br J Psychiatry*. 2011;198(4):295–301.

38. Vo M, Lau J, Rubinstein M. Eating disorders in adolescent and young adult males: presenting characteristics. *J Adolesc Health*. 2016;59(4):397–400.

39. Statuta SM, Asif IM, Drezner JA. Relative energy deficiency in sport (RED-S). *Br J Sports Med*. 2017;51(21):1570–1571.

📶 ADDITIONAL RESOURCES AND WEBSITES

Additional Resources and Websites for Clinicians:

Academy for Eating Disorders. Accessed March 2021—https://www.aedweb.org

The American Academy of Child and Adolescent Psychiatry. Accessed March 2021—http://www.aacap.org/

American Psychiatric Association (APA). Accessed March 2021—https://www.psychiatry.org

Lock J, Le Grange D. *Treatment Manual for Anorexia Nervosa: A Family-Based Approach*. Guildford Press, 2015.

The National Eating Disorders Association (NEDA). Accessed March 2021—http://www.nationaleatingdisorders.org

National Institute of Mental Health—Eating Disorders. Accessed March 2021—http://www.nimh.nih.gov/health/publications/eating-disorders/index.shtml

Society for Adolescent Health and Medicine (SAHM). Accessed March 2021—http://www.adolescenthealth.org/

Additional Resources and Websites for Parents/Caregivers:

Boachie A, Jasper K. *Parent's Guide to Defeating Eating Disorders*. Jessica Kingsley Publishers; 2011.

Bryant-Waugh R. *ARFID Avoidant restrictive Food Intake Disorders: A Guide for Parents and Carers*. Routledge; 2019.

Crosbie C, Sterling W. *How to nourish your child through an eating disorder. A simple plate-by plate approach to rebuilding a healthy relationship with food*. The Experiment; 2018.

F.E.A.S.T. Accessed March 2021—https://www.feast-ed.org/

Katzman DK, Pinhas L. *Help for eating disorders. A parent's guide to symptoms, causes and treatments*. Robert Rose Inc, 2005.

Kelty Eating Disorders. Accessed March 2021—https://keltyeatingdisorders.ca/

Lock J, Le Grange D. *Help Your Teenager Beat an Eating Disorder*. The Guildford Press; 2005.

Maudsley Parents. Accessed March 2021—http://www.maudsleyparents.org/

IX

Functional and Unexplained Medical Conditions

CHAPTER 39

Chronic Noninflammatory Musculoskeletal Pain Disorders

Christina Schutt
Bethany Marston
David M. Siegel

KEY WORDS
- Central sensitization
- Musculoskeletal pain
- Pain amplification
- Somatic symptoms

INTRODUCTION

It is not uncommon for adolescent and young adult (AYA) patients to describe physical pain or other somatic symptoms that lack clear or sufficient historical, laboratory, and/or physical findings to explain the discomfort. These presentations can be challenging because there are many potential explanations for such symptoms, and an accurate diagnosis and effective management plan can be elusive. Chronic primary pain syndromes and mental health diagnoses are important potential diagnostic considerations. This chapter presents a brief discussion of psychiatric diagnoses (as outlined in the *Diagnostic and Statistical Manual of Mental Disorders*, Fifth edition [DSM-5]) followed by a more extensive review of amplified or primary musculoskeletal pain syndromes.

PSYCHIATRIC DIAGNOSES WITH SIGNIFICANT SOMATIC MANIFESTATIONS

Adjustment Disorder

Adjustment disorder is the development of emotional or behavioral symptoms in response to an identifiable stressor with marked distress that is out of proportion to the intensity or severity of the stressor with significant impairment in functioning. Considered in this framework, potential stressors during adolescence and young adulthood that can lead to somatic symptoms include the following:
- Physical changes of puberty
- The cognitive developmental progression from concrete to formal operational thinking
- Changing demands and expectations in the family, and social, academic, and vocational realms

Milder and often more time-limited psychological disequilibrium or emotional distress can also precipitate bodily discomfort and lead to physical complaints such as light-headedness, nausea, headache, abdominal pain, backache, and palpitations. Seeking care for these symptoms may be perceived to be a "more legitimate" reason to see the clinician than overtly expressed psychological distress, the symptoms of which may be less acceptable to the patient and/or family.

Physical Symptoms Associated with Psychological Distress

There are many clinical scenarios in which physical symptoms or medical problems are strongly influenced by psychological factors.

For example, the patient with asthma may experience increased bronchospasm when under emotional stress, leading to greater episodes of coughing, wheezing, and shortness of breath. Managing or preventing symptoms in these circumstances is not usually easily or rapidly accomplished. Helping AYAs and families to understand the connection between the mind and body provides a good foundation for management. The "medical legitimacy" of the primary physiologic disorder (i.e., asthma) represents a common ground of acceptance between clinician and patient/family and provides the clinician with a familiar and well-understood template for medical treatment. In addition to medical treatment, the clinician must explore with adolescents or young adults the sources of stress and anxiety that contribute to inadequate control of the primary disease and its symptoms. This process takes time and may necessitate several visits. Open-ended, thoughtful questions and a trusting relationship between the AYA and clinician are essential. Collaboration with a health psychologist or family therapist is often an important enhancement to the care team.

Somatic Symptom and Related Disorders

Complaints of significant somatic symptoms without identifiable biomedical etiology are common during AYA patient encounters. In the past, this constellation has been classified as somatoform somatization disorder. The DSM-5 introduced a new categorization for these conditions.[1] This revised template provides a more useful set of diagnostic labels and descriptions, recognizing that most of these patients present to medical rather than mental health clinicians. Beginning with the most common, these include the following:

1. Somatic symptom disorder: Persistent (>6 months) somatic symptom(s) that cause psychosocial impairment, with persistent thoughts about the seriousness of symptoms, anxiety about symptoms or general health, or excessive time and energy devoted to symptoms or health concerns. Incorporation of affective, cognitive, and behavioral components rather than just somatic symptoms alone is central to making the diagnosis.

   The criteria for somatic symptom disorder require the presence of a symptom or symptoms with associated excessive or disproportionate thoughts, feelings, or behaviors about these symptom(s). The diagnostic emphasis is placed on the presence of disruptive or maladaptive thoughts or behaviors rather than the absence of an explanation for the AYA's medical complaints.[2] The symptom may be medically "explained" or not. This categorization encompasses most of those patients who, in the past, were diagnosed with somatization disorder, undifferentiated somatoform disorder, or hypochondriasis (a term that was eliminated from the DSM-5 because it is considered stigmatizing). Since the DSM-5 was published, concerns have been raised that the current classification may lead to overdiagnosis of somatic symptom disorder in those individuals with medical illness.[3]

2. Illness anxiety disorder: Persistent (>6 months) preoccupation with having a serious undiagnosed illness, anxiety about health, or excessive health behaviors or maladaptive avoidance of situations perceived as health threats, accompanied by minimal somatic symptoms, and not better explained by another disorder.

3. Conversion disorder (functional neurologic symptom disorder): Neurologic symptoms that are found, after appropriate neurologic assessment, to be incompatible with neurologic pathophysiology.

4. Psychological factors affecting other medical disorders: Presence of one or more clinically significant psychological or behavioral factors that adversely affect a medical condition by increasing the risk for suffering, death, or disability.

5. Factitious disorder: The falsification of medical or psychological signs and symptoms in oneself or others that are associated with the individual taking surreptitious actions to misrepresent, simulate, or cause signs or symptoms of illness or injury in the absence of obvious external rewards. In contrast to somatic symptom disorders, in which symptoms are associated with unconscious conflict, factitious disorders are those of *conscious* falsification of symptoms and signs to create a sick role, thought to be motivated by the need to be cared for. Factitious disorders are serious and are often difficult to distinguish from somatic symptom disorders. This is particularly the case for factitious disorders that are chronic, such as factitious disorder imposed on self (previously, Munchausen syndrome) or factitious disorder imposed on another (previously, Munchausen syndrome by proxy).[4] Factitious disorders need to be distinguished from malingering, in which there is conscious and intentional exaggeration or falsification of symptoms for an obvious secondary gain. Malingering is not considered a psychiatric condition.

The clinical approach to AYA with suspected somatic symptom or related disorders should be informed by a few general principles.

A biopsychosocial assessment, one that assesses the biological, psychological and socials factors that may contribute to the presenting problem should be conducted. Biomedical and psychosocial factors must be evaluated at the onset. The clinician should seek to understand psychological stressors and conflicts, as well as the biomedical elements. This holistic perspective may help the clinician to efficiently narrow the differential diagnosis. It may also help AYAs and families to be more accepting of a diagnosis of a suspected somatic symptom or related disorder, since these have been included among the diagnostic possibilities all along rather than seeming to be a diagnosis of exclusion. Elements of the assessment include the following:

1. Detailed history focused on the presenting symptoms: It is important not to neglect the symptoms that brought the patient and family to the clinician. Focusing on the distressing physical sensations described by the patient conveys that the clinician is taking their concerns seriously.

2. Physical examination focused on symptoms.

3. Laboratory and imaging studies: Studies should be based on the history and physical examination and should be limited to the least number of minimally invasive tests required to clarify the diagnosis or rule out important alternate possibilities.

4. Evaluation for psychiatric disease: Mood disorders (especially major depression), anxiety disorders, and even schizophrenia can all manifest with somatic focused distress; sometimes physical symptoms may be the AYA's only complaints initially. When the evaluation suggests the presence of significant psychiatric illness, formal mental health consultation is warranted.

5. Evaluation for personality disorders: The diagnosis of personality disorders has been debated for adolescents under 18 years old. However, AYAs with enduring attitudes and habitual patterns of response that characterize obsessive–compulsive personality disorder or histrionic personality disorder seem to be at higher risk for developing somatic symptom disorder. In addition, AYAs with personality traits of dependency or neurotic preoccupation with self also have a greater tendency to experience and describe unexplained physical symptoms.

6. Evaluation of environmental factors: Environmental and psychosocial factors may contribute to the emergence and perpetuation of various chronic pain syndromes. Somatic complaints in parents, family members, or peer contacts should be examined as possible models for, and contributors to, the patient's own symptoms and behaviors. Cultural norms and expectations might also reinforce a form of illness and/or an expression of distress that manifests as physical pain. As with other health conditions, social determinants of health certainly influence the presentation and management of chronic pain. An awareness of the patient's cultural milieu may provide important context for understanding unexplained somatic symptoms.

SYNDROMES OF CHRONIC MUSCULOSKELETAL PAIN

Terminology

Syndromes of widespread or regional chronic musculoskeletal pain can occur in patients of any age, but the onset is most common during adolescence and young adulthood. Definitions and terms used to describe these syndromes vary, especially across subspecialties. Fibromyalgia is a common term and is well defined in the adult population. Many pediatric practices prefer to use the term amplified musculoskeletal pain syndrome (AMPS), which is descriptive and does not presume an etiology. This terminology remains generally accepted within the scope of practice of rheumatology and is used in the remainder of this chapter. The nomenclature of pain disorders continues to evolve. The International Association for the Study of Pain (IASP) has advocated for framing chronic pain as its own distinct disorder, and has new terminology including chronic widespread pain and chronic primary and secondary musculoskeletal pain as part of an alternative classification scheme for use within the *International Classification of Diseases*, 11th edition (ICD-11).[5] The IASP framework has not been broadly adopted and there is lack of clear consensus across specialties regarding the ideal terminology. Clinicians should anticipate ongoing changes to diagnostic labels as the pathophysiology and treatment pathways for musculoskeletal pain disorders become better understood.

Some localized pain syndromes, including complex regional pain syndrome (CRPS), have similar features and are described below. Each of these musculoskeletal pain syndromes can be viewed as being on a continuum ranging from milder, more localized pain with limited functional impairment (and likely response to short-term treatment) to more generalized pain with high severity, a significant degree of allodynia, persistent fatigue and possibly mood disorder, and the need for more prolonged and multidisciplinary-based treatment.

Clinical Presentations
Diffuse Amplified Pain Syndromes

Diffuse amplified pain syndromes (termed fibromyalgia, AMPS, and/or chronic widespread pain) are characterized by widespread musculoskeletal pain, localized to joints and/or muscles, and are associated with varying levels of pain-associated disability and other associated symptoms. Some patients may have an identifiable initiating event, but a common feature of these pain syndromes is the lack of specific laboratory, imaging, or tissue pathology that explains the symptoms.

Fibromyalgia and Juvenile Fibromyalgia

1. The predominant complaint is chronic widespread musculo-skeletal pain affecting the upper and lower, as well as left and right sides of the body.
2. Most patients describe poor sleep quality, fatigue, mood disruption, and difficulty concentrating.
3. Many will have other somatic manifestations including headache, irritable bowel or other abdominal symptoms, dysmenorrhea, subjective swelling or skin color changes, dizziness, or multiple chemical sensitivities.
4. Symptoms may accumulate over time, and the diagnosis might not be recognized early on. Many patients present with concerns about arthritis, lupus, or other underlying rheumatologic conditions. Affected AYAs and families are often frustrated when no ready explanation for these symptoms is found on initial routine testing.
5. Although patients' symptoms and function may vary, there are no confirmatory tests for the diagnosis of fibromyalgia. The American College of Rheumatology's revised 2016 classification criteria rely on a thorough and detailed history. These criteria are better studied in adults but are often applied to pediatric populations as well. In the evaluation of patients with widespread pain, it is also important to perform a complete physical examination since a diagnosis of fibromyalgia does not exclude coexistence of another illness. (**Table 39.1**).

Diffuse Pain or Total Body Pain Some pediatric patients with widespread pain who go on in later adolescence/young adulthood to be identified as having fibromyalgia may not meet diagnostic criteria at presentation. Children seeking evaluation and care for their pain earlier in life than adulthood have significant and distressing discomfort, often associated with allodynia or subjective hyperalgesia, but they may have yet to manifest other manifestations of fibromyalgia such as fatigue, poor sleep, and mood changes. Whereas some AYAs with diffuse pain seem to have had an inciting event (e.g., trauma or illness) this is not present in all such patients. It is important to evaluate for and exclude other causes of diffuse pain such as arthritis, hypermobility, or psychiatric illness.

Localized Amplified Pain Syndromes

As the name implies, AYAs with localized amplified pain syndromes have pain characteristics similar to those experienced by patients with diffuse amplified pain syndromes, but the distribution of pain is limited to a body region such as a limb or torso rather than being widespread. Peripheral body areas tend to be more often involved than central body areas. As with diffuse amplified pain, patients can sometimes describe an inciting event, such as a trauma, or illness.

Complex Regional Pain Syndrome Complex regional pain syndrome is a noninflammatory condition that includes regional pain, hyperesthesia or allodynia, vasomotor disturbances including swelling and color change, and eventually can lead to dystrophic changes. Complex regional pain syndrome may be identified by other names, and is sometimes divided into two types:

- Type I (also known as reflex sympathetic dystrophy [RSD]) is characterized by the absence of a definable nerve injury. This type is much more common than type II.
- Type II (formerly known as causalgia) is characterized by the presence of an identifiable nerve injury or lesion.

The diagnosis is usually based on clinical features alone and diagnostic studies are only necessary to resolve any clinical ambiguity.

There are currently no validated confirmatory tests for the diagnosis of CRPS. Markers of autonomic function such as resting sweat output, resting skin temperature, or quantitative sudomotor axon reflex testing have limited diagnostic value and currently are not validated for screening or confirmatory purposes.[6]

TABLE 39.1

Fibromyalgia Criteria—2016 Revision

Criteria

A patient satisfies modified 2016 fibromyalgia criteria if the following three conditions are met:

1. Widespread pain index (WPI) ≥7 and symptom severity scale (SSS) score ≥5 OR WPI of 4–6 and SSS score 9
2. Generalized pain, defined as pain in at least 4 of 5 regions, must be present. Jaw, chest, and abdominal pain are not included in generalized pain definition.
3. Symptoms have been generally present for at least 3 mo.
4. A diagnosis of fibromyalgia is valid irrespective of other diagnoses. A diagnosis of fibromyalgia does not exclude the presence of other clinically important illnesses.

Ascertainment

1. **Widespread pain index**: Note the number of areas in which the patient has had pain over the last week. In how many areas has the patient had pain? Score will be between 0 and 19.

Left upper region (Region 1)	Right upper region (Region 2)	Axial region (Region 5)
Jaw, left[a]	Jaw, right[a]	Neck
Shoulder girdle, left	Shoulder girdle, right	Upper back
Upper arm, left	Upper arm, right	Lower back
Lower arm, left	Lower arm, right	Chest[a]
		Abdomen[a]

Left lower region (region 3)	Right lower region (Region 4)
Hip (buttock, trochanter), left	Hip (buttock, trochanter), right
Upper leg, left	Upper leg, right
Lower leg, left	Lower leg, right

2. **Symptom severity scale score**
Fatigue
Waking unrefreshed
Cognitive symptoms
For each of the three symptoms above, indicate the level of severity over the past week using the following scale:
0 = No problem
1 = Slight or mild problems, generally mild or intermittent
2 = Moderate, considerable problems, often present and/or at a moderate level
3 = Severe: Pervasive, continuous, life-disturbing problems
The SSS score is the sum of the severity scores of the three symptoms (fatigue, waking unrefreshed, and cognitive symptoms) (0–9) plus the sum (0–3) of the number of the following symptoms the patient has been bothered by that occurred during the previous 6 mo:
1. Headaches (0–1)
2. Pain or cramps in lower abdomen (0–1)
3. Depression (0–1)
The final symptom severity score is between 0 and 12.
The fibromyalgia severity (FS) scale is the sum of the WPI and SSS.

The FS scale is also known as the polysymptomatic distress (PSD) scale.
[a]Not included in generalized pain definition.
Reprinted from Wolfe F, Clauw DJ, Fitzcharles MA, et al. 2016 Revisions to the 2010/2011 fibromyalgia diagnostic criteria. *Semin Arthritis Rheum.* 2016;46(3):319–329. With permission from Elsevier.

Imaging studies may be helpful in the evaluation of CRPS, though findings may vary depending on duration of symptoms and severity.

- In early stages, skeletal scintigraphy (bone scan) may reveal increased uptake of technetium-99m on delayed bone images; however, a normal scan does not rule out the diagnosis.
- Plain x-rays are less helpful early in disease, but patchy demineralization within the affected area can be seen in later stages after prolonged symptoms and disuse.

- Magnetic resonance imaging (MRI) can reveal skin thickening and edema or contrast enhancement of soft tissue in early stages of illness. In later stages, changes in skin thickness may persist and changes in muscle such as atrophy may be seen.[7]

Localized Pain without Autonomic Changes Adolescents and young adults may present with severe pain and allodynia localized to a region of the body similar to classic CRPS, but lacking any clear changes in temperature, color, or other neurovascular abnormalities. This may represent an early phase of the disease or may be a variant. Such patients may similarly have an identifiable inciting event such as an injury (which may be minor) or illness, but in many cases they do not.

Epidemiology

Estimates of prevalence vary, but U.S. hospital-based pediatric rheumatology clinics report that 7.6% of new patients seen were diagnosed with fibromyalgia. Community prevalence rates of fibromyalgia have been reported to be 1% to 6%.[8] The incidence of CRPS in adults is approximately 5 to 26 per 100,000.[7] Specific data about the incidence of CRPS in AYAs are lacking.

- The clinical characteristics of juvenile fibromyalgia and fibromyalgia are similar regardless of age, though the developmental and psychosocial differences between adolescence and adulthood have a bearing on the impact of the disease and on some aspects of treatment.
- Amplified pain syndromes are more common in females, with an approximately 4:1 female to male ratio.[9]
- Average age at diagnosis in pediatric studies is about 13 years.[9,10] However, there are reports of diagnosis in children as young as 2 years old.

Pathophysiology

A biopsychosocial model, considering biologic, psychological, and environmental factors, is useful for understanding the effects of AMPS on function and to inform management. Although the factors that cause AMPS are incompletely understood, pain processing appears to be altered in several ways in adult fibromyalgia and related conditions, and much of this research has been conceptually extrapolated to younger patients.[9]

1. The concept of central sensitization may be important in understanding this disorder. Pain results from abnormal pain processing in the brain, leading to a perception of pain at much lower levels of noxious stimuli (e.g., pressure or heat). When compared to normal controls:
   a. Functional MRI has demonstrated increased cortical activity in pain-processing regions in patients with fibromyalgia in response to pressure stimuli.[11]
   b. Patients with fibromyalgia demonstrate increased levels of pain neurotransmitters such as substance P and glutamate, and decreased levels of inhibitory substances such as dopamine, serotonin, and norepinephrine.[12]
2. Peripheral nerve abnormalities may also play a role. Small fiber neuropathy, including altered detection thresholds for temperature, mechanical, and pressure sensation, has been described.[13,14]
3. Genetic, environmental, and family influences are also important in the development of fibromyalgia. Juvenile and adult fibromyalgia are much more common in females than males, and similarly increased in those with affected relatives. Studies posit an association with human leukocyte antigen (HLA) linkages and potential polymorphisms in neurotransmitter genes, but causality remains unclear.[15]
4. Personality and family traits have been shown in some studies to be associated with increased fibromyalgia symptoms or severity, including emotional sensitivity or anxiety, poor family functioning, poor coping responses such as pain catastrophizing, and sedentary behaviors.

Differential Diagnosis

The differential diagnosis can be substantially narrowed in many cases with a careful history and physical examination. Alternate diagnoses often can be confirmed or excluded with laboratory or imaging studies. **Table 39.2** lists differential diagnoses that should be considered based on presenting symptoms.

TABLE 39.2

Differential Diagnosis of Diffuse or Localized Pain by Presenting Symptoms

	Conditions Presenting with Diffuse Musculoskeletal Pain	Conditions Presenting with Localized or Regional Pain, with or Without Vascular Changes
Psychological	Somatic symptom disorder, conversion, factitious disorders, etc.	
Mechanical		Compartment syndrome or chronic compartment syndrome
		Overuse or traumatic injury
		Orthopedic conditions (e.g., Osgood–Schlatter disease, Perthes disease, osteochondritis dissecans, etc.)
	Malignancy or neoplasia, systemic or localized	
	Hypermobility	
Vascular		Raynaud phenomenon or chilblains
		Deep vein thrombosis or thrombophlebitis
		Arterial insufficiency or claudication
Infection		Osteomyelitis
		Cellulitis or localized infection
Neurologic		Thoracic outlet syndrome
		Peripheral neuropathy
		Erythromelalgia
		Restless legs
Rheumatic disease	Rheumatoid or juvenile arthritis	
	Chronic recurrent multifocal osteomyelitis or chronic nonbacterial osteomyelitis	
	Systemic lupus erythematosus	
	Vasculitis	
	Other systemic autoimmune disease	
Other	Thyroid disease	
	Genetic conditions (i.e., Fabry disease)	
	Vitamin D or C deficiency	
		Progressive diaphyseal dysplasia

MANAGEMENT

The management of AMPS differs across medical disciplines and institutions. In the rheumatology community, there is general consensus regarding principles of treatment, which are described below.[16]

Optimal management of AMPS should start with education about the diagnosis for the AYA and, when appropriate, the family. Education should include (1) mechanisms of pain and sensitization, (2) the concept that pain does not always indicate tissue damage, (3) the importance of sleep and sleep hygiene, (4) the effects of physical activity, and (5) the psychological effects of chronic pain. Patients and families should also be made aware that medical or psychological comorbidities and social context may impact symptoms. For example, psychiatric comorbidities such as anxiety and major depressive disorder are common in patients with amplified musculoskeletal pain.[17]

Management should focus on improvements in function and quality of life. Reduction or complete eradication of pain may not be achievable and is likely to be a slower process. Optimal treatment often benefits from a multidisciplinary approach including specialists in physical and occupational therapy, psychology with expertise in amplified pain, and pediatric rheumatology. Nonpharmacologic therapies should be prioritized, particularly in younger patients.

- Exercise therapies based on aerobic and/or strength training approaches are safe and effective in improving physical function, pain, and well-being. Supervised or group exercise programs may be more effective than individual training. In localized syndromes including CRPS, an emphasis should be placed on improving use of the affected limb(s) along with desensitization techniques, in addition to general exercise therapy.
- Cognitive-behavioral therapy (CBT) should be used in most patients to improve coping, reduce pain catastrophizing, and manage symptoms related to depression and anxiety.
- Desensitization therapy of the affected body part, usually done through occupational therapy, is helpful especially for regional pain syndromes and particularly when there is disabling allodynia.
- Other movement-based strategies (e.g., Tai chi, yoga) and mindfulness-based stress reduction, as well as less commonly used interventions (e.g., acupuncture or hydrotherapy) have been shown in some studies to be useful adjunctive therapies for some patients.
- Evidence is lacking or risks outweigh benefits for some interventions including chiropractic care, biofeedback, and magnetic or electrical stimuli.

Pharmacotherapy may be a useful adjunct for symptom management in select patients, especially those with diffuse or severe pain refractory to nonpharmacologic treatment, or for AYAs with severe sleep disturbance, or profound functional disability. Patients with AMPS may experience more medication side effects than healthy peers, which may make it difficult for them to adhere to medication regimens or tolerate adequate doses.[18] Most research on pharmacotherapy for AMPS is limited to adult patients and no specific medications are approved for adolescents in the United States.

- Serotonin–norepinephrine reuptake inhibitors (SNRIs): Duloxetine and milnacipran have been approved to treat fibromyalgia in adults. Venlafaxine may also be helpful. A placebo-controlled trial of duloxetine in adolescents showed efficacy in decreasing pain severity.[19]
- Gamma-aminobutyric acid analog antiepileptics: Pregabalin (approved in adult fibromyalgia) and gabapentin have indications for neuropathic pain, and both are used clinically in diffuse and localized AMPS.
- Tricyclic antidepressants: Amitriptyline at low doses, and the muscle relaxant cyclobenzaprine, which is chemically similar, is used off-label with benefit in some patients, particularly those in whom nonrestorative sleep or muscle spasm are prominent features.
- Tramadol, a weak opioid with SNRI activity may have benefit in some patients, but other opioids should not be used for treatment of amplified pain syndromes because of the risk of both increased pain sensitization and narcotic dependency. Nonsteroidal anti-inflammatory drugs (NSAIDs) generally have little benefit and carry the potential for adverse effects.
- Vitamin D supplementation in those who are deficient can sometimes reduce nonspecific musculoskeletal pain.
- There is evidence that bisphosphonates improve pain in CRPS; however, these medications should be used with caution in AYAs recognizing that definitive efficacy and safety data are lacking in this population. Consideration of bisphosphonates in females of child-bearing age needs to be taken into account due to their long-term release from bone and their ability to cross the placenta.

The following medications have been considered or tested for treatment of AMPS, but are not recommended because of lack of efficacy or risk of adverse effects:

- Selective serotonin reuptake inhibitors (SSRIs) may help with associated mood symptoms but have not been shown to improve pain in adults.
- Monoamine oxidase inhibitors (MAOIs) and antipsychotics should be avoided for safety concerns and lack of demonstrated efficacy.
- Sodium oxybate (gamma hydroxybutyrate) is used for narcolepsy, and has been postulated to treat pain and fatigue in other conditions, but psychoactive effects and safety concerns precluded approval for treatment of fibromyalgia in the United States and Europe.
- Ketamine has some weak evidence for efficacy, particularly in CRPS, but also has concerns for problematic use and adverse effects.[20]
- Corticosteroids and intravenous immune globulin (IVIG) are useful in some forms of neuropathic pain syndromes but are not effective in fibromyalgia. There are data to suggest that systemic corticosteroids have some efficacy in the early stages of CRPS, but trial results are conflicting, and evidence of benefit overall is weak.
- There is increasing interest in the use of cannabinoids to treat fibromyalgia and similar chronic pain syndromes, but high-quality evidence is limited.[21] Similarly, the use of low-dose naltrexone, an opioid antagonist, has been suggested for treatment of fibromyalgia symptoms for several years and has some popular support from patient advocates. There are only small studies of cannabinoids with unclear results, and there are no studies in the pediatric population.[18,22]

OTHER PRIMARY PAIN SYNDROMES

Many AYAs develop primary pain syndromes that are not primarily musculoskeletal (e.g., functional abdominal pain, irritable bowel syndrome, chronic pelvic pain, chronic nonmigraine headache, etc.). These syndromes may frequently overlap with AMPS. A similar approach to management may be useful in these conditions, focusing on education, functional improvement, and management of symptoms and emotional distress. See Chapters 28 and 41 for evaluation and management of these diagnoses.

CHRONIC FATIGUE SYNDROME

While some patients with fibromyalgia syndrome experience profound fatigue along with widespread pain, there are AYAs whose dominant symptom is persistent, overwhelming, and disabling fatigue leading to the diagnosis of chronic fatigue syndrome. This condition is discussed in more detail in Chapter 40.

SUMMARY

Pain is a common presenting symptom for AYAs seeking clinical care. Syndromes of widespread or regional chronic musculoskeletal pain can occur in patients of any age, but the onset is most common during adolescence and young adulthood. Alternative diagnoses should be carefully considered with a full history and physical examination as the diagnosis of AMPS is a diagnosis of exclusion. A complete biopsychosocial assessment of the patient is essential to not only correctly establishing the diagnosis of AMPS but also for designing a treatment approach most likely to be accepted and effective.

Amplified musculoskeletal pain syndromes can be viewed as being on a continuum ranging from mild to more severe pain and can affect the body diffusely or be localized to a single region. Optimal management of AMPS includes a multidisciplinary approach that includes education for patient and family, physical and occupational therapy focused on aerobic and desensitization therapy, and CBT. Judicious use of pharmacotherapy has been studied and evidence is presented to support administration of different agents in select patients. We recommend, however, that the majority of patients with AMPS be managed with a combination of nonmedication strategies.

REFERENCES

1. American Psychiatric Association. *Diagnostic and Statistical Manual of Mental Disorders*. 5th ed. 2013.
2. Dimsdale JE, Creed F, Escobar J, et al. Somatic symptom disorder: an important change in DSM. *J Psychosom Res*. 2013;75(3):223–228.
3. Frances A. DSM-5 somatic symptom disorder. *J Nerv Ment Dis*. 2013;201(6):530–531.
4. Squires JE, Squires RH. A review of Munchausen syndrome by proxy. *Pediatr Ann*. 2013;42(4):67–71.
5. Nicholas M, Vlaeyen JWS, Rief W, et al. The IASP classification of chronic pain for ICD-11: chronic primary pain. *Pain*. 2019;160(1):28–37.
6. Lee HJ, Kim SE, Moon JY, Shin JY, Kim YC. Analysis of quantitative sudomotor axon reflex test patterns in patients with complex regional pain syndrome diagnosed using the Budapest criteria. *Reg Anesth Pain Med*. 2019;44:1026–1032.
7. Urits I, Shen AH, Jones MR, et al. Complex regional pain syndrome, current concepts and treatment options. *Curr Pain Headache Rep*. 2018;22(2):10.
8. Creed F. A review of the incidence and risk factors for fibromyalgia and chronic widespread pain in population-based studies. *Pain*. 2020;161(6):1169–1176.
9. Sherry DD, Sonagra M, Gmuca S. The spectrum of pediatric amplified musculoskeletal pain syndrome. *Pediatr Rheumatol Online J*. 2020;18(1):77.
10. Tan EC, Zijlstra B, Essink ML, et al. Complex regional pain syndrome type I in children. *Acta Paediatr*. 2008;97(7):875–879.
11. López-Solà M, Woo CW, Pujol J, et al. Towards a neurophysiological signature for fibromyalgia. *Pain*. 2017;158(1):34–47.
12. Kashikar-Zuck S, Cunningham N, Peugh J, et al. Long-term outcomes of adolescents with juvenile-onset fibromyalgia into adulthood and impact of depressive symptoms on functioning over time. *Pain*. 2019;160(2):433–441.
13. Üçeyler N, Zeller D, Kahn AK, et al. Small fibre pathology in patients with fibromyalgia syndrome. *Brain*. 2013;136(Pt 6):1857–1867.
14. Cagnie B, Coppieters I, Denecker S, et al. Central sensitization in fibromyalgia? *Semin Arthritis Rheum*. 2014;44(1):68–75.
15. Arnold LM, Fan J, Russell IJ, et al. The fibromyalgia family study: a genome-wide linkage scan study. *Arthritis Rheum*. 2013;65(4):1122–1128.
16. Sherry DD, Brake L, Tress JL, et al. The treatment of juvenile fibromyalgia with an intensive physical and psychosocial program. *J Pediatr*. 2015;167(3):731–737.
17. Cunningham NR, Tran ST, Lynch-Jordan AM, et al. Psychiatric disorders in young adults diagnosed with juvenile fibromyalgia in adolescence. *J Rheumatol*. 2015;42(12):2427–2433.
18. Gmuca S, Sherry DD. Fibromyalgia: treating pain in the juvenile patient. *Paediatr Drugs*. 2017;19(4):325–338.
19. Upadhyaya HP, Arnold LM, Alaka K, et al. Efficacy and safety of duloxetine versus placebo in adolescents with juvenile fibromyalgia: results from a randomized controlled trial. *Pediatr Rheumatol Online J*. 2019;17(1):27.
20. Connelly M, Weiss JE, for the CARRA Registry Investigators. Pain, functional disability, and their association in juvenile fibromyalgia compared to other pediatric rheumatic diseases. *Pediatr Rheumatol Online J*. 2019;17(1):72.
21. Cameron EC, Hemingway SL. Cannabinoids for fibromyalgia pain: a critical review of recent studies (2015-2019). *J Cannabis Res*. 2020;2(1):19.
22. Younger J, Noor N, McCue R, et al. Low-dose naltrexone for the treatment of fibromyalgia: findings of a small, randomized, double-blind, placebo-controlled, counterbalanced, crossover trial assessing daily pain levels. *Arthritis Rheum*. 2013;65(2):529–538.

ADDITIONAL RESOURCES AND WEBSITES

Additional Resources and Websites for Clinicians:

European League Against Rheumatism (EULAR) revised recommendations for managing fibromyalgia—Macfarlane GJ, Kronisch C, Dean LE, et al. EULAR revised recommendations for the management of fibromyalgia. *Ann Rheum Dis*. 2017;76:318–328. https://pubmed.ncbi.nlm.nih.gov/27377815/

Review of Amplified Pain—Sherry D, Clinch J. Pain amplification syndromes. In: Petty R, Laxer R, Lindsley C, et al., eds. *Textbook of Pediatric Rheumatology*. 8th ed. Elsevier; 2021:702–713.e5.

Revision of fibromyalgia diagnostic criteria—Wolfe F, Clauw DJ, Fitzcharles MA, et al. 2016 Revisions to the 2010/2011 fibromyalgia diagnostic criteria. *Semin Arthritis Rheum*. 2016;46(3):319–329. https://pubmed.ncbi.nlm.nih.gov/27916278/

Additional Resources and Websites for Parents/Caregivers:

Information about AMPS and fibromyalgia:

American College of Rheumatology Fact Sheet for patients on fibromyalgia—https://www.rheumatology.org/Portals/0/Files/Fibromyalgia-Fact-Sheet.pdf

American College of Rheumatology Fact Sheet for patients on amplified musculoskeletal pain syndrome—https://www.rheumatology.org/Portals/0/Files/Amplified-Musculoskeletal-Pain-Syndrome-Fact-Sheet.pdf

Arthritis Foundation information for patients concerning fibromyalgia—https://www.arthritis.org/diseases/fibromyalgia

Children's Hospital of Philadelphia information (including videos) on amplified musculoskeletal pain, fibromyalgia, complex regional pain syndrome for patients and families—https://www.stopchildhoodpain.org/juvenile-fibromyalgia/

Information about complex regional pain syndrome:

Arthritis Foundation information for patients on CRPS—https://www.arthritis.org/diseases/complex-regional-pain-syndrome

NIH information for patients and caregivers on CRPS—https://www.ninds.nih.gov/Disorders/Patient-Caregiver-Education/Fact-Sheets/Complex-Regional-Pain-Syndrome-Fact-Sheet

Additional Resources and Websites for Adolescents and Young Adults:

University of Michigan information for patients on chronic pain including a series of self-management modules—https://fibroguide.med.umich.edu/

40

Fatigue and Myalgic Encephalomyelitis/ Chronic Fatigue Syndrome

Peter C. Rowe

KEY WORDS
- Chronic fatigue syndrome
- Fatigue
- Joint hypermobility
- Myalgic encephalomyelitis
- Neurally mediated hypotension
- Orthostatic intolerance
- Postural tachycardia syndrome

INTRODUCTION

Fatigue is a private, subjective experience that, unlike muscle weakness, is difficult to quantify. It usually refers to an unpleasant, overwhelming sense of exhaustion that affects mental and physical activity, and differs from sleepiness or lack of motivation. Acute fatigue is a common symptom in adolescents and young adults (AYAs); 20% to 35% report fatigue of at least moderate severity over the preceding month. Acute fatigue usually is readily explained by factors such as inadequate sleep, excessive work or physical training demands, psychosocial factors, iron deficiency, or self-limited medical conditions. Because it can be the initial sign of a life-threatening underlying medical or psychiatric condition—ranging from vasculitis to severe depression—or associated with more protracted and potentially disabling disorders such as the condition now termed myalgic encephalomyelitis/chronic fatigue syndrome (ME/CFS), the challenge is to differentiate the benign and self-limited from the disabling or dangerous conditions.

CAUSES OF FATIGUE

Fatigue can be associated with virtually any disease of any organ system. Most causes of acute fatigue are readily apparent from the history, physical examination, and simple laboratory studies. Common causes include recent inadequate sleep or poor sleep hygiene, psychological distress, and infection.

Sleep requirements remain constant or increase through adolescence, averaging 9 hours per night, but many biologic, social, and scholastic pressures result in lower average amounts of sleep, closer to 7 hours nightly on weeknights.[1,2] In addition, most AYAs sleep more on weekends than they do during the week. Sleep disorders are increasingly being recognized as a cause of fatigue and/or daytime sleepiness in AYAs (Chapter 25).

Psychological disorders that can be associated with too little sleep and increased fatigue include depression, anxiety, stressful situations, or bipolar disorder. In general, a thorough history from the patient and parent will illuminate symptoms of a mental health disorder that correspond to the onset of excessive fatigue.

Fatigue can also result from medications (including antihistamines, sedatives, antidepressants, psychotropic medications), alcohol, marijuana, or illicit drug use, and infectious diseases such as mononucleosis, hepatitis, SARS-CoV-1 and -2, human immunodeficiency virus, tuberculosis, Lyme disease, or bacterial endocarditis. Finally, endocrine disorders including thyroid disease, adrenal disease, or diabetes mellitus as well as other systemic illnesses (e.g., connective tissue diseases, anemia, neoplasms, congenital heart disease, asthma, inflammatory bowel disease, or kidney or liver failure) will also produce fatigue.

Red flags for more serious conditions include unexpected weight loss, fevers, abnormalities on the neurologic examination, generalized lymphadenopathy, adventitious sounds on the lung examination in someone without asthma, fatigue during exertion, clubbing, orthopnea, bronzing of the skin, and erythematous, swollen joints.

MYALGIC ENCEPHALOMYELITIS/CHRONIC FATIGUE SYNDROME

Myalgic encephalomyelitis/chronic fatigue syndrome is a relatively common disorder affecting AYAs. It has a heterogeneous group of precipitating and perpetuating factors. Despite the absence of white blood cells in the spinal fluid and other classical signs of encephalitis, there is emerging evidence of disturbed central and autonomic nervous system function, notably involving diminished cerebral blood flow.[3] To maximize functioning of affected individuals, symptomatic treatment (e.g., of headaches, insomnia, pain, lightheadedness, etc.) should begin before 6 months of fatigue have elapsed and prior to diagnostic confirmation of ME/CFS.

Definition

In 2015, a report from the Institute of Medicine of the United States National Academy of Science described ME/CFS as a serious, chronic, complex, multisystem disease that often can profoundly limit the health and activities of affected patients.[4] The core symptoms (Table 40.1) should be present at least half the time with at least moderate intensity. These criteria assume that, after careful investigation, no other disorder is identified that could explain the patient's symptoms.

Epidemiology

Population-based studies have shown that ME/CFS affects previously healthy, active individuals from all socioeconomic strata and from all races,[5] although in clinical practice in the United States, Canada, Australia, and other countries, the vast majority of patients are White, even when there are no economic barriers to health care.[6] The prevalence of ME/CFS varies depending on the case definition used, but has been estimated at 1 to 3 per 1,000 in adolescents. While ME/CFS is much more common after age 10 years, when present in younger children, the symptoms are similar to those who are older.[7] Female AYAs are more likely to develop ME/CFS than male AYAs, in a ratio of 2 to 4:1. Across the globe, ME/CFS

TABLE 40.1

Institute of Medicine Criteria for Myalgic Encephalomyelitis/Chronic Fatigue Syndrome

The diagnosis of ME/CFS requires the following three symptoms:

1. A substantial reduction or impairment in the ability to engage in pre-illness levels of occupational, educational, social, or personal activities that persists for more than 6 months and is accompanied by fatigue, which is often profound, is of new or definite onset (not lifelong), is not the result of ongoing exertion, and is not substantially alleviated by rest.
2. Post exertional malaise
3. Unrefreshing sleep

At least one of the following two additional manifestations is required:

a. Cognitive impairment
b. Orthostatic intolerance

is a common reason for home tutoring and prolonged inability to attend regular school classes. The factor that most closely predicts school attendance is physical functioning as opposed to mental health and/or behavioral issues.[8]

Symptoms

Myalgic encephalomyelitis/chronic fatigue syndrome can be recognized by its profound fatigue, a substantial impairment in the activities the individual previously tolerated, unrefreshing sleep, lightheadedness and other symptoms of orthostatic intolerance, and cognitive problems like difficulty with concentration, processing, and short-term memory. Other common symptoms seen in 30% to 70% of patients include headaches, myalgias, arthralgias, nausea, abdominal pain, problems with temperature regulation, sore throat, and chest pain.

Etiology

Infection

The onset of ME/CFS can be abrupt—associated with a flu-like or mononucleosis-like infection—but gradual onset of symptoms is also common.[9] However, no single pathogen has been identified as a cause for all instances of ME/CFS. Finally, evidence of persistent infection has not been detected in those with ME/CFS, although unrecognized and untreated tick-borne infections can cause overlapping symptoms.

- After mononucleosis and certain other acute infections, 10% to 13% of AYA patients can develop CFS; the severity of the initial infection appears to be a main risk factor, not the patient's premorbid behavioral state.[10,11]
- In contrast, ME/CFS can follow relatively mild acute respiratory symptoms of SARS infection.
- Immune abnormalities are variable, and autoimmune phenomena are occasionally present. Antinuclear antibody titers can be present in the absence of signs of recognized rheumatologic disorders, and usually without evidence of elevations in the sedimentation rate, antibodies to double-stranded DNA, or extractable nuclear antibodies.[6] There are no clear features consistent with a classical immunodeficiency disorder.[4]

Orthostatic Intolerance

In AYAs, ME/CFS symptoms (fatigue, lightheadedness, cognitive problems, headaches, and others) are usually made worse by prolonged upright posture.[12–15] This orthostatic intolerance is present in >95% of AYAs with ME/CFS, and is commonly accompanied by the following:

- Postural tachycardia syndrome (POTS), defined as a greater than 40-beat increase in heart rate with standing for adolescents or a 30-beat change in those aged 20 years and older, often with reproduction of orthostatic symptoms (lightheadedness, headache, cognitive difficulties, warmth, nausea), in the first 10 minutes of quiet standing or head-up tilt table testing.[7]
- Varying forms of hypotension, including (a) classical orthostatic hypotension (reductions of 20 mm Hg in systolic or 10 mm Hg

in diastolic pressure in the first 3 minutes upright), (b) delayed orthostatic hypotension (same criteria occurring after the 3-minute point upright), or (c) neurally mediated hypotension characterized by a 25 mm Hg reduction in systolic blood pressure.[7]

- Low orthostatic tolerance, defined by orthostatic symptoms and a reduction in cerebral blood flow in the absence of changes in blood pressure or heart rate. In adult ME/CFS patients, 42% have hypotension or POTS during head-up tilt testing, but importantly 58% have a greater than threefold reduction in cerebral blood flow compared to controls in the absence of hypotension or tachycardia when upright.[3]

Treatment of orthostatic intolerance can be associated with improvements in overall function, including energy and tolerance of activity in those with chronic fatigue and ME/CFS.[7,12]

Allergic Inflammation

Allergies and food sensitivities are more common in adults with ME/CFS than would be expected from population estimates. In affected AYAs, 31% report a triad of upper gastrointestinal symptoms—epigastric pain, reflux, and early satiety—often beginning as the overall symptoms of ME/CFS emerge. These symptoms are consistent with a delayed hypersensitivity to milk protein. These individuals have improved health-related quality of life when consuming a milk-free diet.[16] Mast cell activation syndrome is a recently described condition in which there is a substantial overlap of symptoms with ME/CFS.[17] This diagnosis should be considered when patients have facial flushing, urticaria, pruritus, swelling, or histories characterized by intolerance of multiple medications or foods.

Mental Health

Depression and anxiety disorders must be evaluated carefully to disentangle the presence of these disorders from ME/CFS. Depression shares some clinical features with ME/CFS, including fatigue, nonrestorative sleep, and difficulty concentrating.[7]

- An estimated 25% of AYAs with ME/CFS develop depression at some time during the course of their illness, compared to 18% in a community sample; 30% have anxiety.[6]
- When present in patients with ME/CFS, the severity of depression is usually mild; anhedonia and symptoms of self-reproach are uncommon.
- Among patients with depressive disorders, fatigue is less severe than in those with ME/CFS and often improves with exercise. In contrast, after a period of activity that exceeds their usual baseline, individuals with ME/CFS experience postexertional malaise—a marked exacerbation of fatigue, cognitive dysfunction, pain, and other symptoms, often lasting more than a day.[7]
- Myalgic encephalomyelitis/chronic fatigue syndrome symptoms are present on weekends and summers, thus differentiating ME/CFS from school phobia. While some AYAs improve during the summer months because they can rest and sleep duration can be increased, symptoms do not disappear.
- It is appropriate to provide medication to ameliorate symptoms of depression and anxiety if warranted, but these medications will not relieve or cure the major symptoms of ME/CFS.

● EVALUATION OF MYALGIC ENCEPHALOMYELITIS/CHRONIC FATIGUE SYNDROME

History

First, it is most helpful to ask a patient to list his or her current symptoms to get a sense of the possible areas that will require evaluation. In those with ME/CFS, the symptoms tend to be predictably similar from one patient to another rather than a random collection of somatic complaints. After getting a sense of the onset of the illness and changes since it began, explore the details of each symptom on the list, asking about the frequency, severity, aggravating and relieving factors, and the timing of each in relation to other symptoms. A careful history that includes a HEEADSSS assessment (see Chapter 4) also needs to focus on the following:

- Orthostatic intolerance, which is indicated by the following:
  - Increased fatigue or lightheadedness when standing still, or in a hot shower or bath, or in hot weather
  - Frequent adoption of postural counter-maneuvers (sitting with knees to chest, doing homework in a reclined position, legs crossed when standing, fidgeting)
  - Avoidance of low-impact activities such as shopping
  - Worsening of fatigue after long periods of sitting (such as at the end of a 90-minute class)
- Menstrual periods
  - Does fatigue worsen in the days before the onset of menses?
- Impact on daily life
  - What activities must the individual now limit or avoid?
  - Can they continue to participate in social activities or sports?
- Family history
  - Higher rates of ME/CFS and other similar disorders (fibromyalgia, irritable bowel disease, temporomandibular joint dysfunction, anxiety, hypotension, syncope, POTS, joint laxity, celiac disease, milk protein intolerance) in first-degree relatives of affected patients

Physical Examination

The physical examination should include a careful neurologic examination, measurement of joint hypermobility, and evaluation for postural dysfunctions. Patients with ME/CFS usually have abnormal findings (see below). Orthostatic testing is warranted in all patients with ME/CFS and those with excessive chronic fatigue, especially if they report frequent lightheadedness. Testing can take two forms:

- In-office passive standing tests: 5 minutes supine, then 10 minutes of quiet standing, leaning against a wall. Record changes in heart rate and blood pressure each minute, as well as changes in orthostatic symptoms and fatigue on a 0 to 10 scale between supine and standing. The test must be observed due to the risk of syncope.[7]
- Laboratory head-up tilt table test: Prolonged testing of 40 to 45 minutes is required to identify neurally mediated hypotension. Shorter

10-minute tests will only identify POTS or, less commonly, orthostatic hypotension. Care should be taken in those with more severe impairment, as prolonged orthostatic testing can aggravate symptoms, often for several days; some centers administer 1 to 2 L of intravenous saline after the test to reduce the risk of an exacerbation.

Common abnormalities on physical examination include the following:

- Tachycardia or hypotension during prolonged upright posture, often associated with a purple discoloration in the dependent limbs, termed acrocyanosis.
- Joint hypermobility, which has been reported in 60% of those with ME/CFS.[18] This can be assessed using the Beighton score (Fig. 40.1). Some ME/CFS patients will also meet criteria for Ehlers–Danlos syndrome.
- Postural dysfunctions: Head-forward posture, thoracic kyphosis, lumbar lordosis, limited passive straight leg raise, brachial plexus dysfunction, and accompanying areas of muscle guarding or tenderness, many of which[19] benefit from evaluation and treatment by a physical therapist.

Laboratory Studies

There is no single test to confirm a diagnosis of ME/CFS. However, the clinician should perform the following to exclude other important causes of chronic fatigue:

- Complete blood count, with white blood count and differential and platelet count
- Serum chemistries including electrolytes, urea, creatinine, total protein, albumin, calcium, alanine aminotransferase (ALT), aspartate aminotransferase (AST), and alkaline phosphatase
- Free T4, thyroid-stimulating hormone
- C-reactive protein or erythrocyte sedimentation rate
- Ferritin or other measures of iron deficiency
- Vitamin B12, especially in AYAs who are vegan or those on proton pump inhibitors
- Vitamin D
- Celiac disease screening
- Urinalysis
- Electrocardiogram

Maneuver (1 point for each positive)	L	R	Score
a. Passive dorsiflexion of the fifth finger at the metacarpophalangeal joint > 90°			
b. Passive apposition of the thumb to the flexor aspect of the forearm			
c. Extension of the elbow > 190°			
d. Extension of the knee > 190°			
e. Forward flexion of the trunk with the knees straight so the palms rest flat on the floor			
Beighton score (maximum score=9)			

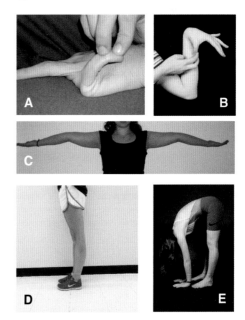

FIGURE 40.1 Assessment of Joint Hypermobility Using the Beighton Score. Examples of each maneuver in the Beighton score are shown in Figure 40.1A–E; the points are assigned as in the scoring sheet. A goniometer is required to accurately measure elbow and knee hyperextension. Beighton scores of 4 or higher have been considered consistent with joint hypermobility, acknowledging that joint hypermobility can be present with lower scores, as the Beighton score does not assess for hypermobility of the shoulders, hips, or ankles. (Reproduced with permission from Roma M, Marden CL, De Wandele I, Francomano CA, Rowe PC. Postural tachycardia syndrome and other forms of orthostatic intolerance in Ehlers-Danlos syndrome. *Auton Neurosc.* 2018;215:91.)

Other testing is dependent on the history and physical examination (e.g., antinuclear antibody testing in someone with a malar rash). The following should be considered:

- Serology for certain infections, including tick-borne diseases in endemic areas. Serology for Epstein–Barr virus and cytomegalovirus can help with categorizing whether the illness might have been initiated by these organisms, but usually does not change management.
- Consider plasma histamine, serum tryptase, chromogranin A (CGA), and other tests for mast cell activation syndrome, especially in those with facial flushing, pruritus, urticaria, or other similar signs and symptoms or allergic inflammation. Do not order CGA as a diagnostic test for mast cell activation in those being treated with proton pump inhibitors, as these medications can independently cause an elevated CGA level.
- Magnetic resonance imaging (MRI) of the brain and cervical spine is not routinely indicated, but important if there is occipital headache, nystagmus, worsening of symptoms on neck movement, or hyperreflexia (chronic fatigue can be a presenting feature of Chiari I malformation and cervical spine stenosis).[20] Dynamic MRI, computerized tomography scan, or x-ray imaging (with flexion, extension, or lateral head and neck rotation) is needed if there is hyper-reflexia, neck pain, and other symptoms suggestive of craniocervical instability (heaviness of the head, a feeling that the head is unsupported).[21]
- Reductions in cerebral blood flow during upright posture can be measured using extracranial Doppler imaging,[3] but this method is not yet widely available.

MANAGEMENT OF MYALGIC ENCEPHALOMYELITIS/CHRONIC FATIGUE SYNDROME

The goal of treatment is to improve function and activity and to ameliorate specific symptoms. While no single pharmacologic agent has been identified to be universally helpful in ME/CFS,[22] many effective treatments for specific symptoms and comorbid conditions are available. While data have demonstrated moderate efficacy for intravenous immunoglobulin (IVIG) in adolescents,[23] the results from adult studies are mixed. Clinicians need to remember that some medications can cause harm, such as corticosteroids, which lead to adrenal insufficiency. Treating the adolescent or young adult with ME/CFS requires careful attention by the patient and the practitioner to the factors that provoke and exacerbate symptoms. Treatment requires a willingness by the patient to try several medications before the best management of symptoms is achieved, and requires the understanding that medications often treat symptoms but will not cure the disorder. The clinician should use an iterative clinical treatment approach that includes the following:

- Develop working hypotheses about the dominant influences on fatigue symptoms.
- Explain and demystify ME/CFS, including how symptoms can be made worse with prolonged orthostatic stress or excessive physical or cognitive activity.
- Initiate nonpharmacologic therapies as listed below.
- Begin pharmacologic treatment as indicated, focusing on the dominant factors influencing the most bothersome symptoms first (e.g., orthostatic intolerance, sleep dysfunction, pain, headache, food and environmental allergies, menstrual dysfunction, low mood, anxiety).
- Reassess at regular intervals (every 1 to 2 months depending on level of severity) and repeat the steps above.

Nonpharmacologic Treatments

Sleep

- Aim for a specified, regular bedtime, recognizing that this is not always possible in those with more challenging reversals of circadian rhythms.
- Eliminate use of electronic devices after "lights out" as these can aggravate fatigue.
- Avoid sleeping more than 12 hours at a time. Longer periods of sleep promote low blood volume and can aggravate orthostatic intolerance.

- If insomnia is impressive and unresponsive to relaxation techniques and standard sleep hygiene measures (e.g., avoiding daytime naps, avoiding caffeine in the evening), pharmacologic treatment may be needed.[7]

Activity and Exercise

- Where possible, encourage gradual increases in daily activity, designed to avoid postexertional malaise.
- Manual physical therapy and treatment of orthostatic intolerance can be bridges to tolerating exercise; recumbent exercise initiated slowly may help, especially in the early days of treatment.
- Emphasize gradual increases in exercise and activities, with specific rest cycles between activities to avoid the "push-crash" cycle of excessive activity on a good day followed by prolonged postexertional collapse.
- Caution is needed with severely affected bed-bound patients, who have been harmed by rigid or too rapid advancement of activity before they have been adequately treated.

Orthostatic Intolerance

- Avoid conditions that aggravate symptoms (prolonged standing, warm environments).
- Increase fluid intake (2 to 3 L daily in most AYAs).
- Increase sodium intake according to taste, supplemented by buffered salt tablets.
- Utilize the muscle pump function of the lower limbs with postural counter-maneuvers: crossing legs and shifting from one leg to the other while standing, sitting with knees higher than hips, and leg muscle contraction exercises before standing.
- Recommend compression garments or support hose at 20 to 30 mm Hg compression (waist-high are more effective than thigh-high, which are more effective than knee-high) and body shaper garments or abdominal binders.

Educational Accommodations

Adolescents and young adults still in school who report orthostatic intolerance are likely to report feeling worse in the morning, when blood volume is lowest, and do somewhat better as the day progresses. Symptoms wax and wane, often unpredictably from day to day, are often worse after vigorous exercise, and persist longer after viral respiratory illnesses. Sample letters explaining the illness and requesting educational accommodations are available in reference 9. These accommodations can include one or more of the following:

- A later start to the school day
- A reduction in course load
- An excuse from gym, or permission to self-modulate exercise
- Salty snacks and water bottle in classroom
- Permission to get up and move around in class and during testing
- Extended time for tests
- Flexibility with assignments and deadlines
- For those with moderate to severe ME/CFS, consider these:
  - A skipped day midweek to rest/recover
  - Half-day attendance
  - Home and hospital teaching

Behavioral Interventions

- Ascertain the level of depressed mood and anxiety, and treat accordingly.
- Counseling can be helpful especially for depression and anxiety, advice for managing a chronic illness, along with relaxation/breathing techniques and distraction.
- Cognitive behavioral therapy is not curative; effect sizes in trials have been modest and unsustained. Cognitive behavioral therapy is no longer recommended as a primary treatment of ME/CFS.[24]

Pharmacologic Treatment

For orthostatic intolerance, medication options are presented in Table 40.2.[7,25,26]

TABLE 40.2

Medications for Managing Orthostatic Intolerance in Adolescents and Young Adults

Medication	Usual Dose	Comments
Vasoconstrictors		
Midodrine	Start at 2.5 mg q4h while awake. Increase every 3–7 d by 2.5 mg to optimal dose or maximum of 10 mg q4h while awake.	Alpha-1 agonist. First-line therapy for those with low blood pressure (BP) (systolic BP <100 or low normal BP). Avoid doses around bedtime. Warn patients to expect scalp tingling, "goose bump" sensation.
Methylphenidate, dextroamphetamine.	Immediate-release form: 5–10 mg b.i.d., increasing gradually to 15–40 mg/d	First-line therapy for those with prominent cognitive dysfunction, personal or family history of attention deficit hyperactivity disorder (ADHD), joint hypermobility. Other stimulants are also effective: use the same doses as would be effective for ADHD.
Volume expanders		
Sodium chloride	Oral: ~1 g in tablet form with meals IV: 0.9% normal saline 1–2 L over 1–2 h	Intravenous (IV) saline is seldom practical over the longer term, but can help restore baseline function after illnesses or as emergency "rescue" therapy.
Fludrocortisone	0.05 mg daily for 1 wk, then 0.1 mg daily. Increase gradually to usual maximum of 0.2 mg daily.	First-line therapy in those with baseline hypotension or increased salt appetite. Add KCl 10 mEq for every 0.1 mg fludrocortisone to prevent hypokalemia. Can aggravate acne. Monitor for the emergence of hypertension, especially when taken with oral contraceptive pills.
Oral contraceptives, Medroxyprogesterone	Most available forms are fine. Conventional dosage or continuous pills for 84 d (one period every 3 mo)	First-line therapy for females with dysmenorrhea or when fatigue and lightheadedness worsen with menses
Desmopressin acetate	0.1 mg at bedtime, increasing to 0.2 mg daily	Useful for those with nocturia. Monitor for hyponatremia.
Heart rate and sympathetic tone modifiers		
Atenolol	12.5–25 mg daily, increase by 12.5-mg increments until optimal effect. Usual dose is 25–50 mg daily.	First-line therapy for those with resting heart rate >100, anxiety, or prominent headache. Higher doses can aggravate fatigue and lightheadedness. Use low doses with caution in patients with asthma.
Propranolol	10–20 mg 3–4 times daily	Other beta blockers can be used as well, starting low and advancing gradually.
Pyridostigmine bromide	Immediate-release form: 30 mg daily, increase by 30 mg every 3–7 d to 60 mg b.i.d.–t.i.d. Sustained-release form: 180 mg daily	Effective in both POTS and neurally mediated hypotension. Can also help with gastrointestinal motility problems. Adverse effects include muscle twitching, nausea, emesis.
Clonidine	0.05 mg at bedtime. Increase after 1 wk to 0.1 mg nightly. Higher doses occasionally tolerated.	Consider in those with anxiety, problems with attention, insomnia, hyperhidrosis. Can improve blood volume.
Ivabradine	2.5–10 mg b.i.d.	Effective for resting heart rate above 100 bpm
SSRI/SNRI		
Escitalopram	Start with 5–10 mg daily for 2 wks, increase gradually up to maximum of 40 mg daily.	Consider in those with dysthymia, depression, or anxiety. SSRI and SNRI medications can help as vasoconstrictors and also as modifiers of central sympathetic tone.
Sertraline	25–100 mg daily	
Duloxetine	Start with 30 mg daily, increase gradually to maximum of 120 mg daily.	Effective in fibromyalgia, so consider if myalgias are prominent.

SSRI, selective serotonin reuptake inhibitor; SNRI, serotonin and norepinephrine reuptake inhibitor.

For headaches and chronic pain, the clinician should consider the following:

- Physical therapy if there is a biomechanical contributor, head-forward posture, slumped shoulders, kyphosis, neck tilt, or other postural dysfunctions.
- Over-the-counter medications that have been demonstrated to be effective for migraine headaches, such as riboflavin 400 mg daily and coenzyme Q10 300 mg daily.
- For severe and chronic migraines, daily medication to prevent headaches may include atenolol, cyproheptadine, topiramate, botulinum toxin, or calcitonin gene-related peptide antagonists.
- For those reporting chronic pain symptoms, tricyclic antidepressants in low doses can be used with caution, but can aggravate lightheadedness.
- Medications used for widespread fibromyalgia pain in adults include gabapentin, duloxetine, pregabalin, and low-dose naltrexone.[7,27]
- For insomnia, consider white noise or meditative telephone apps, melatonin, L-theanine 50 to 200 mg nightly, sedating antihistamines such as cyproheptadine, trazodone, doxepin, clonidine, and others if needed.
- For those with urticaria, facial flushing, and intolerance of foods and medications, consider medications used in the management of allergies and mast cell activation syndrome, including H1 and H2 antihistamines (reserving sedating antihistamines for nighttime use), montelukast, and nasal or oral cromolyn.

Outcomes

Health outcomes for the adolescent or young adult with ME/CFS are thought to be better than that for adults with this disorder. In a large Australian cohort, the duration of illness among those who recovered was 1 to 16 years, with a mean of 5 years.[6] Although not formally studied, a subset of these young people have been observed to have persistent disability. While full recovery is possible, long-term data identify persistent limitations in quality of life even among some of those who report resolution of the illness.[28]

SUMMARY

Myalgic encephalomyelitis/chronic fatigue syndrome is a serious, complex, multisystem disorder that can interfere substantially with normal activities in AYAs, often for many years. It can begin insidiously or following infectious illnesses like mononucleosis, and is readily recognized by the characteristic symptoms of intense fatigue, limited ability to engage in activities that were well tolerated before the illness, unrefreshing sleep, postexertional malaise, cognitive difficulties, and symptoms of orthostatic intolerance. While no laboratory test is available to confirm the diagnosis, a careful physical examination can identify a number of possible abnormalities, including joint hypermobility, postural dysfunctions, and restricted range of motion in the limbs and spine, acrocyanosis, and the provocation of symptoms as well as heart rate and blood pressure abnormalities during standing or head-up tilt. No single pharmacologic agent is available to treat the symptoms, but many treatments for symptoms are available to improve function and quality of life.

ACKNOWLEDGMENTS

The author wishes to acknowledge Martin Fisher, Marvin Belzer, and Lawrence Neinstein for their contributions to previous versions of this chapter.

REFERENCES

1. Caskadon MA. Sleep in adolescents: the perfect storm. *Pediatr Clin North Am.* 2011;58(3):637–647.
2. Fisher M. Fatigue in adolescents. *J Pediatr Adolesc Gynecol.* 2013;26(5):252–256.
3. van Campen CLMC, Verheugt FWA, Rowe PC, et al. Cerebral blood flow is reduced in ME/CFS during head-up tilt testing even in the absence of hypotension or tachycardia: a quantitative, controlled study using Doppler echography. *Clin Neurophysiol Pract.* 2020; 5:50–58.
4. *Beyond Myalgic Encephalomyelitis/Chronic Fatigue Syndrome: Redefining an Illness. Committee on the Diagnostic Criteria for Myalgic Encephalomyelitis/ Chronic Fatigue Syndrome. Institute of Medicine.* The National Academies Press; 2015.
5. Jason LA, Richman JA, Rademaker AW, et al. A community-based study of chronic fatigue syndrome. *Arch Intern Med.* 1999;159(18):2129–2137.
6. Rowe KS. Long term follow up of young people with chronic fatigue syndrome attending a pediatric outpatient service. *Front Pediatr.* 2019;7:21.
7. Rowe PC, Underhill RA, Friedman KJ, et al. Myalgic encephalomyelitis/chronic fatigue syndrome diagnosis and management in young people: a primer. *Front Pediatr.* 2017;5:121.
8. Crawley E, Sterne JAC. Association between school absence and physical function in paediatric chronic fatigue syndrome/myalgic encephalopathy. *Arch Dis Child.* 2009;94(10):752–756.
9. Nijhof SL, Maijer K, Bleijenberg G, et al. Adolescent chronic fatigue syndrome: prevalence, incidence, and morbidity. *Pediatrics.* 2011;127(5):e1169–e1175.
10. Katz BZ, Shiraishi Y, Mears CJ, et al. Chronic fatigue syndrome after infectious mononucleosis in adolescents. *Pediatrics.* 2009;124(1);189–193.
11. Hickie, I, Davenport T, Wakefield D, et al. Post-infective and chronic fatigue syndromes precipitated by viral and non-viral pathogens: prospective cohort study. *BMJ.* 2006;333(7568):575.
12. Bou-Holaigah I, Rowe PC, Kan J, et al. Relationship between neurally mediated hypotension and the chronic fatigue syndrome. *JAMA.* 1995;274(12):961–967.
13. Stewart JM, Gewitz MH, Weldon A, et al. Orthostatic intolerance in adolescent chronic fatigue syndrome. *Pediatrics.* 1999;103(1):116–121.
14. Wyller VB, Due R, Saul JP, et al. Usefulness of an abnormal cardiovascular response during low-grade head-up tilt-test for discriminating adolescents with chronic fatigue from healthy controls. *Am J Cardiol.* 2007;99(7):997–1001.
15. Roma M, Marden CL, Flaherty MAK, et al. Impaired health-related quality of life in adolescent myalgic encephalomyelitis/chronic fatigue syndrome: the impact of core symptoms. *Front Pediatr.* 2019;7:26.
16. Rowe PC, Marden CL, Jasion SE, et al. Cow's milk protein intolerance in adolescents and young adults with chronic fatigue syndrome. *Acta Paediatr.* 2016;105(9): e412–e418.
17. Afrin LB, Molderings GJ. A concise, practical guide to diagnostic assessment for mast cell activation disease. *World J Hematol.* 2014;3:1–17.
18. Roma M, Marden CL, De Wandele I, et al. Postural tachycardia syndrome and other forms of orthostatic intolerance in Ehlers-Danlos syndrome. *Auton Neurosci.* 2018;215:89–96.
19. Rowe PC, Marden CL, Flaherty MAK, et al. Impaired range of motion of limbs and spine in chronic fatigue syndrome. *J Pediatr.* 2014;165(2):360–366.
20. Heffez DS, Ross RE, Shade-Zeldow Y, et al. Clinical evidence for cervical myelopathy due to Chiari malformation and spinal stenosis in a non-randomized group of patients with the diagnosis of fibromyalgia. *Eur Spine J.* 2004;13(6):516–523.
21. Henderson FC, Austin C, Benzel E, et al. Neurological and spinal manifestations of the Ehlers-Danlos syndromes. *Am J Med Genet C Semin Med Genet.* 2017; 175(1):195–211.
22. Smith MEB, Haney E, McDonagh M, et al. Treatment of myalgic encephalomyelitis/ chronic fatigue syndrome: a systematic review for a National Institutes of Health Pathways to Prevention workshop. *Ann Intern Med.* 2015;162(12):841–850.
23. Rowe KS. Double-blind randomized controlled trial to assess the efficacy of intravenous immunoglobulin for the management of chronic fatigue syndrome in adolescents. *J Psychiat Res.* 1997;31(1):133–147.
24. Friedberg F, Sunnquist M, Nacul L. Rethinking the standard of care for myalgic encephalomyelitis/chronic fatigue syndrome. *J Gen Intern Med.* 2020;35(3): 906–909.
25. Miller AJ, Raj SR. Pharmacotherapy for postural tachycardia syndrome. *Auton Neurosci.* 2018;215:28–36.
26. Shen WK, Sheldon RS, Benditt DG, et al. 2017 ACC/AHA/HRS guideline for the evaluation and management of patients with syncope : a report of the American College of Cardiology/American Heart Association Task Force on Clinical Practice Guidelines and the Heart Rhythm Society. *Heart Rhythm.* 2017;14(8):e155–e217.
27. Sarzi-Puttini P, Giorgi V, Marotto D, et al. Fibromyalgia: an update on clinical characteristics, aetiopathogenesis and treatment. *Nat Rev Rheumatol.* 2020;16(11): 645–660.
28. Brown MM, Bell DS, Jason LA, et al. Understanding long-term outcomes of chronic fatigue syndrome. *J Clin Psychol.* 2012;68(9):1028–1035.

ADDITIONAL RESOURCES AND WEBSITES

Additional Resources and Websites for Clinicians:

The following webinars by Dr. Rowe provide a clinical approach to pediatric ME/CFS and more information on managing orthostatic intolerance:

A Clinical Approach to ME/CFS in Adolescents and Young Adults—https://www.youtube.com/watch?v=_WqGmHpL6MI

The International Association for CFS/ME website has links to CFS/ME organizations around the world, as well as to websites of medical specialties related to CFS, and details about their scientific conferences on CFS/ME—https://www.iacfsme.org/

Managing Orthostatic Intolerance—http://www.youtube.com/watch?v=5iF30TVLaRE&playnext=1&list=PLCDC685DB095C02DC&feature=results_video

The following websites have information about managing ME/CFS and some of the more common comorbid conditions. The first three often make webinars available on various topics relevant to ME/CFS.

Dysautonomia International website—http://dysautonomiainternational.org/

Ehlers Danlos Society website—https://www.ehlers-danlos.com/

Solve ME/CFS Initiative—https://solvecfs.org/

These links provide further clinical management advice:

Centers for Disease Control ME/CFS website—https://www.cdc.gov/me-cfs/index.html

U.S. ME/CFS Clinician Coalition—https://mecfscliniciancoalition.org/about-mecfs/

Additional Resources and Websites for Parents/Caregivers:

All of the websites listed above as suitable for health professions include content suitable for parents

The Solve ME/CFS Initiative website lists other resources for patients and caregivers—https://solvecfs.org/research/patient-and-caregiver-resources/

The Solve ME/CFS Initiative also invites individuals to follow them on:

Join us on Facebook at www.Facebook.com/SolveMECFSInitiative

Follow us on Twitter at www.twitter.com/plzsolvecfs

Subscribe to our YouTube Channel at www.youtube.com/solvecfs

The Dysautonomia International website has a specific link to support group resources for parents and patients, including adolescents—http://dysautonomiainternational.org/page.php?ID=24

Additional Resources and Websites for Adolescents and Young Adults:

All of the websites listed above as suitable for health professions include content suitable for teenagers and young adults

The Dysautonomia International website has a specific link to support group resources for parents and patients, including adolescents—http://dysautonomiainternational.org/page.php?ID=24

Standing Up To POTS—http://standinguptopots.org/

CHAPTER 41

Chronic Abdominal Pain

Wael N. Sayej
Paula K. Braverman

KEY WORDS
- Celiac disease
- Chronic abdominal pain
- Disorders of Gut–Brain Interaction
- Functional abdominal pain
- Functional gastrointestinal disorders
- Inflammatory bowel disease
- Irritable bowel syndrome (IBS)
- Lactose intolerance
- Recurrent abdominal pain
- Rome IV criteria

INTRODUCTION

Chronic abdominal pain is a common complaint among adolescents and young adults (AYAs). The differential diagnosis of chronic abdominal pain includes functional gastrointestinal disorders (FGIDs) and organic disorders related to anatomic abnormalities, inflammation, or tissue damage. The Rome IV criteria have been developed to assist in diagnosing and treating FGIDs among different age groups, recently defined, by the Rome Foundation Board of Directors and the Rome IV Committees, as Disorders of Gut–Brain Interaction (DGBI).[1,2] In the new classifications, the committees recognized that the term "functional" has limitations by being nonspecific and potentially stigmatizing. The term "functional" was removed from most of the disorders while also recognizing that it is not possible to completely eliminate the use of FGIDs at this time. The Rome IV criteria provide symptom-based guidelines by which FGIDs can be diagnosed. Functional gastrointestinal disorders are characterized in the Rome IV criteria based on age including neonates/toddlers, child/adolescent (4 to 18 years), and adults (≥19 years).[3] There is ongoing research into the pathophysiology of the gut–brain axis related to FGIDs as well as pharmacologic and dietary treatment options. Efforts to treat chronic abdominal pain can lead to frustration for patients, families, and clinicians alike. The approach to this problem is particularly challenging, and in most cases, there is no specific organic abnormality found. This chapter reviews the epidemiology, pathophysiology, differential diagnosis, clinical approach, and available treatment modalities for chronic abdominal pain with an emphasis on FGIDs.

DEFINITION

Chronic abdominal pain is one of the most common reasons for referral to pediatric and adult gastroenterologists. The differential diagnosis of chronic abdominal pain includes FGIDs and organic disorders related to anatomic abnormalities, inflammation, or tissue damage. Functional gastrointestinal disorders are disorders of the gastrointestinal (GI) system in which symptoms cannot be explained by organic abnormalities but are based on clinical symptoms in children, adolescents, and adults.[1] The Rome criteria are a diagnostic system developed to characterize and standardize the diagnosis of FGIDs. Initially developed in 1994 to guide researchers, the criteria have been revised and evolved over the past three decades with the intent of making them more clinically useful and relevant. Functional gastrointestinal disorders are recognized as DGBI with GI symptoms related to any combination of the following: motility disturbance, visceral hypersensitivity, altered mucosal and immune function, altered gut microbiota, and altered central nervous system processing.[2,3] This chapter will focus on the diagnosis and treatment of chronic abdominal pain with an emphasis on FGIDs.

DIFFERENTIAL DIAGNOSIS AND CLINICAL MANIFESTATIONS OF CHRONIC ABDOMINAL PAIN

Functional Gastrointestinal Disorders

Functional gastrointestinal disorders, characterized by persistent and recurring GI symptoms, include several separate idiopathic disorders that can affect any part of the GI tract.

Epidemiology

The prevalence of FGIDs in AYAs is unknown for several reasons.

1. There may be overlapping symptoms, and individuals may have more than one FGID as defined by the Rome criteria.[2,3]
2. The prevalence of FGIDs differs depending on the version of Rome criteria applied and the population studied, including the geographic region or country, suggesting different perceptions and sociocultural interpretations of symptoms.[2,3]
3. The Rome criteria may not accurately reflect the clinical presentation. This was specifically discussed in the 2012 Multinational Irritable Bowel Syndrome Initiative report indicating that the Rome criteria are not necessarily adequate or most relevant for the clinical diagnosis of irritable bowel syndrome (IBS).[4]

Despite these limitations, the following studies provide some estimates of the prevalence of chronic abdominal pain in children and AYAs.

1. A study in Cali, Colombia utilized the Spanish version of the Questionnaire of Pediatric Gastrointestinal Symptoms-Rome IV (QPGS-IV) to determine the prevalence of FGIDs and the diagnostic accuracy of the QPGS-IV. Of 487 surveyed schoolchildren, aged 10 to 18 years, 20.8% had FGIDs. The QPGS-IV had a sensitivity of 75% and specificity of 90%.[5]
2. A cross-sectional study in the United States, utilizing Rome IV criteria, in which 1,255 mothers of children aged 0 to 18 years completed an online survey about their children's

GI symptoms found that 25% of children and adolescents had FGIDs based on the Rome IV criteria.[6]

3. A systematic review of the worldwide literature assessing IBS among individuals aged 15 years and older found prevalence rates from 7% to 21%, with a pooled prevalence of 11% for those less than age 30 years.[7]

4. A cross-sectional study of 1,002 adult subjects determined the frequency of common FGIDs was 20.7% (n = 207) and 20.9% (n = 209) among subjects based on the Rome III and Rome IV criteria, respectively.[8]

Etiology of Functional Gastrointestinal Disorders

The etiology of FGID is still not well understood; however, recent studies indicate multidimensional causes. Current theories suggest that FGIDs are due to the following:

1. Dysregulation or impairment of the bidirectional communication in the "gut–brain axis" involving[2]:
   a. Neural systems (neurotransmitters, e.g., serotonin, noradrenaline) and the autonomic and enteric nervous systems, which affect motility and secretions
   b. Gut and peripheral immune systems (e.g., cytokines, mast cell activation, T-cell activation)
   c. Endocrine systems (hypothalamic–pituitary–adrenal axis)
2. Visceral hypersensitivity (hyperalgesia) with alteration in the neural processing of visceral stimuli, resulting in lower pain thresholds and/or alterations in pain perception. Possible disturbance in pain processing in patients with IBS and functional dyspepsia is evidenced by brain imaging studies (functional magnetic resonance imaging [MRI] and evoked brain responses) demonstrating activation of certain areas of the brain and structural brain changes (insular cortex, amygdala, and hippocampus).[9]
3. Other factors influencing the gut–brain axis include genetic predisposition, psychological factors (stress, anxiety, trauma, pain, mood, cognitive function, expectation, conditioning), and physical factors (infection, mucosal inflammation, alteration in enteric microbiota).[10]

Diagnostic Criteria

The full Rome IV criteria are available at https://theromefoundation.org/rome-iv/rome-iv-criteria/. The Rome IV criteria include categories for infants/toddlers, children, and adolescents (4 to 18 years) and for adults (≥19 years). A key change from Rome III to Rome IV criteria for FGIDs was the elimination of Rome III's criterion that there is "no evidence of structural disease to explain the symptoms," and replacement with Rome IV's criterion "after appropriate medical evaluation the symptoms cannot be attributed to another medical condition."[2,3] Different FGIDs can co-occur in the same adolescent or young adult.[3] The following are the relevant differences in the Rome IV categories by age group.

1. The child/adolescent components are classified by symptom pattern or area of symptom location, whereas the adult components are divided into six domains (Table 41.1).
2. The Rome IV criteria for adults no longer include functional abdominal pain. This has been replaced with unspecified functional bowel disorder, which is defined as bowel symptoms not attributable to an organic etiology that do not meet criteria for IBS, or functional constipation, diarrhea, or abdominal bloating/distension disorders.
3. The criteria for the same diagnostic category of FGIDs differ by age group. For adult FGIDs, the criteria must be fulfilled for the last 3 months with symptom onset at least 6 months prior to diagnosis. For children/adolescents, many of the categories only require active symptoms for 2 months and do not specify a time frame for onset of symptoms.

Table 41.2 outlines the age-related Rome IV diagnostic criteria for several FGIDs common to both the child/adolescent and adult age group, including IBS and functional dyspepsia.

TABLE 41.1

Rome IV Classification for Functional Gastrointestinal Disorders

Adult Categories	Child/Adolescent Categories

Esophageal disorders
• Functional chest pain
• Functional heartburn
• Reflux hypersensitivity
• Globus
• Functional dysphagia
	Functional nausea and vomiting disorders
	• Cyclic vomiting syndrome
	• Functional nausea and functional vomiting
	  • Functional nausea
	  • Functional vomiting
	• Rumination syndrome
	• Aerophagia

Gastroduodenal disorders
• Functional dyspepsia
  • Postprandial distress syndrome
  • Epigastric pain syndrome
• Belching disorders
  • Excessive supragastric belching
  • Excessive gastric belching
• Nausea and vomiting disorders
  • Chronic nausea vomiting syndrome
  • Cyclic vomiting syndrome
  • Cannabinoid hyperemesis syndrome
• Rumination syndrome
	Functional abdominal pain disorders
	• Functional dyspepsia
	  • Postprandial distress syndrome
	  • Epigastric pain syndrome
	• Irritable bowel syndrome
	• Abdominal migraine
	• Functional abdominal pain—not otherwise specified

Bowel disorders • Irritable bowel syndrome (IBS) • Functional constipation • Functional diarrhea • Functional abdominal bloating/distention • Unspecified functional bowel disorder • Opioid-induced constipation	**Functional defecation disorders** • Functional constipation • Nonretentive fecal incontinence
Centrally mediated disorders of gastrointestinal pain • Centrally mediated abdominal pain syndrome • Narcotic bowel syndrome/opioid-induced hyperalgesia	

Gallbladder and sphincter of Oddi disorders
• Biliary pain
  • Functional gallbladder disorder
  • Functional biliary sphincter of Oddi disorder
• Functional pancreatic sphincter of Oddi disorders	

Anorectal disorders
• Fecal incontinence
• Functional anorectal pain
  • Levator ani syndrome
  • Unspecified functional anorectal pain
  • Proctalgia fugax
• Functional defecation disorders
  • Inadequate defecatory propulsion
  • Dyssynergic defecations	

Adapted from *Rome Foundation.* Accessed March 12, 2021. https://theromefoundation.org/rome-iv/rome-iv-criteria/

TABLE 41.2

Rome IV Diagnostic Criteria for Selected Functional Gastrointestinal Disorders in Children/Adolescents and Adults

Functional Dyspepsia (FD)

Children and Adolescents[a]	Adults[b]
One or more symptoms at least 4 times per month a. Postprandial fullness b. Early satiation c. Epigastric pain or burning unrelated to defecation d. Symptoms not fully explained by other medical condition	One or more of the following symptoms and no evidence of structural disease a. Postprandial fullness b. Early satiation c. Epigastric pain d. Epigastric burning

FD subtypes (One subtype required for adults; subtypes adopted for children and adolescents)

Postprandial distress syndrome: Postprandial fullness, early satiation with following supportive criteria:
a. Postprandial epigastric pain/burning (adults)
b. Bloating, nausea, excessive belching (all ages)

Epigastric pain syndrome: epigastric pain or burning with following supportive criteria:
a. No retrosternal pain (children and adolescents)
b. Postprandial epigastric bloating, belching, nausea (adults)
c. Pain induced or relieved by eating or occurs during fasting (all ages)

Irritable Bowel Syndrome (IBS)

Children and Adolescents[a]	Adults[b]
Abdominal pain at minimum 4 d per month for at least 2 mo and at least 1 of the following: a. Related to defecation b. Change in frequency or form (appearance) of stool c. Pain persists after resolution of constipation d. Symptoms not fully explained by other medical condition	Recurrent abdominal pain at minimum averaging 1 d/wk for previous 3 mo and with at least 2 of the following: a. Related to defecation b. Change in frequency of stool c. Change in form (appearance) of stool.

IBS subtypes:
- IBS with predominant constipation (IBS-C)
- IBS with predominant diarrhea (IBS-D)
- IBS with mixed bowel habits (IBS-M)
- IBS unclassified (IBS-U)

Other Functional Abdominal Pain Disorders

Children and Adolescents	Adults
Abdominal migraine Incapacitating abdominal pain not explained by another medical condition occurring at least twice in previous 6 mo and meeting all of the following criteria: a. Paroxysmal episodes of intense, acute abdominal pain (periumbilical, midline, or diffuse) lasting at least 1 h b. Abdominal pain is the most severe and distressing symptom c. Pain occurs with at least 2 of the following symptoms: anorexia, nausea, vomiting, headache, photophobia, pallor d. Individualized stereotypical patterns or symptoms e. Weeks to months between episodes	**Centrally mediated abdominal pain syndrome** Abdominal pain not explained by another medical condition and meeting all of the following: a. Continuous or nearly continuous abdominal pain b. Absence of or only occasional association of pain with physiologic events (e.g., eating, defecation, or menses) c. Some aspects of daily functioning impacted by pain d. Pain is genuine
Functional abdominal pain—not otherwise specified Abdominal pain not explained by another medical condition and occurring at least 4 times per month in the previous 2 mo and meeting all of the following criteria: a. Episodic or continuous abdominal pain that is not only associated with physiologic events (e.g., eating, menses) b. Does not meet criteria for IBS, FD, or abdominal migraine	**Unspecified functional bowel disorder** Does not meet criteria for IBS; functional constipation or diarrhea; or abdominal bloating/distension disorders.

[a]Children and adolescents (2 to 18 years): Criteria fulfilled for at least 2 months before diagnosis.
[b]Adults (≥19 years): Criterion fulfilled for the last 3 months with symptom onset at least 6 months prior to diagnosis.
Adapted from *Rome Foundation*. Accessed March 12, 2021. https://theromefoundation.org/rome-iv/rome-iv-criteria/

Organic and Other Causes of Chronic Abdominal Pain

Causes of Chronic Pain Commonly Associated with Dyspepsia

Gastroesophageal reflux; peptic ulcer disease; gastroparesis; biliary tract obstruction; gallbladder dyskinesia; chronic pancreatitis; and sphincter of Oddi dysfunction.

Causes of Chronic Pain Commonly Associated with Altered Bowel Pattern

Inflammatory bowel disease (IBD) (Crohn disease, ulcerative colitis [UC], IBD-unclassified); celiac disease; lactose intolerance; colitis; complications of constipation (encopresis, megacolon); and infection (parasites and bacteria)

1. Inflammatory bowel disease is a chronic inflammatory disease of the GI tract. It is an umbrella term for two main disorders—Crohn disease and UC. In 5% to 15% of patients, endoscopic and histologic findings cannot differentiate between Crohn disease and UC and these patients are labeled as IBD-unclassified.[11] Crohn disease can involve any part of the digestive tract from the mouth to the anus, typically with skipped lesions. Ulcerative colitis can be localized to the rectum (proctitis), rectum and sigmoid colon (proctosigmoiditis), left colon (left-sided colitis), or the entire colon (pancolitis). The following manifestations can occur with IBD:
   a. Poor growth, weight loss
   b. Anemia, elevated erythrocyte sedimentation rate (ESR), and elevated fecal calprotectin or lactoferrin[12]
   c. Bloody stools—although stools may be positive for hemoccult without signs of diarrhea
   d. Extraintestinal manifestations, including arthralgias, arthritis, uveitis, episcleritis, primary sclerosing cholangitis, hepatitis, erythema nodosum, and pyoderma gangrenosum
   Diagnosis of IBD involves laboratory blood tests, stool tests, endoscopic evaluation (upper endoscopy and colonoscopy with biopsies and video capsule endoscopy), and imaging studies (Computed tomography [CT] scan, CT or MRI enterography, upper GI series with small bowel follow through).
2. Celiac disease is a chronic autoimmune disease that affects the small intestine in genetically susceptible individuals. It is triggered by exposure to gluten. Also known as celiac sprue, gluten-sensitive enteropathy, or nontropical sprue, celiac disease is one of the most common genetic diseases (human leukocyte antigen [HLA] class II haplotypes DQ2 and DQ8). Studies suggest that the prevalence is increasing worldwide, with current pooled global prevalence of 1.4% in the general population based on positive serologic tests and 0.7% based on biopsies.[13] The prevalence is 5% to 10% in those with an affected first-degree relative and up to 20% in siblings. This disease is often underrecognized and underdiagnosed by clinicians, with only 10% to 15% of those affected having been diagnosed and treated. Celiac disease can be asymptomatic and 70% of affected individuals are not diagnosed until adulthood (>20 years of age).[14] Extraintestinal manifestations become more prevalent with increasing age. Celiac disease is associated with the following signs and symptoms[14]:
   a. Gastrointestinal symptoms include diarrhea, constipation, abdominal pain, anorexia, vomiting, bloating, malabsorption, weight loss, and malnutrition.
   b. Extraintestinal manifestations include fatigue, dermatitis herpetiformis, osteopenia, short stature, delayed puberty, iron deficiency anemia resistant to oral iron, hepatitis, arthritis, aphthous stomatitis, dental enamel hypoplasia, seizures, recurring headache, unexplained infertility in females, and psychiatric disorders (anxiety, panic attacks, depression).[14]
   c. Associated conditions include Type 1 (insulin-dependent) diabetes mellitus (10% prevalence), thyroiditis, IgA deficiency, Addison disease, Down syndrome, and Turner syndrome.[14]
   d. Celiac disease is associated with an increased risk for malignancies, including small bowel adenocarcinoma, esophageal cancer, and non-Hodgkin lymphoma.
   Diagnosis is dependent on clinical suspicion, screening with serologic testing, and small bowel biopsy for confirmation in those with positive serology. Patients with celiac disease may also have FGIDs including IBS, which can contribute to challenges in deciding who to screen.
3. Lactose intolerance is the most common food sensitivity that affects many individuals. Primary lactose intolerance resulting in lactose malabsorption is caused by lactase non-persistence, a genetically programmed reduction in the activity of lactase after weaning in childhood. Lactose malabsorption is rare in infants and young children with lactase activity approaching adult levels by 7 to 10 years of age.[15] Secondary lactose intolerance can occur in the setting of GI disorders such as celiac disease, Crohn disease, gastroenteritis, and peptic ulcer disease, and can be induced by antibiotics.[15]
   a. Gastrointestinal symptoms include bloating, diarrhea, flatus, borborygmi, and cramps.
   b. A systematic review and meta-analysis study in 2017, that included 62,910 children (aged 10 years and older) and adult participants from 84 countries (covering 84% of the world population), determined the global prevalence estimate of lactose malabsorption is 68%.[15]
   c. The most affected populations in North America are Asians (variable, 15% to 100%), Native Americans (79%), African Americans (75%), and Hispanics (51%), whereas Whites (21% nonpersistence), specifically Scandinavians and Northern Europeans (5% to 20%), are the least affected.[16]
   Lactose intolerance is typically diagnosed with (a) hydrogen breath test (lactose challenge induces increase of H2 in exhaled air); (b) lactose intolerance test (lactose challenge induces increase in blood sugar); or (c) lactase activity at the intestinal brush border (biopsy sample collected during endoscopy looks at lactase enzyme activity).[16]

Causes of Chronic Pain Commonly Associated with Paroxysmal Abdominal Pain

Musculoskeletal pain; bowel obstruction; and ureteral obstruction.

Other Causes of Chronic Abdominal Pain

The differential diagnosis includes gynecologic conditions, referred pain from the lungs or spine, systemic conditions such as diabetic ketoacidosis, or sickle cell crisis.

⬤ DIAGNOSIS

In 2005, the American Academy of Pediatrics and the North American Society for Pediatric Gastroenterology, Hepatology and Nutrition (NASPGHAN) Subcommittee on Chronic Abdominal Pain in Children were unable to produce an evidence-based procedural algorithm for the diagnostic evaluation of chronic abdominal pain in children and adolescents. The conclusions drawn by the subcommittee and detailed below continue to provide a framework for evaluating patients with FGIDs.[17,18]

History

1. Some patients have features of more than one FGID.
2. The pain frequency, severity, location, or impact on lifestyle cannot distinguish functional and organic disorders. Timing of the symptoms, including postprandial pain and nighttime awakening, was not found to be helpful.
3. "Alarm symptoms or signs" suggestive of organic disease requiring further diagnostic testing include, but are not limited to,

(a) involuntary weight loss; (b) family history of IBD; (c) deceleration in linear growth; (d) unexplained fever; (e) gastrointestinal blood loss; (f) significant vomiting (cyclical vomiting, bilious vomiting); (g) chronic severe diarrhea; (h) persistent right upper or right lower quadrant pain.

4. Family history: (a) Parental history of anxiety, depression, and somatization is not helpful in distinguishing between functional and organic disorders. (b) Overall family functioning (e.g., cohesion, conflict, marital satisfaction) does not differ between those with FGIDs and healthy families or those with acute illness.

5. Issues regarding the relationship of pain to current stress and emotional and behavioral concerns include (a) a history of anxiety, depression, and more negative life event stress does not distinguish functional from organic abdominal pain; (b) a relationship that exists between daily stress and pain episodes as well as increased negative life events and persistent symptoms; (c) no evidence to support the concept of emotional/behavioral symptoms predicting the severity of pain, course of the pain episode, or response to treatment; and (d) evidence to support that adolescents with FGIDs are at risk for emotional problems and psychiatric disorders (e.g., anxiety and depression) later in life.

Physical Examination

The physical examination of patients with FGIDs is usually normal or characterized by mild tenderness to palpation without rebound usually in the mid- or upper abdomen.

Diagnostic Tests

Testing for Organic Disorders

The following tests should be considered in the evaluation of AYAs for a possible organic disorder.[19,20]

1. Primary screening tests
   a. Complete blood count with differential, ESR, C-reactive protein (CRP), chemistry profile with liver function tests, anti–tissue transglutaminase (tTG IgA), and total IgA
   b. Urinalysis with or without culture
   c. Stool samples obtained for evidence of occult blood, inflammatory markers (fecal calprotectin or lactoferrin), and ova and parasites (including stool for Giardia antigen)

   A prospective cohort study enrolling 193 children (6 to 18 years old) with abdominal pain found that the combination of three tests (CRP [>10 mg/L], hemoglobin [<2 SD for age and sex], and fecal calprotectin [>250 mcg/g]) was a useful strategy to identify patients at high risk for IBD who should be referred for diagnostic endoscopy.[12]

2. If diarrhea is present, additional studies should be considered, including the following:
   a. Stool for *Clostridioides difficile* toxin, and fecal calprotectin or fecal lactoferrin if not already obtained in primary screening tests
   b. Breath tests: Lactose breath test to rule out lactose intolerance; glucose or lactulose breath test to rule out small intestinal bacterial overgrowth
   c. Celiac serologies (anti-tTG IgA, endomysial IgA): Because celiac disease is often undiagnosed, there is discussion in the literature about more widespread screening for this disease in AYAs. The American College of Gastroenterology recommends screening for celiac disease in patients with IBS associated with diarrhea and mixed symptoms.[19]

3. If dyspepsia is present, additional studies to be considered include the following:
   a. Testing for *Helicobacter pylori* (stool antigen or urea breath test)
   b. Serum amylase and lipase

4. Radiologic studies (upper GI series with small bowel follow through; hepatobiliary scintigraphy with cholecystokinin infusion; abdominal, renal, or pelvic ultrasound). In the presence of alarm symptoms, consider MRI or CT enterography to evaluate for IBD and intestinal lymphoma.

5. Referral to a gastroenterologist for possible endoscopy or colonoscopy should be considered for patients with alarm symptoms or specific symptoms such as dyspepsia unresponsive to treatment, right upper quadrant pain, dyspepsia with recurrent vomiting, or symptoms and/or physical examination suggestive of pelvic pathology or urinary tract abnormalities.

6. Referral to a clinician with expertise in gynecology should be considered for patients with symptoms and/or physical examination suggestive of pelvic pathology or urinary tract abnormalities.

Diagnostic Tests—Additional Considerations

The Subcommittee on Chronic Abdominal Pain in Children found the following[17,18]:

1. There is no evidence that ultrasonography of the abdomen or pelvis, endoscopy, biopsy, or pH monitoring in the absence of alarm signals significantly detects organic disease.

2. Functional gastrointestinal diseases can be diagnosed by a primary care clinician when (1) there are no alarm symptoms, (2) the physical examination is normal, and (3) there is a negative stool sample for occult blood. Testing is sometimes necessary to reassure the patient and family, especially when the pain significantly affects the patient's quality of life.

3. Clinical and technical practice guidelines published by the American Gastroenterology Association (AGA) concluded that routine diagnostic testing is not recommended in patients with suspected IBS without alarm symptoms[19,21] with the exception of obtaining stool studies for chronic diarrhea (fecal calprotectin, fecal lactoferrin, and Giardia antigen). The guidelines advised against serologic tests (ESR and CRP) to rule out IBD but endorsed testing for celiac serologies in some patients. The AGA guidelines also concluded that rectal bleeding and nocturnal pain did not discriminate IBS from organic disease, but anemia, weight loss, family history of colorectal cancer, IBD, or celiac disease were important alarm features that warrant further investigation.

4. There is inconclusive evidence that short-chain poorly absorbed carbohydrates may trigger GI symptoms. Lactose intolerance may also mimic or coexist with FGIDs. Although the data are controversial, some individuals also appear to have nonceliac gluten sensitivity (NCGS), a condition in which patients have negative serology and intestinal biopsies but develop celiac-like or IBS-like symptoms when exposed to dietary gluten. Symptoms alone cannot differentiate celiac disease from NCGS.[14]

5. Keeping a pain diary for 1 to 3 weeks may be helpful to document the pattern, timing, severity, precipitating factors, and association with food or beverage. In addition to helping the clinician work through the differential diagnosis, this type of diary provides a way for AYAs to be directly involved in their care plan.

Approach to the Evaluation of Functional Gastrointestinal Disorders

A careful history and physical examination should be performed. If further clarification of the history is needed, AYAs should be asked to keep a pain diary with a follow-up appointment scheduled in 1 to 3 weeks. If there are alarm signals or further diagnostic testing is warranted, appropriate laboratory tests and/or radiologic studies should be obtained. If a careful history and physical examination yield no obvious organic source for the chronic abdominal pain, the practitioner should explain to AYAs that the evaluation seems to indicate an FGID. Although a serious underlying disease is not suspected, AYAs should be assured that the symptoms they are experiencing are real. It is also useful to explain the concepts of visceral hypersensitivity and disordered gut–brain communication in terms that AYAs and families can understand.

TREATMENT OR THERAPEUTIC APPROACH

Functional gastrointestinal disorders are best treated in the context of a biopsychosocial model, which may include psychological interventions, dietary modifications, and specific pharmacologic therapy to reduce the frequency and severity of the symptoms. Pharmacologic therapy should be used judiciously for specific symptomatology and specific functional GI conditions. Psychological and physical pain triggers should be identified so that they can be modified or reversed. The goal of treatment is to restore normal functioning and return to daily activities rather than focusing on the pain itself.

Treatment Options for Functional Gastrointestinal Disorders

The Subcommittee on Chronic Abdominal Pain in Children found a paucity of studies evaluating pharmacologic and dietary treatments in children and adolescents. Many of the studies in adults have focused on IBS. Treatment options are reviewed below.[17,18,22]

Pharmacologic Treatments

The following medications have some evidence of effectiveness from pediatric and adult studies[22]:

1. H2-receptor antagonists or proton-pump inhibitors may relieve some symptoms of ulcer-like dyspepsia.
2. Alosetron, a 5-HT3 antagonist, has been helpful in adult females with severe diarrhea-predominant IBS (IBS-D). Because of potential side effects (severe constipation, ischemic colitis, bowel perforation), it is available only under a restricted prescribing program for females with severe IBS-D that is debilitating.
3. Linaclotide, a guanylate cyclase 2C agonist which increases release of fluid with chloride and bicarbonate into the intestine and accelerates GI transit, is used to treat constipation-predominant IBS (IBS-C) and chronic constipation. It has a black box warning for children due to the risk of severe dehydration.
4. Lubiprostone, a chloride channel-2 agonist, is a bicyclical fatty acid compound that activates chloride-rich fluid secretion in the intestine. It is approved for treatment of chronic idiopathic constipation in adults and IBS-C in females at least 18 years old.
5. Plecanatide, a guanylate cyclase-C agonist, is approved for chronic idiopathic constipation and IBS-C. It results in electrolyte and fluid transport into the lumen of the intestines.
6. Eluxadoline, an opioid receptor agonist and antagonist in the enteric nervous system, is approved by the U.S. Food and Drug Administration for the management of IBS-D. It helps improve global symptoms and stool consistency in IBS-D. Due to risk of pancreatitis, it is contraindicated in patients who had a cholecystectomy, or who have sphincter of Oddi or pancreatic problems.
7. Tricyclic antidepressants (TCAs; e.g., amitriptyline) used at low doses may improve symptoms of abdominal pain in adults with IBS and children/adolescents with IBS and functional abdominal pain. Tricyclic antidepressants have been shown to be more effective than selective serotonin reuptake inhibitors for the treatment of FGIDs in adults and children.[23,24] Tricyclic antidepressants appear particularly useful in cases of functional dyspepsia and IBS with refractory diarrhea in adults.[23] Data in children and adolescents are conflicting. A Cochrane review on the use of antidepressants (amitriptyline or citalopram) in children and adolescents with functional abdominal pain concluded that there may be no difference between antidepressants and placebo.[25]
8. Rifaximin, a newer and minimally absorbed antibiotic, has been shown to be beneficial in IBS with modest efficacy and minimal side effects. Short-term trials have shown that rifaximin is more effective than placebo for symptoms of bloating in adults with IBS.[22]

Other Treatment Options[22]

1. Antispasmodic or anticholinergic agents (e.g., hyoscyamine, dicyclomine, otilonium, pinaverium, cimetropium, drotaverine) may be used for symptomatic relief on short-term basis.
2. Antidiarrheals such as loperamide may reduce stool frequency in IBS-D, but may not improve pain or bloating compared to placebo.
3. Polyethylene glycol (PEG), an osmotic laxative, has demonstrated benefit in the treatment of chronic idiopathic constipation. However, while it may help with constipation, it has not been consistently shown to be beneficial for treatment of pain and bloating symptoms associated with IBS-C.
4. Enteric-coated peppermint oil capsules are thought to have smooth muscle-relaxing properties and may reduce abdominal pain in IBS.
5. Probiotics and prebiotics may improve IBS symptoms in AYAs.
6. Percutaneous electrical nerve stimulation (auricular neurostimulation) has been shown to improve abdominal pain scores and well-being in pediatric patients with IBS.[26]

Diet Therapies in Irritable Bowel Syndrome[22,27]

1. High-fiber diet has been recommended in both IBS-C and IBS-D, as well as functional abdominal pain. If high-fiber foods are unsuccessful, fiber supplements are available over the counter. Soluble fiber (ispaghula/psyllium) has the most scientific support. Insoluble fiber is not effective and may exacerbate pain and bloating in IBS. Excessive fiber should be avoided because it may cause gas and distension as well as exacerbation of constipation and diarrhea.
2. Diet that is low in fermentable oligosaccharides, disaccharides, monosaccharides, and polyols (FODMAP) may provide symptom relief in some individuals because malabsorption of dietary carbohydrates may provoke symptoms. Low-FODMAP diets limit foods with lactose (milk and milk products), sorbitol and mannitol (found in some fruits and vegetables and sometimes added as artificial sweeteners), fructose (found in certain fruits and honey and some high fructose corn syrups), and fructans and galacto-oligosaccharides (found in wheat, rye onions, garlic, legumes, and lentils).
3. Gluten-free diet: Some individuals with NCGS may have symptom improvement on a gluten-free diet, but research on the effectiveness of gluten-free diets is inconclusive.
4. Given the high prevalence of lactose intolerance in Hispanic, Asian, and African American AYAs, testing for lactose intolerance or a trial of lactose-free diet (minimum of 2 weeks) may be helpful in patients who have IBS-like symptoms.

Psychological Factors and Interventions[28,29]

Psychological factors, including stress, anxiety, and depression, are known to cause or contribute to FGIDs in AYAs. Recent literature has shown that somatization, catastrophizing, and ineffective coping mechanisms are predictors of poor outcomes. Counseling consists of reassuring AYAs and their families that the symptoms accompanying FGIDs are real and that no specific organic disease has been found. The practitioner should stress that the pain is not "in the young person's head" but is a real manifestation, which can be exacerbated, by stress. It is important to reassure AYA patients that they are physically healthy and can continue with all activities. Often AYAs with FGIDs miss days of school or work. If this is the case, the family, teachers, school nurse, and employer should work together with AYAs to keep them in school or at work. Significant changes in the type or character of pain should prompt reevaluation.

If significant depression, anxiety, or family stressors are present, AYAs and families may require referral for further psychological or family assessment. However, psychological intervention may be helpful even when symptoms of depression, anxiety, and/or stress are mild or moderate. Cognitive behavioral therapy, hypnotherapy, relaxation therapy, and multicomponent psychological therapy have been shown to be effective in treating functional disorders in AYAs. Guided imagery, which leads to muscle relaxation, has been shown to be beneficial in children. Ultimately, the goal is to reduce the impact of symptoms on the AYAs' daily routine. Prompt recognition and intervention are important. Long-term follow-up studies have shown that children with persistent abdominal pain are at increased risk for developing psychiatric disorders, like anxiety and depression, during adolescence and adulthood.[17,30] Cognitive behavioral therapy, coping strategies, and parental education have become the primary foci for the management of FGIDs to improve outcomes.

SUMMARY

Chronic abdominal pain is a common occurrence in AYAs with a differential diagnosis that includes organic causes and disorders of gut–brain interactions. Cognitive behavioral therapy and coping strategies in conjunction with a growing number of medications, particularly for IBS, can improve the symptoms and impact long-term outcomes of AYAs with FGIDs. It is important for clinicians treating AYAs with FGIDs to validate their symptoms and provide education about the gut–brain interactions which are now understood to be the etiology of FGIDs.

REFERENCES

1. Rome Foundation. Updated March 12, 2021. https://theromefoundation.org/rome-iv/rome-iv-criteria/
2. Drossman DA. Functional gastrointestinal disorders: history, pathophysiology, clinical features and Rome IV. *Gastroenterology*. 2016;150(6):1262–1279.E2.
3. Hyams JS, Di Lorenzo C, Saps M, et al. Functional disorders: children and adolescents. *Gastroenterology*. 2016;150(6):1456–1468.E2.
4. Pimentel M, Talley NJ, Quigley EMM, et al. Report from the multinational irritable bowel syndrome initiative 2012. *Gastroenterology*. 2013;144(7):e1–5.
5. Velasco-Benitez CA, Gómez-Oliveros LF, Rubio-Moreno LM, et al. Diagnostic accuracy of the Rome IV criteria for the diagnosis of functional gastrointestinal disorders in children. *J Pediatr Gastroenterol Nutr*. 2021;72(4):538–541.
6. Robin SG, Keller C, Zwiener R, et al. Prevalence of pediatric functional gastrointestinal disorders utilizing the Rome IV criteria. *J Pediatr*. 2018;195:134–139.
7. Lovell RM, Ford AC. Global prevalence of and risk factors for irritable bowel syndrome: a meta-analysis. *Clin Gastroenterol Hepatol*. 2012;10(7):712–721.e4.
8. Chuah KH, Beh KH, Rappek NAM, et al. The epidemiology and quality of life of functional gastrointestinal disorders according to Rome III vs Rome IV criteria: a cross-sectional study in primary care. *J Dig Dis*. 2021;22(3):159–166.
9. Hong JY, Kilpatrick LA, Labus J, et al. Patients with chronic visceral pain show sex-related alterations in intrinsic oscillations of the resting brain. *J Neurosci*. 2013;33(29):11994–12002.
10. Shin A, Preidis GA, Shulman R, et al. The gut microbiome in adult and pediatric functional gastrointestinal disorders. *Clin Gastroenterol Hepatol*. 2019;17(2):256–274.
11. Lamb CA, Kennedy NA, Raine T, et al. British Society of Gastroenterology consensus guidelines on the management of inflammatory bowel disease in adults. *Gut*. 2019;68(3):s1-s106.
12. Van de Vijver E, Heida A, Ioannou S, et al. Test strategies to predict inflammatory bowel disease among children with nonbloody diarrhea. *Pediatrics*. 2020;146(2):e20192235.
13. Singh P, Arora A, Strand TA, et al. Global prevalence of celiac disease: systematic review and meta-analysis. *Clin Gastroenterol Hepatol*. 2018;16(6):823–836.e2.
14. Al-Toma A, Volta U, Auricchio R, et al. European Society for the Study of Coeliac Disease (ESsCD) guideline for coeliac disease and other gluten-related disorders. *United European Gastroenterol J*. 2019;7(5):583–613.
15. Storhaug CL, Fosse SK, Fadnes LT. Country, regional, and global estimates for lactose malabsorption in adults: a systematic review and meta-analysis. *Lancet Gastroenterol Hepatol*. 2017;2(10):738–746.
16. Jansson-Knodell CL, Krajicek EJ, Savaiano DA, et al. Lactose intolerance: a concise review to skim the surface. *Mayo Clin Proc*. 2020;95(7):1499–1505.
17. Di Lorenzo C, Colletti RB, Lehmann HP, et al. Chronic abdominal pain in children: a technical report of the American Academy of Pediatrics and the North American Society for Pediatric Gastroenterology, Hepatology and Nutrition. *J Pediatr Gastroenterol Nutr*. 2005;40(3):249–261.
18. Di Lorenzo C, Colletti RB, Lehmann HP, et al. Chronic abdominal pain in children: a clinical report of the American Academy of Pediatrics and the North American Society for Pediatric Gastroenterology, Hepatology and Nutrition. *J Pediatr Gastroenterol Nutr*. 2005;40(3):245–248.
19. Carrasco-Labra A, Lytvyn L, Falck-Ytter Y, et al. AGA technical review on the evaluation of functional diarrhea and diarrhea-predominant irritable bowel syndrome in adults (IBS-D). *Gastroenterology*. 2019;157(3):859–880.
20. Menees SB, Powell C, Kurlander J, et al. A meta-analysis of the utility of C-reactive protein, erythrocyte sedimentation rate, fecal calprotectin, and fecal lactoferrin to exclude inflammatory bowel disease in adults with IBS. *Am J Gastroenterol*. 2015;110(3):444–454.
21. Smalley W, Falck-Ytter C, Carrasco-Labra A, et al. AGA clinical practice guidelines on the laboratory evaluation of functional diarrhea and diarrhea-predominant irritable bowel syndrome in adults (IBS-D). *Gastroenterology*. 2019;157(3):851–854.
22. Ford AC, Moayyedi P, Chey WD, et al. American College of Gastroenterology monograph on management of irritable bowel syndrome. *Am J Gastroenterol*. 2018;113(Suppl 2):1–18.
23. Talley NJ, Locke GR, Saito YA, et al. Effect of amitriptyline and escitalopram on functional dyspepsia: a multicenter, randomized controlled study. *Gastroenterology*. 2015;149(2):340–9 e2.
24. Kulak-Bejda A, Bejda G, Waszkiewicz N. Antidepressants for irritable bowel syndrome-a systematic review. *Pharmacol Rep*. 2017;69(6):1366–1379.
25. de Bruijn CMA, Rexwinkel R, Gordon M, et al.. Antidepressants for functional abdominal pain disorders in children and adolescents. *Cochrane Database Syst Rev*. 2021;2:CD008013.
26. Krasaelap A, Sood MR, Li BUK, et al. Efficacy of auricular neurostimulation in adolescents with irritable bowel syndrome in a randomized, double-blind trial. *Clin Gastroenterol Hepatol*. 2020;18(9):1987–1994.e2.
27. Rej A, Avery A, Ford AC, et al. Clinical application of dietary therapies in irritable bowel syndrome. *J Gastrointestin Liver Dis*. 2018;27(3):307–316.
28. Newton E, Schosheim A, Patel S, et al. The role of psychological factors in pediatric functional abdominal pain disorders. *Neurogastroenterol Motil*. 2019;31(6):e13538.
29. Reed B, Buzenski J, van Tilburg MAL. Implementing psychological therapies for gastrointestinal disorders in pediatrics. *Expert Rev Gastroenterol Hepatol*. 2020;14(11):1061–1067.
30. Shelby GD, Shirkey KC, Sherman AL, et al. Functional abdominal pain in childhood and long-term vulnerability to anxiety disorders. *Pediatrics*. 2013;132(3):475–482.

ADDITIONAL RESOURCES AND WEBSITES

Additional Resources and Websites for Clinicians:
American Academy of Pediatrics—https://www.aappublications.org/
American College of Gastroenterology—https://gi.org/guidelines/
https://gi.org/topics/irritable-bowel-syndrome/
https://gi.org/wp-content/uploads/2018/07/IBS-Monograph-2018.pdf
American Gastroenterology Association—https://gastro.org/practice-guidance/practice-updates/
British Society of Gastroenterology—https://www.bsg.org.uk/resource-type/guidelines/
European Society for Paediatric Gastroenterology, Hepatology and Nutrition—https://www.espghan.org/knowledge-center
North American Society for Pediatric Gastroenterology, Hepatology & Nutrition—https://naspghan.org/professional-resources/medical-professional-resources/
https://naspghan.org/professional-resources/clinical-guidelines/
Rome Foundation—https://theromefoundation.org/
World Gastroenterology Organization—https://www.worldgastroenterology.org/guidelines/global-guidelines

Additional Resources and Websites for Parents/Caregivers:
American Academy of Pediatrics—https://www.healthychildren.org/English/health-issues/conditions/abdominal/Pages/Irritable-Bowel-Syndrome-IBS-and-Inflammatory-Bowel-Disease-IBD.aspx
American Gastroenterology Association—https://gastro.org/practice-guidance/gi-patient-center/
Association of Pediatric Gastroenterology and Nutrition Nurses—http://apgnn.org/?esid=patientEd
GI Kids—https://gikids.org/digestive-topics/
IBS Impact—http://www.ibsimpact.com/ibs-children/

Additional Resources and Websites for Adolescents and Young Adults:
American Academy of Pediatrics—https://www.healthychildren.org/English/health-issues/conditions/abdominal/Pages/Irritable-Bowel-Syndrome-IBS-and-Inflammatory-Bowel-Disease-IBD.aspx
American College of Gastroenterology—https://gi.org/patients/
https://gi.org/topics/irritable-bowel-syndrome/
American Gastroenterology Association—https://gastro.org/practice-guidance/gi-patient-center/
Association of Pediatric Gastroenterology and Nutrition Nurses—http://apgnn.org/?esid=patientEd
GI Kids—https://gikids.org/digestive-topics/
IBS Impact—http://www.ibsimpact.com/ibs-children/
World Gastroenterology Organization—https://www.worldgastroenterology.org/education-and-training/educational-programs#ibs

PART XI

Sexuality and Contraception

CHAPTER 42

Adolescent and Young Adult Sexuality

Devon J. Hensel
Jonathon J. Beckmeyer

KEY WORDS
- Romantic relationships
- Sexual behavior
- Sexual health
- Sexuality

INTRODUCTION

Adolescence and young adulthood are important periods in the development of lifelong sexual health.[1] Different key biologic, psychological, social, and behavioral aspects of adult sexuality begin to unfold. Among many changes, adolescents and young adults (AYAs) will experience new sexual feelings and interests, initiate intimate romantic and sexual relationships, and explore a wide range of partnered and solo sexual behaviors. While the large majority of AYAs navigate these changes without issue, some may experience adverse outcomes, such as sexually transmitted infections (STIs) and/or unintended pregnancy.[2] As a result, it can be common to equate the emergence of sexuality with these potential consequences. However, it is important to remember that AYAs need to go through formative experiences in managing sexuality to develop the physical, social, and emotional skills they will need to be sexually independent and responsible adults.[3]

This chapter provides an overview of the key changes in heterosexual AYA sexuality (see Chapters 43 and 44 for additional information on sexuality issues for lesbian, gay, bisexual, transgender, and other sexual minority [LGBT] youth). Using data from different nationally representative studies, we address the development of close relationships in adolescence and young adulthood and the association of these relationships to the emergence of solo and partnered sexual behaviors. This information is intended to improve clinicians' ability to engage in sexuality-related topics directly and regularly with AYA patients and their families, to anticipate initiation of sexual health changes, and to proactively devise counseling strategies that may improve health outcomes.

CLOSE RELATIONSHIPS IN ADOLESCENCE AND YOUNG ADULTHOOD

Close relationships—both romantic and nonromantic—play an important role in the development of sexuality during adolescence and young adulthood. Each partnership's emotional and behavioral characteristics provide a context for young people's ongoing learning and organizing of sexuality. Different relationships can fulfill different needs, such as intimacy, companionship, or sexual behavior(s), at different points in the life course; changes in these relationships help AYAs build the skills to transition from childhood into healthy adult sexuality.[4,5]

Types of Relationships and Meaning

Several studies have articulated changes in the trajectory of young males' and females' close relationships in industrialized countries from early adolescence to early adulthood.[6]

Between pre- and early adolescence:
- Relationship interests shift from same-gender friendship groups to mixed-gender friendship groups in early adolescence to opposite-gender dyadic friendships and romantic interests.
- Romantic crushes emerge and allow youth to explore their romantic interests and ideals.
- Initial romantic partnerships are typically short lived (e.g., "going together"); usually arranged by peers or friends, rather than by the adolescent themselves.
- Early relationships are limited in physical and emotional investment, and typically consist of interactions occurring at school, in groups, or via social media.

During middle adolescence:
- Adolescents and young adults are increasingly aware of their romantic feelings toward specific individuals. As a result, group and dyadic dating become increasingly common forms of romantic socializing.
- These relationships increase in both the importance adolescents ascribe to them and the time adolescents spend with partners.

By late adolescence:
- Most young people have had and/or are in a serious romantic relationship.
- These dyads are associated with the emergence of more adult-like emotional and communication qualities, such as expressing feelings, negotiating conflict, or recognizing sexual satisfaction.
- Young people also make decisions about more involved types of partnered sexual behavior (e.g., genital touching, oral sex, or vaginal sex).

During young adulthood:
- Relationships include increased degree of investment and confidence in the relationship.
- Adolescents and young adults further hone the characteristics of communication with one's partner, greater comfort with one's own sexuality, and increased sexual activity which they established in earlier relationships.
- Although relationship stability is normally a sign of healthy relationships during young adulthood, between 23% and 30% (across studies) of young adults can become stuck in low-quality, unsatisfying partnerships, which undermine their well-being.
- Young females may be more confident than young males in navigating these romantic relationships, as the social dynamics contained in these relationships often mimic those in friendships.

Across the developmental periods, it is critical to acknowledge the complexity of AYA relationship types. Understanding the content and nature of these relationships from the AYA perspective is important to accurately assess their impact on sexuality and sexual health.[7] For example, the range of partnership types can include "friends with benefits" and "hook-ups," "ex" or "old" boyfriend/girlfriends, or "casual" sex partners or "one-night stands."[8] All of these forms have different meanings and implications for the AYA. In addition, relationships with a current/former partner with whom they have a child have a unique status.[9] Sexual activity of different types may or may not occur in any of these relationship formats, and they likely differ in the amount of communication, affection, and commitment an AYA expects.

Developmental Benefits in Relationships

Close partnerships in adolescence and young adulthood help individuals learn the emotional and behavioral skills they will need to manage sexual relationships during their lifetime.[4,5,8] Emotional skills include learning how to develop intimacy, build trust and fidelity, express love and affection, negotiate conflict, resolve conflicting emotions, and successfully end relationships. Behavioral skills include learning about a wide range of "lighter" (e.g., hugging, handholding, and kissing, as well as manual-genital touching) and more involved (e.g., oral sex and penile-vaginal intercourse) partnered sexual acts, understanding and advocating for sexual pleasure, communicating likes and dislikes, and balancing power in relationships.

SOLO AND PARTNERED SEXUAL BEHAVIOR IN ADOLESCENCE AND YOUNG ADULTHOOD

Traditional discussions of AYA sexual behavior commonly center on three partnered behaviors: giving or receiving oral sex, penile-vaginal sex, and penile-anal sex. It is also vital to consider the role of other intimate partnered contact (e.g., kissing, hugging, holding hands, genital touching), any solo behaviors (e.g., masturbation), and the absence of any "behavior" (e.g., sexual abstinence). Understanding specifically what AYAs are (or are not) participating in when they say that they are "having sex" is key to a clinician's being prepared to assess ongoing levels of sexual risk as well as contraceptive and condom use needs.

Sexual "Abstinence"
Overview and Context[10,11]

- Many cultural terms (e.g., "abstinence," "virginity," or "celibacy") are used to describe AYA's nonparticipation in sexual activity.
- Young people sometimes differentiate between "primary" sexual abstinence (an absence of any lifetime sexual intercourse experience, usually penile-vaginal sex) and "secondary" sexual abstinence (first-time sexual experience followed by periods without sexual activity).
- Choosing "primary" and "secondary" sexual abstinence could occur for a variety of reasons:
  - Avoid perceived social or health risks.
  - Uphold moral or religious commitments.
  - Peer or parental pressure
  - Saving sexual experience for one's future spouse
  - Not "ready" for sex (typically seen in younger AYAs)
- A clinician should not assume no sexual contact is occurring if an adolescent or young adult says that they are "sexually abstinent" or "not sexually active." This could mean either:
  - Avoidance of all sexual activity that occurs by one's self, or with partners
  - Avoiding a limited scope of behaviors, such as those that carry a risk of pregnancy or STIs, while still participating in other behaviors. Some abstainers participate in nonpenetrative

partnered sexual behaviors because they believe that behaviors such as kissing, breast fondling, genital stimulation, and oral-genital sex do not "count" as sexual experience.

Prevalence

- The Youth Risk Behavior Survey (YRBS) suggests that 61.6% of high school students have never had sexual intercourse (females: 62.4%; males: 63.8%), with a reported upward trend between 2009 and 2019.[12]

Solo Masturbation
Overview and Context[13–15]

- Solo masturbation is perhaps the most difficult of all sexual behaviors to study, as it has been historically stigmatized and social/gender norms may still proscribe masturbation, particularly among females.
- Solo masturbation serves important functions in developing sexuality, including:
  - Learning about the geography of one's body
  - Learning about sexual response
  - Learning about one's own personal sexual likes and dislikes, and communicating these preferences to partners
- Solo masturbation can be used to experience sexual pleasure in the absence of a partner, when one does not desire to have sex with a partner, as an alternative to avoid STI/pregnancy, or as a follow-up to partnered sexual activities that were not sexually fulfilling.
- Often, clinicians do not ask questions about masturbation.

Prevalence[13,15]

The National Survey of Sexual Health and Behavior (NSSHB) suggests that:
- 62.6% to 80.0% of adolescent males and 43.3% to 58.0% of adolescent females,[16] as well as 86.1% to 94.3% of emerging (e.g., over the age of 18) adult males and 66.0% to 84.6% of emerging adult females have ever masturbated in their lifetime.
- 42.9% to 58.0% of adolescent males, 24.1% to 25.5% of adolescent females, 61.1% to 62.8% of young adult males, and 26.0% to 43.7% of young females have masturbated in the past month.

Partnered Masturbation
Overview and Context

- The term "partnered masturbation" can refer either to two individuals who self-masturbate in the presence of one another or to individuals stimulating the genitals of their partner.
- Partnered masturbation can serve as an important source of partner-focused sexual learning including negotiating sexual needs and desires and understanding shared intimacy and pleasure.
- Partnered masturbation:
  - Often precedes first vaginal sex.
  - Can occur early in the early stages of a relationship, or when a sexual encounter or partner is more casual.
  - May serve as a "safer" behavior choice to avoid STI or pregnancy
  - Maybe one of multiple sexual behaviors enacted with a partner, such as part of "foreplay" prior to vaginal sex, or as the ending behaviors as part of a sexual event.

Prevalence[17]

- The 2015 National Sexual Exploration in America Study suggested that among 18- to 24-year-olds, 21.6% of females and 21.9% of males reported partnered masturbation in the last month.

Oral Sex
Overview and Context[18,19]

- The term "oral sex" can refer to several different sexual practices and can take on a variety of meanings in different contexts for AYAs.

- The most common definition is stimulation of the vaginal (cunnilingus) or penile genital (fellatio) area by use of the mouth, tongue, or teeth, both received from a partner and/or given to a partner. In addition, oral stimulation of the anus (rimming) may also be practiced. Variability in these definitions creates challenges for assessing the prevalence of oral sex.
- Oral sex is practiced during adolescence and young adulthood for a variety of reasons, including:
  - Perception that it is less risky than vaginal sex or anal sex
  - Belief that participating in oral sex may bring social status or popularity
  - Belief that it will "preserve virginity," particularly among younger adolescents
  - To enhance sexual pleasure, intimacy, or as part of foreplay
- It is important that clinicians ask specific questions about oral sexual practices and the motivations surrounding those practices.

Prevalence[16]

The National Survey of Family Growth (NSFG) demonstrates that:
- Among 15- to 17-year-olds, 26.6% of females and 23.3% of males have ever given oral sex while 30.4% of females and 38.1% of males have ever received oral sex.
- Among 18- to 19-year-olds, 56.6% of females and 56.2% of males have ever given oral sex, while 58.6% of females and 64.9% of males have ever received oral sex.

Penile-Vaginal Sex
Overview and Context[20,21]

- Penile-vaginal sex is perhaps the most culturally significant sexual behavior in Western societies as evidenced by being constructed as the traditional way that an individual "loses their virginity" or has their "first sex," and that the first experience may influence people's experiences in the future.
- Penile-vaginal sex is also the behavior most often referenced in association to the concept of "abstinence."
- Adolescents and young adults may choose penile-vaginal sex for a variety of reasons including emotional reasons (e.g., to express love or intimacy), physical reasons (e.g., sexual interest or stress reduction), or social reasons (e.g., increased social status or popularity).
- The frequency of vaginal sex may increase over time in relationships as relationship quality and sexual satisfaction also grow.

Prevalence[17,22]

- The NSFG demonstrates that among 15- to 19-year-olds, 47% of young females and 49% of young males report having vaginal sex; and among 20- to 24-year-olds, 85% of males and 87% of females report ever having vaginal sex.
- The 2015 National Sexual Exploration in America Study suggested that among 18- to 24-year-olds, 52.1% of females and 53.3% of males had penile-vaginal sex in the last year.

Penile-Anal Sex
Overview and Context[20,23–27]

- Penile-anal sex is typically a most difficult sexual behavior to discuss and is stigmatized.
- The difficulty in having a discussion and/or stigma associated with anal sex should not make clinicians think that young people do not participate in anal sex.
- Adolescent and young adult participation in penile-anal sex can vary across different contexts.
- Penile-anal sex occurs in both AYAs' main and casual relationships, as well as in monogamous and nonmonogamous relationships.
- Some AYAs may not consider penile-anal sex as "having sex," and may use it as a means to preserve virginity.

- Some may perceive penile-anal sex to be a "safer" alternative to vaginal sex, as it poses no risk of pregnancy.
- Anal sex may occur as an act of physical pleasure or emotional intimacy with one's partner, in deference to partner requests, or in response to imbalanced relationship power.

Prevalence[28]

- The NSFG shows that among 15- to 19-year-olds, 10.8% of females and 10.5% of males report lifetime experience with penile-anal sex, while among 20- to 24-year-olds, 31.5% of females and 33.6% of males report lifetime experience with penile-anal sex.
- The National 2015 Sexual Exploration in America Study suggested that among 18- to 24-year-old AYAs, 6.7% of females and 2.7% of males had penile-anal sex in the last month, while 17% of females and 24% of males had penile-anal sex in the last year.

Sexting
Overview and Context[29–34]

- Sexting refers to sending and receiving flirtatious or sexually suggestive messages, sexually suggestive images, or videos, and/or seminude or nude images and videos through digital communication tools such as text messages, social media, and email.
- Participation in sexting can be associated with substantial reputational, educational, or legal trouble. Police and prosecutorial interpretation of child pornography statutes may differ across cities, states, provinces, or countries, making it possible that AYAs who participate in sexting could be charged criminally.
- Sexting has been studied as both a relationship behavior and a sexual behavior.
  - Adolescents and young adults may sext with their romantic partners or persons with whom they are exploring a romantic/sexual relationship.
  - Sexting may occur with someone an AYA likes and/or with whom they hope to be in a relationship.
  - Sexting may occur with someone an AYA knows in person, knows online only, and/or does not know well or at all.
  - Sexting can occur because of pressure from others.
  - Sexting can be used to flirt, to connect with someone an AYA likes, to communicate sexual desire, and initiate in-person sexual behavior.
  - Sexting allows for sexual exploration that is free from the risk of STIs and unintended pregnancy.
- Adolescents and young adults recognize that a risk of sexting is having sexts shared beyond the intended recipient. Despite acknowledging that it is inappropriate to share texts beyond the intended recipient, they state that they would share sexts with others.

Prevalence[29–33]

- According to the NSSHB, among adolescents, about 1 in 10 adolescents has participated in sexting. About 40% of young adults have sent a sext, and 41% have received a sext.

OUTCOMES ASSOCIATED WITH SEXUAL BEHAVIOR

While most AYAs participate in sexual behavior without issue, some young people experience adverse sexual outcomes, including unintended pregnancy and STIs. More information associated with the prevalence and organization of these conditions can be found in Chapter 78 (Sexual Violence and Aggression) Chapter 45 (Pregnancy), and Chapters 61 to 67 (STIs).

CLINICIAN RECOMMENDATIONS

Clinicians play a direct and important role in assuring sexual and reproductive health care during adolescence and young adulthood. Sexuality is a recommended dimension of preventative health across the life span, and it intersects with several specific goals in Healthy People 2030.[35] Yet, many clinicians do not address these topics as part of primary care and/or other clinical interactions.[36] Outlined below are some recommendations.

1. All clinically associated visits can and should be used as opportunities to (re)address adolescent or young adult sexual health issues.

2. When discussing sexual health with AYAs, clinicians should also be directing them toward reliable, confidential, and accurate sources of information about sex.

3. Clinicians should remember that regular and complete sexual health assessments are necessary for all AYAs regardless of gender or sexual identity. Clinicians may falsely assume specific patients either do not participate in sex, or that they only choose "low-risk" behaviors.

4. In early adolescence, clinicians may initiate a conversation with patients regarding emerging sexual feelings, which could include normalizing solo masturbation. For example, clinicians can express that many young people express sexual feelings by masturbating or exploring what feel good on their own bodies, and additionally explain that doing so is a normal thing to do. As AYAs become older or enter into close relationships, the conversation can also be used to normalize both solo masturbation as a means of delaying sex, or being able to communicate to a partner about how they liked to be touched.

5. Beginning in early adolescence, clinicians should regularly (re)assess AYAs' close/intimate relationships. Clinicians should expect participation in these relationships to emerge as adolescents enter middle school or junior high, and to begin asking about them as a means of establishing rapport on this topic. It is also important to revisit partnerships mentioned in prior conversations, to gauge changes in the relationship's importance, as well as to get a sense of the types of emotional experiences the adolescent or young adult has had in that relationship. Starting and ending romantic experiences can be stressful for AYAs. How an adolescent feels about a relationship can impact their mental health; thus, it is important for clinicians to ask about both the positive and negative attributes of these relationships.

   Questions to facilitate this early conversation may include the following:

   "Is there anyone you like at school/church/etc.? What do you like about them? What kinds of things do you do together? How often do you see them?" In follow-up visits, clinicians might ask *"What's new with your love life? The last time you were here, you mentioned a person named X. Are they still important to you?"*

6. Asking adolescents about romantic activities broadly is more likely to capture the range of romantic involvements common during adolescence. In addition, if AYAs say that they are not romantically involved with anyone, clinicians should not assume that they are not sexually active.

7. The emotional content in a relationship also provides cues as to when lighter or more involved partnered sexual behaviors may emerge. In the context of every partnership, clinicians should ask specific questions about how and when the young person expresses sexual or physical affection for partners. They should also assess any unintended pregnancy and/or STI risk associated with those activities. Clinicians should also screen for any pressures for sexual coercion and/or unwanted sex.

   Questions may include the following:

   "How do you and X express affection for each other? Do you hold hands? Hug? What other kinds of things do you do with X?" In the context of ongoing assessment, these questions can be amended: *"Last time you were here, you mentioned that you and X liked to (hold hands and kiss). Is that still how you prefer to spend time together? Are (condoms/birth control pills/abstinence) still working for you? How can I help you?"*

8. Clinicians also need to be vigilant about clarifying what an adolescent or young adult means when they say they are "sexually abstinent," including periods when they do and do not have relationships with partners. It would be helpful for clinicians to be equipped to provide appropriate information around any misperceptions AYAs may have about sexual risk reduction in their behavior choices, as well as to support their motivations for remaining abstinent, or changing their approach to abstinence.

   It may be helpful to begin both these conversations with a question related to why they chose abstinence: *"Why is abstinence important for you? What does it provide to you (or you and X)?"* In this manner, the clinician gains a sense of any perceived moral, religious, or safety benefits an adolescent or young adult derives from their version of abstinence and provides appropriate points of risk-reduction counseling.

   Questions or prompts could include: *"You mentioned that (activities X, Y, and Z) are 'safer' and that's why you (or you and X) do them together. Did you know that some of them could actually increase the likelihood that you could...? (get pregnant/catch an STI). I'd like to talk about how we can make sure you protect yourself while you are with X."*

9. Clinicians need to be aware of the changes in AYA relationships, even when an adolescent or young adult has been in, or is currently in, a more "regular" relationship. When two or more partners are mentioned, or a new partner emerges, clinicians can ask patients how well they know their partner's sexual history, what sexual risks they perceive, and what methods they are using to reduce adverse sexual outcomes. Clinicians should also be prepared to adjust their counseling around condom and contraceptive use, as well as sexual refusal strategies, in the context of these partnerships.

   Questions or prompts might include: *"You mentioned you are/were (kissing/holding hands/having oral/vaginal/anal sex) with Y (the last time you were here), but that they weren't your boy/girlfriend. What does that mean? How are you protecting yourself with this partner?"*

10. Encourage open, honest, and direct sexual communication between AYAs and their parents/guardians/caregivers. It may be useful to remind parents/guardians/caregivers that despite increasing independence, their children still need, and value, guidance from them. Reinforce the importance of knowing and asking questions about their child's close relationships and empower parents/guardians/caregivers to check in on the emotional and behavioral content in these relationships. It may be necessary to assure parents/guardians/caregivers that asking about specific experiences will not "cause" their children to participate in them (e.g., vaginal sex), but it will provide parents/guardians/caregivers an ongoing sense of the young person's readiness to manage them. Likewise, help AYAs initiate "tough" conversations with their parents/guardians/caregivers, vetting any advanced concerns they may have about parents/guardians/caregivers' being angry or upset regarding sexual issues. If necessary, provide a neutral space for AYAs and their parents/guardians/caregivers to talk out specific issues, helping to guide the conversation to specific issues, and validating emotions and concerns on both sides.

SUMMARY

Intimate relationships become more important to all adolescents—regardless of gender or sexual identity—as adolescence progresses. These relationships are often the context for first (as well as ongoing) solo and partnered sexual experiences. Clinicians are in a good position to engage, screen, and provide counseling on sexual and reproductive health issues to all AYAs.

REFERENCES

1. Hensel DJ, Fortenberry JD. Lifespan sexuality through a sexual health perspective. In: Tolman DL, Diamond LM, eds. *APA Handbook on Sexuality and Psychology.* APA Press; 2013.
2. Viner RM, Ozer EM, Denny S, et al. Adolescence and the social determinants of health. *Lancet.* 2012;379(9826):1641–1652.
3. Schalet AT. Beyond abstinence and risk: a new paradigm for adolescent sexual health. *Womens Health Issues.* 2011;21(3):S5–S7.
4. Norona JC, Roberson PNE, Welsh DP. "I learned things that make me happy, things that bring me down" lessons from romantic relationships in adolescence and emerging adulthood. *J Adolescent Res.* 2015;0743558415605166.
5. Coyle KK, Anderson PM, Franks HM, et al. Romantic relationships: an important context for HIV/STI and pregnancy prevention programmes with young people. *Sex Education.* 2014;14(5):582–596.
6. Manning WD, Longmore MA, Copp J, et al. The complexities of adolescent dating and sexual relationships: fluidity, meaning(s), and implications for young adults' well-being. *New Dir Child Adolesc Dev.* 2014;2014(144):53–69.
7. Beckmeyer JJ, Jamison TB. Identifying a typology of emerging adult romantic relationships: implications for relationship education. *Fam Relat.* 2020.
8. Beckmeyer JJ, Herbenick D, Fu TCJ, et al. Prevalence of romantic experiences and competencies among 14 to 17 year olds: implications for the primary care setting. *Clin Pediatr.* 2020;59(2):116–124.
9. Hensel DJ, Fortenberry JD. Adolescent mothers' sexual, contraceptive, and emotional relationship content with the fathers of their children following a first diagnosis of sexually transmitted infection. *J Adolescent Health.* 2011;49(3):327–329.
10. Poppi FIM. Pro domo sua: narratives of sexual abstinence. *Sexuality Culture.* 2021;25(2):540–561.
11. Long-Middleton ER, Burke PJ, Cahill Lawrence CA, et al. Understanding motivations for abstinence among adolescent young women: insights into effective sexual risk reduction strategies. *J Pediatric Health Care.* 2013;27(5):342–350.
12. Centers for Disease Control. *Youth risk behavior survey data summary & trends report, 2009–2019.* Published 2020. Accessed. https://www.cdc.gov/healthyyouth/data/yrbs/pdf/YRBSDataSummaryTrendsReport2019-508.pdf
13. Kaestle C, Allen K. The role of masturbation in healthy sexual development: perceptions of young adults. *Arch Sex Behav.* 2011;40(5):983–994.
14. Das A. Masturbation in the united states. *J Sex Marital Ther.* 2007;33(4):301–317.
15. Robbins CL, Schick V, Reece M, et al. Prevalence, frequency, and associations of masturbation with partnered sexual behaviors among US adolescents. *Arch Pediatr Adolesc Med.* 2011;165(12):1087–1093.
16. Holway GV, Hernandez SM. Oral sex and condom use in a U.S. national sample of adolescents and young adults. *J Adolesc Health.* 2018;62(4):402–410.
17. Herbenick D, Bowling J, Fu TCJ, et al. Sexual diversity in the United States: results from a nationally representative probability sample of adult women and men. *PLoS One.* 2017;12(7):e0181198.
18. Vannier SA, O'Sullivan LF. Who gives and who gets: why, when, and with whom young people engage in oral sex. *J Youth Adolesc.* 2012;41(5):572–582.
19. Bay-Cheng LY, Fava NM. Young women's experiences and perceptions of cunnilingus during adolescence. *J Sex Res.* 2011;48(6):531–542.
20. Hensel DJ, Fortenberry JD, Orr DP. Variations in coital and noncoital sexual repertoire among adolescent women. *J Adolesc Health.* 2008;42(2):170–176.
21. Sayegh MA, Fortenberry JD, Shew M, et al. The developmental association of relationship quality, hormonal contraceptive choice and condom non-use among adolescent women. *J Adolesc Health.* 2006;39(3):388–395.
22. Centers for Disease Control and Prevention. Key statistics from the National Survey of Family Growth–sexual activity between opposite-sex partners. Published 2020. Accessed March 21, 2021. https://www.cdc.gov/nchs/nsfg/key_statistics/s-keystat.htm#oppositesexpartners
23. Meston CM, Buss DM. Why humans have sex. *Arch Sex Behav.* 2007;36(4):477–507.
24. Hensel DJ, Fortenberry JD, Orr DP. Factors associated with event level anal sex and condom use during anal sex among adolescent women. *J Adolesc Health.* 2010;46(3):232–237.
25. Houston AM, Fang J, Husman C, et al. More than just vaginal intercourse: anal intercourse and condom use patterns in the context of "main" and "casual" sexual relationships among urban minority adolescent females. *J Pediatr Adolesc Gynecol.* 2007;20(5):299–304.
26. Lescano CM, Houck CD, Brown LK, et al. Correlates of heterosexual anal intercourse among at-risk adolescents and young adults. *Am J Public Health.* 2009;99(6):1131–1136.
27. Maynard E, Carballo-Diéguez A, Ventuneac A, et al. Women's experiences with anal sex: motivations and implications for STD prevention. *Perspect Sex Reprod Health.* 2009;41(3):142–149.
28. Habel MA, Leichliter JS, Dittus PJ, et al. Heterosexual anal and oral sex in adolescents and adults in the United States, 2011–2015. *Sex Transm Dis.* 2018;45(12):775–782.
29. Beckmeyer JJ, Herbenick D, Fu TCJ, et al. Characteristics of adolescent sexting: results from the 2015 national survey of sexual health and behavior. *J Sex Marital Ther.* 2019;45(8):767–780.
30. Klettke B, Hallford DJ, Mellor DJ. Sexting prevalence and correlates: a systematic literature review. *Clin Psychol Rev.* 2014;34(1):44–53.
31. Mitchell KJ, Finkelhor D, Jones LM, et al. Prevalence and characteristics of youth sexting: a national study. *Pediatrics.* 2012;129(1):13–20.
32. Mori C, Cooke JE, Temple JR, et al. The prevalence of sexting behaviors among emerging adults: a meta-analysis. *Arch Sex Behav.* 2020;49(4):1103–1119.
33. Strassberg DS, McKinnon RK, Sustaíta MA, et al. Sexting by high school students: an exploratory and descriptive study. *Arch Sex Behav.* 2013;42(1):15–21.
34. Patchin JW, Hinduja S. It is time to teach safe sexting. *J Adolesc Health.* 2020;66(2):140–143.
35. U.S. Department of Health and Human Services. *Healthy people 2030 objectives.* Published 2020. Accessed December 13, 2020. https://health.gov/healthypeople/objectives-and-data/browse-objectives
36. Hensel DJ, Herbenick D, Beckmeyer JJ, et al. Adolescents' discussion of sexual and reproductive health care topics with providers: findings from a nationally representative probability sample of U.S. adolescents. *J Adolesc Health.* 2020.

🛜 ADDITIONAL RESOURCES AND WEBSITES

Additional Resources and Websites for Clinicians:

American Academy of Pediatrics—*Bright Futures* Guidelines: provides guidance to health care on promoting healthy sexual development and sexuality from birth to young adulthood—https://brightfutures.aap.org/Bright%20Futures%20Documents/BF4_HealthySexuality.pdf

American Academy of Pediatrics—https://www.aap.org/en-us/advocacy-and-policy/aap-health-initiatives/adolescent-sexual-health/Pages/default.aspx

Additional Resources and Websites for Parents/Caregivers:

American Sexual Health Association: This association provides a wealth of resources on sexual health for both men and women, and specific resources directed at parents—www.ashasexualhealth.org/parents/

Answer: Answer provides links to books, organizations, websites, and workshops that support parents in their critical role as sex educators for their children—http://answer.rutgers.edu/page/parentresources

Centers for Disease Control and Prevention: The CDC offers parent and guardian resources to help teens make healthy choices about sex—https://www.cdc.gov/healthyyouth/parents/index.htm

Center for Parent Information and Resources: This resource page addresses development of sexuality for young people with disabilities—http://www.parentcenterhub.org/repository/sexed/

Center for Parent Information and Resources: This resource page addresses development of sexuality for young people with disabilities—http://www.parentcenterhub.org/repository/sexed/

Center for Young Women's Health and **Young Men's Health:** These websites provide resources for parents to communicate to teens about sex and contraceptives—http://youngwomenshealth.org/parents/and http://youngmenshealthsite.org/parents/

Guttmacher Institute: Through research, policy analysis, and public education, the Guttmacher Institute advances sexual and reproductive health and provides resources about adolescents—www.guttmacher.org

Planned Parenthood of America: These tools found on the Planned Parenthood website offer videos, tips, and additional resources on puberty, setting healthy limits, parent-teen relationships, talking to kids about sexuality, and parenting LGBTQ kids
Communication—https://www.plannedparenthood.org/learn/parents
Fact sheets and books—https://www.plannedparenthood.org/learn/parents/resources-parents

PFLAG: This website provides resources for parents, families, friends, and allies of LGBTQ people including publications, educational programs, and advocacy campaigns—https://community.pflag.org/

Sex Positive Families: This webpage provides age-congruent, inclusive, medically accurate, and sex-positive education resources for families—https://sexpositive-families.com/10-best-sex-ed-resources-for-families/

Additional Resources and Websites for Adolescents and Young Adults:

Bedsider: Online birth control support network with information for selection and usage of different birth control methods—http://bedsider.org/

Center for Young Women's Health and Young Men's Health: These websites provide information targeted at adolescents, including guides on a variety of sexual health topics such as contraception, STIs, LGBT health, and puberty—http://youngwomenshealth.org and http://youngmenshealthsite.org

Coalition for Positive Sexuality: This website offers resources and tools for teens to take care of themselves and affirm their decision about sex, sexuality, and reproductive control—http://www.positive.org/

Go Ask Alice!: Large database of questions about a variety of reproductive and sexual health concerns—www.goaskalice.columbia.edu

Love Matters: This website offers a space to talk and ask questions openly and honestly about love, sex, and relationships for young adults around the world—https://lovematters.in/en

MTV, It's Your Sex Life: Using an interactive website, MTV has resources for young adults on pregnancy, STDs and testing, LGBTQ, relationships, consent, and a national hotline—www.itsyoursexlife.com/

Options for Sexual Health: This online resource offers sexual and reproductive health care, information, and education from a feminist, pro-choice, sex-positive perspective—https://www.optionsforsexualhealth.org/

Planned Parenthood Federation of America: Providing up-to-date, clear, and medically accurate information, Planned Parenthood helps both young men and women better understand their sexual health—www.plannedparenthood.org/teens

Safe Teens: Teenagers can use this youth-friendly website to find information on teen pregnancy, STDs, safe sex, relationships, and LGBTQ issues—www.safeteens.org/

Scarleteen: This website provides a wealth of information for teens and young adults about sexuality, sex, and relationships, as well as advice and support, and even a safer sex shop—www.scarleteen.com/

Stay Teen: Using videos, games, quizzes, and a sex education resource center, this website delivers quality information about sex, relationships, abstinence, and birth control for teens—http://stayteen.org/

Teen Health: Adolescents can use this website to learn facts about sexual health including articles about puberty, menstruation, infections, and birth control—http://teenshealth.org/teen/sexual_health/

CHAPTER 43

Sexual Minority Adolescents and Young Adults

Jen Makrides
Errol L. Fields

KEY WORDS

- Bisexual
- Gay
- Lesbian
- Lesbian, gay, bisexual (LGB)
- Men who have sex with men (MSM)
- Queer
- Sexual attraction
- Sexual behavior
- Sexual identity
- Sexual minority
- Sexual minority youth
- Sexual orientation

INTRODUCTION

This chapter reviews diverse sexual orientations in the context of adolescent and young adult (AYA) health and development, addresses the strengths and challenges faced by sexual minority youth (SMY), and describes the role of the clinician in supporting these youth and their families as they transition into adulthood.

It is important for the clinician to recognize that while lesbian, gay, bisexual, transsexual, and queer (LGBTQ) issues are often presented as a group, sexuality and gender are two separate experiences—even for patients who may identify as sexual minorities and gender diverse. Sexual orientation refers to the sexual or romantic attractions, behaviors, and identity/ies that interact to form an individual's sexuality. Gender identity refers to an individual's internal sense and experience of gender, which may include male, female, nonbinary, gender queer, or gender fluid among others. Gender expression refers to how an individual expresses their gender such as through clothing, preferred pronouns, demeanor, and interaction with cultural norms.[1] It is important that clinicians be aware of the distinction between sexual orientation and gender identity. For more information on transgender and gender diverse youth, see Chapter 44.

Terminology

Sexual Orientation

Sexual orientation is a multidimensional construct, which includes at least three components pertinent to our discussion: **sexual identity**, **sexual attraction**, and **sexual behavior**.

Sexual identity describes how an individual thinks of themselves and the language or words they use to describe their sexual orientation. Sexual identity can refer to an individual's self-identification of their sexual orientation, their social identification with others with similar sexual orientations, or both.

There are many sexual identity labels that people may use and preferences for terms may depend on age and cultural context. Below are some examples of current terminology but it is not inclusive. Heterosexual typically refers to individuals who are attracted to individuals of the opposite sex or gender. Lesbian/gay typically refer to women/girls and men/boys who are attracted only to individuals of the same sex or gender, and queer is often used to reference nonheterosexual identities and/or gender diverse identities. Same-gender loving is an identity used among some Black/African American people as a more culturally affirming term for nonheterosexual identities; and Two-Spirit is a Native American term that often refers to a third gender, and may refer to nonheterosexual self-identification.[1] Bisexual typically refers to individuals who are attracted to individuals of both the same and the opposite sex or gender and pansexual refers to individuals who are attracted to individuals regardless of their sex or gender. The term asexual typically refers to individuals who have little or no sexual attractions regardless of gender, although they may seek romantic relationships and engage in sexual activity.

Sexual attraction describes whom one is attracted to and may include females, males, both, neither or gender minorities not captured by the above classifications.

Sexual behavior describes what kind of sex an individual is having, and with whom. For instance, "men who have sex with men (MSM)," is a term that is often used in research to capture behavior rather than the diversity of sexual identities seen within the MSM population.

Taken together, these three aspects—identity, attraction, and behavior—help guide our role in providing developmental and medical guidance to our patients. Clinicians may care for a female patient who identifies as lesbian (sexual identity), is attracted to only women (sexual attraction), and has oral sex with female partners and oral and vaginal sex with male partners (sexual behavior). All of these aspects of her sexuality are important components to a thorough sexual history, which will allow the clinician to support her development into adulthood and identify, address, or preempt potential health risks.

A recent publication from the National Academies of Sciences, Engineering, and Medicine recognizes the difficulty in crafting an inclusive term to delineate individuals who identify as lesbian, gay, bisexual, pan, queer (or a synonym for these identities), are attracted to same-sex individuals, and/or have same-sex partners.[1] For the purposes of this discussion, we will use the term **sexual minority youth (SMY)** as it is more inclusive of the diversity of nonheterosexual orientations and clearly distinguishes sexual orientation from gender identity.

Prevalence of Sexual Minorities

Data from the Youth Risk Behavior Survey (YRBS) indicate that the percentage of youth who identify as nonheterosexual has increased from 11.2% in 2015 to 15.6% in 2019 with 2.5% of adolescents identifying as gay or lesbian, 8.7% as bisexual, and 4.5% as unsure.[2] Data from the National Survey of Family Growth suggests similar increases in reported same-sex sexual attraction and behavior over time.[1] The most recent National College Health Assessment, a survey of young adult college students, reports a nearly twofold increase in students who identify as nonheterosexual between 2014 and 2020, with 19.5% of students in the most recent survey identifying as nonheterosexual, including over 3% who identify as gay or lesbian and nearly 10% who identify as bisexual.[3]

SEXUAL IDENTITY AND DEVELOPMENT

Identity development, the process by which an individual understands how and where they fit in society, is one of the key tasks of adolescence.[4] Sexual identity development is one aspect of identity development and is thought to involve two related processes: identity formation and identity integration. Identity formation occurs through becoming aware of, questioning and exploring one's sexuality, and identity integration occurs through the incorporation of sexuality into one's self-concept. Sexual identity formation is often described as a developmental feature of early adolescence with increasing comfort and integration of sexual identity often occurring in middle to late adolescence.[4] However, as with other aspects of development, sexual identity development is often nonlinear and variable both across and within individuals as well as sociocultural contexts.[4]

HOMOPHOBIA AND HETEROSEXISM

While prejudice and bias against sexual minorities has had an overall decline in the last 20 years,[5] SMY continue to experience attitudes, behaviors, social norms, and systems that can be stigmatizing or discriminatory. Homophobia is a term used to describe bias, prejudice, hatred, or other negative attitudes against persons with sexual minority identities, behaviors, or attractions. Like other types of bias or prejudice, homophobia engenders an assault on one's personhood, or self-identity. Unlike some other forms of prejudice (e.g., racism or xenophobia), the perpetrators of homophobia are more frequently individuals who would otherwise be sources of social support (e.g., parents/caregivers or family) or embedded in groups central to one's identity (e.g., religious or other community groups). Because the process of identity development in AYAs involves seeking affirmation and support from these important referent groups, the experience of homophobia may isolate SMY when interpersonal attachments are critical and have significant negative impacts on developmental and health outcomes. Studies have consistently demonstrated that SMY who experience family rejection are more likely to experience poor mental health outcomes and engage in substance use and sexual risk behaviors than SMY who are accepted and affirmed by their families.[6] Moreover, studies have demonstrated that family acceptance during adolescence can be protective against depression, suicidality, substance use, human immunodeficiency virus (HIV), and sexually transmitted infections (STIs), and associated with higher reported social support, self-esteem, and general health.[6,7] A study from the Family Acceptance Project demonstrated that with increasing levels of family acceptance, the percentage of sexual (and gender) minority youth who believed they could be happy as adults also increased.

Heterosexism is a term that refers to the societal expectation that heterosexuality is the expected norm, while homosexuality, bisexuality, or any other nonheterosexual orientation is treated as abnormal, inferior, or inconsequential. It encompasses internalized or interpersonal attitudes and behaviors that demean or invalidate sexual minority experiences as well as structural and systemic processes that exclude and marginalize sexual minorities (e.g., sexual health curricula that excludes same-sex orientations, antidiscrimination policies that exclude sexual orientation).

Like homophobia, heterosexism can impact health and development of sexual minorities. An analysis conducted shortly before the United States established federal marriage equality demonstrated that state policies favoring same-sex marriages were associated with reduced adolescent suicide attempts. Similarly, studies that have demonstrated antiheterosexist structural policies[8] on college campuses are associated with lower rates of heterosexist or homophobic discrimination, lower psychological distress, and higher self-acceptance among AYA sexual minorities.[9]

MINORITY STRESS, INTERSECTIONALITY, AND THE HEALTH OF SEXUAL MINORITY YOUTH

Minority stress theory and intersectionality are key concepts for understanding how SMY's experience in society interacts with health outcomes.

Minority stress theory explains that "stigma, prejudice, and discrimination create a hostile and stressful social environment that causes mental health problems."[10] It explores how these multiple stressors impact the individual on both distal and proximal levels. Examples of the distal experiences include overt prejudice, such as derogatory comments, and policies that until recently prohibited sexual minorities from marrying under federal law. Proximal minority stress includes the internalization of stigma, the expectation of rejection, and concealment. This might present as a young adult concealing their sexual orientation from their family for fear of rejection and/or, despite having a loving same-sex relationship, feeling there is something wrong with being homosexual (internalized homophobia).[10] Minority stress theory has subsequently been expanded and applied to broad health disparities, ranging from biologic outcomes of chronic stress to behavioral health, including topics such as substance use, HIV and STI risk and rates, pregnancy rates, and mental health.

Intersectionality addresses the impact of multiple minority identities on experience. Crenshaw's seminal work asserted that the experiences of Black women were not included in "single-axis" examinations of race discrimination (which focused primarily on Black men, but not women) or gender discrimination (which focused primarily on White women, but not Black women). She asserted that being Black and a woman created a separate experience of intersecting identities that is not captured by the single-axis model.[11]

Intersectionality is critical to understanding how multiple nondominant identities, such as being Latino and a sexual minority, a young woman and a sexual minority, or a Black adolescent male and a sexual minority, may create challenges (and strengths) unique to that experience. Racial/ethnic minority SMY whose connection to their racial or ethnic identity provides important strength and support may prioritize this connection over "coming out" or sharing their sexual minority identity. This compartmentalization of sexual identity can be protective by preserving existing social supports but may also isolate the youth from developing sexuality-related networks and supports, particularly when those supports are absent in their existing communities.[12] It is imperative that clinicians consider the potential compounding effects of multiple oppressed or marginalized identities on SMY and the impact these multiple minority stressors can have on health-related risk and health disparities.[12]

HEALTH CONCERNS FOR SEXUAL MINORITY YOUTH

Sexual minority youth, like their heterosexual counterparts, are generally healthy and well-adjusted individuals, with rare chronic health issues. While studies in adult sexual minorities have identified disparities in cardiovascular and cancer risk compared to heterosexuals, studies in youth populations have primarily demonstrated health disparities in mental health, substance use, eating disorders, and sexual and reproductive health. Sexual minority youth are disproportionately affected by social conditions that threaten their health and successful transition to adulthood, such as: runaway and homelessness, bullying and victimization, and intimate partner violence (IPV). Sexual minority youth also experience health care disparities that can impact their ability to receive needed care. It is important to recognize that the health and social disparities experienced by SMY are linked to stigma, discrimination, and stressors that disproportionally affect these youth and that supportive families, communities, clinicians, and policies affirming sexual minorities have been shown to be protective and promote healthy adjustment into adulthood.[1] Intersecting identities (i.e., gender, race/ethnicity, socioeconomic status) may have protective or compounding effects on these health disparities.[12]

Mental Health and Suicidality

Sexual minority youth have a higher risk for mental health conditions, including depression, anxiety, posttraumatic stress disorder, suicidal ideation, and suicide attempt than their heterosexual peers.[1] Data from the 2019 YRBS (and the prior two cycles in 2015 and 2017) demonstrated a significantly higher percentage of SMY than heterosexual youth who report persistent feelings of sadness and hopelessness and who report attempting suicide in the preceding 12 months.[2]

Substance Use Disorders

Compared to their heterosexual peers, SMY are at increased risk of substance use disorders during their adolescence, young adulthood, and over their lifespan.[1] Analysis of the YRBS data from 2019 shows that 31.1% of lesbian, gay, and bisexual youth used marijuana and 33.9% had used alcohol within the past 30 days, compared with only 20.9% and 28.8%, respectively, among heterosexual peers.[2] Additional research highlights the impact of intersectionality on risk, demonstrating disparities in substance use by race/ethnicity, male or female sex, and sexual orientation.[1]

Eating Disorders

In a recent literature review, the prevalence of eating disorders was noted as generally higher in SMY as compared to their heterosexual peers.[13] Sexual minority males seem to be at greatest risk. Compared to heterosexual males, sexual minority males have significantly higher rates of eating disorders, while rates among young women are similar across sexual minorities and heterosexuals. There seem to be multiple potential etiologies for the male prominence of this disparity among SMY including differences in sociocultural and psychological risk factors for eating disorders between sexual minority and heterosexual males, sexual minority community norms related to body image and sexual attraction, the impact of minority stress, and overlapping disparities of comorbid mental illnesses that can increase the risk for eating disorders.[14]

Sexual Health: HIV and Other Sexually Transmitted Infections

Adolescent and young adult MSM between the ages of 13 to 24 years represent the second highest rate of new HIV infections in the United States, with the burden unfairly distributed among Black and Latino youth.[1,15] These youth are also at increased risk for syphilis, with rates increasing across the United States and disproportionately borne by MSM. Sexual minority women, including women with only same-sex partners, are also at risk for HIV, human papilloma virus (HPV), and other STIs; however adolescent females with only same-sex partners are much less likely to receive testing than women who have sex with at least some opposite-sex partners.[1] The Centers for Disease Control and Prevention (CDC) advises that having only same-sex partners in not an indication to deny women STI and HIV testing.[16]

Reproductive Health

Sexual minority women are more likely to have mistimed pregnancies throughout their life, including adolescence.[17] A recent analysis found that lesbian youth had twice the risk and bisexual young women had nearly five times the risk of teen pregnancy compared to heterosexual peers, and a significant portion of the increased risk was explained by higher rates of bullying and maltreatment, including physical, emotional, and sexual abuse.[17]

Runaway, Homelessness, and Foster Involvement

Due to a number of factors, including family rejection, physical, emotional, and sexual abuse, and financial and emotional neglect, SMY are often overrepresented in the homeless and foster involved youth population. They account for anywhere from 20% to 40% of homeless youth and are 2.5 times as likely to experience foster care placement relative to heterosexual youth.[18] Compared to their heterosexual peers, they are more likely to experience bias within the systems established to support homeless youth including access to housing, shelter, and welfare.[1] They also experience a disparate burden of policing and involvement with juvenile and criminal justice systems[1] and are at greater risk for human trafficking and involvement in survival sex.[18]

Bullying and Victimization

Bullying and victimization can range from verbal and electronic harassment to physical assault and sexual violence. Recent national surveys of sexual minority and gender diverse youth including the Gay, Lesbian & Straight Education Network 2019 National School Climate Survey,[19] and the Human Rights Campaign 2018 LGBTQ Youth Survey[20] report high rates of verbal and physical harassment, electronic harassment, and sexual harassment among SMY. The 2019 YRBS reported significantly higher odds of feeling unsafe at school, being threatened or injured with a weapon at school, and being bullied at school or bullied electronically among youth who identified as lesbian, gay, or bisexual compared to their heterosexual peers.[2]

Research has found associations between bullying, mental health, and substance use in SMY, and that school-based discrimination and harassment explains much of the disparity in substance use between SMY and heterosexual peers.[21] Both proximal and distal minority stressors, including internalized homophobia, negative reactions to disclosure of sexual orientation, and bullying, among others, can impact the risk of substance use in SMY.[22]

Intimate Partner Violence

Sexual minority youth face an increased risk of IPV and dating violence when compared to their heterosexual peers; the intersection of Black and/or female with sexual minority status further increases the risk of dating violence when compared to White and male peers, respectively.[1] The minority stress model may explain some of the increased risk of IPV for SMY: among sexual minority college students, concealment of identity, and internalized homonegativity were associated with an increased risk of IPV.

The 2019 YRBS data indicates that youth who identify as lesbian, gay, or bisexual youth experienced higher rates of physical and sexual dating violence in the last 12 years than youth who identify as heterosexual, and that rates of lifetime forced sexual intercourse were nearly four times higher among youth who identify as lesbian, gay, or bisexual than among youth who identify as heterosexual.[2] While IPV prevention programs have been studied in heterosexual youth, additional research is needed to inform IPV prevention and intervention programs for SMY and adults, with attention to how race, ethnicity, and gender intersect with sexual minority status.[23]

Reproductive coercion is a form of IPV where one partner limits the other's ability to control their fertility or protect themselves from STIs; this may include limitations on birth control access, pressure or force to become pregnant or father children, or non-consensual condom removal (often referred to as "stealthing"), among other tactics.[24] Although data are limited, studies suggest SMY face higher rates of reproductive coercion and stealthing than their heterosexual peers.[25]

SUPPORTING SEXUAL MINORITY YOUTH: COMBATTING STIGMA AND PROMOTING RESILIENCE

The health risks described above are *incrementally higher* for SMY compared to heterosexual youth but are *not universally higher*. All SMY have the potential to reach adulthood happy and healthy especially when provided with appropriate support. The following protective factors and environmental supports help SMY build resilience in the face of stigma, prejudice, and discrimination: family and parental/caregiver acceptance, safe and inclusive school environments, community and peer supports, and access to affirming, inclusive, and adolescent-friendly health care environments. The impact of family and parental/caregiver acceptance has been described above.

School characteristics that have been described as protective and affirming for SMY include: antibullying policies, supportive teachers and other affirming adults, affirming student organizations and clubs (e.g., Gender & Sexualities Alliances), and sexual health curricula inclusive of same-sex orientations.[1,19] School-based policies to prohibit discrimination based on sexual orientation are associated with less bullying, lower substance use, better mental health, and higher self-esteem for both SMY and heterosexual youth.[1] Community and peer supports such as SMY-serving community organizations and digital or online support networks (e.g., Trevor Chat, Q Chat Space) are important sources of affirmation that help SMY combat stigma and build resilience.[26] Finally, their health care environment and therapeutic relationship with their clinician can be a unique source of support for SMY.

CARING FOR SEXUAL MINORITY YOUTH

Evidence tells us that supportive adults, including parents/caregivers, teachers, mentors, and clinicians, are key players in the development of youth, and SMY are no exception. Like their heterosexual counterparts, SMY highlight the importance of time alone with a clinician, confidentiality, and clinician knowledge and communication as key traits they desire.

Creating an Inclusive Clinical Environment and Engaging Sexual Minority Youth in Care

The American Academy of Pediatrics (AAP) Policy Statement on *Office-Based Care for Lesbian, Gay, Bisexual, Transgender, and Questioning Youth* recommends pediatric offices be teen friendly and welcoming to SMY. Unfortunately, many SMY still report barriers to care such as clinical environments with heterosexist bias and clinicians with limited clinical, cultural, and structural competency in caring for sexual minorities. A recent literature review[27] describes the following important elements of affirming and inclusive care for clinicians to incorporate into their clinical practice:

- Environmental markers of affirmation and inclusion (e.g., rainbow flags; posters, flyers, and pamphlets featuring SMY youth, safe space designations)
- Patient materials that avoid heteronormative assumptions
- Demonstrated knowledge about and sensitivity to specific SMY health care needs
- Approach to all patients that acknowledges and normalizes the diversity of sexuality and gender identity
- Patient–clinician rapport that creates a welcoming and safe environment
- Clear establishment of confidentiality (and the limits of confidentiality) for all AYAs

Addressing Mental and Behavioral Health Needs

Mental health assessments should be routinely practiced in all AYA populations using age-appropriate screening tools. However, given the increased risk of depression, anxiety, substance use disorders, and suicidality in SMY, clinicians should be especially mindful of these patients' potential vulnerability.

While there are a dearth of programs designed specifically for SMY with mental and behavioral health needs, identifying programs and interventions that include the following strategies[1,28] will help SMY cope with these stressors, including:

- Identifying and working to reduce sources of distress in SMY and families
- Supporting SMY's developmental process and age-appropriate milestones (e.g., positive peer relationships, safe exploration of romantic interest and relationships)
- Facilitating adaptive coping (and addressing maladaptive coping) against stigma and discrimination
- Providing developmentally appropriate and affirmative information on sexual orientation
- Reducing internalized negative attitudes towards same-gender attractions, behaviors, and identities
- Incorporating multicultural awareness and cultural competency in supporting youth and families

Importantly, conversion or reparative therapy, an approach designed to change one's sexual orientation or gender identity, is not evidence-based, can be harmful and coercive, and should not be used as a mental or behavioral health approach. It has been discredited by every major medical and mental health professional organization including the AAP, the Society for Adolescent Health and Medicine, the American Psychiatric Association, and the American Psychological Association. It has been legally prohibited as a practice in minors among licensed mental health practitioners in 20 states.

Addressing Sexual and Reproductive Health Needs

For clinicians caring for AYAs, it is critical to assess the components of identity, attraction, *and* behavior for all youth, as these may often be emerging and/or discordant in adolescents. In order to serve all youth, it is important for the clinician to regularly and clearly ask about each of these components of sexual orientation in a private and confidential space. The clinician should address the developmental aspects of becoming a romantically and sexually involved individual and assess patient needs and risks based on their sexual behaviors.

Taking an Inclusive Sexual History

Clinicians should be aware of and practice the following components of taking an inclusive sexual history:

- **Establish and ensure confidentiality:** Any history about sexuality and sexual behaviors should occur during time alone with the clinician; if the topic comes up with parents/caregivers or others in the room, it is important to revisit it when the patient is alone.
- **Be specific when asking about sexual behavior. Exhibit confidence and comfort when asking sensitive questions:** Start by explaining to youth that the sexual history is important for promoting and maintaining sexual health. Introductory comments like "I know this may be embarrassing, but I ask all of my patient's these questions because it's important for your health" can establish a safe space to discuss what may feel like an uncomfortable topic. Direct, nonjudgmental follow-up questions about sexual activity might include: "have you had oral sex (receiving or giving)? Anal sex (receptive or insertive)? Penis–vagina sex?" Following up with direct, nonjudgmental questions about sexual activity will help clinician to effectively counsel about the Six P's (see **Table 43.1**).
- **Make no assumptions about sexual identity, attraction, or behavior:** When speaking with youth about their sexual and

TABLE 43.1

The Six P's: Partners, Practices, Pregnancy, Protection from STIs, Past History of STIs, and Sex Positivity

Partners	• In the past month, 3 mo, 6 mo, 12 mo, how many people have you had sex with? • What is/are the genders of the people you have had sex with? • Is it possible that any of your sex partners had sex with someone else while they were still having sex with you?

Practices	• To understand your risks for STIs, I need to understand the kind of sex you have had recently.
	• Have you had vaginal sex, meaning "penis in vagina sex"?
	• Have you had anal sex, meaning "penis in rectum/anus sex"?
	  • If yes: Did you top—meaning put your penis in your partner's anus, bottom—meaning your partner put his penis in your anus or both?
	• Have you had oral sex, meaning "mouth on penis/vagina/anus"?
	  • If yes: What body parts did you and your partner use?
	• Have you had any kind of sex where you and your partner used sex toys?
	  • If yes: What kind of toys? How did you and your partner use them?
	• For each type of sex and with each partner, do you use condoms or other barriers: never, sometimes, or always?
	  • If never: Why don't you use condoms?
	  • If sometimes: When, with whom, or with what type of sex do you use condoms or other barriers?

Pregnancy desires and prevention	• Do you have plans to have children in the future? • Are you currently trying to conceive or father a child?" • Do you ever have the type of sex that could result in a pregnancy? • If yes: Would you like information about how to prevent unplanned pregnancy?
Protection from STIs	• What are the ways you can protect you and your partner from HIV and STIs? • What strategies do you use? Condoms or other barriers? PrEP? Monogamy? Avoiding specific types of sex?
Past history of STIs	• Have you ever been tested for HIV, or other STIs? • Has your current partner or any former partners ever been diagnosed or treated for an STI? • Have you ever been diagnosed with an STI? • If yes: When? In what body part? How many times? What type of medicine did you get for treatment? • Have you had any symptoms or problems in the body parts you use for sex?
Positivity and pleasure	• When you have sex, do you enjoy it? • Do you ever have pain with sex? • Do you have any concerns about your sexual functioning? • For example, problems with erections, lubrication or wetness, problems or pain with anal sex • Do you (can you) talk to your partner(s) about what you like/dislike sexually? • What questions do you have about sex?

STI, sexually transmitted infections; HIV, human immunodeficiency virus; PrEP, pre-exposure prophylaxis

Source: Adapted from https://www.cdc.gov/std/treatment-guidelines/clinical-risk.htm; https://powertodecide.org/one-key-question

romantic history, it is important to ask questions that invite honest answers and do not presume sexual identity, attraction, the sex of a patient's partners or the types of sex the patient has with them. For instance, one might ask "are you dating anyone" rather than "do you have a girlfriend?" Other clinicians may choose to ask "what genders are you interested in or attracted to?" Following up about who a patient has been intimate with is also critical, as identity and behavior are not always concordant. Clinicians should ask patients the genders of each of their sex partners. The AAP Policy Statement on *Office-Based Care for Lesbian, Gay, Bisexual, Transgender, and Questioning Youth* offers additional guidance on using neutral terms when taking a sexual history.[29] Reminding the adolescent or young adult that your office is a safe space for all sexualities and behaviors, regardless of their response, allows the adolescent or young adult to revisit this conversation and may encourage those who are fearful to disclose their interests to speak with you.

- **Promote healthy sexuality and provide comprehensive, inclusive, nonstigmatizing, and developmentally—appropriate information about sexual and reproductive health and practices:** Most SMY do not receive adequate sex education through school.[19] Clinicians can help fill this gap with evidence-based prevention and risk-reduction strategies (e.g., abstinence, condoms and other barriers, fewer partners, HPV vaccination, partner communication, HIV/STI testing, and Pre-exposure Prophylaxis [PrEP]). This includes:
  - Barrier methods to reduce the likelihood of HIV/STI transmission based on sexual behavior: external and internal condoms for receptive/insertive vaginal, anal, or oral sex with a penis; dental dams for oral–vaginal or oral–anal sex; and appropriate barriers and cleaning of shared sex toys.
  - Asking all youth—including SMY—about their need or desire for contraception, while acknowledging to the patient that this question may not apply to them. Pairing questions about birth control with inquiries about current and future parenting desires acknowledges and normalizes sexual minority family units. Like other youth, many SMY may desire to become parents in the future, and may face additional obstacles associated with minority stress and internalized stigma and heterosexism.[30]
  - Asking about sexual functioning, pleasure and pain/discomfort with sex in order to promote positive sexual experiences. Sex positivity is an important aspect of sexual education and one that all youth, and SMY in particular, are less likely to receive relevant information about.

Table 43.1 reviews the key components of a comprehensive sexual history.

Human Immunodeficiency Virus/Sexually Transmitted Infections: Prevention, Screening, and Treatment

In addition to sexual health prevention, screening and treatment recommendations important for all youth, clinicians should be aware of the following recommendations that may be specific to SMY.

- **Vaccines:** All youth should receive hepatitis A and B (given in early childhood), and HPV vaccines (given in early adolescence), regardless of sexual orientation or behaviors. Catch-up is recommended for all youth who have not completed the series. Specific considerations are summarized in Table 43.2.
- **HIV/STI screening for men who have sex with men:** For MSM, the CDC recommends at least annual testing for HIV, syphilis, gonorrhea, and chlamydia, with more frequent testing at 3- to 6-month intervals for individuals at higher risk. Understanding patients' sexual behaviors is critical. Men who have sex with men with a history of oral or receptive anal sex should receive extragenital gonorrhea and chlamydia screenings in addition to genitourinary screening.[16] Extragenital infections are often asymptomatic, can facilitate ongoing STI transmission, increase risk of HIV acquisition, and would be undetected by genitourinary screening.

TABLE 43.2

Advisory Committee on Immunization Practices (ACIP) Guidelines for Sexually Transmitted Viral Infections

Vaccine	Sexual Minority–Specific Indications	
	Adolescents ≤18	Young Adults 19+
HPV	Indicated for all adolescents	All young adults through age 26 y
HAV	MSM (and anyone with oral–anal contact)	MSM (and anyone with oral–anal contact)
HBV	Indicated for all adolescents	MSM (and those presenting for STI treatment)

Source: https://www.cdc.gov/vaccines/acip/index.html
HPV, human papilloma virus; HAV, hepatitis A virus; HBV, hepatitis B virus.

- Proctitis (inflammation of the distal rectum) and proctocolitis (inflammation of the colonic mucosa) should be in the differential for sexual minority males who have receptive anal intercourse and present with tenesmus, anorectal pain, rectal discharge (proctitis), and/or diarrhea and abdominal cramps (proctocolitis). Patients presenting with these symptoms should be tested for rectal gonorrhea and chlamydia, HSV and syphilis, in addition to screening for HIV at the time of presentation. Presumptive treatment includes 500 mg IM ceftriaxone and 100 mg doxycycline twice daily for 7 days; doxycycline should be extended to 21 days in patients who test positive for chlamydia, have bloody discharge and/or perianal or mucosal ulcers, or who are living with HIV.[16] Visit the CDC website for most up-to-date treatment recommendations.
- HIV/STI screening in women who have sex with women: Women with same-sex partners are at risk for the same STIs and related complications, such as pelvic inflammatory disease (PID), as their peers who have opposite-sex partners. While specific guidelines for women with same-sex partners are not delineated, the CDC advises that sexually active women should be screened for

STIs and HIV regardless of whether they are sexually active with males or females (Table 43.3).[16]

- HIV PrEP: Pre-exposure prophylaxis is currently approved in the form of daily pill for HIV negative persons for the prevention of HIV acquisition. Daily PrEP can reduce risk of HIV acquisition through sex by up to 99%.[31] It was initially approved for adults, but an adolescent indication approved in May 2018 extends use to persons over 35 kg (roughly 77 lb). Pre-exposure prophylaxis is an important prevention tool for all AYAs at risk for HIV, and is highlighted here given HIV disparities impacting racial/ethnic and SMY.

Supporting Parents/Caregivers of Sexual Minority Youth

The role of parental/caregiver and family support cannot be understated. It will help SMY successfully transition to adulthood, combat minority stress and intersectional stigma, develop resilience, and avoid significant health and social disparities. Pediatric and AYA medicine clinicians can play a critical role in helping parents/caregivers understand the impact their affirmation and support can have on their child's well-being. It is recommended that clinicians focus on the following supportive actions:

- Hear and acknowledge parents'/caregivers' fears and concerns. Create a space for parents/caregivers to tell their stories, share concerns, and discuss beliefs.
- Provide parents/caregivers with anticipatory guidance (e.g., importance of parental monitoring, dialogue between child and parent/caregiver, parental advocacy in school and extracurricular settings).
- Share evidence-based medical expertise about parents'/caregivers' roles in supporting their youth.
- Provide appropriate resources (e.g., community resources, affirming individual and family mental health care resources) to assist parents/caregivers and families with the acceptance of their sexual minority children.

SUMMARY

Sexual minority youth have the same potential to develop into happy, well-adjusted adults as their heterosexual peers. Health disparities faced by SMY are modifiable; working to reduce stigma and homophobia in our communities will improve health outcomes for SMY and other youth. Sexual minority youth are a diverse group

TABLE 43.3

CDC's Sexually Transmitted Infection (STI) Screening Guidelines for Sexually Active Adolescents and Young Adults (≤25 Years)

	Sexually Active Women	Heterosexually Active Men	Men Who Have Sex with Men
Chlamydia and gonorrhea	All Retest 3 mo after treatment	Chlamydia: consider in high prevalence clinics or populations Gonorrhea: No recommended screening	Annually at all sites of contact (urethra, rectum, pharynx)* Every 3–6 mo if at increased risk *Testing for *Chlamydia trachomatis* pharyngeal infection is not recommended
Trichomonas	Consider in high-prevalence clinics or with high-infection risk	None	
Herpes	Consider HSV serology in persons presenting for STI evaluation (especially for persons with multiple partners)		Consider HSV serology in persons with prior undiagnosed genital ulcers
Syphilis	Pregnant women		Annually if sexually active Every 3–6 mo if at increased risk
HIV	All (opt-out) All who seek STI evaluation and treatment		Annually if sexually active with negative or unknown status, **and** >1 partner since last test (or partner with multiple partners)

Source: https://www.cdc.gov/std/treatment-guidelines/screening-recommendations.htm
HSV, herpes simplex virus.

of individuals, and clinicians must recognize the unique experiences of each patient. Adolescent and young adult clinicians have the opportunity to educate and support SMY and their families to promote healthy, well-adjusted transitions into adulthood. Clinicians should be comfortable and direct when asking youth about their sexual identity, behavior, and attractions. Further, clinicians should provide comprehensive education about safe sex, pregnancy planning and prevention, and sexual pleasure. Remember that all sexually active youth, regardless of identity and partner, should be screened for STIs and asked about pregnancy planning and/or prevention.

ACKNOWLEDGMENT

The authors wish to acknowledge Eric T. Meininger for contributions to previous versions of this chapter.

REFERENCES

1. White J, Sepúlveda MJ, Patterson CJ. *Understanding the Well-Being of LGBTQI+ Populations*. National Academies Press; 2020. doi:10.17226/25877
2. Centers for Disease Control and Prevention. 2019 Youth Risk Behavior Survey Data. Accessed April 19, 2021. https://www.cdc.gov/yrbs
3. American College Health Association. *American College Health Association-National College Health Assessment III: Reference Group Executive Summary Fall 2020*; 2020. Accessed April 22, 2021. https://www.acha.org/documents/ncha/NCHA-III_FALL_2021_REFERENCE_GROUP_EXECUTIVE_SUMMARY.pdf
4. Mcneely C, Blanchard J. The Teen Years Explained: A Guide to Healthy Adolescent Development.; 2009. https://www.jhsph.edu/research/centers-and-institutes/center-for-adolescent-health/_docs/TTYE-Guide.pdf. Accessed April 22, 2021.
5. Charlesworth TES, Banaji MR. Patterns of implicit and explicit attitudes: I. long-term change and stability from 2007 to 2016. *Psychol Sci*. 2019;30(2):174–192.
6. Russell ST, Fish JN. Mental health in lesbian, gay, bisexual, and transgender (LGBT) youth. *Annu Rev Clin Psychol*. 2016;12:465–487.
7. Ryan C, Russell ST, Huebner D, et al. Family acceptance in adolescence and the health of LGBT young adults. *J Child Adolesc Psychiatr Nurs*. 2010;23(4):205–213.
8. Raifman J, Moscoe E, Austin SB, et al. Difference-in-differences analysis of the association between state same-sex marriage policies and adolescent suicide attempts. *JAMA Pediatr*. 2017;171(4):350–356.
9. Woodford MR, Kulick A, Garvey JC, et al. LGBTQ policies and resources on campus and the experiences and psychological well-being of sexual minority college students: advancing research on structural inclusion. *Psychol Sex Orientat Gend Divers*. 2018;5(4):445–456.
10. Meyer IH. Prejudice, social stress, and mental health in lesbian, gay, and bisexual populations: conceptual issues and research evidence. *Psychol Bull*. 2003;129(5):674–697.
11. Crenshaw K. Demarginalizing the intersection of race and sex: a black feminist critique of antidiscrimination doctrine, feminist theory, and antiracist politics. *Univ Chic Leg Forum*. 1989;1989(1). Accessed March 25, 2021. http://chicagounbound.uchicago.edu/uclf/vol1989/iss1/8
12. Fields E, Morgan A, Sanders RA. The intersection of sociocultural factors and health-related behavior in lesbian, gay, bisexual, and transgender youth: experiences among young black gay males as an example. *Pediatr Clin North Am*. 2016;63(6):1091–1106.
13. Calzo JP, Blashill AJ, Brown TA, et al. Eating disorders and disordered weight and shape control behaviors in sexual minority populations. *Curr Psychiatry Rep*. 2017;19(8):49.
14. Murray SB, Nagata JM, Griffiths S, et al. The enigma of male eating disorders: a critical review and synthesis. *Clin Psychol Rev*. 2017;57:1–11.
15. Gay, Bisexual, and Other MSM | Volume 31 | HIV Surveillance | Reports | Resource Library | HIV/AIDS | CDC. Accessed April 22, 2021. https://www.cdc.gov/hiv/library/reports/hiv-surveillance/vol-31/content/msm.html#age
16. Sexually transmitted infections treatment guidelines, 2021. *MMWR Recomm Rep*. 2021;70(No. RR-4):1–187. Accessed July 27, 2021. https://www.cdc.gov/std/treatment-guidelines/default.htm
17. Charlton BM, Roberts AL, Rosario M, et al. Teen pregnancy risk factors among young women of diverse sexual orientations. *Pediatrics*. 2018;141(4):e20172278.
18. Choi SK, Wilson BDM, Shelton J, et al. *Serving Our Youth 2015: The Needs and Experiences of Lesbian, Gay, Bisexual, Transgender, and Questioning Youth Experiencing Homelessness*. The Williams Institute with True Colors Fund; 2015.
19. Kosciw JG, Clark CM, Truong NL, et al. *The 2019 National School Climate Survey: The Experiences of Lesbian, Gay, Bisexual, Transgender, and Queer Youth in Our Nation's Schools*. 2020. Accessed March 22, 2021. https://www.glsen.org/research/2019-national-school-climate-survey
20. Kahn E, Johnson A, Lee M, et al. 2018 LGBTQ Youth Report. Accessed April 25, 2021. https://www.hrc.org/resources/2018-lgbtq-youth-report
21. Coulter RWS, Bersamin M, Russell ST, et al. The effects of gender- and sexuality-based harassment on lesbian, gay, bisexual, and transgender substance use disparities. *J Adolesc Heal*. 2018;62(6):688–700.
22. Goldbach JT, Tanner-Smith EE, Bagwell M, et al. Minority stress and substance use in sexual minority adolescents: a meta-analysis. *Prev Sci*. 2014;15(3):350–363.
23. Scheer JR, Martin-Storey A, Baams L. Help-seeking barriers among sexual and gender minority individuals who experience intimate partner violence victimization. In: Russel B, ed. *Intimate Partner Violence and the LGBT+ Community: Understanding Power Dynamics*. Springer International Publishing; 2020:139–158.
24. Grace KT, Anderson JC. Reproductive coercion: a systematic review. *Trauma Violence Abuse*. 2018;19(4):371–390.
25. Bonar EE, Ngo QM, Philyaw-Kotov ML, et al. Stealthing perpetration and victimization: prevalence and correlates among emerging adults. *J Interpers Violence*. 2021;36(21-22):NP11577–NP11592.
26. Wagaman MA, Watts KJ, Lamneck V, et al. Managing stressors online and offline: LGBTQ+ youth in the southern United States. *Child Youth Serv Rev*. 2020;110:104799.
27. Laiti M, Pakarinen A, Parisod H, et al. Encountering sexual and gender minority youth in healthcare: an integrative review. *Prim Heal Care Res Dev*.2019;20:e30.
28. Substance Abuse and Mental Health Services Administration, Ending Conversion Therapy: Supporting and Affirming LGBTQ Youth. HHS Publication No. (SMA) 15-4928. Substance Abuse and Mental Health Services Administration, 2015. Accessed April 22, 2021. https://store.samhsa.gov/sites/default/files/d7/priv/sma15-4928.pdf
29. Levine DA, Committee On Adolescence. Office-based care for lesbian, gay, bisexual, transgender, and questioning youth. *Pediatrics*. 2013;132(1):e297–e313.
30. Amodeo AL, Esposito C, Bochicchio V, et al. Parenting desire and minority stress in lesbians and gay men: a mediation framework. *Int J Environ Res Public Health*. 2018;15(10):2318.
31. Centers for Disease Control and Prevention (CDC), US Public Health Service. *Preexposure Prophylaxis for the Prevention of HIV Infection in the United States—2017 Update: A Clinical Practice Guideline*. CDC website. Published March 2018. Accessed June 9, 2021. https://www.cdc.gov/hiv/pdf/risk/prep/cdc-hiv-prep-guidelines-2017.pdf

ADDITIONAL RESOURCES AND WEBSITES

Additional Resources and Websites for Clinicians:

Advocates for Youth—https://www.advocatesforyouth.org/

American Academy of Pediatrics—Adolescent Sexual Health—https://www.aap.org/en-us/advocacy-and-policy/aap-health-initiatives/adolescent-sexual-health/Pages/Sexual-History.aspx

CDC A guide to taking a sexual history—https://www.cdc.gov/std/treatment/Sexual History.pdf

Human Rights Campaign—www.hrc.org
Advocacy and research organization that promotes rights and well-being for all LGBTQ+ individuals

The National LGBT Health Education Center of The Fenway Institute—https://fenwayhealth.org/the-fenway-institute/education/the-national-lgbtia-health-education-center/
Provides educational programs, resources, and consultation to health care organizations with the goal of optimizing quality, cost-effective health care for lesbian, gay, bisexual, transgender, queer, intersex, asexual, and all sexual and gender minority (LGBTQIA+) people

Physicians for Reproductive Health—https://prh.org/medical-education/

SIECUS Sex Ed for Social Change—https://siecus.org/

What Works in Youth IIIV—https://whatworksinyouthhiv.org/strategies/prep-hiv-prevention

Additional Resources and Websites for Parents/Caregivers:

The Family Acceptance Project—http://familyproject.sfsu.edu/ is a research, intervention, education and policy initiative to promote the well-being of LGBTQ+ youth including diverse families amd conservative families to support their sexual and gender minority children.

PFLAG Parents, Families, and Friends of Lesbian and Gays—www.pflag.org is an organization supporting and connecting parents, families and friends of the LGBTQ community. There are over 400 chapters nationwide, in nearly every state. PFLAG provides confidential peer support, education, and advocacy to LGBTQ+ people, their parents and families, and allies.

Additional Resources and Websites for Adolescents and Young Adults:

It Gets Better—www.itgetsbetter.org
Mission is to communicate to LGBTQ youth around the world that it gets better, and to create and inspire the changes needed to make it better for them
Website features a stories page of over 60,000 video messages

Q Chat Space—https://www.lgbtcenters.org/QChatSpace
Professionally facilitated text-based online support groups
Gives youth safe opportunities to connect with each other in spaces moderated by trusted adults

The Trevor Project—www.thetrevorproject.org
Leading national organization providing crisis intervention and suicide prevention services to LGBTQ young people under 25
Resources, including a hotline, text and chat features, to support LGBTQ youth

CHAPTER 44

Transgender Adolescents and Young Adults

Johanna Olson-Kennedy

KEY WORDS
- Gender-affirming medical care
- Gender diverse youth
- Gender dysphoria
- Transgender youth

INTRODUCTION

"Transgender" is a broad term that is used to describe individuals who experience incongruence between their designated sex at birth and their internal sense of "maleness" or "femaleness." For many transgender people, this incongruence causes gender dysphoria, the persistent emotional, psychological, or physical distress about this incongruence. Many transgender people pursue a phenotypic gender transition utilizing hormones and/or surgery to more closely align their bodies with their internal gender identity. The last decade has seen a large increase in the number of transgender youth seeking medical intervention across the United States, Canada, and Europe in early and middle adolescence.[1,2] Unfortunately, little formal education about the care of these extraordinary youth is yet to be incorporated routinely into professional curricula.

Historically, the experience of gender incongruence has been assigned clinical diagnostic codes that fall under the umbrella of psychopathological conditions. The diagnosis "Gender Identity Disorder" was removed from the *Diagnostic and Statistical Manual of Mental Disorders, Fifth Edition* (DSM-5) and replaced by "Gender Dysphoria" in 2013.[3] The transgender experience should not be considered psychopathological, but the distress that results from the incongruence may often lead to functional problems that should be addressed by a team that includes both medical and mental health professionals.

Transgender adolescents and young adults (AYAs) face multiple medical and mental health challenges, including discrimination, harassment, violence, homelessness, eating disorders, anxiety, depression, and suicidality. While gender-affirming health care as well as the rights and protections for transgender individuals are becoming more available across the world, there remain significant challenges for the transgender community regarding access to medical care, legal document changes, victimization secondary to hate crimes and others. Medical interventions, including the use of puberty blockers and gender-affirming hormones (GAHs), can afford a transgender AYA the opportunity to live in a more authentic presentation of self, thereby mitigating some of the anxiety and depression that often accompany gender dysphoria. Parental/caregiver support is linked to lower depression, anxiety, and suicidality among transgender AYAs. Clinicians can offer critical support and affirming care for transgender AYAs and their families and encourage family members to do the same.

TERMINOLOGY

The elements that make up an individual's psychosexual identity include, but are not limited to, designated sex at birth, gender identity, gender expression, and sexual/romantic attraction.

Designated sex at birth is generally determined based on genital anatomy at the time of birth and is recorded on the birth certificate accordingly. In many states across the United States, this can be changed if someone identifies later as a different gender. There are still some states that do not allow this change.

Gender identity is an individual's internal sense and experience of "maleness" or "femaleness." For transgender AYAs, their gender identity is not aligned with their designated sex at birth.

Gender expression includes how an individual presents his/her or their gender with clothing, hair, name, pronouns, and mannerisms. Gender expression also includes gender performance; how an individual acts with respect to the cultural constructs and expectations around gender.

Sexual/romantic attraction refers to whom an individual finds romantically and/or sexually attractive. Sexual attraction is often mistakenly conflated with gender identity. Transgender AYAs have a range of sexual attraction identity labels and should not be assumed to have any particular sexual orientation labels based on their designated sex at birth. For example, an individual designated male at birth, who has a transfeminine identity, might be sexually and romantically attracted to males, females, both, neither, or any-gendered people. From a health care perspective, risk for sexually transmitted infections (STIs) and necessary screening should rely on assessment of specific sexual behaviors and presence of specific body parts.

Gender identity, gender expression, and sexual attraction are not binary. There are an infinite number of places along the spectrum of male → female or masculine → feminine that all people might identify. In addition, they may fluctuate over time, particularly gender expression. Transgender AYAs may make sociocultturally strategic decisions about gender expression in different environments. For younger adolescents, understanding that there is a spectrum of identities that are not limited to the male/female binary is important for them to move forward in their gender exploration process.

While professionals, academics, families, and allies adopt language to define the gender identities of others, it is critical to recognize that individuals should, and do, self-identify their own gender. Clinicians should be cognizant that the lexicon is dynamic, particularly among transgender AYAs, and best approached by asking each individual how they identify themselves before assigning a label. Some AYAs may prefer not to identify themselves as transgender in any way and identify simply as "boy/man" or "girl/woman."

Increasingly common are AYAs presenting to care who identify as "nonbinary." These young people identify outside of the traditional gender binary categories of male and female, and instead consider themselves both, neither, or something else entirely. The approach to nonbinary-identified AYAs requires attention to each individual's needs. Gender diverse or transgender AYAs should be asked about their chosen name and pronoun at each office visit. Inquiring about each young people's identity, name, and pronouns can help foster trust and develop rapport between clinician and patient.

PREVALENCE

There continues to be a lack of information accurately or consistently describing the prevalence of transgender individuals, and studies from around the world report a broad range from 1:200 to 1:100,000.[4–6] While specific prevalence rates are unknown, it is the case that increasing numbers of transgender youth are seeking care in clinics around the world.[1,2] The most recent prevalence data comes from the Williams Institute, and estimates the prevalence to be 0.6% of adults in the United States who identify as a transgender.[7]

ETIOLOGY

Many theories have attempted to explain the cause of gender incongruence ranging from hormone imbalance in utero to parental/caregiver psychopathology or history of trauma.[8,9] To date, no clear etiology has been identified that adequately provides a causal explanation for the transgender experience. The phenomenon of gender incongruence continues to be classified within the mental health domain, and transgender individuals are still in many cases required to complete a comprehensive psychiatric evaluation, as well as live for a certain amount of time in their authentic gender role in order to receive medical intervention for phenotypic transition. In addition, attempts are still made to try and dissuade or change individual's experienced gender identity with "corrective" therapy. While this approach has been repudiated by most medical and mental health professional societies, there are still some institutions that practice this outdated and damaging intervention with transgender people.

COMING OUT PROCESS

Transgender AYAs experience initial awareness about their gender incongruence in many ways. Many recognize from very early childhood that their gender is different than the one they were designated at birth. Some are able to articulate their experience to parents/caregivers, family members, or others in early childhood, and many cannot. Many transgender AYAs describe a history of feeling "different" but not necessarily ascribing that difference to gender incongruence until later in adolescence. Given the lack of information that parents/caregivers and clinicians have about transgender experience, it is common for young people to acquire such information from the internet. In other words, transgender AYAs will turn to the internet for such information. Perhaps it starts with a search for information about why people don't feel like the gender designated to them at birth. This may be followed by a long and arduous exploration of gender, and the development of an online community of other transgender AYAs. Limited data and clinical experience seem to indicate a bimodal distribution of transgender awareness in transgender boys/young men with one peak in early childhood and a second around or shortly after the experience of puberty. Gender dysphoria is commonly exacerbated, or initiated at the time of puberty, as the body begins to develop the permanent secondary sex characteristics of a gender that is misaligned with one's own understanding of their gender. Among transgender girls/

young women, there is more commonly awareness of gender incongruence during early childhood, although later discovery is also not uncommon. This may be due to the societal inability to tolerate those whom they perceive to be "boys in girls' clothing," which might subsequently drive parents/caregivers to seek professional care earlier. For youth who discover their transgender identity in adolescence, disclosure often occurs first to close friends, followed by parent/caregiver and extended family. Parent/caregiver response to the disclosure of transgender identity is critical to the well-being and future of these youth. Multiple studies have demonstrated the positive effect of supportive parents/caregivers. While it is true that many parents/caregivers react to their adolescent's disclosure of transgender identity with surprise, anger, confusion, and disbelief, those who are accepting, open, and supportive help mitigate the multitude of psychosocial challenges faced by transgender youth.[10]

EMOTIONAL AND BEHAVIORAL HEALTH

Mood Disorders and Anxiety

Transgender youth frequently have symptoms of mood disorders and anxiety that are intimately entangled with the experience of gender dysphoria. Many AYAs presenting for medical interventions are already engaged in mental health services and are often prescribed psychotropic medications. However, a diagnosis of depression or other mood disorder should not preclude an adolescent or young adult from initiating puberty suppression or GAH therapy. Anecdotal information suggests that individuals can wean or discontinue psychotropic medications altogether after initiating phenotypic gender transition. Close partnering with mental health professionals is strongly advised in cases where AYAs are experiencing significant mental health morbidities.

Homelessness

Transgender AYAs are disproportionately represented among the population of young people experiencing homelessness. While a broader understanding and greater tolerance of gender diversity is occurring in the United States and other parts of the world, it is still common for gender and sexual minoritized youth to be rejected by their families of origin. Transgender youth in the foster system are much less likely to remain in foster families, and more often placed in group homes. Youth experiencing homelessness are at increased risk for violence, poverty, drug use, human immunodeficiency virus (HIV), survival sex, and exposure to environmental hazards.

Violence

Transgender youth commonly report being victims of violence, hate crimes, sexual assault (see Chapter 78), harassment, bullying, and physical assault in school, communities, places of employment, and, too often, in their own homes. Assessment for history of and exposure to potential violence is an important part of screening at each visit.

Suicide

Suicidal ideation and attempts are extraordinarily high among transgender people compared to the population at large.[11] A recent study reported that 77% of transgender people over the age of 16 had seriously considered suicide, with 43% reporting an attempted suicide. One-third of those who had attempted had done so before the age of 15.[12] Research has demonstrated that parental/caregiver support is protective against depression and suicidality. In addition, a study in 2019 demonstrated a link between exposure in adolescence to reparative therapy and suicidality.[13] Discussing suicidal thoughts, plans, and access to carry out such plans (guns, knives, drugs, medications) with transgender youth is imperative, and should be revisited frequently. Even youth who are undergoing hormone treatment should be frequently queried about suicidal thoughts, plans, and attempts because gender incongruence is a permanent state even if phenotypic gender transition is undertaken. Gender dysphoria and its subsequent sequelae are difficult to predict and fluctuate over time.

HEALTH CONCERNS

Substance Use

Transgender AYAs use drugs and alcohol more than their cisgender (nontransgender) peers to cope with anxiety and distress related to gender dysphoria. Screening and referral for problematic drug use are important in these youth.

Eating Disorders

Clinical reports of eating disorders among transgender AYAs are common. Body dysphoria is pervasive and should be assessed at the initial visit with transgender patients seeking care. Again, the presence of an eating disorder should not preclude initiation of GAH care but needs to be simultaneously addressed by an experienced mental health professional.

Obesity

Intentional weight gain, in order to hide endogenous body shape, is common among both transgender boys/young men, transgender girls/young women and nonbinary young people. Both feminizing and masculinizing hormones can increase appetite; therefore, encouraging youth to have healthy eating habits and advising them to engage in regular exercise should be incorporated into routine anticipatory guidance.

Pregnancy

Specific sexual behaviors and acts should not be assumed in transgender AYAs. Inquiry about specific sexual acts using thoughtful and appropriate language will give clinicians more accurate information about pregnancy risk. In addition, all youth should be counseled that exogenous hormone use is not adequate birth control. Transgender young women/transfeminine AYAs can still impregnate other individuals even while taking feminizing hormones and blockers, and transgender young men/transmasculine AYAs can become pregnant despite using testosterone. Transgender AYAs should be advised to use birth control if they are engaging in sexual behaviors with associated pregnancy risk.

Sexually Transmitted Infections

While there are very few data regarding transmasculine AYAs and STI acquisition, it is important to advise those taking testosterone that are at increased risk for STIs due to thinning and drying of the vaginal walls. Youth should be reminded that if they are having receptive genital sex, adequate lubrication and care will help avoid tearing and undue exposure to infections. Atrophy of the vaginal lining is common and can be addressed with intravaginal estrogen. Human immunodeficiency virus infection rate is increased among transgender young women/transfeminine AYAs due to unprotected sex, survival sex, unmonitored hormone injections, and injection drug use. Transmasculine and nonbinary young people may also engage in survival sex; the concomitant use of needles for injecting hormones and drugs should not be overlooked by the clinician as it represents a significant health risk.

MEDICAL INTERVENTION

The approach to care for transgender youth is dependent on the age and sexual development of youth at presentation, presence of a social support system, medical condition, and the individual needs of youth regarding the presentation of their gender. While there continues to be a lack of consensus about the timing of initiation of GAHs, increasing numbers of gender-specific clinics are adopting a more individualized approach for these timelines. Most individuals accessing gender-affirming medical interventions are in mid-to-late adolescence, although the average age seems to be getting younger. The decision making around initiation of GAHs is one that is best done in conjunction with the youth, the family, and the health care team, which may include a medical and mental health clinician.

Hormones

Adolescents can be administered gonadotropin-releasing hormone analogs (GnRHa) in early puberty (sexual maturity rating [SMR] 2 or 3) to suppress the development of undesired endogenous secondary sexual characteristics.[14] Older AYAs can be prescribed GAHs to induce secondary sexual characteristics that more closely match their internal gender identity. Hormone-scheduling doses and medical monitoring are outlined in the *Endocrine Society's Clinical Care Guidelines*.[14]

Hormone Therapy Risk

GnRH Analogs

For youth who are starting GnRHa, the most concerning issue is slower bone mineral density (BMD) accrual during the period of GnRHa administration. In the earliest studies of youth undergoing pubertal suppression for gender-related concerns, BMD did not diminish during a year of treatment, but was lower than age-matched peers, indicating that BMD accrued at a prepubertal rate during treatment. However, BMD recovered after GAHs were added.[15] In 2020, Schagen et al. examined bone density trends among 78 youth and found that at the start of GnRHa treatment, mean areal bone mineral density (aBMD) and bone mineral apparent density (BMAD) values were within the normal range in all groups. In transfeminine youth, the mean z-scores were well below the population mean. Over 2 years of GnRHa treatment, BMAD stabilized or showed a small decrease, whereas z-scores decreased in all groups. During 3 years of combined administration of GnRHa and GAHs, a significant increase of BMAD was found. Z-scores normalized in transboys but remained below zero in transgirls.[16] More data is being collected to gain a better understanding of the clinical implications of GnRHa use in youth with gender dysphoria. Other clinical reports of emotional instability and weight gain have been reported in youth on GnRH analog treatment. GnRHa use does not impact fertility, but rather, provides a pause on pubertal development. Those youth who discontinue GnRHa and do not go on to GAHs will resume the changes of endogenous puberty a few months after discontinuing GnRHa. The most current Endocrine Society Guidelines recommend monitoring height, weight, sitting height, blood pressure, and Tanner staging every 3 to 6 months, leutinizing hormone (LH), follicle-stimulating hormone (FSH), estrogen/ testosterone, and 25OH vitamin D every 6 to 12 months, and bone density via DEXA scan at baseline, and every 1 to 2 years following initiation of GnRHa.[14]

Gender-Affirming Hormone Use

A growing body of evidence is available for documenting the medical side effects of GAH use in transgender adolescents[17]; however, it remains true that there is more to be learned about the physiologic impact of cross-sex hormones on mental and behavioral health outcomes. Potential side effects may be extrapolated with caution from dissimilar populations.

Estrogen and Androgen Blocker Therapy Estradiol and androgen antagonists may have side effects that include venous thromboembolic events, elevation of transaminases, prolactinoma, gallstones, and hyperkalemia (from spironolactone use). Less dangerous side effects include nausea, mood swings, decreased libido, shrinking of the testicles (often desirable), and decreased muscle mass. Desired changes include breast development, softening of the skin, increased emotions, slowed growth of facial and body hair, and diminished erections. All youth should be counseled about the potential loss of fertility, and if male pubertal development has progressed to SMR 3, sperm banking should be discussed as an option for those young people interested in future biologic offspring. Hormone scheduling doses and medical monitoring are outlined in the *Endocrine Society's Clinical Care Guidelines*.[14]

Testosterone Therapy The following side effects should be considered and discussed with patients initiating testosterone therapy: elevation of transaminases, insulin resistance, changes in lipid profile, and polycythemia. Less dangerous side effects include acne, increased libido, and premature scalp hair thinning/balding. Desired side effects include deepening of the voice, development of facial hair, male pattern body hair, clitoral enlargement, increased muscle mass and strength. While there are transgender men who have discontinued testosterone use, resumed ovulation, and carried and birthed their own children, it is unclear when, or if, fertility is no longer an option in the course of testosterone treatment. Harvesting eggs is expensive and difficult, but should be discussed with patients interested in preserving reproductive tissue for future use. In youth who begin treatment in SMR 2 or 3, viable ova will not have developed and will likely not be suitable for harvesting. A promising new technology includes preservation of ovarian tissue prior to initiation of testosterone use. Hormone scheduling doses and medical monitoring are outlined in the *Endocrine Society's Clinical Care Guidelines*.[14]

Surgery

Transmasculine: Surgical interventions for transgender males/transmasculine AYAs may include male chest reconstruction for those who have undergone female breast development prior to intervention and genital surgery for gender confirmation. Male chest reconstruction is increasingly being performed on minors, but genital surgery is generally delayed until youth reach the age of consent based on their state/province or country of residence.

Transfeminine: For transgender females/transfeminine AYAs, breast augmentation may be required, as well as genital reconstruction for gender confirmation. Genital surgery in transgender young women is usually delayed until youth reach the age of consent based on their state/province or country of residence.

Preintervention Assessment

The current standard of care recommends assessment of AYAs by mental health therapists skilled in gender-related care prior to initiation of medical intervention. While there are varying opinions about this model of care for transgender people, most agree that it is prudent to involve skilled and experienced mental health clinicians prior to, as well as during, the time youth are undergoing gender transition. Mental health therapists provide AYAs with a necessary "toolbox" of resiliency skills necessary to navigate phenotypic gender transition in adolescence or early adulthood. Historically, the role of mental health professionals has been emphasized in the period of time leading up to hormone initiation but recent data and clinical experience indicate that it is the period immediately following initiation of hormones that may be the most challenging and that patients may benefit more from mental health involvement in this time period.

OTHER ISSUES FOR TRANSGENDER ADOLESCENT AND YOUNG ADULTS

Sex-Segregated Facilities

Laws governing the use of appropriate sex-segregated facilities for transgender people vary across the world, and in the United States, across states. Many U.S. college campuses are moving toward supporting transgender people utilizing the sex-segregated facilities that correspond to an individual's gender identity, but this is certainly not universally applied. In addition, there have been a handful of states that have legislated appropriate access to sex-segregated locker rooms and restrooms in the K-12 school setting. These laws are still rare and are not always enforced in every school.

Electronic Records

Most electronic record systems document a gender marker that corresponds to the gender on an individual's birth certificate. This applies to schools as well as health care facilities. There is no consensus, nor systematized approach as to how to address the issue of incongruence between an electronic gender marker and an individual's identity; it becomes the purview of each institution about how to manage this discrepancy. In addition, prior to someone getting their name changed, a birth name of record is often what appears in an electronic documentation system. Transgender AYAs are often challenged with advocating for specific chart notations to be made that alert providers and administrators to use appropriate pronouns and names. This issue, if poorly managed, can lead to an individual's transgender status being inadvertently disclosed. In many states across the United States, birth certificates can be amended and reissued to accurately reflect name and gender with a physician's declaration document. There are currently 11 states, and Washington DC that allow individuals to have a nonbinary gender marker replace a designated birth gender marker on a birth certificate. While there are many countries that allow an individual to have their legal documents changed to reflect a gender marker correctly, some require surgical procedures, and some do not allow a gender marker changed at all.

APPROACH TO THE TRANSGENDER ADOLESCENT AND YOUNG ADULTS AND FAMILY

Transgender AYAs should be treated with the same dignity and respect as any other youth or young adult. Accurate names, pronouns, and use of specific names for body parts that feel most comfortable should be solicited and subsequently honored. Clinicians should model nonjudgmental and compassionate communication with youth in front of parents/caregivers and other family members. The needs of youth with gender dysphoria should be taken seriously, as the sequelae of untreated gender dysphoria can be life-threatening. Positive parental/caregiver engagement has a tremendous impact on a young people's current and future mental and physical health. Parental/caregiver rejection has been linked to depression, use of drugs and alcohol, and high-risk sexual behavior among teens. Because there is such a strong correlation between parental/caregiver support and well-being of transgender youth, parents/caregivers who are struggling to understand and accept their transgender children should be referred to local support groups, family gender conferences, and appropriate literature.

SUMMARY

In summary, increasing numbers of transgender young people are seeking medical intervention in adolescence. Gender affirming care and parental/caregiver support are critical determinants of mental health outcomes for trans and nonbinary youth. While provision of medical care currently remains within the purview of gender specialized clinics (within the United States and Western Europe), adolescent medicine clinicians are uniquely suited to initiate and continue care related to gender dysphoria.

ACKNOWLEDGMENTS

The author wishes to acknowledge Eric Meininger and Gary Ramafedi for their contributions to previous versions of this chapter.

REFERENCES

1. de Vries ALC, Cohen-Kettenis PT. Clinical management of gender dysphoria in children and adolescents: the Dutch approach. *J Homosex.* 2012;59(3):301–320.
2. Spack NP, Edwards-Leeper L, Feldman HA, et al. Children and adolescents with gender identity disorder referred to a pediatric medical center. *Pediatrics.* 2012;129(3):418–425.
3. American Psychiatric Association. *Diagnostic and Statistical Manual of Mental Disorders.* 5th ed. American Psychiatric Publishing; 2013.
4. De Cuypere G, Van Hemelrijck M, Michel A, et al. Prevalence and demography of transsexualism in Belgium. *Eur Psychiatry.* 2007;22(3):137–141.
5. Veale JF. Prevalence of transsexualism among New Zealand passport holders. *Aust N Z J Psychiatry.* 2008;42(10):887–889.
6. Gates G. *How Many People Are LGBT?* UCLA School of Law, Williams Institute. Accessed February 25, 2014. http://williamsinstitute.law.ucla.edu/wp-content/uploads/Gates-How-Many-People-LGBT-Apr-2011.pdf
7. Flores AR, Herman JL, Gates GJ, et al. *How Many Adults Identify as Transgender in the United States?* The Williams Institute; 2016.
8. Meyer-Bahlburg HF. From mental disorder to iatrogenic hypogonadism: dilemmas in conceptualizing gender identity variants as psychiatric conditions. *Arch Sex Behav.* 2010;39(2):461–476.
9. Gooren L. The biology of human psychosexual differentiation. *Horm Behav.* 2006;50(4):589–601.
10. Travers R, Bauer G, Pyne J, et al. Impacts of strong parental support for trans youth: a report prepared for Children's Aid Society of Toronto and Delisle Youth Services. Trans PULSE Project. Accessed February 25, 2014. http://transpulseproject.ca/wp-content/uploads/2012/10/Impacts-of-Strong-Parental-Support-for-Trans-Youth-vFINAL.pdf
11. Clements-Nolle K, Marx R, Katz M. Attempted suicide among transgender persons: the influence of gender-based discrimination and victimization. *J Homosex.* 2006;51(3):53–69.
12. Bauer GR, Pyne J, Francino MC, et al. Suicidality among trans people in Ontario: implications for social work and social justice. *Service Social.* 2013;59(1):35–62.
13. Turban JL, Beckwith N, Reisner SL, et al. Association between recalled exposure to gender identity conversion efforts and psychological distress and suicide attempts among transgender adults. *JAMA Psychiatry.* 2020;77(1):68–76.
14. Hembree WC, Cohen-Kettenis PT, Gooren L, et al. Endocrine treatment of gender-dysphoric/gender-incongruent persons: an endocrine society clinical practice guideline. *J Clin Endocrinology Metabolism.* 2017;102(11):3869–3903. https://doi.org/10.1210/jc.2017-01658
15. Delemarre-van de Waal HA, Cohen-Kettenis PT. Clinical management of gender identity disorder in adolescents: a protocol on psychological and paediatric endocrinology aspects. *Eur J Endocrin.* 2006;155(suppl 1):S131–S137.
16. Schagen SEE, Wouters FM, Cohen-Kettenis PT, et al. Bone development in transgender adolescents treated with GnRH analogues and subsequent gender-affirming hormones. *J Clin Endocrinol Metab.* 2020;105(12):e4252–e4263.
17. Mahfouda S, Moore JK, Siafarikas A, et al. Gender-affirming hormones and surgery in transgender children and adolescents. *Lancet Diabetes Endocrinol.* 2019;7(6):484–498.

ADDITIONAL RESOURCES AND WEBSITES

Additional Resources and Websites for Clinicians:
Gender Spectrum, resources for health professionals—https://www.genderspectrum.org/articles/online-programs-social-and-health
Guidelines for the Primary and Gender-Affirming Care of Transgender and Gender Nonbinary People—https://transcare.ucsf.edu/guidelines
The National LGBT Health Education Center – A Program of the Fenway Institute—https://fenwayhealth.org/the-fenway-institute/education/the-national-lgbtia-health-education-center/
World Professional Association for Transgender Health—https://www.wpath.org

Additonal Resources and Websites for Parents/Caregivers:
Gender Born, Gender Made by Diane Ehrensaft
Gender Spectrum—https://www.genderspectrum.org/articles/understanding-gender
The Transgender Teen by Stephanie Brill and Lisa Kinney
Trans Youth Equality Foundation—http://www.transyouthequality.org

Additional Resources and Websites for Adolescents and Young Adults:
Gender Spectrum—https://www.genderspectrum.org/articles/my-gender-journey
I am J by Chris Beam
Parrotfish by Ellen Whittlinger
Trans Youth Equality Foundation—http://www.transyouthequality.org
You and Your Gender Identity; A Guide to Discovery by Dara Hoffman Fox

CHAPTER 45

Adolescent and Young Adult Pregnancy and Parenting

Joanne E. Cox
Heather M. Bernard

KEY WORDS

- Abortion
- Contraception
- Pregnancy
- Prenatal care
- Parenting
- Unplanned

INTRODUCTION

Adolescent and young adult (AYA) pregnancy rates have significantly declined over the last three decades, yet challenges remain. There are significant regional differences in rates of AYA pregnancies, many of which are unplanned. Successful pregnancy prevention initiatives focus on delaying initiation of adolescent sexual activity, access to contraceptives, and youth-development initiatives. Both decreased sexual activity and improved access and use of contraception have contributed to declining rates. Risk factors for early unplanned pregnancy include poverty, history of trauma, cultural and family values that favor early pregnancy, behavioral health concerns, exposure to sexualized media, and lack of access to contraception. Evaluation of the pregnant AYA requires a nonjudgmental approach and presentation of all pregnancy options. Knowledge of potential pregnancy complications is important. Interventions for adolescent parents and their children that include both medical and social support successfully decrease repeat pregnancy and contribute to positive child and adolescent outcomes. Knowledge about abortion options, prenatal care needs, and pregnancy complications is important.

Although pregnancy rates have declined, since a peak year in 1991, by 81% for adolescents 15 to 19 years old and 66% for young adults aged 20 to 24 years, more AYA experience an unplanned pregnancy in the United States than in other industrialized countries.[1,2] Over 80% of adolescent pregnancies and 70% of pregnancies to unmarried females aged 20 to 24 years are unplanned.[2] Unplanned pregnancies are prevalent, especially in AYAs who are minoritized, of low-income status, and in those who have not completed high school. In 2011, 75% of pregnancies were unplanned in adolescent 15 to 19 years old, whereas in females aged 20 to 24 years, 59% of pregnancies were unplanned, resulting in considerable public cost.[3]

There are significant trends in comparing AYA pregnancy and birth rates (Figs. 45.1, 45.2, and 45.3)

- **Lifetime number of opposite sex sexual partners:** The number of lifetime sexual partners increases with age and is consistently higher among males than females (see Fig. 45.1).
- **Pregnancy rates:** Pregnancy rates increase with age up through age 29. The percentage of pregnancies that end in births increases with age, while the percentage ending in abortions decreases and miscarriages remain constant.
- **Birth rates trends:** In 2019, teen birth rates reached a nadir of 16.7 per 1,000 girls aged 15 to 19 years, compared to 66.6 per 1,000 young adults aged 20 to 24 years in 2019.[1] Trends show a decrease in birth rates among AYAs (see Fig. 45.2). Variables that affect AYA birth rates include race/ethnicity, social determinants of health, and geographic location. Over the last 15 years, Hispanic teens have had the highest teen birth rates.[1] Teen birth rates also vary considerably by state. In 2018, Arkansas had the highest teenage birth rates at 30.4 per 1,000 females aged 15 to 19 years. This compares to Massachusetts, with the lowest teenage birth rate at 7.2 per 1,000 females aged 15 to 19 years.[1] Geographically, teen birth rates declined more in large urban counties than small, medium-sized counties in the United States.[4]

FACTORS CONTRIBUTING TO ADOLESCENT AND YOUNG ADULT PREGNANCY

Poverty: Poverty is strongly associated with adolescent and unplanned young adult pregnancy. Unfortunately, minoritized communities experience poverty at higher rates than nonminoritized communities, contributing to the racial and ethnic disparities seen in adolescent parenthood. Recent evidence suggests that both long-term exposure to poverty and living in impoverished neighborhoods independently increase the risk of adolescent and unplanned pregnancy.[5] For AYAs, living in poverty may be associated with a lack of hope for the present and future, that translates into other risk behaviors and lack of attention for the consequences. A baby can represent success and hope for the future for AYAs faced with economic and educational obstacles.

Rates of sexual activity: There has been a decline in lifetime reports of sexual activity; however, in 2019, the current prevalence rate among 15 to 19 year olds was 29.0% for Black adolescents, 29.7% for Hispanic adolescents, and 27.5% for White adolescents.[6] Males are slightly more likely to be sexually experienced than females; and sexual activity increases with grade among 9th through 12th graders.

Physical and sexual abuse: Abusive relationships are common features in the lives of AYA mothers. Adolescents with a history of child abuse or neglect are twice as likely to experience early pregnancy.[6,7] Reproductive coercion by male partners is also a potential risk factor.

Cultural and family values: Many AYAs live in communities familiar with early parenthood, so they may be less likely to postpone sexual intercourse. Adolescents living in families with variable parental/caregiver support, little restriction of risky behaviors, and poorly defined goals are more likely to become sexually active and likewise to become adolescent parents. Other cultural factors

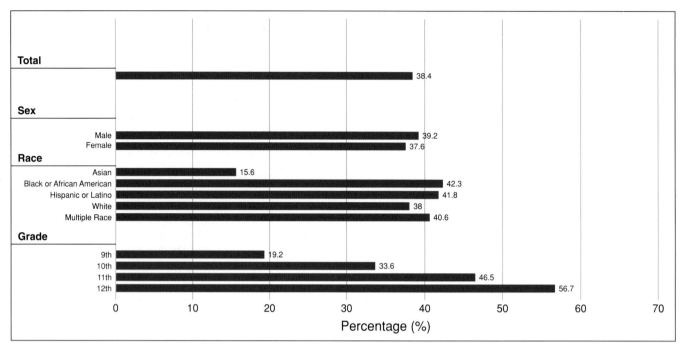

FIGURE 45.1 Prevalence of lifetime sexual intercourse in high school students, by sex, race, and grade level in the United States, 2019. Center for Disease Control and Prevention (CDC). *1991–2019 High School Youth Risk Behavior Survey Data.* Accessed March 28, 2021 http://yrbs-explorer.services.cdc.gov/

that may play a role in decisions to become pregnant include peer pressure, early dating, and lack of religious affiliation. Although more adolescents have delayed pregnancy, they often experience unplanned pregnancy as young adults.

Early initiation of sexual activity is not unusual if other family members have a prior history of becoming pregnant during

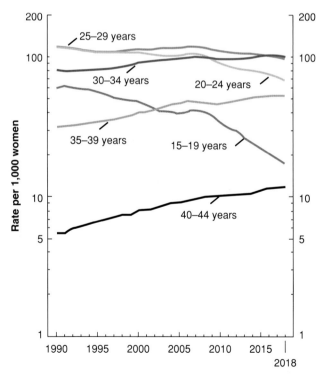

NOTE: Rates are plotted on a logarithmic scale.
SOURCE: NCHS. National Vital Statistics System, Natality.

FIGURE 45.2 Trends in birth rates (per 1,000) by age group of mother, in the United States, 1990 to 2018. From Martin JA, Hamilton BE, Osterman MJK, et al. National vital statistics reports births: final data for 2018. 2019;68(13):1980–2018.

adolescence. For example, adolescent parents may have mothers, sister, or brothers who were teen parents. Pregnancy can result in both joy or excitement and increased stress, which increases or decreases a sibling's risk of pregnancy.

Behavioral health: Although a causal relationship between depression and childbearing has been difficult to establish, mental health remains influential in adolescent parenthood.[8-10] Pregnant and parenting teens have high rates of depression, but they also often have poor social supports and conflicted relationships while living in low-income, violence-prone neighborhoods. These factors and circumstances can predispose them to mental health disorders.[9] Other risk behaviors associated with depression, such as substance use, are associated with concomitant sexual activity.[11]

Early puberty and development: Since 1900, the average age at onset of menarche has significantly decreased. This earlier physical maturation has widened the gap between reproductive capacity and cognitive and emotional development and has increased the risk of unintended pregnancy in this age group.

Many developmental characteristics of adolescents, particularly of younger teens, promote positive decision making regarding sexual activity and the successful use of contraceptives. These characteristics include the ability to plan for the future, foresee the consequences of their actions, or have a sense of personal invulnerability.

Access to and adherence with contraception: Obtaining and adhering to contraceptives remains critical to minimizing the number of unplanned AYA pregnancies. In 2019, about 10.1% of male high school students and 13.4% of female high school students did not use any method to prevent pregnancy during their most recent sexual intercourse. Among those who did use some form of contraception, the condom was most popular. About 60% of males and 49.6% of females used a condom during their most recent sexual intercourse. About 20% of males and 25.7% of females report using a birth control pill during their most recent sexual intercourse.[6]

Between 2015 and 2017, the most common contraceptive method ever used among female adolescents 15 to 17 years old who had ever had sexual intercourse was condoms (975), followed by the withdrawal method (65%), and oral contraceptives (53%). Methods associated with higher efficacy of pregnancy prevention,

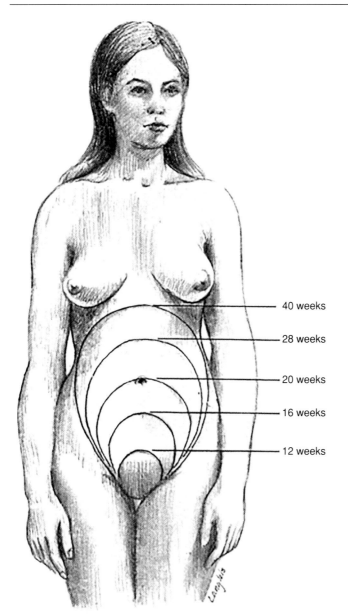

FIGURE 45.3 Uterine size by pregnancy date in weeks. Cox JE, Economy K. Teen pregnancy. In: Emans SJ, Laufer MR, DiVasta AD, eds. *Emans, Laufer & Goldstein Pediatric and Adolescent Gynecology*, 7th ed. Wolters Kluwer; 2019.

such as Depo-Provera (19%), long-acting reversible contraceptives (LARCs) (20%), and the implant (15%) had a lower prevalence of ever being used.[12] Other methods such as the patch and the ring were not commonly reported.[12]

Although positive attitudes toward pregnancy may be a factor in the failure to use contraception, access to confidential counseling and prescriptions are also important. In 1977, the U.S. Supreme Court ruled in favor of the constitutional right to privacy for minors to obtain contraceptives in all states. Currently, however, only 23 states and the District of Columbia explicitly allow all minors to consent to contraceptive services without the need for special circumstances.[13] Access to confidential care is key to the receipt of contraceptive services.[14] Additional barriers include loss of insurance coverage, lack of access to contraceptive care, and poor continuity of care.

Many environmental, social, and psychological barriers interfere with decision making regarding sexual activity and contraception among AYAs. Significant obstacles to successful contraception include inaccurate information, accessibility,

contraceptive acceptability, and pressures from interpersonal relationships. Some young women choose not to use contraception because they desire a baby. Adolescents and young adults may also experience barriers to acquiring contraception from their health providers. Clinicians may not address sexuality and contraception use, and patients may be embarrassed to initiate the discussion. Some clinicians may be overtly judgmental of sexuality and contraception. Clinicians may be unwilling to provide contraception to AYAs without parent consent.[14] Clinicians may be overly concerned about the safety of contraceptives, especially LARC methods such as the intrauterine device (IUD).[15] In a systemic review of youth perspectives on AYA-friendly health care, positive characteristics included readily accessible hours and appointments, positive staff attitudes, AYA-appropriate clinic space, and youth involvement in their health decision making.[16] Since many AYAs continue to see pediatricians through adolescence, the American Academy of Pediatrics Committee on Adolescents provided guidelines for the delivery of sexual and reproductive health services.[17]

REPEAT PREGNANCY

Repeat teen birth has decreased over the past two decades yet accounts for 16.7% of total births to teen mothers. Low-income, minoritized adolescents experience a disproportionate number of repeat births.[13] Between 2004 and 2015, the prevalence of repeat teen births was highest in Hispanic youth at 18.7%.[18] However, the most significant decline in percentage of repeat teen births occurred in non-Hispanic Black youth by 21.8%. Repeat pregnancy often adversely affects parenting by increasing stress and reducing maternal economic and educational outcomes. Inconsistent contraceptive use and high-risk sexual activity are known predictors of repeat pregnancy. Early postpartum use of LARC has demonstrated significant efficacy in preventing repeat pregnancies.[12]

Multiple interventions have been tested to decrease repeat pregnancy. Successful approaches often provide family planning, parenting, and social support elements.[19,20] Teen-tot medical homes, mentoring, motivational interviewing, and home visiting show promise. Adolescent and young adult mothers with a strong sense of control over contraceptive decision making and intent to prevent pregnancy are the most likely to avoid rapid repeat pregnancy.

ADOLESCENT PREGNANCY PREVENTION INTERVENTIONS

Many adolescent pregnancy prevention interventions have been implemented and studied over the last two decades. They generally fall into three categories: (1) clinic-based models with emphasis on counseling and access to contraception; (2) school-based abstinence-only and comprehensive educational programs; and (3) school-linked community programs.[21]

Program designs vary and may be developed by parents, schools, physicians, religious groups, social service agencies, and government departments. Successful programs include elements of abstinence promotion, contraceptive information/availability, sexual education, school completion strategies, job training, and other youth development strategies such as volunteerism and involvement in the arts or sports. Successful programs base program components on the age and developmental stage of the target group. Although abstinence effectively prevents pregnancy and sexually transmitted infections (STIs), abstinence-only education may lead to increased unprotected sexual activity in high school students.[22,23]

Research strongly supports a two-pronged approach to primary prevention by using methods to delay sexual initiation and by providing contraceptive education and availability if necessary. Comprehensive reproductive-health education is not associated with increased sexual behavior or teenage pregnancy. In fact,

IX

comprehensive sexuality programs have been shown to delay the onset of sexual activity, reduce the frequency of sexual activity, reduce the number of sexual partners, and increase the use of contraception.[22] As such, results from the National Survey of Family Growth demonstrate that adolescents aged 15 to 19 years who received comprehensive sexuality education were 50% less likely to report a pregnancy.[22]

EVALUATION AND MANAGEMENT OF THE PREGNANT ADOLESCENT AND YOUNG ADULT

When an adolescent or young adult presents to a health care facility for reproductive health services or advice, it is important to provide a welcoming, comfortable, and confidential environment.

Role of the Clinician

Determining whether a pregnancy is intentional or unintentional is imperative in planning the management of the pregnancy. Both the mother's age and her intentions behind the pregnancy may significantly affect the management of the pregnancy. An unplanned pregnancy can be a crisis for the young woman and her family. The clinician is uniquely positioned to offer guidance and support.

Pregnancy requires that the clinician balance their attention to the pregnant patient's medical issues and counseling needs. The young woman should be granted confidentiality as they discuss choices and plans. The clinician must also be familiar with their local laws on adolescent confidentiality as they vary geographically. In ideal circumstances, the adolescent or young adult's family and partner need to be considered as a plan is formulated to manage the pregnancy. However, the clinician must ascertain whether there has been sexual coercion, history of physical abuse, and whether the potential for abuse exists. Opportunities for intervention include the following:

- Diagnosis of pregnancy and facilitated decision making
- Open, nonjudgmental options counseling and service planning
- Screening for depression, substance use, resource insecurity, and domestic violence
- Management of pregnancy, if the AYA chooses to continue the pregnancy
- Preparation for parenthood, if the AYA chooses to raise the child
- Referrals for subspecialty services, as needed
- Support, if the AYA chooses adoption
- Family planning and safe-sex education

Despite a clinician's personal preferences, the clinician needs to counsel the patient about her options or refer her to a clinician who is comfortable counseling pregnant AYAs. If they are not available within the clinician's health program, appropriate external referrals for care should be made. Timeliness is important because some of the choices are only available during the early weeks of the pregnancy.

Common Presentations of Pregnancy

Adolescents and young adults may present with various complaints that may suggest early pregnancy. The most frequent objective concern is a missed or abnormal menstrual period. Others may report abdominal pain, fatigue, breast tenderness, vomiting, or appetite changes. Patients with such concerns should be queried about sexual activity, contraceptive use, and desire for a pregnancy test. Adolescents may need extra time to discuss their concerns and fears about a possible pregnancy. A flexible approach can allow patients to make healthy decisions for their particular situation.

Pregnancy Tests

The development of sensitive and specific pregnancy tests has significantly facilitated the early diagnosis of pregnancy. Young women are often unsure of their last menstrual period (LMP). This is even more likely in adolescents who may not yet have regular menstrual cycles. Pregnancy tests measure human chorionic gonadotropin (hCG), a glycoprotein that is secreted by invasive cytotrophoblast cells in early pregnancy and implantation. The most common is an immunoassay that detects serum levels of the beta subunit of hCG as low as 7 mIU/mL. Most urine pregnancy tests will detect hCG when levels exceed 25 mIU/mL, thus giving a positive test result around the first missed menstrual period with an accuracy of 93%.[24]

1. Human chorionic gonadotropin levels during pregnancy: The clinician needs to remember that hCG levels change significantly during pregnancy and that the results must be interpreted based on the particular test used (sensitivity and specificity). Serum hCG is detectable 8 days after conception in about 5% of women and by day 11 in more than 98% of women. At 4 weeks gestation, serum hCG doubling times are approximately 2.2 days, but only every 3.5 days by 9 weeks' gestation. Levels peak at 10 to 12 weeks' gestation and then decline rapidly until a slower rise begins at 22 weeks' gestation, which continues until term.
   a. Abnormally elevated levels can indicate either a multiple-gestation pregnancy or a molar pregnancy. In addition, anticonvulsants, phenothiazine, and promethazine may increase serum hCG levels.
   b. Abnormally low levels can indicate a spontaneous abortion or ectopic pregnancy. Low levels may also indicate delayed ovulation or implantation. Diuretics and promethazine can decrease hCG levels.
2. Serum hCG levels after pregnancy: Levels gradually decrease after delivery or abortion, and the initial decrease is quite rapid. After 2 weeks, the serum hCG level should be <1% of the level when the pregnancy was terminated.
   a. Term delivery: Levels should drop to <50 mIU/mL by 2 weeks—undetectable by 3 to 4 weeks.
   b. First-trimester abortion: Initial serum hCG levels are much higher. If the abortion is at 8 to 10 weeks and initial serum hCG levels are more than 150,000 mIU, then levels at 2 weeks can be 1,500 mIU/mL and detectable for 8 to 9 weeks.
3. Types of pregnancy kits
   a. Immunometric tests: These tests are based on enzyme-linked immunosorbent assay (ELISA) techniques that identify two antibodies for hCG, making these tests specific for the beta subunit of hCG. The urine test kits provide an accurate qualitative response within 2 to 5 minutes and measures hCG levels as low as 5 to 50 mIU/mL. These tests provide positive test results as soon as 10 days after fertilization. These are the most common tests used in most family planning and young women's health clinics.
      (1) Home pregnancy testing: Home pregnancy testings are popular because they are convenient, quick, and confidential. Home pregnancy testings are often used in the week after the missed menstrual period. During this period of pregnancy, urine hCG values are highly variable. The problem with this technique is that the young person may not follow instructions and this causes an inaccurate result, that is, performing test too early.
   b. Quantitative β-hCG immunoassay: This expensive, highly sensitive test for specific levels of serum hCG takes 4 hours to complete and is positive 10 to 18 days post conception. However, it has no advantage over the immunometric urine tests for the regular clinical setting. The major use is for identifying an abnormal pregnancy such as ectopic pregnancy or threatened miscarriage by checking the doubling time or hCG disappearance over time.
4. False-positive and false-negative results
   a. False-negative hCG test results most often occur with urine testing due to a misreading or interpretation of color

changes. There may be a hCG concentration below the sensitivity threshold of the test used, a miscalculation of the LMP, delayed ovulation, or delayed menses from early pregnancy loss. In addition, elevated lipids, immunoglobulin levels, and low serum protein levels can interfere with the serum test.

    b. False-positive test results with immunometric tests are rare but can also occur with laboratory error. Very rarely, pregnancy test results are positive from hCG production from a nonpregnancy source such as tumors of the ovaries, breast, and pancreas. For this reason, clinical correlation with the laboratory finding is essential. Should the laboratory result be inconsistent with the clinical presentation, the clinician must verify the pregnancy test result using more sensitive tests.

5. Ultrasound estimated crown-to-rump length is an accurate method for estimating the duration of pregnancy starting between 10 and 14 weeks. It has accuracy plus or minus 5 days.[25] Ultrasound can help confirm gestational age before referral to abortion services or prenatal care.

6. The physical examination is also an essential element of the initial evaluation. The pelvic examination will help determine the gestational age of the fetus and will identify any problems that may require immediate attention.

7. Uterine enlargement indicates the following (Fig. 45.3)
   - 8 weeks of gestation: Uterine enlargement detected.
   - 12 weeks of gestation: Uterus palpated at the symphysis pubis.
   - 20 weeks of gestation: Fundal height at the umbilicus. Fetal movements should be detected. Fetal heart sounds should also be audible by Doppler study.

8. Other signs
   - Reduction in muscle tone of the cervix, known as cervical softening
   - Discoloration of the cervix (it may appear purple or hyperemic)
   - Uterine softness
   - Vaginal bleeding or abdominal pain may indicate pregnancy complications, such as threatened abortion or an ectopic pregnancy, requiring further assessment.

Gestational Age

Most AYAs will want to know the gestational age of the fetus. Clinicians should carefully determine the LMP. Those with regular cycles lasting approximately 28 days can best predict the gestational age, which is calculated by counting the weeks since the LMP. Expected due-date calculators are available online, easily accessible, and helpful for calculating gestational age.

    The expected date of delivery (also called the expected date of confinement) can be obtained from the pregnancy wheel or is estimated using the Nägele rule. Add 7 days to the first day of the LMP, subtract 3 months from the month of the LMP, and add 1 year to the calculated date. If the uterus is smaller than expected by menstrual dates, the clinicians should consider an error in pregnancy test, an ectopic pregnancy, an incomplete or missed-spontaneous abortion, or fertilization occurred later than reported dates suggest. If the uterus is larger than expected, considerations include the following: twins, uterine fibroids, uterine anomaly, hydatidiform mole, or earlier fertilization.

⬤ PREGNANCY COUNSELING

Counseling the pregnant adolescent or young adult about her pregnancy options is perhaps the most important aspect of early pregnancy management. Clinicians who offer pregnancy tests should be prepared to provide such counseling and medical assessment, including pelvic examination for confirmation of gestational age of the fetus, STI screening, and multivitamins prescription with folate supplementation.

Critical elements of counseling the pregnant AYA include the following:

1. Clinical Assessment: Assess the individual's expectations and desires regarding the possible pregnancy. Privacy and confidentiality are critical. Identifying any stressors or safety concerns is useful while counseling the AYA about her test results. A private discussion permits the clinician to consider the AYA independent of others who may become involved with the pregnancy.

2. Confidentiality: The AYA patient is entitled to confidentiality, although family members sometimes disagree. Adolescents and young adults should be reminded that any discussions that occur in a health facility remain confidential unless they wish to inform or include others. This allows AYAs to make their own choices regarding disclosing the pregnancy. Occasionally, there are mental health concerns, such as the threat of suicide, homicide, or abuse that require the involvement of others. The clinician should familiarize themselves with the medical confidentiality laws of their geographic area, particularly regarding statutory rape, parental/guardian consent for termination, and judicial bypass statutes.

3. Support of the partner or concerned adult: The patient may be accompanied by a partner or an adult. In this case, patient should be offered the choice of including this person in a portion of the pregnancy counseling session. If the pregnancy test result is positive, the patient should be encouraged to seek the support of trusted adults (e.g., parents/caregiver, grandparents, or another trusted adult). These adults could form a "core of support" for the adolescent or young adult should she elect to carry the pregnancy to term or decide to terminate the pregnancy. The patient's partner may also share in the decision-making process. However, it is vital to first screen the AYA for safety in both their relationship and family domains.

4. Strength-based approach: The clinician needs to provide the opportunity for open discussion with a focus on strengths when counseling an AYA about a positive-pregnancy test result. The clinician should allow the individual to express her wishes for this pregnancy without imposing their personal values on the patient.

5. Presenting options: The AYA needs to consider the many options for their pregnancy, including:
   - Carrying the pregnancy to term and assuming parental responsibility
   - Family-centered care for the AYA and their new baby, thereby sharing child-care responsibilities with the baby's extended family
   - Placing the baby with adoptive parents after the baby is born
   - Terminating the pregnancy (e.g., induced abortion)

⬤ TERMINATING THE PREGNANCY

Among female AYA 15 to 19 years old, the percent of unintended pregnancies that result in abortion is 38%.[3] This rate is increased in younger populations; almost 49% of unwanted pregnancies result in abortion in girls younger than 15 years. Among women aged 20 to 24 years, 37% of all pregnancies result in abortion. This number increases to 41% when the pregnancy is unintended.[3] The abortion rate for women aged 15 to 44 years has declined from 16.9/1,000 in 2011, reaching a nadir of 11.3/1,000 in 2018.[26] There are many possible explanations for this trend, including fluctuation and variability in the availability and accessibility of abortions nationwide and an overall decrease in the number of pregnancies. Abortions are a service that is frequently offered in free-standing clinics that are separate from the more traditional primary health care programs. Thus, clinicians must often refer patients to another facility for this procedure. Some AYAs lack the skills to negotiate health services alone in a new health facility and may require scaffolding to successfully receive care. Mandatory waiting periods and Medicaid restrictions have decreased access to abortion services.

Clinicians of patients seeking an abortion should be aware that careful follow-up and psychological supports are needed while the AYA explores this option. They should be aware of their local laws governing abortion access and care for adolescents seeking abortion services. For instance, parental notification laws apply in the majority of U.S. states. Careful attention to legal considerations, including the rights of parents/caregiver, will be important as the clinician advocates for the adolescent. Any financial barriers that may interfere with the adolescent's ability to obtain an abortion should also be reviewed prior to referral for additional services.

Patients who are certain about their decision to terminate the pregnancy should be encouraged to do so in the early stages of the pregnancy. Early termination will minimize both the complications and the costs of the procedure. Induced abortions are usually performed within 8 weeks of conception.

After an AYA has decided to end her pregnancy, she may need help in selecting the best method. There are more termination options for those with early pregnancies, but AYAs may delay making this decision until after 15 weeks. Termination methods used in the first 12 weeks are safe and include vacuum aspiration, curettage, and medical terminations with either methotrexate-misoprostol or mifepristone-misoprostol.

Between 12 and 24 weeks, dilation and evacuation, amnioinfusion, and uterotonic/hypertonic techniques are utilized. Most young women have a first-trimester abortion and decide between a medical or surgical method.

Choice of Medical Versus Surgical Early Abortion Methods
Medical Method
Advantages of the medical method are that it avoids surgery and anesthesia, is less painful, may be easier emotionally, provides the patient with more control, is a more private process, and has less risk of infection. Medical methods can be used through the first trimester.[27]

Disadvantages of the medical method include bleeding, cramping and nausea, more waiting and uncertainty, extra clinic visit, limited to pregnancies up to 70 days of gestation, and risk of methotrexate-induced birth defects if abortion is incomplete.

Types of Medical Methods
First Trimester Mifepristone (RU-486) combined with misoprostol is the recommended therapy. Misoprostol alone is less effective.[27]
1. Mifepristone-misoprostol: Mifepristone is a synthetic progesterone antagonist that is an effective abortifacient. The efficacy increases with the addition of a prostaglandin analog such as misoprostol given either orally or vaginally. The earlier in pregnancy that these are used, the higher the efficacy. In women with pregnancies <7 weeks, 97% have a complete abortion.[27] The technique involves at least three visits:
   a. First visit: Mifepristone 200 mg
   b. 24 to 48 hours later: Misoprostol 800 µg. Some abortions are complete before this visit. If not, four 200-µg tablets are given orally. In those who have not aborted, two-thirds occur within 4 hours of the prostaglandin administration.
   c. Two weeks later: Checkup to ensure completed abortion
2. Second trimester
   Medical techniques for second-trimester abortions include hypertonic saline instillation, hypertonic urea instillation, and prostaglandin E₂ suppository insertion. These techniques account for less than 1% of all abortions in the United States. Most of these methods have been replaced by faster, safer, and less expensive dilation and evacuation procedures.

Surgical Method
The advantages of using a surgical method include that only one visit is required, the outcome is more certain, the AYA patient can be less involved, and it can be done under general anesthesia.

Types of Surgical Methods In the United States, surgical methods are the most common method of termination of pregnancy.
1. Vacuum aspiration
   a. The most widely used and standard first-trimester surgical method
   b. Relatively simple technique requiring small cervical dilation
   c. May be performed with local anesthesia
   d. Can be done in an office through 14 weeks' gestation
2. Dilation and evacuation
   a. Most common second-trimester method of abortion
   b. Requires more dilation than the aspiration method. Laminaria or other osmotic dilators are often inserted before the procedure to gradually dilate the cervix. This may be a 1- to 2-day procedure.
   c. Commonly used for procedures between 13 and 16 weeks. Many clinicians use this procedure up through 20-plus weeks.
   d. Para cervical or general anesthesia is used before evacuating the uterus.

Abortion Risks and Complications
Short-Term Postabortion Complications Infection occurs in up to 3% of all women. This is minimized by prior diagnosis and treatment of *Neisseria gonorrhoeae* and *Chlamydia trachomatis* as well as by the use of prophylactic antibiotics. Infection from retained products requires antibiotics and an additional procedure. Intrauterine blood clots occur in <1% of procedures. The use of laminaria and skillful technique lowers the risk of cervical trauma. Young women have lower risks of trauma.

Other complications include bleeding (0.03% to 1%) and failed abortion (0.5% to 1%). The mortality rate is less than 1 per 100,000 abortions.

Long-Term Postabortion Complications
Medical There are no long-term complications of abortion from the most common methods. First-trimester abortion with vacuum aspiration does not appear to affect fertility rates or cause future spontaneous abortions.

Psychological Although some studies report that AYA women may consider abortion a stressful experience, these symptoms are often short-lived and can be mitigated with support before, during, and after the procedure. For example, a population-based longitudinal study comparing women aged 15 years or older who received abortions, to those who were denied, showed that women who received an abortion suffered no increase in symptoms of anxiety and depression over a 2-year follow-up period.[28] It is important to note that postabortion stress may be higher in adolescents under age 18 years, especially if they perceived high levels of conflict with parents/caregiver.

🔴 MEDICAL MANAGEMENT OF THE PREGNANT ADOLESCENT

Prenatal care is a major factor predicting a positive outcome for an AYA birth. Factors associated with adequate prenatal care are increased age, a longer interpregnancy interval, partner/social support, and participation in a specialized pregnancy program. These programs often include a multidisciplinary team including medicine, social work, nursing, and nutrition. The following is a brief guide for the clinician on important areas of prenatal care for the AYA patient.
1. Initial evaluation should include a thorough history, including both a family history and a personal medical history for acute and chronic medical issues. A substance use history for tobacco, alcohol, and other drugs is important. Risk for human immunodeficiency virus (HIV) infection should be assessed. Due to a reluctance to disclose sensitive information during

an initial visit, clinicians should continue to assess risk status throughout the pregnancy as the relationship builds. A complete physical examination and pelvic examination should be performed. Laboratory evaluation should include complete blood cell count, urinalysis, blood type and group, syphilis serology, sickle cell test in patients of African descent, test for Tay–Sachs disease for Mediterranean or Jewish heritage, rubella titer, Papanicolaou test beginning at age 21, gonococcal and chlamydia tests, Hepatitis B serology, and HIV antibody counseling and testing.

2. Topics to be covered on successive visits include physiology of pregnancy, maternal nutrition, substance use, STIs and HIV infection, discussion and referral to a prepared childbirth class, childbirth, breastfeeding and infant nutrition, infant care and development, contraception, sexuality, and postdelivery care needs.

3. Nutrition: Ideal weight gain should be 25 to 40 pounds. The AYA should be advised against dieting during pregnancy. A prenatal vitamin supplement, containing iron and folic acid, should be prescribed. Additional iron is required if iron deficiency is diagnosed. Adolescents and young adults consuming <1,000 mg of calcium per day should be given a calcium and vitamin D supplement. Consumption of fruits and vegetables and avoidance of sugar-sweetened beverages and energy-dense foods should be encouraged.

4. Prenatal visits: Adolescents and young adults should have visits every 2 to 4 weeks, through the 7th month. Visits are every 2 weeks in the 8th month, and weekly thereafter.

5. Psychosocial aspects: It is essential to consider that the pregnant AYA's acceptance of the pregnancy and her relationship with her parents or the father of the child may change during the course of the pregnancy. Depression is common before, during, and after a teen pregnancy. Screenings at every prenatal visit is important.

6. Substance use: Due to the serious consequences of substance use for both mother and infant, a thorough assessment of past and present drug use is necessary at pregnancy diagnosis and throughout the prenatal period. The following is a list of common substances and their effects during pregnancy.
   a. Alcohol: Fetal alcohol syndrome including prenatal and postnatal growth retardation; facial dysmorphogenesis (microcephaly, short palpebral fissures, cleft palate, and micrognathia); abnormalities of the central nervous system (CNS); and increased risk of cardiac defects, joint abnormalities, hepatic fibrosis, mental retardation, and learning difficulties.
   b. Amphetamines: May cause malformations.
   c. Cocaine: Increased risk of spontaneous abortion and premature delivery; neurobehavioral deficits in the newborn; increased prevalence of abruptio placentae; increased risk of genital and urinary tract defects including prune belly syndrome, hypospadias, and hydronephrosis.
   d. Heroin: Intrauterine growth retardation; neonatal abstinence syndrome (infant irritability, tremor, convulsions, or poor feeding due to heroin withdrawal); increased risk of hepatitis, HIV, and other infections in the mother.
   e. Lysergic acid diethylamide: Increased risk of congenital abnormalities including hydrocephalus, spina bifida, and myelomeningocele.
   f. Marijuana: Although more research is needed, evidence suggests that marijuana use during pregnancy is associated with the risk of low birth weight and developmental problems.[29]
   g. Nicotine: Impaired growth; increased risk of spontaneous abortion.

7. Medications and pregnancy: The U.S. Food and Drug Administration classifies drug classes A through D in terms of whether benefits out way risks during pregnancy. Pregnant AYAs should be advised to avoid over-the-counter medications and herbal supplements unless they have been reviewed by their medical clinician.

8. The chronically ill AYAs: Pregnancy in chronically ill patients presents specific challenges and requires coordination with their specialty care providers. In addition, each illness may be associated with specific risks.

9. Human immunodeficiency virus infection: Clinicians should universally offer HIV counseling and testing to pregnant patients. Educational counseling should include the risks of perinatal transmission. Pregnant women infected with HIV should be referred for appropriate treatment and supportive services. Some women may choose to terminate their pregnancy once their HIV status is known. Due to the risks of HIV transmission through breast milk, breast-feeding is not recommended for HIV-infected mothers in the United States. In resource limited countries outside of the United States, the World Health Organization recommends that HIV-positive mothers exclusive breastfeed for the first 6 months. Infants will require treatment after delivery.

10. Domestic violence: Several studies have demonstrated an increased risk for domestic violence during and before a teen pregnancy. Violence can be severe, leading to injuries and death.[30] Battering often starts or becomes worse during pregnancy. Prenatal risk assessment should include specific questions regarding family and partner violence. Clinicians must be knowledgeable about domestic violence–reporting laws in their state and familiar with community resources.

MEDICAL COMPLICATIONS OF PREGNANCY

Adolescents are not at a higher risk of developing complications during early pregnancy. Potential complications for AYAs include the following:

1. Spontaneous abortion: A spontaneous abortion may occur in 20% of all pregnancies. A spontaneous abortion occurring in the first 20 weeks of pregnancy usually results from abnormal chromosomal development in the fetus or abnormalities of the pelvic structure within the AYA.

   Abdominal cramping and vaginal bleeding characterize the early stages of a miscarriage or spontaneous abortion. The term "threatened abortion" refers to pregnancies complicated by bleeding and cramping, but the cervix remains long and closed. Should the condition progress and the pregnancy is nonviable, an abortion is considered "inevitable." Physical changes include a widening of the cervical os and an increase in the bleeding and cramping. A "complete abortion" occurs when all the products of conception have passed. An ultrasound will confirm the absence of the fetus, and physical examination will show that the cervical os is closed. If the miscarriage is considered an incomplete abortion, a dilation and evacuation procedure will be necessary to prevent blood loss and infection.

2. Ectopic pregnancy occurs in 2% of pregnancies. Prior STIs and age over 35 years increase risk. Abdominal cramping and bleeding suggests an ectopic or extrauterine pregnancy.

3. Hydatidiform mole, or gestational trophoblastic disease, may occur in 1 of 1,000 pregnancies each year. Although AYAs commonly experience vaginal bleeding and abdominal cramping with a problem pregnancy, those with a hydatidiform mole usually have severe and profuse bleeding. The uterus is larger than expected given the estimated gestational age of the fetus, and the hCG levels are often >100,000 mIU/mL. Ultrasound of the uterus demonstrates the characteristic "cluster of grapes" appearance of the mass.

An immediate procedure is needed to terminate a molar pregnancy. Although the procedure is complicated because it places the patient at increased risk for severe hemorrhage, treatment with dilation and suction is the treatment of choice. Close follow-up of the serum hCG level is required to ensure that the tumor has been adequately removed. The hCG level should remain <2 mIU/mL for 1 year. If the hCG level remains elevated, it suggests that the tumor has not been sufficiently removed; if the hCG level rises, the tumor may have recurred. The patient should use a reliable method of contraception for the year after the diagnosis of trophoblastic disease.[31]

Adoption

While most AYAs who continue their pregnancy intend to raise their baby, some will express an interest in placing their child in a home with adoptive parents/caregivers. Few consider this option when the pregnancy test is obtained, although it is important that the pregnant AYA be counseled about it alongside other pregnancy options. In most states and the District of Columbia, pregnant minors may legally place their child for adoption without parental involvement. Less than 10% of the babies born to unmarried teens are placed in adoptive homes. Unmarried teen mothers who place their children for adoption are more likely to be White, have higher socioeconomic status and educational aspirations, and be from suburban residences.

OTHER CONSEQUENCES OF ADOLESCENT PREGNANCY

Child Outcomes

For adolescents older than 15 years, pregnancies do not have an increased risk of adverse outcomes if they receive adequate prenatal care. However, there are increased risks for teens <15 years, independent of prenatal care, for prematurity, low birth weight, and mortality. Factors associated with pregnancy outcome are variations in prenatal care, nutritional status, prepregnancy weight, STI exposure, smoking, and substance use.

Although there have been few recent long-term outcome studies, the children of teen mothers may face significant challenges with risks of developmental delay, behavioral problems, school failure, and behavioral health problems.[19] These outcomes are often mediated by the additional socioeconomic and socioemotional challenges that teen mothers face, such as depression, poverty, and lower educational attainment. Sons are at increased risk for incarceration and teen fatherhood and daughters are at increased risk for pregnancy; continuing family cycles of teen pregnancy. The toxic stress associated with poverty and violence exposure experienced in childhood may contribute to poor child developmental and psychological outcomes.[32] Rapid repeat pregnancy is also associated with poorer child developmental outcomes.

Growth and Development

No definitive data suggest that adolescent pregnancy adversely affects growth and development, although some recent studies have suggested small potential decreases in hip-bone mineralization and ultimate height in the very young pregnant adolescents. Young adolescents (e.g., <15 years) may not fully understand the long-term implications of childbirth, particularly in the early stages of the pregnancy.

Education and Socioeconomic Issues

Adolescent parenthood is associated with socioeconomic disadvantage. Mothers, who give birth before age 20, often delay school completion. Factors linked to higher educational attainment for adolescent mothers are older age at first birth, growing up in a smaller family, the presence of reading materials in the home, maternal employment, and higher parental educational level.[19] While 80% of young mothers receive governmental assistance at some point in time, most eventually do not receive public assistance.

Subsequent Childbirth

Adolescent parenting interventions often target repeat pregnancy because short interpregnancy intervals are associated with adverse pregnancy, neonatal, and child outcomes. Second births to adolescent mothers has declined over the past decade. However, within 2 years, approximately 18% of teen mothers become pregnant again.[28] Protective factors against repeat adolescent pregnancy are older maternal age (>16 years), participation in a specialized adolescent parent program, use of effective contraception, school attendance, new sex partner, and avoidance of interpersonal violence.

MALE ADOLESCENTS AND YOUNG ADULTS AS FATHERS

Young fathers rarely receive the same degree of attention and support offered to mothers, yet AYA men are at high risk for unplanned pregnancy. Fathers may not be included in decisions regarding pregnancy options, or establish a long-term supportive relationship with the child's mother. However, child outcomes improve when fathers participate in the child's care. Even if not romantically involved, AYA parents/caregivers need to negotiate their family responsibilities and plan childcare together.

Whenever possible, the clinician should attempt to discuss reproductive health issues with their sexually active male AYA patients. This is easily done during health maintenance visits, but it should also be done during acute visits for STI evaluation. In addition, asking the sexually active male patient about whether he has fathered a child and to inquire about his reproductive life plan is reasonable. Supportive counseling should be available for male AYAs who are actively involved with babies they have fathered and for male AYAs who have pregnant partners.

CARE OF YOUNG PARENTS AND THEIR CHILDREN

Parenting is the most common outcome, yet it is, in many respects, the most challenging because it requires the parenting AYA dyad, to assume long-term responsibility for a baby. A comprehensive care program that is designed to address the health and social needs of pregnant AYAs is optimal. Essential elements for prenatal programs include a complement of medical, psychological, social, and educational services; and linkages to mother/infant programs.[19]

Family-Centered Care for the Mother and Newborn

Because adolescents can rarely assume independence after the birth of a baby, the adolescent's family (or community) should prepare to offer support; young mothers are often lonely with inadequate support systems. Living arrangements may be unpredictable. Clinicians who care for the young parents/caregivers will need to link parenting AYAs to community-based services for extended families. Home-visiting programs can benefit both AYAs.

Adolescent parents benefit from comprehensive postnatal programs that combine medical care for the teens and their children with parenting education and social support. Patient-centered medical home practices or teen-tot clinics provide pregnant and parenting adolescents with integrated primary care and social/mental health services.[33] They can improve infant immunization rates, parenting abilities, and assist with the adolescent's return to school. The medical home should have readily available contraception, especially access to LARCs, immunizations, and well-baby care. Young parents are at increased risk for depression, school failure, poor parenting, and domestic violence and should be screened at each visit. Home-visiting programs can also be effective as well as school-based programs. Program staff should encourage enrollment of children in early childhood education programs such as Head Start. Long-term continuous relationships with caring clinicians are essential to positive outcomes.[19]

SUMMARY

Unplanned pregnancy for AYAs has significantly declined over the last three decades yet significant regional differences persist. Adolescents are overall becoming sexually active later and using more effective contraception. Effective pregnancy prevention programs focus on delaying sexual initiation, increasing the use of effective contraception, and offering youth development opportunities. When assessing a pregnant AYA, it important to use a nonjudgmental approach that includes discussing all pregnancy options. Medical abortions can be used through the first trimester. Significant pregnancy complications include spontaneous abortion, ectopic pregnancy, and hydatidiform mole. When an adolescent or young adult chooses to parent, medical home-based programs can improve outcomes for mother and child.

ACKNOWLEDGMENT

The authors wish to acknowledge Madeline Beauregard for their contributions to previous versions of this chapter.

REFERENCES

1. Martin JA, Hamilton BE, Osterman MJK. Births in the United States, 2019. *NCHS Data Brief*. 2020;(387):1–8.
2. *Power to Decide, the Campaign to Prevent Unplanned Pregnancy*. Accessed February 3, 2021. https://powertodecide.org/
3. Finer LB, Zolna MR. Declines in unintended pregnancy in the United States: 2008–2011. *N Engl J Med*. 2016;374(9):843–852.
4. Romero L, Pazol K, Warner L, et al. Reduced disparities in birth rates among teens aged 15–19 years—United States, 2006–2007, and 2013–2014. *MMWR Morb Mortal Wkly Rep*. 2016;65(16):409–414.
5. Penman-Aguilar A, Carter M, Snead MC, et al. Socioeconomic disadvantage as a social determinant of teen childbearing in the US. *Public Health Rep*. 2013;128(Suppl 1):5–22.
6. Redfield RR, Bunnell R, Greenspan A, et al. *Morbidity and Mortality Weekly Report Centers for Disease Control and Prevention MMWR Editorial and Production Staff (serials) MMWR Editorial Board*. 2020;69;1–80. Accessed March 25, 2021. https://www.cdc.gov/healthyyouth/data/yrbs/index.htm
7. Noll JG, Shenk CE. Teen birth rates in sexually abused and neglected females. *Pediatrics*. 2013;131(6):1181–1187.
8. Siegel RS, Brandon AR. Adolescents, pregnancy, and mental health. *J Pediatr Adolesc Gynecol*. 2014;27(3):138–150.
9. Hodgkinson S, Beers L, Southammakosane C, et al. Addressing the mental health needs of pregnant and parenting adolescents. *Pediatrics*. 2014;133(1):114–122.
10. Brown JD, Harris SK, Woods ER, et al. A longitudinal study of depressive symptoms and social support in adolescent mothers. *Maternal Child Health J*. 2012;16(4):894–901.
11. Centers for Disease Control U, Center for HIV N, Hepatitis V, Prevention T, of Adolescent D, Health S. *Substance Use and Sexual Risk Behaviors Among Youth*. Accessed March 25, 2021. www.cdc.gov/healthyyouth
12. Menon S; Committee on Adolescence. Long-acting reversible contraception: specific issues for adolescents. *Pediatrics*. 2020;146(2):e2020007252.
13. Office of Population Affairs. *Trends in Teen Pregnancy and Childbearing*. https://www.hhs.gov/ash/oah/adolescent-development/reproductive-health-and-teen-pregnancy/teen-pregnancy-and-childbearing/trends/index.html
14. Fuentes L, Ingerick M, Jones R, et al. Adolescents and young adult reports of barriers to confidential care and receipt of contraceptive services. *J Adolesc Health*. 2018;62(1):36–43.
15. Pritt N, Norris A, Berlan E. Barriers and facilitators to adolescents' use of long-acting reversible contraceptives. *J Pediatric Adolesc Gynecol*. 2017;30(1):18–22.
16. Ambresin A-E, Bennett K, Patton GC, et al. Assessment of youth-friendly health care: a systemic review of indicators drawn from young peoples' perspectives. *J Adolesc Health*. 2013;52(6):670–681.
17. Marcell AV, Burstein GR; Committee On Adolescence. Sexual and reproductive health services in the pediatric setting. *Pediatrics*. 2017;140(5):e20172858.
18. Dee DL, Pazol K, Cox S, et al. Trends in repeat births and use of postpartum contraception among teens—United States, 2004–2015. *MMWR Morb Mortal Wkly Rep*. 2017;66(16):422–426.
19. Powers ME, Takagishi J; Committee on Adolescence, Council On Early Childhood. Care of adolescent parents and their children. *Pediatrics*. 2021;147(5):e2021050919.
20. Cox JE, Harris SK, Conroy K, et al. A parenting and life skills intervention for teen mothers: a randomized controlled trial. *Pediatrics*. 2019;143(3):e20182303.
21. Lavin C, Cox JE. Teen pregnancy prevention: current perspectives. *Curr Opin Pediatr*. 2012;24(4):462–469.
22. Breuner CC, Mattson G; Committee On Adolescence, Committee on Psychosocial Aspects of Child and Family Health. Sexuality education for children and adolescents. *Pediatrics*. 2016;138(2):e20161348.
23. Fox AM, Himmelstein G, Khalid H, et al. Funding for abstinence-only education and adolescent pregnancy prevention: does state ideology affect outcomes? *Am J Public Health*. 2019;109(3):497–504.
24. Cole LA, Khanlian SA, Sutton JM, et al. Accuracy of home pregnancy tests at the time of missed menses. *Am J Obstet Gynecol*. 2004;190(1):100–105.
25. Whitworth M, Bricker L, Neilson JP, et al. Ultrasound for fetal assessment in early pregnancy. *Cochrane Database Syst Rev*. 2010;(4):CD007058.
26. Kortsmit K, Jatlaoui TC, Mandel MG, et al. Abortion Surveillance—United States, 2018. *MMWR Surveill Summ*. 2020;69(7):1–30.
27. Creinin MD, Grossman DA; Committee on Practice Bulletins—Gynecology Society of Family Planning Medication. Abortion up to 70 days of gestation. *Obstet Gynecol*. 2020:136(4);e31–e47.
28. Foster DG, Steinberg JR, Roberts SCM, et al. A comparison of depression and anxiety symptom trajectories between women who had an abortion and women denied one. *Psychol Med*. 2015;45(10):2073–2082.
29. Conner SN, Bedell V, Lipsey K, et al. Maternal marijuana use and adverse neonatal outcomes: a systematic review and meta-analysis. *Obstet Gynecol*. 2016;128(4):713–723.
30. Palladino CL, Singh V, Campbell J, et al. Homicide and suicide during the perinatal period: findings from the national violent death reporting system. *Obstet Gynecol*. 2011;118(5):1056–1063.
31. Seckl MJ, Sebire NJ, Fisher RA, et al. Gestational trophoblastic disease: ESMO clinical practice guidelines for diagnosis, treatment, and follow-up. *Ann Oncol*. 2013;24(Suppl 6):vi39–vi50.
32. Siegel BS, Dobbins MI, Earls MF, et al. Early childhood adversity, toxic stress, and the role of the pediatrician: translating developmental science into lifelong health. *Pediatrics*. 2012;129(1):e224–e231.
33. Cox JE, Buman MP, Woods ER, et al. Evaluation of raising adolescent families together program: a medical home for adolescent mothers and their children. *Am J Public Health*. 2012;102(10):1879–1885.

ADDITIONAL RESOURCES AND WEBSITES

Additional Resources and Websites for Clinicians:

Centers for Disease Control and Prevention-Breastfeeding during HIV Infection—https://www.cdc.gov/breastfeeding/breastfeeding-special-circumstances/maternalor-infant-illnesses/hiv.html
This Centers for Disease Control and Prevention site provides all the latest recommendations on breastfeeding in pregnant women.

Centers for Disease Control and Prevention-Reproductive health: Teen Pregnancy—https://www.cdc.gov/teenpregnancy/index.htm
This Centers for Disease Control and Prevention site provides all the latest data on adolescent pregnancy.

U.S. Department of Health and Human Services: Teen Pregnancy Prevention Program—https://opa.hhs.gov/grant-programs/teen-pregnancy-prevention-program-tpp
This website summarizes adolescent pregnancy prevention program funding.

What Works for Disadvantaged and Adolescent Parent Programs: Lessons from Experimental Evaluations of Social Programs and Interventions for Children—https://www.childtrends.org/wp-content/uploads/2013/04/Child_Trends-2012_08_20_WW_ParentPrograms.pdf
This Child Trends article reviews 20 parenting programs for adolescent parents.

Additional Resources and Websites for Parents/Caregivers:

Power to Decide—https://powertodecide.org
This website provides data and latest information on adolescent and young adult unplanned pregnancy prevention.

Youth.gov Office of Adolescent Health—https://youth.gov/federal-agencies/office-adolescent-health
This federal agency provides grant support and information about adolescent pregnancy prevention.

Additional Resources and Websites for Adolescents and Young Adults:

Centers for Disease Control and Prevention—https://www.cdc.gov/teenpregnancy/index.htm
This website provides all the latest data on adolescent pregnancy.

Power to Decide—https://powertodecide.org
This website provides data and latest information on adolescent and young adult unplanned pregnancy prevention.

Youth.gov Office of Adolescent Health—https://youth.gov/federal-agencies/office-adolescent-health
This federal agency provides grant support and information about adolescent pregnancy prevention.

IX

Contraception

Romina Loreley Barral
Melanie A. Gold

KEY WORDS

- Birth control
- Combination hormonal contraception
- Contraception
- Contraceptive implant
- Depot medroxyprogesterone acetate
- Emergency contraception

- Family planning
- Female contraception
- Intrauterine device
- Levonorgestrel
- Long-acting reversible contraception
- Ovulation inhibition
- Unintended pregnancy

INTRODUCTION

In the United States, rates of pregnancy, abortion, and birth among adolescents and young adults (AYAs) started to decline early in the 1990s, reaching historically low numbers due to availability of newer and more effective contraceptive methods. A significant proportion of AYAs switched to longer acting hormonal methods that were introduced to the U.S. market in the early 1990s, including an injectable contraceptive (Depo-Provera) and an implant (Norplant). By 1995, more than one in eight teen contraceptive users (13%) were using a longer acting method.[1] Over the last decade, improved contraceptive methods with more advantages have become available. In spite of an increase in use and availability, there remains an underutilization of the most effective methods in the United States compared to other developed countries.[2]

The unintended pregnancy rate among adolescents in the United States has been declining since the late 1980s. It increased slightly between 2001 and 2008, then declined substantially between 2008 and 2011: among girls aged 15 to 19 years old, 82% of pregnancies were unintended in 2008, compared to 75% in 2011; whereas 64% of pregnancies were unintended among 20 to 24 years old in 2008 and 59% in 2011.[3] More detailed data on unintended pregnancy in adolescents are included in Chapter 45. Despite marked declines over the last three decades, pregnancy rates continue to be higher in the United States than in many other industrialized countries and marked sociodemographic disparities continue to persist.[1]

Sexual Activity and Contraceptive Usage

Use of contraceptive methods has increased worldwide. As per the National Health Statistics Report (NHSR) from the National Survey of Family Growth (NSFG) released in June 2017, contraceptive use overall at last intercourse among never-married sexually active females 15 to 19 years old increased between 1988 (79.9%) to 2002 (83.2%) and 2011 to 2015 (89.9%); 56.5% used a condom, 31.5% used the pill, and 12.6% used other hormonal methods. The NSFG found racial variations with non-Hispanic White female teenagers

reporting NCHS higher percentages of using the pill at last sex (39.3% compared with 20.8% and 13.3% among Hispanic and non-Hispanic Black teenagers, respectively); dual method use (condom plus hormonal method) had the same pattern.

The same report revealed that during 2011 to 2015, the most common method used at first intercourse among 15 to 19 years old in the United States was the condom (76% in 2011 to 2015 trending up from 71% in 2002) followed by the pill (20% in 2011 to 2015 trending up from 15% in 2002). The use of dual methods at first sex increased significantly from 10.4% in 2002 to 19% in 2011 to 2015.[2]

According to the National Center for Health Statistics (NCHS) Data Brief released in May 2020,[4] in 2015 to 2017, 78% of U.S. females and 89% of males, aged 15 to 24 years, who had sexual intercourse before age 20 used a method of contraception the first time they had sexual intercourse. This was more common for those whose coitarche was at ages 15 to 16 (79%) and 17 to 19 (83%) compared with those whose coitarche was at earlier at age 14 (57%).

According to this same report, the most common ever used methods among sexually active 15- to 19-year-old females were the condom (97%), withdrawal (65%), or the pill (53%). Approximately 19% ever used emergency contraception (EC) and 20% of female teenagers ever used long-acting reversible contraception (LARC), including intrauterine device (IUD, 5%) and contraceptive implant (15%).

For current contraception use, the latest NCHS Data Brief for 2017 to 2019 period indicated that approximately 38.7% of women aged 15 to 19 years and 60.9% of those aged 20 to 29 years were using some type of contraceptive.[5] Pill use generally decreased with increasing age with 19.5% of women aged 15 to 19 years and 21.6% of women aged 20 to 29 years currently using the pill compared with 10.9% of those aged 30 to 39 years. Condom use was similar among women aged 20 to 29 years (10.4%) and 30 to 39 years (9.7%); use was lower among women aged 15 to 19 years (5.1%) and 40 to 49 years (6.5%). Use of LARCs was similar among women aged 20 to 29 years (13.7%) and 30 to 39 years (12.7%). Compared with these age groups, LARC use was lower among women aged 15 to 19 years (5.8%) and 40 to 49 years (6.6%).

This same report indicated overall current use of any method of contraception was higher among older women and non-Hispanic White women compared with younger women and Hispanic and non-Hispanic Black women, for ages 15 to 49 years. More specifically, pill use was higher among non-Hispanic White women (17.8%) compared to Hispanic (7.9%) and non-Hispanic Black (8.1%) women. Condom use was lower among non-Hispanic White women (7.0%) compared to Hispanic (10.5%) and non-Hispanic Black (11.0%) women. Current use of LARCs did not significantly differ across the Hispanic-origin and race groups shown, around 10% to 11%.

Although no data are available yet, we anticipate an important negative impact of COVID-19 pandemic on rates of contraception utilization due to decreased access to health care in general.

CONTRACEPTIVE METHODS

Most unintended pregnancies are the result of contraceptive failure or nonuse. Both the effectiveness inherent to each method (perfect use) and how correctly and consistently each method is used (typical use) can affect overall effectiveness of each contraceptive method (Table 46.1). The gap between perfect use and typical use increases with methods that are more user dependent. Adolescents represent a group with higher failure rates for many user-dependent methods as well as higher discontinuation rates compared to adult women. Estimates of contraceptive failure from the 2006 to 2010 NSFG showed that although between 1995 and 2006 to 2010 the overall failure rate declined significantly across most demographic subgroups; women younger than 30 years of age still have a higher probability of contraceptive failure (specifically with pills, condom, or withdrawal) compared to the relevant reference groups (women older than 30) for the first 12 months of use.[6] In addition, adolescents often use contraceptive methods inconsistently (nearly half "take breaks") or discontinue them early (up to half discontinued combination oral contraceptives [COCs] within the first 6 months of use) compared to adult women.

The NSFG report[6] also noted racial and ethnic differences among women 15 to 44 years old: African American (AA) and Hispanic women had significantly higher probabilities of method failure compared to White women for all methods combined (15%/14% vs. 8%) and for condom use (21%, 19%, and 9%, respectively). Pill failure rates also differed between AA and White women (13% vs. 6%), but there were no differences by race or ethnicity for withdrawal. It is important that clinicians remember that social determinants of health shape access and utilization of health care and may explain these differences, rather than assume these differences are due to inherent characteristics of the affected population.

Throughout this chapter, we reference the United States Medical Eligibility Criteria for Contraceptive Use (U.S. MEC),[7] an excellent resource that provides guidance on contraceptive method safety for women with specific medical conditions. Chapters 47 to 49 provide detailed information on specific contraceptive methods.

LONG-ACTING REVERSIBLE CONTRACEPTIVE METHODS

Long-acting reversible contraceptives include intrauterine contraception (IUC) and subdermal contraceptive implants. These are top-tiered contraceptive methods based on effectiveness, with failure rates of less than 0.1% per year for both perfect and typical use (see Chapter 49). These methods have the highest rates of continuation and satisfaction of all reversible contraception among adolescents. The American College of Obstetricians and Gynecologists (ACOG), the American Academy of Pediatrics (AAP), the U.S. Centers for Disease Control (CDC), and the World Health Organization (WHO), all recognize the potential impact of LARCs to reduce unintended pregnancies. Following ACOG recommendations, discussions about contraception should follow a tiered approach, beginning with review of the most effective methods.[8] Tier 1 methods such as LARC, do not rely on the user. Tier 2 methods rely on consistent use daily (pill), weekly (patch), every 3 weeks (vaginal ring), or every 3 months (depo-medroxyprogesterone acetate [DMPA]). Finally, tier 3 methods include those that rely on the user during sexual activity (male and female condom, spermicide, natural family planning), or immediately after EC.

Contraceptive counseling needs to include a reproductive health justice framework given past use of LARCs for fertility control in communities that have been traditionally marginalized. This includes supporting patient autonomy in selecting a method and choosing when to start it, ensuring the provision of equitable care, and avoiding potential coercion.[8] Potential sources of coercion can include parents/caregivers, partners, and peers. A clinician's own enthusiasm for LARCs, could be an inadvertent additional source of coercion.[9] The ACOG Committee Opinion on counseling adolescents about contraception reaffirmed lessons on contraception in 2019: "Patient choice should be the principal factor driving the use of one method of contraception over another, and respect for the adolescent's right to choose or decline any method of reversible contraception is critical."[8]

Long-acting reversible contraception was not used sufficiently among 15 to 19 year olds to make reliable estimates prior to 2006 to 2010. Once they were introduced to this population, the percentage of teenagers who had ever had sexual intercourse and ever used a LARC quickly increased from 3.1% between 2006 to 2010, to 5.8% between 2011 to 2015, and finally 20% between 2015 to 2017.[2,4] Latest estimates of current use indicate 5.8% of teens 15 to 19 years old used LARCs from 2017 to 2019.[5]

The latest NCHS data brief report from NSFC, published in 2020 and with data from 2017 to 2019, revealed LARC use to be similar among women aged 20 to 29 (13.7%) and 30 to 29 (12.7%), but lower among women aged 15 to 19 (5.8%) and 40 to 49 (6.6%). Current use of LARCs was higher for women with some college, but no bachelor's degree (12.5%) and women with a bachelor's degree or higher (13.1%) compared with women with a high school diploma or who have passed the General Educational Development (GED) test (7.9%). Current use was not significantly different from use among women without a high school diploma or GED (9.3%).[5] Current LARC use also did not significantly differ across Hispanic (10.3%), non-Hispanic White (10.9%), and non-Hispanic Black women (10.9%).[5]

In the United States, reasons identified for lack of LARC use, include, but are not limited to:
* women's lack of knowledge about and nonaccepting attitudes toward methods
* pervasive misconceptions about risks and benefits of use
* restrictive counseling and practice patterns of clinicians
* myths and misconceptions among both users and clinicians
* high initial up-front costs associated with initiating methods (despite cost-effectiveness over time)

Long-acting reversible contraception may have another advantage. One cause of unintended pregnancy among AYA women is the rate of sexual assault, which is higher for youth than among any other group. Dating violence among adolescents is also an increasing risk affecting this age group, and strong associations of intimate partner violence (IPV) with unintended pregnancy have been reported. Male partners may attempt to get partners pregnant, by flushing COCs down the toilet, removing contraceptive vaginal rings, and poking holes in condoms. Long-acting reversible contraceptives are ideal for women in these violent or coercive settings to prevent unwanted pregnancies resulting from sexual assault or IPV. In fact, the copper IUD allows for discrete contraception because it is less likely to affect menstrual cycle regularity. Although the removal of an IUD may be more challenging, the strings can be cut high up in the cervical canal if there is a need to hide the presence of the IUD or concern that the partner may feel or pull on the strings.

Intrauterine Devices
Current Use

Data from NHSR[10] found that ever use of an IUD among 15- to 44-year-old women in the United States declined from 1982 (18%) through 2002 (5.8%), but increased between 2002 and 2006 to 2010 (7.7%). Adolescents continue to report using less effective contraceptive methods. Data from the 2012 NHSR showed that between 2006 and 2010, 2.7% of adolescents, aged 15 to 19 years, who used contraception reported using an IUD, compared to 5.6% and 5.9% in women aged 20 to 24 years and 25 to 44 years, respectively. Data published in the 2017 NHSR showed that ever use of an

TABLE 46.1

Percentage of Women Experiencing an Unintended Pregnancy During the First Year of Typical Use and Perfect Use of Contraception and the Percentage Continuing Use at the End of the First Year—the United States

Method	Women Experiencing an Unintended Pregnancy Within the First Year of Use		Women Continuing Use at 1 y[c] (%)
	Typical Use[a] (%)	Perfect Use[b] (%)	
No method[d]	85	85	
Spermicides[e]	21	16	42
Withdrawal	20	4	46
Fertility awareness-based methods	15		47
Ovulation method[f]	23	3	
Two-Day method[f]	14	4	
Standard days method[f]	12	5	
Natural cycles[f]	8	1	
Symptothermal method[f]	2	0.4	
Sponge	17	12	36
Parous women	27	20	
Nulliparous women	14	9	
Diaphragm[g]	17	16	57
Condom[h]			
Female	21	5	41
Male	13	2	43
Combined pill and progestin-only pill (POP)	7	0.3	67
Evra patch	7	0.3	67
NuvaRing	7	0.3	67
Depo-Provera	4	0.2	56
Intrauterine device (IUD)			
ParaGard (Copper-T)	0.8	0.6	78
Skyla (13.5 mg levonorgestrel [LNG])	0.4	0.3	
Kyleena (19.5 mg LNG)	0.2	0.2	
Liletta (52 mg LNG)	0.1	0.1	
Mirena (52 mg LNG)	0.1	0.1	80
Nexplanon	0.1	0.1	89
Tubal occlusion	0.5	0.5	100
Vasectomy	0.15	0.1	100

Emergency Contraceptives: Use of emergency contraceptive pills or placement of a copper intrauterine contraceptive after unprotected intercourse substantially reduces the risk of pregnancy.

Lactational amenorrhea method: LAM is a highly effective temporary method of contraception. However, to maintain effective protection against pregnancy, another method of contraception must be used as soon as menstruation resumes, the frequency of or duration of breastfeeds is reduced, bottle feeds are introduced or the baby reaches 6 months of age.

[a]Among typical couples who initiate use of a method (not necessarily for the first time), the percentage who experience an unintended pregnancy during the first year if they do not stop use for any other reason. Estimates of the probability of pregnancy during the first year of typical use for spermicides, withdrawal, fertility awareness-based methods, the diaphragm, the male condom, the pill, and Depo-Provera are taken from the 2006–2010 NSFG corrected for underreporting of abortion; see the text for the derivation of estimates for the other methods.

[b]Among couples who initiate use of a method (not necessarily for the first time) and who use it *perfectly* (both consistently and correctly), the percentage who experience an unintended pregnancy during the first year if they do not stop use for any other reason. See the text for the derivation of the estimate for each method.

[c]Among couples attempting to avoid pregnancy, the percentage who continue to use a method for 1 year.

[d]This estimate represents the percentage who would become pregnant within 1 year among women now relying on reversible methods of contraception if they abandoned contraception altogether.

[e]150 mg gel, 100 mg gel, 100 mg suppository, 100 mg film.

[f]About 80% of segments of FABM use in the 2006 to 2010 NSFG were reported as calendar rhythm. Specific FABM methods are too uncommonly used in the United States to permit calculation of typical use failure rates for each using NSFG data, rates provided for individual methods are derived from clinical studies. The Ovulation and TwoDay methods are based on evaluation of the cervical mucus. The Standard Days method avoids intercourse on cycle days 8 through 19. Natural Cycles is a fertility app that requires user input and basal body temperature recordings and dates of menstruation and optional LH urinary test results. The symptothermal method is a double-check method based on evaluation of cervical mucus to determine the first fertile day and evaluation of cervical mucus and temperature to determine the last fertile day

[g]With spermicidal cream or jelly.

[h]Without spermicides.

Adapted from Trussell J. Contraceptive efficacy. In: Hatcher RA, Trussell J, Nelson AL, et al., eds. *Contraceptive Technology.* 21th revised ed. Ardent Media; 2018.

IUD between 2011 and 2015 among adolescents aged 15 to 19 years has remained unchanged (2.8%)[2] and between 2015 and 2017 use had increased to 5%.[4]

Although IUDs are extremely effective and safe methods with the lowest adverse side effect profiles, there are multiple myths and misconceptions about their use among both clinicians and users. The most frequently cited misconceptions among patients include fear of the IUD causing an abortion, risk of pelvic inflammatory disease (PID), secondary infertility after IUD removal, ectopic pregnancies, hair loss, as well as osteoporosis and cancer. Patients are also concerned about the quantity of bleeding following IUD insertion, the amount of weight change, and the level of pain during insertion. Further, there remains a misunderstanding that insertion must take place at a particular time during the menstrual cycle. In addition, clinicians have misconceptions regarding the need to obtain parental/caregiver consent and safety for inserting IUDs in nulliparous women, the latter of which has been successful. The CHOICE study showed high acceptance of LARC among teens, and nulliparity is not a contraindication to IUD use (see Chapter 49).[11]

Advantages

Hormonal IUDs are not only effective for contraception, but also provide other noncontraceptive health benefits, such as decreasing dysmenorrhea, menorrhagia, and endometriosis. Intrauterine devices are among the most efficacious contraceptive methods with the advantage of being estrogen free. Both the hormonal and copper IUDs are also the most effective EC methods available (see section on EC at the end of this chapter). Intrauterine devices are also highly effective methods of contraception for patients with contraindication to other hormonal methods. For example, the copper IUD (Category 1), levonorgestrel (LNG) IUD (Category 3), and progestin-only pills (POPs) (Category 3) are highly recommended for patients with autoimmune disorders and positive antiphospholipid antibodies.[12]

Current Availability in the United States

Copper 10 Year Intrauterine Device (Paragard)

The copper IUD (Paragard), manufactured by Cooper Surgical Inc, is one of the most effective EC methods when used within 5 days of unprotected sexual intercourse.

Levonorgestrel-Intrauterine Devices

There are currently four LNG-releasing IUDs available in the United States (Table 46.2).[13] Mirena, Skyla, and Kyleena are manufactured by Bayer. Mirena was the first available LNG containing IUD (U.S. Food and Drug Administration [FDA] approved in 2000), followed by Skyla (2013) and then Kyleena (2016). Skyla and Kylena have smaller, shorter devices with a lower dose of LNG compared to Mirena. Liletta was approved in 2015 and brought to the market as a generic form of Mirena (approved 2016) to lower cost and increase access.

Implants (Etonogestrel Implant or Nexplanon)

Current Use

Contraceptive implants were not used sufficiently among adolescents to make reliable estimates prior to 2006 to 2010. In 2006 to 2010, 0.6% of teenagers had ever used a contraceptive implant. By 2011 to 2015, 5.8% of teenagers had ever used LARC, with 3.0% having used implants.[2] Between 2015 to 2017, 20% of female teenagers had ever used LARC, with 15% of them having used the implant.[4]

Several studies have confirmed the high efficacy, convenience, and cost-effectiveness of the contraceptive implant. However, restricted availability of trained clinicians, limited marketing, and high initial cost have contributed to limited use in the United States. Norplant (FDA approved by 1990) was the first implant and it consisted of six rods containing LNG (FDA approved by 1990). It was eventually removed from the market in 2002 due to complications with insertions and removals and manufacturing issues. Implanon, a 68-mg etonogestrel (ETG) containing implant, was FDA approved in 2006 and provided improved insertion and removal of a single rod.[11] In 2010, it was replaced by Nexplanon or Implanon NXT (Merck & Co.). Identical in size and hormone content to the original Implanon, this implant has a "next-generation applicator" that facilitates subdermal insertion of the implant using one hand and prevents deep or even intravascular insertions. To facilitate in situ localization of the implant, the Nexplanon rod contains 15 mg of barium sulfate, making it radiopaque and detectable by 2-dimensional x-ray imaging and computer tomography. Ultrasound scanning with a high-frequency linear array transducer (10 MHz or greater) or magnetic resonance imaging may be used,

TABLE 46.2
IUD Names and Characteristics[14]

IUD Name	Active Ingredient (Dose)	FDA-Approved Duration of Use (years)	Potential Efficacy Beyond FDA-Approved Duration (years)	Efficacy[a]	Menstrual Impact	Amenorrhea at 1 y (Percentage)	String Color
Paragard	Copper 380-mm wire	10	12	0.80	Cyclical menses, maybe heavier flow with cramps	NA	White
Mirena	Levonorgestrel (LNG) (52 ug)	5 initially, now 6	7	0.20	Lighter, less frequent menses, improved cramps	20	Gray
Liletta	LNG (52 ug)	3 initially, now 6	5	0.20	Lighter, less frequent menses	19	Blue
Kyleena	LNG (19.5 ug)	5	—	0.30	Menses are likely to still be present	12	Blue with silver ring on stem
Skyla	LNG (13.5 ug)	3	—	0.30	Cyclic menses	6	Gray with silver ring on stem

[a]Percentage of women experiencing an unintended pregnancy in the first year of use. FDA, U.S. Food and Drug Administration.

as well.[11] To prevent migration of the implant, the device should be inserted 3 to 5 cm below the biceps' grove to avoid large vessels and nerves. The duration of efficacy for Nexplanon was initially FDA-approved for up to 3 years; more recent data support effectiveness for up to 5 years.[11]

Advantages

Etonogestrel implants provide highly effective, discreet, easy-to-use, convenient, long-acting, estrogen-free contraception. Implants are a particularly good choice for postpartum adolescents and young women whose risk for a blood clot is elevated and for whom estrogen is contraindicated. The ETG implant effectively inhibits ovulation by preventing luteinizing hormone (LH) surge and inhibits endometrial proliferation. These two effects explain its use as an option in the hormonal treatment of endometriosis and dysmenorrhea.[11] The most frequent reason for Nexplanon early discontinuation is frequent bleeding. Despite anecdotal overestimations, U.S. studies indicate only 11% to 14% of users request early removal due to bleeding.[11] Bleeding patterns are usually unpredictable. Studies found that implant users with "satisfactory" bleeding in the first 3 months postinsertion were likely to continue with favorable bleeding patterns. Another third of users develop satisfactory bleeding patterns in the second 3 months, while another third continue to have unsatisfactory bleeding even 6 months postinsertion. Overall, prolonged or frequent bleeding is more common in the early months of implant use.[11]

Current Availability in the United States

Nexplanon, manufactured by Merck & Co., is the only implant currently marketed in the United States; it is a 40- × 2-mm single rod containing 68 mg of ETG, the biologically active metabolite of desogestrel, covered with a rate-controlling membrane of ethylene vinyl acetate that slowly releases ETG.

⬤ INJECTABLES (DEPOT MEDROXYPROGESTERONE ACETATE: DEPO-PROVERA OR DMPA)

Current Use

Depo-Provera or DMPA is a popular contraceptive choice that is widely used among AYAs in the United States. According to NSFG data, the use of DMPA in female adolescents aged 15 to 19 years remained relatively stable between 2002 (20.7%) and 2006 to 2010 (20.3%).[2] Between 2011 to 2015, 17.3% of all female teenagers had ever used injectables (17.2% used Depo-Provera and 0.04% used Lunelle, which was discontinued in 2002).[2] Between 2015 to 2017, 19% of female teenagers 15 to 19 years who had ever had sexual intercourse had ever used DMPA.[4]

Advantages

Advantages of DMPA include the following:
- High effectiveness including a 2-week grace period at the end of the 3 months during which DMPA can be given and contraceptive efficacy remains unchanged; this is ideal for AYA women who have poor adherence to other user-dependent methods.
- Estrogen-free contraceptive
- Convenience and low maintenance, as well as intercourse and partner independent
- Initial cost of approximately $50 per injection for each 12-week interval of use
- Ideal method for breastfeeding women, given its lack of negative impact on lactation and on the infant's growth[11]
- For young women with sickle cell disease, DMPA is particularly beneficial because it reduces the incidence of sickle cell crises.[11]
- Progesterone has anticonvulsant effects by reducing neuronal excitability and DMPA does not have drug interactions with common anticonvulsants that compromise effectiveness of other

oral and implantable contraceptive methods making it ideal for women with seizure disorders.
- Depot medroxyprogesterone acetate leads to very light or absent bleeding by the third dose,[11] and has a long history of clinical use to suppress menses. Amenorrhea is a side effect that is frequently desired by AYA women and can prevent anemia and iron deficiency. This might be particularly useful for developmentally delayed AYAs for whom menstrual hygiene is challenging.
- Other benefits include decreased incidence of primary dysmenorrhea, endometriosis, ovulation pain, improvement of menstrual symptoms (breast tenderness, mood swings, headaches, nausea, and cyclic menstrual cramps), and functional ovarian cysts.[11]
- Depot medroxyprogesterone acetate decreases risk of endometrial cancer by 80% and decreases incidence of uterine fibroids and ectopic pregnancies.
- Because DMPA creates thick mucus and amenorrhea, there is a decreased incidence of PID in adolescents with cervicitis who use DMPA.

Availability in the United States

Depot medroxyprogesterone acetate was approved by FDA in 1992 and is the only injectable preparation for contraception available in the United States. Its intramuscular (IM) formulation consists of 150 mg of medroxyprogesterone acetate in an aqueous suspension administered in the gluteal or deltoid muscle area every 11 to 13 weeks. In December 2004, the FDA approved a micronized formulation of 104-mg DMPA that can be administered subcutaneously in the abdomen or thigh (DMPA-SC). Although currently not widely used, there is potential to expand access to subcutaneous DMPA if an autoinjector for self-administration was available as this would be convenient, especially in circumstances of limited clinical access (e.g., during a pandemic).

⬤ COMBINATION METHODS: COMBINATION ORAL CONTRACEPTIVE PILLS, CONTRACEPTIVE PATCH, AND CONTRACEPTIVE RING

Combined methods include COCs, the combined hormonal patch, and the combined vaginal ring. The combined hormonal patch and vaginal ring are relatively newer contraceptive methods. Combination hormonal contraceptives do not protect against sexually transmitted infections (STIs) or human immunodeficiency virus (HIV) (see Chapter 48).

Combination Oral Contraceptive Pills
Current Use

Combination oral contraceptives have been the most common contraceptive method used by women and their partners in the United States, second only to female sterilization. Among 15- to 19-year-old women, COC pill use decreased from 61% in 2002, to 53% between 2006 to 2010, and remained stable between 2011 to 2015[2] and 2015 to 2017.[4] However, by 2017 to 2019, use dropped to 19.5%.[5]

Advantages

Combination oral contraceptive pills have many noncontraceptive benefits and are first-line off-label therapy for women who experience heavy or prolonged menstrual bleeding, infrequent or painful menses, recurrent luteal phase ovarian cysts, family history of ovarian cancer, personal risk factors for endometrial cancer, acne and hirsutism, and polycystic ovary syndrome (PCOS). Combination oral contraceptives regulate menstrual periods, improve premenstrual syndrome (PMS) and premenstrual dysphoric disorder (PMDD), and decrease anovulatory bleeding and pain caused by ovulation (Mittelschmerz disease syndrome), menstrual migraines, risk of benign breast conditions, episodes of sickle cell crises, catamenial seizures, iron deficiency anemia, symptoms of endometriosis, and risk of uterine fibroids. They have favorable impact on bone health for high-risk women. Extended use of COCs are an off-label for treatment of anemia due to heavy or prolonged menstrual bleeding and control of menses in developmentally delayed women who often struggle with menstrual hygiene. Continuous or extended cycling offers reliable ovulation suppression, decrease in estrogen withdrawal symptoms, and a decrease in unscheduled bleeding episodes with similar compliance to monthly cycling, although it may cause unscheduled bleeding in the initial 3 to 6 months of use.[11]

Availability

Different formulations are available: monophasic, multiphasic, and variable combinations, but they all have similar advantages and effectiveness.[11] Pills can be packaged with 7 days of hormone free intervals (monthly cycling) or a shortened or even eliminated hormone free intervals (extended use or continuous cycle use).

Even though COC components and doses have changed over time with new hormone compounds being introduced, the two chief components remain the same: estrogen and progestin. Ethinyl estradiol (EE) provides the estrogen component in most COCs, while different progestins have been used as the progestin component. There are different progestin classification systems, but the most commonly used categorizes progestins into generations. The first three generations of progestins are derived from 19-nortestosterone and the fourth generation is drospirenone. Newer progestins are hybrids.

Contraceptive Ring and Patch
Current Use

Data for ever use of the contraceptive ring among 15 to 19 year olds are available starting in 2006 to 2010 and remained stable at 5% throughout 2011 to 2015,[2] the latest data analyzed for ever ring use in this age group. Ever use of the contraceptive patch among sexually experienced female adolescents aged 15 to 19 in the United States was reported as 1.5%, 10.3%, 1.8%, and 1% in 2002, 2006 to 2010, 2011 to 2015,[2] and 2015 to 2017,[4] respectively.

Advantages

Ring and patch advantages are similar to COCs, with the benefit that neither method requires daily use nor oral administration and they are verifiable methods (patients can see or feel them), which could facilitate consistent and correct use. Both methods have comparable cycle control to COCs. The ring has excellent cycle control, especially in the first 6 months of use, and is less likely to produce irregular bleeding compared to COC pills. Patch users experience more breakthrough bleeding in the first two cycles of use compared to COC pill users.

Availability

The vaginal contraceptive ring (NuvaRing) was FDA approved in 2001. It is a soft, translucent, and flexible ethylene vinyl acetate copolymer ring with a 4 mm cross-sectional diameter. It releases 120 µg of ETG and 15 µg of EE daily. The ring is designed to be placed vaginally and kept in for 3 weeks, then removed for 7 days to allow a withdrawal bleed before insertion of a new ring. It is commonly used for extended cycling.[11] There is no generic form.

A year-long ring was recently approved by the FDA in August 2018. Annovera is a translucent ethylene vinyl acetate copolymer ring, similar in diameter to NuvaRing (56 mm vs. 54 mm), but twice as thick (8.4 mm vs. 4 mm). It contains 103 mg of segesterone acetate (SA, a new nonoral progestin) and 17.4-mg EE and has daily hormonal release rates similar to NuvaRing of SA 150 mcg/day and EE 13 mcg/day. The ring is designed to be placed vaginally and kept in place for 3 weeks, then removed for 7 days to allow a withdrawal bleed before insertion of *the same* ring. Its package serves as reservoir for safe keeping during the withdrawal week. Unlike NuvaRing,

an unopened package does not require refrigeration. There is no generic form. There are no reported data on use by adolescents.

Progesterone vaginal rings have been approved for medical use since 1998, developed by the Population Council, and available since 2014 in a number of South and Central American countries, but not in the United States.

In 2002, the FDA approved a transdermal contraceptive patch (Ortho Evra), a beige colored 20-cm patch that contains 6 mg of norelgestromin (NGMN) and 0.75 mg of EE, releasing 150 mcg/day of NGMN and 35 mcg/day of EE. The patch is applied to upper arms or torso (excluding the breasts), lower abdomen, or buttocks for 7 days, and replaced weekly for 3 weeks, allowing a patch-free week for withdrawal bleeding before starting the next cycle. In 2005, the FDA required that Ortho Evra's label include a warning about the increased levels of estrogen and increased risk of blood clots in women who are using the patch compared to the pill. The FDA strengthened the warning in 2008 and in 2011, the FDA upgraded that warning to a "black-box" warning. Ortho Evra was discontinued in the United States after the FDA approved Xulane in 2014. Ortho Evra is still available in Canada and Europe. Xulane, a generic hormonal birth control patch, delivers the same levels of estrogen as the Ortho Evra patch and has a black-box warning regarding an increased risk of heart disease, heart attack, and stroke. As per its label, "the risk of VTE may be greater with Xulane in women with a body mass index (BMI) >30 kg/m² compared to women with a lower BMI. Xulane is contraindicated in women with a BMI ≥30 kg/m²." In addition, there is limited and conflicting evidence that contraceptive patches might have lower effectiveness in patients who weigh more than 90 kg.[11]

A new hormonal patch, Twirla, was released by the Agile pharmaceutical company and FDA approved in 2020. This patch works like Ortho Evra and Xulane but is round and slightly larger (28 cm²) than the Xulane (14 cm²) patch. It contains 2.6-mg levonorgestrel and 2.3 mg EE, and releases 120 mcg/day LNG and 30 mcg/day EE, with lower EE daily dose compared to other patches, and with a progestin that has been associated with decrease rates of venous thromboembolism (VTE) compared to other progestins. Its label indicates a contraindication for women with a BMI >30 kg/m² and those who are older than 35 years and smoke tobacco.

Progestin-Only Pills
Current Availability

The progestin dose is lower in POPs compared to the dose in COCs (hence the name "mini-pill"). Until recently in the United States, there was only one available POP containing 0.35-mg norethindrone (Micronor, Ortho-McNeil; Nor-QD, Watson; Nora-BE, Watson; Jolivette, Watson; Camila, Barr; Errin, Barr; Heather, Glenmark). These pill packs contain 28 active pills with no placebo pills or hormone-free week, and, for maximum efficacy must be taken within 3 hours at the same time every day. Progestin-only pills that contain norethindrone do not consistently suppress ovulation; their primary mechanism of action is thickening of cervical mucus.

In 2019, the FDA approved a second POP (Slynd); each pack contains 24 4-mg drospirenone tablets and 4 inert tablets. The primary mechanism of action is suppression of ovulation. The package label allows "a 24-hour missed pill window," compared to the 3-hour window of norethindrone pills. Its label also indicates that while scheduled withdrawal bleeding and spotting decreases with longer duration of use, unscheduled bleeding and spotting remain relatively common in users of this POP. Drospirenone has anti-mineralocorticoid activity comparable to a 25-mg dose of spironolactone and the manufacturer advises checking serum potassium levels during the first treatment cycle in patients on daily, long-term treatment for chronic conditions of diseases with medications that may increase serum potassium concentrations.

Advantages

Since POPs do not contain estrogen, there is no increase in risk of stroke, myocardial infarction, pulmonary embolism, or VTE.[7] Progestin-only pills may also be a good choice when an adolescent or young adult wants an oral contraceptive but cannot tolerate estrogen-related side effects or has estrogen contraindications, such as migraine with aura. Due to the limited duration of action of the "old" POPs compared to COCs, adherence to the narrow time frame acceptable to maintain effective contraceptive coverage may be particularly difficult; nevertheless, POPs are an acceptable alternative that should be offered to adolescents who want an oral progestin-only contraceptive.

STARTING CONTRACEPTION

Most contraceptive methods can be initiated at any time during the menstrual cycle provided that pregnancy or the possibility of pregnancy can be ruled out. The "quick start" method refers to starting a method immediately rather than waiting for the next menstrual period.[11]

HELPING AN ADOLESCENT OR YOUNG ADULT WOMAN SELECT THE CONTRACEPTIVE METHOD THAT IS RIGHT FOR HER

When helping a female adolescent or young adult choose a method of contraception, the method characteristics and patient needs should be considered. On one side, the patient and clinician together should consider method convenience, effectiveness, STI and PID risk reduction, minimizing adverse effects, and maximizing noncontraceptive benefits of each method. On the other side, AYA women must consider many different issues when choosing a method of contraception including access, cost, confidentiality, and age- and life-stage-appropriate medical services, as well as complexities inherent to different adolescent developmental stages (concrete thinking, incomplete understanding of direct consequences of risk-taking behaviors, importance of adherence to medication regimens, lack of independence in terms of financial costs/insurance and transportation issues, etc.). Patients with certain health conditions need particular consideration when selecting a suitable and safe contraceptive. Figure 46.1 summarizes medical eligibility criteria for contraceptive use. For example, estrogen-containing methods are contraindicated for those who have migraine headaches with aura or a history of thromboembolic events. Some methods provide particular noncontraceptive benefits, such as DMPA for those with sickle cell disease or a seizure disorder, or those on concomitant medications that decrease the effectiveness of hormonal contraceptives that go through first-pass metabolism.

All women should be counseled about the full range of effective contraceptive options for which they are medically eligible so that they can pick the optimal method for themselves (Fig. 46.1). Although there are highly effective, reversible methods available such as LARCs, it is important to assess STI, HIV, and PID risk, and discuss with patients that LARCs and other moderately effective hormonal methods do not prevent STIs or HIV. Consistent and correct use of male latex condoms reduces the risk for HIV infection and other STIs, including chlamydia, gonorrhea, and trichomoniasis infections. In addition, it is important to discuss that certain infections, such as herpes simplex virus (HSV), human papillomavirus (HPV), molluscum contagiosum, and pubic lice, can be transmitted despite condom use.

SPECIAL ISSUES IN PROVIDING CONTRACEPTION TO ADOLESCENTS AND YOUNG ADULTS WITH CHRONIC MEDICAL CONDITIONS

The recommendations for contraception use among AYA women who have varying medical conditions are well described in the

U.S. MEC (Fig. 46.1).[7] Included on this website are the initial and updated recommendations, as well as charts in English and Spanish in both MS Word and PDF format. The CDC has an app that includes the U.S. MEC[7] and is available for the iPhone and iPad. The following section includes contraceptive recommendations and considerations in AYAs with psychiatric (depressive disorders are covered in the U.S. MEC) and intellectual disabilities that are not covered in this chart.

Psychiatric Disease and Intellectual Disabilities

Adolescents and young adults with psychiatric conditions frequently have their family planning needs overlooked. Issues arising may include the following:
* Recognition of contraceptive need
* Individual's capacity to give informed consent
* Ability to utilize some of the contraceptive methods

Some individuals with mental illness may have a dual diagnosis, including substance abuse or seizure disorder. Barrier methods provide needed reduction in the risk of acquiring an STI and HIV, but they may not be used consistently. Long-acting reversible contraception methods may be an excellent primary form of contraception, but potential interactions with medications (e.g., seizure medications with implant) need to be considered in this recommendation. Adolescents and young adults with intellectual disabilities in an institutional setting may benefit from a LARC where compliance with other methods may be a problem. This population is potentially vulnerable for exploitation, so both sex education and an effective form of contraception is important. Oral contraceptives in this setting may have low adherence rates.

EMERGENCY CONTRACEPTION

Emergency contraception is the only contraceptive method designed to prevent pregnancy after intercourse. Emergency contraception can provide protection from pregnancy as many as 120 hours after unprotected or inadequately protected penile-vaginal intercourse and should be made available to every AYA female. Every female AYAs receiving clinical treatment for rape and sexual assault occurring within 120 hours should be counseled and offered EC. These recommendations extend to transgender or gender nonbinary (TGNB) AYA, who have the capacity to become pregnant, if they desire pregnancy prevention, present for care within 120 hours of condomless receptive penile-vaginal intercourse or are not using a reliable method of contraception. While testosterone use may be used to stop menstruation, TGNB AYAs taking testosterone may still ovulate and be able to get pregnant; testosterone is not a substitute for contraception, and they should be counseled about and offered EC routinely.

Use of Emergency Contraception by Adolescents and Young Adults

Use of EC among adolescents has been rising over time. The NSFG from 2011 to 2015 found the reported use of EC by teens, ages 15 to 19 years, steadily increased over time from 8.1% in 2002 to 22.9% between 2011 to 2015.[2] The 2015 to 2017 NSFG found that among females aged 15 to 19 years who had ever had sexual intercourse, 19% reported ever using EC.[4]

Advance Prescription and Access

No physical examination or testing is needed before providing oral EC. Clinicians can facilitate access to EC by writing advance prescriptions for oral EC for AYA women or TGNB patients who have the capacity to become pregnant. This can reduce the cost of obtaining EC for those whose insurance covers EC by prescription. Studies have shown that AYA women are more likely to use EC if it has been prescribed in advance of need;[15] these studies also showed

Summary Chart of U.S. Medical Eligibility Criteria for Contraceptive Use

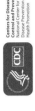

Centers for Disease Control and Prevention
National Center for Chronic Disease Prevention and Health Promotion

Key:
1 No restriction (method can be used)
2 Advantages generally outweigh theoretical or proven risks
3 Theoretical or proven risks usually outweigh the advantages
4 Unacceptable health risk (method not to be used)

Each method has two sub-columns: **I** = initiation of contraceptive method; **C** = continuation of contraceptive method. A single value applies to both unless shown as "I=x, C=y".

Table (first part)

Condition	Sub-Condition	Cu-IUD	LNG-IUD	Implant	DMPA	POP	CHC
Age		Menarche to <20 yrs: 2; ≥20 yrs: 1	Menarche to <20 yrs: 2; ≥20 yrs: 1	Menarche to <18 yrs: 1; 18–45 yrs: 1; >45 yrs: 1	Menarche to <18 yrs: 2; 18–45 yrs: 1; >45 yrs: 2	Menarche to <18 yrs: 1; 18–45 yrs: 1; >45 yrs: 1	Menarche to <40 yrs: 1; ≥40 yrs: 2
Anatomical abnormalities	a) Distorted uterine cavity	4	4				
	b) Other abnormalities	2	2				
Anemias	a) Thalassemia	2	1	1	1	1	1
	b) Sickle cell disease‡	2	1	1	1	1	2
	c) Iron-deficiency anemia	2	1	1	1	1	1
Benign ovarian tumors	(including cysts)	1	1	1	1	1	1
Breast disease	a) Undiagnosed mass	1	2	2*	2*	2*	2*
	b) Benign breast disease	1	1	1	1	1	1
	c) Family history of cancer	1	1	1	1	1	1
	d) Breast cancer‡ i) Current	1	4	4	4	4	4
	ii) Past and no evidence of current disease for 5 years	1	3	3	3	3	3
Breastfeeding	a) <21 days postpartum			2*	2*	2*	4*
	b) 21 to <30 days postpartum — i) With other risk factors for VTE			2*	2*	2*	3*
	ii) Without other risk factors for VTE			2*	2*	2*	3*
	c) 30–42 days postpartum — i) With other risk factors for VTE			1*	1*	1*	3*
	ii) Without other risk factors for VTE			1*	1*	1*	2*
	d) >42 days postpartum			1*	1*	1*	2*
Cervical cancer	Awaiting treatment	I=4, C=2	I=4, C=2	2	2	1	2
Cervical ectropion		1	1	1	1	1	1
Cervical intraepithelial neoplasia		1	2	2	2	1	2
Cirrhosis	a) Mild (compensated)	1	1	1	1	1	1
	b) Severe‡ (decompensated)	1	3	3	3	3	4
Cystic fibrosis‡		1	1*	1*	2*	1*	1*
Deep venous thrombosis (DVT)/Pulmonary embolism (PE)	a) History of DVT/PE, not receiving anticoagulant therapy — i) Higher risk for recurrent DVT/PE	1	2	2	2	2	4
	ii) Lower risk for recurrent DVT/PE	1	2	2	2	2	3
	b) Acute DVT/PE	2	2	2	2	2	4
	c) DVT/PE and established anticoagulant therapy for at least 3 months — i) Higher risk for recurrent DVT/PE	2	2	2	2	2	4*
	ii) Lower risk for recurrent DVT/PE	2	2	2	2	2	3*
	d) Family history (first-degree relatives)	1	1	1	1	1	2
	e) Major surgery — i) With prolonged immobilization	1	2	2	2	2	4
	ii) Without prolonged immobilization	1	1	1	1	1	2
	f) Minor surgery without immobilization	1	1	1	1	1	1
Depressive disorders		1*	1*	1*	1*	1*	1*

Table (second part)

Condition	Sub-Condition	Cu-IUD	LNG-IUD	Implant	DMPA	POP	CHC
Diabetes	a) History of gestational disease	1	1	1	1	1	1
	b) Nonvascular disease — i) Non-insulin dependent	1	2	2	2	2	2
	ii) Insulin dependent	1	2	2	2	2	2
	c) Nephropathy/retinopathy/neuropathy‡	1	2	2	3	2	3/4*
	d) Other vascular disease or diabetes of >20 years' duration‡	1	2	2	3	2	3/4*
Dysmenorrhea	Severe	2	1	1	1	1	1
Endometrial cancer‡		I=4, C=2	I=4, C=2	1	1	1	1
Endometrial hyperplasia		1	1	1	1	1	1
Endometriosis		2	1	1	1	1	1
Epilepsy‡	(see also Drug Interactions)	1	1	1*	1*	1*	1*
Gallbladder disease	a) Symptomatic — i) Treated by cholecystectomy	1	2	2	2	2	2
	ii) Medically treated	1	2	2	2	2	3
	iii) Current	1	2	2	2	2	3
	b) Asymptomatic	1	2	2	2	2	2
Gestational trophoblastic disease‡	a) Suspected GTD (immediate postevacuation) — i) Uterine size first trimester	1*	1*	1*	1*	1*	1*
	ii) Uterine size second trimester	2*	2*	1*	1*	1*	1*
	b) Confirmed GTD — i) Undetectable/non-pregnant β-hCG levels	1*	1*	1*	1*	1*	1*
	ii) Decreasing β-hCG levels	2*	2*	1*	1*	1*	1*
	iii) Persistently elevated β-hCG levels or malignant disease, with no evidence or suspicion of intrauterine disease	2*	2*	1*	1*	1*	1*
	iv) Persistently elevated β-hCG levels or malignant disease, with evidence or suspicion of intrauterine disease	4*	4*	1*	1*	1*	1*
Headaches	a) Nonmigraine (mild or severe)	1	1	1	1	1	1*
	b) Migraine — i) Without aura (includes menstrual migraine)	1	1	1	1	1	2*
	ii) With aura	1	1	1	1	1	4*
History of bariatric surgery‡	a) Restrictive procedures	1	1	1	1	1	1
	b) Malabsorptive procedures	1	1	1	1	3	COCs: 3; P/R: 1
History of cholestasis	a) Pregnancy related	1	1	1	1	1	2
	b) Past COC related	1	2	2	2	2	3
History of high blood pressure during pregnancy		1	1	1	1	1	2
History of Pelvic surgery		1	1	1	1	1	1
HIV	a) High risk for HIV	I=1*, C=1*	I=1*, C=1*	1	1	1	1
	b) HIV infection — i) Clinically well receiving ARV therapy	I=1, C=1	I=1, C=1	If on treatment, see Drug Interactions			
	ii) Not clinically well or not receiving ARV therapy‡	I=2, C=1	I=1, C=2	If on treatment, see Drug Interactions			

Abbreviations: ARV = antiretroviral; C=continuation of contraceptive method; CHC=combined hormonal contraceptive (pill, patch, and ring); COC=combined oral contraceptive; Cu-IUD=copper-containing intrauterine device; DMPA = depot medroxyprogesterone acetate; I=initiation of contraceptive method; LNG-IUD=levonorgestrel-releasing intrauterine device; NA=not applicable; POP=progestin-only pill; P/R=patch/ring; SSRI=selective serotonin reuptake inhibitor; ‡ Condition that exposes a woman to increased risk as a result of pregnancy. *Please see the complete guidance for a clarification to this classification: https://www.cdc.gov/reproductivehealth/contraception/mmwr/mec/appendixd.html

FIGURE 46.1 U.S. Medical Eligibility Criteria that rates the safety of contraceptive methods for women with a variety of underlying medical conditions. From Centers for Disease Control and Prevention (CDC), Division of Reproductive Health, National Center for Chronic Disease Prevention and Health Promotion. *United States Medical Eligibility Criteria (USMEC) for Contraceptive Use, 2016: Summary chart of U.S. Medical Eligibility Criteria for Contraceptive Use.* Updated 2020. https://www.cdc.gov/reproductivehealth/contraception/pdf/summary-chart-us-medical-eligibility-criteria_508tagged.pdf. *(continued)*

IX

Summary Chart of U.S. Medical Eligibility Criteria for Contraceptive Use

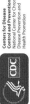

Left Table

Condition	Sub-Condition	Cu-IUD I	Cu-IUD C	LNG-IUD I	LNG-IUD C	Implant I	Implant C	DMPA I	DMPA C	POP I	POP C	CHC I	CHC C
Hypertension	a) Adequately controlled hypertension	1*	1*	1*	1*	1*	1*	2*	2*	1*	1*	3*	3*
	b) Elevated blood pressure levels (properly taken measurements)												
	i) Systolic 140-159 or diastolic 90-99	1*	1*	1*	1*	1*	1*	2*	2*	1*	1*	3*	3*
	ii) Systolic ≥160 or diastolic ≥100‡	1*	1*	2*	2*	2*	2*	3*	3*	2*	2*	4*	4*
	c) Vascular disease	1*	1*	2*	2*	2*	2*	3*	3*	2*	2*	4*	4*
Inflammatory bowel disease	(Ulcerative colitis, Crohn's disease)	1	1	1	1	1	1	2	2	2	2	2/3*	2/3*
Ischemic heart disease‡	Current and history of	1	1	2	3	2	3	3	3	2	3	4	4
Known thrombogenic mutations‡		1*	1*	2*	2*	2*	2*	2*	2*	2*	2*	4*	4*
Liver tumors	a) Benign												
	i) Focal nodular hyperplasia	1	1	2	2	2	2	2	2	2	2	2	2
	ii) Hepatocellular adenoma‡	1	1	3	3	3	3	3	3	3	3	4	4
	b) Malignant (hepatoma)	1	1	3	3	3	3	3	3	3	3	4	4
Malaria		1	1	1	1	1	1	1	1	1	1	1	1
Multiple risk factors for atherosclerotic cardiovascular disease	(e.g., older age, smoking, diabetes, hypertension, low HDL, high LDL, or high triglyceride levels)	1	1	2	2	2*	2*	3*	3*	2*	2*	3/4*	3/4*
Multiple sclerosis	a) With prolonged immobility	1	1	1	1	1	1	2	2	1	1	3	3
	b) Without prolonged immobility	1	1	1	1	1	1	2	2	1	1	2	2
Obesity	a) Body mass index (BMI) ≥30 kg/m²	1	1	1	1	1	1	1	1	1	1	2	2
	b) Menarche to <18 years and BMI ≥ 30 kg/m²	1	1	1	1	1	1	2	2	1	1	2	2
Ovarian cancer‡		1	1	1	1	1	1	1	1	1	1	1	1
Parity	a) Nulliparous	2	2	2	2	1	1	1	1	1	1	1	1
	b) Parous	1	1	1	1	1	1	1	1	1	1	1	1
Past ectopic pregnancy		1	1	1	1	1	1	1	1	2	2	1	1
Pelvic inflammatory disease	a) Past												
	i) With subsequent pregnancy	1	1	1	1	1	1	1	1	1	1	1	1
	ii) Without subsequent pregnancy	2	2	2	2	1	1	1	1	1	1	1	1
	b) Current	4	2*	4	2*	1	1	1	1	1	1	1	1
Peripartum cardiomyopathy‡	a) Normal or mildly impaired cardiac function												
	i) <6 months	2	2	2	2	1	1	1	1	1	1	4	4
	ii) ≥6 months	2	2	2	2	1	1	1	1	1	1	3	3
	b) Moderately or severely impaired cardiac function	2	2	2	2	2	2	2	2	2	2	4	4
Postabortion	a) First trimester	1*	1*	1*	1*	1*	1*	1*	1*	1*	1*	1*	1*
	b) Second trimester	2*	2*	2*	2*	1*	1*	1*	1*	1*	1*	1*	1*
	c) Immediate postseptic abortion	4	4	4	4	1*	1*	1*	1*	1*	1*	1*	1*
Postpartum (non-breastfeeding women)	a) <21 days					1	1	1	1	1	1	3*	3*
	b) 21 days to 42 days												
	i) With other risk factors for VTE					1	1	1	1	1	1	3*	3*
	ii) Without other risk factors for VTE					1	1	1	1	1	1	2	2
	c) >42 days					1	1	1	1	1	1	1	1
Postpartum (in breastfeeding or non-breastfeeding women, including cesarean delivery)	a) <10 minutes after delivery of the placenta												
	i) Breastfeeding	1*	1*	2*	2*								
	ii) Nonbreastfeeding	1*	1*	2*	2*								
	b) 10 minutes after delivery of the placenta to <4 weeks	2*	2*	2*	2*								
	c) ≥4 weeks	1*	1*	1*	1*								
	d) Postpartum sepsis	4	4	4	4								

Right Table

Condition	Sub-Condition	Cu-IUD I	Cu-IUD C	LNG-IUD I	LNG-IUD C	Implant I	Implant C	DMPA I	DMPA C	POP I	POP C	CHC I	CHC C
Pregnancy		4*		4*		NA*	NA*	NA*	NA*	NA*	NA*	NA*	NA*
Rheumatoid arthritis	a) On immunosuppressive therapy	2	1	2	1	1	1	2/3*	2/3*	1	1	2	2
	b) Not on immunosuppressive therapy	1	1	1	1	1	1	2	2	1	1	2	2
Schistosomiasis	a) Uncomplicated	1	1	1	1	1	1	1	1	1	1	1	1
	b) Fibrosis of the liver‡	1	1	1	1	1	1	1	1	1	1	1	1
Sexually transmitted diseases (STDs)	a) Current purulent cervicitis or chlamydial infection or gonococcal infection	4	2*	4	2*	1	1	1	1	1	1	1	1
	b) Vaginitis (including trichomonas vaginalis and bacterial vaginosis)	2	2	2	2	1	1	1	1	1	1	1	1
	c) Other factors relating to STDs	2*	2	2*	2	1	1	1	1	1	1	2	2
Smoking	a) Age <35	1	1	1	1	1	1	1	1	1	1	3	3
	b) Age ≥35, <15 cigarettes/day	1	1	1	1	1	1	1	1	1	1	4	4
	c) Age ≥35, ≥15 cigarettes/day	1	1	1	1	1	1	1	1	1	1	4	4
Solid organ transplantation‡	a) Complicated	3	2	3	2	2	2	2	2	2	2	4	4
	b) Uncomplicated	2	2	2	2	2	2	2	2	2	2	2*	2*
Stroke‡	History of cerebrovascular accident	1	1	2	2	2	3	3	3	2	3	4	4
Superficial venous disorders	a) Varicose veins	1	1	1	1	1	1	1	1	1	1	1	1
	b) Superficial venous thrombosis (acute or history)	1	1	1	1	1	1	1	1	1	1	3*	3*
Systemic lupus erythematosus‡	a) Positive (or unknown) antiphospholipid antibodies	1*	1*	3	3	3*	3*	3*	3*	3*	3*	4*	4*
	b) Severe thrombocytopenia	3*	2*	2*	2*	2*	2*	3*	2*	2*	2*	2*	2*
	c) Immunosuppressive therapy	2*	1*	2*	2*	1	1	2*	2*	2*	2*	2*	2*
	d) None of the above	1*	1*	2*	2*	1	1	2*	2*	2*	2*	2*	2*
Thyroid disorders	Simple goiter/hyperthyroid/hypothyroid	1	1	1	1	1	1	1	1	1	1	1	1
Tuberculosis‡ (see also Drug Interactions)	a) Nonpelvic	1	1	1	1	1	1	1	1	1	1	1	1
	b) Pelvic	4	3	4	3	1	1	1	1	1	1	1	1
Unexplained vaginal bleeding	(suspicious for serious condition) before evaluation	4*	2*	4*	2*	3*	3*	3*	3*	2*	2*	2*	2*
Uterine fibroids		2	2	2	2	1	1	1	1	1	1	1	1
Valvular heart disease	a) Uncomplicated	1	1	1	1	1	1	1	1	1	1	2	2
	b) Complicated‡	1	1	1	1	1	1	1	1	1	1	4	4
Vaginal bleeding patterns	a) Irregular pattern without heavy bleeding	1	1	1	1	2	2	2	2	2	2	1	1
	b) Heavy or prolonged bleeding	2*	1*	1*	2*	2*	2*	2*	2*	2*	2*	1*	1*
Viral hepatitis	a) Acute or flare	1	1	1	1	1	1	1	1	1	1	3/4*	2
	b) Carrier/Chronic	1	1	1	1	1	1	1	1	1	1	1	1
Drug Interactions													
Antiretrovirals used for prevention (PrEP) or treatment of HIV	Fosamprenavir (FPV)	1/2*	1*	1/2*	1*	2*	2*	1*	1*	2*	2*	3*	3*
	All other ARVs are 1 or 2 for all methods.												
Anticonvulsant therapy	a) Certain anticonvulsants (phenytoin, carbamazepine, barbiturates, primidone, topiramate, oxcarbazepine)	1	1	1	1	2*	2*	1*	1*	3*	3*	3*	3*
	b) Lamotrigine	1	1	1	1	1	1	1	1	1	1	3*	3*
Antimicrobial therapy	a) Broad spectrum antibiotics	1	1	1	1	1	1	1	1	1	1	1	1
	b) Antifungals	1	1	1	1	1	1	1	1	1	1	1	1
	c) Antiparasitics	1	1	1	1	1	1	1	1	1	1	1	1
	d) Rifampin or rifabutin therapy	1	1	1	1	2*	2*	1*	1*	3*	3*	3*	3*
SSRIs		1	1	1	1	1	1	1	1	1	1	1	1
St. John's wort		1	1	1	1	2	2	1	1	2	2	2	2

Updated in 2020. This summary sheet only contains a subset of the recommendations from the U.S. MEC. For complete guidance, see: https://www.cdc.gov/reproductivehealth/contraception/contraception_guidance.htm. Most contraceptive methods do not protect against sexually transmitted diseases (STDs). Consistent and correct use of the male latex condom reduces the risk of STDs and HIV.

CS314239-A

Centers for Disease Control and Prevention
National Center for Chronic Disease Prevention and Health Promotion

FIGURE 46.1 (Continued)

no increase in sexual activity or decrease in use of ongoing contraceptive use.[11] Despite this, many practicing pediatricians and pediatric residents do not routinely counsel patients about EC and do not prescribe it. In 2019, the AAP released a policy statement on EC encouraging education of pediatricians on available EC, routine counseling, and advanced prescription of EC as a public health strategy to reduce teen pregnancy (see Additional Resources and Websites). In 2019, the ACOG reaffirmed their 2017 recommendation that obstetrician–gynecologists write advance prescriptions for oral EC to increase awareness and remove barriers, especially for adolescents.[8]

Despite recommendations for advance prescription and universal counseling about EC, access to EC can be challenging for many AYA women, particularly immigrants, non-English speaking women, survivors of sexual assault, those living in areas with few pharmacy choices, and poor women. "Women's health" or family planning clinics should provide comprehensive, respectful, and gender-affirming care with welcoming physical environments, staff training, and policies and procedures for TGNB AYAs. Establishing connections with local transaffirming clinicians who perform IUD insertions for EC may improve TGNB patients' experiences with EC access in a time-sensitive situation.

Transgender or gender nonbinary AYA patients may also encounter challenges in picking up EC pills at pharmacies. Questions may be asked of individuals who present as male or who are listed as "male" on their insurance or identification when they try to fill a prescription. Writing "prescription appropriate for patient's sex" in the pharmacy note when prescribing EC, electronically or on paper, may prevent this problem. There are no requirements for sex or age to purchase LNG-EC over-the-counter in the United States. As such, informed pharmacy staff should provide gender-affirming support for cisgender and TGNB AYAs so that they can avoid unwarranted restrictions to accessing EC. The Guttmacher Institute maintains an up-to-date list of state policies on EC. It is important to educate every AYA patient regarding how to promptly contact their medical provider if they are unable to fill an EC prescription or provide over-the-counter EC.

Relative Effectiveness

The exact effectiveness of emergency contraceptive pills (ECPs) is difficult to measure, and some researchers believe the effectiveness may be lower than that reported on package labels. Overall, the copper IUD is the most effective EC method with one recent study showing that the LNG IUD is noninferior.[16] After the IUD, the most effective methods are ulipristal acetate (UPA, Ella) followed by POPs containing LNG.[11] The use of COCs-EC (Yuzpe method) is no longer a standard of care. When used for EC, the Copper-T IUD is 99% effective in reducing pregnancy risk.[11]

There is no mention of the effectiveness of Ella in the patient package insert or provider label. However, the observed and expected pregnancy rates reported in two Phase III clinical trials suggests effectiveness rates of 60% and 66%. The failure rate has been described as approximately 1.4%.[17] More recently, a prospective, open-label clinical cohort study was conducted with 700 women between May 2011 and March 2014 to determine if UPA had similar efficacy as EC when administered before versus after ovulation.[18] Women requesting EC within 120 hours after a single act of unprotected sexual intercourse were recruited at a community family planning clinic in Hong Kong. Each participant received a single oral dose of UPA 30 mg, and 693 participants completed follow-up. Ovulatory status at the time of UPA administration was determined by serum progesterone level supplemented by menstrual history and ultrasound tracking. The percentage of pregnancies prevented, as a main outcome measure, was significantly higher among participants who were preovulatory (77.6%) compared with those who were postovulatory (36.4%) at the time of UPA administration ($P < 0.0001$). The observed pregnancy rate following UPA

administration was significantly lower than the expected pregnancy rate only in the preovulatory group ($P < 0.0001$), compared to the postovulatory group ($P = 0.281$). The overall failure rate was 1.7% (1.4 vs. 2.1% in the pre- and postovulatory groups, respectively). The efficacy of UPA-EC was significantly better when administered before rather than after ovulation.[11]

The effectiveness listed on the Plan B/Next Choice package is 89%. The failure rate has been described as approximately 2% to 3%.[17] Ulipristal acetate is at least as effective as LNG when used within the first 72 hours after unprotected intercourse. However, UPA is more effective than oral LNG when used between 72 and 120 hours after unprotected intercourse, and, therefore, constitutes a better option for women who require EC on the fourth and fifth days after unprotected intercourse.[11] Two trials comparing UPA 30-mg single dose to LNG 1.5-mg single dose in a meta-analysis found that UPA was more effective compared to LNG within 72 hours after unprotected intercourse, which was significant at a marginal level.[11] When the 72- to 120-hour data from the Glasier 2010 trial were included in the meta-analysis, UPA was associated with lower risk of pregnancy than LNG and the difference was significant.[11]

The published literature on combined progestin-estrogen ECPs estimates a range of effectiveness between 56% and 89% in reducing pregnancy risk. Data clearly show that the progestin-only ECP regimen is more effective than the Yuzpe method.

COPPER INTRAUTERINE DEVICE FOR EMERGENCY CONTRACEPTION (PARAGARD)

The copper IUD or Paragard, when used for EC, should be inserted within 5 days of unprotected intercourse.[11] This method can be used beyond 5 days as long as the time of ovulation can be reasonably determined and insertion occurs no more than 5 days after ovulation.[11] This insertion timing would ensure insertion before implantation, if one is seeking a contraceptive action versus an early abortifacient.[17]

Mechanism of Action

The copper IUD or Paragard prevents pregnancy by causing a foreign body sterile inflammatory process via production of cytotoxic peptides and activation of enzymes leading to inhibition of sperm motility, reducing sperm capacitation and survival, and increasing phagocytosis. Copper also causes an increase in copper ions, enzymes, prostaglandins, and macrophages in uterine and tubal fluids, impairing sperm function and preventing fertilization.[11] The very high effectiveness of the copper-releasing IUD when used for EC implies that it may also act by preventing implantation of the blastocyst.[17]

Advantages

The copper IUD is the only EC that can also provide 10 to 12 years of ongoing highly effective contraception for women with no copper allergy. In addition to being one of the most cost-effective ongoing methods of contraception, it is one of the most effective EC and therefore, one of the best choices when unprotected sexual intercourse occurs around the time of ovulation. Women who have intercourse around ovulation should ideally be offered a copper IUD. It is also one of the best options for women with elevated BMI (>24 kg/m^2), since data show no clinical concern of lower effectiveness with increased BMI[19] as compared to UPA and LNG oral EC methods. The copper IUD should also be considered, as in the case of all IUDs, for patients who have privacy concerns or who have partners who sabotage their contraception.

Side Effects

Menstrual disturbances such as menorrhagia and dysmenorrhea are common with copper IUDs. Menses can have increased length,

IX

flow, and discomfort during the first several cycles after the copper IUD is inserted. Dysmenorrhea and heavy menses are the most frequent reasons for copper IUD early removal.[11] Average blood loses may increase up to 55%, although rarely leading to anemia. Because the copper device does not contain hormones, it does not cause progestin-related side effects seen with LNG-IUDs. Rates of expulsion, perforation, and risk of PID do not differ when a copper IUD is used for EC compared to regular, ongoing use of an IUD for contraception. A study comparing IUD use among nulliparous and parous women found similar rates of complications, discontinuation, and expulsion. This study found that copper IUD users had a rate of PID of 3.5 per 1,000 women-years, rates of (ectopic) pregnancy of 0.6% to 1.1% per year, and rates of expulsion of 0% to 1.2% per year. Nulliparous women did not show more complications compared to parous women. There was not a significantly higher IUD removal rate among nulliparous women compared to parous women. Main reasons for removal were "menstrual problems" and "contraception no longer necessary."[20] A more recent systematic review of randomized controlled trials, and prospective and retrospective observational studies of IUD use, found no differences in rates of infection or expulsions between nulliparous and parous women. Fertility rates among nulliparous women following IUD removal appeared no different from the general population. However, higher rates of insertion difficulty, insertion failure, and pain during insertion were observed among nulliparous women.[21]

The copper IUD is largely underused for EC. Harper et al.[22] conducted a survey among 1,246 clinicians (response rate 65%) in a California State family planning program, where U.S. FDA-approved contraceptives are available at no cost to low-income women. The results showed that the large majority of clinicians (85%) never recommended the copper IUD for EC, and most (93%) required two or more visits for an IUD insertion. Recommendation of the copper IUD for EC is rare, despite its high efficacy and long-lasting contraceptive benefits. Same day insertion of IUDs for EC and ongoing contraception use is ideal clinical practice and could greatly enhance access, especially to young women. This type of service, however, requires clinic flow and scheduling adjustments.

LEVONORGESTREL INTRAUTERINE DEVICE FOR EMERGENCY CONTRACEPTION (MIRENA AND LILETTA)

Previously, only the copper IUD was offered for EC because data were lacking on the efficacy of using an LNG IUD for this purpose. However, in 2021 a randomized noninferiority trial was published comparing the use of LNG IUD to copper IUD for EC among women, 18 to 35 years of age, seeking EC after at least one episode of unprotected intercourse within the prior 5 days. The women were randomized to receive either an LNG 52-mg IUD or a copper T380A IUD while being unaware of group assignment. The primary outcome of the study was a positive urine pregnancy test 1 month after IUD insertion. The prespecified noninferiority margin was 2.5 percentage points. Among the 355 women randomly assigned to receive LNG IUDs and 356 assigned to receive copper IUDs, 317 and 321, respectively, received the interventions and provided 1-month outcome data. Of these, 290 in the LNG group and 300 in the copper IUD group had a 1-month urine pregnancy test. In the modified intention-to-treat and per-protocol analyses, pregnancy rates were 1 in 317 (0.3%; 95% confidence interval [CI], 0.01 to 1.7) in the LNG IUD group and 0 in 321 (0%; 95% CI, 0 to 1.1) in the copper IUD group; the between-group absolute difference in both analyses was 0.3% points (95% CI, −0.9 to 1.8), consistent with the noninferiority of the LNG IUD compared to the copper IUD. The study concluded that LNG IUD was noninferior to the copper IUD for EC.[16]

Mechanism of Action

Like the copper IUD, the LNG IUD device creates a foreign body sterile inflammatory process via production of cytotoxic peptides and activation of enzymes, leading to inhibition of sperm motility, reduced sperm capacitation and survival, and increased phagocytosis. In addition, the LNG component directly interferes with sperm transport, sperm capacitation, the acrosome reaction, and oviduct transport.[16]

Advantages

Like the copper IUD, the efficacy of the LNG IUD for EC does not appear to be affected by higher BMI in contrast to oral LNG or UPA which are both less effective among women with higher BMI. Adolescents tend to prefer the LNG IUD over the copper IUD for ongoing contraception because of its menstrual benefits of decreasing dysmenorrhea and menorrhagia. Finally, like the copper IUD, the LNG IUD for EC avoids the delayed initiation of ongoing hormonal contraception that is recommended when UPA is used for EC.

Side Effects

Among LNG IUD for EC users, 5.2% sought medical care for adverse events in the first month after IUD placement as compared with 4.9% of copper IUD users. The main reasons for seeking medical care included cramping (1.2%), bleeding and cramping (0.9%), pain (0.9%), and bleeding (0.6%).[16] Other reasons for seeking medical care included "concerns related to the IUD" (0.9%) such as confirming that the IUD was still in place, concerns that pain caused by a kidney infection might be related to the IUD, and concerns about string length or about not being able to feel the strings (or both).[16]

ULIPRISTAL ACETATE OR ULIPRISTAL ACETATE (ELLA) FOR EMERGENCY CONTRACEPTION

Ulipristal acetate or UPA is a second-generation progesterone receptor (PR) modulator, which has been marketed in Europe since 2009 and was FDA approved in 2010 as a dedicated product specifically marketed for EC. It is manufactured by Afaxys, Inc. Ulipristal acetate is available in health clinics, and only by prescription in pharmacies in both Europe and the United States, regardless of patient age. Pharmacy prices tend to be $40 to $56, about $5 to $10 more than oral LNG EC products. Since UPA is available only by prescription, it is covered by some private and public insurance. Ella may be ordered from an online prescription service—www.prjktruby.com/products/ella/. The pill is mailed the following day, and the cost of the product plus shipping is $90.

Mechanism of Action

Ulipristal acetate is a derivative of 19-norprogesterone that binds to PRs to produce an antiprogesterone contraceptive effect. Antiglucocorticoid and antiandrogen activities were observed at doses 50-fold greater than that necessary for an antiprogestin effect. One tablet of 30 mg of UPA is taken orally as soon as possible within 120 hours (5 days) of unprotected intercourse or a known or suspected contraceptive failure. Ulipristal acetate has different mechanisms of action, depending on the time of the menstrual cycle when it is administered.[23] A 2016 systematic review found that all the studies in the review conclude that UPA is effective in inhibiting ovulation even when administered shortly before the LH peak.[24] The effects on the fallopian tubes are less clear. Low-dose UPA used for EC has no significant effect on endometrial thickness and on an embryo's attachment, but these results are still a matter of debate. Evidence suggests that UPA modulates human sperm functions but has no effect on an established pregnancy. The majority of the evidence concurs in excluding a postfertilization effect of UPA, even though more studies are needed to clarify its mechanism of action.

Advantages

Clinical trials show that UPA is a well-tolerated and effective method of EC when used within 120 hours of intercourse. Unlike

LNG, UPA's effectiveness does not decline with delay in treatment. Therefore, UPA is an excellent option for women in need of EC who present "late" after unprotected intercourse.[11] Obese and overweight women also have a higher oral EC failure rate. Data from a meta-analysis of two randomized controlled trials comparing the efficacy of UPA showed that the risk of pregnancy was more than threefold greater for obese women (BMI of 30 kg/m^2 or greater, OR = 3.60, CI 1.96 to 6.53; P <0.0001) and more than 1.5 times higher for overweight women (BMI 25 to 30 kg/m^2) when compared with women with normal BMI, regardless of which EC regimen was taken.[19,11] For obese women, the risk of pregnancy was greater for those taking oral LNG compared to UPA users. Levonorgestrel showed a rapid decrease in efficacy with increasing BMI, reaching the point where it appeared no different from pregnancy rates expected among women not taking LNG at a BMI of 26 kg/m^2 compared with 35 kg/m^2 for UPA. For both ECs, pregnancy risk was related to the cycle day of intercourse.

Side Effects

Most side effects are mild or moderate and consist of headaches, dysmenorrhea, nausea, fatigue, dizziness, abdominal pain, and back pain. After EC use, the onset of the next menses occurred a mean 2.1 days (SD 8.2) *later* than expected in the UPA group, but duration of bleeding was not affected by UPA use. In women with available data on cycle length, menses occurred within 7 days of expected time in 769 (76%) of 1,013 women in the UPA group. Based on these data, it is recommended that patients be counseled that onset of menses after UPA use may be later than expected and a pregnancy test is indicated if the patient does not have a period within 3 weeks of taking it. Nausea and vomiting (13% to 29%) are the most frequently reported side effects among women treated with oral LNG or UPA for EC, compared to COC (Yuzpe method) for EC (50% have nausea and 20% have vomiting).[11] Routine use of an antinausea medication, such as meclizine, 1 hour before the first Yuzpe method dose was found to decrease nausea and vomiting; antinausea medication is generally considered unnecessary when using oral LNG or UPA for EC.[11]

Because UPA is an antiprogestin, it can negatively impact quick-starting progestin-containing hormonal contraceptives. Based on several studies, the FDA updated the UPA package label to include warnings regarding the co-administration of UPA and hormonal contraception. The label now states that if a woman wishes to use hormonal contraception after using UPA, she should do so no sooner than 5 days after the intake of UPA and that she should use a reliable barrier method until the next menstrual period. The label also now states that because UPA and the progestin component of hormonal contraceptives both bind to the progesterone receptor, using them together may impair the ability of UPA to delay ovulation. The American Society for Emergency Contraception (ASEC) has a more flexible, patient-centered protocol for providing ongoing contraception after EC (see Additional Resources and Websites). The AAP Committee on Adolescence recommends that ongoing hormonal contraceptives should not be initiated sooner than 5 days after the use of UPA to minimize the risk of interference with UPA activity (see Additional Resources and Websites).

LEVONORGESTREL PILLS FOR EMERGENCY CONTRACEPTION

Types

Over the past decade, the number of oral LNG pills specifically marketed for EC expanded from 3 to 11 name brands manufactured by nine different pharmaceutical companies and generic brands. Originally, all formulations of oral LNG EC contained two tablets, each containing 0.75 mg LNG, with instructions to take one as soon as possible and repeat the dose in 12 hours. Currently, all oral LNG EC is packaged with a single-tablet dose of 1.5-mg LNG with instructions to take one tablet as soon as possible. Although data supports the use of oral LNG EC up to 120 hours, the FDA insert instructions still advise use up to 72 hours after unprotected sex.

Availability

Although oral LNG EC has been approved for over-the-counter sale since 2013 without any age restrictions, major barriers to EC access remain. Oral LNG EC can be purchased from a variety of retail pharmacies. Oral LNG EC is also available from school-based health centers, university health centers, family planning clinics, community health centers, and online at sites like www.afterpill.com. Some universities have vending machines on campus so students can purchase EC 24 hours a day, 7 days a week.

Cost

Prices for oral LNG EC vary greatly. In 2017, the average price of Plan B One-Step was $49 and generics cost about $39 (with little change since 2014).[25] In 2021, name brands range from $40 to $50 while generics range from $11 to $45. Vending machines available at some universities charge approximately $32. Online products such as AfterPill can be purchased for $20 + $5 shipping or $60 + $5 shipping of $65 if buying three units, although the product may not arrive in time for emergency use. Even though oral LNG EC is available over-the-counter, many third-party insurance plans will cover the cost minus the pharmacy co-pay if a prescription is written and, in some states, like New York, Medicaid insurance will entirely cover the cost of LNG EC whether it is obtained as OTC or by prescription.

Specific Advantages

Over-the-counter availability of LNG EC pills has dramatically increased women's access. Pharmacy access reduces barriers in many ways: not requiring appointments; being open on evenings, weekends, and holidays; offering over-the-counter EC to men; providing EC to undocumented women immigrants and women with Medicaid who otherwise cannot afford OTC ECPs; and women needing a prescription for their private insurance to cover the cost of ECPs. More recently, online and vending machine purchasing has further expanded access for women who have credit cards.

Mechanism of Action

Oral LNG EC delays ovulation and fertilization and may inhibit implantation, but it is not effective once implantation has begun. One review[22] of the literature noted that "early treatment with ECPs containing only LNG has been shown to impair the ovulatory process and luteal function."[23] Oral LNG does not impair attachment of human embryos and has no effect on the expression of endometrial receptivity markers. A recent study found 1.5-mg levonorgestrel had no effect on the quality of cervical mucus or on the penetration of sperm in the uterus. The reduced efficacy of oral LNG when treatment is delayed suggests that interference with implantation is not a likely effect.

Side Effects

Studies have shown similar side effects for LNG and for UPA when used for EC. Reported complaints include fatigue, breast tenderness, headache, lower abdominal pain, dizziness, and diarrhea. As mentioned, LNG and UPA cause nausea and emesis, although this is less than what is reported for the Yuzpe method.[11] In the study conducted by Glasier in 2010, the onset of next menses after EC occurred a mean 1.2 days earlier than expected in the LNG group, but duration of bleeding was not affected by EC. In women with available data on cycle length, menses occurred within 7 days of expected time in 731 (71%) of 1,031 women in the LNG group compared to 769 (76%) of 1,013 women in the UPA group.[19] In 69 women with a reported stable menstrual cycle length of 24 to 34 days, bleeding patterns following EC administration in the follicular ($n = 26$), periovulatory ($n = 14$), and luteal ($n = 29$) phase were studied. Data obtained in this limited number of women indicated that EC administered before the onset of the LH surge inhibits ovulation and hastens the end of the current menstrual cycle. Thereafter, the menstrual cyclicity is "reset" and proceeds normally in the subsequent cycle. In contrast, EC administered after the onset of the LH peak has no effect on ovulation and consequently on cycle characteristics.

Emergency Contraception and Weight

Body weight does not impact the efficacy of the Cu-IUD or LNG IUD. Women with BMI >25 kg/m^2 should be offered a copper IUD or LNG IUD as first-line care or UPA if immediate IUD insertion is unavailable or declined by the patient. The CDC[26] recommends that AYA women in need of EC who do not wish to use an IUD or who do not have access to IUD insertion should still be offered an oral EC method regardless of their weight. Even though no clinical trials have specifically evaluated the impact of weight on the effectiveness of oral EC, meta-analyses have suggested that both LNG and UPA may be less effective in AYA women whose BMI is >25 kg/m^2.[11] In response to these data and labeling changes to European EC products, the FDA conducted its own review of the evidence and issued a statement in 2016 indicating that the data regarding BMI and the effectiveness of LNG EC are conflicting and made no labeling changes. The FDA stated that there were no safety concerns that preclude with the use of LNG EC in women with a BMI greater than 25 kg/m^2 or with body weight greater than 165 lb and that the most important factor affecting how well EC works is how quickly it is taken after unprotected intercourse.[27]

Repeated Use

Pregnancy risk increases with repeated acts of unprotected intercourse, especially after EC use. When women have multiple episodes of unprotected sexual intercourse, EC effectiveness decreases even when EC is used after every incident of unprotected intercourse. A copper IUD or LNG IUD provides women with the best protection because all future episodes of intercourse will be protected. Some clinicians have worried that because UPA delays, rather than inhibits ovulation, women might be at greater risk of pregnancy if they have subsequent unprotected intercourse after taking UPA compared to women who take LNG, although not currently supported by evidence.

Ethical Considerations Around Mechanism of Action

Despite EC being available over-the-counter, some clinicians continue to have ethical concerns around its mechanism of action. Medical authorities, including the FDA, National Institute of Health, and ACOG define a pregnancy as beginning with implantation of a fertilized ova. Emergency contraceptive pills do not interrupt implantation. Therefore, ECPs are not abortifacients. When advising women, it is important to clarify that ECPs, like any of the other hormonal contraceptives (including COCs, POPs, DMPA, implant, ring, and patch) as well as breastfeeding, prevent pregnancy primarily by delaying or inhibiting ovulation and inhibiting fertilization. It is not scientifically possible to definitely rule out that any of these methods, including breastfeeding, may inhibit implantation of a fertilized egg in the endometrium. However, the best available evidence is that the mechanism of action of LNG and UPA ECPs to prevent pregnancy can be fully accounted for by mechanisms that do not involve interference with postfertilization events. The very high effectiveness of the emergency insertion of a copper IUD implies a possible postfertilization effect.[23]

SUMMARY

Adolescents and young adults have the ability to make their own reproductive health and contraceptive choices, which should be honored and respected. Contraception is important for prevention for unintended pregnancies. Clinicians should work with AYAs to find a method that best meets their personal needs and that they will be able to adhere to successfully. Adolescents and young adults should have access to a wide range of contraceptive options with LARCs being first-line options due to their greater effectiveness. Contraception counseling must be approached within a reproductive health justice framework and take into account the difficulties and health care disparities faced by AYAs. It is important to incorporate messages about condom use and STI prevention with contraceptive counseling. Clinicians must provide counseling that is developmentally appropriate to the adolescent, acknowledge how they access health care, is culturally sensitive and is not perceived as directive or coercive.

REFERENCES

1. Boonstra H. Teen pregnancy: Trends and lessons learned. New York: Alan Guttmacher Institute; 2002 Feb. Available at https://www.guttmacher.org/sites/default/files/pdfs/pubs/tgr/05/1/gr050107.pdf Last accessed August 28 2022.
2. Abma JC, Martinez GM. Sexual activity and contraceptive use among teenagers in the United States, 2011–2015. National health statistics reports. 2017(104):1–23.
3. Finer LB, Zolna MR. Shifts in intended and unintended pregnancies in the United States, 2001–2008. *Am J Public Health.* 2014;104(Suppl 1):S43–S48.
4. Martinez GM, Abma JC. Sexual activity and contraceptive use among teenagers aged 15–19 in the United States, 2015–2017. *NCHS Data Brief.* 2020;(366):1–8.
5. Daniels K, Abma JC. Current contraceptive status among women aged 15–49: United States, 2017–2019. *NCHS Data Brief.* 2020;(388):1–8.
6. Sundaram A, Vaughan B, Kost K, et al. Contraceptive failure in the United States: estimates from the 2006–2010 National Survey of Family Growth. *Perspect Sex Reprod Health.* 2017;49(1):7–16.
7. Accessed March 8, 2021. https://www.cdc.gov/mmwr/volumes/65/rr/pdfs/rr6503.pdf
8. Committee opinion No. 710 summary: counseling adolescents about contraception. *Obstet Gynecol.* 2017;130(2):486–487. doi: 10.1097/AOG.0000000000002228. PMID: 28742669.
9. Gomez AM, Fuentes L, Allina A. Women or LARC first? Reproductive autonomy and the promotion of long-acting reversible contraceptive methods. *Perspect Sex Reprod Health.* 2014;46(3):171–175.
10. Daniels K, Daugherty J, Jones J. Current contraceptive status among women aged 15–44: United States, 2011–2013. *NCHS Data Brief.* 2014;(173):1–8.
11. Hatcher RA, Nelson AL, Trussell J, et al. *Contraceptive Technology.* 21st revised ed. Managing Contraception, LLC; 2018. *Contraceptive Technology.* Accessed April 1, 2021. http://www.contraceptivetechnology.org/the-book/
12. Sammaritano LR, Bermas BL, Chakravarty EE, et al. 2020 American College of Rheumatology guideline for the management of reproductive health in rheumatic and musculoskeletal diseases. *Arthritis Rheumatol.* 2020;72(4):529–556.
13. ACOG Committee Opinion No. 735: adolescents and long-acting reversible contraception: implants and intrauterine devices. *Obstet Gynecol.* 2018;131(5):e130–e139. doi: 10.1097/AOG.0000000000002632
14. Francis JKR, Gold MA. Long-acting reversible contraception for adolescents: a review. *JAMA Pediatr.* 2017;171(7):694–701.
15. Rodriguez MI, Curtis KM, Gaffield ML, et al. Advance supply of emergency contraception: a systematic review. *Contraception.* 2013;87(5):590–601.
16. Turok DK, Gero A, Simmons RG, et al. Levonorgestrel vs. copper intrauterine devices for emergency contraception. *N Engl J Med.* 2021;384(4):335–344.
17. Cleland K, Zhu H, Goldstuck N, et al. The efficacy of intrauterine devices for emergency contraception: a systematic review of 35 years of experience. *Hum Reprod.* 2012;27(7):1994–2000.
18. Li HWR, Lo SST, Ng EHY, et al. Efficacy of ulipristal acetate for emergency contraception and its effect on the subsequent bleeding pattern when administered before or after ovulation. *Hum Reprod.* 2016;31(6):1200–1207.
19. Glasier AF, Cameron ST, Fine PM, et al. Ulipristal acetate versus levonorgestrel for emergency contraception: a randomised non-inferiority trial and meta-analysis. *Lancet.* 2010;375(9714):555–562.
20. Veldhuis HM, Vos AG, Lagro-Janssen ALM. Complications of the intrauterine device in nulliparous and parous women. *Eur J Gen Pract.* 2004;10(3):82–87.
21. Foran T, Butcher BE, Kovacs G, et al. Safety of insertion of the copper IUD and LNG-IUS in nulliparous women: a systematic review. *Eur J Contracept Reprod Health Care.* 2018;23(5):379–386.
22. Harper CC, Speidel JJ, Drey EA, et al. Copper intrauterine device for emergency contraception: clinical practice among contraceptive providers. *Obstet Gynecol.* 2012;119(2 Pt 1):220–226.
23. Trussell J. Emergency Contraception: Trussell J Raymond EG Cleland K Emerg Contracept Last Chance Prev Unintended Pregnancy 2019 Available Ecprinceton-eduquestionsec-Rev Accessed March 27, 2021:38.
24. Rosato E, Farris M, Bastianelli C. Mechanism of action of ulipristal acetate for emergency contraception: a systematic review. *Front Pharmacol.* 2016;6:315.
25. Accessed April 1, 2021. https://www.americansocietyforec.org/reports-and-fact-sheets
26. CDC US SPR. Accessed March 26, 2021. https://www.cdc.gov/mmwr/volumes/65/rr/pdfs/rr6504.pdf

27. Research C for DE and Plan B (0.75 mg levonorgestrel) and Plan B One-Step (1.5 mg levonorgestrel) Tablets Information. FDA. Published online November 3, 2018. Accessed April 1, 2021. https://www.fda.gov/drugs/postmarket-drug-safety-information-patients-and-providers/plan-b-075mg-levonorgestrel-and-plan-b-one-step-15-mg-levonorgestrel-tablets-information

📶 ADDITIONAL RESOURCES AND WEBSITES

Additional Resources and Websites for Clinicians:

The American Academy of Pediatrics (AAP) and LARCS—https://www.aap.org/en-us/advocacy-and-policy/aap-health-initiatives/adolescent-sexual-health/Pages/Contraception.aspx

The American College of Obstetricians and Gynecologists (ACOG) and LARCs—https://www.acog.org/programs/long-acting-reversible-contraception-larc

American Society for Emergency Contraception. Clinical minute: Emergency contraception for transgender or gender nonbinary patients—https://providers.bedsider.org/articles/clinical-minute-emergency-contraception-for-transgender-or-gender-nonbinary-patients

ARSHEP contraception talk links for providers—https://prh.org/arshep-ppts/

Bedsider: Succinct review on clinical considerations when offering EC to transgender and nonbinary AYA patients—https://providers.bedsider.org/articles/clinical-minute-emergency-contraception-for-transgender-or-gender-nonbinary-patients

The Centers for Disease Control (CDC) and LARCs—https://www.cdc.gov/teenpregnancy/health-care-providers/improving-contraceptive-access.html

Contraceptive Choice Center, Washington University School of Medicine, St Louis, MO—https://contraceptivechoice.wustl.edu/

Crawford-Jakubiak JE, Alderman EM, Leventhal JM; Committee on Child Abuse and Neglect; Committee on Adolescence. Care of the Adolescent After an Acute Sexual Assault. *Pediatrics*. 2017;139(3):e20164243. doi: 10.1542/peds.2016-4243

The Guttmacher Institute: State Policies on Emergency Contraception. Accessed April 1, 2021. https://www.guttmacher.org/print/state-policy/explore/emergency-contraception

Master SO, Gold MA. Emergency contraception. In: Upadhya K, Trent M, Kaul P, eds. *Adolescent Medicine: State of the Art Reviews: Contraception*. American Academy of Pediatrics; 2019; 134–149.

Reproductive health access project. Multiple resources on Sexual and reproductive health—https://www.reproductiveaccess.org/contraception/

Rome ES, Issac V. Sometimes you do get a second chance: emergency contraception for adolescents. *Pediatr Clin North Am*. 2017;64(2):371–380. doi: 10.1016/j.pcl.2016.11.006

Saldanha N. Use of short acting reversible contraception in adolescents: the pill, patch, ring and emergency contraception. *Curr Probl Pediatr Adolesc Health Care*. 2018;48(12):333–344. doi: 10.1016/j.cppeds.2018.11.003

Society for Adolescent Health and Medicine. Emergency contraception for adolescents and young adults: guidance for health care professionals. *J Adolesc Health*. 2016;58(2):245–248. doi: 10.1016/j.jadohealth.2015.11.012

Upadhya KK; Committee on Adolescence. Emergency contraception. *Pediatrics*. 2019;144(6):e20193149. doi: 10.1542/peds.2019-3149.

The World Health Organization (WHO) and LARCs—https://www.familyplanning2020.org/sites/default/files/Global%20Consensus%20Statement%20-%20Expanding%20Contraceptive%20Choice.pdf

Additional Resources and Websites for Parents/Caregivers and Adolescents and Young Adults:

Amaze.org. Multiple audio-visual resources on sexual and reproductive health—https://amaze.org/

American Society for EC. Multiple fact sheets on Emergency Contraception for Transgender and Nonbinary patients; Providing Ongoing Hormonal Contraception after Use of Emergency Contraceptive Pills; and EC in the Covid Era—https://www.americansocietyforec.org/reports-and-factsheets

Bedsider. Succinct review on contraceptive methods for AYA—https://www.bedsider.org/methods

Planned Parenthood. Multiple hands outs on sexual and reproductive health—https://www.plannedparenthood.org/learn/birth-control

Reproductive health access project. Multiple resources on Sexual and reproductive health—https://www.reproductiveaccess.org/

Young Men's Health. Succinct review on sexual health contraceptive methods for AYA—https://youngmenshealthsite.org/

Young Women's Health. Succinct review on sexual health and contraceptive methods for AYA—https://youngwomenshealth.org/

IX

CHAPTER 47

Barrier Contraceptives and Spermicides

Michelle Forcier

KEY WORDS

- Barrier contraception
- Cervical cap
- Cervical shield
- Condoms (external, internal)
- Contraceptive shield
- Diaphragm
- Spermicide
- Sponge

INTRODUCTION

Barrier methods of contraception include external condoms (ECs), internal condoms (ICs), cervical cap and shield, sponge, and diaphragm. The addition of vaginal spermicides in the forms of gel, cream, foam, suppository, and film may offer some additional contraceptive benefits for these barrier methods. Both barrier methods and spermicides have fewer systemic effects than hormonal contraceptive methods, but are significantly less efficacious, and are rarely recommended as the sole method of contraception for patients who wish to avoid an unwanted pregnancy. Barrier methods of contraception are most efficacious when used in addition to significantly more effective long-acting reversible contraceptive (LARC) implants or short-acting reversible contraceptive (SARC) hormonal methods. Dual methods, that include either ECs or ICs, also provide superior protection against sexually transmitted infections (STIs) for adolescents and young adults (AYAs) who elect to be sexually active. Barrier methods may both prevent skin-to-skin contact, as well as retain seminal fluids. This twofold barrier effect prevents STI transmission and sperm from ascending into the uterus and upper tract. Barriers and spermicides are nonprescription and sometimes easier for AYAs to access over-the-counter. When patients elect to use barrier methods as their sole contraceptive, clinicians should offer detailed counseling and prescriptions for emergency contraception to improve potential contraceptive efficacy.

EXTERNAL CONDOMS

External condoms (also called male condoms or condoms placed on the penis) are the oldest and most common method of barrier contraception, still serving as a major form of birth control, despite consistently higher failure rates than most other current contraceptive methods. External condoms are commonly used by AYAs. Data from 2011 to 2015 National Survey of Family Growth (NSFG) indicated that condom use was lower among women aged 15 to 19 years versus those aged 20 to 39 years at 5.3% and 10%, respectively.[1] Further, the NSFG survey reported that condom use rates did not differ by race or ethnicity, but were lowest in women with a general education development (GED) certificate or high school degree. (Most studies referenced in this chapter discuss data that reflect historical concepts of binary demographics of female or male, and are not reflective of more modern concepts of nonbinary and transgender identities. Gender neutral terminology will be used wherever possible throughout the chapter).

This 2015 to 2017 NSFG survey provided data showing that 15 to 19 years old females and males reported condom use "every time" that they had intercourse—35.6% and 53.5%, respectively. Among 20- to 24-year-olds, women and men reported using condoms "every time"—17.9% and 25.9%, respectively. In this same survey, 38.2% and 23.3% of 15- to 19-year-old adolescent females and males, respectively reported "none" or not using any condoms during sex during the past 4 weeks. Older AYAs, including 19- to 24-year-old females and males, reported not using condoms in the past 4 weeks more frequently—65.1% and 40.4%, respectively. Patterns of condom use by age and education were similar for both "every time" and "100% of the time during intercourse over the past 4 weeks," with higher rates in non-Hispanic Black persons, in casual relationships, and with more than a single partner. Approximately 37% and 45% of 15- to 24-year-old females and males, respectively, reported dual use of condoms with hormonal methods. This survey also showed that 29.6% of 15- to 44-year-old women who used a condom in the past 4 weeks reported varying problems with condom use, ranging from "broke or completely fell off" or "only used part of the time," to both (6.5%, 25.8%, and 3%, respectively). An earlier NSFG survey from 2006 to 2010 reported that age did not factor into significant differences in contraceptive failure rates. Black and Hispanic women, with an expected confounder of higher poverty rates, showed higher method failure than White or "other" races for all methods and condoms (15% and 21% versus approximately 8% all methods; 21% and 19% versus 9% and 7% for condoms).[2]

According to the 2017 Youth Risk Behavior Survey (YRBS), among the 28.7% of U.S. high school students reporting being currently sexually active, 53.8% reported condom use at last intercourse.[3] Prevalence of condom use was higher in males than females, across race and grade. Condom use at last intercourse was higher among heterosexual identified youth (56.1%) compared to lesbian, gay, bisexual (LGB) or "not sure" students (39.9% and 44.1%, respectively). Prevalence of condom use was higher among heterosexual males (61.8%) compared to heterosexual females (49.6%). Adolescents and young adults who had sexual contact with both sexes had lower rates of condom use (36.1%) than their heterosexual counterparts (50.3%). Further, 13.8% of the high school students reported not using any method to prevent pregnancy at last intercourse, with a higher prevalence among students who were female, younger than their partner, Black and Hispanic, and in their freshman year. Lesbian, gay, bisexual, and "not sure" youth were less likely to have not used any protection (27.4% and 25.0%) than heterosexual counterparts (11.5%). There appear to be no differences in condom use at "first sexual encounter" by race and ethnicity. Condoms are reported as a dual method in 15% of teens, with non-Hispanic White female teenagers having the highest rates of dual method use. Improved use of dual methods has been also associated with nulliparity, insured status, and later sexual debut.

Among college students, the 2019 National College Health Assessment (NCHA) data showed that 50.3% of college women were engaging in receptive vaginal sex in the past 30 days with 45.7% having a single partner.[4] Sixty-four percent of college males and 55.0% of college females reported using male condoms during last intercourse, while only 1% or less used ICs. Dual method use in college students was reported as 48.% and 44.1% of males and females, respectively.

Condom use during oral and anal sex is relatively uncommon. In one national study, 10.8% and 31.5% of 15- to 19- and 20- to 24-year-old AYAs, respectively, reported anal intercourse, with only 32.0% and 25.0% reporting using a condom at last intercourse.[5] Adolescents and young adults who were 15 to 19 and 20 to 24 years old reported increasing rates of oral sex with age, but only 10.4% and 6.5% used condoms at last oral sex, respectively. The 2021 Centers for Disease Control and Prevention (CDC) STI guidelines recommend condom use, but also advise offering triple screening for gonorrhea and chlamydia in all sexually active AYAs at least annually.[6] The 2011 to 2015 NSFG reported that over half of AYAs engage in oral intercourse, with condom use at last oral sex 8% and 9% for females and males, respectively.[7]

Condoms for Sexually Transmitted Infection Prevention

Condom use has risen since the 1980s, related to public health campaigns to promote human immunodeficiency virus (HIV) prevention. While less efficacious as a contraceptive, condoms are most protective for STIs transmitted in genital fluids that can be exchanged during penile intercourse.[8] Latex and polyurethane condoms are impermeable to *Chlamydia trachomatis, Neisseria gonorrhoeae*, trichomoniasis, syphilis, Hepatitis B and C, and HIV. Consistent use of condoms in heterosexual couples reduced transmission of HIV seroconversion by 80% or incidence 1.14/100 person–years "always" users versus 5.75/100 person–years for "never" users.[9] Condoms also provide some measure of skin-to-skin barrier protection against viruses such as herpes simplex virus (HSV) and human papilloma virus (HPV). Consistent and correct condom use demonstrated a 70% reduction in HPV transmission, improved clearance of HPV infection, decreased risk of genital warts and cervical cancer, and regression of cervical intraepithelial neoplasia.

The 2013 American Academy of Pediatrics (AAP) policy statement on condom use for AYAs recommends that pediatric clinicians address the following issues:

- Encourage communication between parents/caregivers and adolescents about sexual activity and sex education with guidance from the AAP Bright Futures.
- Provide parent/caregiver educational programs to create skills and incentives to talk with adolescents about condom use.
- Improve condom availability in their medical home and in the community.

Uses of External Condoms

Contraceptive Use

1. As a primary method of birth control, alone or in conjunction with a spermicide, a female barrier, hormonal method, or intrauterine contraception
2. As a backup method of contraception during fertile periods, that is, fertility awareness method (FAM), during the first 7 days of initiating contraceptives or in face of a gap in SARC adherence

Noncontraceptive Uses

1. To reduce transmission of STIs—oral, vaginal, anal
2. To blunt sensation, to treat premature ejaculation
3. To reduce cervical antisperm antibody titers in women with associated infertility
4. To reduce allergic reaction in women with sensitivity to sperm

Types of External Condoms

External latex condoms are most commonly used in the United States. These are marketed in a variety of shapes and sizes, but typically measure 170 mm long and 50 mm wide, and 0.03 to 0.10 mm thick. Additional features such as ribbing, lubricants (spermicides, silicone, water-based gels), colors, scents, and tastes are marketing strategies, but are not linked to efficacy. In the past, sex educators promoted a "one-size-fits-all" concept to discourage some males from refusing to wear condoms because of self-reports of large penis size. More recent data suggest that size matters, and improved fit may improve condom use. Many heterosexual men and women report condom fit or feel problems that included decreased sensation, lack of naturalness, condom size complaints, decreased pleasure, and pain and discomfort. Condoms that fit poorly are more than two times more likely to break, slip, or interfere with erection, orgasm, and sexual pleasure. In addition, males with poorly fitting condoms are twice as likely to remove a condom during intercourse than those with well-fitting condoms.

Polyurethane condoms are made with nonbiodegradable materials that are stronger and less likely to be damaged by handling, petroleum lubricants, or shelf life. However, polyurethane condoms continue to be less popular than their latex counterparts as they are more expensive, less elastic and form fitting, and two to five times more likely to break or slip. Despite demonstrated drawbacks, nonlatex condoms remain an important barrier method for persons with true sensitivities or allergies to latex.

Natural or skin (lamb cecum) condoms are as effective as latex or polyurethane condoms for pregnancy prevention, but not recommended for STI protection. Skin condoms have larger pores (up to 1,500 nm in diameter) that may allow HIV and Hepatitis B virus transmission across these membranes. Natural and skin condoms may not prevent STIs and are, therefore, not recommended for AYAs at risk for STIs.

Mechanism of Action

Condoms are sheaths that create a physical barrier and prevent skin to skin contact, as well as contain and prevent exchange of fluids. Condoms are regulated medical devices subject to testing by the U.S. Food and Drug Administration (FDA). Latex condoms manufactured in the United States, can typically last up to 5 years, and are tested electronically for holes before packaging. Consumer Reports regularly tests the U.S.-manufactured condom models for strength, reliability, and perforation. All models passed minimum standards for reliability, holes, and packaging with additional features not affecting failure or score. The reservoir tip allows for pooled semen and decreases the potential for leakage. Oil-based lubricants and "double bagging" (wearing two condoms at the same time) are not recommended as they impact structural integrity of latex condoms and may increase tears.

Effectiveness

Condoms are currently the most efficacious way to prevent STIs in sexually active AYAs, but are inferior with respect to birth control in comparison to LARC and other modes of contraception.[8] The CDC U.S. Medical Eligibility Criteria for Contraceptive use (CDC MEC) does not contain a content section for condoms as a sole method of contraception, continuing to highlight that while effective for STI prevention, condoms remain significantly inferior to other forms of contraception. World Health Organization

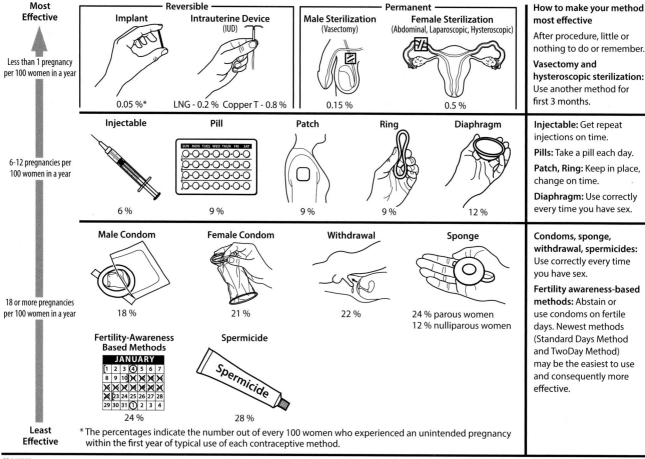

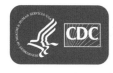

FIGURE 47.1 CDC Effectiveness of Family Planning Methods* Table. Sources: Adapted from World Health Organization (WHO) Department of Reproductive Health and Research, Johns Hopkins Bloomberg School of Public Health/Center for Communication Programs (CCP). Knowledge for health project. Family planning: a global handbook for providers (2011 update). Baltimore, MD; Geneva, Switzerland: CCP and WHO; 2011; and Trussel J. Contraceptive failure in the United States. *Contraception* 2011;83:397–404. *The percentages indicate the number out of every 100 women who experienced an unintended pregnancy within the first year of typical use of each contraceptive method.

Tiered-Effectiveness Counseling recognizes the superior efficacy of LARCs versus SARCs and barriers, promoting use of first-line methods for all AYAs.[10] In their visual effectiveness tool (see Fig. 47.1), condoms are considered Tier 3 or "Less Effective" than other methods estimating more than 13 pregnancies per 100 women in 1 year.

Perfect use (i.e., consistent and always correct) is estimated as two condoms breaking per 100 condoms used. However, real life condom efficacy requires proper technique to avoid slips and breaks, as well as consistent use from start to finish of each and every coitus. Sundaram reported that most contraceptive failures, excluding LARCs, occur in the first 6 months of use; estimated condom specific failure rates ranged from 13% to 18%.[2] Approximately one-third of contraceptive failures occur in months 1 to 3 of use, with two-thirds of failures occurring in the first 6 months of use. Condoms were only slightly less effective than withdrawal (20%). Subgroup analyses indicated that increasing parity, poverty, Black and Hispanic race, and cohabitation predicted higher condom

failure rates. Real-life condom failure typically results from lack of correct and consistent use as opposed to device failure.

Contraception counseling for all sexually active persons optimally focuses on dual methods such as LARCs or SARCs for pregnancy prevention supported by concurrent use of condoms to provide STI protection. The combination optimizes reproductive health outcomes in all sexually active AYAs. Dual method research has focused on AYAs and factors such as sociodemographics (age, race/ethnicity, education), risk perception, types of and duration of relationship, number of partners, partner support of condoms, and exposure to HIV counseling and prevention. Estimates of dual method prevalence vary widely, with U.S. rates consistently lower than Western Europe. Nationwide 8.8% of high school youth, reported dual methods at last sex.[3] Dual methods were more common in students who identified as heterosexual, White, and older ages and those who had sexual contact with only the opposite sex. Studies vary regarding whether LARC use is associated with same or lower condom use and changes in STI rates.

Improving Condom Success

Correct and consistent condom use over time is the key to efficacy. Factors associated with decreased condom use include spontaneous intercourse with more casual sexual partners, not feeling at risk for HIV, lack of family connectedness, lack of parent–teen communication about sex, experience of pornography and interpersonal violence, and use of alcohol or other substances. Of particular importance, as seen in other areas of AYA health, parent/caregiver communication and support is linked to improved health outcomes, including increased condom use. Parent–teen communication about sex is associated with condom use self-efficacy and intention to use.[11,12] Other situational factors that have been linked to improved condom use include peer influence; more favorable attitudes toward contraception; more accurate knowledge about reproductive health, condom use, and STI prevention; easy access to condoms (including carrying condoms on their person), school-based condom availability; and more open communication both with family and partners.[13,14] Educational and behavioral interventions that have been tailored to address motivation, negotiation skills, access to condoms, and cultural characteristics of individual populations have been effective in promoting condom use, but are not effective in promoting abstinence.[15,16]

Systemic disadvantage and racism continues to impact AYAs' right to reproductive justice. Condom availability and accessibility vary according to geographic regions and overall community resources.[17] Adolescents and young adults of color and who live in lower socioeconomic communities are more likely than their White counterparts to live in a "contraception desert," where despite living closer to a pharmacy, pharmacy characteristics make access to condoms more difficult and less likely to be obtained.[18] There are high levels of environmental and physical barriers to obtaining condoms, including few stores, personnel required to access and provide condoms, and the majority of stores offering only a single type of condom.[19] In addition, other vulnerable AYA populations such as women who have sex with women and other sexual minoritized persons, homeless youth, and transgender and nonbinary youth are also at risk for issues with education, access, and suboptimal use of barrier contraceptive.[20,21] Condom counseling, with a diverse community of AYAs, necessitates a culturally respectful approach to listening carefully and openly, establishing a dialogue about goals and priorities, and providing each youth with patient-centered consent-based plan or care.

Improving consistent and correct use of condoms is essential to their ultimate effectiveness. Studies indicate that condom errors vary across time and populations assessed. Common errors that impair effectiveness include using condom during only part of penetrative activities; using incorrect placement techniques, including not squeezing air from the tip or leaving room at the tip; putting a condom on inside out; using lubricants that decrease condom integrity; and not removing the condom correctly. Studies demonstrate common issues with uncomfortable feel or fit, erectile dysfunction, slipping, leaking, or breaking are common and deterrents to regular use.

The following are some recommended tips for discussing *correct and consistent condom use* (Fig. 47.2):

- Ensure safe storage conditions (heat, expiration dates) along with privacy and easy access.
- Plan how to integrate condom use during intercourse.
- Follow techniques for opening and removing the condom from its package, as many as half of condom breaks occur before penetration.
- Correct direction for unrolling condom, pinching tip to allow slack or remove air from reservoir to allow for semen to collect, and unroll condom down over entire length of the erect penis
- Continue to check placement of condom during the whole period of intercourse to assess slippage and integrity of device.
- Use new condom for every act of sex including each orifice (oral, vaginal, anal) and throughout the entire sex act (i.e., from start to finish of sex).

- Use only water-based or silicone lubricants applied to external surface of the condom, vulva, or vagina (petroleum-based lubricants or medications can destroy condom integrity in less than a minute allowing viral or sperm transmission).
- Correct condom removal includes grasping the rim of the condom at the base of a partially erect or firm penis and carefully pulling off the condom making sure that semen does not spill out.
- Inspect for signs of breakage or spillage. If concerned, consider emergency contraception or spermicide.

Advantages

- Readily available without prescription and obtainable in many schools, pharmacies, or retail settings
- Relatively inexpensive costing between $0.50 and $1.50 (U.S. dollars) per condom
- Portable and easily carried by men and women for easy access in many settings
- Male partner is included in contraception and family planning participation.
- Visible proof of protection during each act of coitus
- Most importantly, currently most effective method of STI prevention other than abstinence

Disadvantages

- One of the least effective methods of contraception
- Requires availability and application with each coitus
- May be perceived as invasive, interruptive, and unnatural
- Requires cooperation of male partner
- May diminish sensation and pleasure

Side Effects of External Condoms

While condoms may be less effective than other hormonal or inserted forms of birth control, there are no restrictions on the use of latex condoms with any medical condition except true latex allergy. Although many women report irritation and discomfort with condom use, this is more likely due to lack of lubrication or irritation from spermicide rather than a true latex allergic reaction. True latex allergies are estimated in less than 5% of the general population, but may be higher in clinician and youth with spina bifida. Nonlatex condoms are recommended for those with true latex allergy. There is an increasing number of nonlatex options including polyisoprene (Skyn Condoms) which has more stretch and may provide more sensation.

Future Developments

On a manufacturing level, there are studies evaluating a variety of strategies to improve condom effectiveness. Multipurpose Prevention Technologies (MPTs) are also in the pipeline as combination products that potentially offer both contraception and STI prevention, but are likely years away from FDA approval and availability. Electrospinning, using nanosized medication polymers to create a tightly woven barrier fabric, can be used to create condoms that additionally deliver medication to kill sperm and infectious agents. Nanocoated condoms have demonstrated some potential to prevent or inactivate different STIs.[22] Condoms that create their own lubricant and reduce friction are being studied and demonstrate some initial user satisfaction and potential for greater use.[23] Condoms are being made with thinner materials and more fit options. These condoms meet breakage and safety standards and may add to improved condom adherence.[24] Condoms are not only made in a variety of sizes, but may also be custom sized and come in one of 60 tailored sizes (myOne Perfect Fit). Condoms are also available with an adhesive top that further improves fit.[25]

Additional efforts to improve condoms uptake include easier to use and more aesthetic packaging, such as the Unique Pull Condoms, Lovability Condoms Tin, and Maude Rise Latex Condoms.

The external condom is a sheath of plastic or rubber that fits snugly over the erect penis. It blocks the man's sperm from entering the woman's body. It also covers the penis to help protect the man and the woman from getting sexually transmitted infections from each other. The external condom can be used with other contraceptives. It can be used with other birth control methods such as birth control pills, shots, implants, spermicide, and diaphragms. It should not be used with the female condom. On average, if 100 couples use condoms for a year, 12 will become pregnant. Correct and more consistent use can reduce the risk of pregnancy even more.

♦ Use a condom every time you have sex. Keep a few handy.
♦ Put the condom on before there is any genital contact.
♦ Open the package carefully.
♦ Unroll the condom all the way to the base of the penis.
♦ Squeeze the air out of the top of the condom to make room for the ejaculate.
♦ Make sure your partner is well lubricated. Use spermicide or water-based or silicon-based lubricants. Do *not* use petroleum-based lubricants with latex condoms.
♦ If the condom tears or starts to slip off during sex, grasp the rim of the condom against the penis and withdraw the penis. The man should wash his hands and his penis. The woman should wash her hands and her labia (do *not* douche). If spermicide is available, the woman should insert spermicide into her vagina according to product directions. She should also use emergency contraception as soon as possible. If the couple wants to have sex again, use a new condom.
♦ Right after ejaculation, while the penis is still firm, the rim of the condom could be gently pressed against the penis as it is removed from the vagina.
♦ Check the used condom for any breaks or tears. If breaks or tears are noticed follow instructions above regarding spermicide and emergency contraception. Tie up the end and throw it away.

DOs and DON'Ts:

Do use a new condom each time you have sex	Don't reuse a condom
Do use a condom made of latex or polyurethane	Don't use lambskin or fake plastic condoms
Do change your condom if you have oral or anal sex before you have intercourse	Don't use the same condom for different sex practices or different sex partners
Do check the expiration date of the condom	Don't use a condom after the expiration date
Do place the condom before the penis touches her genitals	Don't let the penis touch her genitals before the condom goes on
Do use water-based lubricants if needed, such as spermicide, K-Y jelly	Don't use the petroleum-based products, such as Vaseline, oils, vaginal creams for infection treatment
Do hold the condom rim against the penis and pull them out together before the penis starts to soften or after ejaculation	Don't let the penis become soft inside her vagina—the condom can fall off
Do check the condom for tears, then tie it off and throw it away	Don't ever wash the condom and recycle it
Do keep emergency contraception and spermicide ready in case something happens and the condom does not work well	Don't wait until you need it, because emergency contraception works better the sooner you use it

FIGURE 47.2 The external condom—patient information sheet.

Adolescents and young adults report that changes in wrapper and applicator design make AYAs more confident that they will not only use condoms, but use them correctly.[26] There are thicker condoms for premature ejaculation prevention (Durex Prolong) and extralarge condoms for penile circumferences up to 56 mm (Glyde Maxi Ultra Thin Extra Large Condom). There are condoms with specialized tips to increase pleasure (One Pleasure Plus Condom) and condoms that use alternates to silicone lubricant and thus are safer to use with silicone toys (Lifestyles Tuxedo Condoms). There are vegan condoms (Good Clean Love Barely There Condoms, Sustain Naturals Ultra-thin Condoms, Glyde Flavored Condoms), and condoms that taste better for oral sex (Glyde Flavored Condoms).

Unique approaches to acceptability and access may also improve condom use. Allbodies digital platform focuses on condoms, gels, and sexual pleasure for nonbinary persons. Both public sector condom distribution initiatives, along with commercial mail order and subscription services can increase access and availability, and for AYAs, decrease embarrassment and risk when having to procure condoms in public spaces.[27,28] One study has indicated that participants would be more likely to use condoms for oral and anal sex if they were FDA approved.[23] In addition, the potential for sex positive approaches to sexual health education and services provides a larger frame normalizing the developmental tasks of AYA sexual development, with a focus on not just risk, but pleasure and intimacy.

INTERNAL CONDOMS

Internal condoms (formerly called female condoms [FC]), came into use in the 1980s, but still only account for less than 1% of all condom use worldwide. In 2018, the FDA renamed female condoms, ICs, with three changes in regulation: renamed as "single-use internal condom"; approved for both vaginal and anal use; and transitioned from Class III to Class II regulation thereby increasing access to further manufacturing developments.[8]

Few adolescents elect to use the IC, with 1.5% reporting ever using. As with ECs, use is inconsistent and often incorrect, decreasing its potential usefulness. Only two FC (FC1 and FC2) have FDA approval in the United States. The FC1 is made from polyurethane, but is no longer produced. The FC2 is made of a nitrile sheath, which is less expensive, as well as less noisy than its earlier counterpart. This 17-cm long, 7.8-cm width device is inserted into the vagina or anus with a flexible external ring outside the orifice entry. Internal condoms are not sensitive to petroleum-based products, and the sheath contains a silicone lubricant on the inside. A version of a natural latex IC is available in other countries, but is not FDA approved in the United States.

Data on the attitudes and use of the IC in AYAs are limited. A focus group of urban youth, ages 15 to 20 years, demonstrated that young women know that IC is woman controlled, while young males' knowledge focused on sexual feeling and pleasure.[29] The authors recommended that focusing on contraceptive effectiveness, lack of side effects, and availability may be important when discussing the IC. The majority of current studies examining pregnancy and STI prevention in AYAs, and sexual or gender minoritized persons, focus on ECs and generally do not include data about vaginal and anal IC use.

Efficacy

Typical first-year failure rates of 21% are considerably higher than the 5% perfect-use failure; this is due to users' ability to use consistently and correctly each time and over time.[30] The IC offers protection against STIs and unintended pregnancy similar to its traditional counterpart and has been of research interest for offering "woman-controlled" methods for sex workers in underdeveloped countries. A 2020 meta-analysis of over 15 studies and almost 7,000 patients determined that the use of dual-condoms, the FC1 and ECs, may be as effective for HIV prevention and even more effective for preventing gonorrhea and chlamydia.[31]

Advantages

- Like the EC, there are usually no contraindications or medically complex conditions that would contraindicate IC use.
- The polyurethane is not sensitive to petroleum-based products. Additional lubrication applied within the condom helps reduce breakage related to friction and allows for less device-related noise.
- For persons whose partners refuse to wear condoms, the IC offers the receptive partner a self-administered protective option, for both anal and vaginal sex.

Disadvantages

- Coitus dependent
- Technically more difficult to insert than ECs
- More expensive than EC

Internal condoms, for understandable reasons, are infrequently used by AYAs. A 2020 study, evaluating the availability of contraception for AYAs at U.S. pharmacies, reported that only eight pharmacies stocked IC.[32] In this caller sample of 1,475 pharmacies, one-third of pharmacies were dismissive, rude, or gave incorrect information about IC to AYA callers. As with ECs, IC may be more difficult for disadvantaged communities to access in relative "contraceptive deserts." The majority of stores in urban areas did not even offer IC.

In addition to being more technically complicated for correct vaginal insertion, persons should check placement throughout the entirety of coitus. Excessive friction can break the condom or invert the condom on withdrawal. Additional lubrication applied within the IC can help reduce this risk. For AYAs, efficacy related to correct and consistent use depends on extensive education, hands-on practice, and significant motivation. As with ECs, clinicians should offer emergency contraception in advance to all IC users.

Instructions for insertion and use are shown (Fig. 47.3). While inserting the IC up to 8 hours before intercourse is acceptable, both partners need to maintain its correct position during sex to prevent it from getting pushed off or into the vagina or anus.

Future Developments

Relatively new models of the IC appear to be noninferior to the FDA-approved FC2 model. Outside of the United States newer models with variations in design were developed to provide users with greater and individual choices. Models available in other countries include Reddy and VA w.o.w Condom, which are latex and use a soft, polyurethane sponge to hold it in place. Oil-based lubricants should not be used with latex-based IC as they can damage latex. PATH's Woman's Condom makes insertion easier using a rounded cap, which dissolves once it is put in place. The Cupid FC condom is WHO approved and available in South Africa, Mozambique, Indonesia, India, and other countries, and is cheaper than the FC2. Internal condom choices are expanding—new models have low failure rates and are acceptable to users. The Natural Sensation Panty Condom is worn like underwear, with the condom built into the panty design. Multifunctional technologies continue to create dual-use devices and are exploring electrospinning technologies that use fibers from liquid spermicides and virobactericides to create IC.

CONTRACEPTIVE SPONGE

The contraceptive sponge was approved in 1983, removed from the United States market in 1994, and then returned in 2005. This device is available over-the-counter, is relatively easy to insert, and can be inserted long before coitus. The sponge is donut-shaped, and a one-size-fits-all, soft polyurethane foam device, inserted over the cervix, and acts as a physical barrier to sperm penetrating the upper tract. The device is moistened with water and then slid back into the posterior vagina where a small concavity fits against the cervix to provide immediate effective contraception. It contains a slow release of 125 to 150 mg of nonoxynol-9 so that no additional spermicides are needed over the 24-hour time frame and may provide protection for multiple acts of coitus. The sponge should stay in place for 6 hours after coitus and then can be removed at any time thereafter. When the woman wishes to remove the sponge, she gently grasps a small polyester loop and pulls it out. Women are warned against leaving the sponge in for great than 24 hours because of risk of toxic shock syndrome.

Mechanism of Action

The primary contraceptive action of the sponge is provided by the spermicidal activity of nonoxynol-9, which is impregnated in the polyurethane foam. The sponge releases 125 to 150 mg of nonoxynol-9 slowly over a 24-hour period. The sponge also traps and absorbs semen and acts as a physical barrier between sperm and the cervical os.

Efficacy

As with any other coitus method, the sponge has higher typical-use failure rates than many other methods. Failure rates of 16% in nulliparous women compared to 32% in parous women are associated with the fit and barrier effect with a more patulous gravid cervix.[30] Nulliparous and parous perfect-use rates are higher at 9% and 20%, respectively. The effectiveness of the sponge as a barrier method can be improved by active use of emergency contraception.[33]

As with other barrier devices, the sponge is available without a prescription, controlled by the female, and may be inserted before and used for multiple acts of sex. Young women electing to use the sponge must intentionally place it before intercourse and be comfortable touching their vagina and inserting and removing the device. Its local action eliminates any concerns regarding systemic hormonal side effects. There are few contraindications to use of the sponge, and these may include allergy to sponge components (polyurethane, metabisulfite, and nonoxynol-9), prior toxic shock syndrome, and current menstruation. Up to 4% of users experience odor, itching, burning, redness, or a rash with its use. Local irritation is most likely due to sensitivity to detergent effects of the spermicide.

Patient Education

Insertion

- Remove the sponge from its package and hold it with the "dimple" side facing up and the loop hanging down.
- Moisten with approximately two tablespoons of water and squeeze the sponge a few times until it becomes sudsy.

The Internal Condom

What is the internal condom?

The internal condom is a thin, soft, loose-fitting pouch with two flexible rigns at either end. One ring helps hold the device in place inside the women's vagina over the end of the womb (cervix), while the other ring rests outside the vagina.

Outer ring lies against the labia (lips of the vulva)

Inner ring is used for insertion; helps hold internal condom in place

How does it work?

The internal condom is made of polyurethane, a type of plastic. The plastic condom covers the inside of the vagina, cervix, and area around the opening to the vagina. The device acts as a barrier to help prevent pregnancy and the transmission of germs that can cause sexually transmitted diseases (STDs), including human immunodeficiency virus (HIV) and acquired immunodeficiency syndrome (AIDS). The device can be inserted by the woman up to 8 hours before sex.

How to insert the internal condom

1. Find a comfortable position. You may want to stand up with one foot on a chair, squat with knees apart, or lie down with legs bent and knees apart.
2. Hold the internal condom with the open end hanging down. Squeeze the inner ring with your thumb and middle finger.
3. Holding the inner ring squeezed together, insert the ring into the vagina and push the inner ring and pouch into the vagina past the pubic bone.
4. When properly inserted, the outer ring will hang down slightly outside the vagina. During intercourse, when the penis enters the vagina, the slack will lessen.

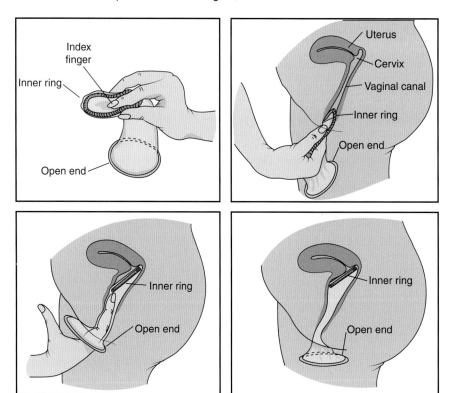

FIGURE 47.3 The internal condom.

Remember:

The internal condom may be hard to hold or slippery at first. Before you use one for the first time during sex, practice inserting one to get used to it. Take your time. Be sure to insert the condom straight into the vagina without twisting the pouch.

During Sex

1. It's helpful to use your hand to guide the penis into vagina inside the internal condom.
2. The ring may move from side to side or up and down during intercource. This is OK.
3. If the internal condom seems to be sticking to and moving with the penis rather than resting in the vagina, stop and add more lubricant to the inside of the device (near the outer ring) or to the penis.

How to remove the internal condom after intercourse

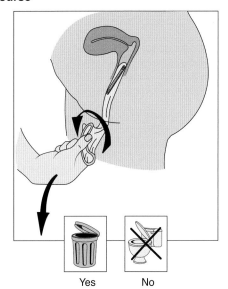

1. Squeeze and twist the outer ring to close it.
2. Pull the internal condom out gently.
3. Throw the condom away in the garbage. Do not flush down the toilet.
4. Do not wash out and use again.

Special Reminders

- Use a new internal condom with every act of intercourse.
- Use it every time you have intercourse.
- Read and follow the directions carefully.
- Do not use a external and internal condom at the same time.
- Be careful not to tear the condom with fingernails or sharp objects.
- Use enough lubricant.

Yes   No

Latex condoms for men are highly effective at preventing STDs, including HIV infection (AIDS), if used properly. If your partner refuses to use a external latex condom, use a internal condom to help protect yourself and your partner.

FIGURE 47.3 (*Continued*).

- Fold the sides of the sponge upward with a finger on each side to support it.
- While in a standing, lying, or squatting position gently introduce the sponge into the vagina and using one or two fingers push the sponge upward as far as it will go.
- Check the position of the sponge by running a finger around the edge of the sponge to make sure that the cervix is covered.

Removal

- Wait 6 hours after the last act of intercourse before removing the sponge.
- Insert one finger into the vagina until the loop is felt.
- If the loop cannot be felt, bear down, lie on your back on the bed with your knees up against your chest, squat down in a low position, or sit on the toilet and tilt your pelvis forward (so that the small of your back is rounded) to bring the sponge closer to the vaginal opening.
- Hook one finger into the loop then gently and slowly pull the sponge out.
- Check to make sure the sponge is intact; if it is torn, remove all pieces from the vagina.
- Discard sponge.

Contraindications

- History of toxic shock syndrome
- Allergy or sensitivity to polyurethane foam, nonoxynol-9, or metabisulfite, or allergy to sulfa
- During menstruation

Advantages

- Lack of hormonal side effects or medical contraindications
- Allows for spontaneity after insertion; can be used over repeated acts of intercourse
- Available without a prescription or fitting by clinicians; one-size-fits-all
- Female-controlled method; does not require partner participation
- May be more comfortable to wear than other barrier methods such as the diaphragm
- Easy to use and not "messy"

Disadvantages

- Relatively high failure rate
- Adolescents and young adults must be comfortable touching genitals in order to insert device.

- Spermicide may cause vaginal, vulvar, or penile irritation. As many as 4% of users will experience a sensitivity reaction to the sponge that can lead to itching, burning, redness, or a rash. Although this may be due to nonoxynol-9, other components of the sponge such as the preservative may be the source of the sensitivity reaction.
- Sponge can become discolored or malodorous in the presence of vaginitis.
- Can be difficult to remove
- Not recommended for use during menses

Future Developments

Three brands of contraceptives sponges are currently marketed: Today (United States), Pharmatex (France, Quebec), and Protectaid (Canada, Europe). Pharmatex and Protectaid are still not approved by the FDA. Protectaid contains active ingredients 6.25 mg of nonoxynol-9, 6.25 mg of benzalkonium chloride, and 25 mg of sodium cholate; Pharmatex contains 60 mg of benzalkonium chloride. Multipurpose Prevention Technologies using sponge-like devices are also in the pipeline as combination products that potentially offer both contraception and STI prevention, but are likely years away from FDA approval and availability.

⬤ CERVICAL SHIELD

The cervical shield (Lea's Shield) (Fig. 47.4) was approved in 2002 and is available by prescription. This cervical shield is a one-size-fits-all device to block sperm from entering the cervix and upper tract. The device is oval with a small concave cup that fits over the cervix, with the remainder of the device filling the proximal vagina. A small one-way valve allows both air and menses to be released from behind the device. This device provides barrier protection by covering the cervix in its entirety, and is even more effective with the additional application of spermicide. The shield differs from its barrier prescription counterparts (cap and diaphragm) in two important ways. First, the shield is held in place by its physical volume and the muscles of the vaginal wall compared to the cap, which is held in place by the cervix, the diaphragm, and the pubic bone. Second, the cervical shield is independent of cervical or vaginal size, and therefore it does not require fitting by a clinician. Because of the one-way valve design, this method can be used as contraception during menses, although some resources advise against this practice. Composed

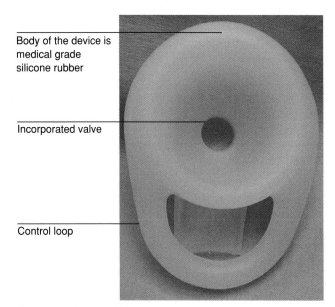

Body of the device is medical grade silicone rubber

Incorporated valve

Control loop

FIGURE 47.4 The Lea's Shield.

of silicone rubber, it is nonallergenic, washable, and reusable for multiple acts of intercourse over a period of 48 hours. It can be worn hours before intercourse and should remain in place for at least 8 hours post-coitus, but correct positioning should be reconfirmed before sex.

Efficacy

Like other barrier methods, efficacy is dependent on correct and consistent use with failure rates up to 15%. Efficacy is also improved by the addition of spermicide with each coitus. Like the sponge, the shield is more effective in nulliparous women, but differs from the diaphragm and cap in that it seems to provide more protection than these methods in multiparous women. Although the shield is not included in the U.S. CDC MEC comparative list for efficacy and continuation, its failure rates are similar.

Insertion of Lea's Shield

Like other barrier methods, women must be comfortable manually inserting and removing the vaginal device. Prior to intercourse, the cup is filled with spermicide and then the device is pushed into the proximal vagina.
- Apply a small amount of spermicide in the bowl of the device.
- Gently squeeze the shield and insert into the vaginal bowl first as high as it will go.
- Check to make sure that the entire cervix is covered by the bowl.

Removal of Lea's Shield

- Insert a finger into the vagina, grasp and twist the control loop to break the suction, and gently remove.
- The shield should be washed thoroughly with mild liquid soap for approximately 2 minutes, dried, and then stored.

Advantages

- There are few contraindications to using this device and no systemic effects.
- Effective for up to 48 hours; additional doses of spermicide are not required for multiple acts of intercourse.
- May be placed early and is usually not detected by the partner
- May offer some reduction of STI risk, especially for cervical and upper genital tract infections

Disadvantages

- Requires a clinician visit to obtain a prescription
- Requires training in placement, removal, cleaning, and storage and may be difficult or uncomfortable to insert and remove
- Replacement every 1 to 3 years

⬤ CERVICAL CAP AND DIAPHRAGM

The cervical cap and diaphragm are prescription-only devices that require fitting by a medical clinician. Like other barrier methods, they block the cervix and prevent sperm from ascending to the upper tract. These methods are rarely used by AYAs, but are of interest to reproductive health scientists because they have the potential to protect against STIs and HIV when used in combination with antimicrobial spermicides.

The cap (FemCap) (Fig. 47.5) is smaller than the diaphragm and made of nonallergenic silicone. It comes in three sizes (22 mm, 26 mm, and 30 mm) that are fit based on obstetrical history, and not by physical examination. The small 22-mm rim is recommended for nulliparous women, the medium for women with prior pregnancy, but no vaginal delivery, and the 30-mm rim for users whose cervix has experienced vaginal delivery. The cap is filled with spermicide, most of it on the side of the cap facing away from the cervix and into the vagina, which may reduce cervical irritation. The device may be used for multiple acts of coitus for up to 48 hours, with checking required to ensure proper placement with each act.

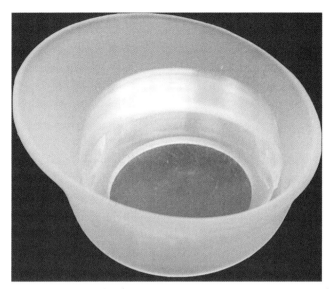

FIGURE 47.5 The FemCap. (Courtesy of FemCap, Inc., and Alfred Shihata, MD.)

The diaphragm is a latex or silicone cup, which is fit with a spring mechanism rim that secures the device and covers the cervix (Fig. 47.6). It has a semiflexible ring that helps hold the device, anchoring it with the pubic bone. Spermicide is placed within the cup on the side that comes in contact with the cervix. PATH designed SILCS diaphragm (Caya R) (Fig. 47.7) is a newer silicone, single-size barrier with a contoured rim that accommodates most women. The preshaped rim sits high in the vaginal vault while a finger cup at the posterior base allows for removal. It is available by prescription in the United States, but designed to be available over-the-counter. The Milex Wide Seal R is another FDA-approved silicone diaphragm, with an arcing spring and extended skirt designed to increase the seal. It comes in sizes 60 to 95 mm. Ortho coil spring, flat spring, and arcing spring diaphragms have been discontinued.

Effectiveness

Effectiveness of the cervical cap is not included in the CDC MEC, but appears to be less effective than its counterpart, the diaphragm. Diaphragm typical-use failure rate is approximately 15%. A diaphragm is more likely to dislodge in women who have extreme uterine ante- or retroversion, as well as in women who prefer to be on top during sex. Diaphragm effectiveness requires additional vaginal spermicide with each act of coitus after that 6-hour window,

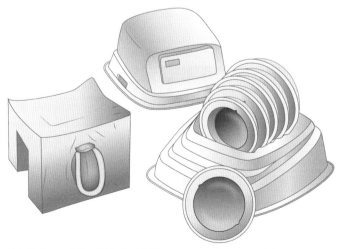

FIGURE 47.6 Milex Wide Seal R Diaphragm and fitting materials.

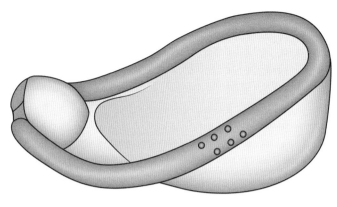

FIGURE 47.7 Caya diaphragm.

with the diaphragm left in place for a full 6 hours after last coitus. Emergency contraception should be considered if a diaphragm is removed or dislodged prior to these 6 hours postcoitus.

Adolescents and young adults can use caps and diaphragms, but are often unable to anticipate intercourse and are more uncomfortable touching the vulva and vagina for correct insertion, making these unusual methods of choice for teens. These devices require additional care and maintenance, with soap and water washes, followed by a soak in an alcohol solution, and cornstarch coating prior to storage in a cool and dry environment.

Contraindications to Use

- History of toxic shock syndrome
- Allergy to latex or spermicidal agents
- Recent pregnancy, before renormalization of anatomy
- Inability of patient to correctly insert and remove diaphragm

Tips to Improve Success of Method

- Correct fitting of device (see later discussion)
- Detailed, hands-on instruction for patient education (see later discussion)
- Careful monitoring of diaphragm between uses to identify any defects (see later discussion)
- Careful selection of patient
  - Offer only to motivated woman willing to touch her genitals and to use the device with *every* act of intercourse.
  - Avoid offering to a woman with a markedly anteverted or retroverted uterus (diaphragm tends to dislodge).
  - Discourage coital positions that compromise stability of diaphragm, particularly the female superior position.

Correct Fitting of Diaphragm

The SILCS diaphragm was developed to increase patient control and access as it does not require fitting at a provider's office. It may be used up to 2 years and then needs replacement. Diaphragms are rarely used today, even in specialized family planning centers. A diaphragm must be fit properly to be effective. The diagonal length of the vaginal canal from the posterior aspect of the symphysis pubis to the posterior vaginal fornix is measured during the bimanual examination and measured against a diaphragm rim. A diaphragm is inserted and checked using the correct size (one size smaller than the first diaphragm felt or perceived by the patient).The diaphragm should touch the lateral vaginal walls, cover the cervix, and fit snugly between the posterior vaginal fornix and behind the symphysis pubis. A diaphragm that is too large may buckle and permit sperm to bypass the diaphragm. A diaphragm that is too small may slip out of place. The clinician should appreciate that the adolescent may be tense during initial fitting, causing the fitting of a smaller diaphragm than would be required if the adolescent were relaxed (Fig. 47.8).

Diaphragm Patient Information and Instructions

The diaphragm is a shallow, dome-shaped cup made of soft rubber. It is inserted into the vagina and placed securely over the cervix. It must be used with spermicidal cream or jelly. The diaphragm prevents pregnancy by providing a barrier between the sperm and uterus.

Instructions to patients

Check diaphragm for tears or holes by holding it up to a bright light and stretching the rubber slightly. Always use with contraceptive cream or jelly. Hold the diaphragm with the dome down and squeeze a tablespoon of cream or jelly into the dome and spread it around the dome and onto the rim with your finger.

To insert your diaphragm, stand with one foot propped up (i.e., on the toilet seat), squat, or lie on your back. Press the edges of the diaphragm together with one hand. With your other hand, spread the lips of your vagina and insert the diaphragm into your vagina. Push the diaphragm downward and back along the back wall of your vagina as far as it will go. Then tuck the front rim of the diaphragm up along the roof of your vagina behind the pubic bone.

Check the placement of your diaphragm by sweeping your index finger across the diaphragm to make sure the cervix is completely covered by the soft rubber dome and that the front rim of the diaphragm is snugly in place behind your pubic bone. (The cervix will feel like the tip of your nose.) When properly placed, the diaphragm will neither cause discomfort nor interfere with sex. The diaphragm and contraceptive cream or jelly can be inserted up to 6 hours before intercourse. If 6 hours have passed since insertion and the time intercourse occurs, put another applicator full of jelly or cream into your vagina without removing the diaphragm.

A new application of spermicidal cream or jelly is necessary with each additional act of intercourse. Do not remove the diaphragm. Use the plastic applicator to insert the jelly or cream in front of the diaphragm.

The diaphragm must be left in place for 6 to 8 hours after the last time you have intercourse, but never leave the diaphragm in place for more than 24 hours. Do not douche.

To remove the diaphragm

To remove the diaphragm, place your index finger behind the front rim of the diaphragm and pull down and out. Sometimes squatting and pushing with your abdominal muscles (i.e., bearing down as though you were having a bowel movement) helps to hook your finger behind the diaphragm. After use, the diaphragm should be washed with soap and water, rinsed thoroughly, and dried with a towel. Store it in its plastic container. You may dust it with cornstarch. Do not use talcum, perfumed powder, Vaseline, baby oil, or contraceptive foam, as they may damage the diaphragm. Inspect the diaphragm (especially around the rim) for holes or defects.

Side effects

Occasionally, the spermicidal cream or jelly has been found to be irritating. Changing to another brand should resolve the problem. Some patients have reported bladder symptoms or urinary tract infections with use of the diaphragm. Rare cases of toxic shock syndrome have been reported in users of the diaphragm. Contact your physician if you have:

- Fever above 38.3° C (101 °F)
- Diarrhea
- Vomiting
- Muscle aches
- Rash (sunburnlike)

FIGURE 47.8 Sample instruction sheet for diaphragms. (Courtesy of Teenage Health Center, Children's Hospital of Los Angeles, Los Angeles, California.)

Patient Education

Insertion of the FemCap

- Apply approximately one to four teaspoon of spermicide in the bowl, spread a thin layer over the outer brim, and insert one to two teaspoon between the brim and dome.
- Gently squeeze the cup and insert it into the vagina with the bowl facing upward and longer brim entering first.
- Push the cap down toward the rectum and back as far as it can go.
- Check to make sure that the cap completely covers the cervix.

Removal of the FemCap

- To remove the cap, squat and bear down.
- Push the tip of a finger against the dome cap to break the suction.
- Grasp the removal strap with the tip of your finger and gently remove the device.
- Wash the cap thoroughly with a mild soap then rinse it with tap water. Allow the cap to air dry or gently pat it dry with a clean, soft towel and store.

Insertion and Removal of Diaphragm

Patient education programs should include the following:

- Demonstration of insertion and removal techniques: after being shown how to place the diaphragm, the teen should insert and

remove it at least once in the office and have the placement checked by the clinician.
- Detailed guidance about use of spermicide
  - Coat the inner surface of the diaphragm with spermicidal gel. One application is effective for up to 6 hours.
  - Add additional spermicide with the applicator if intercourse is delayed beyond 6 hours or if additional acts of coitus are anticipated. Additional doses must be placed into the vagina; the diaphragm should not be removed to add spermicide.
  - Apply an extra dose immediately if the diaphragm is dislodged during intercourse, and consider using emergency contraception.
- Removal instructions
  - Wait at least 6 hours after the last episode of coitus to remove the device.
  - Remove before 24 hours of use to reduce the risk of toxic shock syndrome.
- Concrete instructions about cleaning and storage of device: Recommend washing device in soap and water, then soaking it in an alcohol solution (70% isopropanol or 80% ethanol) for at least 20 minutes after each application. Coat the device with cornstarch or another agent to prevent contamination or cracking, and store it in a dry container.
- Return for refitting of the diaphragm every 1 to 2 years, after every pregnancy, and after any 10% to 20% change in body weight.

Advantages

* Reduced risks of STIs, including HIV
* May be placed in anticipation of coitus

Disadvantages

* Some require professional sizing and all are available only by prescription.
* Requires motivation and extensive education for proper use.
* Requires preparation and access to supplies; therefore, it may limit spontaneity and may not meet the impulsive needs of the adolescent.
* May be considered messy, especially for multiple acts of intercourse.
* Not an acceptable method if either partner is allergic to spermicide or latex
* There is a small risk of toxic shock syndrome associated with poorly timed or prolonged use.
* The diaphragm increases the risk of cystitis by increasing the count of enteric organisms within the vagina.

Future Developments

Animal studies of the BufferGel Duet, a disposable, one-size-fits-all polyurethane spermicidal microbicidal diaphragm, show that it maintains the protective acidity of the vagina and has some efficacy. While not yet approved by the FDA, acidform gels, buffergel, and diaphragm delivery systems have undergone Phase I trials and found to be safe and acceptable, with the majority of participants preferring the Duet over ECs.

⬤ VAGINAL SPERMICIDES

The common active ingredient of spermicides is nonoxynol-9, a surfactant and organic compound used in various cosmetic and cleaning products. Benzalkonium chloride and sodium choate are spermicidal agents active in some contraceptive sponges. The inert base blocks or absorbs sperm, and the chemically active ingredient breaks down sperm cell membranes. Lemon juice, lactic acid, and neem plant oils are anecdotally spermicidal, but there are no data supporting the effectiveness of these methods.

Types of Spermicides

Spermicides come in a variety of forms (gels, films, foams, and suppositories) (Table 47.1). Spermicides vary in application, onset, and duration of use. Most spermicides are active for 1 hour unless used with additional barrier methods. Foam is one of the most commonly used spermicides with the benefit of being instantly efficacious. Gels, films, and suppositories need approximately 15 minutes to coat the cervix and become effective.

Human immunodeficiency virus researchers have long been interested in exploring the in vitro virucidal and bactericidal activity of vaginal spermicides. At present, clinical data do not support its use in this way. A number of studies have consistently demonstrated that nonoxynol-9 does not reduce risk of HIV and other STI transmission. The detergent effects of nonoxynol-9 seem to cause local epithelial irritation and sloughing exposing the submucosal and creating a portal of entry for HIV and other STIs. A case-control study of sex workers in Africa has demonstrated that multiple daily use (>3.5 times/day) increases the risk of HIV.[34] Benzalkonium can likewise work as an irritant in the vagina and negatively impact normal lactobacillus flora.

Efficacy

Typical-use failure rates are estimated at 29%. Less than half of women continue to use this method a year out. Correct and consistent use of spermicides has a slightly lower perfect-use failure rate of 18%. Use with adjunct barrier methods improves effectiveness. Spermicides have low efficacy compared to most other methods. As a nonprescription method, with few systemic side effects and additional local-lubricant effect, spermicides may offer some benefits to AYAs. Messiness, need to apply in advance of each coitus, and changes in odor and taste may be unpleasant for some AYAs. Along with lack of efficacy, the risk for STI transmission risk should make spermicides a less desirable option in this age group. The CDC does not recommend the use of spermicide alone or as a lubricant for condoms. Condoms lubricated with spermicides are no more effective than other lubricated condoms in protecting against the transmission of HIV and other STIs. Use of nonoxynol-9 is associated with breakdown of the protective genital epithelium, which has been associated with increased risk for transmission of HIV infection.

Condoms lubricated with nonoxynol-9 are not recommended for STI and HIV prevention. Spermicide-coated condoms cost more, have a shorter shelf life than other lubricated condoms, and have been associated with urinary tract infection in young women. The CDC does recommend condom use, even with spermicide, if there is no other option available. Petroleum- or oil-based products (e.g., mineral oil, baby oil, vegetable oil, Vaseline, cold creams, hand moisturizers) degrade and weaken latex after as little as a minute of contact. Water- or silicone-based lubricants do not react with latex and can decrease friction, irritation, and breakage, thus making them a relatively more useful adjunct to condoms than spermicides

Mechanism of Action

The components of spermicidal agents include an inert base (foam, cream, or jelly), which holds the spermicidal agent and blocks sperm from entering the cervical os. Spermicides destroy sperm by breaking down the outer cell membrane.

Contraindications

* Allergy or sensitivity to spermicidal agents or to the ingredients in the base
* Inability to use due to vaginal abnormalities or inability to master the insertion technique

Advantages

* No proven systemic side effects
* Readily available without prescription
* Overall, convenient, easy-to-learn method for teenagers
* May be used by women with or without involvement of partner
* May provide lubrication
* May be useful as a backup method for other contraceptives

TABLE 47.1

Examples of Various U.S. Brand Spermicides

Manufacturer	Brand Name of Nonoxynol-9	Delivery System	Dose
Ortho	Conceptrol	Gel	4% 100 mg/applicator
McNeil	Delfen II	Jelly	2% 0.1 g
Blairex Lab.	Encare	Suppository	100 mg
J and J Products	Gyncol II	Jelly	150 mg
Apothecus Pharm	VCF	Film Foam	28% 12.5%

Disadvantages

- Relatively high failure rate
- Considered messy by some teenagers (some forms)
- Must be used only a short time before intercourse is started
- Requires 10 to 15 minutes for activation (some formulations)
- Requires that woman be comfortable with touching her genitals
- Unpleasant taste if oral–genital sex is involved
- May cause a local allergic reaction

Future Developments

The need for vaginal agents that are contraceptive and protective against HIV and other STIs is increasingly compelling. Various additional spermicidal agents, especially those avoiding the surfactant nonoxynol-9 irritant effects, are being studied. One area of research includes evaluation of antimicrobial peptides which may be less damaging to mucosa and may have direct spermicidal effects.[34]

 ## SUMMARY

Barrier methods may offer some measure of contraception for AYAs, but are neither less efficacious nor easier to use than many other forms of birth control, especially implanted LARCs. The most important function of barrier methods for many AYAs may be the protection they offer against STIs, including HIV. When offering sexual health counseling, it may be more beneficial to separate out superior family planning and contraceptive options from barrier methods, which offer most benefit for STI prevention. Dual method use, along with patient readiness and careful partner selection, offers a fourfold approach to more responsible sexual decision making. While improved technologies are important, clinician awareness and ability to address disparities for socially vulnerable AYAs (persons of color, gender and sexual minoritized persons, youth with disabilities and chronic medical conditions, etc.) is key to improving education, access, and appropriate use of barrier methods. Incorporating patient-centered sex-positive counseling can support AYAs in making healthy decisions and empower the ability to consent and preserve sexual and body autonomy.

REFERENCES

1. Daniels K, Abma JC. Current contraception status among women aged 15–19: United States, 2015–2017. *NCHS Data Brief*. 2018;(327), Accessed April 24, 2020. https://www.cdc.gov/nchs/products/databriefs/db327.htm
2. Sundaram A, Vaughan B, Kost K, et al. Contraceptive failure in the United States: estimates from the 2006–2010 national survey of family growth. *Perspect Sex Reprod Health*. 2017;49(1):7–16.
3. Kann L, McManus T, Harris WA, et al. Youth risk behavior surveillance- United States, 2017. *MMWR Surveill Summ*. 2018;67(8):1–114.
4. American College Health Association. *American College Health Association-National College Health Assessment II: Reference Group Executive Summary Spring 2019*. American College Health Association; 2019.
5. Habel MA, Leichliter JS, Dittus PJ, et al. Heterosexual anal and oral sex in adolescents and adult in the United States, 2011–2015. *Sex Transm Dis*. 2018;45(12):775–782.
6. Centers for Disease Control and Prevention. STD Treatment Guidelines 2021. Accessed September 6, 2021. https://www.cdc.gov/std/treatment-guidelines/toc.htm
7. Holway GV, Hernandez SM. Oral sex and condom use in a U.S. national sample of adolescents and young adults. *J Adolesc Health*. 2018;62(4)402–410.
8. Beksinska M, Wong R, Smit J. Male and female condoms: their key role in pregnancy and STI/HIV prevention. *Best Pract Res Clin Obstet Gynaecol*. 2020;66:55–67.
9. Centers for Disease Control and Prevention (CDC). Condom Effectiveness: Fact Sheet for Public Health Personnel. Accessed May 28, 2020. https://www.cdc.gov/condomeffectiveness/latex.html
10. Curtis KM, Tepper NK, Jatlaoui TC, et al. U.S. Medical Eligibility Criteria for Contraceptive Use, 2016. *MMWR Recomm Rep*. 2016;65(3):1–103. Accessed May 14, 2021. http://dx.doi.org/10.15585/mmwr.rr6503a1externalicon.
11. Ritchwood TD, Penn D, Peasant C, et al. Condom use self-efficacy among younger rural adolescents: the influence of parent–teen communication, and knowledge of and attitudes toward condoms. *J Early Adolesc*. 2017;37(2): 267–283.
12. Eversole JS, Berglas NF, Deardorff J, et al. Source of sex information and condom use intention among Latino adolescents. *Health Educ Behav*. 2017;44(3):439–447.
13. Guzzo KB, Hayford SR. Adolescent reproductive and contraceptive knowledge and attitudes and adult contraceptive behavior. Matern *Child Health J*. 2018;22(1):32–40.
14. Wang T, Lurie M, Govidasamy D, et al. The effects of school-based condom availability programs (CAPS) on condom acquisition, use, and sexual behavior: a systemic review. *AIDS Behav*. 2018;22(1):308–320.
15. Gibson LP, Gust CJ, Gillman AS, et al. mechanisms of action for empirically supported interventions to reduce adolescent sexual risk behavior: a randomized controlled trial. *J Adolesc Health*. 2020;67(1):53–60.
16. Whiting W, Pharr JR, Buttner MP, et al. Behavioral interventions to increase condom use among college students in the United States: a systematic review. *Health Educ Behav*. 2019;46(5):877–888.
17. Shacham E, Nelson EJ, Schulte L, et al Geographic variation in condom availability and accessibility. *AIDS Behav*. 2016;20(2):2863–2872.
18. Barber JS, Ela E, Gatny H, et al. Contraception Desert? Black–White differences in characteristics of nearby pharmacies. *J Racial Ethn Health Disparities*. 2019;6(4):719–732.
19. McCool-Myers M. Implementing condom distribution programs in the United States: qualitative inserts from program planner. *Eval Program Plann*. 2019;74:20–26.
20. Everett BG, Higgins JA, Haider S, et al. Do sexual minorities receive appropriate sexual and reproductive health care and counseling? *J Womens Health*. 2019;28(1):53–62.
21. Light A, Wang L-F, Zeymo A, et al. Family planning and contraception use in transgender men. *Contraception*. 2018;98(4):266–269.
22. Yah CS, Simate GS, Hlangothi P, et al. Nanotechnology and the future of condoms in the prevention of sexually transmitted infection. *Ann Afr Med*. 2018;17(2):49–57.
23. Cooper BG, Chin SL, Xiao R, et al. Friction-lowering capabilities and human subject preference for a hydrophilic surface coating on latex substrates. *R Soc Open Sci*. 2018;5(10):180291.
24. Siegler AJ, Rosenthal EM, Sullivan PS, et al. Double-blind single-center, randomized three-way crossover trial of fitted, thin, and standard condoms for vaginal and anal sex: C-PLEASURE Study protocol and baseline data. *JMIR Res Protoc*. 2019;8(4):e12205.
25. Ting CY, Ting RS-K, Lim CJ, et al. Pilot study on functional performance and acceptability of two new synthetic adhesive male condoms (Wondaleaf): a randomized cross-over trial. *Contraception*. 2019;100(1):65–71.
26. Graham CA, Towler LB, Crosby RA. Assessing the perceived benefits of a new condom wrapper/integrated applicator: an exploratory study. *Int J STD AIDS*. 2019;30(4):329–335.
27. Butler SM, Mooney K, Janousek K. The condom fairy program: a novel mail-order service for condoms and sexual health supplies. *J Am Coll Health*. 2019;67(8):772–780.
28. Tibbits M, Ndashe TP, King K, et al. Promoting condom use through a youth-focused community-wide free condom distribution initiative. *Am J Pub Health*. 2018;108(11):1506–1508.
29. Beksinska M, Smit J, Joanis C, et al. Female condom technology: new products and regulatory issues. *Contraception*. 2011;83(4):316–321.
30. Trussell J. Contraceptive efficacy. In: Hatcher RA, Trussell J, Nelson AL, et al., eds. *Contraceptive Technology*. 21st ed. Managing Contraception LLC.2018;833.
31. Wiyeh AB, Mome RKB, Mahasha PW, et al. Effectiveness of the female condom in preventing HIV and sexually transmitted infections: a systemic review and meta-analysis. *BMC Public Health*. 2020;20(1):319.
32. Hsu R, Tavrow P, Uysal J, et al. Seeking the female (internal) condom in retail pharmacies: experiences of adolescent mystery callers. *Contraception*. 2020;101(2):117–121.
33. Black A, Guilbert E, Costescu D, et al. Canadian Contraception Consensus (Part 2 of 4). *J Obstet Gynaecol Can*. 2015;37(11):1033–1039.
34. Madanchi H, Shoushtari M, Kashani HH, et al. Antimicrobial peptides of the vaginal innate immunity and their role in the fights against sexually transmitted diseases. *New Microbes New Infect*. 2019;34:100627.

📶 ADDITIONAL RESOURCES AND WEBSITES

Additional Resources and Websites for Clinicians:

Centers for Disease Control and Prevention—Reproductive Health—https://www.cdc.gov/reproductivehealth/contraception/mmwr/mec/summary.html

Compendium of Sexual and Reproductive Health resources for Healthcare Providers—https://nationalcoalitionforsexualhealth.org/tools/for-healthcare-providers/compendium-of-sexual-reproductive-health-resources-for-healthcare-providers

Office of Population Affairs—Reproductive Health and Teen Pregnancy—https://opa.hhs.gov/adolescent-health/reproductive-health-and-teen-pregnancy-https://www.hhs.gov/ash/oah/resources-and-training/adolescent-health-library/reproductive-health-resources-and-publications/index.html

Reproductive health Access Project—https://www.reproductiveaccess.org/

Reproductive Health Resources—Contraceptive Technology—http://www.contraceptivetechnology.org/reproductive-health-resources/

Additional Resources and Websites for Adolescents and Young Adults and Parents/Caregivers:

Bedsider. Birth Control—https://www.bedsider.org/methods

Planned Parenthood: Birth Control—https://www.plannedparenthood.org/learn/birth-control

Reproductive health Access Project—https://www.reproductiveaccess.org/

Society for Adolescent Health and Medicine: Sexual and reproductive Health Resources for Adolescents and Young Adults—https://www.adolescenthealth.org/Resources/Clinical-Care-Resources/Sexual-Reproductive-Health/Sexual-Reproductive-Health-Resources-For-Adolesc.aspx

CHAPTER 48

Contraceptive Pills, Patches, Rings, and Injections

Anita L. Nelson

KEY WORDS

- Combined hormonal contraceptives
- Contraceptive patches
- Contraceptive vaginal rings
- Depot medroxyprogesterone acetate (DMPA)
- Oral contraceptives
- Progestin-only contraceptives
- Quick Start
- Short-acting contraceptives

INTRODUCTION

Short-acting hormonal contraceptive methods, such as birth control pills, transdermal contraceptive patches, vaginal contraceptive rings, and progestin-only injections are the most frequently used methods for ongoing birth control by sexually active adolescent and young adult (AYA) women. They often switch among methods in this category as they balance side effects, convenience, and privacy, as well as access issues. All noninjectable methods have about equivalent efficacy; their first-year failure rates are 0.3% with correct and consistent use and 7% with typical use. Many of these short-acting hormonal methods also offer considerable noncontraceptive health benefits. Newer short-acting hormonal products have addressed potential shortcomings of earlier options. Widespread adoption of practices that facilitate access that AYA women have to ongoing supplies of these methods is recommended to reduce unintended pregnancies in this vulnerable population. Finally, the needs of special populations within the AYA group deserve mention as many of these methods can help address those needs.

CLINICAL PRACTICES TO ENHANCE CONTRACEPTIVE SUCCESS

The following practices have been recommended by the Centers for Disease Control and Prevention (CDC) and endorsed by most professional organizations prominent in reproductive health.[1]

- Minimize physical examinations and laboratory testing for method initiation. Once the woman's history has qualified her as a candidate for her method (following U.S. Medical Eligibility Criteria [MEC] for Contraceptive Use described in Chapter 46), no further evaluations are needed to initiate progestin-only pills (POPs) or injections; combined hormonal contraceptives (CHCs) require only documentation of a normal blood pressure. Complete well-woman care and comprehensive health counseling are both valuable, but neither is required to initiate any of these methods.
- Quick Start (Same Day Start) of all these methods is preferred. This means that any of these methods can be initiated any day in the woman's cycle when the clinician is reasonably certain from the women's history that she is not pregnant (Table 48.1). Routine urine pregnancy testing is discouraged.
- If the woman has had recent unprotected intercourse, provide oral emergency contraception (EC).
  - For levonorgestrel EC, have her take (EC) immediately and then start on-going hormonal method.
  - For ulipristal acetate, have her take that EC immediately, but delay initiation of hormonal method until 5 days after last intercourse, after all the sperm are dead.
  - Advise her to use barrier methods for contraception until her hormonal method is able to protect her (2 days after starting POPs or 7 days after starting CHCs or depot medroxyprogesterone acetate [DMPA]).
- Prescribe supplies sufficient to last a year (13 cycles) whenever possible, and have the pharmacist dispense all her supplies at once to reduce unintended pregnancy and abortions.[2]
- Counsel about other potential ways to obtain refills if unable to get 1 year supply initially.
  - Online orders can be delivered directly to the patient's home.
  - Depot medroxyprogesterone acetate can be given by pharmacists; subcutaneous (sub-Q) DMPA may be self-administered especially after training.
- Help AYA women plan ahead about where they will store their supplies (especially if privacy is important) and how to remember when to redose (computer/phone apps like https://www.bedsider.org/reminders_app may be especially helpful).
- Offer EC in advance of need to AYA women who use any of these methods to ensure they have EC immediately available when they have unprotected intercourse.
- Reduce return office visits. Many experts recommend a 3-month visit following method initiation for AYA women to monitor their

---

TABLE 48.1

How to Be Reasonably Certain That a Woman Is Not Pregnant[1]

A clinician can be reasonably certain that a woman is not pregnant if she has no symptoms or signs of pregnancy and meets any one of the following criteria:

- Is ≤7 d after the start of normal menses.
- Has not had sexual intercourse since the start of last normal menses.
- Has been correctly and consistently using a reliable method of contraception.
- Is ≤7 d after spontaneous or induced abortion.
- Is within 4 wk. postpartum.
- Is fully or nearly fully breastfeeding (exclusively breastfeeding or the vast majority [≥85%] of feeds are breastfeeds), amenorrheic, and <6 mo postpartum.

success with the new method, but many women would prefer to have virtual visits to ask questions at any time.
- Offer barrier methods with or without pre-exposure prophylaxis (PrEP) for sexually transmitted infection (STI) risk reduction.

OVERVIEW OF HORMONAL METHODS OF CONTRACEPTION

Having hormonal contraceptives with several differences in the constituent hormones, formulations, and delivery systems enables clinicians to meet each woman's contraceptive needs and preferences, to maximize her noncontraceptive benefits and to deal with potential side effects. There are two groups of POPs—one low-dose continuous formulation with norethindrone (offered in many generic brands) and a cyclic formulation with a stronger progestin (drospirenone). There are over 100 named combined oral contraceptives (COCs). The active pills in COCs are available with one of four different estrogens combined with one of five different progestins packaged either in monophasic cyclic formulations of different durations (28 vs. 91 days) or in multiple different multiphasic monthly cyclic formulations. The "hormone-free" interval for different formulations varies from 2 to 7 days; those "placebo pills" can also contain low-dose estrogen and/or other supplements, such as iron or folate. A sixth progestin is used in the injectable contraceptives; and a seventh is used in a new vaginal ring. Other compounds are available internationally. There are two different combined hormonal transdermal contraceptive patches, two different combination vaginal rings, and two different progestin-only injectable contraceptives.

Mechanisms of Action of Sex Steroids

Progestins provide the bulk of contraceptive activity for hormonal methods. All progestins thicken the cervical mucus to block sperm entry into the upper genital tract. They inhibit the onset of uterine contractions from the cervix to the fundus that carry sperm into the upper track at the time of ovulation. They camouflage the gradient of increasing progesterone concentrations that guides the sperm to the awaiting oocyte. Ciliary action in the fallopian tube is slowed by progestin, which disrupts fertilization timing and slows transit time to implantation. Progestins may also affect the function of the corpus luteum (if one forms) and/or the decidualization of the endometrium, which, theoretically, could have interceptive activity. In dose- and potency-related fashions, progestins can effectively suppress ovulation by blocking the luteinizing hormone (LH) surge. For example, the low-dose norethindrone POP suppresses ovulation in 40% to 60% of cycles, while DMPA injections suppress ovulation so potently that fertility does not return on average until 9 months after the final injection.

The first three groups of progestins (outlined below) used in oral contraceptives derive from a C-19 androgen scaffolding, so they express both progestational and varying androgenic impacts. The first group (norethindrone ethynodiol diacetate, norethindrone acetate) is reasonably neutral metabolically except when combined with lower estrogen doses, when stronger androgenic impacts emerge. These progestins all share a relatively short half-life (8 hours). The second major group (norgestrel, levonorgestrel) is more potent, longer acting, and more androgenic; that last property is responsible for both the cosmetic complications (acne, hirsutism) and the progestin's ability to reduce estrogen's stimulation of hepatic protein products, which reduces the risk of estrogen-induced venous thromboembolism (VTE). The newer contraceptive patch, all the hormonal intrauterine devices, and one EC pill use one of these progestins (levonorgestrel). The third group (norgestimate, desogen) is long-acting, but less androgenic. Metabolites of these progestins are used in the generic contraceptive patches, the monthly vaginal rings, and the implant. The fourth progestin (drospirenone) derives from a spironolactone-like compound, has

antimineralocorticoid and antiandrogenic properties and allows complete expression of the estrogen. The new POP utilizes this progestin. Drospirenone may be associated with an increased risk of hyperkalemia in women who take other drugs that increase potassium levels or who have renal insufficiency. The fifth progestin used in oral contraceptives (dienogest) is a unique compound with strong progestational activity, which controls both ovarian and endometrial activity; it also has direct antiangiogenic activity. Progestin-only injectables rely on high-dose deposits of medroxyprogesterone acetate. The new 13-cycle contraceptive vaginal ring utilizes a new nonoral progestin (segesterone acetate) that has high progesterone affinity, but no androgenicity.

Estrogen is added to progestins to provide better cycle control. Estrogen contributes a little to contraceptive activity by providing negative feedback to reduce pituitary release of follicle stimulating hormone (FSH) that triggers recruitment of ovarian follicles. Currently there are four estrogens used in hormonal contraceptives. *Ethinyl estradiol* (EE) is a potent, long-acting estrogen that is found in virtually all combined hormonal methods. It is relatively resistant to hepatic metabolism and can circulate through the liver five to six times before its serum concentration is reduced by 50% enabling it to provide endometrial support needed for once-daily administration. However, each pass through the liver induces production of important carrier proteins (e.g., sex hormone-binding globulin [SHBG], corticosteroid-binding globulin [CBG], and thyroid-binding globulin [TBG]) and prothrombotic factors [such as the extrinsic clotting factors]). Each pass also suppresses antithrombin III production. *Mestranol* is a prodrug that is found in 50-mcg formulations. It requires hepatic metabolism to convert it into EE. This hepatic conversion is variable; 50 mcg of mestranol produces only 35- to 40-mcg EE. *Estradiol (E_2) valerate* is a weak, short-acting estrogen used in one multiphasic formulation that relies on its progestin for good cycle control. The fourth estrogen (*estetrol* or E_4) is the first new estrogen introduced for contraception in 50 years. Estetrol has a long half-time with minimal metabolic impacts. It is antagonistic to estrogen receptor alpha ERα in the cell membrane so it has minimal effect on the liver or breast tissue, but selectively and weakly binds to nuclear ERα. The downstream effects of this selective receptor binding is 1% to 10% that of E_2 and EE. Metabolites of E_4 have negligible estrogenic activity.

ORAL CONTRACEPTIVES

Progestin-Only Pills

Progestin-only methods can be used by virtually every woman. According to the U.S. MEC, the only Category 4 condition (contraindication) to the use of the older, low-dose norethindrone POPs is current or recent breast cancer (see Chapter 46). This makes the traditional POPs a "go-to" pill to offer women whose history may require more investigation or to act as a bridge to another method that requires preauthorization.

Older studies suggest that typical use failure rates for the low-dose norethindrone POP are the same as combined pills (7%), even though ovulation suppression is inconsistent. Because it has an 8-hour half-life, it thickens the cervical mucus for only a limited time. As a result, women have to take the daily pill reliably within 2 hours of the appointed hour or use a back-up method. In this "mini-pill" formulation, every pill is an active pill. This simplifies counseling but results in unpredictable bleeding patterns; amenorrhea and unscheduled spotting/bleeding are not uncommon although they are generally well tolerated.

More recently, a new POP with 4 mg drospirenone has been introduced.[3] This POP is administered in cycles of 24 active pills and 4 placebo pills to induce scheduled bleeding. This pill suppresses ovulation just as well as most COCs. Missed pill rules are the same for this POP as instructions for COCs (**Table 48.2**). Bleeding patterns

TABLE 48.2

Recommendations for Late or Missed Dose(s) of Combined Hormonal Contraceptives

	How Long Late/Missed Dose?		
	≤24 h	**24–48 h**	**≥48 h**
Combined pill	Take 1 pill	Take 2 pills[a]	Take 2 pills[a]
Patch	Reattach current patch OR place new patch	Place new patch	Place new patch
Ring	Replace current ring	Replace current ring	Replace current ring
Back-up needed	No	No	7 d
Levonorgestrel emergency contraception needed if coitus in last 5 d	No	Yes, if missed method earlier in cycle, too	Yes, especially if missed in first wk of use

Note: Vomiting or diarrhea with pill <48 hours require no changes. If gastrointestinal problem persists >48 hours, follow instructions for >48 hours of missed doses and use back-up for 7 days of consecutive method use after symptoms resolve.
[a]May take 2 pills at once.
Modified from Reference 1.

with this POP are improved. Less than 1% of women discontinued due to abnormal bleeding. Because of potassium-sparing properties of drospirenone, women who have renal impairment or adrenal insufficiency are not candidates. Those chronically using potassium-sparing medications need to have potassium levels checked once about 2 weeks into the first pack to rule out hyperkalemia.

Combined Oral Contraceptives

Approximately 53% of at-risk young women aged 15 to 19 years report they have used birth control pills for a time.[4] Episodic use is fairly common, which can increase the risk for VTE and adverse bleeding patterns. Less than one-third of teens use pills for 12 months. Oral contraceptives offer many important noncontraceptive health benefits that may increase a young woman's commitment to their use if she understands that association.

It is possible to use the differences in oral contraceptive formulations to help select one that will address women's contraceptive and noncontraceptive needs. One good starting point is to ask if she wants scheduled bleeding each month or not. Extended cycle formulations are very healthy options for active AYA women and for those with menstrually-related problems.

Some experts recommend using pills with at least 30-mcg EE as initial start pills for young adolescents to prevent adverse effects on bone mineralization, but allow possibility of switching later to lower-dose pills, if needed.[5] It is not clear if the efficacy of oral contraceptives is diminished in users with a higher body mass index (BMI); however, it is clear that failure rates are higher in women in lower socioeconomic groups where obesity rates are very high. Special counseling may be warranted, but obesity is not a contraindication to oral contraceptive use.[6]

VAGINAL CONTRACEPTIVE RINGS

Two different types of vaginal hormonal rings are available. The first group with EE and etonogestrel provides 1 month of contraceptive protection in each ring. The U.S. Food and Drug Administration (FDA) product labeling calls for this ring or its generic version to be placed high in the vaginal vault on the first day of menses, removed after 3 weeks and replaced with a new ring 7 days later. Studies have shown, however, that the use of this ring can be extended to 30 to 31 days to eliminate the hormone-free week altogether. Cycle control with cyclic use of these rings is superior to

that of most oral contraceptives even though area-under-the-curve estrogen exposure is about half that of 30- to 35-mg oral contraceptives. Progestin exposure is the same as found with birth control pills. Efficacy with this ring does not vary by weight or BMI. Venous thromboembolic risks are no different than those found with low-dose oral contraceptives. Vaginal rings may be less susceptible to drug–drug interactions.[7] Vaginal delivery systems are advantageous for women with challenges with oral administration, such as difficulty swallowing pills, malabsorptive bariatric surgery procedures, Crohn disease, irritable bowel syndrome, or eating disorders. Convenience is an important feature for many users.

Ring users must feel comfortable touching the genital area. For those who have any difficulty introducing the ring into the vagina manually, a smooth-rimmed, cardboard tampon insertion tube can be used (after removal of the tampon) to place the ring flat against the vaginal walls anywhere in the upper vagina. In that position, only 30% of women report their partners can detect the ring's presence during coitus and only a fraction of those women need to remove the ring for partner comfort. Pressure sensation with the ring or repeated expulsion generally indicates that the ring was placed too low in the vagina or placed incorrectly across the vagina like a diaphragm. The ring may be removed for no more than 3 hours in any 24-hour period. The pouch that the ring comes in serves as a temporary storage area and should be used to dispose of the ring as solid waste at the end of its useful life. The ring increases vaginal secretions, which can be helpful to provide lubrication during intercourse. It increases lactobacillus numbers, which reduces recurrences of bacterial vaginosis.

The newer contraceptive vaginal ring releases EE and a unique new progestin, segesterone acetate.[8] This progestin has very strong pure progesterone activity and no androgenicity. One ring provides pregnancy protection for up to 1 year with 28-day cyclic use (21 days in and 7 days out). Failure rates in the clinical trial were less than 3%, which is quite low for modern clinical trials of combined hormonal method.[9] Bleeding patterns with the ring are also very satisfactory to users. Only a fraction of the hormones in the ring are released over a 13-cycle use, so extended use of this ring may be feasible once clinical trials have shown it is safe and effective when used this way. Not only does this ring provide the convenience of a once-a-month administration, but it assures that the user has adequate supplies for a full year without requiring any refills.

TRANSDERMAL CONTRACEPTIVE PATCHES

There are two different types of transdermal patches. In the first group, there are two generic versions of the original EE/norelgestromin (a metabolite of norgestimate) patch. The other patch has lower levels of EE and uses levonorgestrel. Currently, all patches are contraindicated for women with BMI ≥30 kg/m² because of higher failure rates and possibly higher risks of thrombosis at higher BMIs. One patch is placed on dry skin on the abdomen, buttock, upper arm, or anywhere on the trunk (except the breasts) at the beginning of the cycle and left in place for 7 days. It is removed and another patch is placed at another eligible site. After three consecutive patches have been used, a patch-free week follows. Patch placement/adhesion should be checked daily to ensure ongoing efficacy. Women with skin disorders that could be exacerbated by patch use or which could affect drug absorption should not use this method. On the other hand, patches are helpful for women with gastrointestinal absorption challenges. Clinical trials have shown that a greater number of women of all ages reported correct use with the patch than with the comparator pill, but the greatest improvement in utilization was found in women aged 18 to 19 years. Many, but not all, studies have found associations between the EE norelgestromin patch and higher risks of VTE. This increased risk is biologically plausible because the 24-hour area-under-the-curve levels of EE with these patches are significantly higher than those found with a 35-mcg oral contraceptive.[10]

The new patch was designed to continue the once-a-week convenience, but with lower estradiol levels (like a 30-mcg EE pill) and with a progestin (levonorgestrel) that has been associated with the lowest increase in VTE risk. Failure rates varied by BMI. Normal weight women had a 2.98% failure rate; that increased to 5.4% in overweight women. There were no episodes of VTE among study participants in the indicated weight range but the numbers were small.[11]

NONCONTRACEPTIVE BENEFITS OF COMBINED HORMONAL CONTRACEPTIVES

Menstrually Related Benefits

Predictable Scheduled Bleeding

Cyclic use of combined hormonal methods induces more predictable bleeding during the hormone-free days so active young women can arrange their activities around their bleeding episodes. For anovulatory women, cycling with CHCs prevents unopposed estrogen stimulation of the endometrium, which can cause prolonged, heavy, and unpredictable bleeding episodes and endometrial hyperplasia.

Lighter Flow

The progestin-dominance of these methods reduces endometrial proliferation and results in thinner endometrial lining to slough during the hormone-free interval. Oral contraceptives are a first-line medical therapy prescribed for heavy menstrual bleeding, often in conjunction with nonsteroidal anti-inflammatory agents (NSAIDs). This is a class effect for all pills, but only one pill (E_2V/Dienogest) carries FDA labeling that is indicated for treatment for heavy and/or prolonged idiopathic menstrual bleeding in women using oral contraceptives for birth control.

Reduction of Dysmenorrhea

One of the leading causes of missed days of school and work is painful menstrual cramping. Whether women suffer primary or secondary dysmenorrhea, the progestin's induction of endometrial pseudodecidualization and its thinning of the endometrial functionalis layer by hormonal contraceptives significantly reduces this problem.

Reduction of Catamenial Disorders

Other conditions flare with menses. Menstrual migraine is the classic, but many other conditions worsen with menses, including catamenial seizures, pneumothorax, sciatica, and asthma. These catamenial exacerbations are best treated by suppressing ovulation (hormonal swings) and by minimizing the frequency of bleeding episodes. Extended cycle use of oral contraceptives or the monthly vaginal contraceptive ring with etonogestrel or with use of injectable DMPA are the most effective options to accomplish those goals. Similarly, premenstrual dysphoric disorder (PMDD) and premenstrual syndrome (PMS) can be treated by eliminating the cyclic hormonal swings with those agents. If scheduled bleeding is desired, the numbers of hormone-free days should be limited to 2 to 4. Low-dose estrogen during those days can cushion impacts of the hormone withdrawal. One formulation (20-mcg EE/3-mg drospirenone in 24/4 formulation) has been shown to be as effective as selective serotonin reuptake inhibitor therapy for PMDD.

Nonmenstrually Related Benefits

Treatment for Acne, Hirsutism, Oily Skin

Oral contraceptives, especially those with higher levels of estrogen and low (or no) androgenicity in the progestins are often particularly helpful to treat these conditions. Estrogen increases SHBG production over time and significantly reduces the levels of unbound androgens in circulation. Three formulations are FDA approved for treatment of mild-to-moderate acne. Because the action is indirect, results may be slow to appear. Maximum improvements for acne are not reached for 6 months; hirsutism results maximize in 2 years.

Reduction in Risk of Anemia

Anemia risks are reduced by reducing menstrual blood loss. Globally, anemia is the number one cause of years lived in disability. Importantly, oral contraceptives have also been found to halve the frequency of sickle cell crises.

Reduction in Risk Endometrial, Ovarian, and Colorectal Cancers

Endometrial cancer is the most common reproductive malignancy. Precursor lesions can develop in young women with anovulatory cycles (infrequent menses), especially if they are obese. Even a few years of COC use can reduce incidence of endometrial carcinoma by 40%; longer-duration use provides greater protection. This protection lasts for 35 years beyond the time of last hormone use.[12] Combined hormonal contraceptives are the only medical intervention that reduces the risk of ovarian carcinoma. Again, this protection is increased with longer duration of use and endures for at least 35 years after last pill use. Prolonged, recent, and ever use of COCs have been shown to reduce the risk of colorectal cancer by 18% to 19%.[13]

Other Health Benefits

Reduction in pregnancies also reduces the risk of ectopic pregnancy.[14] Formation of functional ovarian cysts (especially corpus luteal cysts) and endometrioma is reduced by use of hormonal contraception.

RISKS POSED BY COMBINED HORMONAL CONTRACEPTION

Increased Risk of Thromboembolism

During their use, all estrogen-containing methods increase the risk for both venous and arterial thromboembolism (deep venous thrombosis [DVT], thromboembolism, pulmonary embolism, stroke, and myocardial infarction [MI]). Pharmacologic doses of EE increase hepatic production of clotting factors. Progestins have no direct impact on such production but may modulate estrogen's impact. All FDA package inserts quote VTE incidence of 1 to 5 per 10,000 women-years among nonpregnant, non-CHC users and, 3 to 12 per 10,000 women-years for CHC users. Overall VTE rates are two to three times higher with low-dose oral contraception compared to baseline. The VTE risk (DVT, pulmonary embolism) is greatest during the first year of use following initiation/reinitiation, which means that episodic use increases VTE risk. Venous thromboembolism risk also increases with increasing age and weight.

Arterial thrombosis (MI and stroke) risk is not increased by low-dose oral contraceptive use by healthy, nonsmoking women. Smoking is a risk factor for increased MI risk, but for healthy, normotensive younger women, smoking does not preclude CHC use. Hypertension is an important risk factor for stroke and precludes use of estrogen-containing contraceptives unless the blood pressure is controlled. Another important risk factor for stroke is true vascular headaches (migraine with aura). While the data on low-dose formulations used by women under age 35 who are normotensive nonsmokers with vascular headaches are mixed, stroke morbidity is so great that estrogen-containing products should be avoided in this situation. It should be noted that all these risks are reversible; past users of CHCs do not have any increased long-term risk for cardiovascular disease.

Breast Cancer: Temporarily Increased Risk

The risk of early breast cancer is increased by 20% to 25% with current or recent use of combined hormonal contraception, but returns to baseline within 5 years of CHC cessation in a pattern that is very similar to the increased risks of breast cancer posed by pregnancy.[15] Breast cancer mortality has not been shown to increase among current or past users. Even among women with a family history of breast cancer or those with benign breast disease, CHC use does not seem to further their increase breast cancer risk. Because the risk of breast cancer among AYAs is very low and duration of pill use does not affect breast cancer risk, young women can be reassured that they will not increase their life-time risk of breast cancer mortality by using combined hormonal contraception.[15]

Increased Risk of Cervical Cancer and Dysplasia

Adenocarcinoma and squamous cell carcinoma of the cervix risks have consistently been associated with longer term use of combined hormonal contraception.[16] However, even in the face of cervical dysplasia, the benefits of CHCs outweigh those risks. Screening protocols are no different for CHC users. This issue is of decreasing clinical significance as rates of vaccination for human papillomavirus increase.

SIDE EFFECTS WITH COMBINED HORMONAL CONTRACEPTIVES

Attributable Side Effects

Bleeding Changes

Hormonal contraceptives almost universally change bleeding patterns. Amenorrhea may worry young women who fear it means their fertility has been compromised. Education is key here. In the absence of concerns about pregnancy, reassure women that there is no medical benefit to scheduled bleeding induced by use of combined hormonal contraception. Unscheduled bleeding often results from delayed pill consumption. Missed method rules are shown in Table 48.2. Postcoital bleeding caused by cervicitis should also be ruled out. However, if the unscheduled bleeding and spotting results from hormonal method use, the suggestions in Table 48.3 can help.

Skin Changes

Darkening of facial skin pigment (melasma) can be induced by estrogen. Switching to progestin-only methods can generally remove the ongoing risk, but that "mask of pregnancy" may only partially fade. Sunscreen and hat use can reduce the risk.

TABLE 48.3

Management Suggestions for Unacceptable Unscheduled Bleeding or Spotting

- **Bleeding when using cyclic pills**
  - Check for inconsistent method use, or tobacco use and rule out postcoital bleeding.
  - For bleeding that occurs late in pill pack: provide formulation with higher doses of progestin in last pills.
  - For bleeding that occurs early in pill pack: provide formulation with higher doses of estrogen or lower doses of progestin in first pills in the pack.
  - For midcycle bleeding: shorten pill-free interval (20-mcg EE formulations) or provide triphasic pills with increases in both estrogen and progestin midcycle.
- **Extended cycle pills or vaginal rings options**
  - Consider Ibuprofen 800 mg orally every 8 h for up to 5 d.
  - Allow 2–4 d of method interruption (after 3 wks consistent CHC use). Restart method again once flow started in that 2–4-d window, OR
  - Alternatively, for pills, double up on pills for 1–2 d if not good time to bleed.
- **DMPA options**
  - Recommend Ibuprofen 800 mg orally every 8 h for up to 5 d OR tranexamic acid 650 mg 2 tablets every 8 h for up to 5 d.
  - Shorten interval for reinjection (10 wks) if bleeding occurs late in injection cycle.
  - Consider adding low-dose pills or vaginal rings 1–2 cycles if no contraindications exist to estrogen use.

Other Changes Noted

Dry eye symptoms are mentioned by contact lens users who take oral contraceptives; eye drops can help. Menstrual migraine symptoms may be exacerbated by withdrawal from pharmacologic levels of EE each month. To prevent this withdrawal, use extended cycle formulations or replace placebo pills with low-dose EE. Progestins relax vascular tension so more venous varicosities may be attributed to progestins.

Nocebo Effects at a Population Level
Commonly Attributed Effects

Virtually all the common side effects habitually attributed to CHC use, such as weight gain, nausea, mastalgia, headache, etc., have been shown in randomized double-blind, placebo-controlled studies to occur no more frequently in pill users than in the placebo users.[17] Since there are also excellent data demonstrating that the act of advising a person that a side effect may happen measurably increases the chance that she will suffer that adverse event, clinicians have been advised that such counseling is unwarranted and very likely unethical.[17]

However, recent genetic studies have demonstrated that circulating levels of synthetic hormones may vary up to 12-fold among different users and that those differences can be associated with different clinical experiences.[13] These insights into differences in uptake and metabolism among different women allow clinicians to initially reassure each patient that, as a rule, she should not anticipate any of these side effects, but advise her that if side effects do occur, adjustments can be made to the formulation she has been prescribed. Table 48.4 lists side effects that may be associated with each of the three hormones that commonly found in combined hormonal contraception. This list may enable clinicians to make more effective formulation adjustments if the hormones are involved.

Infectious Diseases

Human immunodeficiency virus (HIV) risk is not increased by use of CHCs, nor is HIV disease progression affected by their use. Oral contraceptive users have lower risk of bacterial vaginosis, but may

TABLE 48.4

Hormones Implicated with Specific Side Effects in Some Women

Estrogen-Related	Progestin-Related	Androgen-Related
Weight gain in breasts, hips, thighs	Cyclic weight gain	Progressive, noncyclic weight change
Telangiectasia	Fatigue	Oily skin
Melasma/chloasma	Bloating	Acne
Cervical eversion	Constipation	Facial hair growth
Nausea/vomiting	Mastalgia	Decreased breast size
Peripheral edema	Varicosities	Increased appetite
	Depression/mood changes	

have higher risk of complicated or recurrent vulvovaginal candidiasis. Chlamydia risk may be higher (due to estrogen-induced cervical eversion), but gonococcal infection risk seems decreased. Pelvic inflammatory disease and resultant tubal infertility are unaffected by use of CHCs.

Depression and Mood Disorders

Findings have been inconsistent. U.S. MEC rates CHC use as Category 1 for women with depression. A large Danish database study reported that hormonal contraceptives were associated with higher risks of first diagnosis of depression, initiation of antidepressants, and suicide attempts. However, a survey of U.S. teens showed no association between current pill use and depression or between pill use and lifetime risk of depressive disorders.[18]

DRUG–DRUG INTERACTIONS

Drugs that induce hepatic enzymes can alter the serum concentrations of estrogen and/or progestin, which may increase failure rates and/or bleeding abnormalities. On the other hand, some women may have excessive levels of circulating hormones, which may cause side effects. Sex steroids can also influence the metabolism of other drugs and alter their efficacy. Other potential mechanisms for drug–drug interactions, such as enterohepatic recirculation or induction of binding globulins, have either no or insignificant clinical impacts compared to the background interindividual variability observed in the absorption and metabolism of these compounds. As new drugs are introduced and older drugs are used for different conditions, the list of drugs that have impacts on these hormonal contraceptives is growing. Below is a summary of the most, but not all, commonly used agents that may interact with CHCs.

Anticonvulsants

Anticonvulsants are the most common class of drugs known to have reciprocal impacts on progestin and estrogen. Many of these drugs are used for other indications, such as treatment of bipolar disease, neuropathic pain, migraines, and posttraumatic stress disorder. Barbiturates (phenobarbital and primidone), phenytoin, carbamazepine, felbamate, rufinamide, oxcarbazepine, and topiramate all decrease circulating levels of both estrogen and progestin in oral contraceptives, pills, and patches. If a COC is desired by a woman using enzyme-inducing anticonvulsants, formulations with at least 35-mcg EE and shortened or no pill-free intervals should be used, and barrier methods should be encouraged. Depot medroxyprogesterone acetate concentrations are not significantly affected by any of these drugs

and may be a better contraceptive option. Many of the newer anticonvulsant drugs (such as clonazepam, ethosuximide, gabalin, pregabalin) do not induce hepatic enzyme activity. Lamotrigine doses need to be increased and clozapine doses need to be reduced when used as monotherapies with estrogen-containing methods.

Antituberculosis Drugs and Antibiotics

Rifampin and related compounds alone or in combination with other antituberculosis agents are very potent inducers of CYP450 enzymes. Ovulation rates in COC users taking rifampin have been noted to be as high as 50%. Liver toxicity is also a concern. Other options, such as DMPA or intrauterine devices (IUDs), are more appropriate. Rifampin is used in some settings to treat methicillin-resistant *Staphylococcus aureus*. No other antibiotics affect unintended pregnancy rates with hormonal contraceptives.

Antiretroviral Agents

As a general rule, the U.S. MEC for contraceptive use rates the nucleoside reverse transcription inhibitors (NRTIs) as Category 1 for all hormonal methods, but the nonnucleoside reverse transcriptase inhibitors (NNRTIs) as Category 2 hormonal methods except DMPA (Category 1). Efavirenz may require higher-dose formulations. Ritonavir-boosted protease inhibitors (PIs) are Category 3 for all hormonal methods except DMPA, which remains Category 1. The CDC has not rated Hepatitis B treatments, but elbasvir and grazoprevir are compatible with hormonal method use, but ombitasvir/paritaprevir/ritonavir is more concerning because of possible abnormal liver-function test results.

Herbal Medicines

The most significant agent to consider in this group is St. John's wort (Hypericum perforation). Even after only a brief exposure, St. John's wort significantly increases both unscheduled bleeding and pregnancy risks for up to 30 days. Depot medroxyprogesterone acetate alone is unaffected by this agent.

Drospirenone

Women who, on a daily basis, use long-term medications that place them at risk for hyperkalemia (e.g., nonsteroidal anti-inflammatory drugs), should have their serum potassium levels tested once about 2 weeks after initiating drospirenone-containing contraceptives. If that potassium level is normal, no further testing is needed.

Other Interactions

Women using high doses of vitamin C or acetaminophen may have higher circulating levels of EE. On the other hand, griseofulvin and modafinil may reduce CHC efficacy. In women using a CHC method, clearance of the following drugs may be reduced, so *higher* systemic levels may result: warfarin, chlordiazepoxide, alprazolam, diazepam, nitrazepam, theophylline, prednisone, caffeine, cyclosporine, and tacrolimus. On the other hand, clearance of the following drugs may be increased in the face of CHC use resulting in *lower* systemic levels: temazepam, salicylic acid, paracetamol, morphine, and clofibric acid. Antifungal agents used episodically do not adversely affect hormone levels.

INJECTABLE HORMONAL CONTRACEPTION: DEPOT MEDROXYPROGESTERONE ACETATE

Overview of Formulations

There are two different formulations of DMPA in the United States—one is administered intramuscularly (IM) (DMPA 150 mg IM) and another is given subcutaneously Depo-SubQ Provera 104. The sub-Q formulation should be injected in the low abdomen and or the lateral thigh. The IM formulation should be injected in a z-pattern into either the deltoid or the gluteus muscle. For women with a BMI >30 kg/m², a spinal needle may be needed to reach the gluteal muscle mass for the IM version, so deltoid injection is preferred. Apply pressure, but do not massage the injection site to assure hemostasis. Generic products exist for the IM version. First year failure rates with correct and consistent use are 0.2% and are 4% in typical use. Efficacy for DMPA is not affected by BMI. Reinjections are scheduled every 11 to 13 weeks for the DMPA-IM and every 12 to 14 weeks for the DMPA sub-Q. However, there is a grace period of at least 2 weeks; patients who return up to 2 weeks late can be treated as if they are on time. The CDC's Selective Practice Recommendations were updated during the COVID-19 pandemic to allow for self-injection of DMPA sub-Q after instruction. Depot medroxyprogesterone acetate prevents pregnancy primarily by suppression of ovulation via inhibition of gonadotropin-releasing hormone pulsatility, but all other progesterone-related mechanisms of action contribute to efficacy. Concerns about increased risk of HIV acquisition have been assuaged by recent studies.[19]

Practice Considerations

Practical tips for providing DMPA are summarized in Table 48.5. The high efficacy, convenience, and privacy of this method are particularly appealing features for AYA women. While there is only one Category 4 condition for these injectables, there are more Category 3 conditions than with POPs. These conditions include complicated diabetes, Stage 3+ hypertension, hepatocellular adenoma, hepatoma, severe cirrhosis, multiple risk factors for atherosclerotic cardiovascular disease, stroke, systemic lupus erythematosus with antiphospholipid antibodies, severe thrombocytopenia, and unexplained abnormal vaginal bleeding. On the other hand, there are very few drug–drug interactions; only aminoglutethimide interferes with DMPA. Discontinuation rates are relatively high, but teens often follow a start-stop-restart pattern.

Benefits of Depot Medroxyprogesterone Acetate

Depot medroxyprogesterone acetate decreases uterine bleeding progressively over time and effectively treats problems of heavy menstrual bleeding, dysmenorrhea, and mittelschmerz. Depot

TABLE 48.5
Depot Medroxyprogesterone Acetate Clinical Pearls

- Use Quick Start/Same Day injection protocol to initiate or reinject.
  - Grace period for reinjection is 2 wks beyond label-recommended date.
    - Administer any day in the cycle when patient not pregnant.
      - Combine with EC, back-up method for 7 d and repeat pregnancy test in 2–3 wks if recent coitus. If Ulipristal acetate used for EC, delay injection of DMPA until 5 d after coitus.
- Routine pregnancy testing is unwarranted if asymptomatic patient returns on time for reinjection.
- Inject IM DMPA with Z pattern. Do **not** massage injection site.
  - Inject in deltoid or gluteus muscles.
    - If obese, use spinal needle if gluteal site is used. Deltoid preferred
- Inject SubQ DMPA in abdomen or lateral thigh
- Consider teaching self-injection but observe for first two injections to rule out severe allergy
  - Warn about possible skin puckering with sub-Q formulations.
- Provide DMPA to identified candidate (U.S. MEC) of any age, for any duration until menopause despite Black Box Warnings limiting duration of use.
- Related issues
  - Provide LNG-EC by advance prescription because many women return late for reinjection.
  - Encourage condoms for STI protection and PrEP, if indicated.

DMPA, depot medroxyprogesterone acetate; EC, emergency contraception; IM, intramuscular; LNG-EC, levonorgestrel emergency contraception; PrEP, pre-exposure prophylaxis; SubQ, subcutaneous; STI, sexually transmitted infection; U.S. MEC, United States Medical Eligibility Criteria.

medroxyprogesterone acetate use reduces seizure episodes (by raising the seizure threshold), the frequency (by 70%) and intensity of sickle cell crises, endometriosis-related pain, anemia, and the risk of pelvic inflammatory disease. Long-term use provides protection from endometrial cancer and possibly ovarian cancer.

Disadvantages of Depot Medroxyprogesterone Acetate
Bleeding Changes

The most prominent disadvantages with injectables are menstrual cycle disturbances, especially prolonged or unscheduled spotting and bleeding with early use. Overall incidence of irregular bleeding is 70% in the first year, which drops as low as 10% in subsequent years. Amenorrhea rates increase, starting at 40% to 50% at 12 months rising to 80% after 5 years. About 20% to 25% of women will discontinue in first year due to menstrual abnormalities. There is no recommendation for treatment of amenorrhea other than reassurance. Tips for helping other bleeding abnormalities are listed on Table 48.3.

Slow Reversibility

Some DMPA metabolites are biologically active and are stored within the adipose tissue. Return to fertility averages 7 to 9 months after injection; it is independent of the number of injections the woman has had but is generally slower in women with more adiposity. This affects not only pregnancy planning, but also time to resolution of any attributable side effects.

Weight Gain

Weight gain may be more likely in teens with high baseline BMIs. In the only prospective, double-blind, placebo-controlled study of DMPA and weight changes, DMPA users showed no weight gain, no change in appetite and no change in resting metabolic rate. However, excessive weight gain has been variably seen in retrospective studies. One important observation is that younger women, who experience at least 5% weight gain with initial DMPA use, are apt to continue gaining weight with continued DMPA use and need at least targeted counseling.[20]

Reversible Bone Loss

The bone density loss that prompted the FDA Black Box warning limiting DMPA use to 2 years has now been found to be reversible and generally not clinically significant for healthy women of any age. However, some experts are still concerned about use in young women near menarche when bone mineral density accumulation is greatest. The World Health Organization suggests no restriction on use of DMPA in women aged 18 to 45 years, but recommends for adolescents <18 that risks and benefits of continued use be reconsidered over time, given the sparse data that are available in this younger age group. Of note, the American College of Obstetricians and Gynecologists does not limit use in younger teens. With DMPA use, teens should be counseled to increase calcium intake and physical activity, since those measures have been shown to blunt its potential adverse impact on BMD in that age group.

Other Impacts

Data on DMPA's impact on mood and depression are limited and conflicting. A history of a current depression is rated as Category 1 condition for DMPA. Users who experience worsening of symptoms while using DMPA may consider discontinuing the method. Anaphylaxis and severe allergic reactions are rare, but clinicians should observe patients after each injection for at least 20 minutes and be prepared to resuscitate. Metabolic impacts are important to consider as possible side effects. There is a temporary adverse impact on lipid profile and changes can be seen in glucose levels. Although DMPA does not have negative impacts of coagulation or inflammation markers, some studies have reported VTE risks may increase as much as 2.2- to 3.6-fold. Women who are carriers of the Factor V Leiden mutations have even higher risks. Past DVT is rated as a Category 2 condition by the U.S. MEC, but some consultants may hesitate to use DMPA in high-risk women.

SPECIAL POPULATIONS

The contraceptive needs of many vulnerable people in this age group deserve special attention. Transgender men may have genital dysphoria that limits the use of IUDs for either contraception or bleeding control while on testosterone. Estrogen containing products may cause more chest dysphoria. Progestin-only methods such as DMPA or stronger POPs may help. Incarcerated women are often deprived of their methods when they enter the system, but have ongoing needs. Extended cycle methods may be more attractive in this setting. Women who are facing abuse or coercion require privacy. Supplies of short-acting methods may be triggers; DMPA may offer the best option for many in this category. Adolescent and young adult women with disabilities require balancing between medical contraindications (limited mobility, drug interactions) and convenience and accessibility issues.

SUMMARY

Short-acting reversible hormonal contraceptives such as pills, patches, and vaginal rings are the most frequently used contraceptive methods by AYAs. However, AYA women tend to use these methods episodically, which can lead to increased health risks and increased failure rates. Clinicians should be prepared for AYA women to experiment with different delivery systems as they learn what fits best into their lives. Practice recommendations have reduced barriers to the successful use of short-acting methods including Quick Start (Same Day Start) protocols, elimination of unnecessary examinations and tests, as well as the provision of ample contraceptive supplies. As described, the introduction of new contraceptive methods has provided incremental improvements important to AYA women. Careful screening for medical eligibility for each of the methods has been streamlined using resources such as the CDC's U.S. MEC and the Selected Practice Recommendations for Contraceptive Use. Clinicians should be aware of the noncontraceptive benefits conferred by hormonal contraceptives including reduction in menstrual disorders, treatment of acne, reduction of hirsutism, and decrease risk of common gynecologic cancers. Further, drug–drug interactions are important to consider, especially with estrogen-containing short-acting methods. Success with short-acting methods requires consistent use. Counseling each AYA woman about how to use the methods and what changes she may expect can improve her success with the method. Equally important is to respond to any concerns the patient may have initially or with later use. Practice tips can be a guide, but speed of response is particularly important to AYA women.

REFERENCES

1. US Selected Practice Recommendations (US SPR) for Contraceptive Use, 2016. https://www.cdc.gov/reproductivehealth/contraception/mmwr/spr/summary.html
2. McMenamin SB, Charles SA, Tabatabaeepour N, et al. Implications of dispensing self-administered hormonal contraceptives in a 1-year supply: a California case study. *Contraception.* 2017;95(5):449–451.
3. Palacios S, Colli E, Regidor P-A. Multicenter, phase III trials on the contraceptive efficacy, tolerability, and safety of a new drospirenone-only pill. *Acta Obstet Gynecol Scand.* 2019;98(12):1549–1557.
4. Martinez GM, Abma JC. Sexual activity and contraceptive use among teenagers aged 15–19 in the United States, 2015–2017. *NCHS Data Brief.* 2020;(366):1–8.
5. Golden NH. Bones and birth control in adolescent girls. *J Pediatr Adolesc Gynecol.* 2020;33(3):249–254.
6. Lopez LM, Bernholc A, Chen M, et al. Hormonal contraceptives for contraception in overweight or obese women. *Cochrane Database Syst Rev.* 2016; 2016(8): CD008452
7. Sunaga T, Cicali B, Schmidt S, et al. Comparison of contraceptive failures associated with CYP3A4-inducing drug–drug interactions by route of hormonal contraceptive in an adverse event reporting system. *Contraception.* 2021;103(4): 222–224.
8. Archer DF, Merkatz RB, Bahamondes L, et al. Efficacy of the 1-year (13-cycle) segesterone acetate and ethinyl estradiol contraceptive vaginal system: results of two multicentre, open-label, single-arm, phase 3 trials. *Lancet Glob Health.* 2019;7(8): e1054–e1064.
9. Trussell J, Portman D. The creeping pearl: Why has the rate of contraceptive failure increased in clinical trials of combined hormonal contraceptive pills? *Contraception.* 2013;88(5):604–610.
10. Cole JA, Norman H, Doherty M, et al. Venous thromboembolism, myocardial infarction, and stroke among transdermal contraceptive system users. *Obstet Gynecol.* 2007;109(2 Pt 1):339–346.
11. Nelson AL, Kaunitz AM, Kroll R, et al. Efficacy, safety, and tolerability of a levonorgestrel/ethinyl estradiol transdermal delivery system: phase 3 clinical trial results. *Contraception.* 2021;103(3):137–143.
12. Michels KA, Pfeiffer RM, Brinton LA, et al. Modification of the associations between duration of oral contraceptive use and ovarian, endometrial, breast, and colorectal cancers. *JAMA Oncol.* 2018;4(4):516–521.
13. Lazorwitz A, Aquilante CL, Dindinger E, et al. Relationship between etonogestrel concentrations and bleeding patterns in contraceptive implant users. *Obstet Gynecol.* 2019;134(4):807–813.
14. Schultheis P, Montoya MN, Zhao Q, et al. Contraception and ectopic pregnancy risk: a prospective observational analysis. *Am J Obstet Gynecol.* 2021;224(2): 228–229.
15. Westhoff CL, Pike MC. Hormonal contraception and breast cancer. *Contraception.* 2018;98(3):171–173.
16. Asthana S, Busa V, Labani S. Oral contraceptives use and risk of cervical cancer–A systematic review & meta-analysis. *Eur J Obstet Gynecol Reprod Biol.* 2020; 247:163–175.
17. Grimes DA, Schulz KF. Nonspecific side effects of oral contraceptives: nocebo or noise? *Contraception.* 2011;83(1):5–9.
18. McKetta S, Keyes KM. Oral contraceptive use and depression among adolescents. *Ann Epidemiol.* 2019;29:46–51.
19. Evidence for Contraceptive Options and HIV Outcomes (ECHO) Trial Consortium. HIV incidence among women using intramuscular depot medroxyprogesterone acetate, a copper intrauterine device, or a levonorgestrel implant for contraception: a randomized, multicentre, open-label trial. *Lancet.* 2019;394(10195):303–313. doi: 10.1016/S0140-6736(19)31288-7.
20. Bonny AE, Secic M, Cromer B. Early weight gain related to later weight gain in adolescents on depot medroxyprogesterone acetate. *Obstet Gynecol.* 2011;117(4): 793–797.

ADDITIONAL RESOURCES AND WEBSITES

Additional Resources and Websites for Clinicians:
The Agency for Healthcare Research & Quality—www.ahrq.gov
The American College of Obstetricians and Gynecologists—www.acog.org
CDC Contraceptive Guidance for Clinicians—https://www.cdc.gov/reproductivehealth/contraception/contraception_guidance.htm
Contraceptive Technology—http://www.contraceptivetechnology.org/
National Clinical Training Center for Family Planning—www.ctcfp.org
The Office of Population Affairs—https://opa.hhs.gov
Reproductive Health National Training Center—www.fpntc.org
Selected practice recommendations for contraceptive use. Third edition 2016—https://www.who.int/reproductivehealth/publications/family_planning/SPR-3/en/
U.S. Medical Eligibility Criteria (U.S. MEC) for Contraceptive Use, 2016—https://www.cdc.gov/reproductivehealth/contraception/mmwr/mec/summary.html

Additional Resources and Websites for Parents/Caregivers:
The American College of Obstetricians and Gynecologists—www.acog.org
American Sexual Health Association—Parents (ashasexualhealth.org)
Bedsider Birth Control Support Network—www.bedsider.org
Emergency Contraception—https://ec.princeton.edu/
Planned Parenthood Federation of American—www.plannedparenthood.org

Additional Resources and Websites for Adolescents and Young Adults:
Bedsider birth control support network—https://www.bedsider.org/
Center for Young Men's Health, Boston Children's Hospital—Young Men's Health (youngmenshealthsite.org).
Center for Young Women's Health, Boston Children's Hospital—Center for Young Women's Health.
Emergency Contraception—https://ec.princeton.edu/
Go Ask Alice!—Go Ask Alice! (columbia.edu).
Planned Parenthood—Birth Control—https://www.plannedparenthood.org/learn/birth-control.
Planned Parenthood Federation of American—www.plannedparenthood.org
Planned Parenthood for Teens—https://www.plannedparenthood.org/learn/teens

49

Long-Acting Reversible Contraception

Michelle Forcier

KEY WORDS

- Contraception
- Hormonal implant
- Intrauterine device (IUD)
- Intrauterine system
- Long-acting reversible contraception (LARC)

INTRODUCTION

Long-acting reversible contraception is an umbrella term for clinician-inserted methods, which once placed, provides the user with exquisite control for their unique family planning needs. Long-acting reversible contraceptives (LARCs), such as IUDs and progestin contraceptive implants, have a major advantage over other birth control methods as they minimize problems with adherence and maximize continuation rates. In addition to contraception, LARCs have demonstrated use for menstrual and related gynecologic problems. Family planning experts have recommended LARCs as a first-line, best-practice contraceptive for persons engaging in sexual activities that involve a risk of pregnancy (i.e., egg and sperm present), including adolescents and nulliparous young persons over 20 years. Even as LARCs clearly offer superior first-line contraception, clinicians incorporating a reproductive justice framework will balance evidence and enthusiasm for LARCs with respectful listening to patient preference, body autonomy, and in the end, ensure patient-centered care. Reproductive justice demands an informed consent model that supports adolescents and young adults (AYAs) in assuming ownership of their body, health, and family planning outcomes.

Many studies, past and present, use broad-based patient or population descriptors predicated on female and male gender binary concepts. This chapter takes gender and sexual diversity in perspective by recognizing that LARC methods can be useful to persons of all genders with uteri. The chapter includes terminology that recognizes anatomy and function without gender monikers, wherever possible. Clinicians who wish to help AYA patients with uteri to avoid early or unintended pregnancy may offer these methods with confidence.

A 2020 U.S. National Survey of Family Growth (NSFG) reported that 20% of AYAs used LARCs, with subdermal implants accounting for most LARC use (15%).[1] The greatest contraceptive trend over time (2008 to 2014) was the use of LARCs, increasing from 6% to 14% across females aged 15 to 44 years.[2] In college-aged persons, studies demonstrate consistent increases in LARC uptake over time; the usage overall is still extremely low compared to less effective methods. In one study, the rate of LARC use among college-aged persons was 2.5%, with 90% electing to use IUD.[3] Condom use in college-aged persons using LARCs is lower than in persons choosing other methods.[4] Long-acting reversible contraception uptake in nulliparous persons has increased, from less than 1% in 2008 to almost 6% in 2014.[5] Thus far, it does not appear that race and ethnicity predict LARC use, but ever experiencing an unintended pregnancy is associated with LARC use in Whites and Hispanics.[6] Rates of LARC use in AYA populations are increasing, but are still underutilized.[7]

TYPES OF LONG-ACTING REVERSIBLE CONTRACEPTION

Long-acting reversible contraception includes a variety of "set it and forget it" rapidly reversible devices that allow for exquisite control over the efficacy and timing of family planning, and are even more effective than permanent sterilization. Long-acting reversible contraceptions have been recommended as a safe and user-friendly top-tier contraceptive for AYAs since 2007 with proven demonstrated reductions in risk of early and unintended pregnancy (see Chapter 47; Fig. 47.1).[8,9]

Because LARCs are functionally user independent, typical and perfect use failure rates are essentially the same, eliminating problems with adherence and misuse (Table 49.1). In addition, LARC users demonstrate consistently higher continuation rates than short-acting reversible contraceptive (SARC) methods across all ages. At present, there are several U.S. Food and Drug Administration (FDA)-approved devices, with many more options available internationally. Intrauterine devices approved by the FDA include levonorgestrel (LNG) intrauterine systems (LNG-IUD) Mirena and Liletta (52 mg, 7 years duration effectiveness), Kyleena (19.5 mg, 5 years), and Skyla (13.5 mg, 3 years). There is a hormone-free copper IUD (CuT380A IUD, Paragard, 1984, [Cu-IUD]) that is effective for up to 12 years. These updated versions of the IUD have been in use and well studied for over 30 years. The etonogestrel (ENG) progesterone-only implant (formerly Implanon, now Nexplanon) was FDA approved in 2006, and is another device that is placed in the subdermal tissues of the nondominant upper arm.

MECHANISM, EFFICACY, AND INSERTION

The ENG is a single 4-cm × 2-mm flexible ethylene vinyl acetate copolymer rod that is inserted subdermally (Fig. 49.1). The newer ENG device, Nexplanon, has an improved inserter that limits placement depth, decreasing procedural variability and risk for deep or intramuscular insertions. Nexplanon contains a single rod with 15 mg barium sulfate, making it radiopaque and easier to detect with

TABLE 49.1

Overview of LARC Devices and Properties

	Implant	IUD			
	Etonogestrel 68 mg	CU	LNG 52 mg	LNG 19.5 mg	LNG 13.5 mg
Brand name	Nexplanon	Paragard	Mirena Liletta	Kyleena	Skyla
Rate unintended pregnancy first year typical use (%)	0.05	0.8	0.2		
Duration (years) Evidence based (FDA package insert)	5 (3)	12 (10)	7 (5)	5 (—)	3 (—)
Device characteristics Strings	—	White	Gray	Blue	Gray
Size horizontal × vertical (mm)	40 × 2	32 × 36	32 × 32	29 × 30	29 × 30
Inserter diameter (mm)		4.01	4.4	3.8	3.8
Initial rate release (mcg/d)	60–70	na	19–20	17.5	14

LARC, long-acting reversible contraception; IUD, intrauterine device; LNG, levonorgestrel.

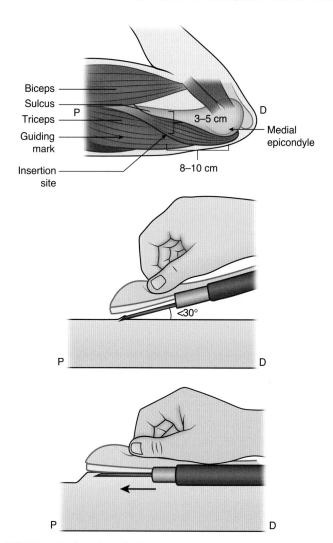

FIGURE 49.1 Insertion of Nexplanon contraceptive device. (Accessed 31 May, 2020. https://www.merck.com/product/usa/pi_circulars/n/nexplanon/nexplanon_pi.pdf)

x-ray if in rare cases the device migrates or is inserted into muscle tissue. Etonogestrel's active ingredient is 68 mg etonogestrel, slow released, with peak serum ENG concentrations reach 800 pg/mL, with a gradual decrease over time. As with other progesterone contraceptive methods, ENG inhibits ovulation, thickens cervical mucus, and thins the endometrial lining. Etonogestrel is very effective with a cumulative pregnancy rate of 0.6 per 100 person-years and no pregnancies reported in a group of over 200 females who used the implant for at least 5 years.[10]

Intrauterine devices are locally acting agents that prevent sperm and egg from coming in contact and prevent fertilization (Fig. 49.2). In general, IUDs are toxic to sperm and oocytes; gametes are rendered inactive or ineffective, and do not fertilize or form viable embryos.[11] Intrauterine devices are not abortifacients and should not be used at present to interrupt an implanted pregnancy. Intrauterine devices do not work by suppressing endogenous estrogen and progesterone hormone production; thus, ovulation and other perimenstrual symptoms may continue. The Cu-IUD T-shaped polyethylene frame is wrapped in copper wire and contains barium sulfate in the stem to render it radiopaque. Copper ions act as a functional spermicide, which both renders gametes inactive and creates an environment unsuitable for fertilization. Copper intrauterine devices create an intrauterine sterile foreign body reaction with cytotoxic inflammatory mediators destroying sperm and ova, inhibiting motility, disconnecting head–tail, inhibiting acrosomal enzyme and capacitation, impairing penetration of the zona pellucida, and with increased local prostaglandin levels, additionally impairing ova fertilizability.

The LNG-IUD creates thick impenetrable mucous, a thin atrophic lining, inflammatory effects, and impaired tubal motility. Levonorgestrel, like its copper counterpart, is a nonsystemic hormonal method, creating a local intrauterine environment hostile to gametes and fertilization. The larger (32-mm × 32-mm) T-shaped polyethylene Mirena or Liletta contain 52 mg LNG, released directly into the uterine body for largely paracrine rather than systemic effects, with Liletta typically available at lower cost than Mirena. Serum progestin levels are about half that of ENG implant users and one-tenth of oral LNG users.[11] Both Kyleena and Skyla IUDs measure 28 mm × 30 mm with release rates of 17.5 mcg/day and 14 mcg/day, and with 5-year and 3-year duration of effectiveness, respectively. Ovulation may be suppressed but is not the

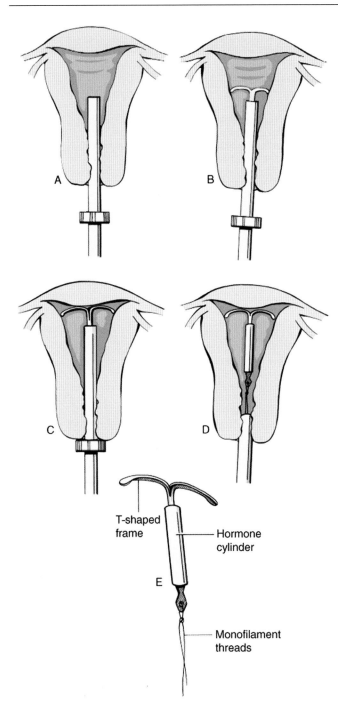

T-shaped
frame

Hormone
cylinder

E

Monofilament
threads

FIGURE 49.2 Image of a Mirena IUD. (Adapted from Gibbs RS, Karlan BY, Haney AF, et al. *Danforth's Obstetrics and Gynecology.* 9th ed. Lippincott Williams & Wilkins; 2003; Curtis M, Linares ST, Antoniewicz L, eds. *Glass' Office Gynecology.* 7th ed. Wolters Kluwer Health; 2014.)

main mechanism of action, with between 45% and 75% of persons ovulating on the 52-mg device, and almost all persons ovulating on the lower-dose LNG-IUDs. Ovulation on the lower-dose LNG-IUDs may result in less amenorrhea and more regular menses, which can be a desired effect for some persons.[11]

Both the implant and IUDs have demonstrated effectiveness far beyond their original FDA study data (**Table 49.1**).[10,12] A 2015 study of over 61,000 persons with newly inserted IUDs calculated 1-year overall Pearl indices of 0.06 and 0.52 for LNG IUDs and Cu-IUDs, respectively.[13] A total of 118 contraceptive failures occurred, with 21 of those diagnosed as ectopic (adjusted hazard ratio for ectopic 0.26 TCu380A and TCu220). Evidence-based data demonstrate longer duration of efficacy than recommended by the FDA Pharmaceutical Inspectorate (PI): Cu-IUD 12 years, LNG (52 mg) 7 years, and LNG (13.5 mg) 3 years. The 52-mg LNG-IUDs remains extremely efficacious through 7 years with a cumulative 7-year pregnancy rate of 0.5 per 100 and may be superior to shorter-acting methods of contraception for up to 9 years.[14] The failure rates for Cu-IUD and LNG (52 mg) are 0.1% and 0.3%, respectively, making the LNG (52 mg) noninferior to the Cu-IUD, allowing both methods to serve as emergency contraception (EC) and extended family planning.[15,16] The less than 1% failure rate for LARCs remains the same across both younger and older age groups, while persons younger than age 21 years using short-acting methods have twice the risk of contraceptive failure, compared to older peers.

● ISSUES AFFECTING EFFICACY—INITIATION

A variety of factors may be associated with AYA's use of LARCs[4,5,17]:
- Earlier age of sexual debut
- Increasing age
- Previous unintended pregnancy, increasing parity, future birth intentions
- Relationship status: Monogamous, cohabitation, or marriage
- Heterosexual orientation
- Attends Title X or hospital-based health center with a primary care provider still in residency training
- Urban over rural geographic location
- Has health insurance, in particular Medicaid or other public health coverage
- English speaking
- Higher education
- High IUD knowledge
- Dissatisfaction with other contraceptive methods

Socioeconomic status and race do not seem to predict LARC use, although data vary across studies. However, studies suggest that lack of knowledge, perceived and actual concerns about side effects (perceived weight gain, irregular bleeding, and long-term health risks), along with parental/caregiver involvement, are significant barriers to initiation of LARCs in AYAs.

As is the case with other health-related decisions, clinician recommendation and confidence is a strong factor when persons select an IUD and ENG for contraception.[6] Despite consistently showing superior efficacy and safety profiles, many clinicians lack awareness of and do not recommend LARC use in AYAs.[18] Many pediatricians still do not counsel, and most do not offer immediate on-site LARC insertion despite the American Academy of Pediatrics (AAP) policy recommending LARCs as first-line contraception. Further, resident physicians report wanting procedural training in LARC insertion, but come up against lack of training opportunities and structural elements in pediatric settings. Higher knowledge about LARCs was associated with female gender, adolescent medicine subspecialty, acknowledging that adolescent pregnancy is a serious problem for patients in their practice, and having read the AAP policy statement.

In addition to reducing clinician-based barriers, improving infrastructure and systems supports, including flexible clinic hours and open appointments, can improve access to LARCs.[19-25] School-based clinics present another opportunity to improve AYAs access to LARCs.[26] **Table 49.2** offers a brief summary of the evidence to support clinician confidence along with answers to expected questions when recommending LARCs to AYAs.

Initiation—Insertion Considerations and Quick-Start

Insertion methods are safe, relatively painless, and simple procedures that are well tolerated in outpatient settings. Side effects are limited, with satisfaction levels consistently higher in LARC

TABLE 49.2

Pros and Cons of LARC: Clinician Highlights for Patient-Centered Counseling

	ENG	LNG-IUD		Cu Intrauterine Device
		52 mg	<20 mg	
Insertion	Upper arm, not require pelvic exam, disposable instruments	Requires pelvic exam, surgical instruments for insertion and that require sterile processing and reuse. Risk of complications decrease with clinician experience (including number of placements/year), ultrasound guidance.		
Removal	Potential for fibrosis make removal more difficult than insertion. Requires surgical instruments (sterilization)	Requires pelvic exam, speculum, and sterile forceps		
Device	5 years superior protection. Expulsion not a risk. Newer insertion techniques have reduced migration concerns.	Efficacy duration to 5, 3–4, and 12 years. Some increase risk of expulsion, with younger nulliparous patients, immediate postpartum or abortion patients, or multiparous patients. Patient and/or partner may remove device		
Pain	Local pain and potential bruising at insertion site. Can minimize pain and bleeding using lidocaine with both bicarb and epinephrine	Pelvic and speculum can be uncomfortable or painful, as it is a more "invasive" exam. Psychological distress related to past sexual trauma, gender dysphoria, and younger age (both cognitive and chronologic)		
Menses Effects	Potential for irregular menses	Results in lighter shorter menses, or amenorrhea.	More likely to have regular, but lighter menses	Regular menses. Potential for heavier, crampier menses
Vaginal Effects	None	Increased potential episodes for vaginitis		
Emergency Contraception	None	Both 52 mg LNG and Cu-IUD very efficacious emergency contraception up to 5 days		
Financial Upfront	$400–$800	$400–$1000		
Financial Over Time	LARCs are the most cost-effective methods, with higher initial cost offset by duration of use over time, efficacy, and reduced pregnancies.			
Insurance	Device, insertion procedure, and clinic visit costs (covered by Medicaid and most insurers)			
Current Procedural Terminology Codes for Clinicians	11981—insert. 11982—remove. 11983—remove reinsert	58300—insert. 58301—remove		

LARC, long-acting reversible contraception; ENG, etonogestrel; LNG-IUD, levonorgestrel intrauterine device.

than SARC users. Determining each young person's family planning needs requires active listening, along with understanding and respecting patient perspectives so as to create a contraceptive plan that addresses that patient's goals; this may or may not include LARCs.[27]

Initiation of LARC contraceptives need not be hindered or delayed depending on patient history and attitudes about pregnancy.[8] The FDA's PI indicates that LARC methods should only be inserted within 5 days of last menstrual period (LMP), with a negative pregnancy test, and reasonable certainty that the patient is not pregnant. Family planning experts offer more flexible guidelines for starting LARCs as long as there is a reasonable certainty that the AYAs are not pregnant, consistent with other "Quick Start Contraception" practices. Overall risk for luteal phase pregnancy with any day initiation of ENG was very low at 0.3%; there was no difference in rates that followed the more rigid PI recommendations.[28]

Determining potential for very early pregnancy that may not be detectable by urine human choriogonadotropin (hCG) hormone

testing includes inquiring about date or time of last sex with potential for sperm and egg contact. If coitus occurred within 5 days, EC may be offered (see Chapter 46). If unprotected sex occurred more than 14 days prior, and the pregnancy test is negative, clinicians may be confident that the patient is currently not pregnant. Patients who are starting LARCs after days 1 to 5 of their LMP should be strongly encouraged to use backup protection or abstain from intercourse for 7 days while the method takes effect. The only exception to this is the use of Cu-IUDs which can both serve as EC and an immediately effective contraceptive.

If there is some possibility of fertilization and/or early implantation, clinicians can offer three options for same-day care:
• Recommend abstinence or 100% condom use for 2 to 4 weeks, and reschedule for repeat urine hCG and LARC insertion.
• Start another SARC, and reschedule urine hCG and LARC. Depot medroxyprogesterone acetate (DMPA) is particularly useful in this case as it does not require self-administration and allows for a 15-week window of coverage and time to return for insertion.

• Provide LARC insertion at time of visit with plan for follow-up pregnancy testing in 3 weeks.

If there are questions about pregnancy status, and concerns that a device could potentially interrupt or harm a pregnancy, subdermal ENG rather than IUD may be inserted, with a follow-up urine hCG in 3 weeks. There are no demonstrated teratogenic effects of progesterone on fetal development. Patients diagnosed as pregnant on ENG most likely became pregnant before or during the first week of ENG activity. Patients who are pregnant can continue the pregnancy with removal of the ENG or terminate while maintaining an ENG implant. In one recent public-sector study, over two-thirds of the clinicians felt that quick-start LARCs in AYAs were safe; rates of clinician confidence in safety was affected by Title X status, previous LARC training, and adolescent specialization.[29]

It is less desirable to insert an IUD if a patient may have a very early pregnancy and would intend on continuing that pregnancy. However, if a young person desires urgent IUD placement, an IUD may be inserted with the understanding and consent that the IUD could affect ongoing pregnancy and increase the miscarriage risk. For patients who are clear that they would elect pregnancy termination, an IUD may be placed with careful follow-up, with subsequent pregnancy testing in 3 to 4 weeks. Abortion suction procedure would remove both the pregnancy and IUD at the same time. Patients could elect to replace their IUD at the time of abortion if they choose.

There are no longer restrictions about the timing of insertion of LARCs. Clinicians can recommend LARC initiation immediately after abortion, postpartum (unless there are concerns about endometrial infection or puerperal sepsis) or postcesarean section. Persons >21 days postpartum or 7 days postabortion require additional backup methods for 7 days following insertion. Counseling pregnant AYAs about these options before delivery or termination can improve access, initiation, and prevent unintended pregnancy.

Issues Affecting Efficacy—Continuation

Adolescents are more likely to stop all contraceptive methods compared to their older adult counterparts, contributing to overall higher contraceptive failure rates in young females. Method failure is much higher for short-acting contraceptives (22-fold greater than LARCs and 2-fold greater for females less than 21 years); this is a compelling argument for universal access for LARCs among AYAs.[30] In one randomized study, LARC continuation rates over a 2-year period were far superior to SARC (64.3% vs. 25.5%), and with lower rates of unintended pregnancy (3.6% vs. 7% to 10%).[31]

ADVANTAGES OF LONG-ACTING REVERSIBLE CONTRACEPTIONS

The most time-intensive aspect of LARCs, as with most other aspects of AYA care including family planning, includes detailed counseling about what to expect and how best to manage side effects. Offering a balanced "risk-in perspective" and focused counseling, begins with discussing the benefits of LARCs as opposed to the risks. This is consistent with strength-based resiliency theory, and may improve patient acceptance, satisfaction, and continuation (see Table 49.2).

Despite persistent misconceptions, IUD safety has been well established over time. Systematic reviews of AYA IUD use found that overall incidence of adverse events related to pregnancy, infection, heavy menses, or perforation was very low. Serious complications such as infection, expulsion, and migration for ENG are also low, and even lower since the switch to Nexplanon (0.92 vs. 1.31 in 1,000 patients).[32] With changes in insertion

site and placement, ENG has reduced risk of migration of these devices.

Additional medical indications, patient factors, and device features may improve recommendation, initiation, and continuation of LARCs. Long-acting reversible contraceptions are particularly useful for patients for whom estrogen-containing products are contraindicated (i.e., patients at risk for venous thromboembolism [VTE] and other coagulopathies, cardiac and valvular anomalies, hormone responsive diseases and malignancies), as well as patients for whom unintended pregnancy could be life-threatening. Other benefits may also help determine method selection for youth anticipating future sexual activity and looking to initiate contraception before first intercourse. Both the 52-mg LNG and Cu-IUDs are essentially equal in efficacy for EC, with more patients potentially electing this method for continuing contraception given the LNG (52-mg) effects on menses.

The overall benefits of LARCs for AYAs include the following:

• Efficacy—<1% failure rate, far superior to all other forms of SARC or barrier contraception.
• Safety—Myths regarding increased risks for sexually transmitted infections (STIs), infertility, and serious morbidity or mortality have long been dismissed.
• Ease of use—Once inserted, patients do not need to "do" anything to ensure contraceptive effectiveness.
• Immediate reversibility—Once removed, LARCs are a quick and completely reversible method of contraception. Return to ovulation and fertility can occur as early as 7 to 14 days after removal. For persons considering LARC removal, effective use of folic acid is ideally started before considering pregnancy. The immediate reversibility and ease of LARCs allows individuals to attempt timing of conception and estimated dates of delivery.

Special Indications for Copper Intrauterine Device

• No hormonal systemic effects—With no-hormonal components, this method addresses some patients' concerns and desire to avoid the use of systemic medications or hormones.
• As a nonhormonal method, Cu-IUD effectiveness is not affected by people with a higher body mass index (BMI) nor does it place patients at risk for increased appetite or weight gain. Copper intrauterine device does not alter the AYA's endogenous estrogen and progesterone hormones. Copper intrauterine device allows for continued menses and supports AYAs who desire monthly menses to reassure themselves about pregnancy or to "feel more natural."
• Longest-acting, reversible contraception—lasting 12 years or more.

Special Indications for Levonorgestrel Intrauterine Device 52 mg (Mirena)

• Menstrual problems including menorrhagia—LNG-IUD (52 mg) can offer relief and is even FDA approved for treatment of menometrorrhagia, including those with bleeding diatheses (see Chapter 53). Local LNG action on the intrauterine lining produces a consistent decrease in overall menstrual volume, with a significant number of patients who experience amenorrhea. Levonorgestrel intrauterine devices may offer relief from dysmenorrhea and endometriosis. Further, LNG-IUDs offer risk reduction for hyperandrogenism and endometrial hyperplasia, relative to local uterine progestin effects.
• Fewer medication interactions—Both Cu- and LNG-IUDs, unlike oral contraceptive pills, have fewer medication interactions. There is no impact on efficacy with antimicrobials and anticonvulsants, including lamotrigine. There are no known interactions between antiretrovirals (ARVs) medications and no impact on human immunodeficiency virus (HIV) shedding, overall complications, infection rates, or morbidity.

Special Indications for Etonogestrel

- Ease of insertion—Subdermal implant in the upper extremity does not require a bimanual, vaginal, and speculum examination for placement, reducing anxiety for patients who have never had a pelvic examination or who are not yet experiencing receptive vaginal intercourse.
- Dysmenorrhea—ENG has an off-label use for management of heavy prolonged menses, with some patients experiencing amenorrhea as a desired side effect.
- Supra–low systemic doses of hormones:
  - Etonogestrel does not appear to affect appetite in the same way that DMPA does in young people with obesity. As weight gain is a concern for many young females starting contraception, lack of impact on appetite and weight gain makes ENG an attractive option. There is a concern that excess weight may have an impact on ENG effectiveness due to its low steady-state delivery; evidence on this issue, however, is inconsistent.[33]
  - Other medical conditions are not affected by this low steady-state dose of ENG including hyperlipidemia, coagulation pathways and disorders, and bone health and risk of osteoporosis.
  - Etonogestrel has no interactions when used with anticonvulsants (e.g., phenytoin, carbamazepine, oxcarbapezine, primidine, topiramate, and barbiturates), and ARV therapy such as ritonavir-boosted protease inhibitors, nonrifampicin, and rifabutin. There is some evidence that anti-HIV drugs, favirenz or nevirapine, and/or specific genotypes may reduce ENG levels.[34]

● DISADVANTAGES OF LONG-ACTING REVERSIBLE CONTRACEPTION

There are few disadvantages to LARCs with the most common side effect being irregular uterine bleeding that patients may not tolerate or desire. Cost may be a consideration in some health care systems.

Contraindications

There are few absolute contraindications for use of LARCs in all people, including adolescents and young nulliparous adults. The Centers for Disease Control and Prevention (CDC) (see Chapter 46; Figure 46.1) and the World Health Organization offer regularly updated Medical Eligibility Criteria for Contraceptive Use for reference when assessing comorbid conditions that may preclude the safe use of LARCs. Absolute contraindications include the following:

- Active pelvic inflammatory disease (PID)—People with active PID should not have a new IUD insertion, but should leave the previously inserted IUD in place and treat around it.
- Ongoing, desired pregnancy—If an IUD user is determined to be pregnant, she must be evaluated for possible ectopic pregnancy. IUDs decrease risk of ectopic pregnancy compared to females not using birth control. However, if a person with an IUD becomes pregnant, it is more likely to be ectopic. People with an intrauterine pregnancy are at risk for spontaneous abortion, septic abortion, preterm delivery, and chorioamnionitis if the IUDs are left in place. Intrauterine device removal decreases these risks somewhat, especially if the IUD strings are visible and the device is removed as soon as possible. Etonogestrel does not impact pregnancy but should be removed if a patient is continuing with a pregnancy plan.
- Allergic reactions to device components
- Wilson disease (Cu-IUD)
- Uterine cavity size (<6 cm or >10 cm) or significant structural abnormalities—IUDs are not typically recommended in people with extremely small or large uteri (<6 cm or >10 cm) or with anatomic uterine abnormalities, as there is a greater risk of expulsion.

Insertion/Removal—Intrauterine Devices

- *Pain*—Clinicians can prepare patients for an IUD insertion by reassuring them that the majority of patients report minimal to moderate pain with insertion. Offering individualized pain management plans can help patients maintain realistic expectations and manage their anxiety.
  - Lidocaine 2% gel, misoprostol, and most NSAIDs have not been shown to significantly reduce pain in most studies. There is no use for misoprostol in softening or decreasing insertion pain. Misoprostol does have significant undesirable gastrointestinal side effects.
  - Effectively injected paracervical lidocaine blocks, tramadol, and naproxen have shown some effect on decreasing pain with cervical dilation and fundal placement of device. For younger adolescents and nulliparous persons, effectively applied paracervical blocks may offer benefit in decreasing the pain of attaching the tenaculum, of dilating a smaller tighter internal os, and in reassuring patients that they can tolerate all aspects of the procedure.
  - Anxiety and pain associated with pelvic, bimanual, and speculum examinations and the potential for medical trauma for patients who have never been sexually active or have genital dysphoria is a very real problem and barrier to insertion. Many patients and parents/caregivers may recognize the potential benefits of an IUD. Therefore, considering insertion under conscious sedation is a realistic and humane option. Various levels of conscious sedation can offer pain and anxiolytic control in certain situations. Conscious sedation may be an option for patients who are younger, immature, developmentally diverse, never experienced receptive vaginal sex, experienced sexual abuse, rape, or trauma, have anxiety disorders or have gender dysphoria.
- *Complications*—Clinicians can minimize insertion errors and complications by being well prepared for most contingencies before and during the insertion. Having the range of potential surgical adjuncts at the bedside during the procedure allows controlled responses to situational factors.
  - Flexible plastic endometrial biopsy catheters are far safer than their larger metal counterparts and effective sounding devices assessing uterine depth prior to insertion.
  - Silver nitrate or monsel solution can help stop bleeding from puncture wounds at tenaculum sites.
  - Cervical dilators, such as Pratt dilators 13 to 21 French, can be helpful in gently enlarging a tight internal os before device placement.
  - A thorough understanding of pelvic anatomy and confidence with assessing the position of the uterus is essential to avoid perforation and assure correct IUD placement.
  - Ultrasound-guided procedures allow for direct visualization of the path of the IUD and assure correct cervical dilation, fundal placement, and can assist in IUD removal when the strings are no longer visible on speculum examination. Ultrasound guidance is not necessary for insertion, but is very useful in training settings as direct visualization can decrease perforation and complications. Intrauterine devices insertion complications are most commonly related to clinician experience and use of rigid metal sounds.
  - Expulsion rates of IUDs are estimated at 5% with increased risk for expulsion associated with higher parity patients, those aged 14 to 19 years, those who experienced previous expulsion, or being placed immediately postabortion or postpartum. Intrauterine device removals are typically easily done using sponge

forceps and gentle traction pulling the string toward the distal vaginal opening. There are some situations that make IUD removal more difficult including nonvisualized strings. The lack of visible strings may be due to the IUD being embedded in the uterine body or cervix or having migrated outside the uterus. These are rare situations that would require advanced clinical referral.

Insertion/Removal—Etonogestrel

- *Pain*—Many younger patients, those who are not yet sexually active, or with trauma or dysphoria may opt for ENG as the insertion procedure does not require a pelvic and speculum exam. Patients may be reassured that ENG insertion is preceded by a local lidocaine block that will be painful for about 10 seconds, but thereafter provide excellent pain control. The insertion time from skin entry to removal of insertion device takes 5 to 10 seconds.
- *Insertion/Removal Complications*—Complications on insertion of an ENG are very rare and most likely related to user experience and supervision. Implant removals may be more complicated and take more time, depending on the depth of placement, encapsulation around the rod, and clinician experience.
  - Lidocaine, with a small amount of epinephrine and bicarb, may help decrease bleeding, bruising, and pain.
  - Fibrosis or capsule formation around the device is the most common removal complication, making removal more time consuming and difficult.
  - Changes in the inserter mechanics, radiopacity, and site of device placement, help limit depth of insertion, avoiding placement deep into the muscle, making it easier to find on imaging and avoiding migration into the vasculature.
  - Etonogestrel is rarely expulsed, but there are reports of device breakage. Younger users of the ENG implant should be counseled against "playing" with their insert as regular flexing and bending of the implant is associated with breakage. Continued efficacy may be an issue if the integrity of the device is impaired.

PREGNANCY PREVENTION DOES NOT EQUAL SEXUALLY TRANSMITTED INFECTION PREVENTION

Most contraceptives are currently not made to offer both STI and pregnancy prevention, although research in multipurpose prevention technologies (MPTs) continues. Despite many years of reliable evidence, some clinicians still refuse to offer LARCs, especially IUDs, to young persons because of concerns regarding increasing PID and infertility risks. Pelvic inflammatory disease risk is only modestly increased 1 to 20 days post insertion when a device is inserted and facilitates movement of the infection to the upper genital track. Intrauterine device users diagnosed with cervicitis or vaginitis should keep their IUDs in place and treat over it. An IUD should only be removed if a patient fails to respond to PID treatment. Unlike combined oral contraceptive pill (COC) users, the vaginal biomes of IUD and DMPA users may show lower lactobacillus counts accounting for some reported increase in bacterial vaginosis.[35] Risk of developing genital STIs and PID with an IUD is the same as the risk without an IUD.[36]

Long-acting reversible contraception users report lower rates of dual contraceptive methods (i.e., barrier methods such as condoms). However, studies do not demonstrate substantial increases in STI/PID rates or morbidity or mortality.[37] Dual use is only slightly less reported with LARCs than SARCs, with factors associated with dual use including age <25 years, lower education, Black race, single relationship status, baseline dual method use, baseline previous experience with STI, greater condom efficacy scores as well as greater partner acceptance of condoms. Dual use among AYAs with new sexual partners is more common than with established partners. Unfortunately, dual use among postpartum AYAs is still low.[38]

GUIDELINES FOR PATIENTS

Counseling and Consent

Preinsertion consent includes reviewing the insertion procedure, and more importantly, counseling on expected benefits and risks, as well as commonly experienced side effects of these long-acting, completely reversible devices. Key elements in counseling and consent include a discussion of the following:

1. Select a method that most meets the patient's needs and goals, while avoiding least desirable side effects using a reproductive justice framework that respects body autonomy and choice.
2. Provide a risk-in perspective model (framing benefits vs. risks); offer balanced consent focusing more on expected outcomes and benefits as opposed to overemphasizing rare adverse events. Make sure the patient understands the difference between common surgical risks of pain, cramping, and abnormal uterine bleeding (AUB) immediately post insertion. Offer reassurance and perspective that rare adverse events of infection, expulsion, perforation, and pregnancy are unlikely.
3. Prepare and reassure the patient regarding the insertion procedure.
4. Use of language during reproductive health counseling is very important. Clinicians can degenderize terminology and be more inclusive using terms such as persons rather than females, people with uteri, and persons engaging in sperm and egg sex for pregnancy. For patients who identity as gender diverse or indicate gender dysphoria, it is important to ask what language about body parts will help them feel most comfortable with the consent and insertion process. Clinicians should continue to check in regarding implicit biases and assumptions about ableism and/or race so that they do not impact patient-centered care.
5. Immediate aftercare can be done orally and in written form so that the patient can refer to the information post procedure.
6. Continue to offer long-term follow-up regarding any concerns that arise, continued STI prevention, and additional anticipatory guidance for safe, healthy sexual and reproductive health.

Clinicians have understandably focused on the risks and adverse outcomes of adolescent sexual activity, including unintended pregnancy, STIs and emotional distress that can arise with romantic relationships. This perspective has begun to broaden to a more developmentally appropriate and inclusive perspective acknowledging that sexual exploration, sexual activity, and a diversity of sexual behaviors are an expected and even desired aspect of AYA development. Sex positive, pro-diversity counseling models for youth and parents/caregivers are helpful as they provide guidance on how to discuss the realities of being an emerging young adult. Youth who are offered open, nonjudgmental opportunities to discuss their sexuality encourages a longitudinal approach for a healthful and satisfying sexuality that extends across the lifespan.

Common and Expected Side Effects—Irregular Uterine Bleeding

Preinsertion counseling on postinsertion changes in menstrual bleeding is likely the most important aspect in preparing young females for continuation of LARCs. Females should be counseled to expect a change in periods and AUB the first 3 months post insertion.

Evaluation and Treatment of Long-Acting Reversible Contraception–Associated Abnormal Uterine Bleeding

- Copper intrauterine device—Persons using the Cu-IUD can expect regular, but heavier menses. For a minority of youth, avoiding amenorrhea and having a regular period make this their method of choice, but more often, the predicted Cu-IUD effect on menstrual periods makes this a less desirable choice for young persons.
- Levonorgestrel intrauterine device—Levonorgestrel 52 mg tends to lessen menses with a 90% reduction in all menstrual bleeding; many patients experience amenorrhea for years post insertion. Levonorgestrel intrauterine device at doses lower than 52 mg may experience more breakthrough bleeding or continuation of regular, lighter periods.
- Etonogestrel—Infrequent bleeding is the most common expected postinsertion effect, follow by amenorrhea, and intermittent prolonged bleeding. The patient's unique menstrual bleeding pattern will usually be established within the first 3 to 4 months and predicts future bleeding patterns.
- While irregular bleeding may be a normal and expected immediate side effect, supporting young females and helping them tolerate this effect is important for continuation rates.
  - Supporting patients who are struggling with post-LARC AUB may include repeating their sexual and gynecologic history with respect to non-LARC sources of bleeding such as pregnancy, STIs, cervicitis or cervical cancer, as well as any potential for acute or chronic anemia with hemodynamic sequelae. Adolescents and young adults are at lower risk than their more mature counterparts for cancers, polyps, and fibroids as a source for AUB. As such, they require a different approach to the evaluation of AUB.
  - For people using a progestogen-only injectable contraceptive who have problematic bleeding, NSAIDs such as naproxen or mefenamic acid 500 mg twice daily for 5 days can offer short-term relief and but will not likely impact long-term bleeding issues.[39] Depot medroxyprogesterone acetate, COCs or progestin-only contraceptive pills may be provided for persons after the initial 3-month start period or when necessary to alleviate episodes of AUB.

Etonogestrel Insertion

- Patient-centered counseling and preparation
  - Serious adverse events are rare, with none judged as drug related.
  - Common complaints are bleeding and pain at insertion site immediately after insertion, which are usually managed with pressure, re-dressing, and oral medication.
- Clinicians must be trained for insertion competency according to FDA guidelines.
- Time for insertion from the skin entry to complete insertion is 1 minute or less. It should be noted that this does not include the time for preparation or anesthetic injection and onset of action. Practical insertion time is from 5 to 10 minutes depending on the situational variables (inserter experience, patient need for reassurance, and clinic infrastructure for preparation).
- The ENG implant comes packaged in a preloaded, sterile, disposable inserter.
- To prevent any risk for unintended pregnancy, the FDA recommends that ENG be inserted during the first 5 days of a female's menstrual cycle, immediately postabortion, or postpartum. As previously stated, Quick-Start methods are highly recommended in the family planning community.
- The device is placed 6 to 8 cm above the medial epicondyle along the medial aspect of the nondominant upper arm, inferior to the sulcus between the biceps and the triceps.
- The skin is cleansed with an antiseptic and 1 to 5 cc of 1% lidocaine (with or without epinephrine) is placed at the trochar

insertion point and can be placed along the planned insertion track of the device.

- The trochar, with implant loaded, is introduced directly under the skin and subdermal layer, tenting the skin until the needle hub is at the level of the skin. Stabilizing the base, the needle is smoothly retracted, leaving the implant behind.
- The implant remains invisible for most persons, but it is easy to palpate. It is important to palpate the area immediately after the removal of the insertion needle to confirm implant placement.
- Pressure is applied to the skin incision site for hemostasis.
- A Steri-Strip is placed to close the incision along with a pressure dressing.
- Routine precautions should be provided for postinsertion care regarding bruising, minor bleeding, and pain after insertion.

Etonogestrel Removal

- Higher rates for removal of ENG were found among patients with amenorrhea, occasional spotting or bleeding, and regular menses than for prolonged or continuous bleeding.
- In clinical trials, ENG showed high contraceptive efficacy, palpability before removal, short removal times, and few removal complications.
- Age, race, BMI, parity, prior contraception method, and postpartum and breast-feeding status did not predict bleeding or removal for bleeding risk.
- The digital extrusion or "pop-out" technique is encouraged for removal. In the "pop-out" technique, the rod is first palpated, marked, and removal site cleansed.
- A small amount of local anesthetic is infused beneath the distal tip of the rod. A 2-mm incision parallel to the rod is made at the distal tip of the implant.
- Then pressure is applied at the proximal end, pushing the rod toward the incision until it pops out, at which time it can be grasped with fingers or forceps.
- Mean removal time is 2 to 4 minutes.
- Instrument removal with noncrushing clamps also may be utilized.
- Removal of ENG implants is distinctly more straightforward than the removal of the LNG capsules (Norplant) for several reasons including single implant, stiffer rod, and less fibrous capsule formation. Fibrosis around the implant is the most common removal complication.

Intrauterine Device Insertion

Intrauterine device insertion requires a pelvic bimanual and speculum exam. Patients may benefit from preinsertion NSAIDs (800 mg ibuprofen or 500 mg naproxen) and even an anxiolytic. Patients benefit from verbal distraction techniques to decrease anxiety and improve procedure tolerance as with other pelvic exam procedures.

- The bimanual examination assesses for uterine size, placement (anteverted, midline, retroverted), and location of cervix. It will also inform the examiner about cervical motion tenderness or other palpable pelvic abnormalities.
- The speculum examination allows for visualization of the external cervical os, paracervical block, and tenaculum grasp for maintaining traction with insertion.
- Insertion requires measuring or sounding the uterus to determine adequate uterine size (6 to 10 cm) and direction of placement.
- Each IUD comes with slightly different inserter devices and techniques, but aim for fundal placement for maximal efficacy.

Intrauterine Device Removal

- Intrauterine device removal is generally a 5- to 10-second procedure by which the strings are grasped with locking forceps and the IUD is gently pulled out from the cervical os.

FUTURE DEVELOPMENTS

Recent developments include use of smaller devices, changes in hormonal content (newer progestins, estradiol) and progesterone antagonists and receptor modulators to block ovulation and prevent follicular rupture. Newer IUD models and MPTs (products that offer both contraception and STI prevention) are exciting new potential developments. The family planning community's contraceptive research provides a long history of consistent data addressing safety, efficacy, and appropriateness of use of LARCs in AYAs. Future developments may recognize the training and service provision discrepancies that are still too common barriers to initiation and offering same-day LARC insertions. A medical education and systems approach to offering primary care clinicians more opportunities to train in LARC counseling, insertion, and removal is an attainable goal.

The extensive use of technology and social media by AYAs puts them at the forefront of learning more about medical, legislative, and legal implications of family planning. Political, legislative, social, and insurance factors impact family planning for all persons. Even with U.S. Affordable Care Act, mandating appropriate medically based counseling and options. and at least one form of birth control covered without cost-sharing does not occur. Clearly, both political and legislative factors can either assure or threaten access and choice.

SUMMARY

Long-acting reversible contraception represents a state-of-the-art, first-line contraceptive option for AYAs. The low failure rates, ease of use, safety, and limited contraindications make LARCs an ideal form of contraception for AYAs. Understanding the consent process, body autonomy, and the right to access top-tier contraceptive methods makes LARCs an essential option for healthy sexuality and attaining reproductive justice. Clinicians are in a unique position to promote and provide access to LARCs with confidence for AYAs. Ongoing research will continue to provide new evidence on the duration of effectiveness of LARCs.

REFERENCES

1. Martinez GM, Abma JC. Sexual activity and contraceptive use among teenagers aged 15–19 in the United States, 2015–2017. *NCHS Data Brief*. 2020;(366):1–8. Accessed May 14, 2020. https://www.cdc.gov/nchs/data/databriefs/db366-h.pdf
2. Kavanaugh ML, Jerman J. Contraceptive method use in the United States: trends and characteristics between 2008, 2012 and 2014. *Contraception*. 2018;97(1):14–21.
3. Logan RG, Thompson EL, Vamos CA, et al. Is long acting reversible contraceptive use increasing? Assessing trends among U.S. college women, 2008–2013. *Matern Child Health J*. 2018;22(11):1639–1646.
4. Walsh-Buhi ER, Helmy HL. Trends in long-acting reversible contraption (LARC) use, LARC use predictors, and dual-method use among a national sample of college women. *J Am Coll Health*. 2018;66(4):225–236.
5. Ihongbe TO, Masho SW. Changes in the use of long-acting reversible contraceptive method among U.S. nulliparous women: results from the 2006–2010, 2011–2013, and 2013–2015 National Survey of Family Growth. *J Women's Health (Larchmt)*. 2018;27(3):245–252.
6. Kramer RD, Higgins JA, Godecker AL, et al. Racial and ethnic differences in patterns of long-acting reversible contraceptive use in the United States, 2011–2015. *Contraception*. 2018;97(5):399–404.
7. Coles CB, Shubkibn CD. Effective, recommended, underutilized: a review of the literature on barriers to adolescent usage of long-acting reversible contraceptive methods. *Curr Opin Pediatr*. 2018;30(5):683–688.
8. ACOG committee opinion no 735: adolescents and long-acting reversible contraception: implants and intrauterine devices. *Obstet Gynecol*. 2018;131(5):e130–e139. DOI: 10.1097/AOG.0000000000002632. PMID: 29683910.
9. Sherin M, Waters J. Long-acting reversible contraceptives for adolescent females: a review of current best practices. *Curr Opin Pediatr*. 2019;31(5):675–682.
10. McNicholas C, Swor E, Wan L, et al. Prolonged use of the etonogestrel implant and levonorgestrel intrauterine device: 2 years beyond Food and Drug Administration–approved duration. *Am J Obstet Gynecol*. 2017;216(6):586.e1–586.e6.
11. Dean G, Schwarz EB. Intrauterine devices (IUDs). In: Hatcher RA, Trussell J, Nelson AL, et al., eds. *Contraceptive Technology*. 21st ed. Managing Contraception LLC; 2018:161–194.
12. Nelson AL, Crabtree Sokol D, Grentzer J. Contraceptive implants In: Hatcher RA, Trussell J, Nelson AL, et al., eds. *Contraceptive Technology*. 21st ed. Managing Contraception LLC; 2018:130–156.
13. Heinemann K, Reed S, Moehner S, et al. Comparative contraceptive effectiveness of levonorgestrel-releasing and copper intrauterine devices: the European Active Surveillance Study for Intrauterine Devices. *Contraception*. 2015;91(4):280–283.
14. Wu JP, Pickle S. Extended use of the intrauterine device: a literature review and recommendations for clinical practice. *Contraception*. 2014;89(6):495–503.
15. Goldstuck ND, Cheung TS. The efficacy of intrauterine devices for emergency contraception and beyond: a systematic review update. *Int J Womens Health*. 2019;11:471–479.
16. Turok DK, Gero A, Simmon RG, et al. Levonorgestrel vs. copper intrauterine devices for emergency contraception. *N Engl J Med*. 2021;384(4):335–344.
17. Bornstein M, Carter M, Zapata L, et al. Access to long-acting reversible contraception among US publicly funded health centers. *Contraception*. 2018;97(5):405–410.
18. Duncan R, Paterson H, Anderson L, et al. "We're kidding ourselves if we say that contraception is accessible": a qualitative study of general practitioners attitudes towards adolescents' use of long-acting reversible contraceptives (LARC). *J Primary Health Care*. 2019;11(2):138–145.
19. Norris AH, Pritt NM, Berlan ED. Can pediatricians provide long-acting reversible contraception? *J Pediatr Adolesc Gynecol*. 2019;32(1):39–43.
20. Davis SA, Braykov NP, Lathrop E, et al. Familiarity with long-acting reversible contraceptives among obstetrics and gynecology, family medicine, and pediatrics residents: results of a 2015 National Survey and Implications for Contraceptive Provision for Adolescents. *J Pediatr Adolesc Gynecol*. 2018;31(1):40–44.
21. Ailigne CA, Phelps R, VanScott JL, et al. Impact of the Rochester LARC initiative on adolescents' utilization of long-acting reversible contraception. *Am J Obstet Gynecol*. 2020;222(4S):S890.e1–S890.e6.
22. Rehring SMA, Reifler LM, Seidel JH, et al. Implementation of recommendations for long-acting contraception among women aged 13 to 18 years in primary care. *Acad Pediatr*. 2019;19(5):572–580.
23. Brittain AW, Tevendale HD, Mueller T, et al. The teen access and quality initiative: improving adolescent reproductive health best practices in publically funded health center. *J Community Health*. 2020;45(3):615–625.
24. Onyewuchi UF, Tomaszewski K, Upadhya KK, et al. Improving LARC access for urban adolescents and young adults in the pediatric primary care setting. *Clin Pediatr*. 2019;58(1):24–33.
25. Espey E, Yoder K, Hofler L. Barriers and solutions to improve adolescent intrauterine device access. *J Pediatr Adolesc Gynecol*. 2019;32(5S):S7–S13.
26. Summit AK, Friedman E, Stein TB, et al. Integration of onsite long-acting reversible contraceptive services into school-based health centers. *J Sch Health*. 2019;89(3):226–231.
27. Hanson RTB, Arora KS. Consenting to invasive contraceptives: an ethical analysis of adolescent decision-making for long-acting reversible contraception. *J Med Ethics*. 2018;44(9):585–588.
28. Richards M, Teal SB, Sheeder J. Risk of luteal phase pregnancy with any-cycle-day initiation of subdermal contraceptive implants. *Contraception*. 2017;95(4):364–370.
29. Morgan IA, Zapata LB, Curtis KM, et al. Health care providers' attitudes about the safety of "Quick-Start" initiation of long-acting reversible contraception for adolescents. *J Pediatr Adolesc Gynecol*. 2019;32(4):402–408.
30. Winner B, Peipert JF, Zhao Q, et al. Effectiveness of long-acting reversible contraception. *N Engl J Med* 2012;366(12):1998–2007.
31. Hubacher D, Spector H, Monteith C, et al. Not seeking yet trying long-acting reversible contraception: a 24-month randomized trial on continuation, unintended pregnancy and satisfaction. *Contraception*. 2018;97(6):524–532.
32. Hindy JR, Souaid T, Larus CT, et al. Nexplanon migration into a subsegmental branch of the pulmonary artery: a case report and review of the literature. *Medicine*. 2020;99(4):e18881.
33. Cohen R, Teal SB. Chapter 5. Implantable contraception. Speroff & Darney's Clinical Guide to Contraception. 2019. Accessed 29 May, 2020. https://books.google.com/books?id=2Pi7DwAAQBAJ&pg=PT183&lpg=PT183&dq=cohen+R+Speroff+and+Darney%27s+clinical+guide+to+contraception&source=bl&ots=xrSbht2AX-&sig=ACfU3U1AkDS0cs8QeiWy5CSt4ijdzLtg8g&hl=en&sa=X&ved=2ahUKEwjKg bDk6NnpAhWElHIEHYMIBdQQ6AEwA3oECAkQAQ#v=onepage&q=cohen%20R-%20Speroff%20and%20Darney's%20clinical%20guide%20to%20contraception&f=false
34. Neary M, Chappell CA, Scarsi KK, et al. Effect of patient genetics on etonogestrel pharmacokinetics when combined with efavirenz or nevirapine ART. *J Antimicrob Chemother*. 2019;74(10):3003–3010.
35. Brooks JP, Edwards DJ, Blithe DL, et al. Effects of combined oral contraceptives, depot medroxyprogesterone acetate and the levonorgestrel-releasing intrauterine system on the vaginal biome. *Contraception*. 2017;95(4):405–413.
36. Mendoza RM, Garbers S, Lin S, et al. Chlamydia infection among adolescent long-acting reversible contraceptive and shorter-acting hormonal contraceptive users receiving services at New York City school-based health centers. *J Pediatr Adolesc Gynecol*. 2020;33(1):53–57.
37. El Ayadi AM, Rocca CH, Kohn JE, et al. The impact of an IUD and implant intervention on dual method use among young women: results from a cluster randomized trial. *Prev Med*. 2017;94:1–6.
38. Kortsmit K, Williams L, Pazol K, et al. Condom use with long-acting reversible contraception vs non-long-acting reversible contraception hormonal methods among post-partum adolescents. *JAMA Pediatr*. 2019;173(7):663–670.
39. FSRH Clinical Effectiveness Unit. *Problematic Bleeding With Hormonal Contraception*. FSRH; 2015. Accessed 28 May, 2020. www.fsrh.org/standards-and-guidance/documents/ceuguidanceproblematicbleedinghormonalcontraception

ADDITIONAL RESOURCES AND WEBSITES

Additional Resources and Websites for Clinicians:

UCSF Intrauterine Devices & Implants: A Guide to Reimbursement—https://larcprogram.ucsf.edu/coding

IX

American Sexual Health Association—http://www.ashasexualhealth.org/understanding-larc/

The American College of Obstetricians and Gynecologists—https://www.acog.org/programs/long-acting-reversible-contraception-larc

Contraceptive Technology—http://www.contraceptivetechnology.org/reproductive-health-resources/

Centers for Disease Control and Prevention Reproductive Health—https://www.cdc.gov/reproductivehealth/contraception/mmwr/mec/summary.html

Reproductive Health Access Project—https://www.reproductiveaccess.org/

Additional Resources and Websites for Parents/Caregivers and Adolescents and Young Adults:

Reproductive Health Access Project—https://www.reproductiveaccess.org/

Bedsiders—https://www.bedsider.org/methods

Society for Adolescent Health and Medicine: Sexual and Reproductive Health Resources for Adolescents and Young adults—https://www.adolescenthealth.org/Resources/Clinical-Care-Resources/Sexual-Reproductive-Health/Sexual-Reproductive-Health-Resources-For-Adolesc.aspx

Planned Parethood—https://www.plannedparenthood.org/learn/birth-control

PART XII

Other Reproductive System and Breast Disorders

50

Gynecologic Examination of the Adolescent and Young Adult

Sarah Pitts
Merrill Weitzel

KEY WORDS
- Gynecologic examination
- Pap test

INTRODUCTION

A gynecologic examination is an essential component of the health care of patients with female genitalia and reproductive organs from birth onward. Reassuring and educating patients about their external anatomy is as important as addressing the concerns and needs of an adolescent or young adult in advance of the first internal gynecologic examination. This chapter reviews the indications for such an examination as well as the necessary aspects of the history and steps of the physical examination that should be taken when conducting a gynecologic examination.

INDICATIONS FOR GYNECOLOGIC EXAMINATIONS

Indications

The indications for a complete or modified gynecologic examination vary and should be guided by patient complaint. A 13-year-old presenting for a physical examination can be reassured that external structures appear healthy. A never sexually active 15-year-old with complaint of white vaginal discharge should be evaluated by obtaining a sample to differentiate physiologic discharge from candidal vaginitis. In contrast, a sexually active 18-year-old with lower abdominal pain and vaginal discharge deserves a complete pelvic examination (Table 50.1).

Clinicians should separate the provision of contraceptive services from gynecologic examinations. A gynecologic examination should not be a barrier to the provision of hormonal contraceptives unless a patient is requesting an intrauterine device (IUD). Patients

TABLE 50.1

Indication for a Modified or Complete Internal Pelvic Examination
Symptoms of vaginal or uterine infection
Menstrual disorders including amenorrhea, dysfunctional uterine bleeding, severe dysmenorrhea, or mild to moderate dysmenorrhea unresponsive to therapy
Undiagnosed lower abdominal pain
Sexual assault (modified to collect the appropriate information and samples)
Suspected pelvic mass
Cervical cancer screening
Request by the adolescent or young adult

and parents/caregivers should also be informed that a gynecologic examination and Papanicolaou test (Pap test) are not the same.[1] Indications for a modified or complete internal pelvic examination vary and are not limited to cervical cancer screening. While external genital examination is routine from birth onward, indications for an internal examination can include symptoms of a vaginal or uterine infection, menstrual disorders, pelvic pain, sexual assault, suspected pelvic mass, cervical cancer screening, or by request of a patient. Finally, a gynecologic examination should be deferred if the patient is resistant or uncomfortable, of if the examination is in conflict with a patient's cultural or religious beliefs.

Cervical Cancer Screening

Cervical cancer screening[2,3] or a Pap test assesses cellular changes of the cervix that may put a patient at risk for cancer. Chapter 55 provides a detailed review of Pap tests including current screening and management recommendations.

Sexually Transmitted Infection Screening

Screening for sexually transmitted infections (STIs)[4] should be conducted once a patient has had a sexual experience, including genital to genital or mouth to genital contact, penetrative vaginal contact (digital, penile, or foreign body), penetrative anal contact, or at a patient's request. While urine-based screening tests for *Chlamydia trachomatis* and/or *Neisseria gonorrhoeae* exist, nucleic acid amplification testing (NAAT) of a vaginal swab is more sensitive.[5] Without a genital complaint, asymptomatic sexually active adolescent and young adult (AYA) females under the age of 25 years do not require an internal gynecologic examination, but a thorough external examination is highly recommended. Screening urine or a vaginal swab for *C. trachomatis*, and also for *N. gonorrhoeae* depending on the local prevalence, is recommended annually in asymptomatic sexually active patients.[5]

OBTAINING THE HISTORY

Building rapport and developing a trusting relationship with the adolescent or young adult prior to examination are important. In order to reduce patient anxiety, it is essential that the office setting be comfortable and friendly.[6] Creating an environment in which private and confidential matters can be discussed without judgment and with reassurance and privacy is of the utmost importance. This may require a special waiting area for AYAs, evening clinic hours, and age-appropriate reading materials. Front desk staff, clinical assistants, nurses, and clinicians should be trained to address confidentiality and the unique psychosocial needs of AYAs. While parents/caregivers are welcome and often essential in providing key pieces of history or support during gynecologic examinations, a separate time and space to interview the patient privately and to answer questions is essential. Confidentiality and its limits, including electronic documentation, must be addressed early in all clinical encounters with patients and parents/caregivers (see Chapter 4)[7-9] to encourage more open communication and better care.

The history should include a gynecologic assessment, general health history, review of systems, and information on risk behaviors. The HEEADSSS or SSHADESS screening framework, as is outlined in Chapter 4, are useful tools. Answers to these questions must be obtained confidentially. Some adolescents, and even some young adults, may feel more comfortable if most of the history is obtained with a parent/caregivers in the room. A few moments of privacy are all that is needed to obtain pertinent positives and negatives about risk behaviors, safety, gender and sexual identity, sexual activity, and prior trauma, and to address any concerns a patient may have that they are more comfortable sharing privately. It is not uncommon for AYAs to feel uncomfortable discussing such topics. Acknowledging this and normalizing questions or concerns about sexual health can put a young person at ease and facilitate the discussion. Should a patient be questioning their gender identity or experiencing gender dysphoria, it is important to know in advance of any discussions about body parts and function. Similarly, knowing that a patient has previously experienced sexual trauma will inform the approach to the gynecologic examination.

It is essential to know what the patient's reason is for the visit and whether there is any expectation, on their part, for a gynecologic examination. If possible, doing this early on in the history can help to allay fears and put the patient at ease if such an examination is not warranted. It is also important to gauge a patient's comfort level with discussing their sexual and menstrual history, as well as their understanding of menstrual periods, sexuality, and genital hygiene. Providing proper education during the interview and normalizing the patient's questions and concerns help build rapport. Establishing a trusting relationship in which a patient feels heard and validated makes the gynecologic examination more comfortable.

It is not uncommon for a patient presenting with one apparent goal of care to report a gynecologic concern later in the encounter or to be in denial of an important gynecologic need. Therefore, the sexual history should be part of a structured line of questioning preceded by the statement, "I routinely ask all my patients these screening questions." Complete gynecologic histories should include the following:

1. Menstrual history—age at menarche and date of last menstrual period; duration of menses and interval between periods or intermenstrual staining, number of pads or tampons changed in a day to assess amount of flow; dysmenorrhea—severity on 10-point scale and extent of missed school, work, or activities; premenstrual symptoms
2. History of vaginal discharge—characteristics and associated symptoms
3. Sexual history—type of sexual contact, consensual versus coerced, number of partners, sex of partners, age at first sexual intercourse; contraceptive methods used, preferences and fertility goals; prior STIs; prior pregnancies
4. Prior Pap test screening—any difficulties with the examination or abnormalities found through testing
5. Family history—any history of uterine abnormalities or gynecologic cancers

GYNECOLOGIC EXAMINATION

An external genital examination should be part of an annual examination for all patients and, indeed, should be offered to every patient. Some patients may decline or defer such an examination to a future visit; such requests should be honored and documented.

For patients who consent, they should be made to feel comfortable and in control with the ability to pause the examination at any point, to ask questions, or, if need be, to stop the examination entirely. A handheld mirror to permit viewing of the genitalia may be helpful and educational for some patients. For a first internal gynecologic examination, the clinician should acknowledge that some patients feel nervous. Explaining that the examination takes only 2 or 3 minutes to perform, discussing the specifics of what to expect, and assuring the patient that the examiner will stop the examination at any point per patient's request can be helpful and reassuring.

Before the examination begins, patients should be given the choice of whether to have a support person in the room during the examination. If a patient declines such support, it is recommended that the steps of the examination be described to them and to their guardian before the guardian leaves the room, insuring that everyone knows what to expect. Some clinical settings require the presence of a trained medical chaperone for sensitive examinations, while others defer to patient preference. If the presence of a chaperone is required by policy, this should be discussed in advance with the patient. It is important to know the chaperone policy in your place of work, and to document in your note whether or not a chaperone or support person was present or declined by the patient.

Having the appropriate gynecologic equipment readily accessible is essential (Table 50.2). Before the patient changes into a gown, indicate the reasons why the gynecologic examination is important for evaluating the chief complaint. It is also good to talk about ways in which the patient might relax and feel in control. The use of imagery, deep breathing, and other relaxation techniques may be helpful for the anxious patient. Patients should also be reassured that adequate drapes will be used to maintain privacy during the examination. Before the examination begins, it is helpful to review the main steps in the examination. Each step will then be explained again as the actual examination is performed.

The steps are as follows for the gynecologic examination:
1. Make sure that the patient has an empty bladder before the examination.
2. Ask the patient to undress privately from the waist down and place a sheet over their lap. If additional examinations are to be performed at the same time, such as a breast examination, then the patient would need to undress completely and wear a gown.

TABLE 50.2

Gynecologic Examination Equipment

Examination table with ankle supports
Gowns, sheets
Light source (speculum light or lamp)
Specula: Metal—Pederson or Huffman or plastic (medium and small)
Chlamydia trachomatis and *Neisseria gonorrhoeae* screening tests (e.g., NAATs for urine, vagina, or cervix)
Cotton swabs
Tubes or slides for wet mounts
10% KOH and saline for wet mounts
pH paper
Spatula and cytobrush (or cytobroom) for Pap test
Pap kits for ThinPrep or other Pap systems
Water-soluble lubricating jelly
Warm water source
Nonsterile gloves
Handheld mirror (use is optional and up to the patient)
Tissues
Tampons and sanitary napkins
Rapid pregnancy test kits
Microscope or access to a laboratory for specimen review

KOH, potassium hydroxide; NAATs, nucleic acid amplification testing.

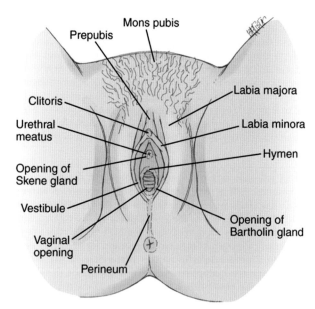

FIGURE 50.1 External genitalia of the pubertal female. (From Weber JR. *Nurse's Handbook of Health Assessment.* 8th ed. Lippincott Williams & Wilkins; 2013.)

3. Cover the patient to the waist with the sheet while the patient lies supine on the examination table, feet resting on the ankle supports. Instruct the patient to bend their knees and slide their buttocks to the end of the table toward their feet. Elevating the head of the table 30 degrees is optional; it can provide the patient with an increased sense of control as it allows improved eye contact with the clinician.

4. Ask the patient to relax their knees to your hands which are held out at either side. Do not pry their legs apart.

5. The sheet should be adjusted so that eye contact is maintained with the patient, the patient's legs are still covered, and the perineum is adequately visualized.

6. Inspect the external genitalia (Fig. 50.1).
   a. Note pubic hair distribution and sexual maturity rating.
   b. Inform the patient before touching the thighs, and then again before grasping each labia lightly between forefinger and thumb and retracting gently in a downward angle, separating the labia to examine the external structures.
   c. Assess for signs of erythema, inflammation, nevi, warts, or other lesions over the perineum, thighs, mons, labia, and perianal region. Check the size of the clitoris, which is typically 2 to 4 mm wide. The Skene glands are two small glands located just inside the urethra and are usually not visible. Bartholin glands are the two small mucus-secreting glands located just outside the hymeneal ring at the 5 and 7 o'clock positions and should not be enlarged, red, or tender.
   d. The hymen should be carefully inspected for estrogen effect (light pink, thickened), for congenital anomalies (septate, imperforate, microperforate), and for transections that might result from consensual or nonconsensual sexual intercourse. With gentle retraction, the anterior vagina may be visible and estrogen effect can be observed—pink mucosa, white vaginal secretions.
   e. Obtaining samples: For patients who have never been sexually active but who need wet mounts to evaluate vaginal discharge, saline-moistened or dry cotton-tipped applicators can be inserted intravaginally to obtain samples without the use of a speculum. Routine NAAT testing in an asymptomatic patient using a vaginal swab can be obtained similarly.

7. Speculum examination: The correct size of speculum should be selected, and metal speculum should be warmed, if possible, before insertion. Depending on the Pap test system used, it may or may not be fine to use a lubricant on the speculum, but warm water is always safe to use. If the hymenal opening is small, a Huffman–Graves pediatric speculum (5/8 inches × 3¾ inches) is used to visualize the cervix. For the sexually active patient, a medium Pederson speculum (1 inches × 4 inches) or a medium Graves speculum (1.5 inches × 4 inches) is often appropriate (Fig. 50.2). A small or medium plastic speculum with an attached light source is also useful for facilitating the examination. For a given patient, the clinician must decide if it would be beneficial and educational to show the patient the speculum prior to use or if it would induce unnecessary fear. A one-finger, gloved (water-moistened) examination performed first may make subsequent speculum insertion and finding of the cervix easier. To avoid surprising the patient during the speculum examination, touch the speculum to the thigh first and tell the patient that you are going to place the speculum into the vagina. The speculum should be inserted posteriorly in a downward direction to avoid the urethra (Fig. 50.3).
   a. Observe the vaginal walls for signs of estrogenization (i.e., pink rather than red epithelium with normal appearing vaginal discharge), inflammation, adherent discharge, or lesions.
   b. Inspect the cervix: The stratified squamous epithelium of the external os is usually a dull pink color. There is often a more erythematous area of columnar epithelium surrounding the cervical os, called a *cervical ectropion*. The junction between the two types of mucosa is called the *squamocolumnar junction*, and it is particularly important that this area be sampled during the Pap test screening. This ectropion may persist throughout the adolescent years, especially in hormonal contraceptive users. Mucopurulent discharge from the cervix characterizes cervicitis, typical of infections with *N. gonorrhoeae*, *C. trachomatis*, and herpes virus. Small, pinpoint hemorrhagic spots on the cervix, so-called "strawberry" cervix, can occur rarely with *Trichomonas vaginalis* infections. The cervix should be examined for any lesions or polyps. Any abnormal growth on the cervix should be referred for further evaluation and colposcopy.
   c. To assess signs and symptoms of vaginitis, swabs for wet mounts and pH can be obtained from the vagina and then rolled in one or two drops of saline on one slide (for *Trichomonas vaginalis*, white cells, or "clue cells") and in one drop of 10% potassium hydroxide (KOH) (for pseudohyphae) on another slide. Roll a swab on a small piece of pH paper and compare the resultant color to the indicator provided with the paper to determine the vaginal pH. Normal vaginal pH is 4.5.[10]
   d. If indicated, obtain a Pap test of the cervix. This should include at least a 360-degree rotation of the spatula in contact with the cervix, with care taken to sample the "transition zone" or squamocolumnar junction. Nylon cytobrushes are also commonly used in addition to the spatula, thereby ensuring the collection of cells from the endocervical canal.
   e. Tests for STIs: Tests for *N. gonorrhoeae* and/or *C. trachomatis* include NAATs, DNA probes, immunoassays, and cultures and may involve cervical or vaginal swabs. See Chapters 61 and 62 for details regarding recommended testing.
   f. Remove the speculum being careful not to pinch the vaginal side walls.
   g. Bimanual examination (Fig. 50.4): The bimanual vaginal–abdominal examination involves the insertion of one or two gloved, lubricated fingers into the vagina while the other hand is placed on the abdomen. If this is a patient's first bimanual examination, it is worthwhile having the patient practice relaxing their abdominal muscles first. Remind the

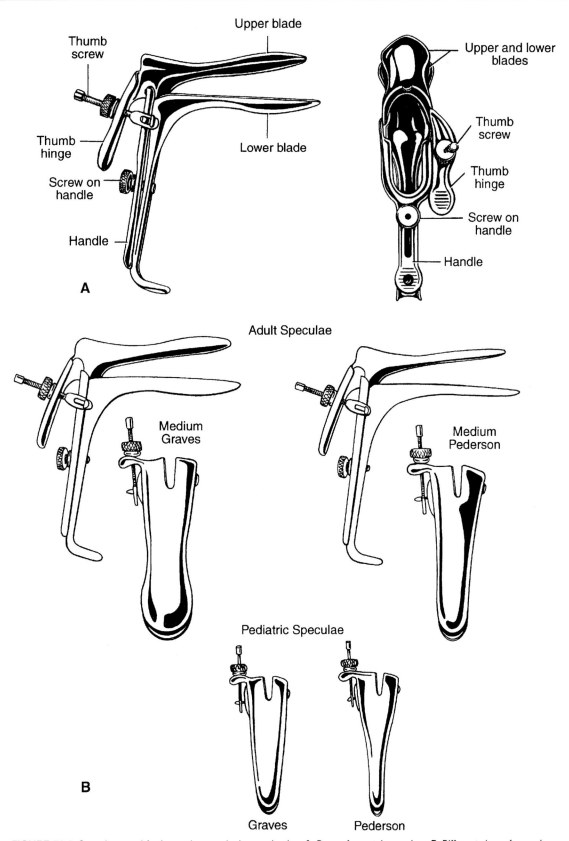

FIGURE 50.2 Speculum used for internal gynecologic examination. **A:** Parts of a metal speculum. **B:** Different sizes of speculuae: Adult speculuae (*top*) and Pediatric speculae (*bottom*). (From Beckmann CRB, Frank W, Swith RP, et al. *Obstetrics and Gynecology*. 5th ed. Lippincott Williams & Wilkins; 2006.)

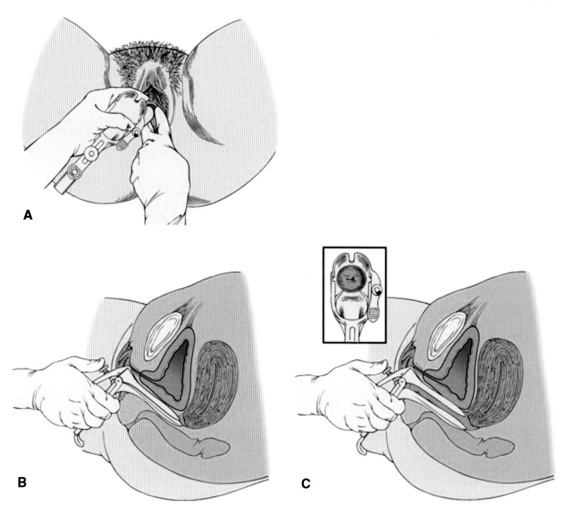

FIGURE 50.3 Insertion of speculum. **A:** With gloved hands, separate the labia and insert the blades of the speculum at a slight angle (10 to 4 o'clock or 2 to 8 o'clock) into the introitus. **B:** Insert the blades of the speculum fully with a slightly downward angle of insertion. **C:** Slowly open the blades of the speculum using the thumb hinge until the cervix is visualized. Depending on the rotation of the uterus, the position of the blades may need to be adjusted internally to see the cervix clearly. (From Weber JR. *Nurse's Handbook of Health Assessment.* 8th ed. Lippincott Williams & Wilkins; 2013.)

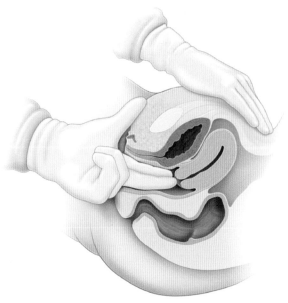

FIGURE 50.4 Bimanual examination. (From Gibbs RS, Karlan BY, Haney AF, et al. *Danforth's Obstetrics and Gynecology.* 10th ed. Lippincott Williams & Wilkins; 2008.)

patient that you will be examining the uterus and ovaries and ask the patient to communicate any feelings of discomfort experienced during the examination.

h. Palpation of the vagina and cervix: Check for masses along the side walls and posterior cul-de-sac, and on the cervix and any tenderness with cervical motion.

i. Palpation of the uterus: Assess the size, the position of the uterus, and any masses or tenderness. Pushing backward on the cervix causes the uterus to move anteriorly, allowing for its palpation with the abdominal hand.

j. Gently explore the posterior fornix and the rectouterine pouch (pouch of Douglas) for masses, fullness, and tenderness.

k. Palpation of the adnexa: Assess for any masses, tenderness, or abnormalities of the ovaries or the adnexal area. To palpate these structures, insert the examining fingers into each lateral fornix, positioning them slightly posteriorly and high. Sweep the abdominal examining hand downward over the internal fingers. Normal ovaries are usually <3 cm long and are rubbery.

l. If there is a history of significant pelvic pain or an adnexal mass is felt, a rectovaginal–abdominal examination can help complete the evaluation of the adnexa or uterus and the rectum, anus, and posterior cul-de-sac. A rectovaginal–abdominal examination is performed with the index finger in the vagina, the middle finger in the rectum, and the other hand on the abdomen. The examination permits evaluation of the uterosacral ligaments and cul-de-sac as well as the mobility of the uterus. It is important to inform the patient that she may experience an urge to defecate, but she will not. The rectovaginal septum should be thin and pliable, and the pelvic floor should be free of masses and tenderness. On indication, stool retrieved can be tested for occult blood.

8. At the completion of the examination, if no abnormalities are found, letting the patient know that they are "healthy" can provide immediate peace-of-mind. Refrain from use of the word "normal" to summarize the gynecologic examination, as such language can be upsetting for some individuals, especially those with gender dysphoria.

9. At the conclusion of the examination, some patients may require assistance sliding up the table before taking their feet out of the ankle supports. Offer the patient tissues to remove any lubrication or secretions from the perineum (to use once the examiner leaves the room). Instruct the patient to dress fully and explain that you will provide privacy to do so. The patient should be in a seated position and draped when the clinician leaves the examining room. Explain that you will return to discuss the clinical findings when they are dressed. If curtains are available, pull the curtain prior to opening the door and exiting the examination room.

During the postexamination discussion, the importance of the findings of the examination (positive or negative) should be discussed in relation to the chief complaint. All questions should be answered, and any therapies or further tests required should be outlined. This is an important time for discussion of the patient's concerns about normal anatomy and physiology, contraception (including emergency contraception), and sexuality. During this discussion, it is important for the examiner to listen carefully, remembering that patients may not communicate all their concerns initially. At the conclusion of the discussion, the parent, guardian, or partner can (with the consent of the patient) be invited to join the clinician and the patient, if they were not already present. Only with the patient's consent should results of the examination and the treatment plan be discussed with another individual. Maintaining confidentiality is essential to preserving the clinician–patient relationship. Parents should be encouraged to ask questions and to voice concerns.

SUMMARY

Helping AYAs through their gynecologic visit sets the stage for reproductive health care throughout life. The gynecologic visit is an ideal opportunity to provide education, listen to concerns, assess medical and psychosocial complaints, and promote a healthy future. The gynecologic examination allows the clinician an opportunity to impart a positive attitude about the body and to stress the importance of health maintenance.

REFERENCES

1. Qin J, Saraiya M, Martinez G, et al. Prevalence of potentially unnecessary bimanual pelvic examinations and Papanicolaou tests among adolescent girls and young women aged 15–20 years in the United States. *JAMA Intern Med.* 2020;180(2):274.
2. U.S. Preventive Services Task Force, Curry SJ, Krist AH, et al. Screening for cervical cancer: U.S. Preventive Services Task Force Recommendation Statement. *JAMA.* 2018;320(7):674–686.
3. Fontham ETH, Wolf AMD, Church TR, et al. Cervical cancer screening for individuals at average risk: 2020 guideline update from the American Cancer Society. *CA Cancer J Clin.* 2020;70(5):321.
4. Barrow RY, Ahmed F, Bolan GA, et al. Recommendations for providing quality sexually transmitted diseases clinical services, 2020. *MMWR Recomm Rep.* 2020; 68(RR-5):1. Accessed February 15, 2021. https://www.cdc.gov/mmwr/volumes/68/rr/rr6805a1.htm
5. Gannon-Loew KE, Holland-Hall C. A review of current guidelines and research on the management of sexually transmitted infections in adolescents and young adults. *Ther Adv Infect Dis.* 2020;7:2049936120960664.
6. American College of Obstetricians and Gynecologists' Committee on Adolescent Health Care. The initial reproductive health visit: ACOG Committee Opinion, Number 811. *Obstet Gynecol.* 2020;136(4):e70.
7. Ford C, English A, Sigman G. Confidential health care for adolescents: position paper of the society for adolescent medicine. *J Adolesc Health.* 2004;35:160.
8. Lewis Gilbert A, McCord AL, Ouyang F, et al. Characteristics associated with confidential consultation for adolescents in primary care. *J Pediatr.* 2018;199:79.
9. Confidentiality in adolescent health care: ACOG Committee Opinion, Number 803. *Obstet Gynecol.* 2020;135(4):e171.
10. Lin YP, Chen WC, Cheng CM, Shen CJ. Vaginal pH Value for Clinical Diagnosis and Treatment of Common Vaginitis. *Diagnostics (Basel).* 2021;11(11):1996. PMC8618584.

📶 ADDITIONAL RESOURCES AND WEBSITES

Additional Resources and Websites for Clinicians:
The American College of Obstetricians and Gynecologists: The Utility of and Indications for Routine Pelvic Examination—https://www.acog.org/clinical/clinical-guidance/committee-opinion/articles/2018/10/the-utility-of-and-indications-for-routine-pelvic-examination
Centers for Disease Control and Prevention: Bimanual Pelvic Exams and Pap Tests among Girls and Young Women—https://www.cdc.gov/cancer/dcpc/research/articles/pelvic-exams-pap-tests.htm

Additional Resources and Websites for Parents/Caregivers:
American Sexual Health Association: Sexual Health Care—https://www.ashasexualhealth.org/sexual-health-care/
The Center for Young Women's Health: Abnormal Pap Tests—https://youngwomenshealth.org/2010/06/10/abnormal-pap-test/
The Center for Young Women's Health: Your First Pelvic Exam—https://youngwomenshealth.org/2013/08/22/pelvic-exam/
Nemours KidsHealth: Female Reproductive System—https://teenshealth.org/en/parents/female-reproductive-system.html?WT.ac=ctg#catbody-basics

Additional Resources and Websites for Adolescents and Young Adults:
American Sexual Health Association: Sexual Health Care—https://www.ashasexualhealth.org/sexual-health-care/
The Center for Young Women's Health: Abnormal Pap Tests—https://youngwomenshealth.org/2010/06/10/abnormal-pap-test/
The Center for Young Women's Health: Your First Pelvic Exam—https://youngwomenshealth.org/2013/08/22/pelvic-exam/
Nemours TeensHealth: Gyn Checkups—https://teenshealth.org/en/teens/obgyn.html?WT.ac=ctg#catgirls
Nemours TeensHealth: Pelvic Exams—https://teenshealth.org/en/teens/pelvic-exams.html#catgirls

XII

CHAPTER

51

Normal Menstrual Physiology

Sari L. Kives
Niamh C. Murphy

KEY WORDS

- Menarche
- Menstruation
- Ovulation
- Puberty

INTRODUCTION

This chapter reviews the normal physiology of the menstrual cycle. The subsequent chapters will discuss common menstrual abnormalities in adolescents and young adults (AYAs).

The initiation of the menstrual cycle is dependent on maturation of the hypothalamic–pituitary–ovarian (HPO) axis which occurs during puberty. This involves a coordinated sequence of events, beginning with the hypothalamic secretion of gonadotropin-releasing hormone (GnRH). In response to GnRH, the pituitary secretes follicle-stimulating hormone (FSH) and luteinizing hormone (LH), and the ovaries secrete estrogen, progesterone, activin, and inhibins.[1] The endometrium of the uterus responds to estrogen and progesterone by initiating endometrial growth and differentiation. In the absence of fertilization, this process culminates in menses.[2]

The first sign of puberty is often an acceleration in growth, followed by thelarche (breast buds), pubarche (development of pubic hair), and finally menarche (the onset of menses).[3] The median age of menarche in developed countries in well-nourished populations has remained relatively stable (between 12 and 13 years) over the past 30 years[4] with the exception being among the non-Hispanic Black population, which has an earlier median age at menarche.[5] In the United States, the median age of menarche is 12.43 years with a mean cycle interval of 32.2 days in the first year.[4] Menarche occurs approximately 2.3 years after thelarche, with anovulatory cycles ranging from 55% to 82% in the first year.[6] Menarche is generally followed by approximately 5 to 7 years of increasing regularity as the cycles shorten to reach the usual reproductive pattern.[3]

The exact trigger of menarche is unknown. It is well understood that both inhibitory and excitatory neurotransmitters, as well as peptides, modulate the activity of the HPO axis. The axis is inactive from late infancy continuing through childhood secondary to central inhibitory mechanisms suppressing GnRH secretion, and to a lesser extent the high sensitivity to low levels of gonadal steroid feedback. At gonadarche, the HPO axis is reactivated in response to metabolic signals from the periphery. Follicle-stimulating hormone and LH levels rise followed by a gradual increase in estrogen concentrations, which stimulates breast development. The increase in pulsatile LH secretion occurs first at night, during sleep, but gradually extends throughout the day. At midpuberty, estrogen production increases sufficiently to stimulate endometrial proliferation, ultimately resulting in menarche.[3] Although controversial, there is

some evidence to suggest that menarche may be associated with achieving a critical body weight of 46 to 47 kg and a minimum body fat level of 17. The maintenance or restoration of menstruation is thought to require a minimum of 21% body fat.[7]

DEFINITION OF MENSTRUAL CYCLE

The duration of a menstrual cycle is from the first day of one menstrual period to the first day of the next period. A typical menstrual cycle has fluctuating levels of pituitary hormones (FSH and LH), stimulating ovarian follicular, ovulatory, and luteal phases, with concurrent growth and differentiation of the endometrium (proliferative and secretory phases) (Fig. 51.1).[8]

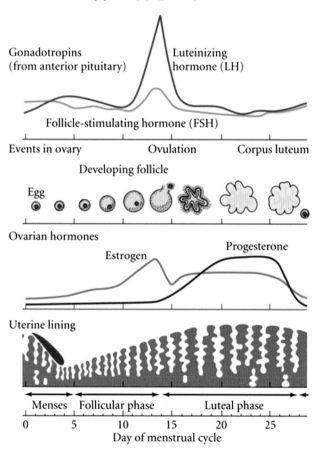

FIGURE 51.1 Normal menstrual cycle. (From Gilbert SF. *Developmental Biology.* 10th ed. Sinauer; 2013, with permission.)

Gonadotropin-releasing hormone is secreted in a pulsatile fashion by a specialized network of hypothalamic neurons termed "the GnRH pulse generator." Gonadotropin-releasing hormone stimulates both LH and FSH synthesis and pulsatile secretion by pituitary gonadotropes.[9] At the beginning of the menstrual cycle, low levels of estrogen initiate positive feedback on hypothalamic GnRH to stimulate pituitary secretion of FSH and LH. At higher levels, estrogen and progesterone provide negative feedback and suppress FSH and LH, thereby preventing further follicular recruitment. Neurotransmitters (e.g., dopamine, norepinephrine) and endorphins (opioids) also play a role in modulating GnRH secretion.[10] Menstrual irregularities that occur with weight loss, stress, exercise, and medications may be secondary to the effect of these entities on the hypothalamus.[11]

The menstrual cycle is best understood by reviewing these three descriptive phases—the follicular phase, the ovulatory phase, and the luteal phase.

Follicular Phase

The duration of the follicular phase is the major determinant of cycle length, usually lasting 14 days (range 7 to 22 days). This phase begins with the onset of menses and ends with ovulation.

1. The corpus luteum from the previous cycle involutes, resulting in decreasing levels of estrogen and progesterone. The low levels stimulate the hypothalamic release of GnRH, which increases the pituitary release of FSH and LH.
2. Follicle-stimulating hormone stimulates the recruitment of ovarian follicles.
3. Luteinizing hormone stimulates ovarian theca cells to produce androgens, which are then converted to estrogens in the ovarian granulosa cells under the influence of FSH. Estrogens (including estradiol) increase FSH binding to granulosa cell receptors, leading to amplification of the FSH effect, allowing one follicle to predominate. Although the gonadotropins act synergistically, FSH primarily affects follicular growth and LH mainly stimulates ovarian steroid biosynthesis.
4. Estradiol drives the proliferative phase of the endometrium and increases the production of growth factors that stimulate proliferation within the glandular and stromal compartments of the endometrium. The height of the endometrium increases from approximately 1 mm at menstruation to 5 mm at ovulation. Estradiol upregulates the number of estrogen and progesterone receptors in endometrial cells.
5. In response to rising estradiol levels in the middle and late follicular phase, FSH release begins to fall.[10]

Ovulatory Phase

The ovulatory phase occurs midcycle, around 2 weeks or so before menstruation starts.

1. An estrogen surge triggers the midcycle LH surge, which induces ovulation approximately 10 to 16 hours later. This is measured as estradiol. An estradiol level ≥200 pg/mL for at least 2 days is needed to induce ovulation. A small preovulatory rise in progesterone is required to induce the FSH surge.
2. A mature follicle releases an oocyte and becomes a functioning corpus luteum.

Luteal Phase

The luteal phase begins with ovulation and ends with the menstrual flow. This phase is more constant, lasting approximately 14 ± 2 days, reflecting the life of the corpus luteum.

1. The corpus luteum produces large amounts of progesterone, as well as increased levels of estrogen, in the form of estradiol. Granulosa cells utilize low-density lipoprotein cholesterol as a substrate for progesterone synthesis. A serum progesterone level >3 ng/mL is presumptive evidence of ovulation. Rising levels of estrogen and progesterone lead to falling levels of FSH and LH.
2. Progesterone antagonizes the action of estrogen by reducing estrogen receptor sites and increasing conversion of estradiol to estrone, a less potent estrogen. Progesterone halts the growth of the endometrium and stimulates differentiation into a secretory endometrium preparing for implantation. Increased tortuosity of the glands and spiraling of the blood vessels histologically characterize the secretory endometrium.
3. Local progesterone suppresses follicular development in the ipsilateral ovary, so that ovulation in the following month may occur in the contralateral ovary.
4. The cervical mucus becomes thick during the luteal phase due to the influence of progesterone.
5. Unless there is fertilization with subsequent production of human chorionic gonadotropin, the corpus luteum involutes after approximately 10 to 12 days. Sloughing of the endometrium occurs secondary to the loss of estrogen and progesterone. Local prostaglandins cause vasoconstriction and uterine contractions.
6. The decreased levels of estrogen and progesterone lead to increased levels of FSH and LH, which provides the positive feedback loop required to initiate another menstrual cycle.

SUMMARY

Menarche is the onset of menses and commencement of cyclic hormonal changes. Normal menstrual cycles require an orchestrated sequence of events to occur between the hypothalamus, pituitary, ovaries, and the endometrium. Abnormal menstrual cycles are not uncommon and require appropriate clinical assessment and evaluation to determine the specific etiology.

ACKNOWLEDGMENTS

This chapter is based on Normal Menstrual Physiology from the 6th Edition authored by Sari L. Kives and Nicole Hubner.

REFERENCES

1. Critchley HOD, Maybin JA, Armstrong GM, et al. Physiology of the endometrium and regulation of menstruation. *Physiol Rev*. 2020;100(3):1149–1179.
2. Berga SL, Johnston-MacAnanny EB. Physiology of the menstrual cycle. In: Bieber EJ, Horowitz IR, Sanfilippo JS, et al., eds. *Clinical Gynecology*. 2nd ed. Cambridge University Press; 2015. 972–984.
3. Taylor HS, Pal L, Seli E, eds. *Speroff's Clinical Gynecologic Endocrinology and Infertility*. 8th ed. Wolters Kluwer Health/Lippincott Williams & Wilkins; 2019.
4. American College of Obstetricians and Gynecologists. Menstruation in girls and adolescents: using the menstrual cycle as a vital sign. Committee Opinion No. 651. *Obstet Gynecol*. 2015;126:e43–46.
5. Al-Sahab B, Ardern CI, Hamadeh MJ, et al. Age at menarche in Canada: results from the National Longitudinal Survey of Children & Youth. *BMC Public Health*. 2010;10(1):736.
6. Emans SJ, Laufer MR, DiVasta A. Emans, Laufer, *Goldstein's Pediatric & Adolescent Gynecology*. 7th ed. Lippincott Williams & Wilkins; 2019.
7. Traboulsi S, Itani L, Tannir H, et al. Is body fat percentage a good predictor of menstrual recovery in females with anorexia nervosa after weight restoration? A systematic review and exploratory and selective meta-analysis. *J Popul Ther Clin Pharmacol*. 2019;26(2):e25–e37.
8. Gilbert SF. *Developmental Biology*. 10th ed. Sinauer Sunderland; 2013.
9. McCartney CR, Gingrich MB, Hu Y, et al. Hypothalamic regulation of cyclic ovulation: evidence that the increase in gonadotropin-releasing hormone pulse frequency during the follicular phase reflects the gradual loss of the restraining effects of progesterone. *J Clin Endocrinol Metab*. 2002;87(5):2194–2200.
10. Neinstein LS. Menstrual problems in adolescents. *Med Clin North Am*. 1990; 74(5):1181–1203.
11. Gordon CM, Ackerman KE, Berga SL, et al. Functional hypothalamic amenorrhea: An Endocrine Society Clinical Practice Guideline. *J Clin Endocrinol Metab*. 2017;102(5):1413–1439.

ADDITIONAL RESOURCES AND WEBSITES

Additional Resources and Websites for Clinicians:
American College of Obstetricians and Gynecologists. Menstruation in girls and adolescents: using the menstrual cycle as a vital sign. Committee Opinion No. 651. *Obstet Gynecol*. 2015;126:e43–e46.
Taylor HS, Pal L, Seli E. *Speroff's Clinical Gynecologic Endocrinology and Infertility*. 8th ed. Wolters Kluwer Health/Lippincott Williams & Wilkins; 2019.

XII

Traboulsi S, Itani L, Tannir H, et al. Is body fat percentage a good predictor of menstrual recovery in females with anorexia nervosa after weight restoration? A systematic review and exploratory and selective meta-analysis. *J Popul Ther Clin Pharmacol.* 2019;26(2):e25–e37.

https://www.uptodate.com/contents/physiology-of-the-normal-menstrual-cycle

Wang YX, Arvizu M, Rich-Edwards JW, et al. Menstrual cycle regularity and length across the reproductive lifespan and risk of premature mortality: prospective cohort study. *BMJ.* 2020;371:m3464.

Additional Resources and Websites for Parents/Caregivers:

AboutKidsHeatlh—Menstruation—https://www.aboutkidshealth.ca/Article?contentid=299&language=English#:~:text=Most%20girls%20get%20their%20period,are%20in%20their%20mid%20teens

Advice for moms: talking to your daughter about menstruation—https://www.thechildren.com/health-info/conditions-and-illnesses/advice-moms-talking-your-daughter-about-menstruation

All about periods—https://kidshealth.org/en/teens/menstruation.html

Menstruation—https://www.aboutkidshealth.ca/article?contentid=299&language=english

Preparing your child for menstruation—https://www.mayoclinic.org/healthy-lifestyle/tween-and-teen-health/in-depth/menstruation/art-20046004

Talking to your child about periods—https://kidshealth.org/en/parents/talk-about-menstruation.html

AboutKidsHeatlh—Menstruation—https://www.aboutkidshealth.ca/Article?contentid=299&language=English#:~:text=Most%20girls%20get%20their%20period,are%20in%20their%20mid%20teens

Additional Resources and Websites for Adolescents and Young Adults:

All about periods—https://kidshealth.org/en/teens/menstruation.html

Menstruation—https://www.aboutkidshealth.ca/article?contentid=299&language=english

Ovulation and the menstrual cycle—https://www.youtube.com/watch?v=WGJsrGmWeKE

When will I get my first period—https://helloclue.com/articles/life-stages/when-will-i-get-my-first-period

Why do women have periods—https://www.youtube.com/watch?v=cjbgZwgdY7Q

52 Dysmenorrhea and Premenstrual Disorders

Paula K. Braverman

KEY WORDS

- Drospirenone
- Dysmenorrhea
- Endometriosis
- Leukotriene
- Nonsteroidal anti-inflammatory drug
- Premenstrual disorders
- Premenstrual dysphoric disorder
- Premenstrual syndrome
- Prostaglandin

INTRODUCTION

Female adolescents and young adults (AYAs) commonly experience menstrual dysfunction. Both dysmenorrhea and premenstrual disorders (PMDs) (premenstrual syndrome [PMS] and premenstrual dysphoric disorder [PMDD]) affect females to some extent during their lifetime. Research into the etiology of these menstrual disorders has led to improved therapies. Experts have also been moving toward consensus opinion for the diagnosis of PMD in order to facilitate clinical diagnosis and research into therapeutic options. This chapter reviews the epidemiology, etiology, clinical presentation, diagnosis, and treatment options currently available for these menstrual disorders.

DYSMENORRHEA

The term "primary dysmenorrhea" refers to pain associated with the menstrual flow, with no evidence of pelvic pathology. "Secondary dysmenorrhea" refers to pain associated with menses secondary to organic disease such as endometriosis or outflow-tract obstruction.[1,2]

Etiology

Prostaglandins and Leukotrienes

The decline in stabilizing progesterone levels during the late luteal phase of ovulatory cycles results in the release of phospholipase A2 and subsequent cascade of prostaglandin and leukotriene (LT) production. Phospholipids from cell membranes are converted by phospholipase A2 into arachidonic acid, the fatty acid precursor for prostaglandin synthesis in the secretory endometrium. Prostaglandin E_2 (PGE$_2$) and prostaglandin F2α (PGF$_2\alpha$), which are formed through the cyclooxygenase pathway, are the key prostaglandins involved in dysmenorrhea. Prostaglandin F$_2\alpha$ induces myometrial contractions, vasoconstriction, and ischemia and mediates pain sensation. Higher PGF$_2\alpha$ levels are correlated with higher intensity of pain. Prostaglandin E$_2$ is associated with platelet disaggregation and, based on receptor interactions, can cause either myometrial contraction or relaxation as well as vasoconstriction or vasodilation. There are two enzymes in the cyclooxygenase system. The COX-1 enzyme has homeostatic functions including gastrointestinal mucosal integrity, renal and platelet function, and vascular hemostasis. COX-2 is induced by inflammation. The upregulation of COX-2 expression and subsequent production of prostaglandin has also been shown to be present in secondary dysmenorrhea caused by endometriosis.[1–3]

Leukotrienes, which mediate the inflammatory response and cause vasoconstriction, are produced from arachidonic acid through the lipoxygenase pathway. Leukotriene receptors are present in uterine tissue.[1–3]

It has been noted that[1–3]:

1. Locally, prostaglandins cause uterine contractions, but are also associated with systemic symptoms including headache, nausea, vomiting, bloating, backache, diarrhea, dizziness, and fatigue.
2. Exogenous administration of PGE$_2$ and PGF$_2\alpha$ produce myometrial contractions and pain, similar to dysmenorrhea, as well as gastrointestinal symptoms.
3. Patients with dysmenorrhea have higher levels of prostaglandins in the menstrual fluid and higher levels of LT C$_4$ and D$_4$ (two types of LT).
4. There is correlation between the timing of peak pain levels (24 to 48 hours postonset of menses) and the highest levels of prostaglandins.
5. Prostaglandin inhibitors decrease dysmenorrhea.

In summary, this evidence supports the hypothesis that primary dysmenorrhea is related to prostaglandins and LTs released in the uterus during ovulatory menstrual cycles and consistent with the observation that primary dysmenorrhea is not usually present in early anovulatory cycles after menarche.[2,3]

Dysmenorrhea is one of the central sensitivity pain syndromes in which there is hypersensitivity to pain. Messages from reproductive organs impact pain perception through neuron excitability in somatovisceral convergent neurons in the spinal cord. It has also been postulated that females with dysmenorrhea may be more sensitive to prostaglandins with PGF$_2\alpha$ sensitizing nerve receptors thereby lowering the pain perception threshold.[1–4]

Other Factors

Risk factors for dysmenorrhea include age (<30 years), low body mass index (BMI), earlier menarche (<12 years), longer cycles, heavy menstrual flow, positive family history, and psychological symptoms. Having a live birth and use of oral contraceptives are inversely associated with dysmenorrhea. Evidence is inconsistent for cigarette smoking, diet, obesity, depression, and abuse and dysmenorrhea.[5]

Epidemiology

Dysmenorrhea is a significant cause of lost work and school hours in female AYAs. Various studies worldwide have shown the following[4–6]:

1. Prevalence: 16% to 91% of reproductive age females have some degree of dysmenorrhea with higher rates of primary dysmenorrhea and lower rates of secondary dysmenorrhea in adolescents versus older females.
2. A review of worldwide studies among 41,140 AYA females published between 2010 and 2015 found:
   a. Prevalence: 34% to 94%
   b. Severe pain: 0.9% to 59.8%
   c. Associated morbidities: Missed school 7.7% to 57.8%; missed social activities: 21.5%
   d. Other activities affected: Sports and sleep disturbance
3. Approximately 10% to 50% of females lose work or school days due to dysmenorrhea, which has socioeconomic impact.

Many AYA females do not report dysmenorrhea symptoms to a clinician.

1. Review of worldwide studies found that less than 50% of AYAs consulted with a clinician. Medical advice was sought by less than 15% in most studies and less than 5% in several studies.[6]
2. Many adolescents use nonpharmacologic self-treatment (rest, heat, exercise, massage, special food or drink, attempts at distraction) and insufficient doses of over-the-counter medications.[4,6–8]

Clinical Manifestations

Primary Dysmenorrhea

Primary dysmenorrhea is associated with the establishment of ovulatory cycles and usually begins within 6 to 12 months of menarche but may occur up to 2 to 3 years later. Although the pain usually begins within a few hours of starting menses, it may also start several days before the onset of menses. Local symptoms include pain that is crampy and episodic in nature in the lower abdomen with radiation to the back and upper thighs. In most cases, the pain resolves within 24 to 48 hours but sometimes the symptoms may persist further into the menstrual cycle. Associated systemic symptoms can include nausea, vomiting, fatigue, mood change, dizziness, diarrhea, backache, headache, and sleep disturbances.[1,2,8,9]

Secondary Dysmenorrhea

Pelvic pathology associated with secondary dysmenorrhea include endometriosis, anatomical abnormalities, pelvic inflammatory disease, benign uterine tumors (fibroids), adenomyosis, cervical stenosis, pelvic adhesions, ovarian cysts, uterine polyps, and pregnancy complications (miscarriage, ectopic pregnancy).[1–3,7,8]

1. **Endometriosis** (Fig. 52.1) is characterized by the presence of endometrial glands and stroma outside of the uterus with implants located in various locations throughout the pelvis. It is the most common cause of secondary dysmenorrhea, as well as the most common pathologic condition in adolescents with chronic pelvic pain. Endometriosis is a progressive disease which can adversely impact future fertility and increases in severity over time. The estimated prevalence is 4% to 17% in postmenarchal females with definitive diagnosis by laparoscopy in at least two-thirds of adolescents being evaluated for dysmenorrhea or chronic pelvic pain not responsive to combined hormonal contraceptives and nonsteroidal anti-inflammatory drugs (NSAIDs).[3,8–10]

   The symptoms of endometriosis in adolescents include chronic pelvic pain, which may be cyclic or acyclic; acyclic pain occurs 28% to 90% of the time.[9] This is in contrast to adults who are more likely to have cyclic pain.[10] Other associated symptoms can include dyspareunia, irregular menses, bowel symptoms such as nausea, constipation, diarrhea, pain on defecation, low back pain, and urinary tract symptoms.[9]

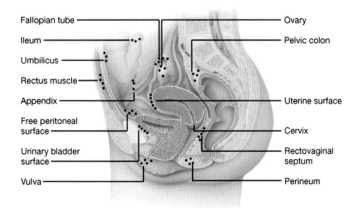

Common sites of endometriosis

FIGURE 52.1 Common sites of endometriosis. (From Endometriosis. In *Lippincott's Nursing Advisor 2012.* Lippincott Williams & Wilkins; 2012.)

On pelvic examination, a tender or nodular cul-de-sac or tender uterosacral ligaments may be found. However, adolescents may not have the classic thickened nodular sacrouterine ligaments and the lesions are difficult to identify on laparoscopy because they have a different appearance (clear or red) than in adults. Endometriosis should be considered in patients with dysmenorrhea who do not respond to a combination of hormonal agents and NSAIDs, as well as those with associated bowel or urinary function symptoms. This diagnosis is also more common when there is a positive family history for endometriosis; there is a high rate of concordance in monozygotic twins. The inheritance is believed to be polygenic and multifactorial.[8–10]

2. **Anatomical abnormalities** include congenital obstructive müllerian malformations and outflow obstruction. Obstructive anomalies enhance retrograde flow and predispose the patient to endometriosis.[10]

Differential Diagnosis

Nongynecologic causes of pelvic pain include gastrointestinal disorders (inflammatory bowel disease, irritable bowel syndrome, constipation, food intolerance), musculoskeletal pain, genitourinary abnormalities (cystitis, interstitial cystitis, calculi), and psychological disorders (history of abuse, mood disorders, somatization).[7,9]

Diagnosis

History

1. **Menstrual history:** Primary dysmenorrhea usually starts 1 to 3 years after menarche while secondary dysmenorrhea should be considered if severe pain starts with the onset of menarche or there are progressively worsening symptoms, abnormal uterine bleeding, acyclic pain, or infertility. Adolescents and young adults should be asked about the degree of pain and the amount of impairment in school, work, and other activities. Any previous use of therapeutic modalities and their effectiveness should be ascertained.[1,7–9]
2. **Other history:** Additional questions should include prior sexually transmitted infections (STIs); sexual activity and dyspareunia; renal or other congenital anomalies; a family history of endometriosis; a review of systems related to the gastrointestinal, genitourinary, and musculoskeletal systems; a psychosocial history to assess stress, mood disorders, and sexual violence; and an assessment of cultural and parent/caregiver modeling regarding menses potentially impacting the reporting or perception of pain. Significant acyclic pain, particularly gastrointestinal and urinary symptoms, raises concern for nongynecologic causes of pain.[1,7–9]

Physical Examination

The clinician should do a pelvic examination for evidence of endometriosis, endometritis, fibroids, uterine or cervical abnormalities, or adnexal masses and tenderness. However, if the teen or young adult is not sexually active and the history is typical for dysmenorrhea, a pelvic examination is indicated only if the symptoms do not respond to standard medical therapy. Examination limited to a cotton swab inserted into the vagina can help rule out a hymenal abnormality or vaginal septum without performing a speculum examination. The musculoskeletal examination should focus on range of motion of the hips and spine to assess for tenderness and limitation in motion.[1,8,9]

Laboratory Tests, Imaging, Laparoscopy

A complete blood count and a determination of the erythrocyte sedimentation rate should be done if pelvic inflammatory disease or inflammatory bowel disease is suspected. Sexually active AYAs should be tested for STIs and pregnancy. A urinalysis and urine culture will help diagnose urinary tract problems. If a müllerian abnormality is suspected, ultrasonography or magnetic resonance imaging will define the anatomy. These imaging modalities are unlikely to assist in the diagnosis of endometriosis in adolescents since endometriomas are less common and superficial lesions are unlikely to be visualized.

If evaluation of the genitourinary, gastrointestinal, and musculoskeletal systems fails to reveal a cause of the pain, and if the pain is severe and intractable despite adherence to treatment with antiprostaglandins and hormonal contraceptives, laparoscopy should be considered. Laparoscopy also presents the opportunity to establish a definitive diagnosis and potentially treat visible lesions or lyse adhesions.[1,7–9] The American College of Obstetricians and Gynecologists (ACOG) recommends evaluation for secondary dysmenorrhea if there is no clinical improvement within 3 to 6 months of empiric therapy for primary dysmenorrhea.[8]

Therapy

The two most effective treatments for primary dysmenorrhea are NSAIDs and hormonal contraceptives.

Education

The patient should be educated and reassured that the problem is physiologic and can be helped. Studies in adolescents have demonstrated that education is important to address knowledge deficits about available treatment modalities and how to use them most effectively.[1,8,9]

Nonsteroidal Anti-Inflammatory Drugs

Nonsteroidal anti-inflammatory drugs are a primary modality of therapy and have been shown to be more effective than placebo for primary dysmenorrhea.[11] Because much of primary dysmenorrhea is secondary to prostaglandin-mediated uterine hyperactivity, prostaglandin inhibitors can alleviate menstrual cramps and associated systemic symptoms. Randomized controlled trials have demonstrated that NSAIDs are effective in alleviating menstrual cramps; there is insufficient evidence to indicate that any individual NSAID is more effective or safer than others. Potential side effects include gastrointestinal symptoms, nephrotoxicity, hematologic abnormalities, and neurologic symptoms (headache, drowsiness).[2,3,11] Some of these drugs and their typical doses are found in Table 52.1. Use of NSAIDs for short periods, with the indicated doses, usually results in minimal side effects.[2] Gastrointestinal and renal side effects may be averted by taking the medication with food and adequate fluid intake respectively.[8]

Over-the-counter ibuprofen and naproxen are available, but because these over-the-counter medications come in lower doses than the prescription formulations, a larger number of tablets may be needed for effectiveness. The medications should be started

TABLE 52.1

Common Nonsteroidal Anti-Inflammatory Medications Used to Treat Dysmenorrhea

Drug	Initial Dose (mg)	Following Dose (mg)
Ibuprofen	800	400–800 every 8 h
Naproxen	500	250–500 every 12 h
Naproxen sodium	440–550	220–550 every 12 h
Mefenamic acid	500	250 every 6 h

Sources: Ferries-Rowe E, Corey E, Archer JS. Primary dysmenorrhea. *Obstet Gynecol.* 2020; 136:1047–1058; Committee on Adolescent Health Care. Dysmenorrhea and endometriosis in the adolescent. *Obstet Gynecol.* 2018;132:e249–e258.

either as soon as possible when the symptoms of dysmenorrhea occur or to coincide with the first sign of menstruation. Efficacy is increased when NSAIDs are initiated 1 to 2 days before the onset of menses and when a loading dose is used followed by regularly scheduled dosing. Usually, these medications are needed only for 2 to 3 days. A trial of a different prostaglandin inhibitor should be tried if the first one does not provide adequate relief of symptoms.[2,3,7,8]

The NSAIDs in **Table 52.1** inhibit both the COX-1 and COX-2 enzymes. However, selective COX-2 inhibitors will have less gastrointestinal side effects and may also be preferred in patients with coagulation disorders related to platelet function. Because of drug recalls, the only COX-2 inhibitor available at the time of this printing is celecoxib. The dosing is 400 mg as a loading dose, followed by 200 mg every 12 hours.[3] These medications are more expensive, potentially more toxic, and not necessarily superior in efficacy to less expensive, nonselective NSAIDs.[11]

Hormonal Therapies

Hormonal contraceptives are another first-line treatment option and can improve dysmenorrhea symptoms in 70% to 80% of females.[2] If the patient wishes contraception or the pain is severe and not responsive to NSAIDs, hormonal contraceptives can be tried alone or in addition to NSAIDs. The maximal effect may not become apparent for several months.[8]

1. Hormonal contraceptives inhibit ovulation and lead to an atrophic decidualized endometrium, resulting in decreased menstrual flow and prostaglandin and LT release. Hormonal contraceptives are also useful in treating both primary dysmenorrhea and secondary dysmenorrhea from endometriosis.[3,8,9]
2. Options include: Combined oral contraceptive pills (COC), intravaginal ring, contraceptive transdermal patch, single-rod progestin implant, depot medroxyprogesterone acetate, and levonorgestrel intrauterine system (LGN IUS)[1,2,7,8]
3. If cyclic hormonal contraception is ineffective, continuous combination hormonal therapy with extended cycling can be tried. Several extended cycling COC formulations are commercially available and both the ring and patch can be used for extended cycling by skipping the withdrawal week. Extended cycling COCs can have superior pain relief compared to cyclic regimens.[1,7–9]
4. After surgical diagnosis of endometriosis, suppression is recommended. Hormonal treatment options commonly used include continuous low-dose hormonal therapy with COC or the vaginal ring, depot medroxyprogesterone acetate, and the LNG IUS.[7,8,10]

Other Hormonal Modalities

1. Gonadotropin-releasing hormone (GnRH) agonists, with utilization of add-back therapy to prevent side effects related to hypoestrogenic state (including bone loss), have been tried in

severe cases of endometriosis unresponsive to other modalities. Caution should be used in patients younger than 16 years because of concerns about compromised bone mineral accrual.[10]

2. A non–U.S. Food and Drug Administration (FDA) approved regimen of continuous norethindrone acetate (5 mg) has been shown to be equivalent to cyclic COCs in young adult females with dysmenorrhea and dosing of 5 to 10 mg has been used in endometriosis.[8,10]

3. Dienogest is a progestin shown to be noninferior to leuprolide acetate for dysmenorrhea caused by endometriosis.[7]

Other Nonhormonal Modalities

Nonhormonal modalities with possible benefit include high-frequency transcutaneous electrical-nerve stimulation, acupressure, exercise, yoga, and topical heat. Acupuncture requires further study.[2,7,8] A Cochrane Review found low-quality, limited evidence with potential benefits from dietary supplements including vitamin B1, fish oil, zinc sulfate, zataria, valerian, ginger, and fenugreek.[12]

PREMENSTRUAL DISORDERS

The term "premenstrual disorders" is used to describe an array of predictable physical, cognitive, affective, and behavioral symptoms, causing significant functional impairment, that occur cyclically during the luteal phase of the menstrual cycle and resolve with menstruation followed by a symptom-free interval until the next time of ovulation.[13–15] Universal classification of PMD has been evolving, and terminology in the literature includes (PMS and PMDD).[15] Although the majority of females have physiologic premenstrual symptoms, they would not be classified as having PMS or PMDD unless those symptoms negatively influence functioning.[13,16] Although there is a growing literature on PMD in adolescents, most of the research has focused on adult females (with females in their 20s commonly included in discussions of females in older age groups). Reference is made in the text when specific information is being discussed about the adolescent or young adult age group.

Epidemiology

The perceived impact of premenstrual symptoms on activities of daily living (ADLs) does not vary significantly across countries or cultures, and the mental and physical symptoms have equal impact.[17] The exact prevalence of PMD is unknown, in part because of differences in definitions and classification. In general, estimates among AYAs and adult females are similar, but PMDD prevalence may be higher in adolescents.[18–20] The age range for peak intensity of PMD symptoms is the 20s to 30s.[17,18] While mild premenstrual symptoms are common among AYAs and adult females, severe symptoms affecting ADLs occur less frequently.

1. About 80% to 95% of menstruating AYAs and adult females have some degree of symptoms before menses, which in many cases are mild physiologic symptoms not significantly affecting ADLs.[13]

2. About 20% to 40% have moderate to severe symptoms affecting ADLs, which meet criteria for PMS.[13,15,18]

3. About 3% to 8% are most severely affected and meet criteria for PMDD.[13,17,18,20]

Risk Factors

1. Possible genetic factors including gene polymorphisms with an estimated 30% to 80% heritability for premenstrual symptoms[15,16,20,21]

2. Association with traumatic events including sexual abuse[15,20]

3. Comorbidities with psychiatric disorders, including depression and anxiety.[15,18,20] There is a strong association between suicidal cognitions and attempts independent of other psychiatric comorbidities.[20,22]

4. In general, personality disorders are not higher among females with PMDD compared to healthy controls, but some studies have found obsessive compulsive disorder and some personality traits occurring more frequently in females with PMD.[20]

5. Other factors associated with PMS include elevated BMI, metabolic syndrome, and use of nicotine cigarettes.[15]

Pathophysiology

The exact mechanism of PMD is unknown. Current hypotheses revolve around gonadal sex steroids and central neurotransmitters, as well as brain function.[15,19,20,23]

1. Alterations in neurotransmitters such as γ-aminobutyric acid (GABA) and serotonin have been implicated:
   a. Females with PMD are thought to have dysregulated allopregnanolone function. Allopregnanolone is a metabolite of progesterone, which positively modulates GABA—the key inhibitory neurotransmitter regulating anxiety and stress. Studies in females with PMDD have found lower levels of cortical and subcortical GABA and possible reduced GABA functional-receptor sensitivity to allopregnanolone. There is also evidence of a possible paradoxical sensitivity to allopregnanolone in which mood and anxiety symptoms are increased rather than inhibited.
   b. Serotonergic function is altered in the luteal phase of females with PMD. Ovarian sex steroids impact serotonergic activity by modulating serotonin transmission. There is evidence of decreased serotonin binding to the serotonin transporter site and lower density of serotonin receptors in PMDD.

2. Brain function: Neuroimaging studies have demonstrated overlap between brain regions involved in PMDD and other mood disorders (major depressive disorder and anxiety). Increased responses in the limbic system (amygdala) to negative stimuli during the luteal phase are linked to lower reactivity in the inhibitory regions of the cortex (anterior cingulate and prefrontal cortices). This would translate into less cognitive control of emotions and negative mood during the luteal phase including impulsivity and impaired executive function.

3. Hormonal factors: There are no differences in the levels of gonadal hormones. Females with PMD are hypothesized to have altered emotional and cognitive processing responses to physiologic cyclical hormonal fluctuations.

Clinical Manifestations

Symptoms described in literature range from mild symptoms to those severe enough to interfere with normal activities. Data analysis from community-based studies of females from 14 countries found that physical symptoms are most commonly reported. Various emotional and physical symptoms include the following[14]:

a. Emotional symptoms: The most prevalent symptom is irritability, followed by depressed mood, anger, mood swings, restlessness, tension, confusion, social withdrawal, sleep disturbances, poor concentration, lack of energy.

b. Physical symptoms: The most prevalent symptoms include abdominal bloating, cramps or abdominal pain, joint–back–muscle pain, breast tenderness, followed by lack of energy, swelling of extremities, weight gain, changes in appetite/food cravings, and headaches.

Diagnosis

The diagnosis relies on the history of cyclic symptoms. No specific physical findings or laboratory tests have proved useful. Three important findings are usually needed to make a diagnosis of PMD:

1. Symptoms must occur in the luteal phase and resolve within a few days of onset of menstruation. Symptoms should not be present in the follicular phase.

2. The symptoms must be prospectively documented over several menstrual cycles and not caused by other physical or psychological problems.
3. Symptoms must be recurrent and severe enough to disrupt normal activities.

The 2011 International Society for Premenstrual Disorders (ISPMD), a consensus group of international experts, published criteria which divided PMD into *Core PMD* and *Variant PMD*. *Core PMD* fulfills the three findings outlined above and includes PMS and PMDD.[13] Symptoms must be prospectively found in at least two menstrual cycles and cause significant distress or impairment in daily functioning such as work, school, and interpersonal relationships. Unlike the Diagnostic and Statistical Manual of Mental Disorders, Fifth Edition (DSM-5) (which requires 5 of 11 specific somatic or affective symptoms with a minimum of 1 affective symptom) there is no delineation of specific symptoms (somatic or psychological) or criteria for the number of symptoms needed to make the diagnosis. *Variant PMD* includes (1) premenstrual exacerbation of underlying psychological or somatic disorders; (2) symptoms occurring with nonovulatory ovarian activity; (3) progesterone-induced symptoms (use of exogenous progestogens); and (4) PMDs without menstruation (hysterectomy with preservation of ovaries). The *Core PMD* are consistent with criteria previously established by ACOG and the Royal College of Obstetricians and Gynaecologists (RCOG). The 2011 ISPMD criteria have been adopted by the RCOG.[18,24]

The DSM-5 specifically includes criteria for PMDD—the most severe form of PMD. The DSM-5 considers mood lability, irritability, dysphoria, and anxiety to be the essential features while the behavioral and physical symptoms accompany the mood symptoms. This is in contrast to PMS which is less severe and may not present with affective symptoms. Symptoms cannot represent exacerbation of an existing medical condition or psychiatric disorder although those disorders may co-occur with PMDD.[16] Symptoms of certain disorders (e.g., seizures, migraine headaches, irritable bowel syndrome, diabetes, asthma, rheumatologic disorders, depression, anxiety) may also be exacerbated during menstruation.[13,18]

While various validated assessment tools have been developed, the prospectively administered Daily Record of Severity of Problems is among the most commonly used tool.[20] The Visual Analogue Scales for Premenstrual Mood Symptoms and Premenstrual Tension Syndrome Rating Scale are other validated options mentioned in the DSM-5.[16] In general, retrospective assessments are not considered diagnostic, but the Premenstrual Symptoms Screening Tool (PSST) has been shown to be useful for initial screening during clinical consultation. This self-rated retrospective questionnaire has been revised for use in adolescents as an adjunct to prospective daily ratings.[25] Prospective recording should be done for at least 2 to 3 months to document that symptoms are occurring cyclically in the luteal phase.

Therapy

Treatment is directed toward the premenstrual affective and physical symptoms. Antidepressant medications and ovulation suppression are the most systematically studied approaches. Studies have yielded conflicting results with other therapies, and most trials have not been well controlled. Treatments have included lifestyle changes, education, stress management, aerobic exercise, vitamin and mineral supplementation, herbal preparations, dietary manipulation, suppression of ovulation, selective serotonin reuptake inhibitors (SSRIs), and medications to suppress physical and psychological symptoms. The choice of treatment should be guided by symptom severity; previous treatment response; need for contraception or plans for pregnancy; and patient preferences.[15,18–20,24,26–30]

Nonpharmacologic Treatment/Complementary Medicine

To date, the strongest evidence for nonpharmacologic/complementary medicine treatment of PMD exists for calcium, chasteberry, and cognitive behavioral therapy (CBT).[27]

1. Calcium (1,200 mg/day in divided doses) has been reported to reduce physical and emotional symptoms of PMS. Calcium homeostasis fluctuates during the menstrual cycle, and hypocalcemia has been associated with affective changes. Higher intake of vitamin D along with calcium has been associated with a reduced risk of PMD.[15,19,20,24,26,27]
2. *Vitex agnus-castus* (chasteberry) has been found to be superior to placebo in reducing somatic and psychological PMD symptoms with few side effects. Currently there is no standard preparation or dosing that can be recommended.[15,19,20,24,27]
3. Cognitive behavioral therapy works by improving coping strategies and modifying maladaptive thinking. Utilizing CBT appears to result in longer long-term efficacy for PMD symptoms than fluoxetine. The RCOG guideline recommends that CBT should be routinely considered as a treatment option for severe PMS since it could potentially prevent the need for pharmacotherapy.[15,19,20,24,27,29]

Other Nonpharmacologic Therapies/Complementary Medicine

1. Lifestyle changes: Although lifestyle changes have not been definitively proven in controlled studies, exercise and stress management practices can improve overall feelings of well-being and aerobic exercise may reduce mood symptoms and bloating.[18,20,27] Education regarding menstrual physiology and the relationship of changing hormones to symptoms can help with understanding of symptoms and may improve self-management.[18,26]
2. Vitamin and mineral supplementation, herbal preparations, and dietary manipulation: There have been some positive outcomes for complementary and alternative therapies. However, although some show promise, more research needs to be carried out to recommend definitively any of these therapies.
   a. *Ginkgo biloba* (ginkgo leaf extract) and *Crocus sativus* (saffron) were cited as deserving additional evaluation by the ISPMD and noted to have potential benefit by the RCOG.[24,27]
   b. Mood and carbohydrate food craving improved in randomized trials evaluating the intake of simple and complex carbohydrates. Increased intake of complex carbohydrates may increase tryptophan, which is a precursor to serotonin.[15,20,27]
   c. Vitamin E, magnesium, and vitamin B_6 have mixed or equivocal results. Although vitamin B_6 was weakly superior in meta-analyses to placebo, the higher study doses used raise concerns about increased risk of peripheral neuropathy.[15,20,24,27]
   d. Evening primrose oil may have some benefit for females with cyclic breast symptoms.[24]
   e. St. John's wort had mixed results and interactions with other drugs is a concern.[19,24]
   f. Other complementary therapies with possible benefit include acupuncture, Qi therapy, reflexology, massage, yoga, biofeedback, guided imagery, krill oil, lavender oil, Chinese and Japanese herbs, transmagnetic stimulation, sleep deprivation, and light therapy.[19,20,27,29]

Suppression of Ovulation

Because PMD appears to be a cyclic disorder of menses occurring in the luteal phase, suppression of ovulation has been used as a therapy.

1. Combined oral contraceptives: Although COC prevents ovulation, data on their effectiveness are mixed and they primarily impact somatic symptoms. Mood symptoms in some individuals with PMD may actually worsen with use of OCP.[24,27] One pill with the progestogen (drospirenone) is approved by the FDA for the severe symptoms of PMDD. Drospirenone has spironolactone antimineralocorticoid and antiandrogenic

XII

properties. The 24/4 formulation OCP containing drospirenone and 20 mcg of ethinyl estradiol demonstrated improvement in both mood and physical-symptom scores in subjects with PMDD. Possible reasons for efficacy of this new formulation include the lower estrogen dose, as well as improved follicular suppression. The maintenance of a more stable hormonal environment due to the longer number of days on hormone may also be helpful (e.g., 24 rather than 21 days).[15,18,20,26,27,29,30]

2. Continuous hormonal therapy with COC can also be considered to suppress cyclic changes and endogenous sex hormone variability; however, studies have shown mixed results.[15,20,30]

3. High-dose estrogen patch or implant: Suppression of ovulation with high-dose estrogens is effective, but must be accompanied by administration of progestogen to prevent endometrial hyperplasia. Since adding progestogen may make PMD symptoms worse, some clinicians have used the LNG-releasing IUS to deliver progesterone to the endometrium and minimize systemic absorption.[18,20,24,28,27]

4. Gonadotropin-releasing hormone: Most studies have shown benefit from the use of GnRH, but the hypoestrogenic effects with loss of bone density are concerning, especially for adolescents, and therefore limit its use. Gonadotropin-releasing hormone with add-back therapy with estrogen and progesterone can be considered when other modalities have failed. However, add-back regimens may cause a recurrence in PMD symptoms.[15,20,24,26,28,30]

5. Bilateral salpingo-oophorectomy would not be considered in adolescents. If done for severe and debilitating symptoms in an adult female, estrogen replacement would be needed until natural menopause would have occurred.[15,19,20,24,27,28]

Medications to Suppress Symptoms

1. *Prostaglandin inhibitors:* Nonsteroidal anti-inflammatory drugs have been used to treat PMS, particularly for the physical symptoms.[18]

2. *Spironolactone,* an aldosterone receptor agonist, may be helpful in patients with breast tenderness and bloating. Doses of 100 mg/day on day 12 of the menstrual cycle until the onset of menses have been used.[18,24]

Psychotropic Medications (Selective Serotonin Reuptake Inhibitors)

Selective serotonin reuptake inhibitors are the drugs of choice and first-line therapy for severe PMS/PMDD in adult females, including young adult females.[24] Efficacy of SSRIs has been shown in randomized placebo-controlled trials and affirmed in a Cochrane Review.[20,24] Fluoxetine, sertraline, and paroxetine are FDA approved for PMDD, and also escitalopram and the serotonin–norepinephrine reuptake inhibitor venlafaxine have also been shown to be effective.[20,24,29] Placebo-controlled studies in adult females have shown that they are effective for 50% to 90% of patients and can improve both physical symptoms and mood.[18,27] Unlike in adults, fluoxetine is not considered first-line therapy for adolescents with PMDD, and there are a paucity of studies in this age group. Further, none of the three SSRIs approved for PMDD are approved for this purpose in the adolescent age group although they could be used in young adult females.[18,26]

1. Selective serotonin reuptake inhibitors used intermittently only during the luteal phase (i.e., 14 days before onset of menses) rather than continuously are equally effective for symptom reduction.[20,24,29] Recent studies have also have demonstrated some success with symptom-onset dosing by taking the SSRI a few days before or with the onset of symptoms and stopping with the onset or a few days after menses start.[19,20,28,30]

2. Unlike treatment for depression, symptoms improve within 48 hours of initiating therapy, and there are no reports of discontinuation symptoms when SSRIs are used intermittently for PMDD.[19,20,30]

TABLE 52.2

Doses of FDA-Approved SSRIs for Premenstrual Dysphoric Disorder

Name of Drug	Dose (mg)
Fluoxetine	20
Sertraline	50–150
Paroxetine CR	12.5–25

Source: Lanza di Scalea T, Pearlstein T. Premenstrual dysphoric disorder. *Psychiatr Clin North Am.* 2017;40:201–216.

3. Low doses are usually effective (**Table 52.2**), although higher doses may be more effective with intermittent dosing.[19]

4. Selective serotonin reuptake inhibitors are usually well tolerated. The most common adverse effects include nausea, somnolence, fatigue, decreased libido, and sweating.[24] Other side effects include dizziness, insomnia, anorgasmia, and gastrointestinal disturbances.[19,29]

Anxiolytics and Other Antidepressants

These medications are second-line therapies that may be useful if there is anxiety and irritability as primary PMD symptoms.[19] Suggested therapies have included benzodiazepines (especially alprazolam), clomipramine, and buspirone. In general, other antidepressants are less effective than SSRIs and studies have had mixed results.[19,20,29] None of these medications would be recommended for routine use in adolescents.

Approach to Treatment of Premenstrual Disorders

Choice of treatment modalities may vary by the age of the patient and severity of symptoms. Several approaches have been outlined by various organizations.

1. The ISPMD consensus statement recommends[28]:
   a. Selective serotonin reuptake inhibitors as first-line treatment
   b. Cognitive behavioral therapy should be routinely considered.
   c. Other treatment options: One or more of the following—COCs, noncontraceptive estrogen preparations, and GnRH analogues
   d. Oral contraceptive pills are recommended for mild to moderate PMD.
   e. Gonadotropin-releasing hormone is reserved for severe cases without improvement on SSRIs.
   f. Evaluation of symptoms while on GnRH analogues should precede bilateral salpingo-oophorectomy.

2. The RCOG recommends the following algorithm[24]:
   a. First line: Exercise, CBT, vitamin B6, COC with drospirenone, continuous or luteal phase SSRI
   b. Second line: Estradiol patches (100 µg) + micronized progesterone (oral or vaginal) or LNG IUS (52 mg)
   c. Third line: Gonadotropin-releasing hormone analogues and add-back hormone replacement therapy (continuous combined estrogen and progesterone)
   d. Fourth line: Surgical treatment ± hormone replacement therapy

3. The following are recommendations for AYAs based on Rapkin[18,19] and Allen[26]:
   a. Adolescents should complete prospective charting; receive education on the menstrual cycle and PMD; and, be informed about supportive therapy including dietary changes, stress reduction, aerobic exercise, CBT, calcium supplements, and possibly chasteberry fruit.

b. A drospirenone containing OCP could be considered first line for hormonal suppression, while high-dose transdermal estrogen along with a progestin can be considered as a first- or second-line choice.

c. When mood symptoms predominate, SSRI therapy is first line in young adult females. In adolescents, although not necessarily first choice, SSRIs can be used with careful monitoring.

d. Gonadotropin-releasing hormone agonists are considered third-line therapy after other steps have failed.

e. Hysterectomy and bilateral oophorectomy would be a choice of last resort and not considered in adolescents.

SUMMARY

Dysmenorrhea and PMD are commonly seen in AYAs. Primary dysmenorrhea presents with the establishment of ovulatory cycles and is caused by production of prostaglandins and LTs. The majority of AYAs will have excellent response to NSAIDs with or without hormonal contraception. Severe symptoms which do not respond to medical therapy require evaluation for secondary amenorrhea with consideration for endometriosis and obstructing genital-tract anomalies. Premenstrual symptoms occur in the majority of AYAs, but a PMD diagnosis requires severity that impacts daily activities. Guidance for diagnosis can be found in the ISPMD consensus guidelines and DSM-5 criteria for PMDD. Research is ongoing regarding the pathophysiology of PMD but current hypotheses include altered responses to normal cyclic hormonal changes and involvement of the neurotransmitters serotonin and GABA. First-line treatment in adults are SSRIs (intermittently or continuously) and/or the drospirenone containing COC. Selective serotonin reuptake inhibitors can be used cautiously in adolescents. Other modalities with the most evidence are CBT, calcium, and chasteberry. Gonadotropin-releasing hormone suppression is considered third-line therapy after exhausting other options while hysterectomy and bilateral oophorectomy is a last resort for adults, but not considered in adolescents.

REFERENCES

1. Rome E, Haines LJ. Dysmenorrhea and premenstrual syndrome. In: Emans SJ, Laufer MR, DiVasta AD, eds. *Pediatric & Adolescent Gynecology.*7th ed. Wolters Kluwer; 2020:466–477.
2. Ferries-Rowe E, Corey E, Archer JS. Primary dysmenorrhea. *Obstet Gynecol.* 2020;136:1047–1058.
3. Harel Z. Dysmenorrhea in adolescents and young adults: an update on pharmacological treatments and management strategies. *Expert Opin Pharmacother.* 2012;13(15):2157–2170.
4. Iacovides S, Avidon I, Baker FC. What we know about primary dysmenorrhea today: a critical review. *Hum Reprod Update.* 2015;21(6):762–778.
5. Latthe PM, Champaneria R. Dysmenorrhea. *BMJ Clin Evidence* 2014;10:813.
6. DeSanctis V, Soliman AT, Elsedfy H, et al. Dysmenorrhea in adolescents and young adults: a review in different countries. *Acta Biomed.* 2016;87:233–246.
7. Burnett M, Lemyre M. No. 345-primary dysmenorrhea consensus guideline. *J Obstet Gynaecol Can.* 2017;39(7):585–595.
8. Committee on Adolescent Health Care. ACOG Committee Opinion No. 760: Dysmenorrhea and endometriosis in the adolescent. *Obstet Gynecol* 2018;132(6):e249–e258.
9. Sachedina A, Todd N. Dysmenorrhea, endometriosis, and chronic pelvic pain in adolescents. *J Clin Res Pediatr Endocrinol.* 2020;12(Suppl 1):7–17.
10. Laufer MR. Gynecologic pain: chronic pelvic pain and endometriosis. In: Emans SJ, Laufer MR, DiVasta AD, eds. *Pediatric & Adolescent Gynecology.* 7th ed. Wolters Kluwer; 2020:489–516.
11. Marjoribanks J, Ayeleke RO, Farquhar C, et al. Nonsteroidal anti-inflammatory drugs for dysmenorrhea. *Cochrane Database Syst Rev.* 2015;7:CD001751.
12. Pattanittum P, Kunyanone N, Brown J, et al. Dietary supplements for dysmenorrhea. *Cochrane Database Syst Rev.* 2016;3(3):CD002124.
13. O'Brien PMS, Backstrom T, Brown C, et al. Towards a consensus on diagnostic criteria, measurement and trial design of the premenstrual disorders: the ISPMD Montreal consensus. *Arch Womens Ment Health.* 2011;14(1):13–21.
14. Dennerstein L, Lehert P, Heinemann K. Global study of women's experiences of premenstrual symptoms and their effects on daily life. *Menopause Int.* 2011;17(3):88–95.
15. Yonkers KA, Simoni MK. Premenstrual disorders. *Am J Obstet Gynecol.* 2018;218:68–74. https://doi.org/10.1016/j.ajog.2017.05.045
16. American Psychiatric Association. *Diagnostic and Statistical Manual of Mental Disorders, DSM-5.* 5th ed. American Psychiatric Publishing; 2013.
17. Dennerstein L, Lehert P, Heinemann K. Epidemiology of premenstrual symptoms and disorders. *Menopause Int.* 2012; 18(2):48–51.
18. Rapkin AJ, Mikacich JA. Premenstrual dysphoric disorder and severe premenstrual syndrome in adolescents. *Pediatr Drugs.* 2013;15(3):191–202.
19. Rapkin AJ, Lewis EI. Treatment of premenstrual dysphoric disorder. *Women's Health.* 2013;9:537–556.
20. Di Scalea TL, Pearlstein T. Premenstrual dysphoric disorder. *Psychiatr Clin N Am.* 2017;40:201–216.
21. McEvoy K, Osborne LM, Nanavati J, et al. Reproductive affective disorders: a review of the genetic evidence for premenstrual dysphoric disorder and postpartum depression. *Curr Psychiatry Rep.* 2017;19(12):94. doi:10.1007/s11920-017-0852-0
22. Osborn E, Brooks J, O'Brien PMS, et al. Suicidality in women with premenstrual dysphoric disorder: a systematic literature review. *Arch Womens Ment Health.* 2020;24(2):173–184. doi:10.1007/s00737-020-01054-8
23. Dubol M, Epperson CN, Lanzenberger R, et al. Neuroimaging premenstrual dysphoric disorder: a systematic and critical review. *Front Neuroendocrinol.* 2020; 57:100838. doi:10.1016/j.yfrne.2020.100838
24. Green LJ, O'Brien PMS, Panay N, Craig M on behalf of the Royal College of Obstetricians and Gynaecologists. Management of premenstrual syndrome. *BJOG.* 2017; 124:e73–e105.
25. Steiner M, Peer M, Palova E, et al. The premenstrual symptoms screening tool revised for adolescents (PSST-A): prevalence of severe PMS and premenstrual dysphoric disorder in adolescents. *Arch Womens Ment Health.* 2011;14(1):77–81.
26. Allen LM, Lam ACN. Premenstrual syndrome and dysmenorrhea in adolescents. *Adolesc Med State Art Rev.* 2013;23(1):139–163.
27. Nevatte T, O'Brien PMS, Backstrom T, et al. ISPMD consensus on the management of premenstrual disorders. *Arch Womens Ment Health.* 2013;16(4):279–291.
28. Ismaili E, Walsh S, O'Brien PMS, et al. Fourth consensus of the International Society for Premenstrual Disorders (ISPMD): auditable standards for diagnosis and management of premenstrual disorder. *Arch Womens Ment Health.* 2016;19(6):953–958.
29. Sepede G, Sarchione F, Matarazzo I, et al. Premenstrual dysphoric disorder without comorbid psychiatric conditions: a systematic review of therapeutic options. *Clin Neuropharmacol.* 2016; 39(5):241–261.
30. Carlini SV, Deligiannidis KM. Evidence-base treatment of premenstrual dysphoric disorder: a concise review. *J Clin Psychiatry.* 2020;81(2):19ac13071. doi:10.4088/JCP.19ac13071

ADDITIONAL RESOURCES AND WEBSITES

Additional Resources and Websites for Clinicians:
American College of Obstetricians and Gynecologists—https://www.acog.org/clinical
https://www.acog.org/clinical/clinical-guidance/committee-opinion/articles/2018/12/dysmenorrhea-and-endometriosis-in-the-adolescent
https://www.acog.org/clinical/journals-and-publications/clinical-updates/2017/09/mood-and-anxiety-disorders
American Psychiatric Association: Diagnostic and Statistical Manual of Mental Disorders (DSM-5)
International Society for Premenstrual Disorders—https://iapmd.org/provider-resources
North American Society for Pediatric and Adolescent Gynecology—https://www.naspag.org/naspag-clinical-recommendations
Royal College of Obstetricians and Gynecologists guideline on PMS—https://www.rcog.org.uk/en/guidelines-research-services/guidelines/gtg48/

Additional Resources and Websites for Parents/Caregivers:
American Academy of Pediatrics—https://www.healthychildren.org/English/health-issues/conditions/genitourinary-tract/Pages/Menstrual-Disorders.aspx
American College of Obstetricians and Gynecologists—https://www.acog.org/womens-health
https://www.acog.org/womens-health/resources-for-you#f:topic=[Menstrual%20Health]
https://www.acog.org/womens-health/faqs/endometriosis
https://www.acog.org/womens-health/faqs/premenstrual-syndrome
https://www.acog.org/womens-health/faqs/dysmenorrhea-painful-periods
Boston Children's Hospital—https://youngwomenshealth.org/
International Society for Premenstrual Disorders—https://iapmd.org/toolkit
North American Society for Pediatric and Adolescent Gynecology—https://www.naspag.org/resources-for-patients
Planned Parenthood—https://www.plannedparenthood.org/learn/health-and-wellness/menstruation

Additional Resources and Websites for Adolescents and Young Adults:
American College of Obstetricians and Gynecologists—https://www.acog.org/womens-health
https://www.acog.org/womens-health/resources-for-you#f:topic=[Menstrual%20Health]
https://www.acog.org/womens-health/faqs/endometriosis
https://www.acog.org/womens-health/faqs/premenstrual-syndrome
https://www.acog.org/womens-health/faqs/dysmenorrhea-painful-periods
Boston Children's Hospital—https://youngwomenshealth.org/
International Society for Premenstrual Disorders—https://iapmd.org/toolkit
North American Society for Pediatric and Adolescent Gynecology—https://www.naspag.org/resources-for-patients
Planned Parenthood—https://www.plannedparenthood.org/learn/teens/puberty/whats-periods

Abnormal Uterine Bleeding

Beth I. Schwartz
Laurie A. P. Mitan

KEY WORDS
- Abnormal uterine bleeding
- Anovulatory bleeding
- Breakthrough bleeding
- Heavy menstrual bleeding

INTRODUCTION

Abnormal uterine bleeding (AUB) is a common menstrual problem during adolescence. This term, AUB, describes any menstrual bleeding of irregular frequency, duration, or flow. When severe, it can result in life-threatening anemia. It is usually both a concern and a nuisance for adolescents and young adults even when mild. The International Federation of Gynecology and Obstetrics classifies AUB in nonpregnant females into etiologic categories of polyps, adenomyosis, leiomyoma, malignancy and hyperplasia, coagulopathy, ovulatory dysfunction, endometrial, iatrogenic, and not yet classified; known by the acronym PALM-COIEN.[1,2] This chapter will focus mainly on the COIEN subtypes, with ovulatory dysfunction being the leading cause in adolescents.

Normally, menstrual cycles occur every 21 to 45 days, with 2 to 7 days of bleeding and 20 to 80 mL of blood loss per cycle.[3] Heavy menstrual bleeding (HMB) is excessive menstrual bleeding interfering with physical health or quality of life and has replaced prior terminologies, including menorrhagia and metrorrhagia.[4] Immaturity of the hypothalamic–pituitary–ovarian (HPO) axis is the leading cause of AUB during adolescence. After menarche, anovulation is associated with 50% to 80% of bleeding episodes during the first 2 years, with decreasing rates over time.[3] Excess estrogen can stimulate the endometrium to proliferate in an undifferentiated manner and shed at irregular intervals without adequate progesterone to provide endometrial stabilization. However, despite these high rates of anovulation with HPO axis immaturity, the negative feedback of estrogen on the HPO axis protects most adolescents from HMB. Even when ovulation does not occur, estrogen production usually declines before the endometrium becomes excessively thickened, and withdrawal bleeding occurs. Therefore, most anovulatory cycles tend to be fairly regular, and the bleeding is limited in duration and quantity. Frequently, polycystic ovary syndrome (PCOS), and less commonly late-onset congenital adrenal hyperplasia, present in this age group (see Chapter 54).

EVALUATION

The evaluation of any patient with bleeding begins with an assessment of hemodynamic stability.

Health providers obtain a detailed history of present illness, past medical history, and family medical history from the patient and, if possible, the parent/caregiver. However, clinicians must be careful to obtain the sexual and reproductive health and relevant social history from the patient alone. Salient information includes age at menarche, cycle regularity, cycle duration, flow, dysmenorrhea, symptoms of anemia, interference with daily activities, including absences from school or work, and the date of the last menstrual period.[3,5] Age at coitarche, use of contraception, risk factors for sexually transmitted infections (STIs), and any history of sexual abuse, genital trauma, or foreign body is also essential to ascertain. Symptoms of possible bleeding disorders include frequent nose bleeds, easy bruising, excessive bleeding after surgery or dental procedures, or HMB resulting in severe anemia at the onset of menarche. Endocrinologic etiologies of AUB are suggested by symptoms of hypothyroidism, hyperthyroidism, hyperandrogenism, or by exogenous hormone use. In addition, some antipsychotic and anticonvulsant medications can lead to AUB through alterations of prolactin levels, medication-induced PCOS, or altered metabolism of contraceptive medications.

Physical examination should include anthropometric measurements, including body mass index (BMI) and vital signs, including the orthostatic measurements of blood pressure and heart rate. Sexual maturity ratings of breasts and pubic hair, and the presence or absence of galactorrhea, should be noted. A complete pelvic examination, or bimanual examination plus vaginal swabs obtained without a speculum, should be considered in sexually active patients to assess for cervicitis due to STIs and pelvic inflammatory disease. A full pelvic examination is unnecessary in nonsexually active teens whose clinical presentation is otherwise consistent with anovulatory bleeding.

Laboratory testing may not be necessary for adolescents with mild anovulatory bleeding as determined by history and clinical examination consistent with physiologic immaturity. Other patients may require some laboratory evaluation (**Table 53.1**).[1]

A urine pregnancy test and screening for STIs (see Chapter 61) should be done in all patients if there is any question of sexual activity. Complete blood-cell count, ferritin, and thyroid stimulating hormone to assess for anemia, thrombocytopenia, iron deficiency, and thyroid dysfunction are recommended for heavy or frequent bleeding. For those who screen positive for a possible bleeding disorder by history, a coagulation screen including fibrinogen, prothrombin time, partial thromboplastin time, and a von Willebrand (vW) profile (vW factor antigen, vW factor/ristocetin cofactor activity, factor VIII activity), should be conducted.[6,7] Hemodynamically unstable patients should have a blood type and cross test performed. Follicle-stimulating hormone, testosterone (total and free), dehydroepiandrosterone-sulfate, and 17-hydroxyprogesterone aid in the evaluation of clinical signs of hyperandrogenism (see Chapter 49). Pelvic ultrasonography may be helpful if structural pathology is

TABLE 53.1

Laboratory Testing for Moderate to Severe AUB

All patients:	In select patients only:	In rare situations:
Urine pregnancy test	Follicle-stimulating hormone	Blood type and cross
Ferritin	Testosterone (total and free)	Platelet function and aggregation testing
Complete blood count including platelet count	Dehydroepiandrosterone-sulfate and/or 17-hydroxyprogesterone	Pelvic ultrasound
Thyroid stimulating hormone	Prothrombin time	
If sexually active: Neisseria gonorrhoeae	Partial thromboplastin time	
Chlamydia trachomatis	Fibrinogen	
	von Willebrand (vW) profile including vW factor antigen, vW factor/ristocetin cofactor activity, factor VIII activity	

suspected or to measure endometrial stripe thickness to help guide more complex cases. An endometrial biopsy may be considered in adults aged 19 to 39 years who fail medical management, especially in patients with conditions associated with endometrial hyperplasia, such as obesity and PCOS.[1] It is not, however, generally indicated for adolescent management.

THERAPY

Acute Abnormal Uterine Bleeding

The severity and cause of the bleeding will guide the management. Severe AUB with hemodynamic instability, regardless of the cause, requires immediate intervention with intravenous fluids or blood transfusion. Adolescents without an underlying cardiovascular disease who have mild to moderate anemia usually respond quickly to intravenous fluids and supplemental iron therapy without transfusion. Adolescents who develop severe anemia over months of abnormal bleeding better tolerate the same level of anemia than

those who develop acute bleeding over hours or days. Bleeding secondary to a systemic problem, such as a bleeding disorder or thyroid dysfunction, may require hormonal therapy identical to that used for the management of anovulatory bleeding until the systemic problem is adequately managed.

The treatment approach to anovulatory AUB depends on the current bleeding status, hemodynamic stability, hemoglobin value, the patient's emotional tolerance, and the potential need for contraception if the teen or young adult is sexually active. Studies comparing medication regimens for bleeding control are limited and have failed to produce clear evidence for one specific regimen. A combination of evidence and clinical experience suggests the following algorithm (Fig. 53.1).

Management is supportive and expectant for those with minimal bleeding and a normal hemoglobin. Oral iron therapy should be prescribed along with a stool softener to prevent constipation. Nonsteroidal anti-inflammatory drugs (NSAIDs) can be adjunctive therapy to decrease bleeding and associated cramping.

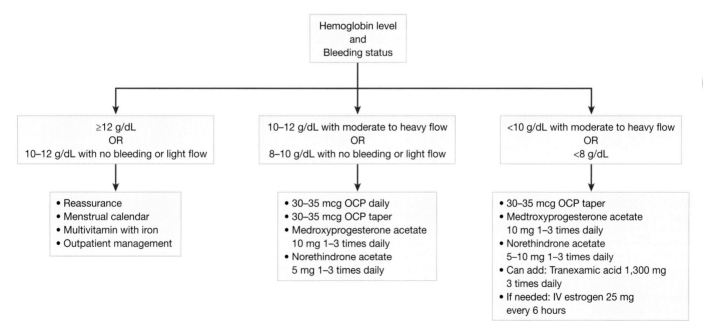

FIGURE 53.1 Algorithm for management of young females with acute AUB based on current hemoglobin and bleeding status.

There is no set regimen when an oral contraceptive pill (OCP) taper is used for management. Patients are commonly prescribed a monophasic pill four times daily for 4 days, then three times daily for 3 days, then two times daily for 2 days, then daily until the follow-up visit. An antiemetic can be prescribed as needed for nausea. Estrogen-containing medications should not be used in patients with contraindications to estrogen therapy, such as hypertension, migraines with aura, or a personal history of venous thromboembolic events or known inherited thrombophilias.[8] Alternatively, progestin-only oral medications can be used to manage active bleeding. Examples of progestin-only regimens include norethindrone acetate 5 mg, given one to three times daily, or medroxyprogesterone acetate 10 mg one to three times daily. These medications are typically used short-term to induce amenorrhea but can be used longer term in patients without contraceptive needs.[9] Medications to treat abnormal bleeding are typically continued for at least 3 to 6 months and until resolution of anemia. They can be continued longer due to patient preference, recurrence of AUB after cessation, or need for contraception in sexually active patients.

Patients who are not hemodynamically stable, have a hemoglobin of <8 g/dL, or have failed outpatient management typically require hospitalization for intravenous hydration and possible blood transfusion until the bleeding stops and the patient is hemodynamically stable. Management is similar to the regimens outlined above. If the bleeding is not improving or the patient is unable to tolerate oral medication, intravenous conjugated estrogen (25 mg every 6 hours for a maximum of 6 doses) may be needed initially, with transition to oral medication once the patient is stable and able to tolerate oral medication. Tranexamic acid can be used as an adjunct therapy, although it should be used with caution in conjunction with estrogen given the increased risk for thromboembolic disease.[9-12] Endometrial curettage or other surgical management is rarely necessary for adolescents.[2]

Chronic Abnormal Uterine Bleeding

Management of chronic AUB is similar to the regimens for mild to moderate AUB as discussed above but with expanded options. Hormonal management options are presented in Table 53.2.[6]

Special Situations

Coagulopathies

Evaluation for common bleeding diatheses, such as vW disease and idiopathic thrombocytopenia (ITP), should be considered as above. Abnormal uterine bleeding also commonly occurs in patients receiving chemotherapy or other interventions that alter bone marrow production, platelet function, or clotting factor synthesis. Input from Hematology should be sought for patients with known bleeding disorders to guide adjunct use of antifibrinolytic or other medications, such as tranexamic acid, aminocaproic acid, or desmopressin.

The management of bleeding in these patients uses the same management strategies above, but often with a longer-term goal of inducing amenorrhea. Oral contraceptive pills can be used in an extended-cycle or a continuous fashion. Prescribing estrogen-containing medications should be done with caution in patients undergoing chemotherapy due to the increased risk of venous thromboembolic events due to malignancy. Depot medroxyprogesterone acetate should be used with caution because initial irregular bleeding is common and intramuscular injections may be contraindicated in patients with severe thrombocytopenia. Gonadotropin-releasing hormone agonists (e.g., leuprolide acetate) can also be used to achieve longer-term amenorrhea in selected patients. However, as they can decrease bone mineral density, use should be reserved for short periods and limited patient populations, such as those undergoing chemotherapy.[17,18] When they are used, add-back therapy should be prescribed by health providers to prevent bone density loss.[19]

TABLE 53.2

Hormonal Management Options for Chronic AUB

Hormonal Methods	Information and Notes
Combined oral contraceptive pills, patches, or vaginal rings	Can be used in cyclic or extended-cycle fashion.
Progestin-only pills	Typical contraceptive doses (norethindrone 35 mcg) rarely used for bleeding management due to high rates of irregular bleeding. Higher-dose versions (i.e., norethindrone acetate 5 mg or medroxyprogesterone acetate 10 mg) can be used to achieve amenorrhea but have not been tested or approved for contraception.
Depot medroxyprogesterone acetate injections	Decreases overall bleeding with increasing amenorrhea rates over time. Due to its high frequency of initial irregular bleeding, this may not be the best option for those who need more acute menstrual management or suppression.
Levonorgestrel 52-mg intrauterine device (IUD)	Decreases overall bleeding with increasing amenorrhea rates over time.[13] Now FDA approved for use in nulliparous females and females under age 18 y; has been successfully used in adolescents for medical indications, even those who are not sexually active.[14] Placement under sedation may be considered if patients cannot tolerate office placement.
Etonorgestrel hormonal implant	Decreases overall bleeding but has only a 20–30% rate of amenorrhea. Irregular bleeding occurs in up to 58% of patients and is a common reason patients request removal.[15,16] May be a good option for bleeding control in sexually active adolescents because it is highly effective contraception.

Iatrogenic Bleeding

Irregular bleeding can also be caused by contraceptive or menstrual management methods, especially progestin-only options due to increased endometrial atrophy. Management of iatrogenic bleeding includes the following:

- Persistent breakthrough bleeding on a 10- to 20-mcg combined OCP pill may be improved by switching to a higher-dose (30- to 35-mcg estrogen) pill.
- Persistent heavy or irregular bleeding on a 30- to 35-mcg pill may require a full withdrawal bleed, especially if being used in an extended-cycle or continuous fashion with consideration of a pill with a different progestin. A 50-mcg pill is rarely needed.
- Breakthrough bleeding with progestin-only contraceptives is due to a combination of irregular endometrial proliferation, especially soon after initiation, and endometrial atrophy. As the initial irregular bleeding with depot medroxyprogesterone acetate and the levonorgestrel intrauterine device (IUD) usually improves over time, expectant management is often appropriate. Irregular bleeding is also a common side effect of the etonorgestrel implant, which may not improve over time.[15] Although there is minimal evidence for effective management of persistent bleeding

on progestin-only contraceptives, multiple regimens have been tried, including NSAIDs; addition of estrogen (conjugated estrogen 1.25 to 2.50 mg daily or micronized estradiol 1 to 2 mg daily); antibiotics (typically doxycycline); mifepristone, or tamoxifen.[20] Although this may stop the bleeding acutely, it may recur.

⬤ SUMMARY

Abnormal uterine bleeding is common during adolescence and often improves over time. Immaturity of the HPO axis is the most common etiology, but other causes should be investigated. There are many hormonal options for management, which should be individualized based on patients' hemodynamic stability, health goals, and preferences.

REFERENCES

1. Committee on Practice Bulletins—Gynecology. Practice Bulletin No. 128: Diagnosis of abnormal uterine bleeding in reproductive-aged women. *Obstet Gynecol.* 2012;120(1):197–206. doi:10.1097/AOG.0b013e318262e320
2. ACOG Practice Bulletin No. 136: Management of abnormal uterine bleeding associated with ovulatory dysfunction. *Obstet Gynecol.* 2013;122(1):176–185. doi:10.1097/01.AOG.0000431815.52679.bb
3. ACOG Committee Opinion No. 651: Menstruation in girls and adolescents: using the menstrual cycle as a vital sign. *Obstet Gynecol.* 2015;126(6):e143–e146. doi:10.1097/AOG.0000000000001215
4. Haamid F, Sass AE, Dietrich JE. Heavy menstrual bleeding in adolescents. *J Pediatr Adolesc Gynecol.* 2017;30(3):335–340. doi:S1083-3188(16)30253-4
5. ACOG Committee Opinion No. 785. Screening and management of bleeding disorders in adolescents with heavy menstrual bleeding: ACOG COMMITTEE OPINION, number 785. *Obstet Gynecol.* 2019;134(3):e71–e83. doi:10.1097/AOG.0000000000003411
6. Committee on Adolescent Health Care, Committee on Gynecologic Practice. Committee Opinion No. 580: Von Willebrand disease in women. *Obstet Gynecol.* 2013;122:1368–1373. doi:10.1097/01.AOG.0000438961.38979.19
7. Mullins TLK, Miller RJ, Mullins ES. Evaluation and management of adolescents with abnormal uterine bleeding. *Pediatr Ann.* 2015;44(9):e218–e222. doi:10.3928/00904481-20150910-09
8. Curtis KM, Tepper NK, Jatlaoui TC, et al. U.S. Medical Eligibility Criteria for contraceptive use, 2016. *MMWR Recomm Rep.* 2016;65(3):1–103. doi:10.15585/mmwr.rr6503a1
9. ACOG Committee Opinion No. 557. Management of acute abnormal uterine bleeding in nonpregnant reproductive-aged women. *Obstet Gynecol.* 2013;121(4):891–896. doi:10.1097/01.AOG.0000428646.67925.9a
10. Bs D, Nanda SK. The role of sevista in the management of dysfunctional uterine bleeding. *J Clin Diagn Res.* 2013;7(1):132–134. doi:10.7860/JCDR/2012/4794.2687.
11. Matteson KA, Rahn DD, Wheeler TL, et al. Nonsurgical management of heavy menstrual bleeding: a systematic review. *Obstet Gynecol.* 2013;121(3):632–643. doi:10.1097/AOG.0b013e3182839e0e
12. Srivaths LV, Dietrich JE, Yee DL, et al. Oral tranexamic acid versus combined oral contraceptives for adolescent heavy menstrual bleeding: a pilot study. *J Pediatr Adolesc Gynecol.* 2015;28(4):254–257. doi:S1083-3188(14)00420-3
13. Schwartz BI, Alexander M, Breech LL. Levonorgestrel intrauterine device use for medical indications in nulliparous adolescents and young adults. *J Adolesc Health.* 2021;68(2):357–363. doi:S1054-139X(20)30297-4
14. Kebodeaux CA, Schwartz BI. Experience with intrauterine device insertion in never sexually active adolescents: a retrospective cohort study. *Am J Obstet Gynecol.* 2018;219(6):600.e1–600.e7. doi:S0002-9378(18)30825-1
15. Mansour D, Korver T, Marintcheva-Petrova M, et al. The effects of implanon on menstrual bleeding patterns. *Eur J Contracept Reprod Health Care.* 2008;13(suppl 1):13–28. doi:10.1080/13625180801959931
16. Berlan E, Mizraji K, Bonny AE. Twelve-month discontinuation of etonogestrel implant in an outpatient pediatric setting. *Contraception.* 2016;94(1):81–86. doi:S0010-7824(15)30130-X
17. ACOG Committee Opinion No. 817. Options for prevention and management of menstrual bleeding in adolescent patients undergoing cancer treatment: ACOG Committee Opinion Summary, number 817. *Obstet Gynecol.* 2021;137(1):e7–e15. doi:10.1097/AOG.0000000000004209
18. Pradhan S, Gomez-Lobo V. Hormonal contraceptives, IUDs, gonadotropin-releasing hormone analogues, and testosterone: menstrual suppression in special adolescent populations. *J Pediatr Adolesc Gynecol.* 2019;32:S23–S29. doi:S1083-3188(19)30180-9
19. Chwalisz K, Surrey E, Stanczyk FZ. The hormonal profile of norethindrone acetate: rationale for add-back therapy with gonadotropin-releasing hormone agonists in women with endometriosis. *Reprod Sci.* 2012;19(6):563–571. doi:10.1177/1933719112438061
20. Zigler RE, McNicholas C. Unscheduled vaginal bleeding with progestin-only contraceptive use. *Am J Obstet Gynecol.* 2017;216(5):443–450. doi:S0002-9378(16)33176-3

🛜 ADDITIONAL RESOURCES AND WEBSITES

Additional Resources and Websites for Clinicians:
American Academy of Family Physicians—www.aafp.org
American Congress of Obstetricians and Gynecologists (ACOG)—www.acog.org
Curtis KM, Tepper NK, Jatlaoui TC, et al. U.S. Medical eligibility criteria for contraceptive use, 2016. *MMWR Recomm Rep.* 2016;65(3):1–103. doi: http://dx.doi.org/10.15585/mmwr.rr6503a1external icon
Emans SJ, Laufer MR, DiVasta AD, eds. *Emans, Laufer, Goldstein's Pediatric & Adolescent Gynecology.* 7th ed. Wolters Kluwer, 2020.
National Heart, Lung, and Blood Institute. 2007, December. *The Diagnosis, Evaluation and Management of von Willebrand Disease* (Full Report) retrieved from https://www.nhlbi.nih.gov/health-topics/all-publications-and-resources/diagnosis-evaluation-and-management-von-willebrand. Accessed September 1, 2022.
North American Society for Pediatric and Adolescent Gynecology (NASPAG)—www.naspag.org

Additional Resources and Websites for Parents/Caregivers:
American College of Obstetricians and Gynecologists—www.acog.org
Healthy Children sponsored by The American Academy of Pediatrics
Kids Health from Nemours Foundation—www.kidshealth.org
Society for Adolescent Health and Medicine—www.adolescenthealth.org
Symptomviewer—HealthyChildren.org

Additional Resources and Websites for Adolescents and Young Adults:
Center for Young Women's Health from Boston Children's Hospital—www.youngwomenshealth.org
Go Ask Alice from Columbia University—www.goaskalice.columbia.edu
Teen's Health from Nemours Foundation—www.teenshealth.org

CHAPTER 54

Amenorrhea, the Polycystic Ovary Syndrome, and Hirsutism

Shannon Fitzgerald
Catherine M. Gordon
Amy Fleischman

KEY WORDS

- Amenorrhea
- Androgens
- Congenital adrenal hyperplasia (CAH)
- Female athlete triad
- Hirsutism
- Hyperandrogenism
- Hypogonadotropic hypogonadism

- Idiopathic hypogonadotropic hypogonadism (IHH)
- Metformin
- Polycystic ovary syndrome (PCOS)
- Primary ovarian insufficiency
- Turner syndrome

INTRODUCTION

Primary amenorrhea is defined by a lack of menses by 14 years, without secondary sexual characteristics, or lack of menses by 15 years. The former definition used 16 years with no menses. Most experts now advocate for using the lower age threshold.[1] Secondary amenorrhea is the lack of menses for 6 months, or the duration of three prior cycles. The causes of primary and secondary amenorrhea include specific genetic abnormalities, enzymatic defects, hormone imbalances, and structural abnormalities. The hypothalamus, pituitary, and/or gonads may be affected. Decreased energy availability due to reduced intake or increased exercise is a common cause of hypothalamic amenorrhea. Polycystic ovary syndrome (PCOS) is another common cause of irregular menses. This syndrome consists of clinical and laboratory hyperandrogenism and dysregulated menses and may include typical ovarian structural changes, although this is no longer a diagnostic criterion. Metabolic abnormalities are commonly associated with this syndrome. Hirsutism, increased body hair in females, is a common clinical manifestation of PCOS, but may also be seen in other conditions causing hyperandrogenism. This chapter will review the causes, evaluation, and treatment of amenorrhea, PCOS, and hirsutism.

AMENORRHEA

Definition

Normal Menstrual Timing

- The average age of menarche for the American adolescent remains at 12.7 years, with a two standard deviation range of 11 to 15 months. However, a recent longitudinal study demonstrated earlier menarche in Black and Hispanic females (12.0 and 11.83 years, respectively) compared to Asian and White females (12.75 and 12.67 years, respectively).[2]
- Ninety-five to ninety-seven percent of females reach menarche by age 16 years and 98% by 18 years.

- There is an average of 2 years between the start of thelarche, the first sign of puberty, and the onset of menarche.
- The onset of menarche is fairly constant in adolescent development, with approximately two-thirds of females reaching menarche at a sexual maturity rating (SMR) of 4. Menarche occurs at SMR 2 in 5% of females, SMR 3 in 25%, and not until SMR 5 in 10%.
- Ninety-five percent of adolescents have attained menarche 1 year after attaining SMR 5.
- Although anovulatory cycles are common in the first 1 to 2 years after menarche, thereafter, menstrual cycles are typically less than 45 days in healthy adolescent females.[3]

Amenorrhea

Primary Amenorrhea

1. No episodes of spontaneous uterine bleeding by the age of 14 years with secondary sexual characteristics absent
2. No episodes of spontaneous uterine bleeding by age 15 years regardless of normal secondary sexual characteristics (chronologic criteria)
3. No episodes of spontaneous uterine bleeding, despite having attained SMR 5 for at least 1 year or despite the onset of breast development 4 years previously (developmental criteria)
4. No episodes of spontaneous uterine bleeding by age 14 years in any individual with clinical stigmata of or genotype consistent with Turner syndrome

Secondary Amenorrhea

After previous uterine bleeding, no subsequent menses for 6 months or a length of time equal to three previous cycles.

Etiology

Primary Amenorrhea without Secondary Sexual Characteristics (Absent Breast Development), but with Normal Genitalia (Uterus and Vagina)

1. Genetic or enzymatic defects causing gonadal (ovarian) insufficiency (hypergonadotropic hypogonadism): A growing number of cases of primary amenorrhea are attributable to a genetic cause.
   - *Turner syndrome, Turner mosaicism, or related genotypes* (45, X; 45, XX/X; 45, XY/X; or structurally abnormal X chromosome): This is the most common genetic cause of hypogonadism. Stigmata are variable, but classically include short stature (height usually <60 in); streaked gonads; hypogonadism; and somatic anomalies (webbed neck, short fourth metacarpal, cubitus valgus, coarctation of the aorta) (see Fig. 54.1).
   - *17α-hydroxylase deficiency with 46, XX karyotype:* These individuals have normal stature, lack of secondary sexual characteristics,

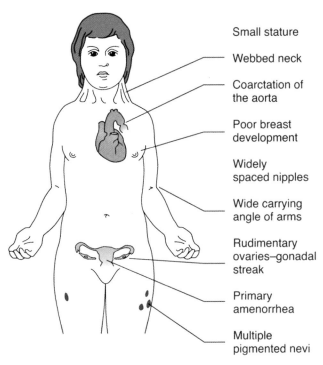

- Small stature
- Webbed neck
- Coarctation of the aorta
- Poor breast development
- Widely spaced nipples
- Wide carrying angle of arms
- Rudimentary ovaries–gonadal streak
- Primary amenorrhea
- Multiple pigmented nevi

FIGURE 54.1 Clinical features of Turner syndrome. (From Rubin R, Strayer DS, Rubin E. *Rubin's Pathology.* 6th ed. Lippincott Williams & Wilkins, 2011.)

hypertension, and hypokalemia. Laboratory test results show an elevated progesterone, low 17-hydroxyprogesterone (17-OHP), and elevated serum deoxycorticosterone level. Mild cases may present without electrolyte abnormalities.

2. *Premature ovarian insufficiency:*
   - Etiologies can include autoimmunity and enzymatic or genetic abnormalities (including Turner syndrome, above); most cases are idiopathic. The etiology may be important in directing further evaluation and in counseling families. For example, a carrier of a premutation in the FMR1 gene (fragile X gene) in a female can manifest as ovarian insufficiency, while future generations would be at risk for severe mental retardation among males. Evidence of autoimmunity, such as ovarian and/or adrenal antibodies, suggests the need to evaluate adrenal status and consider clinical evidence of other autoimmune diseases such as hypothyroidism, hypoparathyroidism, or type 1 diabetes mellitus. Rare mutations have been identified that manifest as premature ovarian insufficiency and thus may play a role in amenorrhea such as EIF4ENIF1, FSHR, GDF9, BMP15, FIGLA, and NOBOX, which are involved with germ-cell development and/or ovarian function, as well as multiple point mutations of the X chromosome.[4]
3. Pituitary/hypothalamic-gonadotropin insufficiency (hypogonadotropic hypogonadism): With the discovery of multiple factors contributing to gonadotropin-releasing hormone (GnRH) activation, idiopathic hypogonadotropic hypogonadism (IHH) (Kallmann, normosmic IHH) has been shown to have multiple genetic contributors. Mutations in KAL1, FGFR1, FGF8, PROK2, PROKR2, and Kisspeptin1, in addition to GnRH1, GnRH receptor, TAC3, TAC3R, and CHD7, among others, have been linked to hypogonadism. This active field continues to evolve, and novel factors and genetic mutations continue to be reported.[5]

Primary Amenorrhea with Normal Breast Development, but Absent Uterus

1. *Complete androgen insensitivity*: In these XY-karyotype individuals, the wolffian ducts fail to develop and external female genitalia are present. The underlying defect is a mutation in the androgen receptor, rendering it insensitive to testosterone's actions. Because müllerian inhibitory factor (MIF) continues to be secreted by the Sertoli cells of male gonads, the müllerian ducts regress, and there is lack of formation of internal female genitalia. Internally, there may be normal male gonads and fibrous müllerian remnants. At puberty, if the gonads remain present, the low levels of endogenous gonadal and adrenal estrogens, unopposed by androgens, may result in breast development. Because of the end-organ insensitivity to androgens, the adolescent develops sparse or absent pubic and axillary hair despite marked elevations in serum testosterone concentrations.

2. *Congenital absence of uterus/agenesis* is often associated with agenesis of the vaginal canal, or Mayer–Rokitansky–Küster–Hauser syndrome. These young females have a 46, XX karyotype and ovaries. They may experience cyclic breast and mood changes. They present with secondary sexual characteristics and normal female testosterone concentrations. They may also have associated renal, skeletal, or other congenital anomalies.

Primary Amenorrhea with No Breast Development and No Uterus

This condition is extremely rare. The individual usually has a 46, XY karyotype, elevated gonadotropin levels, and low-normal female testosterone levels. These individuals produce enough MIF to inhibit development of female internal genital structures, but not enough testosterone to develop male internal and external genitalia. The causes include the following:

1. 17,20-lyase deficiency
2. Agonadism, including no internal sex organs
3. 17α-hydroxylase deficiency with 46, XY karyotype: may present with hypertension.

Primary and Secondary Amenorrhea with Normal Secondary Sexual Characteristics (Breast Development) and Normal Genitalia (Uterus and Vagina)

1. Hypothalamic causes
   - *Idiopathic hypogonadotropic hypogonadism,* as outlined above, may manifest as primary or secondary amenorrhea and in mild cases occur with normal secondary sexual characteristics.
   - *Medications and drugs:* Particularly phenothiazines; oral, injectable, or transdermal contraceptives; glucocorticoids; and heroin
   - *Other endocrinopathies:* Hyperthyroidism or hypothyroidism, prolactinoma, and cortisol excess
   - *Stress:* Common in adolescents and young adults (AYAs) and may relate to family, school, romantic relationships, or peer problems.
   - *Exercise:* Athletes, particularly runners, gymnasts, competitive divers, figure skaters, and ballet dancers, have higher rates of amenorrhea and higher rates of low-energy availability, sometimes associated with disordered eating. Sports that may place athletes at higher risk for this condition include those that emphasize leanness, such as dance or gymnastics, or those that use weight classification, such as martial arts. The "female athlete triad," a term coined in 1992, was defined by the American College of Sports Medicine[6] to include a spectrum of energy availability, menstrual irregularity, and bone health. In 2014, however, due to further evidence and experience, the International Olympic Committee introduced a broader, more comprehensive definition to demonstrate the cause of this syndrome to be an energy deficiency related to imbalance between energy intake and energy expenditure, which they described as "Relative Energy Deficiency in Sport (RED-S)." This more

inclusive definition recognizes the many aspects of physiologic function affected by an energy deficiency, including energy availability, bone health, and menstrual function, as seen in previous definitions, but also including cardiovascular health, protein synthesis, and psychological health. This low-energy availability may be due to undereating, overexercise, or both.[6] The prevalence of secondary amenorrhea in young adult athletes ranges broadly and varies by the sport studied. Secondary amenorrhea is estimated to be present in ~2% to 5% of college females, but increases to 69% among dancers and 65% in long distance runners.[6] The pulsatile nature of luteinizing hormone (LH), and normal menstrual function appears to be dependent on energy availability (caloric intake minus energy expenditure). Low-energy availability (such as RED-S, above) may result in a hypometabolic state that can include metabolic alterations, hypoglycemia, hypoinsulinemia, euthyroid sick syndrome, hypercortisolemia, and suppression of the total secretion and amplitude of the diurnal rhythm of leptin.[3] Leptin, a hormone secreted by fat tissue, has been shown to be a permissive factor in menstruation, likely due to its correlation with adequate fat mass.[3] Although both athletes with amenorrhea and regularly menstruating athletes have reduced LH pulsatile secretions and 24-hour mean leptin levels, runners with amenorrhea have more extreme suppression and disorganization of LH pulsatility. The level of energy availability needed to maintain normal reproductive function is not known for a given individual. However, studies have used 30 kcal/kg of lean body mass, as there are demonstrable metabolic and bone effects that occur and disruptions in LH can be seen after only 5 days below this threshold.[6] Low levels of estradiol (E_2) may be present, which have been implicated as the cause of bone loss, placing these young females at increased risk of stress fractures. The condition may be reversible with weight gain or with lessening of the intensity of exercise. However, there is also evidence that the loss of bone density may be partially irreversible despite resumption of menses, estrogen replacement, or calcium supplementation. There remain many unanswered questions about exercise-induced amenorrhea, especially related to whether hormonal therapy or vitamin/mineral supplementation is beneficial in minimizing skeletal loss in this population. This is an active area of research, with preliminary data suggesting that transdermal estrogen[7] and combined therapy with dehydroepiandrosterone (DHEA) and estrogen/progestin may be beneficial for older adolescents.[7]

- *Weight loss:* Adolescents and young adults with simple weight loss and those with anorexia nervosa may present with amenorrhea. In patients with anorexia nervosa and simple weight loss, the mechanism appears to be hypothalamic derangement. This alteration appears to be more severe in AYAs with anorexia nervosa. The E_2 levels in patients with weight loss and anorexia nervosa can vary from low to normal. Consequently, such individuals may or may not respond to progesterone withdrawal with uterine bleeding. The AYA with amenorrhea and severe weight loss is also at risk for decreased bone density, and treatment of this metabolic consequence in anorexia nervosa is also an active area of research. While often challenging to achieve, treatment of amenorrhea for this population includes weight restoration which often will lead to the spontaneous return of menses.
- *Chronic illnesses:* Certain chronic illnesses can affect the hypothalamic–pituitary axis. Examples include cystic fibrosis, chronic renal disease, and disorders of gastrointestinal absorption (e.g., celiac disease).

- *Hypothalamic failure*
- Lesions: Include craniopharyngioma, tuberculous granuloma, and other tumors and infectious etiologies
- Idiopathic
2. Pituitary causes
   - *Nonneoplastic lesions resulting in hypopituitarism:* Sheehan syndrome (pregnancy related), Simmonds disease (nonpregnancy related), aneurysm, or empty sella syndrome
   - *Tumors:* Adenoma or carcinoma
   - *Infiltrative:* Hemochromatosis
   - *Idiopathic*
3. Ovarian causes
   - *Premature ovarian insufficiency:* Menopause occurring under age 40 years. This diagnosis can have genetic underpinnings (see above section: Amenorrhea), or be associated with autoantibodies directed against ovarian tissue, sometimes in association with thyroid and adrenal autoantibodies (i.e., autoimmune etiology). The diagnosis can also be due to iatrogenic causes, such as in individuals who received chemotherapy and/or radiation therapy for cancer as children or adolescents. Unfortunately, in most cases, the etiology remains unknown.
4. Hyperandrogenism: Polycystic ovary syndrome, congenital adrenal hyperplasia (CAH), or androgen-producing tumor. These etiologies are discussed in detail below.
5. Uterine causes: Uterine synechiae (Asherman syndrome)
6. Pregnancy

Diagnosis

The evaluation of amenorrhea can be pursued with a thorough history, physical examination, and performance of several laboratory tests in a logical sequence. It is essential to rule out the diagnosis of pregnancy before conducting an extensive evaluation. **Figures 54.2** and **54.3** review the evaluation of primary and secondary amenorrhea.

History

History should include the following:

1. Systemic diseases: Diseases associated with secondary amenorrhea include, but are not limited to, anorexia nervosa, systemic illness such as inflammatory bowel disease and diabetes mellitus, as well as central processes such as pituitary adenoma. A history of thyroid dysfunction is particularly important, because even mild thyroid dysfunction can lead to menstrual abnormalities.
2. Family history, including ages of parental growth and development, mother's and sisters' ages at menarche, as well as a family history of thyroid disease, diabetes mellitus, eating disorders, menstrual problems, or fertility issues
3. Past medical history including any significant childhood illnesses
4. Pubertal growth and development, including breast and pubic hair development, and the presence of a growth spurt
5. Menstrual history
6. History of androgen excess such as significant acne or hair growth, suggesting PCOS, or other ovarian or adrenal abnormality
7. Stress, anxiety, depression or other mood concerns
8. Medications: Hormonal therapies (e.g., depot medroxyprogesterone, oral contraceptives, etc.) or illicit drugs (heroin and methadone, for example, can cause menstrual dysfunction)
9. Nutritional status and recent weight changes
10. Exercise history, particularly for sports, and level of activity that may predispose to amenorrhea such as those sports and activities for which leanness may confer an advantage (e.g., dance, gymnastics) or those with weight categories (e.g., wrestling), as outlined above
11. Sexual history, contraception, and symptoms of pregnancy

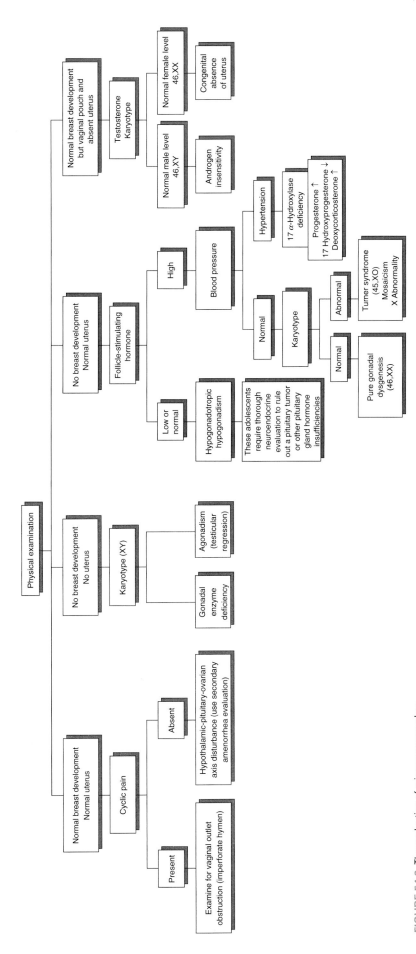

FIGURE 54.2 The evaluation of primary amenorrhea.

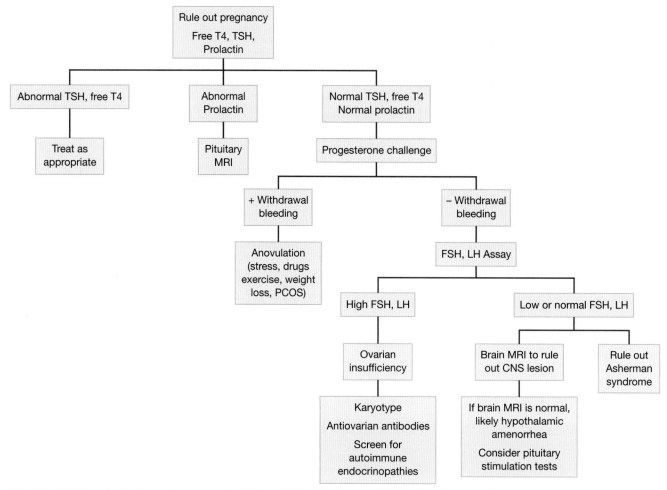

FIGURE 54.3 The evaluation of secondary amenorrhea. TSH, thyroid-stimulating hormone; PCOS, polycystic ovary syndrome; MRI, magnetic resonance imaging; FSH, follicle-stimulating hormone; LH, luteinizing hormone; CNS, central nervous system.

Physical Examination

The physical examination should include the following:

1. Height, weight, and vital signs (blood pressure and heart rate)
2. Signs of systemic disease or malnutrition
3. Signs of androgen excess such as acne or hirsutism
4. Signs of thyroid dysfunction, including examination of the thyroid gland, skin, and hair
5. Signs of insulin resistance such as acanthosis nigricans (hyperpigmented velvety skin changes on neck, axillae, or other intertriginous areas) (Fig. 54.4)
6. Phenotype consistent with Turner syndrome: Webbed neck, low-set ears, broad shield-like chest, short fourth metacarpal, and increased carrying angle of the arms (Fig. 54.1)
7. Test for anosmia in females with primary or secondary amenorrhea when considering anosmic hypogonadotropic hypogonadism (Kallmann syndrome)
8. Sexual maturity rating: This is important for evaluating progress in secondary sexual characteristics, because most adolescents are not menarchal until SMR 4, and 95% are menarchal by 1 year after SMR 5.
9. Breast examination: Check for estrogenized texture and for galactorrhea.
10. Pelvic examination: Search for a stenotic cervix, vaginal agenesis, imperforate hymen, transverse vaginal septum, absent uterus, or enlarged uterus suggesting pregnancy. An external genital examination is a critical component of the workup to assess for evidence of estrogenization or androgen excess

(e.g., clitoromegaly), as well as check for abnormalities of the hymen. A full pelvic examination may not be necessary if the adolescent or young adult is not sexually active, and the history or physical examination reveals the cause of amenorrhea.

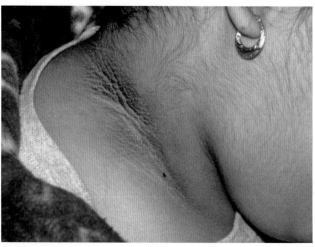

FIGURE 54.4 Acanthosis nigricans. Linear, alternating dark and light pigmentation becomes more apparent when the skin is stretched. (From Goodheart HP. *Goodheart's Photoguide of Common Skin Disorders.* 4th ed. Lippincott Williams & Wilkins, 2015.)

Laboratory Evaluation

The laboratory evaluation for AYAs can begin with evaluation of LH, FSH, and E_2 to establish whether primary hypogonadism or hypogonadotropic hypogonadism is the cause.

1. Evaluation for primary and secondary amenorrhea with normal secondary sexual characteristics:
   a. Pregnancy should always be considered and ruled out.
   b. If evidence of galactorrhea is present, prolactin level should be obtained; this is the most sensitive test for a prolactin producing pituitary microadenomas (see Chapter 60). Rarely, a patient who responds to progesterone withdrawal can have a microadenoma.
   c. If clinical hyperandrogenism is present, further lab testing is warranted (See discussion below on PCOS).
   d. Diabetes mellitus and hypo-/hyperthyroidism should be considered, and if clinically indicated, should be ruled out with measurements of blood glucose and/or thyroid function studies. Thyroid stimulating hormone and a free or total thyroxine with a measure of thyroid binding protein should be measured to rule out the possibility of either primary or central hypothyroidism.
   e. Uterine synechiae, or Asherman syndrome, should be considered if there is a history of dilation and curettage, or endometritis. This condition may cause partial or total obliteration of the uterine cavity. If this problem is suggested by the history, a gynecologic referral for evaluation by hysteroscopy or hysterosalpingography is indicated.

If the results of the aforementioned evaluation do not identify a cause, the workup should proceed as follows:

Administer progesterone withdrawal test or "challenge" (5- to 10-day course)

- A *positive (withdrawal bleed) response to progesterone* correlates with circulating E_2 levels adequate to prime the endometrium, as seen with either hypothalamic–pituitary dysfunction or PCOS. A positive response ranges from minimal brown staining to normal menstrual flow.
- If there is *no response to progesterone*, then either hypothalamic–pituitary dysfunction or ovarian insufficiency is likely. A high FSH level indicates ovarian insufficiency, whereas a normal or low FSH level suggests a hypothalamic–pituitary disturbance. If ovarian insufficiency is suspected, a karyotype, antiovarian/antiadrenal antibodies, and screening for autoimmune endocrinopathies may be done. In addition, more rare causes, such as fragile X-premutation carrier status and galactosemia, should be considered. If hypothalamic–pituitary failure is suspected, magnetic resonance imaging (MRI) scans of the brain, visual fields, and a pituitary hormonal evaluation are warranted. An MRI should always be considered in a female patient with a history of headaches or visual changes.
- Individuals with weight loss, anorexia nervosa, problematic substance use, or excessive exercise may or may not respond to progesterone withdrawal. If they do not experience bleeding within 10 to 14 days of discontinuing the progesterone, it is indicative of low E_2 levels and further evaluation may be warranted.
- Evaluation for primary amenorrhea with either absent uterus or absent secondary sexual characteristics:
  a. A physical examination and potentially radiographic studies would suggest that the AYA falls into one of three categories:
     - Absent uterus, normal breasts
     - Absent breasts, normal uterus
     - Absent breasts, absent uterus

In general, breast development should be at least at stage SMR 4 to be considered indicative of full gonadal function. A breast stage of SMR 2 or SMR 3 may indicate adrenal function alone without full gonadal function.

a. If the examination reveals normal breast development, but an absent uterus and blind vaginal pouch, a karyotype and a test for serum testosterone concentrations are indicated.
   - XX karyotype plus female testosterone concentration: Congenital absence of uterus
   - XY karyotype plus male testosterone concentration: Androgen insensitivity
b. If the examination reveals absent secondary sexual characteristics, but a normal uterus:
   - A low or normal FSH level suggests a hypothalamic or pituitary abnormality, and a full pituitary evaluation is indicated.
   - A high FSH level and a blood pressure within the reference range suggest a genetic disorder or gonadal dysgenesis. A karyotype should be ordered.
   - A high FSH level and hypertension suggest 17α-hydroxylase deficiency. This is confirmed by an elevated progesterone level, low 17α-hydroxyprogesterone level, and an elevated serum deoxycorticosterone level.
c. The absence of both breast development and uterus or vagina is very rare. These findings suggest gonadal failure and the presence of MIF secretion from a testis. This could arise from anorchia occurring after MIF activity was present or an enzyme block, such as a 17,20-lyase defect. The evaluation should include LH, FSH, progesterone, and 17-OHP measurements, and a karyotype.

Treatment

Primary Amenorrhea

Hypogonadotropic Hypogonadism Treatment should be directed towards the potential cause of the amenorrhea, as below. If diagnosed with IHH, therapy should begin with estrogen replacement. A transdermal β-E_2 patch can be used starting at 0.025 mg/day of E_2, or cut to initiate lower doses, and used overnight and advanced slowly over time. Half of the 0.3 mg Premarin pill can also be utilized. Recent studies support improved safety and efficacy with the use of transdermal estrogen preparations, avoiding effects of the first pass through the liver.[7] Patients who have already reached an acceptable adult height can receive up to 0.625 mg/day of conjugated estrogens (Premarin) or 0.05 to 0.1 mg of E_2 via transdermal patch. High doses of estrogen should be avoided during growth to prevent premature epiphyseal closure in females who have not yet reached final adult height.

A typical maintenance schedule would be 0.625 to 1.25 mg/day of conjugated estrogens daily or twice-weekly estrogen patch application of 0.05 to 0.1 mg of E_2, with 10 mg of medroxyprogesterone acetate (Provera) for 10 days of each month to bring on a withdrawal bleed and thereby avoiding endometrial hyperplasia. This schedule can be repeated each month. The dose of estrogen may vary depending on the individual and the estrogen response, but usually does not exceed 1.25 mg/day of conjugated estrogens or 0.1 mg/day of transdermal estrogen. If pregnancy is desired, pulsatile GnRH via pump therapy is a therapeutic option.

Oral contraceptive pills are often used for convenience, but should only be used after pubertal development is complete, as the dosing is too high for pubertal initiation.[7] Oral contraceptive pills should be used for those who are at risk of undesired pregnancy, or transdermal or oral E_2 with a levonorgestrel intrauterine device. Although low risk, some of these patients may still be spontaneously ovulating, so contraceptive options should be considered.

Pituitary Defect Hormonal therapy, as outlined above. Effective treatment may also require supplementation of other pituitary hormones.

Genetic Abnormalities Leading to Gonadal Defects Hormonal therapy, as outlined above. If a Y chromosome is present, gonadal removal is usually necessary because of the risk for developing gonadoblastoma. If a 46, XX karyotype is present, then the gonadal tissue should be visualized to assess if the tissue is at increased risk for tumor progression. With complete gonadal dysgenesis, these individuals are universally sterile. However, with an intact uterus, the individual may be able to bear children after donor oocyte implantation and hormonal support.

Enzymatic Defects

17α-Hydroxylase Deficiency Both glucocorticoid and estrogen–progesterone replacement are needed.

17,20-Lyase Deficiency Estrogen–progesterone replacement is needed.

Androgen Insensitivity All intra-abdominal gonads associated with a Y chromosome have a relatively high potential for malignancy and should be removed. The appropriate timing for removal should be individualized for each patient. After the gonads are removed, maintenance estrogen therapy is needed. The AYA should be informed that she may require vaginoplasty to have normal sexual function. The discussion about infertility and the abnormal sex chromosome should be done with additional counseling support as needed.

Congenital Absence of the Uterus Because these adolescents have normal-functioning ovaries, they do not require hormonal replacement therapy. They may require a vaginoplasty for normal sexual function and an MRI or intravenous pyelogram to rule out associated renal anomalies. These adolescents must be informed that they cannot carry a pregnancy, but may be able to have genetic offspring with the assistance of a surrogate. Therefore, they may require additional support and counseling.

Primary and Secondary Amenorrhea with Normal Secondary Sexual Characteristics

1. Polycystic ovary syndrome (see detailed discussion below)
2. Hypothalamic–pituitary dysfunction
   a. Alleviate the precipitating cause, if known.
   b. Hormonal therapy with progestin to induce uterine bleeding every 1 to 3 months and/or estrogen and progestin therapy is recommended.
3. Hypothalamic–pituitary failure
   a. The cause must be evaluated and corrected if possible.
   b. Replacement therapy with cyclic conjugated estrogens and progestins, as outlined above, is recommended.
4. Ovarian insufficiency
   These AYAs also require cyclic estrogen and progestin therapy, as above.
5. Uterine synechiae: This problem requires referral to a gynecologist for possible transhysteroscopic lysis of the adhesions.

Amenorrhea Associated with Weight Loss

In young females with amenorrhea associated with weight loss, bone mineral density (BMD) loss can occur soon after amenorrhea develops. The safest and most efficacious method for reversing bone loss is weight restoration. However, for those for whom this goal cannot be achieved, the efficacy of estrogen replacement therapy, with provision of transdermal versus oral preparations is an area of continued debate. Transdermal estrogen is likely more beneficial for bone health though some AYAs prefer an oral therapy due to ease of use. Estrogen likely has beneficial effects on bone and other tissues, but other supplemental therapies appear to be needed, in addition to the estrogen replacement in many patients. Experimental therapies, such as low-dose androgen supplementation (DHEA or testosterone), insulin-like growth factor I (IGF-I), or growth hormone, and bisphosphonates, are gaining further support in the literature.[7] Many adolescents who recover from anorexia nervosa at a young age (younger than 15 years) have regional (lumbar spine and femoral neck) bone

deficits. The longer the duration of anorexia nervosa and/or weight loss, the less likely the BMD will return to a normal range.

Relative Energy Deficiency in Sport (RED-S), previously known as "The Female Athlete Triad"

Female AYAs who participate regularly in athletics may develop RED-S,[6] which includes low-energy availability due to a high level of physical activity, accompanied by varying degrees of disordered eating, menstrual dysfunction (typically oligomenorrhea), and decreased BMD.

Treatment considerations for athletes with amenorrhea include the following:
   a. Most bone mineralization in female adolescents occurs by the middle of the second decade of life.
   b. Premature bone demineralization occurs in young females with hypothalamic dysfunction that manifests as either amenorrhea or oligomenorrhea in the setting of participation in athletics or dance, and eating disorders.
   c. Regular menses and fertility should return with a decrease in the intensity of activity. An AYA with significant menstrual dysfunction attributed to exercise should be encouraged to increase her caloric intake and modify excessive exercise activity.
   d. Calcium intake should be increased to 1,300 mg/day (elemental calcium) daily in these young females with efforts made to optimize dietary calcium intake.
   e. Vitamin D deficiency should be avoided, and supplemental vitamin D of 600 to 1,000 IU provided daily.
   f. Hormonal therapy remains an area of active study. Studies have suggested that transdermal estrogen may be more beneficial to bone health in this population[7] compared to oral estrogen therapy. In addition, combined therapy with DHEA and low-dose combined oral contraceptive pills has demonstrated a positive effect on BMD for older adolescents.[7] Androgens, estrogens, growth hormone, IGF-1, and bisphosphonates are being tested in clinical trials, with some demonstrating improvements in bone health.[8]
   g. The practitioner should evaluate these individuals, as outlined previously, to eliminate the possibility of pregnancy, thyroid dysfunction, prolactinoma, or a disorder of androgen excess. It should not be assumed that amenorrhea is simply secondary to exercise.

● THE POLYCYSTIC OVARY SYNDROME AND HIRSUTISM

Definition

Polycystic ovary syndrome is a disorder of the hypothalamic–pituitary–ovarian system, giving rise to temporary or persistent anovulation and androgen excess. The syndrome was originally described in 1935 by Stein and Leventhal as amenorrhea, hirsutism, and obesity associated with enlarged cystic ovaries. For many years, there was an emphasis on the morphologic changes in the ovary. However, enlarged polycystic ovaries may occur in healthy females, in up to 30% to 40% of healthy adolescent females, and in females with other conditions such as Cushing syndrome and CAH. In addition, females with other classic features of PCOS may have ovaries of normal size.

Polycystic ovary syndrome is one of the most common endocrine disorders, affecting approximately 5% to 10% of premenopausal females, and is the most common cause of hyperandrogenism in females and adolescents. True prevalence rates are difficult to study due to referral biases, variable phenotypes, populations studied, and diagnostic criteria used. It is estimated that approximately 6% to 18% of adolescent females meet criteria for PCOS.[9] Polycystic ovary syndrome also negatively impacts health-related quality of life for adolescents.[10]

As there are a spectrum of related signs and symptoms, there have been multiple criteria used in the diagnosis of PCOS. The 1990 U.S. National Institutes of Health Consensus Conference identified key features for the diagnosis of PCOS—menstrual dysfunction, clinical and/or biochemical evidence of hyperandrogenism, and the exclusion of CAH and/or thyroid dysfunction. Probable criteria for PCOS included insulin resistance and perimenarchal onset.

The 2003 Rotterdam consensus workshop defined PCOS more broadly, recognizing ovarian dysfunction as the primary component, without mandatory anovulation. The revised definition included two of the three following criteria with the exclusion of other etiologies of hyperandrogenism:

- Oligo- and/or anovulation
- Clinical and/or biochemical signs of hyperandrogenism
- Polycystic ovaries by ultrasonography

The Androgen Excess and PCOS Society in 2006 broadened the definition to include clinical and/or biochemical hyperandrogenism (most reliably hirsutism and an elevated free testosterone) and ovarian dysfunction. Evaluation of ovarian morphology was suggested and other causes of hyperandrogenism were to be ruled out. The consensus definitions are broad, allowing for a clinical and biochemical diagnosis of a wide spectrum of phenotypes.

As a response to the Endocrine Society recommending the use of the Rotterdam criteria as above for adult females, the Pediatric Endocrine Society developed recommendations in 2015 for the diagnostic criteria for PCOS in adolescents. This guideline included the combination of abnormal uterine bleeding with evidence of hyperandrogenism.[11]

In more recent years, adolescent-specific diagnostic recommendations (including the 2018 International PCOS Guideline) continue to focus on the persistence of oligo/amenorrhea with clinical and/or biochemical hyperandrogenism in diagnosing PCOS in adolescents.[9,12]

More recent research criteria have included abnormal response to GnRH stimulation, dexamethasone suppression testing, and adrenocorticotropic hormone (ACTH) stimulation testing.[11] Reaching an accurate diagnosis is particularly important because PCOS increases metabolic and cardiovascular risks, which are linked to insulin resistance and compounded by obesity. Androgen excess can result in laboratory changes including decreased high-density lipoprotein cholesterol (HDL-C) level. Insulin resistance and its associated risks are also present in females with PCOS who are not obese.

Etiology

Endocrine Findings

Polycystic ovary syndrome is characterized by menstrual irregularities ranging from amenorrhea or oligomenorrhea, to abnormal uterine bleeding. An androgen-excess state is present, leading to hirsutism and acne with rare mild virilization.

Hyperandrogenism

- Androstenedione and dehydroepiandrosterone sulfate (DHEAS): Elevated serum levels
- Testosterone: Often minimally elevated total serum levels are seen, with elevated free (unbound) testosterone

In females with a primary diagnosis of PCOS, the source of excess androgens may be secretion from the ovaries, the adrenal gland, or both. Two other sources contribute to androgen excess:

a. Androstenedione is converted peripherally in adipose tissue to testosterone.

b. There is a decrease in binding of testosterone to sex hormone–binding globulin (SHBG). Healthy females have approximately 96% of their testosterone bound to SHBG, where it is inactive, whereas patients with PCOS have only 92% of their testosterone bound; therefore, there is a larger percentage of free and active testosterone in patients with PCOS.

Pathophysiology

The exact initiating cause of PCOS is not known, but may be related to the following:

1. Abnormal hypothalamic–pituitary function
2. Abnormal ovarian function
3. Abnormal adrenal androgen metabolism
4. Insulin resistance: Insulin resistance may exist in females with PCOS who are of normal weight or who have obesity, and the hyperinsulinism that ensues may promote the hyperandrogenic state.

Factors leading to the development of PCOS include the following:

1. Insulin resistance at the time of puberty contributing to a relative hyperinsulinemic state
2. Insulin and IGF-1 have mitogenic effects on the ovaries, causing theca-cell hyperplasia, which leads to excessive androgen production. Hyperinsulinemia has been directly correlated with a decrease in hepatic production of insulin-like growth factor–binding protein 1 (IGFBP1). The decrease in bound IGF-1 results in an increase in free IGF-1. The increase in IGF-1 and the decrease in IGFBP1 have both been found to correlate with increases in adrenal and ovarian androgens, resulting in the clinical presentation of premature adrenarche and PCOS.[11] Therefore, both high IGF-1 levels and low IGFBP1 levels may correlate with early insulin resistance and be pathophysiologically and clinically linked to the progression to PCOS and insulin resistance.
3. The increased ovarian androgen levels cause follicular atresia, impairing E2 production.
4. The combination of theca cell hyperplasia and arrested follicular maturation constitutes the typical histologic features of PCOS.
5. Because not all adolescents ultimately develop PCOS, it is thought that there is a genetic factor involved. Genetic studies of family clusters have shown a high incidence of affected relatives, with high inheritance rates.[11] Current research has demonstrated that there are approximately 14 genetic loci significantly associated with the development of PCOS. Notably, there are also shared biologic pathways between PCOS and a number of metabolic disorders, menopause, depression, and male-pattern baldness. However, a specific genetic profile has yet to be validated.
6. Valproate can also induce menstrual disturbances, polycystic ovaries, and hyperandrogenism. First described in 1993, it is well documented that females on valproate acid have increased rates of polycystic ovaries and hyperandrogenism. Young ovaries seem more susceptible to this drug.[13]

Clinical Consequences

Polycystic ovary syndrome can present with many signs and symptoms:

1. *Anovulation*: Anovulation is a key feature. Usually, the anovulation in PCOS is chronic and presents as either oligomenorrhea or amenorrhea of perimenarchal onset. Some females who report normal menses may be anovulatory. Few females with PCOS have normal ovulatory function.
2. *Polycystic ovaries*: The ovaries in patients with PCOS are usually enlarged, pearly white, sclerotic with multiple (20 to 100) cystic follicles. Normally, follicles develop to approximately 19 to 20 mm and then ovulation occurs. In AYAs with PCOS, multiple follicles develop, but only to approximately 9 to 10 mm in size. Histologically, the ovaries have the same number of primordial follicles, but the number of atretic follicles is doubled. Also, there is an absence of corpora lutea. The polycystic ovary is a sign, not a disease entity on its own. The typical histologic changes of the polycystic ovary can be seen in ovaries of any size. A sonographic spectrum exists within patients

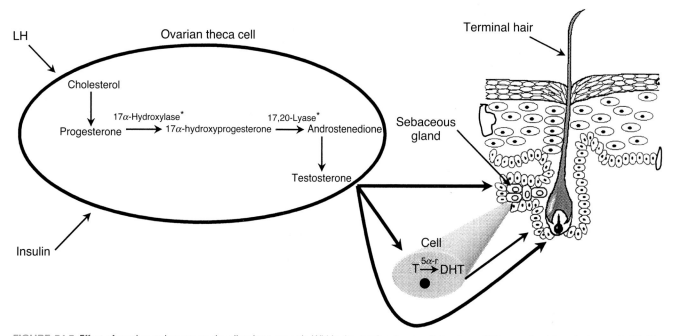

FIGURE 54.5 Effect of ovarian androgens on the pilosebaceous unit. Within the ovarian theca cell, insulin and LH may stimulate cytochrome P-450c17α activity, resulting in increased 17α-hydroxylase and 17,20-lyase activity, as denoted by *asterisks*. These two enzymes comprise the P-450c17α complex. Ovarian testosterone, along with DHT from 5α-reductase within the pilosebaceous unit, stimulates the androgen receptors at the hair follicle and sebaceous glands. Hirsutism and acne can result. (From Gordon CM. Menstrual disorders in adolescents: excess androgens and the polycystic ovary syndrome. *Pediatr Clin North Am.* 1999;46:519–543, with permission.)

with PCOS, and polycystic ovaries on ultrasound are not by themselves sufficient for diagnosis of PCOS.

3. *Hyperandrogenism/hirsutism*: Hyperandrogenism is a key feature of PCOS. Hyperandrogenism in PCOS is caused by a combination of ovarian and adrenal androgens and may include hirsutism, as well as treatment resistant severe acne. Hirsutism is defined as increased growth of terminal (long, coarse, and pigmented) hair in a young female, more than is cosmetically acceptable in a certain culture. The condition commonly refers to an increase in length and coarseness of the hair, in a male pattern, including predominantly midline hair of the upper lip, chin, cheeks, inner thighs, lower back, and periareolar, sternal, abdominal, and intergluteal regions. The effects of sex hormones and other factors on hair development and distribution can be more easily understood by considering the pilosebaceous unit (Fig. 54.5). The clinical manifestations of androgen excess vary depending on end-organ sensitivity to androgens. Hirsutism can result either from overproduction or increased sensitivity of hair follicles to androgens. Terminal hair growth is stimulated by the increased conversion of testosterone to dihydrotestosterone (DHT) from excess 5α-reductase within this unit or the presence of more numerous hair follicles. Androgens are synthesized from the ovary or adrenals from steroidogenic pathways within each gland (Fig. 54.6). Clinical hirsutism may not occur in all females with PCOS, but females with PCOS have elevated blood androgen levels.

4. *Obesity*: Originally, obesity was regarded as a classic feature, but its presence is extremely variable and not mandatory for diagnosis. Approximately 40% to 50% of females and adolescents with PCOS are obese. Obesity in females with PCOS is usually of the android type, with increased waist–hip ratios. Obesity with PCOS also worsens insulin resistance and increases cardiovascular risk. In females with obesity, weight loss may improve and/or cure the signs and symptoms of PCOS.

5. *Infertility*: Although infertility may not be a current concern to the adolescent patient, the risk is significantly elevated due to anovulation.

6. *Cancer risk*: There is an increased risk for cancer of the endometrium due to prolonged unopposed estrogen stimulation of the endometrial lining from chronic anovulation. There may also be an increased risk of breast cancer associated with chronic anovulation during the reproductive years.

7. *Elevated lipoprotein profile*: The abnormalities in females with PCOS include elevated levels of cholesterol, triglycerides, and low-density lipoprotein cholesterol (LDL-C) and lower levels of HDL-C and apolipoprotein A-1. Although hyperandrogenism plays some role in these changes, hyperinsulinemia (insulin resistance) and increased inflammatory cytokines probably have a larger effect.

8. *Insulin resistance and hyperinsulinemia*: Both are well-recognized features of PCOS and associated with many of the late complications of PCOS. Approximately 50% of females with

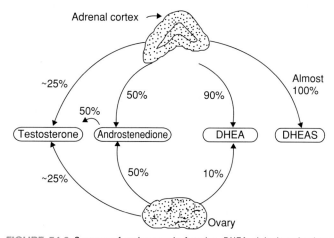

FIGURE 54.6 Sources of androgens in females. DHEA, dehydroepiandrosterone; DHEAS, dehydroepiandrosterone sulfate. (From Emans SJ. Androgen abnormalities in the adolescent girl. In: *Pediatric and Adolescent Gynecology.* 7th ed. Lippincott Williams & Wilkin; 2019, with permission.)

PCOS are insulin resistant. Although insulin resistance is associated with obesity, it can also be found in females with PCOS who are of normal weight.

9. *Impaired glucose tolerance and diabetes*: Females and adolescents with PCOS are at increased risk for impaired glucose tolerance and overt type 2 diabetes mellitus because of the insulin resistance. Similar to insulin resistance, impaired glucose tolerance has been seen in both adolescents with obesity and of normal weight.[14]

10. *Cardiovascular disease*: Because of the prevalence of the risk factors listed previously, females with PCOS may be at long-term risk for increased cardiovascular disease. In addition, it appears these risks start in adolescence with one study demonstrating adolescent females having greater carotid intima–media thickness and stiffer arteries than females without PCOS.[15]

Differential Diagnosis

1. Familial hirsutism and/or increased sensitivity to normal androgen levels
2. Androgen-producing ovarian and adrenal tumors
3. Cushing syndrome: Cushing syndrome is usually excluded by history and physical examination, and if needed, a 24-hour urine collection for free cortisol, midnight salivary cortisol, or an overnight dexamethasone suppression test can be done.
4. Congenital adrenal hyperplasia: A late-onset 21-hydroxylase deficiency can mimic PCOS. The diagnosis of CAH is based on elevated early morning serum 17-OHP level, or level after ACTH stimulation testing.

Diagnosis

Criteria for the diagnosis of PCOS include the following:

1. *Irregular menses:* Chronic anovulation with a perimenarcheal onset of menstrual irregularities is classic and can present as oligomenorrhea, primary or secondary amenorrhea.
2. *Hyperandrogenism with or without skin manifestations:* Biochemical or clinical evidence of androgen excess. Serum-free testosterone level is the best marker for ovarian causes of hyperandrogenism and DHEAS is the best marker of adrenal sources.
3. *Absence of other causes of hyperandrogenism*

The following are not needed for diagnosis, but are supportive evidence of the diagnosis:

1. *Polycystic ovaries*: The Androgen Excess and PCOS Society updated recommendations in 2013 regarding ultrasound evaluation.[11] The meta-analysis and expert opinion concluded that follicle number per ovary in adult females ($\geq$25) was the best diagnostic criteria using high-resolution ultrasound. Ovarian volume should be used if high-resolution studies are not available. The use of anti-müllerian hormone concentrations to assess ovarian function instead of ultrasound has been proposed. However, the lack of standardized assays and variability in adolescents limit the utility at this time. Furthermore, more recent recommendations[9,12] do not support the use of ovarian morphology in the diagnosis of PCOS in adolescents.
2. *Increased body weight*: Body mass index (BMI) >30 kg/m² in adults or >85th percentile in children, based on standardized U.S. Centers for Disease Control and Prevention growth curves.
3. *Elevated LH and FSH levels*: Although LH and FSH levels have been used, the sensitivity and specificity of these hormones are low.
4. Prolactin: Most individuals with PCOS have reference-range levels of prolactin, although 4% to 20% have mildly elevated levels.[16] Prolactin may augment adrenal androgen secretion in this subset of patients.

Therapy

1. Medroxyprogesterone acetate (10 mg) can be given for 10 days every 1 to 3 months to induce withdrawal bleeding, or estrogen and progestins can be given as oral contraceptive pills or E2 patches with progesterone administered orally. Having a withdrawal bleed at least every 3 months prevents endometrial hyperplasia, which could lead to irregular, heavy bleeding.
2. Insulin-sensitizing agents, specifically metformin, should be considered as first-line therapy, particularly in adolescent females with clinical (acanthosis nigricans, Fig. 54.4) or biochemical evidence of hyperinsulinism or dysglycemia.
3. Weight loss in females with PCOS and obesity reduces insulin resistance and insulin levels, thereby reducing testosterone secretion and PCOS symptoms. Lifestyle modification with dietary and activity interventions should be the initial intervention in females with obesity and PCOS. However, weight loss is difficult to achieve. Older AYAs with morbid obesity (BMI >40 kg/m² or BMI >35 kg/m²) and secondary complications, such as hypertension, sleep apnea, cardiovascular disease, and PCOS, may be candidates for medication use and/or surgical weight-loss therapy.
4. Infertility may not always be brought up initially as a concern by an AYA although many may worry about their future fertility.[17] When fertility is desired, clomiphene citrate and/or metformin therapy may be used to stimulate ovulation. Exogenous gonadotropins are also used in research and clinical practice.

Therapy for Hirsutism

Therapies outlined above including estrogen and progestin, weight loss, and metformin may improve hirsutism. Other therapies include:

1. *Cosmetic approaches*: Camouflaging with makeup, bleaching, and removal with physical methods such as shaving, plucking, or waxing may be used by adolescents to hide undesired hair. Chemical depilatories are designed to use on specific body locations. Electrolysis or thermodestruction of the hair follicle retards regrowth for days to weeks and can permanently remove hair. Photothermodestruction with a laser is expensive but can offer long periods between regrowth and can lead to permanent hair loss. All of these methods can cause skin irritation, folliculitis, and pigment abnormalities.
2. *Topical therapy*: Eflornithine hydrochloride 13.9% cream has been approved by the U.S. Food and Drug Administration for the treatment of unwanted facial hair. The agent is an irreversible inhibitor of L-ornithine decarboxylase, an enzyme that is important in controlling hair growth and proliferation, although this treatment is not always covered by insurance as it may be considered a cosmetic treatment. The agent slows and miniaturizes hairs that are present. Side effects can include rash and stinging, and occurred in <10% of patients in early trials.
3. *Antiandrogenic agents:* The addition of spironolactone can be considered for significant clinical hyperandrogenism unresponsive to estrogen/progestin therapy. Spironolactone works primarily by competing at the androgen receptor peripherally, and also inhibits 5α-reductase. The starting dose is usually 50 mg/day and is typically effective between approximately 75 and 200 mg/day. The medication can be increased by 25 mg every 1 to 2 weeks. However, the maximal response is not seen for 6 months to 1 year. Side effects are minimal but can include dry mouth, diuresis, fatigue, menstrual spotting, and may induce hyperkalemia on laboratory evaluation, although this remains an area of investigation.[18] The drug is contraindicated during pregnancy, because it can lead to the feminization of the male fetus. Therefore, a contraceptive should be prescribed simultaneously, which can also help prevent irregular bleeding.

Screening and Therapy for Metabolic Abnormalities

Because of the potential for abnormal glucose tolerance (insulin resistance) and hyperlipidemia, even in individuals of normal weight,[14] it is important to evaluate these factors in AYAs with PCOS and to consider therapeutic interventions. Many clinicians and scientists favor the treatment of insulin resistance in females with PCOS with insulin-sensitizing medications because the reduction of hyperandrogenism by hormonal therapy does not correct the underlying hyperinsulinism. The use of insulin-sensitizing agents such as metformin may reduce the risk of hyperinsulinism, type 2 diabetes, and the metabolic syndrome.[19] In addition, the reduction in hyperinsulinism has been shown to induce ovulation and regulation of menstrual cycling.[19] Studies have shown that the use of metformin in young adolescents with PCOS may regulate menstrual cycling and reduce the clinical hyperandrogenic effects especially in AYAs with PCOS and BMI ≥25 kg/m², as well as high-metabolic–risk groups such as certain ethnicities and individuals at increased risk of type 2 diabetes.[11,12] In addition, metformin may be able to prevent the development of the PCOS phenotype in young females with premature adrenarche.[19] These remain areas of active research.

Young females with PCOS should have their cholesterol, triglycerides, LDL, and HDL measured, according to the guidelines for high-risk children and AYAs. In addition, these females should be checked and followed for impaired glucose tolerance and diabetes. The screening evaluation for abnormal glucose metabolism is an area of continued debate. The current American Diabetes Association recommendations for pediatric diabetes screening include the evaluation of a fasting blood sugar every 2 years, beginning at age 10 years or puberty, in all children who are overweight, as defined by a BMI of greater than the 85th percentile for age and sex, weight for height >85th percentile, or weight >120% of ideal for height plus any one of the designated risk factors:

- Family history of type 2 diabetes mellitus in a first- or second-degree relative
- Maternal history of diabetes or gestational diabetes during the child's gestation
- High-risk race/ethnicity (native American, African American, Hispanic, Asian/Pacific Islander)
- Signs of insulin resistance or conditions associated with insulin resistance (acanthosis nigricans, hypertension, dyslipidemia, PCOS)

Polycystic ovary syndrome is listed as a condition associated with insulin resistance, and therefore, the diagnosis of PCOS in an AYA who is obese and has a family history of diabetes or a high-risk ethnicity meets the criteria for a fasting blood glucose screening. However, there is growing evidence that AYAs who are lean with PCOS may also be at risk for insulin resistance and that both females who are lean and who are obese with PCOS may benefit from oral glucose-tolerance testing (oral glucose challenge of 1.75 g/kg up to a maximum of 75 g). The use of HgbA1C (≥6.5%), as a screening tool for diabetes, was agreed upon by an International Expert Committee in 2009. However, the use of HgbA1C remains an area of research in this population. The absence of obesity and acanthosis nigricans does not rule out insulin resistance in the presence of clinical hyperandrogenism. Diagnosis and continued monitoring of these individuals may reduce the risk of metabolic and cardiovascular disease. Reduction in insulin resistance is important, and diet and exercise are critical first-line steps. Insulin-sensitizing medications, specifically metformin as above, may prove to be beneficial. Current guidelines suggest it be considered for adolescents with PCOS.[9,12] Patients with PCOS should be treated medically for diabetes mellitus and hyperlipidemia, if diagnosed, as standard for AYA patients.

Polycystic ovary syndrome is a common endocrinopathy that often presents during adolescence. Recent guidelines for the diagnosis of PCOS in adolescents focus on irregular menses, and biochemical or clinical evidence of androgen excess in the absence of other causes. Although used frequently in the past, pelvic ultrasound findings are no longer considered a diagnostic criterion for adolescents. As PCOS is often associated with long-term comorbidities and can affect health-related quality of life, early and accurate diagnosis is vital. Treatment for PCOS should be holistic and comprehensive, with a focus on preventing long-term complications while catering to the adolescent's concerns. Associated metabolic abnormalities should also be screened for and appropriately treated.

HIRSUTISM

Differential Diagnosis

The differential diagnosis for hirsutism is presented in **Table 54.1**, with data obtained from a sample of more than 1,000 premenopausal females that had hyperandrogenemia.[20] Note that PCOS is the most common cause of androgen excess and one of the most common endocrine abnormalities in female AYAs. Other causes may include the following:

1. Idiopathic hirsutism
2. Ovarian causes
   a. Tumor: Sertoli–Leydig cell tumor, lipoid cell tumor, hilar cell tumor
   b. Pregnancy: Luteoma
3. Adrenal causes
   a. Congenital adrenal hyperplasia: 21-hydroxylase or 11-hydroxylase deficiency, classic or nonclassic, late onset
   b. Tumors: Adenomas and carcinomas
   c. Cushing syndrome
4. Nonandrogenic causes of hirsutism
   a. Genetic: Racial, familial
   b. Physiologic: Pregnancy, puberty, postmenopausal
   c. Endocrine: Hypothyroidism, acromegaly
   d. Porphyria
   e. Hamartomas
   f. Drug induced: Drugs that cause hirsutism by increasing androgenic activity include testosterone, DHEAS, danazol, corticotropin, high-dose corticosteroids, metyrapone, phenothiazine derivatives, anabolic steroids, androgenic progestin, and acetazolamide. Nonandrogenic drugs that can cause hirsutism include cyclosporine, phenytoin, diazoxide, triamterene-hydrochlorothiazide, hexachlorobenzene, penicillamine and psoralens, and minoxidil. Valproate is also associated with menstrual disturbances and hyperandrogenism.
   g. Syndromes: Hurler syndrome, de Lange syndrome

Indications for Further Evaluation

1. Rapid onset of signs and symptoms
2. Virilization
3. Symptoms suggesting Cushing syndrome (e.g., weight gain, slow linear growth, weakness, or hypertension)

Evaluation

Physical Examination

1. Extent of hirsutism: Grading systems are available that enable a clinician to quantitate the degree of hirsutism in a patient. The Ferriman–Gallwey hirsutism scoring system (Fig. 54.7) enables clinicians to quantify the extent of hirsutism by circling an individual's appearance on a flow sheet and recording the total score on the patient's chart. These scores can be helpful for making comparative assessments between visits and for appraising the efficacy of a particular therapy. Some terminal hair on the lower abdomen, face, and around the areola is normal, but hair on the upper back, shoulders, sternum, and upper abdomen suggests more marked androgen activity.
2. Stigmata of Cushing syndrome (e.g., truncal obesity, striae, posterior fat pad)

TABLE 54.1

Differential Diagnosis of Clinically Apparent/Biochemical Androgen Excess

Diagnosis	Sample	Key History/Examination Findings	Additional Testing
Polycystic ovary syndrome (PCOS)	89%	+/– Irregular menses, slow-onset hirsutism, obesity, infertility, diabetes, hypertension, family history of PCOS, diabetes	Fasting glucose, insulin and lipid profile, blood pressure (BP), ultrasonography positive for multiple ovarian cysts
21-Hydroxylase nonclassic adrenal hyperplasia (late-onset CAH)	6%	Severe hirsutism or virilization, strong family history of CAH, short stature, signs of virilization, more common in Ashkenazi Jews of Eastern European descent	17-OHP level before and after ACTH stimulation test elevated, CYP21 genotyping
Androgenic secreting neoplasm	2%	Pelvic masses, rapid-onset hirsutism or virilization	Pelvic ultrasonography or abdomen/pelvic CT scan
Cushing syndrome	1%	Hypertension, buffalo hump, purple striae, truncal obesity	Elevated BP, positive urinary 24-hour free cortisol, salivary cortisol, and/or dexamethasone suppression test
Others, including:			
Hyperandrogenic insulin-resistant acanthosis nigricans (HAIR-AN)	2%	Brown velvety patches of skin (acanthosis nigricans), obesity, hypertension, hyperlipidemia, strong family history of diabetes	Fasting glucose and lipid profile, BP, fasting insulin level
Hyperandrogenism with hirsutism, normal ovulation		Regular menses, acne, hirsutism without detectable endocrine cause	Elevated androgen levels and normal serum progesterone in luteal phase
Other causes with normal androgen levels:			
Idiopathic hirsutism		Regular menses, hirsutism, possible overactive 5α-reductase activity in skin and hair follicle	Normal androgen levels, normal serum progesterone in luteal phase
Hypothyroidism		Fatigue, weight gain, history of thyroid ablation, and untreated hypothyroidism, amenorrhea	TSH elevated
Hyperprolactinemia		Amenorrhea, galactorrhea, infertility	Prolactin elevated

ACTH, adrenocorticotropic hormone; TSH, thyroid-stimulating hormone; CT, computed tomography; 17-OHP, 17-hydroxyprogesterone.

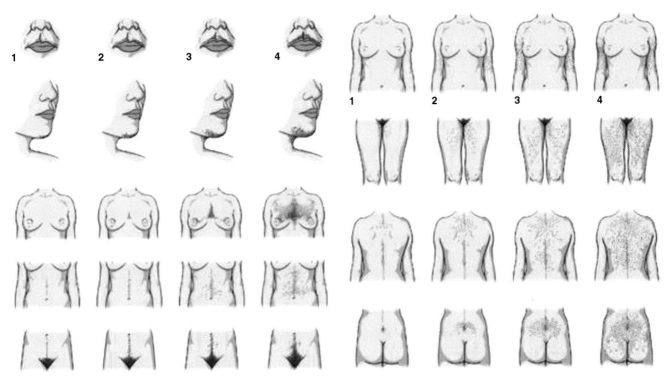

FIGURE 54.7 Ferriman–Gallwey hirsutism scoring system. Each of the nine body areas most sensitive to androgen is assigned a score from 0 (no hair) to 4 (frankly virile), and these separate scores are summed to provide a hormonal hirsutism score. (Reproduced from Hatch R, Rosefield RL, Kim MH, et al. Hirsutism: implications, etiology, and management. *Am J Obstet Gynecol.* 1981;140:815–830, ©Elsevier.)

3. Signs of virilization: Check clitoral diameter or index. A clitoral diameter >5 mm is abnormal. The clitoral index is the product of the vertical and horizontal dimensions of the glans. The normal range is 9 to 35 mm^2; a clitoral index >100 mm^2 suggests virilization. Other signs of virilization may include male-pattern baldness, voice changes, and possibly male-pattern muscular changes.

Laboratory Evaluation

The goals of the laboratory evaluation include demonstrating androgen excess and locating the source of the excess.

1. Measuring androgen excess
   a. Plasma testosterone (free and total)
   b. Dehydroepiandrosterone sulfate: Levels >700 mcg/dL suggest significant adrenal androgen production. An adrenal tumor should be ruled out. However, PCOS, CAH, or an ovarian tumor can result in levels this high.
   c. 17-hydroxyprogesterone: This hormone should only be measured in the morning (ideally between 7 and 9 AM). This is characteristically elevated in patients with CAH due to 21-hydroxylase deficiency. One can also measure 11-deoxycortisol in the morning to rule out 11-hydroxylase deficiency if suspected clinically.
2. Locating the source of androgen excess
   a. If male levels of testosterone or very elevated DHEAS levels are obtained, or a mass is felt on examination, perform an ultrasonography or MRI scan of adrenal glands and ovaries.
   b. If elevated androgen levels and signs suggest hypercortisolism, perform a screening for Cushing syndrome: 24-hour urine for free cortisol or midnight salivary cortisol. This can be followed by a dexamethasone suppression test.
      • An ovarian source is suggested by cortisol suppression, but a lack of androgen suppression. An ultrasonography of the ovaries is helpful in this instance.
      • Cushing syndrome or an adrenal tumor is suggested by lack of cortisol suppression.
   c. If 17-OHP level is elevated but nondiagnostic, an ACTH stimulation test is recommended. This is helpful in differentiating normal and idiopathic hirsute females from those with late-onset CAH due to incomplete 21-hydroxylase deficiency.

To perform the test, measure a baseline 17-OHP and repeat a serum level 60 minutes after 0.25 mg of ACTH is administered intravenously. This test can also be used to rule out less common forms of late-onset CAH due to 11-hydroxylase or 3β-hydroxysteroid dehydrogenase deficiency by measuring the appropriate adrenal hormone values pre- and poststimulation.

Therapeutic considerations for hirsutism are discussed above under PCOS therapy.

◗ SUMMARY

The differential diagnosis of primary and secondary amenorrhea is broad, but can be due to specific genetic abnormalities, enzymatic defects, hormone imbalances, or structural abnormalities. A thorough and thoughtful approach can usually identify the cause and treatment can then be catered to the patient, as needed. Often, decreased energy availability due to reduced intake or increased exercise is a cause of irregular menses in AYAs. Polycystic ovary syndrome is another common cause of irregular menses and consists of clinical and laboratory hyperandrogenism and dysregulated menses. Polycystic ovaries are often associated with the syndrome, although this is no longer a diagnostic criterion in recent guidelines. Metabolic abnormalities are commonly associated with this syndrome and should be screened for and treated appropriately. Hirsutism may be associated with PCOS, but may also be seen in other conditions that cause hyperandrogenism.

REFERENCES

1. Practice Committee of the American Society for Reproductive Medicine. Current evaluation of amenorrhea. *Fertil Steril.* 2006;86(5 Suppl1):S148–S155.
2. Biro FM, Pajak A, Wolff MS, et al. Age of menarche in a longitudinal US cohort. *J Pediatr Adolesc Gynecol.* 2018;31(4):339–345.
3. Gordon CM, Ackerman KE, Berga SL, et al. Functional hypothalamic amenorrhea: An Endocrine Society Clinical Practice Guideline. *J Clin Endocrinol Metab.* 2017;102(5):1413–1439.
4. França MM, Mendonca BB. Genetics of primary ovarian insufficiency in the next-generation sequencing era. *J Endocr Soc.* 2019;4(2):bvz037.
5. Silveira LFG, Latronico AC. Approach to the patient with hypogonadotropic hypogonadism. *J Clin Endocrinol Metab.* 2013;98(5):1781–1788.
6. Mountjoy M, Sundgot-Borgen J, Burke L, et al. The IOC Consensus Statement: Beyond the Female Athlete Triad–Relative Energy Deficiency in Sport (RED-S). *Br J Sports Med.* 2014;48(7):491–497.
7. Klein KO, Phillips SA. Review of hormone replacement therapy in girls and adolescents with hypogonadism. *J Pediatr Adolesc Gynecol.* 2019;32(5):460–468.
8. DiVasta AD, Feldman HA, O'Donnell JM, et al. Impact of Adrenal Hormone Supplementation on bone geometry in growing teens with anorexia nervosa. *J Adolesc Health.* 2019;65(4):462–468.
9. Peña AS, Witchel SF, Hoeger KM, et al. Adolescent polycystic ovary syndrome according to the international evidence-based guideline. *BMC Med.* 2020;18(1):72.
10. Trent ME, Rich M, Austin SB, et al. Quality of life in adolescent girls with polycystic ovary syndrome. *Arch Pediatr Adolesc Med.* 2002;156(6):556–560.
11. Rosenfield RL. The diagnosis of polycystic ovary syndrome in adolescents. *Pediatrics.* 2015;136(6):1154–1165.
12. Witchel SF, Oberfield SE, Peña AS. Polycystic ovary syndrome: Pathophysiology, presentation, and treatment with emphasis on adolescent girls. *J Endocr Soc.* 2019;3(8):1545–1573.
13. Svalheim S, Sveberg L, Mochol M, et al. Interactions between antiepileptic drugs and hormones. *Seizure.* 2015;28:12–17.
14. Flannery CA, Rackow B, Cong X, et al. Polycystic ovary syndrome in adolescence: Impaired glucose tolerance occurs across the spectrum of BMI. *Pediatr Diabetes.* 2013;14(1):42–49.
15. Patel SS, Truong U, King M, et al. Obese adolescents with polycystic ovarian syndrome have elevated cardiovascular disease risk markers. *Vasc Med.* 2017;22(2):85–95.
16. Delcour C, Robin G, Young J, et al.. PCOS and hyperprolactinemia: what do we know in 2019?. *Clin Med Insights Reprod Health.* 2019;13:1179558119871921.
17. Trent ME, Rich M, Austin SB, et al. Fertility concerns and sexual behavior in adolescent girls with polycystic ovary syndrome: implications for quality of life. *J Pediatr Adolesc Gynecol.* 2003;16(1):33–37.
18. Millington K, Liu E, Chan YM. The utility of potassium monitoring in gender-diverse adolescents taking spironolactone. *J Endocr Soc.* 2019;3(5):1031–1038.
19. Carreau AM, Baillargeon JP. PCOS in adolescence and type 2 diabetes. *Curr Diab Rep.* 2015;15(1):564.
20. Elhassan YS, Idkowiak J, Smith K, et al. Causes, patterns, and severity of androgen excess in 1205 consecutively recruited women. *J Clin Endocrinol Metab.* 2018;103(3):1214–1223.

📶 ADDITIONAL RESOURCES AND WEBSITES

Additional Resources and Websites for Clinicians:

Ackerman KE, Singhal V, Baskaran C, et al. Oestrogen replacement improves bone mineral density in oligoamenorrhoeic athletes: A randomized clinical trial. *Br J Sports Med.* 2019;53(4):229–236.

The American College of Obstetricians and Gynecologists Committee Opinion. Primary ovarian insufficiency in adolescents and young women. *Am Coll Obstet Gynecol.* 2014;20(5):245–247.

American Diabetes Association. 2. Classification and diagnosis of diabetes: standards of medical care in diabetes–2021. *Diabetes Care.* 2021;44(Suppl 1):S15–S33.

Bordini B, Rosenfield RL. Normal pubertal development: part II: clinical aspects of puberty. *Pediatr Rev.* 2011;32(7):281–292.

Ferriman D, Gallwey JD. Clinical assessment of body hair growth in women. *J Clin Endocrinol Metab.* 1961;21:1440–1447.

Ibáñez L, Díaz M, García-Beltrán C, et al. Toward a treatment normalizing ovulation rate in adolescent girls with polycystic ovary syndrome. *J Endocr Soc.* 2020;4(5):bvaa032.

Ibáñez L, Oberfield SE, Witchel S, et al. An international consortium update: Pathophysiology, diagnosis, and treatment of polycystic ovarian syndrome in adolescence. *Horm Res Paediatr.* 2017;88(6):371–395.

Weiss Kelly AK, Hecht S; COUNCIL ON SPORTS MEDICINE AND FITNESS. The Female Athlete Triad. *Pediatrics.* 2016;138(2):e20160922.

Additional Resources and Websites for Parents/Caregivers:

Center for Young Women's Health—https://youngwomenshealth.org/

HealthyChildren.org—From the American Academy of Pediatrics—https://www.healthychildren.org/English/Pages/default.aspx

Nemours KidsHealth—the Web's most visited site about children's health—https://kidshealth.org/en/teens/pcos.html

PCOS Awareness Association | Hormone Health Network—https://www.hormone.org/support-and-resources/peer-support-groups/pcos-awareness-association

PCOS Resources | NICHD—Eunice Kennedy Shriver National Institute of Child Health and Human Development—https://www.nichd.nih.gov/health/topics/pcos/more_information/resources

Additional Resources and Websites for Adolescents and Young Adults:

Center for Young Women's Health—https://youngwomenshealth.org/

HealthyChildren.org—From the American Academy of Pediatrics—https://www.healthychildren.org/English/health-issues/conditions/obesity/Pages/Polycystic-Ovary-Syndrome.aspx

Nemours KidsHealth—the Web's most visited site about children's health—https://kidshealth.org/en/teens/pcos.html

Polycystic Ovary Syndrome (PCOS) (for Teens)—Nemours KidsHealth—https://kidshealth.org/en/teens/pcos.html

Polycystic Ovary Syndrome PCOS for Teens | Hormone Health Network—https://www.hormone.org/diseases-and-conditions/polycystic-ovary-syndrome-pcos-for-teens

CHAPTER 55

Cervical Cancer Screening and Management of Abnormal Tests

Anna-Barbara Moscicki

KEY WORDS

- Cervical cancer screening
- Cytology
- Human papillomavirus

INTRODUCTION

Cervical cancer remains the second leading cause of cancer-associated deaths in individuals assigned female at birth worldwide. The burden is mainly in low- to middle-income countries due to lack of adequate screening. This will remain a problem since access to the human papillomavirus (HPV) vaccine is financially unattainable for many affected countries. In comparison, cervical cancer screening in the United States significantly impacted cervical cancer cases. Although screening resulted in dramatic decreases over the last 50 years, screening rates have plateaued over the last two decades. This plateau has been attributed to cytology limitations, which had been considered the mainstay of cervical cancer screening. The approach to screening has changed with a greater understanding of the natural history of HPV and the development of new, more sensitive technologies. In addition, the performance of screening is most likely to be influenced by several factors, specifically the female's HPV vaccination status. The influential role of other factors associated with increased cervical cancer risk, such as smoking cigarettes or prolonged oral contraceptive use, is less clear. This chapter will review (1) the natural history of HPV from infection to the development of precancer lesions to cervical cancer, (2) how cervical cancer screening can be implemented to decrease cervical cancer rates while minimizing false-positive tests resulting in unnecessary procedures, and (3) the current cervical cancer screening strategies and risk-based management of abnormal test results.

PREVALENCE OF ABNORMAL CERVICAL CANCER SCREENING TESTS

The prevalence of abnormal cytology peaks in female adolescents and young adults (AYAs) in the United States, with rates ranging from 3% to 14%.[1] This is not surprising since this parallels the peak prevalence of HPV of around 25% to 41% among females <25 years in the United States and Europe.[2,3] The high rates of HPV and abnormal cytology underscore the vulnerability of AYAs to HPV. It is estimated that over 60% of female AYAs will acquire HPV at least once within 3 to 5 years after the onset of sexual intercourse.[4] Repeated infections are also common in female AYAs, with 70% to 80% acquiring second and third infections within 3 years of the initial infection.[5] Infection with multiple HPV types is also common. Fortunately, most of these infections and their corresponding abnormal cytology spontaneously regress.[1]

The majority of the abnormal cytology is low-grade squamous intraepithelial lesions (LSILs), which are considered benign changes due to HPV infection. These lesions are associated with both low- (nononcogenic) and high- (oncogenic) risk HPV types.[6] High-grade squamous intraepithelial lesions (HSILs) are considered true precancer lesions. Although the rates of HSILs are substantially lower than those of LSILs in AYAs, the prevalence of both of these lesions peaks in female AYAs less than 30 years of age.[1] The prevalence of cytologic LSIL and HSIL among 21- to 24-year-olds is 6.5% and 0.7%, respectively, and among 25- to 29-year-olds is 3.8% and 0.4%.[7] Because of the insensitive nature of cytology, the actual rates of histologic HSIL[8] are higher than reported by cytology. In one large study, the prevalence of histologic (h) HSIL was 1.3% and 2.1% in 21- to 24-year-olds and 25- to 29-year-olds, respectively.[7] Age also influences the natural history of HSIL. High-grade squamous intraepithelial lesions in female AYAs are much more likely to regress spontaneously than in older female patients. One study of female AYAs aged 13 to 24 years showed that 70% of biopsy-proven HSIL regressed over 3 years.[9] Of those HPV 16/18 associated, 50% regressed. Several other studies of female AYAs showed similar results.[10] Although the reasons for this are not completely clear, HSIL likely develops relatively quickly after infection in cells vulnerable to dysplasia. Consequently, HSIL in a young female likely represents a relatively recent abnormality when the chances of clearance are the greatest. High-grade squamous intraepithelial lesions detected in older females are far more likely due to a long-term persistent infection that the immune system fails to clear.[11]

Impact of Human Papillomavirus Vaccination on Abnormal Cytology Rates

Human papillomavirus vaccination has had a profound impact on hHSIL rates. Recent data from a meta-analysis showed that in areas where HPV vaccination programs have been implemented, rates of hHSIL have decreased by 51% in 15- to 19-year-old girls.[12] The most significant reductions observed were in those populations with high vaccine coverage in populations most likely to have not initiated sexual activity as the vaccine is preventative and not therapeutic. For example, a recent publication from Scotland, which implemented vaccination with the bivalent vaccine, found the prevalence of HSIL among a highly vaccinated population to be less than 0.2%.[13] A recent report from Sweden showed a decrease of around 90% in cervical cancer in those vaccinated before age 17 years.[14] Human papillomavirus vaccines were introduced in the United States in 2007. Currently, the vaccine is licensed for females and males aged 9 to 45 years for indications that include prevention of cervical, vulvar, vaginal, anal, and oropharyngeal cancers, and anogenital warts. In the United States, screening is targeted to ages 9 to 12 years with subsequent makeup vaccination for older AYAs aged up to 26 years.

VULNERABILITY OF THE CERVIX TO HUMAN PAPILLOMAVIRUS

The cervical transformation zone (TZ) is critical in cervical cancer development. It is useful to review the formation of this zone and the natural history of HPV in understanding abnormal cervical changes.[15]

In Utero and Prepuberty

During embryologic development, the müllerian ducts give rise to the fallopian tubes, uterus, and vagina. These structures in the fetus are lined by immature cuboidal epithelium (which becomes columnar epithelium) from the uterus to the hymenal ring. The urogenital sinus epithelium grows up the vaginal vault and replaces the native epithelium up to the ectocervix with squamous epithelium. This replacement is usually incomplete, creating an abrupt squamocolumnar junction (SCJ) on the ectocervix. Squamous metaplasia is a process during which undifferentiated columnar cells transform themselves into squamous epithelium. However, the process is relatively quiescent until puberty, resulting in minimal changes to the SCJ during childhood. The area of columnar epithelium seen on the ectocervix is referred to as *ectopy*.

Pubertal Metaplastic Changes

With puberty, the pH level of the vagina drops. This is thought to be secondary to rising levels of estrogen, which enhances glycogen production of the squamous cells and in turn provides a source of energy for the vaginal flora, specifically lactobacilli. Lactobacilli convert glycogen to lactic acids, resulting in a lowered pH level. This new acidic environment most likely contributes to the augmentation of the squamous metaplastic process, resulting in relatively rapid replacement of columnar epithelium by squamous epithelium, hence referred to as the TZ (Fig. 55.1).

The TZ represents the area between the original SCJ and the current SCJ. By the early 30s, most female patients have substantial replacement of their columnar epithelium, resulting in little to

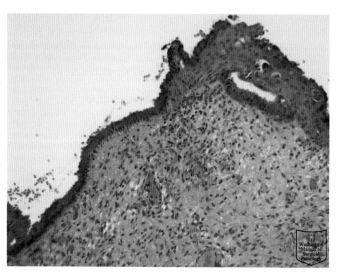

FIGURE 55.1 Replacement of cervical columnar epithelium by squamous epithelium (the transformation zone). (From Pfeifer JD, Dehner PD, Humphrey PA. *Washington Manual of Surgical Pathology*. Lippincott Williams & Wilkins; 2019.)

no visible ectopy. Although squamous metaplasia continues, it is now found well inside the endocervical canal.

Squamous epithelium is generally 60 to 80 cell layers thick and appears smooth and pink, covering the vagina and a portion of the ectocervix. The *columnar epithelium* is a single-layer, mucus-producing, tall epithelium extending between the endometrium and the squamous epithelium. This thin layer results in a red appearance due to its increased vascularity and has an irregular surface with long papillae and deep clefts. During puberty, the TZ is a combination of the squamous and columnar epithelium and metaplastic tissue. The hallmark of metaplasia seen on magnification includes fusion of the villi, causing a loss of translucency to the columnar epithelium. Eventually, the papillary structures are lost, and the new surface takes on a less translucent appearance, more similar to the squamous epithelium. As this process is somewhat piecemeal, the examiner can often see remnants of columnar epithelium in small pockets. When these openings become completely closed by the squamous epithelium, the mucus-secreting epithelium may continue to produce mucus. If that mucus becomes inspissated, the gland dilates, and a *nabothian cyst* results which is benign. However, nabothian cysts eventually self-destruct from the pressure of the inspissated mucus.

Metaplasia and Human Papillomavirus Infections

The vulnerability of the cervix to HPV infections is most likely related to the process of squamous metaplasia, which is most active during adolescents and young adulthood.[16] It is estimated that 75% of causal HPV infections associated with cancer development occur before the age of 30 years.[17] This association reflects the natural life cycle of HPV and its dependence on host-cell proliferation and differentiation, both characteristics of squamous metaplasia. Initial HPV infections require access to basal cells through inflammation or trauma. Recent data suggest that junctional stem cells, which are programmed to undergo the cellular transformation associated with squamous metaplasia are key to the development of cancer in part due to the longevity of these stem cells.[18] Differentiation of these basal cells to well-differentiated squamous epithelial cells supports HPV replication by allowing expression of certain viral proteins at different layers of differentiation. The expression of the oncogenic proteins E_6 and E_7 causes histologic changes, including abnormal cell proliferation, and the appearance of abnormal mitotic figures, both features of SIL. Features that are mild and restricted to the basal and parabasal areas are classified as LSIL. When these features become more extensive and extend into the upper half of the epithelium, the changes are classified as HSIL. These changes coincide with increased expression of the oncogenes E_6 and E_7 throughout the epithelium. Although both LSIL and HSIL are pathologic changes due to HPV infection, HSIL is less likely to regress for reasons not well understood.

CERVICAL DYSPLASIA

Impact of Cofactors

Human papillomavirus infection is the causative factor for cervical SIL and cancer, and sexual behavior is the most significant risk factor for HPV infections, specifically reporting new sexual partner or having a nonmonogamous relationship.[5,19] Acquiring other sexually transmitted infections (STIs) also increases the risk, which may represent a break in the cervical barrier due to inflammation caused by the STI or reflects the "at-risk" partner. Condom use also shows some protection against HPV acquisition, underscoring important counseling messages to female and male AYAs.

The causes of cervical cancer are complex. Because the rates of HPV are 100 to 700 times more common than invasive cancers, it is assumed that HPV is necessary but insufficient for cancer development. Most HPV infections are quickly eliminated by the host's innate and adaptive immune responses.[20,21] Innate responses are likely responsible for rapid clearance, whereas cell-mediated immune responses are important in clearing established infections and offering protection from re-exposure. This immune response is likely responsible for the observation that with age, the prevalence of HPV declines. In comparison, lack of an adequate immune response results in the persistence of HPV infection, and in turn, HPV persistence is a strong risk for the development of HSIL and cervical cancer.[11] In a study of young female research participants, HPV 16 persistence at 2 years was associated with a 50% risk of cervical intraepithelial neoplasia (CIN) 3 within 12 years.[11] Human papillomavirus persistence is a common problem among persons with immunodeficiencies including human immunodeficiency virus (HIV) infection and solid organ transplants.[22,23]

Another factor associated with cancer development is tobacco exposure. Even when adjusted for the number of sex partners, patients who smoke have a higher risk of developing cervical SIL and invasive cancers than nonsmokers.[24] Other risk factors implicated include *Chlamydia trachomatis* infections, multiparity, and history of prolonged oral contraceptive use.[1,25-27] Final events leading to invasive cancer have yet to be defined. Important elements include but are not limited to viral integration into the host genome leading to overexpression of *E6* and *E7* leading to the accumulation of genetic errors resulting in the activation of numerous cancer pathways.[28] Chronic proinflammatory states of cervical tissue may also play a critical role in releasing carcinogens from damaged tissue, accelerating cellular and DNA damage as seen with other cancers.[29] There is emerging evidence that these chronic inflammatory states may be driven by cervical/vaginal microbial dysbiosis.[30-32] The *Lactobacillus crispatus*–dominated microbiome has long been considered a critical part of vaginal health. Many studies have now documented that HPV persistence and HSIL are associated with highly diverse non-*Lactobacillus* dominated microbiome.[30,33]

Cervical Screening Tests

Because HPV infections are common in female AYAs and rarely ever become cancerous before 21 years of age, screening for cervical cancer in this age group (under 21 years) is not cost-effective and leads to inappropriate treatment and potential harm.[34] Because of recent gains in knowledge using molecular markers, changes in these guidelines are undergoing rapid changes. The U.S. Preventive Services Task Force (USPSTF) updated their guidelines in 2018 to recommend using liquid-based cytology (Table 55.1) starting at age 21 years with screening at 3-year intervals.[35] At 30 years of age, screening can also include co-testing—cytology with HPV DNA or primary HPV testing with screening at 5-year intervals. The power of HPV testing is the negative predictive value—if HPV

is not present, then there is no cancer allowing for greater intervals between screening tests. Human papillomavirus testing is not recommended in younger female patients since the high rates of infection and low cancer risk result in a test with an extremely low positive predictive value. With these less frequent screening recommendations, it is essential to continue annual STI screening.

The American Cancer Society (ACS) 2020 cervical cancer screening guidelines slightly differ from the USPSTF in that they recommend screening to start at 25 years of age using U.S. Food and Drug Administration (FDA)-approved primary HPV testing.[36] This recommendation was based on data that shows co-testing with cytology adds little to the sensitivity, and the current birth cohort reaching the screening age of 21 years has exceeded 50% HPV vaccination rates of which herd protection has been demonstrated.[36,37] The rates of cervical cancer remain exceedingly low in those under 25 years of age. The ACS, however, acknowledges that FDA-approved primary HPV tests may not be widely available and therefore, in these cases, recommend co-testing every 5 years or cytology alone every 3 years starting at age 25 years. In addition, a limitation to primary HPV testing is its low positive predictive value which necessitates a triage test. Currently, three triage tests are approved: cytology, HPV genotyping for HPV 16/18, and Ki67/p16 dual staining (CINtec PLUS Cytology). These tests can be assayed from cervical samples collected in liquid-based media. As these recommendations continue to change, accessing the most up-to-date guidelines at the USPSTF, the American Society for Colposcopy and Cervical Pathology (ASCCP), and ACS websites will be important to provide high-quality patient care according to national standards by age group.

The follow-up evaluation required for benign Pap smear findings not associated with neoplastic changes is shown in Table 55.2. In addition, the current triage practices for abnormal cytology changes in female young adults are outlined in the following sections.

TABLE 55.1

Guidelines for Initiation and Frequency of Cervical Cancer Screening: Select U.S. Organizations

Criteria	American Cancer Society (2019)	U.S. Preventive Services Task Force (2018)
Age to begin screening	25 y	21 y
Screening interval for cytology (conventional pap or liquid-based testing)	Primary HPV testing (preferred) or co-testing[a] every 5 y or cytology every 3 y	Cytology every 3 y for <30 y Co-testing[a] or primary HPV testing every 5 y or cytology every 3 y for 30–65 y
Age to end screening	65 y	65 y

HPV, human papillomavirus.
[a]If HPV DNA negative and normal cytology.

TABLE 55.2

Follow-Up Evaluation Recommendations for Nonmalignant Cytology Findings

Pap Smear Finding	Recommendation
Insufficient quantity	Repeat age-based screening in 2–4 mo
Poor specimen	Repeat age-based screening in 2–4 mo
Air-drying artifact	Repeat age-based screening in 2–4 mo
No endocervical cells	Among 21–29-y-old female patients no action is required. If >29 y, HPV testing is preferred. Repeat cytology in 3 y also acceptable
Normal endometrial cells	If premenopausal, no action is required. If postmenopausal, endometrial evaluation is recommended
Trichomoniasis	Recall patient, perform sexually transmitted infection evaluation, and treat patient and partner
Yeast	Review chart; if no symptoms, no need to follow-up
Inflammation	Consider recent coitus, infection
Reactive, reparative changes	Identify irritant, if possible; essentially normal

HPV, human papillomavirus.

For immunocompromised patients (e.g., solid organ transplants, patients living with HIV, patients with autoimmune disorders on immunosuppressive treatments), these recommendations are slightly altered. Currently, primary HPV testing is not recommended, and screening should start at age 21 years with cytology at 12-month intervals. If 3 consecutive cytology are normal screening can occur at 3-year intervals.[23,38] In addition, HPV testing is not recommended for female patients under 30 years of age. However, these guidelines continue to be updated at https://aidsinfo.nih.gov/guidelines.

Management of Abnormal Screening Tests

Recently, guidelines for managing patients with abnormal cytology were updated and are risk based, defined as equal management for equal risk.[39] Thresholds for accepted risk of CIN 3 were established by expert opinion. It is important to understand that these risk thresholds are socially defined (i.e., the threshold in the United States is much lower than that in most other middle- and lower-income countries). In addition, histologic CIN 3 is used to calculate these risks instead of hHSIL, which combines CIN 2 and 3. Most agree that CIN 3 is the true precancer and that CIN 2 has a much more subjective pathologic description. Management includes immediate treatment, referral to colposcopy, increased surveillance, and routine screening based on the degree of risk. With new data and new technologies, these recommendations are likely to change. Current management guidelines can be found at http://www.asccp.org/Guidelines-2/Management-Guidelines-2.

Recommendations for Young Adults

Human Papillomavirus Testing: General Considerations

High-risk (hr) HPV testing is not recommended in AYAs younger than 25 years including triage for atypical squamous cells of undetermined significance (ASCUS) or in follow-up of abnormal cytology. The one exception to this rule is for the follow-up for CIN 2 and 3 (see below).

Atypical Squamous Cells of Undetermined Significance and Low-Grade Squamous Intraepithelial Lesions on Cytology

Atypical squamous cells of undetermined significance/HPV negative patients have an extremely low risk of CIN 3+ in all age groups. In addition, the risk of CIN 3+ among patients with ASCUS not taking HPV status into account was only slightly lower than ASCUS/HPV positive in AYAs. The rate of invasive cancer during this period was 0.03% among the 21- to 24-year-olds, underscoring the rare risk of missing cancer. The similar natural histories for ASCUS and LSIL resulted similar management strategies for both cytology results.

Guidelines recommended that female patients aged 21 to 24 years with ASCUS/HPV negative or positive or LSIL have repeat cytology at 12-month intervals for 2 years. Human papillomavirus testing or immediate referral to colposcopy is not recommended. If at any of the follow-up visits, HSIL or greater is diagnosed, referral to colposcopy is recommended. If at 24 months, the patient has a diagnosis of ASCUS or higher, the patient should be referred for colposcopy.

If the two consecutive cytology visits are negative, the patient can return to routine screening. For patients >25 years, colposcopy referral is recommended for ASCUS/HPV positive. If the HPV testing is negative, the patient can continue routine screening.

Atypical Squamous Cells Suggestive of High-Grade Squamous Intraepithelial Lesions

All patients, regardless of age with ASC suggestive of HSILs (ASC-H) and HSIL cytology reports, are managed by immediate referral to colposcopy. Management of patients <25 years with ASC-H and HSIL differs from older patients in that immediate loop electrocautery excision procedure (LEEP) without histologic confirmation of CIN 3 is not recommended unless an endocervical curettage (ECC) has evidence of CIN and/or the SCJ is not visible. This is because

many patients <25 years are likely to have regression of HSIL. When no lesion is visualized, random biopsy and ECC are recommended.[40]

Primary Human Papillomavirus Testing with Reflex Testing

For patients with a positive primary HPV testing, referral to colposcopy is recommended if the reflex test is positive for HPV 16/18, dual stain positive, or has ASCUS or worse. If the female is positive for non-16/18 hrHPV with a triage cytology of ASCUS or worse or a triage with a dual stain positive, then referral to colposcopy is recommended. If cytology is normal or dual stain is negative, then the HPV test is repeated in 1 year. If the HPV test is negative, then screening in 3 years is recommended.

Previous HPV test results also influence management. As HPV testing is not recommended for patients under 25 years of age, this is in general for patients ≥25 years of age. For example, a patient with hrHPV with ASCUS with a previous HPV negative test is managed by return in 1 year using HPV-based screening instead of referral to colposcopy.

Management of Histologic Low-Grade Squamous Intraepithelial Lesion (Cervical Intraepithelial Neoplasia 1)

Because over 90% of CIN 1 will regress spontaneously in adolescent, young adult, and adult patient, treatment of CIN 1 is not recommended at any age. Follow-up of histologically diagnosed CIN 1 depends on the referral cytology. If CIN 1 is diagnosed after ASCUS/LSIL cytology, follow-up is similar to those recommended for ASCUS/LSIL cytology with cytology at 12-month intervals. ASC-H or HSIL at any visit warrants referral back to colposcopy. Atypical squamous cells of undetermined significance or LSIL can be followed unless persistent at 24 months where referral back to colposcopy is recommended. After two consecutive negative tests, routine screening is recommended. If CIN 1 is diagnosed after ASC-H or HSIL referral and there is adequate colposcopy, observation is recommended by colposcopy and cytology at 12-month intervals up to 24 months, provided the examination is adequate and endocervical assessment is negative or CIN 1. If at any follow-up visit CIN 2, 3 is identified, the female should be managed per CIN 2, 3 guidelines (see below), which can also be an observation. If during follow-up, high-grade lesions are seen on colposcopy or HSIL on cytology persists at 1 year, rebiopsy is recommended. If HSIL persists at the 24-month follow-up by cytology, histology, or colposcopy, a diagnostic excisional procedure is recommended (i.e., LEEP/loop excision of the TZ). A diagnostic excisional procedure is recommended if the colposcopy is inadequate or ungraded CIN or CIN 2+ is seen on endocervical sampling. Patients with two consecutive negative tests (for patients <25 years this is cytology and colposcopy and for patients who become >25 years is colposcopy and HPV-based testing) should be followed with HPV-based testing every 3 years for at least 25 years.

Management of Histologic High-Grade Squamous Intraepithelial Lesions (Cervical Intraepithelial Neoplasia 2, 3)

Since a significant proportion of AYAs will show regression of CIN 2, 3 lesions,[9] it is recommended that if the colposcopy assessment is adequate, observation is preferred and treatment is optional in patients concerned about fertility. Of note, the new histologic terminology uses similar terms as cytology: LSIL for CIN 1 and HSIL for CIN 2 or 3.[8,41] When HSIL/CIN 2 on biopsy is specified, observation is preferred, and when HSIL/CIN 3 is specified or colposcopy is inadequate, treatment is recommended. High-grade squamous intraepithelial lesions not specified as either CIN 2 or 3 observation is acceptable but treatment is preferred. For patients <25 years of age, observation with colposcopy and cytology is recommended and for those ≥25 years, colposcopy and HPV-based testing at 6 and 12 months. If both visits have LSIL or less on cytology and CIN 1 or less on histology, cytology should be performed 12 months later

TABLE 55.3

Cervical Dysplasia Treatment Regimen Response Rates

	Cryotherapy	LEEP
Response rate		
Single (%)	80	95
Repeated (%)	95	95
Advantages	Simple office-based procedure	SCJ on ectocervix
	Inexpensive	Can tailor to lesion
	Only mildly painful	Provides specimen for pathology
Disadvantages	Watery vaginal discharge for 4–6 wk	Expensive, more painful
	Not recommended for lesions that extend into the canal or cover more than 75% of the surface area of the ectocervix, the SCJ or the upper limit of lesion is not fully visualized; endocervical canal sample is diagnosed as CIN 2+ or CIN that cannot be graded, after previous treatment for CIN 2+, if cancer is suspected.	Bleeding complications
		Premature rupture of membrane in future
	No specimen for pathology	
	Stenosis	

LEEP, loop electrocautery excision procedure; SCJ, squamocolumnar junction.

for patients <25 years and HPV-based testing for those ≥25 years. If cytology is then negative, it is recommended that the female be tested with HPV-based testing at 1-year intervals for 3 years. This is one of the exceptions to using HPV-based testing in this age group because of the increased sensitivity of HPV testing compared to cytology. Then using HPV-based tests, test at 3-year intervals for 25 years. If the lesion progresses by colposcopy or HSIL is persistent at the 12-month visit, repeat biopsy is recommended. If at 12 months, biopsy remains CIN 2 or cytology is ASCUS-H or HSIL, colposcopy and cytology for patients <25 years and colposcopy and HPV-based testing for patients ≥25 years is recommended at 6-month intervals. If HSIL by cytology or CIN 2, 3 by histology persist at 24 months, treatment is recommended. If CIN 3 is found at any visit, treatment is recommended.

Therapy for Cervical Dysplasia

The principle in developing a treatment plan is that cervical dysplasia, specifically HSIL, is treated to prevent progression to cancer. If the lesions are confined to the ectocervix, many treatment options are available (Table 55.3).

1. Avoid both diagnostic and treatment steps at the same procedure: One practice to be avoided, in patients <25 years, is to combine the diagnostic and treatment steps by performing colposcopic examination to rule out invasion and excising the T-zone by a LEEP without biopsy confirmation. Approximately 90% of patients <25 years have no HSIL found on the specimen on undergoing a LEEP, and the cost exceeds the benefit for patients without dysplasia with regard to side effects.[42] As can be seen in Table 55.3, each of the major treatment modalities has minimal adverse impacts when used once. However, because recurrent lesions may develop and require further treatment, the cumulative effects of multiple treatments (particularly LEEP) must be considered. A recent meta-analysis

showed that excisional therapy has a higher rate of premature labor and low birth weight.[43] Ablative treatment for small lesions (less than two quadrants) may be preferable in AYAs with adequate colposcopy. Ablative therapy has less risk on future fertility than excisional procedures. Excisional therapy can also target the lesion, thus avoiding large excisions.

2. Screen for STIs: In general, screening for STIs before cryotherapy or LEEP is recommended to avoid the complications such as pelvic inflammatory disease (PID).[44]

3. Smoking cessation advice: All patients with SIL who smoke should be encouraged to stop smoking. Advise them that continued tobacco use increases susceptibility to cancer.

4. Condom use: Condom use decreases HPV acquisition, enhances LSIL regression, and promotes colonization of protective microbiota, so it should be encouraged.[45]

There is no recommendation to stop hormonal contraception during treatment. It is also not recommended to screen male partners of patients with abnormal Pap smears for HPV infections because few studies have demonstrated HPV disease in this group.

Recommendations for treatment of cervical lesions change over time and differ based on the patient's age and other risk factors. Clinicians involved in the treatment of cervical lesions should refer to the ASCCP website where consensus recommendations are updated as they become available at www.asccp.org/asccp-guidelines.

Screening is recommended in patients who received the HPV vaccine, whether this was before or after the onset of sexual activity.

 SUMMARY

Although HPV is the most common STI, the majority of infections will spontaneously clear and only the minority (<10%) that persist are at risk for cervical cancer. The majority of causal infections occur decades prior to the development of cancer. The vulnerability of female AYAs to these infections is thought to be associated with the development of the TZ within the cervix. Co-factors that increase the risk of progression to cancer include smoking cigarettes, prolonged oral contraceptive use, and multiparity. However, the risks associated with these behaviors have minimal impact on the overall risk. Therefore, these behaviors do not influence cervical cancer-screening strategies nor the management of abnormal screening tests. Although cytology has substantially reduced cervical cancer rates, newer technologies, specifically HPV detection are now being favored. Because of its high sensitivity and strong negative predictive value of primary HPV tests, screening intervals have been extended to every 5 years. However, because of its low positive predictive value, primary HPV testing requires a triage testing that includes cytology, HPV genotyping, and Ki67/p16 dual staining. Because HPV vaccination rates have now exceeded 70% in most states, some professional societies have recommended starting cervical cancer screening at age 25 years with primary HPV testing at 5-year intervals. Other professional societies continue to endorse starting at 21 years of age using cytology at 3-year intervals and at age 30 years, recommend switching to co-testing (HPV and cytology) at 5-year intervals. The alignment of recommendations is likely forthcoming, therefore, monitoring key websites is critical for optimizing patient care. Management of abnormal cervical cancer screening test results remains risk based with established thresholds for (a) close surveillance, (b) referral to colposcopy, and (c) immediate treatment.

REFERENCES

1. Moscicki AB, Schiffman M, Burchell A, et al. Updating the natural history of human papillomavirus and anogenital cancers. *Vaccine.* 2012;30(Suppl 5):F24–F33. doi:10.1016/j.vaccine.2012.05.089

2. Kjær SK, Munk C, Junge J, et al. Carcinogenic HPV prevalence and age-specific type distribution in 40,382 women with normal cervical cytology, ASCUS/LSIL, HSIL, or cervical cancer: what is the potential for prevention? *Cancer Causes Control.* 2014;25(2):179–189. doi:10.1007/s10552-013-0320-z

XII

3. Forman D, de Martel C, Lacey CJ, et al. Global burden of human papillomavirus and related diseases. *Vaccine.* 2012;30(Suppl 5):F12–F23. doi: 10.1016/j.vaccine.2012.07.055

4. Winer RL, Feng Q, Hughes JP, et al. Risk of female human papillomavirus acquisition associated with first male sex partner. *J Infect Dis.* 2008;197(2):279–282. doi: 10.1086/524875

5. Moscicki AB, Ma Y, Jonte J, et al. The role of sexual behavior and human papillomavirus persistence in predicting repeated infections with new human papillomavirus types. *Cancer Epidemiol Biomarkers Prev.* 2010;19(8):2055–2065. doi: 10.1158/1055-9965.EPI-10-0394

6. Guan P, Howell-Jones R, Li N, et al. Human papillomavirus types in 115,789 HPV-positive women: a meta-analysis from cervical infection to cancer. *Int J Cancer.* 2012;131(10):2349–2359. doi: 10.1002/ijc.27485

7. Wright TC Jr, Stoler MH, Behrens CM, et al. The ATHENA human papillomavirus study: design, methods, and baseline results. *Am J Obstet Gynecol.* 2012;206(1):46.e1–46.e11. doi: 10.1016/j.ajog.2011.07.024

8. Darragh TM, Colgan TJ, Cox JT, et al. The lower anogenital squamous terminology standardization project for HPV-associated lesions: background and consensus recommendations from the College of American Pathologists and the American Society for Colposcopy and Cervical Pathology. *J Low Genit Tract Dis.* 2012;16(3):205–242. doi: 10.1097/LGT.0b013e31825c31dd

9. Moscicki AB, Ma Y, Wibbelsman C, et al. Rate of and risks for regression of cervical intraepithelial neoplasia 2 in adolescents and young women. *Obstet Gynecol.* 2010;116(6):1373–1380. doi: 10.1097/AOG.0b013e3181fe777f

10. Tainio K, Athanasiou A, Tikkinen KAO, et al. Clinical course of untreated cervical intraepithelial neoplasia grade 2 under active surveillance: systematic review and meta-analysis. *BMJ.* 2018;360:k499. doi: 10.1136/bmj.k499

11. Kjær SK, Frederiksen K, Munk C, et al. Long-term absolute risk of cervical intraepithelial neoplasia grade 3 or worse following human papillomavirus infection: role of persistence. *J Natl Cancer Inst.* 2010;102(19):1478–1488. doi: 10.1093/jnci/djq356

12. Drolet M, Bénard É, Pérez N, et al. Population-level impact and herd effects following the introduction of human papillomavirus vaccination programmes: updated systematic review and meta-analysis. *Lancet.* 2019;394(10197):497–509. doi: 10.1016/S0140-6736(19)30298-3

13. Palmer T, Wallace L, Pollock KG, et al. Prevalence of cervical disease at age 20 after immunisation with bivalent HPV vaccine at age 12–13 in Scotland: retrospective population study. *BMJ.* 2019;365:l1161. doi: 10.1136/bmj.l1161

14. Lei J, Ploner A, Elfström KM, et al. HPV vaccination and the risk of invasive cervical cancer. *N Engl J Med.* 2020;383(14):1340–1348. doi: 10.1056/NEJMoa1917338

15. Moscicki ABSA. The cervical epithelium during puberty and adolescence. In: Jordan JSA, Shafi M, Jones, H III, eds. *The Cervix.* 2nd ed. Blackwell Publishing; 2006. 81–101.

16. Hwang LY, Ma Y, Shiboski SC, et al. Active squamous metaplasia of the cervical epithelium is associated with subsequent acquisition of human papillomavirus 16 infection among healthy young women. *J Infect Dis.* 2012;206(4):504–511. doi: 10.1093/infdis/jis398

17. Burger EA, Kim JJ, Sy S, et al. Age of acquiring causal human papillomavirus (HPV) infections: leveraging simulation models to explore the natural history of HPV-induced cervical cancer. *Clin Infect Dis.* 2017;65(6):893–899. doi: 10.1093/cid/cix475

18. Doorbar J, Quint W, Banks L, et al. The biology and life-cycle of human papillomaviruses. *Vaccine.* 2012;30(Suppl 5):F55–F70. doi: 10.1016/j.vaccine.2012.06.083

19. Moscicki AB, Ma Y, Farhat S, et al. Redetection of cervical human papillomavirus type 16 (HPV16) in women with a history of HPV16. *J Infect Dis.* 2013;208(3):403–412. doi: 10.1093/infdis/jit175

20. Daud II, Scott ME, Ma Y, et al. Association between toll-like receptor expression and human papillomavirus type 16 persistence. *Int J Cancer.* 2011;128(4):879–886. doi: 10.1002/ijc.25400

21. Farhat S, Nakagawa M, Moscicki AB. Cell-mediated immune responses to human papillomavirus 16 E6 and E7 antigens as measured by interferon gamma enzyme-linked immunospot in women with cleared or persistent human papillomavirus infection. *Int J Gynecol Cancer.* 2009;19(4):508–512. doi: 10.1111/IGC.0b013e3181a388c4

22. Moscicki AB, Ellenberg JH, Farhat S, et al. Persistence of human papillomavirus infection in HIV-infected and -uninfected adolescent girls: risk factors and differences, by phylogenetic type. *J Infect Dis.* 2004;190(1):37–45. doi: 10.1086/421467

23. Moscicki AB, Flowers L, Huchko MJ, et al. Guidelines for cervical cancer screening in immunosuppressed women without HIV infection. *J Low Genit Tract Dis.* 2019;23(2):87–101. doi: 10.1097/LGT.0000000000000468

24. Roura E, Castellsagué X, Pawlita M, et al. Smoking as a major risk factor for cervical cancer and pre-cancer: results from the EPIC cohort. *Int J Cancer.* 2014;135(2):453–466. doi: 10.1002/ijc.28666

25. Smith JS, Bosetti C, Muñoz N, et al. Chlamydia trachomatis and invasive cervical cancer: a pooled analysis of the IARC multicentric case-control study. *Int J Cancer.* 2004;111(3):431–439. doi: 10.1002/ijc.20257

26. Smith JS, Green J, Berrington de Gonzalez A, et al. Cervical cancer and use of hormonal contraceptives: a systematic review. *Lancet.* 2003;361(9364):1159–1167. doi: 10.1016/s0140-6736(03)12949-2

27. Arnheim Dahlström L, Andersson K, Luostarinen T, et al. Prospective seroepidemiologic study of human papillomavirus and other risk factors in cervical cancer. *Cancer Epidemiol Biomarkers Prev.* 2011;20(12):2541–2550. doi: 10.1158/1055-9965.EPI-11-0761

28. Galloway DA, Gewin LC, Myers H, et al. Regulation of telomerase by human papillomaviruses. *Cold Spring Harb Symp Quant Biol.* 2005;70:209–215. doi: 10.1101/sqb.2005.70.041

29. De Marco F. Oxidative stress and HPV carcinogenesis. *Viruses.* 2013;5(2):708–731. doi: 10.3390/v5020708

30. Norenhag J, Du J, Olovsson M, et al. The vaginal microbiota, human papillomavirus and cervical dysplasia: a systematic review and network meta-analysis. *BJOG.* 2020;127(2):171–180. doi: 10.1111/1471-0528.15854

31. Kyrgiou M, Mitra A, Moscicki AB. Does the vaginal microbiota play a role in the development of cervical cancer? *Transl Res.* 2017;179:168–182. doi: 10.1016/j.trsl.2016.07.004

32. Ilhan ZE, Łaniewski P, Thomas N, et al. Deciphering the complex interplay between microbiota, HPV, inflammation and cancer through cervicovaginal metabolic profiling. *EBioMedicine.* 2019;44:675–690. doi: 10.1016/j.ebiom.2019.04.028

33. Mitra A, MacIntyre DA, Ntritsos G, et al. The vaginal microbiota associates with the regression of untreated cervical intraepithelial neoplasia 2 lesions. *Nat Commun.* 2020;11(1):1999. doi: 10.1038/s41467-020-15856-y

34. Sasieni P, Castanon A, Parkin DM. How many cervical cancers are prevented by treatment of screen-detected disease in young women? *Int J Cancer.* 2009;124(2):461–464. doi: 10.1002/ijc.23922

35. US Preventive Services Task Force; Curry SJ, Krist AH, Owens DK, et al. Screening for cervical cancer: U.S. Preventive Services Task Force recommendation statement. *JAMA.* 2018;320(7):674–686. doi: 10.1001/jama.2018.10897

36. Fontham ETH, Wolf AMD, Church TR, et al. Cervical cancer screening for individuals at average risk: 2020 guideline update from the American Cancer Society. *CA Cancer J Clin.* 2020; 70. doi: 10.3322/caac.21628

37. Melnikow J, Henderson JT, Burda BU, et al. Screening for cervical cancer with high-risk human papillomavirus testing: updated evidence report and systematic review for the US Preventive Services Task Force. *JAMA.* 2018;320(7):687–705. doi: 10.1001/jama.2018.10400

38. Moscicki AB, Ellenberg JH, Crowley-Nowick P, et al. Risk of high-grade squamous intraepithelial lesion in HIV-infected adolescents. *J Infect Dis.* 2004;190(8):1413–1421. doi: 10.1086/424466

39. Perkins RB, Guido RS, Castle PE, et al; 2019 ASCCP Risk-Based Management Consensus Guidelines Committee. 2019 ASCCP risk-based management consensus fuidelines for abnormal cervical cancer screening tests and cancer precursors. *J Low Genit Tract Dis.* 2020;24(2):102–131. doi: 10.1097/LGT.0000000000000525

40. Khan MJ, Werner CL, Darragh TM, et al. ASCCP colposcopy standards: role of colposcopy, benefits, potential harms, and terminology for colposcopic practice. *J Low Genit Tract Dis.* 2017;21(4):223–229. doi: 10.1097/LGT.0000000000000338

41. Waxman AG, Chelmow D, Darragh TM, et al. Revised terminology for cervical histopathology and its implications for management of high-grade squamous intraepithelial lesions of the cervix. *Obstet Gynecol.* 2012;120(6):1465–1471. doi: 10.1097/aog.0b013e31827001d5

42. Sadler L, Saftlas A, Wang W, et al. Treatment for cervical intraepithelial neoplasia and risk of preterm delivery. *JAMA.* 2004;291(17):2100–2106. doi: 10.1001/jama.291.17.2100

43. Kyrgiou M, Koliopoulos G, Martin-Hirsch P, et al. Obstetric outcomes after conservative treatment for intraepithelial or early invasive cervical lesions: systematic review and meta-analysis. *Lancet.* 2006;367(9509):489–498. doi: 10.1016/S0140-6736(06)68181-6

44. ACOG Committee opinion no. 436: evaluation and management of abnormal cervical cytology and histology in adolescents. *Obstet Gynecol.* 2009;113(6):1422–1425. doi: 10.1097/AOG.0b013e3181ac06e0

45. Hogewoning CJA, Bleeker MCG, van den Brule AJC, et al. Condom use promotes regression of cervical intraepithelial neoplasia and clearance of human papillomavirus: a randomized clinical trial. *Int J Cancer.* 2003;107(5):811–816. doi: 10.1002/ijc.11474

📶 ADDITIONAL RESOURCES AND WEBSITES

Additional Resources and Websites for Clinicians:

ASCCP Risk-Based Management Consensus Guidelines for abnormal cervical cancer screening tests—http://www.asccp.org/Guidelines-2/Management-Guidelines-2

Cancer Stat Facts: Cervical Cancer—https://seer.cancer.gov/statfacts/html/cervix.html

HPV Vaccine for Clinicians—https://youngwomenshealth.org/clinicians/hpv-vaccine-nurses/

U.S. Preventive Services Task Force: Cervical Cancer Screening Recommendations—https://www.uspreventiveservicestaskforce.org/uspstf/recommendation/cervical-cancer-screening

Additional Resources and Websites for Parents/Caregivers:

Centers for Disease Control and Prevention: Human Papillomavirus: For Parents—https://www.cdc.gov/hpv/parents/index.html

Additional Resources and Websites for Adolescents and Young Adults:

AMAZE.org: What is HPV? (video for youth age 11 years and older)—https://amaze.org/video/stds-what-is-hpv/

HPV Vaccine for AYA—https://youngwomenshealth.org/2012/07/03/hpv-vaccine/

Making Sense of Pap Tests, HPV Tests, and the New Landscape of Cervical Cancer Screening—https://www.ashasexualhealth.org/making-sense-pap-tests-hpv-tests-new-landscape-cervical-cancer-screening/

National Cervical Cancer Coalition (for AYA >21 years)—https://www.nccc-online.org/understanding-cervical-cancer-screening/

CHAPTER 56

Vaginitis and Vaginosis

Maria H. Rahmandar
Paula K. Braverman

KEY WORDS
- Bacterial vaginosis
- *Trichomonas vaginalis*
- Vaginitis
- Vulvovaginal candidiasis

INTRODUCTION

The most common causes of vaginal infection and inflammation in postpubertal individuals are bacterial vaginosis, vulvovaginal candidiasis, and *Trichomonas vaginalis*. Bacterial vaginosis is the most frequent cause of abnormal vaginal discharge and odor. Vulvovaginal candidiasis is the second most common cause of vaginitis, with *Candida albicans* as the causative yeast species in the majority of cases. *Trichomonas vaginalis* is a sexually transmitted flagellated protozoan that infects the vaginal mucosa.[1,2] Work-up of vaginitis complaints should include laboratory evaluation, since self-diagnosis or diagnosis based on history and physical alone are often inaccurate.[3] Treatment should be guided by recommendations from the Centers for Disease Control and Prevention (CDC) guidelines.[4]

Historically, studies have been conducted within a gender/sex binary. The full spectrum of the gender experience is not represented in the studies cited in this chapter and the clinical recommendations focus on patients assigned to the female gender at birth. In addition, the racial/ethnic disparities highlighted in this text do not reveal the underlying causes of these health inequities.

VAGINA: NORMAL STATE

Vaginal Flora

Before puberty, the vagina is colonized with various bacterial species ranging from fecal flora to respiratory flora, and has a pH of 6.5 to 7.5.[5] After puberty, the estrogen-stimulated epithelial cells produce more glycogen, and lactobacilli become predominant. Metabolism of glycogen to lactic acid by the lactobacilli contributes to the lowering of the vaginal pH to <4.5 and helps to maintain a vaginal environment that appears to protect the individual from colonization by more pathogenic organisms. Some lactobacilli also produce hydrogen peroxide, a potential microbicide.[6]

Vaginal Secretions

Physiologic discharge may begin before menarche; these secretions may be copious but are not associated with odor or pruritus. During the menstrual cycle, changes can be noted in vaginal secretions, including little to no secretions to sticky white or clear mucoid secretions. These secretions are a normal result of the changing hormonal milieu of the menstrual cycle.[1]

VULVOVAGINITIS IN PREPUBERTAL FEMALES

Vulvovaginitis in prepubertal females often is related to poor hygiene, tight clothing, or nonabsorbent underpants. Patients should be counseled regarding hygienic measures, and antibiotics or antifungals generally are prescribed only if a predominant organism is identified by culture. Usually, the organisms found are normal flora (i.e., lactobacilli, diphtheroids, streptococci, and *Staphylococcus epidermidis*), respiratory pathogens (most commonly *Streptococcus pyogenes*), or gram-negative enteric organisms (i.e., *Escherichia coli*, which may not be pathogenic but overpopulation may contribute to odor/discharge). *Candida* species can be part of the normal vaginal microbiota, and yeast vaginitis typically only occurs if other risk factors are present. Any sexually transmitted infection (STI) should prompt an investigation for sexual abuse.[5]

VULVOVAGINITIS AND VAGINOSIS IN PUBERTAL FEMALES: GENERAL APPROACH

Etiology

The three most common types of vaginitis are bacterial vaginosis, vulvovaginal candidiasis, and *Trichomonas vaginalis*.[2] Other causes of discharge include physiologic discharge, hormonal contraceptives (estrogen effect), chemical irritants, foreign bodies (i.e., tampons), and poor hygiene. From the patient's perspective, vaginal discharge secondary to cervicitis from *Neisseria gonorrhoeae* or *Chlamydia trachomatis* can be indistinguishable from discharge secondary to vaginitis.[1]

Evaluation

1. *History*: Should include type, duration, and extent of symptoms (i.e., discharge, pruritus, odor, dyspareunia, dysuria, rash, pain); relation of symptoms to menses; frequency and type of sexual activity, and number of sexual partners; previous STIs; contraceptive history; medications, especially antibiotics and steroids; use of deodorants, soaps, lubricants, or douches; and history of immunosuppression.
2. *Examination*: Should include inspection of color, texture, origin (vaginal or cervical), adherence to the vaginal wall, and odor of the vaginal discharge; inspection of the perineum, vulva, vagina, and cervix for erythema, swelling, lesions, atrophy, trauma, and foreign bodies; and palpation of the introitus, uterus, and adnexa for tenderness or masses (Fig. 56.1).
3. *Laboratory*: Laboratory evaluation should be completed since relying on history and physical alone often results in misdiagnosis and incorrect treatment.[7] Similarly, self-diagnosis is

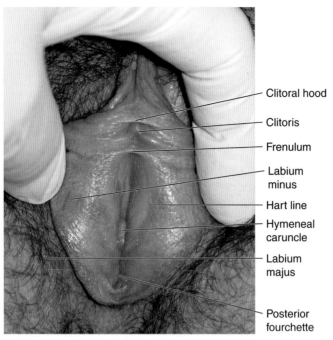

FIGURE 56.1 Normal vulva. (From Edwards L, Lynch PJ. *Genital Dermatology Atlas*. 3rd ed. Lippincott Williams & Wilkins; 2018.)

Clitoral hood
Clitoris
Frenulum
Labium minus
Hart line
Hymeneal caruncle
Labium majus
Posterior fourchette

not recommended due to frequent inaccurate diagnosis and patient-initiated improper treatment.[3]

a. The pH of vaginal secretions is sampled from the lateral vaginal wall. Cervical mucosa should not be sampled due to its higher pH.[6] Measurement of vaginal pH can be key in diagnosis since a value ≤4.5 is in the normal range and also seen in patients with vulvovaginal candidiasis while values >4.5 are found with bacterial vaginosis and *Trichomonas vaginalis*.

b. A saline wet mount should be examined under the high-power lens. Normal findings include <10 white blood cells (WBCs) per high-power field as well as lactobacilli. Abnormal findings include presence of "clue cells" (Fig. 56.2), defined as epithelial cells covered with bacteria and demonstrating indistinct borders, as well as trichomonads. Motility of trichomonads decreases with time; thus, immediate inspection of wet mount is advised, ideally within an hour.[1]

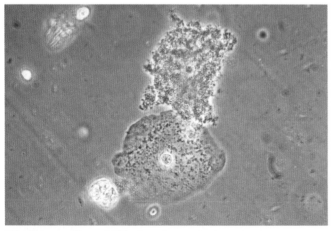

FIGURE 56.2 Clue cell. This photomicrograph of a vaginal smear specimen depicts two epithelial cells, a normal cell, and an epithelial cell with its exterior covered by bacteria, giving the cell a roughened, stippled appearance known as a "clue cell." Clue cells are a sign of bacterial vaginosis. (Image courtesy of M. Rein and the Centers for Disease Control and Prevention Public Health Image Library ID 14574. Available at http://phil.cdc.gov/)

TABLE 56.1

Vaginal Discharge in the Adolescents and Young Adults (AYAs)

Condition	Signs and Symptoms	Diagnosis in the Office Setting
Physiologic discharge	Clear gray discharge, no offensive odor, no burning or itching	Wet prep: Epithelial cells with no or few polymorphonuclear cells; no pathogens
Vulvovaginal candidiasis	Curd-like discharge, intense burning, pruritus, usually no odor, often associated vulvitis	KOH/wet prep: Budding yeast and pseudohyphae
Trichomoniasis	Pruritus; malodorous, frothy, yellow-green discharge; dysuria; rarely, abdominal pain	Wet prep: Pear-shaped organism with motile flagella, point-of-care test
Bacterial vaginosis	Homogenous, malodorous, gray-white discharge; usually mild or no pruritus or burning	Wet prep: Epithelial cells covered with bacteria, few polymorphonuclear leukocytes, pH >4.5
Retained tampon	Malodorous discharge, local discomfort	History and physical examination, history of exposure to deodorant spray or scented tampons
Irritant vaginitis	Vaginal discharge, erythema	History and physical examination

c. A potassium hydroxide (KOH) slide should be prepared, and an immediate fishy, amine odor is called a positive "whiff test," which is suggestive of bacterial vaginosis (or sometimes *Trichomonas vaginalis*). Potassium hydroxide preparation may reveal yeast buds and pseudohyphae.[1,2]

d. Point-of-care tests (POCTs) or laboratory testing for *Trichomonas vaginalis*, vulvovaginal candidiasis, and bacterial vaginosis should be considered particularly when microscopy is not available in the office setting. Newer multiplex nucleic acid amplification test (NAAT) testing which simultaneously detects all three causes of vaginitis is now available. In one study, NAAT was more sensitive than clinician diagnosis when multiple causes of vaginitis were present.[8,9]

e. In sexually active females with discharge, testing for *C. trachomatis*, *N. gonorrhoeae*, and *Trichomonas vaginalis* is advised.[1]

Table 56.1 outlines the causes of vaginitis in adolescents and young adults (AYAs).

Treatment

See specific recommendations for the common causes of vaginitis in the following sections. Probiotics, intravaginal yogurt, and other nonmedical/anecdotal interventions are not recommended for prevention or treatment of vaginitis.[4,10]

● BACTERIAL VAGINOSIS

Bacterial vaginosis is the most frequent cause of vaginitis.[2] However, it is not a true vaginitis as it is not characterized by a marked inflammatory response of the vaginal mucosa (no/few WBCs on wet prep), thus the term "vaginosis."[1]

Etiology

Bacterial vaginosis consists of the replacement of normal lactobacilli in the vagina with *Gardnerella vaginalis*; anaerobic bacteria (i.e., *Bacteroides* sp, *Peptostreptococcus* sp, *Fusobacterium* sp, *Prevotella* sp, *Ureaplasma*, *Mycoplasma*, and *Mobiluncus* sp); more recently identified bacterial vaginosis–associated bacteria (BVAB 1 to 3); and others (i.e., *Atopobium vaginae*, *Leptotrichia/Sneathia* sp, *Megasphaera* sp, and *Eggerthella*-like bacteria.).[1] Hydrogen peroxide and lactic acid producing lactobacilli help maintain an acid pH level that prevents the growth of other bacteria.[6] In bacterial vaginosis, there is loss of lactobacilli, leading to an elevated pH level, and high concentrations of bacterial vaginosis–causing bacteria which produce malodorous amines.[1] *G. vaginalis* forms a biofilm on vaginal epithelium, which provides a surface for anaerobes to adhere, and potentially decreases treatment success and increase recurrence.[11]

Epidemiology

1. Prevalence: The worldwide prevalence of bacterial vaginosis ranges from 23% to 29%. In North America, specifically, Black (33%) and Hispanic (31%) populations have a higher prevalence of bacterial vaginosis compared to White (23%) or Asian (11%) populations.[12]
2. Transmission: There continues to be controversy about the possibility of bacterial vaginosis being transmitted sexually. Although bacterial vaginosis occurs among sexually active females, it can also occur in females who have not been sexually active. In addition, while the use of condoms seems to be a protective factor, treatment of partners does not prevent reoccurrence of the disease process.[1]
3. Predisposing factors: Bacterial vaginosis is associated with douching, cigarette smoking, new and increased number of sex partners, and STIs; whereas condom use and hormonal contraception are protective.[13]

Clinical Manifestations

1. Presentation: At least 50% of cases are asymptomatic.[2] The discharge is classically homogeneous, thin, and grayish-white, with a "fishy" odor.[1,2]
2. Examination may reveal the typical discharge adhering to the vaginal walls and odor.
3. Complications: Bacterial vaginosis is linked to serious sequelae including pelvic inflammatory disease (PID); increased acquisition and transmission of STIs, including human immunodeficiency virus (HIV); irregular bleeding; preterm labor; premature rupture of membranes; and postpartum endometritis.[1,13]

Diagnosis

1. The gold standard has been Nugent scoring from a vaginal Gram stain which identifies the presence or absence of various bacterial morphotypes.[8] However, this is typically used in research settings. The Amsel criteria are commonly used for clinical diagnosis. Three of the four clinical symptoms and signs are required: (1) homogeneous, grayish-white discharge; (2) vaginal pH level >4.5; (3) positive whiff test before or after 10% KOH; and (4) wet prep showing "clue cells," that comprise at least 20% of the epithelial cells.[3,14]
2. Commercial tests are available including Affirm VP III, an automated DNA probe assay for detecting high concentrations of *G. vaginalis*, along with other causes of vaginitis;[15] and OSOM BVBlue,[16] a 10-minute Clinical Laboratory Improvement Amendments (CLIA)-waived chromogenic diagnostic test based on the presence of elevated sialidase enzyme activity which is produced by bacterial pathogens including *Gardnerella*.[16] Sensitivities and specificities for these tests are 95%/100% and 90.3%/96.6% respectively, compared to Gram stain.[15,16]
3. Newer diagnostic tests include NAATs which are multiplex assays utilizing algorithms to assess for the presence of lactobacilli and bacterial vaginosis–associated bacteria as an indication of the dysbiosis associated with bacterial vaginosis. These tests have sensitivities of 90.5% to 99% and specificities of 85.8% to 94% compared to Gram stain/Amsel criteria and also detect the other two common causes of vaginitis (e.g., *Candida* and *Trichomonas vaginalis*) on a single swab.[14] Nucleic acid amplification tests are more costly than other bacterial vaginosis testing options.[9]
4. Pap tests are not reliable for diagnosing bacterial vaginosis with a sensitivity of 49% and specificity of 93%. Symptomatic patients with concerns for bacterial vaginosis on the Pap test should have bacterial vaginosis diagnostic testing prior to treatment and asymptomatic patients do not need evaluation or treatment.[3]

Therapy

1. For nonpregnant patients, recommended regimens are metronidazole 500-mg oral tablet twice daily for 7 days, metronidazole 0.75% gel 5 g intravaginally once daily for 5 days, or clindamycin 2% cream 5 g intravaginally daily for 7 days. Cure rates for all these regimens are approximately 70% to 80%.[14] Alternative treatments include oral tinidazole and either oral or intravaginal (ovule) clindamycin regimens.[4] A newly approved treatment is a single oral dose of 2 g of secnidazole which has clinical cure rates comparable to metronidazole.[3,14] Secnidazole is considered an alternative in the 2021 CDC's STI Treatment Guidelines because of cost and lack of long-term outcome data.[4] Please see the CDC's STI Treatment Guidelines for the most updated information (www.cdc.gov).[4] Clindamycin cream is oil based and might weaken latex condoms and diaphragms for up to 5 days after treatment.[4] The 2021 CDC's STI Treatment Guidelines specifically state that it is not necessary to refrain from alcohol use while taking metronidazole or tinidazole since there is no inhibition of acetaldehyde dehydrogenase to cause the side effects seen with disulfram.[4]
2. Recurrent bacterial vaginosis occurs in over half of females within 1 year.[2] The initial treatment recommended by the CDC is repeating the same treatment or choosing another recommended regimen.[4] For multiple reoccurrences, after initial re-treatment, suppression therapy then follows with at least a 3-month course of intravaginal metronidazole twice a week.[4] Suppression only lasts during the treatment period. Other alternative regimens with some limited data are discussed in the CDC's STI Treatment Guidelines.[4]
3. Symptomatic pregnant females in any trimester can be treated with the recommended regimens for nonpregnant females with oral or vaginal metronidazole or oral clindamycin, 2% clindamycin cream, or clindamycin ovules. Neither tinidazole nor secnidazole should be used since there are limited or insufficient data regarding risk in human studies.[4] It is not recommended to screen asymptomatic females at low risk for premature delivery since adverse outcomes are not reduced with bacterial vaginosis treatment. Evidence is mixed in comparing the risk and benefits of screening or treating asymptomatic females at high risk for premature delivery and therefore, screening is also not recommended for this group.[4]
4. Adolescents and young adults (AYA) with the human immunodeficiency virus (HIV) receive the same regimens as non–HIV-infected AYA.[4]
5. Treatment of asymptomatic females with bacterial vaginosis before hysterectomy and pregnancy termination is recommended by American Congress of Obstetrics and Gynecology.[17]

XII

6. Treatments under investigation include biofilm disrupting agents, probiotics, and vaginal microbiota transplantation.[4,14,18] Studies do not support the efficacy of use of probiotic formulations or use of intravaginal *Lactobacillus* for bacterial vaginosis.[4]

7. Counseling: Patients should be advised to use condoms if sexually active during treatment and avoid douching which is associated with relapse.[4] Treatment of male partners is not helpful, but female sex partners should be aware of symptoms and evaluated if symptomatic. Follow-up is not necessary unless symptoms persist.

VULVOVAGINAL CANDIDIASIS

Vulvovaginal candidiasis is the second most common form of vaginitis. A major issue in diagnosis is distinguishing true infection from nonpathogenic colonization, as colonization is common and is also a prerequisite for infection.[2]

Etiology

Vulvovaginal candidiasis is usually caused by *C. albicans* (90% of clinical cases) and occasionally by other *Candida* species, particularly *Candida glabrata*.[3]

Epidemiology

1. Prevalence: The overall prevalence of vulvovaginal candidiasis is unknown; however, an estimated 75% of females experience at least one episode of vulvovaginal candidiasis during their lifetime; 50% will have a recurrence, and approximately 8% to 10% will have recurrent vulvovaginal candidiasis, defined as ≥3 episodes in a 12-month period.[2,4]

2. Transmission: Yeast likely originates in the gastrointestinal tract. Although vulvovaginal candidiasis is usually not sexually acquired or transmitted, evidence exists that sexual contact plays a role in transmission in some patients.[2] Approximately 20% of male partners have asymptomatic penile colonization.[2] Symptomatic male partners might present with balanitis.[4]

3. Predisposing factors: Immunosuppressive states (e.g., uncontrolled diabetes mellitus, HIV infection, or therapy with steroids or immunosuppressive agents), pregnancy, and use of antibiotics in females colonized with *Candida*; behavioral factors (e.g., orogenital sex); innate host factors, including genetic predispositions and altered local vaginal immune responses (such as those seen with increased immune response to yeast, resulting in inflammation from yeast colonization).[1,2] There is a possible increased risk of infection with contraceptives, including estrogen-containing oral contraceptives, and an intrauterine device (IUD).[2]

Clinical Manifestations

1. Presentation: Patients may experience nonspecific symptoms of vulvar pruritus, intense burning, erythema, external dysuria, dyspareunia, and discharge. The itching may remit with menses, and the discharge classically appears white, odorless, and "cottage cheese–like," but can vary in character.[1,2]

2. Examination may reveal the classic discharge and erythematous vulva with fissures, excoriations, edema, and satellite lesions.[1,2]

3. Vulvovaginal candidiasis is classified as "uncomplicated" when there are infrequent episodes with mild-to-moderate symptoms due to *C. albicans* in nonimmunocompromised females. Vulvovaginal candidiasis is classified as "complicated" when there is recurrent vulvovaginal candidiasis consisting of three or more episodes in 12 months, or severe symptoms, or due to non-albicans species, or in females with diabetes or who are immunocompromised.[3,4]

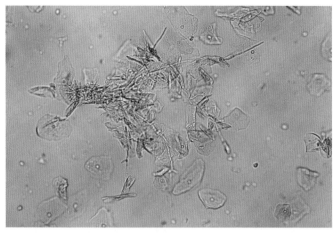

FIGURE 56.3 Vaginal candidiasis. This photomicrograph of a wet-mounted vaginal smear specimen reveals the presence of *C. albicans* in a patient with vaginal candidiasis. (Image courtesy of Dr. Stuart Brown and the Centers for Disease Control and Prevention Public Health Image Library ID 15675. Available at http://phil.cdc.gov/)

4. Recurrent vulvovaginal candidiasis affects <5% of women and 10% to 20% of the time non-*C. albicans* species including *C. glabrata* are found. No apparent risk factors are identified in at least 50% of cases.[2,4] Severe vulvovaginal candidiasis presents with significant erythema as well as edema, fissuring, and excoriation. Both recurrent vulvovaginal candidiasis and severe vulvovaginal candidiasis are not as responsive to the usual courses of therapy.[3,4]

Diagnosis

1. Diagnosis is supported by wet prep or KOH findings of yeast buds, hyphae, and pseudohyphae (Fig. 56.3) (sensitivity 50% to 70%) and a normal pH of <4.5.[2,3]

2. Cultures may be useful in cases of recurrent vulvovaginal candidiasis to identify the yeast species and help guide treatment. However, cultures are not used for routine diagnosis because asymptomatic colonization is common in up to 30% of females.[2,3]

3. A rapid test for *Candida* antigens in vaginal discharge is commercially available. The Affirm VP III is a DNA probe that can provide results for detecting *Candida* in less than 1 hour if run in-house. Sensitivity and specificity are 81% and 98%, respectively.[15]

4. Multiplex NAAT tests identify the *Candida* sp group, and depending on the test, also separately identify other common non-*C. albicans* species including *C. glabrata*, and *Candida krusei*. Sensitivities and specificities for the *Candida* sp group are 86.2% to 90.7% and 93.6% to 98.7%, respectively compared to culture.[9,19] These tests are more costly but simultaneously detect *Trichomonas vaginalis* and bacterial vaginosis as well as *Candida* sp on a single swab.

5. Findings of *Candida* on Pap tests require further confirmatory diagnostic testing for symptomatic patients.[3]

Therapy

1. Uncomplicated cases in nonpregnant patients can be treated by:
   a. Topical, intravaginal agents: Short-course topical formulations of azoles (i.e., regimens of 1 to 3 days) including clotrimazole, miconazole, tioconazole, butoconazole, and terconazole effectively treat uncomplicated vulvovaginal candidiasis. Please see the CDC's STI Treatment Guidelines for a more comprehensive list of topical treatment options (www.cdc.gov).[4]

b. Oral agent: Fluconazole 150-mg oral tablet, one tablet in a single dose. Patients often prefer single-dose oral therapy over intravaginal therapy because of convenience and ease of use.[3,4]

2. Pregnancy: Seven-day therapy with topical azole medications can be used during pregnancy. Oral agents should be avoided.[4]

3. Severe vulvovaginal candidiasis or immunocompromised host: Cases with severe symptoms and signs have lower clinical cure rates with short-course medications. Treating with either 7 to 14 days of topical azoles or oral fluconazole 150 mg once and then repeating the same dose in 3 days is advised.[4]

4. Human immunodeficiency virus infection: Same as non–HIV-infected females. However, cases of clinically severe vulvovaginal candidiasis may be treated as discussed in the section on severe vulvovaginal candidiasis. Though vulvovaginal candidiasis is associated with higher risk of HIV acquisition and higher levels of HIV in the cervicovaginal tissue, it is unclear if treatment of vulvovaginal candidiasis impacts HIV acquisition or transmission.[4] Since recurrence is not uncommon in immunocompetent individuals, HIV testing should only be considered in females with recurrent vulvovaginal candidiasis who have risk factors for HIV infection.[1]

5. Recurrent vulvovaginal candidiasis (three or more symptomatic episodes in 12 months): Predisposing factors for infection should be reduced and vaginal cultures or NAAT obtained to guide therapy. For recurrent *C. albicans* vulvovaginal candidiasis, prescribe the routine short courses for uncomplicated infection or 7 to 14 days of topical treatment or oral therapy every 3 days for three total doses. Maintenance therapy consists of weekly oral medications for 6 months (see CDC guidelines for more details). Culture with susceptibility testing should be considered for patients with persistent symptoms because of possible azole resistance among both *C. albicans* and non-albicans *Candida* infections.[4] About 50% of females will have recurrent disease after maintenance therapy is discontinued.[2]

6. Non-albicans *Candida* species: Optimal treatment is unknown; however, consider 7 to 14 days of a nonfluconazole azole drug (oral or topical) as first-line therapy. For recurrence, CDC recommends 600 mg of boric acid in a gelatin capsule intravaginally daily for 3 weeks. If symptoms recur, consider referral to a specialist.[4]

7. There is a lack of evidence to support probiotics, essential oils, intravaginal yogurt, or dietary changes.[10]

8. Counseling: Partners are not routinely treated unless the male partner has symptoms and signs of balanitis. Follow-up is not necessary for individuals who become asymptomatic after treatment.[4]

TRICHOMONIASIS

Etiology

Trichomonas vaginalis is a motile, flagellated protozoan and is the third most common cause of infectious vaginitis.[1,2]

Epidemiology

1. Prevalence: The prevalence of *Trichomonas vaginalis* in the United States is around 3%. Difference in prevalence varies with the study population examined. Prevalence increases with increasing age to 11% among females aged 40 and above. Racial/ethnic disparities are also seen, with the highest prevalence in non-Hispanic Black females (13.3%) and the lowest in non-Hispanic White females (1.3%).[20] This infection is also associated with poverty and lower education attainment.[4]

2. Transmission: The organism is almost always sexually transmitted, though rare transmission via nonsexual contaminated fomites (i.e., wet washcloths) is possible.[1]

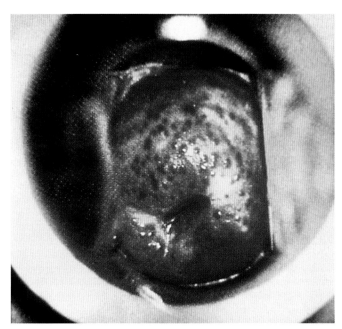

FIGURE 56.4 Strawberry cervix due to a *Trichomonas vaginalis* infection. With *Trichomonas vaginalis*, the cervical mucosa may reveal punctuate hemorrhages with accompanying vesicles or papules, also known as strawberry cervix. (Image courtesy of Centers for Disease Control and Prevention Public Health Image Library ID 5240. Available at http://phil.cdc.gov/)

3. Predisposing factors: Risk factors similar to that of other STIs including high-risk sexual behaviors

Clinical Manifestations

1. Presentation: Most infections (70% to 85%) are asymptomatic and if left untreated can last for months to years.[4,20] In females, *Trichomonas vaginalis* infects the urethra, vulva, vagina, and cervix.[21] Nonspecific symptoms include pruritus, dysuria, dyspareunia, lower abdominal pain, and postcoital bleeding. Discharge is classically diffuse, frothy, yellow or green, and malodorous.[20]

2. Examination may reveal erythema and excoriation of the external genitalia, as well as frothy, yellow-green (or gray-white), foul-smelling vaginal discharge. Cervicitis ("strawberry cervix") (Fig. 56.4) consists of erosions or petechiae of the cervix and is seen in only 2% of cases.[1]

3. Complications: Evidence links *Trichomonas vaginalis* infection to an increased rate of HIV acquisition and transmission, an increased rate of PID in HIV-infected women, and an increase in perinatal morbidity.[20]

Diagnosis

1. Nucleic acid amplification tests are currently recognized as a highly sensitive testing modality, particularly as compared to wet mount microscopy.[3,4] There are a number of NAATs available to detect *Trichomonas vaginalis* from clinician or patient-collected vaginal swabs and clinician-collected endocervical swabs, liquid endocervical cytology media, and urine specimens. Sensitivity ranges from 92.9% to 100% and specificity between 98.2% and 99.7% compared to wet mount and culture.[22] Several of these NAATs can produce results more rapidly in less than 1 hour. Multiplex NAATs which simultaneously test for the other causes of vaginitis (bacterial vaginosis, vulvovaginal candidiasis) demonstrate sensitivities of 96.5% to 96.7% and specificities of 95.1% to 99.1% compared to culture.[9,19]

2. Wet prep is commonly used when a microscope is available in the office setting, but sensitivity is 60% to 70% at best.[2]

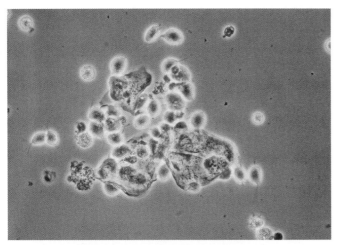

FIGURE 56.5 *Trichomonas vaginalis* protozoan parasites. This photomicrograph of a wet-mounted vaginal discharge specimen reveals numbers of *Trichomonas vaginalis* protozoan parasites. (Image courtesy of Joe Miller and the Centers for Disease Control and Prevention Public Health Image Library ID 14500. Available at http://phil.cdc.gov/)

Trichomonads appear as flagellated pear-shaped motile organisms similar in size to polymorphonuclear leukocytes (Fig. 56.5). The whiff test can be positive on KOH prep with an elevated vaginal pH.[2,3]

3. Cultures: Culture of *T. vaginalis* via Diamond medium or with the use of the InPouch culture system was previously considered gold standard for diagnosis because of high sensitivity and specificity. However, due to the technical challenges of culture and length of time to diagnosis, other testing modalities are commonly used.[3,4]

4. Rapid/POCTs: There are several non–NAAT U.S. Food and Drug Administration-approved methods for more rapid testing of vaginal samples. The OSOM Trichomonas POCT rapid test yields results in 10 minutes, (sensitivity 83%, specificity 99%) compared to wet mount/culture and the Affirm VP III yields results in 60 minutes (sensitivity 89.6% to 92.0% and specificity 99.9% compared to wet mount/culture).[15,23] Other available rapid tests utilize Helicase-dependent amplification (Solana Trichomonas Assay; Amplivue Trichomonas Assay) and have high sensitivity compared to NAAT.[4]

5. Liquid-based cytology versus conventional Pap: Due to their poor sensitivity, neither conventional Pap (50%) nor liquid-based cervical cytology (61%) is ideal for the diagnosis of *Trichomonas vaginalis*.[20] Confirmatory diagnostic testing should be conducted prior to treatment.[3]

Therapy

1. Nonpregnant patients should receive oral metronidazole as a 500-mg tablet twice a day for 7 days. Single-dose metronidazole therapy was found to have a lower cure rate in meta-analysis and a multicenter randomized trial. Single-dose tinidazole 2 g orally is considered an alternative that is equivalent or superior to single-dose metronidazole treatment.[4] Patients allergic to nitroimidazoles should receive desensitization, since no other medication classes are effective.[4] Avoidance of alcohol is no longer considered necessary as discussed in the bacterial vaginosis treatment section.

2. Treatment failure: If there is reexposure to untreated partner, the 7-day course of metronidazole should be repeated. If failure occurs in the absence of reexposure to an untreated partner, the AYA should be retreated with tinidazole or metronidazole 2 g by mouth daily for 7 days. For situations when high-dose treatment for 7 days fails, combinations of simultaneous oral

and vaginal treatment regimens are described in the CDC's STI Treatment Guidelines. Resistance to metronidazole has been found in 4% to 10% of vaginal *Trichomonas vaginalis* cases; one study founds tinidazole resistance in 1% of cases.[4] Any suspicion of resistance to nitroimidazoles should be reported to the CDC for discussion of further susceptibility testing, and treatment recommendations.[4]

3. Pregnancy: *Trichomonas vaginalis* treatment in pregnancy has not been shown to reduce perinatal morbidity prematurity or low birth weight in asymptomatic females. However, treatment of symptomatic females is indicated for symptom relief and prevention of sexual transmission.[4] Recommended treatment is metronidazole orally 500 mg twice a day for 1 week. Data have shown no association between teratogenicity and metronidazole use during pregnancy. Tinidazole should not be used in pregnancy.[4]

4. Human immunodeficiency virus infection: Females should be treated with 500 mg orally twice a day for 7 days.[4]

5. Counseling: Routine treatment of partners is recommended. Patients should also avoid sexual contact until the patient and all partners have completed medications and are asymptomatic. Follow-up is not necessary for individuals who become asymptomatic after treatment. Due to high rates of reinfection, rescreening 3 months after initial treatment is recommended.[4]

OTHER CAUSES OF VAGINAL DISCHARGE

1. Physiologic discharge: Normal overall increase in vaginal secretions before menarche and just before each menses[1]
2. Extravaginal lesions: May cause staining of the underwear and perception of a discharge[5]
3. Irritant vaginitis: Related to soaps, bubble baths, and tight-fitting clothing can contribute to vulvovaginitis[5]
4. Foreign bodies: Forgotten tampons and other foreign objects[1]

SUMMARY

Vaginal complaints are common in postpubertal individuals. Laboratory evaluation can help in providing accurate diagnosis, distinguishing between the most common causes of vaginitis including bacterial vaginosis, vulvovaginal candidiasis, and *Trichomonas vaginalis*, and inform appropriate treatment. Newly available multiplex NAATs enable diagnosis of the three most common causes of vaginitis from a single swab, and provide improved sensitivity over in-office microscopic and nonamplified tests.

ACKNOWLEDGMENTS

This chapter is based on Chapter 51 from the 6th edition, authored by Sherine Patterson-Rose and Paula K. Braverman.

REFERENCES

1. Berlan ED, Emans SJ, DiVasta AD. Vulvovaginal complaints in the adolescent In: Emans SJ, Laufer MR, DiVasta AD, eds. *Emans, Laufer, Goldstein's Pediatric & Adolescent Gynecology*. 7th ed. Lippincott Williams & Wilkins; 2020:251–275.
2. Nyirjesy P. Management of persistent vaginitis. *Obstet Gynecol*. 2014;124(6):1135–1146.
3. Paavonen JA, Brunham RC. Vaginitis in nonpregnant patients: ACOG Practice Bulletin Number 215. *Obstet Gynecol*. 2020;135(5):1229–1230.
4. Workowski KA, Bachmann LH, Chan PA, et al. Sexually transmitted infections treatment guidelines, 2021. *MMWR. Recomm Rep*. 2021;70(4):1–187.
5. French A, Emans SJ. Vulvovaginal problems in the prepubertal child. In: Emans SJ, Laufer MR, DiVasta AD, eds. *Emans, Laufer, Goldstein's Pediatric & Adolescent Gynecology*. 7th ed. Lippincott Williams & Wilkins; 2020:175–193.
6. Powell AM, Nyirjesy P. New perspectives on the normal vagina and noninfectious causes of discharge. *Clin Obstet Gynecol*. 2015;58(3):453–463.
7. Nwankwo TO, Aniebue UU, Umeh UA. Syndromic diagnosis in evaluation of women with symptoms of vaginitis. *Curr Infect Dis Rep*. 2017;19(1):3.
8. Coleman JS, Gaydos CA. Molecular diagnosis of bacterial vaginosis: an update. *J Clin Microbiol*. 2018;56(9):e00342–18.

9. Schwebke JR, Gaydos CA, Nyirjesy P, et al. Diagnostic performance of a molecular test versus clinician assessment of vaginitis. *J Clin Microbiol.* 2018;56(6):e00252-18.

10. Saxon C, Edwards A, Rautemaa-Richardson R, et al. British Association for Sexual Health and HIV national guideline for the management of vulvovaginal candidiasis (2019). *Int J STD AIDS.* 2020;31(12):1124–1144.

11. Verstraelen H, Swidsinski A. The biofilm in bacterial vaginosis: implications for epidemiology, diagnosis and treatment: 2018 update. *Curr Opin Infect Dis.* 2019;32(1):38–42.

12. Peebles K, Velloza J, Balkus JE, et al. High global burden and costs of bacterial vaginosis: a systematic review and meta-analysis. *Sex Transm Dis.* 2019;46(5):304–311.

13. Lewis FMT, Bernstein KT, Aral SO. Vaginal microbiome and its relationship to behavior, sexual health, and sexually transmitted diseases. *Obstet Gynecol.* 2017;129(4):643–654.

14. Muzny CA, Kardas P. A narrative review of current challenges in the diagnosis and management of bacterial vaginosis. *Sex Transm Dis.* 2020;47(7):441–446.

15. Becton Dickinson. *Affirm VPIII microbial identification test (package insert). Secondary Affirm VPIII microbial identification test (package insert).* Accessed March 29, 2021. https://www.bd.com/resource.aspx?IDX=14055

16. Sekisui Diagnostics. *OSOM BVBlue test (product insert). Secondary OSOM BVBlue test (product insert).* Accessed March 29, 2021. https://www.sekisuidiagnostics.com/wp-content/uploads/2018/12/OSOM-BVBlue_DI_3763-12.pdf

17. American College of Obstetricians and Gynecologists. ACOG Practice Bulletin No. 195: prevention of infection after gynecologic procedures. *Obstet Gynecol.* 2018;131(6):e172–e189.

18. Lev-Sagie A, Goldman-Wohl D, Cohen Y, et al. Vaginal microbiome transplantation in women with intractable bacterial vaginosis. *Nat Med.* 2019;25(10):1500–1504.

19. Schwebke JR, Taylor SN, Ackerman R, et al. Clinical validation of the aptima bacterial vaginosis and aptima Candida/Trichomonas vaginitis assays: results from a prospective multicenter clinical study. *J Clin Microbiol.* 2020;58(2):e01643–19.

20. Meites E. Trichomoniasis: the "neglected" sexually transmitted disease. *Infect Dis Clin North Am.* 2013;27(4):755–764.

21. Division of STD Prevention, National Center for HIV, Viral Hepatitis, STD, and TB Prevention, Centers for Disease Control and Prevention. Trichomoniasis—CDC Basic Fact Sheet. Reviewed April 25, 2022. Accessed September 1, 2022. https://www.cdc.gov/std/trichomonas/stdfact-trichomoniasis.htm

22. Association of Public Health Laboratories. *Advances in Laboratory detection of Trichomonas vaginalis (updated).* Accessed March 29, 2021. https://www.aphl.org/aboutAPHL/publications/Documents/ID_2016November-Laboratory-Detection-of-Trichomonas-update.pdf

23. Sekisui Diagnostics. *OSOM Trichomonas rapid test (product insert). Secondary OSOM Trichomonas rapid test (product insert).* Accessed September 1, 2022. https://sekisuidiagnostics.com/product-documents/osom_trich_181_pi.pdf

📶 ADDITIONAL RESOURCES AND WEBSITES

Additional Resources and Websites for Clinicians:
General Information Websites for Clinicians:
American Academy of Pediatrics—https://www.aap.org/
American College of Obstetricians and Gynecologists—https://www.acog.org

American College of Obstetricians and Gynecologists Practice Bulletin on Vaginitis in Nonpregnant Patients—https://www.acog.org/clinical/clinical-guidance/practice-bulletin/articles/2020/01/vaginitis-in-nonpregnant-patients
Centers for Disease Control & Prevention: Sexually Transmitted Diseases information website—http://www.cdc.gov/std
North American Society for Pediatric and Adolescent Gynecology—https://www.naspag.org/
Society for Adolescent Health & Medicine—https://www.adolescenthealth.org/

Additional Resources and Websites for Parents/Caregivers:
ACOG Patient materials—https://www.acog.org/womens-health
HealthyChildren.org from the American Academy of Pediatrics (also in Spanish)
Vaginal Infections—https://www.healthychildren.org/English/health-issues/conditions/genitourinary-tract/Pages/Vaginal-Infections.aspx
Yeast Infections in Girls & Young Women—https://healthychildren.org/English/health-issues/conditions/genitourinary-tract/Pages/Yeast-Infections-in-Girls-and-Young-Women.aspx
Trichomonas vaginalis Infections—https://www.healthychildren.org/English/health-issues/conditions/sexually-transmitted/Pages/Trichomonas-vaginalis-Infections.aspx
North American Society for Pediatric and Adolescent Gynecology Patient Education
Vaginal Discharge—https://www.naspag.org/assets/docs/vaginal_discharge_2020.pdf
Vulvar & Vaginal Hygiene—https://www.naspag.org/assets/docs/vulvar_hygiene_2020.pdf
Prepubertal Vulvovaginitis—https://www.naspag.org/assets/docs/prepubertal_vulvovaginitis_2.pdf
Spanish—https://www.naspag.org/naspag-patient-handouts-spanish
Polish—https://www.naspag.org/naspag-patient-handouts-polish
Russian—https://www.naspag.org/naspag-patient-handouts-russian
Planned Parenthood—https://www.plannedparenthood.org/learn/parents
YoungWomensHealth.org—www.youngwomenshealth.org

Additional Resources and Websites for Adolescents and Young Adults:
ACOG Patient materials—https://www.acog.org/womens-health
Bedsider—https://www.bedsider.org/
CDC—https://www.cdc.gov/std/healthcomm/fact_sheets.htm
NASPAG—https://www.naspag.org/patient-handouts
Planned Parenthood—https://www.plannedparenthood.org/learn/teens
YoungWomensHealth.org
Vulvar and Vaginal Care and Cleaning—https://youngwomenshealth.org/2017/04/19/vulvar-and-vaginal-care-and-cleaning/
Vaginal Infections (Vaginitis)—https://youngwomenshealth.org/2012/11/20/vaginal-infection/
Spanish: https://youngwomenshealth.org/2005/10/06/infecciones-vaginales/
Bacterial Vaginosis—https://youngwomenshealth.org/2012/09/21/bacterial-vaginosis/
Spanish: https://youngwomenshealth.org/2011/03/07/vaginosis-bacteriana/
Yeast Infections (Candidiasis)—https://youngwomenshealth.org/2013/06/19/yeast-infection/
Spanish: https://youngwomenshealth.org/2006/06/26/infecciones-vaginales-por-hongos/
Trichomoniasis (Trichomonal Vaginitis; "Trich")—https://youngwomenshealth.org/2012/12/11/trichomoniasis/
Spanish: https://youngwomenshealth.org/2006/06/28/tricomoniasis/

CHAPTER 57

Pelvic Masses

Paula J. Adams Hillard

KEY WORDS

- Adnexal torsion
- Corpus luteum cyst
- Dermoid cyst
- Follicular cyst
- Functional cyst
- Imperforate hymen
- Müllerian anomalies
- Ovarian cyst
- Paratubal cyst

INTRODUCTION

A pelvic mass may be identified during routine screening examination, evaluation for abdominopelvic pain, or abnormal bleeding. It may also be an incidental finding on imaging for an unrelated medical concern. While adnexal masses may be of ovarian origin, other diagnoses should be considered. While there is overlap, the list of likely diagnoses of a pelvic mass for prepubertal, adolescent, and young adult females is different than for older female patients.[1] Table 57.1 lists conditions associated with the diagnosis of pelvic masses in adolescents and young adults (AYAs). In particular, müllerian anomalies with obstruction typically present in early adolescence due to the accumulation of obstructed menses. Table 57.2 categorizes ovarian masses in AYAs.

TABLE 57.1

Conditions Diagnosed as a Pelvic Mass in Adolescent and Young Adult Females

Urinary	Full urinary bladder
	Urachal cyst
	Pelvic kidney
Uterus	Sharply anteflexed or retroflexed uterus
	Pregnancy
	Intrauterine
	Tubal
	Abdominal
	Obstructed müllerian anomaly
Ovarian or adnexal masses	Functional cysts
	Endometriomas
	Neoplastic tumors
	Benign
	Malignant
	Primary ovarian
	Metastatic
	Borderline
	Inflammatory masses
	Tubo-ovarian complex
	Appendiceal abscess
Other	Peritoneal cyst
	Stool in sigmoid
	Paraovarian or paratubal cysts
Less common or rare conditions in AYAs	Uterine leiomyoma or adenomyoma
	Diverticular abscess
	Carcinoma of the GI tract
	Retroperitoneal tumors (Wilms tumor or anterior sacral meningocele)
	Uterine carcinoma, sarcoma, or other malignant tumors

AYAs, adolescent and young adults; GI, gastrointestinal.

TABLE 57.2

Benign Ovarian Tumors

Functional Cysts
    Follicular
    Corpus luteal
    Theca lutein

Neoplastic Masses
    Germ cell tumors
        Benign cystic teratoma (dermoid)
        Dysgerminoma
        Mixed germ cell tumor
        Endodermal sinus tumor
        Immature teratoma
        Embryonal tumor
        Choriocarcinoma
        Polyembryomas
    Sex cord–stromal tumors
        Sertoli–Leydig cell tumor
        Granulosa cell tumor
        Fibroma
        Adenofibroma
    Epithelial tumors
        Serous cystadenoma
        Mucinous cystadenoma
        Brenner tumor

Other
    Endometrioma

CONGENITAL ANOMALIES

Uterine Defects: Incomplete Lateral Fusion

Anatomical genital anomalies may present as a pelvic mass during adolescence. Though rare, they can have profound implications for future reproductive capability. Obstructing anomalies typically present with pain and a pelvic mass, representing an accumulation

of menstrual fluid within the vagina (hematocolpos) and/or uterus (hematometra).[2] It is uncommon but not unheard of for nonobstructing anomalies to present in young adulthood. Embryologically, the uterus is formed by the fusion of paramesonephric ducts in the midline (Fig. 57.1). If lateral fusion is incomplete, then a uterus didelphys may form with two separate uterine halves (each with a cervix, corpus, attached fallopian tube and ovary, and

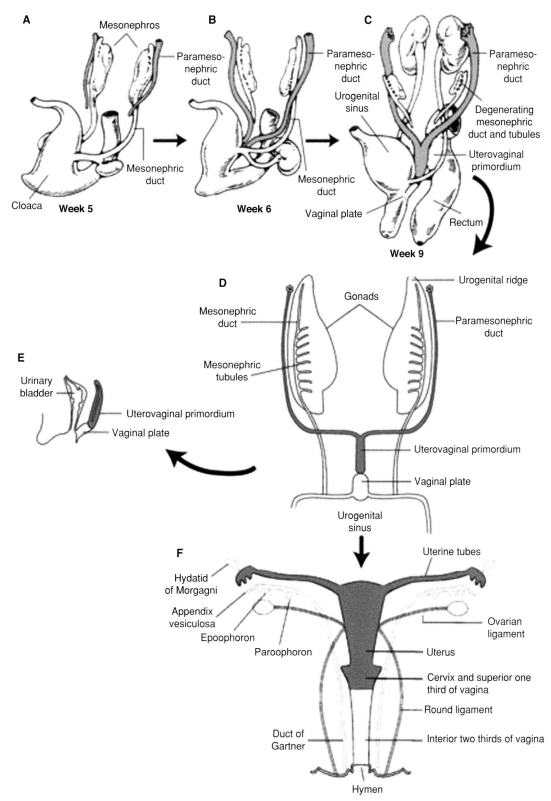

FIGURE 57.1 Development of uterus from paired paramesonephric ducts. (From Dudek RW. *BRS Embryology.* 5th ed. Lippincott Williams & Wilkins; 2010.)

possibly vaginal canal) (Fig. 57.2). On either physical examination or radiologic imaging, the obstructed hemiuterus may be mistaken for an adnexal mass. If uterine fusion is partial, there may be a bicornuate uterus or blind uterine horn. There may be a unilateral obstructed horn, and if functional endometrium is present within this obstructed horn, severe cyclic pain can occur. The diagnosis can be suggested on the basis of a screening pelvic ultrasound examination. If a developmental anomaly is suspected on ultrasound examination, magnetic resonance imaging (MRI) is the best technique for clarifying genital anomalies.[3] Renal and skeletal

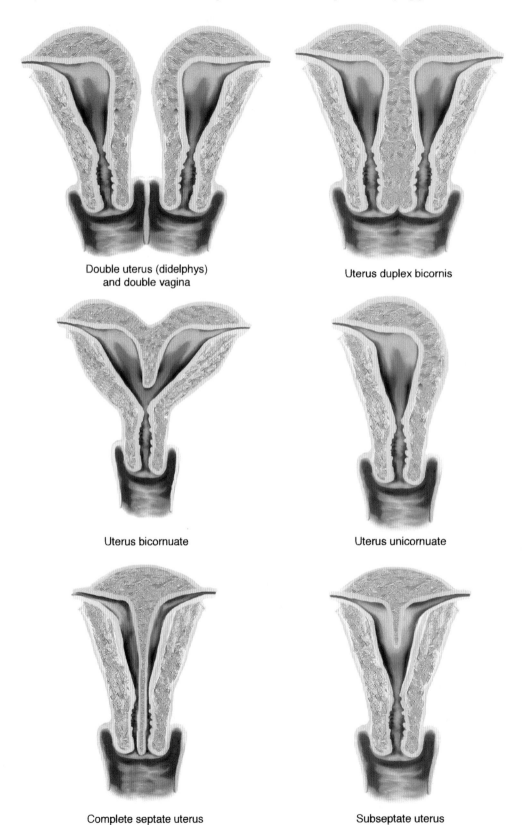

Double uterus (didelphys)
and double vagina

Uterus duplex bicornis

Uterus bicornuate

Uterus unicornuate

Complete septate uterus

Subseptate uterus

FIGURE 57.2 Uterine fusion abnormalities. (From Baggish MS, Valle RF, Guedj H. *Hysteroscopy: Visual Perspectives of Uterine Anatomy, Physiology and Pathology*. 3rd ed. Lippincott Williams & Wilkins; 2007.)

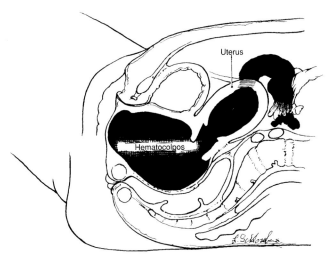

FIGURE 57.3 Hematocolpos, hematometra, hematosalpinx due to imperforate hymen. (From Handa VL, Van Le L. *Te Linde's Operative Gynecology.* 12th ed. Lippincott Williams & Wilkins; 2019.)

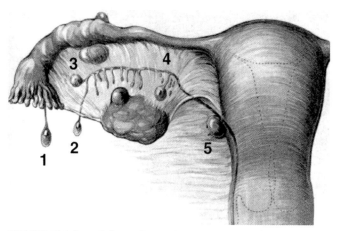

FIGURE 57.4 Paratubal cysts from embryologic remnants. (From Dudek RW. *BRS Embryology.* 5th ed. Lippincott Williams & Wilkins; 2010.)

anomalies are common in conjunction with uterine lateral fusion defects; when renal anomalies, including renal agenesis or dysgenesis, are diagnosed, there should be a high level of suspicion for müllerian anomalies.[4]

The vagina also forms in two parts (cranial and caudad), and defects typically occur as a result of failure of longitudinal fusion or canalization. If the upper and lower vaginal portions do not fuse, then a transverse vaginal septum forms. Similarly, if the solid core of tissue at the junction of the vaginal plate and the urogenital sinus do not canalize completely, an imperforate hymen or vaginal agenesis results. If a uterus with functional endometrium is present with a transverse vaginal septum or imperforate hymen, a hematocolpos or hematometra forms, presenting as a "pelvic mass" (Fig. 57.3). Imperforate hymen is the most frequent obstructive anomaly of the female genital tract, but estimates of its frequency vary from 1 case per 1,000 population to 1 case per 10,000 population.[5]

Uterovaginal Agenesis

Patients with uterovaginal agenesis—Mayer–Rokitansky–Küster–Hauser (MRKH) syndrome—typically present with primary amenorrhea. They may have uterine remnants containing functioning endometrium, which can cause pain, and a mass diagnosed with ultrasonography or MRI.

Müllerian Duct Remnants

Another class of congenital anatomical anomalies that can create pelvic masses arises from remnants of the mesonephric/müllerian duct system or mesovarium that should have degenerated in utero in the presence of antimüllerian hormone. At least 25% of female adults have small remnants of these systems. These remnants can be present in the lateral adnexa as paraovarian cysts or paratubal cysts (Fig. 57.4). They are often multiple and can vary in size from <1 cm to 20 cm or larger. Along the lateral wall of the vagina or uterus, these remnants present as Gartner duct cysts. These müllerian remnants are rarely symptomatic; however, torsion of any adnexal mass, including a paratubal cyst, can occur, and persistent larger masses may be confused with an ovarian neoplasm.

Urachal Cysts and Pelvic Kidneys

Urachal cysts, although rare, can be found along the midline above the bladder and can be confused with other pelvic masses. A pelvic kidney must also be included in the differential diagnosis (Fig. 57.5). Any other structure in the pelvis, such as a full bladder or hard stool in the rectum, can be confused with a pelvic mass.

PREGNANCY PRESENTING AS PELVIC MASS

The possibility of an intrauterine pregnancy enlarging the uterus or an ectopic pregnancy (see Chapter 58) causing an abdominal or adnexal mass must be considered in the differential diagnosis of every young female with secondary sexual characteristics (Fig. 57.6). A sensitive urine pregnancy test can reliably rule out a clinically significant pregnancy. However, in many instances, the test is not ordered because the clinician does not consider it likely that the AYA has been sexually active. Adolescents and young adults may be unwilling or unable to disclose their history of sexual activity for a variety of reasons—they may fear disappointing their parents/caregivers or the clinician; they may have insufficient knowledge or awareness of pregnancy-related symptoms; they may deny the possibility of pregnancy; the clinician may not have established or discussed the provisions of confidentiality; or questions may not have been asked in a sensitive manner in a private setting. Both sexual abuse and early consensual sexual activity may occur, resulting in pregnancy. In the presence of pelvic mass, a pregnancy test should be performed. The consequences of missing a pregnancy-related cause of pain, bleeding, or a pelvic mass justifies pregnancy testing in all female AYAs presenting with pain, amenorrhea, abnormal bleeding, or a pelvic mass.[6]

INFECTION AS A CAUSE OF A PELVIC MASS

Adolescents and young adults have the highest age-specific rates of *Chlamydia trachomatis* and thus are at risk for upper tract

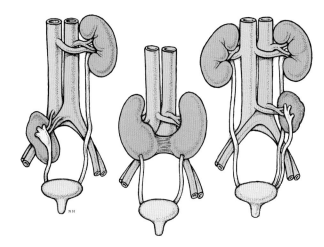

FIGURE 57.5 Pelvic kidney, horseshoe kidney, and supernumerary kidney. (Courtesy of Neil O. Hardy, Westpoint, CT.)

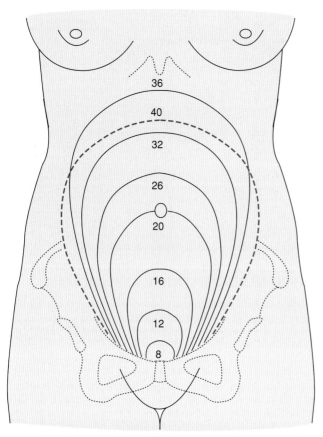

FIGURE 57.6 Pregnancy with fundal height corresponding to gestational age. (From Beckmann CRB, Ling FW, Smith RP, et al. *Obstetrics and Gynecology.* 5th ed. Lippincott Williams & Wilkins; 2006.)

involvement with salpingitis or a pelvic abscess (tubo-ovarian abscess [TOA]) (see Chapter 63).[7] In the acute stage, a pelvic infection may be indolent in its presentation or, alternatively, accompanied by fever, discharge, cervical motion tenderness, and possibly adnexal masses (pyosalpinges or TOAs) (Fig. 57.7). After resolution of the acute infection, the tubes may remain dilated and filled with fluid (hydrosalpinges), particularly if their fimbriae have been

scarred by inflammation and thus sealed. Treated pelvic abscesses may also cause palpable masses due to adhesions—pelvic scarring with matting or agglutination of bowel, ovary, fallopian tube, and other structures. Other infectious causes of pelvic masses include an appendiceal abscess or (rarely in young girls) diverticulitis or Meckel diverticulum.

ADNEXAL TORSION

Adnexal torsion involves the rotation of adnexal structures and is a cause of acute pelvic pain, which is often accompanied by nausea and vomiting. The diagnosis may be missed if the possibility of torsion is not considered.[8] Torsion of the normal adnexa can occur; however, torsion is more likely to occur when an adnexal mass rotates around its vascular pedicle. Once rotated, the venous flow to the mass is obstructed while arterial flow continues, inflating the mass until the arterial flow is compressed (Fig. 57.8). The adnexal structures become edematous and ultimately gangrenous.

Diagnosis

The diagnosis of adnexal torsion is a clinical one, as imaging findings are typically not definitive. A history typically includes acute onset of severe pain, which is often accompanied by nausea and vomiting. Findings on examination include peritoneal signs with rebound tenderness. Typical findings on ultrasound examination with Doppler flow studies include the presence of a mass, edema, adnexal asymmetry, and absent venous and/or arterial flow; unfortunately, these findings are neither perfectly sensitive nor specific, and clinical judgment must be used, including a high index of suspicion. Consultation with a gynecologist is essential, as adnexal torsion is a surgical emergency.

Treatment

Treatment consists of untwisting the adnexa rather than extirpation, even if hemorrhage and apparent necrosis are present, as ovarian preservation is most often possible. Untwisting the adnexa can usually be performed laparoscopically. Excision of the cyst or adnexal mass can be performed laparoscopically, or may be delayed and performed as an interval procedure once edema has resolved. Every attempt should be made to preserve the involved ovary.

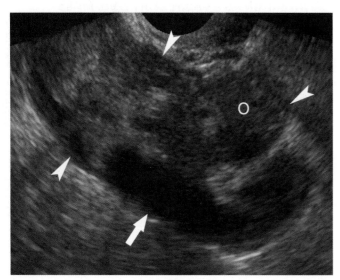

FIGURE 57.7 Tubo-ovarian abscess. Ultrasound of the pelvis shows complex mass (*arrowheads*) around the ovary (O) and dilated tube (*arrow*). (From Klein J; Vinson EN, Brant WE, Helms CA. *Brant and Helms' Fundamentals of Diagnostic Radiology.* Lippincott Williams & Wilkins; 2018.)

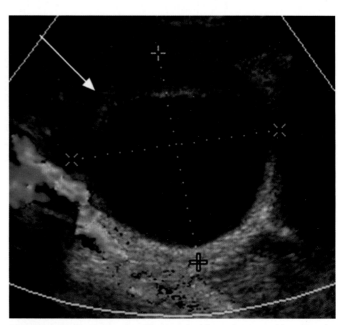

FIGURE 57.8 Ovarian torsion. Ultrasound with ovarian cyst with no Doppler flow. (From Shirkhoda A. *Variants and Pitfalls in Body Imaging.* 2nd ed. Lippincott Williams & Wilkins; 2010.)

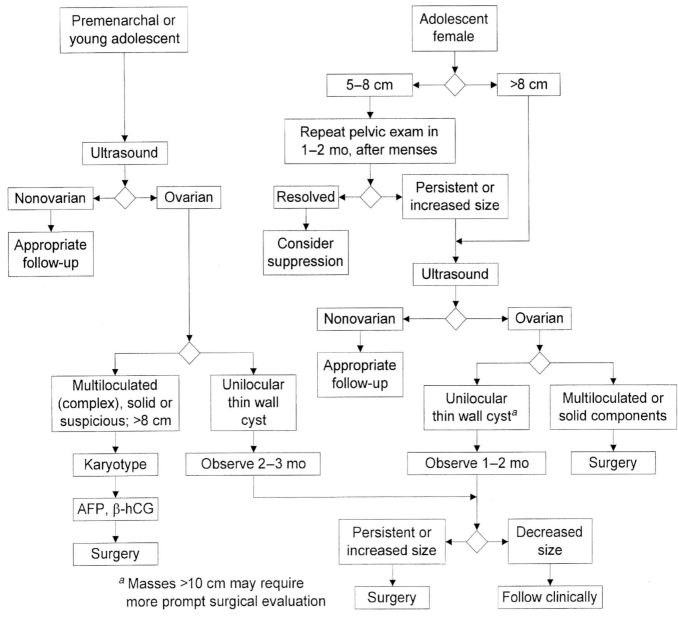

FIGURE 57.9 Management of pelvic masses in prepubertal, adolescent, and young adult females. AFP, α-fetoprotein; hCG, human chorionic gonadotropin.

UTERINE NEOPLASMS

In female AYAs, uterine neoplasms are rare. Benign leiomyomas (fibroids) are rare in adolescence, may be asymptomatic or cause abnormal bleeding, and will be evident on pelvic imaging.

OVARIAN MASSES

Benign ovarian masses include *functional ovarian cysts, endometriomas, and benign ovarian neoplasms*. Whenever an ovarian mass is diagnosed in an AYA female or prepubertal child, every effort must be made to preserve the reproductive function, whether the mass is physiologic or neoplastic, benign, or malignant.[9] Table 57.2 lists ovarian masses. Suspicion of an adnexal mass should prompt a pelvic ultrasound to confirm. A unilocular cyst <8 cm in size is unlikely to be malignant, particularly if asymptomatic.

Figure 57.9 provides a plan for the management of pelvic masses in premenarchal and female AYAs.

Physiologic (Functional) Ovarian Cysts

Functional ovarian cysts include *follicular cysts, corpus luteum cysts, and theca lutein cysts*. All are benign and usually do not cause symptoms or require surgical management. Functional cysts result from the expansion of the cavity of a preovulatory follicle (follicular cyst) or corpus luteum, and are associated with the disordered function of the pituitary–ovarian axis. The incidence of functional ovarian cysts in AYAs is not well established. However, most follicular cysts are asymptomatic, and they are frequently an incidental finding on pelvic imaging (Fig. 57.10A, B). Corpus luteal cysts can be painful, as they result from acute hemorrhage into the cystic corpus luteum cavity. Theca lutein cysts—the least common type of functional cyst—result from human chorionic gonadotropin (hCG) stimulation, producing bilateral follicular cystic ovarian enlargement. They occur in patients with gestational trophoblastic disease (molar pregnancies and choriocarcinoma) and multiple pregnancies and regress with the removal of the pregnancy-associated hCG production.

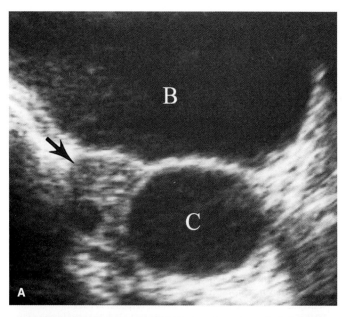

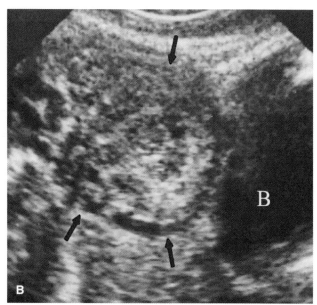

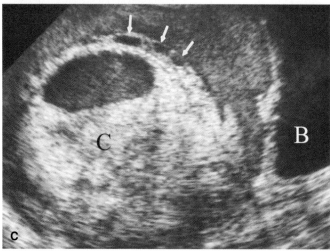

FIGURE 57.10 Ovarian cysts. Ultrasound with (**A**) simple follicular cyst, (**B**) hemorrhage into cyst, and (**C**) hemorrhagic corpus luteal cyst in patient on warfarin. (From Klein J, Vinson EN, Brant, WE, Helms CA. *Brant and Helms' Fundamentals of Diagnostic Radiology.* Lippincott Williams & Wilkins, 2018.)

1. **Follicular cysts**: The most common type of functional ovarian cyst is a follicular cyst. Follicular cysts are unilocular and simple without internal structure and range in size from 3 to 15 cm in diameter but rarely exceed 8 cm (Fig. 57.11). Follicular cysts can be seen in prepubertal girls, and they typically resolve over time. Management depends on symptoms, patient age, menarchal status, cyst size and character, and associated medical conditions. Torsion or rupture may occur, causing pain, and misdiagnosis is common.[10] In AYAs, follicular cysts usually resolve spontaneously in 4 to 8 weeks unless the patient is using progestins (e.g., levonorgestrel intrauterine system or depot medroxyprogesterone acetate [DMPA]), which can slow follicular atresia and require a longer time for resolution. In general, conservative management of cysts smaller than 8 cm in a premenopausal female is recommended. Persistent ovarian masses are more likely to be neoplastic and should prompt consideration of surgical excision. Decisions about whether surgical excision of ovarian masses is required are best made by gynecologic surgeons who have experience with AYA and pediatric patients.[11] Decisions about the type of surgical intervention are guided by the suspicion of malignancy and imaging characteristics of the mass.

2. **Corpus luteal cysts**: A corpus luteal cyst is arbitrarily defined as a "cyst" if it exceeds 3 cm in diameter, but it can reach

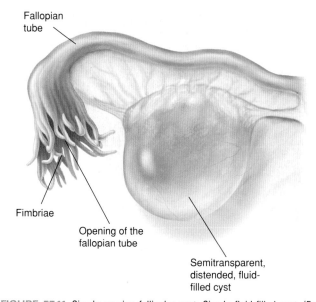

FIGURE 57.11 Simple ovarian follicular cyst. Simple fluid-filled cyst. (From Lippincott. *Pathophysiology Made Incredibly Visual!* 2nd ed. Lippincott Williams & Wilkins; 2011.)

larger dimensions. They may be associated with delayed menses. Corpus luteal cysts are less common than follicular cysts but are clinically more significant because they can be associated with acute pain (due to bleeding into the enclosed cystic space) or rupture, leading to acute hemoperitoneum. This can be a surgical emergency, particularly if the patient is taking an anticoagulant. A cyst may rupture during intercourse late in the cycle (days 21 to 26); although rare, rupture can also follow pelvic examination, strenuous exercise, or trauma. Pain can occur in the absence of trauma. Patients presenting with pain and an adnexal mass on ultrasound examination may require gynecologic consultation to differentiate an unruptured corpus luteal cyst, which should be managed medically, from torsion, hemoperitoneum, or appendicitis—acute surgical emergencies. Typical ultrasonographic findings include a mixed echogenic adnexal mass (Fig. 57.10C). Doppler flow ultrasonographic studies can suggest the possibility of torsion with decreased venous and/or arterial flow. Because oral contraceptives suppress follicular development and ovulation, they reduce the risk of functional cysts in a dose-dependent manner. Administration of oral contraceptives to induce cyst regression is no more effective than an observation period with no hormonal therapy, although it will suppress the development of subsequent functional cysts.[12]

Endometriomas and Endometriosis

Endometriosis is a condition in which ectopic endometrium is present outside of the uterus. The presence of ovarian endometriosis can result in the formation of an ovarian endometrioma. There is a broad range of ultrasound appearances of endometriomas—diffuse, low-level internal echoes occur in most endometriomas, and hyperechoic wall foci and multilocularity also suggest the diagnosis of an endometrioma (Fig. 57.12).

Endometriosis has historically been considered to be a condition affecting adults; however, it is receiving increasing recognition as a cause of pelvic pain in adolescents.[13] Although the prevalence of endometriosis in adolescents is not well established, there is a familial incidence, and endometriosis can be demonstrated in up to 40% to 50% of adolescents undergoing laparoscopy because of chronic pelvic pain unresponsive to the use of oral medications, such as oral contraceptives and nonsteroidal anti-inflammatory

drugs (NSAIDs). Endometriomas are also rare in adolescents, who typically have early-stage or mild disease.

Clinical manifestations include worsening dysmenorrhea, premenstrual or acyclic pelvic pain, and deep dyspareunia. On pelvic examination, findings of diffuse or localized tenderness, particularly in the cul-de-sac posterior to the uterus, diminished uterine motility (a result of adhesion formation particularly between the uterus and the sigmoid), cervical motion tenderness (from adhesions), and possibly an ovarian mass (endometrioma) are suggestive of endometriosis.

Adolescents rarely have the "classic" finding of uterosacral nodularity. Because laparoscopy provides a definitive diagnosis of suspected endometriosis, AYAs with pelvic pain or dysmenorrhea unresponsive to NSAIDs and oral contraceptives should be referred to a gynecologist for surgical confirmation of possible endometriosis.[14]

Benign Ovarian Neoplasms

Benign ovarian neoplasms typically are unilocular and cystic, without solid components, papillations, vascular septae, or ascites.[15] Adolescents and young adults with persistent cystic ovarian masses on ultrasonography following 6 to 8 weeks of observation may have an ovarian neoplasm and should be referred to a gynecologist for surgical management. Benign cystic teratomas (dermoid cysts) are the most common ovarian neoplasm in adolescents. Any female with a plain film x-ray or an ultrasonogram showing characteristics suspicious of a teratoma (bone, teeth, or fat components) should also be referred for gynecologic surgical evaluation (Fig. 57.13). Solid masses of any size are suspicious for a malignant tumor and should lead to prompt referral.

Benign Germ Cell Tumors

Benign cystic teratomas (dermoid cysts) are the most common benign ovarian neoplasm of adolescence and the subsequent reproductive years.[11] Dermoid cysts include all three germ cell layers. They are generally thick-walled cysts and may be filled with sebaceous material and hair; they may also contain cartilage, teeth, or other tissues such as thyroid (Fig. 57.14). These embryologic elements produce characteristic findings on ultrasonography that can suggest the likelihood of a benign cystic teratoma. Malignant transformation occurs in less than 2% of dermoid cysts in female patients of all ages and is rare in AYAs. Dermoid cysts vary in size from millimeters to quite large, but the vast majority of dermoids are smaller than 10 cm. They are unilateral (approximately 10% are bilateral), very mobile, anteriorly positioned, and nontender adnexal masses on examination. Benign cystic teratomas are usually asymptomatic. The risk of torsion with dermoid cysts is approximately 15%.

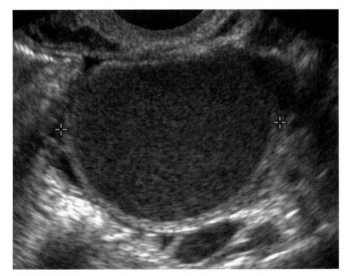

FIGURE 57.12 Endometrioma. Transvaginal sonogram shows adnexal cyst with homogeneous internal echoes. Appearance is similar to a hemorrhagic cyst, but an endometrioma will not resolve over approximately two cycles. (From Klein J, Vinson EN, Brant WE, Helms CA. *Brant and Helms' Fundamentals of Diagnostic Radiology.* Lippincott Williams & Wilkins; 2018.)

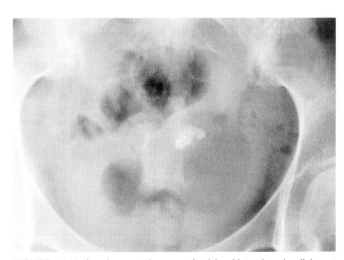

FIGURE 57.13 Anterior–posterior x-ray of pelvis with teeth and radiolucent fat in a benign cystic ovarian teratoma (dermoid cyst). (Courtesy of Hal Grass, DC, Denver, CO.)

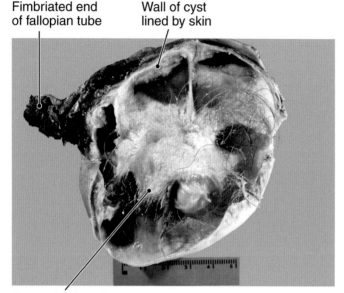

Fimbriated end of fallopian tube | Wall of cyst lined by skin

Mass of hair and sebaceous material

FIGURE 57.14 Benign ovarian cystic teratoma (dermoid cyst). (From McConnell TH. *Nature of Disease.* 2nd ed. Lippincott Williams & Wilkins; 2013.)

It occurs more frequently than in other ovarian tumors in general, perhaps because of the high-fat content of most dermoid cysts, allowing them to "float" within the abdominal and pelvic cavity. An ovarian cystectomy is almost always possible rather than an oophorectomy, even if it appears that only a small amount of ovarian tissue remains. Preserving a small amount of ovarian cortex in a young patient with a benign lesion is preferable to the loss of the entire ovary. Adolescents and young adults with ultrasonography suggesting a dermoid should be referred to a gynecologic surgeon who appreciates the importance of ovarian conservation.

Benign Epithelial Neoplasia

Serous or mucinous cystadenomas account for 10% to 20% of benign ovarian neoplasms in female adolescents. These tumors are typically uni- or multiloculated, fluid-filled cystic masses (Fig. 57.15). Serous cystadenomas may not be recognized as neoplasms; cyst aspiration without removal of the entire cyst (including multiple loculated areas and cyst wall) frequently results in recurrence of

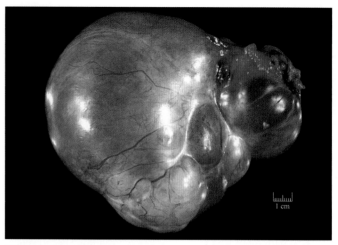

FIGURE 57.16 Mucinous cystadenoma with multiple loculations. (From Reichert RA. *Diagnostic Gynecologic and Obstetric Pathology.* Lippincott Williams & Wilkins; 2011.)

these neoplasms. Benign mucinous cystadenomas have smooth, lobulated surfaces with multiloculations filled with viscous mucoid material (Fig. 57.16); these masses can reach very large dimensions (Fig. 57.17). Surgical removal of these adenomas is necessary for tissue diagnosis and to prevent symptoms from an enlarging mass or torsion.

Sex Cord–Stromal Tumors

Overall, these tumors are relatively rare, but they occur with higher prevalence in premenarchal girls than in AYAs and comprise 10% to 20% of childhood ovarian tumors. They may be hormonally active. Granulosa cell tumors and theca cell tumors produce estrogen, whereas Sertoli–Leydig cell tumors produce androgens with or without estrogen. As a result of this sex steroid production, sex cord–stromal tumors can cause precocious puberty, menstrual abnormalities, endometrial hyperplasia or carcinoma, or hirsutism, acne, and virilization. These signs should prompt pelvic imaging for diagnosis which typically reveals a solid or mixed solid and cystic mass (Fig. 57.18). Pure granulosa cell tumors are highly malignant, whereas mixed tumors behave less aggressively. Prognosis is excellent with unilateral salpingo-oophorectomy and appropriate surgical staging for 95% of tumors that are unilateral.

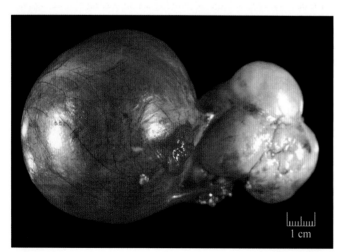

FIGURE 57.15 Intact serous cystadenoma as thin-walled cyst. (From Reichert RA. *Diagnostic Gynecologic and Obstetric Pathology.* Lippincott Williams & Wilkins; 2011.)

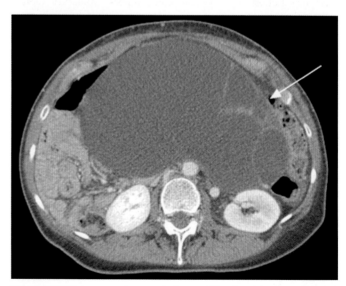

FIGURE 57.17 Large mucinous cystadenoma filling the abdomen on CT imaging. (From Shirkhoda A. *Variants and Pitfalls in Body Imaging.* 2nd ed. Lippincott Williams & Wilkins; 2010.)

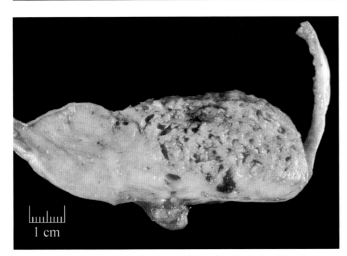

FIGURE 57.18 Granulosa cell tumor with section through solid and spongy portion of cystic and solid ovarian mass. (From Reichert RA. *Diagnostic Gynecologic and Obstetric Pathology*. Lippincott Williams & Wilkins; 2011.)

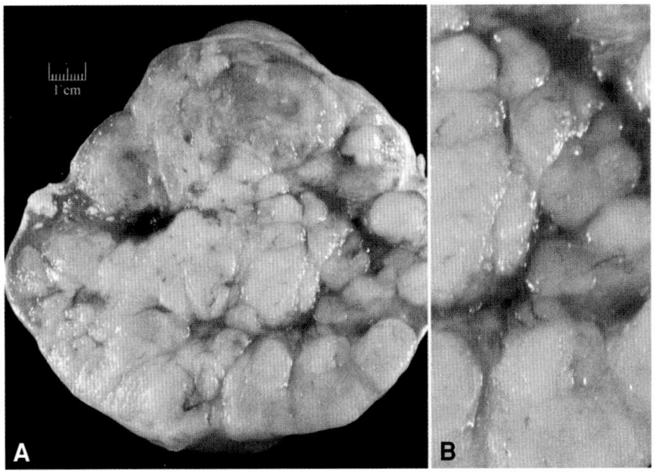

FIGURE 57.19 Dysgerminoma with solid lobulated appearance. (From Reichert RA. *Diagnostic Gynecologic and Obstetric Pathology*. Lippincott Williams & Wilkins; 2011.)

MALIGNANT OVARIAN MASSES

Ovarian cancer is rare in AYAs and younger girls. Only slightly more than 1% of all ovarian cancers occur in female patients younger than 18 years. The incidence of ovarian malignancies in girls 18 years and younger is 5.9/1 million female patients.[16] With increasing age from childhood through young adulthood, there is a progression from germ cell to epithelial cell malignancies.[16] Ultrasound features of an ovarian mass that are a cause of concern for malignancy include solid consistency, large size, complex appearance (not entirely cystic), internal loculations, internal or external excrescences, and ascites. Efforts to preserve fertility are important considerations in the management of ovarian malignancies in adolescents.

Malignant Germ Cell Tumors

In female patients younger than 20 years, one-half to two-thirds of all ovarian tumors are of germ cell origin and one-third of those tumors are malignant. Germ cell tumors of all types, including dermoids, are seen with slightly greater frequency in the third decade of life compared to during adolescence, but secondary malignant change in teratomas remains uncommon in AYAs under age 30 years.[17] Malignant germ cell tumors include dysgerminomas, mixed germ cell tumors, endodermal sinus tumors, immature teratomas, embryonal tumors, choriocarcinomas, and polyembryomas. Because some ovarian neoplasms secrete protein tumor markers, including α-fetoprotein (AFP), hCG, carcinoembryonic antigen (CEA), lactate dehydrogenase (LDH), and others, measurement of these substances can be considered in making a diagnosis of an ovarian tumor and in following up malignant tumors for recurrence and clinical response.[18] Cancer antigen (CA) 125 is a tumor marker for epithelial ovarian cancer, and while useful in evaluating adnexal masses in postmenopausal patients, it is not very specific. In AYAs and premenopausal adults, it may be elevated with many other benign gynecologic conditions. The decision about whether to assess tumor markers in an AYA with an adnexal mass is best left to the gynecologic surgeon, as they will assess the risks of malignancy.

Dysgerminomas comprise 50% of all ovarian germ cell malignancies (Fig. 57.19). About 5% to 10% of these tumors occur in phenotypically female patients with disorders of sex differentiation (DSD). The presence of a Y chromosome is associated with a risk of malignancy, although the degree of risk is related to the type of DSD; bilateral gonadectomy is recommended if the risk is high.[19]

Malignant Epithelial Tumors

Although these tumor types are the most common type of ovarian malignancy in female adults, they are rare in AYAs.[20] Less than 5% of ovarian epithelial tumors in AYAs are invasive malignancies. Appropriate surgical staging, cytoreductive surgery, and chemotherapy are required in these patients, as in adults; conservative management in early-stage disease may allow the preservation of fertility.[21] These patients require ongoing management by a gynecologic oncologist. Included in this group of neoplasias are serous cystadenocarcinomas, mucinous cystadenocarcinomas, and endometrial cystadenocarcinomas. In adolescents, approximately 7% of epithelial tumors will be borderline malignancies, which can be managed in conjunction with a gynecologic oncologist, with conservative surgery (unilateral salpingo-oophorectomy), careful assessment of the contralateral ovary, and appropriate staging procedures.[22] Epithelial borderline tumors become more common in the third decade of life, compared to during adolescence and young adulthood.[17]

Genetic Risk of Epithelial Ovarian Cancers

Approximately 15% of ovarian cancer is associated with genetic mutations in the breast cancer gene 1 (*BRCA-1*), although other cancer susceptibility genes are now being identified.[23] Families with multiple family members with breast and/or ovarian cancer should be offered referral to specific familial cancer centers for genetic counseling and potential testing. Ideally, the family member who has the malignancy should be tested, rather than the adolescent. Although the optimal age at which genetic testing should be performed has not been well established, professional guidelines recommend against testing minors, and many clinicians recommend offering counseling and testing in young adulthood.[24] Some reports of interviews with mutation carriers and their adult offspring indicate that improved health behaviors during adolescence and young adulthood may result from the disclosure of hereditary risks for adult cancers.[25]

Other Carcinomas

In AYAs, the more common metastatic lesions of the ovary include lymphomas and leukemias.

Minimizing the Risks of Ovarian Masses and Malignancies

Hormonal contraception minimizes the risks of functional ovarian masses in a dose-dependent manner.[12] Adolescents and young adults who have had an oophorectomy, an ovarian cystectomy, or an ovarian neoplasm may benefit from the use of combined estrogen–progestin contraceptives (e.g., pills, rings, patches) to minimize the risks of developing a subsequent functional cyst. Combination contraceptives minimize the risks that a sole-remaining ovary will develop a functional ovarian cyst and be vulnerable to surgical extirpation. In AYAs with a previous malignancy who are being monitored for recurrence, the development of a functional cyst will almost invariably lead to patient and parental anxiety, additional diagnostic testing, and even potential surgical exploration. Therefore, suppression of functional ovarian cysts can be particularly beneficial.

Combination contraceptives are associated with a 30% to 60% reduction in the risk of epithelial ovarian malignancies.[26] Preventing ovarian cancer is seldom a motivating factor in the use of hormonal contraception for AYAs; however, when combined with the contraceptive and other noncontraceptive benefits of combination contraceptives, such as decreased acne, dysmenorrhea, menorrhagia, and ovarian cysts, this benefit may provide additional motivation for ongoing oral contraceptive use to teens and their families.

SUMMARY

Pelvic masses in AYAs range from exaggerations of normal physiologic findings (a cystic ovarian follicle or corpus luteal cyst) to complex müllerian anomalies. Pelvic masses may be asymptomatic and found on imaging for unrelated medical concerns, or may present with acute pain, such as with adnexal torsion. Pregnancy may also present an adnexal mass if the pregnancy is ectopic. A pelvic infection (i.e., pelvic inflammatory disease) may present with an adnexal mass, comprised of a TOA. The most common ovarian neoplasm in an adolescent is a benign cystic teratoma (a dermoid cyst). Ovarian conservation should be a priority in management of adnexal masses. Consultation with a gynecologic surgeon who understands the variety of adnexal masses that may present in adolescence or young adulthood and who appreciates the importance of ovarian conservation is imperative in the management of pelvic masses.

REFERENCES

1. Solone M, Hillard PJA. Adult gynecology: reproductive years. In: Berek JS, ed. *Berek & Novak's Gynecology.* 16th ed. Wolters Kluwer; 2020:193.
2. Dietrich JE, Millar DM, Quint EH. Obstructive reproductive tract anomalies. *J Pediatr Adolesc Gynecol.* 2014;27(6):396–402.
3. Church DG, Vancil JM, Vasanawala SS. Magnetic resonance imaging for uterine and vaginal anomalies. *Curr Opin Obstet Gynecol.* 2009;21(5):379–389.
4. O'Flynn O'Brien KL, Bhatia V, Homafar M, et al. The prevalence of müllerian anomalies in women with a diagnosed renal anomaly. *J Pediatr Adolesc Gynecol.* 2021;34(2):154–160.
5. Hillard PA. Imperforate hymen. *Medscape.* Accessed March 7, 2021. https://emedicine.medscape.com/article/269050-overview
6. Hillard PJA. Pediatric and adolescent gynecology. In: Berek JS, ed. *Berek and Novak's Gynecology.* 16th ed. Wolters Kluwer; 2020:181.
7. Workowski KA, Bachmann LH, Chan PA, et al. Sexually transmitted infections treatment guidelines, 2021. *MMWR Recomm Rep 2021.* 2021;70(4):1–187.
8. Childress KJ, Dietrich JE. Pediatric ovarian torsion. *Surg Clin North Am.* 2017;97(1):209–221.
9. Kirkham YA, Kives S. Ovarian cysts in adolescents: medical and surgical management. *Adolesc Med State Art Rev.* 2012;23(1):178–191.
10. Adnexal torsion in adolescents: ACOG Committee Opinion No, 783. *Obstet Gynecol.* 2019;134(2):e56–e63.
11. Hernon M, McKenna J, Busby G, et al. The histology and management of ovarian cysts found in children and adolescents presenting to a children's hospital from 1991 to 2007: a call for more paediatric gynaecologists. *BJOG.* 2010;117(2):181–184.
12. Grimes DA, Jones LB, Lopez LM, et al. Oral contraceptives for functional ovarian cysts. *Cochrane Database Syst Rev.* 2011;9:CD006134.
13. Steenberg CK, Tanbo TG, Qvigstad E. Endometriosis in adolescence: predictive markers and management. *Acta Obstet Gynecol Scand.* 2013;92(5):491–495.
14. Shim JY, Laufer MR. Adolescent endometriosis: an update. *J Pediatr Adolesc Gynecol.* 2020;33(2):112–119.
15. Barroilhet L, Vitonis A, Shipp T, et al. Sonographic predictors of ovarian malignancy. *J Clin Ultrasound.* 2013;41(5):269–274.
16. Wohlmuth C, Wohlmuth-Wieser I. Gynecologic malignancies in children and adolescents: how common is the uncommon? *J Clin Med.* 2021;10(4).
17. Young RH. Ovarian tumors and tumor-like lesions in the first three decades. *Semin Diagn Pathol.* 2014;31(5):382–426.
18. Terzic M, Rapisarda AMC, Corte LD, et al. Diagnostic work-up in paediatric and adolescent patients with adnexal masses: an evidence-based approach. *J Obstet Gynaecol.,* 2021;41(4):503–515.
19. Morin J, Peard L, Vanadurongvan T, et al. Oncologic outcomes of pre-malignant and invasive germ cell tumors in patients with differences in sex development–a systematic review. *J Pediatr Urol.* 2020;16(5):576–582.
20. Hazard FK, Longacre TA. Ovarian surface epithelial neoplasms in the pediatric population: incidence, histologic subtype, and natural history. *Am J Surg Pathol.* 2013;37(4):548–553.
21. Bercow A, Nitecki R, Brady PC, et al. Outcomes after fertility-sparing surgery for women with ovarian cancer: a systematic review of the literature. *J Minim Invasive Gynecol.* 2021; 28(3):527–536.
22. du Bois A, Ewald-Riegler N, de Gregorio N, et al. Borderline tumours of the ovary: a cohort study of the Arbeitsgemeinschaft Gynakologische Onkologie (AGO) Study Group. *Eur J Cancer.* 2013;49(8):1905–1914.
23. PDG Cancer Genetics Editorial Board. Genetics of breast and gynecologic cancers (PDQ®):health professional version. In: *PDQ Cancer Information Summaries.* National Cancer Institute (US); 2002.
24. Emans SJ, Laufer MR, DiVasta A. *Emans, Laufer, Goldstein's Pediatric and Adolescent Gynecology.* 7th ed. Lippincott Williams & Wilkins; 2020.
25. Bradbury AR, Patrick-Miller L, Pawlowski K, et al. Learning of your parent's BRCA mutation during adolescence or early adulthood: a study of offspring experiences. *Psychooncology.* 2009;18(2):200–208.
26. Del Pup L, Codacci-Pisanelli G, Peccatori F. Breast cancer risk of hormonal contraception: counselling considering new evidence. *Crit Rev Oncol Hematol.* 2019; 137:123–130.

ADDITIONAL RESOURCES AND WEBSITES

Additional Resources and Websites for Clinicians:

The American College of Obstetricians and Gynecologists—http://www.ACOG.org

The North American Society for Pediatric and Adolescent Gynecology—http://www.NASPAG.org

Additional Resources and Websites for Parents/Caregivers and Adolescents and Young Adults:

The American College of Obstetricians and Gynecologists—For Patients—https://www.acog.org/womens-health

Center for Young Women's Health—https://youngwomenshealth.org

The North American Society for Pediatric and Adolescent Gynecology-Resources for Patients—https://www.naspag.org/resources-for-patients

58

CHAPTER

Ectopic Pregnancy

Melissa Mirosh

KEY WORDS

- Ectopic pregnancy
- Methotrexate
- Quantitative β-hCG
- Salpingectomy
- Salpingostomy
- Transvaginal ultrasound

INTRODUCTION

Ectopic pregnancy is uncommon in the adolescent population. Teens have not usually had the exposures to infection, intra-abdominal inflammation, or fertility therapy that are typically associated with this condition. However, patients in their 20s are more likely to have encountered these risk factors. Ectopic pregnancy should be a consideration when any reproductive age female presents with new onset of abnormal uterine vaginal bleeding or abdominal/pelvic pain and a positive pregnancy test. This chapter will review the epidemiology, diagnosis, and management of ectopic pregnancy tailored to the unique needs of adolescents and young adults (AYAs).

ECTOPIC PREGNANCY

Incidence and Prevalence

1. *Rate and anatomic location*: The overall risk of ectopic pregnancy is 2%.[1] This is only an approximation because there are many miscarriages, abortions, and medically treated ectopic pregnancies that are not reported. Ectopic pregnancies occur almost exclusively in the oviduct (95%—most of these within the ampulla), while 1.4% are abdominal and approximately 3% are cervical or ovarian. An ectopic pregnancy can also occur with an intrauterine pregnancy, a condition known as a heterotopic pregnancy (1/30,000 spontaneously conceived pregnancies).[2]
2. *Trends*: The risk of dying from an ectopic pregnancy has continued to decline over the past three decades. It accounted for 2.7% of maternal-related deaths in the United States from 2011 to 2013.[3] The risk of death from ectopic pregnancy in the United Kingdom has remained stable from 2011 to 2017.[4]
3. *Race*: Ectopic pregnancies are more frequently seen in minoritized racial/ethnic groups (e.g., Black, Hispanic/Latino, and Native/Indigenous) compared to White female populations. This demographic trend is also seen with respect to overall maternal morbidity and mortality. This discrepancy is likely multifactorial and includes factors such as increased sexually transmitted infection (STI) rates in these populations, socioeconomic status, and access to care.[5]

Etiology and Risk Factors

At least 50% of ectopic pregnancies do not have any associated risk factor.[6] Of the risk factors that have been described, many are associated with mid-to-later reproductive years. These would include fertility therapy, tubal ligation, age, and diethylstilbestrol exposure.[1] The risks that particularly apply to AYAs are fallopian tube pathology due to pelvic infection (untreated or recurrent STIs or pelvic inflammatory disease [PID]), intrauterine device (IUD) use, and smoking.[1,7] Although the absolute risk of ectopic pregnancy is lower with the use of an IUD (explained by low rate of contraceptive failure), the risk of ectopic pregnancy is elevated should a pregnancy occur with an IUD in situ.[8]

Differential Diagnosis

In addition to ectopic pregnancy, the differential diagnosis for an AYA presenting with acute abdominal or pelvic pain is best divided into obstetric, gynecologic, and nongynecologic categories.

1. Obstetric
   a. Normal intrauterine pregnancy
   b. Hemorrhagic corpus luteum
   c. Spontaneous or threatened abortion
2. Gynecologic
   a. Adnexal torsion
   b. Hemorrhagic ovarian cyst
   c. Symptomatic or ruptured ovarian cyst
   d. Pelvic inflammatory disease
3. Nongynecologic
   a. Appendicitis
   b. Renal colic
   c. Inflammatory bowel disease
   d. Gastroenteritis
   e. Severe constipation
   f. Musculoskeletal pain

Clinical Presentation

Symptoms can range from mild cramping and vaginal spotting to hemorrhagic shock. However, the classic triad of vaginal bleeding, delayed menses, and severe lower abdominal pain associated with tubal rupture is less common because early ultrasound diagnosis is more typical.

Acute Presentation: Classic, Ruptured Ectopic Pregnancy

1. The patient who presents with an acutely ruptured ectopic pregnancy would typically exhibit symptoms of pain and hemodynamic instability. Pelvic pain may be extreme, sharp,

or stabbing in nature, and shoulder tip pain can be associated with hemoperitoneum. Dizziness, lightheadedness, and loss of consciousness may occur from hypotension. Some females may present with symptoms related to gastrointestinal distress (e.g., nausea, vomiting, and diarrhea), and these should not be discounted as a possible ectopic pregnancy. Menses may be abnormal or absent, and this may not seem unusual as teens often have irregular bleeding patterns.

2. Classic signs of a ruptured ectopic pregnancy:
   a. Vital signs: The patient may be in shock with rapid thready pulse, hypotension, and change in mental status.
   b. Abdomen will be tender to palpation, possibly even rigid, with marked rebound tenderness.
   c. Bimanual examination: Cervical motion tenderness is apparent with a slightly enlarged and globular uterus. Often, a pelvic mass is not palpable, due to limitations of the examination or because the rupture has eliminated the bulging mass in the fallopian tube.

3. Investigations: Laboratory testing requirements are minimal and are necessary only to confirm pregnancy, prepare for surgery, and rule out other pathologies.
   a. Pregnancy testing: Sensitive qualitative urine pregnancy test results should be positive. A baseline quantitative serum β-human chorionic gonadotropin (β-hCG) will allow monitoring of pregnancy resolution.
   b. The "three Cs of hemorrhage":
      • Complete blood cell (CBC) count—including hemoglobin and hematocrit
      • Crossmatch—blood group and screen to prepare for possible transfusion, as well as Rh typing to determine the need for Rh immunoglobulin
      • Coagulation factors—if blood loss has been significant, patients may have evidence of disseminated intravascular coagulation and consideration should be given to appropriate laboratory testing.
   c. Ultrasonography: If the patient is hemodynamically unstable, an ultrasound is not indicated and should not delay a patient's surgery. If ultrasonography is performed, however, the most remarkable finding will be free fluid and clots in the pelvis; blood may fill the entire abdominal cavity. If there is a positive pregnancy test, a corpus luteum ovarian cyst may be seen and the endometrium thickened with decidual material. In fact, a hemorrhagic corpus luteum cyst is the other main consideration in the differential diagnosis, particularly if the pregnancy is too early to be identified visually. The presence of an intrauterine pregnancy essentially rules out ectopic pregnancy in an adolescent or young adult because heterotopic pregnancy is extremely rare without assisted reproductive technologies. It is not necessary to visualize the pregnancy in the tube, and the absence of a uterine pregnancy on ultrasonography is not necessarily diagnostic of an ectopic pregnancy. In the context of an acute and unstable presentation, the final diagnosis will usually be confirmed at the time of surgery.

4. Therapy: Fluid resuscitation should be started immediately and performed aggressively. Blood transfusion can also be initiated if appropriate. The primary method of management is surgery, both for diagnostic and therapeutic purposes. If the patient is Rh negative, she requires Rh immunoglobulin perioperatively. In the operating room, effort should be made in an AYA to preserve the fallopian tube, if possible. If a hemorrhagic corpus luteum is the cause of the bleeding, then if at all possible the ovary should be preserved. If an oophorectomy is required, progesterone supplementation should be instituted until 10 to 12 weeks gestation if the patient wishes to continue the intrauterine pregnancy.

Subacute Presentations

An adolescent or young adult with a positive pregnancy test result who presents with cramping, abnormal vaginal spotting or bleeding, and lower abdominal/adnexal pain should be suspected of having an ectopic pregnancy, particularly if the diagnosis is supported by physical findings of cervical motion tenderness, a closed cervix, adnexal tenderness, and (possibly) an adnexal mass. The workup and treatment depend on the female adolescent or young adult's risk factors and her pregnancy intentions.

The initial diagnosis of a clinically suspected ectopic pregnancy in the hemodynamically stable patient begins with a complete history and physical examination, lab work, and transvaginal ultrasound (TVUS) imaging. The timing of her last normal menstrual period, positive pregnancy test, or previous ultrasound imaging is potentially helpful; however, the definitive management will be based on current TVUS and serial quantitative β-hCG levels. The lab work should include CBC count (for white blood cell, hemoglobin, and hematocrit), blood typing and screening to determine Rh status, and a serum quantitative β-hCG. The adolescent patient may need an explanation for the role of transvaginal ultrasonography as she may be hesitant to have a probe inserted vaginally.

Laboratory and Imaging Evaluation

The properties and limitations of each diagnostic test should be recognized to appropriately use each of them in the workup.

1. β-Human chorionic gonadotropin: Typically, β-hCG levels will double every 2 days in a normal first-trimester intrauterine gestation. For a patient with an initial β-hCG level under 1,500 mIU/mL, the smallest increase over 48 hours that can still be associated with a continuing intrauterine pregnancy is 53%. This percentage rise increases with increasing β-hCG levels (38% at 3,500 mIU/mL and 33% at 5,000 mIU/mL).[9] If β-hCG measurements are unchanged or increasing abnormally, the pregnancy is nonviable, regardless of location. Pregnancies that have inappropriately low β-hCG levels are more likely to be ectopic. Serial β-hCG measurements can be extremely helpful in determining the fate of these pregnancies.

2. Ultrasonography: Ultrasound studies at appropriate β-hCG levels are usually diagnostic, and often the definitive method of pregnancy dating and localization. Transvaginal ultrasound is highly accurate at identifying ectopic pregnancy, with sensitivities and specificities ranging from 87% to 99%.[10] This may require more than one assessment depending on the clinical picture. A normal intrauterine pregnancy should be visible with TVUS by 5 to 6 weeks gestational age. Ectopic pregnancies have a range of appearances on TVUS, including a mass separate from the ovary, a hyperechoic ring, or, least likely, a gestational sac with or without a fetal pole.[11] The lowest concentration of β-hCG that is associated with a visible normal intrauterine gestation is known as the discriminatory zone. More conservative levels are being used to avoid disrupting a wanted intrauterine pregnancy. The American College of Obstetricians and Gynecologists lists 3,500 mIU/mL as the recommended level for TVUS.[6] If no intrauterine gestation is seen with this level of β-hCG, then an ectopic pregnancy should be strongly suspected.

Outpatient Follow-Up—Using Serial β-Human Chorionic Gonadotropin Levels

1. Declining β-hCG levels: If the β-hCG levels are declining by 50% to 66% every 3 days, it is likely that the patient has experienced a complete resolution of the pregnancy. The β-hCG levels must be followed up until they are undetectable (based on local laboratory values).

2. Increasing β-hCG levels: If the β-hCG levels are increasing by at least 66% every 2 to 3 days, they should be followed up in a mildly symptomatic patient until they reach the discriminatory zone and the diagnosis can be made via ultrasound. If

the patient becomes increasingly symptomatic before reaching the discriminatory zone, a laparoscopic investigation may be considered. It is useful to discuss with the patient whether the pregnancy is wanted. A dilation and curettage can be performed at the time of laparoscopy if the pregnancy is discovered to be intrauterine. If the pregnancy is wanted, consider delaying insertion of the uterine manipulator until an ectopic gestation is confirmed.

3. Abnormally changing β-hCG levels: If the β-hCG levels are declining or rising at an inappropriate rate, the pregnancy (either intrauterine or ectopic) is likely nonviable. However, this does not differentiate between a miscarriage and an ectopic pregnancy.
    a. If her β-hCG levels are above the discriminatory level, an ultrasound should be obtained to localize the pregnancy. If it is not within the endometrial cavity, the pregnancy is likely to be ectopic.
    b. If her β-hCG levels are less than the discriminatory range, it is important to assess the patient's desire for pregnancy. If she does not wish to continue with the pregnancy, medical termination can be offered without definitively locating the pregnancy. This commonly involves methotrexate followed by misoprostol to evacuate the uterus. Some advocate for the use of a dilation and curettage (D&C) to provide a tissue diagnosis of an abnormal intrauterine pregnancy. The presence of trophoblastic villi and a rapid drop in β-hCG levels rule out an ectopic pregnancy.[9]

Management

Issues Unique to Adolescents and Young Adults

1. Access to care and follow-up: There are several factors in the evaluation and treatment of ectopic pregnancy that are unique to, or should be emphasized in, AYA females. These patients may present later in gestation because of denial of pregnancy or fear of consequences. They may have trouble accessing the medical system or are unable to seek help due to lack of transportation or money. Once in your office, establishing an accurate history is often difficult as menstrual cycles can be irregular and these patients may be poor historians.

2. Confidentiality and consent for treatment: One must be aware of the local legislation with respect to informed consent for minors. In many regions, clinicians can provide medical care to an adolescent who understands the nature of the diagnosis and/or treatment, without necessarily involving a parent/caregiver. Teens may have a particular need for confidentiality which must be respected. On the other hand, clinicians should make every effort to negotiate with the teen to involve a parent/caregiver in such an important issue as the diagnosis and treatment of an ectopic pregnancy. Young adults may be able to provide consent, but confidentiality could be an issue particularly with respect to insurance coverage.

Approaches to Management

In the adolescent or young adult with an ectopic pregnancy, treatment should generally be fertility sparing and take into account the challenges that some adolescents may have with follow-up recommendations.

1. *Surgical approach*: Surgery will be the treatment option for patients not meeting criteria for medical or expectant therapy or who decline those options. A minimally invasive approach is preferred although this will depend on surgical skill set, local resources, and patient factors.
    Tube-sparing or salpingectomy: The most common surgical procedures are salpingostomy (tube-sparing) and salpingectomy. Salpingectomy is preferred with intractable hemorrhage, tubal rupture, recurrent ectopic in the same

tube, or request for sterilization. The latter two circumstances seldom occur in AYAs. Removing the tube allows for quick hemostasis, more reliable resolution of the ectopic pregnancy, and removes the increased risk of recurrent ectopic on the affected side.[12]

There is conflicting evidence regarding the benefit for tube-sparing surgery. In theory, the benefit of saving the tube would improve the potential for future fertility (which is crucial in younger patients). However, both randomized controlled trials (RCTs) and meta-analysis have not demonstrated a benefit to future fertility with salpingostomy versus salpingectomy, particularly if the contralateral tube is normal.[12–14] If there is evidence of adhesions or other abnormalities of the contralateral tube, then salpingostomy is preferred as subsequent fertility rates are lower with salpingectomy.[15] Salpingostomy is also associated with the need for ongoing monitoring of β-hCG levels as there is a higher chance of persistent ectopic (7% vs. <1% for salpingectomy) (RR 15.0; 95% CI 2.0 to 113.4).[12]

2. *Medical therapy*: Early diagnosis of ectopic pregnancy using laboratory tests and sensitive imaging techniques has significantly reduced the mortality and morbidity of this condition. It has also enabled the use of outpatient medical therapy in lieu of surgical intervention, which in time has reduced hospitalization costs and surgical complications. Methotrexate has become the established medical method of treatment for patients diagnosed with an unruptured ectopic pregnancy. It is a folic acid antagonist and, therefore, exerts its effect on rapidly dividing cells.

The success rates for methotrexate range from 85% to 95%.[16] Factors that are associated with higher rates of treatment success include β-hCG levels <5,000 mIU/mL, no visible fetus or fetal cardiac activity, and minimal pelvic free fluid or hematosalpinx.[6] Single-dose, double-dose, and multidose protocols are available for methotrexate use. A meta-analysis comparing multidose to single-dose protocols showed a nonsignificant increase of treatment success with a multidose protocol. However, a higher rate of adverse effects and no change in time to resolution of ectopic suggests minimal benefit to a multidose protocol.[17] An RCT comparing single- and double-dose protocols showed no difference in success rates, but did have a decreased time to resolution with the double-dose protocol (31.9 vs. 21.7 days; $P = .025$), which would shorten time needed for follow-up.[18] Patients must be counseled about the possibility of treatment failure (and possible tubal rupture) and the signs and symptoms that may indicate complications and necessitate return to hospital. Because it is common for abdominal pain to occur as the ectopic pregnancy resolves 24 to 48 hours after administration of methotrexate, the differentiation of "normal" from "abnormal" pain can be challenging and may result in additional emergency room visits for reassessment and reassurance.

The dose used for treating ectopic pregnancy, usually 50 mg/m², is much lower than that used for cancer chemotherapy. Many different regimens of methotrexate delivery have been employed for treatment of ectopic pregnancy, including oral, intramuscular, and local injection (under laparoscopic or ultrasound guidance). **Tables 58.1** and **58.2** list exclusion criteria and a logarithm for methotrexate use.

Because the doses are so much lower than that used for chemotherapy, the common side effects of methotrexate observed at higher dosages (e.g., nausea, vomiting, stomatitis, and diarrhea) are rarely seen with doses used to treat ectopic pregnancies. Rarely, reversible leukopenia or transient hair loss may be seen.

3. *Treatment of unusual ectopic pregnancy sites*: As mentioned previously, ectopic pregnancies are rarely located outside the fallopian tubes. Sites may include the ovary, cesarean

TABLE 58.1

Methotrexate Therapy for Ectopic Pregnancy—Exclusion Criteria

Patient characteristics:
  Hemodynamically unstable
  Unable to comply with follow-up visit schedule or to return if
    complications develop
  Immunocompromised (WBC count <3,000)
  Anemia (hemoglobin <8 g/dL)
  Active pulmonary disease
  Renal compromise (creatinine clearance >1.3 mg/dL)
  Hepatic compromise (elevated liver function test results; aspartate
    aminotransferase >50 IU/L)
  Hematologic dysfunction
  Thrombocytopenia

β-hCG characteristics:
  Most institutions exclude levels >10,000 mIU/ng

Ultrasonography findings:
  Gestational sac (maximum density of entire mass) >3.5–4.0 cm[a]
  Fetal cardiac motion[a]
  Excessive fluid in cul-de-sac consistent with hemorrhage

[a]Relative contraindication.
hCG, human chorionic gonadotropin; WBC, white blood cell.

or other surgical scars, cervix, uterine cornua, omentum, or other abdominal sites. Due to their small numbers, there is limited evidence on best management practices. Traditional approaches have included surgical resection in the presence of advanced gestation or hemodynamic instability and methotrexate (either systemic or local injection) for stable patients or a site that would be difficult to access surgically.[19]

4. *Expectant management*: Expectant management is reasonable for a certain subset of young females presenting with ectopic pregnancy. These patients are usually asymptomatic and generally have a β-hCG level below 1,500 mIU/mL, which is falling spontaneously. They also need to be reliable, as losing a patient to follow-up could be disastrous. Under these circumstances, approximately 75% of patients will have successful

TABLE 58.2

Systemic Methotrexate Treatment Algorithm

Treatment Day	Investigation/Management
1	Patient eligible for methotrexate therapy Labs: Quantitative β-hCG, renal function tests, liver function tests, CBC count, blood type, and screen Methotrexate administered in 50 mg/m² dose intramuscularly Patient care instructions, including anticipated symptoms and analgesia
4	Labs: Quantitative β-hCG
7	Labs: Quantitative β-hCG, renal and liver function tests, CBC count Compare β-hCG levels from day 4 and 7: If the decline in value is ≥15%, continue to monitor β-hCG until they resolve. If the decline is <15%, a second methotrexate dose is needed. Consider surgical treatment if the patient becomes hemodynamically unstable, has increasing pain and/or falling hematocrit, or if there is an ineffective response to methotrexate.

hCG, human chorionic gonadotropin; CBC, complete blood cell.

TABLE 58.3

Systemic Methotrexate Follow-Up Instructions

To patients
  Advise patients to avoid:
  • Sexual intercourse (may rupture ectopic pregnancy)
  • Sun exposure (photosensitivity reaction possible)
  • Consuming gas-producing foods—leeks, beans, corn, cabbage
    (abdominal bloating may worsen)
  • Alcohol
  • Nonsteroidal anti-inflammatory agents (NSAIDS) (e.g., aspirin,
    ibuprofen, naproxen)
  • Penicillin
  • Prenatal vitamins or folate supplements

  Advise patients on when to follow-up:
  • Return to clinic in 4 d for clinical assessment and repeat tests of
    the pregnancy hormone—human chorionic gonadotropin

  Advise patients on what to expect:
  • In the next few days, you may experience abdominal pain and
    some cramping. This discomfort should be self-limited, but if you
    feel dizzy or weak, or the pain does not resolve, have someone
    take you to the emergency room immediately. There is a small
    chance that the pregnancy could rupture through the tube, and you
    would need immediate surgery.
  • Your next period may be unusually heavy

To clinicians
  No vaginal or bimanual exam is required during follow-up if the
    patient is well. If they have persistent pain consider urgent pelvic
    US to rule out hemorrhage.

resolution of their ectopic pregnancy without intervention.[20] Unfortunately, the need to assess these patients carefully over the course of several weeks, especially if they develop pain, may result in the need for repeated clinical visits. Adolescents should be considered on an individual basis as candidates for conservative management because for many teens the follow-up and surveillance requirements will be too demanding for optimal adherence. If an adolescent has good parent/caregiver support for clinical follow-up, this may be a reasonable option.

Follow-Up

Females treated with methotrexate or expectant management will require weekly (or more frequent) quantitative β-hCG determinations until the levels become undetectable. Table **58.3** outlines specific guidelines for following up a patient treated with methotrexate. For patients undergoing surgical management, the typical protocol is to check the quantitative β-hCG level on the first postoperative day, followed by weekly tests until the β-hCG level is undetectable (particularly with salpingostomy). With tube-sparing surgery, approximately 7% of females will have persistent trophoblastic tissue; so, it is prudent to ensure that the β-hCG levels return to normal, and another pregnancy should be prevented until that time.[12]

Persistent Disease

If persistent disease is diagnosed, further treatment is necessary. If surgical treatment was used initially, methotrexate should probably be used as second line as long as the patient is not continuing to bleed from the ectopic pregnancy. If methotrexate was used initially, options include surgical treatment or repeat methotrexate. Rarely, expectant management can be considered, but would again require a well-informed, compliant patient.

Contraception

It is important to provide effective contraception during the recovery period, not only to prevent a second pregnancy from complicating the β-hCG results, but also to allow the tubal tissue time to heal, thereby presumably reducing the risk of a second ectopic pregnancy in rapid succession. Waiting until the β-hCG levels "zero out" before starting contraception puts the patient at risk for pregnancy because ovulation often precedes complete β-hCG clearance. Assuming the adolescent or young adult is not seeking to conceive, every effort should be made to offer and provide reliable and acceptable contraception after a failed pregnancy (intrauterine or ectopic) or any pregnancy for that matter. Most contraceptive methods can be started immediately after management of the ectopic pregnancy. A period of abstinence (or backup contraception such as condoms) would be recommended for 2 weeks after initiation of contraception.

Rh Considerations

Unsensitized Rh-negative females should be given an appropriate dose of Rh immunoglobulin promptly (50 to 120 mcg if gestational age <12 weeks; 300 mcg if >12 weeks).[21,22] Although very occasionally the blood type of the "father" is used to determine whether an Rh-negative female receives immunoglobulin, it is always prudent to treat the Rh-negative adolescent anyway, because of the uncertainty that may exist with respect to paternity.

FERTILITY AFTER TREATMENT OF ECTOPIC PREGNANCY

Two RCTs have been published comparing fertility outcomes after medical, tubal-sparing (salpingostomy), and salpingectomy treatments for ectopic pregnancy. No significant difference was found between each method of treatment. The rate of intrauterine pregnancy 2 to 3 years after treatment ranged from 56% to 71%.[12,13] One study comparing medical and surgical treatment of younger females aged 18 to 28 had an intrauterine pregnancy rate of 60% to 69% at 2 years ($P = .942$).[23] Meta-analysis data that includes cohort studies does find a trend toward a higher intrauterine pregnancy rate for females who had salpingostomy, especially if they had additional risk factors for ectopic pregnancy (OR 1.96; 95% CI, 0.88 to 4.35).[15] This would support an attempt to preserve the tube if possible for patients with pelvic disease.

On average, ectopic pregnancies recur in 10% of patients.[6,13] Some studies suggest a higher recurrence rate for patients treated with salpingostomy,[14,15] while others show no difference.[12,13] Given this relatively high rate of recurrence, an early ultrasound is recommended for any subsequent pregnancies to confirm the location of the pregnancy.

Regardless of the method of treatment, AYA patients who have had only one ectopic pregnancy can be reassured that their chances of having an intrauterine pregnancy in the future are excellent. The method of treatment can therefore be tailored to the needs of the individual patient.

SUMMARY

Ectopic pregnancy is fortunately uncommon in AYAs. Risk factors may include smoking, prior PID, and IUD use. The hallmark tests for diagnosis involve TVUS and quantitative β-hCG levels. Most ectopic pregnancies are managed surgically although, for patients who will be reliable for follow-up, medical management with methotrexate or even conservative management may be appropriate. Providing the contralateral tube is normal, future fertility is maintained after treatment of an initial ectopic pregnancy.

REFERENCES

1. Panelli DM, Phillips CH, Brady PC. Incidence, diagnosis and management of tubal and nontubal ectopic pregnancies: a review. *Fertil Res Pract.* 2015;1:15.

2. Chukus A, Tirada N, Restrepo R, et al. Uncommon implantation sites of ectopic pregnancy: thinking beyond the complex adnexal mass. *Radiographics.* 2015;35(3):946–959.
3. Creanga AA, Syverson C, Seed K, et al. Pregnancy-related mortality in the United States, 2011–2013. *Obstet Gynecol.* 2017;130(2):366–373.
4. Knight M, Bunch K, Tuffnell D, et al, eds. *On behalf of MBRRACE-UK. Saving Lives, Improving Mothers' Care—Lessons learned to inform maternity care from the UK and Ireland Confidential Enquiries into Maternal Deaths and Morbidity 2015–17.* National Perinatal Epidemiology Unit, University of Oxford; 2019.
5. Stulberg DB, Cain L, Dahlquist IH, et al. Ectopic pregnancy morbidity and mortality in low-income women, 2004–2008. *Hum Reprod.* 2016;31(3):666–671.
6. American College of Obstetricians and Gynecologists' Committee on Practice Bulletins—Gynecology. ACOG practice bulletin no. 193: tubal ectopic pregnancy. *Obstet Gynecol.* 2018;131(3):e91–e103.
7. Hendriks E, Rosenberg R, Prine L. Ectopic pregnancy: diagnosis and management. *Am Fam Physician.* 2020;101(10):599–606.
8. Heinemann K, Reed S, Moehner S, et al. Comparative contraceptive effectiveness of levonorgestrel-releasing and copper intrauterine devices: the European Active Surveillance Study for Intrauterine Devices. *Contraception.* 2015;91(4):280–283.
9. Barnhart KT, Guo W, Cary MS, et al. Differences in serum human chorionic gonadotropin rise in early pregnancy by race and value at presentation. *Obstet Gynecol.* 2016;128(3):504–511.
10. Kirk E, Bottomley C, Bourne T. Diagnosing ectopic pregnancy and current concepts in the management of pregnancy of unknown location. *Hum Reprod Update.* 2014;20(2):250–261.
11. Scibetta EW, Han CS. Ultrasound in early pregnancy: viability, unknown locations, and ectopic pregnancies. *Obstet Gynecol Clin North Am.* 2019;46(4):783–795.
12. Mol F, van Mello NM, Strandell A, et al. Salpingotomy versus salpingectomy in women with tubal pregnancy (ESEP study): an open-label, multicentre, randomised controlled trial. *Lancet.* 2014;383(9927):1483–1489.
13. Fernandez H, Capmas P, Lucot JP, et al. Fertility after ectopic pregnancy: the DEMETER randomized trial. *Hum Reprod* 2013;28(5):1247–1253.
14. Cheng X, Tian X, Yan Z, et al. Comparison of the fertility outcome of salpingotomy and salpingectomy in women with tubal pregnancy: a systematic review and meta-analysis. *PLoS One.* 2016;11(3):e0152343.
15. Ozcan MCH, Wilson JR, Frishman GN. A systematic review and meta-analysis of surgical treatment of ectopic pregnancy with salpingectomy versus salpingostomy. *J Minim Invasive Gynecol.* 2021;28(3):656–667.
16. Po L, Thomas J, Mills K, et al. Guideline no. 414: management of pregnancy of unknown location and tubal and nontubal ectopic pregnancies. *J Obstet Gynaecol Can.* 2021;43(5):614–630.
17. Yang C, Cai J, Geng Y, et al. Multiple-dose and double-dose versus single-dose administration of methotrexate for the treatment of ectopic pregnancy: a systematic review and meta-analysis. *Reprod Biomed Online.* 2017;34(4):383–391.
18. Song T, Kim MK, Kim ML, et al. Single-dose versus two-dose administration of methotrexate for the treatment of ectopic pregnancy: a randomized controlled trial. *Hum Reprod.* 2016;31(2):332–338.
19. Alalade AO, Smith FJE, Kendall CE, et al. Evidence-based management of nontubal ectopic pregnancies. *J Obstet Gynaecol.* 2017;37(8):982–991.
20. Jurkovic D, Memtsa M, Sawyer E, et al. Single-dose systemic methotrexate vs expectant management for treatment of tubal ectopic pregnancy: a placebo-controlled randomized trial. *Ultrasound Obstet Gynecol.* 2017;49(2):171–176.
21. American College of Obstetricians and Gynecologists. Practice Bulletin No. 181: Prevention of Rh D alloimmunization. *Obstet Gynecol* 2017;130(2):e57–e70.
22. Fung KFK, Eason E. No. 133-prevention of Rh alloimmunization. *J Obstet Gynaecol Can.* 2018;40(1):e1–e10.
23. Turan V. Fertility outcomes subsequent to treatment of tubal ectopic pregnancy in younger Turkish women. *J Pediatr Adolesc Gynecol.* 2011;24(5):251–255.

ADDITIONAL RESOURCES AND WEBSITES

Additional Resources and Websites for Clinicians:
Comprehensive review of ectopic pregnancy (has free registration to read the article)—https://emedicine.medscape.com/article/2041923-overview
Good summary of ectopic pregnancy diagnosis and management—https://www.merckmanuals.com/en-ca/professional/gynecology-and-obstetrics/abnormalities-of-pregnancy/ectopic-pregnancy?query=ectopic%20pregnancy
NICE guidelines for initial diagnosis and management of ectopic pregnancy—https://www.nice.org.uk/guidance/ng126/resources/ectopic-pregnancy-and-miscarriage-diagnosis-and-initial-management-pdf-66141662244037

Additional Resources and Websites for Parents/Caregivers:
American College of Obstetricians and Gynecologists FAQ section on ectopic pregnancy for patients—https://www.acog.org/womens-health/faqs/ectopic-pregnancy
Health Link BC link with patient information on ectopic pregnancy—https://www.healthlinkbc.ca/health-topics/hw144921
Mayo Clinic website with patient information on ectopic pregnancy—http://www.mayoclinic.org/diseases-conditions/ectopic-pregnancy/basics/definition/con-20024262

Additional Resources and Websites for Adolescents and Young Adults:
American College of Obstetricians and Gynecologists FAQ section on ectopic pregnancy for patients—https://www.acog.org/womens-health/faqs/ectopic-pregnancy
Health Link BC link with patient information on ectopic pregnancy—https://www.healthlinkbc.ca/health-topics/hw144921
Mayo Clinic website with patient information on ectopic pregnancy—http://www.mayoclinic.org/diseases-conditions/ectopic-pregnancy/basics/definition/con-20024262

CHAPTER

59

Male Genitourinary Health and Disorders

William P. Adelman

KEY WORDS

- Epididymitis
- Hydrocele
- Male genital examination
- Scrotal masses
- Scrotal swelling
- Spermatocele
- Testicular self-examination
- Testicular torsion
- Urethritis
- Varicocele

INTRODUCTION

A complete examination of the male genitals is a crucial part of the examination of adolescents and young adults (AYAs). It is necessary to assess growth and development, to identify common variants and abnormalities, to address genital symptoms, and is recommended by national organizations as part of AYA primary care.[1-5] It is a relatively easy examination to learn and perform because the male genitalia are readily accessible for palpation and the anatomy is straightforward (Fig. 59.1). Once the anatomy is understood, a history and physical examination are often all that are required to make an accurate diagnosis of a genitourinary

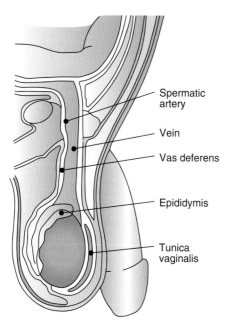

FIGURE 59.1 Male genitalia showing inguinal area, spermatic cord, epididymis, and testis.

Spermatic artery

Vein

Vas deferens

Epididymis

Tunica vaginalis

disorder. If the anatomy of the presenting condition is unclear, due to inability to perform a complete examination or loss of usual landmarks, ultrasonography is a simple, noninvasive method to clarify anatomy. This chapter reviews the male genital examination and outlines an approach to diagnosis and management of common disorders including scrotal masses, cryptorchidism, testis torsion, urethritis, epididymitis, testis cancer, hydrocele, varicocele, and spermatocele.

MALE GENITAL EXAMINATION

Inspection

Inspect the pubic hair area and underlying skin noting sexual maturity rating (SMR).[1-3] Next, inspect the groin and inner aspect of thighs, followed by the penile meatus, prepuce, glans, corona, and shaft (Fig. 59.2). It is best to have the uncircumcised patient retract his own foreskin. Uncircumcised males have higher prevalence rates of pearly penile papules as well as ulcerative sexually transmitted infections (STIs). Pink, pearly penile papules are benign, uniform-sized papules that arise most commonly along the corona, during SMR 2 or 3, in as many as 15% of teenagers[6] (Fig. 59.3). Inspect the scrotum and recognize that contraction of the dartos muscle of the scrotal wall produces folds or rugae, most prominent in the younger adolescent. An underdeveloped scrotum may indicate an ipsilateral undescended testicle. With a retractile testis, the scrotum is normally developed. Finally, inspect the testes—the left testis is usually lower than the right. Check for enlargement (tumor, infection, hydrocele, or hernia) or asymmetry, suggesting atrophy or cryptorchidism on one side or unilateral enlargement as seen with a tumor. Check for a "transverse lie" or "horizontal lie" of the testis, suggesting a "bell clapper deformity" and increased risk for torsion (Fig. 59.4).

Palpation

Palpate the inguinal area, spermatic cord, epididymis, testes, and external inguinal ring. Check for lymphadenopathy or hernia in the inguinal area. To palpate the spermatic cord, apply gentle traction on the testis with the nondominant hand and palpate the structures of the cord with the index or middle finger and thumb of the dominant hand. The vas deferens feels like a smooth, rubbery tube and is the most posterior structure in the spermatic cord. Thickening and irregularity of the vas deferens may be caused by infection. Check for a varicocele (dilated pampiniform plexus of veins) within the spermatic cord. The epididymis lies along the posterolateral wall of the testis. The head of the epididymis attaches at the superior pole of the testis. The epididymis becomes the vas deferens and leaves the testis as part of the spermatic cord. The easiest way

530

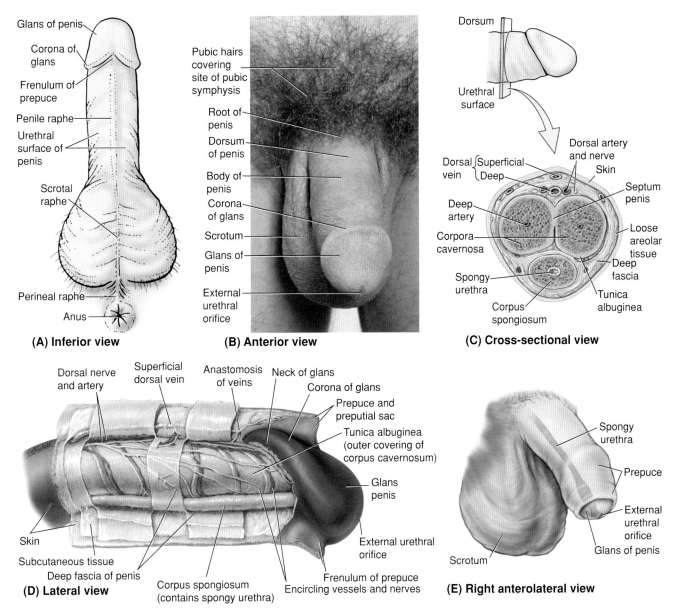

FIGURE 59.2 Penis and scrotum. **A:** The urethral surface of the circumcised penis is shown. **B:** The dorsum of the circumcised penis and the anterior surface of the scrotum are shown. The penis comprises a root, body, and glans. **C:** The penis contains three erectile masses: two corpora cavernosa and a corpus spongiosum (containing the spongy urethra). **D:** The skin of the penis extends distally as the prepuce, overlapping the neck and corona of the glans. **E:** An uncircumcised penis. (From Dalley AF, Agur AMR. *Moore's Clinically Oriented Anatomy*. 9th ed. Wolters Kluwer Health; 2022.)

to find the epididymis is to follow the vas deferens toward its junction with the tail of the epididymis. Tenderness, induration, and swelling in this area usually indicate epididymitis. A well-localized, nontender, spherical enlargement of the epididymal head is a spermatocele. Palpate the testes to check size, shape, and presence of tenderness or masses. The adult testes are approximately 4 to 5 cm long and 3 cm wide but vary from one person to another. Stabilize the testis with the nondominant hand and use the dominant hand's thumb and first two fingers to palpate the entire surface. The testes should be roughly the same size (within 2 mL in volume), and volumes vary according to pubertal stage. Testicular volume could be quantified with the use of an orchidometer or by ultrasound. *Any induration within the testis is suspicious of testicular cancer until proved otherwise.* The appendix testis (a small appendage of normal tissue that is usually located on the upper portion of the testis), present in 90% of males, can sometimes be palpated at the superior pole of the testis. Palpate the external inguinal ring by sliding your index finger along the spermatic cord above the

inguinal ligament while having the patient cough or strain to check for a hernia.

CRYPTORCHIDISM

Cryptorchidism refers to at least one undescended testis that cannot be drawn into the scrotum.[7,8]

Epidemiology

Cryptorchidism is the most common genitourinary disorder of childhood, with a prevalence of 1% of boys by the age of 1 year.

Diagnosis

When a testis is not palpable in the scrotum, gentle massage should be performed along the line of descent from the anterosuperior spine, medially, and downward to the pubic tubercle. If the testis is not truly undescended, it should become palpable in the scrotum. If cryptorchidism is present, the teen should be examined for

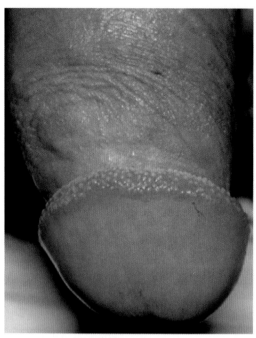

FIGURE 59.3 Pearly penile papules. (Reproduced with permission from Goodheart HP. *Goodheart's Photoguide of Common Skin Disorders.* 4th ed. Lippincott Williams & Wilkins; 2015.)

stigmata of associated disorders (i.e., Noonan, Klinefelter, or Kallmann syndrome or trisomy 13, 18, or 21).[3,8]

Complications

Infertility

Sperm production in the cryptorchid testis may be significantly impaired compared with normal testicular function, regardless of patient age at the time of discovery.

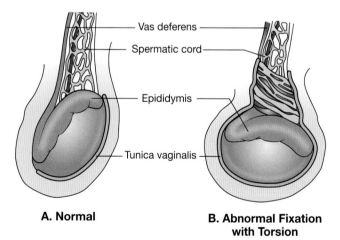

FIGURE 59.4 Bell clapper deformity. The tunica vaginalis attaches to the posterolateral surface of the testes and limits their movement within the scrotum. If the fixation is too high (anterior and cephalad), a bell clapper deformity is present, the testes can move more freely, and torsion is more likely. **A:** Fixation is normal. **B:** Fixation is too high, leading to an abnormal lie of the testis, allowing the testis to rotate transversely and resulting in torsion. (From the Merck Manual Professional Version [Known as the Merck manual in the US and Canada and the MSD Manual in the rest of the world], edited by Robert Porter. Copyright (2021) by Merck Sharp & Dohme Corp., a subsidiary of Merck & Co., Inc., Kenilworth, NJ. Accessed April 1, 2021. http://www.merckmanuals.com/professional)

Malignancy

About 5% to 12% of all malignant testicular tumors occur in males with a history of an undescended testis. The relative risk of tumors in such individuals is increased approximately 10 to 40 times that of a male without cryptorchidism. Moreover, the risk is increased even if the testis is brought down into the scrotum. Orchidopexy performed before puberty decreases the risk of testis cancer compared to those boys with cryptorchidism who undergo orchidopexy after puberty.[8]

Therapy

Therapy for cryptorchidism in teenagers should be corrective surgery. These teens should be aware of the increased risk of testicular cancer and some national organizations recommend they be taught testicular self-examination.[8]

⬤ SCROTAL SWELLING AND MASSES

Evaluation

The general approach to the adolescent or young adult with a scrotal mass or a painful scrotum (Fig. 59.5) includes a directed history, physical examination, and laboratory testing.

History

The adolescent or young adult should be questioned regarding the presence and prior history of genitourinary anomalies, pain, trauma, change in testicular or scrotal size, and sexual activity. Abrupt onset of pain is suggestive of torsion; gradual onset suggests epididymitis or orchitis; lack of pain suggests a tumor or cystic mass. Torsion is often preceded by episodes of mild pain. Reactive hydroceles are common secondary to trauma, orchitis, testicular cancer, and epididymitis, and are noted as changes in the scrotum. Epididymitis in adolescence and young adulthood is usually sexually transmitted.

Physical Examination

Inspection of the testes can differentiate torsion from infection. In torsion, the affected testis is often higher than on the contralateral side. With infections, the affected testis is often lower. In torsion, the affected testis and often the contralateral testis lie horizontally instead of in the usual vertical position, secondary to the congenital defect involved, and the epididymis is usually displaced anteriorly, as the testis twists on its vascular pedicle (see Fig. 59.4). Careful palpation of the testicular surfaces, the epididymis and cord (posterior structures), and the head of the epididymis (superior structure) can further identify the cause of the painful mass. Isolated swelling and tenderness of the epididymis suggest epididymitis. A tender, pea-sized swelling at the upper pole of the testis suggests torsion of the appendix testis. Generalized swelling and tenderness of both the testis and the epididymis can be found in either testicular torsion or epididymitis with orchitis. Presence of a cremasteric reflex makes torsion unlikely. However, it is often present in torsion of the appendix testis. Prehn sign, the relief of pain with elevation of the testis, suggests epididymitis. Lack of pain relief with elevation of the testis is not a reliable test for torsion. Nausea or vomiting with testicular pain is usually caused by torsion.

If a painless mass is present (see Fig. 59.5), palpate to assess its location and then transilluminate the mass. Important findings on physical examination include the following: a mass within the testis is a tumor until proved otherwise; a mass palpable separate from the testis is unlikely to be a tumor; a "bag of worms" or "squishy tube" along the left spermatic cord is a varicocele; a mass located near the head of the epididymis, above and behind the testis is probably a spermatocele; a mass anterior to or surrounding the testis is probably a hydrocele; or a mass that is separate from the

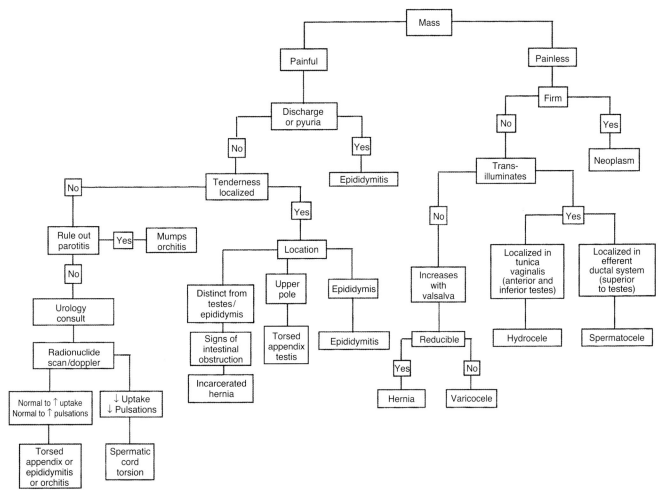

FIGURE 59.5 Diagnostic approach to scrotal masses. (Adapted from Schlossberger N. Male reproductive health: I. Painful scrotal masses. *Adolesc Health Update.* 1992, 4:1; Klein BL, Ochsenschlager DW. Scrotal masses in children and adolescents: a review for the emergency physician. *Pediatr Emerg Care.* 1993;9:351–361.)

testis/epididymis, enlarges with straining (Valsalva), and is reducible is probably a hernia. Transilluminate the mass with a light source. Clear transillumination suggests a hydrocele or a typical spermatocele, whereas absence of transillumination suggests a testicular tumor or, if the mass is separate from the testis/epididymis, a hernia or a large spermatocele.

Laboratory Evaluation

A painful scrotum, or dysuria, in conjunction with a urine dipstick test that is positive for leukocyte esterase, or the presence of leukocytes on microscopy (especially if there are >20 white blood cells/high-power field) is suggestive of epididymitis rather than torsion. If a reasonable suspicion of torsion exists, emergent urology consultation is warranted. One should not delay this referral by ordering time consuming diagnostic tests, as the primary therapy should be surgical exploration.

Differential Diagnosis

When confronted with a painless scrotal mass or swelling (see Fig. 59.5), important conditions to consider include hydrocele, spermatocele, varicocele, hernia, testicular tumor, and idiopathic scrotal edema. When addressing a painful scrotal mass or swelling, the differential diagnosis should include torsion of spermatic cord, torsion of appendix testis, epididymitis, orchitis, trauma with hematoma, incarcerated hernia, Henoch–Schonlein syndrome, cellulitis or infected piercing, hymenoptera sting or insect bite, and testicular tumor with bleeding or infarction.

TORSION

Etiology

Testicular torsion is a twisting of the testis and spermatic cord, which results in venous obstruction, progressive edema, arterial compromise, and, eventually, testicular infarction. Normally, the testes are covered anteriorly with a mesothelial structure, the tunica vaginalis. In some males, the tunica vaginalis is abnormally enlarged and engulfs the testes. This causes the testis to lie like a "bell clapper" in the scrotal cavity (see Fig. 59.4). With this deformity, a testis can twist on the spermatic cord, compromising circulation. Aside from torsion at the spermatic cord, appendages of the testes or of the epididymis can occasionally undergo torsion (Fig. 59.6A).

Epidemiology

Two-thirds of cases occur between 12 and 18 years, with incidence peaking at 15 to 16 years during periods of growth. The risk of developing torsion by age 25 is estimated to be approximately 1 in 160.[9]

Clinical Manifestations

The onset of testicular torsion is usually abrupt, and 50% of teenagers have had brief prior episodes of scrotal pain. Pain may be isolated to the scrotum or may radiate to the abdomen, and nausea or vomiting may occur. Physical examination shows a tender and swollen testis, where the affected side is higher than the

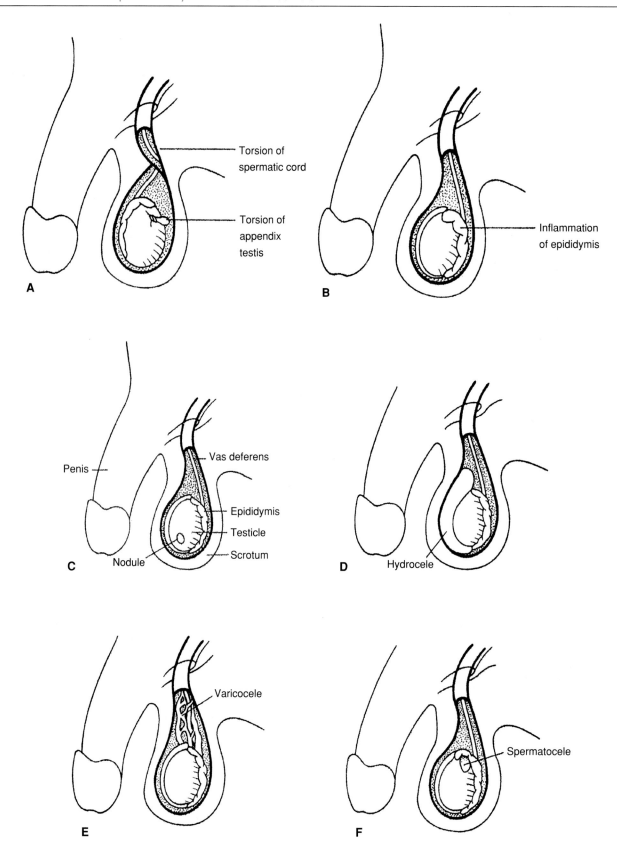

FIGURE 59.6 **A:** Torsion. **B:** Epididymitis. **C:** Testis tumor. **D:** Hydrocele. **E:** Varicocele. **F:** Spermatocele. (From Kapphahn C, Schlossberger N. Male reproductive health: I. Painful scrotal masses. *Adolesc Health Update.* 1992;4:1.)

contralateral side because of the elevation from the twisted spermatic cord. In contrast, in inflammatory conditions, the affected side is often lower.

The epididymis, if palpable, is often out of the usual posterolateral location. The affected testis and often the contralateral testis lie in a horizontal plane rather than in the normal vertical plane. The cremasteric reflex, fever, and scrotal redness are usually absent.

Diagnosis

Testicular torsion is a surgical emergency. The diagnosis of torsion should be suspected in any adolescent or young adult with a painful swelling of the scrotum. If the history (acute onset of pain, nausea or vomiting, prior episodes of pain, lack of fever, lack of dysuria, or urethral discharge) and physical examination (patient in distress, high-riding testis, horizontal position of testis, generalized swelling of the testis) are consistent with torsion, a urology consultation should be obtained immediately, and decisions made for further testing or direct surgical exploration (see Fig. 59.5).

Therapy

Therapy involves immediate surgery. Saving testicular function depends on early surgical intervention. If surgery is performed within 6 hours of symptom onset, recovery is the rule; if surgery is performed between 6 and 12 hours, 62% of patients have recovery of testicular function. After 12 hours, the success rate falls to 20% to 38% and after 24 hours, only up to 11% of testes survive. Regardless of time to presentation, aggressive surgical intervention should ensue.[10]

⬤ URETHRITIS IN MALES

Etiology

Urethritis is an inflammatory condition of the urethra, resulting from infectious and noninfectious causes. Traditionally, infectious urethritis is divided into two categories: gonococcal urethritis, caused by *Neisseria gonorrhoeae*, and nongonococcal urethritis (NGU), caused by organisms other than *N. gonorrhoeae*. The most common cause of NGU in the United Sates is *Chlamydia trachomatis*. A more detailed discussion of these two organisms (including treatment for urethritis presumptively caused by one or both of these organisms) can be found in Chapter 62.

Mycoplasma genitalium is an STI that can cause both acute and chronic urethritis and can present as a challenging clinical syndrome in AYA males. The fastidious nature of this organism and lack of widely available diagnostic tests, makes this a particularly challenging organism in understanding its natural history and pathogenesis. Additionally, widespread empirical treatment and drug-resistant *M. genitalium* further complicate treatment.[11–13]

Epidemiology

The most common causes of NGU in the United States are *C. trachomatis* (15% to 40%), *M. genitalium* (15% to 25%) and less commonly *Trichomonas vaginalis* (1% to 8%), herpes simplex virus, and adenovirus. *Neisseria meningitidis* can be transmitted through oral–penile contact and cause urethritis. Enteric bacteria can also cause urethritis, associated with insertive anal intercourse.[14]

Worldwide, *M. genitalium* is a major cause of nongonococcal urethritis (NGU) but an uncommon sexually transmitted infection in the general population, with a prevalence of about 1%. Prevalence rates peak in males between 25 and 34 at greater than 2%. Some studies suggest a higher prevalence in males than females, but among 16- to 19-year-olds, the rate in females is higher than males. *M. genitalium* is strongly associated with increasing numbers of sexual partners, same sex behaviors among males, and coinfection with other STIs.

Clinical Manifestations

The key symptoms of urethritis include dysuria, urethral discharge, frequency, urgency, and urethral pruritus. Key signs include urethral irritation, erythema, scant or profuse discharge, and in severe cases, meatitis. Many individuals with sexually transmitted urethritis are asymptomatic or have minimal symptoms that can easily be ignored. Among males, the most common clinical manifestation of *M. genitalium* infection is urethritis and *M. genitalium* is now recognized as the dominant organism associated with persistent urethral symptoms following treatment of NGU.

Diagnosis

N. gonorrhoeae and *C. trachomatis* are best diagnosed via nucleic acid amplification tests. *T. vaginalis* can be diagnosed via direct microscopy, rapid antigen, and nucleic acid amplification testing (NAAT). Nucleic acid amplification tests are much more sensitive than microscopy for diagnosis (95% to 100% versus 51% to 65%) and is the preferred modality for trichomonas diagnosis. While NAAT for trichomonas is not approved by the Food and Drug Administration (FDA) for males, several large national labs have performed the necessary Clinical Laboratory Improvement Amendments validation for urine based NAAT for trichomonas. In areas of high prevalence of *T. vaginalis*, males who have sex with females may be presumptively screened and treated when presenting with NGU. In contrast to *T. vaginalis*, *M. genitalium* is more challenging to diagnose. The organism does not possess a cell wall and so cannot be seen on Gram stain. It is fastidious to culture, requiring weeks to months to grow, and conventional methods of drug sensitivity testing are not possible. Serology testing of antibodies is not specific and is affected by cross reactivity to other mycoplasmas, such as *Mycoplasma pneumoniae*. Nucleic acid amplification tests for *M. genitalium* exist and are FDA cleared for use with urine and urethral, penile meatal, endocervical, and vaginal swab samples, but are not yet widely utilized. Males with recurrent NGU should be tested for *M. genitalium* using an FDA-cleared NAAT. In clinical practice, if testing is unavailable, the diagnosis is suspected with persistent or recurrent urethral symptoms despite an appropriate first-line course of treatment.[11–14]

Therapy

Treatment for urethritis presumed caused by *M. genitalium* is challenging due to growing worldwide antimicrobial resistance, and nations differ in their recommended treatments. In the United States, the Centers for Disease Control and Prevention recommends treatment regimens tailored to availability of macrolide resistance testing. If *M. genitalium* is macrolide sensitive, the recommended regimen is doxycycline 100 mg orally twice per day for 7 days, followed by azithromycin 1 g orally for the initial dose then 500 mg orally daily for three additional days. For macrolide-resistant *M. genitalium* or if resistance testing is not available, the recommended regimen is doxycycline 100 mg orally twice per day for 7 days, followed by moxifloxacin 400 mg orally once daily for 7 days.[14] First-line treatment with single-dose macrolides for *M. genitalium* should not be used.[11–14]

⬤ EPIDIDYMITIS

Etiology

Epididymitis is an inflammation of the epididymis caused by infection or trauma. In sexually active males younger than 35 years, it is most frequently caused by *C. trachomatis* or *N. gonorrhoeae*. Epididymitis due to *Escherichia coli* or other bowel flora can be secondary to unprotected insertive anal intercourse. Sexually transmitted epididymitis usually is accompanied by urethritis, which often is asymptomatic.[14] Non–sexually transmitted epididymitis may be caused by instrumentation, surgery, catheterization,

TABLE 59.1

Differentiating Torsion from Epididymitis

Symptoms and Other Findings	Torsion	Epididymitis
Pain	Severe	Severe
Onset	Sudden/abrupt	Hours to days
Prior episodes	50% of cases	Usually not
Nausea or vomiting	Frequent	Less frequent
Time to presentation	Short (<24 h)	Longer (>24 h)
Cremasteric reflex	Usually absent	Usually present
Epididymal abnormality	Obscured or anterior	Palpable and tender
Prehn sign	Absent: No relief of or increase in pain with elevation of the scrotum	Present: Pain relief with elevation of the scrotum
Urethral symptoms	Absent	May have dysuria, discharge
Urethral Gram stain	Negative	May be positive for gram-negative intracellular diplococci or white blood cells
Urinalysis	Usually negative	First-catch urine positive for white blood cells and/or leukocyte esterase

or anatomical abnormalities. Epididymitis can be difficult to differentiate from torsion (Table 59.1).

Epidemiology

Epididymitis is usually caused by an STI.[14] It is rare in prepubertal and non–sexually active males without a history of genitourinary tract abnormalities. In these populations, a postviral infectious phenomenon is the most likely explanation.[15]

Diagnosis

The diagnosis is suggested when a sexually active adolescent or young adult presents with subacute onset of pain in the hemiscrotum, inguinal area, or abdomen, with epididymal swelling and tenderness, a reactive hydrocele, urethral discharge, dysuria, possibly fever, and pyuria (see Fig. 59.6B). Approximately two-thirds of individuals see a clinician after 24 hours of pain—later than those who have testicular torsion. Swelling of the epididymis alone is more common with epididymitis than with torsion of the testes (59% vs. 15%). The laboratory evaluation should include a nucleic acid amplification test on a urine sample or an intraurethral swab for *N. gonorrhoeae* and *C. trachomatis* or a culture of intraurethral exudate. Examination of a first-void urine for leukocytes and testing for syphilis and human immunodeficiency virus (HIV) are appropriate.

Absence of urethral discharge, leukocytes on a Gram-stained endourethral swab specimen, or pyuria (including a negative urine dip for leukocyte esterase) would necessitate an urgent urology consultation, as the likelihood of torsion increases. If one of the preceding tests is abnormal but the teen or young adult has any risk factors suggesting torsion (i.e., prepubertal or non–sexually

active teen, elevated or rotated testes, history of prior pain episodes, or acute onset with rapid progression), an immediate urology consultation should be obtained, and further testing may be considered. Orchitis can cause similar symptoms, but it usually occurs without dysuria or urethral discharge. Mumps infection is the most common cause. Mumps orchitis is usually unilateral and can occur without a history of parotitis. Other viruses (e.g., adenovirus, Coxsackie virus, ECHO virus, Epstein–Barr virus) may also cause orchitis, but less commonly.

Therapy

Information on treatment of STIs is available from the Centers for Disease Control and Prevention at https://www.cdc.gov/std/treatment-guidelines/default.htm (see also Chapters 61 to 67).[14] Scrotal support, bed rest, and analgesics are an adjunct to antimicrobial therapy. If infection with either *N. gonorrhoeae* or *C. trachomatis* is the most likely cause, a single dose of ceftriaxone (500 mg) intramuscularly (IM) is administered with doxycycline (100 mg) orally twice a day for 10 days. If the infection is thought to be caused by enteric organisms only then the recommended treatment regimen is monotherapy with levofloxacin 500 mg orally once daily for 10 days, and if the infection is likely caused by *C. trachomatis*, *N. gonorrhoeae*, or enteric organisms then the recommended regimen is ceftriaxone 500 mg IM in a single dose plus levofloxacin 500 mg orally once daily for 10 days. Failure to improve within 3 days requires reevaluation. All partners should be treated. In HIV/acquired immunodeficiency syndrome (AIDS) infection or for other immunocompromised states, therapy is the same and clinicians should be aware that other opportunistic, including fungal and mycobacterial infections, are more common than in immunocompetent patients.

TESTICULAR TUMORS

Etiology

Most testicular neoplasms are malignant and of germ cell origin (95%). Seminomas are the most common testicular cancer of a single cell type (40% of germ cell tumors), with a peak incidence in the 25- to 45-year age group; nonseminoma tumors (embryonal cell, choriocarcinoma, teratoma, yolk sac, and mixed forms) peak in the 15- to 30-year age group (see Fig. 59.6C).[16,17]

Epidemiology

Testicular tumors are the most common solid tumor in males aged 15 to 35 years, with an incidence of 1.4 to 12 per 100,000 males. Testicular cancer is 4.5 times more common among White men compared to African American men, and more than twice as common compared to Asian American men. The risk for Hispanics is between that of Asians and non-Hispanic Whites. The risk of a testicular tumor is increased 10 to 40 times in a teenager with a history of cryptorchidism.

Diagnosis

The diagnosis of tumor should be suspected in any male with a firm, circumscribed, painless area of induration within the testis that does not transilluminate. Swelling is noted in up to 73% of cases at presentation, but is usually considered asymptomatic by the patient. Testicular pain is the presenting symptom in 18% to 46% of patients who have germ cell tumors. Scrotal ultrasound and serum tumor markers (alpha-fetoprotein, human chorionic gonadotropin, and lactate dehydrogenase) are sufficient to make the diagnosis prior to orchiectomy.

Therapy

Therapy is based upon staging and confirmative diagnosis and cell type. Definitive therapy involves a coordinated effort among the urologist, the primary care specialist, and the oncologist.

TESTICULAR EXAMINATION AND SELF-EXAMINATION

The benefit of a genital exam for cancer screening in *asymptomatic* AYAs is unknown as randomized clinical trials are lacking. The U.S. Preventive Services Task Force (USPSTF), citing "moderate certainty that screening for testicular cancer has no net benefit,"[18] recommends *against* screening for testicular cancer by means of testicular self-examination or clinician examination due to the low incidence of disease and high cure rates of treatment, even in patients who have advanced disease. Additionally, there are potential harms associated with screening, which include false-positive results, anxiety, and harms from diagnostic tests or procedures.[18] In contrast, The American Cancer Society recommends that asymptomatic males with risk factors for testis cancer such as cryptorchidism, previous testicular cancer, or family history of testicular cancer should *consider* monthly self-examination.[19] The European Association of Urology recommends that males *perform* testicular self-exam if they have clinical risk factors,[20] and the American Urologic Association advises patients who had cryptorchidism to perform monthly self-examination after puberty to potentially help find cancer early.[8]

HYDROCELE

Etiology

This mass is a collection of fluid between the parietal and visceral layers of the tunica vaginalis, which lies along the anterior surface of the testis and is a remnant of the processus vaginalis—the embryonic sleeve through which the testes descend. If the processus vaginalis remains fully open, an inguinal hernia will result. If a small opening remains, a hydrocele will form in the scrotum (see Fig. 59.6D). If an opening remains proximally but is closed distally before the scrotum, a hydrocele of the spermatic cord will form.

Diagnosis

A hydrocele is usually a soft, painless, fluctuant, scrotal mass that is anterior to the testis, transilluminates, and appears cystic on ultrasonography. Hydroceles often decrease in size by morning and increase in size by evening. Long-standing hydroceles are usually benign. The presence of a new hydrocele should alert the examiner to check for a possible underlying cause such as a hernia, testicular tumor, trauma, or infection.

Therapy

No therapy is required for an asymptomatic long-standing hydrocele. Treatment of the underlying condition is required for a new onset or reactive hydrocele. Indications for surgical treatment include a painful or tense hydrocele that might reduce circulation to the testis, a bulky mass that is uncomfortable, an embarrassment for the adolescent or young adult, or a hydrocele associated with a hernia (a communicating hydrocele).

VARICOCELE

Etiology

A varicocele, or dilated scrotal veins, results from increased pressure and incompetent venous valves in the internal spermatic veins (see Fig. 59.6E), and is most often noted on the left side.

Epidemiology

Varicocele is common in the 10- to 20-year age group, with a prevalence of 15%. Eighty-five percent of varicoceles are clinically evident on the left side, and 15% are noted bilaterally.

Diagnosis

Varicoceles are detected either on routine examination or secondary to a patient's self-discovery. Occasionally, a patient complains of an ache or pain from the varicocele. Most varicoceles are found on physical examination. Varicoceles have been divided into three grades based on physical examination:

* Grade 1—The varicocele is only felt when the patient bears down. It may feel like a thickened or asymmetric spermatic cord. The distension usually decreases when the patient lies down.
* Grade 2—The varicocele is palpable but not visible.
* Grade 3—The varicocele is large enough to be visible. It has a "bag of worms" appearance and can be palpated above the testes.

Therapy

A patient with a normal semen analysis need not be referred for treatment of his varicocele. However, semen analysis is not often a practical test to perform on teenage boys. In those cases where semen analysis is not practical, loss of testicular volume or failure of the testis to grow during puberty is a traditional indication for surgical correction of a varicocele during adolescence. Referral to a urologist for varicocele repair may be considered in the following instances[21]: (1) results of semen analysis are abnormal; (2) testicular size is smaller by two standard deviations when compared with normal testicular growth or an asymmetry exists such as the volume of the left testis is at least 3 mL less than that of the right, or if serial ultrasounds are performed, then a difference exists of >2 mL in testicular volume; (3) response of either luteinizing hormone (LH) or follicle-stimulating hormone (FSH) to gonadotropin-releasing hormone stimulation is supranormal, or nonstimulated LH and FSH levels are abnormal; (4) bilaterally palpable varicoceles are detected; or (5) a large, symptomatic varicocele or scrotal pain is present.

SPERMATOCELE

A spermatocele is a retention cyst of the epididymis that contains spermatozoa. Most are small (<1 cm in diameter), painless, cystic, freely movable, and will transilluminate (see Fig. 59.6F). If large, the patient may present complaining of a "third testicle," and turbidity from increased spermatozoa may prevent transillumination. It is usually felt as a smooth, cystic sac located above and posterior to the testis, at the head of the epididymis. No therapy is indicated, unless it is large enough to annoy the patient, in which case a urologist may excise it.

SUMMARY

The male genital examination is straightforward and important to assess growth and development, to identify common variants and abnormalities, and to address genital symptoms. With an organized approach to the male genital examination, the clinician can complete a comprehensive assessment, address genitourinary health, and diagnose male genitourinary disorders.

REFERENCES

1. Hagan JF, Shaw JS, Duncan PM, eds. *Bright Futures: Guidelines for Health Supervision of Infants, Children, and Adolescents.* 4th ed. American Academy of Pediatrics; 2017. Accessed March 1, 2021. www.aap.org/en-us/professional-resources/practice-support/Pages/PeriodicitySchedule.aspx
2. Adelman WP. Adolescent preventive counseling (generic). BMJ Best Practice (US Version). *British Medical Journal.* 2020. Accessed March 19, 2021. http://bestpractice.bmj.com/
3. Marcell AV, Bell DL, Joffe A; SAHM Male Health Special Interest Group. The male genital examination: a position paper of the Society for Adolescent Health and Medicine. *J Adolesc Health.* 2012;50(4):424–425.
4. Marcell AV, Burstein GR; Committee on Adolescence. Sexual and reproductive health care services in the pediatric setting. *Pediatrics.* 2017;140(5):e20172858.
5. Grubb LK, Powers M; AAP Committee on Adolescence. Emerging issues in male adolescent sexual and reproductive health care. *Pediatrics.* 2020;145(5):e20200627.
6. Honigman AD, Dubin DP, Chu J, et al. Management of pearly penile papules: a review of the literature. *J Cutan Med Surg.* 2020;24(1):79–85.

7. Braga LH, Lorenzo AJ. Cryptorchidism: a practical review for all community healthcare providers. *Can Urol Assoc J.* 2017;11(1–2Suppl 1):S26–32.
8. Kolon TF, Herndon CDA, Baker LA, et al. Evaluation and treatment of cryptorchidism: AUA guideline. *J Urol.* 2014;192:337–345.
9. Schick MA, Sternard BT. Testicular torsion. [Updated November 20, 2020]. In: StatPearls [Internet]. StatPearls Publishing; 2021. Accessed March 19, 2021. https://www.ncbi.nlm.nih.gov/books/NBK448199/
10. Mellick LB, Sinex JE, Gibson RW, et al. A systematic review of testicle survival time after a torsion event. *Pediatr Emerg Care.* 2019;35(12):821–825.
11. Gnanadurai R, Fifer H. Mycoplasma genitalium: a review. *Microbiology.* 2020;166:21–29.
12. Horner PJ, Martin DH. Mycoplasma genitalium infection in men. *J Infect Dis.* 2017;216(Suppl_2):S396–S405.
13. Conway R, Cook S, Soni S. Antibiotic treatment of Mycoplasma genitalium infection. *Pharm J.* 2019;303(7928). doi:10.1211/PJ.2019.20206592
14. Workowski KA, Bachmann LH, Chan PA, et al. Sexually transmitted infections guidelines, 2021. *MMWR Recomm Rep.* 2021;70(4):1–187.
15. Gkentzis A, Lee L. The aetiology and current management of prepubertal epididymitis. *Ann R Coll Surg Engl.* 2014;96:181–183.
16. Smith ZL, Werntz RP, Eggener SE. Testicular cancer: epidemiology, diagnosis, and management. *Med Clin N Am.* 2018;102:251–264.
17. Stevenson SM, Lowrance WT. Epidemiology and diagnosis of testis cancer. *Urol Clin N Am.* 2015;42:269–275.
18. U.S. Preventive Services Task Force. Screening for testicular cancer: U.S. Preventive Services Task Force reaffirmation recommendation statement. *Ann Intern Med.* 2011;154:483–486. Accessed March 19, 2021. https://www.uspreventiveservicestaskforce.org/uspstf/recommendation/testicular-cancer-screening
19. American Cancer Society. *Testicular cancer.* Accessed March 19, 2021. https://www.cancer.org/cancer/testicular-cancer.html
20. European Association of Urology. *Testicular cancer.* Accessed March 19, 2021. https://uroweb.org/guideline/testicular-cancer/
21. Garcia-Roig ML, Kirsch AJ. The dilemma of adolescent varicocele. *Pediatr Surg Int.* 2015;31:617–625.

ADDITIONAL RESOURCES AND WEBSITES

Additional Resources and Websites for Clinicians:
Adelman WP, Joffe A. The adolescent male genital examination: what's normal and what's not. *Contemp Pediatr.* 1999;16:76.
Adelman WP, Joffe A. Genitourinary issues in the male college student: a case-based approach. *Pediatr Clin North Am.* 2005;52:199–216.
American Urological Association. Male GU Exam—http://www.auanet.org/meetings-and-education/for-medical-students/male-gu-exam
Bell DL, Breland DJ, Ott MA. Adolescent and young adult male health: a review. *Pediatrics.* 2013;132:535–546.
Partnership for Male Youth. Health Provider Toolkit for adolescent and young adult males available at http://ayamalehealth.org/index.php
Pinto-Sander N. Mycoplasma genitalium infection. *BMJ.* 2019;367:i5820. doi: 10.1136/bmj.i5820
Sexual and Reproductive Health Resources for Adolescents and Young Adults compiled by the Society for Adolescent Health and Medicine including online resources, Apps and tech services, advocacy, healthcare resources and helplines—https://www.adolescenthealth.org/Resources/Clinical-Care-Resources/Sexual-Reproductive-Health/Sexual-Reproductive-Health-Resources-For-Adolesc.aspx

Additional Resources and Websites for Parents/Caregivers:
Sexual and Reproductive Health
Sexual and Reproductive Health Resources for Adolescents and Young Adults compiled by the Society for Adolescent Health and Medicine including online resources, Apps and tech services, advocacy, healthcare resources and helplines—https://www.adolescenthealth.org/Resources/Clinical-Care-Resources/Sexual-Reproductive-Health/Sexual-Reproductive-Health-Resources-For-Adolesc.aspx
Testicular Disorders—http://www.nlm.nih.gov/medlineplus/testiculardisorders.html.
A comprehensive review of testicular disorders
Varicocele—https://urology.ucsf.edu/patient-care/children/genital-anomalies/adolescent-varicoceles

Additional Resources and Websites for Adolescents and Young Adults:
Sexually Transmitted Infections—http://www.advocatesforyouth.org/topics-issues/stis?task=view
http://www.cdc.gov/std/healthcomm/fact_sheets.htm
http://www.positive.org/ Coalition for Positive Sexuality
Testicular Cancer and Health—https://www.cancer.org/cancer/testicular-cancer.html
Testicular Disorders—http://www.nlm.nih.gov/medlineplus/testiculardisorders.html
A comprehensive review of testicular disorders
Testicular exams—http://kidshealth.org/teen/sexual_health/guys/testicles.html
A teenage-focused approach to many questions regarding the male health examination
Testicular torsion—http://kidshealth.org/teen/sexual_health/guys/torsion.html#cat20016
http://www.childrenshospital.org/health-topics/conditions/testicular-torsion
Varicocele—https://urology.ucsf.edu/patient-care/children/genital-anomalies/adolescent-varicoceles

CHAPTER 60

Breast Disorders and Gynecomastia

Amy Desrochers DiVasta

KEY WORDS

- Breast cyst
- Breast development
- Breast imaging
- Fibroadenoma
- Galactorrhea
- Gynecomastia
- Macromastia
- Mastalgia
- Mastitis
- Prolactinoma

INTRODUCTION

While serious breast disorders are rare during adolescence and young adulthood, breast complaints and anxiety regarding normal development are common (**Table 60.1**). Clinicians must understand normal breast development and its variations, how to manage common breast complaints, and warning signs of serious disease. When evaluating breast complaints, key historical features assist the clinician (**Table 60.2**).

NORMAL DEVELOPMENT

Breast tissue begins as ectoderm-derived mammary bands apparent in embryos 4 mm in length. Breast glands in newborns are still rudimentary. Male and female breast development are equivalent until puberty. During puberty, the breast develops and changes in response to an increase in sex hormones (Chapter 2).

The milk-producing alveolus, or terminal duct, is the primary unit of the breast. Ten to 100 alveoli make up a lobule, which drains into lactiferous ducts that merge to form a sinus beneath the nipple. Fibrous tissue stroma surrounds and supports the lobules and ducts. Other structures in the breast include lymphatics, fat tissue, and nerves.

TABLE 60.1

Common Breast Complaints in Female Adolescents

Congenital Anomalies	Disorders of Development	Acquired Breast Disease
Polythelia	Asymmetry	Mastalgia
Polymastia	Macromastia	Nipple discharge
Supernumerary breast	Tuberous breast deformity	Mastitis/abscess
Amastia		Gynecomastia
		Breast mass

CONGENITAL ANOMALIES

Accessory Nipples or Breasts

Failure of the primordial milk crest to regress leads to the persistence of breast tissue along the "milk line," from the axilla to the groin. This condition occurs in 1% to 6% of females, and can be familial.

1. *Polythelia*: Accessory nipple(s); the most common congenital breast anomaly in males and females
2. *Polymastia*: Presence of accessory breast tissue

Usually, no treatment or excision is needed unless the accessory breast increases in size or the patient has cosmetic concerns. These conditions can be associated with other congenital anomalies, particularly renal malformations; genitourinary ultrasonography could be considered.

Absence of Breast Tissue

Primary amastia, the congenital absence of breast tissue, results from complete involution of the mammary ridge. Amastia is a rare, usually unilateral abnormality. Iatrogenic amastia can occur if the

TABLE 60.2

Key Factors for the Evaluation of Breast Complaints in Adolescent/Young Adult Females

1. History of symptoms: Duration, timing, relationship to menses. Any breast pain, and if so, exacerbating and alleviating factors? Any breast discharge, skin change, trauma, or change in breast size? Unilateral or bilateral?
2. Change in size of mass: Masses that change in size with menstrual cycles may be cysts; those that do not are more likely solid masses. Sudden increase in growth is a concerning sign.
3. Medication history: Recent initiation of certain medications could explain mastodynia or nipple discharge.
4. Pubertal timing and menstrual history
5. Past medical history: Certain factors increase the risk of malignancy. Chest wall radiation increases the risk of subsequent breast cancer. A history of malignancy that can metastasize to the breast (lymphoma, rhabdomyosarcoma) should raise concern. Any patient with a history of cancer must be followed up carefully for evidence of recurrence, including breast-cancer recurrence.
6. Family history: First-degree family members affected by cancer increase a patient's risk; the age of these family members should be carefully documented. Screening for breast disease should begin 10 y before the age at which the youngest close relative was diagnosed. Patients with strong family histories of breast cancer, especially if bilateral disease or in conjunction with ovarian or endometrial cancer, should be referred for genetic counseling.

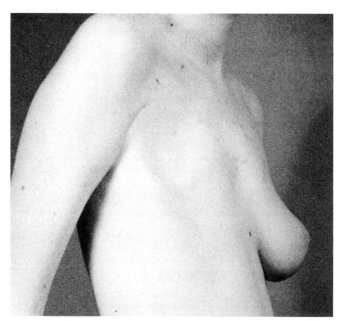

FIGURE 60.1 A 14-year-old girl with Poland syndrome. Note the right-sided amastia. (From Shamberger RC. Chest wall deformities. In: Shields TW, ed. *General Thoracic Surgery*. 4th ed. Williams & Wilkins; 1994:529–557.)

developing breast bud is disturbed by surgery or invasive procedures. *Poland syndrome* presents with amastia, absence of the pectoralis major muscle, rib anomalies, webbed fingers, and radial nerve palsies. Amastia can be extremely disturbing to adolescents and young adults (AYAs), but can be surgically corrected (Fig. 60.1). Athelia is the absence of the nipple on one or both sides, and can be corrected surgically.

DISORDERS OF BREAST DEVELOPMENT

Breast Asymmetry

Some degree of breast asymmetry and differential rates of breast growth are normal. Breast asymmetry may also be caused by a large mass that distorts the normal breast tissue, such as a giant fibroadenoma; these masses are typically evident during a routine breast examination. Pseudoasymmetry is also a possibility, resulting from deformities of the rib cage such as a pectus excavatum.

If the physical examination is normal other than the asymmetry, the appropriate treatment is reassurance and supportive counseling. Most asymmetry seen during early puberty will resolve completely by adulthood. After sexual maturity rating (SMR) 4, however, significant asymmetry is unlikely to resolve on its own. Surgical correction can be offered to those who have completed breast growth, who have marked asymmetry or significant distress, and who understand the risks and benefits of the procedure. The clinician must be sensitive to the adolescent's desire to be "normal" and not appear different than her peers. Breast asymmetry is associated with poor self-esteem, regardless of asymmetry severity.[1]

Macromastia

Macromastia, or breast overgrowth, can be associated with many physical and psychological symptoms. The cause of macromastia is not well understood, but may include an abnormal response of the breast to normal estrogen stimulation. Obesity and macromastia are closely related, but the relationship is complex.

1. Clinical manifestations: Physical complaints include back and shoulder pain, postural changes, breast discomfort, mood disturbances, intertrigo, and limited ability to participate in physical activity. Adolescents are also concerned about self-image, difficulty finding clothing that fits, and unwanted social attention. Eating-disordered behaviors and diminished self-esteem are both associated with macromastia.[2]
2. Diagnosis: Evaluation should include a thorough examination and ultrasound if needed to rule out any underlying mass.
3. Management: Patients should be fit for a supportive, comfortable bra. Weight loss may help to improve symptoms for patients living with obesity. For persistent symptoms, reduction mammaplasty is performed in adolescents who have completed breast growth to prevent the need for a second procedure. Adolescents report a high rate of both satisfaction and symptom relief following surgery. Neither younger age nor obesity increases the risk of complications from reduction mammaplasty.[3]

Tuberous Breast Deformity

Tuberous breast deformity is a rare disorder of breast development leading to underdeveloped and unusually shaped breasts. Patients present with a narrow breast, underdevelopment of the breast mound, and overdevelopment of the nipple-areolar complex (Fig. 60.2). The treatment of choice is plastic surgery; reassurance is also an option for milder cases.

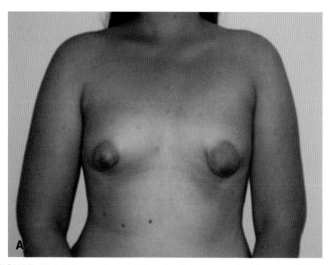
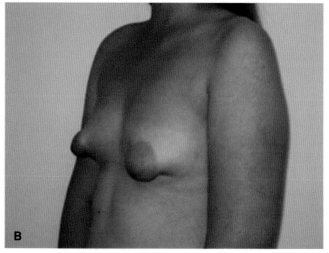

FIGURE 60.2 Tuberous breast deformity. Note the overdevelopment of the superior aspect and nipple–areolar complex with minimal inferior development on the right.

BENIGN BREAST DISEASE

Mastalgia

Mastalgia, or breast pain, can be a distressing problem and affects up to 40% of reproductive-age young females. Mastalgia can be cyclic (worse immediately before menses) or noncyclic. Common causes include premenstrual fibrocystic changes, exercise, early pregnancy, or medications such as combined hormonal contraceptives (CHCs). The evaluation should include a breast examination and a pregnancy test. Once the diagnosis of mastalgia has been made, treatment includes analgesics (topical or oral nonsteroidal anti-inflammatory drugs), good bra support (both night and day if needed), and reassurance. Most breast pain resolves spontaneously within 3 to 6 months. Combined hormonal contraceptives may improve or worsen breast pain, possibly in a dose-related manner. Evening primrose oil, chamomile extract, and vitamin E taken orally (PO) have shown some efficacy in small trials.

Mastitis

Mastitis (breast infection) or breast abscesses present with acute breast tenderness, erythema, and swelling. Predisposing conditions include pregnancy, lactation, breakdown of the nipple skin, preexisting cyst/ductal ectasia (see below), breast hair removal, nipple piercing, and breast trauma.

1. Clinical manifestations: Constitutional symptoms (malaise, fever) may occur. Physical examination reveals an edematous, erythematous breast, possibly with purulent discharge (Fig. 60.3). A discrete abscess may be palpated as an area of fluctuance.
2. Diagnosis: Any purulent breast drainage or nipple discharge should be sent for culture. An abscess can be confirmed with ultrasound if necessary.
3. Management: For simple mastitis, treat with antibiotics for 7 to 10 days and warm compresses. Antibiotic therapy should be targeted at the most likely pathogens (*Staphylococcus aureus,* streptococci, enterococcus). Dicloxacillin or amoxicillin–clavulanic acid provides adequate coverage of most skin pathogens. For penicillin-allergic patients, clindamycin is a good alternative. If patients are breast-feeding, expression of milk from the affected side should continue to prevent milk stasis. Infants can continue breast-feeding from the affected side.
4. Abscess: Patients should be reexamined within several days to confirm response to treatment. Persistent infection despite antibiotic therapy should be evaluated with reexamination of the breast, consideration of methicillin-resistant *S. aureus* (MRSA), and ultrasonography for an underlying

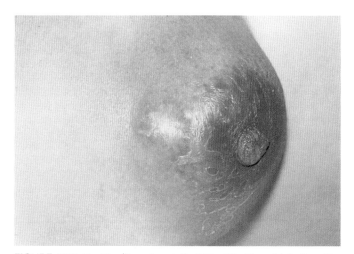

FIGURE 60.3 Mastitis. (From Sweet RL, Gibbs RS. *Atlas of Infectious Diseases of the Female Genital Tract.* Lippincott Williams & Wilkins; 2005.)

abscess. Abscess drainage can be attempted in the office with a large-bore needle. If needle aspiration is unsuccessful or if the abscess reaccumulates, the patient should be referred for incision and drainage or surgical management. Incisions should be as small as possible to limit resulting distortion. Patients who fail to respond to adequate antibiotic therapy should be screened for underlying immunosuppressive disease that may interfere with their ability to clear the infection, like diabetes mellitus or human immunodeficiency virus infection.

Nipple Discharge

Nipple discharge can have many causes, including infection, endocrine disorders, and breast pathology. The first step in the evaluation is to determine the type of discharge. Milky, white discharge suggests galactorrhea. Nonmilky discharge (watery, serous, purulent, serosanguineous, bloody) usually indicates an underlying breast or nipple problem. Even bloody discharge is usually not related to underlying carcinoma in this age group. The following etiologies are most common in AYAs:

1. Contact dermatitis: Local contact dermatitis of the nipple can cause serous, purulent, or bloody discharge. Culprits may include soap, clothes, clothing detergent, or lotion. Treatment is identification and discontinuation of the offending agent, with topical steroid cream for symptom relief. Breastfeeding pads will prevent the nipple from adhering to the bra or clothing, which can lead to further nipple trauma and a recurrence of symptoms.
2. Infection: Purulent discharge indicates infection. Treatment is as outlined above for mastitis.
3. Montgomery tubercles: The periareolar glands of Montgomery will occasionally drain fluid through ectopic openings on the areola. Discharge is usually serous or serosanguineous. Ultrasound can confirm the clinical suspicion through visualization of the retroareolar cyst. Discharge will resolve spontaneously.
4. Mammary duct ectasia: Ductal ectasia refers to dilation of the mammary ducts as well as periductal inflammation. No clear etiology is known. Discharge is usually serous or serosanguinous. Ultrasound can confirm the diagnosis. Treatment includes reassurance and supportive care; mastitis risk may be slightly increased.
5. Intraductal papilloma: These rare, benign, proliferative tumors often present with bloody discharge from a single duct. They represent a focal hyperplasia of the ductal epithelium invaginating into the duct on a vascular stalk. Disruption of this stalk leads to the bloody discharge. If the proliferation of duct epithelium grows large enough, it creates a palpable mass. Although an infrequent finding in AYAs, a palpable mass associated with a bloody nipple discharge has a high probability of being an intraductal papilloma, even in teens. Ultrasound and potentially ductogram should be performed. Any abnormality found should be excised.

GALACTORRHEA

Galactorrhea is the secretion of milk or a milk-like fluid from the breast in the absence of parturition or beyond 6 months postpartum in a nonbreast-feeding person. It is usually bilateral, may occur intermittently or persistently, and may be spontaneous or expressed.

Prolactin secretion from lactotrophs (cells that produce prolactin in response to hormonal signals) of the anterior pituitary gland (Fig. 60.4) is necessary for normal lactation. Dopamine binds to lactotrophs, and inhibits prolactin secretion. Transection or compression of the pituitary stalk increases prolactin secretion by interfering with dopaminergic pathways. Prolactin secretion is also increased by stress, suckling, sleep, and intercourse.

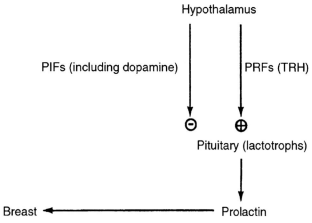

FIGURE 60.4 Schema of prolactin control. PIFs, prolactin-inhibiting factors; PRFs, prolactin-releasing factors; TRH, thyrotropin-releasing hormone.

TABLE 60.4
Interpretation of Serum Prolactin Concentrations

Prolactin Concentration (ng/mL)	Suggested Diagnosis
<25	Normal

25–150	Nonprolactin-secreting tumor
	Dysfunction of dopaminergic
	  pathway
	Microprolactinoma
	Medication-induced
	  hyperprolactinemia

150–250	Microprolactinoma
>500	Macroprolactinoma

Etiology

In females, most galactorrhea is caused by hyperprolactinemia from prolactinomas (benign anterior pituitary neoplasms that secrete prolactin through lactotroph hyperplasia) or secondary to medications. Less common causes of hyperprolactinemia include[4]:

1. Hypothalamic and infundibular lesions, including craniopharyngiomas, infiltrative disorders, and damage to the infundibulum from surgery or head trauma (inhibition of counter-regulatory dopamine release)
2. Primary hypothyroidism (increased thyrotropin-releasing hormone stimulates lactotrophs)
3. Acromegaly or Cushing disease
4. Renal failure (decreased prolactin clearance) or liver failure (decreased dopamine synthesis)
5. Infrequently, galactorrhea can occur with normal prolactin concentrations in females with unexplained hypersensitivity to prolactin, or those who engage in frequent breast stimulation.

Medication-Induced Hyperprolactinemia

A full medication list should be queried to identify any potential pharmacologic causes (Table 60.3). If possible, the offending drug should be discontinued. Alternative medications with lower potential to elevate prolactin levels should be considered. If prolactin levels fail to decrease within 2 weeks after discontinuation, an intracranial mass should be considered. In patients with antipsychotic-induced hyperprolactinemia, dopamine agonist therapy is not recommended. Prolactin levels are less likely

TABLE 60.3
Medications Causing Hyperprolactinemia

Antipsychotics Risperidone Olanzapine Haloperidol Phenothiazines	**Antihypertensive agents** Verapamil α-Methyldopa Reserpine
Antidepressants Tricyclic antidepressants Monoamine oxidase inhibitors Selective serotonin reuptake inhibitors	**Gastrointestinal medications** Metoclopramide Domperidone **Other medications** Opiates and opiate antagonists Estrogens Anesthetics Anticonvulsants Antihistamines (H2) Dopamine-receptor blockers

to normalize in this setting, and the underlying psychosis may be exacerbated. Patients with hypogonadism or low bone mass related to medication-induced hyperprolactinemia should be treated with estrogen or testosterone if the causative medication cannot be stopped.

Diagnosis

Evaluation should start with a carefully drawn serum prolactin level. Prolactin secretion is pulsatile, and is augmented by stress, eating, and breast stimulation. Levels should be drawn in the morning in a fasting, nonexercised state, without prior breast manipulation (no tight-fitting clothes or breast examination). If results are abnormal, the test should be repeated and confirmed (Table 60.4).

Additional evaluation includes a pregnancy test, thyroid-stimulating hormone (TSH), alanine aminotransferase (ALT), and serum creatinine.[4,5] Persistent hyperprolactinemia with no known underlying etiology requires a pituitary brain magnetic resonance imaging (MRI) with contrast to evaluate for an intracranial lesion. Patients who are asymptomatic but have incidentally discovered elevated prolactin levels should be assessed for macroprolactinemia. Macroprolactin is a large-molecule circulating prolactin that is less bioactive, and often does not require further diagnostic testing or treatment. If a discrepancy exists between a large pituitary tumor and mildly elevated prolactin levels, blood samples should undergo serial dilution to eliminate a laboratory artifact that can occur with certain assays that leads to falsely low prolactin levels (the "hook effect").

Classification of Prolactinomas

1. Microadenomas are <10 mm in diameter and do not cause any local symptoms. They rarely grow (<10% chance of increasing in size). Treatment is not needed if estradiol levels are within the reference range, menses are normal, galactorrhea is absent/tolerable, and fertility is not currently desired. Restoration of gonadal function and prevention of decreased bone mineral density (BMD) can be accomplished with a dopamine agonist to lower prolactin levels or estrogen replacement therapy.[5]
2. Macroadenomas are >10 mm in diameter and can cause visual field defects, headaches, neurologic deficits, and loss of anterior pituitary function. They have a significant potential for growth, and initial treatment with dopamine agonists is recommended. Neurosurgical consultation should also be obtained.

Treatment of Prolactinomas

1. Dopamine agonists decrease prolactin secretion and synthesis. Therapeutic goals include resolution of galactorrhea, correction of visual field defects, reversal of amenorrhea, improvement of sexual function, and resolution of infertility.

a. Cabergoline is the most effective medication for normalizing prolactin levels and shrinking pituitary tumors. The Endocrine Society recommends cabergoline as first-line therapy for prolactinomas.[5] Initial doses of 0.25 mg PO twice weekly should be prescribed, increasing to 0.5 to 1 mg twice weekly as needed. Only 3% of patients are unable to tolerate the drug because of side effects, which include headache, dizziness, and nausea. While high doses of cabergoline (≥3 mg daily) have been associated with an increased risk of cardiac-valve regurgitation, standard doses of cabergoline for hyperprolactinemia do not appear to cause clinically significant valve disease.[6] Although there are no known detrimental fetal effects, current recommendations are to discontinue the drug 1 month before attempting conception.

b. Bromocriptine is also effective in lowering prolactin levels and reducing tumor size, although less so than cabergoline. Initial dosing is 1.25 mg PO at bedtime, increased to 2.5 to 5 mg twice a day as needed. Side effects are more common (12% of patients) and include nausea, vomiting, and dizziness. When bromocriptine is used to restore fertility, and stopped when pregnancy is confirmed, there is no increased risk of spontaneous abortions, ectopic pregnancies, or congenital malformations.

2. Combined estrogen/progestin hormonal contraceptives: Females with a microadenoma who are amenorrheic may be treated with CHCs in lieu of dopamine agonist therapy. Combined estrogen/progestin hormonal contraceptives restore menses and prevents hypogonadal effects. Tumor size has not increased in patients treated with CHCs for 2 years.[7]

3. Transsphenoidal surgery is rarely required and reserved for AYAs who are resistant to or intolerant of dopamine-receptor agonists, or who have invasive macroprolactinomas with compromised vision.[5] After surgical intervention, prolactin levels normalize in approximately 70% of all patients with microprolactinomas and in 30% with macroprolactinomas. However, the recurrence risk is 20% to 50%.

4. Radiation has been used rarely in patients with aggressive tumors that do not respond to dopamine agonists or surgery.

Monitoring of Prolactinomas

1. Estrogen status should be closely monitored because of the known risk of low BMD associated with hypoestrogenic amenorrhea. Patients with hyperprolactinemia may experience decreased BMD and an increased risk of fractures.[8] Baseline BMD measurement by dual-energy x-ray absorptiometry (DXA) should be considered in patients with hyperprolactinemia and amenorrhea.

2. Periodic prolactin measurements should begin 1 month after therapy initiation to guide dosing, and be repeated every 1 to 3 months after each change in dosage. Once normal prolactin levels are achieved, prolactin should be measured every 6 to 12 months.[5]

3. A dedicated pituitary MRI should be done 1 year after diagnosis for microadenomas, or 3 months after diagnosis for macroadenomas. Repeat MRI with any increase in symptoms or serum prolactin level.

4. Visual field examinations should be performed for all patients with a macroadenoma potentially impinging on the optic chiasm.

5. If a patient wishes to conceive, bromocriptine should be the initial treatment to induce ovulation. Barrier contraceptives should be used until two normal menstrual cycles have occurred. Bromocriptine should be discontinued after the first missed menstrual cycle/confirmation of pregnancy. Microadenomas rarely grow during pregnancy; macroadenomas that do not undergo surgery or irradiation prior to pregnancy

enlarge in 31% of cases. Monitoring of serum prolactin is not recommended during gestation, given the expected changes in prolactin during pregnancy.[5] Similarly, routine pituitary MRI is not recommended during pregnancy unless new symptoms (headache, visual change) develop. If symptomatic growth of prolactinomas occurs during pregnancy, bromocriptine therapy is recommended.

6. Once patients achieve 2 to 3 years of normal prolactin levels and no visible tumor remains on MRI, dopamine agonist withdrawal may be attempted. The risk of recurrence after withdrawal is 18% to 80%, and correlates with the degree of prolactin elevation at diagnosis as well as tumor size. Recurrence is most likely in the first year after therapy is stopped. Serum prolactin should be measured every 3 months for the first year, and annually thereafter or if symptoms recur. Pituitary MRI should be repeated if the prolactin increases.

BREAST MASSES IN FEMALES

While the presence of a breast mass typically causes concern, the majority of breast masses during adolescence and young adulthood are benign (Table 60.5). Malignancies comprise less than 1% of excisional biopsies performed. In addition to appropriately establishing the cause of a breast mass, clinicians must reassure AYAs and their parents/caregivers that malignant disease is highly unlikely.

Evaluation of a Breast Mass

Evaluation should include a detailed history outlining the location, duration, growth pattern, and characteristics of the mass (see Table 60.2). Family history will help the clinician determine if there is a predisposition to breast problems. Physical examination should characterize the mass: size, shape, firmness, location, and associated findings. Ultrasound is indicated for lesions that are irregular, firm, immobile, difficult to assess, or associated with overlying skin changes.[9] Mammography is not indicated in AYA females; the dense breast tissue of these patients obscures pathologic findings. Current strategies seek to establish a diagnosis without surgical excision, saving patients with benign lesions from an unnecessary surgery.

Fibroadenomas

1. Fibroadenomas are the most common breast mass in AYAs, comprising 44% to 94% of biopsied breast lesions. These well-circumscribed, fibroepithelial lesions are uniformly smooth and sharply demarcated from surrounding tissue. Fibroadenomas are most common during later adolescence, and occur more frequently in African Americans than Caucasians.[10]

2. Clinical manifestations: Round or oval, rubbery mass, distinct from the rest of the breast. Can be multiple and/or bilateral

3. Diagnosis can be made clinically. Ultrasound can be used to confirm a fibroadenoma, which appears as a hypoechoic lesion with smooth round distinct borders, wider than tall.

4. Management: The natural history is slow growth and possible regression. Surveillance is a reasonable and preferable

---

TABLE 60.5

Breast Masses in Adolescence

Benign Breast Masses—Common	Benign Breast Masses—Rare	Malignant Breast Masses—Extremely Rare
Fibroadenoma	Intraductal papilloma	Rhabdomyosarcoma
Cyst	Juvenile papillomatosis	Neuroblastoma
Abscess	Phyllodes tumor	Lymphoma
		Phyllodes tumor
		Adenocarcinoma

therapeutic option for many patients. Expectant management includes serial examination and perhaps ultrasonography every 6 months. Fibroadenomas do not appear to confer increased breast cancer risk later in life.[11] If the lesion is large, if symptoms are present, or the patient/family is anxious, fibroadenomas can be removed via excision or cryoablation.

5. Giant fibroadenomas: A separate, uncommon variant in which the fibroadenoma undergoes markedly rapid growth to a large size (>5 to 10 cm). The patient presents with a rapidly enlarging breast. These lesions occur more frequently in African American teens. Giant fibroadenomas may distort the affected breast and typically require surgical removal.

Breast Cysts

1. Breast cysts can present as multiple breast masses, or increasing size or tenderness of a mass associated with menses.
2. Clinical manifestations: A firm, well-circumscribed mass distinct from the surrounding breast is found.
3. Diagnosis: Ultrasonography reveals a round, well-demarcated hypoechoic structure with fluid content.
4. Management: Cysts will usually resolve spontaneously over weeks to months. If a breast cyst persists and is symptomatic, it can be treated with fine-needle aspiration (FNA) of fluid and resolution of the mass. Simple cysts can recur and can easily be reaspirated. Symptomatic cysts that recur after multiple aspirations should be referred for simple excision.

Fibrocystic Breast Changes

1. Fibrocystic breast changes occur in approximately 50% of all females clinically. The mean age at diagnosis is 15 to 17 years. The pathophysiology is unknown, but may be related to an imbalance of estrogen/progesterone. Risk factors include consumption of animal fats and alcohol and higher body weight.[12]
2. Clinical manifestations: Fibrocystic changes are often associated with complaints of multiple masses. Tenderness and swelling are more common a week before menstruation, and are often relieved by menstruation. Nodularity and lumpiness are apparent on examination, most commonly in the upper outer quadrant of the breasts. The examination will change over time.
3. Diagnosis: Primarily by clinical examination. Ultrasonography is not helpful, as it will reveal normal breast tissue.
4. Management: Mild analgesics (topical or oral nonsteroidal anti-inflammatory drugs), supportive bras, and low-dose CHCs have been effective for reducing symptoms. While oral danazol or tamoxifen have been utilized in adults with severe symptoms, these medications have not been studied in teens.

Juvenile Papillomatosis

1. Juvenile papillomatosis is a rare, benign proliferative tumor. It presents as a firm, well-circumscribed mass with multiple cysts separated by fibrous septa, usually affecting patients <30 years of age.
2. Clinical manifestations: Patients present with a unilateral, solitary, painless breast mass clinically similar to a fibroadenoma.
3. Diagnosis: Ultrasonography can help distinguish juvenile papillomatosis from fibroadenoma. On ultrasound, the lesions are ill-defined, with multiple peripheral anechoic cystic spaces (lending juvenile papillomatosis the name "Swiss cheese disease").
4. Management: Although it's a benign lesion, the clinical significance of juvenile papillomatosis involves controversy over whether it is associated with concurrent or subsequent carcinoma. The patients at highest risk of an associated carcinoma are those who have one of the following: positive family history of breast cancer, atypical histology, bilaterality, multifocality, or recurrence.[13] For these reasons, treatment is complete surgical excision and close clinical follow-up of both the patient and family members.

Phyllodes Tumors

1. Phyllodes tumors are fibroepithelial tumors that can be either benign or malignant. They comprise only 1% of breast neoplasms in AYAs, but are the most common malignant lesions in this age group.
2. Clinical manifestations: A painless, rapidly growing mass that is large (>5 cm) upon presentation. Skin changes overlying the mass are common.
3. Diagnosis: On ultrasound, a phyllodes tumor can be difficult to distinguish from a fibroadenoma. An MRI may help to differentiate between the two.
4. Management: Given the difficulty in distinguishing between a phyllodes tumor and large fibroadenoma, surgical excision of lesions >5 cm is recommended. Wide local resection with achievement of negative margins is the surgical goal, to prevent recurrence.

BREAST MALIGNANCY

Primary breast cancer is extremely rare in AYAs. Data from the Surveillance Epidemiology and End Results program of the National Cancer Institute from 1972 to 2008 suggest a rate of 0.08 new breast cancers per 100,000 girls younger than age 20 years in the United States. Other population studies estimate an annual age-adjusted incidence of breast cancer of 3.2 per million in patients younger than 25 years (with all documented cases occurring in those aged 20 to 24 years).[14] Rather than primary breast cancer, the more common malignant tumors found in the breast tissue of AYAs are secondary or metastatic, including rhabdomyosarcoma, neuroblastoma, or lymphoma.

Striking family clusters of breast cancer can occur in families carrying mutations of BRCA1 and BRCA2, which account for almost 80% of hereditary breast cancer and approximately 5% to 6% of all breast cancers. Although these mutations are rare in the general population, they occur in approximately 1% of Ashkenazi Jewish females. For individuals whose personal or family history suggests a hereditary predisposition to breast cancer, genetic screening should be considered. Decisions around genetic screening are difficult, and should be carried out with the help of a qualified genetic counselor.[15] Screening for mutations should not occur until the information obtained would be helpful in guiding management. While an 18 year old can legally pursue genetic testing, neither screening nor follow-up recommendations will change regardless of the results, as cancer risk associated with BRCA1/2 rarely manifests before the late 20s. Based on consensus recommendations, at age 25 years, annual mammography, breast MRI, and clinical breast examinations should begin for surveillance. Thus, the optimal time to pursue genetic testing time is at this age.

Patients with a history of radiation therapy to the chest are at increased risk of developing a second primary cancer of the breast, and require careful monitoring. Estrogen-containing contraceptives should be avoided when possible in patients with a history of chest radiation. Recent data support an association between a slightly increased risk of breast cancer when comparing current or recent users of hormonal contraception to never users (relative risk 1.2).[16] This relative risk translates into one additional case of breast cancer for every 7,690 users of hormonal contraception. For AYAs (who have an extremely low baseline risk of breast cancer) the absolute increase in risk was only two additional breast cancer diagnoses/100,000 females <35 years using hormonal contraception per year.[16] While risk increases with longer duration of hormonal contraception use, the risk of breast cancer returns to baseline after discontinuation of hormonal contraception.[16]

It is important to note that many variables known to be associated with breast cancer risk were not included in this study, such as alcohol consumption, physical activity, age of first menses, and breast screening practices.[17] Risks may be balanced by the marked reduction in other cancer types seen with hormonal contraception use. Studies of breast cancer risk with hormonal contraception use in carriers of the BRCA1 and 2 mutations are mixed.[18]

PHYSICAL EXAMINATION OF THE BREAST

A thorough and careful breast examination is essential to the evaluation of any breast complaint. Clinicians must be sensitive to the patient's potential feelings of embarrassment or modesty. The patient should be informed of the parts of the examination, and given the opportunity to be accompanied by a parent/caregiver or friend. If the patient declines, a chaperone should be offered by the examiner. Optimal examination occurs within a week of completion of menses, when the breast is least tender. If an examination is indeterminate, repeating it at a different point in the menstrual cycle may be informative.

Inspection should be performed with the AYA in an upright position to assess for asymmetry, breast distortion, or skin conditions. Palpation should occur in a systematic manner to cover the entire breast in an orderly fashion. Regional lymph nodes should also be assessed. The areola should be compressed to elicit nipple discharge; if found, note the color and from where it appeared (nipple, periphery of areola). Masses should be measured, and their consistency and mobility evaluated. The analogy of a clock face can be used to describe the area of breast abnormality.

Breast Self-Examination

Breast self-examinations (BSE) can help AYAs to understand their body and improve comfort with clinical examinations. The American Cancer Society notes that research has not shown a clear benefit of regular breast examinations, but also states that females should be familiar with their breasts and report changes to their clinician right away. However, we believe BSE is beneficial for establishing a lifelong habit of patients investing in their own breast health. Breast self-examinations should be taught during adolescence to patients with history of previous radiation to the chest, a history of malignancy that may metastasize to the breast, or a family history of BRCA1/2 mutations. Clinician breast examinations are recommended as routine part of clinical care every 1 to 3 years starting at age 20 years.

BREAST IMAGING AND BIOPSY

Breast Imaging

Ultrasonography is superior in characterizing masses in AYAs, and can distinguish a cystic mass from a solid one. It cannot definitively distinguish a benign solid mass from a malignant one, but can help guide patient management by providing a noninvasive means of monitoring the size and interval growth of palpable masses. Magnetic resonance imaging may offer additional characterization of breast masses above that of ultrasound, but indications for MRI are still being determined. Mammography is of limited utility in the AYA breast. The dense fibroglandular tissue leads to poor-quality images and poor sensitivity. Mammography should not be used in patients aged <30 years unless specifically recommended for follow-up of other imaging by a radiologist skilled in evaluating ultrasound and MRI images obtained from AYAs.

Breast Biopsy

Clinical observation and serial examinations are the mainstay of treatment for most adolescent breast masses.[19] However, FNA and core-needle biopsy may be considered in rare circumstances, such as AYAs with a history of chest radiation or malignancy, hard masses with irregular borders, axillary lymphadenopathy, or a persistent solid mass with concerning features on ultrasound or MRI. Fine-needle aspiration is also used to manage breast cysts. If an aspiration obtains nonbloody fluid, the lesion is a benign cyst and no further treatment is needed. Cytology on the cyst fluid is not indicated unless it is bloody. If FNA reveals a solid mass, a core biopsy can be obtained to characterize the mass. Given the rarity of the need for these procedures even in young adults, patients should be referred to a breast center with experience treating AYAs.

GYNECOMASTIA

Gynecomastia refers to an increase in the glandular and stromal tissue of the male breast. When identified during puberty, it is usually benign and transient. Gynecomastia can also be due to a serious underlying disorder, or can persist long enough that the adolescent seeks treatment.

Epidemiology

Transient gynecomastia affects 40% to 60% of adolescent males.[20] It usually occurs at SMR 3 or 4 genital development, and peaks in prevalence at ages 11 to 14 years. Approximately 4% of males will have severe gynecomastia (breast tissue >4.0 cm in diameter or the size of an average, midpubertal female breast) that persists into adulthood.

Etiology

The exact etiology of gynecomastia remains unknown. A common hypothesis is that a temporary imbalance of increased free estrogen compared to free androgens exists, with stimulation of breast development. With progression of puberty, androgen concentrations increase and the imbalance resolves.

Mechanisms to account for an increase in estrogen or a decrease in androgen activity include[20]:
1. Increase in serum estrogen concentrations
   a. Increased estradiol secretion from testes (e.g., Leydig cell tumors) or adrenal tumors
   b. Excessive conversion of androgens to estrogens by aromatase (enhancement of extraglandular aromatase activity due to hyperthyroidism, liver disease, increased body fat, medication/drug use)
   c. Increased estrogen bioavailability (limited estrogen bound to sex hormone–binding globulin [SHBG])
   d. Exogenous estrogen intake (oral intake or use of topical estrogens)
2. Decrease in serum androgen concentrations
   a. Impairment of testicular production: Primary hypogonadism (anorchia, Klinefelter syndrome), secondary hypogonadism (disordered hypothalamus or pituitary), congenital enzyme defects, drug-induced inhibition of enzymes needed in testosterone synthesis, or chronic stimulation of Leydig cells by high levels of human chorionic gonadotropin (hCG) from tumor
   b. Hyperestrogenic states suppressing luteinizing hormone (LH) and testosterone secretion
   c. Increased hepatic clearance of androgens
   d. Decreased bioavailability of testosterone due to increases in SHBG with liver disease or hyperestrogenic states
3. Alterations of estrogen and androgen receptors
   a. Androgen-receptor deficiency states (androgen insensitivity syndromes)
   b. Drug interference with androgen receptors (spironolactone, flutamide, or cimetidine)
   c. Drugs that mimic estrogens and stimulate estrogen-receptor sites (digoxin and phytoestrogens in some marijuana preparations)

Clinical Manifestations

Most cases of gynecomastia are bilateral. Gynecomastia ranges from Type I (subareolar nodule) to Type III (large amount of glandular tissue, resembles SMR 3 breast development in females). Tenderness on palpation is common. True gynecomastia should be distinguished from pseudogynecomastia caused by adipose tissue over the pectoral muscles in some obese males, and from breast masses due to cancer, dermoid cysts, lipomas, hematomas, or neurofibromas.

Physical Examination

Examine the patient in the supine position, with his hands behind his head; the examiner then places the thumb and forefinger at opposing margins of the breast. In gynecomastia, as the fingers are brought together, rubbery or firm breast tissue can be felt as a freely movable, and occasionally tender, disk of tissue concentric to the areola. In pseudogynecomastia, no discrete mass is felt. In other conditions such as a lipoma or dermoid cyst, the mass is usually eccentric to the areola. Physical examination should also include a testicular examination to exclude other causes of gynecomastia including hypogonadism, testicular mass, or atrophy.

Diagnosis

Pubertal gynecomastia can be presumed as the etiology of the breast enlargement in adolescents who (a) present with a unilateral or bilateral, subareolar, rubbery or firm mass; (b) are not using any medications or drugs possibly associated with gynecomastia (Table 60.6); (c) have a normal testicular examination; and (d) lack any evidence of renal, hepatic, thyroid, or other endocrine disease. If these criteria are met, no further tests are necessary. The patient should be reevaluated in 6 months. If medication or drug use is suspected, the substance should be discontinued and the adolescent reexamined in 1 month. At that time, breast tenderness, if present, and breast size should decrease.

Pathologic gynecomastia should be suspected if the patient is prepubertal, glandular tissue >4 cm, development is rapid, or the patient has other abnormalities on examination (hypertension, severe acne, abnormal testes, galactorrhea). Evaluation for pathologic causes of gynecomastia should include measurement of serum hCG, estradiol, testosterone, LH. If galactorrhea is present, measure prolactin, as well. Manage abnormal results as follows:

1. Elevated hCG concentration: Perform testicular ultrasonography. The presence of a mass suggests a testicular germ-cell

tumor. A normal sonogram suggests an extragonadal germ-cell tumor or hCG-secreting neoplasm. A chest film and abdominal computed tomography (CT) are indicated.
2. Decreased testosterone and elevated LH concentrations suggest primary hypogonadism, including Klinefelter syndrome or testicular atrophy caused by mumps orchitis.
3. Decreased testosterone and normal/low LH concentrations suggest secondary hypogonadism. Prolactin should be measured and a pituitary MRI obtained if prolactin is elevated.
4. Elevated testosterone and LH concentrations suggest androgen resistance, although TSH should also be measured as hyperthyroidism can increase LH concentrations.
5. Elevated estradiol with low/normal LH concentrations: Perform testicular ultrasonography. A testicular mass indicates a likely Leydig or Sertoli cell tumor. The absence of a mass should prompt an adrenal CT scan or MRI to assess for adrenal neoplasm. If none are found, an increase in extraglandular aromatase activity is likely.
6. Normal concentrations of hCG, LH, testosterone, and estradiol indicate idiopathic gynecomastia.

Management

Underlying causes of gynecomastia should be treated as appropriate, including discontinuation of causative medications. In most individuals with mild to moderate pubertal gynecomastia, only reassurance is needed. Most cases (90%) will improve or resolve within 12 to 18 months, while the remainder may persist into adulthood. There has been no proven relationship between gynecomastia and the development of breast cancer in males.

Medical therapy should be reserved for those individuals who have severe gynecomastia and who are significantly concerned about the condition. Options trialed for medical management include androgens (testosterone, dihydrotestosterone, and danazol), antiestrogens (clomiphene, tamoxifen, and raloxifene), and aromatase inhibitors (testolactone, anastrozole, letrozole, and formestane). No drug is approved by the U.S. Food and Drug Administration for the treatment of adolescent gynecomastia, and studies using these medications in adolescents are limited.[21] Surgical treatment is preferable for older adolescents with moderate to severe gynecomastia associated with psychological sequelae, or in patients with persistent gynecomastia >1 year in whom spontaneous resolution is unlikely. Surgical treatment of gynecomastia significantly improves quality of life for adolescents, with measurable improvements in physical and psychosocial functioning.[22]

 SUMMARY

Breast complaints in AYAs commonly include discomfort (mastalgia), developmental variations (asymmetry), developmental anomalies, nipple discharge, and gynecomastia. Medications are common causes of both galactorrhea and gynecomastia. Clinicians should reassure AYAs and their families regarding the spectrum of normal development, and appropriately intervene when anomalies occur. Clinicians should not hesitate to involve mental health experts and plastic surgeons when appropriate. Masses in this age group are common; malignant masses are rare. Persistent masses require evaluation. Physical examination and ultrasound imaging provide diagnostic information in a minimally invasive manner.

TABLE 60.6	
Medications Causing Gynecomastia	

Hormones	*Cardiovascular drugs*
Estrogens	Verapamil, nifedipine
Testosterone	α-Methyldopa
Anabolic steroids	Digoxin
Chorionic gonadotropin	Captopril, enalapril
Antiandrogens	Minoxidil
Spironolactone	*Antibiotics*
Flutamide	Ketoconazole
Cyproterone	Metronidazole
Psychoactive agents	*Gastrointestinal agents*
Phenothiazines	Cimetidine
Atypical antipsychotic agents	Ranitidine
Tricyclic antidepressants	Omeprazole
Diazepam	Metoclopramide
Haloperidol	*Others*
Drugs of Abuse	Antiretroviral drugs
Marijuana	Cancer chemotherapeutics
Alcohol	Phenytoin
Amphetamines	Penicillamine

REFERENCES

1. Nuzzi LC, Cerrato FE, Webb ML, et al. Psychological impact of breast asymmetry on adolescents: A prospective cohort study. *Plast Reconstr Surg.* 2014;134(6):1116–1123.
2. Cerrato F, Webb ML, Rosen H, et al. The impact of macromastia on adolescents: a cross-sectional study. *Pediatrics.* 2012;130(2):e339–346.
3. Xue AS, Wolfswinkel EM, Weathers WM, et al. Breast reduction in adolescents: indication, timing, and a review of the literature. *J Pediatr Adolesc Gynecol.* 2013;26(4):228–233.

4. Huang W, Molitch ME. Evaluation and management of galactorrhea. *Am Fam Physician.* 2012;85(11):1073–1080.

5. Melmed S, Casanueva FF, Hoffman AR, et al. Diagnosis and treatment of hyperprolactinemia: an Endocrine Society clinical practice guideline. *J Clin Endocrinol Metab.* 2011;96(2):273–288.

6. Vroonen L, Lancellotti P, Garcia MT, et al. Prospective, long-term study of the effect of cabergoline on valvular status in patients with prolactinoma and idiopathic hyperprolactinemia. *Endocrine.* 2017;55(1):239–245.

7. Testa G, Vegetti W, Motta T, et al. Two-year treatment with oral contraceptives in hyperprolactinemic patients. *Contraception.* 1998;58(2):69–73.

8. Di Filippo L, Doga M, Resmini E, et al. Hyperprolactinemia and bone. *Pituitary.* 2020;23(3):314–321.

9. Salzman B, Fleegle S, Tully AS. Common breast problems. *Am Fam Physician.* 2012;86(4):343–349.

10. Lee M, Soltanian HT. Breast fibroadenomas in adolescents: current perspectives. *Adolesc Healt. Med Ther.* 2015;6:159–163.

11. Nassar A, Visscher DW, Degnim AC, et al. Complex fibroadenoma and breast cancer risk: a Mayo Clinic Benign Breast Disease Cohort Study. *Breast Cancer Res Treat.* 2015;153(2):397–405.

12. Frazier AL, Rosenberg SM. Preadolescent and adolescent risk factors for benign breast disease. *J Adolesc Health.* 2013;52(5 Suppl):S36–40.

13. Valeur NS, Rahbar H, Chapman T. Ultrasound of pediatric breast masses: what to do with lumps and bumps. *Pediatr Radiol.* 2015;45(11):1584–1599; quiz 1581–1583.

14. Simmons PS, Jayasinghe YL, Wold LE, et al. Breast carcinoma in young women. *Obstet Gynecol.* 2011;118(3):529–536.

15. Werner-Lin A, Hoskins LM, Doyle MH, et al. "Cancer doesn't have an age": genetic testing and cancer risk management in BRCA1/2 mutation-positive women aged 18–24. *Health (London).* 2012;16(6):636–654.

16. Mørch LS, Skovlund CW, Hannaford PC, et al. Contemporary hormonal contraception and the risk of breast cancer. *N Engl J Med.* 2017;377(23):2228–2239.

17. Schneyer R, Lerma K. Health outcomes associated with use of hormonal contraception: breast cancer. *Curr Opin Obstet Gynecol.* 2018;30(6):414–418.

18. Moorman PG, Havrilesky LJ, Gierisch JM, et al. Oral contraceptives and risk of ovarian cancer and breast cancer among high-risk women: a systematic review and meta-Analysis. *J Clin Oncol.* 2013;31(33):4188–4198.

19. McLaughlin CM, Gonzalez-Hernandez J, Bennett M, et al. Pediatric breast masses: an argument for observation. *J Surg Res.* 2018;228:247–252.

20. Guss CE, DiVasta AD. Adolescent Gynecomastia. *Pediatr Endocrinol Rev.* 2017;14(4):371–377.

21. Lapid O, Van Wingerden JJ, Perlemuter L. Tamoxifen therapy for the management of pubertal gynecomastia: a systematic review. *J Pediatr Endocrinol Metab.* 2013;26(9–10):803–807.

22. Nuzzi LC, Firriolo JM, Pike CM, et al. The effect of surgical treatment for gynecomastia on quality of life in adolescents. *J Adolesc Health.* 2018;63(6):759–765.

ADDITIONAL RESOURCES AND WEBSITES

Additional Resources and Websites for Clinicians:

DiVasta AD, Weldon CB, Labow BI. The breast: Examination and lesions. In: Emans SJ, Laufer MR, DiVasta AD, eds. *Emans, Laufer, Goldstein's Pediatric and Adolescent Gynecology,* 7th ed. Wolters Kluwer; 2020.

American College of Obstetricians and Gynecologists—https://www.acog.org/clinical/clinical-guidance/practice-advisory/articles/2018/01/hormonal-contraception-and-risk-of-breast-cancer

Breast fibroadenomas in adolescents: current perspectives—https://www.ncbi.nlm.nih.gov/pmc/articles/PMC4562655/pdf/ahmt-6-159.pdf

Management of adolescent gynecomastia: An Update—https://www.ncbi.nlm.nih.gov/pmc/articles/PMC6166145/pdf/ACTA-88-204.pdf

Additional Resources and Websites for Parents/Caregivers and Adolescents and Young Adults:

https://www.everydayhealth.com/womens-health/the-girls-guide-to-healthy-breasts.aspx

https://kidshealth.org/NicklausChildrens/en/parents/az-fibroadenoma.html?WT.ac=ctg

https://www.livescience.com/36562-breast-growth-disorder-harms-teen-girls-health.html

https://www.stanfordchildrens.org/en/topic/default?id=breast-conditions-in-young-women-90-P01589&sid=

https://www.tigerlilyfoundation.org/for-girls/

https://youngwomenshealth.org/2014/02/27/buying-a-bra/

https://youngwomenshealth.org/2014/02/27/breast-health/

https://youngwomenshealth.org/2014/02/27/breast-self-exam-and-cancer-risks/

XII

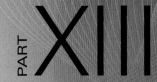

PART XIII

Sexually Transmitted Infections

Overview of Sexually Transmitted Infections

Lea E. Widdice

KEY WORDS

- Adolescent development
- Sexually transmitted infections (STIs)
- STI clinical services
- STI diagnosis
- STI laboratory services
- STI management
- STI prevention
- STI syndromes

INTRODUCTION

Sexually transmitted infections (STIs), also known as sexually transmitted diseases (STDs), are caused by a variety of bacteria, viruses, protozoa, and ectoparasites, which spread predominantly through sexual activity and intimate physical contact. A majority of STIs are initially asymptomatic, yet may still be transmissible. When present, the signs and symptoms caused by STIs can be nonspecific. Advancements in biomedical research have made it possible to identify the causative microbial agents resulting in improved treatments. When left untreated, many STIs can lead to chronic and life-altering sequelae.

Sexually transmitted infections caused by bacteria include chlamydia (*Chlamydia trachomatis),* gonorrhea (*Neisseria gonorrhoeae),* syphilis and condyloma latum (*Treponema pallidum*), chancroid (*Haemophilus ducreyi*), granuloma inguinale or Donovanosis *(Klebsiella granulomatis)*, and infections caused by *Mycoplasma genitalium.* Sexually transmitted infections caused by viruses include herpes (herpes simplex viruses [HSV] 1 and 2), genital warts and human papillomavirus (HPV) associated diseases, and human immunodeficiency virus (HIV). Among some nonpediatric populations, hepatitis B and hepatitis C are transmitted primarily through sexual contact. The most common protozoal STI is trichomoniasis (*Trichomonas vaginalis*). Ectoparasitic STIs include pubic lice and scabies.

Recognition and categorization of infections as STIs can change over time based on developments in biomedical research and epidemiology. In addition, infections categorized as STIs can have important, nonsexual modes of transmission, including mother-to-child transmission for many bacterial and viral STIs; syringe and needle transmission seen in some individuals with HIV; and nonsexual, person-to-person contact for scabies. Some infections may be categorized as STIs in some populations but not others. For example, in adults, hepatitis B is often categorized as an STI whereas in children, hepatitis B is commonly transmitted mother-to-child and not categorized as an STI. Finally, some infections with known sexual transmission are not categorized as STIs because other modes of transmission are more important, such as Zika virus and Ebola.

This chapter provides a general overview of the clinical manifestations, epidemiology, prevention, diagnosis, and treatment of STIs among adolescents and young adults (AYAs). Please see pathogen-specific chapters and other STI-related topics in this book.

CLINICAL MANIFESTATIONS OF SEXUALLY TRANSMITTED INFECTIONS

Sexually transmitted infections, when symptomatic, cause a wide variety of nonspecific symptoms determined by the biology of the etiologic agent and the anatomical location of infection. Table 61.1 lists common presenting symptoms of STIs and their infectious agents. Common syndromes caused by STIs include cervicitis, urethritis, vulvovaginitis, vaginosis, genital ulcers, pelvic inflammatory disease (PID), prostatitis, epididymitis, hepatitis, and STI-related enteric infections. Complications and sequelae following infection are the cause of significant disease burden including PID and ectopic pregnancy among females; urethral strictures and phimosis among males; abscesses; sepsis; and infertility, as well as acquired immunodeficiency syndrome (AIDS) and HPV associated cancers.

BURDEN OF DISEASE AND ESTIMATES OF INCIDENCE IN ADOLESCENTS

The high burden of STIs in AYAs is associated with high incidence and prevalence for some infections and the potential to cause chronic disease. Estimates of prevalence and incidence of STIs are determined through public health surveillance programs and epidemiologic studies. When comparing prevalence and incidence between adolescents and adults, it is worth noting that the estimates are most often calculated for the entire population, not the sexually active population. Therefore, the burden of STIs is even greater among AYAs than population estimates indicate.

In estimates based on 2018 public health data from noninstitutionalized, nonincarcerated, civilians in the United States, AYAs aged 15 to 24 years account for nearly one-fifth (19%) of the prevalence and almost one-half (46%) of the incidence of STIs.[1] Chlamydia and gonorrhea continue to disproportionately occur among adolescents. Among 15- to 39-year-old males and females, two-thirds of the incident urogenital chlamydia and one-half of the incident urogenital gonorrhea infections occurred in 15- to 24-year-olds; approximately 2.6 million chlamydia and 800,000 gonorrhea incident infections occurred among 15- to 24-year-olds. Among 14- to 49-year-olds, 16% of incident syphilis infections (approximately 24,000 infections) occurred in 15- to 24-year-olds. No national estimates of incident infections for *M. genitalium* are available. Among 15- to 59-year-olds, 16% of incident trichomoniasis infections (approximately 1.1 million infections)

TABLE 61.1

Sexually Transmitted Infections by Presenting Symptom

1. Abnormal vaginal discharge
   Vaginal site of infection or disrupted normal flora:
   a. *Candida* species
   b. *Trichomonas vaginalis*
   c. Bacterial vaginosis
   Cervical site of infection:
   a. *Neisseria gonorrhoeae*
   b. *Chlamydia trachomatis*
   c. Herpes simplex viruses types 1 and 2
   d. *Mycoplasma genitalium*

2. Urethral discharge and/or dysuria
   a. *N. gonorrhoeae*
   b. *C. trachomatis*
   c. *Ureaplasma urealyticum*
   d. Herpes simplex viruses types 1 and 2
   e. *T. vaginalis*
   f. *M. genitalium*
   g. Epstein–Barr virus
   h. Adenoviruses

3. Vulvar pruritus or burning, painful lesions, external dysuria
   a. Herpes simplex viruses types 1 and 2
   b. *Candida* species
   c. *T. vaginalis*

4. Foul or fishy odor of vaginal discharge
   a. Bacterial vaginosis
   b. *T. vaginalis*

5. Genital ulcer and/or lymphadenopathy
   a. Herpes simplex viruses types 1 and 2
   b. *Treponema pallidum*
   c. *Haemophilus ducreyi* (chancroid)
   d. *C. trachomatis* (LGV strains)
   e. *Klebsiella granulomatis* (granuloma inguinale, Donovanosis)

6. Genital growths
   a. Human papillomavirus (genital warts)
   b. Molluscum contagiosum
   c. Condyloma latum (secondary syphilis)
   d. *Klebsiella granulomatis* (granuloma inguinale, Donovanosis)

7. Abdominal/pelvic pain
   a. pelvic inflammatory disease

8. Anorectal pain/discharge/bleeding
   a. *N. gonorrhoeae*
   b. *C. trachomatis*
   c. *Shigella* species
   d. *Campylobacter* species
   e. *Entamoeba histolytica*
   f. *Giardia lamblia*

9. Scrotal pain
   a. *N. gonorrhoeae*
   b. *C. trachomatis*
   c. Coliform/enteric bacteria

10. Throat pain/Pharyngitis
    a. *N. gonorrhoeae*
    b. *C. trachomatis*
    c. Epstein–Barr virus

11. Hepatitis
    a. Hepatitis A and B virus
    b. Cytomegalovirus
    c. *T. pallidum*

12. Arthralgia and/or arthritis
    a. *N. gonorrhoeae* (disseminated gonococcal infections)
    b. *C. trachomatis* (reactive arthritis)
    b. Hepatitis B virus

13. Pruritus
    a. *Pthirus pubis*
    b. *Sarcoptes scabiei*
    c. *T. pallidum*

14. Flu-like or mononucleosis syndrome
    a. Cytomegalovirus
    b. Epstein–Barr virus
    c. Human immunodeficiency virus (HIV)
    d. Herpes simplex viruses types 1 and 2
    e. Hepatitis A and B virus

15. Rash
    a. *T. pallidum*
    b. *N. gonorrhoeae* (disseminated gonococcal infections)
    c. *C. trachomatis* (reactive arthritis)
    d. Hepatitis B virus
    e. Epstein–Barr virus
    f. Herpes simplex viruses types 1 and 2
    g. HIV

occurred in 15- to 24-year-olds. Among 15- to 49-year-olds, nearly half (42%) of the approximate 572,000 HSV type 2 incident infections occurred in 15- to 24-year-olds. Among individuals older than 12 years of age, 22% of the new sexually transmitted HIV infections occurred among 13- to 24-year-olds (approximately 7,200 infections).[1] Approximately 9 million 15- to 24-year-olds had ≥1 HPV type detectable by laboratory testing. Overall, the estimates of incident STIs in the United States clearly indicate that the burden of disease among AYAs is high. Among AYAs, special populations share an undue burden of STIs, including women,

men who have sex with men (MSM), and immunocompromised individuals.

TRANSMISSION OF SEXUALLY TRANSMITTED INFECTIONS

The probability of transmission of STIs depend on relationships between infection and disease symptoms, duration of infection, and infectiousness of the specific STI. Chlamydia, gonorrhea, syphilis, chancroid, and trichomoniasis are curable, short-lived infections with high transmission probabilities and individuals are susceptible to reinfection. The long asymptomatic periods of chlamydia, gonorrhea, and trichomoniasis result in these infections being widespread, whereas the higher likelihood of symptoms with syphilis and chancroid result in these infections being more prevalent in populations with higher-risk behaviors. Viral STIs are longer lasting, with longer asymptomatic periods, longer infectious periods but lower transmission probabilities than bacterial STIs.

ACQUISITION OF SEXUALLY TRANSMITTED INFECTIONS

Risks associated with acquisition of STIs include behavioral factors. Sexual behaviors that reduce exposure to infectious partners, including delayed sexual debut, and lower number of sexual partners, can decrease the risk of STI acquisition. Similarly, behaviors that reduce exposure to infectious tissue and bodily fluid can reduce the risk of some STIs. Consistent and correct external (formerly male) condom use can reduce the risk of HIV, hepatitis B, chlamydia, gonorrhea, and trichomoniasis. Internal (formerly female) condoms are less well studied but appear to reduce the risk of acquisition of STIs. Dental dams are recommended for prevention of STIs transmitted through oral sex, but few studies have examined their effectiveness. Choice of sexual acts affects the risk of STI acquisition. Engaging in sexual acts with less risk of microscopic and macroscopic trauma to the mucosal epithelium through physical and chemical trauma reduces the risk of STI acquisition.

Host defenses against STIs increase throughout puberty which may account for some of the increased risk of STI among adolescents compared to adults. In response to increasing estrogen throughout puberty, vaginal epithelial thickens, offering increased physical protection from infection. The presence of cervical ectopy, which decreases as females age, increases the risk of STI acquisition, including chlamydia, gonorrhea, and HPV. Cervical mucus production increases and thickens, providing a barrier to infection. Vaginal epithelial glycogen production increases throughout puberty, leading to changes in the vaginal flora that results in a protective decrease in vaginal pH. Hormonal changes in epithelium also lead to increased immune protection. Inflammation and ulceration from STI can increase the risk of acquiring other STIs.

Incongruence between adolescents' physical and psychological, cognitive, and social development can present challenges as adolescents navigate their emerging sexual and reproductive lives and protect themselves from STIs. During middle adolescence (usually ages 12 to 16 years for female and 14 to 17 years for males), secondary sexual characteristics have developed and interest in sexual activity is present. Socially, adolescents are exploring increasing independence from family along with increasing attachments to peer groups and experimenting with relationships and sexual behaviors. Cognitively, adolescents are developing abstract and long-term thinking. As young adolescents explore potentially risky behaviors, their ability to conceptualize the long-term risks from higher-risk sexual acts may not be fully developed. Thus, adolescents who are physically ready to engage in sexual activity may have a hard time planning for condom use, negotiating for preventive behaviors with sexual partners, or accessing prevention and treatment services. Parental/caregiver monitoring and communication and clinician counseling can help adolescents reduce risk-taking behaviors.[2]

PREVENTION OF SEXUALLY TRANSMITTED INFECTIONS

Sexually transmitted infection prevention efforts include protection of individuals from acquisition of STIs, interruption of transmission of STIs, and prevention or reduction of complications from STIs. Effective interventions necessarily differ based on the biology and epidemiology of each STI and characteristics of individuals,

networks, and populations. Prevention efforts evolve with developments in biomedical research and changes in epidemiology, human behavior, and cultural, social, and political environments.

Vaccines

Historically, vaccines have been the best method for preventing and even eradicating infectious diseases. Effective prophylactic vaccines are currently available for HPV and hepatitis B. Clinical trials to assess vaccines to prevent HIV infection are ongoing. Prophylactic vaccines to prevent primary HSV infection and therapeutic vaccines to reduce recurrences and viral shedding are being evaluated in clinical trials. Development and clinical trials of vaccines to prevent gonorrhea, syphilis, and chlamydia are national and World Health Organization priorities.

Behavioral Interventions

Behavioral counseling to encourage prevention of STIs is recommended for sexually active AYAs.[3,4] Behaviors recommended by the Centers for Disease Control and Prevention (CDC) to prevent STIs include condom use, limiting the number of sexual partners, practicing mutual monogamy, and abstinence from sexual activity. The U.S. Preventive Services Task Force (USPSTF) recommends intensive behavioral counseling for sexually active AYAs to reduce the risk of STIs. Effective behavioral interventions are tailored to an individual's risks and situations and personal goal setting and can be in-person, or web-based, single or multiple sessions, individual or group, and primary care setting or counseling setting. Interventions that include group counseling, involve more than 120 minutes of counseling, and are delivered over several sessions have the strongest effect in preventing STIs.[5] Less resource intensive interventions tailored to the clinical setting and population may also be effective.[4]

Antimicrobial-Based Interventions

Prophylaxis for Human Immunodeficiency Virus

Pre-exposure prophylaxis (PrEP) is recommended for AYAs at risk for HIV as part of HIV prevention strategies.[6] Successful use of PrEP requires an ongoing therapeutic relationship between the AYAs and their clinicians to maintain medication adherence and monitor for toxicities, side effects, and acquisition of other STIs. Adolescent's access to PrEP is affected by legal considerations, involvement of parents/caregivers, availability of confidential services, and cost of treatment. Clinical models to promote success of PrEP use by adolescents are being developed.

Postexposure prophylaxis for HIV can be effective in preventing infection from sexual transmission. It is used for prevention of infection after infrequent exposure, such as after a sexual assault. It should be initiated within 72 hours and as soon as possible after exposure.

Partner Management

Management of partners of patients with STIs is longstanding prevention intervention. In general, those with a STI(s) should notify their partners and encourage them to seek medical treatment and evaluation. Clinicians can encourage partner management by providing patients with written information to share with partners and providing partners with easily accessible STI services. Encouraging patients to notify their partners is associated with increased partner notification rates and reduced reinfection. Clinicians should be mindful of the potential risk of intimate partner violence when encouraging partner notification. Barriers to patient-initiated partner notification identified by AYAs include fear of retaliation or loss of their relationship, lack of concern or understanding of STI complications, social stigma, and embarrassment. Barriers to partners obtaining evaluation identified by AYAs include lack of transportation to a health care site and partner's fear of test results.[7]

XIII

Expedited partner therapy (EPT) or patient-delivered partner treatment is an adjunct to partner management for chlamydia and gonorrhea. For male partners of infected females, patient-delivered treatment has been shown, in randomized controlled studies, to be as effective or more effective than patient-initiated partner referral for STI evaluation.[8] When delivering treatment, patients should provide information to their partner on how to seek appropriate health care and evaluation. Expedited partner therapy for gonorrhea or chlamydial infection among MSM is not routinely recommended because of the potential for other STIs and warrants testing for HIV and other bacterial STIs.[4] Existing data suggest that EPT has a limited role in partner management for trichomoniasis. There are no data to support the use of EPT in the routine management of syphilis.

Asymptomatic Screening and Treatment

Screening for asymptomatic STIs can identify patients in need of curative treatment for bacterial STIs and suppressive treatment for viral STIs. The development of improved laboratory testing technology in the 1990s made widespread screening for many STIs possible. The CDC and USPSTF provide screening recommendations for which patient populations to screen, organisms to test for, anatomical sites to sample, and laboratory tests to use, as well as frequency of screening.[9] Local public health departments also develop screening recommendations based on local epidemiology. Professional organizations and subspecialty group guidelines may be pertinent to special populations or certain settings.

Clinicians must identify patients' sexual risk behaviors so that they can identify whom to screen for which infections at which anatomical sites. Due to clinicians' and patients' biases and comfort with discussing sexuality and sexual behaviors, communication about sexual risk behaviors can be challenging. Training is available for clinicians to gain competency in communication with AYAs to assess the need for STI screening.[10–13] Successful screening programs also require health care systems that account for social, emotional, legal, and cultural barriers experienced by AYAs in accessing care and disclosing risk behaviors.

⬤ DIAGNOSIS OF SEXUALLY TRANSMITTED INFECTIONS

Accurate diagnosis improves treatment for STIs. Because symptoms of STIs are nonspecific and overlapping (see **Table 61.1**), accurate diagnosis can be challenging. Accurate histories and directed physical examinations remain essential for the diagnosis of STIs and related syndromes. A physical examination can clarify location of symptoms and the appearance of abnormalities when patients and clinicians may lack a shared vocabulary or understanding of anatomy and signs and symptoms of disease. In addition, patients may be reluctant to describe physical abnormalities or not recognize signs of an STI. Details of physical examination findings for specific STIs and STI-related syndromes can be found in pathogen- and syndrome-specific chapters. Training on engaging adolescent patients and their parents/caregivers in consenting to and involvement in the physical examination is necessary to ensure patient's comfort and well-being.[10–13] Policies and guidelines should be in place to ensure clinicians and their assistants conduct examinations in culturally and legally appropriate ways.[14,15]

Advances in biomedical technology have led to an increasing number of diagnostic tests for STIs. Guidance on which diagnostic tools to have available in generalist clinical settings and STI specialist clinical settings is provided by the CDC.[16] Diagnostic tests marketed for clinical care in the United States must be cleared by the U.S. Food and Drug Administration (FDA). Clinical laboratories can validate "home grown" or "in-house" tests for clinical use.

Understanding test performance characteristics (sensitivity, specificity, positive predictive value, negative predictive value) is important for clinical decision making especially, when a diagnosis

is unclear, the response to treatment is inadequate, or changes to sample collection have occurred. The positive and negative predictive values provide guidance on how likely a patient is to have the disease if the test is positive or how likely the patient is to not have the disease if the test is negative. Performance characteristics of tests can be obtained by contacting the laboratory personnel as well as reviewing the test's package insert. The peer-reviewed biomedical literature is the source of information for performance of diagnostic tests in specific populations.

Appropriately and adequately collected samples that have been prepared and transported properly are critical for reliable diagnostic test results. Information about test performance for different sample types, for example, urine, vaginal, cervical, urethral, penile meatal, anal, pharyngeal, serum, and whole blood is available in package inserts and, sometimes, is available in peer-reviewed literature. Self-collected samples, that is, samples collected by the patient rather than a clinician, are well accepted and standard of care for vaginal samples used to test for chlamydia, gonorrhea, trichomoniasis, and *M. genitalium*. Growing evidence supports the acceptability of self-collected rectal and pharyngeal samples. Patient instructions for self-collected samples are available from clinical laboratories or manufacturers' websites. Self-collected penile meatal swabs have excellent diagnostic performance characteristics, but this sample type has not been widely adopted by diagnostic test manufacturers or laboratories.

Point-of-care tests can provide results rapidly and are simple to operate so that individuals without specialized training in laboratory techniques can operate the test. These tests can be used at the location (point) of patient care. Wet mount with normal saline, potassium hydroxide (KOH), and urine dip tests are well established point-of-care tests. Further, reliable, accurate, FDA-cleared point-of-care tests to detect chlamydia, gonorrhea, trichomoniasis, HIV, and syphilis are available for clinical use. Point-of-care tests have the potential to improve STI treatment, prevention, and antibiotic stewardship and will require implementation of new clinical pathways for test operation, result notification, patient education, treatment, and partner notification and treatment.

⬤ TREATMENT OF SEXUALLY TRANSMITTED INFECTIONS

Authoritative treatment recommendations for STIs and STI-related syndromes are addressed in the *Sexually Transmitted Diseases Treatment Guidelines* from the CDC.[4] Updates to the guidelines are available on the CDC website and published in the Morbidity and Mortality Weekly Report (https://www.cdc.gov/std/treatment/). The guidelines address treatment goals, strategies, and practices for specific etiologies of STIs and syndromes for the general population as well as special and vulnerable populations, including adolescents. Treatment guidelines for other countries and geographical areas are also available from professional organizations.[17] When treating STIs in adolescents, clinicians should be mindful of challenges and complications adolescents might face due to lack of privacy, autonomy combined with lack of experience with the health care system and taking prescribed medications. Adolescents and young adults experience barriers to accessing care, and following through on recommended treatments might be accentuated by the desire to maintain confidentiality and fear of punishment or retaliation if the need for treatment is disclosed. In addition, adolescents' stage of cognitive development may affect how they understand the goals of treatment and accept treatment recommendations.

⬤ EMERGING ISSUES

Mycoplasma Genitalium

Mycoplasma genitalium was recognized as an STI after isolation from two males with nongonococcal urethritis in the 1980s.[18] It is a recognized cause of nongonococcal urethritis in males but its role in rectal symptoms and proctitis is less clear. Infection in females is associated with cervicitis, PID, spontaneous abortion, and infertility. Lack of a cell wall confers low susceptibility to common antibiotics. In addition, it rapidly acquires antibiotic resistance. Macrolide resistance developed in at least 12% of *M. genitalium* infections treated with 1 g of azithromycin. Although prevalence in the general population has not been established, prevalence, among males and females seeking STI services, is similar to chlamydia. The role of asymptomatic infection in development of disease and adverse sequelae are unknown. Prospective trials to determine if screening and treating asymptomatic individuals prevents adverse reproductive sequelae in females, and persistent urethritis and sequelae in males, have not been reported. Currently, asymptomatic screening is not recommended in the United States. Testing for *M. genitalium* with resistance testing is recommended for males with recurrent urethritis and females with recurrent cervicitis and may be considered in females with PID.[4]

Testing and Treatment in Nontraditional Settings

Sexually transmitted infection diagnostic and treatment services are increasingly available outside of the traditional health care setting. This has the potential to increase access to STI services, but requires caution about the quality of testing and attention to linkage with care. Nontraditional settings' provision of STI screening, testing, and treatment in mobile care clinics and pop-up sites is intended to extend the reach of established STI clinicians. Internet-based testing and over-the-counter testing with mail-in samples is becoming increasingly available. Sample collection kits are sent to the individual's home or purchased over-the-counter and returned to a laboratory for testing. The process for linkage to treatment differs between internet testing sites and companies. Some internet sources of testing and treatment are reliable.[19] However, caution about the quality of these services is required, including the use of recommended tests and validation of diagnostic tests with shipped samples. These services should readily provide information to clinicians about the tests used and validation of shipped samples. Other nontraditional settings for STI screening and testing that are being developed include pharmacy-based testing and over-the-counter testing using point-of-care tests.

SUMMARY

Sexually transmitted infections and STI-related syndromes are a natural, although unwelcome, part of adolescence and young adulthood. Prevention, diagnosis, and treatment of STIs during adolescence and young adulthood are important for the development of lifelong sexual health.

ACKNOWLEDGMENT

This chapter was based on Chapter 56, Overview of Sexually Transmitted Infections published in the previous edition written by J. Dennis Fortenberry.

REFERENCES

1. Kreisel KM, Spicknall IH, Gargano JW, et al. Sexually transmitted infections among US women and men: prevalence and incidence estimates, 2018. *Sex Transm Dis.* 2021;48(4):208–214.
2. Dittus PJ, Michael SL, Becasen JS, et al. Parental monitoring and its associations with adolescent sexual risk behavior: a meta-analysis. *Pediatrics.* 2015; 136(6):e1587–1599.
3. U. S. Preventive Services Task Force, Krist AH, Davidson KW, et al. Behavioral counseling interventions to prevent sexually transmitted infections: US Preventive Services Task Force Recommendation Statement. *JAMA.* 2020;324(7):674–681.
4. Workowski KA, Bachmann LH, Chan PA, et al. Sexually Transmitted Infections Treatment Guidelines, 2021. *MMWR Recomm Rep.* 2021;70(4):1–187.
5. Henderson JT, Senger CA, Henninger M, et al. Behavioral counseling interventions to prevent sexually transmitted infections: updated evidence report and systematic review for the US Preventive Services Task Force. *JAMA.* 2020;324(7):682–699.
6. Tanner MR, Miele P, Carter W, et al. Preexposure prophylaxis for prevention of HIV acquisition among adolescents: clinical considerations, 2020. *MMWR Recomm Rep.* 2020;69(3):1–12.
7. Reed JL, Huppert JS, Gillespie GL, et al. Adolescent patient preferences surrounding partner notification and treatment for sexually transmitted infections. *Acad Emerg Med.* 2015;22(1):61–66.
8. Gannon-Loew KE, Holland-Hall C, Bonny AE. A review of expedited partner therapy for the management of sexually transmitted infections in adolescents. *J Pediatr Adolesc Gynecol.* 2017;30(3):341–348.
9. U.S. Preventive Services Task Force. *Recommendation Topics*, Published. [cited 2021 October 4].
10. Centers for Disease Control and Prevention. *A Guide to Taking a Sexual History*. October 4, 2021. https://www.cdc.gov/std/treatment/sexualhistory.pdf
11. American Sexual Health Association. *Resources for Health Care Providers*. [cited October 4, 2021]. https://www.ashasexualhealth.org/
12. Centers for Disease Control and Prevention. *Sexually Transmitted Diseases (STDs) Training*. February 26, 2021 [cited 2021 October 4]. https://www.cdc.gov/std/training/default.htm
13. American Academy of Pediatrics. *Adolescent Sexual Health*. 2021. https://www.aap.org/en-us/advocacy-and-policy/aap-health-initiatives/adolescent-sexual-health/Pages/Sexual-History.aspx
14. Committee on Practice and Ambulatory Medicine. Use of chaperones during the physical examination of the pediatric patient. *Pediatrics.* 2011;127(5):991–993.
15. Committee on Child Abuse and Neglect. Protecting children from sexual abuse by health care providers. *Pediatrics.* 2011;128(2):407–426.
16. Barrow RY, Ahmed F, Bolan GA, et al. Recommendations for providing quality sexually transmitted diseases clinical services, 2020. *MMWR Recomm Rep.* 2020;68(5):1–20.
17. International Union Against Sexually Transmitted Infections. IUSTI Treatment Guidelines (Europe). June 30, 2021. https://iusti.org/treatment-guidelines/
18. Peel J, Bond S, Bradshaw C, et al. Recent advances in understanding and combatting *Mycoplasma genitalium*. *Fac Rev.* 2020;9:3.
19. Huang W, Gaydos CA, Barnes MR, et al. Cost-effectiveness analysis of Chlamydia trachomatis screening via internet-based self-collected swabs compared with clinic-based sample collection. *Sex Transm Dis.* 2011;38(9):815–820.

🛜 ADDITIONAL RESOURCES AND WEBSITES

Additional Resources and Websites for Clinicians:

American Sexual Health Association (ASHA)—https://www.ashasexualhealth.org
ASHA has been providing resources and information for over one hundred years and has excellent youth-focused material.

CDC Recommendations for Providing Quality Sexually Transmitted Diseases Clinical Services, 2020—https://www.cdc.gov/mmwr/volumes/68/rr/rr6805a1.htm
This report provides CDC recommendations to US health care providers regarding quality clinical services for STIs for primary care and STI specialty care settings. These recommendations complement CDC's Sexually Transmitted Diseases Treatment Guidelines, 2021.

CDC Sexually Transmitted Diseases—https://www.cdc.gov/std/default.htm
This webpage contains links to information about STIs in AYAs; key resources such as STI surveillance information, STI Treatment Guidelines, STI Fact Sheets for patients and other patient education tools; data and statistics; laboratory information; prevention; program management and tools; and training. It also contains links to information about specific diseases and conditions.

CDC Sexually Transmitted Infections Training—https://www.cdc.gov/std/training/default.htm
This webpage contains links to a variety of online and webinar STI training courses, links to a national network of STI/HIV prevention training centers for regional expertise and learning opportunities.

The National Academies of Sciences, Engineering, and Medicine, Sexually Transmitted Infections: Adopting a Sexual Health Paradigm (2021)—https://www.nap.edu/catalog/25955/sexually-transmitted-infections-adopting-a-sexual-health-paradigm
This report is a review of the current state of STIs in the United States and offers recommendations for future public health programs and policy and research in STI prevention and control.

National Institutes of Allergy and Infectious Diseases—https://www.niaid.nih.gov/diseases-conditions/sexually-transmitted-diseases
Information about national priorities in research to develop effective prevention and treatment approaches to control STIs.

U.S. Preventive Services Task Force Published Recommendations—https://www.uspreventiveservicestaskforce.org/uspstf/topic_search_results?topic_status=P
This webpage is searchable for current screening guidelines, including gonorrhea, chlamydia, syphilis, HIV, HSV serologic testing, hepatitis B, hepatitis C as well as recommendations for HIV pre-exposure prophylaxis.

Additional Resources and Websites for Parents/Caregivers:

American Sexual Health Association (ASHA)—https://www.ashasexualhealth.org
CDC Parent Information—https://www.cdc.gov/parents/teens/index.html
Reliable public health information about sexually transmitted infections and sexual health

iwannaknow.org—http://www.iwannaknow.org; Spanish-language version—https://www.quierosaber.org
Web sites designed specifically for adolescents, parents, and educators to offer information on sexual health for teens and young adults. Adolescents and caregivers can find facts, support, resources to answer questions and get access to in-depth information about sexual health, sexually transmitted infections (STIs), and healthy relationships.

Office of Disease Prevention and Health Promotion, Talk with Your Teen About Preventing STDs—https://health.gov/myhealthfinder/topics/health-conditions/hiv-and-other-stds/talk-your-teen-about-preventing-stds

The Office of Disease Prevention and Health Promotion has useful information in English and Spanish about STIs, including sections on talking to teens about preventing STIs.

Society for Adolescent Health and Medicine—https://www.adolescenthealth.org/Resources/Resources-for-Adolescents-and-Parents.aspx

This webpage contains links to resources for sexual and reproductive health for adolescents and parents as well as confidentiality resources for adolescents, young adults, and parents.

Additional Resources and Websites for Adolesents and Young Adults:

American Sexual Health Association (ASHA)—https://www.ashasexualhealth.org

CDC Sexually Transmitted Diseases—https://www.cdc.gov/std/default.htm

iwannaknow.org—http://www.iwannaknow.org; Spanish-language version—https://www.quierosaber.org

Web sites designed specifically for adolescents, parents, and educators to offer information on sexual health for teens and young adults. Adolescents and caregivers can find facts, support, resources to answer questions and get access to in-depth information about sexual health, sexually transmitted infections (STIs), and healthy relationships.

ParaSociety for Adolescent Health and Medicine—https://www.adolescenthealth.org/Resources/Resources-for-Adolescents-and-Parents.aspx

This webpage contains links to resources for sexual and reproductive health for adolescents and parents as well as confidentiality resources for adolescents, young adults, and parents.

Neisseria Gonorrhoeae and Chlamydia Trachomatis

Catherine Silva
Renata Arrington Sanders

KEY WORDS

- Cervicitis
- Chlamydia trachomatis
- Extragenital infections
- Neisseria gonorrhoeae
- Pelvic inflammatory disease
- Urethritis

INTRODUCTION

Infections with Neisseria gonorrhoeae (N. gonorrhoeae) and Chlamydia trachomatis (C. trachomatis) are genital and oral sexually transmitted infections (STIs) frequently diagnosed in adolescents and young adults (AYAs). Biologic, behavioral, and psychosocial factors contribute to the high rates observed in this population. Screening and adequate treatment prevent transmission between partners and serious complications for the affected patient.

ETIOLOGY

Neisseria gonorrhoeae is an aerobic, oxidase-positive, diplococci bacteria found intracellularly, within, or associated with polymorphonuclear leukocytes. Its success as a human pathogen is the result of several virulence factors: (1) membrane proteins (that adhere and invade cellular membranes and prevent bactericidal activity); (2) porin B protein (insertion into host cell membrane); (3) lipooligosaccharide (LOS) (tissue toxin); (4) Opa protein (binding with cells); and (5) pili (adherence to host tissue).[1]

The first step in pathogenesis for N. gonorrhoeae is adhesion via the pili and Opa protein. Pili are long, hair-like appendages that help them attach to the host's mucosal epithelial cell surfaces. The Opa protein strengthens the attachment and initiates the invasion of epithelial cells. Pilin proteins are antigenically different and inhibit phagocytosis. This tight adhesive mechanism prevents the bacteria from being washed away by urine or vaginal discharge. The LOS and porin proteins are secondary mediators of adhesion.[2] Once adhesion is completed, colonization occurs. The porin protein acts as a nutrition channel. The LOS protein promotes the invasion of epithelial cells and can change to escape immune cell recognition. Lipooligosaccharide proteins can change to evade recognition from immune cells. Sialylation of the LOS allows N. gonorrhoeae to resist bactericidal activity.[2]

Reinfection occurs due to the lack of immunity with N. gonorrhoeae, partially due to the antigenic variation among the pili proteins. Cell wall proteins are their primary virulence factors that mediate the adhesion of bacterium within colonies, augment attachment to host cells, and cause antiphagocytosis. The release of IgA protease by N. gonorrhoeae can cleave IgA of mucosa and help organisms evade the effects of IgA. Neisseria gonorrhoeae

also produce beta-lactamase, which destroys penicillin and has a remarkable capacity to alter its antigenic structure to adapt to changes in the new microenvironment, which is why it has developed resistance to numerous antibiotics.

Chlamydia trachomatis is a gram-negative, obligate intracellular bacteria. Chlamydia trachomatis serovars can be divided into three groups—serovars A, B, and C are the leading cause of noncongenital blindness in developing nations; serovars D through K are commonly found in the urogenital tract and cause STIs; and serovars L1, L2, and L3 cause lymphogranuloma venereum (LGV), an invasive urogenital or anorectal infection.[3] Chlamydial serovars are assigned based on their immune response to the outer membrane protein and their associated symptoms, immune response, reinfection risk, and infection duration.[4] The immune response against C. trachomatis consists of both a neutralizing antibody and a T-cell–mediated immune response. The long-term pathologic immune response to C. trachomatis heat shock protein (cHSP60) can result in long-term tissue damage to the fallopian tube in females with pelvic inflammatory disease (PID) or repeat infections.[4]

Chlamydia trachomatis has a unique developmental cycle lasting between 48 and 72 hours, with initial attachment and ingestion of the infectious particle (the elementary body) into the host cell. The elementary body changes into an active form, called the reticulate body, within 6 to 8 hours, and these forms create large inclusions within cells.[3] These reorganize into small elementary bodies, released within 2 to 3 days from ruptured cells, infecting new epithelial cells. The intracellular nature of the pathogen and the inert nature of the elementary body eliminate the possibility for the evolution of surface components and the development of antibiotic-resistant mutations.[3] The lack of response may also explain the asymptomatic nature of most chlamydial infections. Therefore, antibiotics capable of intracellular penetration targeting both the intracellular and intravacuolar phases of the organism's life cycle must be used for a prolonged course or have a long half-life to ensure adequate levels.

EPIDEMIOLOGY

Neisseria Gonorrhoeae

Incidence and Prevalence

The World Health Organization (WHO) estimates that approximately 87 million new gonococcal infections occurred among 15- to 49-year-olds in 2016, with incidence highest in the WHO African Region, the Americas, and Western Pacific, and the lowest incidence in the European region.[5] Neisseria gonorrhoeae is the second most notifiable condition in the United States. In 2018, there were 583,405 cases reported to the Centers for Disease Control and

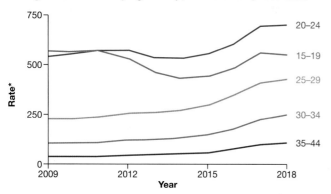
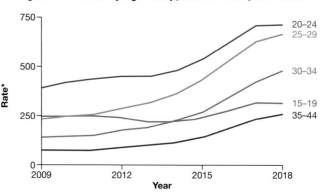

Gonorrhea — Rates of Reported Cases Among Females
Aged 15–44 Years by Age Group, United States, 2009–2018

Gonorrhea — Rates of Reported Cases Among Males
Aged 15–44 Years by Age Group, United States, 2009–2018

* Per 100,000.

FIGURE 62.1 Line graphs of prevalence of Gonorrhea by age and sex in the United States from 2009 to 2018. Graphs are adapted from the CDC.

Prevention (CDC)—179.1 cases per 100,000.[6] This is an increase of 5% from 2017 and 82.6% since 2009. In addition, *N. gonorrhoeae* rates have increased among males and females in all regions of the United States and among all racial groups.[6] The following section will describe rates of *N. gonorrhoeae* by sex, age, and race.

Sex The prevalence among females was highest in the WHO African region (1.9%), followed by the Americas (0.9%) and the Western Pacific region (0.9%), and was lowest in the European region (0.3%). Among males, the prevalence was highest in the African region (1.6%), the Americas (0.8%) and Western Pacific (0.7), and lowest in Europe (0.3%).[7] The rate of reported *N. gonorrhoeae* cases among females in 2018 compared to 2017 increased by 3.6%, approximately 119 to 213 cases per 100,000. For males, the rate increased by 6%, 201 to 213 cases per 100,000[6] (Fig. 62.1).

Age Worldwide, AYAs continue to have disproportionately higher rates of *N. gonorrhoeae* than other age groups. For example, in the United States in 2018, females aged 15 to 19 years and 20 to 24 years had the highest rates, while males aged 20 to 24 years and 25 to 29 years had the highest rates. Overall, the rates increased in most age groups for males and females except for 15- to 19-year-olds; both females and males slightly decreased, 1.7% and 0.9%, respectively (Fig. 62.1).[6]

Race Although *N. gonorrhoeae* rates increased among all racial groups, there is a persistent disparity by race/ethnicity. The rates

among non-Hispanic Black, American Indian/Alaska Native, Native Hawaiian/Other Pacific Islander, and Hispanic populations were disproportionately higher than non-Hispanic Whites in the 2018 CDC Sexually Transmitted Disease (STD) Surveillance Report. Non-Hispanic Black and American Indian/Alaska Native populations had 7.7 and 4.6 greater rates of *N. gonorrhoeae* than non-Hispanic Whites, respectively. Non-Hispanic Black females aged 15 to 19 years and 20 to 24 years had 8.88 and 6.9 times the rate as their non-Hispanic White counterparts.[8] Similar disparities were noted among non-Hispanic Black males. In the American Indian/Alaska Native population, the female rate of *N. gonorrhoeae* was 6.3 times that of non-Hispanic White females.[8]

Chlamydia Trachomatis
Incidence and Prevalence
Chlamydia trachomatis is the most prevalent bacterial STI in the world. The 2018 WHO report on global STI surveillance estimated 127 million cases in 2016.[9] A recent meta-analysis demonstrated that the prevalence of *C. trachomatis* in the general population was 2.9% (95% CI, 2.4% to 3.5%), with the highest prevalence in the Americas, followed by Europe, Africa, and the Western Pacific regions, while South-East Asian populations have the lowest prevalence. *Chlamydia trachomatis* infections were the most commonly reported bacterial STI in the United States in 2018, with 1,758,668 cases, corresponding to 539.9 cases per 100,000. There was an increase of 2.9% compared to 2017, from 524.6 to 539.9 cases per 100,000[6] (Fig. 62.2).

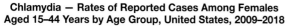
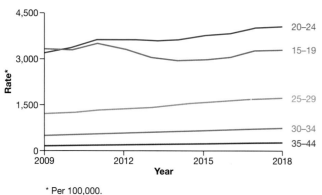
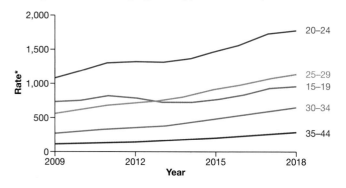

Chlamydia — Rates of Reported Cases Among Females
Aged 15–44 Years by Age Group, United States, 2009–2018

Chlamydia — Rates of Reported Cases Among Males
Aged 15–44 Years by Age Group, United States, 2009–2018

* Per 100,000.

FIGURE 62.2 Line graphs of prevalence of Chlamydia by age and sex in the United States from 2009 to 2018. Graphs are adapted from the CDC.

Sex Pooled estimates from countries in different parts of the world indicate that female prevalence is higher than male prevalence; 3.1% for females (95% confidence interval (CI), 2.5% to 3.8%) versus 2.6% for males (95% CI, 2.0% to 3.2%). This may be due to more females being screened, diagnosed, or reported to have *C. trachomatis* than males (Fig. 62.2). Among females in the United States, *C. trachomatis* rates increased by 11.4% from 2014 to 2018. In 2018, there were 692.7 cases per 100,000 among females.[6,10] Among males, there was a 37.8% increase in the incidence of *C. trachomatis* from 2014 to 2018. In 2018, there were 380.6 cases per 100,000 among males.

Age Adolescents and young adults who are 15 to 24 years old continue to have the highest rates of reported cases of *C. trachomatis* worldwide. In the Unites States, in 2018, 15- to 19-year-olds had 2,110.6 cases per 100,000, and 20- to 24-year-olds had 2,899.2 cases per 100,000.[6] From 2014 to 2018, the rate among females increased by 12.1% in 15- to 19-year-olds and by 11.9% in 20- to 24-year-olds. Similar increases in trends have been noted among males from 2014 to 2018; 15- to 19-year-olds had an increase of 32.8%, and 20- to 24-year-olds increased by 31.1%.[6]

Race The rates of *C. trachomatis* increased in all racial and Hispanic ethnic groups from 2014 to 2018. The rate of reported cases among non-Hispanic Black females was five times the rate among non-Hispanic White females. Non-Hispanic Black males had 6.8 times the rate of non-Hispanic White males.[8] Non-Hispanic Black males and females aged 15 to 24 years have higher rates of reported *C. trachomatis* cases than their non-Hispanic White counterparts of the same age group. American Indians/Alaska Native and Native Hawaiian/Other Pacific Islander populations have 3.7 and 3.3 times the rate, respectively, compared to the non-Hispanic Whites.[8]

Geography

The rates of reported cases of *C. trachomatis* in the United States by state in 2018 ranged from 198.2 cases per 100,000 in West Virginia to 832.5 cases per 100,000 in Alaska.[6] The District of Columbia reported 1,298.9 cases per 100,000 population.[6] In 2018, 70 counties and independent cities reported 44% of all chlamydia cases; 67.1% were located in the South and West.[6] Similar to *N. gonorrhoeae*, most states having the highest reported *C. trachomatis* case rates in males and females 15 to 24 years of age were in the South.[6] The rate ratios of *N. gonorrhoeae* and *C. trachomatis* varied by geographic location and race/ethnicity (Fig. 62.3).

Gay, Bisexual, and Other Men Who Have Sex with Men

Data suggest that gay, bisexual, and other men who engage in insertive or receptive anal sex with men are at increased risk for STIs, including *N. gonorrhoeae* and *C. trachomatis* in areas outside the urogenital tract. For example, data from a sample of 2,075 males in the National Human Immunodeficiency Virus (HIV) Behavioral Surveillance (NHBS) found that one in eight had *N. gonorrhoeae* and *C. trachomatis* in at least one of two extragenital sites (pharynx or anus).[11] *Neisseria gonorrhoeae* and *C. trachomatis* at extragenital sites are frequently asymptomatic, contribute to gonococcal antimicrobial resistance, and increase the individual risk for acquisition of HIV.

Factors Contributing to Neisseria Gonorrhoeae and Chlamydia Trachomatis

Biologic, behavioral, and psychosocial factors contribute to sexually active AYAs being at higher risk of acquiring STIs. Adolescent females are more prone to getting STIs due to cervical ectopy. Cervical ectopy is a normal finding among adolescent girls where during development, the columnar cells of the endocervix are exposed to the vaginal environment facilitating the attachment of sexually transmitted organisms. Other factors, such as rectal douching in young men who have sex with men (YMSM), may increase susceptibility for chlamydia and gonorrhea transmission through sloughing rectal epithelium.[12]

Multiple psychosocial factors contribute to high STI rates in AYAs. Social factors including not having insurance, transportation, or access to STI prevention and treatment services can contribute to the high prevalence of *N. gonorrhoeae* and *C. trachomatis* among adolescents. Some adolescents are more likely to have multiple, sequential, or overlapping sex partners, use barrier protection inconsistently or incorrectly, and exist in sexual networks that predispose them to STIs.[6] Those who initiate sex early in adolescence or engage in transactional sex (sex for money, goods, or a place to stay) are also at higher risk of STIs.[13] There is also the concern of confidentiality of services and the stigma or embarrassment of seeking STI services. Minoritized youth may fear and distrust health care institutions due to systemic racism, personally mediated clinician bias, or language barriers.[8] All of these factors can negatively impact sexual health care–seeking behaviors.

Screening for Neisseria Gonorrhoeae and Chlamydia Trachomatis

According to the CDC's 2021 STI Treatment Guidelines, annual routine screening for *N. gonorrhoeae* and *C. trachomatis* is recommended for all sexually active females less than 25 years old and females 25 years and older who are at increased risk for infection.

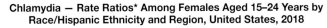

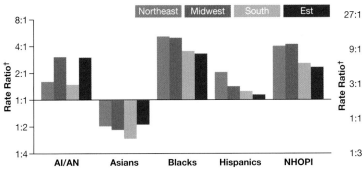

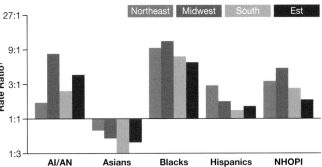

* For the rate ratios, Whites are the reference population.
† Y-axis is log scale.
NOTE: See Section A1.5 in the Appendix for information on reporting STD case data for race/Hispanic ethnicity.
ACRONYMS: AI/AN = American Indians/Alaska Natives; NHOPI = Native Hawaiians/Other Pacific Islanders.

FIGURE 62.3 Bar charts of the rate ratios of Chlamydia and Gonorrhea in the United States in 2018 by race and region. Graphs are adapted from the CDC.

In addition, the American Academy of Pediatrics Bright Futures Guidelines recommend screening for sexual activity annually starting at the 11-year-old well visit.[14] The 2021 U.S. Preventive Services Task Force (USPSTF) recommendations recommend screening for *N. gonorrhoeae* and *C. trachomatis* in all sexually active females aged 24 years and younger and in females aged 25 years or older are at increased risk.[15] Risk factors include new or multiple sex partners, a sex partner with concurrent partners, a sex partner with an STI, inconsistent condom use if not in a mutually monogamous relationship, previous or concurrent STI, and exchanging sex for money or drugs. Currently, there is insufficient evidence to recommend annual routine screening in males.[15] However, screening is warranted in sexually active males in clinical settings that serve populations with a high prevalence of *N. gonorrhoeae* and *C. trachomatis*. These clinical settings include AYA clinics, correctional facilities, and public STI clinics.

Sexually active YMSM should also be screened at least annually with specimen collections from all exposure sites (pharynx, urethra, rectum) regardless of condom use.[13,16] Men who have sex with men who are at increased risk of *N. gonorrhoeae* infection or HIV should be screened at all exposure sites every 3 to 6 months.[16] The CDC recommends screening for urethral infection for *N. gonorrhoeae* and *C. trachomatis* in males who have had insertive intercourse in the prior year. Screening for rectal infection should occur annually in MSM who have had receptive anal intercourse in the prior year. A test for pharyngeal infection for *N. gonorrhoeae* should occur for males who have had receptive oral sex in the prior year. Routine screening for *C. trachomatis* pharyngeal infection is not recommended. Instead, more frequent screening (every 3 to 6 months) is indicated based on sexual risk behavior and new sexual or multiple partners.

Other screening and testing recommendations vary based on population. Screening for youth living with HIV should occur at the first HIV evaluation and then at least annually. Young cisgender women who have sex with cisgender women and transgender/gender diverse youth may also be at risk for STIs. Clinicians should assess transgender and gender diverse youth's STI-related risk based on anatomy and sexual behaviors. Transmission risk is determined by the specific STI and sexual practice (e.g., oral–genital sex; vaginal or anal sex using hands, fingers, or penetrative sex items; and oral–anal sex). Digital–vaginal or digital–anal contact, particularly with shared penetrative sex items, has contributed to sexual transmission.[17] The prevalence and incidence estimates for STIs in gender-diverse youth are often based on data from convenience samples. However, in one study of adults living with HIV, MSM with HIV had an STI incidence of 20%.[18] Overall, clinicians should screen for asymptomatic STIs based on the sexual behaviors described by the patient.[13]

The CDC and USPSTF recommend using nucleic acid amplification tests (NAAT) for *N. gonorrhoeae* and *C. trachomatis* screening in both males and females. Sensitivity of urogenital NAAT specimens in females ranges from 72% to 100% with slight variations based on collection methods—clinician collected, self-collected, or urine collection.[19] For males, sensitivity ranges from 89% to 100% for urethral, meatal, and urine specimens. With NAAT screening, rectal and pharyngeal gonorrhea and rectal chlamydia have 89% to 93% sensitivity. Pharyngeal chlamydia has 69% sensitivity. The specificity for various sites ranged from 90% to 100% for both infections in males and females.[19] According to pooled evidence from the 2021 USPSTF report, self-collected vaginal specimens have similar sensitivity to physician-collected specimens for asymptomatic chlamydial (90% to 100%) and gonococcal infections (100%).[20] No studies were included in this report for males due to inclusion criteria. However, other studies have demonstrated the accuracy of extragenital self-collected samples in individuals who engage in receptive oral or anal sex and have shown high acceptability.[21]

Clinical Manifestations of Neisseria Gonorrhoeae and Chlamydia Trachomatis

This section provides an overview of the sex-specific clinical manifestations for *N. gonorrhoeae* and *C. trachomatis*. Both can present similarly, and coinfections can occur within the same individual.

Chlamydia trachomatis has an incubation period from 5 to 14 days following infection. *Neisseria gonorrhoeae* has an incubation period from 2 to 7 days.

Clinical Syndromes of the Female Genital Urinary Tract

1. *Urethritis*: Chlamydial or gonococcal infections of the urethra may not result in specific symptoms. Persons with infection may report urinary symptoms such as frequency and dysuria, and the urinalysis will be consistent with pyuria. Not all cases, however, will have organisms present on Gram stain or bacterial culture.

2. *Cervicitis*: Chlamydial infections of the cervix are often asymptomatic, which is why routine annual screening of young sexually active females is recommended. Symptoms are usually nonspecific and include an increase or change in vaginal discharge, vaginal pruritus, intermenstrual bleeding (defined as uterine bleeding at irregular intervals), and postcoital bleeding. Abnormal examination findings include mucopurulent endocervical discharge, easily induced endocervical bleeding, or edematous ectopy.

   Gonococcal infection of the cervix is frequently less asymptomatic than chlamydial infections (70% vs. 85%, respectively).[16] Symptoms usually develop approximately 10 days after infection, and females can present with vaginal pruritus, intermenstrual bleeding, and/or a mucopurulent discharge. Examination findings may show a normal cervix, or it may often be friable with mucopurulent discharge.

3. *Pelvic Inflammatory Disease*[17]: *Pelvic inflammatory disease* is an inflammatory disorder of the upper female genital tract. Sexually transmitted organisms, including *N. gonorrhoeae* and *C. trachomatis* are often implicated, with 50% of cases attributable to these organisms. However, other anaerobic organisms commonly result in a diagnosis of PID. Acute PID can be difficult to diagnose due to variable symptoms and signs associated with the condition. Symptoms can include urinary frequency, abnormal vaginal discharge, postcoital bleeding, lower abdominal/pelvic pain, and intermenstrual bleeding. Pelvic inflammatory disease can also be missed in clinical practice because some cases are subclinical and present with no symptoms. Signs of PID on examination include cervical motion, uterine or adnexal tenderness, and purulent endocervical and vaginal discharge. Females with PID caused by *N. gonorrhoeae* may appear more acutely ill and more likely to be febrile (see Chapter 63). Potential complications of PID include the following:

   a. Chlamydial and gonorrheal infections can ascend to the upper reproductive tract, presenting with adnexal mass or enlargement. Pelvic ultrasound is typically the first-line imaging study to evaluate an adnexal mass or enlargement.

   b. *Tubo-ovarian abscess (TOA)*: *Neisseria gonorrhoeae* and *C. trachomatis* infection can cause a complex infectious mass of the adnexa, called a tubo-ovarian abscess. Classically, a TOA presents with an adnexal mass, fever, elevated white-blood cell count, lower abdominal/pelvic pain, and vaginal discharge; however, presentations of this disease can be variable.

   c. *Perihepatitis (Fitz–Hugh–Curtis syndrome)*: Occasionally, *N. gonorrhoeae* and *C. trachomatis* infection can spread to the Glisson capsule surrounding the liver and cause perihepatitis or inflammation of the liver capsule. Most commonly caused by *C. trachomatis*, perihepatitis can be associated with PID. Symptoms include sharp pleuritic pain in the right upper quadrant, nausea, vomiting, and fever. Liver function tests are frequently normal or mildly elevated.

   d. Tubal infertility, ectopic pregnancy, and chronic pelvic pain can occur in females who have asymptomatic or symptomatic infections.

4. *Bartholinitis*: *Neisseria gonorrhoeae*, *C. trachomatis*, and other nonsexually transmitted pathogens may lead to the inflammation of the Bartholin glands. Most patients will have asymptomatic involvement of the Bartholin gland. Symptoms, if present, include perilabial pain and discharge. On examination, there may be edema of the labia, enlargement, and tenderness of the gland.

Clinical Syndromes of the Male Genital Urinary Tract

1. *Urethritis*: *Chlamydia trachomatis* is the most common cause of nongonococcal urethritis in persons with male genitalia and can present with dysuria and mucoid or watery urethral discharge. The discharge is often scant or clear and noted with the milking of the urethra or stained undergarments. The incubation period for chlamydial urethritis is 5 to 10 days after exposure. Gonococcal urethritis has an incubation period of 2 to 5 days after exposure, although some studies have shown incubation of up to 2 weeks after exposure.

2. Epididymitis: The most common cause of epididymitis in sexually active persons with male genitalia less than 35 years old is *N. gonorrhoeae* and *C. trachomatis*. Acute epididymitis is the pain, swelling, and inflammation of the epididymis lasting less than 6 weeks. Usually, the presentation consists of unilateral testicular pain, swelling, and tenderness. Epididymitis is generally diagnosed with concurrent urethritis, but some individuals may have asymptomatic urethritis. Additional imaging may be required to distinguish from other causes. Ultrasound findings may be normal or may show epididymal hyperemia and swelling. Gram stain of urethral secretions and urine microscopy showing polymorphonuclear leukocytes can help with the diagnosis. All suspected cases should be tested for *N. gonorrhoeae* and *C. trachomatis* by NAAT.[16]

Other Clinical Syndromes

1. *Conjunctivitis*: Direct inoculation of the epithelial cells of the conjunctiva with infected genital secretions can lead to conjunctivitis. Chlamydia serovars D through K are the genital disease resulting in conjunctivitis. Symptoms consist of nonpurulent erythematous injection of the epithelial surface of the conjunctiva and can develop a cobbled appearance. Gonococcal conjunctivitis usually occurs in infants born to untreated mothers. However, there are some case reports of autoinoculation from an anogenital source.[16] Gonococcal conjunctivitis symptoms can range from mild-to-aggressive purulent discharge, periorbital edema, and conjunctival injection.[16] Patients with gonococcal conjunctivitis should be evaluated emergently by an ophthalmologist.

2. *Pharyngitis*: *Neisseria gonorrhoeae* and *C. trachomatis* have been detected in the pharynx and are mostly asymptomatic. Symptoms may include sore throat, pharyngeal exudates, and cervical lymphadenitis.

3. *Proctitis*: Sexually transmitted gastrointestinal syndromes include proctitis, proctocolitis, and enteritis. In patients presenting with proctitis or proctocolitis, *N. gonorrhoeae* and *C. trachomatis* should be considered.[16] Proctitis is the rectal inflammation usually presenting with anorectal pain, tenesmus, or rectal discharge. Proctocolitis is when the inflammation extends into the colonic mucosa and presents with proctitis, diarrhea, or abdominal cramps. Fecal leukocytes can be found in stool specimens depending on the pathogen. Lymphogranuloma venereum serovars of *C. trachomatis* are possible pathogens for proctocolitis.[16] Anorectal–gonococcal

infections can occur in anyone who engages in anal sex but are commonly seen in MSM who engage in receptive anal sex. Anorectal gonorrhea can be the only site of infection in up to 40% of MSM.[16] Gonococcal proctitis is associated with an increased risk of HIV infection.

4. *Lymphogranuloma venereum*: Lymphogranuloma venereum is caused by *C. trachomatis* serovars L1, L2, and L3. It is a predominantly lymphatic tissue disease that spreads to causing lymphangitis, inflammation of the lymphatic system. It can lead to areas of necrosis in lymph nodes and abscess formation. Lymphogranuloma venereum is primarily endemic in heterosexual individuals residing in East and West Africa, India, South-East Asia, and the Caribbean.[16] However, there have been increasing reports among MSM with outbreaks in Western Europe and North America.[16,22] There are three stages of infection:

   a. Primary infection presents with a genital ulcer or mucosal inflammatory reaction at the inoculation site that spontaneously heals within a few days.

   b. Secondary infection usually occurs 2 to 6 weeks later and manifests as either an inguinal syndrome or anorectal symptoms. Inguinal syndromes are more common in males and involve the development of unilateral buboes or painful inguinal lymph nodes. Anorectal syndrome results from an inflammatory mass in the rectum and retroperitoneum. Symptoms are similar to proctocolitis with rectal discharge, anal pain, constipation, fever, and tenesmus.

   c. Late LGV occurs if the earlier stages of the disease go untreated, resulting in fibrosis and strictures of the anogenital tract, leading to genital elephantiasis, anal fistula, and infertility.

5. *Reactive Arthritis Triad (RAT)*: The RAT consists of arthritis, conjunctivitis or uveitis, and urethritis or cervicitis. Although a rare syndrome, it can occur following an STI, most commonly with *C. trachomatis* infection. Individuals with a history of chlamydia-induced arthritis warrant evaluation for recurrent urogenital infections with *C. trachomatis* and initiation of appropriate treatment.

Treatment

The following recommended treatment regimens are based on the 2021 CDC STI Treatment Guidelines.[16]

Uncomplicated Urogenital Infections

Uncomplicated urogenital chlamydial infections' first-line treatment is:
- Doxycycline 100 mg twice daily for 7 days
  Alternative Regimens:
- Azithromycin 1 g single dose (observed treatment if possible)
  OR
- Levofloxacin 500 mg orally (PO) once daily for 7 days

When administering doxycycline, clinicians must counsel patients on the importance of adherence to the 7-day regimen. Delayed-release doxycycline 200 mg daily for 7 days is just as effective and better tolerated but costlier. Doxycycline is contraindicated in pregnant patients. When nonadherence is a concern, azithromycin should be administered preferably with direct observation of therapy.[16]

According to the CDC's 2021 updated STI treatment guidelines, a high-dose intramuscular (IM) regimen of ceftriaxone is recommended for gonococcal urogenital infections. The dosing of ceftriaxone depends on the patient's weight.
- <150 kg—ceftriaxone 500 mg IM single dose
- 150 kg—ceftriaxone 1 g IM single dose

Previous CDC treatment guidelines recommended a second agent, but this is no longer the recommendation due to increased gonococcal resistance to azithromycin. If *C. trachomatis* coinfection has not been excluded, then presumptive treatment for

C. trachomatis should be prescribed. Although the CDC treatment guidelines no longer recommend azithromycin for the presumptive treatment of *C. trachomatis* infection, clinicians should determine if there are concerns for nonadherence that would warrant the use of 1 g of azithromycin instead of doxycycline.

Epididymitis

Sexually active male patients under 35 years presenting with acute epididymitis should receive empiric treatment. The recommended regimen for epididymitis likely caused by *N. gonorrhoeae* and *C. trachomatis* is a single dose of ceftriaxone IM (500 mg if weight <150 kg, 1 g if weight ≥150 kg) PLUS doxycycline 100 mg twice daily for 10 days.[13,23] If there is suspicion that epididymitis may involve enteric organisms based on the patient's report of engagement in insertive anal sex, fluoroquinolones should be used instead of doxycycline. The alternate fluoroquinolone regimens are either ofloxacin (300 mg twice daily for 10 days) or levofloxacin (500 mg daily for 10 days); these offer coverage against *C. trachomatis* as well.

Proctitis

Treatment for patients with asymptomatic chlamydial rectal infection is doxycycline 100 mg twice daily for 7 days. Studies have shown that doxycycline is more efficacious for rectal *C. trachomatis* infection than azithromycin.[16] For uncomplicated gonococcal infection of the rectum, treatment is a single dose of ceftriaxone IM (500 mg if weight <150 kg, 1 g if weight ≥150 kg).[16] If the patient is presenting with symptoms of proctitis, then empiric treatment for both *C. trachomatis* and *N. gonorrhoeae* is indicated. Empiric treatment consists of a single dose of ceftriaxone IM (500 mg if weight <150 kg, 1 g if weight ≥150 kg) PLUS doxycycline 100 mg twice daily for 3 weeks.[23]

Pelvic Inflammatory Disease

Outpatient treatment for mild to moderate PID in females includes a single dose of ceftriaxone IM (500 mg if weight <150 kg, 1 g if weight ≥150 kg) PLUS doxycycline 100 mg twice daily for 14 days PLUS metronidazole 500 mg twice daily for 14 days.[13,23] All outpatients should be reexamined within 72 hours to ensure clinical improvement. While PID in pregnancy is rare, doxycycline for treatment of PID is contraindicated. Therefore, alternative regimens with less risk to the fetus should be utilized. The CDC recommends hospitalization for pregnant patients with PID as well as those who have severe disease (e.g., severe abdominal pain, fever, nausea/vomiting), tuboovarian abscess, surgical emergency, or are unable to follow and outpatient treatment regimen. (See Chapter 56).

Oropharyngeal Infection

The clinical significance of oropharyngeal chlamydia infection is not clear. Current literature suggests *C. trachomatis* infection from the oropharynx can be sexually transmitted to genital sites.[24] Current treatment recommendations are either azithromycin (1 g PO as a single dose) or doxycycline (100 mg twice daily for 7 days).[13]

For *N. gonorrhoeae* oropharyngeal infection, a single high dose of ceftriaxone IM is recommended, 500 mg if weight is <150 kg, and 1 g if weight is ≥150 kg. For patients with a beta-lactam allergy, ceftriaxone can still be considered depending on the type of allergy and thorough assessment of the allergic reaction with either a test dose procedure or skin test. An infectious disease consultation is recommended if the patient has a severe allergic reaction or anaphylaxis to ceftriaxone.[23]

Conjunctivitis

Treatment for gonococcal conjunctivitis is a single 1 g dose of ceftriaxone IM and presumptive treatment for *C. trachomatis* infections. Since conjunctivitis due to *N. gonorrhoeae* and *C. trachomatis* is uncommon in adolescents and adults, there is limited data on treatment. Infectious disease and ophthalmology consultations are recommended.[16]

Lymphogranuloma Venereum

The preferred treatment for all stages of LGV infection for patients who are not pregnant is a 21-day course of doxycycline 100 mg PO twice a day.[13] Patients will need close follow-up to monitor adherence and resolution of symptoms. An alternative regimen for patients who cannot take doxycycline is azithromycin 1 g PO once a week for 3 weeks. If the patient is pregnant, erythromycin 500 mg four times a day for 21 days is recommended. Azithromycin has been effective in pregnancy; however, there is no published evidence to support the efficacy of azithromycin for the treatment of LGV during pregnancy.[13]

Treatment Considerations for Pregnant Females

For uncomplicated *N. gonorrhoeae* infections, females should receive the preferred treatment of high-dose ceftriaxone. For presumptive *C. trachomatis* infections, doxycycline is contraindicated and the recommended treatment is a single dose of 1 g of azithromycin.

Expedited Partner Therapy

Expedited Partner Therapy (EPT) is a treatment approach where a clinician gives a patient who has tested positive for an STI treatment for their sex partners in the absence of medical evaluation. The CDC has recommended EPT since 2006 to help reduce *C. trachomatis* and *N. gonorrhoeae* reinfection rates.[25] Under the current guidelines, EPT should be considered for heterosexual partners of patients diagnosed with *C. trachomatis* and *N. gonorrhoeae* who are unlikely to access evaluation and treatment. However, EPT is not recommended for MSM due to the risk of coexisting infections, especially HIV in their partners. Clinicians can verify local regulations regarding EPT on the CDC website (www.cdc.gov/std/ept).

According to the 2021 CDC STI Gonococcal Treatment Guidelines, if *C. trachomatis* infection has been excluded, partner treatment can be a single 800 mg dose of cefixime.[16,25] If it has not been excluded, partner treatment should include cefixime and doxycycline 100 mg twice daily for 7 days. The recommended EPT regimen for isolated *C. trachomatis* infection is a single dose of azithromycin 1 g or doxycycline 100 mg twice daily for 7 days.[13]

Retesting

All patients with a positive *N. gonorrhoeae* or *C. trachomatis* infection should be retested 3 months after treatment or at the first visit thereafter within 12 months of treatment. A "test of cure" is only indicated in pregnant patients with chlamydia, patients with persistent symptoms, or those treated with an inferior treatment regimen based on cure rates, such as erythromycin and amoxicillin. Treatment with doxycycline, azithromycin, levofloxacin, or ofloxacin has a greater than 95% cure rate in compliant, nonpregnant patients. Patients who need retesting should have it performed no earlier than 3 weeks after treatment due to the risk of a false positive due to the presence of dead organisms. A test of cure is recommended for all pharyngeal gonococcal infections, regardless of the treatment regimen used to ensure eradication given the challenges to effective treatment on infections at this site.[16,23]

Antibiotic Resistance

The CDC-sponsored Gonococcal Isolate Surveillance Project (GISP) monitors trends in drug resistance of *N. gonorrhoeae* in the United States. The GISP and other global surveillance programs have shown increased resistance to multiple antibiotics, including penicillins, tetracyclines, macrolides, and fluoroquinolones. The most alarming trend has been a progressive decrease in susceptibility to cephalosporins and azithromycin in *N. gonorrhoeae*.[23]

Previously dual therapy with ceftriaxone and azithromycin were recommended for gonococcal infections. The GISP and global surveillance data have shown an increasing minimum inhibitory concentration (MIC) trend, indicating decreased susceptibility to

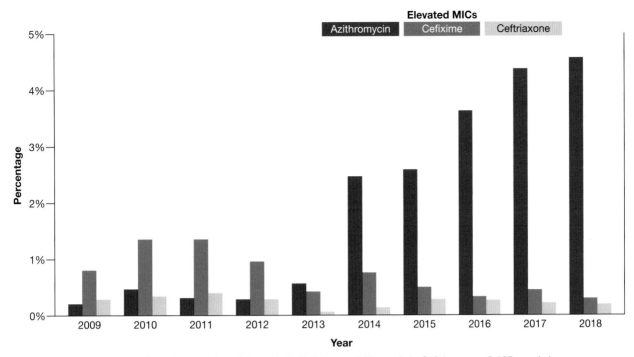

NOTE: Elevated MIC = Azithromycin: ≥ 2.0 mcg/mL; Cefixime: ≥ 0.25 mcg/mL; Ceftriaxone: ≥ 0.125 mcg/mL.

FIGURE 62.4 Bar graph showing percentage of *N. gonorrhea* isolates with elevated minimum inhibitory concentrations to azithromycin, cefixime, and ceftriaxone from 2009 to 2018. Graph is adapted from the CDC.

ceftriaxone and cefixime (Fig. 62.4).[23] Dual therapy with azithromycin has contributed to the emergence of resistance and is no longer recommended.[23] Azithromycin resistance increased from 0.6% in 2013 to 4.6% in 2018. *Neisseria gonorrhoeae* isolates from MSM have also had higher resistance than males who have sex with females only.[26] Antibiotic resistance has resulted from a combination of frequent *N. gonorrhoeae* pharyngeal infections, underscreening, and wide variability of ceftriaxone concentrations in the pharynx. Ceftriaxone dosage has increased as a result of change in resistance and because of the longer treatment duration needed to reach above the MICs necessary to inhibit *N. gonorrhoeae* growth in vitro.

Special Circumstances

When in-person clinical examinations are limited, clinicians may need to implement phone or telemedicine appointments to ensure clinical care. In April 2020, the CDC provided guidance on management when patient access to in-person clinical examinations was limited.[27] Self-collected mail-in samples are recommended alternative methods for testing. The recommended treatment for penile discharge or urethritis is cefixime 800 mg plus azithromycin 1 g taken PO or cefpodoxime 400 mg PO every 12 hours for two doses plus azithromycin 1 g taken PO. Treatment of proctitis includes cefixime 800 mg once, plus doxycycline 100 mg taken twice daily for 7 days PO, or cefpodoxime 400 mg PO every 12 hours for two doses plus doxycycline 100 mg taken twice daily for 7 days PO. In addition, clinicians should manage concerns for PID or vaginal discharge related to *N. gonorrhoeae* or *C. trachomatis* infection in person.

Prevention

There are multiple ways for at-risk AYAs to prevent *N. gonorrhoeae* and *C. trachomatis*. Delaying the onset of sexual intercourse or abstaining from sex can effectively limit exposure. If used consistently and correctly, male latex condoms are 98% effective against *N. gonorrhoeae* and *C. trachomatis* infections.[28] Female condoms are 95% effective when used correctly during each sex act.[29] Other prevention methods include limiting the number of sex partners and avoiding sex while intoxicated or impaired by alcohol or other substance use.

SUMMARY

In summary, the high prevalence of *N. gonorrhoeae* and *C. trachomatis* infections occur worldwide, especially among AYAs. Biologic factors, such as cervical ectopy, psychosocial factors, and sociobehavioral factors such as concurrent and serial sexual partners and unknowingly being in a high prevalence sexual network, contribute to high rates. Screening recommendations vary by gender, age, and the sexual behaviors of the AYA. Timely treatment is needed to prevent the development of resistant organisms, transmission between partners, and the potential for serious complications. Expedited partner therapy is recommended for sexual partners who are unable or unwilling to seek care after notification by index patients.

REFERENCES

1. Chakraborty P. Neisseria and Moraxella Catarrhalis. In: *A Textbook of Microbiology*. New Central Book Agency; 2020.
2. Quillin SJ, Seifert HS. Neisseria gonorrhoeae host adaptation and pathogenesis. *Nat Rev Microbiol*. 2018;16(4):226–240. doi:10.1038/nrmicro.2017.169
3. Elwell C, Mirrashidi K, Engel J. Chlamydia cell biology and pathogenesis. *Nat Rev Microbiol*. 2016;14(6):385–400. doi:10.1038/nrmicro.2016.30
4. Menon S, Timms P, Allan JA, et al. Human and pathogen factors associated with chlamydia trachomatis-related infertility in women. *Clin Microbiol Rev*. 2015;28(4):969–985. doi:10.1128/CMR.00035-15
5. Rowley J, Hoorn SV, Korenromp E, et al. Chlamydia, gonorrhea, trichomoniasis and syphilis: global prevalence and incidence estimates, 2016. *Bull World Health Organ*. 2019;97(8):548–562P. doi:10.2471/BLT.18.228486
6. Center for Disease Control and Prevention. *Sexually Transmitted Disease Surveillance 2018*. 2019. doi:10.15620/cdc.79370
7. Kirkcaldy RD, Weston E, Segurado AC, et al. Epidemiology of gonorrhea: a global perspective. *Sex Health*. 2019;16(5):401–411. doi:10.1071/SH19061
8. Centers for Disease Control and Prevention. Sexually Transmitted Disease Surveillance 2019. Atlanta: U.S. Department of Health and Human Services.
9. Report on global sexually transmitted infection surveillance, 2018. Geneva: World Health Organization; 2018. Licence: CC BY-NC-SA 3.0 IGO.
10. Huai P, Li F, Chu T, et al. Prevalence of genital Chlamydia trachomatis infection in the general population: a meta-analysis. *BMC Infect Dis*. 2020;20(1):589. doi:10.1186/s12879-020-05307-w

XIII

11. Jones MLJ, Chapin-Bardales J, Bizune D, et al. Extragenital Chlamydia and Gonorrhea among community venue–attending men who have sex with men—five cities, United States, 2017. *MMWR Morb Mortal Wkly Rep.* 2019;68(14):321–325. doi:10.15585/mmwr.mm6814a1

12. Li P, Yuan T, Fitzpatrick T, et al. Association between rectal douching and HIV and other sexually transmitted infections among men who have sex with men: a systematic review and meta-analysis. *Sex Transm Infect.* 2019;95(6):428–436. doi:10.1136/sextrans-2019-053964

13. Frieden TR, Jaffe HW, Rasmussen SA, et al. *Morbidity and Mortality Weekly Report Sexually Transmitted Diseases Treatment Guidelines, 2015 Centers for Disease Control and Prevention MMWR Editorial and Production Staff (Serials) MMWR Editorial Board*; 2015.

14. AAP Bright Futures. *Bright Futures Medical Screening Reference Table for Adolescence Visits (11 Through 21 Years)*; 2018.

15. U.S. Preventive Services Task Force. *Recommendation: Chlamydia and Gonorrhea: Screening | United States Preventive Services Taskforce.* Published 2014. Accessed March 4, 2021. https://www.uspreventiveservicestaskforce.org/uspstf/recommendation/chlamydia-and-gonorrhea-screening

16. Workowski KA, Bachmann LH, Chan PA, et al. *Morbidity and Mortality Weekly Report Sexually Transmitted Infections Treatment Guidelines, 2021 Centers for Disease Control and Prevention MMWR Editorial and Production Staff (Serials) MMWR Editorial Board.* 2021;70(4):1–187.

17. Muzny CA, Harbison HS, Pembleton ES, et al. Sexual behaviors, perception of sexually transmitted infection risk, and practice of safe sex among southern African American women who have sex with women. *Sex Transm Dis.* 2013;40(5):395–400. doi:10.1097/OLQ.0b013e31828caf34

18. Patel P, Bush T, Mayer K, et al. Routine brief risk-reduction counseling with biannual STD testing reduces STD incidence among HIV-infected men who have sex with men in care. *Sex Transm Dis.* 2012;39(6):470–474. doi:10.1097/OLQ.0b013e31824b3110

19. Nelson HD, Zakher B, Cantor A, et al. Screening for Gonorrhea and Chlamydia: Systematic Review to Update the U.S. Preventive Services Task Force Recommendations. Agency for Healthcare Research and Quality (US); 2014 Sep. Report No.: 13-05184-EF-1.

20. *Recommendation: Chlamydia and Gonorrhea: Screening | United States Preventive Services Taskforce.* Accessed March 29, 2021. https://uspreventiveservicestaskforce.org/uspstf/recommendation/chlamydia-and-gonorrhea-screening

21. Lunny C, Taylor D, Hoang L, et al. Self-collected versus clinician-collected sampling for Chlamydia and Gonorrhea screening: a systemic review and meta-analysis. *PLoS One.* 2015;10(7):e0132776. doi:10.1371/journal.pone.0132776

22. European Centre for Disease Prevention and Control. Lymphogranuloma venereum—ECDC Annual Epidemiological Report for 2018;2020.

23. St. Cyr S, Barbee L, Workowski KA, et al. Update to CDC's treatment guidelines for gonococcal infection, 2020. *MMWR Morb Mortal Wkly Rep.* 2020;69(50):1911–1916. doi:10.15585/mmwr.mm6950a6

24. Ribeiro S, De Sousa D, Medina O, et al. Prevalence of gonorrhea and chlamydia in a community clinic for men who have sex with men in Lisbon, Portugal. *Int J STD AIDS.* 2019;30(10):951–959. doi:10.1177/0956462419855484

25. *CDC—Guidance on the Use of Expedited Partner Therapy in the Treatment of Gonorrhea.* Published 2021. Accessed March 31, 2021. https://www.cdc.gov/std/ept/gc-guidance.htm

26. Wind CM, De Vries E, Van Der Loeff MFS, et al. Decreased azithromycin susceptibility of Neisseria gonorrhoeae isolates in patients recently treated with azithromycin. *Clin Infect Dis.* 2017;65(1):37–45. doi:10.1093/cid/cix249

27. Center for Disease Control and Prevention. *Guidance and Resources During Disruption of STD Clinical Services.* Published 2020. Accessed November 1, 2021. https://www.cdc.gov/std/prevention/disruptionGuidance.htm

28. Holmes KK, Levine R, Weaver M. *Effectiveness of Condoms in Preventing Sexually Transmitted Infections.* Vol 82; 2004. http://www.who.int/bulletin

29. Gallo MF, Kilbourne-Brook M, Coffey PS. A review of the effectiveness and acceptability of the female condom for dual protection. *Sex Health.* 2012;9(1):18–26. doi:10.1071/SH11037

📶 ADDITIONAL RESOURCES AND WEBSITES

Additional Resources and Websites for Clinicians:

The CDC—Gonorrhea—https://www.cdc.gov/std/gonorrhea/arg/default.htm

The CDC—Gonorrhea and Expedited Partner Therapy—https://www.cdc.gov/std/ept/gc-guidance.htm

Jones MLJ, Chapin-Bardales J, Bizune D. Extragenital Chlamydia and Gonorrhea among community venue–attending men who have sex with men—Five Cities, United States, 2017. *MMWR Morb Mortal Wkly Rep.* 2019;68(14);321–325.

Recommendation Statement: Chlamydia and Gonorrhea: Screening | United States Preventive Services Taskforce—https://www.uspreventiveservicestaskforce.org/uspstf/recommendation/chlamydia-and-gonorrhea-screening

St. Cyr S, Barbee L, Workowski KA, et al. Update to CDC's treatment guidelines for gonococcal infection, 2020. *MMWR Morb Mortal Wkly Rep.* 2020;69(50):1911–1916. doi:10.15585/mmwr.mm6950a6

Workowski KA, Bachmann LH, Chan PA, et al. Sexually transmitted infections treatment guidelines, 2021. *MMWR Morb Mortal Wkly Rep.* 2021;70(4):1–187.

Additional Resources and Websites for Parents/Caregivers:

Be an Askable Parent. American Sexual Health Association—https://www.ashasexualhealth.org/parents/

Resources for Parents. Planned Parenthood—https://www.plannedparenthood.org/learn/parents/resources-parents

Sexually Transmitted Infections—https://www.healthychildren.org/English/health-issues/conditions/sexually-transmitted/Pages/Sexually-Transmitted-Infections-Prevention.aspx

Talking to Your Kids About STDs (for Parents). Kids Health—https://kidshealth.org/en/parents/stds-talk.html

Talking with Your Teens about Sex: Going Beyond "the Talk"—https://www.cdc.gov/healthyyouth/protective/pdf/talking_teens.pdf

Additional Resources and Websites for Adolescents and Young Adults:

CDC Fact Sheet: Information for Teens and Young Adults: Staying Healthy and Preventing STDs—https://www.cdc.gov/std/life-stages-populations/life-stages-populations/stdfact-teens.htm

Fact Sheets and Brochures. American Sexual Health Association—http://chlamydiacoalition.org/patient-education-materials/

Healthy Relationships, Healthy Life: College Workshops Empower Students to Protect Their Own Sexual Health—https://www.cdc.gov/std/products/success/HealthyRelationshipsSuccessStory.pdf

It's Your Future. You can Protect It—https://www.cdc.gov/teenpregnancy/pdf/teen-condom-fact_sheet-english-march-2016.pdf

Your Safer Sex Toolbox. American Sexual Health Association—https://www.ashasexualhealth.org/safer-sex-toolbox/

63 Pelvic Inflammatory Disease

Lydia A. Shrier

KEY WORDS

- Infertility
- Pelvic inflammatory disease
- Pelvic pain
- Perihepatitis
- Sexually active
- Sexually transmitted
- Tubo-ovarian abscess

INTRODUCTION

Pelvic inflammatory disease (PID) is a clinical syndrome resulting from ascending polymicrobial infection of the female upper genital tract and includes endometritis, parametritis, salpingitis, oophoritis, tubo-ovarian abscess (TOA), peritonitis, and perihepatitis. Pelvic inflammatory disease is most commonly caused by sexually transmitted pathogens (e.g., *Chlamydia trachomatis* and/or *Neisseria gonorrhoeae*). Female adolescents and young adults (AYAs) are the age–sex groups at highest risk for infection with *C. trachomatis* and *N. gonorrhoeae*, and therefore at highest risk for PID. Other risk factors for PID include early coital debut, sexual intercourse without a condom, multiple sexual partners, history of sexually transmitted infection (STI), douching, and smoking. The diagnosis of PID is clinical, based on the presence of nonspecific signs and symptoms in a sexually active young female AYA and the exclusion of other causes, and regardless of test results for genitourinary *C. trachomatis* or *N. gonorrhoeae*. For most cases, treatment for PID can be administered effectively in the outpatient setting, provided that the patient presents for one dose of parenteral cephalosporin and completes a 14-day course of oral antimicrobial therapy. Sexual partners from the 60 days prior to diagnosis should be treated for both *C. trachomatis* and *N. gonorrhoeae*. Pelvic inflammatory disease can result in serious reproductive health sequelae, including chronic pelvic pain, ectopic pregnancy, and tubal infertility. Because the presentation of PID is most commonly mild to moderate, there can be delays in diagnosis and treatment, increasing the risk of sequelae. Clinicians should have a high index of suspicion for PID in a sexually active AYA with lower abdominal or pelvic pain. Screening for *C. trachomatis* and *N. gonorrhoeae* may reduce the incidence of PID.

ETIOLOGY

Pelvic inflammatory disease most commonly results from an STI that ascends from the lower to the upper genital tract. Pelvic inflammatory disease may also develop as a postpartum, postabortion, or postsurgical infection. Although rare, PID can be seen in adolescent females who have not had sexual contact (e.g., with ruptured appendicitis, Hirschsprung disease, or obstructing genitourinary anomaly).

Epidemiology

Adolescents and young adults account for up to one-third of cases of PID. By age 24, approximately 3% of sexually experienced females have been diagnosed with PID.[1] Adolescents and young adults of Black race seen in U.S. emergency departments have twice the rate of PID diagnosis as their White counterparts[2]; the disproportionate burden of STIs among Black adolescents[3] and other health care–related disparities may contribute to this finding. Females of lower socioeconomic status are more likely to report receipt of treatment for PID.[4]

Risk Factors

Factors confer risk for PID primarily by influencing exposure to pathogens, size of inoculum, and susceptibility of host. Adolescent and young adult females have the highest rates of *C. trachomatis* and *N. gonorrhoeae*,[3] the STI pathogens most frequently associated with PID. Many adolescents have a cervical ectropion, in which the transitional zone between the columnar and squamous epithelium is external to the cervical os; this mucosal tissue is highly susceptible to STIs. Adolescents lack local protective antibodies to STI pathogens because they have not had prior exposure, and therefore they may be more susceptible to ascending infection and resultant PID when they have a first STI. Risk of PID is higher among females who had younger age at coitarche and those who have had sex with multiple partners.[1] Inconsistent or lack of condom use increases risk of STIs and PID.[5] Pelvic inflammatory disease is also associated with history of STI and smoking.[1,6] Vaginal douching may increase the risk of PID by resulting in endometrial infection with organisms associated with bacterial vaginosis (BV).[7]

Contraception has not been consistently shown to increase or decrease risk of STI or PID. There has been no, inconclusive, or mixed evidence for oral contraceptive pill (OCP) or depot medroxyprogesterone acetate (DMPA) use and increased risk of incident *C. trachomatis* and *N. gonorrhoeae* infection.[8,9] The PID Evaluation and Clinical Health (PEACH) study did not find that PID was associated with OCPs or DMPA.[5] The rate of PID is low following intrauterine device (IUD) insertion, even in the presence of an STI (≤1%).[10]* Based on the current evidence, hormonal and intrauterine methods of contraception are safe and do not substantively alter risk of STI or PID. Contraceptive counseling for AYAs should focus on maximizing efficacy for pregnancy prevention while accommodating individuals' health conditions and preferences, as well as encouraging correct and consistent condom use for STI prevention.

Note. An IUD should not be placed if there are frank signs of infection (e.g., mucopurulent discharge from the cervical os).

Microbiology

Pelvic inflammatory disease is a polymicrobial infection; *N. gonorrhoeae*, *C. trachomatis*, genital mycoplasmas (e.g., *Mycoplasma genitalium*), and aerobic and anaerobic bacteria comprising endogenous vaginal flora (and identified in BV) have been associated with PID. *Neisseria gonorrhoeae* and *C. trachomatis* have been identified in the lower or upper genital tract in up to three-fourths of PID cases[11]; adolescents with PID are more likely than adults to be infected with these organisms.[12] Pelvic inflammatory disease incidence following infection with *N. gonorrhoeae* or *C. trachomatis* is difficult to estimate owing to a variety of factors, including asymptomatic infection, insufficient screening, and missed PID diagnoses. In a predominantly AYA sample, almost one in five of those who were diagnosed with *N. gonorrhoeae* and/or *C. trachomatis* infection were diagnosed with acute PID within 30 days.[13] According to estimates based on AYA data, just under 5% of *M. genitalium* infections progress to PID and just under 10% of PID is attributable to *M. genitalium*.[14] In the PEACH study, females with BV-associated organisms in the endometrium were at elevated risk of endometritis, persistent endometritis after recommended PID treatment, and recurrent PID.[15] Subclinical PID is 2.7 times more common in females with versus without BV.[16] More than 60% of females with PID have evidence of upper tract infection with anaerobic organisms (e.g., *Bacteroides* species).[17] Other endogenous vaginal flora, such as colonizing respiratory or enteric pathogens (e.g., *Escherichia coli*, *Haemophilus influenzae*, and *Streptococcus* species), have also been found in a minority of cases of PID.

Pathogenesis

Following lower tract infection, commonly with *N. gonorrhoeae* or *C. trachomatis,* anaerobes, facultative bacteria, and genital mycoplasmas supplant vaginal lactobacilli. Inflammatory disruption of the cervical barrier facilitates ascension of the inciting pathogens and other microorganisms from the vagina into the normally sterile uterus. Retrograde menstruation and sexual intercourse can further aid movement of organisms from lower to upper genital tract.

Inflammation can lead to decreased tubal motility, resulting in collection of fluid (hydrosalpinx) or pus (pyosalpinx) within one or both tubes. Spillage of infected contents from the tubes into the peritoneal cavity may result in peritonitis or perihepatitis (Fitz–Hugh–Curtis syndrome). Typically, Fitz–Hugh–Curtis syndrome occurs when infected material tracks along the right paracolic gutter, causing inflammation of the hepatic capsule and diaphragm. Less commonly, lymphatic spread (e.g., from parametritis following a procedure such as IUD placement) or hematogenous spread (e.g., in tuberculosis) can result in Fitz–Hugh–Curtis syndrome. Tubo-ovarian abscess develops if resolution of upper genital tract infection is delayed or if previous scarring occludes the tube. The abscess can form in the tube or between the tube and ovary. Tubo-ovarian abscess may be less likely to occur in younger versus older females, possibly due to a greater number of pathogenic organisms or lower recognition of PID as a cause of abdominal pain in older females.[18] Pelvic inflammatory disease can result in loss of ciliated epithelial cells within the fallopian tubes, impeding ovum movement and resulting in infertility and ectopic pregnancy. Inflammatory response to infection can lead to adhesions, bands of scar tissue in the tubes, between the tubes and the ovaries, or in the peritoneal cavity. Adhesions can result in partial or complete obstruction of the tubes, further contributing to infertility and ectopic pregnancy, and causing chronic abdominal or pelvic pain.

PRESENTATION

Because PID has variable microbiology, progression, affected organs, and severity, the presentation can be highly variable and, at times, subtle. Even in the absence of symptoms (i.e., subclinical PID), PID still confers risk for adverse reproductive health

outcomes, including infertility.[16] Acute PID may present with abrupt or gradual onset of lower abdominal pain (generally bilateral) or pelvic pain, often developing within 1 week of menses; the pain is constant, cramping or dull, and exacerbated by walking and intercourse. Additional symptoms can include malodorous, discolored, or otherwise abnormal vaginal discharge; painful, irregular, prolonged, postcoital, and/or heavy uterine bleeding; dyspareunia; dysuria; and urinary frequency. Patients with Fitz–High–Curtis syndrome may present with inspiratory dyspnea; sharp, pleuritic right upper quadrant pain; and/or referred right subscapular pain. An ileus may result in anorexia, nausea, or vomiting. Fever, tachycardia, and ill appearance are uncommon and indicative of more severe PID, including TOA.

EVALUATION AND DIAGNOSIS

The diagnosis is based on nonspecific clinical criteria and therefore the evaluation of an AYA female with suspected PID hinges on gathering information that may further support the diagnosis of PID and exclude or confirm other diagnoses. The differential diagnosis is broad (**Table 63.1**). Correct diagnosis of PID relies on a properly performed pelvic examination, including speculum examination, bimanual examination, and (ideally) microscopy of vaginal fluid. An abdominal examination is useful in the consideration of alternative diagnoses, such as appendicitis. However, abdominal tenderness in PID may be mild or absent and with or without rebound tenderness (more common in severe PID). Prompt diagnosis and treatment is essential to decreasing risk of adverse reproductive health outcomes. It is also important to evaluate alternative diagnoses carefully and examine additional criteria to avoid consequences of misdiagnosing PID (e.g., delayed appropriate treatment, unnecessary antibiotics, psychological stigma, clinician bias toward future PID diagnosis, and financial burden).

The Centers for Disease Control and Prevention (CDC) recommends that treatment for PID be initiated in a sexually active young female who has lower abdominal or pelvic pain without an alternative explanation or who meets at least one of the following minimum criterion on bimanual examination: cervical motion tenderness *or* uterine tenderness *or* adnexal tenderness (**Table 63.2**).[19]

TABLE 63.1

Differential Diagnosis of Lower Abdominal/Pelvic Pain in addition to PID

Gastrointestinal	Gynecologic
Appendicitis	Corpus luteum cyst
Cholecystitis	Dysmenorrhea
Cholelithiasis	Ectopic pregnancy
Constipation	Endometriosis
Diverticulitis	Mittelschmerz
Gastroenteritis	Ovarian
Hernia	Cyst
Inflammatory bowel disease	Torsion
Irritable bowel syndrome	Tumor
Urologic	Pregnancy (intrauterine or
Cystitis	ectopic)
Nephrolithiasis	Spontaneous, septic, or
Pyelonephritis	threatened abortion
Urethritis	Postabortion endometritis
Musculoskeletal	Rheumatologic/Autoimmune
Sprain or strain	Hypermobility disorders (e.g.,
Fracture	Ehlers–Danlos syndrome)
Infection (e.g., myositis,	Psychiatric
fasciitis, osteomyelitis, or	Somatization disorder
septic arthritis)	Hematologic/Oncologic
	Sickle cell disease
	Thrombosis
	Malignancy

TABLE 63.2

CDC Diagnostic Criteria for PID

Initiate treatment for PID in sexually active young females and other females at risk for STIs if they have
- Pelvic or lower abdominal pain without an alternative explanation, *or*
- One or more of the minimum clinical criteria on pelvic examination

Minimum criteria
- Cervical motion tenderness, *or*
- Uterine tenderness, *or*
- Adnexal tenderness

Additional criteria
- Oral temperature >38.3 °C (>101 °F)
- Abnormal cervical mucopurulent discharge or cervical friability
- Presence of abundant numbers of WBCs on saline microscopy of vaginal fluid
- Elevated ESR
- Elevated CRP
- Laboratory documentation of cervical infection with *N. gonorrhoeae* or *C. trachomatis*

More specific criteria
- Endometrial biopsy with histopathologic evidence of endometritis
- Transvaginal sonography or magnetic resonance imaging techniques demonstrating thickened, fluid-filled tubes with or without free pelvic fluid or tubo-ovarian complex, or Doppler studies suggesting pelvic infection (e.g., tubal hyperemia)
- Laparoscopic findings consistent with PID

WBC, white blood cells; ESR, erythrocyte sedimentation rate; CRP, C-reactive protein.

Adnexal tenderness may be unilateral or bilateral and an adnexal mass may be palpated. Clinicians must consider that AYAs may not disclose sexual activity or may have had nonconsensual sexual contact. Because presentation of PID is highly variable and often mild, requiring both lower abdominal or pelvic pain and tenderness on bimanual examination to make the diagnosis is inadequately sensitive. Additional clinical findings that increase the specificity of the minimum criteria include abnormal (e.g., mucopurulent) vaginal or cervical discharge; friable, inflamed cervix; and abundant white blood cells (WBCs) seen on saline microscopy ("wet prep") of vaginal fluid. If the vaginal or cervical discharge looks normal and no white blood cells are seen in the vaginal fluid, then PID is not likely to be the diagnosis. Wet prep is also used to detect conditions such as BV and trichomoniasis.

Laboratory test findings can further enhance the specificity of the clinical criteria for PID diagnosis (Table 63.2).[19] White blood count may be normal or elevated in PID; the absence of leukocytosis or neutrophilia may be most useful in excluding alternative infectious diagnoses such as appendicitis. Elevated erythrocyte sedimentation rate (ESR) or C-reactive protein (CRP) level increases the likelihood of PID and may be particularly high in females with Fitz–Hugh–Curtis syndrome (perihepatitis), severe PID, or TOA. Vaginal (preferable), endocervical, or urine specimens should be evaluated using nucleic acid amplification tests (NAAT) for *N. gonorrhoeae* and *C. trachomatis*; a positive result, indicating lower genital tract infection, supports the diagnosis of PID. However, females can meet diagnostic criteria for PID—and should receive treatment—without a positive STI test result. Females with possible PID should have a pregnancy test and be evaluated for ectopic pregnancy if the test is positive. Pelvic inflammatory disease can occur in pregnancy; pregnant patients with lower abdominal or pelvic pain should be evaluated for PID. Urinalysis and urine culture are used to evaluate for urinary tract infection, pyelonephritis, and nephrolithiasis. Human immunodeficiency virus and syphilis testing should be performed as part of a complete STI evaluation. In

patients from communities with high prevalence of trichomoniasis, and in patients with lower genital tract symptoms (e.g., vulvovaginal itching, burning, irritation, odor, or discharge) and wet prep testing is negative or unavailable, NAAT testing for *T. vaginalis* may be conducted, which can often be done simultaneously with *N. gonorrhoeae* and *C. trachomatis* testing.

Pelvic ultrasonography is helpful if the clinician cannot adequately assess the adnexa, palpates an adnexal mass, or suspects ectopic pregnancy or TOA. The transvaginal approach is optimal for visualization of the pelvic organs, particularly the adnexa. Ultrasonographic evidence of PID includes thickened, fluid-filled tubes and tubal hyperemia on Doppler testing; the cogwheel-sign—appearance of thickening of the longitudinal folds in the endotubal walls on cross-sectional imaging is 95% to 99% specific for PID.[20] Free pelvic fluid or tubo-ovarian complex (inflamed, edematous ovary adherent to the tube) may also be observed. A TOA will appear as a complex, multilocular, cystic and solid mass in the adnexa, with multiple fluid levels. The ultrasound can be normal or nonspecific in PID. Ultrasonography is useful to evaluate conditions other than PID and TOA, such as ectopic pregnancy; ovarian cyst, tumor, or torsion; and appendicitis. Other forms of imaging are not routinely used in diagnosis of PID.

Laparoscopy may be indicated to elucidate the diagnosis in the patient who does not respond to antibiotic therapy or to evaluate for other diagnoses such as endometriosis in the patient with chronic or recurrent "PID." Laparoscopy is highly specific for PID if tubal erythema, edema, or adhesions; purulent tubal exudate or cul-de-sac fluid; or abnormal tubal fimbriae is seen; however, laparoscopy can miss endometritis and tubal inflammation. Laparoscopy may also be used in the management of TOA and for lysis of adhesions from PID. Endometrial biopsy may be undertaken rarely to obtain definitive histologic evidence of endometritis in a female with suspected PID and negative findings on laparoscopy.

TREATMENT

Empirical treatment should be initiated promptly in AYA females who are diagnosed with PID, using a CDC-recommended antimicrobial regimen.[19] Broad-spectrum antibiotics are required to treat the polymicrobial infection. Treatment regimens include coverage for *N. gonorrhoeae* and *C. trachomatis* (regardless of test results), as well as anaerobes (Table 63.3).[19] In a randomized controlled trial, females treated for acute PID with metronidazole in addition to ceftriaxone and doxycycline had decreased endometrial anaerobes, *M. genitalium,* and pelvic tenderness, compared to females treated with ceftriaxone and doxycycline.[21] Recommended intramuscular/oral regimens now include metronidazole along with doxycycline and a third-generation cephalosporin.[19] Adverse gastrointestinal effects (e.g., nausea, vomiting, and diarrhea) can affect three in four females receiving PID treatment;[21] rates of gastrointestinal effects are similar between regimens that do and do not include metronidazole and inclusion of metronidazole does not appear to reduce adherence.[21,22]

In most cases, PID treatment can be accomplished in the outpatient setting. In the PEACH trial, long-term reproductive health outcomes did not differ between females with mild-to-moderate PID randomized to initiate treatment in the inpatient setting versus receive exclusively outpatient treatment.[11] Clinical judgment is used to select initial treatment setting, informed by the CDC criteria for hospitalization: surgical emergencies (e.g., appendicitis) cannot be excluded; TOA; pregnancy; severe illness, nausea, and vomiting, or high fever; inability to follow or tolerate outpatient oral treatment; lack of clinical response to oral antimicrobial therapy.[19] Other reasons to consider hospitalization in AYAs with suspected PID include age <15 years, abortion or gynecologic surgery within previous 14 days, previous PID, immunodeficiency, and medical or social circumstances that may delay or preclude

XIII

TABLE 63.3

CDC Treatment Regimens for PID

Parenteral Regimens
Recommended
    Ceftriaxone 1 g IV every 24 h <u>plus</u> doxycycline 100 mg PO or IV every
        12 h <u>plus</u>
            metronidazole 500 mg PO or IV every 12 h
    or
    Cefotetan 2 g IV every 12 h <u>plus</u> doxycycline 100 mg PO or IV every 12 h
    or
    Cefoxitin 2 g IV every 6 h <u>plus</u> doxycycline 100 mg PO or IV every 12 h
Alternative
    Ampicillin–sulbactam 3 g IV every 6 h <u>plus</u> doxycycline 100 mg PO or
        IV every 12 h
    or
    Clindamycin 900 mg by IV every 8 h <u>plus</u> gentamicin loading dose by
        IV or IM (2 mg/kg body weight), followed by a maintenance dose
        (1.5 mg/kg body weight) every 8 h. Single daily dosing (3–5 mg/kg
        body weight) can be substituted.
Parenteral therapy can be discontinued within 24–48 h of clinical
improvement. Therapy should be continued with doxycycline 100 mg
PO twice a day and metronidazole 500 mg PO twice a day to complete
a total of 14 d of therapy. If the alternative parenteral regimen of
clindamycin plus gentamicin is used, therapy can be continued with
clindamycin 450 mg PO four times a day *or* doxycycline 100 mg PO
twice a day to complete the 14 d of therapy.

Intramuscular/Oral Regimens
Recommended
    Ceftriaxone 500 mg IM in a single dose <u>plus</u> doxycycline 100 mg PO twice
        a day for 14 d <u>with</u> metronidazole 500 mg PO twice a day for 14 d
    or
    Cefoxitin 2 g IM and probenecid 1 g PO concurrently in a single dose
        <u>plus</u> doxycycline 100 mg PO twice a day for 14 d <u>with</u> metronidazole
        500 mg PO twice a day for 14 d
    or
    Another parenteral third-generation cephalosporin (e.g., ceftizoxime
        or cefotaxime) <u>plus</u> doxycycline 100 mg PO twice a day for 14 d
        <u>with</u> metronidazole 500 mg PO twice a day for 14 d

appropriate outpatient treatment. Adolescents are more likely than clinicians to endorse hospitalization for patients with suspected PID who are young, are homeless, are afraid to inform a partner, or have parents/caregivers unaware of the diagnosis.[23] Ideally, clinicians determine need for hospitalization in a shared decision-making process with the AYA patient.

If inpatient treatment is required, intravenous ceftriaxone with metronidazole (intravenous or oral), or intravenous cefotetan or cefoxitin, should be used to optimize activity against anaerobes.[19] These regimens also include doxycycline, which is preferably administered orally secondary to pain and venous sclerosis associated with infusion. Nonsteroidal anti-inflammatory drugs such as ibuprofen or naproxen can be used for pain management. If an IUD is in situ, it does not need to be removed. Regardless of treatment setting or test positivity, patients need to complete the full course of antibiotics. Adherence to oral medications for PID can be low, particularly among adolescents. Azithromycin and fluoroquinolones are not recommended for the treatment of PID owing to concerns for antimicrobial resistance of *M. genitalium* and *N. gonorrhoeae*, respectively. All sex partners within the preceding 60 days require treatment for *C. trachomatis* and *N. gonorrhoeae* infections, regardless of patient or partner microbiologic test results. Patients and their partners should be advised to abstain from sexual intercourse until they both have completed treatment and their symptoms have resolved. Clinicians may wish to recommend 3 to 4 weeks to aid adolescents in fully understanding the extent of the duration of abstinence.

Adolescent and young adult females being treated with an appropriate inpatient or outpatient regimen should demonstrate clinical improvement, including defervescence and decreased tenderness on abdominal and bimanual pelvic examination, within 72 hours. If inpatient management is initiated, the parenteral component of the therapy may be discontinued 24 to 48 hours after clinical improvement, and oral doxycycline continued and metronidazole added to complete a 14-day course. Patients who do not improve as expected require further evaluation, additional parenteral antibiotic therapy, and/or surgical intervention. Obtaining a pelvic ultrasound, if not already done, may reveal a TOA. Diagnostic laparoscopy may be considered to evaluate for alternative diagnoses. Patients diagnosed with PID who have a positive test result for *C. trachomatis* or *N. gonorrhoeae* should be retested 3 months following treatment.

Diagnosis of a TOA should prompt hospitalization. Medical management is the appropriate initial treatment in patients who are hemodynamically stable, have an abscess ≤5 cm, and do not have physical or imaging evidence of TOA rupture. Parenteral treatment should be continued for at least 24 hours or until clinical improvement is observed, including resolution of fever and leukocytosis, and substantial reduction in pain and tenderness. The abscess should be stable or decreasing in size on imaging. At this point, the patient can be transitioned to an oral regimen of doxycycline and either clindamycin or metronidazole (to enhance coverage of anaerobes) to complete at least 14 days of therapy and the TOA has completely resolved in imaging. Tubo-ovarian abscesses that are >5 cm or do not improve with medical management may require drainage, preferably using minimally invasive techniques.

⬤ SEQUELAE

Females who have had PID are at increased risk of PID (recurrence), infertility, ectopic pregnancy, and chronic abdominal/pelvic pain; AYAs who have had PID may be at higher risk for adverse reproductive health outcomes compared with adults.[24,25] More than one in five females with an episode of PID will experience a recurrence.[12] Risk is inversely correlated with treatment of contacts. Pelvic inflammatory disease is the most common cause of tubal factor infertility. In the U.S., almost one in four females with a history of PID treatment report infertility, 1.8 times the prevalence in females with no such history; among 18- to 29-year-old females, PID treatment is associated with four times the prevalence of infertility.[24] In a nationwide, population-based study of Taiwanese females, PID was associated with more than twice the risk of subsequent ectopic pregnancy; adolescents had a higher risk of ectopic pregnancy than adults.[25] More than 40% of females with mild-to-moderate PID experience subsequent chronic abdominal/pelvic pain.[12] Females with recurrent PID have more than four times the risk of chronic pelvic pain, compared to females with a single episode.[26]

Close follow-up, behavioral counseling, STI screening, and effective contraceptive management are essential to preventing adverse reproductive health outcomes in AYAs diagnosed with PID. Use of comprehensive and creative approaches, such as community nursing visits and text messages,[27] may be required to support adherence in AYAs. In the PEACH study, compared to adults with PID, adolescents had shorter time to pregnancy and to recurrent PID.[12] Although it is important to counsel an adolescent about the risk of infertility from PID, clinicians should be aware that the adolescent may assume that the patient is unable to conceive and not use effective contraception. Placing discussion of infertility risk in the broader context of PID sequelae (i.e., the other risks of recurrence, ectopic pregnancy, and chronic pelvic pain) and sexual and reproductive health (e.g., disease prevention and family planning) may aid the clinician in navigating the nuances of this counseling.

PREVENTION

Primary prevention involves STI prevention education, screening, and prompt treatment. Consistent condom use lowers the risk for PID two- to threefold.[5] Across four trials, the risk of PID was 32% lower in the 12 months following a single chlamydia test.[28] U.S. national guidelines recommend annual screening for *C. trachomatis* and *N. gonorrhoeae* in all sexually active females under the age of 25.[19] More frequent counseling and screening is warranted for AYA females with multiple or new partners, a history of chlamydia or gonorrhea, or new diagnosis of another STI.[29] If *C. trachomatis* or *N. gonorrhoeae* is detected, appropriate treatment should be immediately provided to prevent incident PID.[19,28]

Secondary prevention focuses on preventing or ameliorating complications and sequelae among AYAs who have been diagnosed with PID. Prompt and appropriate treatment for suspected PID improves reproductive health outcomes. Partner counseling and treatment is essential to mitigating the spread of PID-causing STIs. Sexual partners from the 60 days prior to the patient's PID diagnosis should be treated for both *C. trachomatis* and *N. gonorrhoeae*. Expedited partner therapy (EPT), providing patients with medications or prescriptions for their sexual partners, is an effective tool for the prevention of STIs and their sequelae if it is unlikely that the partners would obtain prompt evaluation and treatment.[30] Expedited partner therapy is legally permissible in nearly all U.S. states.[30] Expedited partner therapy prescriptions are often not filled, especially if given to adolescent patients, suggesting that AYAs should be provided with medications for EPT.[31] Because the only recommended treatment for gonorrhea—ceftriaxone by injection—is not feasible as EPT, clinicians should provide EPT for PID in the form of a single oral dose of cefixime 800 mg and oral doxycycline 100 mg twice a day for 7 days.[30]

Tertiary prevention seeks to decrease the risk of morbidity following an episode of PID. Consistent condom use reduces the risk of recurrent PID and infertility by 50% and 60%, respectively.[32] Optimizing screening for subsequent STIs is important in preventing PID sequelae, especially chronic pelvic pain.[12,26]

SUMMARY

Pelvic inflammatory disease is a clinical syndrome that usually results from a polymicrobial infection of sexually transmitted pathogens and vaginal flora ascending to the female upper genital tract. As a result of biologic, behavioral, and epidemiologic factors, female AYAs are at highest risk for PID. Diagnosis of PID is clinical, based on the presence of nonspecific signs and symptoms in a sexually active young females and the exclusion of other causes, and regardless of test results for genitourinary chlamydia and/or gonorrhea. Clinicians must have a high index of suspicion for PID in a sexually active female adolescent with lower abdominal or pelvic pain.

In most cases, treatment for PID can be administered effectively in the outpatient setting using one dose of parenteral cephalosporin and a 14-day course of oral therapy with doxycycline and metronidazole. Treatment of sexual partners from the 60 days prior to diagnosis is essential to mitigating transmission of infection, sequelae to partners, and reinfection of the patient.

Pelvic inflammatory disease can result in serious reproductive health sequelae, including chronic pelvic pain, ectopic pregnancy, and infertility. Counseling to reduce STI risk and screening to detect asymptomatic STIs is essential to reducing the incidence of PID.

REFERENCES

1. Kreisel K, Torrone E, Bernstein K, et al. Prevalence of pelvic inflammatory disease in sexually experienced women of reproductive age—United States, 2013–2014. *MMWR Morb Mortal Wkly Rep.* 2017;66(3):80–83.

2. Goyal M, Hersh A, Luan X, et al. National trends in pelvic inflammatory disease among adolescents in the emergency department. *J Adolesc Health.* 2013; 53(2):249–252.

3. Centers for Disease Control and Prevention. *Sexually Transmitted Disease Surveillance 2018.* U.S. Department of Health and Human Services; 2019.

4. Leichliter JS, Chandra A, Aral SO. Correlates of self-reported pelvic inflammatory disease treatment in sexually experienced reproductive-aged women in the United States, 1995 and 2006–2010. *Sex Transm Dis.* 2013;40(5):413–418.

5. Ness RB, Soper DE, Holley RL, et al. Hormonal and barrier contraception and risk of upper genital tract disease in the PID Evaluation and Clinical Health (PEACH) study. *Am J Obstet Gynecol.* 2001;185(1):121–127.

6. Li M, McDermott R. Smoking, poor nutrition, and sexually transmitted infections associated with pelvic inflammatory disease in remote North Queensland Indigenous communities, 1998–2005. *BMC Womens Health.* 2015;15:31.

7. Gondwe T, Ness RB, Totten P, et al. Novel bacterial vaginosis-associated organisms mediate the relationship between vaginal douching and pelvic inflammatory disease. *Sex Transm Infect.* 2020;96(6):439–444.

8. Deese J, Pradhan S, Goetz H, et al. Contraceptive use and the risk of sexually transmitted infection: systematic review and current perspectives. *Open Access J Contracept.* 2018;12:91–112.

9. McCarthy KJ, Gollub EL, Ralph L, et al. Hormonal contraceptives and the acquisition of sexually transmitted infections: an updated systematic review. *Sex Transm Dis.* 2019;46(5):290–296.

10. Birgisson NE, Zhao O, Secura GM, et al. Positive testing for Neisseria gonorrhoeae and Chlamydia trachomatis and the risk of pelvic inflammatory disease in IUD users. *J Womens Health.* 2015;24(5):354–359.

11. Ness RB, Soper DE, Holley RL, et al. Effectiveness of inpatient and outpatient treatment strategies for women with pelvic inflammatory disease: results from the Pelvic Inflammatory Disease Evaluation and Clinical Health (PEACH) randomized trial. *Am J Obstet Gynecol.* 2002;186(5):929–937.

12. Trent M, Haggerty CL, Jennings JM, et al. Adverse adolescent reproductive health outcomes after pelvic inflammatory disease. *Arch Pediatr Adolesc Med.* 2011;165(1):49–54.

13. McKee DL, Hu Z, Stahlman S. Incidence and sequelae of acute pelvic inflammatory disease among active component females, U.S. Armed Forces, 1996–2016. *MSMR.* 2018;25(10):2–8.

14. Lewis J, Horner PJ, White PJ. Incidence of pelvic inflammatory disease associated with Mycoplasma genitalium infection: evidence synthesis of cohort study data. *Clin Infect Dis.* 2020;71(10):2719–2722.

15. Haggerty CL, Totten PA, Tang G, et al. Identification of novel microbes associated with pelvic inflammatory disease and infertility. *Sex Transm Infect.* 2016;92(6):441–446.

16. Wiesenfeld HC, Hillier SL, Meyn LA, et al. Subclinical pelvic inflammatory disease and infertility. *Obstet Gynecol.* 2012;120(1):37–43.

17. Sweet RL. Treatment of acute pelvic inflammatory disease. *Infect Dis Obstet Gynecol.* 2011;2011:561909.

18. Lee SW, Rhim CC, Kim JH, et al. Predictive markers of tubo-ovarian abscess in pelvic inflammatory disease. *Gynecol Obstet Invest.* 2016;81(2):97–104.

19. Workowski KA, Bachmann LH, Chan PA, et al. Sexually transmitted infections treatment guidelines, 2021. *MMWR Recomm Rep.* 2021;70(4):1–187.

20. Romosan G, Valentin L. The sensitivity and specificity of transvaginal ultrasound with regard to acute pelvic inflammatory disease: a review of the literature. *Arch Gynecol Obstet.* 2014;289(4):705–714.

21. Wiesenfeld HC, Meyn LA, Darville T, et al. A randomized controlled trial of ceftriaxone and doxycycline, with or without metronidazole, for the treatment of acute pelvic inflammatory disease. *Clin Infect Dis.* 2021;72(7):1181–1189.

22. Savaris RF, Fuhrich DG, Maissiat J, et al. Antibiotic therapy for pelvic inflammatory disease. *Cochrane Database Syst Rev.* 2020;8(8):CD010285.

23. Trent M, Recto M, Qian Q, et al. Please be careful with me: Discrepancies between adolescent expectations and clinician perspectives on the management of pelvic inflammatory disease. *J Pediatr Adolesc Gynecol.* 2019;32(4):363–367.

24. Anyalechi GE, Hong J, Kreisel K, et al. Self-reported infertility and associated pelvic inflammatory disease among women of reproductive age--National Health and Nutrition Examination Survey, United States, 2013–2016. *Sex Transm Dis.* 2019;46(7):446–451.

25. Huang C, Huang C, Lin S, et al. Association of pelvic inflammatory disease (PID) with ectopic pregnancy and preterm labor in Taiwan: a nationwide population-based retrospective cohort study. *PLoS One.* 2019;14(8):e0219351.

26. Trent M, Bass D, Ness RB, et al. Recurrent PID, subsequent STI, and reproductive health outcomes: findings from the PID evaluation and clinical health (PEACH) study. *Sex Transm Dis.* 2011;38(9):879–881.

27. Trent M, Perin J, Gaydos CA, et al. Efficacy of a technology-enhanced community health nursing intervention vs. standard of care for female adolescents and young adults with pelvic inflammatory disease: a randomized clinical trial. *JAMA Netw Open.* 2019;2(8):e198652.

28. Low N, Redmond S, Uusküla A, et al. Screening for genital chlamydia infection. *Cochrane Database Syst Rev.* 2016;9(9):CD010866.

29. Hay PE, Kerry SR, Normansell R, et al. Which sexually active young female students are most at risk of pelvic inflammatory disease? A prospective study. *Sex Transm Infect.* 2016;92(1):63–66.

30. Centers for Disease Control and Prevention. *Expedited Partner Therapy website.* Accessed March 29, 2021. https://www.cdc.gov/std/ept/default.htm

31. Slutsker JS, Tsang L-YB, Schillinger JA. Do prescriptions for expedited partner therapy for Chlamydia get filled? Findings from a multijurisdictional evaluation, United States, 2017–2019. *Sex Transm Dis.* 2020;47(6):376–382.

32. Ness RB, Randall H, Richter HE, et al. Condom use and the risk of recurrent pelvic inflammatory disease, chronic pelvic pain, or infertility following an episode of pelvic inflammatory disease. *Am J Public Health.* 2004;94(8):1327–1329.

XIII

Explanations for references older than 10 years:

5. PEACH trial, large randomized trial, no study since has provided information similar to that cited in this chapter.
11. PEACH trial, large randomized trial, results provided basis for treatment guidelines used in current practice.
31. PEACH trial, large randomized trial, no study since has provided information similar to that cited in this chapter.

📶 ADDITIONAL RESOURCES AND WEBSITES

Additional Resources and Websites for Clinicians:

Centers for Disease Control and Prevention—https://www.cdc.gov/std/treatment-guidelines/toc.htm

ACOG Committee Opinion No. 737: Expedited Partner Therapy. *Obstet Gynecol* 2018;131:e190–e193. https://www.acog.org/clinical/clinical-guidance/committee-opinion/articles/2018/06/expedited-partner-therapy

Addison J, Shrier LA. Sexually Transmitted Infections: Chlamydia, Gonorrhea, Pelvic Inflammatory Disease, and Syphilis. In: Emans SJ, Laufer MR, DiVasta AD, eds. *Emans, Laufer and Goldstein's Pediatric and Adolescent Gynecology.* 7th edition. Lippincott Williams & Wilkins; 2019. https://www.cochranelibrary.com/cdsr/doi/10.1002/14651858.CD010285.pub3/full

Centers for Disease Control and Prevention. Expedited Partner Therapy website—https://www.cdc.gov/std/ept/default.htm

Centers for Disease Control and Prevention. Sexually Transmitted Diseases Tools & Materials, including brochures, fact sheets, infographics, provider pocket guides, videos and podcasts, webinars, and other resources for providers and patients—https://www.cdc.gov/std/treatment-guidelines/provider-resources.htm

Essential Sexual Health Questions to Ask Adults. Essential Sexual Health Questions to Ask Adolescents. Pocket cards for health care providers. National Coalition for Sexual Health, 2018—https://nationalcoalitionforsexualhealth.org/tools/for-healthcare-providers/body/Provider-Postcard_Combo_3.15.19.pdf

LeFevre ML; U.S. Preventive Services Task Force. Screening for Chlamydia and gonorrhea: U.S. Preventive Services Task Force recommendation statement. *Ann Intern Med.* 2014;161:902–910. https://jamanetwork.com/journals/jama/fullarticle/2769474

Savaris RF, Fuhrich DG, Maissiat J, Duarte RV, Ross J. Antibiotic therapy for pelvic inflammatory disease. *Cochrane Database of Systematic Reviews.* 2020;8:CD010285. doi: 10.1002/14651858.CD010285.pub3. Accessed 28 March 2021. https://www.acpjournals.org/doi/10.7326/M14-1981?url_ver=Z39.88-2003&rfr_id=ori:rid:crossref.org&rfr_dat=cr_pub%20%200pubmed

U.S. Department of Health and Human Services. 2020. Sexually Transmitted Infections National Strategic Plan for the United States: 2021–2025. Washington, DC—https://www.hhs.gov/sites/default/files/STI-National-Strategic-Plan-2021-2025.pdf

U.S. Preventive Services Task Force, Krist AH, Davidson KW, et al. Behavioral counseling interventions to prevent sexually transmitted infections: U.S. Preventive Services Task Force Recommendation Statement. *JAMA* 2020;324:674–681.

Workowski KA, Bachmann LH, Chan PA, et al. Sexually transmitted infections treatment guidelines, 2021. *MMWR Recomm Rep.* 2021;70(4):1–187.

Additional Resources and Websites for Parents/Caregivers:

Webpages for parents with information on pelvic inflammatory disease, sexually transmitted diseases, and talking with your child about sexually transmitted diseases (in English and some in Spanish).

Nemours Children's Health—https://kidshealth.org/en/parents/pelvic-inflammatory-disease.html?ref=search

https://kidshealth.org/en/parents/stds-talk.html?WT.ac=ctg#catstd and https://kidshealth.org/es/parents/stds-talk-esp.html?WT.ac=pairedLink#catstd

https://kidshealth.org/en/parents/talk-child-stds.html?WT.ac=catstd and https://kidshealth.org/es/parents/talk-child-stds-esp.html?WT.ac=pairedLink#catstd

Additional Resources and Websites for Adolescents and Young Adults:

Webpages and videos on pelvic inflammatory disease, sexually transmitted diseases, and talking with your partner about sexually transmitted diseases (in English and some in Spanish).

Center for Young Women's Health, Boston Children's Hospital—https://youngwomenshealth.org/2013/02/21/pelvic-inflammatory-disease/

https://kidshealth.org/en/teens/std-pid.html?ref=search

https://www.cdc.gov/std/pid/stdfact-pid.htm and https://www.cdc.gov/std/spanish/eip/PID-FS-Sp-July-2017.pdf

https://www.cdc.gov/std/life-stages-populations/stdfact-teens.htm

https://kidshealth.org/en/teens/stds-talk.html and https://kidshealth.org/es/teens/stds-talk-esp.html?WT.ac=t-ra#catstds

https://kidshealth.org/en/teens/the-talk.html?WT.ac=ctg#catstds and https://kidshealth.org/es/teens/the-talk-esp.html?WT.ac=pairedLink#catstds

https://www.youtube.com/watch?v=-grwthAl4Qs&list=PLJvP6pW6mcXps0SxFeq5mD4LZHMKijzdd&index=1, https://www.youtube.com/watch?v=L-BJrpFIaUo&list=PLJvP6pW6mcXps0SxFeq5mD4LZHMKijzdd&index=2, https://www.youtube.com/watch?v=-rlTHdkm_-4&list=PLJvP6pW6mcXps0SxFeq5mD4LZHMKijzdd&index=3, https://www.youtube.com/watch?v=s1OCAO9S0VU&list=PLJvP6pW6mcXps0SxFeq5mD4LZHMKijzdd&index=4

KABI Chronicles. Brief animated videos on STI prevention and testing. Centers for Disease Control and Prevention, 2018. https://www.youtube.com/watch?v=ZPNk6FNsvng

What is Pelvic Inflammatory Disease (PID)? Brief animated video on PID. CMcC Narratives, 2018.

CHAPTER 64

Syphilis

Teresa A. Batteiger

KEY WORDS
- Latent syphilis
- Neurosyphilis
- Nontreponemal tests
- Primary syphilis
- Reverse sequence syphilis screening
- Secondary syphilis

INTRODUCTION

Syphilis is an acute, localized sexually transmitted infection (STI) leading to systemic infection and chronic disease if untreated. The causative agent of syphilis is *Treponema pallidum*. Syphilis is sometimes asymptomatic, but often is associated with localized signs of primary infection such as an ulcer at the infection site, or evidence of disseminated secondary infection manifested by symptoms such as skin rash, lymphadenopathy, fever, or mucocutaneous lesions. The disease caused by syphilis has been divided into stages based on clinical signs and symptoms, which guide therapy and follow-up. Outbreaks among adolescents and young adults (AYAs) are common, often through connected social and sexual networks.[1]

EPIDEMIOLOGY

1. Syphilis is caused by *T. pallidum*, a motile, spiral microorganism (spirochetes) 6 to 20 μm in length and about 0.20 μm in diameter.[2]
2. Most infections are contracted by sexual contact, including kissing, oral–genital, penile–vaginal, and penile–anal intercourse. Nonsexual transmission from direct contact with cutaneous or mucous membrane lesions is rare. Other transmission modes include maternal–fetal transplacental congenital infections, peripartum infection of newborns by contact with maternal genital lesions, and transfusion–related transmission.[3] The estimated rate of transmission after sexual exposure to a person with primary or secondary syphilis is 30% or higher.[4]
3. Syphilis in the United States waxes and wanes in 7- to 10-year cycles. Rates of primary and secondary syphilis in the general population have increased nearly every year since 2001. In 2019, rates again increased (to 11.9 cases per 100,000 population), when 38,992 cases of primary and secondary syphilis were reported in the United States. Of these, 1,708 (4.4%) were 15- to 19-year-olds, and 6,325 (16.2%) were among 20- to 24-year-olds. In 2019, 22 cases of syphilis were reported among 10- to 14-year-olds.[5]
    a. Global rates: Reported estimated incident cases of syphilis in 2016 were 6.3 million.[6] Prevalence rates of syphilis in pregnant females vary between low- and middle-income countries compared with high-income countries. High-income countries have high rates of antenatal testing with low positivity rates while low- and middle-income countries have lower antenatal testing rates but higher positivity rates.[4] In 2019, 78 countries reported data to the World Health Organization with an average of 3.2% (range 1.1% to 10.9%) of individuals attending antenatal care clinics testing positive.[7] Global pooled prevalence in men with male sex partners (MSM) from 2000 to 2020 was 7.5%, with a range from 1.9% in Australia and New Zealand (1.0% to 3.1%) to 10.6% in Latin America and the Caribbean (range 8.5% to 12.9%).[8]
4. Syphilis epidemiology demonstrates the extreme health disparities associated with many STIs.[5]
    a. Geographic disparity: Syphilis has substantial geographical concentration, with approximately 50% of primary and secondary cases reported from 1.4% of U.S. counties. In 2019, the highest rates of reported cases of primary and secondary syphilis were in the West (16.9 cases per 100,000 population) followed by the South (12.2 cases per 100,000 population). Rates increased across all regions from 2018 to 2019.
    b. Racial disparity: In 2019, primary and secondary syphilis rates remained highest among Blacks. Reported cases of primary and secondary syphilis in 2019 were 734 cases in Blacks 15- to 19-year-olds compared to 318 cases in Whites 15- to 19-year-olds. Reported cases in 20 to 24 years old were 2,517 and 1,486 for Black and for White youth, respectively.
    c. Gender disparity: During 2018 to 2019, the rates of primary and secondary syphilis in males increased from 18.6 to 20.1 cases per 100,000, and in females from 3.0 to 3.9 cases per 100,000. Since 2015, the rate among males has increased from 13.6 to 20.1 cases per 100,000 males, and the rate among females has increased from 1.4 to 3.9 cases per 100,000 females. In 2019, rates among 15 to 19-year-old male adolescents was 11.2 compared with 4.9 in female adolescents. Rates among 20- to 24-year-old male adults were 45.2 compared with 11.6 in female adults.
    d. Sex partner disparity: Men with male sex partners (MSM) account for the majority of cases of primary and secondary syphilis in the United States from 2018 to 2019, 47.1% of all reported primary and secondary syphilis cases were in MSM (41.6% of cases were in MSM only, and an additional 5.5% of cases were in men who have sex with men and women). This is slightly decreased from 2018, where 53.5% of reported cases were in MSM (48.2% in MSM only, and an additional 5.3% of cases were in MSM and women). In contrast, reported cases in women and in men who have sex with women only (MSW) increased. In MSW, reported cases increased from 15.4% in 2018 to 18.7% in 2019. In women, reported cases increased from 14.2% in 2018 to 16.7% in 2019.

PATHOGENESIS

Treponema pallidum produces an immediate localized inflammatory response, associated with regional lymphadenopathy. Antibody responses can be detected within 1 to 2 weeks of infection. A delayed hypersensitivity response clears most—but not all—organisms in local lesions within about 14 days.[2] Inflammation and local tissue necrosis cause the characteristic induration and ulcer formation of primary syphilis. Dissemination via blood and lymphatics occurs within a few days of infection. Dysregulation of the delayed hypersensitivity response is associated with gumma formation characteristic of late syphilis.[9]

CLINICAL MANIFESTATIONS

Clinical manifestations of syphilis depend on the stage of infection and the specific body areas and organs infected. The stages of syphilis are identified as: primary, secondary, early latent, late latent, latent of unknown duration, and late syphilis. Late syphilis (other than late congenital syphilis) is not seen in AYAs and is not additionally considered in this chapter. Neurosyphilis has various manifestations and can occur at any stage.[10]

Primary Syphilis

Syphilis should be considered for any ulcerating lesion of the genitals, cervix, anus, or lips/mouth, but lesions of fingers, arms, and breasts are not rare. Primary lesions appear after an incubation period of 10 to 90 days (average is 21 days).[11] Characteristics of primary syphilis are:

1. Ulcer characteristics (Fig. 64.1)
   a. Single lesions are 1 to 2 cm in size but multiple lesions are common. Lesions may also appear as "kissing lesions," adjacent ulcers across a fold of skin.
   b. Ulcers are typically painless and described as having a punched out, clean appearance, with slightly elevated, firm margins. However, ulcer characteristics are an unreliable basis for the diagnosis of syphilis.[12]

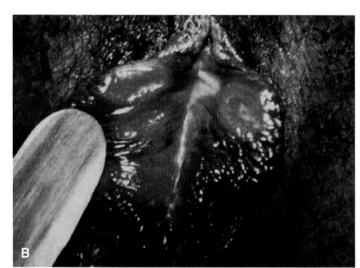

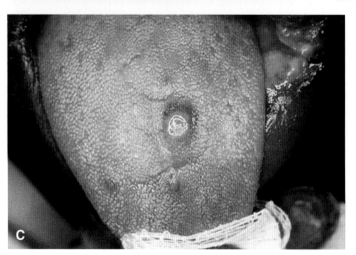

FIGURE 64.1 Primary syphilis chancre. Location of the chancre is dependent on the site of inoculation. **Panel A**. A cleanly bordered ulcer on the penile shaft. (Courtesy of Arthur Eisen, MD.). **Panel B**. An ulcer on the left labium. (From Sweet RL, Gibbs RS. *Atlas of Infectious Diseases of the Female Genital Tract*. Lippincott Williams & Wilkins; 2005.) **Panel C**. An ulcer on the tongue. (Centers for Disease Control and Prevention.)

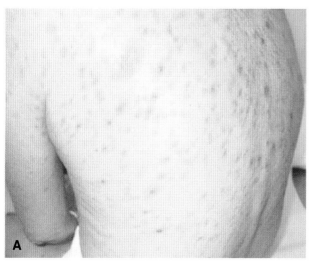
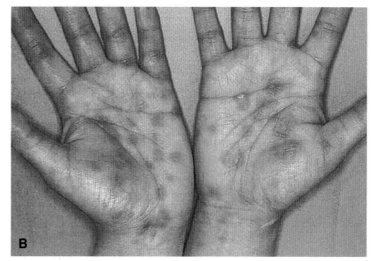

FIGURE 64.2 Secondary syphilis. The rash of secondary syphilis involves the trunk and extremities (**panel A**) with predilection for palms and soles (**panel B**). (Modified after Potts SR. Images in clinical medicine. *N Engl J Med*. 1993:329:176.)

2. Bilateral regional lymphadenopathy, with firm, nonsuppurative, usually nontender nodes
3. Ulcers typically heal within 3 to 6 weeks.
4. Systemic symptoms such as fever, myalgia, or malaise are uncommon.

Secondary Syphilis

Secondary syphilis appears 6 to 8 weeks after infection and 4 to 10 weeks after the appearance of the primary ulcer. *Treponema pallidum* can be identified in lesions and body fluids.[13]

Signs and symptoms:

1. Rash (occurs in about 90% of individuals with secondary syphilis)
   a. Involves the trunk and extremities with predilection for palms and soles. Lesions on palms and soles may be scaly and hyperkeratotic (Fig. 64.2).
   b. Rashes are bilateral and symmetrical and tend to follow the lines of cleavage.
   c. Sharply demarcated lesions, 0.5 to 2.0 cm in diameter, with a reddish-brown hue

   d. Rash is most commonly macular, papular, maculopapular, annular, or pustular but almost any type of rash can be reported, including acneiform lesions, herpetiform lesions, and lesions similar to psoriasis. Lesions in intertriginous areas may erode and fissure, especially in the nasolabial folds and near the corners of the mouth.
   e. Lesions are typically nonpruritic, but pruritus has been reported in up to 40% of individuals.[14]
   f. Rash typically lasts a few weeks (2 to 6 weeks) and will resolve even without treatment.
2. Condylomata lata can occur in warm, moist areas. They appear as moist, gray to white, wart-like growths (Fig. 64.3).
3. Mucous patches occur in the mouth, on the tongue, or on the anogenital mucosa. They appear as oval-shaped macules or erosions, with a gray to white coloration.
4. General or regional lymphadenopathy (~70%)
   a. Rubbery, nonpainful nodes, without suppuration
   b. Occasional hepatosplenomegaly
5. Flu-like syndrome (~50%)
   a. Sore throat, fever, and malaise most common
   b. Headaches
   c. Lacrimation and nasal discharge
   d. Arthralgia and myalgia
6. Alopecia (uncommon): Moth eaten–appearing alopecia of the scalp and eyebrows (Fig. 64.4)

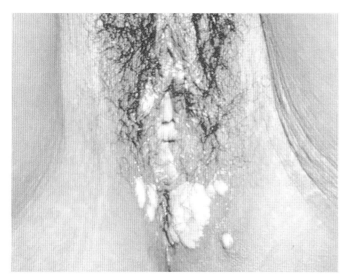

FIGURE 64.3 Secondary syphilis. Condyloma lata appear as moist, gray to white, wart-like growths and are highly infectious. (From Goodheart HP. *Goodheart's Photoguide of Common Skin Disorders*, 4th ed. Lippincott Williams & Wilkins; 2015.)

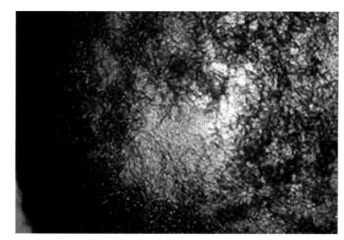

FIGURE 64.4 Secondary syphilis. Moth eaten–appearing alopecia. (Courtesy Centers for Disease Control and Prevention. Phil #17887.)

7. Other rare manifestations
   a. Arthritis, bursitis, periostitis
   b. Hepatitis (subclinical elevations in liver enzymes occur in up to 50% of individuals)[15]
   c. Iritis and anterior uveitis, as well as other ocular manifestations including optic neuritis
   d. Glomerulonephritis

Latent Syphilis

Latent syphilis is characterized by the following:
1. Absence of clinical signs and symptoms of syphilis
2. Positive serologic tests for syphilis, including both nontreponemal and treponemal tests

Two stages of latent syphilis are differentiated to guide treatment. *Early latent syphilis* is defined as infection duration of 12 months or less, without clinical evidence of syphilis. For treatment purposes, early latent syphilis is grouped with primary and secondary syphilis. *Late latent syphilis* refers to infection duration of greater than 12 months, and requires a different treatment regimen. The term *latent syphilis of unknown duration* is used when the timing of seroconversion cannot be established.[16]

Neurosyphilis

Clinically significant neurosyphilis develops in up 20% of patients with untreated early syphilis but abnormal cerebrospinal fluid (CSF) can be found in a much higher proportion of patients with early syphilis. Neurosyphilis in AYAs is usually asymptomatic but may manifest as acute meningitis. Meningovascular syphilis is rare. Late presentations of neurosyphilis include parenchymatous disease, which is divided into general paresis and tabes dorsalis.[10]

1. Asymptomatic neurosyphilis: This is the most common form where patients do not have any signs or symptoms of neurologic disease
   a. Characterized by abnormal CSF, including pleocytosis, elevated protein, and positive CSF-venereal diseases research laboratory (VDRL) test
   b. Rates of asymptomatic neurosyphilis decrease as the duration of infection increases
2. Acute syphilitic meningitis results in inflammation of the meninges.
   a. Usually occurs during secondary syphilis or the early latent period
   b. Common symptoms: Fever, headache, photophobia, and meningismus
   c. Less frequent symptoms: Confusion, delirium, and seizures
   d. Common findings include cranial nerve palsies and abnormal CSF (increased protein, lymphocytic pleocytosis, and lowered glucose).
3. Meningovascular syphilis
   a. Rare in AYAs (occurs 5 to 12 years after initial infection)
   b. Symptoms and signs result from an endarteritis producing local areas of infarction
   c. Symptoms: Headache, dizziness, mood changes, and memory loss
   d. Signs: Hemiparesis, hemiplegia, focal or generalized seizures, aphasia
4. Parenchymatous neurosyphilis
   a. Symptoms and signs result from destruction of nerve cells.
   b. General paresis results from cortical involvement and results in personality changes; affect changes; hyperactive reflexes; Argyll Robertson pupils (accommodation, but not reactive to light); delusions; decreased memory, judgment, and insight; and slurred speech.

   c. Tabes dorsalis results from spinal cord damage, primarily involving the posterior column and dorsal roots. This results in the development of wide-based, ataxic gait with foot slap. Paresthesias, shooting pains, bladder disturbances, and peripheral neuropathy can also occur.

Congenital Syphilis

Adolescents and young adults with congenital syphilis bear the stigmata of early disease and may develop additional manifestations of syphilis.[17]
1. Early congenital syphilis parallels secondary syphilis among adults and occurs before the age of 2 years. The most common abnormalities include:
   a. Skeletal abnormalities, including osteochondritis (up to 90% of those affected)
   b. Hepatomegaly or splenomegaly (~50%)
   c. Petechiae; hemolytic anemia and thrombocytopenia (35% to 40%)
   d. Skin lesions (~40%)
   e. Persistent rhinitis (snuffles) (~20%)
   f. Neurosyphilis (~25%)
2. Late congenital syphilis corresponds to late syphilis in adults, and often presents during puberty. Most infections (60%) are latent, but new findings include:
   a. Abnormal faces including saddle nose and frontal bossing (~85%)
   b. Palatal deformity (~75%)
   c. Dental deformities including Hutchinson incisors and mulberry molars (~55%)
   d. Interstitial keratitis (up to 50%)
   e. Clutton joints: Symmetrical, painless swelling of knees (30% to 45%)
   f. Sensorineural eighth nerve deafness (3% to 4%)
   g. Neurosyphilis (up to 5%)

DIFFERENTIAL DIAGNOSIS

Primary Syphilis

Sexually Transmitted Genital Ulcer Diseases

The most common sexually transmitted genital ulcer is genital herpes. Fewer than 20 cases of chancroid were reported in the past 5 years in the United States[18]; ulcers due to lymphogranuloma venereum and granuloma inguinale are also rare.
1. Herpes simplex (Chapter 65): Painful, multiple lesions beginning as vesicles on an erythematous base. Primary lesions may be extensive, and associated with tender adenopathy, and recurrent lesions are usually unilateral without significant adenopathy.
2. Chancroid (Chapter 67): Painful lesions with a deep purulent base and often erythematous borders. Local lymph nodes are often fluctuant and tender.
3. Lymphogranuloma venereum (Chapter 67): Nonindurated, herpetiform ulcer that heals rapidly. Many patients present with advanced disease including fever and massive regional adenopathy.
4. Granuloma inguinale (donovanosis) (Chapter 67): Nontender, fleshy, beefy-red, easily bleeding ulcers.

Nonsexually Transmitted Causes of Genital Ulcers
1. Traumatic lesions
2. Candida balanitis
3. Behçet syndrome
4. Aphthous ulcer

Secondary Syphilis
1. Psoriasis
2. Pityriasis rosea

3. Drug associated rash
4. Tinea versicolor
5. Alopecia areata
6. Lichen planus
7. Lupus erythematosus
8. Scabies
9. Pediculosis
10. Rosacea
11. Infectious mononucleosis
12. Condyloma acuminatum (the differentiation is to condyloma lata)

DIAGNOSIS

Diagnosis of syphilis requires a combination of clinical and laboratory criteria and is dependent on stage. *Treponema pallidum* cannot be cultured, so laboratory diagnosis requires direct detection of the organism in clinical samples (i.e., dark-field examination) or a reactive serologic test. Syphilis serologic screening is routine during pregnancy and often performed as part of evaluation for other STIs, including human immunodeficiency virus (HIV). Routine syphilis screening is recommended for youth with high-risk markers such as commercial sex work, injection drug use, and males with multiple same-sex partners; however, routine syphilis screening for AYAs is not recommended.[19]

Laboratory Findings

Screening and diagnostic algorithms for syphilis have undergone substantial changes in recent years; clinicians are advised to review and understand the algorithm used in local laboratories.

Dark-Field Examination

The dark-field examination allows immediate diagnosis but requires specialized equipment and training and is not widely available (Fig. 64.5). Technique is as follows:
1. Clean lesion with saline and gauze.
2. Abrade gently with dry gauze. Avoid inducing bleeding.

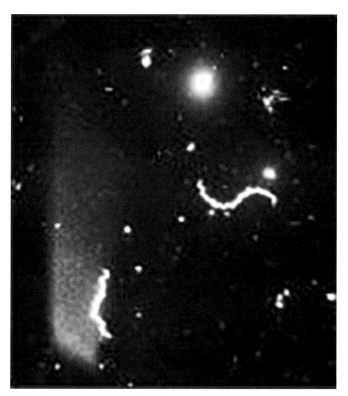

FIGURE 64.5 Appearance of *T. pallidum* on dark-field microscopy.

3. Squeeze lesion to express serous transudate.
4. Place a drop of transudate on a slide.
5. Place a drop of saline on transudate and cover with a cover slip.
6. Examine under dark-field microscope for typical motile, corkscrew shaped organisms.
7. For internal lesions, a bacteriologic loop can be used to transfer the fluid to a slide.

Serologic Tests

1. Nontreponemal antibody tests assess anticardiolipin antibodies formed to surface lipids on *T. pallidum*.
   a. Rapid Plasma Reagin (RPR) is visually assessed by agglutination.
   b. Venereal Diseases Research Laboratory (VDRL) is assessed by flocculation seen by microscopy.
   c. Nontreponemal tests are used for screening and to monitor response to treatment. Nontreponemal test titers correlate with disease activity and decrease, usually to nondetectable levels, within 12 months of treatment. Peak titers are seen within 2 to 4 weeks of initial treatment, and subsequently decline. A fourfold change in titer, equivalent to a change of two dilutions (e.g., from 1:8 to 1:32 or 1:16 to 1:4), demonstrates a substantial change. Rapid Plasma Reagin and VDRL are equally valid but quantitative titers cannot be directly compared.
2. Treponemal antibody tests:
   a. Fluorescent Treponemal Antibody–Absorbed (FTA-ABS) is used to confirm a positive result from RPR or VDRL.
   b. *Treponema pallidum* particle agglutination (TP-PA) test is widely used as the treponemal test to confirm a positive nontreponemal test and to resolve discrepant results of reverse sequence syphilis screening algorithms (see 2e below and Fig. 64.6).
   c. Enzyme immunosorbent assay (EIA) and chemiluminescence immunoassay (CIA) are treponemal tests, with high specificity but cannot be titered.
   d. Treponemal tests remain positive for life, limiting their usefulness in distinguishing new from previously treated infections.
   e. Advances in laboratory technology have led to reverse sequence syphilis screening algorithms (Fig. 64.6).[20] This approach uses automated, high-throughput EIA or CIA as the screening test, with confirmation by a nontreponemal test. Advantages include improved laboratory efficiency and increased detection of latent and late infections (although potentially with increased rates of false-positive tests).
3. Sensitivity[21,22]:
   a. The sensitivity of nontreponemal tests in primary syphilis depends on the duration of infection. In primary syphilis, sensitivity of nontreponemal tests ranges from 62% to 78%. In secondary syphilis, sensitivity approaches 100%. In early latent syphilis, sensitivity ranges from 82% to 100%. Sensitivity decreases in late latent and tertiary syphilis.
   b. Sensitivity of treponemal tests is 70% to 100% in primary syphilis, and approaches 100% in secondary syphilis.
4. Biologic false-positive (BFP) tests: This is defined as a reactive nontreponemal test and a nonreactive treponemal test. The proportion of BFPs is dependent on the prevalence of syphilis. However, the overall prevalence of BFP results in the general population is ≤1.5%.[21] Most false-positive nontreponemal test results show a low titer (dilution <1:8), and the probability of a false-positive finding decreases with increasing titer.[23] The causes of false-positive test results include the following:
   a. Acute infection: Viral infections, chlamydial infections, Lyme disease, *Mycoplasma* infections, nonsyphilitic spirochetal infections, and various bacterial, fungal, and protozoal infections
   b. Autoimmune diseases

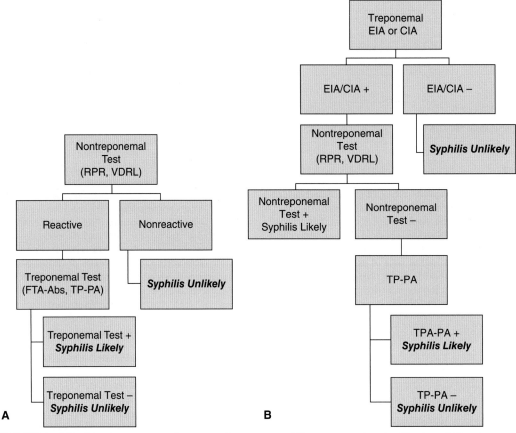

FIGURE 64.6 Traditional nontreponemal–treponemal sequence syphilis sero-screening algorithm (**panel A**) and reverse sequence syphilis screening algorithm (**panel B**).

c. Narcotic addiction
d. Aging
e. Hashimoto thyroiditis
f. Sarcoidosis
g. Lymphoma
h. Leprosy
i. Cirrhosis of the liver
j. Human immunodeficiency virus infection: Can lead to unusually high, unusually low, or fluctuating titers
5. False-positive treponemal tests occur but most are reported as borderline and not positive.

Polymerase Chain Reaction Detection of Treponema Pallidum

Polymerase chain reaction (PCR) can increase the types of specimens available for detection of *T. pallidum*, although it has been found to be most useful in ulcerative disease. The sensitivity and specificity are reported at approximately 80% and 95% respectively, when using genital ulcer specimens.[24] However, there are no currently available U.S. Food and Drug Administration-approved tests.

Diagnosis by Stage[19]

Primary Syphilis

1. Presence of chancre(s).
2. Identification of spirochetes by dark-field examination of ulcer transudate.
3. A positive nontreponemal test result with a high titer (1:8 or higher) or rising titer (two or more than two dilutions) *and* a positive treponemal test result (e.g., FTA-ABS or TP-PA).

Adolescents and young adults with a positive dark-field examination should be treated, as should those with a typical lesion and a positive serologic test result. If the initial serologic test result is

negative, it should be repeated 1 week, 1 month, and 3 months later in suspected cases. A treponemal test should be used to confirm a positive nontreponemal test result.

Secondary Syphilis

1. Examination findings consistent with secondary syphilis
2. Dark-field examination of material from lesions or lymph nodes
3. Serodiagnosis with combination of nontreponemal and treponemal tests

Treatment should be provided if the dark-field examination result is positive or for typical findings of secondary syphilis and a positive nontreponemal test that is confirmed with a treponemal test.

Early and Late Latent Syphilis

Both an RPR/VDRL and a FTA-ABS/TP-PA (or other treponemal) test should be performed. Treponemal tests are essential in latent and late syphilis because the nontreponemal tests can be as low as 80% sensitive in these states. Patients should be treated if the treponemal test result is positive and there is no documentation of appropriate prior treatment. A decision about a lumbar puncture in these instances should be done in consultation with an expert in this area.

Neurosyphilis

A positive CSF-VDRL is diagnostic of neurosyphilis, especially when accompanied by CSF pleocytosis. The CSF-VDRL cannot be replaced by other nontreponemal tests (such as the RPR) even if those tests are used to monitor serologic response to treatment.[25] A CSF FTA-ABS can be evaluated if the CSF-VDRL is negative, as neurosyphilis is highly unlikely with a negative CSF FTA-ABS.[26]

1. Central nervous system infection occurs in patients with primary or secondary syphilis, although not all develop symptomatic disease.
2. Cerebrospinal fluid examination is not routine in early syphilis without neurologic signs or symptoms.
3. Indications for CSF examination continue to be refined, but the following apply regardless of disease stage[27]:
   a. Neurologic or ophthalmologic signs or symptoms
   b. Treatment failure
   c. Serum nontreponemal test titer is greater than or equal to 1:32
   d. Nonpenicillin therapy is planned
   e. Human immunodeficiency virus infection

Syphilis in Pregnancy

Pregnant AYAs should be screened early in pregnancy. When access to prenatal care is suboptimal or if follow up is uncertain, testing should be performed at the time that pregnancy is confirmed.[19] Seropositive patients are considered infected unless treatment is documented and serologic titers have appropriately declined. Screening should be repeated in the third trimester and again at delivery in areas or populations with a high prevalence of syphilis. Syphilis should be considered for pregnancy loss after 20 weeks of gestation.[28]

Syphilis and Human Immunodeficiency Virus

Ulcerative lesions increase the risk of HIV acquisition and transmission. Treponemal and nontreponemal serologic tests for syphilis are accurate for most individuals with both syphilis and HIV infection. Human immunodeficiency virus–infected individuals with neurologic symptoms or failure to respond to antibiotic treatment should be evaluated for neurosyphilis.[19]

THERAPY[19]

Penicillin is the antibiotic of choice for syphilis treatment: the formulation, dosage, and duration of therapy depends on the stage of syphilis. For individuals with a history of penicillin allergy, skin testing and desensitization, if indicated, are recommended. Few data are available on nonpenicillin regimens, especially among AYAs.[19] Clinicians should always review the Centers for Disease Control and Prevention's (CDC) STI guidelines available at: https://www.cdc.gov/std/treatment/default.htm

Primary and Secondary Syphilis

1. Benzathine penicillin G: The total recommended dose is a single injection of 2.4 million units intramuscularly (IM).
2. Penicillin-allergic nonpregnant patients:
   a. Doxycycline 100 mg orally (PO) two times a day for 14 days, or
   b. Tetracycline 500 mg PO four times a day for 14 days is recommended.
   c. Limited data suggests that ceftriaxone 1 g IM or intravenously (IV) for 10 days is effective for treatment of early syphilis, but the optimal dose and duration have not been defined.
   d. Azithromycin 2 g as a single oral dose. However, treatment failure due to acquired azithromycin resistance of *T. pallidum* is reported. This treatment should be used only if other options are unavailable and careful follow-up is assured.
   e. Use of any alternative therapies in HIV-infected persons has been insufficiently studied.
   f. Patients who cannot tolerate an alternative therapy should be referred for penicillin desensitization.
   g. Pregnancy: Penicillin desensitization and penicillin treatment according to stage.

3. Other considerations
   a. Patients with syphilis should be tested for HIV. For high-risk patients or in high-prevalence areas, patients with primary syphilis should be retested for HIV after 3 months.
   b. Patients with signs or symptoms of neurologic or ophthalmic disease should be evaluated by CSF analysis and/or slit-lamp examination.
4. Follow-up
   a. Infected individuals should be reexamined clinically, and serologic test results should be rechecked at 6 and 12 months but can be evaluated more frequently if follow-up is uncertain or there is concern for reinfection. Nontreponemal antibody titers should be used for follow-up. If nontreponemal antibody titers have not decreased fourfold by 6 to 12 months, this may be indicative of treatment failure. These individuals should have additional clinical evaluation, serologic testing, and be evaluated for HIV infection. If follow-up cannot be ensured, retreatment is recommended. Additionally, these individuals should be considered for CSF examination to assess for neurosyphilis.
   b. For those individuals with treatment failure, retreatment should include three weekly injections of benzathine penicillin G 2.4 million units IM unless neurosyphilis is identified.

Latent Syphilis

There are two regimens for nonpenicillin allergic patients:
1. Early latent syphilis: Benzathine penicillin G 2.4 million units IM in a single dose
2. Late latent syphilis or latent syphilis of unknown duration: Benzathine penicillin G 7.2 million units total, administered as three weekly doses of 2.4 million units IM each
3. Penicillin-allergic patients: There is limited data regarding the effectiveness of alternative regimens to penicillin for treatment of latent syphilis. Only acceptable regimens are doxycycline 100 mg PO two times a day or tetracycline 500 mg PO four times a day. Either is given for 14 days for individuals with early latent syphilis or 28 days for others. Patients with abnormal CSF examinations should be treated for neurosyphilis.
4. Other considerations
   a. Patients with latent syphilis should be tested for HIV.
   b. Patients with signs or symptoms of neurologic disease should be evaluated for neurosyphilis with CSF examination.
5. Follow-up
   a. Nontreponemal serologic titers should be assessed at 6, 12, and 24 months after treatment. If titers increase fourfold or initial high titers (1:32 or greater) fail to decrease fourfold (two dilutions) within 12 to 24 months, or if signs or symptoms of syphilis occur, the individual should be evaluated for neurosyphilis and re-treated appropriately.

Neurosyphilis

1. Recommended regimen for neurosyphilis, ocular syphilis, or otosyphilis in individuals not allergic to penicillin: Aqueous crystalline penicillin G 18 to 24 million units daily administered as 3 to 4 million units IV every 4 hours or as a continuous infusion for 10 to 14 days.
   a. Alternative regimen: Procaine penicillin G IM 2.4 million units daily, plus probenecid 500 mg PO four times a day, both for 10 to 14 days
   b. Some experts add benzathine penicillin G 2.4 million units IM after completion of either of these two regimens for individuals with late latent syphilis to provide comparable total duration of therapy.
2. Penicillin-allergic patients: Patients should be desensitized to penicillin and treated with penicillin. No alternatives have been adequately evaluated. Some specialists recommend ceftriaxone 2 g daily IM or IV for 10 to 14 days.

3. Other management considerations: All patients with neuro-syphilis should be tested for HIV.
4. Follow-up: In immunocompetent patients or patients with HIV on appropriate antiretroviral therapy (ART), normalization of the serum RPR is predictive of normalization of the CSF parameters following treatment. Therefore, repeated CSF examinations in these populations with normalization of the serum RPR is not necessary.

Syphilis in Pregnancy[19]

Pregnant females should receive penicillin doses appropriate for the stage of syphilis. Penicillin is effective in preventing transmission to the fetus and in treating fetal infections. Some experts recommend additional therapy, such as a second dose of benzathine penicillin G 2.4 million units IM given 1 week after the first dose for females who have primary, secondary, or early latent syphilis. During the second half of pregnancy, syphilis treatment may be adjusted by sonographic fetal evaluation for congenital syphilis. Pregnant females with a history of an allergy to penicillin should be skin tested and either treated or desensitized.

Management of Sex Partners[19]

1. Sex partners of persons with primary, secondary, or early latent syphilis within the preceding 90 days should be tested for syphilis but treated presumptively, even if seronegative. Treatment is the same as for primary syphilis. If exposure occurred more than 90 days before examination, the individual should be treated presumptively if serologic test results are not immediately available and follow-up is uncertain. If serologic testing is negative, no treatment is needed.
2. Partners should be notified and treated if the affected patient has syphilis of unknown duration with high nontreponemal serologic test titers (1:32 or greater).
3. Sex partners of patients with late syphilis should be evaluated both clinically and serologically for syphilis.
4. Identification of at-risk sex partners: Time periods used to identify partners at risk are as follows:
   a. Three months plus duration of symptoms for primary syphilis
   b. Six months plus duration of symptoms for secondary syphilis
   c. One year for early latent syphilis

Human Immunodeficiency Virus-Infected Individuals[19]

1. Penicillin regimens should be used whenever possible. Skin testing and desensitization can be used as appropriate.
2. Primary and secondary syphilis in HIV-infected patients: The CDC recommends no change in therapy for early syphilis in HIV-infected patients. Some experts recommend adding multiple doses of benzathine penicillin G, similar to the dosages used to treat late syphilis.
   a. All individuals with HIV infection should have a thorough neurologic examination to determine need for CSF examination. Cerebrospinal fluid examination should be reserved for patients with an abnormal neurologic examination. If CSF examination is consistent with neurosyphilis, patients should be treated according to the recommendations for individuals with neurosyphilis without HIV infection.
   b. Follow-up: HIV-infected AYAs should have follow-up serologic testing at 3, 6, 9, 12, and 24 months. Those individuals with treatment failure should have a CSF examination and be retreated similarly to those who are not HIV infected. If the CSF is normal, most experts would retreat with benzathine penicillin G 7.2 million units as three weekly doses of 2.4 million units each.
3. Late latent syphilis:
   a. Individuals with HIV infection with latent syphilis should be treated as individuals without HIV infection.

Jarisch–Herxheimer Reaction

Jarisch–Herxheimer reaction occurs within 2 hours of treatment in 50% of patients with primary syphilis, in 90% of those with secondary syphilis, and in 25% of those with early latent syphilis.[29] The reaction consists of the following:
1. Headache, fever, chills, myalgias
2. Elevated neutrophil count
3. Tachycardia

These symptoms may last up to 24 hours, and resolve with reassurance, rest, and antipyretics. The reaction can induce transient uterine contractions in pregnant females.

 SUMMARY

In conclusion, syphilis continues to be problematic in the United States and globally. Rates have been increasing despite ongoing control efforts. There are disparities between geographic locations, races, gender, and sex partner choices. Syphilis causes a myriad of signs and symptoms, so clinicians must maintain a high index of suspicion for screening and diagnosis. Testing for syphilis relies heavily on indirect testing measures as *T. pallidum* cannot be cultured. Further study is needed for improving methods for the diagnosis of syphilis. Finally, penicillin remains the treatment of choice for syphilis, although there are acceptable alternatives in specific cases.

ACKNOWLEDGMENT

The author would like to acknowledge Dennis Fortenberry, MD, for his contribution to the previous version of this chapter.

REFERENCES

1. Brewer TH, Schillinger J, Lewis FMT, et al. Infectious syphilis among adolescent and young adult men: implications for human immunodeficiency virus transmission and public health interventions. *Sex Transm Dis.* 2011;38(5):367–71.
2. Lafond RE, Lukehart SA. Biological basis for syphilis. *Clin Microbiol Rev.* 2006;19(1):29–49.
3. Stoltey JE, Cohen SE. Syphilis transmission: a review of the current evidence. *Sex Health.* 2015;12(2):103–109.
4. Kojima N, Klausner JD. An update on the global epidemiology of syphilis. *Curr Epidemiol Rep.* 2018;5(1):24–38.
5. Centers for Disease Control and Prevention (2021). *Sexually transmitted disease surveillance 2019 [Internet].* U.S. Department of Health and Human Services. Accessed August 4, 2021. Available from: https://www.cdc.gov/std/statistics/2019/default.htm
6. Rowley J, Hoorn SV, Korenromp E, et al. Chlamydia, gonorrhea, trichomoniasis, and syphilis: global prevalence and incidence estimates, 2016. *Bull World Health Org.* 2019;97(8):548–562P.
7. World Health Organization. *The Global Health Observatory: Data on syphilis 2021* [updated 7/21/2020, accessed 11/15/2021]. Available from https://www.who.int/data/gho/data/themes/topics/topic-details/GHO/data-on-syphilis
8. Tsuboi M, Evans J, Davies EP, et al. Prevalence of syphilis among men who have sex with men: a global systematic review and meta-analysis from 2000–20. *Lancet Glob Health.* 2021;9(8):E1110–E1118.
9. Carlson JA, Dabiri G, Cribier B, et al. The immunopathobiology of syphilis: the manifestations and course of syphilis are determined by the level of delayed-type hypersensitivity. *Am J Dematopathol.* 2011;33(5):433–460.
10. Ghanem KG. Neurosyphilis: a historical perspective and review. *CNS Neurosci Ther.* 2010;16(5):e157–e168.
11. Golden MR. Marra CM, Holmes KK. Update on syphilis: resurgence of an old problem. *JAMA.* 2003;290(11):1510–1514.
12. DiCarlo RP, Martin DH. The clinical diagnosis of genital ulcer disease in men. *Clin Infect Dis.* 1997;25(2):292–298.
13. Mullooly C, Higgins SP. Secondary syphilis: the classical triad of skin rash, mucosal ulceration and lymphadenopathy. *Int J STD AIDS.* 2010;21(8):537–545.
14. Chapel TA. The signs and symptoms of secondary syphilis. *Sex Transm Dis.* 1980;7(4):161–164.
15. Ridruejo E, Mordoh A, Herrera F, et al. Severe cholestatic hepatitis as the first symptom of secondary syphilis. *Dig Dis Sci.* 2004;49(9):1401–1404.
16. Shockman S, Buescher LS, Stone SP. Syphilis in the United States. *Clin Dermatol.* 2014;32(2):213–218.
17. Chakraborty R, Luck S. Managing congenital syphilis again? The more things change. *Curr Opin Infect Dis.* 2007;20(3):247–252.
18. Centers for Disease Control and Prevention. *Sexually Transmitted Disease Surveillance 2018.* U. S. Department of Health and Human Services; 2019. doi: 10.15620/cdc.79370. Available from cdc.gov/std/stats18/STDSurveillance2018-full-report.pdf
19. Workowski KA, Bachmann LH, Chan PA, et al. Sexually transmitted infections treatment guidelines, 2021. *MMWR Recomm Rep.* 2021;70(4):1–187.

20. Lipinsky D, Schreiber L, Kopel V, et al. Validation of reverse sequence screening for syphilis. *J Clin Microbiol.* 2012;50(4):1501.

21. Tuddenham S, Katz SS, Ghanem KG. Syphilis laboratory guidelines: performance characteristics of nontreponemal antibody tests. *Clin Infect Dis.* 2020;71(Suppl 1): S21–S42.

22. Cantor AG, Pappas M, Daeges M, et al. Screening for syphilis: Updated evidence report and systematic review for the US preventative services task force. *JAMA.* 2016;315(21):2328–2337.

23. Matthias J, Klingler EJ, Schillinger JA, et al. Frequency and characteristics of biological false positive test results for syphilis reported in Florida and New York City, USA, 2013 to 2017. *J Clin Microbiol.* 2019;57(11):e00898–19.

24. Gayet-Ageron A, Lautenschlager S, Ninet B, et al. Sensitivity, specificity, and likelihood ratios of PCR in the diagnosis of syphilis: a systematic review and meta-analysis. *Sex Transm Infect.* 2013;89(3):251–256.

25. Marra CM, Tantalo LC, Maxwell CL, et al. The rapid plasma reagin test cannot replace the venereal disease research laboratory test for neurosyphilis diagnosis. *Sex Transm Dis.* 2012;39(6):453–457.

26. Harding AS, Ghanem KG. The performance of cerebrospinal fluid treponemal-specific antibody tests in neurosyphilis: a systematic review. *Sex Transm Dis.* 2012;39(4):291–297.

27. Ghanem KG, Moore RD, Rompalo AM, et al. Lumbar puncture in HIV-infected patients with syphilis and no neurologic symptoms. *Clin Infect Dis.* 2009;48(6):816–821.

28. Gomez GB, Kamb ML, Newman LM, et al. Untreated maternal syphilis and adverse outcomes of pregnancy: a systematic review and meta-analysis. *Bull World Health Organ.* 2013;91(3):217–226.

29. Myles TD, Elam G, Park-Hwang E, et al. The Jarisch–Herxheimer reaction and fetal monitoring changes in pregnant women treated for syphilis. *Obstet Gynecol.* 1998;92(5):859–864.

ADDITIONAL RESOURCES AND WEBSITES

Additional Resources and Websites for Clinicians:

The American Sexual Health Association (ASHA). Provides an array of youth-focused information and resources for clinicians—http://www.ashastd.org

Centers for Disease Control and Prevention (CDC). The Centers for Disease Control and Prevention site with recent statistics, treatment guidelines, and a free downloadable STI treatment guideline—http://www.cdc.gov/STD/treatment

E-medicine. Website on syphilis—https://emedicine.medscpe.com/article/969023-overview

National Institute of Allergy and Infectious Diseases (NIAID). NIAID information from the National Institutes of Health (NIH). Useful for research updates—https://www.niaid.nih.gov/diseases-conditions/syphilis

Additional Resources and Websites for Parents/Caregivers:

Kids/Teens Health from Nemours. Kids' health site on syphilis and STI in general—http://kidshealth.org/teen/infections/stds/std_syphilis.html

Additional Resources and Websites for Adolescents and Young Adults:

The American Sexual Health Association (ASHA). The American Sexual Health Association has sites designed specifically for adolescents and young adults. General information on STIs, including sexuality and STI prevention for adolescents are directly and explicitly addressed: English: http://iwannaknow.org ; Spanish: http://www.quierosaber.org. There is also a section for parents: http://www.iwannaknow.org/parent.html

Similar information is available at: https://www.ashasexualhealth.org/

Centers for Disease Control and Prevention (CDC). A plain language summary of syphilis—https://www.cdc.gov/std/syphilis/STDFact-syphilis.htm

Health central. Information about sexual health and prevention of STI, including syphilis—http://www.healthcentral.com/sexual-health/safesex.html?ic=506012

XIII

Herpes Genitalis

Christine Johnston

CHAPTER **65**

KEY WORDS
- Genital herpes
- Genital ulcer disease
- Herpes simplex virus

INTRODUCTION

Herpes genitalis, or genital herpes, is caused by herpes simplex virus type 1 (HSV-1) and HSV type 2 (HSV-2), which cause a chronic infection with intermittent reactivations that result in painful, self-limited mucosal or cutaneous ulcerations. Herpes simplex virus types 1 and 2 are related DNA viruses that are highly prevalent in humans, with 66.6% of the world's population aged 0 to 49 years infected with HSV-1 and 13.2% aged 15 to 49 years infected with HSV-2.[1] During primary genital infection, symptoms can be severe with multiple ulcerations in the anogenital region and systemic symptoms such as fever and headache, while reactivations are typically localized and not associated with systemic symptoms. Herpes simplex virus type 1 classically causes oral ulcerations (gingivostomatitis and cold sores), but it has become a more prominent cause of first-episode genital herpes, particularly among adolescents and young adults (AYAs).[2] Herpes simplex virus type 2 is associated with more symptomatic genital infection compared to HSV-1. Both HSV-1 and HSV-2 may be shed from the genital tract and transmitted in the absence of symptoms. Since the infection is persistent throughout the lifespan and disclosure to sexual partners is strongly recommended, a diagnosis of genital herpes may have significant implications for sexual and mental health, particularly for AYAs.

EPIDEMIOLOGY

Prevalence and Incidence

Seroprevalence studies have given us insight into the very high prevalence of HSV-1 and HSV-2. Importantly, HSV-1 seroprevalence reflects both oral and genital infection, whereas HSV-2 seroprevalence reflects genital infection. In 2016, 66.6% of the world's population aged 0 to 49 years was HSV-1 seropositive, with an estimated 140 million people aged 15 to 49 years with genital HSV-1 infection.[1,3] An additional 491.5 million people aged 15 to 49 years have genital HSV-2 infection (13.2% global prevalence), with over 77 million infections in AYAs between 15 to 24 years old.[1] The most recent United States National Health and Nutrition Examination Surveys (NHANES) conducted in 2015 to 2016 showed the prevalence of HSV-1 was 47.8% and of HSV-2 was 11.9% among persons 14 to 49 years of age.[4] The prevalence of HSV-1 has significantly decreased

from 59.4% in 1999 to 2000 to 48.1% in 2015 to 2016. Herpes simplex virus type 2 seroprevalence has also declined over time, from 18.0% in 1999 to 2000 to 12.1% in 2015 to 2016. In the United States, 65% of prevalent genital herpes infections were in females.[5] Similar to other sexually transmitted infections (STIs), there are significant health disparities in HSV seroprevalence among racial groups in the United States, with HSV-1 seroprevalence highest in Mexican-Americans.[4] In 2007 to 2010, HSV-2 seroprevalence among Black non-Hispanic females aged 14 to 49 years was 49.9%, 3.3-fold higher compared to White non-Hispanic females, who had a seroprevalence of 15.3%.[6] These differences in seroprevalence reflect disparities in determinants of health and socioeconomic factors, rather than differences in sexual behavior.[6–8]

The prevalence of both HSV-1 and HSV-2 increases with age and acquisition occurs frequently in AYAs. For example, of an estimated 572,000 incident genital infections in the United States in 2018, 42% occurred in 18- to 24-year-olds.[5] Therefore, clinicians should be aware that AYAs may present with primary or undiagnosed recurrent genital herpes. Recent data suggest that incident genital HSV-1 has become more common than genital HSV-2 among AYAs. In a clinical trial of a prophylactic HSV vaccine, healthy, HSV-1/2 seronegative females aged 18 to 30 years were followed for 20 months for HSV acquisition.[9] The rate of new infections as measured by seroconversion to HSV-1 was 2.5/100 person-years, more than twice that of HSV-2 (1.1/100 person-years), and HSV-1 infections in the genital area appeared three times more frequently than HSV-2 genital infections.[2] In some sexual health clinic settings, HSV-1 has surpassed HSV-2 as the most common cause of first-episode genital herpes,[10] and genital acquisition of HSV-1 is predicted to continue to increase over the coming decades.[11]

Transmission

Herpes simplex virus types 1 and 2 are transmitted through direct contact of skin or mucosal surfaces with infected secretions. Transmission may occur through genital–genital, genital–anogenital, or oral–genital/anogenital contact. The virus does not survive on surfaces and therefore transmission through fomites does not occur. Biologic factors place people with vaginas at greater risk for HSV-2 acquisition than people with penises. The mucosal surface of the vagina and cervix has more exposed vascular, mucosal surface compared to the penile urethral meatus.

Although viral shedding is highest while genital lesions are present, most genital transmission occurs on days when the source partner has no visible genital lesions, during periods of asymptomatic shedding. Transmission often occurs from partners who are unaware that they have HSV infection. The decreasing seroprevalence of HSV-1 among AYAs results in increased susceptibility to incident genital HSV-1 infections upon initiation of sexual activity.

PATHOGENESIS

Herpes simplex virus types 1 and 2 are large neurotropic DNA viruses that infect skin and mucosal surfaces and establish latent infection in neuronal ganglia. Humans are the only hosts for HSV-1 and HSV-2. Chronic infection is mostly quiescent with periodic reactivations that cause self-limited ulcers. Virus particles can be intermittently detected in cervical, urogenital, and anorectal secretions of persons with genital HSV infection. The virus is transmitted through close contact with infected secretions at mucosal or epithelial skin surfaces. Upon infection, the virus replicates in the epidermal and dermal cells of a susceptible host. After replication, the virus spreads through contiguous cells to mucocutaneous projections of sensory nerves. The virus then travels to the sacral ganglia, where the virus persists for the lifetime of the host.[12]

Chronic viral infection is characterized by periods of latency, in which the virus has restricted expression of genes and is contained in the sacral ganglia, and lytic infection. During lytic infection, the virus reactivates, replicates, and travels through nerves to skin and mucosal surfaces. The neuronal transport of the virus is thought to cause prodrome symptoms of tingling and itching.[12] The virus is then shed from mucosal or skin surfaces, which may result in recurrent, self-limited genital lesions or asymptomatic shedding. Importantly, the virus can be transmitted during periods of asymptomatic shedding. The host factors that lead to viral reactivation are not well understood, and there is a wide spectrum of clinical recurrences, from asymptomatic to frequent reactivations. Reactivation can be triggered by a variety of stimuli, such as ultraviolet light, immunosuppression, fever, stress, and local trauma. In addition, immunocompromised hosts have more frequent recurrences.

Infections by Serologic Type

During primary infection, it is not possible to differentiate between HSV-1 and HSV-2 infection clinically, as both viruses can cause either mild infection with a single ulceration or severe infection with multiple ulcerations and systemic symptoms. However, it is important to differentiate between HSV-1 and HSV-2 due to significant differences in natural history (**Table 65.1**). For example, simultaneous oral and genital HSV-1 acquisition may occur, resulting in lesions at both sites, whereas symptomatic oral HSV-2 infection is rare.

TABLE 65.1

Clinical Features of Genital Herpes Caused by HSV-1 and HSV-2

	HSV-1	HSV-2
Acquisition from oral source	Yes	No
Acquisition from genital source	Yes	Yes
Can also cause oral ulcers	Yes	Very rare
Median recurrences/year[a]	0–1	4
Average proportion of days virus is detected from genital tract	3–7%	20%
Cause of neonatal HSV	Yes	Yes
Increases risk of HIV acquisition	Unknown	Yes
Suppressive therapy prevents transmission to susceptible partners	Unknown	Yes

HIV, human immunodeficiency virus; HSV, herpes simplex virus.
[a]>1 year after first episode.

Herpes simplex virus type 1 infection in the genital tract is associated with much less frequent recurrences and subclinical shedding than with genital HSV-2 infection (**Table 65.1**).

CLINICAL MANIFESTATIONS

Definition of Terms

1. Primary infection: Virologic evidence of genital herpes in a patient seronegative for antibodies to HSV-1 and HSV-2
2. First clinical episode: First clinical manifestations due to HSV-1 or HSV-2 infection. This term includes both primary infections and nonprimary first episodes (first episode in patient with HSV-1 or HSV-2 antibody).
3. Recurrent clinical episode: Recurrence of genital HSV lesions in a patient with a previously documented symptomatic genital herpes episode

Primary Infection

Clinical manifestations of primary genital herpes begin approximately 1 week (range 2 to 12 days) following initial infection. Primary genital HSV infection involves both systemic and local symptoms.[13] Local symptoms may include painful lesions, dysuria, pruritus, vaginal, urethral, or rectal discharge, and tender inguinal adenopathy. Herpetic lesions can be extensive and may involve the vulva, perineum, vagina, perianal area, and cervix or large areas of the penis or anorectum. Pharyngeal involvement may be seen in HSV-1.

Lesions usually begin as small papules or vesicles on an erythematous base that coalesce and ulcerate (Fig. 65.1). Pain and irritation from lesions usually peak between days 7 and 11 of disease in the absence of antiviral medication and heal during the second week. Crusting and reepithelialization occur in the penile and mons area, but crusting does not occur on mucosal surfaces. Scarring is uncommon. Lesions typically heal by the end of the third week of disease without antiviral therapy.

Systemic symptoms including fever, headache, malaise, and myalgias occur over the first week of illness in more than half of infected symptomatic individuals. Complications of primary genital HSV infection can include aseptic meningitis and other neurologic complications (such as autonomic nervous system dysfunction and transverse myelitis), extragenital lesions (buttock, groin, or thigh areas), hepatitis, and disseminated disease. In addition, proctitis may occur in people who have receptive anal sex and is characterized by severe tenesmus and anal ulceration. In one study, anal ulceration occurred in one-third of patients with HSV proctitis; therefore, clinicians must have a high index of suspicion.[14]

First Clinical Episode

First episodes of genital herpes are more often associated with systemic symptoms and a prolonged duration of lesions and viral shedding and are more likely to involve multiple genital and extragenital sites compared to recurrent episodes. Some persons with first clinical episode of symptomatic genital herpes have serologic evidence of prior HSV-1 or HSV-2 infection. Because some people do not have genital herpes symptoms at the time of viral acquisition, it is difficult to know when the infection was acquired. Persons with prior oral HSV-1 infection remain at risk of genital HSV-2. However, prior HSV-1 infection may diminish the severity of first-episode genital HSV-2. It is not clear if genital HSV-1 protects against genital HSV-2 infection.

Recurrent Episodes

During recurrent episodes of genital herpes, clinical manifestations are localized to the genital region and are of mild to moderate severity compared to primary infection. Patients may have prodromal symptoms that can range from mild paresthesias to shooting

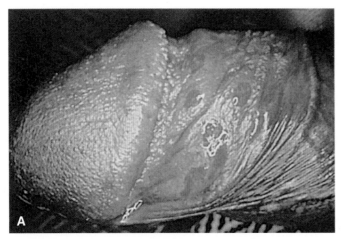

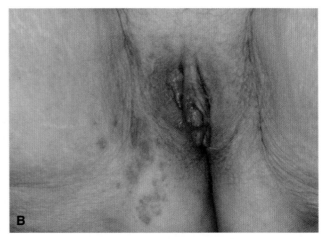

FIGURE 65.1 Genital herpes lesions **(A)** on the penis and **(B)** on the vulva. (A: From Goodheart HP. *Goodheart's Photoguide of Common Skin Disorders.* 4th ed. Lippincott Williams & Wilkins; 2015. B: © Dr. P. Marazzi/Photo Researchers, Inc.)

pains in the buttocks, legs, or hips. Genital lesions typically last 6 to 12 days without antiviral therapy and may resolve much more quickly with therapy. Lesions in recurrent episodes occur on predominantly epithelialized skin, are often unilateral with a much smaller area of involvement and associated with fewer lesions compared to the first episode (Figs. 65.2 and 65.3). The frequency and duration of recurrences vary considerably between episodes in the same individual and among different individuals. After the first year, genital recurrences tend to decrease in frequency for both HSV-1 and HSV-2. Genital HSV-2 recurs more frequently than genital HSV-1 (Table 65.1). In addition to classic genital ulcerations, recurrent HSV episodes may present with genital pruritus, papules or fissures, dysuria, and urethritis.

DIFFERENTIAL DIAGNOSIS

Herpes genitalis lesions must be differentiated from early syphilis, lymphogranuloma venereum, excoriations, allergic and irritant contact dermatitis, intercourse-associated trauma, and genital lesions of Behçet syndrome. In addition, fixed drug eruption or

inflammatory bowel disease can cause genital ulcerations. Chancroid and granuloma inguinale cause genital ulcerations but are rarely seen in the United States.

DIAGNOSIS

Genital herpes is the most prevalent infectious cause of genital ulcers in the United States. However, clinical diagnosis of genital herpes is both insensitive and nonspecific. The classic painful, multiple vesicular, or ulcerative lesions are absent in many infected persons. The clinical diagnosis of genital herpes should be confirmed by type-specific viral testing collected from genital lesions, since the prognosis and counseling depend on the type of HSV causing genital herpes.[15]

Laboratory Evaluation

Herpes simplex virus infection can be diagnosed by detecting the virus from genital lesions ("virologic" tests) or detecting antibodies to HSV proteins in blood ("serologic" tests). Both virologic and serologic tests should be type-specific, meaning that they can differentiate between HSV-1 and HSV-2. If genital ulcers are present, they should be sampled for definitive diagnosis of HSV-1 or HSV-2 using virologic tests. Herpes simplex virus polymerase chain reaction

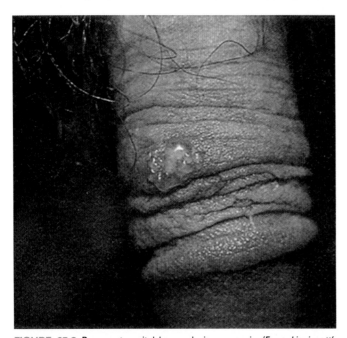

FIGURE 65.2 Recurrent genital herpes lesion on penis. (From *Lippincott's Nursing Advisor 2013.* Lippincott Williams & Wilkins; 2013.)

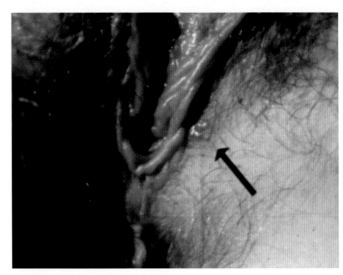

FIGURE 65.3 Recurrent genital herpes lesion on vulva. (From Nettina SM. *Lippincott Manual of Nursing Practice.* 11th ed. Lippincott, Williams & Wilkins; 2018.)

(PCR) performed on a lesion swab is the most sensitive test for detection of HSV and is preferred when available.[15] Several type-specific assays with high sensitivity and specificity are now available.[16] Viral culture sensitivity is much lower than PCR, particularly for recurrent and healed lesions, but this may be the only virologic test available in some settings. Tzanck preparations, direct fluorescence antigen (DFA), and cervical Pap smears are insensitive and nonspecific diagnostic methods and should not be used for HSV diagnosis.

If genital ulcers are not present, HSV serologic tests are used to diagnose genital herpes infection. Both type-specific and type-common antibodies to HSV develop during the first several weeks following infection and persist indefinitely. Immunoglobulin M (IgM) HSV testing is strongly discouraged, because it is not type specific and may be positive with recurrent HSV episodes.[17]

Accurate type-specific HSV immunoglobulin G (IgG) antibody assays are based on the HSV-specific glycoprotein G2 for the diagnosis of HSV-2 infection and glycoprotein G1 for HSV-1 infection. Currently, the U.S. Food and Drug Administration (FDA)-approved gG-based type-specific assays are laboratory-based and point-of-care tests that provide results for HSV-2 antibodies from capillary blood or serum.

The sensitivities and specificities of these glycoprotein G type-specific tests for the detection of HSV-2 antibody vary. The most studied test, HerpeSelect HSV-1 and HSV-2 enzyme-linked immunosorbent assays (ELISA), may be falsely positive at low index values (1.1 to 3.5), and falsely negative for HSV-1. For instance, a recent study compared HSV enzyme immunoassay (EIA) test results to the gold standard Western Blot results in 864 persons, and reported the sensitivity for HSV-1 was 70.2% and 91.6%, respectively.[18] In contrast, the EIA had high sensitivity (91.9%) but poor specificity for HSV-2 (57.4%), particularly at EIA index values <3.0, when only 39.8% of results were confirmed with the Western Blot. The risk of false-positive HSV-2 EIA results was significantly higher in people with HSV-1 antibody.[18] Therefore, low EIA values should be confirmed with another test, such as Biokit or the Western blot,[19] analogous to two-step testing for syphilis diagnosis. These confirmatory tests may be difficult to find. Most persons with HSV-2 antibody by type-specific testing have acquired anogenital HSV infection, which may be asymptomatic. Clinicians must be aware of the potential for false-positive tests, particularly among AYAs who have a low overall HSV-2 seroprevalence and should be prepared to confirm low-positive test results with a second assay. Because positive HSV-1 antibody tests may indicate an acquired oral HSV infection in childhood, HSV-1 serologic testing is of limited utility for the diagnosis of genital HSV-1 infection. Adolescents and young adults with HSV-1 infection remain at risk for HSV-2 acquisition.

Type-specific HSV-2 serologic assays may be useful in the following clinical situations:
- Recurrent or atypical genital symptoms with negative HSV cultures

- A clinical diagnosis of genital herpes without laboratory confirmation
- A patient with a sex partner with genital herpes

Herpes simplex virus type 1 or 2 serologic screening among asymptomatic persons is not recommended by the U.S. Preventive Services Task Force due to potential harm with high rate of false-positive test results and lack of clear benefit from testing.[20]

THERAPY

Principles of Genital Herpes Management

Counseling regarding the natural history of genital herpes, sexual and perinatal transmission, and methods to reduce transmission is integral to management. Antiviral medications offer clinical benefits to persons with symptomatic infections used on an episodic basis or when used as daily suppressive therapy.

Systemic antiviral drugs decrease the duration and complications of genital herpes when used to treat first clinical episodes and recurrent episodes and can prevent recurrences and transmission when used as daily suppressive therapy. However, these drugs neither eradicate latent virus nor affect the risk, frequency, or severity of recurrences once the drug is discontinued. There are three FDA-approved antiviral medications for treatment of genital herpes: acyclovir, valacyclovir (the prodrug of acyclovir), and famciclovir. Valacyclovir has the benefit of less frequent dosing due to a longer half-life compared to acyclovir. Acyclovir is a guanosine analogue that is phosphorylated by viral thymidine kinase—therefore it is active only in infected cells and is very safe and well tolerated.[21] All three medications are effective to decrease the duration of first episode and recurrent genital herpes and decrease the time to first recurrence when used as suppressive therapy. Topical therapy with antivirals for genital HSV offers minimal clinical benefit and is not recommended.

First Clinical Episode of Genital Herpes

Although AYAs with first-episode herpes may present with mild clinical manifestations, severe or prolonged symptoms can develop. Given the excellent safety profile of the antiviral medications, it is recommended that antivirals are empirically started at the time of clinical evaluation and lesion swab collection if genital herpes is suspected.

The Centers for Disease Control and Prevention (CDC)-recommended regimens for first clinical episodes are shown in Table 65.2. Treatment is recommended for 7 to 10 days but may be extended if healing is incomplete after 10 days of therapy. All antivirals are effective to decrease time for healing compared to placebo, and they have not been compared to each other head-to-head. Therefore, the choice of antiviral therapy may depend on patient preference, cost, or dosing preferences. On occasion, severe first-episode genital herpes may require hospitalization and IV acyclovir therapy.

TABLE 65.2

Treatment for Genital Herpes

Medication	First Episode Therapy Treat for 7–10 d	Episodic Therapy for Recurrent Genital Herpes	Suppressive Therapy for Recurrent Genital Herpes
Acyclovir	400 mg t.i.d.	400 mg t.i.d. × 5 d or 800 b.i.d. × 5 d or t.i.d. × 2 d	400 mg b.i.d.
Valacyclovir	1 g b.i.d.	500 mg b.i.d. × 3–5 d or 1 g b.i.d. × 5 d	500 mg q.d. or 1 g q.d. (if >9 recurrences/y)
Famciclovir	250 mg t.i.d.	125 mg b.i.d. × 5 d or 1 g b.i.d. × 1 d or 500 mg × 1 then 250 b.i.d. × 2 d	250 b.i.d.

Suppressive Therapy for Recurrent Genital Herpes

Suppressive therapy reduces the frequency of genital herpes recurrences, even among those who have infrequent outbreaks, and decreases the risk for genital HSV-2 transmission to susceptible partners by 50%. Quality of life is often improved in patients with frequent recurrences who receive suppressive compared with episodic treatment. The frequency of recurrent outbreaks diminishes over time in many patients, and the patient's psychological adjustment to the disease may change. Therefore, the need to continue therapy should be discussed periodically during suppressive treatment (e.g., once a year). Ease of administration and cost also are important considerations. There is no laboratory monitoring required and antiviral resistance is very rare in immunocompetent hosts. Since HSV-1 recurrences are infrequent and the impact of suppressive therapy on genital HSV-1 transmission is unknown, the benefits of suppressive therapy may be fewer for patients with genital HSV-1 as compared to HSV-2. However, for patients with frequent recurrences of genital HSV-1, suppressive therapy should be considered. See Table 65.2 for recommended suppressive dosing regimens for acyclovir, valacyclovir, and famciclovir.

Episodic Therapy for Recurrent Genital Herpes

Episodic treatment of recurrent genital herpes is most effective if given within 1 day of lesion onset, or during the prodrome that precedes some outbreaks. In those with known genital infection, a supply of drug or a prescription can be provided with instructions to self-initiate treatment immediately when symptoms begin. The CDC-recommended regimens for episodic therapy are shown in Table 65.2.

Management of Sex Partners

The sex partners of AYAs who have genital herpes may benefit from evaluation and counseling. Symptomatic sex partners should be evaluated and treated in the same manner as persons who have genital lesions. Asymptomatic sex partners of patients who have genital herpes should be assessed for a history of past genital lesions and offered HSV type-specific serologic testing. Disclosure of genital herpes status to sexual partners is recommended and has been shown to decrease the risk of transmission to partners. However, disclosure may be anxiety provoking for AYAs. A recent small study showed that persons of younger age were less likely to disclose genital herpes status than those who were older, although relationship factors, such as relationship commitment and time in relationship also significantly influenced the likelihood of disclosure.[22] Strategies for disclosure may be discussed with clincians.

COUNSELING

Below are counseling messages that should be provided to AYAs diagnosed with genital HSV. Genital HSV counseling has many nuances but taking time to empathetically explain these concepts to patients may help them cope with the diagnosis of a stigmatized infection that can have a lasting impact on sexual health. A comprehensive counseling guide is available.[23]

1. The sexual transmission of HSV can occur during asymptomatic periods. Persons with active lesions or prodromal symptoms should abstain from oral, vaginal, and anal contact with uninfected partners until the lesions are clearly healed.
2. Since viral shedding can occur in the absence of lesions, consistent and correct condom use should be recommended to any person who has had a genital herpes episode. Male latex condoms can reduce, but not eliminate, the risk of HSV.
3. Herpes simplex virus type 1 infection can be transmitted to the oral or genital tract during oral sex.

4. Many patients newly diagnosed with HSV develop psychological distress due to shame, stigma, and having to live with an incurable infection that could substantially interfere with future relationships. Clinicians can address these concerns by encouraging patients to recognize that herpes is a manageable condition by (1) giving information, (2) providing support resources, and (3) helping define treatment options.
5. Since a genital herpes diagnosis may affect perceptions about existing or future sexual relationships, it is important for patients to understand how to talk to sexual partners about STIs.
6. Herpes simplex virus type 2 discordant couples should be encouraged to consider suppressive antiviral therapy as part of a strategy to prevent transmission, in addition to consistent condom use and avoidance of sexual activity during recurrences.
7. Research on HSV therapeutic and preventive vaccines is ongoing, as is research to cure HSV infection. At the time of writing the chapter, there were no approved vaccines or cure strategies for HSV infection. Herpes simplex virus type 2 infection increases the risk for human immunodeficiency virus (HIV) acquisition, particularly after incident infection. Consideration of HIV pre-exposure prophylaxis (PrEP) should be considered for those who are at risk of HIV infection.

COMPLICATIONS

A new diagnosis of genital herpes may be associated with significant psychological distress. Patients may note shock, fear, guilt, social isolation, or anger. Anxiety and depression can also occur and may persist. Some persons have concerns about how herpes will impact their future sex life and relationships. There can be considerable embarrassment, shame, and stigma associated with a herpes diagnosis and this can substantially interfere with a patient's relationships.

Local complications of genital herpes include secondary bacterial infection of lesions, phimosis (males), or labial adhesions (females). During primary infection, urinary retention, constipation, and impotence may occur. Sacral radiculopathy can also occur, causing paresthesias in the lower extremities.

Neonatal HSV is one of the most feared complications of genital HSV infection. Herpes simplex virus can be transmitted to neonates during delivery. Most birthing persons of infants who acquire neonatal herpes lack histories of clinically evident genital herpes or have acquired HSV infection during pregnancy. Pregnant patients should be screened for a history of genital lesions and symptoms.

Neurologic complications of genital HSV include recurrent aseptic meningitis, which is typically associated with HSV-2 infection.

SUMMARY

Herpes genitalis is a very common chronic infection caused by HSV-1 or HSV-2. Symptoms include recurrent self-limited genital ulcerations and periodic viral shedding from skin and mucosal surfaces that can be associated with transmission to sexual partners. The symptoms can be controlled with safe and effective antiviral therapy. Due to stigma associated with the infection, psychological distress may be the most prominent complication of genital herpes among AYAs. Accurate counseling and education can provide patients with needed tools to optimize sexual and mental health after a diagnosis of genital herpes.

ACKNOWLEDGMENTS

The author wishes to acknowledge Gale R. Burstein and Kimberly A. Workowski for their contributions to previous versions of this chapter.

REFERENCES

1. James C, Harfouche M, Welton NJ, et al. Herpes simplex virus: global infection prevalence and incidence estimates, 2016. *Bull World Health Organ*. 2020; 98(5):315–329.
2. Bernstein DI, Bellamy AR, Hook EW 3rd, et al. Epidemiology, clinical presentation, and antibody response to primary infection with herpes simplex virus type 1 and type 2 in young women. *Clin Infect Dis*. 2013;56(3):344–351.
3. Looker KJ, Magaret AS, May MT, et al. Global and regional estimates of prevalent and incident herpes simplex virus type 1 infections in 2012. *PLoS One*. 2015;10(10):e0140765.
4. McQuillan G, Kruszon-Moran D, Flagg EW, et al. Prevalence of herpes simplex virus type 1 and type 2 in persons aged 14-49: United States, 2015-2016. *NCHS Data Brief*. 2018;304:1–8.
5. Spicknall IH, Flagg EW, Torrone EA. Estimates of the prevalence and incidence of genital herpes, United States, 2018. *Sex Transm Dis*. 2021;48(4):260–265.
6. Fanfair RN, Zaidi A, Taylor LD, et al. Trends in seroprevalence of herpes simplex virus type 2 among non-Hispanic blacks and non-Hispanic whites aged 14 to 49 years—United States, 1988 to 2010. *Sex Transm Dis*. 2013;40(11):860–864.
7. Stebbins RC, Noppert GA, Aiello AE, et al. Persistent socioeconomic and racial and ethnic disparities in pathogen burden in the United States, 1999–2014. *Epidemiol Infect*. 2019;147:e301.
8. Hill AV, De Genna NM, Perez-Patron MJ, et al. Identifying syndemics for sexually transmitted infections among young adults in the United States: a latent class analysis. *J Adolesc Health*. 2019;64(3):319–326.
9. Belshe RB, Leone PA, Bernstein DI, et al; Herpevac Trial for Women. Efficacy results of a trial of a herpes simplex vaccine. *N Engl J Med*. 2012;366(1):34–43.
10. Dabestani N, Katz DA, Dombrowski J, et al. Time trends in first-episode genital herpes simplex virus infections in an urban sexually transmitted disease clinic. *Sex Transm Dis*. 2019;46(12):795–800.
11. Ayoub HH, Chemaitelly H, Abu-Raddad LJ. Characterizing the transitioning epidemiology of herpes simplex virus type 1 in the USA: model-based predictions. *BMC Med*. 2019;17(1):57.
12. Smith G. Herpesvirus transport to the nervous system and back again. *Annu Rev Microbiol*. 2012;66:153–176.
13. Corey L, Adams HG, Brown ZA, et al. Genital herpes simplex virus infections: clinical manifestations, course, and complications. *Ann Intern Med*. 1983;98(6):958–972.
14. Bissessor M, Fairley CK, Read T, et al. The etiology of infectious proctitis in men who have sex with men differs according to HIV status. *Sex Transm Dis*. 2013; 40(10):768–770.
15. Wald A, Huang ML, Carrell D, et al. Polymerase chain reaction for detection of herpes simplex virus (HSV) DNA on mucosal surfaces: comparison with HSV isolation in cell culture. *J Infect Dis*. 2003;188(9):1345–1351.
16. Binnicker MJ, Espy MJ, Duresko B, et al. Automated processing, extraction and detection of herpes simplex virus types 1 and 2: a comparative evaluation of three commercial platforms using clinical specimens. *J Clin Virol*. 2017;89:30–33.
17. Jung S, Theel ES. Overutilization of IgM serologic assays for herpes simplex virus. *J Appl Lab Med*. 2020;5(1):241–243.
18. Agyemang E, Le QA, Warren T, et al. Performance of commercial enzyme-linked immunoassays for diagnosis of herpes simplex virus-1 and herpes simplex virus-2 infection in a clinical setting. *Sex Transm Dis*. 2017;44(12):763–767.
19. Workowski KA, Bolan G; Centers for Disease Control and Prevention. Sexually transmitted diseases treatment guidelines, 2015. *MMWR Recomm Rep*. 2015; 64(RR-03):1–137.
20. Feltner C, Grodensky C, Ebel C, et al. Serologic screening for genital herpes: an updated evidence report and systematic review for the US preventive services task force. *JAMA*. 2016;316(23):2531–2543.
21. De Clercq E. Selective anti-herpesvirus agents. *Antivir Chem Chemother*. 2013; 23(3):93–101.
22. Myers JL, Buhi ER, Marhefka S, et al. Associations between individual and relationship characteristics and genital herpes disclosure. *J Health Psychol*. 2016; 21(10):2283–2293.
23. Steben M, Fisher WA. *Genital herpes counselling tool 2019*. https://www.canada.ca/en/public-health/services/infectious-diseases/sexual-health-sexually-transmitted-infections/canadian-guidelines/sexually-transmitted-infections/genital-herpes-counselling-tool.html

ADDITIONAL RESOURCES AND WEBSITES

Additional Resources and Websites for Clinicians:
CDC STD Resources—https://www.cdc.gov/std/default.htm
Gnann JW Jr, Whitley RJ. Clinical practice: genital herpes. *N Engl J Med*. 2016; 375(7):666–674.
Johnston C, Corey L. Current concepts for genital herpes simplex virus infection: diagnostics and pathogenesis of genital tract shedding. *Clin Microbiol Rev*. 2016;29(1):149–161.
National Network of STD Clinical Prevention Training Centers Clinical Consultation Network—https://www.stdccn.org/render/Public
National STD Curriculum—https://www.std.uw.edu/
Steben M, Fisher WA. *Genital herpes counselling tool 2019*. https://www.canada.ca/en/public-health/services/infectious-diseases/sexual-health-sexually-transmitted-infections/canadian-guidelines/sexually-transmitted-infections/genital-herpes-counselling-tool.html

Additional Resources and Websites for Parents/Caregivers:
American Sexual Health Association: I Wanna Know: How Does Herpes Testing Work—http://www.iwannaknow.org/how-does-herpes-testing-work/
Centers for Disease Control: Genital Herpes Fact Sheet—https://www.cdc.gov/std/herpes/stdfact-herpes-detailed.htm
Dawson, Ella. STIs aren't a consequence. They're inevitable. TEDxConneticutCollege. May 11, 2016—https://www.youtube.com/watch?v=Ycll-hclrLI
Ebel C, Wald A. *Managing Herpes: How to live and love with a chronic STD*. American Social Health Association; 2002.
Park I. Killing the scarlet h: stigma and scandal in the world of genital herpes. In: Park I, ed. *Strange Bedfellows. Adventures in the Science, History, and Surprising Secrets of STDs*. FlatIron Books; 2021.
Warren, T. *The Good News About the Bad News: Herpes* (Everything you need to know). New Harbinger Publications, Inc.; 2009.
Wessel L. Flawed herpes testing leads to false positives and needless suffering. STAT (statnews.com). Accessed January 26, 2017.

Additional Resources and Websites for Adolescents and Young Adults:
American Sexual Health Association: I Wanna Know: How Does Herpes Testing Work—http://www.iwannaknow.org/how-does-herpes-testing-work/
Centers for Disease Control: Genital Herpes Fact Sheet—https://www.cdc.gov/std/herpes/stdfact-herpes-detailed.htm
Dawson, Ella. STIs aren't a consequence. They're inevitable. TEDxConneticutCollege. May 11, 2016—https://www.youtube.com/watch?v=Ycll-hclrLI
Ebel C, Wald A. *Managing Herpes: How to Live and Love with a Chronic STD*. American Social Health Association; 2002.
Park I. Killing the scarlet h: stigma and scandal in the world of genital herpes. In: Park I, ed. *Strange Bedfellows. Adventures in the Science, History, and Surprising Secrets of STDs*. FlatIron Books; 2021.
Warren, T. *The Good News About the Bad News: Herpes (Everything You Need to Know)*. New Harbinger Publications, Inc.; 2009.
Wessel L. Flawed herpes testing leads to false positives and needless suffering. STAT (statnews.com). Accessed January 26, 2017.

66 Human Papillomavirus Infection and Anogenital Warts

LaKeshia N. Craig
Jessica A. Kahn

KEY WORDS
- Anogenital warts
- External genital warts
- Human papillomavirus
- Human papillomavirus vaccines
- Management
- Oral human papillomavirus
- Sexually transmitted infection
- Treatment

INTRODUCTION

Human papillomaviruses (HPVs) are small, nonenveloped, double-stranded deoxyribonucleic acid (DNA) viruses of the Papillomaviridae family. More than 200 HPV types have been identified, approximately 40 of which can infect the anogenital and oropharyngeal mucosa. Genital HPV types infect the squamous epithelium and are classified as low risk and high risk.[1] Low-risk types, including HPV 6 and 11, most commonly cause anogenital warts, but may also cause mild vulvar intraepithelial neoplasia (VIN), vaginal intraepithelial neoplasia (VaIN), cervical intraepithelial neoplasia (CIN), penile intraepithelial neoplasia (PeIN), and anal intraepithelial neoplasia (AIN). High-risk types, including HPV 16, 18, 31, 33, 35, 39, 45, 51, 52, 56, 58, and 59, may cause mild, moderate, or severe VIN, VaIN, CIN, PeIN, and AIN; vulvar, vaginal, cervical, penile, and anal cancers; and oropharyngeal cancer. Mild, moderate, and severe cervical intraepithelial neoplasias have been classified as 1, 2, and 3, respectively (e.g., CIN1, CIN2, or CIN3). Current understanding of the biology of anogenital HPV infection suggests that it is more appropriate to classify HPV-associated preinvasive intraepithelial squamous lesions in two instead of three tiers, as noted in consensus recommendations.[2] These include low-grade squamous intraepithelial lesion (LSIL), indicating self-limited HPV infection that is commonly diagnosed, transient, and highly unlikely to progress to carcinoma, and high-grade squamous intraepithelial lesion (HSIL) that is more likely to be persistent and may progress to invasive carcinoma.[2] These two tiers may be further classified using the appropriate -IN or intraepithelial neoplasia terminology, specifying the location (e.g., CIN3 for an –IN 3 lesion of the cervix, and VaIN 3 for an -IN 3 lesion of the vagina).

Epidemiology

Prevalence

Human papillomavirus infection is extremely common, and prevalence peaks during adolescence and young adulthood. Prior to HPV vaccine introduction, it was estimated that the average lifetime probability of acquiring HPV among those with at least one opposite-sex partner was 84.6% (range, 53.6% to 95.0%) for females and 91.3% (range, 69.5% to 97.7%) for males.[3] Since the introduction of preventative HPV vaccines, the prevalence of vaccine-type HPV, CIN, and anogenital warts has decreased markedly.

A systemic review and meta-analysis using data from multiple countries demonstrated that 5 to 8 years after HPV vaccine introduction:

- prevalence of HPV 16 and 18 decreased by 83% among 13- to 19-year-old females and by 66% among 20- to 24-year-old females.[4]
- prevalence of HPV 31, 33, and 45 decreased by 54% among 13- to 19-year-old females.
- diagnosis of anogenital warts decreased by 67% among 15- to 19-year-old females, by 54% among 20- to 24-year-old females, by 48% among 15- to 19-year-old males, and by 32% among 20- to 24-year-old males.

The meta-analysis also demonstrated that 5 to 9 years after vaccine introduction, CIN2/3 decreased by 51% among screened 15- to 19-year-old females and by 31% among 20- to 24-year-old females. Furthermore, since HPV vaccine introduction, there has been an estimated 88.2% reduction in prevalence of oral HPV infection with types 6, 11, 16, and 18 in vaccinated versus unvaccinated 18- to 33-year-olds in the United States.[5] The current decrease in prevalence of HPV and CIN is expected to translate into substantial reductions in cervical and other HPV-related cancers in the future.

Transmission

Human papillomavirus transmission occurs primarily through sexual contact, including oral–genital, digital–genital, and genital–genital (e.g., penile–anal, penile–vaginal) contact. Adolescents and young adults (AYAs) typically acquire HPV infection soon after sexual initiation.[6] Vertical transmission of HPV 6 or 11 from mother to child during delivery may cause recurrent respiratory papillomatosis (RRP) in young children, though RRP is uncommon.[7]

Risk Factors

The primary risk factor for HPV infection is number of sexual partners, both lifetime and recent. Additional factors that have been associated with HPV infection include earlier age of sexual initiation, inconsistent condom use, cigarette smoking (also a cofactor in cervical carcinogenesis), immunosuppression including human immunodeficiency virus (HIV) infection, history of sexually transmitted infections (STIs), and male partner's lack of circumcision.[6]

Pathophysiology and Natural History of Human Papillomaviruses Infection

Human papillomavirus initially infects the basal layer of epithelial cells through microabrasions in the skin or mucosa. Infected cells migrate to the suprabasal layers, where viral gene expression, viral replication, and particle formation occur. Although HPV infection

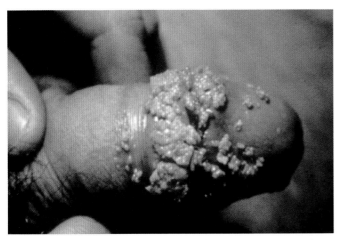

FIGURE 66.1 Condylomata acuminata (penis). (From Goodheart HP. *Goodheart's Photoguide of Common Skin Disorders*. 4th ed. Lippincott Williams & Wilkins; 2015.)

is extremely common in AYAs, the vast majority of infections do not progress to anogenital warts, precancers, or cancers and resolve spontaneously.[8]

Clinical Manifestations

Types of Anogenital Warts

External genital warts or condylomata are very common, and 90% are caused by HPV 6 or 11.[9] Types include the following.

1. Condylomata acuminata: Exophytic growths with a granular, irregular surface, and finger-like projections. They usually have highly vascular cores that produce punctuated or looplike patterns unless obscured by overlying keratinized surfaces (Figs. 66.1 and 66.2).
2. Papular warts: Smooth, skin-colored, well-circumscribed papules that are usually 1 to 4 mm in diameter and have a round, slightly hyperkeratotic, or smooth surface (Fig. 66.3).
3. Keratotic warts: These have a thick, horny (crust-like) layer; they resemble common warts or seborrheic keratoses (Fig. 66.4).
4. Flat-topped macules: These are subclinical lesions that are difficult to detect without techniques such as treatment with a weak acetic acid solution.

Location

Typical sites for anogenital warts in females include the cervix, vagina, vulva, urethra, and anus, but are most common in the external genital areas such as the vaginal introitus. Typical sites in males include under the foreskin of the uncircumcised penis, on the shaft of the circumcised penis, and on the scrotum and anus. Condylomata can be multifocal or multicentric. Condylomata acuminata tend to occur on partially keratinized, non–hair-bearing ("moist") skin; keratotic and papular warts tend to occur on fully keratinized (hair-bearing or non–hair-bearing) skin; and flat-topped warts may occur on either skin surface.

Color

Pink, red, tan, brown, or gray.

Symptoms

Anogenital warts are typically asymptomatic but may cause pruritus, burning, pain, urethral or vaginal discharge, urethral bleeding, or postcoital bleeding.

Exacerbating Factors

Exacerbating factors include pregnancy, skin moisture, and/or vaginal or urethral discharge.

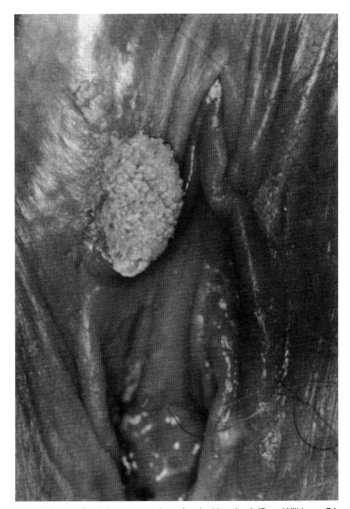

FIGURE 66.2 Condylomata acuminata (vaginal introitus). (From Wilkinson EJ, Stone IK. *Atlas of Vulvar Disease*. Williams & Wilkins; 1994, Figure 17.9a.)

Clinical Course

Lesions usually appear 2 to 3 months after infection, with a range of approximately 3 weeks to 8 months. Warts may regress spontaneously, persist, or increase in size or number. Over a period of months to years, most anogenital warts resolve. Risk factors for persistence include immunosuppression, high-risk HPV infection, and older age.

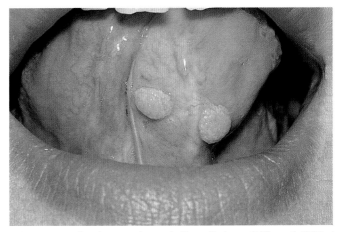

FIGURE 66.3 Papular warts (tongue). (From *Lippincott Williams & Wilkins' Comprehensive Dental Assisting*. Lippincott Williams & Wilkins; 2011.)

XIII

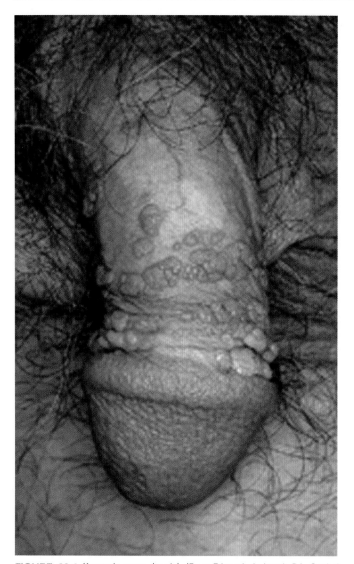

FIGURE 66.4 Keratotic warts (penis). (From Edwards L, Lynch PJ. *Genital Dermatology Atlas*. 2nd ed. Lippincott Williams & Wilkins; 2010.)

Differential Diagnosis

The differential diagnosis for anogenital warts includes micropapillomatosis labialis of the labia minora, pearly penile papules, seborrheic keratosis, other benign genital lesions (skin tags, fibromas, lipomas, hidradenomas, and adenomas), condylomata lata (secondary syphilis) (see Fig. 66.5), molluscum contagiosum, granuloma inguinale, and high-grade intraepithelial lesions, and cancer (Bowen disease, Bowenoid papulosis, dysplastic nevi, VIN, VaIN, PeIN, AIN, and squamous cell carcinoma).

Diagnosis

Human Papillomaviruses Detection

Human papillomavirus detection methods may be categorized in two ways: HPV genotyping and identification of HPV DNA physical integration into cervical cells.[10] Molecular techniques for HPV DNA detection include nucleic acid hybridization, signal amplification, and target amplification methods. Research and clinical laboratories primarily use polymerase chain reaction (PCR)-based assays to detect HPV DNA as they are easily automated, have high reproducibility and specificity, and allow for identification of multiple HPV genotypes at relatively low cost. Several real-time PCR-based assays have been developed in recent years, which have a lower risk of contamination and are more sensitive and reproducible

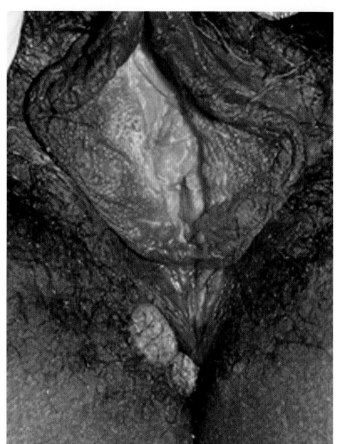

FIGURE 66.5 Condylomata lata (perineum). (From Edwards L, Lynch PJ. *Genital Dermatology Atlas*. 2nd ed. Lippincott Williams & Wilkins; 2010.)

than conventional PCR. In-situ DNA hybridization (ISH) is a signal amplification assay that detects HPV DNA (HPV-ISH) in cells or tissue specimens. Several techniques are available to identify HPV-DNA that has been physically integrated into cells, including the fluorescence in-situ hybridization (FISH) assay and PCR-based assays such as the detection of integrated papillomavirus sequences (DIPS) method, quantitative real-time PCR, and next-generation sequencing (NGS) technology which has the capacity to perform whole genome sequencing of individual samples and examine multiple individual samples concurrently. Human papillomavirus may also be detected using serologic assays—typically with virus-like particle enzyme immunoassays—but these are not used clinically.

Cervical Cancer Screening

In the United States, there are three major organizations that publish cervical screening guidelines: the American Cancer Society, the United States Preventive Services Task Force (USPSTF), and the American College of Obstetricians and Gynecologists (ACOG). The American Cancer Society recommends that individuals with a cervix (including transmasculine individuals) initiate cervical cancer screening at age 25 years and undergo primary HPV testing every 5 years through age 65 years.[11] If primary HPV testing is not available, then individuals aged 25 to 65 years should be screened with co-testing (HPV testing and cytology) every 5 years or cervical cytology alone every 3 years. The USPSTF and ACOG recommend cytology alone in females 21 to 29 years of age, and one of these options for females 30 to 65 years of age: cytology alone every 3 years, high-risk HPV testing alone every 5 years, or co-testing with high-risk HPV testing and cytology every 5 years.[12,13] Screening may be indicated at a younger age or more frequently for young females who are immunocompromised. Cervical cancer screening and management of abnormal results are discussed in more detail in Chapter 55.

Genital Warts

Genital warts can usually be diagnosed using direct visual inspection with a bright light and, if necessary, magnification.[14] A speculum examination is helpful in AYAs with a cervix with external genital warts to evaluate for vaginal and cervical warts. An otoscope and small spreader are helpful to inspect the male urinary meatus. Anoscopy should be considered for immunosuppressed males and females with recurrent perianal warts and a history of anoreceptive intercourse, and urethroscopy should be considered for males with gross hematuria or an altered urinary stream. Because individuals with external anal warts also have intra-anal warts, inspection of the anal canal by digital examination, standard anoscopy, or high-resolution anoscopy should be considered. Acetowhite testing, HPV DNA testing, and biopsy are not recommended routinely for diagnosis. However, patients with anogenital warts who are not responsive to therapy or have features suggestive of neoplasia (e.g., blue or black discoloration, induration, bleeding, ulceration, increased pigmentation, rapid growth, or fixation to underlying structures) should be referred to a specialist for further evaluation and possible biopsy.

Treatment

General Considerations

No treatment is recommended for asymptomatic HPV infection. Management of LSIL and HSIL is described in Chapter 55. This chapter focuses on treatment for anogenital warts. The goal of therapy is to eradicate or reduce the size of clinically apparent anogenital warts in order to ameliorate clinical symptoms or cosmetic concerns.[14] However, it is reasonable not to begin treatment unless the warts persist or enlarge because anogenital warts may resolve spontaneously and it is not clear whether treatment of anogenital warts alters the natural history of the infection or decreases future viral transmission. Treatment should be guided by the patient's preferences, extent and type of lesion, the clinician's experience, potential for adverse effects, and available resources.

Treatments for external genital warts are classified as patient applied or clinician administered. Patient-applied therapies require that the patient can adequately visualize the lesions to be treated and adhere to the specified treatment schedule. There is no definitive evidence that any one treatment is more effective than another. Treatment strategies are presented in **Table 66.1**. Anogenital warts usually respond within 3 months of therapy, though immunosuppression and nonadherence to treatment may affect response. If one treatment strategy fails, another may be tried. However, if anogenital warts persist, then patients should be referred to a specialist. The use of more than one treatment modality at the same time has not been shown to be effective and may increase the risk of side effects. Partner evaluation is valuable if feasible, in that it provides an opportunity for the clinician to screen partners for anogenital

---

TABLE 66.1

Recommended Treatment Options for External Genital Warts

Treatment Option	Mechanism of Action	Instructions for Use	Advantages	Disadvantages
Patient applied				
Imiquimod 3.75% or 5% cream	Topically active immune enhancer that stimulates production of interferon	The cream is provided in individual packets and pump bottles. Apply the 3.75% cream every night for up to 8 wks, or the 5% cream three times per week for up to 16 wks, until all lesions have disappeared. Both are left on overnight (6–10 h), then washed off with soap and water. Wash off before sexual intercourse.	May be applied at home. Can be applied to new warts as they appear	Local erythema, erosion, itching, and burning; rarely, may worsen autoimmune skin disorders. May weaken condoms/diaphragms. Takes up to 16 wks to treat. Safety during pregnancy has not been established
Sinecatechins 15% ointment	Botanical quantified extract from green tea leaves consisting of more than 85% catechins—an active ingredient that exhibits specific antioxidant, antiviral, antitumor, and immunostimulatory properties	Apply 0.5-cm strand of ointment to each wart using a finger to ensure coverage with a thin layer of ointment until complete clearance of warts. Use three times daily for a maximum of 16 wks. Do not wash off after use.	May be applied at home	May cause erythema, pruritus/burning, pain, ulceration, edema, induration, and vesicular rash. May weaken condoms/diaphragms. Sexual contact should be avoided while the ointment is on the skin. Not recommended for immunocompromised persons or those with clinical genital herpes. Safety during pregnancy is unknown
Podophyllotoxin/ podofilox 0.5% solution or gel	Antimitotic	Using a cotton swab for the solution or a finger for the gel, apply to genital warts twice daily for 3 d, followed by 4 d of no therapy. The cycle can be repeated up to four times if needed. Total wart area treated should not exceed 10 cm², and total volume of podofilox should not exceed 0.5 mL/d. Allow to dry after treatment, and patients should wash their hands before and after each application.	Widely available. Inexpensive. Easy to apply. May be applied at home	May cause local erosion, burning, pain, and itching. Not useful for cervical, mucosal lesions, or extensive disease. Podofilox is contraindicated during pregnancy

(continued)

TABLE 66.1

Recommended Treatment Options for External Genital Warts (*Continued*)

Treatment Option	Mechanism of Action	Instructions for Use	Advantages	Disadvantages
Clinician applied				
Trichloroacetic acid (TCA) or bichloracetic acid (BCA) 80–90%	Caustic agent—chemical coagulations of proteins	Clinician first applies occlusive ointment to the healthy tissue surrounding lesion, or treats the area with a topical anesthetic (e.g., benzocaine topical solution). The back or front end of a cotton swab is used to apply the solution sparingly until the lesions blanch (frost). The solution should air-dry before the patient resumes a normal position. If necessary, sodium bicarbonate, soap, or talc may be applied to remove unreacted acid. Avoid contact with normal skin. Repeat weekly for up to 6 wks until warts have resolved.	Inexpensive Easy to apply Safe in pregnancy	Destroys normal tissue if overapplied
Cryotherapy with liquid nitrogen or cryoprobe	Thermal-induced cytolysis	Liquid nitrogen can be used to treat vaginal warts, but use of a cryoprobe is not recommended because of the risk of vaginal perforation or fistula formation. A cotton applicator designed for cryotherapy is placed in liquid nitrogen briefly and then quickly applied with gentle pressure for 2–3 s to the wart to be treated as well as 2–3 mm of surrounding skin. The surface of the wart should briefly turn white and then return to its normal color. Process can be repeated every 1–2 wks.	Well tolerated Safe in pregnancy No anesthesia needed though local anesthetics may facilitate treatment if the area is large Minimal risk of scarring	May cause pain, necrosis, blistering Overapplication may lead to complications, while underapplication may lead to poor results.
Surgical procedures		These procedures may include excision with a scalpel, curettage, or scissors; electrosurgery; and laser therapy.	Useful for extensive disease, intraurethral warts, or lesions resistant to other therapies Safe in pregnancy Rapid resolution of condylomata	Requires hospital setting, clinician expertise, appropriate equipment, and anesthesia Expensive With surgical excision, scarring and bleeding are possible Laser is not readily available, and intact DNA may be liberated into the air with laser

BCA, bichloracetic acid; DNA, deoxyribonucleic acid; TCA, trichloroacetic acid.

warts and other STIs and to educate partners about HPV and genital warts.

Specific Treatment Recommendations and Considerations (www.cdc.gov/std/treatment)

- *Patient-applied treatments* for external genital warts, including warts of the vulva, perineum, penis, scrotum, external anus, and perianus (Table 66.1), include imiquimod 3.75% or 5% cream, podophyllotoxin/podofilox 0.5% solution or gel, and sinecatechins 15% ointment. If possible, the clinician should apply the first treatment to demonstrate both the application technique and the warts to be treated.
- *Clinician-administered treatments* for external genital warts (Table 66.1) include bichloracetic acid (BCA) or trichloroacetic acid (TCA) 80% to 90% solution, cryotherapy with liquid nitrogen or cryoprobe, and surgical removal by tangential

scissor excision, tangential shave excision, curettage, laser, or electrosurgery.

- *Treatment by location:* Patients with cervical warts may be treated with cryotherapy with liquid nitrogen, surgical removal, or TCA or BCA 80% to 90% solution, but should be managed with a specialist and exophytic warts should be biopsied to exclude an HSIL prior to treatment. Patients with vaginal warts may be treated using cryotherapy with liquid nitrogen (but not a cryoprobe due to a risk of perforation and fistula formation), TCA/BCA 80% to 90% solution, or surgical removal. Recommended regimens for patients with urethral meatus warts are cryotherapy with liquid nitrogen or surgical removal. Recommended regimens for intra-anal warts are cryotherapy with liquid nitrogen, TCA/BCA 80% to 90% solution, or surgical removal. They should be managed in consultation with a colorectal specialist. Oral warts may be treated with cryotherapy or surgical removal.

Those with external anal or perianal warts may also have intra-anal warts; therefore, they may benefit from an inspection of the anal canal by digital examination or anoscopy.

• *Treatment in patients with special conditions:*

a. Pregnancy: Several factors associated with pregnancy, such as hormonal factors and relative immunosuppression, may promote growth of anogenital warts. The only treatments recommended during pregnancy are BCA/TCA, cryotherapy, electrocautery, and surgical excision. Cesarean delivery is indicated for females with genital warts if the pelvic outlet is obstructed or if vaginal delivery would result in excessive bleeding; a cesarean delivery should not be performed solely to prevent transmission of HPV to the newborn. Pregnant females with anogenital warts should be counseled concerning the low risk for RRP.

b. Immunosuppression: Adolescents and young adults who are immunosuppressed due to HIV infection, organ transplantation, or other conditions may have more extensive genital warts, may not respond to treatment as well as immunocompetent AYAs, and may have more frequent recurrences. In addition, squamous cell carcinomas originating in or resembling genital warts occur more frequently among immunocompromised patients. Therefore, evaluation by a specialist should be considered.

Counseling

Clinicians should educate patients with anogenital warts about HPV infection, its transmission, and its clinical consequences. Key messages are as follows: genital warts are caused by specific HPV types that are usually different from the types that cause cervical cancer; genital warts may recur after treatment; it is unclear whether treatment reduces transmission of HPV to partners; condom use may reduce transmission of HPV and acquisition of genital warts but is not fully protective against transmission of HPV; during treatment, AYAs should avoid sexual activity; anogenital warts do not affect fertility; and a vaccine is available to prevent genital warts but it will not treat existing HPV or warts. Clinicians should provide information about available treatment options for anogenital warts, their prognosis, and strategies to prevent HPV-related disease and other STIs (e.g., abstinence, limiting number of sexual partners, and using condoms consistently and correctly). It is not necessary to perform Pap testing more frequently in those with genital warts. The HPV vaccine does not treat existing HPV or genital warts, but can prevent most cases of genital warts in individuals who have not been exposed to the HPV types that cause warts at the time of vaccination.

Clinicians should make sure that patients being treated for external genital warts can visualize their warts, especially those who are using patient-applied therapies. Patients should be advised to examine the areas being treated for signs of inflammation or infection (such as redness, swelling, or discharge) regularly and report these immediately to the clinician. General perineal care may promote healing, including sitz baths and keeping the area clean and dry. During treatment and after visible warts have resolved, follow-up visits are helpful to monitor for complications of therapy; educate AYAs about signs of recurrence, and reiterate prevention messages. Clinicians should provide support and when necessary, refer patients to support groups or for individual counseling.

Human Papillomavirus Vaccines

Prophylactic HPV vaccines consist of virus-like particles, which are recombinant viral capsids that are identical to HPV virions morphologically, but do not contain viral DNA. Therefore, they cannot replicate and pose no infectious or oncogenic risk. The three licensed vaccines are an HPV 16, 18 vaccine (2vHPV, Cervarix, GlaxoSmithKline), an HPV 6, 11, 16, 18 vaccine (4vHPV, Gardasil,

Merck & Co., Inc.), and an HPV 6, 11, 16, 18, 31, 33, 45, 52, 58 vaccine (9vHPV, Gardasil 9, Merck and Co., Inc.). The only vaccine currently available in the United States is the 9vHPV vaccine. Clinical trials of the 2vHPV, 4vHPV, and 9vHPV vaccines have demonstrated that they are safe, well tolerated, and highly effective (close to 100%) in preventing vaccine type–related persistent HPV infections and CIN2/3 in young females in clinical trials.[15,16] The 4vHPV vaccine has demonstrated high efficacy (approximately 99%) in preventing genital warts. Ongoing surveillance has demonstrated that vaccine effectiveness remains high at least 10 to 12 years after vaccination.

The Advisory Committee on Immunization Practices of the U.S. Centers for Disease Control and Prevention recommends routine HPV vaccination for all adolescents 11 to 12 years of age. The vaccine series may be started as early as age 9 years. Catch-up vaccination is recommended for males and females up to 26 years of age.[17] A two-dose series is recommended for those who receive the first dose before the 15th birthday (0-, 6- to 12-month schedule) and a three-dose series is recommended for those who receive the first dose after the 15th birthday and for those with immunocompromising conditions (0-, 1- to 2-, and 6-month schedule). Human papillomavirus vaccines are not recommended for use in pregnant females (though a pregnancy test is not required prior to vaccinating) but can be used for breastfeeding or lactating individuals. Vaccination is not contraindicated for those who have a history of sexual activity, anogenital warts, or HIV infection but is contraindicated for those who have experienced a severe allergic reaction (e.g., anaphylaxis) to a vaccine component or following a prior dose of HPV vaccine.

Vaccine uptake has been suboptimal despite availability of the first HPV vaccine in the United States since 2006, the high efficacy of all HPV vaccines in preventing HPV infections and related diseases, and the fact that HPV vaccination is a key strategy for reducing the enormous economic and humanistic burden of cervical cancer and other HPV-associated cancers globally. In 2020, cervical cancer remains the fourth most common cancer among females worldwide.[18] Approximately 35,900 cancers are caused by HPV in the United States each year, including an estimated 14,000 oropharyngeal cancers among males and females, 11,000 cervical cancers among females, and 6,500 anal cancers among males and females.[19] However, in 2019, only 71.5% of adolescents in the United States aged 13 to 17 years had received ≥1 dose of HPV vaccine, and only 54.2% had completed the HPV vaccination series.[20] These rates still fall short of the Healthy People 2030 goal of 80% complete vaccination of 13- to 15-year-olds. The World Health Organization launched a global strategy to accelerate the elimination of cervical cancer in 2018: (1) 90% of females fully vaccinated with the HPV vaccine by the age of 15 years; (2) 70% of females screened for cervical cancer using a high-performance test by the age of 35 years and again by the age of 45 years; and (3) 90% of females with precancer treated and 90% of females with invasive cancer managed.

Evidence-based strategies to maximize HPV vaccine uptake include clinician- and system-level interventions. At the clinician level, clinicians should utilize key messages that drive parents'/caregivers' and AYAs' decisions about vaccination.[21] These messages should include the following: the clinician strongly supports vaccination (e.g., "I recommend we give Sarah her first HPV vaccine today; it's important that she gets this vaccine to prevent cervical cancer later in her life"); HPV vaccines are safe, effective, and should prevent most HPV-associated anogenital cancers; HPV is very common and adolescents are often infected soon after sexual initiation; it is important to vaccinate patients at the recommended age (11 to 12 years) before they are exposed to HPV; it is important to complete the vaccine series; and vaccination does not lead to riskier sexual behaviors. In vaccine-hesitant parents/caregivers and AYAs, motivational interviewing and presumptive recommendations (i.e., informing parents/caregivers that vaccines are due instead of asking what the parent/caregiver thinks about vaccines) have been shown to increase vaccine acceptance.[22,23] Administering HPV vaccines at the same visit as other age-appropriate vaccines (e.g., tetanus, diphtheria, and acellular pertussis [Tdap] and meningococcal vaccines) and recommending it in the same way as other vaccines (e.g., "Now that Isaiah is 12 years old, we will be giving him three vaccines that will protect him from meningitis, cancers caused by HPV, and pertussis.") is important in maximizing acceptance and uptake. Clinicians should explain that HPV vaccines do not prevent STIs other than HPV, and that Pap testing is still recommended after vaccination. System-level strategies to improve vaccination rates include promotion of preventative health visits, vaccinating at every office visit, implementing quality improvement efforts to improve vaccination, patient reminder and recall efforts, standing orders for vaccination, and electronic health record alerts. Vaccination in alternative settings including pharmacies and schools is also effective for improving vaccination.

SUMMARY

Human papillomavirus is a virus, transmitted primarily through sexual contact, which can cause anogenital warts and both oral and anogenital cancers. With the introduction of safe and highly effective HPV vaccines, the prevalence of HPV and associated diseases have been decreasing; however, HPV vaccine uptake is suboptimal. Anogenital warts are typically diagnosed by visual inspection, and treatment regimens are classified as patient-applied or clinician-applied. Clinicians should educate patients about HPV infection, its transmission, and its clinical consequences, as well as the importance of vaccination prior to infection.

ACKNOWLEDGMENT

The authors would like to acknowledge the valuable contributions made by Dr. Shelly Ben Harush Negari to a previous edition of this chapter.

REFERENCES

1. Magalhães GM, Vieira ÉC, Garcia LC. Update on human papilloma virus—part I: epidemiology, pathogenesis, and clinical spectrum. *An Bras Dermatol*. 2021; 96(1):1–16.
2. Darragh TM, Colgan TJ, Cox JT, et al. The lower anogenital squamous terminology standardization project for HPV-associated lesions: background and consensus recommendations from the College of American Pathologists and the American Society for Colposcopy and Cervical Pathology. *Arch Pathol Lab Med*. 2012;136(10):1266–1297.
3. Chesson HW, Dunne EF, Hairi S, et al. The estimated lifetime probability of acquiring human papillomavirus in the United States. *Sex Transm Dis*. 2014;41(11):660–664.
4. Drolet M, Bénard É, Pérez N, et al. Population-level impact and herd effects following the introduction of human papillomavirus vaccination programmes: updated systemic review and meta-analysis. *Lancet*. 2019;394(10197):497–509.
5. Chaturvedi AK, Graubard BI, Broutian T, et al. Effect of prophylactic human papillomavirus (HPV) vaccination on oral HPV infections among young adults in the United States. *J Clin Oncol*. 2018;36(3):262–267.
6. El-Zein M, Ramanakumar AV, Naud P. Determinants of acquisition and clearance of human papillomavirus infection in previously unexposed young women. *Sex Transm Dis*. 2019;46(10):663–669.
7. Derkay CS, Bluher AE. Update on recurrent respiratory papillomatosis. *Otolaryngol Clin North Am*. 2019;52(4):669–679.
8. Doorbar J, Egawa N, Griffin H, et al. Human papillomavirus molecular biology and disease association. *Rev Med Virol*. 2015;25(Suppl 1):2–23.
9. Yanofsky VR, Patel RV, Goldenberg G. Genital warts: a comprehensive review. *J Clin Aesthet Dermatol*. 2012;5(6):25–36.
10. Tsakogiannis D, Gartzonika C, Levidiotou-Stefanou S, et al. Molecular approaches for HPV genotyping and HPV-DNA physical status. *Expert Rev Mol Med*. 2017; 19:e1.
11. Fontham ETH, Wolf AMD, Church TR, et al. Cervical cancer screening for individuals at average risk: 2020 guideline update from the American Cancer Society. *CA Cancer J Clin*. 2020;70(5):321–346.
12. Curry SJ, Krist AH, Owens DK, et al; US Preventive Services Task Force. Screening for cervical cancer: US Preventive Services Task Force recommendation statement. *JAMA*. 2018;320(7):674–686.
13. American College of Obstetricians and Gynecologists. *Practice advisory: updated cervical cancer screening guidelines*. Accessed October 18, 2021. https://www.acog.org/clinical/clinical-guidance/practice-advisory/articles/2021/04/updated-cervical-cancer-screening-guidelines
14. Workowski KA, Bachmann LH, Chan PA, et al. Sexually transmitted infections treatment guidelines, 2021. *MMWR Recomm Rep*. 2021;70(4):1–187.
15. Huh WK, Joura EA, Giuliano AR, et al. Final efficacy, immunogenicity, and safety analyses of a nine-valent human papillomavirus vaccine in women aged 16–26 years: a randomized, double-blind trial. *Lancet*. 2017;390(10108):2143–2159.
16. Meites E, Szilagyi PG, Chesson HW, et al. Human papillomavirus vaccination for adults: updated recommendations of the advisory committee on immunization practices. *MMWR Morb Mortal Wkly Rep*. 2019;68(32):698–702.
17. Meites E, Kempe A, Markowitz LE. Use of a 2-dose schedule for human papillomavirus vaccination—updated recommendations of the advisory committee on immunization practices. *MMWR Morb Mortal Wkly Rep*. 2016;65(49):1405–1408.
18. Ferlay J, Ervik M, Lam F, et al. *Global Cancer Observatory: Cancer Today*. International Agency for Research on Cancer; Accessed April 1, 2021. https://gco.iarc.fr/today/home
19. Data abstracted from Centers for Disease Control and Prevention webpage (https://www.cdc.gov/cancer/hpv/statistics/cases.htm, accessed April 1, 2021) which are derived from the Surveillance, Epidemiology, and End Results (SEER) Program of the National Cancer Institute (https://seer.cancer.gov/statfacts/html/cervix.html, accessed April 4, 2021).
20. Elam-Evans LD, Yankey D, Singleton JA, et al. National, regional, state, and selected local area vaccination coverage among adolescents aged 13–17 years — United States, 2019. *MMWR Morb Mortal Wkly Rep*. 2020;69(33):1109–1116.
21. Rosen BL, Shepard A, Kahn JA. US health care clinicians' knowledge, attitudes, and practices regarding human papillomavirus vaccination: a qualitative systematic review. *Acad Pediatr*. 2018;18(2S):S53–S65.
22. Dempsey AF, Pyrzanowski J, Campagna EJ, et al. Parent report of provider HPV vaccine communication strategies used during a randomized, controlled trial of a provider communication intervention. *Vaccine*. 2019;37(10):1307–1312.
23. Reno JE, Thomas J, Pyrzanowski J, et al. Examining strategies for improving healthcare providers' communication about adolescent HPV vaccination: evaluation of secondary outcomes in a randomized controlled trial. *Hum Vaccin Immunother*. 2019;15(7–8):1592–1598.

ADDITIONAL RESOURCES AND WEBSITES

Additional Resources and Websites for Clinicians:
American Cancer Society—https://www.cancer.org/health-care-professionals/hpv-vaccination-information-for-health-professionals.html
American College of Obstetricians and Gynecologists—https://www.acog.org/programs/immunization-for-women/physician-tools/human-papillomavirus-frequently-asked-questions-for-providers
Centers for Disease Control and Prevention—https://www.cdc.gov/hpv/hcp/index.html
National Foundation for Infectious Diseases—https://www.nfid.org/infectious-diseases/hpv-and-healthcare-professionals/
2021 Sexually Transmitted Infections Treatment Guidelines—https://www.cdc.gov/std/treatment-guidelines/STI-Guidelines-2021.pdf

Additional Resources and Websites for Parents/Caregivers:
American Cancer Society—https://www.cancer.org/healthy/hpv-vaccine.html
Centers for Disease Control and Prevention—https://www.cdc.gov/hpv/index.html
https://www.cdc.gov/vaccines/parents/diseases/hpv.html
Centers for Disease Control and Prevention (Spanish)—https://www.cdc.gov/hpv/parents/about-hpv-sp.html
https://www.cdc.gov/hpv/parents/vaccine/six-reasons-sp.html
https://www.cdc.gov/vaccines/parents/by-age/years-11-12-sp.html
https://www.cdc.gov/vaccines/parents/diseases/hpv-sp.html
https://www.cdc.gov/vaccines/parents/diseases/hpv-basics-color-sp.pdf
Immunization Action Coalition (Spanish)—https://www.immunize.org/catg.d/p4310-01.pdf
https://www.immunize.org/catg.d/p4250-01.pdf
Nemours Health—https://teenshealth.org/en/parents/hpv-vaccine.html?WT.ac=p-ra#catstd
https://teenshealth.org/en/parents/genital-warts.html?ref=search

Additional Resources and Websites for Adolescents and Young Adults:
American Sexual Health Association—https://www.ashasexualhealth.org/human_papilloma_virus/
Centers for Disease Control and Prevention—https://www.cdc.gov/std/hpv/stdfact-hpv.htm
Center for Young Women's Health—https://youngwomenshealth.org/2012/07/05/hpv/
https://youngwomenshealth.org/2012/07/03/hpv-vaccine/
Immunization Action Coalition (Spanish)—https://www.immunize.org/catg.d/p4251-01.pdf
Nemours Health—https://teenshealth.org/en/teens/hpv-vaccine.html?ref=search
https://teenshealth.org/en/teens/std-warts.html?ref=search#catstd

Other Sexually Transmitted Infections Including Genital Ulcers, Pediculosis, Scabies, and Molluscum

Mandakini Sadhir

Sinduja Lakkunarajah

M. Susan Jay

KEY WORDS

- Chancroid
- Emerging sexually transmitted infections (STI)
- Granuloma inguinale
- Lymphogranuloma venereum (LV)
- Molluscum
- Pubic lice
- Scabies

INTRODUCTION

Chancroid, lymphogranuloma venereum (LGV), and granuloma inguinale constitute the classic minor ulcerative sexually transmitted infections (STIs) and should be considered in the differential diagnosis of genital ulcers (see Table 67.1). In the United States, the most common causative agent of genital ulcers is the herpes simplex virus (HSV) (see Chapter 65 on HSV), followed by syphilis. Approximately 3% to 10% of these patients will have more than one infection. There is also an increased risk of human immunodeficiency virus (HIV) infection associated with these ulcerative infections.[1] Other potential STIs include scabies, pediculosis, and molluscum contagiosum. Finally, pathogens such as the Zika and hepatitis A viruses and bacteria such as *Shigella flexneri* and *Neisseria meningitidis* have been identified as sexually transmissible pathogens and should be considered by clinicians if risk factors are identified.

CHANCROID

Etiology

Chancroid is caused by the gram-negative facultative anaerobic coccobacillus, *Haemophilus ducreyi*.[4]

Epidemiology

This disease is uncommon in the United States but highly prevalent in southern, central, and eastern Africa. According to the Centers for Disease Control and Prevention (CDC), reported cases of chancroid in the United States have fallen dramatically.[5] There is concern that the reduction in cases may be due to the difficulty in culturing the causative agent. Chancroid is a known risk factor for HIV and enhances disease transmission. Co-infection with syphilis or herpes simplex may also occur.[6]

Clinical Manifestations

The incubation period is generally 3 to 10 days. Classically, chancroid presents as a tender inflammatory papule on the genitalia that becomes pustular and then ulcerates in 1 to 2 days. The characteristic ulcer is painful, soft, friable, and nonindurated with ragged undermined margins, a granulomatous base, and a foul-smelling yellow or gray, necrotic purulent exudate (Fig. 67.1). Males may present with inguinal pain or ulcers located on the prepuce, coronal sulcus, or frenulum. In females, multiple lesions may be present on the vulva, clitoris, cervix, or perianal region. Females may be asymptomatic or present with dysuria, dyspareunia, vaginal discharge, pain with defecation, and rectal bleeding. Rarely, extragenital sites may be involved (inner thighs and fingers).[7]

Painful unilateral inguinal lymphadenitis—known as a *bubo*—develops in as many as 50% of patients. Complications may result in a secondary bacterial infection leading to further ulceration, rupture, or phimosis in males.[7]

Diagnosis

Probable diagnosis of chancroid can be made using CDC criteria (Table 67.1). Accuracy of clinical diagnosis ranges from 33% to 80%. A "school of fish" is what is described on the Gram stain. Gram stain identifies about 10% of culture-positive cases and hence should not be used alone for diagnosis. Culture is the "gold standard" for diagnosis, with a sensitivity of 35% to 75% and specificity of 94% to 100%. Culture material may be obtained from the base or margin of the genital ulcers or the aspirates of buboes, although intact buboes tend to be sterile. Laboratories should be notified in advance for receipt of the specimens.[2] There are no U.S. Food and Drug Administration (FDA)-approved nucleic acid amplification tests (NAAT) for this organism, but these tests can be performed in laboratories that have developed their own NAAT and have conducted Clinical Laboratory Improvement Amendment (CLIA) verification studies on specimens obtained from genital sites.[2]

Treatment

Treatment is outlined in Table 67.2.

Other Management Considerations

Clinical improvement should be seen within 3 to 7 days. Failure to improve should raise the possibility of an incorrect diagnosis or co-infection with another STI such as HIV. Large ulcers may require more than 2 weeks to resolve; fluctuant lymphadenopathy heals even more slowly. Adenopathy may progress to fluctuation despite successful therapy and does not represent treatment failure.

LYMPHOGRANULOMA VENEREUM

Etiology

Lymphogranuloma venereum is caused by the obligate intracellular organism *Chlamydia trachomatis*. Chlamydia has 18 serovars associated with disease; serovars L_1, L_2, and L_3 cause LGV. Lymphogranuloma venereum strains can cause a systemic infection that, if untreated, can lead to colorectal fistulas and strictures and

TABLE 67.1

Differential Diagnosis of Genital Ulcers[1-3]

Infection	Clinical Manifestation	Diagnosis

Chancroid
Cause: *Haemophilus ducreyi*
	• Painful, shallow, friable, nonindurated genital ulcer with ragged undermined margins, granulomatous base, and foul-smelling yellow or gray, necrotic purulent exudate
	• Painful inguinal adenopathy known as "buboes" present
		• Culture of lesion (not widely available) or positive nucleic acid amplification test for *H. ducreyi*
		• CDC criteria for "probable" diagnosis (all four need to be present):
		  a. ≥1 painful genital ulcer(s)
		  b. No evidence of syphilis infection on dark-field examination or serologic test performed at least 7–14 d after onset of ulcer
		  c. Typical clinical presentation of a genital ulcer and regional lymphadenopathy
		  d. Negative HSV-1 or HSV-2 NAAT or negative HSV culture of ulcer exudate or fluid

Lymphogranuloma venereum Cause: *Chlamydia trachomatis*	• Painful inguinal and/or femoral lymphadenopathy. "Groove" sign is pathognomonic • Self-limited genital ulcer or papule at site of inoculation	Genital lesion swab or lymph node aspirate tested using NAATs, immunofluorescence
Granuloma inguinale Cause: *Klebsiella granulomatis*	• Painless, slowly progressive ulcerative lesions on genitals or perineum; bleed easily on contact • Regional lymphadenopathy uncommon	Identification of Donovan bodies within histiocytes of granulation tissue smears or biopsy specimens
Syphilis Cause: *Treponema pallidum*	• Primary chancre: Painless ulcer with indurated raised border and "punched out" appearance • Regional lymphadenopathy may occur	• Screen: Nontreponemal tests (RPR, VDRL) • Confirm: Treponemal tests (FTA-ABS or TPPA) • Dark-field microscopy showing spirochetes
Genital herpes Cause: HSV 1 and 2	• Painful vesicular lesions developing into ulcers • Constitutional symptoms present in primary infection	Viral culture or PCR for HSV DNA
Nonsexually transmitted genital ulcers	• Painful, well-demarcated ulcer • Constitutional symptoms may be present if viral in etiology (CMV, EBV)	Negative for HSV or other STIs

CDC, Centers for Disease Control and Prevention; CMV, cytomegalovirus; EBV, Epstein–Barr virus; FTA-ABS, fluorescent treponemal antibody-absorbed; HSV, herpes simplex virus; NAAT, nucleic acid amplification tests; PCR, polymerase chain reaction; RPR, rapid plasma reagin; STI, sexually transmitted infection; TPPA, treponema pallidum particle agglutination; VDRL, venereal diseases research laboratory.

chronic pain.[2,8] These lesions can become superinfected with other STIs or pathogens.

Epidemiology

Lymphogranuloma venereum is endemic in parts of Africa, India, South America, and the Caribbean. Outbreaks have been reported in Europe among men with HIV infection who have sex with men (MSM).[9]

Clinical Manifestations

The incubation period is 3 to 30 days (usually 7 to 12). Infection occurs in three stages:

a. *Primary stage*: The initial lesion begins as a small, painless papule or pustule at the site of inoculation that can erode into an asymptomatic herpetiform ulcer that often heals without scarring within a week. Lesions are typically found on the penis, urethral glans, and scrotum in males and on the vulva, vaginal wall, fourchette, and cervix in females. Oral ulcers can occur.[2] Rectal lesions occur in both sexes from receptive anal intercourse and can be associated with diarrhea, rectal discharge, and tenesmus; however, rectal LGV can be asymptomatic.[2] Mucopurulent cervicitis and urethritis may also occur. Women usually have primary involvement of the rectum, vagina, and cervix.

b. *Secondary or inguinal stage:* This stage typically occurs 2 to 6 weeks after the appearance of the primary lesion and involves painful inflammation of the inguinal and femoral lymph nodes. Inguinal adenopathy is unilateral in 70% of cases and is more common in males (Fig. 67.2). The "groove" sign is the result of enlarged inguinal nodes above and femoral nodes below Poupart ligament; this is considered pathognomonic for LGV (Fig. 67.3). Nodes can become matted and fluctuant and produce the characteristic bubo.[8] Buboes may rupture in one-third of patients or develop into hard, nonsuppurative masses. Most buboes eventually heal, but some will form sinus

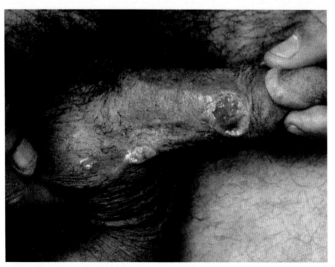

FIGURE 67.1 The lesions in chancroid are painful and more irregular appearing than in syphilis. (From Craft N, Taylor E, Tumeh PC, et al. *VisualDx: Essential Adult Dermatology*. Lippincott Williams & Wilkins; 2010.)

TABLE 67.2
Treatment of Chancroid[2,3,7]

CDC Recommended Treatments	Other Management Considerations	Follow-Up
Azithromycin 1 g orally in a single dose or Ceftriaxone 250 mg IM in a single dose or Ciprofloxacin 500 mg orally twice daily × 3 d or Erythromycin base 500 mg orally 3 times daily × 7 d	Persons with HIV infection: May require longer or repeated treatment due to treatment failures and slow healing. Use single-dose therapies only when close follow-up assured Pregnancy/lactation: Ciprofloxacin contraindicated Uncircumcised males: Higher treatment failure rates and slower healing especially if ulcers under foreskin Sex partners: Examine and treat sex partners who had sexual contact with patient in the 10 d preceding the patient's onset of symptoms	Within 3–7 d of start of therapy Weekly follow-up until resolution of lesions and symptoms If no improvement: • test for other STIs including HIV and treat if positive • review adherence to treatment Test for HIV and syphilis at the time of diagnosis and repeat testing in 3 months if initial tests were negative. Consider offering more frequent testing and pre-exposure prophylaxis (PrEP) to those at an increased risk for HIV infection

Buboes (fluctuant adenopathy): Treat by aspiration for symptomatic relief and to prevent rupture or by incision and drainage with wound packing (more definitive).
Clinical resolution of fluctuant lymphadenopathy is slower than that of ulcers.
CDC, Centers for Disease Control and Prevention; HIV, human immunodeficiency virus; STI, sexually transmitted infection.

tracts. Bubonic relapse occurs in 20% of untreated cases. Constitutional symptoms may occur with the inguinal buboes and be associated with systemic spread of chlamydia, leading to arthritis, hepatitis, and pneumonitis.

c. *Tertiary or genito-anorectal syndrome (uncommon):* This stage occurs more often in females and in males who have receptive anal intercourse.[10] Patients initially develop symptoms of proctocolitis (anal pruritus, rectal discharge, rectal pain, tenesmus, and fever). Subsequent manifestations include perirectal abscesses, rectovaginal and anorectal fistulas, rectal strictures, and rectal stenosis. Chronic untreated LGV can lead to repetitive scarring and fistulous tract formation in the genital region.

Diagnosis

Diagnosis of LGV is definitively made only with polymerase chain reaction (PCR)-based genotyping, but this test is not widely available, and results would not be available in a timely manner. Hence, the diagnosis is usually based on clinical findings and "a positive" NAAT for *C. trachomatis* (which does not identify LGV serovars specifically) from symptomatic anatomic sites. If a patient presents with proctocolitis, they should be tested for chlamydia with a NAAT obtained from a rectal specimen.[2]

Treatment

Patients with a clinical syndrome consistent with LGV should be treated presumptively for LGV before the results of NAAT are known (see **Table 67.3**).

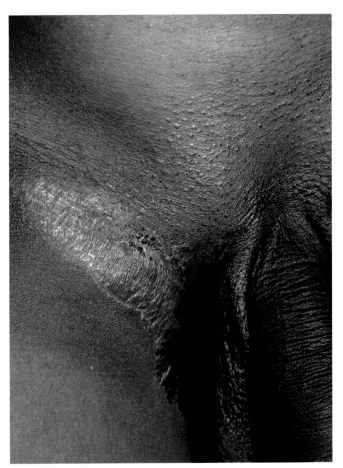

FIGURE 67.3 Lymphogranuloma venereum with groove sign of swelling above and below the inguinal fold. (From Lugo-Somolinos A, McKinley-Grant L, Goldsmith LA, et al. *VisualDx: Essential Dermatology in Pigmented Skin*. Lippincott Williams & Wilkins; 2011.)

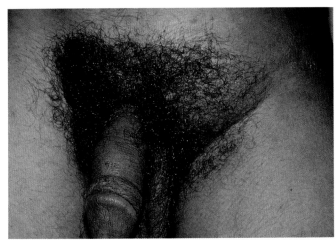

FIGURE 67.2 Lymphogranuloma venereum. Painful inguinal lymphadenopathy in a male infected with *Chlamydia trachomatis*. (Image from Rubin E, Farber JL. *Pathology*. 3rd ed. Lippincott Williams & Wilkins; 1999.)

XIII

TABLE 67.3

Treatment of Lymphogranuloma Venereum (LGV)[2,11]

CDC Recommended Treatment	Alternative Treatments	Other Management Considerations	Follow-Up
Doxycycline 100 mg orally twice daily × 21 d	Azithromycin 1 g orally once weekly for 3 wks or Erythromycin base 500 mg orally 4 times a day for 21 d	Persons with HIV infection: May require prolonged treatment due to delayed resolution of symptoms Pregnancy/lactation: Use erythromycin first line; azithromycin may be used as an alternative although safety and efficacy data are lacking. Avoid using doxycycline during the 2nd and 3rd trimesters Sexual Contacts: Examine, test, and treat contacts in the 60 d prior to onset of patient's symptoms. For asymptomatic contacts, use a chlamydia regimen (doxycycline 100 mg orally twice daily × 7 d)	Monitor until signs and symptoms resolve Test for other STIs, especially HIV, gonorrhea, and syphilis

CDC, Centers for Disease Control and Prevention; HIV, human immunodeficiency virus; STI, sexually transmitted infection.

GRANULOMA INGUINALE

Etiology

Granuloma inguinale, or Donovanosis, is caused by *Klebsiella granulomatis*, an intracellular gram-negative bacillus.[4]

Epidemiology

Granuloma inguinale is considered endemic in Papua, New Guinea, southeast India, South Africa, central Australia, Brazil, and the Caribbean. It is extremely rare in the United States and Western Europe.[2,8] It is transmitted primarily through sexual contact; autoinoculation can also lead to spread of the disease.

Clinical Manifestations

Infection can result in granulomatous and destructive ulcers on the genital, inguinal, and perineal skin and should be included in the differential diagnosis of chronic progressive genital ulcers. Lesions are typically localized without accompanying constitutional symptoms. The genital area is involved in 90% of cases and the inguinal area in the remainder. Extragenital lesions occur in 6% of cases secondary to autoinoculation. Lesions are more common in uncircumcised males with poor genital hygiene, and occur on the coronal sulcus, prepuce, frenulum, glans penis, and anus. In females, the labia minora and fourchette are commonly affected. Infection of the cervix and upper genital tract can mimic cervical cancer. The ulcerovegetative or ulcerogranulomatous form is the most common clinical presentation.[8] It produces large, extensive, nonindurated ulcerations with beefy-red, highly vascular, and friable granulation tissue (Fig. 67.4). True inguinal lymphadenopathy does not occur with granuloma inguinale unless bacterial superinfection develops. However, subcutaneous granulomas near the inguinal nodes (pseudobuboes) can mimic inguinal enlargement.

Diagnosis

The organism is difficult to culture. Tissue smears or crush biopsies of the lesions are used to diagnose granuloma inguinale. Tissue smears are obtained by firmly rolling a cotton swab across the base of a nonbleeding ulcer and then across a slide. "Crush biopsies" involve removing tissue from the advancing surface of the ulcer and "crushing" or smearing the specimen between two slides. Giemsa or Wright stain is used to identify the dark-staining, safety pin–shaped intracytoplasmic inclusion bodies within large mononuclear cells or histiocytes known as donovan bodies.[8]

Treatment

Treatment is outlined in **Table 67.4**. If treatment is successful, there will be symptomatic improvement within 3 days and objectively within 7 days.

PEDICULOSIS AND SCABIES

Pediculosis and scabies are ubiquitous and highly contagious parasitic skin infections that occur both in individuals and in clusters of individuals such as school children, homeless people, hospital staff, and immunocompromised individuals.

Pediculosis Pubis

Etiology

Pediculosis pubis (pubic lice) is caused by the pubic or crab louse, *Pthirus pubis*, an obligate human parasite (Fig. 67.5).

Epidemiology

1. Transmission: Infestations are most common among adolescents and young adults (AYAs). Transmission occurs as a result of close bodily contact, primarily through sexual contact. Condoms do not prevent transmission, and infestations frequently coexist with other STIs.[14] Pediculosis pubis can be transmitted by infected clothing, towels, and bedding. There is no current evidence linking ectoparasites to transmission of HIV.

2. Life cycle: The female crab louse lives for 3 to 4 weeks. Each day, it lays about three nits that are cemented firmly to the hair shaft in areas of dense hair terminals. The nits hatch in 6 to 8 days as nymphs and mature into adult lice in 10 to 14

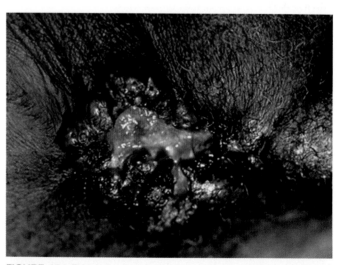

FIGURE 67.4 This perianal ulceration with heaped-up borders is typical of granuloma inguinale (Donovanosis). (Courtesy of Jack Mosley. In: Edwards L, Lynch PJ, eds. *Genital Dermatology Atlas.* 2nd ed. Lippincott Williams & Wilkins; 2010.)

TABLE 67.4

Treatment of Granuloma Inguinale[2,12,13]

CDC Recommended Treatment	Alternative Treatments	Other Management Considerations	Follow-Up
Azithromycin 1 g orally once per week or 500 mg daily for at least 3 wks and until all lesions have completely healed[a]	Use all medications below for at least 3 wks and until all lesions healed Doxycycline 100 mg orally twice a day[a] or Erythromycin base 500 mg orally 4 times daily[a] or Trimethoprim-sulfamethoxazole one double-strength (160 mg/800 mg) tablet orally twice daily[a]	Persons with HIV infection: Should be treated the same as those without HIV Pregnancy/lactation: Erythromycin or azithromycin; Avoid doxycycline during the 2nd and 3rd trimester Sexual contacts: Examine and offer treatment to all contacts exposed 60 d prior to the onset of symptoms in the infected partner	Follow until resolution of all lesions Test for other STIs, including gonorrhea, chlamydia, herpes, syphilis, HIV, and hepatitis B if not clinically improving

CDC, Centers for Disease Control and Prevention; HIV, human immunodeficiency virus; STI, sexually transmitted infection.
[a]Consider adding another antibiotic if no improvement within the first few days of initial therapy.

days. The parasite spends its life on skin and feeds on blood. It dies approximately 24 hours after being off its human host; lower environmental temperatures can prolong survival. Adult lice can live on the skin for approximately 1 month.

Clinical Manifestations

Symptoms occur 2 or more weeks after contact and occur more rapidly with subsequent infections. Once symptoms are present, the infection is usually well established. Common areas of infection include hair on the chest, axilla, abdomen, thighs, genitals, and occasionally the male beard. It has even been noted on eyelashes and scalp hair. Pruritus, the main symptom, is probably a hypersensitivity reaction to the louse bite. Small blue spots known as maculae ceruleae may appear on the thighs and abdomen after prolonged infestations and represent feeding sites of the louse.

Diagnosis

Diagnosis of pediculosis pubis is made by direct visualization of lice and/or nits (eggs) on the hair shafts (Fig. 67.6). Lice appear as tiny, tan to grayish-white oval insects. Nits can be seen as small yellowish-white, glistening oval kernels attached to hair shafts. Dermoscopic examination is used to confirm the presence of lice and nits in vivo.

Treatment

Pubic lice do not transmit systemic disease. The goals of treatment are symptomatic relief, prevention of reinfestation and transmission, as well as getting rid of the active infection. Topical treatments are more effective when applied to dry hair so as to decrease percutaneous absorption. Embryos may survive initial treatment, requiring a second treatment in 7 to 10 days (Table 67.5).

Additional Management Considerations[15]

1. Clothing or bed linens worn or used within 2 days of diagnosis should be machine washed at 130 °F to 140 °F and machine dried using the hot cycle for at least 20 minutes, or dry-cleaned. Clothing that cannot be decontaminated as above should be bagged for at least 72 hours (preferentially for 2 weeks) to allow newly hatched lice to die. Fumigation is not necessary.
2. Residual nits should be removed with a fine comb. A solution of vinegar and water can be used to loosen them.
3. Patients with pediculosis pubis should be evaluated for syphilis, gonorrhea, chlamydia, and HIV. All sexual contacts within the past month should be treated and sexual contact avoided until both patient and partner(s) are reevaluated for persistent infection.

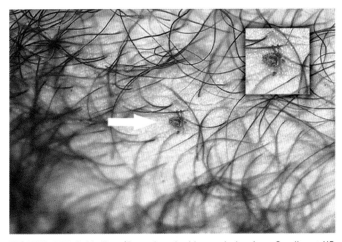

FIGURE 67.5 Pubic lice. (Reproduced with permission from Goodheart HP. *Goodheart's Photoguide of Common Skin Disorders.* 4th ed. Lippincott Williams & Wilkins; 2015.)

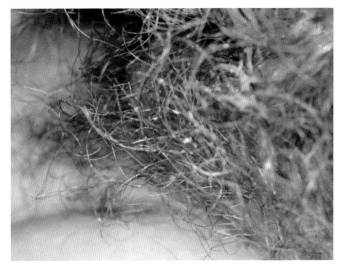

FIGURE 67.6 Multiple nits on pubic hairs suggestive of pubic lice infestation. (From Craft N, Taylor E, Tumeh PC, et al. *VisualDx: Essential Adult Dermatology.* Lippincott Williams & Wilkins; 2010.)

XIII

TABLE 67.5

Treatment of Pediculosis[6,15]

Drug	Application Instructions/Dosing	Warnings/Precaution	Other
CDC Recommended Regimens			
Permethrin 1% cream rinse[a]	Apply to affected areas and wash off after 10 min. Avoid eyes	Pruritus, erythema, burning, and stinging	Can be used in pregnancy
Pyrethrins with piperonyl butoxide[a]	Apply to affected areas and wash off after 10 min. Avoid eyes	Pruritus, burning, and stinging	Can be used in pregnancy
CDC Alternative Regimens			
Malathion 0.5% lotion	Apply to affected areas for 8–12 h and wash off	Bad odor, potentially flammable, toxic if ingested; avoid eyes	FDA approved only for treatment of head lice
Ivermectin	250 mcg/kg orally, repeat in 7–14 d	Take on an empty stomach. Human data suggest low risk in pregnancy and probably compatible with breastfeeding. Inadequate safety data for use in children <15 kg. Potential for neurotoxicity; useful in multiple parasitic infections; avoid eyes	Not FDA-approved treatment

[a]After washing the cream or product off, fingers, a nit comb or tweezers should be used to remove the nits.
CDC, Centers for Disease Control and Prevention; FDA, U.S. Food and Drug Administration.

4. Persons with HIV infection: Treat the same as for noninfected AYAs.
5. Pediculosis of eyelashes: Apply occlusive ophthalmic-grade petrolatum ointment (prescription only) to the eyelid margins two to four times a day for 10 days to smother lice and nits.

Scabies

Etiology

Scabies is a highly contagious, ectoparasitic infection caused by *Sarcoptes scabiei* var *hominis*, a small mite; it is host specific to humans.

Epidemiology

1. Transmission: The mite is transmitted by prolonged (10 to 20 minute) skin-to-skin contact.[16] Sexual transmission is common, as is nonsexual spread in family groups. Transmission can occur before the patient is symptomatic and throughout the infestation as long as it remains untreated. Scabies is frequently found in institutional settings.
2. Life cycle: Female mites burrow into the epidermal layer of the skin laying two to four eggs per day for 4 to 5 weeks. The adult female then dies within the burrow. After 3 to 5 days, the eggs hatch, and the larvae return to the skin surface to mature in 10 to 17 days. Only 10% of eggs become adults.[17] Away from the host, human mites have been shown to survive up to 72 hours.

Clinical Manifestations

Symptoms occur 3 to 6 weeks after first exposure and 1 to 4 days after reexposure, resulting in an intensely pruritic, papular eruption associated with eczematous lesions and areas of excoriation (Fig. 67.7).[16] Pruritus is often worse at night or after a hot bath and is caused by a cell-mediated immune reaction to the mite and its by-products. Burrows (Fig. 67.8), if seen, appear as short wavy lines a few millimeters to 1 cm in length. Skin lesions are typically seen between finger webs, on the flexor surfaces of the wrists, in the axillary folds, and on the nipples, waist, umbilicus, buttocks, thighs, knees, ankles, and genital areas. Scabies usually spare the face, neck, and scalp except in children.

Crusted or Norwegian scabies is a rare and aggressive form of scabies found in immunodeficient, debilitated, or malnourished patients. This infection is characterized by an extremely large number of mites that leads to a concomitant inflammatory and hyperkeratotic reaction. This is due to the host's immune system inability to control the mite replication. The thick, crusted scales are highly contagious. Treatment failures occur frequently, and septicemia is a common complication.

Scabies can lead to secondary staphylococcal or streptococcal infections (impetigo, ecthyma, paronychia, and furunculosis).[16] In countries where scabies is seen in large numbers, there has been an association with poststreptococcal glomerulonephritis and chronic kidney disease as well as rheumatic fever and heart disease.[18]

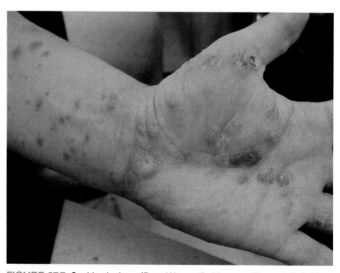

FIGURE 67.7 Scabies lesions. (From Werner R. *Massage Therapist's Guide to Pathology.* 5th ed. Lippincott Williams & Wilkins; 2012.)

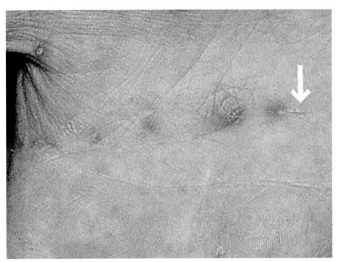

FIGURE 67.8 Burrow of scabies—a person with scabies has intense itching. Skin lesions include small papules, pustules, lichenified areas, and excoriations. With a magnifying lens, look for the burrow of the mite that causes it. A burrow is a minute, slightly raised tunnel in the epidermis and is commonly found on the finger webs and on the sides of the fingers. It looks like a short (5 to 15 mm), linear or curved, gray line and may end in a tiny vesicle. (From Goodheart HP. *Goodheart's Photoguide of Common Skin Disorders*. 4th ed. Lippincott Williams & Wilkins, 2015.)

Diagnosis

1. Diagnosis is usually made on the basis of the distribution of lesions and a history of intense itching and similar symptoms in family members or sexual partners. Definitive diagnosis requires microscopic identification of mites, eggs, or feces from skin scrapings of papules or burrows using videodermatoscopy, videomicroscopy, or dermoscopy. These modalities have a higher sensitivity and specificity when used by an experienced operator.[2] Burrows are virtually pathognomonic for human scabies, but are often difficult to demonstrate.

2. Isolation of mite: Best results are obtained using a no. 15 scalpel blade to scrape the leading edge of an intact burrow or affected areas under the fingernails. Visibility of burrows can be enhanced by applying mineral or immersion oil, saline, or ink to the skin. Scrapings are examined under oil or saline on low power for the presence of eggs, feces, or mites. Alternately, punch or shave biopsies of inflamed lesions can be used with varying results. In resource-poor areas, handheld dermatoscopes and adhesive tape (placed over lesions, pulled off rapidly, and transferred to a slide) have been used to identify mites and burrows.[19,20]

Treatment

Treatment is outlined in **Table 67.6**.

Additional Management Considerations[2,7,17]

1. Environmental control: Bedding and clothing worn during the 4 days preceding treatment should be machine washed, dried using the hot cycle, dry-cleaned, or set aside in a sealed plastic bag for at least 72 hours. Fumigation is not necessary.
2. Follow-up: Pruritus may persist for up to 2 weeks after treatment. Symptoms persisting longer may be due to medication resistance, incorrect scabicidal application, poor skin penetration in crusted scabies, reinfection, or other allergies. Consideration can be given to retreatment with a different regimen after 1 to 2 weeks, although some specialists recommend this only with confirmation of live mites.
3. Sex partners as well as close personal and household contacts from within the previous month should be treated.
4. Persons with HIV infection: Treat the same as noninfected individuals. However, persons with HIV infection are at increased risk for crusted scabies, which should be managed in consultation with a specialist.
5. Crusted scabies: Requires combination treatment with oral ivermectin plus a topical scabicide (5% permethrin cream or 25% benzyl benzoate). An individual may benefit from additional doses of ivermectin on days 22 and 29 of therapy if the case is severe.[2]

TABLE 67.6
Treatment of Scabies[2,20,21]

Medication	Application/Dosing	Warnings/Precautions	Other
CDC Recommended Regimens			
Permethrin cream 5%	Apply neck down and wash off after 8–14 h, including fingernails and skin folds. Can apply at bedtime and wash off in AM.	Pruritus, Erythema, Burning and stinging	FDA approved for use in pregnant and lactating females and children ≥2 y of age
Ivermectin	200 mcg/kg orally, repeat in 2 wks	Not for use with crusted scabies	Not FDA approved, safety not established in pregnant or lactating females. Consider for use in epidemics
CDC Alternative Regimens			
Lindane 1% (infants and young children aged <10 y should not be treated with lindane)	Apply 1 oz of lotion or 30 g of cream in thin layer from neck down and wash off after 8 h, including web spaces and beneath nails	Neurotoxic. Reports of aplastic anemia. Do not apply after bathing due to absorption, do not use with extensive dermatitis, seizure disorders, or in pregnant or lactating females	Resistance has been reported. Only use when recommended treatments fail or are not tolerated

CDC, Centers for Disease Control and Prevention; FDA, U.S. Food and Drug Administration.

MOLLUSCUM CONTAGIOSUM

Etiology

Molluscum contagiosum is caused by a large double-stranded DNA virus of the genus *Molluscipoxvirus* in the family *Poxviridae*.

Epidemiology

Humans appear to be the only known host. Transmission occurs by direct person-to-person contact, fomites, or autoinoculation. Sexual contact is the most common form of transmission in AYAs. Activities such as swimming may be associated with disease spread through use of contaminated fomites. Individuals with atopic dermatitis may be at increased risk for infection.[22,23]

Clinical Manifestations

The incubation period varies from 2 weeks to 6 months. Lesions commonly occur on the face, trunk, and extremities. In sexually active AYAs, the lesions are commonly seen on the genitals, abdomen, and inner thighs. These may be more widespread in immunocompromised individuals.[4] Lesions present as smooth, firm, dome-shaped, flesh-colored, and semitranslucent papules with central umbilication (Fig. 67.9). Immunocompetent hosts typically have fewer than 20 lesions that are 2 to 5 mm in diameter. Persons with HIV infection and immunocompromised patients may develop hundreds of lesions that may occur in clusters (Fig. 67.10) or can present with "giant molluscum" up to 15 mm in diameter that are difficult to eradicate and are easily spread. Most lesions are asymptomatic; however, 10% of patients may have an encircling eczematoid reaction.[4]

Diagnosis

The clinical appearance of the lesion is usually diagnostic. Wright or Giemsa staining of the caseous material within the core demonstrates intracytoplasmic inclusion bodies known as molluscum bodies.

Treatment

Molluscum contagiosum has a self-limiting course in immunocompetent individuals. Lesions usually resolve in 2 to 6 months, but untreated infections may last for 12 months and even up to 4 years. Treatment may be indicated to prevent spread of disease via autoinoculation and further transmission in sexually active individuals. Immunocompromised individuals are also at greater risk of

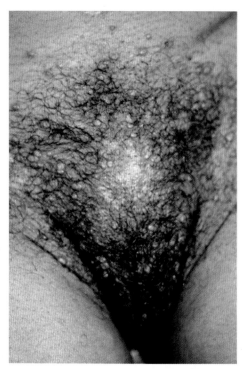

FIGURE 67.10 Molluscum contagiosum in a female with human immunodeficiency virus infection: typical umbilicated papules are shown. (From Kroumpouzos G. *Text Atlas of Obstetric Dermatology*. Lippincott Williams & Wilkins; 2013.)

secondary inflammation and bacterial infection. Currently, treatment for molluscum is controversial but, the overall opinion is that those with extensive disease or have cosmetic complaints should be treated.[24] Various treatment options are described in **Table 67.7**. When lesions are not resolving, a consultation to dermatology is indicated.

Persons With Human Immunodeficiency Virus Infection/ Immunosuppressed Patients

Molluscum contagiosum is considered an opportunistic infection in HIV disease and as a marker for advanced infection. Persons with HIV infection have high treatment failure rates with almost all standard therapies. The antiviral agent cidofovir used topically or systemically has been shown to be beneficial. Other experimental treatments using photodynamic, electron beam, and contact immunotherapy with diphencyprone have shown some improvement in persons with HIV infection. Interferon α has been used with success in immunocompromised individuals.[24]

FOLLOW-UP

Patients should watch for the development of new lesions after several weeks that may have been incubating at the time of the initial treatment. Patients should refrain from sharing clothing or towels with others. Lesions should be kept clean and covered with clothing or watertight bandages, especially before participating in contact sports or sharing equipment (swimming pools).

EMERGING SEXUALLY TRANSMITTED INFECTIONS

As sexual behaviors continue to evolve and travel is becoming more common, infections not typically associated with sexual activity are becoming more prevalent. A careful history that includes both a detailed travel and sexual history becomes more important when obvious causes or routes of infection are not evident. Examples of these "nonclassic" STIs include enteric infections like hepatitis

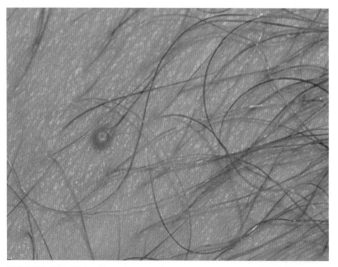

FIGURE 67.9 This skin-colored, shiny papule with a central dell is typical of molluscum contagiosum. (From Edwards L, Lynch PJ. *Genital Dermatology Atlas*. 3rd ed. Lippincott Williams & Wilkins, 2017.)

TABLE 67.7

Treatment of Molluscum Contagiosum[24,25]

	Method	Side Effects	Comments
Mechanical			
Curettage/needle extraction	Lesions scraped away after using topical anesthetic	Pain, bleeding, scarring	• Works best when there are few lesions • Safe in pregnancy
Cryotherapy	Liquid N_2 applied for 10–20 s in 2 freeze–thaw cycles. Repeat in 1 wk as needed	Pain, blistering, scarring, hyper- or hypopigmentation	• Effective and preferred for large single or few lesions
Pulse dye laser (585 nm)	Single pulse to each lesion after topical anesthetic. May repeat in 2–3 wks if needed	Minimal pain, transient hyperpigmentation	Option for recalcitrant lesions
Chemical			
Trichloroacetic acid (TCA) (100%)	Applied to the lesion(s) once weekly for 4–6 wks	Mild pain, irritation, and scarring	• Safe in pregnancy • Can be used in recalcitrant lesions
Cantharidin (0.7%)	Applied sparingly to lesion(s) and washed off in 4 h (2–6 h). May be repeated in 2–4 wks	Pain, blistering	• Not FDA approved • Not recommended for use on face or genitalia
Podophyllotoxin (0.5%)	Apply twice daily for 3 d, wait 4 d, and repeat weekly up to 4 wks	Erythema, pruritus, irritation, inflammation	
Retin A (0.025%, 0.05%, or 0.1%)	Apply 1–2 times daily for 4 wks	Mild erythema, irritation	• Data limited to case reports • Not for use in pregnancy
Potassium hydroxide aqueous solution (5–10%)[17]	Applied with a cotton swab twice daily until lesions cleared	Erythema, stinging, hyper- or hypopigmentation	
Salicylic acid gel (12%)	Apply to each lesion 1–2 times a week until cleared	Stinging	
Immunomodulators			
Topical 5% imiquimod	Apply 3 times/wk for 8 h (overnight), wash off in the AM. Use for 4–12 wks	Erythema, pain, itching, burning sensation, blistering, pigmentary changes	Not for use in pregnancy
Intralesional *Candida* antigen injection	0.2–0.3 mL injected directly into lesion or diluted at 50% with lidocaine every 3 wks	Pain	Single study reported with 93% response rate
Oral cimetidine	Prescribe dose at 25–40 mg/kg/d		More effective in nonfacial lesions

FDA, U.S. Food and Drug Administration.

A virus or Shigella, and newly identified infections noted to be associated with sexual contact such as the Zika virus.[26] The first reported outbreak of the Zika virus was in 2007.[27] Reports in 2013 demonstrated that the virus was detectable in the semen and urine of a male patient and hence could be sexually transmitted. In 2015, *N. meningitidis* became a concern as a nonclassic STI due to a large outbreak of urethritis due to this organism at a U.S. clinic.[26] Outbreaks involving hepatitis A and Shigella were most commonly seen in MSM. In certain populations (e.g., persons with HIV infection), hepatitis A vaccine immunity may wane over time, placing individuals at increased risk if exposed.[26] (See Chapters 35 and 36.)

 SUMMARY

There are a number of uncommon STIs that clinicians need to consider when AYAs present with genital lesions/ulcers. Eliciting detailed information about recent travel and sexual behaviors may provide important diagnostic clues for STIs caused by the hepatitis A and Zika viruses as well as Shigella and *N. meningitidis*. While

treatment is key to alleviating symptoms, patients should be counseled that, despite adherence to treatment, significant time may be required for lesions to resolve fully.

 ACKNOWLEDGMENT

We would like to acknowledge Dr. Wendi Ehrman for her contributions to previous editions of this chapter.

REFERENCES

1. Cohen MS, Council OD, Chen JS. Sexually transmitted infections and HIV in the era of antiretroviral treatment and prevention: the biologic basis for epidemiologic synergy. *J Int AIDS Soc*. 2019;22(suppl 6):e25355.
2. Workowski KA, Bachmann LH, Chan PA, et al. Sexually transmitted infections treatment guidelines, 2021. *MMWR Recomm Rep*. 2021;70(4):1–187.
3. Kemp M, Christensen JJ, Lautenschlager S, et al. European guideline for the management of chancroid, 2011. *Int J STD AIDS*. 2011;22(5):241–244.
4. Committee on Infectious Diseases, American Academy of Pediatrics. Chancroid and cutaneous ulcers. In: Kimberlin DW, Barnett ED, Lynfield R, et al., eds. *Red Book: 2021 Report of the Committee on Infectious Diseases*. American Academy of Pediatrics; 2021.
5. Division of STD prevention, National Center for HIV/AIDS, Viral Hepatitis, STD, and TB Prevention, Centers for Disease Control and Prevention. Accessed April 6, 2021. https://www.cdc.gov/std/treatment-guidelines/chancroid.htm

6. Mookerjee AL, Newell GC. Chancroid. In: Lebwohl M, Heymann WR, Berth-Jones J, et al., eds. *Treatment of Skin Disease: Comprehensive Therapeutic Strategies*. 4th ed. Saunders; 2014:133–134.

7. Roett MA, Mayor MT, Uduhiri KA. Diagnosis and management of genital ulcers. *Am Fam Physician*. 2012;85(3):254–262.

8. Edwards L, Lynch PJ, Neill SM. *Genital Dermatology Atlas*. 2nd ed. Lippincott Williams & Wilkins; 2011.

9. Haar K, Spiteri G, Sfetcu O, et al. P3.136 epidemic of lymphogranuloma venereum (LGV) in Europe. *Sex Transm Infect*. 2013;89(suppl 1):A190.

10. Ceovic R, Gulin SJ. Lymphogranuloma venereum: diagnostic and treatment challenges. *Infect Drug Resist*. 2015;8:39–47.

11. Pereira FA. Lymphogranuloma venereum. In: Lebwohl M, Heymann WR, Berth-Jones J, et al., eds. *Treatment of Skin Disease: Comprehensive Therapeutic Strategies*. 4th ed. Saunders; 2014:428–429.

12. Guidry JA, Rosen T. Granuloma inguinale. In: Lebwohl M, Heymann WR, Berth-Jones J, et al., eds. *Treatment of Skin Disease: Comprehensive Therapeutic Strategies*. 4th ed. Saunders; 2014:286–287.

13. O'Farrell N, Moi H. 2016 European guideline on donovanosis. *Int J STD AIDS*. 2016;27(8):605–607.

14. Salavastru CM, Chosidow O, Janier M, et al. European guidelines for the management of pediculosis pubis. *J Eur Acad Dermatol Venereol*. 2017;31(9):1425–1428.

15. Centers for Disease Control and Prevention. Parasites. Accessed February 12, 2021. https://www.cdc.gov/parasites/lice/pubic/health_professionals/index.html

16. Hay RJ, Steer AC, Engelman D, et al. Scabies in the developing world—its prevalence, complications, and management. *Clin Microbiol Infect*. 2012;18(4):313–323.

17. Centers for Disease Control and Prevention. Parasites-scabies. Accessed February 12, 2021. https://www.cdc.gov/parasites/scabies/biology.html

18. Chung SD, Wang KH, Huang CC, et al. Scabies increased the risk of chronic kidney disease: a 5-year follow-up study. *J Eur Acad Dermatol Venereol*. 2014;28(3):286–292.

19. Walter B, Heukelbach J, Fengler G, et al. Comparison of dermoscopy, skin scraping, and the adhesive tape test for the diagnosis of scabies in a resource-poor setting. *Arch Dermatol*. 2011;147(4):468–473.

20. Gunning K, Pippitt K, Kiraly B, et al. Pediculosis and scabies: treatment update. *Am Fam Physician*. 2012;86(6):535–541.

21. Strong M, Johnstone P. Cochrane review: interventions for treating scabies. *Evid-Based Child Health*. 2011;6(6):1790–1862.

22. Chen X, Anstey AV, Bugert JJ. Molluscum contagiosum virus infection. *Lancet Infect Dis*. 2013;13(10):877–888.

23. Olsen JR, Gallacher J, Piguet V, et al. Epidemiology of molluscum contagiosum in children: a systematic review. *Fam Pract*. 2014;31(2):130–136.

24. Meza-Romero R, Navarrete-Dechent C, Downey C. Molluscum contagiosum: an update and review of new perspectives in etiology, diagnosis, and treatment. *Clin Cosmet Investig Dermatol*. 2019;12:373–381.

25. Enns LL, Evans MS. Intralesional immunotherapy with candida antigen for the treatment of molluscum contagiosum in children. *Pediatr Dermatol*. 2011;28(3):254–258.

26. Williamson DA, Chen MY. Emerging and reemerging sexually transmitted infections. *N Engl J Med*. 2020;382(21):2023–2032.

27. World Health Organization. *Zika virus*. Accessed January 07, 2021. https://www.who.int/news-room/fact-sheets/detail/zika-virus

🛜 ADDITIONAL RESOURCES AND WEBSITES

Additional Resources and Websites for Clinicians:
CDC: Diseases characterized by genital, anal, or perianal ulcers—https://www.cdc.gov/std/treatment-guidelines/genital-ulcers.htm
CDC: Molluscum contagiosum—https://www.cdc.gov/poxvirus/molluscum-contagiosum/
CDC: Pubic lice—https://www.cdc.gov/parasites/lice/pubic/
CDC: Scabies—https://www.cdc.gov/parasites/scabies/
NIH: Sexually transmitted infections—https://www.niaid.nih.gov/diseases-conditions/sexually-transmitted-diseases
WHO: Sexual and reproductive health and research including the Special Programme HRP—https://www.who.int/teams/sexual-and-reproductive-health-and-research

Additional Resources and Websites for Parents/Caregivers and Adolescents and Young Adults:
American Sexual Health Association (ASHA)—http://www.ashasexualhealth.org/
American Sexual Health Association (ASHA). STDs A to Z—https://www.ashasexualhealth.org/stds_a_to_z/
American Sexual Health Association (ASHA) website for teen and young adult sexual health. I wanna know!—http://www.iwannaknow.org/teens/index.html
CDC—https://www.cdc.gov/std/spanish/default.htm
Boston Children's Hospital: Center for Young Women's Health—http://www.youngwomenshealth.org/sexuality_menu.html#stds
CDC—http://www.cdc.gov

PART XIV

Substance Use and Substance Use Disorders

CHAPTER 68

Adolescent and Young Adult Substance Use

Holly Schroder
Jillian R. Hagerman
Leslie R. Walker-Harding

KEY WORDS

- Addiction
- Adolescent brain development
- Alcohol
- Drug use
- Drug use prevention
- Generational forgetting
- Marijuana
- Opioid use disorder
- Risk and protective factors
- Substance use disorder
- Vaping

INTRODUCTION

Adolescent and young adult (AYA) use of alcohol, marijuana, tobacco, and other illicit drugs (AMTOD) is a major public health problem. The last two decades have brought new complexity to drug use in the United States. Legalization of marijuana for medicinal and/or general adult use continues to increase with only six states where marijuana is still fully illegal and in a recent Gallup poll from 2020, 68% of Americans believe that marijuana should be legal.[1] As the next decade unfolds, the impact in the AYA community of this shift in acceptance and legality, will become clearer. In addition, the last two decades have been marked by an increasingly visible opioid use crises with the increase in nonprescription use of opioids in the adult and AYA population. In adolescents, after a peak in heroin and narcotic use in 2001, a steady decrease in initiation of use is documented in the Monitoring the Future survey 2020 (2020 MTF) prevalence estimates.[2] The continued use of prescription and synthetic drugs for recreational purposes continues to be a national concern. In the short term, drug use is associated with significant morbidity and mortality in the AYA population. In the long term, much of the adult morbidity and mortality attributed to AMTOD use can be traced to behaviors that began during adolescence. Alcohol, tobacco, and marijuana are the three drugs most used by the AYA age groups. Other drugs wax and wane in popularity and their use, following a predictable pattern. A phenomenon called generational forgetting contributes to the popularity of a particular drug over time. Generational forgetting occurs in the absence of knowledge; otherwise, Drug "X" is perceived as safer than other drugs, and its use increases. As use increases, the drug's negative effects become more widely known, and use of Drug "X" is perceived as increasingly risky. This increased perception of risk causes the popularity of Drug "X" to wane, leading to Drug X's replacement by a different drug that is perceived as being of lower risk. Decades later, when the risk of Drug "X" is no longer common knowledge, it again becomes popular.

In addition to generational forgetting which has played a role in the current selection of substances the AYA population is using beyond alcohol, tobacco and marijuana, this last decade has seen a dramatic increase in electronic vaporizer device use (vaping) to consume tobacco and marijuana, in particular. While this chapter will discuss the trends in vaping use, it is important to note that the increase in vaping nicotine, reversed years of successful efforts to lower tobacco and nicotine initiation in the AYA population. According to 2020 MTF, some of this increase has leveled off in nicotine use but vaping use with marijuana has continued to increase.[2]

It is important to highlight that increased marketing of vaping devices, marijuana products, and alcohol to the AYA population in various media settings that they frequent, has played a role in the acceptability and choices the AYA populations have made in initiation and use of substances in the past decade.[3,4]

EPIDEMIOLOGY

Middle and High School Youth

The best data on adolescent substance use come from the *MTF study*, conducted by the Institute for Social Research at the University of Michigan (http://www.monitoringthefuture.org/). This school-based study began in 1975, and currently surveys a nationally representative sample of 8th, 10th, and 12th graders. Because the anonymous surveys are conducted in schools, MTF data do not reflect drug use by out-of-school youth (including youth who dropout, are homeless, or incarcerated), whose use is typically higher. The sample in 2020 consists of 11,821 youth in 112 secondary schools nationwide. The 2020 MTF data collection was stopped prematurely due to the COVID-19 pandemic. The completed surveys represented 25% of a typical year's data collection, although results were still gathered from a broad geographic and representative sample and the data were statistically weighted to provide national numbers.[2] Since this data was collected before the COVID-19 pandemic it does not reflect the impact of social distancing and virtual school on adolescent substance use. We will have to wait for future research to help us understand the effects of life in a pandemic. The most important findings from the 2020 MTF survey are discussed in the following section.

Overall trends in drug use among 8th, 10th, and 12th graders have fluctuated since 1975, with peak use in 1981 when 66% of MTF adolescents reported use of an illicit drug in their lifetime. After reaching a low of 29.8% in 1992, lifetime drug use then increased to a peak level of 43.3% in 1997; use decreased again to a low of 32.6% in 2008. From 2013 to 2016 use fluctuated between 36% and 32%. After 2016, lifetime illicit drug use has increased slightly each year to a high of 34.8% in 2019, mostly driven by increasing rates of marijuana use. In 2020, rates of lifetime illicit drug use remained stable at 34.7%. One of the more concerning trends over the last several years in the MTF samples has been the change of perception of risk

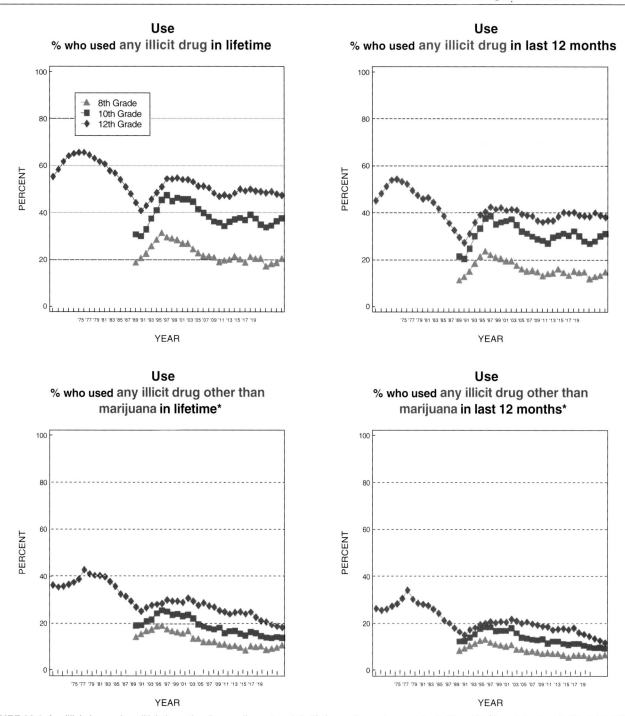

FIGURE 68.1 Any illicit drug and any illicit drug other than marijuana: trends in lifetime and annual use grades 8, 10, and 12. (From Johnston LD, Miech RA, O'Malley PM, et al. *Monitoring the Future national survey results on drug use, 1975–2020: 2020 Overview, key findings on adolescent drug use.* Institute for Social Research, The University of Michigan, 2021. Accessed March 26, 2021. Available at http://www.monitoringthefuture.org//pubs/monographs/mtf-overview2020.pdf) *In 2001, a revised set of questions on other hallucinogen use and tranquilizer use were introduced. In 2013, a revised set of questions on amphetamine use was introduced. Data for any illicit drug other than marijuana were affected by these changes.

of substances. Over the last decade, there has been a decline in perceived risk for marijuana, which can foreshadow future increases in drug use in this cohort. The MTF survey categorizes use across a continuum by asking about lifetime use (ever used), annual use (any use in the last year), 30-day use (a measure of regular use), and daily use. The data are then able to give an estimate of chronicity of use for 8th, 10th, and 12th graders. Figure 68.1 shows trends in lifetime use of various drugs. **Table 68.1** shows prevalence of lifetime, annual, past 30 days, and daily use of various drugs for 8th, 10th, and 12th graders in 2020.

In general, the 2020 MTF data showed continued low levels of most forms of illicit substance use among teens. Notably, both alcohol and marijuana are illicit for this age group, although alcohol is included in its own category in MTF and not included in rates of illicit drug use. One of the most important trends in 2020 was related to rates of nicotine and marijuana vaping. Starting in 2017, questions about vaping nicotine and marijuana were added to the MTF survey (previously the questions were about vaping in general) and each year the number of teenagers who reported using these substances increased significantly. In 2020, for the first time since these

TABLE 68.1

Prevalence of Use of Various Drugs for 8th, 10th, and 12th Graders, 2020

	Lifetime			Annual			Past 30 d			Daily		
	8th	10th	12th	8th	10th	12th	8th	10th	12th	8th	10th	12th
Approximate Weighted N[a]	15,100	15,000	13,700	15,100	15,000	13,700	15,100	15,000	13,700	15,100	15,000	13,700
Any Illicit Drug	18.5	36.8	49.1	13.4	30.1	39.7	7.7	18.5	25.2	-	-	-
Any Illicit Drug Other Than Marijuana	8.7	14.9	24.1	5.5	10.8	17.0	2.5	5.0	8.4	-	-	-
Any Illicit Drug Including Inhalants	25.1	40.0	50.3	17.0	31.5	40.2	9.5	19.3	25.2	-	-	-
Marijuana/Hashish	15.2	33.5	45.2	11.4	28.0	36.4	6.5	17.0	22.9	1.1	3.5	6.5
Synthetic Marijuana	-	-	-	4.4	8.8	11.3	-	-	-	-	-	-
Inhalants	11.8	9.9	7.9	6.2	4.1	2.9	2.7	1.4	0.9	-	-	0.1
Hallucinogens	2.8	5.2	7.5	1.5	3.5	4.8	0.6	1.2	1.5	-	-	0.1
Hallucinogens, Adjusted	-	-	7.9	-	-	-	-	-	1.8	-	-	-
LSD	1.3	2.5	3.8	0.8	1.7	2.4	0.3	0.5	0.8	-	-	0.1
Hallucinogens Other Than LSD	2.3	4.5	6.6	1.3	3.0	4.0	0.5	0.9	1.3	-	-	0.1
PCP	-	-	1.6	-	-	0.9	-	-	0.5	-	-	0.1
Ecstasy (MDMA)	2.0	5.0	7.2	1.1	3.0	3.8	0.5	1.0	0.9	-	-	0.1
Salvia	-	-	-	1.4	2.5	4.4	-	-	-	-	-	-
Cocaine	1.9	3.3	4.9	1.2	2.0	2.7	0.5	0.8	1.1	-	-	0.1
Crack	1.0	1.4	2.1	0.6	0.8	1.2	0.3	0.4	0.5	-	-	0.1
Other Cocaine	1.6	3.0	4.4	1.0	1.8	2.4	0.3	0.7	1.0	-	-	0.1
Heroin												
Any Use	0.8	1.1	1.1	0.5	0.6	0.6	0.2	0.4	0.3	-	-	0.1
With a Needle	0.6	0.7	0.7	0.4	0.4	0.4	0.2	0.2	0.3	-	-	0.1
Without a Needle	0.5	0.8	0.8	0.3	0.4	0.4	0.1	0.2	0.2	-	-	0.1
Narcotics Other Than Heroin	-	-	12.2	-	-	7.9	-	-	3.0	-	-	0.2
OxyContin	-	-	-	1.6	3.0	4.3	-	-	-	-	-	-
Vicodin	-	-	-	1.3	4.4	7.5	-	-	-	-	-	-
Amphetamines	4.5	8.9	12.0	2.9	6.5	7.9	1.3	2.8	3.3	-	-	0.3
Ritalin	-	-	-	0.7	1.9	2.6	-	-	-	-	-	-
Adderall	-	-	-	1.7	4.5	7.6	-	-	-	-	-	-
Methamphetamine	1.3	1.8	1.7	1.0	1.0	1.1	0.5	0.6	0.5	-	-	-
Crystal Methamphetamine (Ice)	-	-	1.7	-	-	0.8	-	-	0.4	-	-	0.2
Bath Salts (Synthetic Stimulants)	-	-	-	0.8	0.6	1.3	-	-	-	-	-	-
Selective (Barbiturates)	-	-	6.9	-	-	4.5	-	-	2.0	-	-	0.1
Selective, Adjusted	-	-	7.2	-	-	4.5	-	-	2.1	-	-	0.3
Methaqualone	-	-	0.8	-	-	0.4	-	-	0.3	-	-	0.3

TABLE 68.1

Prevalence of Use of Various Drugs for 8th, 10th, and 12th Graders, 2020 (*Continued*)

	Lifetime			Annual			Past 30 d			Daily		
	8th	10th	12th	8th	10th	12th	8th	10th	12th	8th	10th	12th
Approximate Weighted N[a]	15,100	15,000	13,700	15,100	15,000	13,700	15,100	15,000	13,700	15,100	15,000	13,700
Tranquilizers	3.0	6.3	8.5	1.8	4.3	5.3	0.8	1.7	2.1	-	-	0.1
Any Prescription Drug	-	-	21.2	-	-	14.8	-	-	-	-	-	-
Over-the-Counter Cough/Cold Medication	-	-	-	3.0	4.7	5.6	-	-	-	-	-	-
Rohpnol	1.0	0.8	-	0.4	0.5	1.5	0.1	0.2	-	-	-	-
GHB	-	-	-	-	-	1.4	-	-	-	-	-	-
Ketamine	-	-	-	-	-	-	-	-	-	-	-	-
Alcohol												
Any Use	29.5	54.0	69.4	23.6	48.5	63.5	11.0	27.6	41.5	0.3	0.1	2.5
Been Drunk	12.8	34.5	54.2	8.5	28.2	45.0	3.4	14.5	28.1	0.1	0.4	1.5
Flavored Alcoholic Beverages	23.5	46.7	60.5	17.0	37.8	45.0	3.5	14.5	28.1	0.1	0.4	1.5
Alcoholic Beverages Containing Caffeine	-	-	-	10.9	19.7	25.4	-	-	-	-	-	-
5+ Drinks in a Row in Last 2 wks	-	-	-	-	-	-	-	-	-	5.1	15.5	23.7
Cigarettes												
Any Use	15.5	27.7	39.5	-	-	-	4.9	10.8	17.1	1.9	5.0	9.3
1/2 Pack+/Day	-	-	-	-	-	-	-	-	-	0.6	1.5	4.0
Kreteks	-	-	-	-	-	3.0	-	-	-	-	-	-
Tobacco Using a Hookah	-	-	-	-	-	18.3	-	-	-	-	-	-
Small Cigars	-	-	-	1.0	1.6	1.6	-	-	-	-	-	-
Dissolvable Tobacco Products	-	-	-	2.4	6.9	7.9	-	-	-	-	-	-
Snuff	8.1	15.4	17.4	-	-	-	2.8	6.4	7.9	-	-	-
Smokeless Tobacco	1.2	1.3	1.8	0.6	0.8	1.3	0.3	0.4	0.9	-	-	-

Trends in annual prevalence of an illicit drug use index for 8th, 10th, and 12th graders. (From Johnston LD, Miech RA, O'Malley PM, et al. *Monitoring the Future national survey results on drug use, 1975–2020: 2020 Overview key findings on adolescent drug use.* Institute for Social Research, The University of Michigan, 2021. Accessed March 26, 2021. Available at http://www.monitoringthefuture.org//pubs/monographs/mtf-overview2020.pdf)

[a]For more information on Approximate Weighted N, please see http://monitoringthefuture.org/pubs/monographs/mtf-vol1_2020.pdf

questions were asked, the percentage of teenagers who reported vaping nicotine and marijuana leveled off. Another notable finding from the 2020 MTF survey was that among 8th graders, past 12-month use of inhalants increased from 3.8% in 2016 to 6.1% in 2020, representing a 64% increase. This stands in contrast to 12th graders who in 2020 reported an all-time low use of inhalants at 1.1%.

It is also important to note that for all other measured reports of illicit drug use, the overall combined use rates are much more consistent than is the rate of use of a particular drug by year or decade. This again illustrates generational forgetting and the perceived risk of particular drugs waxing and waning over time. However, it also illustrates that the number of youth interested in other illicit drugs remains relatively stable over time (see Fig. 68.1).

Monitoring the Future does not report comprehensive data for all race and ethnic groups, but they do include information about the three largest racial and ethnic groups including Whites, African Americans, and Hispanics. For many years, White students had higher rates of illicit drug use than did African American and Hispanic students, but the differences have narrowed in more recent years mostly as a result of increasing marijuana use among African American and Hispanic students, coupled with slight decrease in use in White students. In 2018 the MTF reported on last year use of any illicit drug by race and of the 12th graders surveyed, 39.5% of White Students, 38.8% of African American students, and 37.2% of Hispanic students reported last year use of any illicit drug. African American students have historically had significantly lower use of alcohol and

XIX

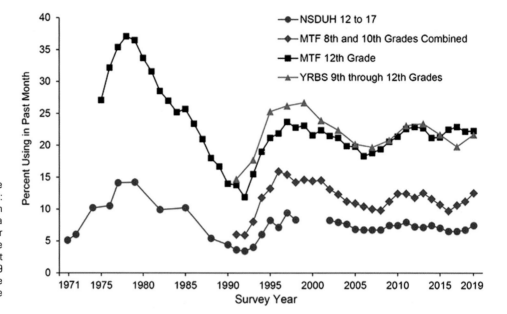

FIGURE 68.2 Past-month marijuana use among youths in NSDUH, MTF, and YRBS: 1971–2019. Substance Abuse and Mental Health Services administration. Note: NSDUH data for youths aged 12 to 17 are not presented for 1999 to 2001 because of design changes in the survey. These design changes preclude direct comparisons of estimates from 2002 to 2019 with estimates prior to 2019. MTF, Monitoring the Future; NSDUH, National Survey on Drug Use and Health; YRBS, Youth Risk Behavior Survey.

cigarettes than White and Hispanic students, especially in the upper grades. In the 2018 MTF, 38% of White 12th graders, 21.2% of African American 12th graders, and 26.4% of Hispanic 12th graders reported past 30-day use of alcohol. Rates of drug use among Hispanic students have generally put them in between African American and White students, but more recently Hispanic students in 12th grade have had the highest use rates for several substances including synthetic marijuana, cocaine, crack, cocaine other than crack, and crystal methamphetamine. White students continue to have the highest rates of misuse of any prescription drug compared to African American and Hispanic students. In 2018, 11.4% of White 12th graders reported prescription drug misuse, while only 6.4% of African American 12th graders, and 8.5% of Hispanic 12th graders reported past-year use. Despite lower levels of substance use, African American adolescents are more likely to have been arrested for drug-related behaviors than White adolescents, likely due to biased treatment of minority youth.[5] Historically, youth who identify as Asian tend to have lower drug use in all categories.[6] American Indian and Alaska Native youth generally have high rates of substance use (*National Survey on Drug Use and Health* [NSDUH 2019]). A survey comparing substance use among American Indian Youths on or near reservations to the MTF data of the same year, found that lifetime and past 30-day substance use rates were substantially higher than for other youth for nearly all illicit substances.[7] It is important to remember that all data must be interpreted in the context in which it occurs, and taking cultural differences and beliefs about substance use as well as environmental differences and structural racism into account when looking at epidemiologic data will provide a deeper understanding of trends. Differences in race/ethnicity data are markers for further evaluation as to the cause and should not be attributed to race identification itself.

Other surveys that track adolescent substance use to varying degrees are the *Youth Risk Behavior Surveillance System* (YRBSS), also administered in schools (www.cdc.gov/HealthyYouth/yrbs/index.htm) and the NSDUH (https://www.cdc.gov/healthyyouth/data/yrbs/index.htm). The latter survey, administered in the home, includes out-of-school youth, but may result in underreporting if parents/caregivers are present. Drug use estimates from the MTF surveys consistently yield higher estimates than the NSDUH. See Figure 68.2 for a comparison of past-month marijuana use among youth from the MTF, NSDUH, and YRBSS surveys.

Alcohol

Alcohol continues to be the drug most used by adolescents. Since 1975, the MTF study has reported a continued decline in alcohol use, however the 2020 data show a slowing of the gradual decline with approximately 20.5% of 8th graders, 40.7% of 10th graders, and 55.3% of 12th graders reporting use in the last year. The number of teenagers who reported having been drunk in the past year reached historic lows in 2019, with 6.6% of 8th graders, 20.2% of 10th graders, and 32.8% of 12th graders reporting having been drunk. Rates slightly increased in 2020 to 7.5% of 8th graders, 23.1% of 10th graders, and 36.9% of 12th graders reporting that they had been drunk in the past year. Historically, males have reported higher rates of alcohol use, including binge drinking, however in the past decade, the difference has narrowed significantly to where there is either no gender difference or slightly higher rates of use for females in some surveys. According to the NSDUH survey since 2012, for persons aged 12 to 20 years, alcohol use among females has been greater than males in lifetime, past-year, and past-month use. Males continue to have slightly higher rates of heavy alcohol use. It is important that changes in use by gender are better understood in the AYA age range.

The 2020 *European School Survey Project on Alcohol and Other Drugs* (ESPAD) reported on data collected in 2019 on substance use in 35 European countries and regions among 15- to 16-year-old students. This study permits the comparison of alcohol use between the United States, where the legal age for alcohol consumption is 21 years, and European countries, most of which have legal drinking ages below 21 years. When comparing binge drinking (five or more drinks in a row), the 2019 ESPAD data indicated that on average 34% of students in European countries report binge drinking at least once in the past month compared to 8.7% of individuals in the United States who reported consuming five or more drinks in a row in the past 2 weeks on the MTF survey of the same year. Alcohol use has decreased in many of the countries surveyed for ESPAD, but use remains high with 79% of students surveyed reporting lifetime use of alcohol, compared to 44% in the United States according to the MTF. These differences underscore that increased restrictions on underage drinking in the United States have resulted in lower levels of reported alcohol use compared to countries with less restrictive policies.

Marijuana

Marijuana use is undergoing change nationally, and as of November 2020, 36 states had legalized the use of marijuana for medicinal purposes and 15 states and the District of Columbia had legalized adult use. These changes have coincided with a significant decrease in adolescents' perceived risk of use, which is reflected in both the MTF and YRBSS surveys. Currently marijuana, both inhaled and ingested, is illegal for use in every state in young people under the age of 21; medicinal use age limits vary by state. Well before changes in state laws regarding this drug, the MTF showed that marijuana is the second most used drug during adolescence. Since 2010, there has been a significant increase in daily use in all grades, however in 2020, the MTF study reported no significant change from rates in 2019 in any of the three grades for lifetime use, past 12-month use, past 30-day use, or daily use. In 2020, the lifetime prevalence of marijuana use was 14.8% in 8th grade, 33.3% in 10th grade, and 43.7% in 12th grade. Historically, there has been a long-standing gender difference in annual marijuana use with males reporting slightly higher rates of use than females, but this difference has been eliminated in all age groups. The gender convergence is due to sharp declines among male users and some increase in female use.

Vaping

There has been a rapid rise in vaping marijuana and nicotine among adolescents in the past few years. Vaping is the use of an electronic device to inhale and exhale a vaporized substance. In the MTF survey, the percentage of teenagers who reported vaping nicotine in the past year doubled across all age groups from 2017 to 2019. For 8th graders, the percentage increased from 7.5% to 16.5%, for 10th graders from 15.8% to 30.7%, and for 12th graders from 18.8% to 35.5%. The rates of vaping marijuana also increased across all age groups and categories from 2017 to 2019. From 2018 to 2019, the percentage of 12th graders vaping marijuana in the past month increased from 7.5% to 14%, which was the second largest 1-year increase for any drug use ever recorded in the 45-year history of the MTF survey. In addition to the alarmingly rapid increase in vaping, this data is concerning because little is still known about the health and safety of inhaling tetrahydrocannabinol (THC) at such high concentrations, and over the past 2 years a significant number of serious lung illnesses and deaths have been linked to vaping devices, the majority of whom vaped THC. Although rates remained high in the 2020 MTF survey, the rapid rise in use seems to have leveled off. Past-year rates for vaping nicotine remained stable at 16.6% for 8th graders, 30.7% for 10th graders, and 34.5% for 12th graders. Past-year vaping of marijuana also remained steady in 2020 at 8.1% of 8th graders, 19.1% of 10th graders, and 22.1% of 12th graders. This is likely related to a slight increase in perceived risk of vaping since 2018. Figure 68.3 shows trends in 30-day vaping use for 8th, 10th, and 12th graders from 1975 to 2019.

Nonmedical Prescription Drug Use

After alcohol, marijuana, and vaping, nonmedical prescription drug use (NMPDU), when taken together, is the next most common form of drug use in adolescence. In the 2020 MTF survey, 14.2% of 12th graders reported lifetime use of prescription medications for nonmedical purposes which is an all-time low since the question was initially asked in 2005. Nonmedical prescription drug use encompasses using medications without a prescription, in addition to using a prescription in a manner inconsistent with prescriber instructions. This typically includes nonmedical use of pain relievers, stimulants, tranquilizers, and sedatives. According to the 2019 NSDUH, rates of past-year NMPDU of pain relievers declined from 3.9% in 2015 to 2.3% in 2019, although rates for prescription pain relievers remain high as compared to prescription misuse of stimulants, tranquilizers, or sedatives. Past-year opioid use for 12- to 17-year-olds has also decreased over the past several years according to the 2019 NSDUH data. This category includes nonmedical use of prescription opioids as well as the use of heroin. This decrease in adolescent use will hopefully translate into less opioid use in the young adult and adult population in the future. It is also important to consider gender in characterizing youth substance

use. Research published in 2017 which focused on transgender youth found that transgender youth were 2.5 times more likely to use cocaine and amphetamines in their lifetime and 2 times as likely to report NMPDU than nontransgender youth. As with other groups subject to societal bias and discrimination, it is important that we begin to understand the context in which this occurs.[8]

Young Adults

Young adult (aged 18 to 25 years) substance use trajectories after high school can include continued abstinence, initiation, or a decrease, increase, or maintenance of past levels of use. Data for young adults do not have uniform age brackets, with some studies including 19- to 24-year-olds and others using 18- to 25-year-olds. Nonetheless, these data show concerning trends in young adult use in the United States. In describing this age group, overall use of AMTOD is higher than among adolescents and older adults. For those over age 21, who can legally purchase alcohol (and perhaps marijuana, depending on the state), controls for use no longer exist. However, even for those between the ages of 18 and 21 (who cannot purchase alcohol legally in the United States), the vast majority have used alcohol.

In the young adult population, females historically reported significantly less illicit drug use than males; however, female use has been increasing. Asian and African American young adults report lower levels of drug use compared to White and Latino young adults, similar to patterns seen among adolescents. Over the past several years, rates of marijuana use in lesbian, gay, and bisexual young adults have increased significantly and to a greater degree than in the overall population of young adults while past-month alcohol use and opioid misuse rates have decreased.[6]

Alcohol and Marijuana

Alcohol remains the most commonly used drug in the young adult population. In the 2019 NSDUH data, approximately 72% of 18- to 25-year-olds reported past-year use of alcohol, with 54.3% reporting consumption of alcohol in the last 30 days. Marijuana is the second most commonly used drug by young adults and in 2019, the percentage of young adults who reported past-year marijuana use was the highest it has been since 2002. According to the 2019 NSDUH survey, 35.4% of young adults between the ages of 18 and 25 reported past-year marijuana use. These rates were higher than what was seen from 2002 to 2016, but similar to estimates from 2017 to 2018.

Cigarettes and Vaping

Among young adults, cigarette use reached an all-time low in 2019 with an annual prevalence of 22%, 30-day prevalence of 12%, and half-pack a day prevalence of 3.1%. Although cigarette use has decreased in the young adult population over the past several years, vaping marijuana and nicotine rates have increased significantly, similar to the trend seen in adolescents. In the 2019 MTF survey, annual and 30-day prevalence of vaping both substances was the highest among 19- to 22-year-olds with 24% to 25% reporting vaping marijuana in the past year and 14% to 15% in the past 30 days, and 32% to 34% of 19- to 22-year-olds reporting vaping nicotine in the past year, and 19% to 22% reporting 30-day use. The annual and 30-day use increases in vaping marijuana and nicotine among 19- to 22-year-olds seen in 2019 are among the largest increases seen for any substance in the history of the MTF survey.

Trends in Illicit Drug Use

Annual use of illicit drugs (other than marijuana) among young adults reached a low point in 1991 and then began to trend upward, peaking in 2001. Levels remained relatively stable from 2003 to 2013 and more recently have decreased from 2014 to 2019. In 2019 MTF survey, 19% of young adults (aged 19 to 28 years) reported using any illicit drug other than marijuana in the past year. Other

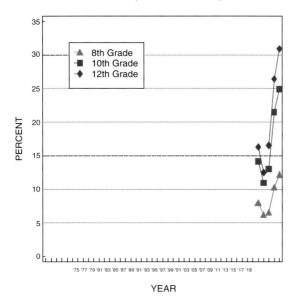

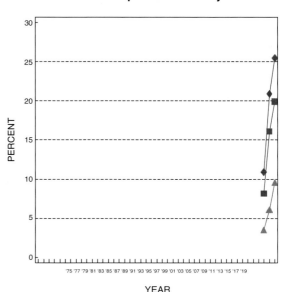

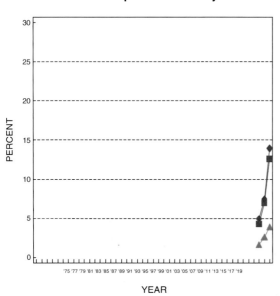

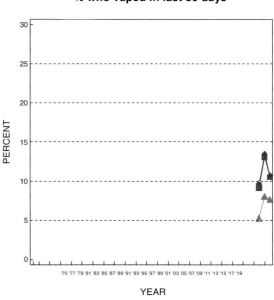

FIGURE 68.3 Vaping: Trends in 30-day use, grades 8, 10, 12. Monitoring the Future national survey results on drug use 1975–2019: Overview, key findings on adolescent drug use. (From Johnston LD, Miech RA, O'Malley PM, et al. *Monitoring the Future national survey results on drug use, 1975–2019: 2019 Overview key findings on adolescent drug use.* Institute for Social Research, The University of Michigan, 2020. Accessed January 29, 2021. Available at http://www.monitoringthefuture.org//pubs/monographs/mtf-overview2020.pdf) *In 2017, the survey switched from asking about vaping in general to asking separately about vaping nicotine, marijuana, and just flavoring. Beginning in 2017, data presented for any vaping are based on these new questions.

notable findings regarding illicit drug use among young adults are as follows:

1. Opiates: Over the past several years there has been a significant decline in opioid use in young adults while use has continued to increase in adults over 25 years of age.[6] Annual use of heroin peaked in 2009 at 0.6% and rates have decreased since then. Most recently, 0.2% of the young adult population reported annual use of heroin in the 2019 MTF study. Use of narcotics, other than heroin by young adults, peaked at 9.1% between 2006 and 2008 and has declined since that time. In 2019, 2.6% of young adults reported annual use of narcotics other than heroin. Notably, use of Vicodin showed a significant 5-year decline to just 1.6% in 2019 and OxyContin use has also leveled off at a very low prevalence over the past 5 years with 1.9% of young adults reporting use in 2019. In general, there appear to be two main types of pain reliever NMPDU: self-treatment (of unmanaged pain or underlying psychiatric issues) and recreational use.[9] While recreational use is more indicative of other risky behaviors, increases in the misuse of pain relievers are linked to increased heroin use and increased

mortality according to the Centers for Disease Control and Prevention.

2. Amphetamines: The recent MTF survey found that 8.1% of college students compared to 5.9% of young adults in general reported using amphetamines. Historically, college students report higher rates of amphetamine use without a doctor's prescription than noncollege youth. The higher rates of non-prescribed use seen in college students may be due to a desire to increase academic performance or increase alertness. Several studies have linked amphetamine prescription misuse with unhealthy weight loss, increased anxiety and impulsivity, increased use of other substances, and other psychiatric issues.[9,10]

3. Cocaine: Cocaine use reached a nadir in 1994. Among the young adult population rates of use increased through 2004 and then decreased through 2013 to a low of 3.9%. Since then, there has been a steady 5-year increase in annual prevalence of cocaine use. Most recently in the 2019 MTF study, 6.5% of young adults reported cocaine use in the past year.

4. 3,4-Methylenedioxy-N-methylamphetamine (MDMA): In the 1990's MDMA ("ecstasy") use grew rapidly in popularity among college students with peak use occurring in 2001 followed by a rapid decline after that. In 2019 MTF survey, after a steady decrease in use over the past 5 years, the annual prevalence of MDMA use in the young adult population (college and noncollege students) was 3.7%.

LONG-TERM OUTCOMES OF DRUG USE

Over the last 10 years, advances in neuroimaging technology and longitudinal studies provide evidence that use of drugs, especially if initiated in early to midadolescence, is associated with significant long-term consequences. The cognitive effects of marijuana use are examined below:

1. A longitudinal study from New Zealand, which followed toddlers into middle adulthood, showed that permanent cognitive impairment and loss of intelligence quotient could occur in persistent marijuana users.[11]

2. The research examining the correlation between schizophrenia and marijuana use continues to grow. Smith et al.[12] found that the younger a person is when they begin to use marijuana heavily and consistently, the more brain abnormalities are seen. Furthermore, those abnormalities resemble the same abnormalities seen in schizophrenia. Another study, controlling for childhood psychotic symptoms and other drug use, found that those who smoked marijuana by age 15 were 7.2 times more likely to develop psychotic symptoms at age 26 than controls.[13]

ADOLESCENT BRAIN DEVELOPMENT AND SUSCEPTIBILITY TO DRUG USE AND DRUG-ASSOCIATED BRAIN DAMAGE

From a developmental perspective, adolescence is characterized by many physical, emotional, and social changes that can make them more vulnerable to substance use.[14] Advances in neuroimaging techniques as well as research using animal models have provided a better understanding of adolescent brain development and help to shed more light on the neurobiology behind the increased pleasure-seeking and risk-taking behaviors of adolescence. One hypothesis behind these behaviors is related to differing rates of development of the emotional center of the brain relative to the executive control center.[15]

Longitudinal studies using functional magnetic resonance imaging have shown that the prefrontal cortex doesn't reach full maturation until age 25.[16] Observed changes in the prefrontal cortex are consistent with neuropsychological studies that show that frontal lobes are involved with emotional regulation, planning, organizing, and response inhibition (the latter three constituting "executive functioning") and adolescents tend to perform poorly in tasks that involved inhibitory control when compared to adults.[16]

In contrast, the limbic and subcortical regions responsible for motivation, reward, and emotional processes, such as the ventral striatum, develop and reach maturation earlier.[16] One neuroimaging study of children, adolescents and adults engaging in reward-based tasks found that the activity within the reward center, specifically the nucleus acumens, in the adolescent brain was similar to that of an adult; however, the activity in the frontal cortex more closely resembled that of a child.[17]

In fact, the dopaminergic system of the brain is functioning at peak performance during adolescence.[18] Studies in rats show that mesolimbic dopamine synthesis in the nucleus accumbens is lower in preadolescent than adolescent rats, which in turn are lower than in adult rats. Dopaminergic and noradrenergic systems have heightened excitability and larger increases in neurotransmitter levels in response to rewarding stimuli.[19] The combination of hyperactive reward center and immature control center in the adolescent brain may contribute to the increase in reward-seeking and risk-taking behaviors experienced by adolescents, particularly regarding substance use.

In addition to adolescents being uniquely susceptible to substance use due to developmental changes, adolescents may also face increased neurologic consequences with substance use. One recent study revealed that the brains of adolescents who were heavy drinkers for at least 1 year (<20 drinks/month) showed significantly decreased gray matter and functioning.[20] Brown et al.[21] found that alcohol-dependent adolescents showed distinct deficits when retrieving verbal and nonverbal information compared to healthy peers. Given the significant brain changes that occur during adolescence, including frontal lobe changes linked to impulse control and decision making, and the areas involved in the brain's reward circuitry, it is not surprising that adolescents may be uniquely susceptible to the harmful effects of drug use, including dependence or addiction.

PROGRESSION OF SUBSTANCE USE

It is clinically useful to conceptualize AYA substance use as occurring across a continuum. Diagnostic criteria for substance use disorders in the fifth edition of the *Diagnostic and Statistical Manual of Mental Disorders (DSM-5)* involve classifying problematic use as "mild," "moderate," and "severe," with individuals moving back and forth through this continuum. Individuals are considered in "early remission" once abstinence is achieved for 3 to 12 months and considered in "sustained remission" when continuous abstinence is maintained for 1 year. However, along the spectrum, relapses can be frequent, cycling the individual back to earlier points in use patterns.

It is useful to consider the various transition points that occur in substance use behaviors for AYAs. The National Institutes of Health currently recognizes six distinct transition points that mark progression toward problematic use and potential remission: opportunity to use, initiation of use, problematic substance use, substance dependence, remission from problematic substance use, and remission from dependence. It is important to note that the age at which each of these transitions initially occur is strongly linked to continued progression to problematic use and dependence. These transition points are described in more detail below, adapting seminal research from MacDonald and later work by Swendenson et al.[22]

No Substance Use

During this period, the adolescent is not subject to any health risks posed by their own use, and they have not yet encountered situations in which they have the ability or choice to use

XIX

substances. Lack of availability of substances, family norms of nonuse, and lack of access to peers who use substances are key protective factors during this point of development. For clinicians, the primary focus for these adolescents involves universal prevention techniques aimed at preventing and delaying initiation of use.

First Opportunity to Use (Median Age of Onset, 16 Years)

At this point, the adolescent is still not subject to any health risks posed by their own use. However, the adolescent is subject to risks from use of substances by friends (e.g., riding with an impaired driver, sexual assault in association with substances, being in a fight with an intoxicated individual). For clinicians, the primary focus is on safety, praising and normalizing abstinence, and prevention of initiation (refusal skills).

Initiation of Use (Median Age of Onset, 17 Years)

The age of substance use initiation has been linked to the development of substance use problems later in life.[23] Following initiation of use of one drug, adolescents may try various other drugs, typically out of curiosity or to fit in with friends. The most commonly used drugs at this point are alcohol, marijuana, and tobacco. Once adolescents initiate substance use, they place themselves at risk for the health risks associated with this use. Even a single episode or very sporadic use can involve significant risk—even death—depending on the circumstances of use and the substances used. Some adolescents may cease using substances for a time, having found the experience unpleasant. Other adolescents will continue to experiment with substances, trying different types of substances with increasing frequency. Use typically occurs in social settings, and positive or pleasurable experiences generally outweigh negative consequences, though this may change as use continues to increase. For clinicians, the primary focus (using motivational interviewing [MI] techniques) should be on reviewing risks of substance use, assessing the adolescent for risk factors associated with use progression, safety, encouraging and normalizing abstinence, and practicing refusal skills.[24]

Problematic Substance Use (Median Age of Onset, 18 Years)

At this point, adolescents will actively seek out substances and begin to organize their lives around assuring a supply. They will actively seek out settings where substances are likely to be and avoid ones where substance use is unlikely. They may buy or perhaps sell substances to assure a supply. The types of substances used continue to expand. The social network will largely consist of using peers. Nonusing friends may become less desirable and distant. Behavioral changes may become apparent. The hallmark of this point in substance use progression is the increasing amount of negative consequences associated with substance use. In addition, the adolescent will need to be increasingly vigilant to hide substance use. Often, individuals who progress to problematic substance use continue on to dependence; this transition typically takes less than 1 year. For clinicians, the focus should be on MI, reviewing risks, safety, assessing increasing problems, and increasing adolescent ambivalence about use and promoting change behaviors.[24] Adolescents at this stage will need careful follow-up and treatment. Involvement of parents/caregivers may be necessary despite protestations from the adolescent.

Substance Use Disorder (Median Age of Onset, 19 Years)

The hallmark of this period is continued use despite experiencing significant negative consequences. At this point, AYAs will often use substances in order to feel normal, and negative consequences continue to increase. Any adolescent in this stage requires a comprehensive evaluation and intensive treatment.

Remission from Problematic Substance Use (Median Age of Onset, 26 Years) and Remission from Substance Use Disorder (Median Age of Onset, Young Adult)

Though some adolescents who have problematic substance use continue to use, others progress toward remission. In these cases, problematic substance use typically persists for a mean of 5 years prior to remission. Similarly, for adolescents who are dependent, dependence typically persists for a mean of 7 years prior to remission of use. In each case, length of substance use prior to abstinence varies greatly based on type of substance and history of substance use. For clinicians, the focus should be on involving the adolescents in evidence-based treatments of substance use disorders, such as cognitive behavioral therapy, contingency management, motivational enhancement therapy, 12-step facilitation therapy, functional family therapy, and multisystemic therapy.

PREVENTION

Factors Influencing Substance Use in Adolescents and Young Adults

Research on the prevention of substance use in AYAs has made significant strides in the past four decades. Prevention science is based on understanding risk and protective factors. *Risk factors* include individual, family, peer, school, and community characteristics (both malleable and unchanging) that precede problem behaviors (e.g., substance use) and contribute to an individual's likelihood of developing problems. At the same time, *protective factors* buffer individuals from the effects of these risks, decreasing an individual's likelihood of developing problems. Substance use prevention is based on the premise that substance use may be prevented by reducing an individual's malleable risk factors and reinforcing an individual's protective factors. Ultimately, adolescent substance use is a complex phenomenon; no single risk factor predicts with certainty that an adolescent will use substances or develop problematic substance use, nor does the presence of a single protective factor offer reassurance that no use will occur. Rather, substance use or nonuse results from a combination of these factors.

A small list of risk factors has consistently emerged as significantly contributing to substance use. Interestingly, many of these risk factors overlap with risk factors for other problematic behaviors, such as delinquency, teen pregnancy, school dropout, and violence. This convergence of risk factors suggests that adolescents who are at greater risk for substance use may also be at risk for developing other problems. **Table 68.2** lists the risk factors identified by the *Substance Abuse and Mental Health Services Administration (SAMHSA)*. To summarize, the more that various substances are readily available and that use of these substances is visible and perceived to be safe and accepted within communities, the more likely AYAs are to use substances.

In addition, at a population level, perception of the risks of substance use is linked to the prevalence of use. For example, according to the MTF study, over the last 30 years, the prevalence of marijuana use rose and fell according to risk perception. The percentage of 12th graders who perceived "great risk" in regular marijuana use reached a nadir (approximately 35%) in 1979. In that same year, reported use of marijuana in the past year by 12th graders peaked at approximately 50%. Perceived risk then began to rise, peaking in 1992. Not surprisingly, use fell to its lowest level at the same time. Following that, perceived risk then began to fade, and use began to rise. Perception of risk not only differs by historical time point, but also by age. According to research done by SAMSHA, young adults aged 18 to 25 years have the highest rates of marijuana use and the lowest perception of risk, compared to any other age group.

While adolescents are exposed to multiple risk factors, they typically have some protective factors in place. Protective factors for substance use are broadly conceptualized as centered around two

TABLE 68.2

Risk Factors: Adolescent Problem Behaviors

Community	Substance Abuse	Delinquency	Teen Pregnancy	School Dropout	Violence
Availability of Drugs					•
Availability of Firearms					•
Community Laws and Norms Favorable Toward Drug Use, Firearms, and Crime	•	•			•
Media Portrayals of Violence					•
Transitions and Mobility	•	•		•	
Low Neighborhood Attachment and Community Disorganization	•	•			•
Extreme Economic Deprivation	•	•	•	•	•
Family					
Family History of the Problem Behavior	•	•	•	•	•
Family Management Problems	•	•	•	•	•
Family Conflict	•	•	•	•	•
Favorable Caretaker Attitudes and Involvement in the Problem Behavior	•	•			•
School					
Academic Failure Beginning in Late Elementary School	•	•	•	•	•
Lack of Commitment to School	•	•	•	•	•
Peer and Individual			•		
Early and Persistent Antisocial Behavior	•	•	•	•	•
Rebelliousness	•	•			
Friends who Engage in the Problem Behavior	•	•	•	•	•
Gang Involvement	•	•			•
Favorable Attitudes Toward Problem Behavior	•	•		•	
Early Initiation of the Problem Behavior	•	•			•
Constitutional Factors	•	•			•

From Adolescent Problem Behaviors. Social Development Research Group. (n.d.). Communities that care: social development strategy chart & risk factor checklist. Accessed January 13, 2014. Available at http://www.sdrg.org/ctcresource/Community%20Building%20and%20Foundational%20Material/Building_Protection_Social_Dev_Strategy_Chart.pdf

concepts: strong social bonding and clear standards for behavior. In general, the more bonded adolescents are to their family, prosocial peers, school, and community, the more likely adolescents are to abide by the behavioral standards of their family and community. By offering opportunities for prosocial involvement and rewarding prosocial participation, parents/caregivers, educators, and community members can increase the bonding young people experience in their families, schools, and communities. A recent study on emerging adults transitioning from high school to college found that having prosocial peers who did not frequently use substances protected young adults from experiencing increasing alcohol and marijuana use rates with their transition to college.[25] Similarly, young adults who reported higher rates of parental monitoring while in high school reported less heavy drinking and marijuana use when they transitioned to college.[25] Additional protective factors can include social skills, refusal skills, belief in the moral order, and religiosity. Table 68.3 shows primary protective factors. Prevention programs are most effective if they specifically target malleable risk factors within communities, while simultaneously, bolstering the protective factors in young people's lives.

XIV

TABLE 68.3

Protective Factors for Preventing Drug Use

Domain	Protective Factors
Individual	High intelligence Achievement oriented Positive self-esteem Optimistic view of future Good coping skills Prosocial orientation High religiosity
Family	Clear messages about no use Parents/caregivers model appropriate alcohol/drug use Strong family–youth attachment Moderate-to-high levels of parental monitoring Supportive parents/caregivers
Peers	Peers do not use drugs Peers have prosocial/conventional values
Schools	Offer opportunities for success and involvement Students feel connected to school School personnel perceived as fair and caring
Community	Recreational activities offered Strong community institutions Media realistically portrays harms associated with drug use Counter marketing media

Prevention Interventions

Early efforts at substance use prevention focused on providing knowledge of the harmful effects of substance use. Evaluation of these programs failed to show an effect; some studies showed an increase in use following the programs. Other unsuccessful efforts relied on the use of authority figures (e.g., police) to deliver anti-drug messages. Beginning in the 1980s, prevention efforts became more sophisticated, recognizing the multiple risk factors of drug use. Today, prevention programs focus on reducing community, school, family, or individual risk factors.

Community or structural prevention interventions typically intercede at county or state levels and often involve policy and media work. These interventions include increased taxes on alcohol and tobacco, raising the minimum legal drinking age, and graduated licensing policies. Increasing taxes on alcohol is linked to lowered mortality rates, fewer traffic crash fatalities, and lower rates of sexually transmitted infections, violence, and crime. Similarly, increasing the minimum drinking age is linked to decreased rates of drinking in AYAs and to decreased mortality rates in vehicular crashes. Additional structural prevention programs involve media campaigns, which can increase health behaviors when targeted and well executed.

Family-based prevention programs typically target parent/caregiver and child interactions and span child development. Early interventions, such as the Nurse Family Partnership, focus on prenatal health up to 2 years, and increasing parenting skills for low-income, single, first-time mothers. Though this intervention occurs early in a child's life, it has been linked with reduced substance use when the children reach the age of 15.[25] Other interventions include the Strengthening Families and Guiding Good Choices programs, for parents/caregivers and early adolescents aged 10 to 14 years. These programs involve five to seven parent/caregiver-training sessions that focus on family management skills, conflict resolution, refusal skills, and parent/caregiver–child bonding. Both programs have been shown to reduce substance initiation and

substance use years after participation. Many of these programs could be successfully initiated in the health care setting and ongoing efforts are focused on scaling these evidence-based prevention interventions for parents/caregivers in health care settings.

Most school interventions are delivered in primary and secondary education settings, and they target school risk factors by teaching skills to students and bolstering teacher instructional and management skills.[25] Programs, such as the Seattle Social Development Project, increase teachers' skills by promoting interactive styles, cooperative learning strategies, and proactive classroom management. This program also facilitates parent/caregiver classes to equip parents/caregivers with skills to help their children succeed in an academic environment. This program showed a decrease in substance use, criminal activity, and mental health problems at 21 years.[26]

In addition to these programs, some prevention interventions focus on peer and individual risk factors. These interventions typically occur in school-based settings or involve community agencies. Life Skills Training is a 3-year prevention curriculum designed for implementation in middle school. The modules focus on decision making, goal setting, anger management, communication, stress reduction, media, peer pressure, and consequences of drug use.[27] Three years after receiving these classes, students had reduced substance use compared to controls, including cigarette smoking, binge drinking, and illicit drug use.[28,29] For a more comprehensive review of drug prevention programs, see the review by Catalano et al.[29]

SUMMARY

Adolescent and young adult use of AMTOD is a major public health problem. The last two decades have brought increasing complexity to substance use in this population with legalization of marijuana, an increasingly visible opioid use crisis, and the emergence of vaping. Alcohol remains the most commonly used substance in AYAs, but marijuana use has risen significantly over the past decade and year over year increases in the percentage of youth who report vaping marijuana and nicotine has increased faster than almost any other substance in the history of the national surveys. The long-term outcomes of substance use disorders impact the life span of an individual. The earlier a person begins to use substances, the more likely they will be to develop a substance use disorder. Decades of research on how to prevent drug and alcohol initiation in childhood and adolescence is available to help communities and parents/caregivers address these threats to adolescent health.

ACKNOWLEDGMENT

The authors wish to acknowledge Erin Harrop for her contributions to previous versions of this chapter.

REFERENCES

1. GALLUP News website. Accessed January 3, 2021. https://news.gallup.com/poll/323582/support-legal-marijuana-inches-new-high.aspx
2. Johnston LD, Miech RA, O'Malley PM, et al. *Monitoring the future: national survey results on drug use 1975–2020: 2020 overview key findings on adolescent drug use.* Institute for Social Research, University of Michigan. http://www.monitoringthefuture.org//pubs/monographs/mtf-overview2020.pdf
3. Ilakkuvan V, Johnson A, Villanti AC, et al. Patterns of social media use and their relationship to health risks among young adults. *J Adolescent Health.* 2019;64(2):158–164.
4. Roditis M, Delucchi K, Chang A, et al. Perceptions of social norms and exposure to pro-marijuana messages are associated with adolescent marijuana use. *Prev Med.* 2016;93:171–176.
5. Kakade M, Duarte CS, Liu X, et al. Adolescent substance use and other illegal behaviors and racial disparities in criminal justice system involvement: findings from a US national survey. *Am J Public Health.* 2012;102(7):1307–1310.
6. Substance Abuse and Mental Health Services Administration website. Accessed January 3, 2021. https://www.samhsa.gov/data/report/2019-nsduh-detailed-tables
7. Swaim RC, Stanley LR. Substance use among American Indian youths on reservations compared with a national sample of US adolescents. *JAMA Netw Open.* 2018;1(1):e180382.
8. De Pedro KT, Gilreath TD, Jackson C, et al. Substance use among transgender students in California public middle and high schools. *J Sch Health.* 2017;87(5):303–309. https://doi.org/10.1111/josh.12499

9. Zullig KJ, Divin AL. The association between non-medical prescription drug use, depressive symptoms, and suicidality among college students. *Addict Behav.* 2012;37(8):890–899.

10. Jeffers A, Benotsch EG, Koester S. Misuse of prescription stimulants for weight loss, psychosocial variables, and eating disordered behaviors. *Appetite.* 2013;65:8–13.

11. Meier MH, Capsi A, Ambler A, et al. Persistent cannabis users show neuropsychological decline from childhood to midlife. *Proc Natl Acad Sci U S A.* 2012;109(40):E26 57–E2664.

12. Smith MJ, Cobia DJ, Wang L, et al. Cannabis-related working memory deficits and associated subcortical morphological differences in healthy individuals and schizophrenia subjects. *Schizophr Bull.* 2014;40(2):287–299.

13. Arseneault L, Cannon M, Poulton R, et al. Cannabis use in adolescence and risk for adult psychosis: longitudinal prospective study. *BMJ.* 2002;325(7374):1212–1213.

14. Edalati H, Afzali MH, Conrod PJ. Poor response inhibition and peer victimization: a neurocognitive ecophenotype of risk for adolescent interpersonal aggression. *J Abnorm Psychol.* 2018;127(8):830–839. https://doi.org/10.1037/abn0000380

15. Crews FT, Robinson DL, Chandler LJ, et al. Mechanisms of persistent neurobiological changes following adolescent alcohol exposure: NADIA consortium findings. *Alcohol Clin Exp Res.* 2019;43(9):1806–1822.

16. Arain M, Haque M, Johal L, et al. Maturation of the adolescent brain. *Neuropsychiatr Dis Treat.* 2013;9:449–461.

17. Galvan A, Hare TA, Parra CE, et al. Earlier development of the accumbens relative to orbitofrontal cortex might underlie risk-taking behavior in adolescents. *J Neurosci.* 2006;26(25):6885–6892.

18. Sharma B, Bruner A, Barnett G, et al. Opioid use disorders. *Child Adolesc Psychiatr Clin N Am.* 2016;25:473–487. http://dx.doi.org/10.1016/j.chc.2016.03.002

19. Karkhanis AN, Leach AC, Yorgason JT, et al. Chronic social isolation stress during peri-adolescence alters presynaptic dopamine terminal dynamics via augmentation in accumbal dopamine availability. *ACS Chem Neurosci.* 2019;10(4):2033–2044.

20. Squeglia LM, Tapert SF, Sullivan EV, et al. Brain development in heavy-drinking adolescents. *Am J Psychiatry.* 2015;172(6):531–542, Published online: 18 May 2015, https://doi.org/10.1176/appi.ajp.2015.14101249

21. Brown SA, Tapert SF, Granholm E, et al. Neurocognitive functioning of adolescents: effects of protracted alcohol use. *Alcohol Clin Exp Res.* 2000;24(2):164–171.

22. Swendsen J, Anthony JC, Conway KP, et al. Improving targets for the prevention of drug use disorders: sociodemographic predictors of transitions across drug use stages in the national comorbidity survey replication. *Prev Med.* 2008;47(6):629–634

23. McGue M, Irons D, Iacono WG. The adolescent origins of substance use disorders: a behavioral genetic perspective. *Nebr Symp Motiv.* 2014;61:31–50.

24. Jensen CD, Cushing CC, Aylward BS, et al. Effectiveness of motivational interviewing interventions for adolescent substance use behavior change: a meta-analytic review. *J Consult Clin Psychol.* 2011;79(4):433–440.

25. White HR, McMorris BJ, Catalano RF, et al. Increases in alcohol and marijuana use during the transition out of high school into emerging adulthood: the effects of leaving home, going to college, and high school protective factors. *J Stud Alcohol.* 2006;67(6):810–822.

26. Leslie LK, Mehus CJ, Hawkins JD, et al. Primary health care: potential home for family focused preventive interventions. *Am J Prev Med.* 2016;51(4 Suppl 2):S106–S118.

27. Catalano RF, Fagan AA, Gavin LE, et al. Worldwide application of prevention science in adolescent health. *Lancet.* 2012;379(9826):1653–1664.

28. Hawkins JD, Kosterman R, Catalano RF, et al. Promoting positive adult functioning through social development intervention in childhood: long-term effects from the Seattle Social Development Project. *Arch Pediatr Adolesc Med.* 2005;159(1):25–31.

29. Botvin GJ, Griffin KW. Life skills training: preventing substance misuse by enhancing individual and social competence. *New Dir Youth Dev.* 2014;2014(141):57–65.

ADDITIONAL RESOURCES AND WEBSITES

Additional Resources and Websites for Clinicians:

European School Survey on Alcohol and Other Drugs—http://www.espad.org/espad-report-2019

Key Substance Use and Mental Health Indicators in the United States: Results from the 2019 National Survey on Drug Use and Health—https://store.samhsa.gov/product/key-substance-use-and-mental-health-indicators-in-the-united-states-results-from-the-2019-national-survey-on-Drug-Use-and-Health/PEP20-07-01-001

Monitoring the future—https://www.drugabuse.gov/drug-topics/trends-statistics/monitoring-future

Youth Risk Behavior Surveillance System—https://www.cdc.gov/healthyyouth/data/yrbs/index.htm

Additional Resources and Websites for Parents/Caregivers:

Get Smart About Drugs: A DEA resource for parents, educators, and caregivers—https://www.getsmartaboutdrugs.gov/content/national-take-back-day

NIH Parents: Facts about Drug Use—https://teens.drugabuse.gov/parents

SAMHSA Parent Resources—https://www.samhsa.gov/underage-drinking/parent-resources

Substance Use Resource Center—AACAP—https://www.aacap.org/AACAP/Families_and_Youth/Resource_Centers/Substance_Use_Resource_Center/Home.aspx

Additional Resources and Websites for Adolescents and Young Adults:

Youth Friendly Substance Use Online Resources

Kelty Mental Health Resource Centre: Resources are available on this website for youth and teens about substance use, including in-depth information on various substances and concurrent disorders, as well as steps to seek help—http://keltymentalhealth.ca/substance-use

Partnership for Drug-Free Kids: This website works to reduce substance abuse among adolescents by supporting families and engaging with teens—http://www.drugfree.org/

Truth Campaign: This campaign provides information and uses videos and social media to engage youth in taking action against tobacco and tobacco companies—http://www.thetruth.com/

Your Room: This website offers information about alcohol and a wide range of drugs, their effects, withdrawal, and how to get help for yourself or for anyone else who needs it—http://yourroom.com.au/

Substance Use Resource Institutes

National Council on Alcohol and Drug Dependence: This informational website provides support to those who need assistance confronting the diseases of alcoholism and drug dependence—http://ncaddms.org/

National Institute of Alcohol Abuse and Alcoholism: NIAAA supports and conducts research on the impact of alcohol use on human health and wellbeing. They provide resources directed toward young people to evaluate your drinking and tools to stay in control—http://rethinkingdrinking.niaaa.nih.gov/

NIDA for Teens: NIDA provides a wealth of knowledge and resources including easy-to-read guides about various drugs. Their website for adolescents includes videos, blog posts, and drug facts—http://teens.drugabuse.gov/

Treatment Service Locators

Behavioral Health Treatment Services Locator: Find treatment facilities for substance abuse/addiction and/or mental health problems—https://findtreatment.samhsa.gov/

Buprenorphine Treatment Physician Locator: Find physicians authorized to treat opioid dependency with buprenorphine by state—http://www.samhsa.gov/medication-assisted-treatment/physician-program-data/treatment-physician-locator

Opioid Treatment Program Directory: Search opioid treatment programs by state—http://dpt2.samhsa.gov/treatment/directory.aspx

Sober Nation Treatment Locator: An extensive directory of recovery centers—http://www.sobernation.com/

Support Groups

Al-Anon Family Groups for Teens: A website with support and resources for teens affected by someone else's alcoholism—https://al-anon.org/newcomers/teen-corner-alateen/AlcoholAnonymous: The AA website can help young people find AA meetings near them and has brochures directed at young people—http://www.aa.org/pages/en_US

Narcotics Anonymous: The NA website can help young people find NA meetings near them and has resources including brochures for young addicts—http://www.na.org/

Smart Recovery: SMART Recovery is a leading self-empowering addiction recovery support group. The website provides resources for teens and youth support programs, meeting locations, and an online community—http://www.smartrecovery.org/teens/

Helplines

Crisis Call Center: Visit http://crisiscallcenter.org/, call 1-800-273-8255, or text "ANSWER" to 839863

Crisis Text Line: Visit www.crisistextline.org/ or text "START" to 741-741

National Suicide Prevention Lifeline: Visit www.suicidepreventionlifeline.org/ or call 1-800-273-TALK (8255)

SAMHSA's Helpline: Visit www.samhsa.gov/find-help/national-helpline or call 1-800-662-HELP (4357)

Alcohol

Rachel H. Alinsky
Scott E. Hadland

KEY WORDS

- Alcohol
- Alcohol intoxication
- Alcohol use
- Alcohol use disorder
- Alcohol use disorder treatment
- Binge drinking
- Screening and brief intervention
- Underage drinking

INTRODUCTION

Alcohol is the most widely used substance in the United States. It is readily available and inexpensive. Alcohol is a central nervous system (CNS) depressant that increases brain activity in areas that produce endorphins and in those that activate the dopaminergic reward system. In terms of physiology and metabolism, alcohol is a nonionized lipid-soluble compound that is completely miscible in water. It is rapidly absorbed from the gastrointestinal tract and is distributed throughout the total body water. It easily penetrates the CNS because of its lipid solubility. In most jurisdictions, alcohol intoxication is legally defined as a blood alcohol concentration (BAC) of 0.08 g/dL or greater.[1] Physiologically, alcohol intoxication depresses the CNS, noticeably altering mood as well as physical and mental abilities. Factors that modulate the effects of alcohol include body weight/body habitus, functional tolerance, medication use, illness, and food consumption, as well as the rate of consumption and the alcohol content of each drink. Given differences in alcohol metabolism by body weight, body habitus, and other physiologic variables, specific BAC levels will have different intoxication effects across individuals (Table 69.1).[2]

The principal ingredient of all alcoholic beverages is ethanol. A standard drink in the United States contains approximately 14 g of "pure" ethanol; however, levels of alcohol vary by type of alcoholic beverage.[1] For instance, a standard drink of beer is 12 oz (which contains about 5% alcohol), whereas wine is 5 oz (containing about 12% alcohol), and distilled spirits are 1.5 oz (containing about 40% alcohol).

The U.S. Department of Health and Human Services recommended in its 2020 to 2025 Dietary Guidelines for Americans that individuals under the legal drinking age of 21 years not consume any alcohol, and that adults aged 21 years and over limit their intake to one drink per day or less for females, and two drinks per day or fewer for males.[3] **Heavy drinking** is defined as alcohol consumption above these levels (8 or more drinks per week for females, 15 or more drinks per week for males). **Binge drinking** is defined as consuming four or more alcoholic beverages per occasion for females or five or more per occasion for males.

EPIDEMIOLOGY OF ALCOHOL USE AMONG ADOLESCENTS AND YOUNG ADULTS

The following highlights epidemiologic data on alcohol use among adolescents and young adults (AYAs) from standard national surveys. Overall, the prevalence of alcohol use and binge drinking has decreased over the past decade.[4]

Adolescents

Youth Risk Behavior Survey

The U.S. Centers for Disease Control and Prevention's (CDC's) 2019 Youth Risk Behavior Survey (YRBS) reveals the following

TABLE 69.1

Typical Effects of Alcohol Consumption in Individuals without High Tolerance

Blood Alcohol Concentration (BAC)	Typical Effects
0.02% About 2 alcoholic drinks	• Some loss of judgment • Relaxation • Slight body warmth • Altered mood
0.05% About 3 alcoholic drinks	• Exaggerated behavior • May have loss of small-muscle control (e.g., focusing your eyes) • Impaired judgment • Usually good feeling • Lowered alertness • Release of inhibition
0.08% About 4 alcoholic drinks	• Muscle coordination becomes poor (e.g., balance, speech, vision, reaction time, and hearing) • Harder to detect danger • Judgment, self-control, reasoning, and memory are impaired
0.10% About 5 alcoholic drinks	• Clear deterioration of reaction time and control • Slurred speech, poor coordination, and slowed thinking
0.15% About 7 alcoholic drinks	• Far less muscle control than normal • Vomiting may occur (unless this level is reached slowly, or a person has developed a tolerance for alcohol) • Major loss of balance

regarding alcohol use among high school–aged adolescents in the United States.[5]

- *Incidence:* 15.0% of high school students in the United States reported that they had their first drink of alcohol (other than a few sips) before the age of 13 years.
- *Current prevalence:* 29.2% reported that they currently drank alcohol (had at least one drink of alcohol during the past 30 days).
- *Binge drinking:* 13.7% met binge drinking criteria (as defined above) during the past 30 days.

Monitoring the Future

Data from the 2020 Monitoring the Future (MTF) survey reveal the prevalence of lifetime, current, and binge drinking across 8th, 10th, and 12th grade levels[6]:

- *Lifetime prevalence:* The prevalence of lifetime alcohol use for 8th, 10th, and 12th graders in 2020 was 25.6%, 46.4%, and 61.5%, respectively. The percentage reporting ever having been drunk across all three grade levels was 26.4%.
- *Current prevalence:* The prevalence of current alcohol use (drinking in the 30 days before the survey) was 9.9% for 8th graders, 20.3% for 10th graders, and 33.6% for 12th graders. Overall, the current prevalence in the past month across all three grades in 2020 was 20.9%.
- *Binge drinking:* The percentage of 8th, 10th, and 12th graders reporting binge drinking during the preceding 2 weeks was 5%, 10%, and 17%, respectively. Overall, the current prevalence of recent binge drinking across all three grades was 10.1%.

National Survey on Drug Use and Health

Data from the National Survey on Drug Use and Health (NSDUH) (2019) survey also provide insights on current, binge, and heavy alcohol use among adolescents in the United States.[7] The NSDUH defines current (past month) use as at least one drink in the past 30 days; binge use as five or more drinks on the same occasion (i.e., at the same time or within a couple of hours) in the past 30 days; and heavy use as five or more drinks on the same occasion on each of 5 or more days in the past 30 days.

- *Current use:* Of the approximately 24.3 million adolescents aged 12 to 17 years in the United States, 9.4% had used alcohol in the past month, with 1.7% meeting criteria for an alcohol use disorder (AUD) in the past year. Rates of current alcohol use were lowest for youth aged 12 or 13 years (1.7%) and increased with age (7.3% for 14- to 15-year-olds and 19.3% for 16- to 17-year-olds).
- *Binge drinking:* Rates of binge alcohol use followed trends similar to current use, with rates lowest for youth aged 12 to 13 years (0.5%) and increasing to 3.2% for 14- to 15-year-olds and 10.8% for 16- to 17-year-olds.

Young Adults and College Students

In the United States, the minimum alcohol drinking age is set at 21 years. Even so, research shows that patterns of drinking behavior are a major concern among 21- to 24-year-olds, especially college students, and national data reflect that many students come to college with already established drinking habits, as highlighted above.[6]

Monitoring the Future

Patterns of alcohol use among young adults in and out of college (i.e., all 18- to 25-year-olds) in the 2019 survey[6] were as follows:

- *Lifetime prevalence:* Lifetime prevalence of alcohol use for young adults increased with age: 67.6% for 19- to 20-year-olds; 84.7% for 21- to 22-year-olds; 89.9% for 23- to 24-year-olds; and 92.3% for 25- to 26-year-olds.
- *Current use:* The rates of current alcohol use (past 30-day use) for young adults also increased with age: 45.6% for 19- to 20-year-

olds; 68.4% for 21- to 22-year-olds; 73.8% for 23- to 24-year-olds; and 75.0% for 25- to 26-year-olds.

- *Binge drinking:* The proportion of young adults who reported binge drinking (i.e., having five or more drinks in a row at least once in the prior 2 weeks) was lower for 19- to 20-year-olds (21%) compared to 21- to 22-year-olds (36%), 23- to 24-year-olds (34%), and 25- to 26-year-olds (38%).

National Survey on Drug Use and Health

Patterns of alcohol use among young adults aged 18 to 25 years in the United States from the 2019 NSDUH data are summarized below.[7]

- *Current use:* The rate of past month's alcohol use was 54.3%.
- *Binge drinking:* Rates of binge drinking ranged from 22.9% among 18- to 20-year-olds to 41.6% for those aged 21 to 25 years. Figure 69.1 shows that young adults aged 18 to 25 years have the highest prevalence of binge drinking in the United States (estimated at 34.3%).
- *Heavy drinking:* Rates of heavy alcohol use were 4.7% for young adults aged 18 to 20 years and 10.8% for those aged 21 to 25 years. Overall, heavy alcohol use was reported by 8.4% of young adults aged 18 to 25 years.

American College Health Association

- According to Fall 2020 data from the American College Health Association's National College Health Assessment (NCHA) survey,[8] the percentage of young adult college students who reported any alcohol use within the past 3 months was 55.8% (57% for females and 54% for males).

Global Epidemiology of Alcohol Use

The World Health Organization (WHO) has compared rates of youth alcohol use throughout the world and found that regional rates among youth typically parallel rates among adults. Compared to American AYAs where 38.2% of 15- to 19-year-olds report drinking alcohol, the highest rates of youth alcohol use in the world are found in Europe, where 43.8% of youth aged 15 to 19 years report drinking.[9] Conversely, the lowest rate of youth drinking in the world is found in the Middle East, where only 1.2% of 15- to 19-year-olds report drinking alcohol.[9] The prevalence of heavy episodic drinking among youth aged 15 to 19 years is highest in Europe (24.1%), the Western Pacific including Australia (18.8%), and the Americas (18.4%), and then peaks in the 20- to 24-year-old age group at rates of 33.9% among Europeans, 28.2% among Western Pacific youth, and 28% among Americans.[9]

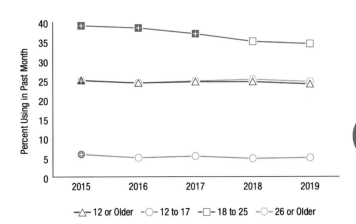

+ Difference between this estimate and the 2019 estimate is statistically significant at the .05 level.

FIGURE 69.1 Past month binge alcohol use among people aged 12 years and older by age groups in the United States. Results from the 2019 National Survey on Drug Use and Health: Summary and National Findings.

Sociodemographic Trends of Alcohol Use among Youth

Gender and Race

Lifetime Prevalence 2019 YRBS data show that the prevalence of current alcohol use for females is higher than for males (31.9% vs. 26.4%, respectively).[5] Current prevalence of alcohol use was highest among youth described as non-Hispanic White (34.2%), followed by non-Hispanic American Indian or Alaskan Native (32.6%), Hispanic (28.4%), multiracial (26.0%), Black (16.8%), and Asian (13.9%).

Binge Drinking According to the YRBS (2019), current binge drinking was more common among female than male adolescents (14.6% vs. 12.7%, respectively). Current binge drinking was most common among non-Hispanic White adolescents (17.3%), followed by Hispanic adolescents (12.4%), and non-Hispanic Black adolescents (6.2%).[5]

Puberty

Pubertal timing has been identified as a potential factor in understanding alcohol use among youth. Girls who become physically mature earlier than their same-aged peers are at risk for younger onset of alcohol use than girls who mature later.[9] The situation for boys is less clear, but there is some evidence that early development may also be linked to increased levels of alcohol consumption.

Risk Factors for Alcohol Use among Adolescents and Young Adults

Many factors contribute to alcohol initiation, use, and alcohol-related problem behaviors among AYAs, and can be categorized as genetic or environmental. Many of these factors are similar to the ones for substance use disorders in general, outlined in Chapter 68. Studies have demonstrated that genetics are more strongly associated with the risk of problem alcohol use than environmental factors, likely related to a number of specific genes that facilitate the transition from regular alcohol use to alcohol dependence.[10] On the other hand, environmental factors rather than genetics more strongly influence the timing of initiation of use.[10] In regard to patterns of use, having friends who use alcohol is a significant risk factor for youth use, as 80% of youth who drink alcohol do so in social situations such as house parties rather than while alone.[10]

Parental Alcohol Use and Alcohol Use Disorder

Various studies have suggested that children of individuals with AUD are more susceptible to AUDs than other youth. Studies of twins and adopted children, for example, indicate that alcohol initiation arises from genetic, shared, and nonshared environmental contributions.[11]

Parental/Caregiver Drinking Standards

Problem alcohol use can be shaped by environmental exposures in the home such as the socialization patterns of parents/caregivers.[12] Parents/caregivers who provide structure around drinking (i.e., rules and communication) foster better regulatory skills in their children, including increased self-control and less risk for alcohol use–related problem behaviors.[12] Youth perceptions of parental/caregiver approval of alcohol use and parents'/caregivers' use of alcohol have been identified as risk factors for youth initiation of drinking behaviors. Studies have shown, for instance, that if parents/caregivers are perceived as being permissive toward drinking, youth are at higher risk of early initiation.[12] Early onset of alcohol use (before age 14 years) has been identified as a risk factor for the later development of alcohol-related problems and disorders in adulthood. For example, studies have found that youth who started drinking before age 13 years are nine times more likely to engage in problem drinking, such as binge drinking, than youth who initiated drinking later.[13]

Media/Advertising of Alcohol

Media influences on the use of alcohol by young people are substantial. Research studies have characterized the extensive marketing efforts of the alcohol industry to promote their products to youth, including advertisements and depictions in entertainment outlets, television, and online.[14] Such advertising has been a powerful medium for setting and reinforcing existing prosocial trends and attitudes about alcohol use within youth culture. Other media, including television, movies, social media, and other internet sites, are known to be influential in promoting alcohol use through attractive portrayals of use without mention of associated negative consequences. Extensive research has demonstrated a consistent strong positive relationship between youth exposure to alcohol marketing and the level of youth alcohol consumption, with exposure to alcohol marketing associated with early alcohol initiation, hazardous drinking, and binge drinking among youth.[14,15] Litt and Stock reported that youth had greater willingness to drink alcohol after viewing experimenter-generated Facebook pages portraying alcohol use as normative among older peers.[16] Developmentally, this is concerning since it can create social norms that drinking is a standard and accepted practice in the community (part of the culture), which can have a strong influence over youth behavior, especially the early initiation of alcohol use and progression from use to an AUD.[16] Jernigan et al. performed a systematic review of cohort studies involving more than 35,000 youth and found that youth who reported greater exposure to alcohol content were more likely to initiate drinking as well as report hazardous or binge drinking at follow-up.[15]

CONSEQUENCES OF ALCOHOL USE AMONG YOUTH

The costs of problematic alcohol consumption in the United States are substantial. The costs of alcohol use likely exceed \$200 billion annually from losses in productivity, health care costs, crime, and other expenses, with one-tenth of costs attributed to underage drinking.[17] Mortality tied to alcohol consumption in the U.S. accounts for approximately 95,000 deaths per year, with young people under age 21 years accounting for more than 3,500 of those deaths.[18] Leading causes of alcohol-related mortality in young people include motor vehicle crash injuries, suicide, and homicide. According to the National Institute on Alcohol Abuse and Alcoholism (NIAAA),[19] morbidity and mortality from alcohol use are substantial among college students aged 18 to 24 years, among whom each year an estimated:

- 1,519 die from alcohol-related unintentional injuries, including motor vehicle crashes.
- 696,000 are assaulted by another student who has been drinking.
- 97,000 are victims of alcohol-related sexual assault or date rape.

Drinking and Driving

According to the 2019 YRBS survey,[5] 5.4% of high school–aged youth reported that they "drove after drinking alcohol" during the past 30 days, while 16.7% reported riding "with a driver who had been drinking alcohol" during the past 30 days. Motor vehicle collisions caused by driving under the influence of alcohol are among the leading causes of injuries for those under age 21 years. According to the most recent NCHA data from Fall 2020,[8] 10.5% of college students reported driving after having any alcohol in the last 30 days.

The U.S. Department of Transportation found that a total of 2,375 youth between age 13 and 19 years (1,577 males) died in alcohol-related motor vehicle crashes in 2019.[20] Overall, national risk estimates for being seriously injured (including death) while driving under the influence of alcohol are significantly higher among 16- to 20-year-olds[21] compared to other youth groups reported. According to the NSDUH (2019), roughly 1 in 13 persons aged 16 years or older (7.8%) drove under the influence of alcohol at least once in the past year.[7] Young people aged 21 to 25 years have the highest rate (11.8%) of driving under the influence of alcohol among persons aged 16 years or older (compared to 3.2% of 16- to 20-year-olds and 7.8% of those 26 years old or older).[22]

Drinking and High-Risk Behaviors

Alcohol use is linked to several other risky behaviors. According to data from the NCHA survey,[8] college students who drank alcohol reported experiencing the following problems in the last 12 months when drinking alcohol:

- Did something you later regretted (36.5%)
- Forgot where you were or what you did (32.3%)
- Got in trouble with the police (3.0%)
- Someone had sex with me without my consent (2.1%)
- Had sex with someone without their consent (0.6%)
- Had unprotected sex (20.4%)
- Physically injured yourself (14.9%)
- Physically injured another person (1.8%)
- Seriously considered suicide (2.5%)
- Reported one or more of the above (53.4%)

Data from the 2019 YRBS also show the co-occurrence of drinking and high-risk sexual behaviors among youth, as 21.2% of high school students in the United States reported drinking alcohol or using drugs before their last sexual intercourse.[5]

Drinking and Disordered Eating/Energy Drinks

The mixing of alcohol with energy drinks (which contain caffeine, plant-based stimulants, and sugar) is a common practice among adolescents, with 10% of high school students and 32% of young adults reporting this behavior.[23] The CDC notes that mixing alcohol with energy drinks is especially dangerous because youth may drink more alcohol than they realize because the caffeine masks the sedating effects of alcohol, leading to greater impairment and a higher risk of driving while intoxicated, sustaining alcohol-related injuries, or having unwanted or unprotected sex.[23] In 2010, the U.S. Food and Drug Administration (FDA) halted the production of caffeinated alcoholic beverages in an attempt to decrease youth consumption of combined caffeine and alcohol. However, youth continue to mix the two on their own.[23] A systematic review in 2020 demonstrated that energy drink consumption among adolescents was associated in cohort studies with increased alcohol use.[24]

Neurotoxicity of Alcohol Use among Youth

Alcohol is considered a neurotoxin. Its full effects on the developing youth brain are not yet known. The dynamic developing brain is potentially susceptible to damage due to problematic alcohol consumption, especially binge drinking and heavy alcohol use patterns among young people. To date, research demonstrates the following neurologic, structural, and cognitive effects of alcohol on the developing brain system among youth[25]:

- Youth are relatively resistant to the sedative effects of alcohol. They show less ataxia and social impairment and fewer acute withdrawal effects than adults. They are more sensitive, however, to the social facilitation that may encourage alcohol consumption.
- Imaging studies of youth with significant alcohol use show reduced hippocampal volumes and abnormalities of the corpus callosum, as well as subtle white matter microstructure abnormalities, particularly in the splenium of the corpus callosum.
- Functional magnetic resonance imaging shows decreased functional activity of the frontal and parietal areas of the right hemisphere, areas responsible for spatial memory.
- Studies show a disruption in learning and memory, especially memory retrieval, and in visual-spatial functioning.
- Neurocognitive testing of youth who use alcohol shows decreased visuospatial motor speed and impaired reading recognition, total reading, and spelling on IQ testing.

- Increased alcohol consumption is associated with decreased memory, abstract thought, and language.
- Youth with more than 100 lifetime drinking episodes show decreased verbal and nonverbal retention when compared to nondrinking controls.
- Withdrawal from alcohol also has neurocognitive effects. An increased number of withdrawal episodes is associated with a decrease in visuospatial function and poorer retrieval of verbal and nonverbal information.
- Alcohol use also disrupts the sleep–wake cycle, resulting in increased sleep latency and increased daytime sleepiness.

Alcohol Withdrawal

Withdrawal from alcohol can be life-threatening. Signs and symptoms can include autonomic hyperactivity, tremor, psychomotor agitation, anxiety, nausea/vomiting, and insomnia. These can progress to hallucinations and seizures. Youth suspected of experiencing withdrawal should be immediately referred for emergency management, which commonly includes the use of benzodiazepines.

ALCOHOL USE DISORDERS AMONG YOUTH

Screening for Alcohol Use and Alcohol Use Disorder

The American Academy of Pediatrics and Bright Futures recommends universal screening of adolescents for substance use as part of routine care.[26] The U.S. Preventive Services Task Force recommends screening everyone aged 18 years and older for alcohol use (Grade B recommendation),[27] but concludes there is not sufficient evidence to make recommendations for or against screening in adolescents aged 12 to 17 years (Grade I recommendation).

Screening, brief intervention, and referral to treatment (SBIRT) has been nationally recognized as an evidence-based approach to prevent and reduce substance use, by identifying substance use "risk" and providing a tailored intervention.[26] Screening, brief intervention, and referral to treatment appears effective in identifying and reducing substance use risk in numerous settings, including emergency departments, primary care offices, dental clinics, and mental health practices.[26]

There are several widely available screening instruments to guide clinicians in identifying AYAs who use alcohol. Screening tools can be administered by the professional as part of the general health interview, although computer- or smart device–administered screening tools are increasingly available and may have better accuracy since youth may be less inclined to provide socially desirable answers to questions about substance use.[28] To be practical, screening tools must be easy to remember, administer, and score. Widely used and recommended youth-specific screening tools are described below.[29]

CRAFFT

The *CRAFFT* is a validated, behavioral health screening tool (see http://crafft.org/get-the-crafft/). CRAFFT is a mnemonic acronym of the first letters of keywords in six screening questions that should be asked exactly as written (see below). Before being asked the CRAFFT questions, the AYA is asked to answer the following three questions: "During the past 12 months, on how many days did you: (1) Drink more than a few sips of beer, wine, or any drink containing alcohol? (2) Use any marijuana (weed, oil, or hash by smoking, vaping, or in food) or 'synthetic marijuana' (like 'K2,' 'Spice')? (3) Use anything else to get high (like other illegal drugs, prescription or over-the-counter medications, and things that you sniff, huff, or vape)?"

Notably, the questions in this screening tool, and several that follow, ask "on how many days" an AYA used substances in the past year, rather than asking "whether" they used substances; this approach is likely to produce more affirmative responses (i.e., has higher sensitivity). If an AYA responds "zero" to all three questions, they should be asked only the CAR question (see below), whereas

XIV

if they answer ≥1 to any one or more of the three, they should be asked all six CRAFFT questions.

C: Have you ever ridden in a CAR driven by someone (including yourself) who was "high" or had been using alcohol or drugs?

R: Do you ever use alcohol or drugs to RELAX, feel better about yourself, or fit in?

A: Do you ever use alcohol or drugs while you are by yourself, or ALONE?

F: Do you ever FORGET things you did while using alcohol or drugs?

F: Do your family or FRIENDS ever tell you that you should cut down on your drinking or drug use?

T: Have you ever gotten into TROUBLE while you were using alcohol or drugs?

Each "Yes" response is scored as one point. A score of ≥2 signifies a "positive" screen and indicates that the AYA is at high risk for having a substance use disorder and should receive further assessment. Newer versions of the CRAFFT screen that probe e-cigarette use and vaping are undergoing validation.

Screening to Brief Intervention

Screening to Brief Intervention (S2BI) is a screening tool that has not only been validated in youth but also can identify moderate/severe substance use disorders based on the frequency of past-year substance use (see https://www.drugabuse.gov/ast/s2bi/#/). Screening to Brief Intervention asks, "In the past year, how many times have you used (1) Tobacco? (2) Alcohol? (3) Marijuana?" with possible answers including "Never", "Once or twice", "Monthly", or "At least weekly." If an AYA has not used any substances, the screen stops; if they respond affirmatively to use of any substances, the clinician then asks about other substances: "(4) prescription drugs that were not prescribed for you (such as pain medication or Adderall)?, (5) illegal drugs (such as cocaine or Ecstasy)?, (6) inhalants (such as nitrous oxide)?, and (7) herbs or synthetic drugs (such as salvia, 'K2', or bath salts)?" As with the CRAFFT, newer versions of the S2BI currently undergoing validation probe e-cigarette use and vaping.

The advantage of the S2BI is that it can identify the presence of an AUD based on frequency of use. Using a cutoff of monthly or more frequent alcohol consumption, the S2BI has 53.3% sensitivity and 94.2% specificity for identifying any AUD (positive predictive value, 21.6%; negative predictive value, 98.5%). The same threshold has 100% sensitivity and 93.6% specificity for identifying moderate or severe AUD.[30]

Brief Screener for Tobacco, Alcohol, and Other Drugs

The *Brief Screener for Tobacco, Alcohol, and Other Drugs (BSTAD)* is another screening tool validated in youth that asks about alcohol use alongside the use of other substances (see https://www.drugabuse.gov/ast/bstad/#/). Similar to the CRAFFT and S2BI, it opens with three questions about tobacco, alcohol, and marijuana, and probes the number of days of use: "In the PAST YEAR, on how many days did you (1) smoke cigarettes or use other tobacco products? (2) have more than a few sips of beer, wine, or any drink containing alcohol? (3) use marijuana (weed; blunts)?" Adolescents and young adults who respond ≥1 to any of the three questions are then asked a series of detailed questions about other substances.

Drug Abuse Screen Test

The *Drug Abuse Screen Test (DAST-10)* is an adapted version of the *DAST* 28-item instrument that takes less than 8 minutes to complete. The *DAST-10* was designed for brief clinical screening and treatment evaluation and can be used with older youth (see https://cde.drugabuse.gov/instrument/e9053390-ee9c-9140-e040-bb89ad433d69).

Alcohol Use Disorders Identification Test

The *Alcohol Use Disorders Identification Test (AUDIT)* was developed by the WHO as a simple way to screen and identify AYAs who are at risk of developing alcohol problems (see https://www.who.int/publications/i/item/audit-the-alcohol-use-disorders-identification-test-guidelines-for-use-in-primary-health-care). The AUDIT includes 10 multiple-choice questions that focus on preliminary signs of hazardous drinking and mild dependence experienced within the last year (including questions on quantity and frequency of alcohol consumption, drinking behaviors, and alcohol-related problems or reactions to problems). It is one of the most accurate alcohol screening tests available, rated 92% effective in detecting hazardous or harmful drinking. The test has been modified into the AUDIT-C, which is a simple three-question screen for hazardous or harmful drinking that can be used in isolation or as part of a general health assessment (see https://cde.drugabuse.gov/instrument/f229c68a-67ce-9a58-e040-bb89ad432be4).

Alcohol, Smoking and Substance Involvement Screening Test

The *Alcohol, Smoking and Substance Involvement Screening Test (ASSIST)* is another standardized, scripted screening tool developed by the WHO (see http://www.who.int/substance_abuse/activities/assist_test/en/). The ASSIST has been studied cross-culturally in eight countries. This interview-guided screening tool provides a detailed assessment of both alcohol and substance use. Originally developed for use in primary care, it has been increasingly applied in other settings, including trauma centers, mental health practices, and college health centers.

The NIAAA developed a program for screening youth aged 9 to 18 years, described in its guide for practitioners (see https://www.niaaa.nih.gov/alcohols-effects-health/professional-education-materials/alcohol-screening-and-brief-intervention-youth-practitioners-guide). Briefly, it consists of two questions about the number of drinks consumed over the past year by the patient and their peers, with questions varying based on the AYA's age. Individuals are assigned to low-, moderate-, or high-risk categories and potential brief interventions are discussed.

Brief Interventions and Referrals to Treatment

After clinicians quantify an AYA's alcohol and other substance use, they should provide appropriate interventions. Most of the screening tools listed above provide specific guidance for clinicians about what to say to the AYA, often including scripted statements. For example, in the CRAFFT, AYAs who report no use of alcohol or drugs and have not ridden in a car driven by someone using substances should receive positive reinforcement. Those who report any use of alcohol or drugs but have a CRAFFT score <2 are encouraged to stop using substances and should receive brief advice regarding the adverse health effects of substance use (e.g., "As your doctor, I recommend that you cut back or stop drinking" and/or "Teens who drink alcohol often end up in risky situations."). The NIAAA's Alcohol Screening and Brief Intervention Guide for Youth has extensive alcohol-focused recommendations for practitioners.

Adolescents and young adults with evidence of a possible AUD should undergo additional evaluation. Importantly, a safety assessment should be conducted, including ensuring that the AYA is not drinking and driving or engaging in other unsafe practices such as condomless sex. Any youth who report dangerous behaviors should receive appropriate interventions to mitigate risk. (In the case of drinking and driving, Students Against Destructive Decisions [SADD] has created a "Contract for Life", which clinicians can use as a guide for ensuring safety; https://www.sadd.org/resources). Clinicians should screen for comorbid mental health problems such as depression, anxiety, and attention-deficit/hyperactivity disorder and ensure that appropriate treatment and/or referrals are provided for these conditions.

Ideally, primary care clinicians should assess and treat substance use problems and provide comprehensive treatment for AUDs in the medical home. However, since addiction training and experience in most settings is poor, many clinicians continue to refer AYAs with alcohol-related problems to outside treatment programs. Locating an AYA-focused substance use treatment program can be difficult in many locations, but in the United States, the Substance Abuse and Mental Health Services Administration (SAMHSA) maintains an updated directory that clinicians can access at https://findtreatment.samhsa.gov. Clinicians should become familiar with local treatment programs to enhance continuity of care across settings.

Diagnosis of Alcohol Use Disorder

In the *Diagnostic and Statistical Manual for Mental Disorders (DSM-5)*, the conditions formerly known as "alcohol abuse" and "alcohol dependence" are now combined into a single entity, "alcohol use disorders." According to the *DSM-5* (**Table 69.2**), anyone

TABLE 69.2
DSM-5 Criteria for Diagnosis of Alcohol Use Disorder

Alcohol use disorder DSM-5[a]

Alcohol is often taken in larger amounts or over a longer period than was intended

There is a persistent desire or unsuccessful efforts to cut down or control alcohol use

A great deal of time is spent in activities necessary to obtain alcohol, use alcohol, or recover from its effects

Craving, or a strong desire or urge to use alcohol

Recurrent alcohol use resulting in a failure to fulfill major role obligations at work, school, or home

Continued alcohol use despite having persistent or recurrent social or interpersonal problems caused or exacerbated by the effects of alcohol

Important social, occupational, or recreational activities are given up or reduced because of alcohol use

Recurrent alcohol use in situations in which it is physically hazardous

Alcohol use is continued despite knowledge of having a persistent or recurrent physical or psychological problem that is likely to have been caused or exacerbated by alcohol

Tolerance, as defined by either of the following:
a. A need for markedly increased amounts of alcohol to achieve intoxication or desired effect
b. A markedly diminished effect with continued use of the same amount of alcohol

Withdrawal, as manifested by either of the following:
a. The characteristic withdrawal syndrome for alcohol (see criteria A and B below)[b]
b. Alcohol (or a closely related substance, such as a benzodiazepine) is taken to relieve or avoid withdrawal symptoms

[a]The presence of at least 2 of these symptoms indicates an Alcohol Use Disorder (AUD). The severity of the AUD is defined as:
　Mild: The presence of 2–3 symptoms
　Moderate: The presence of 4–5 symptoms
　Severe: The presence of 6 or more symptoms
[b]Alcohol withdrawal-Criteria A and B
A. Cessation of (or reduction in) alcohol use that has been heavy and prolonged
B. Two (or more) of the following, developing within several hours to a few days after Criterion A:
　(1) Autonomic hyperactivity (e.g., sweating or pulse rate greater than 100)
　(2) Increased hand tremor
　(3) Insomnia
　(4) Nausea or vomiting
　(5) Transient visual, tactile, or auditory hallucinations or illusions
　(6) Psychomotor agitation
　(7) Anxiety
　(8) Grand mal seizures

meeting any two of the 11 diagnostic criteria for abuse and dependence during the same 12-month period would receive a diagnosis of AUD. Alcohol use disorders are now characterized as mild, moderate, and severe, depending on the number of criteria met.[31] Broadly speaking, an AUD consists of persistent use of alcohol despite negative consequences and loss of control over substance use. Additional criteria include alcohol cravings, tolerance, and withdrawal.

In 2019, approximately 1.7% of adolescents aged 12 to 17 years and 9.3% of young adults aged 18 to 25 years in the United States had an AUD. Research shows that most people with an AUD do not receive treatment. In 2019, for instance, only 66,000 adolescents aged 12 to 17 years and 339,000 young adults aged 18 to 25 years received treatment for an AUD.[32] In 2019, of the 1.7% of 12- to 17-year-olds classified as needing AUD treatment, only 4.6% received treatment at a specialty facility. In 2019, of the 9.5% of 18- to 25-year-olds classified as needing AUD treatment, only 5.8% received treatment at a specialty facility.

Many AYAs with alcohol use and AUD also have anxiety, depression, or other mental health disorders. It is important for clinicians to assess for and address other comorbid mental health conditions when evaluating youth with AUD. Although the components of a full evaluation are outside the scope of this chapter, clinicians should also ensure general health needs are addressed, including reproductive health needs, to mitigate against alcohol-related negative health consequences (e.g., unplanned pregnancy, sexually transmitted infection).[33]

Treatment for Alcohol Use Disorder

Treatment for AUDs is a growing field. Typical treatments include medications and/or behavioral health supports. There are three FDA-approved medications for the treatment of AUD.[34] All three are only approved for adults aged ≥18 years but are often used off-label for the treatment of adolescents aged <18 years. Medications are considered first-line in adults.[35] They may be helpful in adolescents, but further studies are needed.

Naltrexone is an opioid antagonist that may decrease cravings for alcohol and that decreases risk of relapse to alcohol use and of binge drinking. It is available in a long-acting, injectable formulation, administered monthly, which promotes adherence, as well as a daily pill.

Acamprosate is a medication that reduces excitatory glutamate neurotransmission in the brain and increases inhibitory gamma-aminobutyric acid neurotransmission; as such, it can decrease cravings and some symptoms of alcohol withdrawal in some individuals. It is available as an oral pill that must be taken three times a day, which likely limits adherence. It can be given in addition to naltrexone in individuals with severe AUD incompletely responsive to a single medication.

Disulfiram is an inhibitor of aldehyde dehydrogenase and causes levels of acetaldehyde to rise when an individual consumes alcohol, leading to headache, flushing, nausea, and sweating. This adverse reaction is meant to deter further use; however, in practice, individuals can stop taking the medication and resume drinking, so adherence can be problematic.

There has also been substantial progress in research on behavioral treatments for adults aged 18 years and older with AUDs. To date, evidence-based treatments for reducing alcohol problems include motivational enhancement therapy, cognitive behavioral therapy, and the adolescent community reinforcement approach. Overall, treatment requires that AYAs pursue substitute activities that provide pleasures and rewards to replace drug use. These activities should be realistic and attainable and facilitate the development of a healthy support system.

Although acute alcohol withdrawal is most commonly managed in inpatient medical units given its potential severity, follow-up addiction treatment does not necessarily need to be delivered in a higher level of care than outpatient treatment.[33] Although residential, partial hospitalization, or intensive outpatient treatment settings may be helpful for AYAs whose AUD is severe or accompanied by comorbid psychiatric diagnoses that could be better managed in a "dual diagnosis" program, or whose home environment is not conducive to recovery, most AYAs can receive AUD treatment from their primary care physician (e.g., for medication management) and a behavioral therapist. Ensuring that AYAs receive care in the least restrictive environment also allows them to pursue other important aspects of their recovery, such as education, employment, and prosocial activities.

Peer support (e.g., Alcoholics Anonymous) may be helpful for some AYAs. Treatments that include family components have been shown to be effective with younger youth, particularly if other family members have struggled with alcohol use. Clinicians can also suggest Al-Anon or Alateen, which are 12-step self-help groups for family members of individuals with substance use disorders, that are helpful for some individuals.

SUMMARY

Alcohol is one of the most widely used substances in the United States. The U.S. Department of Health and Human Services recommends that individuals under age 21 years not consume any alcohol, and that adults aged 21 years and over limit their intake to one drink per day or less for females, or two drinks per day or fewer for males. Although the prevalence of alcohol use and binge drinking have decreased among AYAs over the past decade, alcohol use remains widely prevalent with 29% of high school students reporting drinking alcohol in the past 30 days, and 13.7% reporting binge drinking in the past 30 days. Among young adults aged 18 to 25 years, 54.3% report current alcohol use. Children of individuals with AUD are more susceptible to AUD than other youth due to genetic and environmental contributions including parental drinking standards. The costs of problematic alcohol consumption in the United States are significant, including 3,500 deaths annually among youth under age 21 years as well as high rates of injuries, including from motor vehicle collisions involving alcohol, assaults, and sexual assaults. Alcohol is a neurotoxin and can cause damage to the developing adolescent brain, affecting learning, memory, and IQ. The American Academy of Pediatrics recommends universal screening of adolescents for substance use with a validated tool such as the CRAFFT, S2BI, BSTAD, DAST-10, AUDIT-C, ASSIST, or NIAAA two-question screener. Youth who screen positive for substance use should receive brief intervention and potential referral to treatment. Youth diagnosed with AUD based on DSM-5 criteria should receive treatment with medication (naltrexone, acamprosate, or disulfiram) and/or behavioral health supports.

ACKNOWLEDGMENT

This chapter is based on "Chapter 64: Alcohol" from the 6th Edition, authored by Rachel Gonzales-Castaneda and Martin M. Anderson.

REFERENCES

1. Centers for Disease Control and Prevention. *Alcohol use and your health. Learn the facts.* Published February 23, 2021. Accessed March 23, 2021. https://www.cdc.gov/alcohol/fact-sheets/alcohol-use.htm
2. Centers for Disease Control and Prevention. *Impaired driving: get the facts | motor vehicle safety.* Published August 24, 2020. Accessed March 23, 2021. https://www.cdc.gov/transportationsafety/impaired_driving/impaired-drv_factsheet.html
3. US Department of Agriculture, US Department of Health and Human Services. *Dietary Guidelines for Americans, 2020–2025.* 2020:164. DietaryGuidelines.gov
4. Clark Goings T, Salas-Wright CP, Belgrave FZ, et al. Trends in binge drinking and alcohol abstention among adolescents in the US, 2002–2016. *Drug Alcohol Dependence.* 2019;200:115–123.
5. Centers for Disease Control and Prevention. *Youth Risk Behavior Surveillance—United States, 2019.* MMWR Suppl 2020;69(1).
6. Johnston LD, Miech RA, O'Malley PM, et al. *Monitoring the Future: National Survey Results on Drug Use 1975–2019: 2019 Overview Key Findings on Adolescent Drug Use.* Institute Social Research, University Michigan. Published online January 2020. Accessed July 9, 2020. http://www.monitoringthefuture.org/pubs/monographs/mtf-overview2019.pdf
7. Substance Abuse and Mental Health Services Administration. *Key Substance Use and Mental Health Indicators in the United States: Results from the 2019 National Survey on Drug Use and Health.* Center for Behavioral Health Statistics and Quality, Substance Abuse and Mental Health Services Administration; 2020. https://www.samhsa.gov/data/
8. American College Health Association. *American College Health Association-National College Health Assessment (ACHA-NCHA III).* American College Health Association; 2020. Accessed March 23, 2021. https://www.acha.org/documents/ncha/NCHA-III_Fall_2020_Reference_Group_Data_Report.pdf
9. World Health Organization. Global Status Report on Alcohol and Health 2018. WHO Press; 2018.
10. Verhoef M, van den Eijnden RJJM, Koning IM, et al. Age at menarche and adolescent alcohol use. *J Youth Adolesc.* 2014;43(8):1333–1345.
11. Quigley J, Committee on substance use and prevention. Alcohol use by youth. *Pediatrics.* 2019;144(1):e20191356.
12. Trucco EM, Madan B, Villar M. The impact of genes on adolescent substance use: a developmental perspective. *Curr Addict Rep.* 2019;6(4):522–531.
13. Koning IM, van den Eijnden RJJM, Engels RCME. Why target early adolescents and parents in alcohol prevention? The mediating effects of self-control, rules and attitudes about alcohol use. *Addiction.* 2011;106(3):538–546.
14. Foxcroft DR, Tsertsvadze A. Universal alcohol misuse prevention programmes for children and adolescents: Cochrane systematic reviews. *Perspect Public Health.* 2012;132(3):128–134.
15. Radesky J, Chassiakos YLR, Ameenuddin N, et al; COUNCIL ON COMMUNICATION AND MEDIA. Digital advertising to children. *Pediatrics.* 2020;146(1):e20201681.
16. Jernigan D, Noel J, Landon J, et al. Alcohol marketing and youth alcohol consumption: a systematic review of longitudinal studies published since 2008. *Addiction.* 2017;112(Suppl 1):7–20.
17. Litt DM, Stock ML. Adolescent alcohol-related risk cognitions: the roles of social norms and social networking sites. *Psychol Addict Behav.* 2011;25(4):708–713.
18. Sacks JJ, Gonzales KR, Bouchery EE, et al. 2010 national and state costs of excessive alcohol consumption. *Am J Prev Med.* 2015;49(5):e73–e79.
19. Centers for Disease Control and Prevention. Alcohol-Related Disease Impact (ARDI) Application. Published July 30, 2020. Accessed March 23, 2021. https://nccd.cdc.gov/DPH_ARDI/default/default.aspx
20. National Institute on Alcohol Abuse and Alcoholism. *Fall semester—a time for parents to discuss the risks of college drinking.* Published August 2020. Accessed March 23, 2021. https://www.niaaa.nih.gov/publications/brochures-and-fact-sheets/time-for-parents-discuss-risks-college-drinking
21. Insurance Institute for Highway Safety. *Fatality facts 2019: teenagers.* Published March 2021. Accessed March 26, 2021. https://www.iihs.org/topics/fatality-statistics/detail/teenagers
22. National Highway Traffic Safety Administration. *Traffic safety facts: 2011 data: young drivers (DOT HS 811–744).* Published online 2013. http://www-nrd.nhtsa.dot.gov/Pubs/811744.pdf
23. Neinstein LS. *The New Adolescents: An Analysis of Health Status.* 2013. https://www.rhyclearinghouse.acf.hhs.gov/sites/default/files/docs/21928-The_New_Adolescents.pdf
24. Centers for Disease Control and Prevention. Alcohol and Caffeine. Published January 14, 2021. Accessed March 23, 2021. https://www.cdc.gov/alcohol/fact-sheets/caffeine-and-alcohol.htm
25. Yasuma N, Imamura K, Watanabe K, et al. Association between energy drink consumption and substance use in adolescence: a systematic review of prospective cohort studies. *Drug Alcohol Depend.* 2021;219:108470.
26. National Institute on Alcohol Abuse and Alcoholism, U.S.Department of Health and Human Services. *Underage Drinking.* http://www.niaaa.nih.gov/alcohol-health/special-populations-co-occurring-disorders/underage-drinking
27. Levy SJL, Williams JF; COMMITTEE ON SUBSTANCE USE AND PREVENTION. Substance use screening, brief intervention, and referral to treatment. *Pediatrics.* 2016;138(1):e20161211.
28. US Preventive Services Task Force; Curry SJ, Krist AH, Owens DK, et al. Screening and behavioral counseling interventions to reduce unhealthy alcohol use in adolescents and adults: US Preventive Services Task Force Recommendation Statement. *JAMA.* 2018;320(18):1899–1909.
29. Harris SK, Knight JR, Van Hook S, et al. Adolescent substance use screening in primary care: validity of computer self-administered versus clinician-administered screening. *Subst Abus.* 2016;37(1):197–203. Published online March 2015.
30. Toner P, Böhnke JR, Andersen P, et al. Alcohol screening and assessment measures for young people: a systematic review and meta-analysis of validation studies. *Drug Alcohol Depend.* 2019;202:39–49.
31. Levy S, Weitzman ER, Marin AC, et al. Sensitivity and specificity of S2BI for identifying alcohol and cannabis use disorders among adolescents presenting for primary care. *Subst Abus.* 2021;42(3):388–395. Published online August 19, 2020:1-8.
32. National Institute on Alcohol Abuse and Alcoholism, U.S. Department of Health and Human Services. Alcohol use disorder: a comparison between DSM–IV and DSM–5. *NIH Publication.* Published online November 2013. http://pubs.niaaa.nih.gov/publications/dsmfactsheet/dsmfact.htm
33. National Institute on Alcohol Abuse and Alcoholism, U.S. Department of Health and Human Services. *Alcohol Use Disorder.* http://www.niaaa.nih.gov/alcohol-health/overview-alcohol-consumption/alcohol-use-disorders
34. Hadland SE, Yule AM, Levy SJ, et al. Evidence-based treatment of young adults with substance use disorders. *Pediatrics.* 2021;147(Suppl 2):S204–S214.
35. Kranzler HR, Soyka M. Diagnosis and pharmacotherapy of alcohol use disorder: a review. *JAMA.* 2018;320(8):815–824.

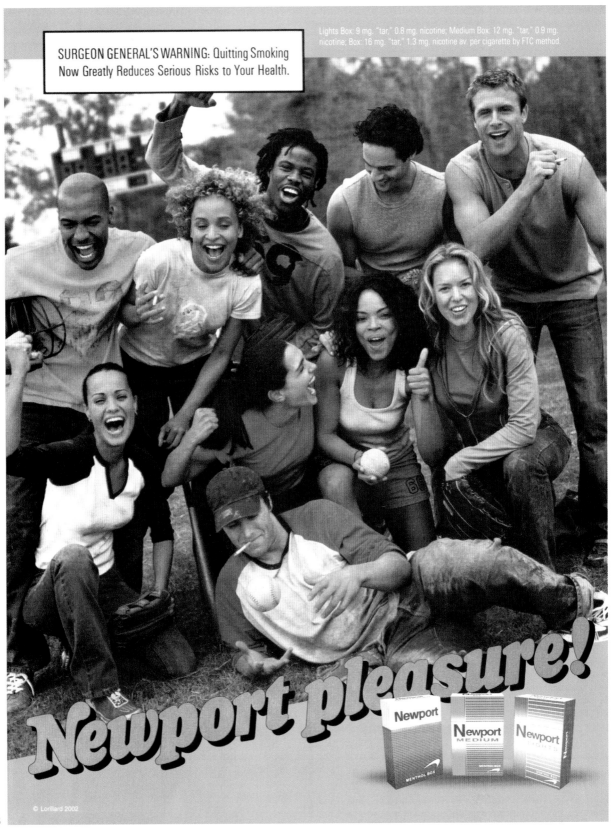

B

FIGURE 70.3 (*Continued*)

regulate impulses and emotion.[14] As a consequence, adolescents are highly vulnerable to drug experimentation and addiction and experience symptoms of dependence at lower levels of nicotine exposure than adults.[13] Functional magnetic resonance imaging (fMRI) examining the neural circuitry involved in nicotine craving and addiction has documented that adolescents who smoke display a hyporesponsivity to the anticipation of nondrug reward (i.e., financial reward) relative to nonsmokers, and this hyporesponsivity becomes more severe with increased smoking.[15] There also is evidence that adolescents who smoke five or fewer cigarettes per day display attenuated responses to other nondrug rewards, including pleasurable food images, relative to nonsmokers, in areas including the insula and inferior frontal region.[16] The implication of these studies is that the use of extremely rewarding drugs, such as nicotine, decreases the perception of the pleasure obtained from nondrug rewards. Furthermore, such changes in the brain occur in the early phases of smoking. The younger one starts smoking cigarettes, the greater the risk of stronger physiologic addiction to nicotine, and early onset smoking is significantly associated with heavier and longer smoking careers compared to late onset.[13]

Modes of Action

Nicotine seems to function as a positive reinforcer through its actions on nicotinic acetylcholine receptors in the mesocorticolimbic dopamine pathway. Stimulation of brain dopamine systems is of great importance for the rewarding and dependence-producing properties of nicotine.[17] Abstinence from nicotine is associated with depletion of dopamine and other neurotransmitters, which may cause numerous withdrawal symptoms including anxiety, irritability, and cravings.[17] There are likely genetic factors (e.g., genetic variants in the CYP2A6 gene that influence the rate at which the body clears nicotine) in an individual's susceptibility to tobacco addiction and response to the various pharmacologic treatments.[18] A recent review of research on adults concluded that faster nicotine metabolism is associated with greater likelihood of nicotine dependence, greater cravings and other withdrawal symptoms, and lower effectiveness of nicotine replacement therapy.[19] This is an active area of ongoing research.

Nicotine Pharmacology

One cigarette contains 6 to 11 mg of nicotine, of which about 1 mg is absorbed, and a typical pack delivers a total of 20 mg of nicotine when smoked. While e-cigarettes vary greatly in design and delivery, 5% JUULpods, which have become very popular among young people in the United States,[20] equate to about one pack of cigarettes in nicotine delivery.[21] JUUL uses patented nicotine salt technology to deliver more nicotine than early-generation e-cigarettes delivered. Each dose of nicotine acts on the user within seconds of being inhaled into the lungs. Plasma concentrations of nicotine decline in a biphasic manner. Typically, the initial half-life of nicotine is 2 to 3 minutes, and the terminal half-life is 30 to 120 minutes. Most nicotine is metabolized in the liver to cotinine. Cotinine has a plasma half-life that varies from approximately 16 to 20 hours. Nicotine and its metabolites are excreted by the kidneys; approximately 10% to 20% of the nicotine is eliminated unchanged in the urine.[17]

Effects of Other Compounds in Cigarettes

In addition to nicotine, cigarettes contain tar—a toxic compound. Cigarettes usually contain thousands of other chemicals, many poisonous and cancer-causing, including arsenic, ammonia, benzene, cadmium, carbon monoxide, cyanide, formaldehyde, lead, nitrosamines, polonium-210, and polynuclear aromatic hydrocarbons. E-cigarettes also can expose users to volatile organic compounds (e.g., formaldehyde, acrolein), metals, and other potentially toxic substances, though typically at much lower levels than combustible cigarettes.[22]

Systemic Effects of Tobacco

The 2014 U.S. Surgeon General's report[23] (marking the 50th anniversary of the first Surgeon General's report on smoking and health in 1964) updated the list of diseases related to tobacco use and concluded that smoking is even more dangerous than previously thought. Use of tobacco products can adversely affect virtually every organ system in the body. Adverse effects include the following:

- Cardiovascular disease—coronary heart disease, stroke, atherosclerotic peripheral vascular disease, aortic aneurysm, early abdominal aortic atherosclerosis in young adults
- Cancers—oropharynx, larynx, esophagus, trachea, bronchus, lung, stomach, pancreas, kidney, ureter, bladder, cervical, colorectal, and acute myeloid leukemia
- Diminished bone density and hip fractures
- Pulmonary effects— chronic obstructive pulmonary disease and worsening asthma
- Gastrointestinal effects—gastroesophageal reflux and peptic ulcer disease
- Cataracts, blindness, and age-related macular degeneration
- Premature wrinkling of the skin
- Periodontitis
- Weakening effect on immune system
- Reproductive effects in females—reduced fertility, ectopic pregnancy, spontaneous abortion, and low–birth-weight babies
- Erectile dysfunction (impotence) in males

Smokeless Oral Tobacco

Smokeless oral tobacco products are classified as either chewing or dipping (also known as snuff) tobacco. Chewing tobacco, including loose leaf, plug, and twist, is chewed or held in the cheek or lower lip. Snuff, further categorized as moist or dry, has a much finer consistency than chewing tobacco and is typically held in place without chewing in the mouth. Smokeless tobacco use increases the risk of oral, prostate, pancreatic, and cervical cancers and is associated with numerous dental, periodontal, and oral soft tissue problems, including gingival recession, periodontal attachment loss, tooth staining, halitosis, and leukoplakia.[24]

Another smokeless tobacco product that has been increasingly used in the United States since its introduction in 2011 is snus. Snus originated in Sweden from a variant of dry snuff. Portion snus, the original and most common form, comes in small teabag-like sachets that are placed under the upper lip, delivering nicotine for an extended period of time without the need for spitting. Snus is viewed as an alternative to smoking, chewing, or dipping tobacco, with evidence of lower harm, although pancreatic cancer rates appear higher in users than nonusers.[25] Other new products in the U.S. market are oral tobacco-free nicotine pouches (e.g., Zyn, On!, Velo) and heated tobacco products (i.e., HTPs with brands like IQOS). Heated tobacco products are battery-powered like e-cigarettes but heat tobacco (not e-liquid) for inhalation, and unlike a lit paper wrapped cigarette, there is no combustion. Swedish Match snus was the first tobacco product granted modified risk orders from the U.S. Food and Drug Administration (FDA), and IQOS recently received FDA approval as a reduced exposure product, but not a reduced risk product. The FDA emphasizes that the tobacco products are not safe, and young people should not start using them.

Secondhand Smoke

Secondhand smoke (SHS) is a mixture of side-stream smoke, which comes from the lit end of a combusted tobacco product, and mainstream smoke, which is exhaled when smoked. Because the cigarette is burning at a lower temperature when it is not being smoked, the combustion is less complete, and the side-stream smoke is richer in toxic chemicals than the inhaled mainstream smoke. Relative to mainstream smoke, side-stream smoke also has smaller particles, which make their way more easily into the lungs and the body's cells. Even though nonsmokers receive a much lower total dose of these chemicals (because the smoke is diluted in the air before nonsmokers inhale it), the effects on blood vessels, blood, and the heart are surprisingly substantial. Living with someone who smokes or working where smoking is permitted is associated with about a 30% increase in the risk of heart disease or death (about one-third the effect of active smoking).[26]

Despite the tobacco industry's efforts to cast doubt on the link between SHS and health risks, few scientists and clinicians would deny that SHS is harmful. Major conclusions of the 2006 Surgeon General's report *The Health Consequences of Involuntary Exposure to Tobacco Smoke*[26] are:

1. Secondhand smoke causes premature death and disease in children and adults who do not smoke.
2. Exposure of adults to SHS has immediate adverse effects on the cardiovascular system and causes coronary heart disease and lung cancer.
3. The scientific evidence indicates that there is no risk-free level of exposure to SHS.
4. Many millions of Americans, both children and adults, are still exposed to SHS in their homes and workplaces despite substantial progress in tobacco control.
5. Eliminating smoking in indoor spaces fully protects nonsmokers from exposure to SHS. Creating separate smoking and nonsmoking sections, cleaning the air, and ventilating buildings cannot eliminate exposures of nonsmokers to SHS.

Intervening directly with young people who are exposed to SHS is a novel approach that shows promise. A text message intervention that included education and behavioral methods for avoiding exposure was found to be feasible and acceptable in a pilot study with adolescents.[27]

PREVENTION AND TREATMENT

The 2020 Surgeon General's Report on *Smoking Cessation* concluded that even brief clinician interventions (<3 minutes) can promote tobacco cessation.[28] Busy practitioners can feasibly address tobacco use in a meaningful way in a short period of time. Given the medical problems associated with SHS and that family members are important role models for young people, clinicians also should provide tobacco cessation referrals and/or treatment for family members who smoke.

Clinical Interventions for Tobacco Prevention and Treatment

Anticipatory guidance should always include tobacco-use counseling. Tobacco exposure may start in utero and first tobacco use may occur in the early school-age years, hence clinical attention to tobacco should start with the prenatal visit and continue throughout childhood, adolescence, and into early adulthood. More than 70% of people who use tobacco visit a clinician each year, creating valuable opportunities for intervention. The National Cancer Institute created the 5-A framework (Ask, Advise, Assess, Assist, and Arrange Follow-up, summarized in Fig. 70.4) to support clinicians in intervening:

1. *Ask* all patients at each visit systematically about all forms of tobacco product use (including cigars, mini cigars, smokeless products, and e-cigarettes) and exposure to SHS. A question about tobacco exposure can be added to the electronic medical record or intake assessment. Including assessment of tobacco exposure as a vital sign provides a simple and effective patient-

---

STEP One: ASK about Tobacco Use

➲ Suggested Dialogue

✓ Do you ever smoke or use other types of tobacco or nicotine, such as e-cigarettes?

– I take time to talk with all of my patients about tobacco use—because it's important.

✓ Condition X often is caused or worsened by exposure to tobacco smoke. Do you, or does someone in your household smoke?

✓ Medication X often is used for conditions linked with or caused by smoking. Do you, or does someone in your household smoke?

STEP Two: ADVISE to Quit

➲ Suggested Dialogue

– Quitting is the most important thing you can do to protect your health now and in the future. I have training to help my patients quit, and when you are ready I would be more than happy to work with you to design a treatment plan.

– Prior to imparting advice, consider asking the patient for permission to do so – e.g., "May I tell you why this concerns me?" [then elaborate on patient-specific concerns]

STEP Three: ASSESS Readiness to Quit

➲ Suggested Dialogue

– For current tobacco users: What are your thoughts about quitting? Might you consider quitting sometime in the next month?

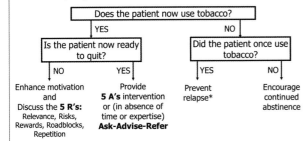

* Relapse prevention interventions are not necessary if patient has not used tobacco for many years and is not at risk for re-initiation.

Fiore MC, Jaén CR, Baker TB, et al. *Treating Tobacco Use and Dependence: 2008 Update.* Clinical Practice Guideline. Rockville, MD: U.S. Department of Health and Human Services. Public Health Service. May 2008.

STEP Four: ASSIST with Quitting

✓ **Assess Tobacco Use History**
• Current use: type(s) of tobacco, amount, time to first cigarette
• Past use:
  – Duration of tobacco use
  – Recent changes in levels of use
• Past quit attempts:
  – Number of attempts, date of most recent attempt, duration
  – Methods used previously—What did or didn't work? Why or why not?
  – Prior medication administration, dose, adherence, duration of treatment
  – Reasons for relapse

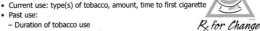

✓ **Discuss Key Issues** (for the upcoming or current quit attempt)
• Reasons/motivation for wanting to quit (or avoid relapse)
• Confidence in ability to quit (or avoid relapse)
• Triggers for tobacco use
• Routines and situations associated with tobacco use
• Stress-related tobacco use
• Concerns about weight gain
• Concerns about withdrawal symptoms

✓ **Facilitate Quitting Process**
• Discuss methods for quitting: pros and cons of the different methods
• Set a quit date: ideally, less than 2 weeks away
• Recommend Tobacco Use Log
• Discuss coping strategies (cognitive, behavioral)
• Discuss withdrawal symptoms
• Discuss concept of "slip" versus relapse
• Provide medication counseling: adherence, proper use, with demonstration
• Offer to assist throughout the quit attempt

✓ **Evaluate the Quit Attempt** (at follow-up)
• Status of attempt and engagement in quitting program; "slips" and relapse
• Medication compliance, extent to which nicotine withdrawal is being alleviated with current regimen, and plans for discontinuation of medication(s)

STEP Five: ARRANGE Follow-up Counseling

✓ Monitor patients' progress throughout the quit attempt. Follow-up contact should occur during the first week after quitting. A second follow-up contact is recommended in the first month. Additional contacts should be scheduled as needed. Counseling contacts can occur face-to-face, by telephone, or by e-mail. Keep patient progress notes.
✓ Address temptations and triggers; discuss strategies to prevent relapse.
✓ Congratulate patients for success and reinforce need for continued support.

TOBACCO CESSATION COUNSELING GUIDESHEET

XIV

Copyright © 1999-2021 The Regents of the University of California. All rights reserved.

FIGURE 70.4 Tobacco cessation counseling guide. (Copyright © 1999–2021 The Regents of the University of California. All rights reserved.)

centered, prohealth message at the beginning of the visit, prompts the clinician to discuss the issue, and helps increase the chances of patients quitting or never using tobacco. Use status and readiness to quit can change quickly in young people. Tobacco use should be assessed at every office visit, regardless of the chief complaint. When asking about newer tobacco products, attention must be paid to terminology, which can differ by age group. Adolescents commonly refer to e-cigarette use as "vaping," while adults are more likely to use the term "electronic cigarette" or "e-cigarette."[29] The frequency of adolescent e-cigarette use and dependence can be assessed with two questions—how many days per month they vape, and how addicted they are to e-cigarettes or nicotine vapes on a scale from 0% (not addicted) to 100% (extremely addicted), both of which have been found to correlate significantly with nicotine exposure as measured in urine.[30] Assessment of tobacco use among youth also has relevance for detection of other risk behaviors and other substances used, given the high rates of co-occurrence.

2. Strongly *Advise* all nonusers not to start and all patients and family members who use tobacco to quit. Advice that is clear, personally relevant, and developmentally appropriate is most effective. Clinicians are viewed as experts, even by teens, and giving a consistent cessation message is important. Those who do not use tobacco products should be praised and their behavior normalized, as youth may overestimate tobacco use among their peers. Clinicians can encourage continued nonuse: "Keep making smart choices."

   For someone who is considering using tobacco and who lives in an environment with frequent exposure to tobacco, offer praise for nonuse to date, encourage healthy alternatives (e.g., physical activity, involvement in school clubs), and role-play methods of gracefully declining to use tobacco among peers. For example, the teen may refuse opportunities to smoke or vape by saying, "No thanks, one of my relatives died of heart disease" or "I don't want to get hooked." For someone who is experimenting or regularly using tobacco, immediate cessation should be encouraged.

3. *Assess* patients' willingness to make a quit attempt to facilitate a tailored approach to counseling. Have they tried to quit in the past year? Are they intending to quit in the near future (i.e., next 6 months) and if so, are they interested in quitting in the next month? Patients who are uninterested in quitting (called "precontemplators") may be in that stage for any number of reasons—lack of knowledge of the health effects (though less likely); low confidence in their perceived ability to quit (self-efficacy); use of tobacco by peers or role models; stress or high levels of nicotine addiction and withdrawal; or more globally, the perceived benefits of vaping or smoking (pros) outweighing the risks or harms (cons). Patients who are interested in quitting, but not immediately, are called "contemplators." These individuals typically are aware that smoking or vaping is a problem, and they want to quit, but they also perceive a number of barriers (e.g., withdrawal effects on stress, mood, concentration, and weight gain). With support and collaborative problem-solving around barriers to quitting, patients may move into the preparation stage, with intention to quit in the next 30 days.

4. *Assist* patients in quitting tobacco, tailoring your strategy to their degree of readiness to quit.
   a. Assisting Patients Not Ready to Quit (Precontemplators and Contemplators): A quick and easy method to encourage patients to generate their own reasons for quitting is to ask: "On a scale from 1 to 10, how important is it for you right now to quit using tobacco?" With the value they report, ask "Why is it an X (e.g., 2) and not a 1?" This question gets patients to identify factors important to them (e.g., cost,

smell of smoke). Next ask, "On a scale from 1 to 10, how confident are you that you could quit right now and not go back to using tobacco?" Then ask, "what would it take to get your confidence to a 10?" The answer to this question identifies barriers to change and presents an opportunity to address them. Instead of lecturing patients about how bad tobacco is for their health (which most patients know), asking these two questions effectively encourages patients to self-identify their own benefits and barriers to quitting. The interaction, though brief, sets up a collaborative process targeted at quitting tobacco.

   b. Assisting Patients Ready to Quit (those in Preparation): Setting a quit date (usually 2 to 4 weeks away) and preparing are important first steps in becoming tobacco-free. Preparation to quit tobacco has physical, psychological, and emotional components. For example, in getting ready to quit (before the quit date), patients should record when, why, and how much tobacco they use, and any triggers for tobacco use, such as drinking coffee or alcohol. Encourage chewing gum, using a toothpick, or drinking a glass of water in place of tobacco use; many patients will notice that nicotine cravings subside within a few minutes. Hard candies, sunflower seeds, or carrot sticks also can be used as substitutes. By the quit date, the patient's environment should be rid of tobacco cues such as ashtrays, lighters, and tobacco products. Clothes, living spaces, and the inside of the patient's car should be cleaned to eliminate the smell of tobacco. Patients should spend time in tobacco-free spaces and avoid places where tobacco use occurs. Patients need to think of themselves as tobacco-free and remind themselves of the benefits of being tobacco-free when coping with cravings. Provide education that withdrawal symptoms are common but transient and that pharmacotherapy is available if needed. Physical activity can help attenuate withdrawal symptoms. As a positive reinforcer, suggest that patients start a money jar with the money saved from not buying tobacco products. The money will accrue quickly, will provide a visual reminder of the money saved, and eventually can be spent on alternative tobacco-free reinforcers. Support from clinicians has been shown to lead to more successful quit attempts. For additional support, patients should be encouraged to call the toll-free tobacco quitline (1-800-QUIT-NOW) and sign up with the National Cancer Institute's website and texting support (http://teen.smokefree.gov/).

   Concerns about postcessation weight gain can be an impediment to quitting tobacco. Strict dieting may reduce success with quitting tobacco and patients should instead be encouraged to engage in physical activity (e.g., walking, biking), eat a healthy diet with planned meals and high-fiber foods, increase water intake, chew sugarless gum, and select nonfood rewards.

   Cessation pharmacotherapy—including nicotine replacement products (e.g., patch, gum, lozenge, inhaler, nasal spray), bupropion (Zyban), and varenicline (Chantix)—is recommended for people aged 18 years and older. Cessation medications with the best evidence are varenicline and combination nicotine replacement therapy (i.e., nicotine patch plus nicotine gum, lozenge, nasal spray, or inhaler). To date, cessation medications tested in adolescents have demonstrated only limited success and are not FDA-approved for use with youth.[28,31] For youth who smoke cigarettes regularly (i.e., >5 cigarettes/day), clinicians may consider prescribing a cessation medication (prescribing instructions for these medications can be found in Fig. 70.5). In the United States, nicotine patches, gum, and lozenges are available over-the-counter for adults 18 years of age and older, but are available only by prescription for youth under age 18.

5. *Arrange* follow-up: Cessation rates significantly improve with regular follow-up. For example, a call, email, or text message can be sent to patients on their quit date to affirm their effort, followed by in-person or telehealth visits every 1 to 2 weeks during the first 3 months of the quit attempt—the time of greatest risk of relapse. Clinician contacts can be augmented or replaced by follow-up arranged via tobacco quitlines, local groups, or emerging social media cessation supports. If patients are able to stay tobacco-free for 6 months, they are more likely to successfully quit permanently.

Most people try to quit tobacco many times before succeeding. Patients should be advised that it is a learning process and that the longer they can remain tobacco-free with each attempt, the more likely they are to quit for good. Irritability, dysphoric mood, and sleep disturbance may occur during quit attempts and patients should be asked about mood changes. For those with numerous unsuccessful quit attempts, referral to an evidence-based cessation group may be helpful. Developed by the American Lung Association, the school-based Not On Tobacco (NOT) Teen Smoking and Vaping Cessation program (https://www.lung.org/quit-smoking/helping-teens-quit/not-on-tobacco) is one of the most popular and effective teen-specific tobacco cessation programs. More effective behavioral therapies for young people are listed in the 2012 and 2016 Surgeon General's Reports.[7,13] In addition, 12-step programs, such as Nicotine Anonymous, may help, although they have not been rigorously evaluated in young people.

OFFICE PRACTICES

Office practices that can ensure systematic and time efficient tobacco use assessment, treatment, and referrals, include the following:

1. *Adopt an "Opt-Out" approach to treating tobacco* that involves automatic referral of all patients identified as using tobacco for evidence-based tobacco cessation treatment or implements such treatment without referral. The opt-out model enhances the reach of tobacco cessation services.[28] Patients who are not interested have the option to opt-out.

2. *Identify a clinic champion and advocate for tobacco-free clinic policies.* If your health care setting still permits tobacco use onsite, develop a plan for going tobacco-free that includes cessation treatment services for staff members who use tobacco.

3. *Place tobacco prevention and treatment posters and informational materials* in your waiting and examination rooms. Free resources are highlighted below.

4. *Eliminate all tobacco advertising from your waiting room,* either by not subscribing to magazines that carry tobacco advertisements or by writing over tobacco ads or placing stickers with counter-messages such as, "Don't fall for this."

FDA-APPROVED MEDICATIONS FOR ADULTS OVER 18 YEARS OF AGE FOR SMOKING CESSATION

Rx for Change

	NICOTINE REPLACEMENT THERAPY (NRT) FORMULATIONS					BUPROPION SR	VARENICLINE
	GUM	**LOZENGE**	**TRANSDERMAL PATCH**	**NASAL SPRAY**	**ORAL INHALER**		
PRODUCT	Nicorette[1], Generic OTC 2 mg, 4 mg original, cinnamon, fruit, mint (various)	Nicorette[1], Generic Nicorette[1] Mini OTC 2 mg, 4 mg; cinnamon, cherry, mint	Habitrol[2], NicoDerm CQ[1], Generic OTC 7 mg, 14 mg, 21 mg (24-hr release)	Nicotrol NS[3] Rx Metered spray 10 mg/mL nicotine solution	Nicotrol Inhaler[3] Rx 10 mg cartridge delivers 4 mg inhaled vapor	Generic (formerly Zyban) Rx 150 mg sustained-release tablet	Chantix[3] Rx 0.5 mg, 1 mg tablet
PRECAUTIONS	■ Recent (≤ 2 weeks) myocardial infarction ■ Serious underlying arrhythmias ■ Serious or worsening angina pectoris ■ Temporomandibular joint disease ■ Pregnancy[4] and breastfeeding ■ Adolescents (<18 years)	■ Recent (≤ 2 weeks) myocardial infarction ■ Serious underlying arrhythmias ■ Serious or worsening angina pectoris ■ Pregnancy[4] and breastfeeding ■ Adolescents (<18 years)	■ Recent (≤ 2 weeks) myocardial infarction ■ Serious underlying arrhythmias ■ Serious or worsening angina pectoris ■ Pregnancy[4] and breastfeeding ■ Adolescents (<18 years)	■ Recent (≤ 2 weeks) myocardial infarction ■ Serious underlying arrhythmias ■ Serious or worsening angina pectoris ■ Underlying chronic nasal disorders (rhinitis, nasal polyps, sinusitis) ■ Severe reactive airway disease ■ Pregnancy[4] and breastfeeding ■ Adolescents (<18 years)	■ Recent (≤ 2 weeks) myocardial infarction ■ Serious underlying arrhythmias ■ Serious or worsening angina pectoris ■ Bronchospastic disease ■ Pregnancy[4] and breastfeeding ■ Adolescents (<18 years)	■ Concomitant therapy with medications/conditions known to lower the seizure threshold ■ Hepatic impairment ■ Pregnancy[4] and breastfeeding ■ Adolescents (<18 years) ■ Treatment-emergent neuropsychiatric symptoms[5] **Contraindications:** ■ Seizure disorder ■ Concomitant bupropion (e.g., Wellbutrin) therapy ■ Current or prior diagnosis of bulimia or anorexia nervosa ■ Simultaneous abrupt discontinuation of alcohol or sedatives/benzodiazepines ■ MAO inhibitors in preceding 14 days; concurrent use of reversible MAO inhibitors	■ Severe renal impairment (dosage adjustment is necessary) ■ Pregnancy[4] and breastfeeding ■ Adolescents (<18 years) ■ Treatment-emergent neuropsychiatric symptoms[5]
DOSING	*1st cigarette ≤30 minutes after waking:* 4 mg *1st cigarette >30 minutes after waking:* 2 mg Weeks 1–6: 1 piece q 1–2 hours* Weeks 7–9: 1 piece q 2–4 hours* Weeks 10–12: 1 piece q 4–8 hours* *while awake ■ Maximum, 24 pieces/day ■ During initial 6 weeks of treatment, use at least 9 pieces/day ■ Chew each piece slowly ■ Park between cheek and gum when peppery or tingling sensation appears (~15–30 chews) ■ Resume chewing when tingle fades ■ Repeat chew/park steps until most of the nicotine is gone (tingle does not return; generally 30 min) ■ Park in different areas of mouth ■ No food or beverages 15 minutes before or during use ■ Duration: up to 12 weeks	*1st cigarette ≤30 minutes after waking:* 4 mg *1st cigarette >30 minutes after waking:* 2 mg Weeks 1–6: 1 lozenge q 1–2 hours* Weeks 7–9: 1 lozenge q 2–4 hours* Weeks 10–12: 1 lozenge q 4–8 hours* *while awake ■ Maximum, 20 lozenges/day ■ During initial 6 weeks of treatment, use at least 9 lozenges/day ■ Allow to dissolve slowly (20–30 minutes) ■ Nicotine release may cause a warm, tingling sensation ■ Do not chew or swallow ■ Occasionally rotate to different areas of the mouth ■ No food or beverages 15 minutes before or during use ■ Duration: up to 12 weeks	*>10 cigarettes/day:* 21 mg/day x 4–6 weeks 14 mg/day x 2 weeks 7 mg/day x 2 weeks *≤10 cigarettes/day:* 14 mg/day x 6 weeks 7 mg/day x 2 weeks ■ Rotate patch application site daily; do not apply a new patch to the same skin site for at least one week ■ May wear patch for 16 hours if patient experiences sleep disturbances (remove at bedtime); before recommending, rule out other factors that might be contributing (e.g., drug interaction between caffeine and tobacco smoke, other medications, and lifestyle factors) ■ Duration: 8–10 weeks	1–2 doses/hour* (8–40 doses/day) One dose = 2 sprays (one in **each** nostril); each spray delivers 0.5 mg of nicotine to the nasal mucosa *while awake ■ Maximum – 5 doses/hour or – 40 doses/day ■ During initial 6-8 weeks of treatment, use at least 8 doses/day ■ Gradually reduce daily dosage over an additional 4–6 weeks ■ Do not sniff, swallow, or inhale through the nose as the spray is being administered ■ Duration: 12 weeks	6–16 cartridges/day Individualize dosing; initially use 1 cartridge q 1–2 hours* *while awake ■ Best effects with continuous puffing for 20 minutes ■ During initial 6 weeks of treatment use at least 6 cartridges/day ■ Gradually reduce daily dosage over the following 6-12 weeks ■ Nicotine in cartridge is depleted after 20 minutes of active puffing ■ Inhale into back of throat or puff in short breaths ■ Do NOT inhale into the lungs (like a cigarette) but "puff" as if lighting a pipe ■ Open cartridge retains potency for 24 hours ■ No food or beverages 15 minutes before or during use ■ Duration: 3–6 months	150 mg po q AM x 3 days, then 150 mg po bid ■ Do not exceed 300 mg/day ■ Begin therapy 1–2 weeks **prior** to quit date ■ Allow at least 8 hours between doses ■ Avoid bedtime dosing to minimize insomnia ■ Dose tapering is not necessary ■ Duration: 7–12 weeks, with maintenance up to 6 months in selected patients	Days 1–3: 0.5 mg po q AM Days 4–7: 0.5 mg po bid Weeks 2–12: 1 mg po bid ■ Begin therapy 1 week **prior** to quit date ■ Take dose after eating and with a full glass of water ■ Dose tapering is not necessary ■ Dosing adjustment is necessary for patients with severe renal impairment ■ Duration: 12 weeks; an additional 12-week course may be used in selected patients ■ May initiate up to 35 days before target quit date OR may reduce smoking over a 12-week period of treatment prior to quitting and continue treatment for an additional 12 weeks

FIGURE 70.5 FDA-approved medications for adults over 18 years of age for smoking cessation. (Copyright © 1999–2021 The Regents of the University of California. All rights reserved.) (*continued*)

XIV

	NICOTINE REPLACEMENT THERAPY (NRT) FORMULATIONS					BUPROPION SR	VARENICLINE
	GUM	**LOZENGE**	**TRANSDERMAL PATCH**	**NASAL SPRAY**	**ORAL INHALER**		

ADVERSE EFFECTS	▪ Mouth and throat irritation
	▪ Jaw muscle soreness
	▪ Hiccups
	▪ GI complaints (dyspepsia, nausea)
	▪ May stick to dental work
	
	▪ Adverse effects more commonly experienced when chewing the lozenge or using incorrect gum chewing technique (due to rapid nicotine release):
	  – Lightheadedness/dizziness
	  – Nausea/vomiting
	  – Hiccups
	  – Mouth and throat irritation
		▪ Mouth and throat irritation
		▪ Hiccups
		▪ GI complaints (dyspepsia, nausea)
			▪ Local skin reactions (erythema, pruritus, burning)
			▪ Sleep disturbances (abnormal or vivid dreams, insomnia); associated with nocturnal nicotine absorption
				▪ Nasal and/or throat irritation (hot, peppery, or burning sensation)
				▪ Ocular irritation/tearing
				▪ Sneezing
				▪ Cough
					▪ Mouth and/or throat irritation
					▪ Cough
					▪ Hiccups
					▪ GI complaints (dyspepsia, nausea)
						▪ Insomnia
						▪ Dry mouth
						▪ Nausea
						▪ Anxiety/difficulty concentrating
						▪ Constipation
						▪ Tremor
						▪ Rash
						▪ Seizures (risk is 0.15%)
						▪ Neuropsychiatric symptoms (rare; see PRECAUTIONS)
							▪ Nausea
							▪ Sleep disturbances (insomnia, abnormal/vivid dreams)
							▪ Headache
							▪ Flatulence
							▪ Constipation
							▪ Taste alteration
							▪ Neuropsychiatric symptoms (rare; see PRECAUTIONS)

ADVANTAGES	▪ Might serve as an oral substitute for tobacco ▪ Might delay weight gain ▪ Can be titrated to manage withdrawal symptoms ▪ Can be used in combination with other agents to manage situational urges ▪ Relatively inexpensive	▪ Might serve as an oral substitute for tobacco ▪ Might delay weight gain ▪ Can be titrated to manage withdrawal symptoms ▪ Can be used in combination with other agents to manage situational urges ▪ Relatively inexpensive	▪ Once-daily dosing associated with fewer adherence problems ▪ Of all NRT products, its use is least obvious to others ▪ Can be used in combination with other agents; delivers consistent nicotine levels over 24 hours ▪ Relatively inexpensive	▪ Can be titrated to rapidly manage withdrawal symptoms ▪ Can be used in combination with other agents to manage situational urges	▪ Might serve as an oral substitute for tobacco ▪ Can be titrated to manage withdrawal symptoms ▪ Mimics hand-to-mouth ritual of smoking ▪ Can be used in combination with other agents to manage situational urges	▪ Twice-daily oral dosing is simple and associated with fewer adherence problems ▪ Might delay weight gain ▪ Might be beneficial in patients with depression ▪ Can be used in combination with NRT agents ▪ Relatively inexpensive (generic formulations)	▪ Twice-daily oral dosing is simple and associated with fewer adherence problems ▪ Offers a different mechanism of action for patients who have failed other agents ▪ Most effective cessation agent when used as monotherapy
DISADVANTAGES	▪ Need for frequent dosing can compromise adherence ▪ Might be problematic for patients with significant dental work ▪ Proper chewing technique is necessary for effectiveness and to minimize adverse effects ▪ Gum chewing might not be acceptable or desirable for some patients	▪ Need for frequent dosing can compromise adherence ▪ Gastrointestinal side effects (nausea, hiccups, heartburn) might be bothersome	▪ When used as monotherapy, cannot be titrated to acutely manage withdrawal symptoms ▪ Not recommended for use by patients with dermatologic conditions (e.g., psoriasis, eczema, atopic dermatitis)	▪ Need for frequent dosing can compromise adherence ▪ Nasal administration might not be acceptable or desirable for some patients; nasal irritation often problematic ▪ Not recommended for use by patients with chronic nasal disorders or severe reactive airway disease ▪ Cost of treatment	▪ Need for frequent dosing can compromise adherence ▪ Cartridges might be less effective in cold environments (≤60°F) ▪ Cost of treatment	▪ Seizure risk is increased ▪ Several contraindications and precautions preclude use in some patients (see PRECAUTIONS) ▪ Patients should be monitored for potential neuropsychiatric symptoms[4] (see PRECAUTIONS)	▪ Patients should be monitored for potential neuropsychiatric symptoms[4] (see PRECAUTIONS) ▪ Cost of treatment
COST/DAY[5]	2 mg or 4 mg: $1.90–$5.49 (9 pieces)	2 mg or 4 mg: $2.97–$4.23 (9 pieces)	$1.52–$3.49 (1 patch)	$9.64 (8 doses)	$16.38 (6 cartridges)	$0.72 (2 tablets)	$17.20 (2 tablets)

[1] Marketed by GlaxoSmithKline.
[2] Marketed by Dr. Reddy's.
[3] Marketed by Pfizer.
[4] The U.S. Clinical Practice Guideline states that pregnant smokers should be encouraged to quit without medication based on insufficient evidence of effectiveness and theoretical concerns with safety. Pregnant smokers should be offered behavioral counseling interventions that exceed minimal advice to quit.
[5] In July 2009, the FDA mandated that the prescribing information for all bupropion- and varenicline-containing products include a black-boxed warning highlighting the risk of serious neuropsychiatric symptoms, including changes in behavior, hostility, agitation, depressed mood, suicidal thoughts and behavior, and attempted suicide. Clinicians should advise patients to stop taking varenicline or bupropion SR and contact a health care provider immediately if they experience agitation, depressed mood, or any changes in behavior that are not typical of nicotine withdrawal, or if they experience suicidal thoughts or behavior. If treatment is stopped due to neuropsychiatric symptoms, patients should be monitored until the symptoms resolve. Based on results of a mandated clinical trial, the FDA removed this boxed warning in December 2016.
[6] Approximate cost based on the recommended initial dosing for each agent and the wholesale acquisition cost from Red Book Online. Thomson Reuters, January 2021.

Abbreviations: MAO, monoamine oxidase; NRT, nicotine replacement therapy; OTC, over-the-counter (nonprescription product); Rx, prescription product.
For complete prescribing information and a comprehensive listing of warnings and precautions, please refer to the manufacturers' package inserts.
Copyright © 1999-2021 The Regents of the University of California. All rights reserved. Updated January 19, 2021.

FIGURE 70.5 (*Continued*)

5. *Have your office celebrate the "Great American Smoke-out"* the Thursday before Thanksgiving, and *"World No-Tobacco Day"* on May 31st. These are high-profile public events to encourage tobacco cessation.

Health Plan Employer Data and Information Set (HEDIS) Standards and Billing Issues

Tobacco prevention and cessation counseling is considered standard of care, and formal ratings of health plans and individual clinicians commonly consider these efforts. The National Committee on Quality Assurance (NCQA: www.ncqa.org) issues annual reports on the state of health care quality. Related to this, reimbursement for tobacco cessation services facilitates implementation and sustainment. Of note, if tobacco cessation is not covered, other related medical issues may be billed, such as asthma, bronchitis, cough, pharyngitis, or upper respiratory infections. The Affordable Care Act expanded coverage of tobacco cessation treatment. For example, Medicare and Medicaid cover FDA-approved tobacco cessation medications. Many plans also cover counseling.[32]

Educational Materials

Tobacco prevention and cessation educational materials are available from a variety of sources either free or for nominal fees. The Centers for Disease Control and Prevention's Office on Smoking and Health (www.cdc.gov/tobacco) summarizes national trends in youth tobacco use and provides educational materials, posters, hypertext links, and other information. RxforChange is a turnkey interdisciplinary tobacco treatment curriculum with patient materials that are available online for free (http://rxforchange.ucsf.edu). Local chapters of the American Cancer Society (www.cancer.org), the American Lung Association (www.lung.org/stop-smoking/), the American Academy of Pediatrics (www.aap.org), the National Cancer Institute (https://teen.smokefree.gov/), and the Agency for Health Care Research and Quality (www.ahcpr.gov) provide tobacco treatment educational materials for clinicians and patients. E-cigarette cessation resources are available from the Truth Initiative (text "DITCHVAPE" to 88709, www.BecomeAnEx.org) and the National Cancer Institute (https://teen.smokefree.gov/quit-vaping).

ADVOCACY ISSUES

Successful tobacco control involves a number of concerted actions, including:

• Increasing the cost of tobacco products through higher taxes and bans on price discounts

- Banning advertising of tobacco products in youth-oriented media, including social media and video games, and youth-frequented activities such as sporting events
- Enforcing laws that ban the sale of tobacco products to people under 21 years of age
- Banning cigarette-vending machines
- Promoting adoption of clean indoor air laws and establishment of smoke-free facilities such as schools, day-care centers, office buildings, restaurants, and bars
- Restricting the sale of flavored tobacco products that appeal to youth
- Limiting the number of retailers in an area that can sell tobacco products
- Limiting the sale of tobacco products to adult-only retailers

Also under consideration is regulatory action to reduce the nicotine content in tobacco products to minimal or nonaddicting levels.

Organizations such as Action on Smoking and Health (http://www.ash.org), Americans for Nonsmokers' Rights (www.nosmoke.org), and the Campaign for Tobacco-Free Kids (www.tobaccofreekids.org) advocate for public policies that prevent young people from using tobacco, help people quit tobacco, and protect all from SHS exposure. The sites have many useful fact sheets, educational materials, and up-to-date information. The Truth Initiative (www.truthinitiative.org), founded as part of the master settlement agreement between the states and the tobacco industry, has involved youth in its counter-advertising campaigns. The University of California, San Francisco (industrydocuments.ucsf.edu/tobacco) provides online access to previously secret internal corporate documents of the tobacco industry, state-by-state reports on tobacco industry activities, and information on smoking in the movies.

AREAS OF RESEARCH

Areas of active research concerning tobacco use prevention and cessation in young people include the following:

1. What defines nicotine addiction in adolescents, how does it differ across tobacco products, and how is nicotine addiction similar to and different from that in adults?
2. What are the best methods, and in which settings, are programs and clinicians best able to help prevent and treat tobacco use in young people?
3. Is there a role for pharmacologic aids for adolescents quitting smoking? Are pharmacologic aids helpful for quitting nicotine vaping?
4. What role will e-cigarettes play in the future landscape of tobacco use? Are e-cigarettes a useful form of harm reduction or are they a gateway into tobacco smoking for young people?
5. What are the long-term health effects of e-cigarette use?

SUMMARY

Tobacco products are addictive and can lead to lifelong use with harmful consequences. Clinicians are in a unique position to help prevent tobacco use initiation and intervene early to stop tobacco use by young people and their families. The landscape, however, is evolving and emerging tobacco products, their health effects, and likelihood for addiction warrant continued attention.

ACKNOWLEDGMENTS

The authors wish to acknowledge Dr. Seth D. Ammerman and Dr. Mark Rubinstein for their contributions to previous versions of this chapter.

REFERENCES

1. Adams J. Surgeon general's advisory on e-cigarette use among youth. In: *U.S. Department of Health and Human Services*; 2018.
2. Ahern CH, Batchelor SM, Blanton CJ, et al. Youth tobacco surveillance—United States, 1998–1999. *MMWR Morb Mortal Wkly Rep*. 2000;49(SS10):1–93.
3. Centers for Disease Control and Prevention. Tobacco use among high school students–United States, 1997. *MMWR Morb Mortal Wkly Rep*. 1998;47(12):229–233.
4. Gentzke AS, Wang TW, Jamal A, et al. Tobacco product use among middle and high school students—United States, 2020. *MMWR Morb Mortal Wkly Rep*. 2020;69(50):1881–1888.
5. Wang TW, Neff LJ, Park-Lee E, et al. E-cigarette use among middle and high school students—United States, 2020. *MMWR Morb Mortal Wkly Rep*. 2020;69(37):1310–1312.
6. Cornelius ME, Wang TW, Jamal A, et al. Tobacco product use among adults—United States, 2019. *MMWR Morb Mortal Wkly Rep*. 2020;69(46):1736–1742.
7. U.S. Department of Health and Human Services. *E-Cigarette Use Among Youth and Young Adults: A Report of the Surgeon General*. U.S. Department of Health and Human Services, Centers for Disease Control and Prevention, National Center for Chronic Disease Prevention and Health Promotion, Office on Smoking and Health; 2016.
8. Burrows DS, Marketing DD. Younger adult smokers: strategies and opportunities. In: *Marketing to Youth MSA Collection*; 1984: Bates No. 501928462–501928550. https://www.industrydocuments.ucsf.edu/tobacco/docs/#id=hjhj0045
9. Teague CE. Research planning memorandum on some thoughts about new brands of cigarettes for the youth market. In: *RJ Reynolds Records; Minnesota Documents; Master Settlement Agreement*; 1973:Bates No. 502987357–502987368. https://www.industrydocuments.ucsf.edu/tobacco/docs/#id=ylnx0096
10. National Cancer Institute. *The Role of the Media in Promoting and Reducing Tobacco Use*. Vol 19. U.S. Department of Health and Human Services, National Institutes of Health, National Cancer Institute; 2008.
11. Lovato C, Watts A, Stead LF. Impact of tobacco advertising and promotion on increasing adolescent smoking behaviors. *Cochrane Database Syst Rev*. 2011; 2011(10):CD003439.
12. Kessler G. United States of America v. Philip Morris USA, Inc., et al., Civil Action no. 99–2496, Final Opinion. 2006.
13. U.S. Department of Health and Human Services. *Preventing Tobacco Use Among Youth and Young Adults: A Report of the Surgeon General*. U.S. Department of Health and Human Services, Centers for Disease Control and Prevention, National Center for Chronic Disease Prevention and Health Promotion, Office on Smoking and Health; 2012.
14. Giedd JN. Structural magnetic resonance imaging of the adolescent brain. *Ann NY Acad Sci*. 2004;1021:77–85.
15. Peters J, Bromberg U, Schneider S, et al. Lower ventral striatal activation during reward anticipation in adolescent smokers. *Am J Psychiatry*. 2011;168(5):540–549.
16. Rubinstein ML, Luks TL, Dryden WY, et al. Adolescent smokers show decreased brain responses to pleasurable food images compared with nonsmokers. *Nicotine Tob Res*. 2011;13(8):751–755.
17. Benowitz NL. Nicotine addiction. *New Engl J Med*. 2010;362(24):2295–2303.
18. Rubinstein ML, Shiffman S, Moscicki A-B, et al. Nicotine metabolism and addiction among adolescent smokers. *Addiction*. 2013;108(2):406–412.
19. Delijewski M, Bartoń A, Delijewska P, et al. Genetically determined metabolism of nicotine and its clinical significance. *Acta Biochim Pol*. 2019;66(4):375–381.
20. Wang TW, Gentzke AS, Creamer MR, et al. Tobacco product use and associated factors among middle and high school students—United States, 2019. *MMWR Surveill Summ*. 2019;68(12):1–22.
21. Prochaska JJ, Vogel EA, Benowitz N. Nicotine delivery and cigarette equivalents from vaping a JUULpod. *Tob Control*. 2021;tobaccocontrol-2020-056367.
22. National Academies of Sciences E, Medicine, Health, et al. *Public Health Consequences of E-Cigarettes*. National Academies Press (US). Copyright 2018 by the National Academy of Sciences. All rights reserved.; 2018.
23. U.S. Department of Health and Human Services. *The Health Consequences of Smoking—50 Years of Progress: A Report of the Surgeon General*. 2014. https://www.ncbi.nlm.nih.gov/books/NBK179276/pdf/Bookshelf_NBK179276.pdf
24. IARC Working Group on the Evaluation of Carcinogenic Risks to Humans. Smokeless tobacco and some tobacco-specific N-nitrosamines. *IARC Monogr Eval Carcinog Risks Hum*. 2007;89:1–592.
25. Boffetta P, Hecht S, Gray N, et al. Smokeless tobacco and cancer. *Lancet Oncol*. 2008;9(7):667–675.
26. U.S. Department of Health and Human Services. *The Health Consequences of Involuntary Exposure to Tobacco Smoke: A Report of the Surgeon General*. 2006. https://www.ncbi.nlm.nih.gov/books/NBK44324/
27. Nardone N, Giberson J, Prochaska JJ, et al. A mobile health intervention for adolescents exposed to secondhand smoke: pilot feasibility and efficacy study. *JMIR Form Res*. 2020;4(8):e18583.
28. U.S. Department of Health and Human Services. *Smoking Cessation. A Report of the Surgeon General*. U.S. Department of Health and Human Services, Centers for Disease Control and Prevention, National Center for Chronic Disease Prevention and Health Promotion, Office on Smoking and Health; 2020.
29. Young-Wolff KC, Klebaner D, Folck B, et al. Do you vape? Leveraging electronic health records to assess clinician documentation of electronic nicotine delivery system use among adolescents and adults. *Prev Med*. 2017;105:32–36.
30. Vogel EA, Prochaska JJ, Rubinstein ML. Measuring e-cigarette addiction among adolescents. *Tob Control*. 2020;29(3):258–262.
31. Gray KM, Rubinstein ML, Prochaska JJ, et al. High-dose and low-dose varenicline for smoking cessation in adolescents: a randomized, placebo-controlled trial. *Lancet Child Adolesc Health*. 2020;4(11):837–845.
32. American Lung Association. Tobacco Cessation Treatment: What is Covered? *American Lung Association*. Updated December 10, 2020. Accessed 3/31/2021. https://www.lung.org/policy-advocacy/tobacco/cessation/tobacco-cessation-treatment-what-is-covered

XIV

ADDITIONAL RESOURCES AND WEBSITES

Additional Resources and Websites for Clinicians:

2018 National Academies of Sciences Public Health Consequences of E-cigarettes—https://nap.nationalacademies.org/catalog/24952/public-health-consequences-of-e-cigarettes

RxforChange Clinician Tobacco Treatment Curricula—https://rxforchange.ucsf.edu/

2020 Surgeon General Report (SGR) on Smoking Cessation full report, executive summary & provider fact sheet—https://www.cdc.gov/tobacco/sgr/2020-smoking-cessation/index.html

2016 SGR E-cigarette Use Among Youth & Young Adults full report, executive summary & provider fact sheet—https://e-cigarettes.surgeongeneral.gov/documents/2016_SGR_Full_Report_non-508.pdf

Additional Resources and Websites for Parents/Caregivers:

Campaign for Tobacco Free Kids Resources for Parents—https://www.tobaccofreekids.org/protectkids/

Centers for Disease Control & Prevention (CDC) Quick Facts on E-cigarettes—https://www.cdc.gov/tobacco/basic_information/e-cigarettes/Quick-Facts-on-the-Risks-of-E-cigarettes-for-Kids-Teens-and-Young-Adults.html

CDC E-cigarette Infographic, E-cigarette Fact Sheet & E-cigarette PSA—https://www.cdc.gov/tobacco/basic_information/e-cigarettes/index.htm

National Cancer Institute's (NCI) Smokefree Program in English & Spanish, for Women, Veterans, & Adults age 60+—https://www.cancer.gov/about-cancer/causes-prevention/risk/tobacco/help-quitting-fact-sheet

2016 SGR E-cigarette Use Among Youth & Young Adults Tips for Parents—https://e-cigarettes.surgeongeneral.gov/documents/2016_SGR_Full_Report_non-508.pdf

2020 SGR on Smoking Cessation Consumer Guide & Infographic—https://www.cdc.gov/tobacco/sgr/2020-smoking-cessation/index.html

2018 Surgeon General Advisory on the E-cigarette Epidemic among Youth Advisory—https://e-cigarettes.surgeongeneral.gov/documents/surgeon-generals-advisory-on-e-cigarette-use-among-youth-2018.pdf

Truth Initiative website—https://truthinitiative.org/

Additional Resources and Websites for Adolescents and Young Adults:

American Lung Association Not-on-Tobacco Teen Smoking & Vaping Cessation Program—https://www.lung.org/quit-smoking/helping-teens-quit/not-on-tobacco

CDC A Youth Guide to E-cigarettes—https://www.cdc.gov/tobacco/basic_information/e-cigarettes/youth-guide-to-e-cigarettes-presentation.html

NCI's Smokefree Teen Program—https://teen.smokefree.gov/

Truth Initiative Quit Smoking & Vaping Tools—https://truthinitiative.org/what-we-do/quit-smoking-tools

CHAPTER 71

Marijuana

Jesse D. Hinckley
Kevin M. Gray

KEY WORDS

- Cannabidiol (CBD)
- Cannabis
- Cannabis-induced psychosis
- Cannabis use disorder
- Cognitive behavioral therapy
- Delta-9-tetrahydrocannabinol (THC) potency
- e-cigarette or vaping use-associated lung injury (EVALI)
- Endocannabinoid system
- Marijuana
- Medical marijuana
- Synthetic cannabinoids (cannabimimetics)

INTRODUCTION

Marijuana is the most commonly used illicit substance among adolescents and young adults (AYAs) in the United States and the world. Its psychoactive and pharmacologic effects are well characterized, but variations in potency and composition, as well as many other individual and environmental variables, may influence these effects. Herein we will review cannabinoid pharmacology, trends in potency and use, changing risk perceptions, behavioral and physiologic effects, diagnosis and treatment of cannabis use disorder, and medical marijuana.

PHARMACOLOGY AND THE ENDOCANNABINOID SYSTEM

Cannabis originates from the taxonomic term *Cannabaceae*, the family of plants from which marijuana and hemp products are derived. The most common species are *Cannabis sativa* and *Cannabis indica*. Cannabis is composed of approximately 70 distinct cannabinoid compounds and approximately 500 total chemical constituents, including various terpenes and flavinoids.[1] The relative concentrations and potencies of cannabinoids vary significantly across plant strains and preparations. Delta-9-tetrahydrocannabinol (THC) is the primary psychoactive cannabinoid and is associated with the euphoria or high experience of marijuana intoxication. Cannabidiol (CBD), another primary cannabinoid, is not associated with the intoxicating effects of marijuana and is of particular interest for potential medicinal uses (see "Medical Marijuana" below). While often used interchangeably with cannabis, marijuana is the product derived from these plants with adequate THC concentrations to be intoxicating. Hemp, on the other hand, consists of products with higher CBD concentrations and relatively low (nonintoxicating) THC levels.

Cannabinoids exert their effects through the endocannabinoid system (ECS), an evolutionarily conserved signaling system that modulates multiple functions and consists of cannabinoid receptors, endocannabinoids (eCBs), and several enzymes involved in the synthesis and degradation of eCBs.[1] Two eCBs have been characterized to date: anandamide (*N*-arachidonoyl-ethanolamide [AEA]) and 2-arachidonoylglycerol (2-AG). The primary targets of cannabinoids and eCBs are the CB1 receptor (CB1R) and CB2 receptor (CB2R), G-protein–coupled receptors that mediate intracellular signaling pathways. The central effects of exogenous cannabinoids are primarily mediated through CB1R, which is expressed by neurons in the brain, peripheral nervous system, and enteric nervous system. CB2 receptor is predominantly expressed in immune cells, and both CB1R and CB2R are expressed by various other peripheral tissues, including the cardiovascular system, gastrointestinal tract, and reproductive system, implicating the ECS in several disease processes and as a target for therapeutics.

Functions of CB1R-mediated signaling include neurodevelopment, cognition, learning, memory, regulation of appetite and food intake, and sleep. CB1 receptor–mediated ECS signaling also regulates long-term potentiation and synaptic pruning, functions fundamental to neurodevelopment, which completes around age 25 years. The role of the ECS in modulating neurodevelopment and cognitive functioning is of primary concern in cannabis use during this period (see "Chronic Effects"). The ECS via CB1R is also implicated in reward and addiction, anxiety, and depression.

Synthetic Cannabinoids

Synthetic cannabinoids (cannabimimetics) are compounds with chemical structures similar to THC and other naturally occurring cannabinoids. The appeal of these products is twofold: (1) users may be attracted to their novelty and the opportunity for a new, distinct "high" and (2) users may wish to avoid detection of marijuana use by routine urine drug testing. The constituency and potency of these products may be highly variable. Several case reports and series suggest that many young people using synthetic cannabinoids experience significant adverse effects, including anxiety, agitation, paranoia, hallucinations, tachycardia, nausea and vomiting, and diaphoresis. Recent regulatory efforts banning synthetic cannabinoids as a class have helped limit availability and distribution.

TRENDS IN PREPARATIONS, POTENCY, AND USE

Over the past two decades, legalization and commercialization of marijuana have resulted in significant changes in THC potency, THC:CBD ratio, and modes of use.[2] Smoking flowers (joints or blunts) remains the most common mode of use, in addition to smoking through a pipe ("bowl") or water pipe ("bong"). Notably, though, THC potency has increased significantly from around 5% to over 20%. Slang terms for marijuana preparations include "weed," "pot," "bud," "grass," and "herb," often emphasizing status as a "natural" substance. Other colloquial terms include "dope" and "Mary Jane." Several concentrates are now also widely available, including oils for vaping; wax or shatter for dabbing; capsules for oral use, suppositories, and creams; and edibles. Dabbing may also be physically dangerous. Wax or shatter, which are solidified high-concentrate THC products, must be flash-vaporized, typically with a butane torch, and the fumes are inhaled to deliver the drug. Among concentrates, there has also been a sharp increase in mean concentration of THC from 6.7% to 55.7%, and as high as 95%.[3] Up to one-third of adolescents now ingest edibles or dab, and approximately 20% report vaping, with similar increases in concentrate use observed among young adults. Notably, the recent rise in vaping (nicotine or THC) is the highest year-over-year increase in any substance used in the past several decades. Young males are more likely to use concentrates, including vaping, dabbing, and ingesting edibles. Edible use is more common among youth who use marijuana at a public event or school.

CHANGING RISK PERCEPTIONS

Marijuana presents a unique challenge, with complementary decreases in perception of harm and disapproval and an increase in perceived benefit from use. Marijuana is often described as natural and many AYAs view it as less harmful or addictive than other substances. Of all substances with legal status for adult consumption, only marijuana has received approval for medical purposes through a political process. While statutory indications include HIV, spasticity, seizure disorders, cancer, and pain, among others, dispensaries promote use for a much wider array of conditions, including anxiety, depression, insomnia, and posttraumatic stress disorder. Unlike the U.S. Food and Drug Administration (FDA)-regulated pharmaceutical advertisements, dispensaries do not simultaneously list harmful or adverse effects of marijuana use. Coincidentally, many AYAs view marijuana as less harmful than antidepressants or anxiolytics.

Another contributor to perceived risk and changes in modes of use may be a changing perception around the risk of combustible marijuana products. Smoked marijuana contains several known carcinogens, some of which are also present in cigarette smoke. While association with lung cancer remains equivocal and unclear, there is evidence of bronchitis in chronic marijuana smoking. A recent survey of young adults found combustible marijuana products are perceived as more dangerous than other forms, while the risk of other adverse effects of concentrate use was perceived to be lower than the health risks of consuming combustible marijuana.[4]

BEHAVIORAL AND PHYSIOLOGIC EFFECTS

Acute Effects

The immediate, short-term effects of marijuana vary significantly based on a number of factors including THC potency, constituency of other cannabinoids, quantity used, and route of administration, in addition to the user's expectations, chronicity of use, and setting of use. When smoked or vaped, THC is rapidly absorbed, and the subjective and physiologic effects begin almost immediately and typically last for 2 to 3 hours.[5] Orally ingested THC absorption is more variable, often over minutes to hours, with the most rapid absorption from capsules and the slowest absorption from baked goods.[6] Marijuana is most often used recreationally to achieve a mild euphoria or "high," to experience pleasant distortions of ordinary experiences, and to facilitate social interactions.

Acute consequences of marijuana use include impaired short-term memory, attention, judgment, cognition, coordination, and balance. Physiologic changes include increased heart rate and orthostatic and supine hypertension. Users frequently experience injected, erythematous sclera and conjunctiva, and dry mouth. Naive users are more likely to report adverse acute experiences, including anxiety or panic, paranoia, and hallucinations. The high potency of edible marijuana products and unclear "serving size" have also resulted in

an increase in unintentional overdoses, with predominant symptoms including nausea, emesis, somnolence, and altered mental status.

Impact on driving

Up to 20% of AYAs have driven while or after using marijuana or ridden in a vehicle driven by someone who has been using marijuana. While overall effects on driving performance appear more modest than those associated with alcohol intoxication, epidemiologic and experimental studies have demonstrated that marijuana use does substantially increase the risk of motor vehicle collisions (MVC).[7] Acute marijuana use affects attention, reaction time, and motor skills, increasing the risk of MVC.[8] Driver impairment has been demonstrated at blood THC levels as low as 2 to 5 ng/mL or after ingesting more than 10 mg of THC orally (the equivalent of one "edible" serving in the state of Colorado), and the impact of driving impairment is up to 6 hours for smoking and up to 8 hours for oral ingestion. Even less-than-weekly use is associated with increased driving impairment and risk of MVC.[9]

Chronic Effects

Parsing the causality and directionality of associations between marijuana use and general health, psychiatric, and psychosocial outcomes is challenging, given the myriad potentially confounding factors (e.g., shared associations) and variations in use (e.g., age of onset, frequency, potency). **Table 71.1** presents the current consensus of the effects of chronic marijuana use.[10]

The impact of chronic marijuana use on the developing brain and cognitive functioning is an urgent concern. Marijuana use is most consistently associated with impairments in attention, processing speed, declarative memory (recall and retrieval), and cognitive control.[11] Cognitive impairments among marijuana users include struggling to learn from mistakes, and monitor and adjust behaviors, all neurodevelopmental tasks fundamental to learning and executive functioning. Greater cognitive impairments are associated with earlier onset of use, chronicity of use, and higher THC potency and quantity used. While cognitive improvements in a number of domains have been noted with sustained abstinence, significant impairment may persist long term.[12]

Adolescent and young adult marijuana use is associated with a number of adverse psychosocial outcomes including impaired school performance, school dropout, unemployment, impaired interpersonal relationships, and life dissatisfaction.[13] Pre-existing

TABLE 71.1	
Effects of Chronic Marijuana Use[a]	
Effect	**Level of Confidence**
Addiction to marijuana and other substances	High
Diminished lifetime achievement	High
Motor vehicle collisions	High
Symptoms of chronic bronchitis	High
Abnormal brain development	Medium
Progression to use of other drugs	Medium
Schizophrenia	Medium
Depression or anxiety	Medium
Lung cancer	Low

[a]Adapted from Volkow ND, Baler RD, Compton WM, et al. Adverse health effects of marijuana use. *N Engl J Med.* 2014;370(23):2219–2227.

risk, negative peer affiliation, shared vulnerabilities, and adverse effects of marijuana on cognition are all potential contributors to adverse psychosocial outcomes. Adolescents and young adults who use marijuana also have higher rates of conduct disorder, attention deficit hyperactivity disorder, major depressive disorder, and generalized anxiety disorder. Marijuana use is also associated with psychosis or schizophrenia and early-onset bipolar disorder. When considering risk factors for suicide, substance use is one of the few consistent predictors, and adolescents who use marijuana regularly are up to six times more likely to attempt suicide.[13]

Cannabinoid Hyperemesis Syndrome

An emerging physiologic consequence of chronic marijuana use is cannabinoid hyperemesis syndrome (CHS), which is characterized by cyclic nausea and vomiting associated with daily to weekly cannabis use.[14] Cannabinoid hyperemesis syndrome is associated with chronicity of use and THC potency. One notable feature of CHS is symptomatic relief from taking hot showers; this behavior often becomes compulsive. While symptomatic relief is possible, CHS resolves after stopping marijuana use.

Cannabis-Induced Psychosis

With increasing THC potency and prevalence of concentrates, a confluence of evidence demonstrates marijuana conveys a risk of developing early-onset schizophrenia and cannabis-induced psychosis. The mechanism of cannabis-induced psychosis is unknown, though most AYAs who use cannabis will not develop signs or symptoms of psychosis. The highest vulnerability appears to be those with familial risk (genetics) of psychosis in a dose-dependent fashion.[15] Other risk factors include increased THC potency, using marijuana more frequently, and starting marijuana use at a younger age, particularly before age 16 years.[16] While the prognosis and clinical course appear variable, marijuana use is associated with lower treatment compliance, higher rate of relapse, and poorer functional outcomes compared to other individuals with schizophrenia who do not use marijuana.

Marijuana-Related Lung Injuries

Another area of concern are marijuana-related lung injuries in AYAs. Of a recent multistate outbreak of electronic cigarette or vaping product use–associated lung injury (EVALI) cases associated with THC vape cartridges, over half of patients were younger than 25 years old.[17] Electronic cigarette or vaping product use–associated lung injury differs from cigarette-associated lung disease perhaps most notably in its acuity, affecting otherwise healthy individuals and often requiring intensive care and intubation. Severity ranges from self-limited injury similar to a chemical burn to chronic loss of pulmonary function and death. Contaminants identified in THC cartridges include talcum, formaldehyde, phencyclidine, and vitamin E acetate.

● DIAGNOSIS AND TREATMENT OF CANNABIS USE DISORDER

Repeated use of marijuana over time is associated with a number of adverse outcomes, particularly among young people. Significant among these is development of a maladaptive pattern involving continued marijuana use despite associated impairment and adverse consequences. Prior editions of the *Diagnostic and Statistical Manual of Mental Disorders (DSM)* included the diagnosis of cannabis abuse and cannabis dependence, whereas the current edition *Diagnostic and Statistical Manual of Mental Disorders, Fifth Edition (DSM-5)* utilizes the term "cannabis use disorder," with three levels of severity.[18] (See Chapter 68 for review of substance use disorder criteria, which also defines cannabis use disorder.) In the U.S. population, 3.6% of adolescents aged 12 to 17 years and 7.5% of young adults aged 18 to 25 years meet criteria

for cannabis use disorder, compared to 2.3% of those aged 26 and older.[19] Tolerance to marijuana's effects occurs over repeated use, and a marijuana withdrawal syndrome has been well characterized and observed in adults and adolescents.[20]

Clinical assessment of marijuana use may include clinical interview for symptoms of *DSM-5* cannabis use disorder, physical examination for signs of intoxication (see Acute Effects) or withdrawal, and toxicology testing for marijuana metabolites. Urine testing is the most commonly available method, though in chronic, frequent, heavy users, urine cannabinoid tests may remain "positive" up to 6 weeks after discontinuing use.

Supportive care may be provided in the event of acute marijuana intoxication. Observation is often indicated to evaluate the acuity versus chronicity of adverse effects such as anxiety/panic and psychosis. In some cases, psychosis may be restricted to the intoxication event, but in other cases marijuana use, particularly in youth, may "unmask" or hasten the onset of a psychotic disorder in a vulnerable individual.

Marijuana withdrawal is common in chronic, daily users, and symptoms are similar in severity to those of nicotine withdrawal. Specific symptoms vary by individual, but often include increased anger/aggression, anxiety, depressed mood, irritability, restlessness, sleeping difficulty and vivid/unusual dreams, decreased appetite, and weight loss. Symptoms typically occur within 1 day of cessation, peak within 1 week, and last up to 2 weeks. Sleep difficulties may persist longer than other symptoms. Investigation of medications targeting marijuana withdrawal in adults is underway, but at present no specific pharmacotherapies are indicated. Withdrawal is often markedly unpleasant and is a clear factor associated with continued use and relapse in chronic users. Developing cognitive and behavioral skills to manage withdrawal symptoms and avoid using/relapsing is an important component of psychosocial marijuana cessation treatment.

An expanding evidence base is available to guide treatment of young people with substance use disorders in general, and cannabis use disorder in particular. The majority of evidence involves the use of individual- or group-delivered motivational enhancement therapy and cognitive behavioral therapy and/or family-based therapies.[21] While these treatments are often associated with reduced marijuana use and marijuana-associated adverse outcomes, few treatments have reliably yielded sustained abstinence outcomes. Recent developments indicate that additional modalities may augment other treatments to enhance outcomes. One is contingency management, in which rewards are provided based on substance abstinence (e.g., gift cards contingent upon negative urine cannabinoid tests).[22] This may be a key component of treatment for youth who are poorly motivated for cessation and only reluctantly engaged in treatment. In addition, the glutamate-modulating medication N-acetylcysteine may augment behavioral marijuana cessation treatment in adolescents.[23]

Delta-9-tetrahydrocannabinol is highly lipophilic and is rapidly distributed into tissues. With chronic use, THC accumulates in tissues and is slowly excreted over time. Thus, the pharmacokinetics of THC and effects differ between occasional and frequent users. Delta-9-tetrahydrocannabinol metabolites are typically detectable in urine for 1 to 3 days after acute use and may remain detectable for more than 6 weeks in chronic, heavy users. The prolonged excretion of THC, the primary metabolite tested in urine drug screens, complicates clinical monitoring during early abstinence and evaluating new marijuana use.

● MEDICAL MARIJUANA

There is growing interest in marijuana for medicinal purposes. The ECS affects several organ systems, including the central nervous, cardiovascular, gastrointestinal, and immune systems.[24] Three pharmaceutical-grade cannabinoids have been approved by the FDA: one formulation of CBD for seizures associated with Lennox–Gastaut or Dravet syndrome in individuals 2 years of age or older and two formulations of THC for anorexia associated with adults with acquired immunodeficiency syndrome, though it is used off label in children as young as 6 years old.[25] Clinical trials are ongoing investigating the efficacy of pharmaceutical CBD in other seizure disorders, as well as for use in neuropsychiatric disorders in children and adolescents, including autism spectrum disorder and Prader–Willi syndrome. A recent study showed pharmaceutical CBD also significantly reduced tuberous sclerosis complex–associated seizures.[26] Marijuana and cannabinoid derivatives, neither of which are approved by the FDA, have shown potential for appetite regulation, nausea, pain, and spasticity.[27]

The American Psychiatric Association,[28] American Academy of Child and Adolescent Psychiatry (AACAP),[29] and the American Academy of Pediatrics[30] oppose the use of marijuana as medicine due to lack of scientific evidence, unclear dosage guidelines, lack of FDA regulation, and most common route of consumption (smoking). However, AACAP encourages scientific evaluation to determine if there are medicinal indications for pharmaceutical-grade cannabinoids in children and adolescents.[29,30]

SUMMARY

As marijuana policy has evolved, notable increases in potency and changes in modes of use have been observed in youth. Young people appear to be particularly prone to adverse effects of chronic marijuana use, most notably including cannabis use disorders and cognitive impairments. With increasing potency, emerging public health concerns include cannabis-induced psychosis, EVALI, and the impact on driving. In addition, AYA marijuana use is associated with adverse psychiatric and social outcomes. An expanding evidence base is available to guide efficacious treatments for AYAs with problematic marijuana use. The majority of evidence supports motivational enhancement, cognitive behavioral therapy, and family-based therapies, while new findings suggest that contingency management as well as the pharmacotherapy N-acetylcysteine may enhance abstinence outcomes. On the other hand, there is growing interest in medicinal uses of marijuana and pharmaceutical-grade cannabinoids. More work is needed to understand the impact of high potency marijuana and to optimize strategies to prevent and treat cannabis use disorders in young people, especially in an evolving public policy setting in which adolescents may be more prone to view marijuana favorably and initiate use.

REFERENCES

1. Zou S, Kumar U. Cannabinoid receptors and the endocannabinoid system: signaling and function in the central nervous system. *Int J Mol Sci.* 2018;19(3):833.
2. Chandra S, Radwan MM, Majumdar CG, et al. New trends in cannabis potency in USA and Europe during the last decade (2008–2017). *Eur Arch Psychiatry Clin Neurosci.* 2019;269(1):5–15.
3. Orens A, et al. *Marijuana Equivalency in Proportion and Dosage: An Assessment of Physical and Pharmacokinetic Relationships in Marijuana Production and Consumption in Colorado.* Colorado Department of Revenue; 2015.
4. Popova L, McDonald EA, Sidhu S, et al. Perceived harms and benefits of tobacco, marijuana, and electronic vaporizers among young adults in Colorado: implications for health education and research. *Addiction.* 2017;112(10):1821–1829.
5. Huestis MA, Smith ML. Cannabinoid markers in biological fluids and tissues: revealing intake. *Trends Mol Med.* 2018;24(2):156–172.
6. Poyatos L, Pérez-Acevedo AP, Papaseit E, et al. Oral administration of cannabis and delta-9-tetrahydrocannabinol (THC) preparations: a systematic review. *Medicina (Kaunas).* 2020;56(6):309.
7. Hartman RL, Huestis MA. Cannabis effects on driving skills. *Clin Chem.* 2013;59(3):478–492.
8. Aydelotte JD, Mardock AL, Mancheski CA, et al. Fatal crashes in the 5 years after recreational marijuana legalization in Colorado and Washington. *Accid Anal Prev.* 2019;132:105284.
9. Colorado Department of Public Health & Environment. *Monitoring Health Concerns Related to Marijuana in Colorado: 2020 Report Summary.* 2020:41.
10. Volkow ND, Baler RD, Compton WM, et al. Adverse health effects of marijuana use. *N Engl J Med.* 2014;370(23):2219–2227.
11. Randolph K, Turull P, Margolis A, et al. Cannabis and cognitive systems in adolescents. *Adolescent Psychiatry.* 2013;3:135–147.
12. Meier MH, Caspi A, Ambler A, et al. Persistent cannabis users show neuropsychological decline from childhood to midlife. *Proc Natl Acad Sci U S A.* 2012;109(40):E2657–2664.
13. Silins E, Horwood LJ, Patton GC, et al. Young adult sequelae of adolescent cannabis use: an integrative analysis. *Lancet Psychiatry.* 2014;1(4):286–293.
14. Sorensen CJ, DeSanto K, Borgelt L, et al. Cannabinoid hyperemesis syndrome: diagnosis, pathophysiology, and treatment—a systematic review. *J Med Toxicol.* 2017;13(1):71–87.
15. Kendler KS, Ohlsson H, Sundquist J, et al. Prediction of onset of substance-induced psychotic disorder and its progression to schizophrenia in a Swedish national sample. *Am J Psychiatry.* 2019;176(9):711–719.
16. Di Forti M, Sallis H, Allegri F, et al. Daily use, especially of high-potency cannabis, drives the earlier onset of psychosis in cannabis users. *Schizophr Bull.* 2014;40(6):1509–1517.
17. Perrine CG, Pickens CM, Boehmer TK, et al. Characteristics of a multistate outbreak of lung injury associated with e-cigarette use, or vaping—United States, 2019. *MMWR Morb Mortal Wkly Rep.* 2019;68(39):860–864.
18. American Psychiatric Association, *Diagnostic and Statistical Manual of Mental Disorders, 5th Edition: DSM-5.* American Psychiatric Publishing; 2013.
19. Substance Abuse and Mental Health Services Administration, *Key substance use and mental health indicators in the United States: Results from the 2019 National Survey on Drug Use and Health.* Center for Behavioral Health Statistics and Quality, Substance Abuse and Mental Health Services Administration; 2020.
20. Preuss UW, Watzke AB, Zimmermann J, et al. Cannabis withdrawal severity and short-term course among cannabis-dependent adolescent and young adult inpatients. *Drug Alcohol Depend.* 2010;106(2–3):133–141.
21. Tanner-Smith EE, Wilson SJ, Lipsey MW. The comparative effectiveness of outpatient treatment for adolescent substance abuse: a meta-analysis. *J Subst Abuse Treat.* 2013;44(2):145–158.
22. Stanger C, Ryan SR, Scherer EA, et al. Clinic- and home-based contingency management plus parent training for adolescent cannabis use disorders. *J Am Acad Child Adolesc Psychiatry.* 2015;54(6):445–53.e2.
23. Gray KM, Carpenter MJ, Baker NL, et al. A double-blind randomized controlled trial of N-acetylcysteine in cannabis-dependent adolescents. *Am J Psychiatry.* 2012;169(8):805–812.
24. National Academies of Sciences, E., and Medicine. *The Health Effects of Cannabis and Cannabinoids: The Current State of Evidence and Recommendations for Research.* The National Academies Press; 2017.
25. United States Food and Drug Administration. *FDA Regulation of Cannabis and Cannabis-Derived Products, Including Cannabidiol (CBD).* Updated January 22, 2021. Accessed September 09, 2022. Available from: https://www.fda.gov/news-events/public-health-focus/fda-regulation-cannabis-and-cannabis-derived-products-including-cannabidiol-cbd
26. Thiele EA, Bebin EM, Bhathal H, et al. Add-on cannabidiol treatment for drug-resistant seizures in tuberous sclerosis complex: a placebo-controlled randomized clinical trial. *JAMA Neurol.* 2020;78(3):285–292.
27. Whiting PF, Wolff RF, Deshpande S, et al. Cannabinoids for medical use: a systematic review and meta-analysis. *JAMA.* 2015;313(24):2456–2473.
28. American Psychiatric Association. *Position statement in opposition to cannabis as medicine.* 2019. https://www.psychiatry.org/File%20Library/About-APA/Organization-Documents-Policies/Policies/Position-Cannabis-as-Medicine.pdf
29. American Academy of Child and Adolescent Psychiatry, *Medical marijuana.* 2012. https://www.aacap.org/aacap/Policy_Statements/2012/AACAP_Medical_Marijuana_Policy_Statement.aspx
30. Committee on Substance Abuse, Committee on Adolescence. The impact of marijuana policies on youth: clinical, research, and legal update. *Pediatrics.* 2015;135(3):584–587.

ADDITIONAL RESOURCES AND WEBSITES

Additional Resources and Websites for Clinicians:
American Academy of Child and Adolescent Psychiatry (2014, updated 2017). Policy Statement on Marijuana Legalization. Available online at—https://www.aacap.org//AACAP/Policy_Statements/2014/AACAP_Marijuana_Legalization_Policy.aspx
American Academy of Pediatrics. Counseling Parents and Teens About Marijuana Use in the Era of Legalization of Marijuana (2017). Available online at—https://pediatrics.aappublications.org/content/139/3/e20164069
American Academy of Pediatrics (2015). Technical Report—The Impact of Marijuana Policies on Youth: Clinical, Research, and Legal Update. Available online at—https://pediatrics.aappublications.org/content/135/3/e769
Canadian Centre on Substance Use and Addiction. The Effects of Cannabis Use during Adolescence (2015). Available online at—https://www.ccsa.ca/effects-cannabis-use-during-adolescence-report
National Institute on Drug Abuse (NIDA). Marijuana DrugFacts. (December 24, 2019). Available online at—https://www.drugabuse.gov/publications/drugfacts/marijuana

Additional Resources and Websites for Parents/Caregivers:
American Academy of Child and Adolescent Psychiatry. Facts for Families: Marijuana and teens. Available online at—https://www.aacap.org/AACAP/Families_and_Youth/Facts_for_Families/FFF-Guide/Marijuana-and-Teens-106.aspx
NIDA. Family Checkup: Positive Parenting Prevents Drug Use. Available online at—https://www.drugabuse.gov/sites/default/files/family_checkup_2019.pdf
NIDA. Marijuana: Facts Parents Need to Know. Available online at—https://www.drugabuse.gov/sites/default/files/mj_parents_facts_brochure.pdf
Partnership to End Addiction: Marijuana Talk Kit: What you need to know to talk with your teen about marijuana. Available online at—https://drugfree.org/wp-content/uploads/2017/02/Marijuana_Talk_Kit.pdf
Partnership to End Addiction. Preventing Drug Use: Connecting and Talking with Your Teen. Available online at—https://drugfree.org/article/connecting-with-your-teen/

Additional Resources and Websites for Adolescents and Young Adults:
NIDA. Marijuana DrugFacts (October 7, 2020). Available online at—https://teens.drugabuse.gov/drug-facts/marijuana
NIDA. Marijuana Facts for Teens. Available online at—https://teens.drugabuse.gov/sites/default/files/marijuana_teens.pdf
NIDA. Teen Brain Development (video). Available online at—https://teens.drugabuse.gov/videos/teen-brain-development-0
Scholastic. Heads Up: Real News About Drugs and Your Body for Students. Available online at—http://headsup.scholastic.com/
Substance Abuse and Mental Health Services Administration. Tips for Teens: The Truth About Marijuana. Available online at—https://store.samhsa.gov/product/Tips-for-Teens-The-Truth-About-Marijuana/PEP19-05

CHAPTER 72

Psychoactive Substance Use

Diana D. Deister
Sharon Levy
William Riccardelli

KEY WORDS

- Barbiturate
- Benzodiazepine
- Cathinone ("bath salts" or "plant food")
- Cocaine
- D-Lysergic acid diethylamide (LSD)
- Inhalant
- Methamphetamine
- Methylenedioxymethamphetamine (MDMA)
- Opioid
- Phencyclidine (PCP)

INTRODUCTION

Use of drugs, chemicals, plants and herbs, mushrooms, and other agents continues to be a major cause of mortality and morbidity for adolescents and young adults (AYAs). All psychoactive substances can have toxic effects, and their use may result in overdose, serious injury, or death. Chronic drug use results in a variety of long-term developmental and health consequences. In this chapter, we review the clinical toxicology and management of the effects of commonly used psychoactive substances other than alcohol, nicotine, and cannabis. Adolescents and young adults may use several drugs and chemicals concurrently, so that the consequent toxic effects may not be those classically associated with one class of substances.

COCAINE

Medical Use

Cocaine is used medically to provide local anesthesia and hemostasis (via vasoconstriction) in surgery.

Preparation and Dose

Cocaine (benzoylmethylecgonine) is a stimulant made from an alkaloid contained in the leaves of the coca bush. The "powder" cocaine commonly available is the hydrochloride salt. Most cocaine is impure or "cut" by adding an inexpensive substance with similar appearance, leading to significant variability in concentration and potency, and pulmonary embolization may result when certain compounds are used in this process. Levamisole, a veterinary antihelminthic medication is commonly used to dilute cocaine and is known to have significant adverse health effects in humans. The increasing use of synthetic opioids, such as fentanyl, as an adulterant has contributed to a rise in overdose deaths in users of cocaine, methamphetamine, and other illicit substances.[1] Sporadic cocaine use may lead to fatal opioid overdose. The risk is especially high for youth who do not have opioid use disorder (OUD) and thus do not have tolerance.

"Crack" is cocaine hydrochloride that has been converted to a freebase by extraction with baking soda, heat, and water. It is usually smoked with cannabis in a tobacco cigarette or cigar or in a crack pipe resulting in a "high" that lasts about 20 minutes. Crack cocaine can also be injected.

Physiology and Metabolism

Nasal insufflation is the most common method of ingestion, resulting in a "high" that lasts 60 to 90 minutes. Cocaine hydrochloride easily dissolves in water for injection, resulting in a faster onset but shorter duration of the high. Cocaine in any form may also be inserted in orifices of the body where it produces both local and systemic effects.

Cocaine is a *stimulant* of the central and peripheral nervous systems; it has *local anesthetic* activity, and it is a *vasoconstrictor*. Central nervous system (CNS) effects are via three distinct actions:

1. Stimulation of D1 and D2 presynaptic dopamine receptors, causing the release of dopamine (primarily), serotonin, and norepinephrine into the synaptic cleft
2. Blockade of neurotransmitter reuptake, causing synaptic entrapment and leaving an excess of neurotransmitters in the synapse
3. Increase in the sensitivity of the postsynaptic receptor sites

The dopamine reuptake transporter controls the level of the neurotransmitter in the synapse by carrying dopamine back into nerve terminals. Because cocaine effectively blocks this transporter, dopamine levels remain high in the synapse, affecting adjacent neurons and perpetuating the classic "high" associated with the drug. Depletion eventually occurs as enzymes break down entrapped neurotransmitters. This leaves the user dysphoric, with feelings of irritability, restlessness, and depression when the transporter resumes normal function. The "low" can be so intense that it leads to craving and repeated use to overcome the dysphoria. The study of the neurochemical pathways underlying these neuroadaptations is facilitating new approaches to treatment, such as N-methyl-D-aspartate (NMDA) receptor antagonists that block both dopaminergic and reinforcing effects.

Cocaine also blocks neuronal reuptake of norepinephrine and stimulates release of epinephrine, leading to what has been described as an "adrenergic storm" stimulating the neurologic, respiratory, and cardiovascular systems. Cocaine is similar to methamphetamine in that both drugs achieve their reinforcing effects via profound stimulation of the mesolimbic/mesocortical dopaminergic neuronal system. Repeated exposure results in either sensitization or tolerance and causes "neuroadaptation" or progressively decreasing sensitivity of neurons, a process that explains many aspects of addiction.

Cocaine is metabolized by hepatic esterases, and, to a lesser degree, by plasma cholinesterase to ecgonine methyl ester, which is hydrolyzed to form benzoylecgonine (BE). Between 5% and 10% of cocaine is metabolized into norcocaine, an active metabolite with greater vasoconstrictive and neurologic activity than cocaine. Progesterone increases hepatic-N-demethylation, resulting in increased formation of norcocaine, potentially increasing toxic effects in females. Increased cocaine levels occur under conditions of decreased hepatic perfusion.

The half-life of cocaine is 30 to 60 minutes. All metabolites of cocaine are excreted by the kidneys making urine testing ideal to identify recent use. Benzoylecgonine is the most predominant urine metabolite and can be detected from the first void after use up to 4 days post use.

Effects of Intoxication

Signs of cocaine intoxication include hyperalert state, increased talking, restlessness, elevated temperature, tachycardia, hypertension, anorexia, nausea, vomiting, dry mouth, dilated pupils, sweating, dizziness, tremors, and hyperactive reflexes.

Adverse Effects

1. Psychiatric/neurologic: Toxic psychosis, hallucinations, delirium, formication, body image changes, agitation, anxiety, irritability, seizures, paresthesias, hyperactive reflexes, tremor, pinprick analgesia, facial grimaces, headache, cerebral hemorrhage, cerebral infarctions, cerebral vasculitis, disruption of thermoregulation, hyperthermia, and coma
2. Skin: Excoriations, rashes, secondary skin infections (Fig. 72.1)
3. Cardiovascular: *Acute:* Vasoconstriction, increased myocardial oxygen demand, tachycardia, angina, arrhythmias, chest pain, aortic dissection, hypertension, stroke, myocardial infarction, and cardiovascular collapse. Dysrhythmias and conduction disturbances range from sinus tachycardia or bradycardia to bundle branch block or a Brugada pattern, to complete heart block, idioventricular rhythms, Torsades de pointes, ventricular tachycardia or fibrillation, or sudden asystole. Cocaine and metabolites (BE and cocaethylene) contribute to von Willebrand factor release by endothelium, which may explain increased thrombosis. *Chronic:* Accelerated atherosclerosis and thrombosis, endocarditis, myocarditis, cardiomyopathy, coronary artery aneurysms, bacterial endocarditis
4. Gastrointestinal: Acute ischemia, gastropyloric ulcers, perforation of the small and large bowel, colitis, hepatocellular necrosis
5. Respiratory: *Acute:* Cough, hemoptysis, bronchospasm/asthma exacerbation, pneumothorax, pneumomediastinum, pneumopericardium, pulmonary edema, cocaine-induced eosinophilic lung disease, bronchiolitis obliterans, pulmonary hemorrhage,

tracheobronchitis, and respiratory failure. *Chronic:* Ischemic necrosis of upper airways, interstitial lung damage, talcosis, silicosis, pulmonary hypertension
6. Musculoskeletal: Rhabdomyolysis, which may lead to acute renal failure, disseminated intravascular coagulation, and multiorgan failure
7. Endocrine: *Acute:* Activation of the hypothalamic–pituitary–adrenal axis, elevation in plasma adrenocorticotropic hormone and cortisol levels, increased release of catecholamines, hyperglycemia which may result in diabetic ketoacidosis and hyperosmolar nonketogenic hyperglycemia. *Chronic:* Hyperprolactinemia secondary to depletion of dopamine
8. Renal: Glomerular, tubular, vascular, and interstitial injury, acute kidney injury, acute renal failure (ARF), malignant hypertension, renal infarction, chronic kidney disease
9. Infectious disease transmission: Increased risk of transmission of sexually transmitted and blood-borne infections; transmission of Hepatitis B and C can occur in noninjecting drug users (cocaine, heroin, methamphetamine) through sharing of drug paraphernalia
10. Obstetric: Low birth weight, prematurity, microcephaly, placental abruption, preeclampsia, spontaneous abortion, fetal death, congenital neurologic, genitourinary, and cardiovascular abnormalities; increased risk of urinary tract infections in infants born with prenatal cocaine exposure, fetal vasoconstriction in utero, neonatal seizures, and sudden infant death syndrome
11. Developmental effects in infants and children prenatally exposed to cocaine: Executive functioning deficits, language development delays, increased externalizing behaviors, increased impulsivity. Increased risk of substance use, earlier initiation of sexual activity, increased involvement with juvenile justice system

Acute Overdose and Treatment

Cocaine is a short-acting drug, and overdose treatment is similar to that for other cardiovascular and respiratory emergencies.

Initial Management

The primary response is to support respiratory and cardiovascular functions, monitor vital signs and cardiac rhythm, and establish intravenous (IV) access. Screening of both urine and blood for drugs and other psychoactive substances should be done to confirm cocaine use and to check for other substances. Electrocardiographic (ECG) monitoring, cardiac isoenzymes, and a chest x-ray are other useful studies. Blood creatine kinase, urinalysis, and renal function tests may be necessary in patients suspected of having significant rhabdomyolysis.

Overdose Treatment

All residual cocaine should be removed from the patient's nostrils. If ingestions are suspected, or if the patient is a "body packer" or "stuffer" (see below), activated charcoal should be administered orally or by gastric tube. If the patient presents with altered mental status, check for and treat hypoglycemia. Hyperthermia is life-threatening and can be treated with antipyretics, a cooling blanket, and iced saline lavage. Seizures can be treated with benzodiazepines or other standard anticonvulsants. Cocaine-associated chest pain should be treated with nitroglycerin, calcium-channel blockers, and aspirin. Beta-blockers should not be used alone but can be used if combined with alpha-blockade due to the action of cocaine on cardiac receptors. Thrombolysis should be considered if the symptoms and signs of toxicity, an ECG, and cardiac enzymes suggest acute myocardial infarction. Blood pressure elevations may be the result of direct CNS stimulation (treated with benzodiazepines), or peripheral alpha-agonist effects (treated with either vasodilators or an alpha-adrenergic antagonist). Agitation and psychosis may be treated with haloperidol or droperidol with consideration given to QTc prolongation from these medications and cocaine itself.

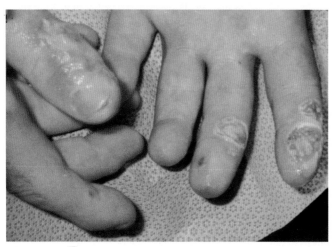

FIGURE 72.1 Crack pipe smoker's callus. (From Berg D, Worzala K. *Atlas of adult physical diagnosis.* Lippincott Williams & Wilkins; 2006.)

Body Stuffer Syndrome

Body stuffers and packers swallow bags of drugs and are at risk of drug overdose if bags leak or break. Abdominal computed tomography may be necessary to rule out residual packets prior to hospital discharge.

Chronic Use

Cocaine is irritating to the mucosa, skin, and airways, and chronic use is associated with erosion of dental enamel, gingival ulceration, keratitis, chronic rhinitis, perforated nasal septum, midline granuloma, altered olfaction, optic neuropathy, osteolytic sinusitis, rashes, burns, and local skin necrosis. People addicted to cocaine also frequently experience anorexia, weight loss, sexual dysfunction, and elevated blood prolactin levels. Cocaine can enhance some cognitive functions in acute use; however, chronic use leads to diminished abilities in most cognitive domains.

Tolerance and Withdrawal

Repeated cocaine use leads to rapid development of tolerance, though no tolerance develops to the cardiovascular side effects. Symptoms of cocaine abstinence or withdrawal include depression, anhedonia, irritability, aches and pains, restless but protracted sleep, tremors, nausea, weakness, intense cravings for more cocaine, slow comprehension, suicidal ideation, lethargy, and hunger. There is currently no widely accepted treatment for cocaine withdrawal or cocaine use disorders, and relapse rates are very high.

Cocaethylene

When alcohol is used with cocaine, cocaethylene is formed in the liver. The half-life of cocaethylene is 2 hours, compared with 30 to 60 minutes for cocaine. Cocaethylene can block dopamine reuptake, thereby augmenting the euphoria and extending the period of intoxication and toxicity and increasing the risk of sudden cardiac death, hepatoxicity, and seizures.

⬤ AMPHETAMINE (AMPHETAMINE, METHAMPHETAMINE, METHYLPHENIDATE, KHAT)

Medical Use

Amphetamines are used to treat attention deficit hyperactivity disorder, narcolepsy, binge eating disorder, and obesity. Appropriate stimulant treatment does not increase the risk of developing a substance use disorder (SUD) but rather may be protective.[2] Methylphenidate and its enantiomer dexmethylphenidate are nonamphetamine stimulants with similar actions and lower potential for misuse. Lisdexamfetamine is a prodrug; neither nasal insufflation nor IV use results in rapid CNS amphetamine levels.

Preparation and Dose

The term "amphetamine" refers to a class of drugs containing an amphetamine base, available either in prescription form or illicitly manufactured, mainly in the form of methamphetamine. Methamphetamine differs structurally from amphetamine by the addition of one methyl group. Methamphetamine can be produced in clandestine "labs," using over-the-counter medications as starting materials, though most illicit methamphetamine enters the United States through international drug cartels. The D-isomer (D-methamphetamine) is cortically more active than the L-isomer and has high bioavailability by any route of administration. Illicit methamphetamine may be mixed with other drugs, including cocaine and fentanyl. Look-alikes containing combinations of caffeine, ephedrine, and phenylpropanolamine require a much larger dose to achieve the same level of cortical stimulation, and cause greater cardiovascular stimulation increasing the risk for stroke, myocardial infarction, or hypertensive crisis.

Prescription amphetamines are typically ingested orally or via nasal insufflation; illicit methamphetamine is usually smoked. Either preparation may be injected intravenously. Smoking methamphetamine produces higher concentrations in the brain for a shorter period.

Physiology and Metabolism

Amphetamines are CNS stimulants that work as sympathomimetic drugs by releasing neurotransmitters from presynaptic neurons, stimulating postsynaptic catecholamine receptors, preventing reuptake of neurotransmitters, and inhibiting monoamine oxidase (MAO).

Effects of Intoxication

Amphetamines have effects similar to cocaine, but last much longer. Symptoms of amphetamine intoxication include hyperalertness, anxiety, confusion, irritability, aggression, delirium, dry mouth, tachycardia, hypertension, tachypnea, jaw clenching, bruxism, reduced appetite, sweating, and psychosis. Amphetamine-related deaths may arise from direct physiologic effects or behavioral impairments.

Adverse Effects

1. Psychiatric/neurologic: Aggressiveness, delirium, psychosis, postuse dysphoria, and suicidal ideation due to depletion of monoamines, seizures, choreoathetoid movements, cerebrovascular accidents, cerebral edema, cerebral vasculitis, hyperthermia
2. Cardiovascular: Tachycardia, hypertension, atrial and ventricular arrhythmias, cardiac ischemia, coronary artery vasospasm, myocardial infarction, necrotizing angiitis, arterial aneurysms, aortic dissections
3. Gastrointestinal: Ulcers, ischemic colitis, hepatocellular damage
4. Musculoskeletal: Muscle contractions, tremors, rhabdomyolysis
5. Respiratory: Pneumomediastinum, pneumothorax, pneumopericardium; acute noncardiogenic pulmonary edema, pulmonary hypertension
6. Renal: Acute tubular necrosis, acute renal failure due to rhabdomyolysis
7. Dental: Xerostomia, maxillary artery vasoconstriction, and poor dental hygiene lead to "meth mouth": chronic gingivitis, extensive dental caries, severe dental abscesses and necrosis (Fig. 72.2)

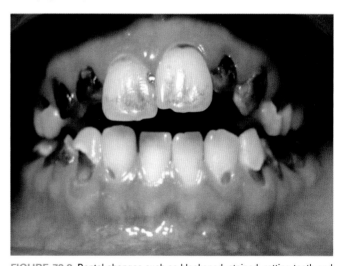

FIGURE 72.2 Dental changes such as blackened, stained, rotting teeth and tooth loss, referred to collectively as "meth mouth," are the result of abusing methamphetamine. (Photo by Dozenist, University of Tennessee Health Science Center, College of Dentistry, Memphis, Tennessee. In: Timby BK, Smith NE, eds. *Introductory Medical-Surgical Nursing.* 12th ed. Lippincott Williams & Wilkins; 2017.)

XIV

Overdose and Emergency Treatment

Complications of amphetamine overdose resemble those of cocaine, although amphetamines do not affect nerve conduction. Emergency treatment is directed toward cardiovascular and respiratory stabilization and control of seizures. Agitation and suicidal ideation are common among youth who have used methamphetamine. Antipsychotics and/or benzodiazepines may be used for agitation, though haloperidol should be used with caution as it causes excitotoxicity and neuronal death in animal models. Chlorpromazine can cause hypotension, anticholinergic crisis, or seizures.

Chronic Use

Chronic use can produce severe psychiatric and physical problems, including loss of executive function, delusions, hallucinations, long-term personality changes, and formication, leading individuals to tear and damage their skin. Choreoathetoid movements and other movement disorders are common and may persist after cessation of drug use. Chronic use is associated with loss of gray matter volume in the frontal cortex. Methamphetamine use by AYAs alters normal development of many brain structures involved in reward processing, such as enlargement of the nucleus accumbens (NAc), a finding that is associated with increased risk-taking and higher reward value.[3]

Tolerance and Withdrawal

Tolerance causes users to escalate the dose or change the route of administration to maintain the desired effect. Symptoms of withdrawal include irritability, agitation, depression, fatigue, sleep problems, increased appetite, headaches, and drug cravings; these symptoms may begin as soon as the high ends, can last up to 7 to 10 days, and are treated supportively.

Cathinone (Khat) and Cathine, "Bath Salts," "Plant Food"

Cathinone is chemically similar to D-amphetamine; cathine is a form of cathinone with less psychoactive effect. These compounds are the active ingredients in khat leaves (*Catha edulis*), which are used as a tea or chewed for their euphoriant and stimulant effects by persons in Africa, the Middle East, and corresponding immigrant and refugee communities in developed nations. Outside the US, khat is used within cultural norms and is not commonly associated with symptoms of SUD. Synthetic cathinones have been marketed with names such as "bath salts," "plant food," and "glass cleaner." Synthetic cathinones have been associated with hyperthermia, violent unpredictable behavior, seizures, and multisystem organ failure: cardiac, gastrointestinal, neurologic, renal, and psychiatric and fatal outcomes.[4]

ECSTASY/MDMA/MOLLY (METHYLENEDIOXYMETHAMPHETAMINE)

Medical Use/Current State of Research

Methylenedioxymethamphetamine (MDMA) was first patented in 1912 as an appetite suppressant but was never manufactured or sold commercially. Beginning in the 1970s the therapeutic applications, including augmenting empathy and the ability to bond with others, reducing fear and facilitating the processing of trauma were investigated. By the 1980s, recreational use of MDMA, sold under the name of Ecstasy, became a fad resulting in an exponential rise in rates of use, and in 1985, the Drug Enforcement Administration in the United States made it a category I substance.[5] In the past decade, small-scale, open-label studies have reported beneficial results in adults with treatment-resistant posttraumatic stress disorder (PTSD). "Breakthrough Therapy" designation was granted by the U.S. Food and Drug Administration (FDA) for MDMA-assisted psychotherapy.[6]

Preparation and Dose

Most MDMA tablets are produced in Europe and smuggled into the US. The drug is sold as a tablet or capsule, often with a symbol printed on it. Tablets sold as MDMA may actually contain methylenedioxyamphetamine (MDA), methyldiethanolamine (MDEA), or something entirely unrelated to the drug, such as D-lysergic acid diethylamide (LSD), caffeine, pseudoephedrine, synthetic cathinones, or dextromethorphan. The drug can be snorted, smoked, or injected, but is usually taken orally. Oral doses take 30 to 60 minutes for onset of effect and duration of action is 3 to 6 hours. Many recreational users begin with a low dose (40 to 70 mg) and gradually add more pills until they experience the desired effect (common dosage range is 75 to 125 mg), this practice is known as "rolling." "Stacking" is the simultaneous ingestion of MDMA with other substances.

Physiology and Metabolism

Methylenedioxymethamphetamine binds to the serotonin transporter in vesicles and the plasma membrane and stimulates release of serotonin into the synapse where excess serotonin binding to postsynaptic receptors results in its effects. Repeated use of MDMA causes serotonin depletion, after which further doses have little or no effect. Methylenedioxymethamphetamine also increases levels of dopamine and norepinephrine in the synaptic cleft.

Effects of Intoxication

Methylenedioxymethamphetamine has both stimulant and hallucinogenic effects. Users describe feelings of enhanced well-being and introspection, empathy, love, affection, and increased energy and ability to bond with others.

Adverse Effects

Methylenedioxymethamphetamine-related emergency department visits and fatalities are commonly due to hyperthermia and cardiovascular effects.

1. Psychiatric/neurologic: Confusion, depression, fatigue, sleep problems, anxiety, seizures, paranoia, spasms, bruxism, hyperthermia, sweating, syndrome of inappropriate antidiuretic hormone (SIADH), blurred vision, faintness, chills, excessive sweating, hyponatremia, hyponatremic dehydration, serotonin syndrome; damage to serotonin transporter neurons
2. Musculoskeletal: Muscle rigidity, rhabdomyolysis
3. Cardiovascular: Myocardial hypertrophy, tachycardia, hypertension, arrhythmias, cardiovascular failure, asystole, sudden cardiac death
4. Gastrointestinal: Nausea, severe hepatic damage requiring transplantation. Methylene dioxymethamphetamine enhances hepatic damage of alcohol by inhibiting aldehyde dehydrogenase 2, resulting in accumulation of toxic acetaldehyde.
5. Developmental: Antenatal exposure results in psychomotor retardation in infancy; learning and memory are impaired in animal models.

Overdose and Emergency Treatment

The most common reaction to MDMA overdose is a syndrome of altered mental status, tachycardia, tachypnea, flushed appearance, profuse sweating, and hyperthermia; this syndrome is similar to the sympathomimetic effects of acute amphetamine overdose. Methylenedioxymethamphetamine should be suspected if a routine urine screen for amphetamines is negative. Delirium, seizures, and profound coma are more frequent with the combination of MDMA and other substances. Adolescents and young adults who present to the emergency room late at night and have clinical manifestations of sympathetic overactivity and increased temperature ("Saturday night fever") should be suspected of using stimulants, and MDMA in particular. Patients chronically taking selective serotonin reuptake inhibitors (SSRIs) or MAO inhibitors for depression risk fatal drug interactions when they ingest MDMA.

Treatment of toxic ingestions of MDMA is supportive, including support of airway, breathing, and circulation; assessment and treatment of cardiac arrhythmias; and monitoring of vital signs and level of consciousness. There is no specific antidote for MDMA toxicity. Close monitoring of serum electrolytes and fluid balance is required to detect SIADH secretion and/or water loading–induced hyponatremia. Hyperthermia should be treated with cooling blankets and IV fluids; muscle relaxants, anticonvulsants, and sedatives, particularly benzodiazepines, may be indicated. Methylene dioxymethamphetamine can be lethal due to hyperthermia, disseminated intravascular coagulation, rhabdomyolysis, renal failure, cardiac arrhythmias and sudden asystole, hyponatremia, seizures, serotonin syndrome, hepatic failure, cerebral infarction, and cerebral hemorrhage.

Chronic Use

Chronic use is associated with long-term cognitive impairments. Impairments in sleep, vision, and cortisol metabolism are well documented. Long-lasting impairment of the 5-hydroxytryptamine (5-HT) system may be more prominent in females and may be reversible in some patients.

Withdrawal Syndrome

Withdrawal is similar to that for other stimulants. The most common symptoms include depression, anxiety, panic attacks, sleeplessness, paranoia, and delusions. Treatment is supportive.

OPIOIDS (OPIUM, HEROIN, MEPERIDINE, OXYCONTIN, OXYCODONE, FENTANYL, SUFENTANIL, DESOMORPHINE)

Medical Use

Opioids are potent antitussives, antidiarrheals, and extremely potent pain relievers. Oral medications with extended half-lives are a tremendous asset in the field of pain management, but also come with the significant risk of addiction, particularly if use results in euphoria. Synthetic narcotics such as fentanyl, which is 80 times more potent than morphine, pose an increased danger of death by overdose. Fentanyl contamination of many different street drugs has increased the proportion of multiple drug overdose.[7]

Preparation and Dose

Opioid refers to all drugs, natural and synthetic, that bind to opioid receptors. Naturally occurring opiates (morphine, codeine, and heroin) are prepared from the opium poppy, *Papaver somniferum*. Synthetic opioid pain relievers such as oxycodone, hydrocodone, and oxymorphone are pharmaceutical products that are diverted and sold illegally.

Illicit synthetic opioids such as fentanyl and desomorphine ("krokodil") are highly potent and may be attractive to individuals who have developed tolerance to other opioids. Use of krokodil, which is easily synthesized from codeine and household chemicals, was a large public health problem in Russia and Ukraine; use has now spread to other countries throughout Europe. Fast onset and short duration of action make this drug highly addictive.

Routes of Administration

Opioids can be ingested, insufflated nasally ("snorting"), smoked, or injected intravenously or subcutaneously. Most AYAs first use prescription pain medications either orally or by nasal insufflation. "Long-acting" formulations can be crushed, making the entire dose available at once. Because of the rapid development of tolerance, individuals may switch to more potent preparations over time.

Heroin, or diacetylmorphine, is a semisynthetic drug that quickly crosses the blood–brain barrier and is metabolized to morphine. It is produced illicitly and commonly mixed with additives. The relatively pure heroin available today can be smoked, insufflated nasally, injected intravenously, or rarely injected subcutaneously ("skin popping"). The ability to use heroin without needles has lowered the barriers to initiation. The effects of intravenous heroin last 3 to 6 hours; tolerant individuals often must use heroin 2 to 4 times a day to avoid withdrawal.

Physiology and Metabolism

There are four opioid receptors in humans. Mu, kappa, and delta are G-protein–coupled receptors that also activate other biochemical pathways; a fourth receptor, sigma, is in a unique class. Mu is the major opioid receptor in the brain and is responsible for the majority of neurologic effects, including euphoria and pain relief. The kappa receptor is found primarily in the brain stem and spinal cord and contributes to pain relief and sedation. Delta receptors are located in the limbic system and are believed to be responsible for affective and emotional changes associated with opioid use. Sigma-1 receptors bind inactive opioids and modulate action of mu, kappa, and delta receptors as well as dozens of other proteins; their contributions to plasticity, reinforcement, and addiction are still being explored. They also bind cocaine, methamphetamine, and dextromethorphan.

Naloxone is a synthetic opioid antagonist that is FDA approved for treatment of opioid overdose. It binds to mu, kappa, and delta opioid receptors with greater affinity than other opioids, resulting in reversal of effect and sudden withdrawal. Because more potent opioids such as fentanyl require more naloxone for reversal, higher dose formulations are now reaching the market.

Methadone was introduced in the 1970s as one of the first medication treatments for OUD. It is an opioid agonist with a long half-life and so can be used to gently stimulate the CNS and prevent the peak and trough levels that occur with shorter-acting opioids. Extensive research has demonstrated the effectiveness of methadone in reducing opioid use and improving outcomes in patients with OUD. Methadone can only be prescribed by specially licensed programs that are restricted from taking patients under age 18 years with few exceptions.

Buprenorphine is a synthetic opioid partial agonist approved for use as therapy for opioid addiction and can be prescribed from a general medical setting. It has intermediate avidity for the opioid receptor, between that of naloxone and other opioids. Because it is a partial agonist, use does not result in the high peaks and low troughs that full agonists do. Buprenorphine is approved for the treatment of OUD in patients aged 16 years and over. The American Academy of Pediatrics recommends medication treatment for AYAs with OUD.[8] In addition to the original sublingual form, newer formulations include intramuscular injection and long-lasting implant. A toolkit produced by the state of Massachusetts is available for prescribing buprenorphine to treat OUD in AYAs.[9]

Naltrexone is an opioid antagonist that has a longer half-life than naloxone and has been approved as a treatment for alcohol and OUDs. A large multisite trial found that it was difficult for patients to initiate since it requires waiting until opioid withdrawal symptoms have passed, and as such, buprenorphine is preferred over naltrexone as first line among patients who need detoxification from opioids.[10]

Effects of Intoxication

Opioids produce analgesia and euphoria. Symptoms of intoxication include anxiety, slow comprehension, euphoria, floating feeling, flushing, hypotonia, pinpoint pupils, skin picking, sleepiness, poor appetite, and constipation. The analgesia produced by opioids dissociates the perception of pain from the emotional response.

Adverse Effects

1. Psychiatric/neurologic: Sedation, apathy, dysphoria, psychomotor agitation or retardation, impaired judgment, delirium, stupor, diminished reflexes, miosis, pinprick analgesia, ataxia, hypothermia, hypotonia, coma
2. Cardiovascular: Circulatory collapse, hypotension, hypothermia, thrombosis, phlebitis, and endocarditis
3. Respiratory: Blocked cough reflex, bradypnea, respiratory failure, pulmonary edema
4. Gastrointestinal: Constipation
5. Skin: Rashes, allergic reactions, secondary bacterial infections, abscesses, cellulitis
6. Neonatal: Low birth weight, neonatal withdrawal, and respiratory compromise

Overdose and Emergency Treatment

Opioid overdose results in coma, respiratory depression or failure, and circulatory collapse. Treatment begins with support of respiratory and circulatory function, protection of the airway to prevent aspiration, and treatment of hypoglycemia if present. Patients should receive naloxone (0.4 to 2 mg) intravenously every 2 to 3 minutes until a response occurs or up to a maximum dose of 10 mg. Naloxone administration must be repeated every 20 to 60 minutes or given by IV infusion to cover the patient for the duration of the overdose. Close observation for reemergence of sedation and respiratory failure is necessary. Naloxone does not reverse hypotension caused by opiate-induced histamine release. Nasal naloxone has been successfully deployed in community health programs for administration by friends and family members of patients with opioid addiction, significantly reducing rates of opioid overdose deaths. Patients with OUD should be given a prescription for naloxone; some states do not require a prescription.

Chronic Use

Problems related to chronic use of opioids are primarily due to impurities, complications of injection or insufflation, and behaviors associated with addiction. Complications include the following:

1. Skin: Abscesses and cellulitis
2. Vascular: Arteritis and thrombosis of the pulmonary vessels
3. Infectious: Lung abscesses with resulting pulmonary fibrosis and pulmonary hypertension; endocarditis and secondary septic emboli; osteomyelitis, septic arthritis, tetanus, HIV, and hepatitis C from injecting infectious organisms directly into a vein
4. Liver and kidney: Hepatitis and glomerulonephritis from injecting foreign material (talc, sugar) into a vein
5. Respiratory: Recurrent aspiration pneumonia from respiratory suppression and blocking of the cough reflex, pulmonary edema, and arrhythmias caused by quinine
6. Myositis ossificans: Extraosseous metaplasia of muscle caused by needle manipulation

Tolerance and Withdrawal

Tolerance, dependence, and addiction occur very quickly, and patients must constantly increase dose and frequency to avoid withdrawal symptoms. Opioid withdrawal presents with flu-like symptoms, which can be extremely unpleasant, but are generally not life threatening in otherwise healthy individuals. Symptoms include anxiety, irritability, yawning, restlessness, sleep disturbances, muscle aches, chills and sweating, piloerection, hyperthermia, lacrimation and nasal secretions, abdominal cramps with vomiting and diarrhea, paresthesias, tremors, mydriasis, hypertension, and tachycardia. The Clinical Opiate Withdrawal Scale, http://www.naabt.org/documents/cows_induction_flow_sheet.pdf, was developed to quantify the symptoms of opioid withdrawal and may be useful clinically during buprenorphine induction. Induction is started once a sufficient number of opioid receptors are available in order to avoid precipitating the rapid withdrawal that occurs when the partial opioid agonist replaces a full agonist on the receptor.

Treatment for opioid withdrawal is supportive, and includes symptomatic treatment of aches and pains with nonsteroidal anti-inflammatory medications, abdominal cramping with dicyclomine and reassurance. The alpha-2 adrenergic agonists clonidine and lofexidine improve tolerability of opioid withdrawal. Buprenorphine can also be used to manage withdrawal symptoms.

NONNARCOTIC CENTRAL NERVOUS SYSTEM DEPRESSANTS

Central nervous system depressants include barbiturates, benzodiazepines, g-hydroxybutyrate (GHB), flunitrazepam, major tranquilizers (phenothiazines), and carbamates such as meprobamate. Physical symptoms of sedative-hypnotic intoxication include slurred speech, incoordination, unsteady gait, nystagmus, decreased reflexes, impaired attention or memory, and stupor or coma. Psychiatric symptoms of intoxication include inappropriate behavior, mood lability, impaired judgment, and impaired social and occupational functioning.

Barbiturates

Medical Uses

Barbiturates are sedative/hypnotic drugs that are used as sleep aides, anticonvulsants, sedative-hypnotic anesthesia, for preinduction of anesthesia, and to reduce intracranial pressure and cerebral ischemia after head trauma or stroke. Their medical use has decreased, being replaced by benzodiazepines for several indications due to less respiratory depression and higher therapeutic index.

Physiology and Metabolism

Over 10 types of barbiturates are used medically in the US; duration of action ranges from minutes to days. Seventy-five percent of phenobarbital is hydroxylated in the liver (with 25% being excreted unchanged in urine); 99% of secobarbital and butabarbital undergo hepatic metabolism.

Barbiturates are g-aminobutyric acid-A (GABA-A) receptor agonists with a unique binding site and have three major effects: they enhance binding of GABA *and* benzodiazepines to their unique sites; they open the chloride ion channel of the GABA receptor even in the absence of GABA; and they increase the duration of channel opening. Increased chloride conductance reduces neuron firing, thus the antiseizure effects. Together, these effects make barbiturates potent drugs with a narrow window of safety. The mesencephalic reticular activating system, which contributes to homeostasis, is particularly sensitive to barbiturates. Lesser-known actions include blocking voltage-gated Ca^{2+} channels, decreasing Ca^{2+} influx at NMDA receptors, and decreasing cellular respiration in neuronal mitochondria. Barbiturates are metabolized by the liver and enhance liver metabolism, shortening the half-life of other drugs and reducing their clinical effectiveness.

Effects of Intoxication

Barbiturates are CNS depressants: low doses result in mild sedation; higher doses result in hypnosis; and still higher doses result in anesthesia and death. Symptoms of intoxication include sleepiness, yawning, slowed comprehension, slurred speech, lateral nystagmus, anorexia, dizziness, and orthostatic hypotension. When barbiturates are used in combination with other depressants such as alcohol, benzodiazepines, or opioids, the effects of both are potentiated and lethal overdoses can occur more easily.

Adverse Effects

1. Psychiatric/neurologic: Fatigue, euphoria or depressed mood, irritability, violent behavior, toxic psychosis, ataxia, slowed

comprehension, diplopia, dizziness, dysmetria, hypotonia, poor memory, lateral nystagmus, and slowed speech
2. Skin: Cutaneous lesions, urticarial rashes, and bullae
3. Respiratory: Respiratory depression, acidosis, respiratory failure

Overdose and Emergency Treatment

Signs and symptoms of overdose include miosis, hypotension, hypothermia, respiratory depression, and decreased gastrointestinal motility. Coma, shock, and death are possible. The presentation is indistinguishable from opiate or other sedative overdose on clinical examination. Urine toxicology can be helpful for diagnosis, but quantitative levels are not predictive of the clinical course. Ingestion of more than 3 g or a blood level of more than 2 mg/dL is the lethal dose for short-acting barbiturates; ingestion of more than 6 to 9 g or a blood level greater than 11 to 12 mg/dL is the lethal dose for long-acting forms. Treatment is primarily supportive, with support of airway, breathing, and circulation. Unabsorbed barbiturate should be removed by gastric lavage followed by activated charcoal. In severe, life-threatening barbiturate poisoning, extracorporeal methods of drug removal, such as hemodialysis, might be considered. Central nervous system stimulants should be avoided.

Tolerance and Withdrawal

If physiologic dependence is suspected, detoxification must be done under close medical supervision, as withdrawal can be life-threatening. Withdrawal symptoms include anxiety, delirium, hallucinations, irritability, mydriasis, sleep disturbance, seizures, headaches, weakness, hyperactive reflexes, tremor, abdominal cramps, flushing, nausea, sweating, and increased temperature. Orthostatic hypotension may also occur, in contrast to benzodiazepine withdrawal, which typically presents with hypertension. Barbiturate withdrawal is treated with replacement by phenobarbital followed by a slow taper until the patient is drug free.

Benzodiazepines
Medical Use

Medical use of benzodiazepines became widespread in the 1970s, and they continue to be used clinically as anxiolytic, antiemetic, hypnotic, anticonvulsant, and antispasmodic medications (Table 72.1). They are also used to treat alcohol withdrawal, neuroleptic malignant syndrome, serotonin syndrome, and catatonia. First thought to be free of negative consequences, benzodiazepines are now known to carry the risk of dependence, withdrawal, and negative side effects. Illicit benzodiazepines are readily available in the United States, and may be obtained by diverting prescriptions or theft from pharmaceutical supplies.

Route of Administration

Benzodiazepines are most often taken orally, though some users may snort them or inject them intravenously. Preparations that cross the blood–brain barrier more quickly have a higher potential for misuse than those that cross more slowly.

Designer Benzodiazepines The use of novel psychoactive substances has been a growing international problem for the last two decades; so-called "designer" benzodiazepines (DBZD) form a dangerous subcategory. Data from the U.S. National Poison Data System indicate the use of DBZP increased over 300% from 2014 to 2017.[11] These substances are generally inexpensive and easily obtained online without a prescription, providing easy access for AYAs.

Chemically, DBZPs may be metabolites or structural manipulations of prescription benzodiazepines or pharmaceutical compounds that were developed for medicinal use but failed to be approved.[12] Many are highly potent and may be adulterated, which increases harm. As a result of their clandestine production and novel status, there is a dearth of information about their safety or toxicologic parameters.

Physiology and Metabolism

Benzodiazepines bind to a unique site on the GABA-A receptor and enhance the inhibitory effects of GABA. Like barbiturates, benzodiazepines enhance the binding of GABA to its receptor and increase the frequency of chloride channel opening. Unlike barbiturates, however, benzodiazepines do not open the ion channel of the GABA receptor in the absence of GABA. This makes benzodiazepines relatively milder in effect and safer to use than barbiturates.

The liver metabolizes benzodiazepines. The duration of the clinical effect is determined by the half-life of active metabolites, and they are often classified this way. Diazepam is highly lipophilic and is rapidly absorbed, with an elimination half-life ranging from 18 to 100 hours. Shorter-acting benzodiazepines have elimination half-lives of about 6 hours. Benzodiazepines and their metabolites may accumulate in adipose tissue, resulting in a delayed appearance of adverse reactions and continued clinical effects beyond discontinuation of the drug. Unlike the barbiturates, benzodiazepines do not induce the metabolism of other drugs.

Effects of Intoxication

Benzodiazepines are CNS depressants. They produce drowsiness, dizziness, weakness, sedation, and a sense of calmness.

Adverse Effects

1. Psychiatric/neurologic: Disinhibition, paradoxical aggression, anxiety, delirium, agitation, visual hallucinations, ataxia, memory loss, impaired psychomotor function, slurred speech, blurred vision
2. Cardiovascular: Mild hypotension
3. Respiratory: Dose-dependent depressant effect on spontaneous breathing, particularly when combined with alcohol or opioids or if underlying lung disease such as chronic obstructive lung disease is present.

Overdose and Emergency Treatment

Benzodiazepine overdose typically presents with dizziness, confusion, drowsiness or unresponsiveness, and blurred vision. Some patients may present with anxiety and agitation. Physical examination signs include nystagmus, slurred speech, ataxia, weakness or hypotonia, hypotension, and respiratory depression.

Treatment for benzodiazepine overdose is primarily supportive, including securing the airway, and cardiovascular and respiratory stabilization. Flumazenil is a benzodiazepine receptor antagonist/partial agonist capable of reversing the sedative effects of benzodiazepines. To treat coma from severe benzodiazepine overdose, flumazenil is given in incremental doses over a few minutes. If a clinical effect is not seen after five spaced doses, it is unlikely that higher doses will be helpful. Flumazenil has a shorter action than many benzodiazepines and may require repeated doses to prevent

TABLE 72.1
Major Pharmacologic Actions of Various Benzodiazepines

Benzodiazepine	Major Pharmacologic Action
Diazepam, chlordiazepoxide, oxazepam, clorazepate, lorazepam, prazepam, alprazolam, halazepam	Anxiolytic
Flurazepam, temazepam, flunitrazepam, triazolam, midazolam	Sedative-hypnotic
Diazepam, clonazepam	Anticonvulsant
Diazepam	Muscle relaxant

XIV

return of symptoms. Flumazenil is contraindicated in mixed overdoses involving seizure-causing agents, because it can counteract anticonvulsant protection conferred by benzodiazepines. It is also relatively contraindicated in individuals who are physically dependent on benzodiazepines because it can precipitate acute benzodiazepine withdrawal.

Chronic Use, Tolerance, and Withdrawal

Benzodiazepines have a high potential for misuse. Care should be used in prescribing benzodiazepines, particularly among patients with SUDs or who are prescribed barbiturates. In addition, they are relatively contraindicated in AYAs with alcohol or OUD.

If physiologic benzodiazepine dependence is suspected, withdrawal must be carefully supervised. Patients who abruptly stop taking benzodiazepines can develop life-threatening, protracted seizures. Patients with a prior seizure history are at much greater risk and medically supervised withdrawal is recommended. Other symptoms of benzodiazepine withdrawal include anxiety, agitation, confusion, sleep disturbance, and flu-like symptoms, including fatigue, headache, muscle pain and weakness, sweating, chills, nausea, vomiting, and diarrhea.

There is an extensive literature on benzodiazepine detoxification. It may be done in an inpatient or outpatient setting, by utilizing one of three approaches: using a benzodiazepine taper and/or benzodiazepine symptom-triggered protocol; using anticonvulsants with baclofen augmentation; or by using a combination of low-dose flumazenil coupled with clonazepam replacement.[13]

Gamma-Hydroxybutyrate (Precursors: 1,4 Butanediol, Gamma-Butyrolactone, Gamma-Valerolactone)

Gamma-hydroxybutyrate (GHB), is a CNS depressant that acts through a metabolite of the inhibitory neurotransmitter GABA and can function as a neurotransmitter itself. Gamma-hydroxybutyrate triggers the release of an opiate-like substance and can modulate sleep cycles, temperature regulation, memory, and emotional control. Subjective effects include relaxation, anxiolysis and mood elevation, euphoria, increased libido, and facilitation of communication. In some countries, GHB is used as an anesthetic and to treat narcolepsy. Gamma-hydroxybutyrate is available as a clear, odorless liquid with a slightly salty taste or white powder and is rapidly absorbed after oral ingestion. Onset of effects is within 15 to 30 minutes and symptoms of intoxication last from 3 to 6 hours. Mixing it with other substances is common; when taken with alcohol, there is an increase in toxic effects of both substances.

Gamma-hydroxybutyrate stimulates protein synthesis and the release of growth hormone, and may be used by bodybuilders to increase lean body mass. It is used as a euphoriant by people attending raves and due to its disinhibiting and sexual enhancing properties is known to be used by men who have sex with men (MSM). Cytochrome P450 inhibitors such as the HIV drugs ritonavir and saquinavir increase GHB bioavailability, putting this population at greater risk.[14] It is also considered to be a "date rape" drug because it has been used to incapacitate victims and is difficult to detect.

Adverse effects include sialorrhea, bradycardia, increased or decreased blood pressure, respiratory depression with acidosis, vomiting, and mild hyperglycemia. Neurologic effects include hypothermia, dizziness, weakness, ataxia, vertigo, nystagmus, short-term amnesia, coma, tonic–clonic seizures, and myoclonus. Confusion, sedation, aggression, impaired judgment, and hallucinations may lead to accidental injury.

Overdose results in the toxidrome of coma, bradycardia, and myoclonus. Co-ingestion with alcohol enhances respiratory depression. Sudden, spontaneous resolution of coma that has no clear etiology with brief myoclonic jerking movements is considered pathognomonic for GHB toxicity. There is no antidote for GHB overdose; the treatment is supportive care. Regular GHB users are known to quickly develop tolerance to it. Withdrawal effects include tachycardia, insomnia, anxiety, tremors, sweating, auditory or visual hallucinations, and may be complicated by rhabdomyolysis and acute renal failure. Acute withdrawal is potentially life-threatening due to seizures, delirium, and autonomic instability.

Baclofen and Muscle Relaxants

Muscle relaxants, clinically used to treat muscle spasticity in children, adolescents, and adults, are diverse in chemical structure and actions; they include such drugs as baclofen, tizanidine, carisoprodol, meprobamate, orphenadrine, and methocarbamol. Muscle relaxants can induce drowsiness, coma, muscle flaccidity, cardiac dysrhythmias, and respiratory depression or sudden respiratory arrest. Psychosis, other psychiatric manifestations, and encephalopathy are common with baclofen toxicity; catatonia has been described following a baclofen overdose.[15] Treatment of patients who overdose on muscle relaxants includes oral decontamination with activated charcoal, close monitoring of neurologic and cardiovascular status, and supportive care. Intubation and mechanical ventilation may be necessary in cases of severe poisoning. Withdrawal symptoms are well documented after acute cessation; symptoms include altered mental status, sedation, insomnia, perceptual disturbances, seizures, hyperthermia, respiratory insufficiency, and muscle spasticity. Prompt reinstatement of the muscle relaxant is required for amelioration of the withdrawal syndrome. Gradual dosage tapering is recommended to prevent onset of withdrawal phenomenon.

INHALANTS

Preparation and Routes of Administration

The majority of inhalants are common household substances that are easily accessed, making them particularly popular among younger children. Of the myriad of products and substances used as inhalants, toluene is the most common and is found in spray paint, airplane glues, rubber cement, cleaning fluids, permanent markers, and lacquer thinner (Table 72.2). "Fad" use of inhalants is common, such that misuse of a specific product may gain short-term popularity in a particular school or town based on word-of-mouth reports among teens. Substances are typically inhaled from a plastic bag ("bagging") or through a saturated cloth ("huffing").

Identifying Inhalant Use

Inhalant use can be difficult to detect. Parents/caregivers may report finding fluid-saturated clothes, empty spray paint cans or plastic bags, or unusual chemicals in a bedroom or among personal

TABLE 72.2
Classes of Inhalants, Chemical Examples, and Toxicity

Class of Inhalant	Product/Chemical Examples	Toxicity
Volatile products	Glues, gasoline, spray paints, butane, paint thinner	Cardiac arrhythmias, respiratory failure, coma, pneumothorax
Gases	Nitrous oxide	Simple asphyxia
Anesthetics	Ether	Coma, respiratory failure
Nitrates	Amyl nitrate, butyl nitrate	Cardiovascular failure, coma, methemoglobin

items where they would not usually be stored. Users may have a distinctive chemical odor to their breath, hair, or clothing, and may appear disheveled.

Physiology and Metabolism

Inhalants are lipophilic, and their effects are felt within minutes due to rapid absorption into the blood and then the brain. The initial effect is stimulation and excitation, which then progresses to a depressant effect on the CNS. Peak effects occur within minutes and excretion is rapid, resulting in very brief periods of intoxication, usually lasting 15 to 30 minutes.

Effects of Intoxication

Inhalant use results in euphoria, decreased inhibition, and decreased judgment. Symptoms of inhalant use include heavy-lidded glazed eyes, slowed reflexes, slurred speech, lacrimation, rhinorrhea, salivation, and irritation of the mucus membranes. Anesthesia is common with drowsiness, stupor, or even obtundation, accompanied by respiratory depression. Users report spinning or floating sensations, exhilaration, and mild delirium.

Adverse Effects

Common adverse effects include gastrointestinal complaints such as anorexia, vomiting, and abdominal pain associated with gastritis. Neurologic effects accompanying inhalant abuse include sleepiness, headaches, dizziness, ataxia, incoordination, and diplopia. Defatting properties of solvents may lead to perinasal and perioral skin rashes and nosebleeds. Respiratory irritation may cause a chronic dry cough, new-onset wheezing, and shortness of breath.

Overdose of inhalants can result in life-threatening complications, including seizures, loss of consciousness, arrhythmias, respiratory failure, or cardiopulmonary arrest (**Table 72.3**). Death can occur, either directly from respiratory or cardiac toxicity or from trauma from risk-taking behaviors and poor judgment. The "sudden sniffing death syndrome" occurs when halogenated hydrocarbons are inhaled, directly sensitizing the bundle of His and cardiac electrical system. The patient, in an excited state, then starts running or dancing and has an adrenergic surge, provoking a fatal arrhythmia.

Chronic Use

Inhalant use is notable for rapid escalation in frequency, strong cravings, and binge behaviors, due to the short duration of intoxication. Chronic effects are characterized by irreversible damage to target organs including brain, kidneys, heart, and liver. Fatty brain tissues such as myelin, axons, and neuronal cell bodies can be damaged or destroyed, leading to diffuse cerebral atrophy. The developing brain is more susceptible to damage. In addition to cognitive decline, chronic inhalant users are more likely to attempt or complete suicide, have mood or anxiety disorders, and have other SUDs.

Diagnosis

Many inhalants are so quickly metabolized and/or excreted that they cannot be detected by the time the patient arrives in the emergency department. Standard toxicologic screening tests of the blood or urine do not include such chemicals as hydrocarbons or nitrites. However, some products, such as paint thinners or glue, may leave chemical signatures behind. For example, heavy toluene exposure can be detected by elevated urinary hippuric acid levels.

Treatment

Treatment is supportive, and aimed at control of arrhythmias, and respiratory and circulatory support. Epinephrine should be avoided since it may provoke cardiac irritability in patients who have inhaled halogenated hydrocarbons. Intubation and mechanical ventilation may be necessary in severely affected patients.

Nitrous Oxide

Nitrous oxide (N_2O), also known as laughing gas, may be used by AYAs for its mind-altering, anxiolytic, and anesthesia-like effects. It is most commonly sold in small balloons or inhaled from whipped cream cans ("whippets"), in which it is used as a propellant. Deaths have occurred after prolonged inhalation of 100% N_2O in a closed space due to displacement of oxygen in the blood with subsequent suffocation. Nitrous oxide is known to deplete vitamin B12, and many patients who present with psychiatric and neurologic symptoms following exposure also have vitamin B12 deficiency.[15,16] Chronic nitrous oxide use has been associated with elevated levels of homocysteine in the blood and urine (secondary to vitamin B12 deficiency) which can lead to a hypercoagulable state and other forms of cardiovascular disease including myocardial infarction, deep vein thromboses, and pulmonary emboli in both acute and chronic users.[16–19]

Nitrites

Amyl, butyl, and isobutyl nitrites are examples of nitrites, referred to as "poppers." These are volatile liquids used for their vasodilatory action, enhancement of sexual pleasure, and subjective feeling of light-headedness. The use of inhaled nitrates is common in MSM, and it is an established risk factor for unsafe sexual behaviors and HIV infection in this same group.[20–22] Amyl nitrite requires a prescription and is currently indicated as an antidote to cyanide poisoning. Butyl and isobutyl nitrite are available over the counter as a room deodorizer, cologne, or liquid incense. The most common side effects are a result of smooth muscle relaxation: severe headache, dizziness, orthostatic hypotension, and occasionally syncope. These effects are enhanced when used together with other hypotensive agents including alcohol or phosphodiesterase inhibitors and make syncope more common. Nitrites can rarely cause clinically significant methemoglobinemia. Frequent users may develop crusty yellow skin lesions on the face that can be misdiagnosed as impetigo or seborrheic dermatitis. Inhaled nitrite-induced maculopathy with visual loss has also been observed.[23]

HALLUCINOGENS

The hallucinogen class of drugs is broad and includes both naturally occurring and synthetic compounds. D-lysergic acid diethylamide, phencyclidine (PCP), psilocybin ("mushrooms"), peyote, mescaline, dimethyltryptamine (DMT), ketamine, Ayahuasca, Ibogaine, morning glory seeds, Jimson weed, dextromethorphan, MDMA, MDA, and MDEA, and salvia are all considered hallucinogenic substances. Organically derived hallucinogens have been

TABLE 72.3

Agent-Specific Toxicities of Inhalant Chemicals

Inhalant Chemical	Agent-Specific Toxicity
Toluene	Renal damage, embryopathy
Amyl and butyl nitrites	Methemoglobinemia, hypotension
Gasoline	Lead poisoning, benzene-induced leukemia
Carbon tetrachloride, trichloroethylene	Hepatitis, cirrhosis
Nitrous oxide	Vitamin B_{12} deficiency
Methylene chloride (paint thinner)	Carbon monoxide poisoning

used in many parts of the world for cultural and religious practices due to their intrinsic ability to produce altered states of consciousness with mystical overtones. The term *hallucinogen* ("producer of hallucinations") is actually a misnomer because prototypical hallucinogens such as LSD, mescaline, and psilocybin at typical dosage levels do not cause hallucinations but rather illusions or sensory distortions. Hallucinogen-persisting perception disorder (HPPD) is a disorder defined by recurrent fleeting distortions, illusions, or other perceptual disturbances, which may be referred to as "flashbacks", following discontinuation of the use of hallucinogens. It has a higher prevalence after the use of LSD compared to other hallucinogens and may occur after sporadic or even one-time ingestion. There is no FDA-approved treatment for HPPD, though use of presynaptic alpha-2 adrenergic agonists (clonidine), and benzodiazepines (clonazepam) is supported in the literature.[24]

Types of Hallucinogens

Table 72.4 contains the subgrouping of hallucinogens based on distinctive psychoactive effects and structure–activity relationship similarities.

Phencyclidine

Medical Use, Preparation, and Dose

Phencyclidine is an arylamine 1-(1-phenylcyclohexyl)piperidine introduced in the 1950s as a general anesthetic but due to adverse effects during surgical recovery, it was discontinued as a medication in 1965. Phencyclidine may be packaged as a liquid, powder, tablet, leaf mixture, or rock crystal. It can be used intravenously, intramuscularly, or orally, or it can be snorted or smoked.

Physiology and Metabolism

The hydrogen chloride salt of PCP is a dissociative anesthetic structurally related to ketamine with stimulant, depressant, and hallucinogenic properties. Its major psychiatric effects are thought to be the result of noncompetitive antagonism of glutamatergic NMDA receptors leading to increased production of dopamine and reuptake inhibition. Phencyclidine is rapidly inactivated by hepatic metabolism with renal excretion. Phencyclidine is fat-soluble,

TABLE 72.4

Types of Hallucinogens and the Psychoactive Effects They Produce

Category	Psychoactive Effect	Examples
Psychedelics	Prominent hallucinations and synesthesias with mild distortion of time and reality, impaired attention/concentration, mild disruption in ego structure	• Indolealkylamines: LSD, psilocybin, DMT • Phenylalkylamines: mescaline
Entactogens	Structural similarities to psychedelics (mescaline) and amphetamines; unique psychoactive characteristics include improved communication, empathy with others, and positive mood enhancement	MDMA, MDA, MDEA
Dissociative anesthetics	Causes anesthesia, emergence reactions, and "out of body" experiences	PCP, ketamine

LSD, D-lysergic acid diethylamide; DMT, dimethyltryptamine; MDMA, methylenedioxymethamphetamine; MDA, methylenedioxyamphetamine; MDEA, methyldiethanolamine; PCP, phencyclidine.

TABLE 72.5

PCP-Induced Intoxication States

Acute intoxication	Delusion, disinhibition, dissociation ("out of body" experience)
Acute or prolonged delirium	Disorientation, clouded consciousness, and abnormal cognition
Schizophreniform psychosis	Hallucinations, thought disorder, and delusions
Mania	Hallucinations, elevated mood, elevated self-attitude, feelings of omnipotence
Depressive reactions	Dysphoria, social withdrawal, paranoia, isolation

easily crosses the blood–brain barrier, and its half-life ranges from 7 to 57 hours; enterohepatic circulation effects result in some users remaining intoxicated for weeks or months. Urinary excretion is highly dependent on urine pH, with significantly higher excretion rates at an acidic pH.

Effects of Intoxication

The clinical symptoms of PCP vary with the dose, route of administration, and experience of the user (Table 72.5).

Phencyclidine causes a characteristic vertical nystagmus but may also cause horizontal or rotatory nystagmus. Its use should be suspected in all AYAs with a distorted thought process, especially when accompanied by analgesia or nystagmus. Open-eye coma, horizontal and vertical nystagmus, hypertension, and rigidity are pathognomonic. Due to PCP's low cost and easy synthesis, it is often sold in addition to or instead of other street drugs, so many users may not be aware they have taken it.

Adverse Effects

Adverse effects associated with PCP use are dose related (see Table 72.6).

Overdose and Emergency Treatment

Use of PCP may result in generalized motor seizures either early in the course of intoxication or delayed in appearance. Death can occur from hyperthermia, injuries sustained during periods of analgesia and aggression, suicide, seizures, or cerebral hemorrhage.

Reduction of Stimuli Extreme caution is necessary when treating patients with PCP overdose. Patients are unpredictable and often have little awareness of the consequences of their behavior. Reducing the levels of light, sound, and other external stimuli can rapidly calm a patient who has used PCP; if possible, patients should not be touched or engaged in conversation. In an emergency, covering the intoxicated patient with a blanket may be helpful. All hazards should be removed from the environment. Restraints are not recommended; they may cause the patient to harm himself or herself in an attempt to escape and can increase the risk of rhabdomyolysis if the patient struggles.

Supportive Care Treatment for PCP overdose is largely supportive. In addition to basic cardiopulmonary resuscitation, it is essential to check for signs of head, neck, back, and internal injuries, which can occur from trauma while the patient is under the behavioral effects of the drug. Because PCP travels through enterohepatic

TABLE 72.6

Adverse Effects of PCP by Dose

Low dose (<5 mg)

Physical: Horizontal and vertical nystagmus, blank stare, ataxia, hypertension, increased deep tendon reflexes, decreased proprioception and sensation, miosis or midposition reactive pupils, diaphoresis, flushing

Cognitive and behavioral: Disorganized thought processes, distortion of body image and of objects, amnesia, agitated or combative behavior, unresponsiveness, disinhibition of underlying psychopathology, schizophrenic reactions, catalepsy, catatonia, illusions, anxiety, and excitement

Moderate dose (5–10 mg)

Physical: Vertical and horizontal nystagmus, hypertension, myoclonus, midposition pupil size, dysarthria, diaphoresis, fever, hypersalivation

Cognitive and behavioral: Amnesia, mutism, anxiety, excitement, delusions, stupor or extreme agitation, violent or psychotic behavior

High dose (>10 mg)

Physical: Eyes that may remain open during coma, hypertension, arrhythmias, increased deep tendon reflexes, muscle rigidity, decerebrate posturing, convulsions, spontaneous nystagmus, miosis, decreased urine output, dysarthria, diaphoresis and flushing, fever

Cognitive and behavioral: Unresponsive, immobile state, amnesia, mutism

Extremely high dose (>500 mg)

Physical: Prolonged coma, rigidity, extensor (decerebrate) posturing, seizures, hypoventilation, hypertension or hypotension

Cognitive and behavioral: Prolonged and fluctuating confusional state after recovery from coma

circulation, repeated doses of activated charcoal may be beneficial regardless of how PCP was used.

Medications Medication use is relatively contraindicated, but, if necessary, IV diazepam or lorazepam can be used to treat seizures. Phencyclidine-induced dystonia does not respond to diphenhydramine.[25] Severe agitation and psychosis caused by PCP can be treated with haloperidol.

Recovery Recovery usually occurs within 24 hours but, depending on the dose, can take days. During the recovery phase, patients may require short-term inpatient psychiatric care to manage paranoia, regressive behavior, and a slow phase of reintegration. With higher doses, the coma can last 5 to 6 days and can be followed by a prolonged recovery period marked by behavioral disorders. Cognitive, memory, and speech disorders may last up to one year after the last use of PCP. Flashbacks may occur, as with LSD.

Ketamine

Ketamine is an arylcycloalkylamine chemical congener of PCP; it is similar to PCP pharmacologically. It is a rapid-acting dissociative anesthetic that combines sedative–hypnotic, analgesic, and amnesic effects with the maintenance of pharyngeal reflexes and respiratory function at normal doses. Like PCP, ketamine is an NMDA receptor antagonist and is used as a human and veterinary anesthetic and occasionally produces unpleasant reactions, anxiety, dysphoria, and hallucinations. Users are attracted to the "dreamy" state of mild hallucinations and "out of body" experiences induced by light ketamine anesthesia. Adverse effects include a cataleptic state, with nystagmus, excessive salivation, involuntary tongue and limb movements, and hypertonus. Laryngospasm, seizures,

apnea, and respiratory arrest have all been reported with ketamine-induced anesthesia. Overdose treatment is supportive, with attention to neurologic, cardiovascular, and respiratory monitoring; ventilatory support may be necessary. Treatment of agitation related to an emergence reaction entails dim lighting, reduction of extraneous external stimuli, and administration of a benzodiazepine. For idiosyncratic dystonic reactions, IV diphenhydramine may be of benefit.

D-Lysergic Acid Diethylamide

D-Lysergic acid diethylamide (LSD) was first formulated in 1938; by the 1950s, LSD was marketed under the name "Delvsid" for the treatment of mental illness and alcoholism and palliation of terminal cancer. By the mid-1960s no significant medical benefits of the drug had been found, and development stopped. D-Lysergic acid diethylamide became illegal in the United States in 1968 due to safety concerns, political beliefs, and its potential for illicit use. In the early 2000s, a resurgence of interest in the therapeutic benefits of hallucinogenic compounds occurred.

Preparation and Dose

Because the production of LSD from rye ergot fungus (e.g., *Claviceps purpurea*) is difficult, much of the LSD sold on the street is either adulterated or contains no LSD.

The drug is extremely potent, with doses measured in micrograms. Low doses of LSD (50 to 75 mcg) produce euphoria while higher doses result in typical LSD illusions or "trips." The current average dose of 20 to 80 mcg is an order of magnitude lower than the 1960s doses of up to 500 mcg. There is clearly a disregard for, and underestimation of, the dangers of LSD due to less frequent aversive effects with lower doses. Even at lower doses, users remain at risk for chronic psychiatric problems, acute physical trauma, and other consequences of risk-taking behaviors that might occur under the influence of the drug.

D-Lysergic acid diethylamide is commonly distributed as a soluble, colorless powder or liquid, sold as colored cylindrical tablets or gelatin squares, or applied to small pieces of paper. These preparations, known as "microdots," "windowpanes," or "blotters," are placed on the oral mucosa for absorption. It is also sold as colorful decals or stickers, some with cartoon characters, which may be appealing to young children. The drug can be mixed with foods or liquids for oral consumption, or delivered in eye drops; it cannot be smoked as it is destroyed by heat.

Physiology and Metabolism

D-Lysergic acid diethylamide is rapidly absorbed, binds to receptors throughout the CNS, and has onset of action in 30 to 40 minutes and a half-life of about 3 hours. The neurologic effects of LSD are not fully understood. D-Lysergic acid diethylamide is similar in chemical structure to the serotonin molecule; it has inhibitory effects through binding to serotonin 5-HT1 receptors, and stimulatory effects through serotonin 5-HT2A receptors. The latter results in glutamate release, alterations in cortical function, and likely the hallucinogen effects.[26]

Effects of Intoxication

Intoxication results in euphoria and sensory illusions that may give rise to hallucinations. Depersonalization and loss of body image are frequently reported and distinguish LSD psychosis from schizophrenia. "Mystical experiences" are also reported. Synesthesias, "trails", and loss of time sense are hallmarks of LSD use.

Adverse Effects

1. Psychiatric/neurologic: Visual and auditory hallucinations, acute psychosis or exacerbation of pre-existing psychotic symptoms, unpredictable and dangerous behavior in uncontrolled settings, synesthesias, depersonalization, loss of sense of time,

loss of ego boundaries, impairment of attention, motivation and concentration, anxiety, depression, paranoia, confusion, flashbacks, flushing, hyperthermia, piloerection, dizziness, paresthesia, dilated pupils, photophobia, blurred vision, conjunctival injection, lacrimation, hyperactive reflexes, ataxia and tremor, loss of muscle coordination and pain perception, restlessness, and sleep disturbances

2. Cardiovascular: Hypertension and tachycardia
3. Gastrointestinal: Anorexia, nausea, dry mouth

Overdose and Emergency Treatment

Overdose may result in grand mal seizures, circulatory collapse, coagulopathies, and coma. Some users experience "bad trips," which terrify the user and may produce a sense of panic, fragmentation, fear of "going crazy," or fear of being intoxicated forever.

Treatment is supportive. Physical restraints and emergency medications are discouraged. Important components of treatment include providing a peaceful, calm environment and reassurance that unusual sensations will cease when the drug wears off. Frequent cycling between lucidity and periods of intense reactions to the drug occur early during intoxication and slow down over time.

History of hallucinogen use is often unreliable; adulteration and misrepresentation of the substances are common. In the case of a patient with clouded sensorium and fever, even with a history of ingestion of LSD, the differential diagnosis must include CNS infection, endocrine disorder, drug or alcohol withdrawal syndrome, and ingestion of a different toxin. The drug can be readily detected in urine by thin layer chromatography or other analytical techniques.

Chronic Use

Chronic adverse effects may include psychosis, depression, and personality changes. The use of a hallucinogen should be considered in the differential diagnosis of an adolescent or young adult who presents with new-onset psychosis.

Tolerance and Withdrawal

Tolerance to LSD develops rapidly but is short-lived. Some daily users of LSD describe the practice of doubling the previous day's dose when using on consecutive days. No withdrawal syndrome has been described.

Dextromethorphan

Dextromethorphan (DXM), the dextro isomer of the codeine analog, levorphanol, has a chemical structure resembling a synthetic opiate. While it lacks an opiate's potent analgesic and sedative properties it is capable of inducing euphoria at very high doses and because of this, it is used recreationally by AYAs in an attempt to experience its psychotropic effects. It does not bind to the mu opioid receptor, but does bind to the opioid sigma receptor. The drug's prominent antitussive properties make it a common ingredient in nonprescription cough and cold syrups. With more than 140 over-the-counter cold and cough products on the market, DXM has surpassed codeine as the most widely used antitussive.

To experience euphoria, users may take five times the maximum daily dose or more.[27] Effects are dose dependent. Over-the-counter products often contain other active ingredients that can be toxic in overdose, making mixed ingestions common. The volume of cough syrup required to experience euphoria has led adolescents to order the pure, highly concentrated powder from internet sources, or to purchase high-concentration dextromethorphan-containing tablets.

Physiology and Metabolism

Dextromethorphan binds to opioid sigma receptors, which may account for some of its sedative and psychomimetic properties. The drug is metabolized to an active metabolite, dextrorphan,

which interacts with the PCP and ketamine receptor in the NMDA neurotransmitter complex. Antagonism of NMDA receptors may be responsible for some of the adrenergic effects seen clinically with large doses of dextromethorphan due to inhibition of catecholamine reuptake. The drug undergoes secondary conjugation in the liver to inactive glucuronide and sulfate esters, and has an elimination half-life of about 3.3 hours.

Intoxication

Dextromethorphan can induce euphoria and produce dissociative effects. The actions of dextrorphan may explain dextromethorphan's PCP-like symptoms in overdose. It can produce mydriasis, nystagmus, blurred vision, cortical blindness, stupor, somnolence and ataxia, coma, slurred speech, hallucinations, toxic psychosis, dysphoria, nystagmus, dystonia, tachycardia, and elevated blood pressure. Dextromethorphan also blocks presynaptic serotonin reuptake and has dopaminergic properties. It interacts with other drugs, including SSRIs, MAO inhibitors, neuroleptics, and tricyclic antidepressants, to produce movement disorders, serotonin syndrome, or neuroleptic malignant syndrome.

Diagnosis and Treatment

Repeated use of dextromethorphan results in rapid development of tolerance. Withdrawal symptoms may occur with regular use and include lethargy, apathy, constipation, anxiety, and insomnia.

Evidence-based guidelines for treatment of DMX poisoning recommend prehospital use of naloxone in patients with decreased consciousness, coma, or respiratory depression. Oral activated charcoal may be indicated. Since DMX is formulated as a hydrobromide salt, overdose with the drug can produce toxic effects similar to those seen with bromism toxicity, such as somnolence, cognitive impairments, neuromuscular changes, and dermal lesions.[28]

Psilocybin

Mushrooms containing psilocybin and psilocin produce effects similar to those of the other hallucinogens. Users reportedly experience euphoria, prominent visual and auditory hallucinations, and synesthesias. The mushrooms are ingested orally, and the onset of effects occurs in 20 to 40 minutes. The effects peak at 90 minutes and usually abate within 5 or 6 hours. Hallucinogenic effects occur at doses above 15 mg of orally ingested psilocybin. Since many other mushroom species can be confused with true *psilocybe* mushrooms, ingestion of misidentified, toxic non-*psilocybe* species can pose a special danger to users.

As with MDMA and LSD, specialty centers for psychedelic research have been established to examine the potential therapeutic psychiatric effects of psilocybin; positive results have been documented for adults with terminal cancer and those with treatment-refractory depression.[29–32] Investigations on using psilocybin as a treatment for tobacco use disorder[33] and alcohol use disorder[34] have yielded preliminary promising findings but the use of psilocybin remains confined to research at this time and no trials have included children or adolescents.

Jimson Weed

Jimson weed (*Datura stramonium*) grows wild in parts of North America and the West Indies. The plant has strong anticholinergic and mildly hallucinogenic properties. Atropine and scopolamine occur in high concentrations in its leaves and seeds though all portions of the plant are potentially toxic. Users eat or make tea from the seeds, or smoke cigarettes made from Jimson weed. Multiple reports of adolescents with severe anticholinergic toxicity secondary to this poisonous, native herb have been published. White, trumpet-shaped flowers or green pods filled with small round seeds can assist in diagnosis of Datura toxicity when anticholinergic toxidrome is present. Serum assays for toxic alkaloids may yield positive results.

unprotected sex. The AAP and National Behavioral Health Council both recommend that adolescents receive general advice to avoid alcohol and drug use. In the United States, while alcohol use is legal for young adults over age 21 years, heavy episodic ("binge") drinking remains common in young adulthood and is associated with a wide variety of health risks (see Chapter 69). Therefore, brief advice including the health risks associated with this pattern of drinking is recommended.

High Risk for Substance Use Disorders

Many AYAs with SUDs have already begun experiencing problems associated with their use of substances, and may respond to a "brief intervention." Brief interventions are based on motivational interviewing—a counseling technique that uses a nonjudgmental, empathetic, clinician-guided exploration of a behavior, identifies ambivalence about the behavior, and works toward resolving the ambivalence through behavior change.

Effectiveness

Brief interventions reduce "unhealthy" drinking by adults. Work with adolescents has found that brief interventions can decrease tobacco initiation and increase quit attempts, decrease perceptions of peer substance use,[11,12] decrease intentions to use substances, reduce cannabis use,[12,13] and improve engagement in SUD treatment. In a large study, adolescents who received a brief intervention were less likely to meet criteria for a SUD 3 years later.[9] Globally, the number of investigations using traditional counseling approaches to addressing substance use, such as motivational interviewing, has grown gradually over the past 20 years.

Method

A key principle of brief interventions is that the patient is in charge of making decisions. The patient is encouraged to make a concrete behavior change plan that may include abstaining completely, reducing quantity or frequency of use, and/or avoiding high-risk behaviors such as driving or having sex while impaired. Other assistance, including medications to suppress cravings or withdrawal symptoms, and laboratory testing may help to support AYAs in making a behavior change (see below).

Follow-Up

Follow-up is an important component to brief interventions. Recording the details of the behavior change plan and asking the AYAs to return after a few weeks to evaluate how well they were able to follow the plan is recommended. If the patient is not willing to return, following up the next time they return to the office for any reason is recommended.

⬤ SCREENING AND TREATING ADOLESCENTS AND YOUNG ADULTS WITH CHRONIC MEDICAL CONDITIONS

In the United States, one in four AYAs has a chronic medical condition such as diabetes, asthma, or arthritis that requires long-term follow-up by a regular care team. Adolescents and young adults or youth with chronic medical conditions (YCMC) share a number of attributes that may be adversely impacted by substance use, including the need to follow a medication regimen, participate in regular clinical monitoring, self-monitor/manage their condition, and manage sleep, diet/meals, and activity levels. Prevalence rates of alcohol, cannabis, and nicotine use are similar among younger YCMC and their healthy peers; however, YCMC are more likely to progress to heavy and problematic substance use by young adulthood,[14] and most do not receive clear advice regarding substance use from their medical teams.[15] Among YCMC, use of alcohol and cannabis are associated with a nearly twofold risk for treatment (medication) nonadherence.[16] Adverse effects of substance use on these issues and attendant risks for poor health outcomes are vital topics to discuss and may be anchor points for screening and brief intervention. Youth with chronic medical conditions may also be prone to using substances to treat pain or other symptoms of their condition. Youth with chronic medical conditions who use cannabis to treat symptoms initiate at younger ages, use more frequently, and report more nicotine use compared to YCMC who use cannabis recreationally, making them a high-risk group for SUD.[17] Frequent interactions with a clinical care team to address underlying health issues may provide physicians with opportunities for SBIRT, leveraging the strong patient–clinician bonds established by long-term clinical management of pediatric onset chronic illness.

Referral to Treatment for Severe Substance Use–Related Problems and Addiction

Addiction is a chronic, relapsing neurologic condition that results from a "rewiring" of the brain's reward system in the nucleus accumbens resulting from exposure to psychoactive substances. Patients with addiction lose control over their use of substances, and will often continue substance use even after severe problems have developed and use no longer results in euphoria. Brain development that occurs during adolescence appears to make this age-group particularly vulnerable to developing addiction. Adolescents and young adults with the clinical picture of addiction may respond to brief interventions (see above). For this group, in addition to reducing use and high-risk behaviors, the target of the intervention should also include ongoing treatment.

Referral to treatment consists of two distinct clinical activities. The first is a brief intervention that recommends seeking treatment for a SUD (see above). The second component involves determining the appropriate treatment format (**Table 73.2**) and level of care (**Table 73.3**), identifying a referral source, and facilitating referral completion. This second component may be particularly challenging as it requires alignment between patient, parent/caregiver (if appropriate), insurance provider, community resources, and availability; insurance and community resource availability is dependent on geographic location.

As with other disorders, patients with addiction should be treated in the least restrictive environment that meets their needs. There are, however, a range of treatment settings including outpatient, intensive outpatient, partial hospital programs, acute residential treatment programs, and long-term residential care (**Table 73.3**). Outpatient treatment can be supported in the medical home. For most, outpatient programs are adequate, though enrollment may be challenging. Outpatient treatment, particularly intensive outpatient or partial hospitalization, often requires daily transportation and could interfere with school, work, and/or parents'/caregivers' work schedules. However, the rapid dissemination of virtual health care associated with the COVID-19 pandemic may result in a permanent increase in the availability of remote programming.

Some AYAs with addiction can benefit from residential treatment. In particular, adolescents who do not or cannot respond to house rules and parental/caregiver limit setting, who are triggered to use substances by their home and/or school environments, and those with frequent contact with peers who use or sell substances may respond better to residential treatment. Adolescents and young adults in unstable housing, at risk of homelessness, or without available parents/caregivers to partner in treatment may also be better served in residential treatment.

The AAP has published guidelines on the criteria for addiction programs serving youth (**Table 73.4**).[21] Some treatment facilities offer specialized programs for young adults. Patients aged 18 to 25 years may prefer these settings, which focus on the typical substances, use patterns, and problems for this age group and facilitate peer support with those of similar age.

An AYA may be unwilling to engage in treatment for addiction even when ongoing drug use poses a serious threat to safety—such

XIV

TABLE 73.2

Psychosocial Formats and Counseling Modalities for Substance Use Disorder Treatment

Psychosocial Formats

Individual counseling	Adolescents with substance use disorders (SUDs) should receive specific treatment for their substance use; general supportive counseling may be a useful adjuvant but should not be a substitute. Several therapeutic modalities (motivational interviewing, cognitive behavioral therapy, contingency management, etc.) have all shown promise in treating adolescents with SUDs.
Group therapy	Group therapy is a mainstay of substance use disorder treatment for adolescents with SUDs. It is a particularly attractive option because it is cost-effective, and takes advantage of the developmental preference for congregating with peers. However, group therapy has not been extensively evaluated as a therapeutic modality for this age group, and existing research has produced mixed results.
Family therapy	Family-directed therapies are the best validated approach for treating adolescent SUDs. A number of modalities have all been demonstrated effective. Family counseling typically targets domains that figure prominently in the etiology of SUDs in adolescents—family conflict, communication, parental monitoring, discipline, child abuse/neglect, and parental SUDs.

Counseling Modalities

Motivational interviewing (MI)	MI is a counseling style frequently used in primary care to support behavior change. The main premise of MI is that motivation to make and sustain a behavior change is not an intrinsic character trait, but rather a constantly changing state that is influenced by others—both positively and negatively. In MI, the counselor facilitates the patient's exploration of the benefits of a current behavior compared to the potential benefits of behavior change and in so doing helps a patient bring out his or her own inner motivation to change.[12]
Cognitive behavioral therapy (CBT)	CBT is a structured, goal-oriented counseling style designed to teach patients specific skills that will help them remain abstinent by training patients to identify thoughts and feelings that precede drug use in order to learn either to avoid the situation or to substitute behaviors other than drug use. CBT is most effective when a patient is willing to practice newly acquired skills. CBT can be used in individual, family, or group therapy settings. It may be used alone or in combination with MI.[12]
Dialectical behavior therapy (DBT)	DBT is very similar to CBT. In this modality, patients are taught to regulate both emotion and behavior by identifying triggers that precede changes in emotional states that lead to dysregulated behavior. DBT is particularly effective for patients with co-occurring mental health disorders.[18]
Contingency management	Contingency management is a treatment model that relies on reinforcement of desirable behaviors. It is often combined with drug testing (negative drug tests result in rewards or positive drug tests result in loss of privileges), though contingency management can be used with other target behaviors, such as participating in treatment, as well. Rewards may be gift certificates, small amounts of money, or in some cases approbation from a parent/caregiver or counselor. Contingency management has been found to be effective in treating adolescents with SUDs and is a mainstay of drug courts, though few models using this modality have been developed for use in SUD treatment programs.[19,20]

as ongoing intravenous drug use. In some states, family members may seek an order for mandatory (involuntary) stabilization through the court system. Voluntary treatment is always preferable to involuntary placement; counseling from a primary care clinician and close follow-up may be appropriate over a short period of time in an attempt to encourage an AYA in need of a higher level of care to accept a treatment referral.

Table 73.2 describes treatment modalities and formats that are the most commonly used in treatment for SUDs. Regardless of the setting, most programs will include elements from these modalities and formats. Systematic reviews and meta-analyses consistently show that family therapy has the strongest empirical support for SUD treatment engagement and outcomes among teens. Similarly, interventions focused broadly on concerned significant others have proven effective at increasing SUD treatment engagement and outcomes across the lifespan. A conceptual framework for including parents/caregivers of AYAs in substance use treatment has been proposed.[22] Few AYAs are able to successfully navigate identifying, entering, and continuing treatment without support from parents/caregivers. Parent/caregivers participation also improves outcomes, though family involvement in treatment and recovery supports is currently the exception rather than the rule.

Pharmacologic Treatment

Pharmacologic treatment may be a useful adjuvant to psychosocial support and counseling (aimed at helping patients identify and avoid triggers, learn new methods for coping with stress and other difficult emotions, improve communication skills, cope with cravings, and other long-term recovery skills) for AYAs with nicotine, alcohol, or opioid use disorders. A full description of pharmacologic treatments in AYAs with SUD is beyond the scope of this chapter. However, medications may be beneficial for selected AYAs with specific SUDs and include (1) medications to treat intoxication and withdrawal, (2) medications to decrease the reinforcing effects, (3) medications to prevent relapse, and (4) medications to treat comorbid psychiatric disorders.

⬤ BEYOND SCREENING: EVALUATING ADOLESCENTS AND YOUNG ADULTS WHO PRESENT WITH BEHAVIORAL OR MENTAL HEALTH SYMPTOMS

Substance use disorders may present with nonspecific signs and symptoms, such as change in school performance, loss of interest in hobbies or extracurricular activities, inability to keep a job, excessive moodiness, irritability, or other mental health symptoms. When

TABLE 73.3

Levels of Care for Substance Use Disorder Treatment

Outpatient Treatment Settings

Outpatient treatment	Ideally, outpatient treatment combines medical management (which could include medication treatment, laboratory testing, and routine medical follow-up and advice) with regular counseling. This level of care can be achieved in a primary care setting.
Intensive *outpatient* program (IOP)	IOP serves as an intermediate level of care for patients who have needs that are too complex for outpatient treatment, but do not require inpatient services. These programs allow individuals to continue with their daily routine and practice newly acquired recovery skills both at home and at work. IOPs generally consist of a combination of supportive group therapy, educational groups, family therapy, individual therapy, relapse prevention and life skills, 12-step recovery, case management, and aftercare planning. The programs range from 2–9 h per day, 2–5 times a week, and last 1–3 mo. These programs are appealing because they provide a plethora of services in a relatively short period of time.
Partial hospital programs	Partial hospitalization is a short-term, comprehensive outpatient program in affiliation with a hospital that is designed to provide support and treatment for patients with SUDs. The services offered at these programs are more concentrated and intensive than regular outpatient treatment as they are structured throughout the entire day and offer medical monitoring in addition to individual and group therapy. Participants typically attend sessions for 7 or 8 h a day at least 5 d a week for 1–3 wks. As with IOPs, patients return home in the evenings and have a chance to practice newly acquired recovery skills.

Inpatient/Residential Treatment Settings

Medically managed withdrawal	Medically supervised withdrawal is indicated for any adolescent who is at risk of withdrawing from alcohol or benzodiazepines and may also be helpful for adolescents withdrawing from opioids, cocaine, or other substances. Support during withdrawal may be an important first step but is not considered definitive treatment. Patients who are discharged after withdrawal management should then begin either an outpatient or residential addiction treatment program.
Acute residential treatment (ART)	ART is a short-term (days–weeks) residential placement designed to stabilize patients in crisis, often before entering a longer-term residential treatment program. ART programs typically target adolescents with co-occurring mental health disorders.
Residential treatment	Residential treatment programs are highly structured live-in environments that provide therapy for those with severe substance use disorder, mental illness, or behavioral problems that require 24-h care. The goal of residential treatment is to promote the achievement and subsequent maintenance of long-term abstinence as well as equip each patient with both the social and coping skills necessary for a successful transition back into society. Residential programs are classified by length of stay: less than 30 d is considered short term while long term is considered longer than 30 d. Residential programs generally consist of individual and group therapy sessions, plus medical, psychological, clinical, nutritional, and educational components. Residential facilities aim to simulate real living environments with added structure and routine in order to provide individuals with the framework necessary for their lives to continue drug and alcohol free upon completion of the program.
Therapeutic boarding school	Therapeutic boarding schools are educational institutions that provide constant supervision for their students by a professional staff. These schools offer a highly structured environment with set times for all activities, smaller more specialized classes, social and emotional support. In addition to the regular services offered at traditional boarding schools, therapeutic schools also provide individual and group therapy for adolescents with mental health or SUDs.

SUD, substance use disorder.

any of these changes are reported by a patient or parent/caregiver, the clinician should be alert to the possibility of a SUD. In addition, any concerns about alcohol or drug use expressed by parents/caregivers, school officials, coaches, employers, or other adults should be taken seriously, even if a patient denies substance use. For young adults, a substance use evaluation may be mandated by the police or university. In these cases, the patient's report, including a thorough history that reviews the outside presenting concerns, collateral history from a parent/caregiver if available, physical examination, and, in some cases, drug test results should all be triangulated to formulate a differential diagnosis. Even if a SUD is "ruled out," new-onset behavioral or emotional symptoms should be fully evaluated as they may signal onset of a serious mental health disorder.

Co-Occurring Mental Health Disorders

Co-occurring mental health disorders are common and a full mental health evaluation is recommended. In some cases it may be difficult to determine whether the symptoms are solely the result of drug use and the question of a co-occurring disorder cannot be fully resolved until the patient has had a period of complete abstinence.

Severe symptoms, symptoms that antedate drug use, or positive family history of a similar disorder all suggest a co-occurring disorder, and concurrent treatment should be considered. In contrast, symptoms that began after the onset of drug use may resolve completely with abstinence, and patients may be observed and reassessed as necessary if symptoms are mild.

Medical Conditions Associated with Substance Use

Substance use disorders are associated with an elevated risk of early mortality throughout the lifespan, even among those with access to integrated medical and SUD services.[23] Chronic disorders and medical conditions that are thought of as problems of middle and older adulthood can have an earlier onset among those who use substances. For example, use of cocaine, amphetamines, and cannabis are all associated with increased risk of acute myocardial infarction among 15- to 22-year-olds.[24] Enhancing primary-care–based services for patients with SUDs may improve health outcomes because of its integrative capabilities to screen for and treat both medical and substance use problems, and to determine the appropriate timing of referral to a specialized SUD treatment.[23]

TABLE 73.4

Criteria for the Selection of a Substance Use Disorder Treatment Program[21]

1. View drug and alcohol use as a primary disease rather than a symptom.
2. Include a comprehensive patient evaluation and a developmentally appropriate management and treatment referral plan for associated medical, emotional, and behavioral problems identified.
3. Maintain rapport with the patient's primary care provider to facilitate seamless aftercare and primary care follow-up.
4. Adhere to an abstinence philosophy. Drug use is a chronic disease, and a drug-free environment is essential. Tobacco use should be prohibited, and nicotine cessation treatment should be provided as part of the overall treatment plan. Continued tobacco, alcohol, or other drug use should be viewed as a need for more treatment rather than discharge or refusal to treat.
5. Maintain a low patient-to-staff ratio.
6. Employ treatment professionals who are knowledgeable in both addiction treatment and child and adolescent behavior and development.
7. Ensure that professionally led support groups and self-help groups are integral parts of the program.
8. Maintain separate treatment groups for individuals at varying developmental levels (adolescents vs. young adults vs. older adults).
9. Involve the entire family in the treatment, and relate to the patients and their families with compassion and concern. Strive to reunify the family whenever possible.
10. Ensure that follow-up and continuing care are integral parts of the program.
11. Offer patients an opportunity to continue academic and vocational education and assistance with restructuring family, school, and social life. Consider formal academic and cognitive skills assessment, because unidentified weaknesses may contribute to emotional factors contributing to the substance use.
12. Keep the family apprised of costs and financial arrangements for inpatient and outpatient care and facilitate communication with managed-care organizations.
13. Be located as close to home as possible to facilitate family involvement, even though separation of the adolescent from the family may be indicated initially.

Physical Examination

A physical examination is an important part of a complete assessment of new-onset behavioral or mental health problems. Signs of chronic drug use are rare in AYAs, but should be noted if present. See Chapter 72 for more detail on physical findings associated with acute intoxication, withdrawal, and chronic substance use.

Drug Testing

Drug testing is a complicated procedure that can be useful as part of an assessment for a SUD, or for monitoring AYAs who are in treatment for a SUD, similar to using biomarkers such as a hemoglobin A1C for following other chronic disorders. While universal drug-testing programs are controversial, the procedure can be useful when indicated. If drug testing is to be used, it is important that the clinician, adolescent, and parent(s)/caregiver(s) discuss who will receive results and how they will be managed. If the adolescent is not willing to share results with parents/caregivers, determining whether the test is worthwhile is a serious consideration, as an adolescent may have little incentive to make a behavioral change, engage in treatment, or accept a referral for further evaluation if parents/caregivers do not receive results. However, even drug test results that are not shared with parents/caregivers can give clinicians an objective understanding of the types of substances and the frequency with which they are being used and can help clinicians adjust treatment and determine the appropriate level of care for patients. The AAP has produced drug-testing guidelines that may be useful to clinicians who use this procedure.[25]

THE ROLE OF PARENTS/CAREGIVERS

Parents/caregivers play a vital role in the prevention and treatment of AYA substance use. Clinicians should encourage parents/caregivers to set clear family rules prohibiting substance use and set a good example by consuming alcohol only in moderation, never driving after drinking, and avoiding illegal drug use.

Some AYAs with SUDs will not engage in treatment despite symptoms of a severe SUD. In these cases, family or parent/caregiver support counseling may be useful, even if the patient refuses to participate. Parents/caregivers can be advised to set firm but logical limits. Limit setting refers to consequences designed by the parents/caregivers, such as suspending privileges to spend time alone with friends, attend parties, or drive. For young adults, parents/caregivers can insist on abstinence as a condition of supporting educational expenses. Logical consequences should be directly related to the substance use behaviors rather than be punitive. For example, a parent/caregivers may take away a cell phone or text service if an adolescent is using the phone to obtain drugs. Because substance use is heavily promoted in U.S. culture, some parents/caregivers may understand use as a normal developmental trope and feel conflicted about enforcing rules and consequences. The clinician can support them by reminding them that it is the "job" of all parents/caregivers to help positively influence their children when they engage in dangerous, unhealthy, or illegal behavior.

Parents/caregivers may unintentionally promote a child's drug use by giving unclear messages (such as, "if you use cannabis, don't get into trouble with it"), or providing resources that a child is not using responsibly. A review of sources of money, communication, and transportation may help parents/caregivers identify targets for logical consequences. If parents/caregivers are unable to enforce their home rules with their minor children, they may seek assistance from the court system, which can mandate services, including drug testing and counseling. It is important for parents/caregivers to emphasize that consequences are intended to support the parents' rules, including "no drug use" and are not intended as punishment.

Ensuring that patients and parents/caregivers feel welcome to return to their clinician to seek help whenever they are ready, may go a long way to ultimately assisting teens and families to get the help they need. A supportive word may stay with the teen and encourage him or her to return for assistance in finding appropriate treatment even after a period of time.

TELEHEALTH

The COVID-19 pandemic forced widespread implementation of telehealth services, and research has established patient, parent/caregiver, and clinician satisfaction with remote care.[26,27] Telehealth services relieve several barriers that are particularly problematic for AYAs seeking substance use treatment. By removing transportation needs, telehealth allows AYAs greater independence in negotiating their own health care and enables individuals who live in remote areas to participate. Removing transportation time also allows participation with minimal disruption to school, work, and other activities. Telehealth may also afford a greater sense of privacy for discussing sensitive topics. Taken together, these factors can facilitate treatment engagement. In the best case, this may create an "on-ramp" for adolescents who would typically forgo recommended treatment. There are also limitations. Physical examination is limited, and subtle information such as facial expressions, body language, and emotional state may be more challenging to assess. Thoughtful approaches that triangulate information from self-report with collateral reports from parents/caregivers or other adults and laboratory monitoring for substance use can provide supplementary information. Adolescents and young adults who are victims of child maltreatment or domestic violence may find it difficult to have a private conversation at home using telehealth, which could compromise their care without the clinician's realizing it. Careful referral procedures from clinicians who are familiar with the patient and family and safety protocols for clinicians of virtual visits can be used to reduce risk. On the other hand, telehealth visits may allow assessment of factors which cannot be assessed in a traditional visit, such as a glimpse of the home environment or visualization of prescription bottles to ensure correct medications are being taken, though it is important to use information gleaned in this manner sensitively as patients may find this look into their home life as invasive.

EQUITY, DIVERSITY, INCLUSION

In 2019, Americans who identify as a race or ethnicity other than non-Hispanic White made up 40% of the country's population, and this proportion is growing. Furthermore, members of Lesbian, Gay, Bisexual, Transgender, Questioning, Intersex, and Two-Spirit (LGBTQI2S+) represent 5% to 7% of youth in the general population and this group endures significant challenges to substance use treatment including minority stigma, fear of judgment, homelessness, social isolation, lack of insurance, and targeted marketing that glorifies alcohol and other drug use within these communities. While each minoritized group faces unique challenges, they have in common a higher burden of SUDs, less access to treatment, and greater health consequences. These factors reduce the number of potential intervention points for substance use treatment, which makes medical outreach more necessary. Even when AYAs do seek SUD care, approximately one-third leave treatment before completion, with minoritized adolescents having significantly lower completion rates. The increasingly diverse population in the United States highlights the importance of investing in research to understand the unique patterns of substance use and prevalence rates by race, ethnicity, gender, and sexual orientation and evaluating whether culturally responsive adaptations are needed for different patient populations. For example, a recent randomized trial of group substance use treatment for a sample of Latino adolescents demonstrated improved outcomes in the culturally accommodated versus standard treatment group.[28]

Diversity in the health care workforce is correlated with quality of care for minoritized populations.[29] One of the foremost strategies for reducing health care disparities is to create a diverse health care workforce, and likewise, efforts to improve access to high quality, culturally responsive substance use treatment begins with addressing inequity in admissions to health professions schools.[30] If the current pattern of underrepresentation in the health professions workforce persists, individuals from historically underserved communities will continue to be disproportionately affected. A more diverse health care professional pipeline may be one of the best strategies for reducing the burden of addiction in the population.

SUMMARY

Substance use disorders are common among AYAs and most can be effectively treated in primary care. Screening, Brief Intervention, and Referral to Treatment is a useful framework for identifying SUDs, and guiding an appropriate conversation. Beyond SBIRT, a range of tools and treatments, including anticipatory guidance and medical advice, medications to treat withdrawal and suppress cravings and laboratory testing can be used to round out services in primary care. Together with integrated behavioral health care, placing treatment services in primary care where AYAs can reliably access them may be one of the most important expansions of health care for this age group.

REFERENCES

1. United Nations. World drug report 2019. Accessed August 11, 2021. https://wdr.unodc.org/wdr2019/en/index.html
2. Levy S, Weiss R, Sherritt L, et al. An electronic screen for triaging adolescent substance use by risk levels. *JAMA Pediatr.* 2014;168(9):822–828. doi:10.1001/jamapediatrics.2014.774
3. Kelly SM, Gryczynski J, Mitchell SG, et al. Validity of brief screening instrument for adolescent tobacco, alcohol, and drug use. *Pediatrics.* 2014;133(5):819–826. Accessed November 24, 2014. https://pediatrics.aappublications.org/content/133/5/819
4. McNeely J, Wu L-T, Subramaniam G, et al. Performance of the tobacco, alcohol, prescription medication, and other substance use (TAPS) tool for substance use screening in primary care patients. *Ann Intern Med.* 2016;165(10):690–699. doi:10.7326/M16-0317
5. National Institute on Alcohol Abuse and Alcoholism. *Alcohol Screening and Brief Intervention for Youth: A Practitioner's Guide*; 2011. Accessed August 31, 2022. https://www.niaaa.nih.gov/sites/default/files/publications/NIAAA_AlcoholScreening_Youth_Guide.pdf
6. Knight JR, Sherritt L, Shrier LA, et al. Validity of the CRAFFT substance abuse screening test among adolescent clinic patients. *Arch Pediatr Adolesc Med.* 2002;156(6):607–614. http://www.ncbi.nlm.nih.gov/entrez/query.fcgi?cmd=Retrieve&db=PubMed&dopt=Citation&list_uids=12038895
7. Saunders JB, Aasland OG, Babor TF, et al. Development of the alcohol use disorders identification test (AUDIT): WHO collaborative project on early detection of persons with harmful alcohol consumption–II. *Addiction.* 1993;88(6):791–804. Accessed November 21, 2014. http://www.ncbi.nlm.nih.gov/pubmed/8329970
8. McCabe SE, Boyd CJ, Cranford JA, et al. A modified version of the drug abuse screening test among undergraduate students. *J Subst Abuse Treat.* 2006;31(3):297–303. doi:10.1016/j.jsat.2006.04.010
9. Sterling S, Kline-Simon AH, Jones A, et al. Health care use over 3 years after adolescent SBIRT. *Pediatrics.* 2019;143(5):e20182803. doi:10.1542/peds.2018-2803
10. Harris SK, Csémy L, Sherritt L, et al. Computer-facilitated substance use screening and brief advice for teens in primary care: an international trial. *Pediatrics.* 2012;129(6):1072–1082. doi:10.1542/peds.2011-1624
11. D'Amico EJ, Parast L, Shadel WG, et al. Brief motivational interviewing intervention to reduce alcohol and marijuana use for at-risk adolescents in primary care. *J Consult Clin Psychol.* 2018;86(9):775–786.
12. Fadus MC, Squeglia LM, Valadez EA, et al. Adolescent substance use disorder treatment: an update on evidence-based strategies. *Curr Psychiatry Rep.* 2019;21(10):96. doi:10.1007/s11920-019-1086-0
13. Dembo R, Robinson RB, Schmeidler J, et al. Brief intervention impact on truant youths' marijuana use: 18-month follow-up. *J Child Adolesc Subst Abuse.* 2014;23(5):318–333. Accessed March 26, 2021. http://www.ncbi.nlm.nih.gov/pubmed/25642126
14. Wisk LE, Weitzman ER. Substance use patterns through early adulthood: results for youth with and without chronic conditions. *Am J Prev Med.* 2016;51(1):33–45. doi:10.1016/j.amepre.2016.01.029
15. Lunstead J, Weitzman ER, Harstad E, et al. Screening and counseling for alcohol use in adolescents with chronic medical conditions in the ambulatory setting. *J Adolesc Health.* 2019;64(6):804–806. doi:10.1016/j.jadohealth.2019.02.011
16. Weitzman ER, Ziemnik RE, Huang Q, et al. Alcohol and marijuana use and treatment nonadherence among medically vulnerable youth. *Pediatrics.* 2015;136(3):450–457. Accessed February 9, 2016. http://www.ncbi.nlm.nih.gov/pubmed/26668849
17. Kossowsky J, Magane KM, Levy S, et al. Marijuana use to address symptoms and side effects by youth with chronic medical conditions. *Pediatrics.* 2021;147(3):e2020021352. doi:10.1542/peds.2020-021352
18. Flynn D, Joyce M, Spillane A, et al. Does an adapted dialectical behaviour therapy skills training programme result in positive outcomes for participants with a dual diagnosis? A mixed methods study. *Addict Sci Clin Pract.* 2019;14(1):28. doi:10.1186/s13722-019-0156-2
19. Schuster RM, Hanly A, Gilman J, et al. A contingency management method for 30-days abstinence in non-treatment seeking young adult cannabis users. *Drug Alcohol Depend.* 2016;167:199–206. doi:10.1016/j.drugalcdep.2016.08.622
20. Godley MD, Godley SH, Dennis ML, et al. A randomized trial of assertive continuing care and contingency management for adolescents with substance use disorders. *J Consult Clin Psychol.* 2014;82(1):40–51. Accessed July 9, 2015. https://www.ncbi.nlm.nih.gov/pmc/articles/PMC3938115/
21. Levy SJL, Williams JF; Committee on Substance Use and Prevention. Substance use screening, brief intervention, and referral to treatment. *Pediatrics.* 2016;138(1):e20161211. doi:10.1542/peds.2016-1211
22. Hogue A, Becker SJ, Fishman M, et al. Youth OUD treatment during and after COVID: increasing family involvement across the services continuum. *J Subst Abuse Treat.* 2021;120:108159. doi:10.1016/j.jsat.2020.108159
23. Bahorik AL, Satre DD, Kline-Simon AH, et al. Alcohol, cannabis, and opioid use disorders, and disease burden in an integrated health care system. *J Addict Med.* 2017;11(1):3–9. doi:10.1097/ADM.0000000000000260
24. Patel RS, Manocha P, Patel J, et al. Cannabis use is an independent predictor for acute myocardial infarction related hospitalization in younger population. *J Adolesc Health.* 2020;66(1):79–85. doi:10.1016/j.jadohealth.2019.07.024
25. Levy S, Siqueira LM, Ammerman SD, et al; Committee on Substance Abuse. Testing for drugs of abuse in children and adolescents. *Pediatrics.* 2014;133(6):e1798–e1807. Accessed October 16, 2014. http://pediatrics.aappublications.org/content/early/2014/05/20/peds.2014-0865
26. Myers KM, Valentine JM, Melzer SM. Feasibility, acceptability, and sustainability of telepsychiatry for children and adolescents. *Psychiatr Serv.* 2007;58(11):1493–1496. doi:10.1176/ps.2007.58.11.1493
27. Pooni R, Pageler NM, Sandborg C, et al. Pediatric subspecialty telemedicine use from the patient and provider perspective. *Pediatr Res.* 2022;91(1):241–246. doi:10.1038/s41390-021-01443-4
28. Burrow-Sánchez JJ, Hops H. A randomized trial of culturally accommodated versus standard group treatment for latina/o adolescents with substance use disorders: posttreatment through 12-month outcomes. *Cultur Divers Ethnic Minor Psychol.* 2019;25(3):311–322. doi:10.1037/cdp0000249
29. Huerto R. Minority patients benefit from having minority doctors, but that's a hard match to make. M Health Lab. Accessed May 25, 2021. https://labblog.uofmhealth.org/rounds/minority-patients-benefit-from-having-minority-doctors-but-thats-a-hard-match-to-make-0

XIV

30. Muppala VR, Janwadkar RS, Rootes A, et al. Creating a pipeline for minority physicians: medical-student-led programming. *Cureus.* 2021;13(4):e14384. doi:10.7759/cureus.14384

🛜 ADDITIONAL RESOURCES AND WEBSITES

Additional Resources and Websites for Clinicians:

American Academy of Pediatrics (AAP)—https://www.aap.org/en-us/advocacy-and-policy/aap-health-initiatives/Substance-Use-and-Prevention/Pages/home.aspx

American Society of Addiction Medicine (ASAM)—https://www.asam.org/

Behavioral Health Equity Information—https://www.samhsa.gov/behavioral-health-equity

Centers for Disease Control and Prevention (CDC)—https://www.cdc.gov/ncbddd/fasd/features/teen-substance-use.html

Find Treatment—https://www.samhsa.gov/find-treatment

National Institute on Alcohol Abuse and Alcoholism (NIAAA)—https://www.niaaa.nih.gov/alcohols-effects-health/professional-education-materials/alcohol-screening-and-brief-intervention-youth-practitioners-guide

The National Institute on Drug Abuse (NIDA)—https://www.drugabuse.gov/

Substance Abuse and Mental Health Services Administration (SAMHSA)—https://www.samhsa.gov/ebp-resource-center

Additional Resources and Websites for Parents/Caregivers:

Centers for Disease Control and Prevention (CDC)—https://www.cdc.gov/ncbddd/fasd/features/teen-substance-use.html

Healthy Children.org

English version—https://www.healthychildren.org/English/ages-stages/teen/substance-abuse/Pages/default.aspx

Spanish version—https://www.healthychildren.org/spanish/ages-stages/teen/substance-abuse/paginas/default.aspx

NIDA for Teens—https://teens.drugabuse.gov/parents

Partnership to End Addiction—https://drugfree.org/

Resources in Spanish—https://drugfree.org/recursos-en-espanol/

Harvard Health Blog: "Blown up in smoke: Young adults who vape at greater risk of COVID symptoms"—https://www.health.harvard.edu/blog/blown-up-in-smoke-young-adults-who-vape-at-greater-risk-of-covid-symptoms-2020082820859

Additional Resources and Websites for Adolescents and Young Adults:

NIDA for Teens—https://teens.drugabuse.gov/teens

SAMHSA for Teens—https://www.samhsa.gov/brss-tacs/recovery-support-tools/youth-young-adults

SAMHSA National Helpline: 1-800-662-HELP (4357)

Smoke Free Teen—https://teen.smokefree.gov/

Quit line: Text "QUIT" to 47848 or Call 877-44U-QUIT (877-448-7848) for live support from trained counselors

quitSTART Application (app)—https://smokefree.gov/tools-tips/apps/quitstart

Truth Initiative—https://truthinitiative.org/

Quit line: Text "DITCHJUUL" to 88709

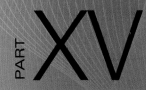

Mental Health

CHAPTER 74

Depression and Anxiety Disorders

Daphne J. Korczak
Suneeta Monga

KEY WORDS

- Adjustment disorder
- Anxiety
- Depression
- Generalized anxiety disorder
- Psychopharmacology
- Psychotherapy
- Social anxiety disorder

INTRODUCTION

Depression and anxiety disorders are highly prevalent among adolescents and young adults (AYAs): 75% of all lifetime cases will have started by age 24 years.[1] Social withdrawal, substance use, poor academic performance, decreased concentration, fatigue, and other somatic complaints may all indicate a new onset of a mental health issue. Adolescents and young adults, collectively referred to as *youth* in this chapter, may also have limited awareness of the severity or functional impact of their symptoms, because of symptom chronicity or reluctance to acknowledge a mental health problem. Thus, clinicians working with youth must have a high index of suspicion for mental health disorders among this population. This chapter reviews the most frequently encountered mood and anxiety disorders of adolescence and young adulthood, and discusses the key causes, assessments, and diagnoses of, and treatments for, these conditions.

DEPRESSION IN YOUTH

Epidemiology

- According to the World Health Organization (WHO), depression is a leading cause of disability globally.
- Prior to the pandemic, clinically significant depressive illness occurred in about 5% to 8% of adolescents in the United States, Canada, and Europe. However, during the first year of the pandemic, approximately 25% of youth reported clinically significant depressive symptoms, with higher prevalence rates in older youth, females, and later in the pandemic.[2]
- Depressive symptoms are widely reported in community studies of youth. In one community survey of 9,863 adolescents in the United States, 18% of participants in early to middle adolescence reported depressive symptoms.
- About 25% to 50% of depressed youth have comorbid anxiety disorders; about 10% to 15% of anxious youth have depression.
- Gender: By midadolescence, the female predominance noted in adult samples is established, with the ratio of affected female youth to affected male youth reaching 2:1.

- Age of onset: Although the mean age of onset of a first depressive episode is mid-20s, this age is decreasing with each generation; the prevalence of the preadult age of onset of major depressive disorder (MDD) is increasing. Many children experience subsyndromal and syndromal symptoms for years before coming to medical attention. Early identification of depression is important for healthy psychosocial and cognitive development and improved health outcomes among youth.
- Onset of depression in adolescence is more likely to remain undetected for a longer period of time than onset in young adulthood or adulthood.
- Clinicians treating youth with depression play a critical role in altering lifelong developmental trajectories.

Course of Illness

The onset of depression in adolescence is associated with a more severe course of illness than onset in young adulthood or adulthood.[3] Affected adolescents are at greater risk of more depressive episodes, more severe episodes, increased suicidality, increased likelihood of dropping out of high school, poorer academic, occupational, and social outcomes, and greater psychiatric comorbidity than those who first experience depression as young adults or adults.

- About 60% to 70% of those who have a depressive episode in adolescence will have a recurrence within 5 years.
- Increased risk of recurrence is associated with greater episode severity, chronicity of symptoms, incomplete recovery, presence of dysthymia, comorbid anxiety, persistence of stressful life events, and parental history of depression.
- Early in the course of depression, a psychosocial stressor is frequently present and identified as a precipitant for the depressive episode. In contrast, depressive episodes later in adulthood may occur without any discernible precipitating stressful event.

Risk Factors

A number of biologic, psychosocial, and social factors have been associated with increased risk of depression among youth (**Table 74.1**).

Biologic

Children of parents with a history of depression are at increased risk of developing depression.

- Twin-study estimates of the heritability of MDD range from 0.36 to 0.70.[4]
- Family studies[5] estimate a 10% to 25% risk of MDD in first-degree relatives of MDD probands, two to three times higher than that in controls.

TABLE 74.1

Risk Factors for Depression among Youth

Biologic Factors
- Female sex
- Older age
- Parent/family history of depression
- Comorbid chronic illness (e.g., diabetes, anxiety disorder, attention deficit hyperactivity disorder)
- Past history of depression
- Comorbid learning disorders
- Genetics (presence of specific serotonin-transporter gene variants)
- Certain medications (e.g., prednisone, isotretinoin [Accutane])
- Substance use

Psychosocial Risk Factors
- Family or peer conflict (e.g., bullying)
- Childhood neglect or abuse (physical, emotional, sexual)
- Poverty
- Recent loss, (e.g., death of a loved one, break up of romantic relationship)
- Academic difficulties or failure of the child
- Discrimination and social exclusion
- Poor (e.g., conflictual) home–school relationships
- Poor-quality (e.g., high conflict, low community support) neighborhoods

- Youth with depression are more likely than adults to have a family history of depression in a first-degree relative.
- Offspring of parents with early-onset depression have about a four to five times higher risk of developing MDD (25% to 40% risk of MDD) than controls.
- An adopted person's risk of developing depression is increased if his or her biologic parent had depression.

Psychological

Psychological factors that may contribute to the development of depression include:
- A tendency to respond to stress with unpleasant emotions, although many people with depression do not have strong emotional responses before the onset of depression.
- A tendency to interpret emotionally neutral events as negative.

The experience of depressive illness during adolescence and young adulthood disrupts normative developmental growth of personality characteristics.

Social

A number of social factors also are risk factors for development of depression among youth:
- Bullying
- Poverty
- Poor physical health
- Social isolation. Research conducted during the COVID-19 pandemic showed that decreased in-person social interactions and activities were strongly associated with depressive symptoms among both previously healthy adolescents, as well as those with a history of mental illness.
- Perceived discrimination within the household (i.e., the perception of having less access to material and emotional supports than other children in the home)
- Increased daily-life stresses (e.g., excessive work or chores, academic difficulties)
- Early-life stress, such as childhood abuse and neglect. Evidence indicates that early-life stress can induce persistent changes in the responsiveness of the hypothalamic–pituitary–adrenal (HPA) axis to stress later in life that is associated with depression (see below).

Causality

The origin of depression is multifactorial: neurobiologic, pathophysiologic, psychological, and social factors contribute to the genesis of MDD.
- *Neurobiologic.* Abnormalities of several brain structures are found in people with MDD, including the hippocampus, the hypothalamus, the amygdala, and the nucleus accumbens. Both structural and functional abnormalities have been described. Several neurotransmitter systems (serotonin, norepinephrine, dopamine) have also been implicated in the dysfunction reported in individuals with MDD, forming the basis for the use of the medication in treatment, as described below.
- *Pathophysiologic.* Possible underlying pathologic processes causing depression include dysfunction of the HPA axis, increased proinflammatory cytokines, and oxidative stress.
- *Psychological.* Numerous psychological theories about the basis of depression have been proposed. Both cognitive and interpersonal theories have led to specific treatment modalities for depressed youth (see Treatment for depression). It is important that clinicians using psychotherapeutic treatment modalities are well versed in the psychological theories pertaining to the basis of depression and the treatment modality that they intend to employ.

ASSESSMENT

In contrast to the transitory aspects of a normal depressed mood in youth, depressive illness is characterized by the persistence of depressed mood, irritability, or anhedonia, and associated features. Pessimism, reduced ability to experience pleasure, and decreased energy and motivation are also frequently present. Experiences of helplessness, hopelessness, or worthlessness may occur. Together with associated depressive symptoms, the condition interferes with the ability to function at school, at home, and with friends.

Important Elements in the Assessment of Depression

Interviews and Collateral Information

Individual clinical interview of the youth and interviews with the parents/caregivers (whenever possible) to obtain collateral information are essential in order to assess symptoms and their functional impact. This should include depressive symptoms, assessment of suicidality and self-harm behaviors, elucidation of precipitating stressors (e.g., breakup of a romantic relationship, bullying, new disclosure of sexual orientation or gender identity concerns), and presence of additional symptoms (psychotic, anxious) or behaviors (substance use) required to ascertain an accurate diagnostic impression.

Youth must be made aware of the limits of confidentiality in this interview when disclosures may have a potential impact on the safety of the patient or others. Youth may downplay or misunderstand the basis of these symptoms and attribute them to problems with nerves, being physically unfit, or intrinsic characterologic deficits. Sleep disturbance and loss of energy or motivation are the most uniformly reported of depressive symptoms after depressed mood. Sadness may be denied at first, but later elicited through clinical interview or inferred from facial expression.

Assessment of Illness Characteristics

The severity of the current depressive episode (mild, moderate, or severe), the presence of associated illness specifiers (e.g., presence of psychotic features), and the nature of the overarching mood disorder (bipolar or unipolar) must be determined as these have important treatment implications.

Consideration of Cultural Background

Cultural background may affect the type and intensity of affective expression.[6] Symptoms of depression share many similarities across cultures, but culture may affect the symptoms emphasized and the idioms used to describe distress.[6] For example, poor eye contact may be a symptom of emotional distress in cultures that stress individual autonomy, but may be a sign of respect in cultures that stress deference. In addition, patients may report symptoms of considerable suffering, but their restrained expression of distress may strain the credibility of the report. Conversely, they may describe symptoms in a highly expressive manner that seems exaggerated. In some cultures, somatic symptoms may constitute the presenting complaint.

Screening Tools for Depression

A number of self-report and clinician-administered instruments have been evaluated and validated for use in the screening and monitoring of depressive symptoms among youth. Self-report measures, have wide appeal because of their ease of administration, patient acceptability, and ability to translate symptom dimensions into quantifiable scores for evaluation. Although these instruments may be helpful supplementary tools for screening and monitoring depressive symptoms, they are not diagnostic instruments and cannot substitute for clinical assessment of depression. Although some measures have been validated in non–English-speaking youth, clinicians must be aware of individual cultural differences, intellectual or cognitive impairments, and comorbidity of depression with psychiatric and other chronic illnesses that may be pertinent and limit the generalizability of the measure's utility for their patient.

Commonly used depression-specific measures, with demonstrated reliability and validity in the populations outlined below, include (but are not limited to) the following:

Beck Depression Inventory-II

Beck Depression Inventory-II (BDI-II) is a 21-item self-report instrument that takes 10 to 15 minutes to complete by individuals 13 years of age and older. Each question is scored from 0 to 3. Higher scores indicate more severe depressive symptoms.

Children's Depression Inventory

Children's Depression Inventory (CDI-2) is a 28-item scale derived from the BDI used to assess depressive symptoms in children and adolescents. Questions from the BDI were modified to make them more appropriate for younger ages. The CDI-2 is a self-report measure that takes 15 to 20 minutes to complete by patients 7 to 17 years of age. Each item is scored from 0 to 3. In addition, two-scale (emotional problems and functional problems) and four-subscale scores can be computed. Higher scores indicate more severe depressive symptoms.

Centre for Epidemiologic Studies Depression Scale for Children

The Centre for Epidemiologic Studies Depression Scale for Children (CES-DC) is a 20-item self-report measure for 8- to 18-year-olds. Items are rated from zero to three and assess depressive symptoms over the past week. Total sum scores range from zero to 60; higher scores indicate greater severity of depression. Scores of 15 or higher indicate a positive screen for clinically significant depressive symptoms.

Patient Health Questionnaire

This questionnaire consists of nine self-report items that takes the adolescent or young adult about 5 to 10 minutes to complete. Originally developed for adults over 18 years of age, psychometric validity data also support its use among adolescents in primary care and pediatric hospital settings.

⬤ DEPRESSIVE DISORDERS AND THE DIAGNOSTIC AND STATISTICAL MANUAL OF MENTAL DISORDERS, FIFTH EDITION

Major Depressive Episode[7]

- Five (or more) of the following nine symptoms must be present during the same 2-week period.

- Symptoms must either be newly present or have clearly worsened when compared with those present before the person's current episode.
- Symptoms must persist for most of the day, nearly every day, for at least two consecutive weeks.
- At least one of the symptoms must be either (1) depressed mood or (2) loss of interest or pleasure.
- Depressed mood, as indicated by either subjective or objective report, most of the day, nearly every day. For adolescents, the mood may be irritable.
- Markedly diminished interest or pleasure in all, or almost all, activities most of the day, nearly every day
- Significant weight loss when not dieting, weight gain, or change in appetite
- Insomnia or hypersomnia nearly every day
- Psychomotor agitation or retardation nearly every day, observable by others, not merely subjective feelings of restlessness or of being slowed down
- Fatigue or loss of energy nearly every day
- Feelings of worthlessness or excessive or inappropriate guilt (which may be delusional) nearly every day (not merely self-reproach or guilt about being sick)
- Diminished ability to think or concentrate, or indecisiveness, nearly every day
- Recurrent thoughts of death (not just fear of dying), recurrent suicidal ideation without a specific plan, suicide attempt, or a specific plan for committing suicide
  Note: symptoms must cause clinically significant distress or impairment in social, occupational, or other important areas of functioning. The episode cannot be attributable to the physiologic effects of a substance or to another medical condition. All of these criteria must be met to represent a major depressive episode.

Adjustment Disorder

See Chapter 39.

Persistent Depression (Dysthymia)[7]

- Depressed mood that occurs for most of the day, for more days than not, for at least 2 years (or 1 year for adolescents). Youth whose depressed mood resolves consistently during the summer months, for example, do not have a persistent depressive disorder.
- At least two of six associated depressive neurovegetative or cognitive symptoms must be present.
- At times, the patient may have also experienced a major depressive episode.
- People with this disorder often describe years of feeling sad. Some youth may be unable to remember a time when they did not feel this way or attribute the experience to part of their personality.
- Youth with persistent depressive symptoms are at high risk of developing comorbid psychiatric illness, including substance use disorders and personality disorders. As a result, they may require treatment for these in addition to management of their depressive disorder.

Bipolar Depression[7]

Bipolar depression is differentiated from unipolar depressive illnesses by the presence of one or more periods of hypomania or mania during the course of illness. That is, bipolar depression refers to a major depressive episode that occurs within the context of bipolar disorder.

- Youth with bipolar disorder, despite having suffered a hypomanic or manic episode in their lifetime, frequently experience much of the illness' morbidity as the result of either syndromal or subsyndromal depressive symptoms.

- A major depressive episode in adolescence or young adulthood may be the index mood episode of bipolar disorder; the mean age of onset of the first mood episode is about 18 years of age.
- The presence of psychotic features, profound psychomotor retardation, or a family history of bipolar disorder should alert the clinician to the possibility of bipolar depression.
- Clinicians considering the diagnosis of bipolar depression should request psychiatric consultation to assess the potential of an underlying bipolar diathesis and obtain management suggestions because treatment algorithms are substantially different from those for unipolar depressive illness.

Youth with depressive disorders may also suffer from comorbid psychiatric illness (particularly anxiety, substance use, attention deficit hyperactivity disorder [ADHD], and conduct disorders). These disorders must also be identified to ensure safe and appropriate recommendations for treatment are made.

 TREATMENT

General Considerations

Ensure Safety

The single most important consideration in determining a treatment plan for depressed youth is to *assess for the risk for suicide* (Chapter 75) and ensure safety. Clinicians must first decide whether the patient should be hospitalized or can be safely managed as an outpatient before proceeding with other treatment recommendations.

Provide Psychoeducation

Communication of the diagnosis of depression, eliciting patient and family conceptualizations of the illness, and the provision of psychoeducation about the symptoms, course, and treatments available for depression are key components to undertake before determining a treatment plan.

Identify and Address Stressors and Psychiatric Comorbidity

Additional components of a comprehensive treatment plan include discussing stressors that may be perpetuating depressive symptoms (e.g., ongoing family or peer conflict), and screening for and addressing comorbid psychiatric illness (e.g., substance use or anxiety disorders), as appropriate. It may be necessary to involve parents/caregivers in order to address these factors.

Mild Depression

- For youth with mild depression, addressing perpetuating factors, providing active support, scheduling regular visits, and monitoring symptoms may help alleviate symptoms.
- Providing active, supportive strategies (e.g., encouraging involvement in enjoyable activities, ensuring sound sleep–hygiene routines, promoting routine physical activity, advocating for patients when they are having difficulties with academics or bullying at school) may relieve symptoms in as many as 20% of depressed youth.[8]
- Patients who do not respond to these strategies should begin a depression-specific treatment.

Moderate to Severe Depression

- Youth with moderate or severe depression should be referred to a specialist for assessment and management recommendations.
- Once assessed, primary care physicians may undertake management plans alone or in collaboration with a mental health specialist.
- Youth with moderate to severe symptoms are less likely to experience symptom remission without psychotherapy, medication, or combination treatment.

Psychotherapy

Cognitive Behavioral Therapy

Cognitive behavioral therapy (CBT) is a manualized treatment modality that can be delivered either individually or in groups, and administered in primary care settings. Cognitive behavioral therapy is based on the cognitive theory of depression, which describes how people's perceptions of, or spontaneous thoughts about, situations influence their emotional, behavioral (and often physiologic) reactions. Perceptions are often distorted when people are depressed, and a stream of seemingly spontaneous negative thoughts, called *automatic thoughts* may be experienced. Depressive automatic thoughts fall into one of three categories: negative thoughts about the self, the world or environment, and the future.

- Cognitive behavioral therapy is an effective stand-alone treatment for depression in adolescents and a first-line treatment for depression of mild to moderate severity.[9]
- The combination of CBT and pharmacotherapy is reportedly more efficacious than either treatment modality alone for the treatment of adolescent depression.[10]
- The largest randomized placebo-controlled study to date, the Treatment for Adolescents with Depression Study,[10] compared placebo, CBT alone, fluoxetine alone, and combination fluoxetine plus CBT. Adolescent participants in the medication arms demonstrated significantly greater improvement in their depressive symptoms than those in either the CBT-alone or placebo arms. In this investigator-initiated study, patients with more severe and persistent depression benefited equally from medication alone or from combined medication and CBT. Another study,[8] however, found that the addition of CBT to antidepressant medication and routine specialist care did not further reduce depressive symptoms for more severely depressed adolescents.

Cognitive behavioral therapy has been adapted for the treatment of depression by focusing on correcting cognitive distortions such as depressive negative self-cognitions (e.g., "I am worthless," "nobody likes me"), utilizing mood diaries to monitor symptoms, and expanding the behavioral component to include behavioral activation strategies (e.g., exercise, participation in group activities).

Interpersonal Therapy

Interpersonal therapy (IPT) is based on the interpersonal theory of depression, which suggests that people who are prone to depression are more likely to seek excessive reassurance in relationships. This support-seeking behavior tends to elicit support-giving behavior, which reinforces the depressive symptoms. The model further posits that this style of interpersonal communication may also occur more commonly in people with deficient social skills. People who excessively seek reassurance and may have poor social skills are theorized to have more interpersonal difficulties, including rejection, within their relationships, which further increases their depressive symptoms. As IPT was originally developed for the treatment of depression in adults, much of the evidence for its effectiveness comes from studies of adult populations, including young adults.

- Interpersonal therapy has since been adapted for administration in adolescents (interpersonal therapy for adolescents [IPT-A]).
- The central tenet of IPT is that depressive symptoms and interpersonal relationships are intertwined.
- Connections are made between the person's depressive symptoms and the practical life events that either precipitate or follow from the onset of the illness.
- Patients must be assessed as having one of four relational areas as a central theme to inform the therapy: role transitions (e.g., graduation, moving away to school), grief, role disputes (having conflictual relationships with important people in their lives), or interpersonal deficits (difficulty forming relationships with peers).
- Similar to CBT, IPT and IPT-A are structured, short-term, manualized therapies.
- In contrast to CBT for the treatment of adolescent depression, data supporting the efficacy of IPT-A is more limited.

- Comparison of the use of IPT-A to medication or in combination with medication to examine its comparative benefit has not been studied.

Nonspecific Psychotherapies

Cognitive behavioral therapy and IPT (or IPT-A) are psychotherapies that may be indicated specifically for treatment of depressive symptoms among youth. Youth with depression may also have *comorbid* psychiatric conditions or symptoms that are functionally impairing and highly problematic in their lives. The clinician may wish to consider using a psychotherapeutic modality that specifically targets these concerns, despite its lack of specificity for depressive symptoms, based on the difficulties that are the most distressing or impairing for the patient. For example, youth with highly conflictual family relationships may benefit from family therapy; those struggling with ongoing themes of past trauma may require a trauma-focused therapy. Motivational interviewing may address comorbid substance use. Dialectical behavior therapy (DBT) may be required to address impulsive anger or persistent thoughts and urges to engage in self-harm or suicidal behavior. Although these psychotherapies are not specific for the treatment of depression, the amelioration of the potentially perpetuating stressors or symptoms may have nonspecific benefits in improving depressive symptoms.

Medication

Antidepressant medications are classified on the basis of their specific relation to brain neurotransmitters. Selective serotonin reuptake inhibitors (SSRIs) are a class of medications that include fluoxetine, sertraline, citalopram, escitalopram, fluvoxamine, and paroxetine (Table 74.2). Selective serotonin reuptake inhibitors inhibit serotonin transporters, blocking reuptake, and increasing the concentration of the serotonin neurotransmitter within the synapse. Within the broader class of SSRIs, specific medications may also influence other neurotransmitter systems (e.g., dopamine, norepinephrine), affecting the effectiveness and adverse effects of various SSRIs.

Laboratory Investigations

Laboratory investigations may be necessary to:
- Rule out alternate underlying causes of the presenting symptoms (e.g., hypothyroidism),
- Assess comorbid medical conditions (e.g., hepatic impairment), or
- Monitor therapeutic drug levels of medications used in combination with SSRIs (e.g., valproic acid).

However, laboratory investigations are not routinely required before initiating or maintaining SSRIs. Psychiatry consultation should be considered when the patient has a comorbid chronic medical illness or requires treatment with SSRIs in combination with other medications.

Evidence and Medication Use

In the United States, the Food and Drug Administration (FDA) has approved fluoxetine and escitalopram for the treatment of depression for adolescents. Health Canada (HC) has not approved antidepressants (including SSRIs) for the treatment of depression for adolescents. It is important, therefore, that, when prescribing SSRIs for patients under the age of 18 years, physicians document relevant issues carefully.

- Randomized double-blind placebo-controlled trials and systematic reviews suggest that SSRIs are effective for the treatment of adolescent depression; response rates range from 40% to 70%.[11,12]
- Response rates for patients receiving placebo are also considerable (30% to 60%). This indicates that the design of the study is important when evaluating the efficacy of antidepressant medications among youth.
- Clinical trials of fluoxetine have found the greatest difference between active drug and placebo.[11,13]
- Two randomized controlled trials (RCTs) showed the efficacy of escitalopram for the treatment of adolescent depression.[14,15]
- A single positive RCT for each of citalopram[16] and sertraline[17] reported greater benefits for these medications over placebo for the treatment of adolescent depression. A second RCT of citalopram demonstrated negative results in the treatment of adolescent depression.[18]
- Examination of paroxetine's efficacy in the treatment of child and adolescent depression has yielded negative results in three RCTs.
- Among patients older than 18 years, several additional medications, including serotonin and norepinephrine reuptake inhibitors (e.g., venlafaxine), norepinephrine and dopamine reuptake inhibitors (e.g., bupropion), and others, have evidence for efficacy in the treatment of depression.[19]
- Based on efficacy data, aripiprazole (an atypical antipsychotic medication) has been approved by the FDA as adjunctive therapy for MDD in adults (>18 years old).

Adverse Effects of Medications

- Selective serotonin reuptake inhibitors are generally well tolerated. Common short-term side effects include gastrointestinal symptoms (e.g., stomach aches, nausea), sleep changes (either insomnia or somnolence, and sleep disturbances, including vivid dreams), restlessness, headaches, appetite changes, and sexual dysfunction.
- An increase in agitation or impulsivity (behavioral activation) may occur. If youth experience behavioral activation, then the clinician must ensure that early signs of hypomania are eliminated from the differential diagnosis.[20]
- Selective serotonin reuptake inhibitors have rarely been associated with increased risk of bleeding and syndrome of inappropriate secretion of antidiuretic hormone.
- Serotonin syndrome may occur as a result of toxicity (e.g., overdose ingestion) and can include changes in mental status, myoclonus, ataxia, diaphoresis, fever, and autonomic dysregulation.
- Both HC and the FDA have issued a health advisory or drug-safety communications about dose-dependent QT-interval prolongation and risk of arrhythmia with citalopram dosages of greater than 40 mg/day and escitalopram dosages greater than 20 mg/day.[21,22] They recommend that clinicians not exceed this dose. Further, patients with congenital long QT syndrome should not be treated with either citalopram or escitalopram. Patients with underlying heart disease or hepatic impairment (affecting citalopram metabolism), including a predisposition to cardiac arrhythmia because of electrolyte disturbances, should be

TABLE 74.2
SSRI Medications: Half-Life and Dosing Schedules

Medication (Trade Name)	Mean Half-Life (h)	Dosing Schedule
Fluoxetine (Prozac)	96	Daily
Sertraline (Zoloft)	26	Daily
Fluvoxamine (Luvox)	15	Daily
Citalopram (Celexa)	35	Daily
Escitalopram (Cipralex)	30	Daily
Paroxetine (Paxil)	21	Daily

SSRI, selective serotonin reuptake inhibitor.

treated with caution if receiving citalopram or escitalopram and monitored closely for cardiac adverse effects, including torsades de pointes.[21]

* Adverse effects of adjunctive aripiprazole treatment include constipation, akathisia, insomnia, fatigue, restlessness, and blurred vision.

Suicide and Selective Serotonin Reuptake Inhibitors

When used appropriately, the potential benefits of SSRIs use outweigh the potential harms of untreated depression for youth with moderate to severe depression.

* Untreated moderate to severe depression is more likely to result in harm than appropriate SSRI use.
* Close initial monitoring, along with careful documentation of symptoms and adverse effects, is required.
* Suicidality lessens with effective treatment and improvement of depressive symptoms.[23]

Monitoring of Medications

For youth who begin a course of SSRI treatment, the goal should be to achieve the minimum effective dosage in 1 to 2 weeks of taking the starting dose. The FDA suggests clinical monitoring of patients at the following time points:

1. Weekly (at least) for the first 4 weeks after initiation of SSRI medication
2. Then, every 2 weeks for the next 2 weeks
3. Then, at 12 weeks
4. Then, as clinically indicated beyond the 12-week point

The FDA notes that additional contact by telephone may be appropriate between face-to-face visits. Guidelines from the American Academy of Child and Adolescent Psychiatry[20] also encourage clinicians to follow the FDA monitoring schedule, although highlight the lack of evidence supporting an association between weekly face-to-face visits and suicide risk. Monitoring assessments should include evaluation of suicidal thoughts and behaviors, and the potential adverse medication effects described above. Overall adherence to medication should also be assessed over time; an abrupt discontinuation of SSRI medications (except fluoxetine) may lead to withdrawal symptoms and an abrupt worsening of depressive symptoms, including suicidality.

Maintenance of Medications

The goal of treatment is to achieve full remission of depression symptoms.

* Once an effective dosage is reached, symptoms should be reassessed at 4-week intervals to evaluate the effectiveness and tolerability of the current dosage and to determine the need to increase the dose.
* Once complete response is achieved, the medication should be continued for a minimum of 6 to 12 months to decrease the risk of depressive relapse.[20]
* Discontinuing an SSRI should consist of a slow taper of medication and occur during a relatively stress-free time (e.g., the summer months).
* For youth with a history of multiple depressive episodes, comorbid psychiatric illnesses, or complicated depressive episodes (e.g., with psychotic features), psychiatric consultation may be warranted before discontinuing medication.
* The presence of psychiatric comorbidity, including substance use disorders, may warrant further psychiatric assessment before embarking on a treatment plan.
* The relationship between ongoing substance use and depressive or anxious symptoms is frequently bidirectional. A substance use disorder should not necessarily exclude patients from receiving appropriate treatment for comorbid depression or anxiety disorders.

ANXIETY DISORDERS IN YOUTH

Anxiety disorders must be delineated from the normative experience of anxiety and stress. Anxiety disorders are diagnosed when the anxiety is *excessive*, *persistent*, and *interferes* with day-to-day functioning. Youth presenting with an anxiety disorder are typically unable to control or stop the worries and/or the worries prevent participation in activities such as school, work, and extracurricular or other social activities.

* Anxiety can be normative; there are specific developmental phases where specific fears or worries may be expected transiently. As such, clinicians must evaluate the degree of anxiety in the context of normative development.
* Anxiety disorders are persistent, unlike transient anxiety, which is often stress-induced, therefore, each anxiety disorder has time-based DSM-5 criteria (e.g., more than 6 months).
* Each anxiety disorder is defined by the main worry expressed by the individual.

Epidemiology

Anxiety disorders are the most common psychiatric disorders in youth, although they are not easily recognized and are often missed or undiagnosed especially in younger age groups.

* Prevalence rates for anxiety disorders are typically in the range of 10% to 20% for all youth.[24,25]
* Comorbidity among the anxiety disorders is the norm.[24] Many youth have symptoms for more than one anxiety disorder, although they may not meet full diagnostic criteria for each of the anxiety disorders.
* Comorbidity between anxiety disorders and other mental health conditions such as ADHD, depression, and substance use is also common.[24]
* In general, most studies suggest that anxiety disorders are more common in females than in males (ratio about 2:1).[24]
* Most anxiety disorders develop in early childhood (median age is 6 years) although they may not be recognized or diagnosed until later. Many individuals, however, may develop anxiety disorders for the first time during adolescence or young adulthood.

Course of Illness

* Anxiety disorders are chronic disorders, although the symptoms may wax and wane overtime.
* Evidence suggests that adolescents meeting criteria for an anxiety disorder have a moderate to high risk to meet criteria for an anxiety disorder in young adulthood.[24,25]
* Additionally, anxiety disorders may progress into mood (depression and bipolar disorder) or substance use disorders.

Risk and Prognostic Factors

Common risk factors for all anxiety disorders can be classified into three broad categories:

Temperamental Factors

Temperament describes the way in which a child approaches and reacts to the world, and interacts and behaves with others. Inborn traits such as a child's innate activity level, adaptability, response to new situations, sensitivity to surroundings, distractibility, and persistence are used to categorize children into various temperamental categories. *Behavioral inhibition* characterized by shyness, timidity, withdrawal, and fear of the unfamiliar appears to be relatively stable over the course of childhood and into adulthood and has been identified as a risk factor for selective mutism (SM), social anxiety disorder (SAD), and generalized anxiety disorder (GAD).[24,26] It is important to note that many children with behavioral inhibition, however, do not develop an anxiety disorder.

Environmental Factors

- Nonspecific environmental factors including various life stress, such as parental divorce, immigration, entry to a new school or neighborhood, experience of loss (e.g., the death of a relative or pet), have all been associated with the development of anxiety disorders.
- As a result of COVID-19 pandemic, adolescents have experienced social isolation, specifically decreased in-person social interactions and activities that have been associated with anxiety symptoms among both previously healthy adolescents and those with a history of mental illness.
- Interpersonal stressors, negative experiences with illicit or prescription drugs, and smoking are risk factors for panic attacks and development of panic disorder.

Parental factors such as overprotection and intrusiveness have been associated with separation anxiety disorder and GAD. Parental modeling of social hesitation or other symptoms of social anxiety are considered risk factors for the development of SAD.[24,26]

Genetic Factors

Evidence suggests that anxiety disorders are heritable disorders with involvement of multiple genes.

- Relatives of probands with anxiety disorders have strong family histories of both anxiety and mood disorders.
- Offspring of individuals with anxiety, depression, and bipolar disorders have increased risk for the development of anxiety disorders.
- Studies suggest that anxious youth are more likely than nonanxious youth to have a parent/caregiver with an anxiety disorder.
- Behavioral inhibition appears to have a strong genetic influence and is strongly associated with a variety of anxiety disorders, most commonly SAD and SM.[24,26]

Causality

- In general, the neurobiology and causes of anxiety disorders are less well understood than depression.
- Current neural system models emphasize the amygdala and related structures.
- Agents such as sodium lactate, caffeine, isoproterenol, yohimbine, carbon dioxide, and cholecystokinin more frequently provoke panic attacks in people with panic disorder than in healthy controls.
- Cigarette smoking and the use of various illicit and prescription drugs may precipitate panic attacks.

ASSESSMENT

Anxiety disorders are often missed and/or not recognized by clinicians and parents/caregivers. Even youth themselves may not recognize that their level of anxiety and/or worry is excessive. For a diagnosis of an anxiety disorder to be made, the anxiety must interfere with the individual's day-to-day functioning and/or cause significant distress to the individual. Anxiety disorder assessments should assess for the main worry experienced; the level of anxiety or worry and whether it is excessive; the impact or interference with day-to-day functioning; and the causes of significant distress.

Important Elements in the Assessment of Anxiety Disorders

Discussion of Confidentiality

As with depression, confidentiality is an essential component in the assessment of young people with an anxiety disorder (see above).

Interviews and Collateral Information

Similar to the assessment of mood disorders, individual clinical interviews with the youth and separate interviews with parents/caregivers (whenever possible) to obtain collateral information are helpful in order to assess for anxiety symptoms and functional impairment. It is important to ascertain an understanding of the impact of, or the interference from, the anxiety symptoms.

Assessment of Illness Characteristics

The assessment of an anxiety disorder should also include the presence of:

- *Medical conditions or factors* that could contribute to the anxiety symptoms (e.g., thyroid disease, excessive caffeine intake). Presence of such factors need to be managed first with subsequent reassessment of the anxiety symptoms before making a diagnosis of an anxiety disorder.
- *External stressors* such as psychosocial stressors (e.g., family conflict); school stressors (e.g., learning or language difficulties); social stressors (e.g., bullying or teasing); other medical stressors (e.g., hearing or visual difficulties) that may contribute to increased stress or transient anxiety. It is essential to determine whether the anxiety presents first or whether it is secondary to a stressor. For example, adolescents with undiagnosed learning issues may experience excessive anxiety and worry about their marks and academic performance, which, given their learning issues, could be normative or expected. When the anxiety is secondary to stressors, anxiety management is not helpful until the primary cause is addressed. Similarly, if the anxiety is secondary to other stressors such as family conflict or bullying, these stressors must be addressed first, before anxiety management strategies can be effectively implemented.
- *Physical symptoms* associated with anxiety (stomachaches, headaches, shortness of breath, dizziness or lightheadedness, nausea and/or vomiting, diarrhea, tingling, numbness, tightness in chest, back, or neck, etc.)
- *Specific worries and thoughts* to help identify the type of anxiety disorder
- The *level of interference* and the persistence of the anxiety, in the context of developmentally normative worries

Consideration of Cultural Background

Clinicians should consider cultural context when diagnosing anxiety disorders. For example, clinicians should be mindful of the value some cultures may place on interdependence among family members; the different cultural views on the role of adolescents; the potentially normative role of parental co-sleeping in some cultures; or expectations that adolescents be quiet and less interactive with their elders or other adults in other cultures.

Assessment of Comorbidity

There is a high comorbidity among young people with anxiety disorders with about half (40% to 60%) of anxious youth meeting criteria for more than one anxiety disorder.[24]

- Comorbidity with other mental health disorders is also high and therefore clinicians should conduct a comprehensive evaluation for comorbid externalizing disorders (e.g., ADHD, oppositional defiant disorder [ODD]); mood disorders (e.g., MDD, dysthymia); and substance use disorders, all of which have implications for treatment.

Screening Tools for Anxiety Disorders

Self-report instruments may be quite helpful in assessing distress and the level of interference experienced by youth with anxiety disorders. These screening tools are generally well received by youth and are easy to administer; however, they are not diagnostic in and of themselves. Commonly used anxiety-specific measures, with demonstrated reliability and validity in the populations outlined below, include (but are not limited to) the following:

Beck Anxiety Inventory

The Beck Anxiety Inventory (BAI) is a 21-item self-report developed for adults that targets the severity of anxiety symptoms experienced during the previous week. Higher total scores indicate more severe anxiety symptoms. The BAI has good internal consistency and good 1-week test–retest reliability.[27] It is most useful in older AYAs.

Multidimensional Anxiety Screen for Children

The Multidimensional Anxiety Screen for Children Second Edition (MASC 2) is a 50-item self-report targeted for youth 8 to 19 years of age that uses a 3-point rating scale.

Screen for Child Anxiety-Related Emotional Disorders/Parent Version and Child Version

The Screen for Child Anxiety Related Disorders (SCARED) is a 41-item self-report instrument for parents/caregivers and youth (targets children and adolescent 8 to 18 years old). Using a three-point scale, the SCARED consists of five factors that screen for panic disorder, GAD, separation anxiety disorder, SAD, and school refusal. The parent and child SCARED demonstrate good internal consistency, good test–retest reliability, and discriminates among the various anxiety disorders and between anxiety disorders and mood disorders.[28]

● ANXIETY DISORDERS AND THE DIAGNOSTIC AND STATISTICAL MANUAL OF MENTAL DISORDERS, FIFTH EDITION

Anxiety disorders are classified by the main fear or worry expressed (Table 74.3).

Generalized Anxiety Disorder

Generalized anxiety disorder is characterized by excessive anxiety and worry (apprehensive expectation) about numerous things for more than 6 months. Youth with GAD can be conceptualized as *"worriers"* as they worry about "anything and everything." The intensity, duration, and frequency of the anxiety/worry are out of proportion to that expected. Controlling the worry is difficult and the worry thoughts interfere with psychosocial functioning. In addition to excessive worry, additional symptoms of restlessness,

easy fatigue, difficulty concentrating, irritability, muscle tension, and/or sleep disturbance are required for the diagnosis of GAD. Adult GAD requires the presence of three or more of these additional symptoms, whereas child and adolescent GAD requires the presence of only one of these additional symptoms.

- Typical worries of GAD include worries about academics (e.g., marks or grades), catastrophic events (e.g., earthquakes, storms, world events), the future, the past (e.g., things said or done). Adolescents with GAD worry more about their competence (e.g., marks), quality of their performance, and punctuality, whereas adults worry more about finances, and job performance. Worries tend to shift over the course of time.
- Normative worries of youth are distinguished from GAD by the level of intensity and frequency of the worries (e.g., those without GAD can put the worry aside, or are otherwise able to manage day-to-day functions despite their worries). The greater the number of worries, the more likely the diagnosis of GAD.
- Compared with normative anxiety, the majority of youth with GAD describe themselves as "being anxious all the time."
- Generalized anxiety disorder is a chronic disorder; although symptoms may wax and wane over time, while full remission is rare.
- Youth with GAD tend to be perfectionistic, overly conforming, and often need to redo things because of dissatisfaction with their performance. They often require excessive reassurance from parents/caregivers and other adults.

Specific Phobias

Specific phobias are characterized by a fear of a specific object, which is often referred to as the phobic stimulus. Several subcategories of specific phobias exist including animal, natural environment, blood–injection–injury, and situation phobias. Other phobias such as fear of vomiting or costumed characters are often subsumed under the subcategory of *other phobias.* Phobias typically develop in childhood with waxing and waning severity of symptoms; persistence of symptoms into young adulthood suggests low probability of remittance. Specific phobias are rarely seen in medical clinical settings in the absence of other psychopathology; however, clinicians should screen for their presence when completing a thorough anxiety assessment and developing a management plan.

Social Anxiety Disorder

Social anxiety disorder is characterized by excessive or intense fear or anxiety about social situations. The specific worry is about *being embarrassed or humiliated or being laughed at,* in front of others.

- In adolescents, the fear or worry must occur during interactions with same-aged peers and not only with adults.
- For a diagnosis of SAD, the social situation must always cause fear or anxiety, although the degree and level of worry or fear may vary from situation to situation. Anticipatory anxiety may begin weeks before the actual event. Youth with SAD will avoid the social situation they fear or endure it with intense fear or anxiety.
- Difficulties such as eating in front of others, having their picture taken, performing in front of others, completing oral presentations, speaking in public or having a conversation are common.
- Over time, individuals with SAD may become more socially withdrawn and isolated as they lose contact with peers and have difficulties forming new relationships. Development of depression and substance abuse disorders may be a sequelae of SAD.
- Clinician judgment is important to determine whether the anxiety, especially in adolescents, is out of proportion to the situation, given the normative preoccupation of adolescents with their peer groups and their often overestimation of the negative consequences of social situations.

TABLE 74.3

Overview of the Different Anxiety Disorders

Anxiety Disorder	Main Worry Thought
Generalized anxiety disorder	Excessive worry about a number of things for 6 mo or longer. Often referred to as "worrywarts." Additional symptoms must be present.
Panic disorder	Recurrent, unexpected attacks of anxiety— often "out of the blue"
Social anxiety disorder/ social phobia	Worry about being laughed at or embarrassed or doing something humiliating in front of others
Selective mutism	Excessive anxiety or inhibition about speaking to the point of mutism. Conceptualized as a variant of social anxiety
Specific phobias	Consuming fear of a specific object. A variety of subcategories exist.
Separation anxiety disorder	Worry that something 'bad' will happen to them or their parent or primary caregiver when not together

- The development of SAD tends to be bimodal with a first peak in preschoolers and a second peak typically developing in early adolescence. Although the disorder tends to emerge out of a history of shyness or social inhibition, it may follow a stressful or humiliating experience.

Selective Mutism

Selective mutism was added to the anxiety disorders in DSM-5 and is currently viewed as a developmental variant of SAD. There is high comorbidity (50% to 100%) with SAD.[26] Due to debilitating levels of anxiety, individuals with SM are unable to speak in social situations despite having normal language and communication skills. Most individuals with SM are able to speak comfortably in their own home; however, are unable to speak outside of the home with peers or adults—they may not even be able to speak to less familiar relatives.

- The lack of speech with teachers and peers causes impairments in academic achievement and social relationships.
- Typical age of onset of SM is prior to age 5; however, given its association with SAD, it is important for clinicians working with older youth to inquire about the possibility of a previous diagnosis or remaining symptoms of SM when assessing for SAD.
- Long-term consequences of SM are unknown. The assumption is that children outgrow the disorder overtime; however, the symptoms or full diagnosis of social anxiety may persist.

Panic Disorder with and without Agoraphobia

- *Panic disorder* is defined as the recurrence of panic attacks with at least one month or more of persistent concern or worry about having additional panic attacks or a significant maladaptive change in behavior related to the attacks.
- A *panic attack* is the occurrence of at least four physical and/or cognitive symptoms developing abruptly and reaching a peak within a few minutes. Panic attacks can occur in the context of any anxiety disorder or other mental health disorder and even some medical disorders. *Expected panic attacks* have an obvious cue or trigger, whereas *unexpected panic attacks* have no obvious cue or trigger and seem to occur for no reason or *"out of the blue."*
- The median age of onset of panic disorder is 20 to 24 years. Onset after age 45 years is unusual.
- A chronic course with waxing and waning of symptoms is typical. Comorbidity with other anxiety and mood disorders is common. Panic attacks and panic disorder are associated with higher rates of suicide attempts and suicidal ideations in the previous 12 months, even when other suicide risk factors are taken into account. Therefore, it is *critical to ask about suicidal ideations* in individuals presenting with panic disorder.
- *Agoraphobia* is characterized by marked fear or anxiety triggered by the risk of exposure to at least two of five situations, including using public transportation; being in open spaces; being in enclosed spaces; standing in line; being in a crowd; or being outside of the home.
- Individuals with agoraphobia usually avoid such situations although varying amounts of anxiety may be seen with different situations and proximity to the situation.
- Individuals with severe agoraphobia may become homebound.

Separation Anxiety Disorder

Separation anxiety disorder is typically seen as an anxiety disorder of childhood in which the child's primary fear or worry is that *"something bad will happen to themselves or their parents/primary caregivers"* when not together.

- Although the full diagnostic criteria are uncommon in older AYAs, features of the disorder may be present, or even develop de novo in this age group at times of stress—for example, when young adults leave the home to go to postsecondary school, enter into a romantic relationship, or become parents themselves.
- Some evidence suggests that children with separation anxiety disorder may develop panic disorder as adolescents or young adults. This highlights the importance of asking about previous separation anxiety disorder diagnoses and/or symptoms when completing a full anxiety assessment of youth, especially those presenting with panic symptoms.

TREATMENT

General Considerations
Ensure Safety

Ensuring safety is important in the management of anxiety disorders, especially given the high comorbidity between anxiety disorders and mood disorders and/or substance abuse disorders.

Psychoeducation

Psychoeducation about anxiety and anxiety disorders is the first step in the management of anxiety disorders. It is important for youth and their families to understand what an anxiety disorder is and the impact it has on day-to-day functioning prior to the development of any management plan. Parental modeling of anxiety and/or facilitation of avoidance of situations causing anxiety must be curtailed. Youth and their families need to understand the importance of facing fears and learning coping strategies to do so, in order to manage and treat the anxiety disorder.

Identify and Address Stressors and Psychiatric Comorbidity

Identification and treatment of other psychiatric comorbidities may take priority over the treatment of the anxiety disorder. For example, adolescents with untreated ADHD may benefit from management of the attentional difficulties before engaging in therapy for the anxiety. Similarly, youth with comorbid depression may require a safety assessment and management of the depressive symptoms before starting therapy for the anxiety symptoms. Youth and families must be informed about substances that can exacerbate anxiety and they must learn to avoid use of these substances.

Mild Anxiety Disorders

Youth with mild anxiety disorders may be functioning quite well. They may benefit from psychoeducation and psychotherapy such as CBT. Cognitive behavioral therapy has the strongest evidence base for the treatment of youth anxiety disorders.[24,29,30,31]

Moderate to Severe Anxiety Disorders

Youth with moderate to severe anxiety disorders may benefit from a referral to a specialist for assessment and management recommendations. In addition to psychotherapy, youth with moderate to severe anxiety disorders may benefit from the addition of medications such as SSRIs.

Psychotherapy
Cognitive Behavioral Therapy

Cognitive behavioral therapy focuses on identifying, challenging, and reframing anxious thoughts into more adaptive ones. Cognitive behavioral therapy is a focused, time-limited therapy that can be conducted in individual or group formats. Therapy is focused on the "here and now," clearly focusing on the specific problems being worked on. Each hour-long session (usually in a series of 8 to 15 sessions) is structured so that skills are built incrementally on skills learned in previous sessions.

Therapy begins with psychoeducation, followed by support for recognizing and understanding feeling states and cues or triggers for anxiety. Relaxation strategies such as muscle-tension relaxation, diaphragmatic breathing, and imagery are taught to target autonomic arousal and physiologic reactivity. Often an anxiety hierarchy or ladder of fears from least to most feared is created to allow for graduated, controlled exposure to these feared situations and stimuli, thereby helping to decrease and eliminate avoidant behaviors. Thought records are often used to help youth identify their automatic thoughts in various situations and learn to challenge these thoughts. Manualized treatments are available and used for youth. Strong evidence supports the use of CBT for youth.[24,29,30]

Exposure Therapy

Exposure therapy, also known as exposure-response–prevention (ERP) therapy, can be used as a stand-alone treatment, although it is often incorporated into a more general CBT approach. Exposure therapy involves learning to become less sensitive to a feared situation or phobic stimulus by gradually exposing the affected person to the stimulus over time.

Acceptance and Mindfulness-Based Therapies

Acceptance and commitment therapy focuses on teaching skills to accept unwanted thoughts, feelings, and sensations; place them in a different context; develop greater clarity about personal values; and commit to needed behavior change. In contrast to changing thoughts, mindfulness-based therapies encourage living in the moment and experiencing things without judgment, thereby seeking to change the relationship between the anxious person and his or her thoughts.

Other Psychotherapies

Increasingly, other therapies, including yoga and various forms of mindfulness and relaxation therapies, are being developed and used to treat anxiety disorders although there is limited evidence-base for their use. Various nonspecific psychotherapies may treat anxiety disorders in youth, such as family-based therapy for families who have high-tension or high-conflict relationships; behavioral and parent/caregiver-management therapies to treat comorbid ODD or ADHD; and trauma-focused CBT for trauma-based anxiety. Supportive and psychodynamic psychotherapies may be beneficial for some cases of anxiety.

Medication

Selective Serotonin Reuptake Inhibitors

The mainstay of medication management for anxiety disorders is the use of SSRIs, which can effectively alleviate anxiety in youth. The Child/Adolescent Anxiety Multimodal Study,[31] a large multisite, RCT, demonstrates that the most effective treatment for moderate to severe anxiety is the combination of medication (SSRIs) and CBT.

Guidelines for the use and monitoring of SSRIs for anxiety disorders are similar to those for depressive disorders (see above for more details regarding adverse effects and suicide risk). The side effects profile and dosing for anxiety are similar to those for depressive disorders, although slow titration is critical in the treatment of anxiety disorders as lower doses are often quite effective in the management of youth anxiety disorders. The goal of treatment is to achieve remission of anxiety symptoms. Once an effective dose of the medication is reached, symptoms should be reassessed at 4-week intervals to evaluate the effectiveness and tolerability of the current dosage, and to determine whether increased doses are necessary. Once complete response is achieved, medication should be continued for a minimum of 6 to 12 months to decrease the risk of relapse. Discontinuing an SSRI should consist of a slow tapering of medication and, as with depression, should occur during a relatively stress-free time (e.g., the summer months).

Benzodiazepines

Benzodiazepines have been used as an acute, short-term treatment for a variety of anxiety disorders primarily in adults. Although benzodiazepines can be helpful in the short-term management of severe cases of anxiety disorders (e.g., in the time frame before an SSRI becomes effective or in the initial stages of CBT), they have concerning side effects, including addiction and misuse. Some individuals experience withdrawal symptoms, especially if the benzodiazepines are not tapered slowly. In addition, discontinuation of the benzodiazepines may cause return of the anxiety symptoms. Side effects include sedation and cognitive impairment; as well as, behavioral disinhibition and, rarely, agitation. As a result, benzodiazepines should only be used for short-term, acute management of anxiety disorders, and only with an awareness and understanding of the potential adverse effects of these medications.

SUMMARY

Depression and anxiety are serious, common mental health disorders of adolescence and young adulthood. It is critical that clinicians working with these individuals screen for these conditions. Comorbidity between mood disorders and anxiety is common; clinicians should assess youth for the presence of both conditions. Treatment approaches should include ensuring safety, providing psychoeducation about the disorder, and considering psychotherapy and pharmacotherapy management that is appropriate for the individual patient and family.

REFERENCES

1. Kessler RC, Berglund P, Demler O, et al. Lifetime prevalence and age-of-onset distributions of DSM-IV disorders in the National Comorbidity Survey Replication. *Arch Gen Psychiatry.* 2005;62(6):593–602. doi:10.1001/archpsyc.62.6.593
2. Racine N, McArthur BA, Cooke JE, et al. Global prevalence of depressive and anxiety symptoms in children and adolescents during COVID-19: a meta-analysis. *JAMA Pediatr.* 2021;175(11):1142–1150.
3. Korczak DJ, Goldstein BI. Childhood onset major depressive disorder: course of illness and psychiatric comorbidity in a community sample. *J Pediatr.* 2009; 155(1):118–123.
4. Wray NR, Gottesman II. Using summary data from the danish national registers to estimate heritabilities for schizophrenia, bipolar disorder, and major depressive disorder. *Front Genet.* 2012;3:118. doi:10.3389/fgene.2012.00118
5. Lieb R, Isensee B, Hofler M, et al. Parental major depression and the risk of depression and other mental disorders in offspring: a prospective-longitudinal community study. *Arch Gen Psychiatry.* 2002;59:365–374.
6. Korczak DJ, Beiser M. Depression. In: Barozzino T, Hui C, eds. *Caring for Kids new to Canada.* Canadian Paediatric Society; 2013.
7. American Psychiatric Association. *Diagnostic and Statistical Manual of Mental Disorders.* 5th ed. American Psychiatric Publishing; 2013.
8. Goodyer IM, Dubicka B, Wilkinson P, et al. A randomised controlled trial of cognitive behaviour therapy in adolescents with major depression treated by selective serotonin reuptake inhibitors. The ADAPT trial. *Health Technol Assess.* 2008;12(14):iii–iv, ix-60.
9. Korczak DJ. Use of selective serotonin reuptake inhibitor medications for the treatment of child and adolescent mental illness: Position Statement of the Canadian Pediatric Society. *Paediatr Child Health* 2013;18(9):487–491.
10. Emslie G, Kratochvil C, Vitiello B, et al. Treatment for Adolescents with Depression Study (TADS): safety results. *J Am Acad Child Adolesc Psychiatry.* 2006;45(12):1440–1455. doi:10.1097/01.chi.0000240840.63737.1d
11. Bridge JA, Iyengar S, Salary CB, et al. Clinical response and risk for reported suicidal ideation and suicide attempts in pediatric antidepressant treatment: a meta-analysis of randomized controlled trials. *JAMA.* 2007;297(15):1683–1696. doi:10.1001/jama.297.15.1683
12. Cheung AH, Emslie GJ, Mayes TL. Review of the efficacy and safety of antidepressants in youth depression. *J Child Psychol Psychiatry.* 2005;46:735–754. doi:10.1111/j.1469-7610.2005.01467.x
13. March J, Silva S, Petrycki S, et al. Fluoxetine, cognitive-behavioral therapy, and their combination for adolescents with depression: Treatment for Adolescents With Depression Study (TADS) randomized controlled trial. *JAMA.* 2004;292:807–820. doi:10.1001/jama.292.7.807
14. Emslie GJ, Ventura D, Korotzer A, et al. Escitalopram in the treatment of adolescent depression: a randomized placebo-controlled multisite trial. *J Am Acad Child Adolesc Psychiatry.* 2009;48:721–729. doi:10.1097/CHI.0b013e3181a2b304
15. Wagner KD, Jonas J, Findling RL, et al. A double-blind, randomized, placebo-controlled trial of escitalopram in the treatment of pediatric depression. *J Am Acad Child Adolesc Psychiatry.* 2006;45:280–288. doi:10.1097/01. chi.0000192250.38400.9e
16. Wagner KD, Robb AS, Findling RL, et al. A randomized, placebo-controlled trial of citalopram for the treatment of major depression in children and adolescents. *Am J Psychiatry.* 2004;161:1079–1083.
17. Wagner KD, Ambrosini P, Rynn M, et al. Efficacy of sertraline in the treatment of children and adolescents with major depressive disorder: two randomized controlled trials. *JAMA.* 2003;290:1033–1041. doi:10.1001/jama.290.8.1033
18. Von Knorring A-L, Olsson GI, Thomsen PH, et al. A randomized, double-blind, placebo-controlled study of citalopram in adolescents with major depressive disorder. *J Clin Psychopharmacol.* 2006;26:311–315. doi:10.1097/01.jcp.0000219051. 40632.d5

XV

19. Lam RW, Kennedy SH, Grigoriadis S, et al. Canadian Network for Mood and Anxiety Treatments (CANMAT) clinical guidelines for the management of major depressive disorder in adults. III. Pharmacotherapy. *J Affect Disord.* 2009;117 (suppl 1):S26–S43. doi:10.1016/j.jad.2009.06.041

20. Birmaher B, Brent D; AACAP Work Group on Quality Issues, et al. Practice parameter for the assessment and treatment of children and adolescents with depressive disorders. *J Am Acad Child Adolesc Psychiatry.* 2007;46:1503–1526. doi:10.1097/chi.0b013e318145ae1c

21. Food and Drug Administration website. Accessed February 7, 2021. http://www.fda.gov

22. Health Canada Antidepressant Cipralex (escitalopram): updated information regarding dose-related heart risk. 2012. http://www.healthycanadians.gc.ca/recall-alert-rappel-avis/hc-sc/2012/13674a-eng.php

23. Sakolsky D, Birmaher B. Developmentally informed pharmacotherapy for child and adolescent depressive disorders. *Child Adolesc Psychiatr Clin N Am.* 2012;21:313–325, viii.

24. Walter HJ, Bukstein OG, Abright AR, et al. Clinical practice guideline for the assessment and treatment of children and adolescents with anxiety disorders. *J Am Acad Child Adolesc Psychiatry.* 2020;59(10):1107-1124.

25. Copeland WE, Angold A, Shanahan L, et al. Longitudinal patterns of anxiety from childhood to adulthood: the Great Smoky Mountains Study. *J Am Acad Child Adolesc Psychiatry.* 2014;53(1):21–33.

26. Monga S, Benoit D. *Assessing and Treating Anxiety Disorders in Young Children:* The Taming Sneaky Fears Program. Springer Nature; 2018.

27. Leyfer OT, Ruberg JL, Woodruff-Borden J. Examination of the utility of the Beck Anxiety Inventory and its factors as a screener for anxiety disorders. *J Anxiety Disord.* 2006;20(4):448–458.

28. University of Pittsburgh. *Screen for Child Anxiety Related Emotional Disorders (SCARED).* Accessed February 1, 2021. Available at https://www.pediatricbipolar.pitt.edu

29. Compton SN, March JS, Brent D, et al. Cognitive-behavioral psychotherapy for anxiety and depressive disorders in children and adolescents: an evidence-based medicine review. *J Am Acad Child Adolesc Psychiatry.* 2004;43(8):930–959.

30. Wang Z, Whiteside SPH, Sim L, et al. Comparative effectiveness and safety of cognitive behavioral therapy and pharmacotherapy for childhood anxiety disorders: a systematic review and meta-analysis. *JAMA Pediatr.* 2017;171(11):1049–1056.

31. Compton SN, Walkup JT, Albano AM, et al. Child/Adolescent Anxiety Multimodal Study (CAMS): rationale, design, and methods. *Child Adolesc Psychiatry Ment Health.* 2010;4:1.

ADDITIONAL RESOURCES AND WEBSITES

Additional Resources and Websites for Clinicians:

AACAP Clinical Practice Guideline for the Assessment and Treatment of Children and Adolescents With Anxiety Disorders—https://www.jaacap.org/action/showPdf?pii=S0890-8567%2820%2930280-X

American Academy of Child and Adolescent Psychiatry (AACAP)—www.aacap.org/AACAP/Resources_for_Primary_Care/Home.aspx

Anxiety and Depression Association of America—www.adaa.org

British Columbia guidelines for diagnosis and treatment of depression and anxiety disorders in children and youth—https://www2.gov.bc.ca/gov/content/health/practitioner-professional-resources/bc-guidelines/anxiety-and-depression-in-youth

NICE guidelines for depression identification and management—https://www.nice.org.uk/guidance/ng134

Additional Resources and Websites for Parents/Caregivers:

AACAP's Anxiety and Children—https://www.aacap.org/AACAP/Families_and_Youth/Facts_for_Families/FFF-Guide/The-Anxious-Child-047.aspx

AboutKidsHealth—www.aboutkidshealth.ca/mentalhealth

American Academy of Child and Adolescent Psychiatry—https://www.aacap.org/AACAP/Families_and_Youth/Facts_for_Families/FFF-Guide/The-Depressed-Child-004.aspx

Anxiety Canada—www.anxietycanada.com

HealthLinkBC—https://www.healthlinkbc.ca/health-topics/ty4640

Child Mind Institute—www.childmind.org

Society for Adolescent Health and Medicine—https://www.adolescenthealth.org/Resources/Clinical-Care-Resources/Mental-Health/Mental-Health-Resources-For-Parents-of-Adolescents.aspx

Additional Resources and Websites for Adolescents and Young Adults:

AboutKidsHealth—www.aboutkidshealth.ca/mentalhealth

Kids Help Phone—https://kidshelpphone.ca/topic/emotional-well-being/depression-sadness/

National Institute of Mental Health—https://www.nimh.nih.gov/health/publications/teen-depression/

CHAPTER 75

Suicide and Suicidal Behaviors in Adolescents and Young Adults

Lisa M. Horowitz
Annabelle M. Mournet
Maryland Pao

KEY WORDS

- Lethal means safety counseling
- Nonsuicidal self-injury
- Protective factors
- Risk factors
- Safety planning
- Suicide assessment
- Suicide attempt
- Suicide risk screening
- Warning signs

INTRODUCTION

Suicide is the second leading cause of death among adolescents and young adults (AYAs).[1] Moreover, the suicide rate among youth aged 10 to 24 years continues to rise, with the rate of suicide for this age cohort increasing by 56% between 2007 and 2017.[2] This chapter provides standard definitions for types of suicidality, an overview of the most recent suicide epidemiology, information on psychological and medical comorbidities of suicide, racial, and gender disparities in suicide, and guidelines and recommendations on suicide risk prevention, screening, assessment, and intervention.

DEFINITIONS

The definitions below are derived from the consensus of widely accepted sources[3,4]:

- *Suicide* is a fatal self-inflicted injury with stated or inferable intent to die.
- *Suicide attempt* refers to a nonfatal self-inflicted injury with stated or inferable intent to die.
- *Interrupted suicide attempt* refers to a suicide attempt wherein the person is engaging in preparatory behavior of a suicide attempt and another individual intervenes prior to the occurrence of the injury.
- *Aborted suicide attempt* refers to a suicide attempt wherein the person begins to make a suicide attempt but stops themselves prior to experiencing injury.
- *Suicidal ideation* is thoughts about one's own death. Ideation ranges from "passive ideation," which refers to thinking about one's death without any plan, to "active ideation" where an individual has an explicit plan and active intent to act on their suicidal thoughts. Regardless of level of intent and plan to act on suicidal thoughts, any level of suicidality is a significant marker of emotional distress, especially in youth.
- *Nonsuicidal self-injury* (NSSI) is purposeful or deliberate, and often repetitive self-injury with a motivation other than death, such as relief from emotional pain, self-punishment, or to gain attention.

It is important to note that phrases such as "committing suicide" or "successful suicide" are no longer considered appropriate terms. Such phrases are discouraged as they carry blaming connotations and mislabel suicidal behavior as something that may be successfully accomplished. Instead phrases such as "died by suicide" or "completed suicide" are more acceptable.[3,4]

EPIDEMIOLOGY

Suicide

Suicide is the second leading cause of death among AYAs (Fig. 75.1).[1] There is a myth that younger children do not engage in suicidal thoughts and behaviors; however, children under the age of 12 years think about, attempt, and die by suicide.[1,5] The rate of suicide increases incrementally with each year of increasing age from 10 to 24 years.[1] In 2019, among youth in the United States aged 10 to 14 years, 15 to 19 years, and 20 to 24 years, the suicide rate per 100,000 was 2.57, 10.50, and 17.31, respectively.[1] Overall deaths for youth aged 10 to 24 years decreased in 2018 from 2017, however, the percentage that died by suicide increased; 27% of all youth deaths in the United States are from suicide.[1]

Rates of suicide also vary by gender and race/ethnicity. The suicide rate among males aged 10 to 24 years (16.48 per 100,000) is nearly four times that of females aged 10 to 24 years (4.57 per 100,000).[1] Males are two to four times more likely than females to die by suicide whereas females are twice as likely as males to make a nonfatal suicide attempt.[6] Significant racial disparities in suicide rates among youth have also been detected. Bridge and colleagues[7] found that Black children under the age of 12 years die by suicide at higher rates than White children; this trend reverses at age 13 years, where White teenagers die by suicide at higher rates, though limited data has explained this racial disparity in the suicide rate. Recent trends show that suicide rates among Black youth are increasing faster than any other race/ethnic group.[1] "Ring the Alarm," a report from the Congressional Black Caucus, shows that there is limited funding toward research that is investigating or seeking to address these disturbing rates.[8] Indigenous populations, such as young American Indians/Alaska Natives (AI/AN) are also at increased risk of suicide, as evidenced by one-third of all deaths among AI/AN youth being attributable to suicide.[1]

Suicidal Ideation and Behaviors

Suicidal behaviors and suicide ideation are even more prevalent than deaths by suicide. According to the most recent Youth Risk Behavior Survey,[9] 8.9% of high school students attempted suicide one or more times in the past year. Moreover, 18.8% of high

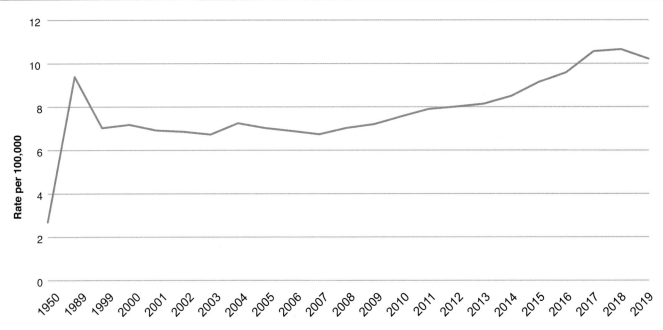

FIGURE 75.1 Suicide death rate among U.S. youth aged 10 to 24 years.

school students reported having seriously considered attempting suicide in the previous year.[9] Since these are "self-reports" of youth in schools, we assume they are underestimates. In addition to the demographic risk factors for suicide discussed above, there are considerable disparities in the rates of suicidal ideation and behaviors among sexual and gender minority youth. Among lesbian, gay, or bisexual (LGB) identified students, 46.8% reported seriously considering suicide and 23.4% of LGB students reported having attempted suicide.[10] Suicide attempt rates among transgender youth are also considerably elevated, with 50.8% of transgender men in a large sample of gender minority youth reporting a previous suicide attempt.[11]

RISK FACTORS, WARNING SIGNS AND PROTECTIVE FACTORS

Risk Factors

There are a number of psychosocial risk factors that may increase an individual's risk of suicide.
- Past suicidal ideation and behavior—the most potent risk factor for future suicidal behavior is previous suicidal thoughts and behaviors.[9]
- Nonsuicidal self-injury—while one's motivating reason for engagement in NSSI is often different than one's reason for engaging in suicidal thoughts and behaviors, NSSI remains a strong predictor for future suicide attempts.[12]
- Mental illness, especially major depressive disorder—depression and suicidal thoughts and behaviors are often co-occurring, with suicidal ideation representing a common symptom of depression. Although depression and suicide often co-occur, they are not synonymous, as evidenced by depression screening being insufficient for identifying suicide risk.[13]
- Adverse childhood experiences (ACEs)—ACEs, such as being in the child welfare system, incarceration, abuse, neglect, parental death, and a family history of suicidality, significantly increase an individual's risk of suicide.[14,15]
- Health risk behaviors—suicidal behaviors are associated with numerous other health risk behaviors, including behaviors that involve access to lethal means (e.g., weapon carrying).[16]

- Military experiences—young adults with military experience may be at increased risk for suicide as the suicide rate among individuals in the U.S. military has increased steadily in recent years and has exceeded the suicide rate of the general population.[17]
- Other psychological characteristics and behaviors—including substance use, disordered eating, sleep disturbance, hopelessness, anxiety, and/or impulsivity.
- Medical comorbidity also represents a significant, but often overlooked, risk factor for suicide. Medically ill youth with asthma, epilepsy, chronic pain, and other conditions are at increased risk for suicide.[18] Moreover, a majority of youth who attempt and die by suicide visited a clinician in the months, and even weeks, leading up to their suicide attempt or death by suicide.[19] This poses a critical opportunity for clinicians to identify and intervene with youth at risk for suicide in the medical setting.

Warning Signs

Most people who have risk factors for suicide will not die by suicide, because risk factors are broad and overinclusive of people at risk. However, what is more important to attend to are warning signs that someone may be at imminent risk for suicide. Talking about "wanting to die" or "not wanting to live anymore," seems like an obvious warning sign, but suicidal talk, especially among young people, is often overlooked and sometimes even dismissed. Yet, many who die by suicide have reported these feelings to an adult before they died. All talk of suicide should be taken seriously and followed up with conversations and professional help if needed. Suicide warning signs fall into the categories of behaviors, mood, and things someone talks about.
- Behaviors: Sleeping too much or too little, aggression, withdrawing from activities, acting recklessly, increased use of alcohol or drugs, isolating from family and friends, looking for a way to kill themselves (online for materials or means), giving away prized possessions, visiting or calling people to say goodbye.
- Mood: Depression, anxiety, rage, humiliation, irritability, loss of interest or pleasure
- Things someone talks about: Killing themselves, being a burden to others, having no reason to live, feeling trapped, experiencing unbearable pain.

Protective Factors

While identifying warning signs and risk factors as important ways to detect suicide risk and intervene, fostering suicide protective factors, such as social connectedness and resilience among AYAs at risk for suicide is also of considerable importance.

Social connectedness is a key suicide protective factor. Connectedness to family, school, peers, and community lower suicidal ideation and suicide attempt rates.[20] Moreover, religion has been shown to be a protective factor against suicide, in part by providing access to a community.[21]

Clinicians can have an important role in helping AYAs and their families foster resilience by promoting the development of independence, social competence, problem-solving skills, adaptability, and other factors that lead to resilience.

SCREENING

There is a misconception that asking patients about suicide will put the thought in someone's head, however, this myth has been refuted.[22] In order to improve detection of patients who are at risk for suicide, several tools have been developed to aid clinicians in screening effectively and to make difficult conversations easier. The Ask Suicide-Screening Questions (ASQ; Fig. 75.2)[23] tool is an example of an effective validated suicide risk screening tool for youth aged 8 years and above. The ASQ is brief, evidence based, and easy to use such that it can be administered by nonmental clinicians. There is also an ASQ Toolkit (www.nimh.nih.gov/ASQ) that can be used by clinicians who want to implement suicide risk screening.

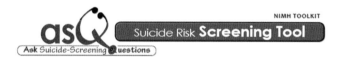

FIGURE 75.2 The Ask Suicide-Screening Questions (ASQ).

ASSESSMENT

When a patient screens positive for suicide risk, it is essential to follow-up with further assessment. Youth suicide risk screening clinical pathways were developed to provide clinicians with step-by-step implementation instructions.[24] The pathways begin with administering the ASQ as a brief screen, followed by the administration of a brief suicide safety assessment (BSSA) using the Columbia-Suicide Severity Rating Scale (C-SSRS)[25] or the ASQ Brief Suicide Safety Assessment (ASQ BSSA).[26] The BSSA is a critical step intended to further assess suicidal thoughts and behaviors, other mental health symptoms, and protective factors in order to determine the patient's disposition and effectively manage their risk. If necessary, a full mental health evaluation is administered following the BSSA. The pathways are meant to be individualized and adapted to meet the needs of each institution's culture, and if implemented thoughtfully, can make screening more feasible and spare unnecessary utilization of limited mental health resources.

The assessment should include, at a minimum, documentation of the following[26]:

Suicidal ideation and behavior
- Frequency and acuity of current and past suicidal ideation
- Presence of a suicide plan, including level of intent, planned methods, and access to means
- Past suicidal behavior; ask "How? When? Why?" and assess level of intent and level of lethality of attempt

Risk factors
- Depression
- Anxiety
- Impulsivity/recklessness
- Hopelessness
- Anhedonia
- Isolation
- Irritability
- Substance use and alcohol use
- Sleep pattern
- Appetite
- Medical illness

Social support and other stressors
- Connection with trusted adults (e.g., parent/caregiver, teacher), friends, and school
- Reasons for living
- Cultural or religious beliefs
- Pressure at school
- Peer victimization/bullying.
- Parent/caregiver discord
- Parent/caregiver mental health (depression, substance use, history of suicidality)
- Abuse, neglect, or exposure to domestic violence
- Access to lethal means

TREATMENTS AND INTERVENTIONS

There are several evidence-based treatments, including psychopharmacologic treatments, available for AYAs at risk for suicide. The treatment for adolescents depression study (TADS)[27] initially provided evidence for the tolerability and efficacy of combining fluoxetine and cognitive behavioral therapy (CBT) to treat adolescent depression. However, the evidence for the use of selective serotonin reuptake inhibitors in adolescents for depression is primarily limited to fluoxetine.[28] In 2004, the U.S. Food and Drug Administration issued a "black-box" warning for antidepressants in children and adolescents due to the concern of increased suicidality. Meta-analyses of antidepressant clinical trials demonstrated a slight increase in suicidality in those receiving antidepressants versus those treated with a placebo leading to the warning being extended in 2007 for young adults aged 25 years

XV

and under.[29] In a recent review, no specific antidepressant agent could be identified as specifically responsible for the increased suicidality incidence.[28] The relationship between antidepressants and suicidality remains controversial and physicians are encouraged to monitor closely for suicidal ideation and behavior when starting antidepressants.

Psychotherapy treatments include CBT, which was shown to reduce suicide reattempts by 50% over an 18-month period compared to treatment as usual.[30] Similarly, dialectical behavior therapy reduced suicide attempts by 50% over 24 months, compared to community treatment.[31]

Clinicians have a renewed interest in collaborative care models of integrated mental health. Models of care include (1) integration of general practitioners and mental health specialists working at separate facilities with separate clinical systems; (2) co-located care within a practice which fosters better communication; and (3) fully integrated medical and behavioral health systems with a team-based approach and shared treatment planning. Telehealth is also an emerging method of managing mental health problems, its feasibility reinforced as a result of the severe acute respiratory syndrome coronavirus 2 (SARS-CoV-2) pandemic.

CLINICAL APPROACH

Development of a Treatment Plan

When a patient is found to be at risk for suicide, the clinician must consider the level of acuity, as this will inform how to proceed with next steps safely. For patients who are found to be experiencing a suicidal crisis, a chain analysis, or a detailed moment-by-moment analysis, can be initiated to review the events, thoughts, behaviors, and other factors that led to the patient's suicidal state. Through a chain analysis, inflection points for de-escalation can be identified to establish a list of possible strategies and interventions. The clinician can collaborate with the patient and a trusted support person to develop coping strategies and safety plans for managing intense suicidal states.

Safety Planning and Lethal Means Safety Counseling

With the guidance of their clinician, all patients that are identified as "at risk for suicide" should create a safety plan to help when they are having thoughts of suicide. This plan should review how to safely store or remove lethal means from the home. Safety planning includes developing coping strategies for times of crisis; recognizing one's own warning signs and triggers; identifying family members, peers, or professionals who can be contacted for help; and providing geographically specific contact information for crisis and prevention online services. Examples in the United States include the National Suicide Lifeline (1-800-273-8255) and the Crisis Text Line (text "start" to 741741).[32] In assessing for suicide risk, clinicians have a unique opportunity to help youth struggling with emotional distress by highlighting their strengths and fostering resilience. Conversations about lethal means in the home and how to remove or safely store them during times of suicidal crises are critical and should ideally be done in collaboration with the patient's parent/caregiver or other people they live with.

Case Example

An 18-year-old female without apparent risk factors for suicide presented with a parent to an outpatient pediatric primary care practice with fatigue and malaise. At the time, the practice was only screening for suicide risk during well visits, however, the patient's nurse had a "bad feeling" that something was "not right" with this patient and screened them for suicide risk. Of note, this was a young female who was doing well in school, popular among her peers, and involved in many extracurricular activities. When screened with the ASQ, the patient endorsed three of the four items

which included: passive and current thoughts of suicide. Following the practice's suicide risk screening system, the patient's physican conducted a BSSA. He found that the young female was recently in trouble for underage drinking and therefore in jeopardy of losing her college scholarship. The physician spoke with the patient, developed a safety plan, engaged in lethal means safety counseling with the patient and her parent to ensure that she would be safe at home, and provided the patient with a mental health referral. The patient reported feeling more "hopeful" upon leaving the office after having spoken about her suicidal thoughts, which she had reported to no one until this nurse screened her. The lesson learned from this case is that while this nurse most likely saved this teenager's life, the nurse relied on intuition. Making suicide risk screening more systematic and universal would obviate reliance on individual clinicians' feelings and guesses and afford young people struggling with suicidal thoughts the opportunity to be recognized in settings that can bridge them to mental health care.

SUMMARY

Adolescent and young adult suicide and suicidal behavior is a major public health problem, affecting millions of young people and their families. Clinicians in medical settings and venues that serve youth, such as schools and college counseling centers, are well positioned to identify AYAs at increased risk for suicide. Using standardized and validated screening and assessment tools, clinicians can detect suicide risk that may otherwise go unnoticed and link patients to evidence-based treatments and interventions. Every adult that comes in contact with youth in schools, college campuses, and medical settings can start the difficult conversation that could save a young person's life.

ACKNOWLEDGMENTS

This work was supported in part by the Intramural Research Program of the NIMH (Annual Report Number ZIAMH002922).

REFERENCES

1. Centers for Disease Control and Prevention. *Web-Based Injury Statistics Query and Reporting System*. National Center for Injury Prevention and Control, CDC; 2018. Accessed December 1, 2020. https://www.cdc.gov/injury/wisqars/index.html
2. Curtin SC, Heron M. Death rates due to suicide and homicide among persons aged 10–24: United States, 2000–2017. *NCHS Data Brief*. 2019;(352):1–8.
3. Silverman MM, Berman AL, Sanddal ND, et al. Rebuilding the Tower of Babel: a revised nomenclature for the study of suicide and suicidal behaviors. Part 2: suicide-related ideations, communications, and behaviors. *Suicide Life Threat Behav*. 2007;37(3):264–277.
4. Nock MK, Borges G, Bromet EJ, et al. Suicide and suicidal behavior. *Epidemiol Rev*. 2008;30(1):133–154. doi:10.1093/epirev/mxn002
5. Burstein B, Agostino H, Greenfield B. Suicidal attempts and ideation among children and adolescents in U.S. emergency departments, 2007–2015. *JAMA Pediatr*. 2019;173(6):598–600.
6. Schrijvers DL, Bollen J, Sabbe BGC. The gender paradox in suicidal behavior and its impact on the suicidal process. *J Affect Disord*. 2012;138(1-2):19–26.
7. Bridge JA, Horowitz LM, Fontanella CA, et al. Age-related racial disparity in suicide rates among U.S. youths from 2001 through 2015. *JAMA Pediatr*. 2018;172(7):697–699.
8. Congressional Black Caucus Emergency Taskforce on Black Youth Suicide and Mental Health. Ring the alarm: the crisis of black youth suicide in America. In: Congressional Black Caucus, ed2019.
9. Cha CB, Franz PJ, ME Guzmán, et al. Annual research review: suicide among youth—epidemiology, (potential) etiology, and treatment. *J Child Psychol Psychiatry*. 2018;59(4):460–482. doi: 10.1111/jcpp.12831
10. Ivey-Stephenson AZ, Demissie Z, Crosby AE, et al. Suicidal ideation and behaviors among high school students—Youth Risk Behavior Survey, United States, 2019. *MMWR Suppl*. 2020;69(1):47–55.
11. Toomey RB, Syvertsen AK, Shramko M. Transgender adolescent suicide behavior. *Pediatrics*. 2018;142(4):e20174218. doi:10.1542/peds.2017-4218
12. Nock MK. Why do people hurt themselves? New insights into the nature and functions of self-injury. *Curr Dir Psychol Sci*. 2009;18(2):78–83. doi:10.1111/j.1467-8721.2009.01613.x
13. Horowitz LM, Mournet AM, Wharff EA, et al. Screening pediatric medical patients for suicide risk· is depression screening enough? *J Adolesc Health*. 2021;68(6):1183–1188. doi:10.1016/j.jadohealth.2021.01.028
14. Thompson MP, Kingree JB, Lamis D. Associations of adverse childhood experiences and suicidal behaviors in adulthood in a U.S. nationally representative sample. *Child Care Health Dev*. 2019;45(1):121–128. doi: 10.1111/cch.12617

15. Ruch DA, Steelesmith DL, Warner LA, et al. Health services use by children in the welfare system who died by suicide. *Pediatrics.* 2021;147(4):e2020011585. doi:10.1542/peds.2020-011585
16. Bridge JA, Goldstein TR, Brent DA. Adolescent suicide and suicidal behavior. *J Child Psychol Psychiatry.* 2006;47(3-4):372–394. doi:10.1111/j.1469-7610.2006.01615.x
17. Nock MK, Deming CA, Fullerton CS, et al. Suicide among soldiers: a review of psychosocial risk and protective factors. *Psychiatry.* 2013;76(2):97–125. doi:10.1521/psyc.2013.76.2.97
18. Rodway C, Tham SG, Ibrahim S, et al. Suicide in children and young people in England: a consecutive case series. *Lancet Psychiatry.* 2016;3(8):751–759. doi:10.1016/s2215-0366(16)30094-3
19. Ahmedani BK, Simon GE, Stewart C, et al. Health care contacts in the year before suicide death. *J Gen Intern Med.* 2014;29(6):870–877. doi:10.1007/s11606-014-2767-3
20. Foster CE, Horwitz A, Thomas A, et al. Connectedness to family, school, peers, and community in socially vulnerable adolescents. *Child Youth Serv Rev.* 2017;81:321–331. doi:10.1016/j.childyouth.2017.08.011
21. Lawrence RE, Oquendo MA, Stanley B. Religion and suicide risk: a systematic review. *Arch Suicide Res.* 2016;20(1):1–21. doi:10.1080/13811118.2015.1004494
22. DeCou CR, Schumann ME. On the iatrogenic risk of assessing suicidality: a meta-analysis. *Suicide Life Threat Behav.* 2018;48(5):531–543. doi: 10.1111/sltb.12368
23. Horowitz LM, Bridge JA, Teach SJ, et al. Ask suicide-screening questions (ASQ): a brief instrument for the pediatric emergency department. *Arch Pediatr Adolesc Med.* 2012;166(12): 1170–1176. doi:10.1001/archpediatrics.2012.1276
24. Brahmbhatt K, Kurtz BP, Afzal KI, et al; PaCC Workgroup. Suicide risk screening in pediatric hospitals: clinical pathways to address a global health crisis. *Psychosomatics.* 2019;60(1):1–9.
25. Posner K, Brown GK, Stanley B, et al. The Columbia–Suicide Severity Rating Scale: initial validity and internal consistency findings from three multisite studies with adolescents and adults. *Am J Psychiatry.* 2011;168(12):1266–1277.
26. National Institute of Mental Health. *Ask Suicide-Screening Questions (ASQ) Toolkit.* Accessed December 1, 2020. https:www.nimh.nih.gov/ASQ
27. March JS, Silva S, Petrycki S, et al. The Treatment for Adolescents with Depression Study (TADS): long-term effectiveness and safety outcomes. *Arch Gen Psychiatry.* 2007;64(10):1132–1143.
28. Vitiello B, Ordóñez AE. Pharmacological treatment of children and adolescents with depression. *Expert Opin Pharmacother.* 2016;17(17):2273–2279.
29. Morrison J, Schwartz TL. Adolescent angst or true intent? Suicidal behavior, risk, and neurobiological mechanisms in depressed children and teenagers taking antidepressants. *Int J Emerg Ment Health.* 2014;16(1):247–250.
30. Brown GK, Have TT, Henriques GR, et al. Cognitive therapy for the prevention of suicide attempts: a randomized controlled trial. *JAMA.* 2005;294(5):563–570.
31. Linehan MM, Comtois KA, Murray AM, et al. Two-year randomized controlled trial and follow-up of dialectical behavior therapy vs therapy by experts for suicidal behaviors and borderline personality disorder. *Arch Gen Psychiatry.* 2006;63(7):757–766.
32. Stanley B, Brown GK. Safety planning intervention: a brief intervention to mitigate suicide risk. *Cogn Behav Pract.* 2012;19(2):256–264.

ADDITIONAL RESOURCES AND WEBSITES

Additional Resources and Websites for Health Professionals:
American Academy of Child and Adolescent Psychiatry (AACAP) Suicide Resource Center—https://www.aacap.org/AACAP/Families_and_Youth/Resource_Centers/Suicide_Resource_Center/Home.aspx
American Academy of Pediatrics (AAP) Suicide Prevention—https://www.aap.org/en-us/advocacy-and-policy/aap-health-initiatives/child_death_review/Pages/Suicide-Prevention.aspx
American Academy of Pediatrics (AAP) Blueprint for Youth Suicide Prevention—https://www.aap.org/suicideprevention
American Foundation for Suicide Prevention (AFSP) Suicide Prevention Resources—https://afsp.org/suicide-prevention-resources#emergency-resources
American Psychiatric Association (APA) Suicide Prevention—https://www.psychiatry.org/patients-families/suicide-prevention
American Psychological Association (APA) Suicide Prevention—https://www.apa.org/advocacy/suicide-prevention
National Institute of Mental Health (NIMH) Ask Suicide-Screening Questions (ASQ) Toolkit—https://www.nimh.nih.gov/ASQ
Fostering Resilience—http://www.fosteringresilience.com/7cs_professionals.php
The Joint Commission Suicide Prevention—https://www.jointcommission.org/resources/patient-safety-topics/suicide-prevention/
National Suicide Prevention Lifeline—https://suicidepreventionlifeline.org/
Zero Suicide Toolkit—https://zerosuicide.edc.org/toolkit

Additional Resources and Websites for Parents/Caregivers:
Fostering Resilience—http://www.fosteringresilience.com/7cs_parents.php
National Institute of Mental Health (NIMH) Shareable Resources on Suicide Prevention—https://www.nimh.nih.gov/health/education-awareness/shareable-resources-on-suicide-prevention.shtml
National Institute of Mental Health (NIMH) Suicide Prevention—https://www.nimh.nih.gov/health/topics/suicide-prevention/index.shtml
National Suicide Prevention Lifeline—https://suicidepreventionlifeline.org/
Seize the Awkward—https://seizetheawkward.org/
Substance Abuse and Mental Health Services Administration (SAMHSA) Suicide Prevention—https://www.samhsa.gov/find-help/suicide-prevention
Suicide Prevention Resource Center (SPRC) Family Members and Caregivers—https://www.sprc.org/settings/family-members-and-caregivers

Additional Resources and Websites for Adolescents and Young Adults:
Crisis Text Line—https://www.crisistextline.org/
The Jed Foundation—https://www.jedfoundation.org/
National Suicide Prevention Lifeline—https://suicidepreventionlifeline.org/
Seize the Awkward—https://seizetheawkward.org/
The Trevor Project—https://www.thetrevorproject.org/get-help-now/

CHAPTER 76

Neurodevelopmental Differences and Disorders in Adolescents and Young Adults

Celia B. Neavel
Ellen Stubbe Kester
Kassandra Gonzalez

KEY WORDS

- Attention deficit hyperactivity disorder
- Autism
- Education
- Future planning
- Genetic syndromes
- Intellectual disabilities
- Interdisciplinary care
- Learning disabilities
- Legal information
- Neurodevelopmental disorders
- Neurodiversity

 ## INTRODUCTION

Recognizing the strengths and needs of adolescents and young adults (AYAs) is crucial in forming meaningful and effective therapeutic alliances and treatment plans, whether they are seen in primary care, consultative care, or other settings. This chapter reviews general approaches to the evaluation and intervention of attention deficit hyperactivity disorder (ADHD), autism spectrum disorder (ASD), learning disabilities (LD), intellectual disabilities (ID), and communication and sensory processing disorders. In addition, the chapter focuses on select syndromes exemplifying known etiologies and comorbid associations: fetal alcohol spectrum disorders (FASDs), fragile X syndrome (FXS), and 22q11.2 deletion syndrome (22q11.2DS).

 ## TERMINOLOGY

There are numerous terms used to describe individuals with neurologic differences. These terms evolve over time with changes in societal and scientific understanding. The terms neurotypical and neuroatypical are used to describe those within and without the range considered normal, respectively. Neurodiversity or neurodivergent connote that differences are valuable aspects of human variation, which need to be supported.

Neurodevelopmental disorders and disabilities refer to neurologically-based conditions interfering with acquisition, application, or retention of skills, such as learning, attention, memory, perception, motor coordination, language, problem solving, and social interaction. These disorders may change in affected individuals but are not considered medically curable. Appropriate diagnosis, accommodations, medical care, and interdisciplinary interventions can promote optimal outcomes.

When describing people with neurodevelopmental differences, it is most accepted to use person-first language (e.g., youth with intellectual disability). However, some individuals prefer identity-first language, such as "autistic" instead of "individual with autism." As language is generational and cultural, a good approach

is to ask the involved AYA or family what they prefer. Examples of neurodevelopmental diagnoses and their prevalence are listed in **Table 76.1**.

 ## EVALUATION

Evaluating neurodevelopmental disorders is a multistep process consisting of clinical interview, review of medical history and current concerns, physical examination, psychosocial assessment, and acquiring further testing or information as needed. An evaluation may occur over multiple visits.

Clinical Interview

It is important to consider the functional ability of the adolescent or young adult. Verbal and nonverbal communication skills are important to assess. Clinicians can observe AYA interactions with accompanying adults to assess vocabulary, grammar, and social interactions. Initial clinical impressions may change as more information is gathered. As with all AYA visits, speaking to and focusing on the patient as much as possible is preferred.

Past and Current Essential Information

Obtaining information can occur through several formats such as questionnaires, speaking to parents/caregivers and AYAs separately, requesting outside records, and, with permission, contacting school or other personnel directly. Information should include the following:

- A three-generation family history focusing on neurodevelopmental, academic, mental health, and congenital disorders
- Pre- and postnatal history with any exposures to substances or environmental contaminants, prematurity, congenital abnormalities, birth trauma, or neonatal illness
- Developmental milestones and temperament with any behavior or sensory processing differences
- Medical history, including the involvement of other medical specialists
- Comprehensive evaluations including those from a speech–language pathologist (SLP), occupational therapist (OT), or physical therapist (PT)
- Mental health history and any interventions
- Education history and the results of any previous psychoeducational or neuropsychiatric testing
- Current or past medications, including complimentary or alternative treatments
- A comprehensive review of systems with emphasis on sleep, neurologic, sensory, or motor deficits

TABLE 76.1

Select Neurodevelopmental Disorder Prevalence in the United States[a]

Disorder	Prevalence	Approximate Rate	Other Information
Any developmental disability	19.73% in 12–17 y	1 in 5	Approx. 2× more males than females[1]
Learning disabilities	9.71% in 12–17 y	1 in 11	Can be in one or more areas[1]
Attention deficit hyperactivity disorder (ADHD)	12.3% in 12–17 y	1 in 8 children	Approx. 2× more males than females Increased steadily over the past 2 decades[1]
Any communication disorder	7.7%	1 in 12	Prevalence decreases with age[2]
Developmental coordination disorder	5–6%	1 in 20	Higher prevalence if born preterm[3]
Autism spectrum disorder (ASD)	1.85%	1 in 54 children	4.3× more likely in boys (2.66%) than girls (0.78%)[3]
Intellectual disability	1.41% in 12–17 y	1 in 71	Approx. 2× more males than females[1]
Fetal alcohol spectrum disorders (FASD)	0.2–5%	0.2–9 in 1,000 1 in 100–1 in 25	Fetal alcohol syndrome[3] Fetal alcohol spectrum disorders
Tourette syndrome	0.6%	1 in 162	Approx. 3× more males than females[3]
Cerebral palsy	0.35% in 12–17 y	1 in 345	Most common motor disability of childhood Higher prevalence if born preterm More common in Black children than White and Hispanic[1]
Down syndrome	0.14%	1 in 700	Most common chromosomal condition[3] 95% trisomy 21 from spontaneous mutation 3% translocation with 1% hereditary; 2% mosaicism Mild-to-moderate ID, some severe Recognizable but variable phenotype; increased risk of ASD
Fragile X syndrome	0.025–0.009% 0.1%	1 in 4,000–7,000 males 1 in 6,000–11,000 females	Most common heritable cause of intellectual disabilities.[4]
22q11.2 deletion syndrome (DiGeorge syndrome, velocardiofacial syndrome)	0.016–0.05%	1 in 2,000 to 1 in 6,000	Most common chromosomal deletion disorder[5]

[a]Individuals can have more than one listed disorder.

Physical Examination

Height, weight, blood pressure, and heart rate may give an indication of underlying abnormalities and are tracked if medications are prescribed. Any hearing or vision impairments should be identified. The physical examination in diagnoses such as ADHD and ASD may be normal or there may be overt or subtle neurologic differences. Observing for dysmorphic features and being aware of organ system anomalies is important. Macrocephaly may be seen in ASD and neurofibromatosis. Skin examinations may show neurocutaneous abnormalities such as in tuberous sclerosis.[6] Sexual maturity rating (SMR) may be important depending on age and underlying diagnosis. A thorough neurologic examination should include observations for any abnormal movements or tics as well as an assessment of strength, sensation, reflexes, hyper- or hypotonicity, balance, and coordination.

Psychosocial Assessment

Although cultural variations in social interactions should be considered, pragmatic language skills, such as turn-taking in conversations and topic maintenance, articulation skills, and consistency of verbal output can be observed during the physical examination.

Ability to follow sequential directions and maintain eye contact and joint attention should be noted. Further, speech tone, prosody, voice modulation, and stress patterns also should be observed.

Pubertal and somatic changes, psychosocial development, and cognitive capacity do not always develop synchronously within any given individual. For example, AYAs may appear older or younger than their functioning ability. Functioning abilities may be disparate in different areas such as communication skills, motor development, and emotional regulation. Asking involved parents/caregivers to estimate the functioning age level of their child in different domains is useful.

The semistructured psychosocial HEEADSSS interview with parents/caregivers and AYAs together and independently can be adapted as in Table 76.2.

Depending on the adolescent or young adult's age and functioning level, having them draw a picture of a person can yield information about fine motor control, visual-motor ability, and attention to task. This further allows an opportunity to engage the adolescent or young adult in conversation and projective testing as they describe their drawing.

XV

TABLE 76.2

HEEADSSS Neurodevelopmental Screening

HOME

Stability, parents/caregivers, increased family conflict or stress on parents/caregivers, how communicate with each other, financial hardships, challenges with insurance, future planning (legal, housing, caretakers)

EDUCATION

Complete educational history preschool on; interventions, grades repeated, best learning modality (auditory, visual, tactile), attention and task completion, comprehensive testing, accommodations, special education services, advocacy, goals for future

EATING

Sensory issues, physical difficulties with eating, difficulty maintaining weight or overweight, (un)able to sit through meal, (un)able to prepare meals, putting nonfood items in mouth

ACTIVITIES

Physical ability; exercise and being outdoors; fine and gross motor coordination, sports, socialization; interests (limited, obsessions); independence engaging in preferred activities, amount of screen time, legal trouble

DRUGS

Prescribed medications, substance use, drug diversion, self-medicating, effect on underlying diagnosis, supplements

SEXUALITY

Pubertal timing, menstrual history and hygiene, history of or risk for abuse, how expresses sexuality, understanding of sexual norms, reproductive life plan, risk transmission with genetic disorders, birth control options depending on underlying diagnoses such as any medical contraindications or if unable to remember or plan ahead, any teratogenic medications

SUICIDE/DEPRESSION

Quality and duration of sleep, self-esteem, behavior changes especially if poor communication skills, increased risk of suicidal ideation or attempts in ADHD/ASD, counseling support

SAFETY

Victim of bullying, driving expectations, bolting or wandering, seizure risk, self-abuse, accidents, poor stranger awareness, ability to manage emotions

Further Diagnostic Information

Clinicians should use norm-based or criterion-referenced screening tools (Table 76.3) to inform their diagnoses. These tools vary in age range and literacy levels, and include self-report, teacher-report, and guardian-report screening tools for global and specific functioning and differences.

Referrals for speech, occupational, and/or physical therapy assessments, psychoeducational testing, and other medical specialists such as developmental–behavioral pediatricians, psychiatrists, neurologists, or geneticists may be indicated to help in diagnostic assessment. Some diagnoses and understanding of more complex patients can only evolve over time.

HEALTH CARE DELIVERY

The Medical Home

A medical home that provides care coordination and is responsive to AYAs and their families results in fewer unmet needs.[6] Adolescents and young adults with neurodevelopmental differences may take longer to feel comfortable with medical settings and clinicians. More frequent, shorter visits within a medical home offer opportunities to decrease anxiety and promote communication. Virtual visits can play a role in increasing access and comfort with health care.

Observation of the biologic, neurologic, and psychological development of adolescents or young adults within a medical home is ideal. Clinicians who know the patient, their functional abilities, and their support system will better be able to address their health care. Adolescents and young adults with neurodevelopmental differences need to receive the routine preventive care provided to their typically developing peers.

Recommended treatments and interventions for neurodevelopmental disorders often have burdens of time and cost. Adolescents and young adults may see multiple subspecialists and therapists and have multiple medical and school reports. Families and AYAs frequently seek out complimentary or alternative treatments in the hopes of improving or even curing underlying conditions. (See Chapter 8) Having a medical home allows clinicians and AYAs and their families to prioritize what interventions are evidence based and can reasonably be afforded and managed. Developing self-advocacy skills should be emphasized whenever possible. Medical homes can promote use of health passports or Emergency Information Forms as part of care coordination. (See Additional Resources and Websites)

Collating health information also can be part of medical transition planning that should start during adolescence (see Chapter 10) Clinicians must determine their own role in the transition process. Clinicians, families, and AYAs may have developed close relationships due to the chronic, pervasive nature of neurodevelopmental differences. Depending on the circumstances, patients may transition into more adult-focused care with the same clinicians, to new clinicians within the same institution or clinical organization, to new health care settings, or a combination.

Got Transition is a program of the National Alliance to Advance Adolescent Health. It reviews Six Core Elements of Health Care Transition (Care Policy/Guide, Tracking and Monitoring, Readiness, Planning, Transfer of Care, and Transition Completion), as well as other necessary information for clinicians, AYAs, and parents/caregivers. (See Additional Resources and Websites).

Integrated Behavioral Health

Patient outcomes are improved with an integrated behavioral health (IBH) approach, defined as "both behavioral health and medical providers functioning together as members of the primary care team."[7] It is critical to have systems in place to connect AYAs and their families with behavioral specialists, social workers, psychologists, psychiatrists, licensed professional counselors, marriage and family therapists, and other clinicians as needed. This increases access to services for families and contributes significantly to ongoing care and targeted interventions for AYAs with neurodevelopmental disorders.

Reproductive Health

Adolescents and young adults with disabilities are three times more likely than typically developing peers to be sexually abused and are more likely to exhibit inappropriate sexual behaviors. Education about reproductive health, sexuality, healthy relationships, sexual abuse prevention, pregnancy risk, and expectations for fertility is important when treating AYAs with disabilities or genetic syndromes.[8] Adolescents and young adults need education and shared

TABLE 76.3

Clinician Toolkits and Screening Instruments

Attention deficit hyperactivity disorder	American Academy of Family Practice National Research Network ADHD Screeners and Quality of Life Assessments for Adults https://www.aafp.org/dam/AAFP/documents/patient_care/adhd_toolkit/adhd19-assessment-screeners.pdf
	American Academy of Pediatrics ADHD: Quality Improvement Resources & Tools (webinar, slides, articles included) https://www.aap.org/en-us/professional-resources/quality-improvement/quality-improvement-resources-and-tools/Pages/adhd.aspx
	Children and Adults with ADHD (CHADD) Clinical Practice Tools https://chadd.org/for-professionals/clinical-practice-tools/
	Conner's Continuous Performance Test 3rd Edition; 8+ y https://storefront.mhs.com/collections/conners-cpt-3
	Conner's Rating Scales; 6–18 y, 18+ https://storefront.mhs.com/search?query=Conners#/products/Conners/0/score/desc/
	Test of Variable Attention; 4+ y https://www.tovatest.com/
	Vanderbilt Assessment Scales; 6–12 y; caregiver/teacher complete https://www.nichq.org/sites/default/files/resource-file/NICHQ_Vanderbilt_Assessment_Scales.pdf
	World Health Organization Adult ADHD Self-Report Scale; 18+ y https://www.hcp.med.harvard.edu/ncs/asrs.php
Autism spectrum disorder	Autism-Spectrum Quotient; Adults & adapted for adolescents; Self-complete https://psychology-tools.com/test/autism-spectrum-quotient and multiple sites
	Caring for Children With Autism Spectrum Disorder: A Practical Resource Toolkit for Clinicians, 3rd edition https://toolkits.solutions.aap.org/autism/home
	Social Communication Questionnaire; 4 y (mental age 2 y) +; caregiver completes https://www.wpspublish.com/scq-social-communication-questionnaire
	Social Responsiveness Scale 2nd Edition; 2.5–18 y, 19+; caregiver/teacher completes https://www.wpspublish.com/srs-2-social-responsiveness-scale-second-edition
Fetal alcohol spectrum disorder	Fetal Alcohol Spectrum Disorder Toolkit https://www.aap.org/en-us/advocacy-and-policy/aap-health-initiatives/fetal-alcohol-spectrum-disorders-toolkit/Pages/default.aspx
General	Adult Self-Report & Adult Behavior Checklist; 18+ y https://aseba.org/adults/
	American Academy of Child and Adolescent Psychiatry Toolbox of Forms (intake, baseline, and monitoring forms) https://www.aacap.org/AACAP/Member_Resources/AACAP_Toolbox_for_Clinical_Practice_and_Outcomes/Forms.aspx
	Child Behavior Checklist 6–18 y; caregiver completes https://store.aseba.org/CHILD-BEHAVIOR-CHECKLIST_6-18/productinfo/201/
	Youth Self Report; 11–18 y https://store.aseba.org/YOUTH-SELF-REPORT_11-18-50-per-Package/productinfo/501/

decision making commensurate with their functional level, with caregiver involvement as indicated. Individuals with disabilities often receive inadequate sexual health information.[9] Education should include building skills to navigate sexual feelings, cues, and relationships. Explicit education regarding when and where sexual behaviors are appropriate may be necessary. This is critical as impulsive or inappropriate sexual behaviors can lead to harm or even into the criminal justice system.

The Sexuality section outlined in Table 76.2 outlines important information that can enable clinicians to explore sexual parameters and identify specific risks. Some individuals with neurodevelopmental differences may show less interest in sexuality, but conversations with parents/caregivers and AYAs remain important.

Clinicians should be aware of local education resources and existing curricula. As well, it is important for clinicians to counsel or refer when underlying disorders may affect pubertal timing, fertility, or genetic disease transmission.[8,9]

CAREGIVER, FAMILY, AND COMMUNITY SUPPORT

Parents/Caregivers and Family

Adolescents and young adults with neurodevelopmental differences can pose complex parenting/caregiver challenges that are likely to impact caregiver health and well-being. Thus, reviewing parent/caregiver self-care is an important component, especially if

XV

they have other children at home. Feeling supported may help parents/caregivers set healthier boundaries and promote appropriate developmental autonomy in their AYAs.

Some parents/caregivers may observe that their child's neurodevelopmental diagnoses become less apparent with time, or that their maturing AYA comprehends their neurodevelopmental differences, develops resiliency, and is able to self-advocate. Other parents/caregivers, however, will experience worsening of their child's situation. Some AYAs with more awareness of their differences may develop mood disorders, participate in risky behaviors, or act out at home, which can be difficult for those around them. Most challenging for caretakers and families are diagnoses associated with declining abilities or severe behavioral problems. The clinician should work with parents/caregivers in seeking support, dispelling guilt, realistic planning, and learning advocacy as appropriate for each situation.

Family and financial stress can be burdensome if the AYA has complex disabilities. Parents/caregivers may be forced to miss work to care for or attend frequent medical or school appointments with their adolescent or young adult. Clinicians practicing in the United States should be aware of the Families Medical Leave Act (FMLA) which entitles eligible employees to take unpaid, job-protected leave for specified family and medical reasons if eligibility requirements are met. (See Additional Resources and Websites.)

As AYAs reach new life stages that are different from their more typically developing peers, families and parents/caregivers may experience grief similar to when they learned of their child's diagnosis. Clinicians should encourage parents/caregivers to allow a level of separation as is appropriate. Respite programs and camps are beneficial for parents/caregivers, siblings, and AYAs. Clinicians can play a role in making recommendations and completing necessary medical evaluations to access these programs. Siblings of AYAs often need support, education, and access to resources and groups as they face their own challenges.[6]

It is well documented that there is a shortage of adequate services across the United States for youth with neurodevelopmental differences. Too often, AYAs end up in the criminal justice system, especially individuals of color.[10] Clinicians should be aware of their specific geographic, national, and local organizations and nonprofit groups that help AYAs and families connect with services and support networks.

EDUCATIONAL SUPPORT

Adolescents and young adults with neurodevelopmental differences benefit from clinicians' understanding educational processes since school services can have a significant impact on future goals, mental health, and overall well-being. Each country will have specific legislation, policies, and programs to support AYAs. This section focuses on what is available in the United States.

For those whose diagnoses interfere with their ability to learn accommodations, modifications, and supports are available as explained below. See **Table 76.4**.

Section 504

The 504 Plan allows students to learn alongside their peers in the general education classroom. A 504 coordinator at the school or district will facilitate a meeting to develop and implement accommodations. This civil rights law applies to college and work environments, as well.

Special Education

Under the Individuals with Disabilities Education Act (IDEA), teaching environments can range from mainstream to self-contained classrooms to residential schools. What is considered a least restrictive environment (LRE), can change over time. The Individuals with Disabilities Education Act can allow for further educational training and transition benefits.

Clinician advocacy and referral to outside organizations can help AYAs receive optimal interventions. Clinicians can write letters of support to schools and workplaces for specific accommodations. (See Additional Resources and Websites.)

Comprehensive Educational Evaluation

If an appropriate, comprehensive assessment (Full and Individual Evaluation [FIE]) has not occurred, parents/caregivers and AYAs have the legal right to request it in writing through the public school. Depending on the area(s) of concern, testing may be completed by a school psychologist, educational diagnostician, SLP, OT, PT, vision specialist, and/or hearing specialist. Clinicians may initiate or may be asked by educators to sign necessary forms attesting to certain medical diagnoses. See **Table 76.4**. The Individuals with Disabilities Education Act includes legal timelines.

The FIE determines whether students are eligible for special education. Evaluators use assessment tools that yield standard scores based on a normative sample and nonstandardized information to make diagnostic decisions. Different states use different eligibility criteria. Figure 76.1 provides information on how to understand standard score interpretation.

Clinicians need to recognize that students with language and cultural differences may not have scores on traditional normative tests that truly reflect their abilities. In those situations, qualitative descriptive information is essential in identifying strengths and needs. Test bias or lack of training in evaluating youth of color and those from diverse backgrounds can result in students not receiving needed services, receiving unneeded services, or receiving inappropriate services (such as services for emotionally disturbed instead of an ADHD with language delay).

Once categories are identified (**Table 76.4**), educational teams, including AYAs and parents/caregivers, meet to develop plans. Clinicians can offer recommendations to be considered such as preferential seating, dietary and bathroom needs, and specific therapies.

Families who are not native English speakers can ask for translators for school meetings. If an inaccurate academic diagnosis is suspected, an Independent Educational Evaluation (IEE) paid by the school district can be requested. Families can file complaints to their state education agency (**Table 76.4**).

Schools should offer transition planning as part of Individualized Education Plans (IEPs). Transition planning begins at age 14 or 16 years, depending on the state. Clinicians can ensure that postsecondary education, job training, life skills acquisition, community programs, adult day activities, and other needs are addressed and submit important diagnostic information.

LEGAL SUPPORT AND PLANNING

Adolescents and young adults and their families benefit from their clinicians being knowledgeable about their legal rights. Knowledge about disability and legal transition to adulthood is important. Involving advocates, attorneys, legal aid organizations, or other resources may be necessary to optimize health outcomes.

Disability Benefits and Financial Planning

In the United States, AYAs with neurodevelopmental disabilities may receive Title XVI disability support through the Social Security Administration (SSA). The Social Security Administration may request (and pay for) additional information from clinicians.

If receiving benefits, AYAs will need an Age 18 Redetermination, during which SSA determines if adult standards for benefits are met. Losing disability benefits may result in losing Medicaid coverage in nonexpansion Medicaid states (12 states as of this writing).

TABLE 76.4

Definitions and Eligibility Categories for School Service Determination

Definitions

Full and individual evaluation (FIE)	An evaluation conducted by school personnel to determine if a student has a disability and what the impact of that disability is on educational attainment.
Gifted and talented (GT)	Students who demonstrate evidence of high achievement capability in intellect, creativity, art, and/or leadership that result in an educational need beyond the general education curriculum. GT programs in some states fall under the umbrella of special education.
Independent educational evaluation (IEE)	An educational evaluation conducted by someone who is not a part of the school district or agency that will be providing the educational services.
Individuals with Disabilities Act (IDEA)	A federal law requiring public schools to provide free, appropriate, and public education in the least restrictive environment for students from early childhood (0–5 y) through public high school or transition programs for qualifying adults up to age 22 y.
Individualized education program/plan (IEP)	A plan for specialized instruction and related services designed to help students with disabilities access their educational curriculum
Least restrictive environment (LRE)	A guiding principle that students with disabilities should receive education to the maximum extent possible with their typically developing peers.
Section 504/504 Plan	Part of the Rehabilitation Act of 1973, a civil rights law, that lays out a plan of accommodations for individuals with disabilities outside of special education. 504 accommodations apply to educational institutions receiving federal funds and work settings

Special Education Eligibility Categories

Autism spectrum disorder (ASD)	A developmental disability affecting a child's social and communication skills. Behavior is often impacted as well
Deaf–blindness	Concomitant visual and hearing impairments
Deafness	A severe hearing impairment that affects linguistic processing with or without amplification.
Emotional disturbance (ED)	Conditions impacting mental health, such as anxiety disorder, schizophrenia, bipolar disorder, obsessive-compulsive disorder, and depression
Hearing impairment (HI)	A hearing loss not covered by the definition of deafness
Intellectual disability (ID)	Below average intellectual disability, as indicated by tests of intellectual abilities *and* measures of adaptive behavior
Multiple disabilities	More than one condition covered by IDEA
Orthopedic impairment[a] (OH)	Conditions affecting physical function, such as cerebral palsy or spina bifida
Other health impairment[a] (OHI)	Includes conditions that limit a child's strength, energy, or alertness, including diagnoses such as developmental coordination disorder, ADHD, asthma, and other chronic medical conditions that impact educational attainment
Specific learning disability (SLD or LD)	Learning challenges that affect a child's ability to read, write, listen, speak, reason, or do math, including conditions such as dyslexia and dysgraphia
Speech or language impairment (SI)	Includes disorders in the areas of receptive language, expressive language, pragmatic language, fluency, voice, articulation, and phonology
Traumatic brain injury[a] (TBI)	A brain injury caused by an accident or physical force
Visual impairment (VI)	Eyesight problems, including partial sight and blindness, that cannot be corrected by eyewear

ADHD, attention deficit hyperactivity disorder.
[a]Diagnosed by physician.

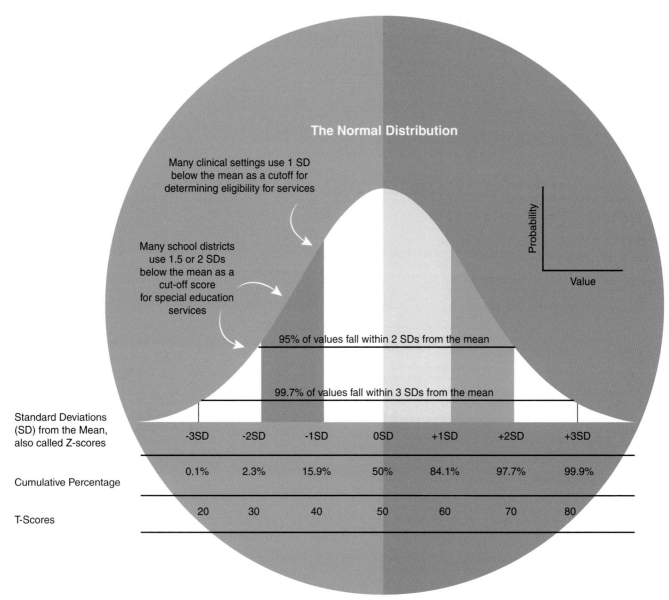

The Normal Distribution

Many clinical settings use 1 SD below the mean as a cutoff for determining eligibility for services

Many school districts use 1.5 or 2 SDs below the mean as a cut-off score for special education services

Probability

Value

95% of values fall within 2 SDs from the mean

99.7% of values fall within 3 SDs from the mean

Standard Deviations (SD) from the Mean, also called Z-scores	-3SD	-2SD	-1SD	0SD	+1SD	+2SD	+3SD
Cumulative Percentage	0.1%	2.3%	15.9%	50%	84.1%	97.7%	99.9%
T-Scores	20	30	40	50	60	70	80

FIGURE 76.1 Normal distribution curve for knowledge, learning, cognitive, and other ability testing.

Adolescents and young adults and families can appeal if disability benefits are discontinued.

To maintain public benefits and stay within income guidelines, AYAs and their families may be able to open a financial trust or an Achieving a Better Life Experience Act account, referred to as an ABLE account. (See Additional Resources and Websites.)

Guardianship and Alternatives

Unless some legal action has occurred, all 18-year-olds can legally enter contracts, make life decisions, consent for medical care, and limit access to school records. Clinicians seeing patients who are 18 years or older with neurodevelopmental disorders should determine if the young person or someone else has legal authority for medical consent. Any legal documentation, such as court orders or formal, signed paperwork should be added to the medical record.

Since some AYAs with neurodevelopmental diagnoses may need ongoing caregiver support, clinicians should encourage a consultation with an attorney or legal aid before the AYA's 18th birthday, if possible. Not doing so can result in health-harming medical, legal, or financial consequences. (See Additional Resources and Websites.)

Guardianship

In the United States, a court can order guardianship when it determines that a person is legally incapacitated. Before a court orders a guardianship, a physician must provide a written letter or certificate stating that a physical examination and estimation of competency was completed. A physician's letter or certificate may include a determination of intellectual disability, which can help a court with its determination. Physicians can review outside records to help in their attestations.

Guardianship Alternatives

While full guardianship can be warranted, less restrictive options exist.

Declaration for mental health treatment: Addresses convulsive therapy, psychoactive medication, and emergency psychiatric treatment in the event of a mental health episode that prevents a young adult (YA) from making decisions as determined by a court. (Varies by state.)

Medical power of attorney: Addresses who can make medical decisions in event that a YA cannot.

Durable power of attorney: Addresses who can make legal decisions for and in accordance with the YA.

Supported decision-making agreement: Addresses who can act as a supporter for YA decisions. Laws for supported decision-making agreements do not exist in all states, but the model is useful.

⬤ PREVALENT CONDITIONS

Attention Deficit Hyperactivity Disorder

Diagnosis and Associated Features

The most prevalent neurodevelopmental disorder is ADHD, which is characterized by deficits in executive function, including inattention, disorganization, hyperactivity, and impulsivity, which can range in severity. Executive function impacts planning and organization, working memory, initiation, task monitoring, self-monitoring, inhibition, emotional control, and the ability to shift easily from one activity to the next. Brain maturation can be delayed for years in this area, requiring coaching and structure.

A neurodiversity approach highlights positive attributes of ADHD such as creativity, the ability to hyperfocus on projects, and the synthesis/association of various types of information into useful connections.[11]

Attention deficit hyperactivity disorder can be a complex disability necessitating careful evaluation for diagnostic criteria outlined in the Diagnostic and Statistical Manual of Mental Disorders, fifth edition (DSM-5).[12-14] Validated screeners and toolkits exist to help in the diagnosis of ADHD (see **Table 76.3**). Collection of objective data and multiple reporters is necessary to establish baseline, monitor progress, and ensure that AYAs are not accessing stimulant medications inappropriately.[13] Clinical practice guidelines are available for diagnosing and treating ADHD[14] and algorithms exist for assessing and treating complex ADHD.[15] See Figure 76.2.

Attention deficit hyperactivity disorder itself may be part of broader diagnoses such as ASD or a genetic complex such as the triad of ADHD, obsessive–compulsive disorder (OCD), and Tourette syndrome (TS).[16] Comorbidities, such as mood disorders and other mental health disorders, communication disorders, and cognitive impairments, exist in 44% to 80% of AYAs with ADHD.[17] Youth with ADHD are at greater risk for legal problems, substance use, aggression, motor vehicle accidents, and suicide attempts.[13,17] Adolescents and young adults with ADHD can exhibit impulsive behaviors and be socially awkward, resulting in low self-esteem.[13] Attention deficit hyperactivity disorder associated with oppositional defiant disorder (ODD) and conduct disorder (CD) worsens prognosis.

The majority of youth diagnosed with ADHD continue to exhibit symptoms and impairment into adulthood. Increased rates of academic underachievement, unemployment, financial problems, and social disruptions occur.[13]

Interventions

Effective interventions are multimodal. Educating AYAs and their families to support their understanding of the diagnosis, including both strengths and needs, and evidence-based treatments is foundational.[15] Clinicians can offer handouts and resources that apply to each AYA's situation, with frequent reviews to check for understanding. (See Additional Resources and Websites.)

Psychosocial treatment can include social skills training, parent/caregiver training, peer intervention, cognitive behavioral therapy, and mindfulness training. Tailored, evidence-based behavioral approaches are needed for ODD and CD. Some strategies that are helpful for addressing executive function difficulties include using verbal and visual prompts for multistep projects and transitions from one activity to another, using visual organization systems, maintaining a consistent structure or routine, breaking tasks into smaller pieces so they seem less overwhelming, and using visual or

other timers to help maintain focus. It will depend on the individual youth (i.e., age and functioning level) as to how much external school, work, and caregiver support is needed versus supporting the AYA in developing their own strategies.

School supports are provided through IEPs or Section 504.[13,14] Clinicians can support AYAs by writing letters confirming the ADHD diagnosis and listing specific recommendations, such as longer test time in a quiet setting or more frequent breaks. (See Additional Resources and Websites.)

Physical Exercise Physical exercise, thought to increase norepinephrine, dopamine, and serotonin levels in the prefrontal cortex, hippocampus, and striatum,[18] benefits cognitive, behavioral, and physical symptoms of ADHD. Encouraging exercise, while being aware of possible motor coordination deficits or DCD with ADHD, is recommended. Opportunities for physical activity and being outside can be requested as part of IEP and Section 504 modifications. "No pass no play" (a state law requiring public school students who participate in extracurricular activities to maintain a minimum grade-point average) may be particularly harmful for youth with ADHD.

Sleep Regulation Sleep problems have been linked to ADHD and may further worsen function. Beneficial interventions can include improving sleep hygiene, promoting exercise earlier in the day, decreasing caffeine, delaying school/work start times, adjusting stimulant medication dosing, and monitoring electronic device usage.[19] Adolescents with ADHD spend twice as much time playing video games daily than their peers without ADHD. Clinicians can screen for daytime sleepiness and make recommendations on reducing technology use.[13] Sleep medication (melatonin, diphenhydramine, alpha agonists, trazodone, and others) may be warranted in some situations. Clinicians should consider other etiologies such as obstructive sleep apnea that require further evaluation and specialty referral.

Nutrition Dietary interventions, such as omega-3 supplementation and exclusion of artificial dyes, have been found to have small beneficial effects, but their role in treating core ADHD symptoms needs further research.[20] Clinicians should address structured, healthy meal planning; appetite suppression resulting from medications; or overeating from sensory seeking and impulsive behaviors. School and work accommodations can include meal planning.

Medication Medication is a key component of evidence-based care for AYAs with ADHD and is effective in reducing symptoms and improving function in 90% of individuals.[14] When prescribing medication or any other treatment recommendations, shared decision making is important.[21] The need for shared decision making has been shown to be important in promoting ongoing development and self-efficacy, enhancing ADHD medication adherence, and optimizing long-term outcomes. Clinicians need to be aware that AYAs and their parents/caregivers bring past experiences, cultural differences, and sometimes misunderstandings about medications. Furthermore, AYAs may have preferences about medication format (liquid, sprinkles, capsules, tablets, patches), duration (few hours to all day), and timing.

Medications for ADHD can seem complicated with new formulations frequently appearing in the marketplace. A recommended resource that can be printed and kept in the office is the ADHD Medication Guide https://www.adhdmedicationguide.com.

Stimulants The most studied and effective stimulant medications are methylphenidate and amphetamines. Neuroimaging confirms that they enhance dopamine neurotransmission.[22] Some AYAs will respond better to one or the other. Stimulant medications work "like a pair of glasses," which means they help when they're on/taken and don't help when they're off/wear off.

XV

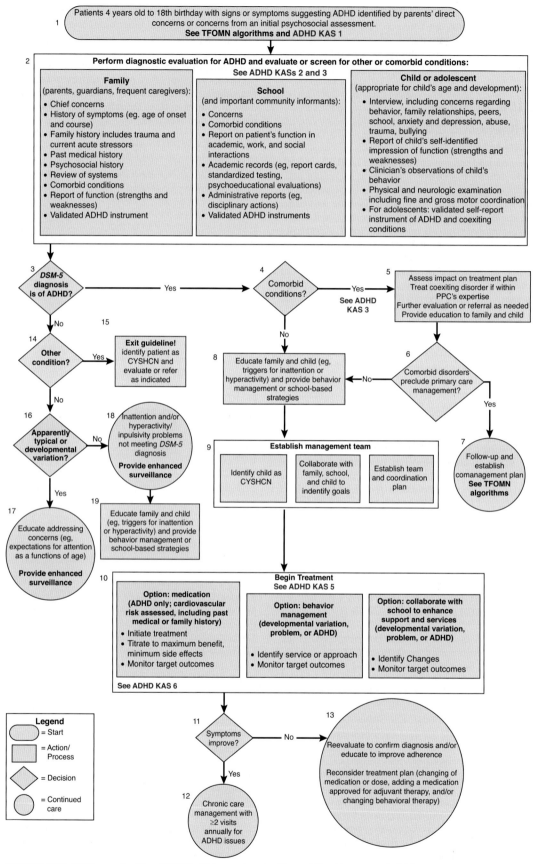

FIGURE 76.2 ADHD care algorithm. CYSHCN, children and youth with special health care needs. KAS, key action statements available in the cited text. (Used with permission from Wolraich M, Hagan JF. *Clinical Practice Guideline for the Diagnosis, Evaluation, and Treatment of Attention-Deficit/Hyperactivity Disorder in Children and Adolescents.* The American Academy of Pediatrics; 2019.).

The most common side effects of stimulant medications include headache, stomachache, appetite suppression, weight loss, and trouble sleeping, which is minimized by taking it with food and earlier in the day. Agitation, irritability, and rarely psychotic symptoms might occur. Stimulants may unmask comorbid bipolar disorder if not previously diagnosed.[14] Tics may appear or worsen with stimulants, so should be monitored and discussed. However, tic disorders are not a contraindication to stimulant medications as the ADHD symptoms may be worse than the tics. Stimulants do not increase sudden cardiac death, although heart rate and blood pressure can have modest elevations which should be monitored.[14] If there is a history of structural cardiac disease or cardiac concerns, cardiology clearance should be obtained.

Misuse and drug diversion to another person by selling, trading, or giving to another happens with up to 30% of AYAs prescribed stimulants. This requires that clinicians directly address such possibilities, including explaining the potential legal consequences. Research continues to explore if prescribing ADHD medications protects from substance use in AYAs with ADHD.[13] Longer acting stimulants (once-daily dosing) may decrease drug diversion or use and enhance adherence. Medication review visits also give the clinician an opportunity for ongoing education with AYAs about ADHD, review of legal rights for school/work accommodations, resource availability, and comorbidity screening.

Nonstimulants Nonstimulant medications also have a role in treating ADHD and comorbidities. The U.S. Food and Drug Administration (FDA) approved guanfacine and clonidine which are alpha-2 noradrenergic receptor agonists, and atomoxetine and viloxazine, which enhance dopamine and norepinephrine cortical transmission.[22]

These medications can be used independently when stimulants have intolerable side effects or are contraindicated, or in conjunction with stimulants. They require daily use with the full benefit becoming apparent after several weeks. Alpha agonists can be helpful with comorbid tic disorders, hyperarousal, anxiety, and poor sleep. Once AYAs are on steady doses, medicine should not be stopped suddenly due to risk of rebound tachycardia and hypertension. Atomoxetine may also help with anxiety and be used if there is a concern about problematic substance use. Atomoxetine has the same black box warning as selective serotonin reuptake inhibitors (SSRIs) and rarely causes liver enzyme elevation. Bupropion has been used off-label for adults with ADHD and can co-treat depression, anxiety, and smoking cessation.

When medication and interventions are stable, follow-up can be every 3 to 6 months. Repeating screening tools and monitoring school/work progress when making treatment changes and at least yearly is suggested.

Adolescents and young adults with complex comorbidities and other mental health diagnoses, or those who do not respond to usual treatment, can be referred to developmental–behavioral pediatricians or psychiatrists.

Autism Spectrum Disorders
Diagnosis and Associated Features

Autism spectrum disorder is a developmental condition with core deficits involving communication, socialization, interpersonal interactions, and behavior patterns that are restrictive or repetitive.[6,23] The degree of impairment in functioning varies between individuals. The DSM-5 criteria for ASD diagnosis include severity rating information.[12] Individuals with social language impairments but not restrictive or repetitive behaviors are diagnosed with social pragmatic communication disorder.[12]

Research indicates multiple genetic and environmental factors that increase the risk for ASD, since the disorder is complex with variable symptoms and severity. It is estimated that intellectual

disability accompanies ASD in approximately 30% of patients.[6] Some individuals with ASD may have more advanced splinter skills such as hyperlexia or exceptional memory. In other individuals, there are regressive syndromes associated with ASD such as Rett syndrome, in which overall function and ability decline over time.

Determining the presence or extent of cognitive impairment in individuals with more moderate to severe ASD can be difficult. Clinicians should ensure that a multidisciplinary team–based assessment is utilized for determining intellectual ability.

Sleeping, eating, and gastrointestinal problems, difficulty with motor planning, and seizures can be associated with ASD.[6] Clinicians should screen for these initially and continue surveillance.

Over 85% of 12- to 17-year-olds with ASD have one or more mental health problems including behavior/conduct (60.8%), anxiety (39.5%), ADHD (48.4%), and depression (15.7%).[24] Increased susceptibility to being bullied can occur. A retrospective study found increased suicide risk for females and young adults with ASD.[25] Aggression in youth with severe ASD and intellectual impairment can become even more challenging as they go through puberty and increase in body size.

There is an increased co-occurrence of ASD with gender nonconformity. Awareness can help in recognizing this association when caring for AYAs with ASD or AYAs who are transgender or nonbinary. Initial clinical guidelines have been developed. Having ASD is not a contraindication to treating gender dysphoria.[26] However, consent issues may need consideration for youth who are minors, have some level of cognitive impairment, are in the foster care system, or have assigned legal decision makers.

Early childhood screening for ASD is considered standard of care, but more mildly affected, lower socioeconomic, Latino or Black youth may not be diagnosed until later. Lack of access, cultural differences, and mistrust of health care systems may be barriers.[6] If a new ASD diagnosis is suspected, referral for thorough diagnostic evaluation and multidisciplinary assessment is recommended.

Referral for genetic evaluation and genetic counseling should be considered if the adolescent or young adult with ASD has not participated in this process recently, especially if dysmorphic features or cognitive impairment are present. The recurrence risk rate of ASD and other neurodevelopmental disorders in families is elevated.[23] Fragile X syndrome testing is recommended for all individuals with ASD. If the etiology remains unknown, a chromosomal microarray is recommended. Knowledge about genetic risk and any genetic findings is important for affected individuals and biologic family members. Other medical evaluations such as electroencephalogram (EEG) and neuroimaging are not routine but depend on history and physical examination.[6]

Prognosis for AYAs with ASD depends on the extent of deficits and comorbidities. Early interventions, supportive family and community, higher intelligence quotient (IQ), and decrease in repetitive behaviors are mitigative.[6,23] Nine percent of adults who were diagnosed with ASD in childhood may no longer meet ASD criteria as adults.[6]

While much of the ASD research focuses on deficits, neurodiversity can also be viewed as advantageous.[27] There are books, blogs, websites, and social media written by and about people with ASD that promote the importance of inclusion and diversity.

Sensory Processing

Clinicians, families, and AYAs may be exposed to the controversy of diagnosing a separate sensory processing disorder (SPD or sensory integration dysfunction). Diagnostic and Statistical Manual of Mental Disorders, fifth edition includes "Hyper- or hyporeactivity to sensory input or unusual interest in sensory aspects of the environment" under Part B of diagnosing ASD[12] and these characteristics can be found in other neurodevelopmental conditions. While research is ongoing, the DSM-5 did not establish a stand-alone diagnosis of SPD. Checklists, questionnaires, and tests exist which evaluate for types of sensory processing differences.

Interventions

Depending on the needs of the youth, treatment focuses on reducing deficits in social communication, maximizing functional independence, and reducing problem behaviors. These services can be time-intensive, expensive, and not uniformly covered by school districts or insurance companies. The clinician's role can involve helping families access services and possibly residential supports to maintain safety when needed. Physicians may be asked to write prescriptions for specific speech and language therapy, occupational therapy, physiotherapy, behavioral therapy and others. Adolescents and young adults may need referrals to psychologists, psychiatrists, or developmental pediatricians.[6]

Most evidence-based interventions for individuals with moderate to severe ASD are based on principles of applied behavioral analysis (ABA) or learning theory. Highly structured programs have been found to result in individuals achieving optimal developmental outcomes, but their basis in behaviorism has become controversial with some AYAs with ASD and other advocates. Relationship-focused interventions are developmentally based approaches that teach individuals to engage in joint attention and social engagement. Parent/caregiver-focused approaches, such as parent/caregiver-mediated treatment and parent/caregiver management training, teach parents/caregivers to target core symptoms of ASD or other behaviors using ABA techniques in a natural setting. Individuals with ASD may receive a combination of approaches through certified therapists.[6] The most severely impaired AYAs with ASD will need persistent, intensive, multidisciplinary care.

Medications Risperidone and aripiprazole are FDA-approved atypical antipsychotics that have been shown to improve irritability, hyperactivity, aggression, and stereotypy. These medications are prescribed for 14% to 23% of youth with ASD. The adverse effects of weight gain and diabetes risk with atypical antipsychotics can be improved by addition of metformin.[28] A table of randomized controlled trials of a broad range of psychotropic medications used in ASD is available.[23] Stimulant and nonstimulant medication may help with ADHD symptoms. Selective serotonin reuptake inhibitors may help with anxiety and depression.

Communication and Language Disorders

Diagnosis and Associated Features

Communication and language-based differences can occur independently or be associated with dyslexia, ID, ASD, ADHD, and other diagnoses. Since communication is one of the most basic human needs, deficits can lead to frustration, undesired behaviors, academic problems, and difficulty socializing, even if cognitive impairment is not present. This is especially true during the AYA developmental stage. Adolescents and young adults may or may not have received speech–language services when they were younger. However, clinician observation or awareness of past struggles should prompt further diagnostic assessment.

Speech difficulties include articulation, phonology, fluency, voice, and dysphagia disorders. Childhood apraxia of speech (CAS) is an example of a neurodevelopmental disorder that causes impairment in planning and/or programming of movement sequences needed for speech. Language disorders can be receptive and/or expressive and can impact content (vocabulary and cohesiveness of messages), form (sentence structure and word endings), and/or use or pragmatics (social appropriateness of interactions). Of 11- to 17-year-olds with communication disorders, 25.4% have multiple types, 24.4% have speech only, 23.2% have language only, 14.5% have swallowing only, and 12.5% have voice only problems.[2]

Interventions

An SLP should be consulted as soon as communication deficits are noted. Speech interventions may occur 1:1, in groups, and as co-treatments. Youth may receive services in the school setting and the clinical setting. Some AYAs with neurodevelopmental disabilities benefit from signing, picture boards, tablets, or other augmentative communication devices that allow for enhanced social interactions in their daily lives. School and work should adopt appropriate accommodations and ensure that any augmentative communication needs are met as AYAs age out of the school system.

Developmental Coordination Disorder

Diagnosis and Associated Features

Developmental coordination disorder (DCD) is a DSM-5 diagnosis and affects psychomotor, sensorimotor, and perceptual-motor abilities.[12] There can be gross and fine motor deficits such as postural control problems, clumsiness, slowness, and developmentally delayed motor learning which can affect quality of life and education. Dysgraphia (delays in production of writing) occurs in half of those with DCD. Clinicians should be aware that AYAs with DCD tend to be poor at sports and physically awkward contributing to limited activity that can lead to weight gain. Further, these young people are known to be bullied, lack school motivation, and have low self-esteem. Other neurodevelopmental disorders and learning problems described in this chapter can be associated with DCD, such as ASD, ADHD, LD, and others. Developmental coordination disorder may be difficult to diagnose but screening history and physical examination can be helpful. Normed assessment tools can be used in the office such as Rey–Osterrieth Complex Figure test and Developmental Coordination Disorder Questionnaire (DCDQ), but referral to OT allows for more thorough evaluation.[29] Clinicians should consider this diagnosis in their AYA patients.

Interventions

Clinicians, educators, OT, and PT can provide recommendations for treatment and accommodations. Clinicians can support AYAs by promoting services through Other Health Impaired (OHI) or section 504 in school settings. Referral for periodic or ongoing OT outside of school also can be helpful. Adolescents and young adults should understand their diagnosis and its impact. Treatment goals are to improve activities of daily living, improve school and physical participation, support lifelong planning, and diminish mental health sequelae.[29]

Intellectual Disability

Diagnosis and Associated Features

Intellectual disability (formerly referred to as mental retardation) is a disability characterized by deficits in intellectual functioning and adaptive behavior.[12] Intellectual disability is associated with global delays in many domains, generally with IQ and adaptive scores below 70.

Diagnosticians, psychologists, educational psychologists, and neuropsychologists diagnose ID using a combination of standardized cognitive and adaptive functioning tests and observations across settings. Even formal testing can be imprecise as testing instruments have different biases and there may be scatter in the subtest results. Given the variability in testing youth, more frequent and comprehensive assessments ensure more valid results. Clinicians should determine that AYAs have recent enough testing that an ID diagnosis is confirmed and accurate.

In some situations, AYAs with mild or even moderate ID may not be obvious to the clinician in casual conversation, especially if the AYA has good social skills and no other associated diagnosis. In other situations, ID may be more apparent or suspected. Adolescents and young adults with more severe and profound ID are more likely to have a genetic etiology.

Clinicians should request and review any records of cognitive evaluation or should help AYAs and families in obtaining needed testing. See Figure 76.1 for information on interpreting standardized tests.

Interventions

Adolescents and young adults with ID require additional supports to augment learning. This can include therapies and other approaches that use touch, movement, and visuals. Educational goals under IDEA will depend on level of severity such as life skills classes. Clinician awareness of cognitive impairment is important in using best approaches for communication with AYAs with ID in the office, and with supporting future planning.

Learning Disabilities

Diagnosis and Associated Features

Learning disabilities are disorders in one or more (but not all) psychological processes, including auditory and visual perception, integration of information, memory, language, or motor skills, that result in difficulty in learning. Dyslexia, dyscalculia, and dysgraphia are specific learning disabilities that impact reading, math, and writing, respectively. The DSM-5 diagnosis requires symptoms that persist for greater than 6 months, despite interventions, start in childhood, and are not better accounted for by other disorders.[12] Learning disabilities may not be apparent until later school years.

Determining LD involves standardized cognitive and achievement testing that demonstrates below average or less than expected cognitive processing in a specific area or areas. Adolescents and young adults with LD will have a gap or measurable difference between their overall IQ and a skill such as reading.

Interventions

Learning disabilities are addressed through remediation and accommodations, considering the type and severity. Examples of accommodations include increased font size, adaptive pens or paper, use of tools such as rulers, keyboards, or graphic organizers, extra tutoring, and information given in different, multisensory ways. Special education teachers and OT, PT, and ST services can recommend and support accommodations. Resource teachers can provide individual or small group lessons in regular or separate classrooms. Students with LD may be served under Section 504 or IDEA. Specialized schools exist for some types of LD.

Clinicians should support AYAs getting testing or repeat testing if academic struggles exist. Distinguishing between ID and LD and quantifying the type and severity of cognitive differences is essential.

Adolescents and young adults with LD may feel stigmatized. Some may experience bullying. Clinicians can help AYAs understand their LD, and help families understand when specialized education is needed. As well, health information should be presented in a way that takes the LD into account.

⬤ ETIOLOGIC CONSIDERATIONS IN NEURODEVELOPMENTAL DISORDERS

Clinicians may diagnose specific neurodevelopmental disorder etiologies when there is abnormal gene identification, known neurologic insult, or toxic exposures. The Environmental Protection Agency lists multiple potential environmental chemicals as concerns for neurologic development.[30]

The majority of AYAs, however, will have variable combinations of environmental, genetic, and biopsychosocial risk factors that result in their diagnoses. Genetic and brain imaging research continues to unveil more biologic factors. One developmental psychopathology framework that may better explain the many overlapping disorders and apparent comorbidities suggests a dynamic, interactive process that involves heritable vulnerabilities in neural circuitry interacting with complex environmental forces. These etiologic variations combined with individual differences result in disorders presenting differently across individuals, especially during biopsychosocial changes, such as those experienced during the adolescent period. Interventions and protective factors may mitigate risk, resulting in improved resiliency and functioning.[13]

Below are examples of complex neurodevelopmental disabilities that have known etiologies. Interventions and medications are based on associated comorbidities, behaviors, and specific medical findings.

Fetal Alcohol Spectrum Disorders

Diagnosis and Associated Features

Fetal alcohol spectrum disorders, which include fetal alcohol syndrome, partial fetal alcohol syndrome, fetal alcohol effect, alcohol-related neurodevelopmental disorder, alcohol-related birth defects, and neurodevelopmental disorder associated with prenatal alcohol exposure (ND-PAE incorporated into DSM-5[12]), are the most common preventable and identifiable cause of developmental and intellectual disorders. Fetal alcohol spectrum disorders are characterized by physical changes, brain and central nervous system problems, and social and behavioral issues.[30]

The American Academy of Pediatrics stresses that no amount of alcohol consumption is considered safe during pregnancy.[30] A clinician should explore prenatal alcohol exposure with the biologic family if available. In cases of adoption or youth in foster care, this may not be possible.

For diagnostic evaluation see Figure 76.3. Multidisciplinary team participation is recommended. Chromosomal microarray testing can help rule out another cause of dysmorphic findings.

Other physical findings of prenatal alcohol exposure can include orthopedic deformities, frequent ear infections, seizures, slow physical growth, vision and/or hearing deficits, cardiac defects, and renal disorders.[30]

Attention deficit hyperactivity disorder was found to be the most common (50%) comorbid neurodevelopmental disorder among children 8 to 11 years old, followed by ID (23.3%), LD (19.9%), ODD (16.3%), psychotic disorders (12.3%), and other mood disorders. Youth with FASD also have higher exposure to neglect, abuse, and being in foster care which may contribute to mental health disorders.[31] A prospective sample of young adults with prenatal alcohol exposure (PAE) found those *less physically* affected by PAE showed more problem behavior, substance use, and legal problems than those cognitively affected.[32]

Protective factors that help reduce sequelae include early diagnosis, appropriate services, caring and stable home environments, and lack of exposure to violence.[32] Adults with FASD can have increased legal trouble, worsening mental health, suicide risk, and victimization.[30]

Interventions

Medications used to improve co-occurring symptoms should be monitored carefully; medication effects may not always act in a manner similar to that of individuals without FASD.[30]

Fragile X Syndrome

Diagnosis and Associated Features

Fragile X syndrome is a genetic condition that causes a range of problems including intellectual impairment, language differences, learning disabilities, and specific behavior profiles, that have variable penetrance depending on the sex and the individual's genetic profile. Individuals with FXS may also have ASD, ADHD, and anxiety. This syndrome is X-linked; males are more severely affected compared to females.[33]

Clinical features can include long faces, connective tissue-like abnormalities, cardiac disease, and, in postpubertal males, macroorchidism. Additional findings can include hypotonia, other orthopedic problems, seizures, ocular disorders, sleep problems,

FASD diagnostic algorithm

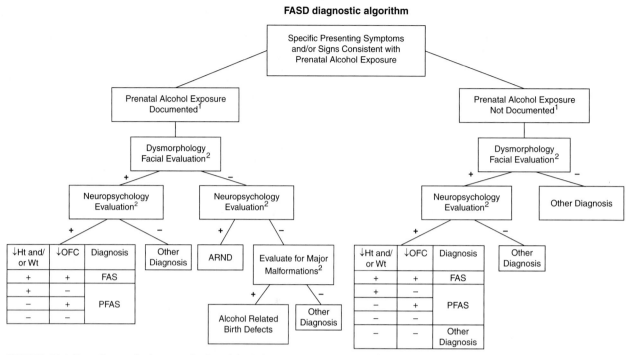

FIGURE 76.3 Flow diagram for home evaluation of fetal alcohol spectrum disorders (FASD). (Used with permission from The American Academy of Pediatrics. Hoyme HE, Kalberg WO, Elliott AJ, et al. Updated clinical guidelines for diagnosing fetal alcohol spectrum disorders. *Pediatrics.* 2016;138(2):e20154256. doi: https://doi.org/10.1542/peds.2015-4256).

and gastrointestinal disorders. Other medical complications may include tremor/ataxia syndrome and premature ovarian insufficiency.[33,34] Overall IQ declines by adolescence and adulthood.

Fragile X syndrome is caused by a mutation of the FMR1 gene located on Xq27.3. The FMR1 gene makes the fragile mental retardation protein (FMRP), and this is decreased or shut down (methylated) by abnormal DNA expansions (CGG repeats) in individuals with FXS. Loss or shortage of this protein disrupts the nervous system and results in the signs and symptoms of FXS.[33,34]

Southern blot analysis and polymerase chain reaction testing are available. Clinicians should consider testing AYAs for FXS based on family history, clinical features, ASD, intellectual disability, or learning disabilities of unknown cause.[33,34]

Interventions

With recent research, targeted pharmacotherapeutic approaches are being tried for the neurobiologic disorders found in FXS.[35] Clinicians should ensure that genetic counseling is available for AYAs with FXS, as well as permutation carriers.

The majority of adults with FXS continue to live at home requiring some level of support. Clinicians caring for AYAs with FXS should monitor health conditions over time.[36]

22q11.2 Deletion Syndrome

Diagnosis and Associated Features

22q11.2 deletion syndrome (22q11.2DS), also known as DiGeorge syndrome or velocardiofacial syndrome, is an autosomal dominant contiguous gene deletion syndrome. The deletion is de novo in 90% of individuals and inherited from a heterozygous parent in 10% of individuals.[37] The diagnosis is established on chromosomal microarray analysis.

Many individuals with 22q11.2DS have cardiac disease (74%), endocrine problems (>50%), immune deficiency, learning difficulties (70% to 90%), speech, neurologic, renal, skeletal, and/or behavior difficulties and characteristic facial features (90%). The craniofacial anomalies can result in velopharyngeal dysfunction

(VPD) and feeding difficulties.[37,38] Psychiatric illness is common in patients with 22q11.2DS including schizophrenia, ASD, and ADHD.[38]

Interventions

Since 22q11.2DS can affect every body system, it is important that AYAs be treated by a multidisciplinary team who can identify the physical and psychosocial needs. Coordination of medical subspecialty care often is warranted. Craniofacial abnormalities, if present, can require multiple surgeries starting as early as in utero and sometimes lasting through young adulthood. The prognosis for 22q11.2DS is highly variable and depends on the nature and degree of associated medical findings. Intelligence quotient is variable, but typically borderline and can decline in AYAs.[37,38]

Research is focusing on cognitive remediation and pharmacology interventions. Currently, the use of psychotropic medication is targeted to specific behaviors, with cardiovascular clearance sometimes needed depending on the medication.[38]

SUMMARY

Clinicians need to follow diagnostic criteria for neurodevelopmental disorders with the understanding that these sometimes can be imprecise, evolving, and overlapping. Environmental, genetic, and lived experiences influence how individual AYA present. Knowledge about identifiable disorders and syndromes, and the collection and review of collateral information (previous assessments, medical records, interventions, and school information), will help in diagnoses and treatment recommendations. Clinicians should assess family and AYA needs, with awareness of SDOH, to maximize AYA development. Accurate diagnostic descriptions can determine school and work accommodations and legal rights. Specific medical diagnoses require monitoring for known or potential organ system involvement and psychiatric comorbidities. Co-occurrence of neurodevelopmental diagnoses is common. Appropriate medical subspecialty and interdisciplinary referrals, care coordination, and the

TABLE 77.1

Assessing Risk within the Family, Peer, School, and Community Domains

Family	Peer	School	Community
History of parental mental illness or substance use	Violent and antisocial behavior of peers	Negative school climate	Violence in the community
Parent/caregiver conflict and violence within the family	Gang involvement	Overcrowding and poorly managed classrooms	Extreme poverty and related forms of disadvantage
Conduct problems by siblings		High incidence of bullying and peer harassment	Availability of drugs and alcohol
Availability of firearms in the home		Lax and ineffective policies related to school safety	Availability of firearms

risk factors by interviewing the adolescent or young adult and other informants and by reviewing archival materials, such as psychiatric reports or, for older AYA, juvenile justice records. There are several structured risk assessment instruments that can be used for the purposes of assessing youth directly.[27] One such tool is the Structured Assessment of Violence Risk in Youth (SAVRY),[27] which offers a manualized, checklist-type assessment of 24 different risk indicators over three domains–historical, social–contextual, and individual–clinical. Clinicians are asked to incorporate multiple sources of information (e.g., personal interviews, reviews of records, consultation with information) to generate ratings of risk status on each item. Once completed, the assessed information can help guide professional judgment in very specific ways.

A variety of other similar instruments exist, some of which permit inferences from clinical "cut scores" (e.g., the Early Assessment Risk List [EARL][28]) and others that utilize an unscored but structured format similar to the SAVRY (e.g., Historical Clinical Risk Management-20 [HCR-20]).[29] A general risk assessment approach is typically used in cases where a youth's behavior has risen to a level of concern, but not yet to a level where immediate intervention to address safety risks is required.

In a targeted risk assessment, there are usually discernible, sometimes immediate threats of violence made by an adolescent or young adult that require immediate action on the part of a clinician. In such cases, the first step is to gauge the level of risk involved and the likelihood an adolescent or young adult will carry through on a threat he or she has made. One model[30] for this type of risk assessment focuses on 10 areas of inquiry: (1) motivation for the referral behavior; (2) method of communicating threats; (3) "unusual interest" in targeted violence; (4) evidence for "attack-related behaviors and planning"; (5) mental status; (6) level of "cognitive sophistication" as applied to planning and executing a targeted violent act; (7) recent losses, including losses of status; (8) coordination of violent communications and related behaviors; (9) concern from collateral contacts about individual's propensity for violence; and (10) contextual and situational factors that increase or decrease the individual's propensity for violence. As with a general risk assessment approach, clinicians who conduct targeted risk assessments can use a variety of information sources to help formulate their plans (interviews, informant reports, etc.). However, in the case of targeted assessments, all information-gathering is predicated on concerns of immediate threat, often when plans to carry out the threat have also been voiced.

It is important to note that assessing an AYA's risk or propensity for violence can be a daunting task for the clinician and carries with it significant responsibilities, both legal and ethical. Those charged with assessing youth who have displayed disordered conduct and violence must not only assess and stabilize the individual involved, but may need to notify law enforcement when there are credible threats of violence. Clinicians that assess a youth's experience of domestic violence and child abuse might similarly need to file reports with authorities so that the safety of everyone involved can be assured. Thus, clinicians must be aware of the legal, ethical, and professional responsibilities that is specific to their discipline and geographic area and trained on the protocols for accurately identifying and efficiently acting on threats of violence.

Prevention and Intervention

Reducing risk factors and strengthening protective factors is fundamental to public health prevention.[31] An understanding of the risk and protective factors most consistently related to youth violence is important to the design and delivery of any program that focuses on prevention. In designing preventive interventions, even knowledge of predictors that are not malleable (e.g., gender, race, and ethnicity) can be useful because it helps to establish for whom prevention services are most needed.

Violence prevention strategies, implemented at a group or population level typically are organized around a public health model (Fig. 77.1), which incorporates many of the risk and protective factors in the community, family, school, peer, and individual

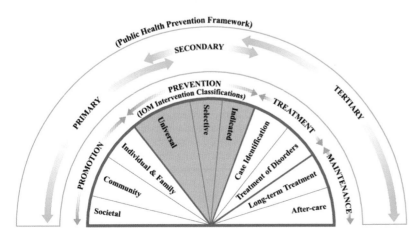

FIGURE 77.1 The Public Health Prevention Framework.[33] Overlap of two prevention models: The Institute of Medicine (IOM) intervention classifications and the public health prevention framework. (Sources: Institute of Medicine, 1994 (IOM Intervention Classifications); Katz and Ali, 2009 (Public Health Prevention Framework); adapted from National Academies of Sciences, Engineering, and Medicine. *Promoting Positive Adolescent Health Behaviors and Outcomes: Thriving in the 21st Century.* N.F. Kahn and R. Graham, eds. National Academies Press; 2020.)

domains.[31] Public health prevention has traditionally been discussed using the terms primary, secondary, and tertiary prevention to designate where in the developmental progression of a problem and for which population a prevention program is most intended. The terms *universal, selected,* and *indicated prevention* are now used to refer to levels of risk and need within different segments of the general population. *Universal* prevention programs focus on all AYAs regardless of their level of risk or need. The intent of these programs is to inoculate every young person against the influences most likely to cause violence. *Selected* programs focus on AYAs at somewhat higher risk for violence. Also, *indicated* programs focus on those at highest risk for violence, including those who have already begun committing violent acts. To the extent that AYAs in this category have not yet engaged in the most serious forms of violence, they are still considered candidates for prevention.[32]

Prevention programs are commonly implemented at the community, school, and family levels, and less so at the individual youth level. This is because it is recognized that individual predispositions and tendencies toward the use of violence are typically only acted upon when the social environment is conducive to that behavior, as is the case in dysfunctional (e.g., abusive and highly aversive) families, or in schools or community settings in which norms support violence and control strategies are ineffectual.

Individual-based clinical prevention interventions targeting individual young people, such as psychotherapy for AYAs diagnosed with conduct disorder, have proven mostly ineffective if not combined with other interventions that focus also on the social environment.[25] Evidence suggests there are greater benefits to youth when a combination of intervention modalities and multicomponent strategies attend to several individual, social, and environmental risk factors.[25,34] Indeed, when cognitive–behavioral therapy and social skills training programs (individual-level interventions) are embedded in programs that also attend to environmental influences related to families and peers, results are far more promising.[25]

Research on programs like multisystemic therapy (MST), a rigorously evaluated, evidence-based program, shows that well-designed interventions directed at older, high-risk, and violence-prone youth in the middle- and high-school grades can in some cases change behavior for the better, even diverting delinquent youth from the criminal justice system.[35] For the individual clinician, the goal following assessment, is, therefore, to become well acquainted with what the research shows about evidence-based prevention programs and to assist as much as possible in helping broker connections between families and service systems so that AYAs have access to the best available options for intervention. A review of evidence-based programs in youth violence prevention, including MST, can be found at the Blueprints for Healthy Youth Development website (http://www.blueprintsprograms.com), which summarizes the goals and components of each program in some detail, their impacts on behavior, and also their benefits and financial costs.

Community-based prevention programs include a variety of approaches to reducing risk factors and enhancing protective factors for youth. Programs can include community mobilizing and community policing, youth mentoring, and employment.[36] While promising in several ways, community-level prevention programs have proved difficult to evaluate because of the complex service delivery systems that surround youth programming in these contexts.[32,36] As a result, the field has amassed relatively little data to help guide program and policymakers to evidence-based models. There is, however, emerging evidence that certain approaches to crime reduction and prevention, like problem-oriented policing, can impact violence.[37]

Prevention and intervention programs focused on gang involvement are often organized at the community level, yet the dynamics of gangs are such that very specialized intervention approaches can be required.[38] Evidence-based practices shown to benefit violent and gang-involved youth tend to focus on reducing the violent behavior more so than extracting the youth from the gangs. Models like the Office of Juvenile Justice and Delinquency Prevention's Comprehensive Gang Model provide some very specific guidance on strategies to engage gang-involved youth using outreach and other forms of social engagement to link youth to needed services and to expand their opportunities for education and employment. Unfortunately, when youth are involved in gangs, the very behaviors that are likely to harm others (and the youth involved) are precisely those that are encouraged and reinforced by gang culture.[39] Consequently, the effects of interventions that do not target gang involvement for violent youth are very likely to fall short of their intended goals related to reducing violence and improving public safety.[40]

According to one comprehensive review of programs,[36] *school-based* violence prevention programs include classroom-based cooperative learning, small-group instruction, proactive classroom management, interactive teaching, and peer learning to create conditions that are conducive to positive behaviors and academic achievement among students. Social and emotional learning programs are also grouped under this general header. Meta-analytic reviews of school-based violence prevention programs have generally shown effects on violence, aggregated across studies, pointing to relatively robust effects of these particular programs.[41] School-based prevention programs implemented with fidelity to the original design of a program model are typically more effective at preventing violence than those implemented with less fidelity, likely because there is a reduction in the quality of implementation that occurs when programs stray from their original design.[41] In addition, program duration is also important; programs that continue over long periods of time generally produce more positive results with respect to a reduction in violence than do those of a shorter duration, all other factors being equal.

Family-based violence prevention approaches can include early childhood education, parent/caregiver training strategies, or programs to help build supports around families to lessen the burden of one or various stressors. Parent training programs are perhaps the most common in this domain. These programs focus on helping parents/caregivers develop the knowledge and skills to think constructively about their adolescent or young adult's behaviors, providing appropriate discipline, monitoring their whereabouts, and openly communicating with their adolescent or young adult to avoid hostile conflicts that can escalate to violence. Findings from systematic and meta-analytic reviews of well implement approaches are generally favorable.[36]

SUMMARY

There is a considerable amount of information on the scope, causes, and consequences of AYA violence and strategies to assess and prevent violence in young people. Understanding risk and protective factors related to violence provides a starting point for developing preventive interventions to reduce risks and enhance protection for youth at-risk, as well as those in the general population, so that patterns of violence that can occur within families, schools, and communities can be broken and lives saved as a result. Universal programs are necessary to attend to risks that all AYAs of a particular region or neighborhood experience, lessening the risk for violence by shifting broad social and environmental factors away from violence and toward more prosocial ways of relating. In addition, the use of evidence-based practices and programs in youth violence prevention is critical to addressing the problem and to reducing costs associated with ineffective, poorly implemented, and low-quality programs. For clinicians, having knowledge of which programs and approaches work best to prevent violence in real world settings is an important goal.[34]

REFERENCES

1. Centers for Disease Control and Prevention, N.C.f.I.P.a.C. Preventing youth violence factsheet. 2022. https://www.cdc.gov/violenceprevention/youthviolence/fastfact.html
2. World Health Organization. Youth violence. 2020 [cited 2020 July 22]; https://www.who.int/news-room/fact-sheets/detail/youth-violence#:~:text=Worldwide%20an%20estimated%20200%20000,people%20in%20this%20age%20group.&text=For%20example%2C%20one%20in%20eight,also%20common%20among%20young%20people
3. David-Ferdon C, Vivolo-Kantor AM, Dahlberg LL, et al. *A Comprehensive Technical Package for the Prevention of Youth Violence and Associated Risk Behaviors.* National Center for Injury Prevention and Control, Centers for Disease Control and Prevention; 2016.
4. Centers for Disease Control and Prevention, N.C.f.H.S. Compressed mortality file, 1999–2016, on CDC WONDER online database. 2017. https://wonder.cdc.gov/cmf-icd10.html
5. Cunningham RM, Walton MA, Carter PM. The major causes of death in children and adolescents in the United States. *N Engl J Med.* 2018;379:2468–2475.
6. Centers for Disease Control and Prevention. Web-based injury statistics query and reporting system (WISQARS). 2016. http://www.cdc.gov/injury/wisqars/
7. Carney JV. Perceptions of bullying and associated trauma during adolescence. *Professional School Counseling.* 2008;11(3):2156759X0801100304.
8. Turner HA, Shattuck A, Finkelhor D, et al. Polyvictimization and youth violence exposure across contexts. *J Adolesc Health.* 2016;58(2):208–214.
9. Woodrow Cox J, et al. More Than 240,000 Students Have Experienced Gun Violence at School Since Columbine. The Washington Post; 2021.
10. Centers for Disease Control and Prevention. Web-based Injury Statistics Query and Reporting System (WISQARS). 2019. https://webappa.cdc.gov/sasweb/ncipc/mortrate.html
11. Centers for Disease Control and Prevention, N.C.f.H.S. "Nonfatal Injury Reports 2000–2019" in Web-based Injury Statistics Query and Reporting System (WISQARS). 2019; Available from: https://webappa.cdc.gov/sasweb/ncipc/nfirates.html
12. Puzzanchera C, Chamberlin G, Kang W. Easy access to the FBI's supplementary homicide reports: 1980–2011. 2013.9.
13. Sheats KJ, Irving SM, Mercy JA, et al. Violence-related disparities experienced by Black youth and young adults: opportunities for prevention. *Am J Prev Med.* 2018;55(4):462–469.
14. Harrell E, *Black Victims of Violent Crime; Bureau of Justice Statistics Special Report.* United States Department of Justice, Office of Justice Programs; 2007.
15. Michigan.gov. Michigan executive order no. 2020-04. Michigan.gov. 2020.
16. Herrenkohl TI, Maguin E, Hill KG, et al. Developmental risk factors for youth violence. *J Adolesc Health.* 2000;26(3):176–186.
17. Ruback RB, Shaffer JN, Clark VA. Easy access to firearms: juveniles' risks for violent offending and violent victimization. *J Interpers Violence.* 2011;26(10):2111–2138.
18. Steffgen G, Recchia S, Viechtbauer W. The link between school climate and violence in school: a meta-analytic review. *Aggression and violent behavior.* 2013;18(2):300–309.
19. Schmidt CJ, Rupp L, Pizarro JM, et al. Risk and protective factors related to youth firearm violence: a scoping review and directions for future research. *J Behav Med.* 2019;42(4):706–723.
20. Herrenkohl TI, Fedina L, Roberto KA, et al. Child maltreatment, youth violence, intimate partner violence, and elder mistreatment: a review and theoretical analysis of research on violence across the life course. *Trauma Violence Abuse.* 2022;23(1):314–328.
21. Decker MR, Wilcox HC, Holliday CN, et al. An integrated public health approach to interpersonal violence and suicide prevention and response. *Public Health Rep.* 2018;133(1_suppl):65S–79S.
22. Kim YS, Leventhal B. Bullying and suicide. a review. *Int J Adolesc Med Health.* 2008;20(2):133–154.
23. Chassin L, Piquero AR, Losoya SH, et al. Joint consideration of distal and proximal predictors of premature mortality among serious juvenile offenders. *J Adolesc Health.* 2013;52(6):689–696.
24. Hawkins JD, Jenson JM, Catalano R, et al. Unleashing the power of prevention. *American Journal of Medical Research.* 2016;3(1):39–74.
25. Connor DF. *Clinical assessment, case formulation, and treatment planning. In: Connor DF, ed. Aggression and Antisocial Behavior in Children and Adolescents.* The Guilford Press; 2002:302–326.
26. McMahon RJ, Frick PJ. Evidence-based assessment of conduct problems in children and adolescents. *J Clin Child Adolesc Psychol.* 2005;34(3):477–505.
27. Borum R, Verhaagen DA. *Assessing and Managing Violence Risk in Juveniles.* The Guilford Press; 2006.
28. Augimeri LK, Walsh M, Enebrink P, et al. *Early Assessment Risk List for Boys: EARL-20B, Version 2.* Earlscourt Child and Family Centre; 2001.
29. Douglas KS, Hart SD, Webster CD, et al. *HCR-20V3: Assessing Risk for Violence: User Guide.* Mental Health, Law, and Policy Institute, Simon Fraser University; 2013.
30. Reddy LA, Goldstein AP., Aggression replacement training: a multimodal intervention for aggressive adolescents. *Residential Treatment for Children & Youth.* 2001;18(3):47–62.
31. Institute of Medicine, Mrazek PJ, Haggerty RJ. *Reducing Risks for Mental Disorders: Frontiers for Preventive Intervention Research. National Academies Press;* 1994.
32. Fagan AA, Catalano RF. What works in youth violence prevention: a review of the literature. *Research on social work practice.* 2013;23(2):141–156.
33. National Academies of Sciences, Engineering, and Medicine. *Promoting Positive Adolescent Health Behaviors and Outcomes: Thriving in the 21st Century.* N.F. Kahn and R. Graham, eds. National Academies Press; 2020.
34. Herrenkohl TI, Aisenberg E, Williams JH, et al. *Violence in Context: Current Evidence on Risk, Protection, and Prevention.* Oxford University Press; 2011.
35. Weiss B, Han S, Harris V, et al. An independent randomized clinical trial of multisystemic therapy with non-court-referred adolescents with serious conduct problems. *J Consult Clin Psychol.* 2013;81(6):1027–1039.
36. Jenson JM, Powell A, Forrest-Bank S., *Effective violence prevention approaches in school, family, and community settings. In:* Herrenkohl TI, Aisenberg E, Williams JH, et al, eds. *Violence in Context: Current Evidence on Risk, Protection, and Prevention.* Oxford University Press; 2011: 130–170.
37. Development Services Group, I., "Community-and problem-oriented policing." Literature review. 2010.
38. Arciaga M, Sakamoto W, Jones EF. *Responding to Gangs in the School Setting.* US Department of Justice, Bureau of Justice Assistance and Office of Juvenile Justice and Delinquency Prevention; 2010.
39. Boxer P. Negative peer involvement in multisystemic therapy for the treatment of youth problem behavior: exploring outcome and process variables in "real-world" practice. *J Clin Child Adolesc Psychol.* 2011;40(6):848–854.
40. Pyrooz DC, Decker SH. Motives and methods for leaving the gang: understanding the process of gang desistance. *Journal of Criminal Justice.* 2011;39(5): 417–425.
41. Wilson SJ, Lipsey MW. School-based interventions for aggressive and disruptive behavior: update of a meta-analysis. *Am J Prev Med.* 2007;33(2 Suppl):S130–S143.

ADDITIONAL RESOURCES AND WEBSITES

Additional Resources and Websites for Parents/Caregivers and Clinicians

Blueprints for Healthy Youth Development—https://www.blueprintsprograms.org/

CDC Youth Violence webpage—https://www.cdc.gov/violenceprevention/youthviolence/index.html

CDC Technical Package on Youth Violence—https://www.cdc.gov/violenceprevention/pdf/yv-technicalpackage.pdf

Futures Without Violence Start Strong Initiative—http://startstrong.futureswithoutviolence.org

National Center for School Safety—https://www.nc2s.org/

Additional Resources and Websites for Parents/Caregivers and Adolescents and Young Adults

Futures without Violence That's Not Cool webinar—public education effort on TDV—https://www.futureswithoutviolence.org/thats-not-cool-teen-dating-violence-healthy-relationships-digital-age/

Love is Respect (youth focused)—https://www.loveisrespect.org

XV

Evaluating and Supporting Adolescents and Young Adults Who Have Experienced Sexual Violence

Constance M. Wiemann
Elizabeth Miller
Mariam R. Chacko

KEY WORDS

- Forensic evaluation
- Prostitution
- Rape
- Sex trafficking
- Sexual abuse
- Sexual assault
- Sexual exploitation
- Survival sex
- Testifying
- Trafficking
- Victimization

INTRODUCTION

Sexual violence (SV) among adolescents and young adults (AYAs) is of particular concern because of its high prevalence in this population, its infrequent disclosure, and the significant health consequences associated with this type of violence. While SV is experienced by AYAs in cultures around the world, this chapter focuses on SV experienced by AYAs in the United States specifically. Rates of SV are higher among subpopulations including females, those experiencing poverty and unstable housing, and among gender nonconforming AYAs. A history of SV exposure not only makes it more difficult for individuals to develop healthy intimate relationships as adults, but it is also significantly associated with multiple negative health outcomes, including human immunodeficiency virus (HIV), sexually transmitted infections (STIs), unintended pregnancy, depression, anxiety, suicidal ideation, and substance use disorder.[1] Clinicians play a key role in prevention education, early identification of victims of SV, and prevention of subsequent negative health outcomes. Clinician-initiated routine discussion with all AYA patients about healthy sexual relationships and provision of SV-related resources can help prevent SV and facilitate disclosure. A trauma-informed, strength-based approach is recommended. Screening and reporting guidelines vary by state and there are established protocols for obtaining reliable medical and forensic evidence.

Definitions

The terms used to describe the range of experiences included in SV are sometimes used interchangeably, frequently unclear, and require definition. These labels have legal ramifications and reporting requirements that impact prevalence and incidence rates. Below is a summary of common terminology associated with SV:

- "Sexual assault" or "sexual violence" is an inclusive term that refers to any form of forced or inappropriate unwanted sexual contact. This would include, for example, situations in which the victim is unable to consent because of intoxication or inability to understand consequences.
- "Rape" is a legal term with a definition that varies widely. In general, this term implies unlawful nonconsensual sexual activity carried out forcibly or under threat of injury against the will of the victim. Nonconsensual sex is divided into two categories— *stranger rape* is perpetrated by a stranger and *acquaintance rape* is perpetrated by someone known to the individual. *Date rape*, occurring between two people in a romantic relationship or potential sexual relationship, is a subset of acquaintance rape.
- "Sexual abuse" typically refers to the sexual victimization of a minor and is primarily a legal term. In certain contexts, the term can include consensual sex between minors or a minor and an adult (*statutory rape*).
- "Sex trafficking," as it pertains to children and adolescents, includes trafficking a minor for the purpose of sexual exploitation, exploiting a minor through commercial sex, and exploiting a minor though survival sex.[2]
- "Transactional sex" typically refers to sex in exchange for money. For those who are minors, it is often called "commercial sexual exploitation of children."
- "Survival sex" is the exchange of sex for food, money, shelter, drugs, or other wants/needs.

Epidemiology

On average, more than 425,000 individuals ages 12 and older experience SV in the United States each year.[3] About two-thirds of sexual assaults are committed by someone the AYA knows. Risk factors for SV include female gender; history of abuse (sexual or other); alcohol use by perpetrator or victim, especially in a dating situation; and dating relationships that include verbal or physical abuse. Gender-specific risk factors include younger age at menarche, greater number of dating and/or sexual partners, and a sexually active peer group for females and homelessness and disability (physical, cognitive, psychiatric) for males.

Male SV is significantly underreported and male adolescents who have experienced SV are often overlooked and underserved. Since most perpetrators of SV against adolescent males are male themselves, these victims may remain silent due to the homosexual nature of the assault. In addition, clinicians may fail to recognize and pursue this possibility because of their lack of awareness of this problem.

Incidence

1. Rates of SV are four times higher among female-identified AYAs ages 16 to 24 years compared to females in all other age groups; across all age groups, Black and Hispanic females experience the highest rates of SV.[4]
2. About 6% of AYAs report that they have been forced to have sexual intercourse; among AYAs who identify as sexual minority (lesbian, gay, or bisexual), these percentages are about 19%.[5]

3. About 26% of females and about 5% of males will experience some form of SV before they turn 18 years.[6]
4. A vast majority of victimizations are perpetrated by peer acquaintances.
5. Adolescents ≤18 years who experience sexual victimization are twice as likely to experience a future assault during their college years.
6. In 2019, sexual abuse, SV that occurs among minors, accounted for almost 10% of all substantiated claims of child victimization, totaling 65,984 cases, 29 of which resulted in death.[7]

Sequelae

The occurrence of SV during childhood has been linked to a variety of psychological and emotional problems during adolescence, with some continuing into adulthood. Sequelae include depression, suicidal ideation and attempts, substance use, posttraumatic stress disorder (PTSD), eating disorders, and precocious sexual behaviors (e.g., earlier age at first coitus and greater number of lifetime partners). In addition, childhood sexual abuse for females has been linked to acquaintance and date rape in adolescence or young adulthood.

Sexual violence during adolescence can have long-lasting effects on one's sense of self-worth and identity. During adolescence, individuals learn to navigate feelings of sexual arousal, develop new forms of intimacy and autonomy, experience intimate interpersonal relationships, and build skills to consider and control consequences of sexual behavior. A first or early sexual experience involving SV may undermine a young person's confidence in negotiating sexual relationships, communicating consent, and making decisions. Adolescents and young adults with prior SV experiences often engage in higher-risk sexual behaviors, have poorer attitudes and beliefs regarding sex, and demonstrate a greater prevalence of consequences from sexual activity, that is, unintended pregnancies and STIs. They also experience significantly higher levels of anxiety, depression, suicidal ideation and attempts, and decreased life satisfaction.

The first 2 months following the SV experience is a time of particular vulnerability for severe depression. Signs of PTSD are common within the first year. Common responses to SV include phobias, self-blame, loss of appetite, sleep disturbances, somatic responses, and drug and alcohol use. Somatic responses can manifest as chronic pelvic pain or recurrent abdominal pain. Sequelae particular to date rape may include self-blame, decreased self-esteem, a difficult time maintaining relationships, and the potential for retraumatization by family, friends, and clinicians.

Indicators that should alert the clinician to suspect abuse include the following:

1. Sexually transmitted infections in a prepubertal adolescent or any adolescent with no history of sexual intercourse.
2. Recurrent somatic complaints, particularly involving the gastrointestinal, genitourinary, or pelvic areas.
3. Behavioral indicators, including significant changes in mood, withdrawal from usual family, school, and social activities; patterns of disordered eating; running away from home; suicidal and self-injurious gestures; rapid escalation of alcohol and/or drug abuse; onset of sexual activity before age 13 years; onset of promiscuous sexual activity; early adolescent pregnancy.

SEX TRAFFICKING

Sex trafficking of AYAs for prostitution and other forms of sexual exploitation is an often-overlooked form of SV. Sex trafficking of minors occurs globally and can lead to serious long-term consequences for victims as well as their families, communities, and society.[2] Sex trafficking can include commercial sex work (prostitution, exotic dancing, and pornography) as well as personal service (domestic or sexual servitude). This criminal endeavor is fast growing and is fueled by a growing demand by customers who pay for illicit sex. Female-identifying AYAs (including transfeminine and gender fluid young people) are a particularly vulnerable group for international and domestic sex trafficking.[8] Many traffickers now use online social medial platforms to recruit targets of trafficking.

Human trafficking victims, who tend to be younger than survivors of other forms of SV, are at increased risk for developing health problems due to substandard living conditions as well as physical, sexual, and emotional trauma. Risk factors or warning signs for possible sex trafficking include those for victims of other forms of SV (see Epidemiology above) as well as homelessness and/or chronic running away; presence of an older boyfriend or age disparity in an intimate or sexual relationship; tattoos (used to mark victim as property of a particular pimp); travel with an older male who is not a parent/caregiver; access to material things that the AYAs cannot afford; <18 years and involved in or history of prior prostitution; and not attending school, frequent absences, or academic failures. Sex trafficking is complicated by the fact that many adolescents are trafficked by individuals who they consider to be their boyfriend/girlfriend, fiancée, or lover. In fact, adolescents may continue to have an intimate relationship with their trafficker as they are trafficked.[2] For this reason, before asking the AYAs any sensitive questions, clinicians should ensure that patients are in a private, confidential space without accompanying persons in the examination room.

INCREASED RISK OF SEXUAL VIOLENCE AMONG POPULATIONS EXPERIENCING MARGINALIZATION

Marginalized populations experience discrimination and exclusion because of unequal power relationships across economic, political, social, and economic dimensions. Multiple structural inequities such as poverty, geographic isolation (including tribal reservations), unstable housing, and community violence increase vulnerability for exposure to SV. The prevalence of SV exposure is higher for certain groups including those who identify as Black, indigenous, and people of color. Systemic racism, intersecting with sexism, classism, homophobia, ableism, and transphobia, all contribute to spheres of marginalization that both increase the likelihood of exposure to SV and limited access to supports and resources. Furthermore, the health care system, social services, and law enforcement, due to longstanding histories of oppression, may not be perceived as safe or trustworthy by AYAs experiencing marginalization, resulting in limited care seeking and receipt of services (see Chapter 85).

Homeless/Street Adolescents and Young Adults

Rates of SV among AYAs who are unstably housed in the United States are also far greater than that of AYAs in the general population.[9] As the housing instability may be due to being pushed out the home and disrupted relationships with family and other social supports, AYAs who are homeless (including those who are living on the street, couch surfing or 'doubled up') are particularly vulnerable to SV, especially sex trafficking. This population is more likely to be offered money, drugs, shelter, or food for sex, increasing their risk for exploitation through survival sex. Although rates of survival sex in this population vary across studies, higher rates of engagement in survival sex are consistently reported by sexual and gender minority AYAs (who make up over a quarter of the unstably housed AYAs and young adult population) compared to heterosexual AYAs.[9] Decisions made by AYAs who are unhoused or living on the street about whether or not to seek care and report occurrences of SV are often compounded by limited trust in health and social service systems, low-perceived problem severity and barriers to access and engagement with health and support services (see Chapter 81).

XV

Lesbian, Gay, Bisexual, Transgender, Gender Diverse, and Gender Nonconforming Adolescents and Young Adults

There are significantly higher rates of childhood sexual abuse among individuals who identify as lesbian, gay, and bisexual (LGB).[1] Over the lifetime, gay and bisexual men were five times more likely to be sexually assaulted than heterosexual men, and lesbian and bisexual women were twice as likely to be assaulted than heterosexual women.[10] While most research suggests that there is no direct *causal* link between experiencing sexual abuse as a child and developing a nonheterosexual orientation in adulthood, recent studies have reported that there is a 25% to 50% higher prevalence rate of childhood sexual abuse among nonheterosexual individuals.[1] Sexual minority youth may experience polyvictimization in childhood and adolescence including greater bias-based discrimination and disproportionate exposure to family violence that may contribute to isolation, fewer supports, and greater vulnerability to SV exposure in adolescence and young adulthood (see Chapter 43).

"Transgender" is a term used to describe individuals whose gender identity is different from their sex assigned at birth. "Gender diverse" and "gender fluid" are more inclusive terms that recognize that AYAs may not perceive their gender identity or expression on a male/female binary. Gender identity and sexual orientation are two different constructs, and being transgender or gender fluid does not predict the gender(s) of the persons to whom they are sexually attracted. A large survey of transgender and nonbinary U.S. adolescents in Grades 7 to 12 revealed a 26.5% prevalence of sexual assault in the past year among transgender males, 27% among nonbinary youth assigned female at birth, 18.5% in transgender females and 17.6% in nonbinary youth assigned male at birth. Adolescents and young adults whose restroom and locker room use was restricted to their sex assigned at birth were more likely to experience SV compared with those without such restrictions.[11] (see Chapter 44).

Childhood gender nonconformity has been associated with increased prevalence of childhood sexual abuse, likely related to bias-based discrimination.[12] In addition to SV, children who are gender nonconforming in behavior or appearance may also be experiencing bullying, physical or emotional abuse at home, depressive symptoms, and other responses to victimization. Therefore, these children should be assessed not only for SV, but also for bullying, other types of abuse, and mental health concerns.[12]

Adolescents and Young Adults with Disabilities

Adolescents and young adults with disabilities are at significantly higher risk for SV than those without disabilities, and those with severe disabilities are at highest risk.[13] Factors that increase vulnerability of AYAs with disabilities to SV include decreased decision-making capacity, physical limitations, communication deficits, limited social networks, disempowerment of the disability community, poor or nonexistent sex education, misunderstanding of rights, and an increased volume of "touch" contact with others (especially if dependent on others for personal hygiene and basic care). Individuals with severe communication impairments might also experience extreme challenges when attempting to communicate their abuse to professionals. It is important to note that perpetrators of SV against AYAs with disabilities are often family members, acquaintances, service providers, personal care staff, mental health, or residential care staff. Therefore, speaking privately with AYAs who have disabilities is vital to ensure that AYAs are aware of their rights and resources available to them (see Chapter 76).

◉ SCREENING AND REPORTING

Healing-Centered Approaches to Sexual Violence Assessment and Support

Despite recommendations for routine, confidential assessment for SV among AYAs and evidence of acceptability of such discussions among AYAs seeking care, routine inquiry for SV does not occur, especially among sexual and gender minority youth. Clinician-initiated routine discussion with all AYA patients about healthy sexual relationships and provision of SV-related resources represents an important public health strategy to overcome the difficulty that some AYAs face when disclosing these violent events. Most of the SV that clinicians will encounter when treating AYAs has been perpetrated by an acquaintance, date, or a significant other. As a result, spontaneous disclosure by the AYA experiencing SV is not likely because AYAs may not perceive what happened as sexual assault, are embarrassed, fear the consequences of disclosure, or believe it is their own fault. Confidentiality, universal education, empowerment, and support (CUES) is a research-informed approach that shifts away from disclosure-driven practice and prioritizes offering information and resources about SV and healthy relationships to all AYAs during clinical encounters.[14] Encouraging AYAs to share this information with people they know normalizes the conversation and creates opportunities for empowering them to help others in their social network (see Chapter 4).

Information about a SV experience may be revealed in the emergency room in close proximity to the sexual assault or it may be revealed weeks, months, or years after the assault. This lapse leaves clinicians with an obligation to inquire about past and present SV experiences in as sensitive a manner as possible, focusing less on disclosure and more about providing information and support in a nonstigmatizing and welcoming way. Asking AYAs about their strengths and social supports can enhance resiliency while building a trusting relationship. A trauma-informed, strength-based approach to assessment is recommended. This approach shifts the focus from "What's wrong with you?" to "What happened to you"? This approach helps to reduce stigma and establish discussion of healthy relationships as a normal part of clinical practice.[15] Identifying a safe, supportive adult with whom they can communicate is important for all AYAs. Adolescents and young adult without a caring adult, or those whose access to one is limited (i.e., a parent who is incarcerated, a young person who is unstably housed), should be offered additional connections to an AYA-serving community mentor and additional supports.

Information pamphlets designed to help AYAs learn about dating and SV or to increase awareness of sexual health are helpful. Some clinicians also find *anticipatory guidance,* a conversation centering on sexual health and signs of healthy relationships can help promote AYA resiliency and serve AYA needs. Within the patient/clinician conversation, AYAs should be provided with *accurate information* about the help they can receive from their social network, protective agencies, victim service agencies (including rape crisis centers), and AYA-relevant hotlines. See for example, https://www.futureswithoutviolence.org/hanging-out-or-hooking-up-teen-safety-card/.[16]

It is recommended that the discussion around sexuality and violence exposure always takes place in *a private, quiet space* where only the clinician and the AYA are present. The concept of *limited confidentiality* should be introduced to the patient in a manner that conveys the legal obligations of the clinician, should any disclosure occur. Some clinicians choose to use a direct but nonthreatening statement similar to,

> "Generally, what you say in here stays in here, but there are some exceptions. If I feel that you may hurt yourself or someone else, or that you have been abused by someone, I will need to talk to others to help make sure you get all the care you need."

Special attention must be paid to communicate with transgender and gender diverse AYAs (see Chapter 44).

An example of an icebreaker that prepares the AYA for some of the questions they will be asked is,

"Because I want to help my patients, I talk to all my patients about topics that may be sensitive or may make you uncomfortable. Here is some information about healthy relationships that I would like to review with you, if you would like? Some young adults come to my office having been hurt by people around them, and I want to make sure that all young people have the right information and know that this is a safe place to talk about things like this."

While disclosure is not the goal, a clinician can follow providing universal education about healthy relationships and SV resources with: "Is any of this part of your story?"

Consistently asking AYAs about their sexual health, even if negative answers were received in prior instances, can allow for this part of the examination to become routine.

Reporting

Sexual violence disclosure requires prompt medical and psychological intervention. When a forensic examination is needed, clinicians who are willing to devote the time and support needed (and have received appropriate training or have ready access to a trained professional) should examine the patient. The clinician should be familiar with trauma-sensitive practices and appropriate protocols for intervention, including client-centered clinical care, connection to advocacy supports, and legal requirements.

The following professional guidelines have been endorsed regarding assessment for and reporting of sexual victimization of adolescents.[15,17]

1. Sexual activity and sexual abuse are not synonymous. It should not be assumed that adolescents under the age of 18 years who are sexually active are, by definition, being abused. In addition, the age of consent for sex varies from state to state.
2. Physicians and other clinicians must know the laws in their geographic areas and report cases of sexual abuse to the proper authority (i.e., child welfare and/or law enforcement) after discussion with the adolescent (and parent/caregiver as appropriate). Whenever possible, the adolescent should be present and participate in completing reports to the relevant authorities so that they can help guide a safer and supportive response.
3. In the United States, federal and state laws should affirm the authority of physicians and other clinicians to exercise appropriate clinical judgment in reporting cases of sexual abuse.

LEGAL ISSUES RELATED TO REPORTING OF SEXUAL VIOLENCE

In the United States, every state mandates reporting of a reasonable suspicion of child abuse, including sexual abuse, to a designated authority. Mandated reporters of child abuse include virtually all clinicians involved in the care of adolescents under the age of 18 years. In addition, reporting is required when there is reasonable suspicion of a vulnerable young adult being sexually abused. A "vulnerable adult" is a person 18 years or older whose ability to perform the normal activities of daily living or to provide for his or her own care or protection is impaired due to a mental, emotional, physical, or developmental disability. The abuse does not need to be proven before being reported; failure to report can result in civil liability or criminal penalties.

An area of potential confusion and controversy is the reporting of "statutory rape." Although this term does not appear in most states' laws, it is generally used to refer to sexual intercourse that is illegal even if it is consensual, and can refer either to sexual contact between two minors or between a minor and an adult. There are a variety of considerations that can have a bearing on when sexual activity, especially in a young adolescent, must be reported. These include use of coercion or pressure, force or threat of force, or a wide age difference between partners even if the adolescent and parent(s)/caregiver(s) consider the current relationship consensual and nonabusive. It is essential that clinicians consult their local legal and medical authorities regarding laws for their state and be aware of their institution's policies.

EVALUATION OF SEXUAL ABUSE AND ASSAULT: MEDICAL AND FORENSIC ASPECTS[18]

Medical Evaluation

Facilitating an Appropriate Medical Evaluation

The AYA will need to consent to the specific purpose and procedures involved in the medical evaluation, including the steps of evidence collection for a rape kit. The age at which an AYA has the ability to consent legally to a forensic medical examination varies by state.[19] Young adults have the right to refuse any or all parts of the examination. The AYA may want to have *a family member or friend* present. The clinician can help the AYA regain a sense of control over their body by encouraging the AYA to make decisions during the examination. It is crucial that the AYA be informed that he or she is in control of what will be done and can refuse treatment or stop the examination.

A physical injury that requires immediate attention takes priority over the examination for evidence collection. Most jurisdictions define "acute" to reflect an event that occurred in the past 72 hours and some as far out as 7 to 10 days.[18] The medical evaluation must reliably obtain medical and forensic evidence and the knowledge based on the findings must be interpreted in an expert form so as to provide a legal defense regardless of whether a rape kit has been completed. Medical professionals who conduct a forensic examination must have advanced training and clinical experience and are advised to use a team approach to providing trauma-centered care.[20] Sexual assault nurse examiner (SANE) programs provide prompt access to emergency medical care by providing a dedicated examination room, a specially trained forensic examiner who is competent in collection of evidence for the investigation, expert witnesses, and a collaborative team approach. Sexual assault nurse examiner programs also provide synchronous telehealth consultation services to clinicians with high patient consent for a SANE on a video-monitor during the examination.[21]

Individual jurisdictions determine the maximum time interval (36 hours to 1 week) in which evidence may be collected. Changing clothes, showering, and brushing teeth can change the yield of the forensic examination. If the AYA declines a forensic examination, a speculum examination to obtain STI tests should not be undertaken until after 96 hours as a speculum examination conducted prior to forensic work will call into question the accuracy of evidence that may later be collected.

General Physical and Anogenital Trauma—Gender-Specific Considerations

Females[22-24]

* Findings of physical or extragenital trauma (extremities, head, and trunk) are three times more common than genital trauma in AYAs. Strangulation has been identified as a lethality indicator in interpersonal violence.
* Genital injury is significantly more likely to be seen in adolescents 13 to 17 years who have no prior history of sexual activity (52%) versus those with a prior history (19%). These injuries are more frequently located on the hymen, labia minora, posterior fourchette, and fossa navicularis and less frequently on the clitoris, vagina, urethra, labia majora, and cervix. The most common genital injuries in adults are small lacerations in the posterior fourchette. Evidence of such injuries is more likely to be identified the earlier the examination occurs.
* Complete hymenal clefts with no evidence of acute injury are not commonly associated with tampon use. No hymenal changes

have been seen with gymnastics, horseback riding, and other vigorous sports. Possible explanations for a single cleft (between the 4 to 8 o'clock position) are painful or difficult insertion in adolescent females from consensual sexual intercourse, tampon use, digital or object penetration during masturbation or by a partner, and childhood accidental injury. Two or more hymenal clefts are more likely to be explained by sexual intercourse. Thus, clinicians should interpret data to the court in the context of recent history of damage or healing. When the history is long in the past, the information should be reviewed with other corroboratory evidence with adequate and detailed history.

- Estrogen affects the adolescent hymen by making it elastic and thereby permitting penile penetration without tearing. Therefore, while posterior hymenal clefts strongly suggest trauma to the area, absence of hymenal clefts should not exclude the possibility of penile–vaginal penetration.

Males[25,26]

- Evidence of trauma is reported in 20% to 37% of adolescent male sexual abuse/assault survivors. Injuries to AYA males have been characterized as mild (46%), moderate (10%), and serious (1.4%). About 42% have no evidence of general body injuries. The most common body injury sites in order of frequency are arm, head, torso, legs, mouth, and neck.
- Most injuries from abuse and assault involve the anus, rectum, and penis with significantly fewer injuries occurring in the perineum, scrotum, or testes. Anal penetration is most commonly from penetration of a penis; penetration from a finger(s) and other objects are also reported. Stranger assaults are more likely to result in anal injuries. Complete anal penetration results in lacerations, injury of the anal canal, perianal injury, and bruising. Anal and rectal lacerations from sexual abuse or assault tend to be located at the 1, 5, 7, and 11 o'clock positions. Complete oral penetration can result in oral injuries including bruising of the soft palate and mixed injuries of the rest of the mouth.

Transgender and Gender Diverse Adolescents and Young Adults

- There is limited published information on the types of physical injuries sustained by transgender and gender diverse AYAs as a result of SV. Examinations and findings should be based on the patient's current anatomy. Transgender AYAs may experience discomfort during a physical examination because of ongoing dysphoria or negative past experiences. The pelvic examination may be a traumatic and anxiety-inducing procedure in transgender males and other transmasculine persons. Therefore, a supportive chaperone should be provided.
- Patients who are taking gender-affirming medications and/or have undergone surgeries may have varying physical examination findings depending on the procedures performed. The anatomy of a neovagina created in a postoperative transgender female is a blind cuff, lacks a cervix or surrounding fornices, and may have a more posterior orientation. Using an anoscope may be a more anatomically appropriate approach for a visual examination. Transgender males who still have ovaries and a uterus can become pregnant even when on testosterone and/or not menstruating. Thus, emergency contraception should be considered.

Facilitating Appropriate Forensic Procedures[27]

The *rape kit* enables collection of evidence such as semen, saliva, clothing, and debris for forensic examination. The earlier an examination is performed, the more likely the evidence of trauma will be noted. Some jurisdictions, particularly those in rural and remote areas, are beginning to use interactive video consultation to support examiners conducting examinations.[28]

The availability of deoxyribonucleic acid (DNA) amplification technology using polymerase chain reaction (PCR) is now used to identify assailants more accurately and allows for collection

of evidence up to five days after the assault and possibly longer.[28] Research on the time frames for evidence collection based on the type of assault has shown: vaginal up to 120 hours; anal up to 72 hours; oral up to 24 hours and; bite marks/saliva on skin up to 96 hours.[27] As consensus on time limitations for forensic evidence is lacking, it is best to consult individual jurisdictions to determine the maximum time interval in which evidence may be collected.

Photography

The Department of Justice recommends photographs to supplement forensic documentation as they record significant genital injuries and fresh trauma (e.g., bloody tears and complete hymenal clefts) that can change due to healing. If photographs are taken, written consent must be obtained, the procedure explained, and photographs taken in a sensitive manner. Forensic protocols on patient identification procedures, correct camera date, number and orientation of shots, ruler for size reference, and a secure and legal filing and storage system should be in place. Photographs should be taken prior to collection of specimens but are not a substitute for notes and diagrams. Photographs should be well composed, in focus, with most of the picture filled with the injury in question. In addition, the image should correspond closely to the description provided by the examiner. Findings such as erythema, swelling, or small labial tears are too subtle and may not be visualized by photographs.

Conducting the Medical History

Key features of conducting the medical history are identified in Table 78.1.

Physical Examination

Prior to examining the AYA, the examiner should provide a step-by-step explanation of the procedure to be followed and why, with reassurance that the AYA will be in control. The AYA may request someone to be present during the physical examination. If an evidence collection kit is to be completed, written consent is needed for the forensic examination, treatment, collection of evidence, and release of medical records. Collection of legally mandated tests for the rape kit has to be synchronized with the general physical examination, pelvic or genital examination, and hospital laboratory tests. It is important to maintain eye contact with the patient throughout the examination. Proceed slowly with verbal directions to allow the patient to relax.

General Physical Findings

- Record the AYA's general appearance, orientation, emotional state, and behavior.

TABLE 78.1

Conducting the Medical History

- A brief description of the incident including body parts touched, orifices penetrated, the geographic location of the assault, identity of the assailant or alleged perpetrator (if known), whether a condom was used, whether any bleeding was noted from contact sites at the time of the assault, and method by which the assailant left the scene.
- Whether a weapon was used and any injuries sustained at the time of attack.
- Whether any illicit drugs or alcohol were used voluntarily or involuntarily (the latter may have been used to render the victim helpless and develop memory loss).
- For biologic females, date of last menses and use of sanitary pads and/or tampons.
- Date and time of last voluntary and involuntary coitus and other recent sexual experiences.
- History of previous STIs, prior pregnancy, and use of contraception.
- Any significant actions after alleged assault, such as showering or douching, rinsing of mouth, and brushing of teeth.

- Observe and document the condition of the AYA's clothing.
- Explore all areas of the body for signs of trauma, especially at the neck, breasts, upper arms, where petechiae and bruises resulting from forced restraint are apt to appear.
- Observe for hoarseness and examine the throat.
- Check for abdominal crepitus; this may signify vaginal or rectal laceration with intra-abdominal bleeding.
- Conduct a genital examination for evidence of trauma.

Genital, Pelvic, and Rectal Examination

- Position: A pelvic examination on AYA is performed in the lithotomy position. Young and petite adolescent females and males can be examined in the knee-chest position for easier visualization of the anogenital area. The anal area in the larger and older male AYAs should be visualized with the AYAs lying in the lateral position and with one or both knees flexed.
- External genitalia: Note and record signs of blood secretions and sites of bruising, hematoma, ecchymoses, abrasions, lacerations and redness, and swelling in the external genitalia, including the hymen. Application of toluidine blue in the female will highlight local injuries of the fossa navicularis, posterior fourchette, and hymenal membrane. While this technique is not accepted by all the U.S. jurisdictions, it has not been found to interfere with DNA analysis. Colposcopic examination can enhance the ability to visualize milder genital trauma.
- Hymen: The hymen can be observed by using a cotton applicator swab moistened with water. Gently stretch the hymen all around to clearly define any partial or complete fresh hymenal tears and the amount of hymenal tissue present, especially at the 6 o'clock position of the posterior rim where acute hymenal tears are more likely to be found. The absence of tears does not rule out previous penetration; therefore, the term "intact" hymen should be avoided.
- Anus: When anal penetration is reported in cisgender or transgender females or males, the perianal and anal area need to be inspected carefully for swelling with bluish discoloration consistent with bruising (not hemorrhoids), sphincter tears, fissures, scars, and distortion of the anus. Recurrent anal penetration should be suspected when there is marked anal laxity with distortion and dilatation. This observation is made when stool is absent in the vault. However, currently there is no consensus on the significance of anal laxity. An anoscopy or a proctoscopy is recommended when internal trauma and pathology (warts) are suspected. Internal trauma should be suspected when rectal bleeding, fever, or signs of an acute abdomen are present.
- Internal examination: An internal pelvic and rectal examination must be performed if there is pain, bleeding, a history of vaginal or rectal penetration, or signs of injury. A primary responsibility of the clinician is to avoid further trauma to the patient in performing this part of the examination. General anesthesia may be indicated. In the young peripubertal adolescent, a small-sized metal speculum is preferred for easier insertion and visualization. Injuries such as ecchymoses and tears to the vagina and cervix must be noted.

  Treatment for all significant trauma, including soft tissue injury as well as injury to the genital area, should precede collection of medicolegal information.
- Description of injuries: Injuries such as abrasions, bruises, bite marks and lacerations, stab wounds or gunshot wounds must be described by site, size, depth, border, shape, pattern, surrounding tissue, color, content (any foreign material in the would like glass or dirt), and any evidence of healing. Without accurate documentation and expert interpretation of injuries, any conclusions drawn about how injuries occurred might be seriously flawed. This will have profound consequences for both the victim and the accused.

Collection of Specimens—Rape Kit[27]

- To avoid compromising evidence, maintain the "chain of evidence" when collecting forensic specimens by strictly following jurisdictional policies, rape kit protocols, and instructions.
- Use a maximum of two swabs per site to concentrate and recover foreign DNA material.
- Legally mandated tests for evidence collection for DNA testing include specimen collection from various parts of the body. To reduce contamination of DNA, masks and nonpowdered gloves should be used by all those involved in the collection and packaging of evidence.
- After evidence for the kit is collected, the sealed box is handed over to a police officer according to legal procedure. The time limit given for this transfer varies by state.

Hospital Laboratory Tests

Table 78.2 describes specific laboratory tests that may be required based on findings from the genital, pelvic. and rectal examination.

Interpretation of Findings

An approach to interpreting findings in the pubertal child and mature adolescent can also be applied to young adults with no prior history of sexual activity. Adolescents and young adults with prior sexual activity may have evidence of trauma.

- Findings that are diagnostic of sexual abuse/assault[29]: Pregnancy that correlates with the date of the assault and semen identified in forensic specimens taken directly from the victim.
- Infections transmitted by sexual contact[30]: Genital, rectal, or pharyngeal *Neisseria gonorrhoeae* infection; syphilis, genital or rectal *Chlamydia trachomatis* infection; *Trichomonas vaginalis* infection; and HIV, provided transmission by blood transfusion has been ruled out.

TABLE 78.2

Laboratory Tests that May Be Required Based on Findings from the Genital, Pelvic and Rectal Examinations

- Sexually transmitted infection tests: Trichomoniasis, bacterial vaginosis, chlamydia, and gonorrhea are the most common infections identified in a survivor of sexual assault. Nucleic acid amplification tests for chlamydia and gonorrhea infection should be obtained from the endocervix, rectum, and pharynx. Nucleic acid amplification tests are also available and acceptable for trichomonas in many settings.
- Wet mount of vaginal secretions should be prepared and examined for evidence of trichomonas, bacterial vaginosis, and candidiasis. If sperm are identified, the laboratory technician validates these findings with the examiner and/or a senior pathologist. The forensic examiner does not do the wet mount to detect sperm.
- Urine pregnancy test should be conducted on all peripubertal and postmenarcheal females and preoperative transgender males.
- A serum sample should be obtained for (1) syphilis serology as a baseline test and repeated within 6–8 wks; (2) Human immunodeficiency virus antibody/antigen (depending on the test available) at baseline and repeated at 4–6 wks, 3 mo, and 6 mo; and (3) hepatitis B surface antigen and antibody.
- Routine toxicology screen is not recommended. However, the circumstances where urine or blood testing would be indicated include medical condition (including lack of recollection of events) suggesting alcohol or drug ingestion and reports from accompanying peers or adults that the victim may have been drugged. Date-rape drugs, such as flunitrazepam and other commonly prescribed benzodiazepines and antihistamines, may not be included in standard drug screening panels. If use is suspected the clinician must contact the laboratory to inquire about the test to order.
- Laboratory specimens from genitalia in a transgender person may cause confusion for laboratory personnel. State clearly that samples provided are indeed from a vagina in a transgender male who has retained their birth name.

- Injuries indicative of acute or healed trauma to the genital/anal tissues[30]: Bruising, petechiae, or abrasions on the hymen or acute laceration of the hymen; partial or complete vaginal laceration; perianal lacerations with exposure of tissues below the dermis; healed hymenal transaction/complete hymen cleft, defined as a defect in the hymen between 4 o'clock and 8 o'clock that extends to the base of the hymen, with no hymenal tissue discernible at that location, and a defect in the posterior (inferior) half of the hymen wider than the transaction with an absence of hymenal tissue extending to the base of the hymen.

Management

Clinicians must be sensitive to the likelihood of gastrointestinal side effects that can occur from multiple oral medications prescribed following a sexual assault evaluation. Treatment should begin with emergency contraception and intramuscular medication for gonorrhea. Medications for other common STIs can begin after the emergency contraception regimen is completed.

- Patient instructions for managing any injuries including those to the genital area.
- Tetanus toxoid 0.5 mL intramuscularly (IM) (plus tetanus immune globulin if dirty wound) is indicated for severe or penetrating trauma.
- Sexually transmitted infection prophylaxis: Since compliance with follow-up visits is poor, prophylactic treatment for gonorrhea, chlamydia, and trichomonas infections should be provided. Recommended regimens include ceftriaxone 500 mg IM in a single dose (1 g IM in persons weighing >150 kg) *plus* doxycycline 100 mg orally twice a day for 7 days *plus* metronidazole 500 mg orally twice a day for 7 days.[29] For penicillin allergy, a single 240-mg IM dose of gentamicin *plus* a single 2-g oral dose of azithromycin is an option. The 7-day treatment regimen is better than a single dose of metronidazole.
- Prevention of pregnancy: Emergency contraception must be offered in all postmenarcheal females (including transmasculine individuals who have a uterus) and may be provided without a speculum examination as long as the pregnancy test at the acute forensic visit is negative. If the AYA has not been using prescription methods of contraception, emergency contraception within 5 days of an incident should be discussed. A single-dose 30-mg tablet of ulipristal acetate (Ella) is approved by the U.S. Food and Drug Administration (FDA) for emergency contraception within 5 days of an incident. The levonorgestrel (progestin-only) pill (1.5 mg) is approved by the FDA for emergency contraception within 3 days of an incident: Plan B One Step (1.5-mg single-dose levonorgestrel) and other generic formulations (My Way, Take Action, Next Choice One Dose), which are available over the counter are preferred. Currently there are no official statements by national organizations on decreased effectiveness of Plan B in females with a BMI is >30 kg/m², as the data are limited and conflicting.[31] If a clinician has concerns, the most practical option is Ulipristal acetate (Ella). Although the copper intrauterine device (Cu-IUD) is the most effective method of emergency contraception, immediate access and placement would be a challenge. If ulipristal acetate is not readily available, Plan B is the only option and should be recommended. Doubling the dose of Plan B dose for females with obesity is not recommended. When hospitals and physicians do not offer or prescribe emergency contraception on religious and ethical grounds, the clinician should refer the young person to a hospital or a physician that does dispense or prescribe emergency contraception.
- Hepatitis B infection: The Centers for Disease Control and Prevention (CDC) recommend postexposure hepatitis B vaccine without hepatitis B immune globulin (HBIG) at the initial examination if the vaccine has not been received previously. Empiric treatment for hepatitis B with HBIG following sexual assault is controversial. Its efficacy in AYAs who are already immunized against hepatitis B infection is unknown.

- Human papillomavirus vaccine: The vaccine is recommended in all AYAs with any history of SV if they have not received or completed the series.
- Human immunodeficiency virus post exposure prophylaxis (PEP): It is difficult to discuss PEP issues in the acutely traumatized survivor, and while HIV seroconversion has occurred in persons whose only risk factor is SV, the frequency is low. The medical decision to recommend PEP is based on (1) the likelihood that the assailant has HIV; (2) any exposure characteristics that might increase risk for HIV transmission; (3) the time lapsed after the event; and (4) the potential benefits and risks associated with PEP. Determination of HIV status of the assailant at the time of the examination is determined on a case-by-case basis. The CDC recommends the following approach to the risk assessment: (1) whether the assailant is a male who has sex with males, uses injection drugs, or crack cocaine; (2) the local epidemiology of HIV/AIDS; and (3) exposure characteristics of the assault.
- Exposure characteristics of the assault when HIV status of the assailant is unknown involves whether (1) vaginal or anal penetration occurred; (2) ejaculation occurred on mucous membranes; (3) multiple assailants were involved; (4) mucosal lesions were present on the assailant or the victim; or (5) any other characteristics of the assault, victim, or the assailant that might increase risk for HIV transmission. Consult a specialist in HIV treatment in your local area if PEP is considered.
- Post exposure prophylaxis is best started within 4 hours of the assault and should not be started after 72 hours post sexual assault (see Chapter 36).
- If the AYA is eligible for PEP, discuss antiretroviral prophylaxis, including toxicity and unknown efficacy.
- Compliance with PEP is reported to be low (15% to 25%). Therefore, a family's ability to fill the prescription, obtain and afford medication refills, and keep follow-up appointments must be an integral part of starting PEP. Family support and follow-up by a social worker should be a standard of care.
- If the AYA accepts PEP, the best approach would be to provide enough medication to last until the follow-up appointment in 3 to 7 days to assess tolerance of medication. Baseline complete blood count and serum chemistry should be obtained.
- Sleep aids: Over-the-counter medication, such as diphenhydramine, hydroxyzine, and melatonin, and behavioral strategies to help with sleep hygiene have been recommended. Prescription medication may be needed if the above strategies do not work.
- Medical follow-up: An appointment with a clinician with expertise in sexual assault medical follow-up should be scheduled as indicated or within 14 to 21 days after the assault. A follow-up examination has been reported to change the interpretation of trauma likelihood in 15% of AYAs who have experienced SV, and 5% were diagnosed with a new STI. A third visit may be scheduled at 8 to 12 weeks to repeat initial serologic studies, including tests for syphilis, hepatitis B, or HIV infection. The AYA should also be followed and evaluated for psychological symptoms (i.e., PTSD, depression, and/or anxiety). Clinicians should determine the appropriate supports and treatment required.
- Written materials: Written materials regarding victims' rights, the rape experience, reporting rape, feelings about rape, and special reactions (the teenage victim, male victim, and the disabled victim) should be given before leaving the hospital. Clinicians can obtain this information from websites and their local District Attorney's Office. In addition, many urban centers have resources and organizations dedicated to providing support for sexual assault victims, but tend to be adult focused.

The Legal Investigative Process and Outcomes[32]

The effort to prosecute sexual assault perpetrators has its own requirements. A single, dedicated individual who can ensure an unbroken chain of evidence during the forensic examination and is able to follow through with detailed, immediate documentation is essential for providing factual testimony in court.[20] The clinician conducting the medical and forensic examination should anticipate that they may be called to testify if a case is prosecuted.

Due to disclosure barriers and insufficient evidence, only a small proportion of cases involving AYAs move to prosecution and about 50% of those result in conviction or guilty plea. Adolescent minors with caregivers who are supportive of the case moving forward are more likely to have the case investigated and prosecuted. Among adults, severe assaults are prosecuted more vigorously, which suggest the strongest cases move through the legal system. A witness assistance program can help victims navigate through the legal process.

Some males experience an erection and ejaculation while being sexually assaulted, which can be misrepresented by a jury as evidence that they somehow consented or enjoyed the experience. Erections are not under voluntary control and can be provoked by a reflex reaction during high anxiety or anal stimulation. This type of interpretation discourages disclosure and can promote feelings of guilt.

SUMMARY

Structural inequities such as poverty, geographic isolation, unstable housing, and community violence increase vulnerability for exposure to SV, with females of all race and ethnic groups and gender nonconforming AYAs experiencing highest rates overall. Clinicians should be familiar with trauma-sensitive practices and appropriate protocols for intervention, including client-centered clinical care, connection to advocacy supports, and legal reporting requirements. Medical and physical examinations should follow established protocols to reliably obtain medical and forensic evidence. Medical professionals who conduct a forensic examination must have advanced training and clinical experience and are advised to use a team approach to providing trauma-centered care.

ACKNOWLEDGMENTS

The authors wish to acknowledge Vaughn I. Rickert, PsyD and Dillon J. Etter, PA-C for their contributions to a previous version of this chapter.

REFERENCES

1. Walker MD, Hernandez AM, Davey MP. Childhood sexual abuse and adult sexual identity formation: intersection of gender, race, and sexual orientation. *Am J Fam Ther.* 2012;40:385–398.
2. Clayton E, Krugman R, Simon P. *Confronting Commercial Sexual Exploitation and Sex Trafficking of Minors in the United States.* National Academies Press; 2014.
3. Department of Justice, Office of Justice Programs, Bureau of Justice Statistics. *Criminal Victimization in the United States, 2019 Statistical Tables.* Accessed April 1, 2021.
4. Centers for Disease Control and Prevention. Web-based injury statistics query and reporting system (WISQARS) (Online), 2019.
5. Centers for Disease Control and Prevention. Youth Risk Behavior Surveillance-United States, 2019. *MMWR* 2019;69(1):1–88.
6. Finkelhor D, Shattuck A, Turner HA, et al. The lifetime prevalence of child sexual abuse and sexual assault assessed in late adolescence. *J Adolesc Health.* 2014;55(3):329–333.
7. US Department of Health and Human Services. Administration for children and families. Administration on children youth and families. Children's bureau. Child maltreatment 2019. Accessed March 30, 2021. http://acf.hhs.gov/cb/report/child-maltreatment-2019
8. U.S. Department of Justice. National Strategy to Combat Human Trafficking. 2017. Accessed March 30, 2021. https://www.justice.gov/humantrafficking/page/file/922791/download
9. Heerde J, Scholes-Balog KE, Hemphill SA. Associations between youth homelessness, sexual offenses, sexual victimization, and sexual risk behaviors: a systematic literature review. *Arch Sex Behav.* 2015;44(1):181–212.
10. Balsam KF, Rothblum ED, Beauchaine TP. Victimization over the life span: a comparison of lesbian, gay, bisexual, and heterosexual siblings. *J Consult Clin Psychol.* 2005;73(3):477–487.
11. Murchison GR, Agenor M, Reisner SL, et al. School restroom and locker room restrictions and sexual assault risk among transgender youth. *Pediatrics.* 2019;143(6):e20182902.
12. Roberts AL, Rosario M, Corliss HL, et al. Childhood gender nonconformity: a risk indicator for childhood abuse and posttraumatic stress in youth. *Pediatrics.* 2012;129(3):410–417.
13. Harrell E. *Crime Against Persons With Disabilities, 2009–2015—Statistical Tables.* Bureau of Justice Statistics, US Department of Justice; 2017.
14. Miller E, McCaw B. Intimate Partner Violence. *N Engl J Med.* 2019;380(9): 850–857.
15. The American College of Obstetricians and Gynecologists, Sexual Assault, Committee Opinion, Number 777. April 2019. Accessed January 23, 2021. https://www.acog.org/clinical/clinical-guidance/committee-opinion/articles/2019/04/sexual-assault
16. FUTURES without violence. Hanging out or hooking up: Teen safety card. https://www.futureswithoutviolence.org/hanging-out-or-hooking-up-teen-safety-card/.
17. American Academy of Family Physicians, American Academy of Pediatrics, American College of Obstetricians and Gynecologists, and Society for Adolescent Medicine. Protecting adolescents: ensuring access to care and reporting sexual activity and abuse. *J Adolesc Health* 2004;35:420–423.
18. Crawford-Jakubiak JE, Alderman EM, Leventhal JM, et al. Care of the adolescent after an acute sexual assault. *Pediatrics.* 2017;139(3):e20164243.
19. Center for Adolescent Health and the Law. *State Minor Consent Laws: A Summary.* 3rd ed. Center for Adolescent Health and the Law; 2010. Accessed January 22, 2021. www.freelists.org/archives/hilac/02-2014/pdftRo8tw89mb.pdf
20. U.S. Department of Justice Office on Violence Against Women. National training standards for sexual assault medical forensic examiners. 2nd ed. August 2018. Accessed February 2, 2021. https://www.ncjrs.gov/pdffiles1/ovw/213827.pdf
21. Walsh WA, Meunier-Sham J, Re C. Using Ttelehealth for sexual assault forensic examinations: a process evaluation of a national pilot project. *J Forensic Nurs.* 2019;15(3):152–162.
22. Emans SJ, Woods ER, Allred EN, et al. Hymenal findings in adolescent women: impact of tampon use and consensual sexual activity. *J Pediatr.* 1994;125(1):153–160.
23. Goodyear-Smith F, Laidlaw TM. Can tampon use cause hymen changes in girls who have not had sexual intercourse? A review of the literature. *Forensic Sci Int* 1998;94(1-2):147–153.
24. Zilkens RR, Smith DA, Phillips MA, et al. Genital and anal injuries: a cross-sectional Australian study of 1266 women alleging recent sexual assault. *Forensic Sci Int.* 2017;275:195–202.
25. Kadish HA, Schunk JE, Britton H. Pediatric male rectal and genital trauma: accidental and nonaccidental injuries. *Pediatr Emerg Care.* 1998;14(2):95–98.
26. Zilkens RR, Smith DA, Mukhtar SA, et al. Male sexual assault: physical injury and vulnerability in 103 presentations. *J Forensic Leg Med.* 2018;58:145–151.
27. U.S. Department of Justice, Office of Justice Programs, National institute of Justice. National best practices for sexual assault kits: a multidisciplinary approach, August 2016. https://www.ojp.gov/pdffiles1/nij/250384.pdf. Accessed January 22, 2021.
28. US Department of Justice Office on Violence Against Women. A national protocol on the sexual assault medical forensic examinations, adults/adolescents, 2013. Accessed January 23, 2021. https://www.ncjrs.gov/pdffiles1/ovw/241903.pdf
29. Workowski KA, Bachmann LH, Chan PA, et al. Sexually transmitted infections treatment guidelines, 2021. *MMWR Recomm Rep.* 2021;70(4):1–187. doi: 10.15585/mmwr.rr7004a1
30. Adams JA, Kellogg ND, Farst KJ, et al. Updated guidelines for the medical assessment and care of children who may have been sexually abused. *J Pediatr Adolesc Gynecol.* 2016;29(2):81–87.
31. Jatlaoui TC, Curtis KM. Safety and effectiveness data for emergency contraceptive pills among women with obesity: a systematic review. *Contraception.* 2016;94(6):605–611.
32. Palusci VJ, Cox EO, Cyrus TA, et al. Medical assessment and legal outcome in child sexual abuse. *Arch Pediatr Adolesc Med.* 1999;153(4):388–392.

ADDITIONAL RESOURCES AND WEBSITES

Additional Resources and Websites for Clinicians:

The American College of Obstetricians and Gynecologists resources on promoting health relationships in adolescents—https://www.acog.org/clinical/clinical-guidance/committee-opinion/articles/2018/11/promoting-healthy-relationships-in-adolescents

Brief on Dating Violence Among Adolescents—https://www.mchlibrary.org/professionals/datingviolence.php

Centers for Disease Control and Prevention–Dating Matters Toolkit—https://vetoviolence.cdc.gov/apps/dating-matters-toolkit/#/

Centers for Disease Control and Prevention–preventing teen dating violence—https://www.cdc.gov/violenceprevention/intimatepartnerviolence/teendatingviolence/fastfact.html

Futures without Violence–Hanging out or hooking up: Clinical guidelines on responding to adolescent relationship abuse: An integrated approach to prevention and intervention—https://www.futureswithoutviolence.org/hanging-out-or-hooking-up-clinical-guidelines-on-responding-to-adolescent-relationship-abuse-an-integrated-approach-to-prevention-and-intervention/

Futures without Violence helps support advocates, survivors and their families—https://www.futureswithoutviolence.org/

National Center for Victims of Crime—http://victimsofcrime.org

Rape, Abuse & Incest National Network (RAINN)—https://www.rainn.org

Additional Resources and Websites for Parents/Caregivers:

Centers for Disease Control and Prevention–Dating Matters Toolkit—https://vetoviolence.cdc.gov/apps/dating-matters-toolkit/#/

Centers for Disease Control and Prevention–preventing teen dating violence—https://www.cdc.gov/violenceprevention/intimatepartnerviolence/teendatingviolence/fastfact.html

Futures without Violence helps support advocates, survivors and their families—https://www.futureswithoutviolence.org/

XV

Me too movement—https://metoomvmt.org

National Center for Victims of Crime—http://victimsofcrime.org

National Human Trafficking Hotline—https://www.acf.hhs.gov/otip/victim-assistance/national-human-trafficking-hotline

Rape, Abuse & Incest National Network (RAINN)—https://www.rainn.org

Additional Resources and Websites for Adolescents and Young Adults:

Centers for Disease Control and Prevention–Dating Matters Toolkit—https://vetoviolence.cdc.gov/apps/dating-matters-toolkit/#/

Centers for Disease Control and Prevention–preventing teen dating violence—https://www.cdc.gov/violenceprevention/intimatepartnerviolence/teendatingviolence/fastfact.html

Futures without Violence adolescent dating safety card—https://www.seahec.org/wp-content/uploads/2012/12/Adolescent_Safety_Card_English.pdf

Futures without Violence helps support advocates, survivors and their families—https://www.futureswithoutviolence.org/

Healthy and Unhealty Relationships—https://www.loveisrespect.org

Me too movement—https://metoomvmt.org

National Center for Victims of Crime—http://victimsofcrime.org

National Human Trafficking Hotline—https://www.acf.hhs.gov/otip/victim-assistance/national-human-trafficking-hotline

Rape, Abuse & Incest National Network (RAINN)—https://www.rainn.org

TeensHealth–Signs of an abusive relationship—https://kidshealth.org/en/teens.html

PART XVI

Special Populations

CHAPTER 79

College Health

Sarah A. Van Orman
James R. Jacobs

KEY WORDS

- College health
- College students
- Medical home
- National College Health Assessment
- Student affairs
- Student health
- Student health services

INTRODUCTION

As of 2018, the 4,495 colleges and universities in the United States enrolled more than 19 million students, 60% in the 14- to 24-year-old age group. College students comprise almost half the young adult population aged 18 to 24 years.[1] They are a unique population with specific health-related assets and vulnerabilities. While students are generally healthy, mental health conditions, chronic illnesses, substance use and injuries represent significant health issues. The college campus is a unique health environment that creates risks and opportunities including efficient and effective delivery of health care services as well as opportunities for prevention through health promotion and public health initiatives. Colleges and universities, collectively referred to as institutions of higher education (IHEs), are important settings for the provision of health care as well as preventing or reducing health risks and enhancing well-being among a large portion of the young adult population. Understanding the campus environment and resources is critical when providing care for a college student. As care for college students is often shared between an on-campus student health service (SHS) and a hometown clinician, strong communication and collaboration are required to ensure the best possible care. Clinicians caring for precollegiate adolescents have significant opportunity to help the student and their family with the transition to college and navigation of health care for the emerging young adult. This chapter focuses on college health in the United States. While some of the content may be applicable to the health care of students attending institutes of higher education globally, significant differences in the structure of higher education and health care delivery systems throughout the world limit generalizability.

On-campus SHSs have as their mission to improve the health and well-being of college students, support student academic success and retention, reduce institutional risk, and create healthier adults in the future. The actual number of college campuses that provide health services is unknown, but some level of basic mental health and medical services is common. What specific services are offered varies widely in the United States, ranging from part-time nurses providing triage and referral to comprehensive ambulatory health care centers providing medical and mental health care, public health, education and prevention services, and occasionally, disability and recreational services. Today's exemplary SHSs provide direct medical and mental health services, undertake population-based initiatives through health promotion and education, and guide campus health policy. Their overarching role is to create a healthy and safe campus environment, one that helps make possible the learning, research, and teaching to which the institution is dedicated and which promotes student success. Student health services seek to reduce risk and reinforce behaviors that create health for the individual and for the community. The best practices in college health continually assess the student population on the particular campus to track their health status and identify service needs. This may involve assessing health status and promoting health in students who may never visit the SHS, through population-based primary prevention programs such as mandatory prematriculation alcohol education and vaccination outreach programs. Student health service professionals frequently advise and help shape campus health policies, such as tobacco-free college campuses, and conduct surveillance of and lead responses to public health concerns.

Issues of college health are important to clinicians serving adolescents and young adults (AYAs) for many reasons, including the following:

- Clinicians often perform precollege examinations or provide care during college years.
- Clinicians may communicate and collaborate with SHS providers and other student affairs professionals regarding the health care needs of a college student.
- Student health service providers may be a source of ongoing referrals to other clinicians of patients needing hospitalization or secondary and tertiary care consultations.
- Noncollege health providers providing care to college students must recognize the college environment has unique occupational and health risks.
- Significant opportunities exist within SHSs for both teaching and research as well as employment and career opportunities.
- Collaboration among SHS clinicians, other clinicians, insurance providers, local public health officials, and student affairs professionals can benefit all parties and especially students.

DATA SOURCES ON COLLEGE STUDENTS AND COLLEGE HEALTH

American College Health Association Institutional Profile

The American College Health Association (ACHA) annually surveys its membership with the ACHA Institutional Profile Survey about the utilization, staffing, and services available at SHS.

While the number of campuses participating is small (approximately 160) and overly representative of medium and large campuses, it does provide the only available limited data regarding the scope and nature of on-campus health services.

Morbidity Data

Comprehensive data on college students are limited in many areas; although age group is identified in most data sets, current college enrollment is not always collected as part of standard demographic data.

The American College Health Association-National College Health Assessment

One source of data regarding the health of the college student population is the ACHA-National College Health Assessment Survey (ACHA-NCHA). This survey began in the spring of 2000. Since its inception, over 2 million students have completed the NCHA (2000 to 2008), the NCHA II (2008 to 2019), and the NCHA III (2019 to present). While the students sampled on any given campus are selected in a randomized manner, the participating IHEs do not represent a random sample and the response rate is low (mean response rate 14% in spring 2020). The NCHA data throughout the rest of this chapter are from the NCHA's Undergraduate Students Reference Group Data Report Spring 2020 completed prior to the COVID-19 pandemic. All NCHA surveys are available at http://www.achancha.org/.

National College Health Assessment Spring 2020 Undergraduate Data Set

* Survey includes 75 IHEs that chose randomly selected students ($N = 39,602$).
* Size of institution: Twenty-two had more than 20,000 students; 15 had between 10,000 and 19,999; 13 had between 5,000 and 9,999; 16 had between 2,500 and 4,999; and 9 had less than 2,500.
* Gender: The sample of students was 66.7% female, 29.1% male, and 3.9% nonbinary.
* Ethnicity: The ethnicity of the students was 73.1% White, 6.1% African American, 11.6% Hispanic, 13.6% Asian, 3.1% Native American/Alaskan Native/Native Hawaiian, 4.6% biracial or multiracial, and 1.2% identity not listed.

Surveys of College Student Substance Use and Mental Health

* Monitoring the Future Study (since 1975) (http://monitoringthefuture.org/)
* Healthy Minds Study (since 2007) (http://healthymindsnetwork.org/)
* Center for Collegiate Mental Health (https://ccmh.psu.edu/)
* Core Alcohol and Drug Survey (since 1989) (http://core.siu.edu/)

KEY ASPECTS OF STUDENT HEALTH SERVICES

Key aspects of the college student population inform care at SHSs:
* College student populations are generally young and healthy; 90% of students surveyed reported their health as good, very good, or excellent.[2]
* College students are very mobile and often have several residences throughout the year, including in their hometown, on campus, and perhaps in another country or near a summer job or internship, with the potential of fragmenting health care.
* The primary disease burden affecting students while in college is mental health conditions and unintentional injuries often associated with alcohol use.
* Short-term goals are student academic and personal success. The longer-term goal is the primary prevention of the diseases of later adulthood, including obesity and tobacco-related illnesses.[3]

* An estimated one-third of young adults enter college with chronic diseases.[2] While some have medical conditions such as asthma, diabetes, and physical disabilities, the most common are students with mental health disorders, learning disabilities, and pervasive developmental disabilities. Students with these chronic diseases need comprehensive services and case management to meet the goals of not only good health and functioning, but also optimal long-term academic, vocational, and personal success.
* Many college students engage in behaviors that place them at increased health risk, including unhealthy alcohol use, marijuana use, and nonmedical prescription drug use, failure to engage in recommended physical activity, poor nutrition, failure to protect themselves against sexually transmitted infections (STIs), and high-risk recreational and vocational activities such as international travel.
* Relationship difficulties and interpersonal violence are frequently reported.[4]
* Mental health conditions and psychosocial stressors are frequent impediments to academic success. Of the top 10 self-reported impediments to academic success, physical illnesses are much less common than issues such as procrastination, stress, anxiety, depression, sleep difficulties, and financial worries (**Table 79.1**).[2]

COLLEGE STUDENT DEMOGRAPHICS

In the fall of 2018, there were 16.6 million undergraduate college students and 3.0 million students in postbaccalaureate programs in the United States. Enrollment increased substantially between 2000 and 2010: undergraduate enrollment increased 37% (13.2 million to 18.1 million) and postbaccalaureate enrollment 36% (2.2 million to 2.9 million). Between 2010 and 2018, this trend has reversed: undergraduate enrollment decreased 8% and is predicted to grow only 2% in the next decade. Postbaccalaureate enrollment grew only 3% from 2010 to 2018 and is expected to grow by an additional 3% in the next decade.[1] College populations have become more diverse, including enrollment of more first-generation students as well as both students of color and international students.

TABLE 79.1

Top 10 Impediments to Academic Performance

Health Issue	Percentage of Surveyed Students Reporting Impact
Procrastination	47.2
Stress	41.7
Anxiety	31.8
Depression	25.3
Sleep difficulties	24.6
Cold/virus or other respiratory illness	17.4
Finances	14.2
Intimate relationships	12.2
Headaches/migraines	11.5
Career	10.6

Impediments reported on the National College Health Assessment. (Used with permission from American College Health Association. *American College Health Association-National College Health Assessment III: Reference Group Executive Summary Spring 2020.* American College Health Association; 2020.)

Trends

Data and extensive tables regarding higher education enrollment are available from the national center for education statistics at http://nces.ed.gov/programs/coe

- Gender: Female enrollment has risen from 29% in 1947, to 38% in 1961, 42% in 1971, 52% in 1981, 55% in 1991, 56% in 2001, and 57% in 2012 and 2018.
- Age: Between 2000 and 2010, the number of 18- to 24-year-olds in the United States enrolled in college increased from 36% to 42%, but over the past decade, this percentage has not changed substantially.
- Racial and Ethic Diversity: Between 1976 and 2018, the racial and ethnic diversity of college students has changed dramatically:
  - Hispanic: Increased from 4% to 20% of enrolled students
  - Asian/Pacific Islanders: Increased from 2% to 7% of enrolled students
  - Black: Increased from 10% to 13% of enrolled students
  - Native American/Alaska Native: Remained unchanged at <1% of enrolled students
  - White: Decreased from 84% to 55% of enrolled students
- International students: After significant increases between 2000 and 2010, the international student population has remained relatively stable over the past 5 years and in 2018 was 992,000 students.

 HEALTH CARE SERVICES

Medical Care

Student health services may provide a range of medical services:

- Acute medical conditions such as minor infections (Epstein–Barr virus infections, genitourinary tract infections, upper respiratory tract infections, and acute gastroenteritis), musculoskeletal injuries, minor trauma, and skin problems are the most frequent conditions seen.
- Reproductive issues are common, including screening, diagnosis, prevention and treatment of STIs, contraceptive management, routine gynecology, and unintended pregnancies.
- Provision of gender-affirming care for transgender students is common.
- Most SHSs have active immunization programs, and many offer pretravel counseling and vaccinations.
- College undergraduate and graduate students receive care at the SHS for chronic medical conditions, including asthma, diabetes, seizure disorders, thyroid disorders, hypertension, eating disorders, and malignancies.
- Integration of routine screening, brief intervention, and referral to treatment for depression, unhealthy alcohol use, eating disorders, history of trauma and adverse childhood experiences (ACEs) and tobacco use during all encounters, including acute care visits for minor conditions, has been a growing trend. These strategies should now be considered an emerging standard of care for the college student population.

Mental Health Care

The prevalence and severity of college student mental health concerns have significantly increased in the past two decades. Mental health symptoms, particularly depression and anxiety, are a frequently reported impediment to academic success, and are significant predictors of lower grade point average (GPA) and dropping out of college.[4] Common diagnoses in this population include stress-related symptoms, anxiety, depression, eating disorders, suicidality, myalgic encephalomyelitis/chronic fatigue syndrome, unhealthy substance use, and other disorders affecting academic performance such as attention deficit disorder. Approximately 50% of NCHA respondents reported moderate to serious psychological distress and over 50% screened positive for significant loneliness.[2]

Between 2007 and 2017, data from the Healthy Minds Survey of 155,026 students at 196 institutions showed an increasing prevalence of mental health concerns as well as treatment. The percentage of students with a lifetime diagnosis of a mental health condition increased from 21.9% to 35.5%, a positive depression screen from 24.8% to 29.9%, and suicidal ideation in the past year from 5.8% to 10.8%. Among students with a diagnosis, rates of treatment in the past year increased from 18.7% to 33.8% with almost 10% of students reporting using on-campus mental health services.[5] Despite increases in treatment, inequities in access remain. Students of color are less likely to engage in treatment and often have higher levels of symptoms on presentation.[6] Gender minority students are more than four times more likely to report mental health problems compared with cisgender students.[7]

Given the significant impact of mental health on student well-being and academic success, almost all IHEs offer some level of mental health services. Services may be available through a stand-alone counseling service or integrated into a larger umbrella unit that provides medical and mental health care services. College mental health services have historically been based on a developmental model that focused on academic support and developmental concerns. As mental health disorders have increased in both severity and prevalence and campus threats of violence have become more common, the field has undergone a significant transition. Common now is the availability of psychiatric consultation and the creation of campus teams ("threat" assessment or behavioral intervention) with procedures to share information and develop interventions such as mandated mental health assessments for when students display behaviors of concern and are felt to pose a risk to self or others.[8]

Unmet mental health needs are a frequently cited concern of SHS providers and IHE staff. Most on-campus mental health services operate from a short-term model, referring students with complex or long-term needs to community providers. Lack of insurance coverage and a shortage of community providers are frequent barriers to students receiving care. Students are often encouraged or required to leave campus and take a leave of absence to receive treatment. To meet the needs of students on campus, many SHSs are embracing novel approaches, including more closely integrating medical and mental health services. Behavioral health programs offer brief, solution-focused mental health counseling integrated into primary care to address high-risk behaviors such as alcohol or tobacco use, stress and sleep disturbances, or as a bridge to more comprehensive mental health care. Delivered within the medical setting, these services are often acceptable to underserved students, male students, international students, and students of color.[9] Universities are also increasingly creating programs which can coordinate or provide services such as intensive outpatient or posthospitalization programs for students with chronic and high-risk mental health conditions while the student remains on campus and enrolled.[10]

Health Promotion, Wellness, Prevention

The campus environment presents a unique opportunity to use prevention strategies for optimal individual health and student academic success. Often referred to by the term "health promotion," most campuses have specific programs which advance student well-being through individual education and wellness programming as well as using environmental strategies such as broad health campaigns and changes to campus health policy. These health promotion and wellness functions are typically part of the SHS or also may be a part of a closely aligned unit such as Division of Student Affairs or Student Life. These programs also conduct population-level assessments to determine areas of greatest need to focus their activities.

Healthy Campus 2020 is an example of a framework for improving the overall health status of a campus population. Universities have an opportunity to extend beyond traditional interventions of education, diagnosis, treatment, and health care within clinical settings and encourage collaborations between academic and student affairs and administrative colleagues. An ecologic approach uses individual and community interventions to improve population health.[11]

Public Health and Communicable Disease Control

The close living and working conditions of a college campus create a high-risk environment for communicable disease outbreaks. The academic calendar brings the movement of large populations to and from campus from throughout the nation and world over a short period.

Well-described communicable disease outbreaks in IHE settings have included the following:

- COVID-19: Colleges and universities were uniquely impacted by the COVID-19 pandemic. Outbreaks developed at many universities despite aggressive mitigation measures and in some cases may have contributed to spread within the surrounding community.[12]
- Influenza and other upper respiratory viruses: These cause significant morbidity among college students, including increasing health care utilization and impacting academic performance.
- Meningococcal disease: First-year students residing on campus are at increased risk. Recent outbreaks have been associated with the Group B serotype.
- Pertussis: A potentially significant issue in young adults.
- Other vaccine-preventable disease outbreaks have included mumps, measles, and varicella. Mumps outbreaks have been common on campuses over the past 10 years, with most cases in fully vaccinated individuals.
- Norovirus: This can be particularly difficult to contain and has led to outbreaks on many campuses of hundreds and in some cases thousands of cases in a short period of time.
- Viral and bacterial conjunctivitis.
- Staphylococcus: Methicillin-resistant *Staphylococcus aureus* outbreaks have been particularly associated with athletic teams and recreational sports facilities.
- Pneumonia: Recent outbreaks of *Mycoplasma pneumoniae* have occurred on several campuses.

Detection and control of communicable diseases, therefore, is one of the most critical roles played by SHSs and the SHS functions as a public health agency on many campuses. Roles of the SHS in communicable disease control include primary prevention through immunization and health education campaigns, active surveillance for diseases, and detection of individual cases or suspect cases. For example, many SHSs are part of the Centers for Disease Control and Prevention sentinel influenza surveillance network. During an active outbreak or when managing individual cases of communicable diseases, the SHS may assist or have primary responsibility along with local public health authorities for case management and contact tracing. Student health services advise or coordinate public information campaigns for the campus community. Public health approaches also address a variety of other chronic diseases and health risks among student populations, including unhealthy alcohol use, mental health, interpersonal violence, and obesity.

● BEHAVIORAL AND OTHER RISK FACTORS

Similar to other young adult populations, college students have a range of risk factors that health professionals must consider when delivering health care. Screening and appropriate intervention can reduce short- and long-term health risks. In the United States, behavioral risk factors are common in emerging young adults 18 to 25 years old.

Alcohol

Alcohol remains one of the most serious public health problems facing college students in the United States, although overall rates of risky drinking and students who consume alcohol regularly have been declining over the past decade. College students are more likely than their noncollege peers to engage in heavy episodic drinking, also known as binge drinking, defined as four or more drinks in one setting for females and five or more drinks for males. While college students are not more likely to experience alcohol use disorders than their noncollege peers, their alcohol use places them at risk for unintentional injury, victimization, and other health and personal consequences such as academic and legal difficulties.[13]

The NCHA and Monitoring the Future (2019) surveys of college students consistently demonstrate high levels of alcohol use among undergraduates and its attendant consequences.

- Over 60% of students report any use within the past 30 days.[2,13]
- Approximately 30% report binge drinking within the past 2 weeks.[2,13]
- Of students who reported alcohol consumption, over 30% reported one or more consequences from their consumption within the past 12 months. Most commonly reported were doing something they later regretted, forgetting where they were or what they did, or having unprotected sex.[2]
- Fifteen percent report moderate- or high-risk use patterns.[2]
- Rates of alcohol use vary widely among college students and among individual IHEs. Male, White, and lesbian, gay, bisexual, transgender, and queer (LGBTQ) students drink more heavily and frequently compared with other college students.

Marijuana

Marijuana use is now at historic levels among AYAs. Monitoring the Future (2019) showed 43% of college students reporting use in the past year and 5.9% daily or near-daily use. Marijuana vaping is common: 14% in the past 30 days.[13] Of the students who reported having used cannabis in the preceding 30 days on the NCHA survey, 38.9% indicated they drove within 6 hours of use.[2] Institutions of higher education are grappling with issues of medical marijuana use and legalization and are struggling to develop new campus policies to address medical marijuana use, use of marijuana within residence halls, and other emerging issues. Marijuana use disorders among students are increasingly common.

Tobacco

While 7.9% of students report use of combustible cigarettes within the last 30 days, daily use is infrequent (2.5% of students).[2,13] Use of electronic nicotine delivery systems (ENDS) or e-cigarettes for nicotine consumption is much more common (22.1% in the past 30 days) as students perceive their health risks to be low.[13] Young adult ENDS users may have never smoked combustible cigarettes, but view ENDS as safer and more attractive.

Other Drugs

Other important drugs include prescription stimulants, benzodiazepines, and opioids. When compared with their same age-group noncollege peers, drug usage among college students in 2019 was similar, with 47% of college students reporting any drug use in the past 12 months. Amphetamine use continues to remain higher among college than noncollege students.[13]

According to the Monitoring the Future (2019) study, the following drugs were reported being used in the past 12 months by students who were not prescribed these medications[13]:

- 8.1% report use of stimulants (amphetamine/dextroamphetamine, methylphenidate): As the number of students on stimulant prescriptions has risen, diversion of stimulants has emerged as a troubling problem. Nonmedical use of prescription stimulants occurs in two distinct patterns, as a study aid and combined with alcohol to reduce its sedating effects in social settings.
- 5.3% report use of hallucinogens.

- 1.5% report use of prescription opioids (e.g., hydrocodone, oxycodone, codeine).
- 3.0% report use of sedatives or tranquilizers (e.g., alprazolam, lorazepam).
- 5.6% report use of cocaine.

Novel substances and new patterns of substance use are not uncommon and can spread quickly through individual campuses, as well as locally, regionally, and nationally. Clinicians caring for college students need to be aware of trends and practices in their local area.

Sexual Assault, Dating Violence, and Stalking

Interpersonal violence including sexual assault, dating violence, and stalking remains part of a common and devastating reality on college campuses. Surveys conducted by the Association of American Universities (AAU) in 2015 and 2019 provide one of the largest sets of data on prevalence of sexual assault and misconduct and experiences of college students. It is estimated that one in four females will experience nonconsensual sexual contact during college, most commonly during their first semester.[14] Female, transgender, nonbinary, gender-queer, and gender nonconforming students are at significantly greater risk than other students. Stalking is reported by 5.1% of undergraduate female students.[2] Despite investments in prevention and response, these numbers are not declining and have actually increased slightly over the past 5 years in the AAU surveys.[14] Research suggests that serial offenders frequently perpetrate these crimes.[15] Alcohol can facilitate these crimes by reducing the capacity of a victim to respond as well as reducing the awareness of bystanders. It is estimated that less than 10% of assaults are reported and in even fewer cases are the perpetrators held responsible.[14] Students who experience sexual assault are at risk for long-term physical and mental health problems. They may leave school and not complete their education. Sexual assault on college campuses has been the focus of national attention and there have been federal efforts to make campuses safer through prevention, survivor response, and holding perpetrators responsible for over a decade. Institutions of higher education are subject to multiple federal requirements, including the Clery Act and Title IX, to provide comprehensive prevention of, response to, and disclosure of these crimes.

Relationship difficulties are also common among college students, with over 12% of students reporting an adverse academic impact in the past 12 months from a relationship difficulty. Abusive relationships are of particular concern: 10.1%, 2.6%, and 2.9% of college students report being in an emotionally, physically, or sexually abusive intimate relationship, respectively, within the past 12 months.[2]

Nutrition and Physical Activity

Poor nutrition, physical inactivity, overweight, obesity, and eating disorders are prevalent in college student populations. In the NCHA survey, 44% of college students report meeting recommendations for physical activity.[2] Eating disorders may present during late adolescence and disordered eating patterns are common. The transition from adolescence to young adulthood is frequently associated with weight gain, and weight gain is common during the early and mid-20s. While the concept of the "freshman fifteen" is overstated, studies suggest that students gain a mean of 3.9 lb (1.8 kg) during the first 3 to 4 months in college. On average, females have been estimated to gain 3.8 lb (1.7 kg) from freshman to senior year and males to gain 9.8 lb (4.5 kg).[16] Dietary factors in the college setting which can contribute to excess weight gain include all you can eat on-campus dining facilities, greater intake of low-density nutrition ("junk") food, and frequent snacking (especially during late night hours where many college students consume a fourth meal). Students may not have access to cooking facilities, lack basic cooking skills, and/or eat many meals out in fast-food restaurants. Physical activity levels decline at the transition to college and continue to decline throughout college. Alcohol intake can be an important contributor to overall calorie intake, and many students, especially female-identified, engage in patterns of restricting food intake to compensate for the calories they anticipate consuming when drinking alcohol. Addressing these patterns are important during the college years as research suggests that this is a critical time for the establishment of long-term health patterns and behaviors.

Food insecurity is a growing concern among student populations. Estimates are that 40% to 50% of college students surveyed may be food insecure.[2,17] Students with food insecurity may be at risk for poor nutrition and overall poorer health as well as disruption to academic progress and lower academic performance. Many campuses have established food banks and other on-campus resources to support student access to nutrition.

Injury Prevention

As the leading cause of death among college students, unintentional injuries should remain a focus of prevention efforts. Alcohol-related fatalities most often result from motor vehicle accidents, but falls, cold exposure, and drowning are also important mechanisms. In some urban campuses, bicycle injuries are a particular problem as riders are often inexperienced, riding without helmets, not observing traffic rules, and texting while riding.

Sexual and Reproductive Health

College students are at risk for STIs and unintended pregnancy. Nearly 60% of college students report having at least one sexual partner in the past 12 months, with a mean number of 2.4 partners. Only 43.1% of students reported using a condom most of the time or always with vaginal intercourse and only 27.8% with last anal intercourse. The most common forms of birth control reported by students are male condoms followed by birth control pills. Inadequate birth control, however, is common, with nearly 10% of students reporting not using a method of birth control the last time they had penile-vaginal intercourse. Nearly 19% of sexually active college students or their female partners reported use of emergency contraception within the past 12 months. Long-acting reversible contraceptives (LARCs) such as intrauterine devices (IUDs) and contraceptive implants are becoming increasingly popular and provide highly effective contraception; 13.5% of undergraduate females reported using an IUD in 2020 and 8.2% a birth control implant.[2] Preexposure prophylaxis (PREP) should be routinely offered to students at risk for human immunodeficiency virus (HIV) infection and is offered at most SHSs.

Sexual and Gender Minority Students

Sexual and gender minority students encompass populations included in the acronym LGBT (lesbian, gay, bisexual, transgender), as well as those who may not self-identify as LGBT (e.g., queer, questioning, asexual, men who have sex with men, gender variant). In a recent survey from Gallup, 5.6% of all persons surveyed and 15.9% of those of traditional college age, born between 1997 and 2002, identified as LGBT.[18] Structural discrimination results in health disparities for these college students. Sexual and gender minority youth much more commonly experience bullying and personal violence than their corresponding sexual and gender majority peers. Family rejection can have physical, emotional, and financial ramifications. As a result, sexual and gender minority students report higher rates of depression, suicide attempts, unhealthy substance use, and high-risk sexual behaviors. Family and community acceptance along with a safe school environment are important protective factors.

While reduction in overall societal stigma for some young people has resulted in young adults "coming out" at younger ages, often before starting college, many students feel comfortable disclosing their identity only after the age of 18 years. College is therefore an important time for many sexual and gender minority students when they are first able to develop romantic relationships, be open in their community regarding their identities, and seek medical and mental health care confidentially. Sexual and gender minority students are at risk for receiving inadequate health services unless clinicians and their staff provide an open and safe environment with providers knowledgeable and prepared to address their mental health and medical concerns.

Clinicians caring for college students should be prepared to counsel and provide referrals to medical and mental health professionals knowledgeable and skilled in gender-affirming care as many students first seek care during college. Many SHSs have providers skilled in providing gender-affirming medical care including hormone treatment. Many young adults reject a binary notion of gender and may prefer the use of gender-neutral pronouns and language or pronouns based on their preferred identity. Verbal questions and written questionnaires should be gender-neutral, and clinicians should address students based on their preference.

Sleep

Similar to other adult populations, college students frequently do not get adequate sleep. Only 8.7% reported getting enough sleep to feel rested in the morning on 6 or more days in the past week.[2] Chronic sleep deprivation can lead to decreased cognitive performance, mood disturbance, and physical symptoms. It can be a risk factor for alcohol and marijuana use as well as poor academic performance.[19] Many aspects of campus and college life contribute to altered sleep patterns and put college students at risk for poor sleep hygiene. These include the cyclic nature of academic requirements leading to all-night study sessions, the adaptation to personal responsibility for sleep schedules when moving away from the family home, the highly stimulating social environment in an on-campus residence facility, a varied daily schedule, and frequent alcohol consumption.

While the most common sleep disorder in college students is inadequate sleep hygiene from challenges of sleeping in a college residential environment, delayed sleep phase disorder (dysregulation of an individual's circadian rhythm) commonly has its onset in young adulthood and should be considered in a college student with sleep concerns.[20]

Vocational Health Risks

College students in many fields may encounter health and safety risks that typically would fall under the category of occupational risks. The largest at-risk group is health care students engaged in health care settings in a professional or preprofessional capacity. This includes medical, nursing, allied health professional, pharmacy, dental, physical therapy, and athletic training students. It has been estimated that nearly one-quarter of students in the health professions experience a blood or body fluid exposure during their training and many of these events are unreported.[21] Other students at unique risk include veterinary students who experience frequent biologic exposures and physical injury, students engaged in laboratory research and study where biologic agents and/or chemical toxins are present, music students who are at risk for auditory damage and musculoskeletal injuries, architecture students with sharp injuries, and art students whose materials may contain toxins.

Because student employees are not classified as employees by IHEs, they are outside the protection provided through the Occupational Safety and Health Administration, even though they are often working within the same settings as employees. Similarly, they are often not covered by on-site employee health and occupational health services. Trainees may also be at higher risk due to a lower skill level when performing procedures, as well as possible fear of reporting accidents and injuries to their instructors. Over

40% of full-time and 80% of part-time undergraduates report being employed in 2018.[22] Younger workers typically experience more work-related injuries than their older counterparts in similar jobs. In one study of college students, 20% of working students had experienced an injury at work.[23]

Clinicians should consider incorporating an occupational risk assessment related to a student's course of study as well as any part-time or other employment and consider occupational and vocational hazards when evaluating injuries and illnesses. Health care students should receive the same preexposure immunizations, postexposure medical care, and training as other health care personnel. These include hepatitis B vaccination; screening for immunity to measles, mumps, rubella, and varicella; annual influenza vaccination; periodic tuberculosis screening; pertussis vaccination; and blood-borne pathogen and infection control training.

International Study

International study is an important part of today's college curriculum and participation in study abroad programs continues to grow. Nearly 350,000 U.S. students studied abroad in 2018 to 2019. Slightly over half of students study in Europe followed by Latin America (13.8%) and Asia (11.7%), Oceania (4.4%), Africa (3.9%), and the Middle East (2.3%). Nearly 11% of U.S. undergraduates overall and over 16% of bachelor's students will study abroad during their degree program. Roughly 65% of students will stay for less than 8 weeks and 33% for approximately one semester, with a few students studying for an entire academic year.[24] The duration and nature of their travel means college students studying abroad are at risk not only for common travel-related illnesses, but also face unique risks. Students often reside in an apartment within the community or with a local family rather than a hotel and engage in different activities than a typical tourist. Young adults who stay abroad for extended periods are more likely to have new sexual partners, a significant risk factor for contracting an STI. Alcohol and drug use can endanger safety and place a student at legal risk. In some countries, services are poor or nonexistent for survivors of sexual violence, and sometimes there is legal peril for even reporting the events; likewise, there are locations where gay, transgender, and other nonbinary identities and behaviors are illegal or dangerous. Occupational exposures such as needle sticks may occur in health professions students, a particular concern in countries with a high prevalence of HIV infection and limited access to postexposure prophylaxis. The greatest risk of serious illness and injury is from motor vehicle accidents and drowning. Another period of high risk is during academic breaks, especially spring break, when both international and domestic travel are combined with alcohol and drug use, high-risk sexual activity, and other behaviors that can lead to significant mortality and morbidity.

A clinician with special skills in travel medicine and familiar with extended travel should evaluate students participating in study abroad experiences. Students should receive information about health and safety in their travel destination including food- and waterborne illnesses; STIs; insect-borne and other infectious diseases in the area; avoidance of unknown animals to reduce rabies risk; personal safety including crime prevention; food, and dietary customs (including availability of special diets); alcohol, tobacco, and other drug customs and laws; vehicular safety and injury/injury prevention; and availability of local medical and mental health care. In addition to standard travel prescriptions and immunizations, college students should receive birth control when appropriate and advance prescription of postexposure medications for HIV if working in a high-risk situation or engaging in high-risk sexual activity.

Previously stable mental health and medical conditions can worsen under the stress associated with life while abroad and access to local health care may be limited. Students with chronic illnesses, including mental health illnesses, should work with their clinician to develop treatment plans, including what to do during exacerbations during extended study abroad. Arrangements should be made for any prescription medications, medical supplies, and medical care. Most study abroad programs will have limited capability to assist students in managing chronic medical and mental health conditions and may not be able to accommodate all reported individual needs or circumstances.

Clinicians should be alert for the development of post-travel illnesses in college students by inquiring about foreign travel particularly during the evaluation of febrile, dermatologic, and gastrointestinal illnesses. Returning student travelers may not recognize the connection to current symptoms when several months have passed and may not provide a travel history unless questioned directly.

FUNDING AND STUDENT HEALTH INSURANCE

In the United States, SHSs are funded through a combination of institutional or tuition support, designated SHS fees paid directly to IHE from students, out-of-pocket service fees, and/or billing of students' private health insurance. At some IHEs, a portion of health services is provided at or by a contracted noncampus clinician billed through traditional private insurance. This can reduce the risk associated with and resources dedicated by campus administrators to manage their own SHS, potentially provide access to more comprehensive services, and provide needed investments in facilities and information technology. Contracted services have typically included only medical services, while both mental health services and health promotion/prevention services have remained with on-campus providers.

If services are outsourced or insurance billing is the primary source of funding, the unique needs of the college student population must be considered:
- Provisions for uninsured and underinsured students to avoid disenfranchising them.
- Students with primary insurance coverage through geographically limited health care networks and limited access to services in the areas where they live, study, and work.
- Accessibility on or near campus.
- Preservation of student confidentiality and reduction of administrative barriers when receiving sensitive services such as reproductive or mental health care.
- Support for population health. Student health services create a healthier student population through public health, prevention, and health promotion efforts that address risks such as communicable diseases, high-risk alcohol use, violence, obesity, nutrition, and mental health. Insurance billing does not provide a reliable funding mechanism for population health measures at the campus level. An additional funding stream for on-campus population-based measures and public health will be necessary. Traditional medical service providers may not have the expertise to provide these services for the campus community.

Student Health Insurance

Prior to the passage of the Affordable Care Act (ACA), estimates were that approximately 20% of college students were uninsured. While this is lower than the rate of the overall population of 19- to 29-year-olds, part-time students, students of color, and students from families with lower incomes were more likely than average to be uninsured. Under a key early provision of the ACA implemented in 2010, families were able to continue coverage of their dependent children until age 26. This provision had an immediate impact on health insurance coverage of young adults.[25] In addition to remaining covered through a family health insurance policy, students may also choose individual policies through the health care marketplace, select a student health insurance benefit plan (SHIP), or may be eligible for state-based Medicaid. Health insurance issues for college students include high deductible plans with impact on student access, cost to families to insure young adults through family plans, geographic and other network limitations potentially limiting coverage in the area in which students attend school or are residing for a job, internship, or study abroad and elimination of the individual mandate. It is possible that many young adults in college will choose not to have health insurance. Student health insurance benefit plans offered on many campuses typically include a broad national network. Student health insurance coverage may be less expensive than individual plans purchased through the marketplace.

OTHER ON-CAMPUS STUDENT SERVICES

Institutions of higher education provide a range of services to support student growth and development and their physical, mental, and emotional well-being. These services, collectively known as student services, student life, or student affairs, vary based on the size, type, and location of an institution. Student health services are often one of these services, and although organization varies widely between campuses, many SHSs institutionally report to a Chief Student Affairs Officer. Student health services as part of or in partnership with a comprehensive student affairs unit are often extensively involved in student affairs programs such as residential life, recreational sports, and orientation. The best practice of college health seeks such educational opportunities and promotes learning not just during the medical or mental health visit but also throughout the campus culture. Other on-campus student affairs professionals are also often extensively involved when developing plans for serving students with disabilities on campus. Students with concerns such as a severe eating disorder, mental health crisis, or a substance use disorder may first come to the attention of a student affairs professional outside the SHS, who may refer and coordinate intervention.

Common student affairs departments that support student health and well-being include the following:
- Academic services, including academic advising, career development, and judicial affairs. Judicial affairs (sometimes called student conduct) enforces community standards and campus codes of conduct, and may include ethical programs/education, disciplinary procedures, and mediation for academic or behavioral concerns.
- Campus life services, including campus safety/police, the student union, student activities, leadership, community service, parent programs, and Greek life.
- Diversity and inclusion, including multicultural affairs, lesbian, gay, bisexual, transgender, queer, intersex, and asexual (LGBTQIA+) student services, international student services, spirituality, faith, or religious services, and disability support services. Disability support services typically coordinate services related to compliance with the Americans with Disabilities Act (ADA).
- Health and wellness, including SHSs, counseling services, sexual assault and violence prevention, prevention of unhealthy alcohol and other drug use, and wellness education.
- Residence life (housing) and food services.
- New student enrollment and enrollment services, including admissions, student orientation, and financial aid.
- Sports and recreation, including intercollegiate athletics, club and intramural sports, recreation, wellness, and fitness programs.

DISEASE-SPECIFIC CONSIDERATIONS

For many specific circumstances, shared responsibility between the hometown clinician, the SHS, other campus resources, and other community health care resources will ultimately provide the best experience for the student-patient. Students with chronic (e.g., diabetes) and subacute (e.g., rehabilitation following ortho-pedic surgery) medical conditions will face challenges, including resource limitations or policies of the SHS, availability of and trans-portation to specialists, out-of-network restrictions of the family's health insurance, the stresses of campus life, and the trials of emer-gence as an independent young adult. The hometown clinician is uniquely positioned to help the student and his or her family to negotiate many of these transitions, and the goal of this section is to provide insights about some of the specific challenges.

- **Allergy immunotherapy:** Many, but certainly not all, SHSs will administer allergy shots, but few will initiate therapy, and fewer still have an allergist on staff. Students initiate therapy with the home allergist (the first and second injections) and then transfer the regimen to the SHS for subsequent injections, under orders submitted by the home allergist, who will also continue to supply sera as needed. Students will often transfer sera back and forth between the SHS and the home allergist during summers and other extended breaks from campus.
- **Food allergies:** Campus dining services are increasingly sophis-ticated in their ability to accommodate food allergies and other dietary needs (e.g., Kosher or vegan). Requests from the family or the clinician to release the student from a required on-campus meal plan are typically not accepted or necessary, but if negotia-tion on this (or housing assignments) is intended, they should commence months in advance of matriculation.
- **Attention deficit hyperactivity disorder (ADHD):** Due to con-cerns about nonmedical use of stimulant medications, SHSs have become increasingly restrictive in initiating stimulant prescriptions and in continuing existing prescriptions. Student health services' expectations for disease documentation might, at minimum, be a letter from a psychiatrist or neurologist certifying the diagnosis and treatment history or, at the more extensive end of the spectrum, documentation of a formal (and preferably recent) psychoeducational assessment using standard evaluation, including raw test results. A letter from the student's hometown clinician describing empiric diagnosis and several years of successful treatment will not usually be accepted. Stu-dents using stimulants and other controlled medications should be encouraged to investigate whether the residence hall or other living situation includes a lockbox or similar fixture where the medication can be secured. Students who take stimulants should be counseled regarding the legal and ethical ramifications of sell-ing or giving away their medications.
- **Chronic pain:** Chronic pain patients attending college who require opioid medications may encounter significant obstacles. Few, if any, SHSs will prescribe long-acting opioids, again owing in at least a small part to overall campus concerns about mis-use and diversion of such medications, but also because this is regarded in many communities as within the purview of pain medicine and other specialists.
- **Disabilities:** Students with physical and mental health disabili-ties, including ADHD, requesting campus or academic accom-modations under the ADA will typically be required to submit appropriate documentation, in accordance with federal require-ments. In general, the SHS (and/or counseling center) will not get involved in certifying disabilities because there is an inher-ent conflict of interest. Students and families should make requests for accommodations early as documentation needs may be extensive and updated testing and evaluation is some-times requested. Educational accommodations required under the ADA are generally handled through a dedicated disabilities service office on campus. Other needs, such as a personal care attendant, which fall outside of the ADA requirements may not be provided through the school. The SHS can be helpful in locat-ing community resources for these types of needs.
- **Asthma:** Many young adults underestimate the severity of their asthma or overestimate their degree of symptom control and

arrive at college ill prepared for the bronchospasm that may ensue from changes in housing, allergens, temperatures, and cli-mate. They may discover that the inhaler they last used 2 years ago has expired. Even the patient with rare exercise-induced wheezing deserves cautionary education and a new rescue inhaler prior to heading off to college.
- **Diabetes:** College students with insulin-dependent diabetes will be challenged by myriad opportunities for food and drink, irregu-lar sleep, academic and professional stressors, and possibly even stigma. Students should be prepared with action plans for antici-pated periods when blood glucose control becomes difficult. As a very practical matter, the student needs to determine campus options for sharps containers and appropriate disposal and a source for medication and supplies. Consider instructing your patient to educate their roommate and/or other close friends about diabetes and hypoglycemic events, with an invitation to intervene in the case of an emergency.
- **Physical therapy:** Even small minimally resourced SHSs often offer in-house physical therapy. This can be a convenient option, for example, for students who undergo an anterior cruciate liga-ment repair or other surgical procedure at home but who need to continue rehabilitation while at school.
- **National Collegiate Athletic Association (NCAA) athletes:** Ath-letic programs often have sports medicine resources that are for the exclusive use of athletes and which are administratively wholly separate from the SHS. The culture and logistics of the athletic program will typically include written or unwritten rules about where the student-athlete should go for medical care. For example, female athletes might be directed to use the SHS for gynecologic services but to utilize the sports medicine depart-ment for all other medical needs. Relevant to this chapter is that for students participating in NCAA athletics, there might be yet another set of clinicians among which the student must navigate.
- **Bipolar and psychotic disorders:** Most SHSs will provide pri-mary care management for mood disorders such as anxiety and depression, including medication management, ideally in col-laboration with the on-campus counseling center or a commu-nity therapist. Few, however, will manage multidrug regimens or have resources to manage bipolar illnesses and psychotic dis-orders. Furthermore, on-campus access to a psychiatrist may be extremely limited, even when the SHS shares a campus with a major academic medical center. Students and their families should begin looking for resources early. While long-term care may not be available through the SHS or on-campus counseling center, these offices are often a good source for referrals and are knowledgeable about local resources.
- **Eating disorders:** Students with eating disorders can be particu-larly challenged by a campus environment. Resources on cam-pus or within the local community may be limited. While many students with eating disorders are anxious to start college and to remain enrolled, this can be detrimental to their recovery. Stu-dents with eating disorders who are significantly underweight, are newly diagnosed, or those who exhibit high levels of eating disorder behaviors frequently require more intensive treatment and support than what is possible as an enrolled student, par-ticularly on a residential campus. Recovery is extremely chal-lenging in this setting. To optimize the student's prospects for collegiate success and safety, patients with eating disorders entering college or returning to college after treatment should have achieved a significant level of recovery and have demon-strated an extended period of stability. When a student with an eating disorder is entering or re-entering the IHE environments, a thoughtful and realistic case management plan should be nego-tiated between the patient, the family, the treating clinicians, and the student health and counseling centers.
- **Substance use disorder recovery:** There are increasing numbers of adolescents who have already endured significant substance

use disorders problems and who have entered recovery prior to arrival at college. The risk of relapse upon entering the collegiate environment is significant. Some campuses are addressing this issue directly, facilitating access to Alcoholics Anonymous, Narcotics Anonymous, and similar programs. Some campuses have created specific programs, Collegiate Recovery Communities, which offer academic and social support and, in some cases, residential housing. Prospective students in recovery may consider preferentially applying to a college with such a program.

- **Infusion medications:** The current era of immune modulators available for rheumatoid arthritis, asthma, psoriasis, inflammatory bowel disease, and other conditions can provide remarkable clinical benefits, but there are challenges for the patient on campus, especially if the medication is administered intravenously or if the formal labeling recommends administration in a specialty setting. Even for more familiar medications such as antibiotics, the SHS might have a policy prohibiting intravenous injections or might not have the expertise to infuse through a peripherally inserted central catheter (PICC line) or through a subcutaneous port. Whether in regard to acute or long-term administration of intravenous medications, each of the topics listed previously, or any of many other examples, the home provider or family should consult with the SHS well in advance of matriculation to determine whether the capacity exists on campus for administration of specialty medications or to enlist the SHS in helping to develop an alternative strategy that will meet the patient's need.

- **Chronic medical conditions:** In addition to diabetes and other disease states listed above, there are numerous additional chronic medical conditions that the late adolescent might be coping with as they enter college, including seizure disorders, organ transplants, cancer, cystic fibrosis, and inflammatory bowel disease. Although the SHS will usually be well able to provide episodic ambulatory care for many of these students, specialty care rarely will be available in the SHS, typically necessitating a relationship with a local specialist. The SHS will know the local specialty resources and will gladly make recommendations, but it is also desirable for the home provider or specialist to make a provider-to-provider connection.

ONGOING ENGAGEMENT WITH THE COLLEGE STUDENT

It is anticipated that many hometown clinicians who care for AYAs will have an ongoing (if sporadic) relationship with their patients during their college years. The final section of this chapter is orientated toward these providers who both prepare their patients to come to campus as well as continue to provide and coordinate care with campus resources including SHS providers.

Prematriculation

In addition to performing precollege physical examinations and signing vaccination compliance forms, there are many ways for the clinician to engage with the patient preparing to enter college.

- **Managing ongoing health care while at college:** Importantly, there is also opportunity—ideally starting at least 1 year prior to any actual prematriculation visit—to engage in conversation about how the patient plans to manage ongoing health conditions while in college. Are the student and his or her family including medical considerations as they develop a short list of favorite colleges? What medical and counseling services are available on campus? Are appropriate specialists available in the community? The patient should be advised to ask such questions during campus visits. Student health services are generally happy to receive questions along the lines of "My daughter is considering your university to start as a freshman in the fall. Can she get allergy shots in your clinic?" "What about injections of omalizumab?" "Is there a psychologist with whom she can

talk with every week about her eating disorder?" "Is there a psychologist near campus whom you can recommend for long-term counseling?"

- **Discussion of substance use and reproductive health:** There is of course opportunity, and possibly parental expectation, for the clinician to engage the patient in prematriculation conversation and counseling regarding use of alcohol and other drugs, sexual identity and safer sexual practices, and the importance of medication adherence (e.g., anticonvulsants, insulin, antidepressants). A useful pamphlet produced by the Society for Adolescent Health and Medicine has been developed to review these key issues (https://www.adolescenthealth.org/SAHM_Main/media/Clinical-Care-Resources/Healthy-Student-Brochure/HSB_Brochure_2012_FNL_wtrmrk.pdf).

- **Accommodation issues:** Once the choice of school is finalized, clinicians may be asked to write letters requesting special accommodations. In some cases, the requests from a student or his or her parents/caregivers are not related to a documented disability, "He or she needs to be assigned a dormitory near the business school." "He or she needs to be granted special permission to have a car on campus." In considering writing such letters, be prepared for most such recommendations to be denied, as the university usually has philosophical, legal, and pedagogical reasons for randomized roommate assignments and so forth. Hometown clinicians might be asked to write letters endorsing emotional support animals and vaccine exemptions. Rules on these topics can vary widely from school to school and some states are increasingly monitoring writers of vaccine exemptions. Requests for accommodations should be sent to the on-campus disability service center.

- **Common health care access issues:** There is also a compelling need to begin mentoring the patient (and his or her parents/caregivers) as a soon-to-be independent consumer of health care. Key topics might include the following:
  - Keeping a medication list
  - Carrying an insurance card
  - In the United States, turning 18 and the implications for confidentiality
  - Scheduling appointments
  - Filling a prescription
  - Providing a clinician your family and personal medical history. Encourage young adults during their last year of high school to take responsibility for scheduling their own medical appointments, picking up prescriptions, and adhering to medication schedules. It is easier to learn these skills while they are still residing at home. Finally, when sending a patient with a complex medical history off to college, providers should write a comprehensive medical summary letter or equivalent documentation (e.g., copies of medical records) that the student can provide to the SHS and any other care providers they encounter.

- **Health insurance:** Discuss with parents/caregivers and soon-to-be college students their plans for health insurance coverage. Students should be able to access nonemergency care in the area where they will be attending school, if needed. Health insurance that may provide excellent coverage in the home community may be problematic if it does not cover care in the area where the student will be attending school. An insurance plan with no local in-network primary or specialty care may result in health compromise and much distress when the student cannot afford to obtain services until they go home for a school break.

- **Consent and confidentiality:** Finally, in the United States, most students starting college will be over the age of 18 years, with implications for confidentiality; laws governing confidentiality in adolescent health vary from country to country. Most SHSs will not accept an authorization signed a priori providing parent's/caregiver's wholesale access to the student's future medical record at the SHS. A college student's rapid development and growth makes this inappropriate. A student who signs such a release in August may feel very differently a few months later. This might seem frustrating for parents/caregivers, but parents/caregivers should be encouraged to allow their student to handle communications with clinicians independently, asking for advice and assistance from parents/caregivers when needed. That being said, most SHS clinicians are willing and desirous to communicate with parents/caregivers after obtaining student consent.

Matriculated Students

The ongoing connection of the hometown clinician with a matriculated college student will likely depend on the nature of the pre-matriculation relationship, availability of health care resources at or near the school, proximity of the school to the practice, the nature of the student's health care issues, and the level of parental involvement.

Typically, the student will use the campus and home health care locations (and possibly others) to best advantage, relying on the SHS for episodic care and some primary care during the academic terms and returning home for ongoing specialty or primary care during school breaks. As an upperclassman and graduate student, the student will likely become increasingly dependent on the SHS and other clinicians in the community close to campus, as internships and other curricular demands limit the time available for trips home. Flexibility to use one site or another will also be influenced by the funding structure of the SHS (e.g., health fee vs. fee-for-service), the restrictions of the student's health insurance coverage, and the relative incentive to use on-campus resources incorporated into health insurance plans offered by the university.

Negotiating this can be confusing, especially for students early in their undergraduate careers. Consider the example of the student who has an incidental visit to an emergency department proximate to his or her college and upon discharge receives the ubiquitous instruction to "follow-up with your primary care provider." The student might well consider his or her provider at home 1,000 miles away to be the "primary care provider" and is tentative about how to incorporate the SHS, especially at centers with admittedly limited resources.

This can be conceptualized as the student navigating a "virtual medical home," where the home is not defined by geography or mutual participation within an identified health system but rather that use of the right resource at the right time results in the best experience for the student-patient. Unfortunately, this virtual medical home does not come with a shared health record, a shared philosophy, or, as suggested in this chapter, a universally standardized menu of on-campus services. The efficacy of this medical home depends on effective, proactive professional communication and collaboration and on an appreciation for the resources and roles provided by the various players.

In a common scenario, the SHS clinician identifies a medical condition in early November to which the student's response is, "I talked with my folks and they want me to wait to follow-up with my regular doctor at home during Thanksgiving break." The SHS has a responsibility to provide the student with copies of relevant imaging studies or laboratory reports to have available for the home clinician and to encourage the student (or his or her parent/caregiver) to immediately get that appointment scheduled, since, almost by definition, such visits will occur around holidays, when the home practice also has limited availability. Likewise, significant interventions made by the home clinician should be communicated back to the SHS if there is an expectation that there will be continuity of care when the student returns to campus. Most SHSs with laboratory or x-ray capabilities will gladly accept "outside" orders from a home clinician if, for example, the patient desires for the home clinician to have ongoing responsibility for monitoring thyroid-stimulating hormone or HgbA1C levels. A corollary of this

is that the SHS will gladly do suture removal, dressing changes, and other primary care follow-up for procedures performed by a home clinician, but it always goes more smoothly when there is a copy of a clinic note or other notification.

The student and his or her family will often have a long-standing relationship with the primary care provider at home and will hold him or her in a place of respect. This may relegate the SHS to a lesser position. The typical scenario is that of a student with an upper respiratory tract infection who is seen in the SHS and does not receive the antibiotic prescription he or she was anticipating. Rather than following the treatment plan offered by the college health clinician and follow-up if needed, the immediate response may be to contact the hometown clinician to request a sight unseen, long distance antibiotic prescription, the assumption being that the SHS was wrong. Clearly, there are many opportunities for the various teams of clinicians to support each other and thereby provide optimal care for the mutual patient and his or her family. Clinician-to-clinician communication can often prevent such situations. Please call the SHS—they want to collaborate in the care of the mutual patient.

Leave of Absence

As a final consideration, the home clinician is an important voice in helping a student or their family to come to peace with a decision to take a medical (understood to be inclusive of mental health concerns) leave of absence. Whether because of acute decompensation of an eating disorder, motor vehicle trauma requiring 2 weeks of hospitalization and then acutely limited mobility, or newly diagnosed insulin-dependent diabetes, there are times when the stressors of catching up with and sustaining school work will exacerbate the clinical condition and detract from participation in the treatment regimen. All of these factors can hinder academic performance and further increase the student-patient's stressors. It is very difficult for a student to remain academically productive while simultaneously managing a severe or chronic medical condition that is newly diagnosed or has become unstable. There are times when the best course is to take a leave for the rest of the semester. Although the student and their family will also be receiving advice and options from the school, the family may look to the trusted home clinician for endorsement of these difficult decisions.

More and more, universities are offering leave-of-absence insurance to refund some portion of tuition when a student takes a medical leave, which is another consideration to suggest during prematriculation counseling with patients with potentially labile medical conditions. Further, in some cases, the best advice might extend past a recommendation to take leave for the remainder of the current semester to include a recommendation to consider transferring to a school closer to home, to a campus in a contained urban setting rather than a sprawling rural setting, to a school with more extensive on-campus access to mental health services, or to one with better access to a subspecialist.

● SUMMARY

College students represent a significant portion of young adults. During the college years, students lay the foundations of their adult health habits and behaviors. Successful management of medical and mental health conditions along with mitigation of behavioral risk factors have a direct impact on students' educational and personal success. Strong partnerships with collaboration and communication between on-campus SHSs, student life professionals, students and their families, and outside clinicians combine direct medical and mental health care with population-based interventions. This comprehensive approach can significantly affect the short- and long-term health of these young adults as they complete this transition to adulthood.

REFERENCES

1. Digest of Education Statistics. *Total Fall Enrollment in Degree-Granting Institutions, by Attendance Status, Sex, and Age: Selected Years, 1970 Through 2029.* Institute of Education Sciences. National Center for Education Statistics. Prepared April 2020. Accessed February 27, 2021. https://nces.ed.gov/programs/digest/d19/tables/dt19_303.40.asp

2. American College Health Association. *American College Health Association-National College Health Assessment III: Undergraduate Student Reference Group Executive Summary Spring 2020.* American College Health Association; 2020.

3. Global Health Data Exchange. *The global burden of disease* 2019. Accessed February 27, 2021. http://www.healthdata.org/united-states

4. Eisenberg D, Golberstein E, Hunt JB. Mental health and academic success in college. *J Econ Anal Policy.* 2009;9(1):1–37.

5. Lipson SK, Raifman J, Abelson S, et al. Gender minority mental health in the U.S.: results of a national survey on college campuses. *Am J Prev Med.* 2019;57(3):293–301.

6. Lipson SK, Kern A, Eisenberg D, et al. Mental health disparities among college students of color. *J Adolesc Health.* 2018;63(3):348–356.

7. Lipson SK, Lattie EG, Eisenberg D. Increased rates of mental health service utilization by U.S. college students: 10-year population-level trends (2007–2017). *Psychiatr Serv.* 2019;70(1):60–63.

8. Higher Education Mental Health Alliance. Published 2012. http://hemha.org/wp-content/uploads/2019/01/campus-teams-balancing-safety-support-campus-jed-guide.pdf

9. Substance Abuse and Mental Health Services Administration. Accessed March 14, 2021. https://www.samhsa.gov/integrated-health-solutions

10. Morris MR, Feldpausch NI, Inga Eshelman MG, et al. Recovering in place: creating campus models of care for the high-risk college student. *Curr Psychiatry Rep.* 2019;21(11):1–8.

11. American College Health Association. *Healthy campus.* Accessed February 1, 2021. http://www.acha.org/healthycampus/

12. Leidner AJ, Barry V, Bowen VB, et al. Opening of large institutions of higher education and county-level COVID-19 incidence – United States, July 6-September 17, 2020. *MMWR Morb Mortal Wkly Rep.* 2021;70(1):14–19.

13. Schulenberg, JE, Johnston, LD, O'Malley, PM, et al. *Monitoring the Future: National Survey Results on Drug Use, 1975–2019. Vol. II. College Students and Adults Ages 19–60.* Institute for Social Research, University of Michigan; Published July 2020.

14. Cantor D, Fisher B, Chibnall S, et al. Report on the AAU campus climate survey on sexual assault and misconduct. Westat. Published January 17, 2020. https://www.aau.edu/sites/default/files/AAU-Files/Key-Issues/Campus-Safety/Revised%20Aggregate%20report%20%20and%20appendices%201-7_(01-16-2020_FINAL).pdf

15. Swartout KM, Koss MP, White JW, et al. Trajectory analysis of the campus serial rapist assumption. *JAMA Pediatr.* 2015;169(12):1148–1154.

16. Vella-Zarb RA, Elgar FJ. The 'freshman 5': a meta-analysis of weight gain in the freshman year of college. *J Am Coll Health.* 2009;58(2):161–166.

17. Nikolaus CJ, An R, Ellison B, et al. Food insecurity among college students in the United States: a scoping review. *Adv Nutr.* 2020;11(2):327–348.

18. Gallup. Accessed February 28, 2021. https://news.gallup.com/poll/329708/lgbt-identification-rises-latest-estimate.aspx

19. Kloss JD, Nash CO, Horsey SE, et al. The delivery of behavioral sleep medicine to college students. *J Adolesc Health.* 2011;48(6):553–561.

20. Prichard JR. Sleep predicts collegiate academic performance: implications for equity in student retention and success. *Sleep Med Clin.* 2020;15(1):59–69.

21. Kessler CS, McGuinn M, Spec A, et al. Underreporting of blood and body fluid exposures among health care students and trainees in the acute care setting: a 2007 survey. *Am J Infect Control.* 2011;39(2):129–134.

22. National Center for Education Statistics. *The Condition of Education 2020. Chapter: 2/Postsecondary Education Section: Postsecondary Students.* College Student Employment; 2020. Accessed March 7, 2021. https://nces.ed.gov/programs/coe/pdf/coe_ssa.pdf

23. Balanay JAG, Adesina A, Kearney GD, et al. Assessment of occupational health and safety hazard exposures among working college students. *Am J Ind Med.* 2014;57(1):114–124.

24. Open Doors. Accessed February 28, 2021. https://opendoorsdata.org/fast_facts/fast-facts-2020/

25. Breslau J, Stein BD, Han B, et al. Impact of the affordable care act's dependent coverage expansion on the health care and health status of young adults: what do we know so far? *Med Care Res Rev.* 2018;75(2):131–152.

🛜 ADDITIONAL RESOURCES AND WEBSITES

Additional Resources and Websites for Clinicians:

Roberts LW. *Student Mental Health: A Guide for Psychiatrists, Psychologists, and Leaders Serving in Higher Education.* 1st ed. American Psychiatric Association Publishing; 2018.

Vaughn JA, Viera AJ. *Principles and Practice of College Health.* 1st ed. Springer Nature; 2021.

https://www.acha.org/

https://www.jedfoundation.org/

https://www.naspa.org/

https://nirsa.net/nirsa

https://store.samhsa.gov/product/Behavioral-Health-Among-College-Students-Information-and-Resource-Kit/SMA19-5052

https://collegiaterecovery.org/recovery-resources/

Additional Resources for Parents/Caregivers:

http://www.ulifeline.org/

https://www.adolescenthealth.org/SAHM_Main/media/Clinical-Care-Resources/Healthy-Student-Brochure/HSB_Brochure_2012_FNL_wtrmrk.pdf

https://www.collegedrinkingprevention.gov/parentsandstudents/parents/default.aspx

https://store.samhsa.gov/product/Talking-With-Your-College-Bound-Young-Adult-About-Alcohol/sma18-4897

https://www.apa.org/pi/disability/resources/parent-college-guide

Additional Resources for Adolescents and Young Adults:

http://www.ulifeline.org/

https://www.crisistextline.org/

https://www.activeminds.org/

https://www.halfofus.com/

https://collegediabetesnetwork.org/

Youth and Young Adults in the Military

Patricia E. Kapunan
William P. Adelman

KEY WORDS

- Civilian
- Deployment
- Military
- Military anticipatory guidance
- Military eligibility
- Military service
- Reserves
- Reserve Officer Training Corps (ROTC)
- Resilience

INTRODUCTION

The U.S. military community centers around adolescents and young adults (AYAs), whose service to their country as a family member or member of the Armed Forces affords them unique opportunities and may present certain challenges. Approximately half a million adolescents between the ages of 12 and 22 have a parent/guardian serving in the military. Nearly 880,000 individuals 25 years old and younger serve across the branches of the all-volunteer military workforce. This age group comprises 52.3% of the active-duty enlisted force, and 91.0% of new recruits.[1,2] As most young adults who join the military do not continue for a full career, military service often serves as a transition between childhood in their original communities and adulthood in higher education and the labor market.[3,4]

A strong emphasis on core values, service, and professionalism, underlies a military culture which exerts great influence on AYAs during a critical time of personal development. The requirements of military service, and the demands of military life, have both positive and negative implications for health, well-being, and resilience. An appreciation and understanding of the unique experience of military-affiliated youth in the context of emerging issues of young adulthood allows the clinician to provide optimal care.[5,6]

This chapter highlights special characteristics and health considerations of military-affiliated youth, including those AYAs preparing for a career in the military. The health data and resources included are specific to the U.S. military and may not be applicable to all countries. While elements of military culture and experience are common to other nations' militaries, individual countries may differ with respect to the societal role and cultural value of military participation, and the resources available to support military members and their families.

THE NEW RECRUIT

Clinicians may be asked to support youth considering or preparing for military service. Supporting older adolescents in their postsecondary educational and vocational plans is a key strategy to promote healthy adolescent development and successful transition to adulthood.[7] The clinician can assist the potential service member and family with an assessment of military service suitability as a potential path to adult independence. Patient-centered anticipatory guidance for those entering military service combines knowledge of AYA medicine with an understanding of the military recruitment and accession process.

Anticipatory Guidance for Military Service

Clinicians can guide youth considering military service through four steps: educate, articulate, navigate, and matriculate.[8]

Educate. Adolescents and young adults should learn about the different military service branches and enlistment processes using information from multiple sources, such as official online resources, discussion with current or previous service members, and through recruiters. If possible, the young person should speak to trusted friends or relatives with military experience.

Articulate. After researching their service of interest, the AYA should be able to articulate what the military offers for them and what the military expects in return. They should be able to explain their choice of service and complete the sentence, "I plan to join the military because…"; or "I decided against the military because…."

Navigate. The third step is to determine the best individual path to service, particularly whether to enlist after high school or seek an officer commission after higher education. Before signing an enlistment contract, youth interested in a specific military occupation should take the armed services vocational aptitude battery (ASVAB), which measures aptitude in verbal, math, science/technical, and spatial content domains.[9] This standardized exam is used to determine enlistment eligibility and guide job classification and can assist applicants in gauging their potential for acceptance into a preferred specialty or vocation. Adolescents and young adults interested in commissioning as officers may apply to a service academy or for a ROTC scholarship at a participating college.

Matriculate. Finally, the AYA should matriculate after discussion with their family, and after reviewing options with a service branch-specific recruiter who can facilitate the administrative and logistical elements of their route to service.

Requirements for Service Entry

In addition to qualifying through aptitude testing or equivalent training, applicants to the U.S. military must meet physical standards and pass a health screening.[10,11] Adolescents and young adults interested in joining the military and their clinicians must be aware of the physical requirements for enlistment, and common medical indications for disqualification.

Height and weight standards are service branch specific. Applicants to all branches undergo medical screening, including physical examination, at a Military Entrance Processing Station (MEPS). Department of Defense Instruction 6130.03 details medically disqualifying conditions for entrance to general military service.[11]

In 2017, the top three diagnostic categories for medical disqualification were[12]:

* Other nutrition, endocrine, and metabolic disorders (20.5%, most commonly weight-related disqualification due to overweight);
* Visual defects (12.3%); and
* Allergic reactions (9.1%).

Medical disqualifications are classified as temporary or permanent. Temporary disqualification is for medical conditions that can be corrected (e.g., weight exceeding entry standards). Some permanently disqualifying medical conditions may be considered for medical exception waivers through which applicants are cleared for service after a more detailed medical evaluation confirms their fitness for duty performance despite the condition. From 2013 to 2018, of nearly 1.2 million applicants for active-duty enlisted service, 13.9% had a condition meriting permanent medical disqualification. Of the 67.5% considered for a medical waiver, 67.6% received a waiver approval.[2]

Adolescents and young adults considering military service should be aware of personal conditions that may be disqualifying and of diagnoses that will not generally receive a waiver. Some common medically disqualifying conditions have time-related specifications (e.g., history of asthma with symptoms after age 13, or history of attention deficit hyperactivity disorder requiring treatment with medications in the previous 24 months).[11] Waiver approval varies by service and medical condition. In 2017, the top two diagnoses for which Army applicants applied for waiver, vision defects, and allergic reactions, had approval rates of >80%, while applicants requesting waivers for ADHD or asthma were approved at lower rates (66.1% and 41.9%, respectively).[12] **Table 80.1** lists

TABLE 80.1
Medical Conditions Disqualifying for Military Service

Psychological
* Bipolar disorder
* Severe personality disorders
* Drug and/or alcohol use disorders or diagnosed substance dependence
* Eating disorders
* Major depression, recurrent
* History of suicidality
* Schizophrenia

Systemic conditions
* Diabetes mellitus type I or type II
* History of cancer with treatment within 5 y (except basal cell carcinoma)
* Severe allergic reaction (anaphylaxis) to insects or food
* Single kidney

Musculoskeletal
* Loss of an arm, leg, or eye
* Prosthetic replacement of joints
* Severe orthopedic injuries that result in functional limitations secondary to residual muscle weakness, paralysis, or marked decreased range of motion

Neurologic
* Headaches, recurrent and severe, which require prescription medication and/or interfere with daily activity
* Seizure disorder with seizure and/or medication within 5 y
* Severe head injury within the past 5 y

Infectious diseases
* AIDS, AIDS-related complex (ARC), HIV antibody positive, or history of any of the above
* Hepatitis, chronic: hepatitis B or hepatitis C carrier

Gastrointestinal
* Inflammatory bowel disease
* History of bariatric surgery

IDS, acquired immunodeficiency syndrome; HIV, human immunodeficiency virus.

several disqualifying conditions unfavorable to military service, that are unlikely to receive a waiver. Figure 80.1 shows the most common pre-existing medical conditions associated with early discharge from service (within 180 days).

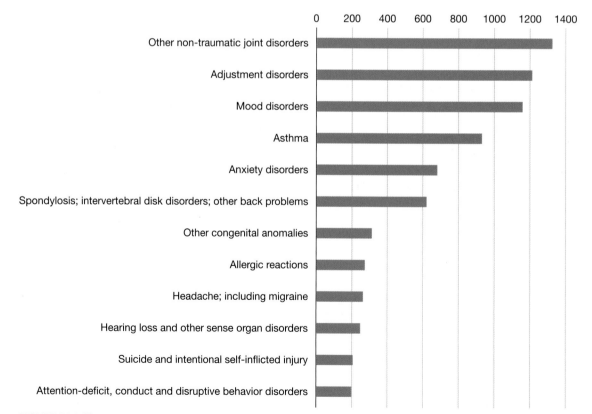

FIGURE 80.1 Most common pre-existing medical conditions associated with early discharge by number of enlisted member discharges in all service branches, 2013–2018. (Source: Accession Medical Standards Analysis & Research Activity (AMSARA). 2019 Annual Report: FY 2013–2018 Applicants, Accessions and Outcomes.)

New applicants to the Armed Forces must also meet legal requirements.[10] The minimum age for enlistment is 17 years; minimum age for officer commission varies by service. Though a high school diploma is desirable, individuals without a high school diploma are considered based on their score on the Armed Forces Qualification Test (AFQT), which is calculated based on the results of the four math and verbal sections of the 10-subtest ASVAB. All applicants are screened with a background check to detect felonies and serious financial problems. Though a waiver may be possible for civic issues, most applicants with a criminal record are disqualified. Applicants who give false information prior to entry may be dishonorably discharged after joining the service.

Recommendations for Clinicians Working with New Recruits

Clinicians without military expertise may refer to the resources listed in this chapter when providing anticipatory guidance to AYAs considering military service. Important aspects of care include encouraging AYAs to research and speak openly about the role of military service in their educational and vocational plans and addressing health considerations that may impact service eligibility and readiness, including weight standards and potentially medically disqualifying conditions. Clinicians can support youth in safely attaining weight or fitness standard goals, and by helping those with potentially disqualifying conditions set realistic health goals and professional expectations.

RESERVE OFFICER TRAINING CORPS STUDENTS

College students enrolled in an Reserve Officer Training Corps (ROTC) scholarship program participate in military training while pursuing a college degree at a participating school. In return, they receive tuition benefits and guaranteed employment after graduation, when they enter military service as an officer in the Active or Selected Reserve components. Students must meet academic performance thresholds as well as the physical fitness standards required of active-duty service members. In addition to their college workload, they participate in physical fitness training, dedicated military coursework, and intensive summer training camps. The Army, Air Force, and Navy each conduct service-specific ROTC programs. Some programs permit extracurricular participation without a military commitment or in preparation for scholarship application; scholarship recipients are expected to continue to meet the academic and physical demands of the ROTC program as a condition of their scholarship.

Recommendations for Clinicians Working with Reserve Officer Training Corps Students

Clinicians working with college-aged youth should be aware of the additional demands and requirements of participation in an ROTC program. Reserve Officer Training Corps scholarship students may be at increased risk for certain health conditions related to their physical fitness training and weight requirements, including musculoskeletal injuries and disordered eating.[13,14] Clinicians working with high school or college students considering applying for an ROTC scholarship can use the same principles of anticipatory guidance to support AYAs in planning to commit to military service through this higher education route.

THE YOUNG ADULT SERVICE MEMBER

More than 2 million individuals serve in the U.S. military. 45.7% of active-duty service members are ≤25 years old, compared to 38.3% in the Selected Reserve. "Active duty" refers to full-time service members in the Army, Navy, Marine Corps, Air Force, and Coast Guard. Unless called to active duty, Selected Reserve members are not full-time, but train periodically throughout the year and participate in annual training exercises. Selected Reserve components include the Army National Guard, Army Reserve, Navy Reserve, Marine Corps Reserve, Air National Guard, Air Force Reserve, and Coast Guard Reserve.[1] Most young adults in the military are enlisted personnel in the active-duty component (Fig. 80.2).

The military is predominately male, representing 83.1% of active-duty members and 79.4% of the Reserve and Guard members. Non-White minorities comprise 31.2% and 26.4% of active duty and Selected Reserve, respectively. Demographics also vary by service branch and officer versus enlisted rank.[1]

Health Considerations for Young Adult Service Members

Young adult service members negotiate the demands of late adolescence while adapting to a military-unique environment and its associated challenges. Risk behaviors and health risks in military members are generally comparable to their nonmilitary peers in the same age group. The 2015 Department of Defense Health-Related Behaviors Survey (HRBS) found that, compared to older age groups, service members ages 17 to 24 years were more likely to text while driving, use tobacco products, or exhibit dangerous drinking behaviors (binge-drinking, heavy or hazardous drinking). In the prior year, they were more likely to have had multiple sex partners, had sex with a new partner without using a condom, been diagnosed with a sexually transmitted infection, or reported an unintended pregnancy. Service members <25 years old were more likely than any other age group to engage in nonsuicidal self-injury, experience suicidal ideation, and to attempt suicide, and were less likely to receive mental health services.[15] Direct comparison of military members' health risk behaviors with age-matched peers is challenging given disparate methodologies in global surveys, but data suggest that military service serves as a protective factor for

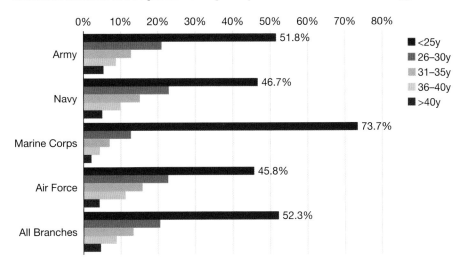

FIGURE 80.2 Age distribution of enlisted active-duty U.S. military personnel. (Source: Office of the Deputy Assistant Secretary of Defense for Military Community and Family Policy. *2019 Demographics: Profile of the Military Community.* Department of Defense; 2020.)

some behaviors (Table 80.2). Fear of disciplinary action for engaging in or reporting risk behaviors, increased health screening and access to health services, and professional performance requirements may explain these trends.

In 2015, 16.9% of HRBS respondents reported any lifetime history of unwanted sexual contact, a negative health outcome not impacted by age group but disproportionately reported by females (46.1%) and lesbian, gay, bisexual, or transgender (LGBT) service members (39.9%).[15] It is important to screen young service members for a history of sexual violence, and those at highest risk in particular, as comprehensive services are available through the Department of Defense Sexual Assault Prevention and Response Program.[16]

Injuries, musculoskeletal problems, and mental health conditions were the top three reasons active service members sought medical care in 2019. Mental health diagnoses were the leading cause of hospital admission and psychiatric admissions were more frequent in younger age groups. Conversely, the frequency of ambulatory care for mental health conditions increased with advancing age.[17–19]

Active-duty, Reserve, and National Guard members may all experience health risks associated with combat exposure and deployment. Acute combat injuries and overuse injuries from combat or training are common and may have significant and/or persistent impacts on the service member's ability to serve and thus their quality of life. Traumatic brain injuries (TBIs), such as those caused by improvised explosive devices, were more commonly seen in recent conflicts and can have long-lasting sequelae. Deployment-related negative health impacts also include excess substance use; mental health risks including depression, posttraumatic stress disorder (PTSD), and suicidality; and chronic somatic symptoms. These risks tend to be more profound with higher combat exposure and comorbid TBI.[6,15]

Screening Considerations

Military culture values discipline, loyalty, and hard work, with high value placed on self-sacrifice, courage, and physical fitness. When these cultural influences combine with the perceived invulnerability and developing critical thinking typical of adolescence, medical conditions may be minimized or hidden from the clinician. Young service members may underplay a health condition or behavior, especially if they fear it will negatively influence military advancement, fitness for duty, or unit reputation.[5] Therefore, clinician must be diligent when collecting a culturally sensitive and careful history.

A modified psychosocial review of systems screening that also addresses military stressors, coping and resilience may be used for young adult military members (Table 80.3).[20]

Recommendations for Clinician Working with Young Adult Service Members

Clinicians should be aware of the specific physical and emotional traumas that may accompany military service and utilize developmentally-appropriate strategies to collaboratively address these health impacts. A culturally sensitive approach and modified psychosocial review of systems can aid in addressing health risks and behaviors. Military-specific supports can be leveraged to support coping and resilience (e.g., unit leaders, unit peer support, chaplaincy services, dedicated health resources).

While active-duty members have essentially free and unlimited access to health services in the military health system, Reserve and National Guard members' benefits are limited to periods of activation to duty, or when care is specifically related to duty performance or duty-related injury. Adolescents and young adults in the Reserve or National Guard living outside predominantly military communities may have fewer social supports and practical resources to support them in balancing military professional demands with civilian life, or to fully address service-related health issues. Clinicians caring for youth in the Reserve or National Guard should be proactive in assessing the specific impacts of military experience and patients' knowledge of and access to military-specific resources.

ADOLESCENTS AND YOUNG ADULTS IN MILITARY FAMILIES

Military family life is characterized by change, service, and sacrifice. Experiences vary widely as military families traverse multiple geographic locations and community types, while negotiating stressors that are unique to military service like deployments and mandatory relocations. Duty-related family separations, combat exposure stress, and service-related injury or illness are among the well-recognized factors impacting military family well-being. Combat-related PTSD, depression and suicidality, TBI, and severe physical injuries can have critical and lasting impact on a service member's family. Also significant for family members are chronic stressors like interruptions of school and work life brought on by multiple moves and the challenges of having to repeatedly establish new support systems, often far from extended family or in a remote or foreign location. In the face of these challenges, military

---

TABLE 80.2

Comparison of Risk-Taking Behaviors in Civilian versus Military Youth and Young Adults

	Civilian (age)	Military (age)	Source
Contraception			
Current use– any birth control	37.2% (15–19 y) 61.9% (20–29 y)	85.4% (17–24 y) 83.1% (25–34 y)	Civilian: NSFG – "Current use of any contraceptive method" Military: HRBS "Use of any contraception at last sex"
Current use– condoms	5.3% (15–19 y) 11.6% (20–29 y)	31.5% (17–24 y) 23.1% (25–34 y)	Civilian: NSFG "Current use of condoms" Military: HRBS "Use of condoms at last sex"
Alcohol Use			
Heavy alcohol drinkers	2.4% (12–17 y) 11.3% (18–25 y)	9.5% (17–24 y)	Civilian: NSDUH– Alcohol use disorder Military: HRBS Frequent binge drinking/Alcohol use disorder
Cigarette Use	4.2% (12–17 y) 26.2% (18–25 y)	19.5% (17–24 y) 12.5% (25–34 y)	Civilian: NSDUH–Past month cigarette use Military: HRBS–Current cigarette use
Marijuana Use	12.6% (12–17 y) 32.4% (18–25 y)	1.0% (17–24 y) 0.8% (25–34 y)	Civilian: NSDUH–Any use in past year Military: HRBS–Any use in past year

HRBS: Meadows SO, Engel CC, Collins RL, et al. *Department of Defense Health Related Behaviors Survey (HRBS).* RAND Corporation; 2018; NSFG: Daniels K, Abma JC. *Current Contraceptive Status Among Women Aged 15–49: United States, 2015–2017. NCHS Data Brief.* National Survey of Family Growth; 2018. https://www.cdc.gov/nchs/nsfg/index.htm; NSDUH: U.S. Department of Health and Human Services. *Substance Abuse and Mental Health Services Administration, Center for Behavioral Health Statistics and Quality.* National Survey on Drug Use and Health; 2018. 2014–2016. https://datafiles.samhsa.gov/

TABLE 80.3

Additional History Questions for Military-Affiliated Youth

Young Adult Service Members	Adolescent or Young Adult Military Family Members
Home and Family Tell me about your unit/squad/crew. Do you feel like a valued member of your unit? Who do you trust most in your unit? Who do you live with? How is life for you in the barracks? What is it like for you, being away from home/family?	**Home and Family** How many places have you lived? Any recent or pending moves? Who is in the military in your family? Do they have to be away a lot? Do you see your extended family? What is your role at home? How is everyone getting along? Who else helps out?
Education and Employment What is your job? Do you like it? Do you have career or education plans for the future? How long are you planning to serve in the military? How is your command? Do you feel supported by your leaders? Have you been involved in any disciplinary actions?	**Education and Employment** Have moves interrupted school or caused academic hardship? Has moving caused other kinds of problems for you or your family? Are you considering joining the military? Why or why not?
Eating Are you trying to lose or gain weight? Do you use supplements or diet aids? Why? Do you stress out about weight standards? What do you do to make weight?	**Activities** Are you or your family involved in any community groups or activities? Do you keep in touch with your friends? How has moving affected your relationships with people?
Activities What do you do on the weekend/on leave? What do you do for fun? Do you have friends or activities outside the military?	**Substance Use** Are you worried about the health or safety of anyone close to you? Do you worry about your own or others' use of alcohol, prescription medications, or other substances?
Suicide/Depression Have you had any experiences that affect your life now? Do you have anyone you can talk to? Do you own a weapon? Have you ever thought about suicide? Have you been deployed? How many times?	**Suicide/Depression** Who could you go to if you felt stressed, down or overwhelmed? Do you worry about family members' stress level or coping? **Safety** Are there weapons in your home? How are they secured? Have you ever felt scared for your own physical safety? Have you ever been hurt?

families can exhibit extraordinary resilience. It is notable that military youth are twice as likely to join the military, compared to their civilian counterparts.[6]

Health Considerations for Adolescents and Young Adults in Military Families

In 2019, of the greater than 1.6 million children in Department of Defense families, less than one-third were in the 12- to 22-year-old age group (30.1% for all military families, 25.8% for active-duty families).[1] As younger service members transition out of the military, families with older children are fewer and tend to represent "career" families with years of accumulated military experience (Fig. 80.3). By the 12th grade, military teenagers have changed schools 6 to 9 times, with an average relocation rate of one move every 2 to 3 years. They experience a higher number of deployments or other family separations, and more frequent disruptions of peer relationships compared to youth from younger military and nonmilitary families.

The negative impact of deployment on psychological well-being may include emotional or behavioral problems. Adolescents from military families are like civilian peers in psychosocial function, and may exhibit fewer risk-taking behaviors, but both psychological well-being and risk behaviors can be negatively influenced by deployment. Teenagers with a deployed family member may exhibit more substance use, disordered eating, or sexual risk behaviors. They may also experience deployment differently from younger siblings, often assuming a greater or more parent-like family role during deployment, and more difficulty when family roles shift again when the deployed service member returns.[21-24]

Evidence-based interventions exist which promote resilience through support of parents/caregivers, family relationships, and family functioning. Dedicated social support is a key strategy for adolescents, through peer groups with shared experiences, community connectedness, or supportive relationships with other trusted adults.[6,21]

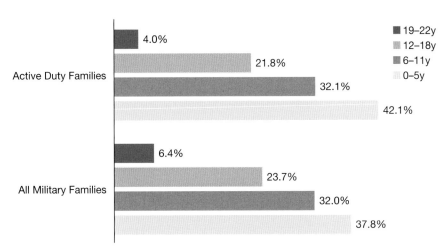

■ 19–22y
■ 12–18y
■ 6–11y
■ 0–5y

FIGURE 80.3 Age distribution of children of active-duty U.S. military families and all U.S. military families. (Source: Office of the Deputy Assistant Secretary of Defense for Military Community and Family Policy. *2019 Demographics: Profile of the Military Community*. Department of Defense; 2020.)

Screening Considerations

Adolescents and young adults with a family member in military service may present with physical or psychological complaints that may or may not be related to their military life experience. Psychosocial screening must consider military experience as a potential source of distress, and preventive health screening should acknowledge the stressors common to military life (**Table 80.3**).

Recommendations for Clinicians Working with Adolescents and Young Adults in Military Families

Clinicians working with AYAs from military families should be aware of factors that may influence health and function. Screening for negative impacts of frequent and mandatory moves, concern for military family members' well-being, and military-related events like deployments, is required to proactively address risk in this population. Evidence supports promoting parent/caregiver well-being, family unit functioning, and connecting youth with resources for social support.[6,21]

Adolescents and young adults in Reserve or National Guard families move less frequently due to service needs but may live in areas where military-specific resources are less accessible. Active-duty families are more likely to live in communities with shared military experience and have access to resources including health care, but frequent moves can make service continuity challenging. Military adolescents typically demonstrate great resilience in the face of these challenges and are more likely than nonmilitary peers to continue a military lifestyle in adulthood. In addition to uncovering risk, helping youth articulate their military family experience acknowledges their service and sacrifice, capacity for resilience, and may help them better negotiate present and future challenges.

 SUMMARY

Military-affiliated AYA negotiate adolescence while coping with the stressors of military life and military professional demands. Developmentally typical behavioral factors interact with the military environment to create unique health risks. Clinicians can better care for this special population by employing anticipatory guidance and risk screening strategies that acknowledge the challenges and opportunities of military experience.

ACKNOWLEDGMENT

This chapter is based on Chapter 80 "Youth and Young Adults in the Military" from *Neinstein's Adolescent and Young Adult Health Care: A Practical Guide*, sixth edition, authored by Jeffrey W. Hutchinson and William P. Adelman.

REFERENCES

1. Office of the Deputy Assistant Secretary of Defense for Military Community and Family Policy. 2019 *Demographics: Profile of the Military Community*. Department of Defense; 2020. https://www.militaryonesource.mil/data-research-and-statistics/military-community-demographics/2019-demographics-profile/
2. Accession Medical Standards Analysis & Research Activity (AMSARA). 2019 Annual Report: FY 2013–2018 Applicants. Accessions and Outcomes. https://www.wrair.army.mil/collaborate/amsara/knowledge-products
3. Robinson CA, Hutchinson JW, Adelman WP. Military service: military culture and the adolescent. In: Elzouki AY, ed. *Textbook of Clinical Pediatrics*. 2nd ed. Springer; 2011:3897—3900.
4. Institute of Medicine, National Research Council. *Investing in the Health and Well-Being of Young Adults*. The National Academies Press; 2014.
5. Hutchinson JW, Greene JP, Bryant CM, et al. Helping those who serve: care of the young adult veteran. *Adolesc Med State Art Rev*. 2013;24(3):553–572.
6. National Academies of Sciences, Engineering, and Medicine. *Strengthening the Military Family Readiness System for a Changing American Society*. The National Academies Press; 2019.
7. Hagan JF, Shaw JS, Duncan PM, eds. *Bright Futures: Guidelines for Health Supervision of Infants, Children and Adolescents*. 4th ed. American Academy of Pediatrics; 2017.
8. Adelman WP. Basic training for the pediatrician: how to provide comprehensive anticipatory guidance regarding military service. *Pediatrics*. 2008;121(4):e993–e997.
9. Official Site of the ASVAB Enlistment Testing Program. Accessed March 6, 2021. https://www.officialasvab.com/
10. Office of the Under Secretary of Defense for Personnel and Readiness. *Qualification Standards for Enlistment, Appointment, and Induction (DoDI 1304.26)*. Department of Defense; 2015. https://www.esd.whs.mil/DD/
11. Office of the Under Secretary of Defense for Personnel and Readiness. *Medical Standards for Military Service: Appointment, Enlistment, or Induction (DoDI 6130.03)*. Department of Defense; 2018. https://www.esd.whs.mil/DD/
12. Accession Medical Standards Analysis & Research Activity (AMSARA). 2018 Annual Report: Attrition & Morbidity Data for 2017. Accessions. https://www.wrair.army.mil/collaborate/amsara/knowledge-products
13. Smith A, Emerson D, Winkelmann Z, et al. Prevalence of eating disorder risk and body image dissatisfaction among ROTC Cadets. *Int J Environ Res Public Health*. 2020;17(21):8137.
14. Radzak KN, Sefton JM, Timmons MK, et al. Musculoskeletal injury in Reserve Officers' Training Corps: a report from the athletic training practice-based research network. *Orthop J Sports Med*. 2020;8(9):2325967120948951.
15. Meadows SO, Engel CC, Collins RL, et al. *Department of Defense Health Related Behaviors Survey (HRBS)*. RAND Corporation; 2018.
16. Official Site of the United States Department of Defense Sexual Assault Prevention and Response. Accessed August 2, 2021. https://www.sapr.mil/.
17. Armed Forces Health Surveillance Center. *MSMR, 27(05). Absolute and Relative Morbidity Burdens Attributable to Various Illnesses and Injuries, Active Component*. US Armed Forces; 2019. https://www.health.mil/Military-Health-Topics/Health-Readiness/AFHSD/Reports-and-Publications/Medical-Surveillance-Monthly-Report
18. Armed Forces Health Surveillance Center. *MSMR, 27(05). Hospitalizations, Active Component*. US Armed Forces; 2019. https://www.health.mil/Military-Health-Topics/Health-Readiness/AFHSD/Reports-and-Publications/Medical-Surveillance-Monthly-Report
19. Armed Forces Health Surveillance Center. *MSMR, 27(05). Ambulatory Visits, Active Component*. US Armed Forces; 2019. https://www.health.mil/Military-Health-Topics/Health-Readiness/AFHSD/Reports-and-Publications/Medical-Surveillance-Monthly-Report
20. Hutchinson JW, Greene JP, Hansen SL. Evaluating active-duty risk-taking: military home, education, activity, drugs, sex, suicide, and safety method. *Mil Med* 2008;173(12):1164–1167.
21. Milburn NG, Lightfoot M. Adolescents in wartime US military families: a developmental perspective on challenges and resources. *Clin Child Fam Psychol Rev*. 2013;16(3):266–277.
22. Klein DA, Adelman WP, Thompson AM, et al. All military adolescents are not the same: sexuality and substance use among adolescents in the U.S. military health-care system. *PLoS One*. 2015;10(10):e0141430.
23. Neyland MKH, Shank LM, Burke NL, et al. Parental deployment and distress, and adolescent disordered eating in prevention-seeking military dependents. *Int J Eat Disord*. 2020;53(2):201–209.
24. Hernandez BF, Peskin MF, Markham CM, et al. Associations between parental deployment, relocation, and risky sexual behaviors among a clinic-based sample of military-dependent youth. *J Prim Prev*. 2015;36(5):351–359.

ADDITIONAL RESOURCES AND WEBSITES

Additional Resources and Websites for Clinicians:
Military Accession Standards
Medical Standards for Military Service: Appointment, Enlistment, or Induction—https://www.health.mil/About-MHS/OASDHA/HSPO/Accessions-and-Medical-Standards
Military Community Resources
The official website of the Military Health System—https://health.mil/
Military OneSource resource hub—https://www.militaryonesource.mil/
National Resource Directory—https://nrd.gov/
Resources for Veterans
Health, wellness, and career services for wounded veterans—https://www.woundedwarriorproject.org/
U.S. Department of Veterans Affairs website: VA Benefits for Service Members—https://www.va.gov/service-member-benefits/

Additional Resources and Websites for Parents/Caregivers and Adolescents and Young Adults:
Recruitment Information—https://www.airforce.com/
https://www.goarmy.com/
https://www.gocoastguard.com/
https://rmi.marines.com/
https://www.navy.com/
Reserve Officer Training Corps (ROTC) College Scholarship Programs—https://www.goarmy.com/rotc
https://www.goarmy.com/rotc/parents-and-advisors/faq.html
https://www.netc.navy.mil/Commands/Naval-Service-Training-Command/NROTC/Requirements/
Military Family Resources
Health and coping resources for children from military families—https://militarykidsconnect.health.mil/
Comprehensive family resources for military spouses and children including employment help, scholarships, summer camp, and family retreats—https://www.militaryfamily.org/
Military Child Education Coalition's resources for military-connected students, their parents and education professionals—https://www.militarychild.org/
Program providing support for youth from National Guard or Reserve families impacted by deployment or serious injury—https://www.ourmilitarykids.org/

CHAPTER 81

Youth Experiencing Homelessness

Meera S. Beharry
Lauren Bretz
Colette (Coco) Auerswald
Curren W. Warf

KEY WORDS

- Couch surfing
- Health status
- Homeless youth
- Literally homeless youth
- Rough sleeping
- Runaways
- Street youth
- Systems youth
- Throwaways
- Trafficked youth
- Youth experiencing homelessness (YEH)

INTRODUCTION

Youth experiencing homelessness (YEH) are extraordinarily resilient and possess immense potential. Relative to their stably housed peers, they face additional challenges as they approach the typical developmental tasks of adolescence.[1-3] This chapter focuses on the unique needs of unaccompanied minors and youth up to age 26 who are experiencing homelessness. Topics addressed in this chapter include etiology of homelessness, terminology, demographic data, and specific health concerns along with general suggestions and approaches to addressing the needs of YEH.

The Path to the Street

With varied paths to the streets and unique individual experiences, YEH are not a homogeneous population.[4] Many have disproportionately experienced a variety of adverse childhood experiences (ACEs) including poverty; early childhood loss (parental separation or incarceration of a household member); parental substance use and domestic violence; mental illness; emotional, physical, and/or sexual abuse and/or neglect; and foster care placement.[1-8]

Definitions and Terms

Youth homelessness is inconsistently defined in the medical literature and in federal legislation.[6] The McKinney-Vento Homeless Education Assistance Act defines youth as homeless when they lack "a fixed, regular, and adequate nighttime residence" offering the definition most reflective of the range of youth's lived experiences of unstable housing.[9]

The literature employs multiple overlapping terms to describe YEH. As noted in Figure 81.1, the umbrella term YEH, includes *runaways*, *throwaways*, those who are *rough sleeping*, and have also been defined by the terms *literally homeless youth* or *street youth*, as well as youth who are staying in shelters. The term also includes those who are *unstably housed* and *couch surfing* by migrating from one unstable housing situation to another. Youth often move from one category to another: for example, a young person who reports that they are couch surfing at one visit, may be in a

shelter by the next. We employ the term *youth experiencing homelessness (YEH)* for all of these youth, recognizing that many youth perceive the term "homeless youth" as deeply stigmatizing.[1,4]

Population Size and Demographics

Data regarding the actual size of the population of YEH nationally and in local jurisdictions are poor.[1,6,7,10] Obstacles to an accurate count include variability in definitions of the terms "homelessness" and "youth"; considerable methodologic challenges to counting a largely hidden population; intermittent nature of youth homelessness; youths' avoidance of services because of fear of the authorities; and reluctance to identify as homeless due to stigma.[10,11] In 2017, Morton et al. estimated the population of unstably housed youth (ages 13 to 25 years) to be 4.16 million for a 12-month period. They estimated that 1 in 30 adolescents 13 to 17 years of age and nearly 1 in 10 young adults 18 to 25 years of age experienced homelessness in a single year.[10]

Though research on structural factors and youth homelessness is still unfolding, there is a broad understanding among clinicians as well as an emerging body of evidence, that homelessness does not result from personal deficits, but from structural factors, including structural racism, homophobia, and transphobia. Structural racism leads to disproportionate poverty, family trauma, and family homelessness among Black, Indigenous and other People of Color

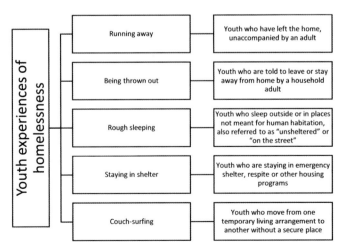

FIGURE 81.1 Terms describing youth experiences of homelessness. The different terms attempt to capture the range of youth experiences that contributed to homelessness and the variety in living situations. Living situations are fluid. (From Gewirtz O'Brien JR, Auerswald C, English A, et al. Youth experiencing homelessness during the COVID-19 pandemic: unique needs and practical strategies from international perspectives. *J Adolesc Health.* 2021;68(2).)

(BIPOC).[12,13] Homophobia, transphobia, and other forms of stigma are both significant causes of homelessness and barriers to gender and sexual minority youth attempting to leave homelessness. This is reflected in the relative rates of homelessness among youth from these backgrounds. Morton et al documented an increased relative risk of experiencing homelessness for youth who reported their identity as African American (1.8 times), Latino (1.3 times), and lesbian, gay, bisexual, transgender (LGBT) (2.2 times) (Fig. 81.2).

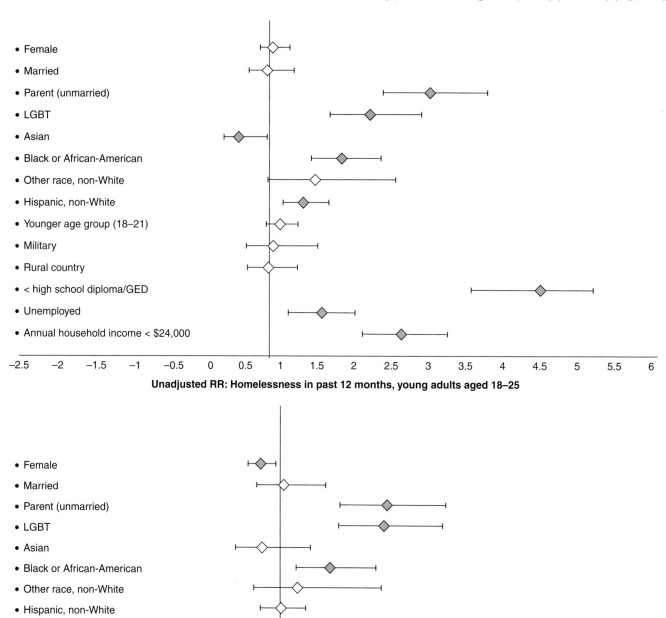

FIGURE 81.2 Relative risk of experiencing homelessness by key demographic characteristics. Unadjusted relative risks (RR) scores calculate risk based only on one demographic variable. The adjusted relative risk control for all other variables in the model. Diamonds represent the RR with extending lines on either side of the diamonds representing corresponding 95% CIs. Filled diamond indicates that the RR is statistically significant ($p < .05$). An RR of 1.0 means that risk is even between two groups. (From Morton MH, Dworsky A, Matjasko JL, et. al. Prevalence and correlates of youth homelessness in the United States. *J Adolesc Health.* 2018;62(1).)

In addition, and importantly for interventions, homelessness was 4.5 times as likely among youth without a high school diploma, 3 times as likely among unmarried youth with children, and 2.6 times as likely in impoverished families with a household income less than $24,000 per year.[10]

RISKY BEHAVIORS, MORBIDITY, AND MORTALITY

Risky Behaviors and the Health of Youth Experiencing Homelessness

Given their lack of familial support, society's failure to provide for them, and their underlying vulnerability, YEH have limited options to meet their basic needs for food, shelter, safety, emotional support, and health care. Although adolescence is a developmental stage during which experimentation and exploration are normative (see Chapter 3), YEH often engage in behaviors considered particularly risky by clinicians in order to meet their basic needs (such as "survival sex": exchanging sex for food, clothing, shelter, or drugs); to gain peer acceptance (use of illegal substances, criminal activities) or to self-medicate.[1,3,4] Although this may be seen as dangerous within a medical paradigm, these behaviors may be quite rational from the standpoint of a youth's survival. To reduce their risk, youth require alternative means to meet these basic needs. Programs serving YEH may engage youth by providing for some of their basic needs and facilitating linkages to drop-in centers, food, education, more stable housing, or opportunities for employment.

Violence and Abuse

Youth experiencing homelessness are not only more likely than housed peers to have experienced trauma prior to experiencing homelessness, they are also at far greater risk than housed youth of experiencing additional episodes of violence, physical abuse, or sexual exploitation once homeless. In a multicity study of YEH, Bender and colleagues found that 79% of youth recruited from agencies that serve YEH reported multiple types of childhood abuse and 29% reported street victimization, that is, having experienced physical or sexual assault while homeless.[14] Lesbian, gay, bisexual, transgender youth report particularly high rates of victimization.[15] Youth may resist reporting or refuse services because of prior trauma resulting from the disclosure of past abuse (such as separation from family and removal from home), or because of economic dependence on a current abuser (e.g., a "pimp" or drug dealer). Clinicians should be guided by local laws and regulations to ensure youth's safety (see Chapter 7). Furthermore, for minors who are being sexually exploited, guidelines regarding trafficked youth also apply.[16]

Substance Use and Mental Health Concerns

Alcohol, tobacco, and other problematic drug use are more prevalent among YEH than among housed youth. Injection drug use (IDU) is far more common among YEH than among housed youth, as are its adverse effects. A longitudinal cohort study of Canadian street-involved youth found that progression from experimentation to regular IDU was associated with prior regular use of the drug first injected, a history of childhood physical abuse, and having a sexual partner present at injection initiation.[17] Community-based naloxone distribution has been found to be a life-saving measure.[18] Harm-reduction strategies that make clean syringes and drug-use paraphernalia available reduce the risk of negative consequences of IDU, including transmission of human immunodeficiency virus (HIV) and hepatitis C.[19]

Youth experiencing homelessness are more likely than their housed counterparts to suffer from psychiatric morbidity, including mood disorders (particularly depression and bipolar disorder), anxiety disorders (particularly generalized anxiety disorder), posttraumatic stress disorder, and suicidality.[3,6,14] Similarly, mortality of YEH is significantly higher than among housed youth, especially females, largely due to preventable causes, particularly suicide, drug overdose, and accidental trauma.[20]

The diagnosis of psychiatric disorders is often clouded by concurrent substance use, which may be an attempt at self-medication.[21] Substance use treatment may be an important first step in the management of underlying mental health disorders. Mental health services should not be deferred while youth continue to engage in drug or alcohol use.

Infectious Diseases, Including Sexually Transmitted Infections

Youth experiencing homelessness are at greater risk for infectious diseases associated with their marginalized status. Youth experiencing homelessness can also unknowingly be a vector of infection as they move from shelter to shelter. In a study of illicit drug-using street-involved youth in Vancouver, the seroincidence of hepatitis C was 10.9 per 100 person-years among females and 5.1 per 100 person-years among males.[22] Similarly, YEH are at significantly increased risk of acquiring HIV infection with some studies indicating that 2% to 11% of YEH are living with HIV. This is 4 to 20 times the rate in the general youth population. Much of this risk is associated with increased risk behaviors such as engaging in survival sex, IDU, and sharing of needles. In reviewing studies from 2000 to 2015, Caccamo and colleagues found significant variability in rates of sexually transmitted infections. Rates for chlamydia and gonorrhea from tested samples ranged from 4.6% to 11.6% and 0.4% to 11%, respectively.[23] Condoms, rapid testing, immediate linkage to care with no-cost antibiotics, and expedited partner therapy, as indicated, should be made available.[3,24,25] In a study evaluating knowledge and attitudes about pre-exposure prophylaxis (PrEP) among YEH (ages 18 to 26) across seven U.S. cities, Santa Maria et al. found that 59% reported being likely or extremely likely to take PrEP.[26] Patients with continued high-risk behaviors for HIV should be provided PrEP and encouraged to continue to use condoms.

Youth experiencing homelessness are also susceptible to dermatologic infections associated with poor hygiene, IDU, or both, including cellulitis and abscesses. Methicillin-resistant *Staphylococcus aureus* should be strongly considered in this population.[27]

Youth experiencing homelessness are also more likely to contract parasitic infections, such as lice and scabies.[3,6,27]

More recently, the COVID-19 pandemic amplified the structural disparities that youth face in trying to stay healthy and presented unique challenges for YEH who were unable to follow quarantine recommendations while unstably housed.[28,29] In addition, outbreaks of isoniazid-resistant tuberculosis among residents of homeless shelters emphasize the challenges of preventing the spread of respiratory infections in this population.[30]

Therefore, YEH should routinely be screened for HIV, hepatitis C, chlamydia, gonorrhea, syphilis, and tuberculosis. A history of IDU, survival sex or trafficking, and/or of men having sex with men may further increase youth's risk and alter the frequency of indicated screening tests, as per current screening guidelines.[24,25]

Reproductive Health

Youth experiencing homelessness require no-cost, on-demand access to the full range of effective contraceptive methods, including long-acting reversible contraception (LARC), emergency contraception, and abortion. Youth who are homeless commonly have difficulties reliably storing medications such as birth control pills, and may benefit from LARC such as medroxyprogesterone acetate injectable contraception, an intrauterine device, or a contraceptive implant. Young women also need access to emergency (or post coital) contraception, which can include the use of higher doses of conventional oral contraceptives within 72 hours of unprotected coitus or the copper IUD in addition to the levonorgestrel products which are marketed specifically as emergency contraception or "morning after pills." All youth should have ready and discreet access to condoms with education about their use. All service clinicians for YEH need to be capable of providing timely access to reproductive health services.[3]

Youth experiencing homelessness are far more likely than housed youth to experience an unintended pregnancy.[6] In some circumstances, pregnancy in a teen who is experiencing homelessness may enable her to move toward reconciliation with her family of origin. For other teens, a pregnancy may have contributed to leaving or being thrown out of their family's home. Women choosing to continue their pregnancy need prompt access to prenatal care, housing stabilization, counseling regarding the fetal risks of alcohol and other substance use, education about infant care and early childhood development, and family reconciliation when possible.[2] A pregnancy can expedite a departure from the street for the adolescent and their child, as women and young children who are experiencing homelessness are usually given a higher priority status for housing.

Sexual Assault

Adolescents aged 12 to 17 years have the highest rates of being sexually assaulted of any age group; this is particularly true for youth who have left their family and are living on the streets or couch surfing.[31] Youth commonly do not initially disclose a sexual assault given that the assailant may be well known to the youth or the family, or even be a family member. Sexual abuse or a sexual assault in the home may have been a key factor in the youth running away (see Chapter 78).

Other Medical Problems

Youth experiencing homelessness have higher rates of common medical problems such as asthma, diabetes, and obesity. They often have not had routine screening for vision and dental problems.[6] In addition, their ACEs put YEH at higher risk of poor health which may be mitigated by stable housing or family support.[8]

⬤ PRINCIPLES AND APPROACH TO CARE

Notwithstanding the trauma and lack of support they have faced, YEH often demonstrate great resilience and, at this critical developmental stage, commonly respond well to caring relationships with adults.[3]

Guidelines for Clinicians

- Though it may seem minor in the eyes of clinicians, the *chief complaint* can serve as an opening to address issues of housing, education, mental health, and social services.
- Recognize that *youth may avoid accessing care for multiple reasons*, including fear of being judged or treated disrespectfully, anxiety about the implications of a health problem, past negative experiences in the health care system, fear of being reported to child protective services (for minors), and concern regarding lack of coverage or inability to pay for care (for young adults). Experiences with rejection, trauma, and loss may leave them with difficulty in trusting others and accepting services. Thanking the young person for coming in and addressing their concerns can help to alleviate fear and anxiety while building rapport.
- Initially, health care clinicians may assume that YEH are more independent, or even more mature, than similarly aged youth since they seem to be engaged in behaviors more commonly encountered by adults, such as drug and alcohol use and sexual activity. The reality, however, is that they are much less prepared to negotiate the challenges of adult life and are highly vulnerable.
- *Foster trust and respect* through a nonjudgmental positive stance toward the adolescent or young adult to maximize the

potential for follow-up. When screening for high-risk behaviors which are more prevalent among YEH, such as IDU and survival sex, clinicians should take a careful history that is respectful of the responses of the patient.[7] Clinicians may erode any trust and rapport by assuming that a young person experiencing homelessness is sexually active or abusing substances.[3]

- *Employ a strengths-focused, trauma-informed, harm-reduction approach* to encourage youth to reduce their risk behaviors to the degree they are able to minimize negative consequences. Speaking about "home" may be difficult for YEH. Clinicians should respect the young person's autonomy and avoid retraumatization by allowing them to keep private any information they are not yet ready to share.
- *Help youth identify their own goals and strengths* to assist them in moving incrementally toward engagement, greater safety, and stability. Employing the strategies of "meeting them where they are" and motivational interviewing are essential in working with YEH.
- *Utilize clinical encounters as opportunities to link youth to available resources* to address their needs, particularly housing, education, employment, and mental health services. Partnerships with schools and other key stakeholders provide a safety net and community of care.

Guidelines for Clinics and Other Programs

- Concerns regarding *confidentiality, reporting, and consent* may be significant obstacles that both prevent youth from presenting for care and clinicians from making care available to YEH. In some U.S. states, such as California, homelessness status alone is not, in and of itself, sufficient basis to report child abuse or neglect.[32] In most states, minors are entitled to confidentiality except when having an intent to die by suicide, commit homicide, or when they disclose physical, sexual, or severe emotional abuse. Placing hotline numbers in the general areas of the clinic, such as the bathrooms, helps to provide information to youth who may not be comfortable discussing their needs directly with a clinician.
- *Low barrier, no-cost health care* must be available to all YEH, including those who are immigrants.
- Due to the lack of continuity in their care and the scarcity of stable and trustworthy adults in their lives to guide their access to medical care, YEH need *intensive case management*.
- Provide *drop-in and evening/weekend hours*, and praise youth for presenting for care without penalizing them for missing appointments. In addition, providing cell phone chargers and places for their pets can help with making a more welcoming environment for YEH.
- Clinic staff serving YEH should be knowledgeable about local drop-in centers, emergency shelters for youth, housing programs, substance abuse programs, mental health and counseling resources, schools, and community resources. Clinic relationships with local child protective services can connect youth to critical resources and when possible and safe, can help foster family reconciliation. If a young person expresses an interest in a particular resource, it is important to quickly facilitate a linkage.
- Many YEH continue to be enrolled in public schools or community colleges. Being a student may enable them to obtain care at school-based health centers including general health care evaluations, dental evaluations, and vision screening. Some well-resourced school-based clinics can provide access to social workers and nurses and may be well situated to engage parents/caregivers or other supportive adults.
- Engage youth in developing and designing programs that build their own skills and leadership capabilities, promote positive social relationships and connections to promote positive self-esteem. Observe, note, and identify positive attributes and contributions. Youth contribute their own valuable insights and experiences and challenge adults to be more responsive.

- Support youth by providing opportunities for employment or mentorship. Youth can serve as members of youth advisory boards or panel discussions. They can also work as staff in "point-in-time" counts or other projects assessing the needs of those experiencing homelessness.

Guidelines for Communities

The U.S. Interagency Council on Homelessness (USICH) report "Preventing and Ending Youth Homelessness, A Coordinated Community Response"[33] has developed a comprehensive strategy with the following points:

- Prevent youth from becoming homeless by identifying and working with families who are at risk of fracturing.
- Effectively identify and engage youth at risk for, or actually experiencing, homelessness and connect them with trauma-informed, culturally appropriate, and developmentally and age-appropriate interventions.
- Intervene early when youth do become homeless and work toward family reunification, when safe and appropriate.
- Develop coordinated entry systems to identify youth for appropriate types of assistance and to prioritize resources for the most vulnerable youth.
- Ensure access to safe shelter and emergency services when needed.
- Ensure that assessments respond to the unique needs and circumstances of youth and emphasize strong connections to and supported exits from mainstream systems when needed.
- Create individualized services and housing options tailored to the needs of each youth, and include measurable outcomes across key indicators of performance, including education and employment.[33]

To address the health of YEH, communities can address structural factors at the legislative, programmatic, and policy levels.[6,33]

- Provide housing on demand to youth as quickly as possible regardless of their engagement in services, as well as access on demand to developmentally appropriate substance use and mental health services.
- Provide a range of options for housing youth, including but not limited to:
  - Youth Shelters: Temporary safe housing with meals, showers, and respite from the streets. Staff can provide referrals and assistance with reuniting with families, returning to school, and preparing for employment.
  - Host Homes: An innovative model to provide safe voluntary emergency shelter or longer-term transitional living with a trained community host. Youth can continue school, prepare for employment and find permanent housing, and can remain in their communities.
  - Transitional Living/Housing: Time-limited supportive housing for youth not ready for independent living. Models are varied from congregate housing with supervision to clustered housing units to shared apartments.
  - Kinship Care: Housing for youth with their biologic or chosen families, who may not otherwise be able to shelter them if they did not receive financial support and wraparound services.
- Implement *cash transfer programs for YEH*, in order to directly address their lack of resources.[34]
- Ensure *youth's access to social services to which they are entitled*, such as housing, case management, education, vocational services, primary, and subspecialty health care.
- Promote *continuity of care* through collaboration among local and regional clinicians for YEH and access to a portable electronic records and documents system.
- Extend foster care services into young adulthood, including access to transitional housing, and extend such services to other transition-aged youth.

- Oppose laws that criminalize homelessness (sit-lie or panhandling ordinances), minor offenses (such as marijuana possession), or informal care for the homeless by extended family or friends.
- Increase awareness of human trafficking, and encourage law enforcement to prosecute traffickers rather than youth.
- Eliminate rules that exclude youth and young adults from the Housing Choice Voucher Program Section 8, commonly referred to as Section 8 (https://www.hud.gov/program_offices/public_indian_housing/programs/hcv/about). or other subsidized housing or family shelters.
- Provide services tailored to the needs of specific high-risk populations, including LGBT and immigrant youth.
- Support the creation of more affordable housing options for all members of the community as a strategy to prevent homelessness.

SUMMARY

While the risks and challenges facing YEH are significantly greater than that of their stably housed counterparts, their needs are similar: strong, stable connections to caring and supportive adults who can provide opportunities for them to learn, grow, and develop into healthy young adults. Clinicians, programs, and communities can improve the experiences and outcomes for YEH through partnerships that include the input and voices of youth while using a strengths-focused, trauma-informed, harm-reduction approach.

ACKNOWLEDGMENT

The authors wish to thank Kirstin Sepulveda, RN for assistance in writing this chapter.

REFERENCES

1. Society for Adolescent Health and Medicine. The healthcare needs and rights of youth experiencing homelessness. *J Adolesc Health*. 2018; 63(3): 372–375.
2. Institute of Medicine and National Research Council. *Investing in the Health and Well-Being of Young Adults*. The National Academies Press; 2014. Accessed April 13, 2021. https://www.ncbi.nlm.nih.gov/books/NBK284787/. doi: 10.17226/18869
3. Warf C, Grant C, eds. *Clinical Care for Homeless, Runaway and Refugee Youth: Intervention Approaches, Education and Research Directions*. Springer International Publishing; 2020.
4. Hickler B, Auerswald CL. The worlds of homeless White and African American youth in San Francisco, California: a cultural epidemiological comparison. *Soc Sci Med*. 2009;68(5):824–831.
5. Embleton L, Lee H, Gunn J, et al. Causes of child and youth homelessness in developed and developing countries: a systematic review and meta-analysis. *JAMA Pediatrics*. 2016;170(5):435–444.
6. Beharry MS, Christensen R. Homelessness in pediatric populations. *Pediatr Clin North Am* 2020; 67(2):357–372.
7. Dawson-Rose C, Shehadeh D, Hao J, et al. Trauma, substance use, and mental health symptoms in transitional age youth experiencing homelessness. *Public Health Nurs*. 2020;37(3):363–370.
8. Barnes AJ, Gower AL, Sajady M, et al. Health and adverse childhood experiences among homeless youth. *BMC Pediatr*. 2021; 21:164.
9. McKinney-Vento Homeless Assistance Act. 42 USC 11434a: Definitions (2015). https://uscode.house.gov/view.xhtml?req=(title:42%20section:11434a%20edition:prelim)#11434a_1
10. Morton MH, Dworsky A, Matjasko JL, et. al. Prevalence and correlates of youth homelessness in the United States. *J Adolesc Health*. 2018; 62:14–21.
11. Auerswald C, Lin J, Petry L, et al. *Hidden in Plain Sight: an Assessment of Youth Inclusion in Point-in-Time Counts of California's Unsheltered Homeless Population*. California Homeless Youth Project; 2013.
12. Bogard K, Murray VM, Alexander C, eds. *Perspectives on Health Equity and Social Determinants of Health*. National Academy of Medicine; 2018.
13. Trent M, Dooley DG, Douge J, et al. American academy of pediatrics, section on adolescent health. The impact of racism on child and adolescent health. *Pediatrics*. 2019;144(2):e2019176515.
14. Bender K, Brown SM, Thompson SJ, et al. Multiple victimizations before and after leaving home associated with PTSD, depression, and substance use disorder among homeless youth. *Child Maltreat*. 2015;20(2):115–124.
15. Keuroghlian AS, Shtasel D, Bassuk EL. Out on the street: a public health and policy agenda for lesbian, gay, bisexual, and transgender youth who are homeless. *Am J Orthopsychiatry*. 2014;84:66–72.
16. National Research Council. *Confronting Commercial Sexual Exploitation and Sex Trafficking of Minors in the United States*. The National Academies Press; 2013.
17. Debeck K, Kerr T, Marshall BDL, et al. Risk factors for progression to regular injection drug use among street-involved youth in a Canadian setting. *Drug Alcohol Depend*. 2013;133(2):468–472.

18. Goldman-Hasbun J, DeBeck K, Buxton JA, et al. Knowledge and possession of take-home naloxone kits among street-involved youth in a Canadian setting: a cohort study. *Harm Reduct J*. 2017;14(1):79.

19. Vancouver Coastal Health. Insite—Supervised Consumption Site website. Accessed April 20, 2021. http://www.vch.ca/Locations-Services/result?res_id=964

20. Auerswald CL, Lin JS, Parriott A. Six-year mortality in a street-recruited cohort of homeless youth in San Francisco, *California. PeerJ*. 2016; 4:e1909.

21. Narendorf SC, Cross MB, Santa Maria D, et al. Relations between mental health diagnoses, mental health treatment, and substance use in homeless youth. *Drug Alcohol Depend*. 2017;175:1–8. doi: 10.1016/j.drugalcdep.2017.01.028

22. Puri N, DeBeck K, Feng C, et al. Gender influences on hepatitis C incidence among street youth in a Canadian setting. *J Adolesc Health*. 2014;55(6):830–834.

23. Caccamo A, Kachur R, Williams SP. Narrative review: sexually transmitted diseases and homeless youth—what do we know about sexually transmitted disease prevalence and risk? *Sex Transm Dis*. 2017;44(8):466–476.

24. Bonin E, Brehove T, Carlson C, et al. *Adapting Your Practice: General Recommendations for the Care of Homeless Patients. Nashville: Health Care for the Homeless Clinicians' Network*. National Health Care for the Homeless Council, Inc.; 2010.

25. Centers for Disease Control and Prevention. Expedited partner therapy website. Accessed April 20, 2021. http://www.cdc.gov/STD/ept/default.htm

26. Santa Maria D, Flash CA, Narendorf S, et al. Knowledge and attitudes about pre-exposure prophylaxis among young adults experiencing homelessness in seven U.S. cities. *J Adolesc Health*. 2019;64(5):574–580.

27. Strashun S, D'Sa S, Foley D, et al. Physical illnesses associated with childhood homelessness: a literature review. *Ir J Med Sci*. 2020;189(4):1331–1336.

28. Gewirtz O'Brien JR, Auerswald C, English A, et al. Youth experiencing homlessness during the COVID-19 pandemic: unique needs and practical strategies from international perspectives. *J Adolesc Health*. 2021;68(20):236–240.

29. UC Berkeley School of Public Health. For the good of us all: Addressing the needs of our unhoused neighbors during the COVID-19 pandemic. 2020. Accessed April 19, 2021. https://publichealth.berkeley.edu/news-media/video-room/uc-berkeley-school-of-public-health-releases-new-report-on-covid-19-homeless-response/

30. Holland DP, Alexander S, Onwubiko U, et al. Response to isoniazid-resistant tuberculosis in homeless shelters, Georgia, USA, 2015–2017. *Emerg Infect Dis*. 2019;25(3):593–595

31. Planty M, Langton L, Krebs C, et al. *Female victims of sexual violence, 1994–2010*. US Department of Justice, Office of Justice Programs, Bureau of Justice Statistics; 2013. Accessed April 13, 2020. https://bjs.ojp.gov/content/pub/pdf/fvsv9410.pdf

32. California Legislative Information. Child abuse and neglect reporting act: homeless children, AB652 (2013). Accessed April 20, 2021. http://leginfo.legislature.ca.gov/faces/billNavClient.xhtml?bill_id=201320140AB652

33. United States Interagency Council on Homelessness. Preventing and ending youth homelessness: a coordinated community response. 2015. Accessed on April 20, 2021. https://www.usich.gov/tools-for-action/coordinated-community-response-to-youth-homelessness/

34. Morton, M. H., Chávez, R., Kull, M. A., et al. *Developing a Direct Cash Transfer Program for Youth Experiencing Homelessness: Results of a Mixed Methods, Multi Stakeholder Design Process*. Chapin Hall at the University of Chicago; 2020.

🛜 ADDITIONAL RESOURCES AND WEBSITES

Additional Resources and Websites for Clinicians:
American Academy of Pediatrics: How to Care For and Support Runaway Youth—https://www.healthychildren.org/English/news/Pages/Caring-for-Runaway-Youth.aspx
Fostering Resilience (For Professionals)—http://fosteringresilience.com/professionals/
National Center for Homeless Education—https://nche.ed.gov/
National Healthcare for the Homeless Council—https://nhchc.org/
The US Interagency Council on Homelessness—https://www.usich.gov/

Additional Resources and Websites for Parents/Caregivers and Adolescents and Young Adults:
Child Welfare Information Gateway: Runaway and Homeless Youth—https://www.childwelfare.gov/topics/systemwide/youth/interventions/homeless-runaway/
Fostering Resilience (For Parents)—http://www.fosteringresilience.com/index_parents.php
National Alliance to End Homelessness—https://endhomelessness.org/
National Network for Youth—https://nn4youth.org/
National Runaway Safeline—https://www.1800runaway.org/
National Safe Place Program—https://www.nationalsafeplace.org/homeless-youth

CHAPTER 82

Youth in and Emancipated from Out-of-Home Care

Heather Taussig
Scott B. Harpin
William R. Betts
Gretchen J. Russo
James Kaferly
Renée Marquardt

KEY WORDS

- Behavioral health
- Child abuse and neglect
- Disparity
- Emancipation
- Foster care
- Kinship care
- Mental health
- Out-of-home care
- Transition care
- Trauma

INTRODUCTION

Over 100,000 adolescents in the United States are in out-of-home care (which includes nonrelative foster care, kinship care, and residential care) on any given day and approximately 20,000 youth emancipate from care each year.[1] Adolescents in out-of-home care, the vast majority of whom have experienced maltreatment, are at increased risk for physical and mental health problems throughout the developmental spectrum and are overrepresented in multiple service systems including juvenile justice, mental health, and special education. For young adults who have emancipated from out-of-home care, the transition to independence may be especially challenging, as these young adults demonstrate high rates of substance use, unplanned pregnancy, significant physical and mental health problems, criminal justice involvement, victimization (including trafficking), economic hardship, and homelessness. The consequences of maltreatment, early life instability, and trauma are far-reaching, often involving a recurring cycle of maltreatment and placement in out-of-home care. Despite the many obstacles facing young people in out-of-home care, there are opportunities to promote resilience through strength-based approaches that promote positive youth development and proactive coordination across systems of care.

While the assessment and treatment of health problems for adolescents in out-of-home care is similar to that of the general population, the clinician must be cognizant of special and more prevalent health issues in this group, including abuse and neglect, infectious diseases, and behavioral health problems. Further, clinicians must navigate a number of additional challenges in assessing the health of young people in out-of-home care and intervening effectively, including: (1) obtaining thorough health histories, (2) inaccurate and missing records, (3) consent and confidentiality issues, (4) interfacing with multiple systems, (5) managing medication and treatment adherence, (6) working with parents/caregivers, (7) navigating the child welfare system, and (8) cultural considerations.

EPIDEMIOLOGY

General Out-of-Home Care Statistics

- Each year, approximately 6 to 8 million youth in the United States are referred to social services for maltreatment and 2 to 3 million have an investigated report. This represents about 3% of all youth ages 0 to 18 years.[1]
- More than 400,000 youth are in out-of-home care each year, which includes placement in nonrelative foster care (46%), kinship/relative care (32%), residential (congregate) care (10%), and other arrangements (12%).[1]
- Almost a third of those in out-of-home care are 12 years or older.[1]
- There is a fairly equal sex distribution among youth in out-of-home care, but African American and multiracial youth are overrepresented relative to the U.S. population.[1]
- Neglect is the most common type of maltreatment precipitating out-of-home care placement, followed by physical abuse. Of note, many youth experience multiple forms of maltreatment, including emotional abuse.[2]

Emancipating Youth

- Approximately 20,000 adolescents "age out" of out-of-home care each year.[1]
- These young adults are at high risk for unemployment, receipt of public assistance, incarceration, substance dependence, early childbearing, and significant mental health problems.[3]
- While some states allow young people to remain in out-of-home care until age 21 years, and some allow youth to return to out-of-home care after 18 years, three-quarters of emancipating youth do not take advantage of these opportunities.[4]
- The Affordable Care Act (ACA) required all states to provide Medicaid coverage for youth who emancipate from out-of-home care at age 18 years or older. This coverage lasts until the age of 26.[5]
- Although many "independent living" programs exist to help emancipating youth with the transition to young adulthood, none have demonstrated effectiveness through rigorous evaluation.[6]

Health and Associated Problems

- Chronic health conditions (e.g., asthma, neurologic problems, and vision and hearing loss) are the most prevalent health problems among youth in foster care; 10% are medically fragile or complex and many have a history of prenatal substance use exposure.[7]
- The most frequent mental health diagnoses for adolescents in out-of-home care are attention deficit hyperactivity disorder

(ADHD) and conduct disorder. In addition, mood, anxiety, and adjustment disorders are 2 to 3 times more common than among non-out-of-home youth who receive Medicaid.[8]

- Adolescents in out-of-home care are more likely to use outpatient and inpatient mental health services and are more likely to be prescribed psychotropic medications.[8]
- Approximately 30% to 50% of youth in out-of-home care are in special education classes.[9]
- Despite high rates of service use in this population, many youth in out-of-home care do not receive needed physical health, mental health, or educational services.[10]

ASSESSMENT AND TREATMENT

Current guidelines suggest that health assessments and preventive services for adolescents entering out-of-home care should align with general recommendations for all youth.[10,12]

- **Initial Assessment:** An initial assessment should be conducted immediately after entry into out-of-home care to screen for infectious diseases, acute and chronic illnesses, substance use, evidence of abuse or neglect (including sex trafficking), and mental health issues including suicidality. Clinicians should address any problems that are identified, including those that may require immediate treatment, and remain vigilant for evidence of recent or past injuries, dental caries and pain, hygiene and nutritional problems, untreated congenital and chronic conditions, missing immunizations, and developmental delays.
- **Comprehensive Assessment:** A comprehensive assessment, including a complete health history and evaluation of the youth's adjustment to care, is recommended within 30 days of placement. Standardized screening tools for mental health problems, including substance use and psychological trauma, should be administered. Confidential assessment of the youth's sexual history, including risk for sexually transmitted infections (STIs) and need for contraception, is also essential. Adolescents with behavioral, learning, or cognitive challenges should be screened for fetal alcohol spectrum disorders, which are commonly missed contributing diagnoses. Any history of possible in utero exposures should be explored and further evaluation completed when prior alcohol exposure is suspected. Of note, physical signs may or may not be present.[12]
- **Laboratory Studies:** Comprehensive STI testing for all youth with a history of sexual activity is strongly recommended. Youth with obesity should be screened for comorbidities such as hypertension, diabetes mellitus, and dyslipidemia. If indicated by nutritional history, anemia and vitamin D screening should also be performed.
- **Immunizations:** Immunization records should be reviewed during each clinical encounter and any needed vaccines administered. Immunization records may be obtained through prior medical clinicians, from school and child care records, or state immunization registries. Youth may have incomplete or missing immunization records despite these efforts, and should be immunized according to standard guidelines.
- **Follow-Up Assessment and Ongoing Care:** A follow-up visit after comprehensive assessment is recommended within 90 days of placement. In addition to identifying acute and chronic health conditions, reviewing behavioral health findings, administering appropriate immunizations, and providing additional health education, clinicians should assess current stressors and the relational fit between the adolescent and the parent/caregiver. Adolescents in care should be seen at least every 6 months to monitor for and address any physical or mental health issues that may arise while in placement.[11]
- **Behavioral Health:** Chronic exposure to trauma adversely impacts behavioral health.[12,13] Screening for mental health problems, including substance use and suicidality, should be conducted at every visit, as youth in out-of-home care have often experienced trauma and toxic stress which are associated with these challenges. Due to the pervasive nature of trauma, clinicians should practice trauma-informed care, and seek to minimize the risk of inadvertently retraumatizing the adolescent during encounters. The impact of trauma is not always recognized, and adolescents often receive other diagnoses including ADHD, oppositional defiant disorder, major depressive disorder, bipolar disorder, generalized anxiety disorder, and reactive attachment disorder. Treatment for these disorders can be challenging because trauma-related problems require clinical approaches that specifically target these aspects. These youth and young adults with mental health needs should be referred to clinicians who have been trained in providing trauma-informed care.[11] Evidence-based treatments such as trauma-focused cognitive behavioral therapy with or without psychotropic medication have been shown to be superior to psychotropic medication alone. Given concerns about overprescription of psychotropic medications, youth in care should only be prescribed these after a trauma-informed mental health assessment has been conducted.[13]

SPECIAL CONSIDERATIONS

There are many unique issues that make health assessments and interventions for adolescents in out-of-home care and young adults with a history of out-of-home care substantially more challenging. They include:

- **Barriers to Obtaining a Health History:** Obtaining a health history may be challenging when services are being provided in the context of an open child welfare case in which permanency determinations are still being made. This impacts youths' and families' willingness to disclose information or candidly report symptoms. Family members and current or previous parents/caregivers may be unwilling or unable to provide information about health issues, medications, or medical supplies and equipment. Sometimes the adolescent or young adult also may be hesitant to share personal information or may report incomplete or inaccurate information.
- **Inaccurate and Missing Records:** Demographic and other identifying information may be incorrect or may change due to adoption. Medical and school records are often incomplete or missing. In addition, it may be difficult to identify previous clinicians due to transitions from one placement to another and inadequate documentation. Due to the fragmentation of health care that often happens in the child welfare system, many youth in out-of-home care and young adults who grew up in out-of-home care do not have access to their health records.
- **Consent and Confidentiality Issues:** Youth may change placements and custody frequently, making it difficult for clinicians to know who has legal authority to make care decisions. Youth may seek confidential services without caseworker or parent/caregiver approval. States differ on the age of consent for different services, determination of who has decision-making power over different types of procedures and treatments, and who may access the results of testing and other health information.
- **Systems of Care Issues:** Because many youth are involved in multiple systems (e.g., child welfare, legal, educational, mental health, or juvenile justice), coordinating services and communication among multiple clinicians is critical but challenging. Clinicians and services may change abruptly due to placement changes or for legal reasons. Young adults may be unwilling to continue supportive services beyond the age of majority even when these services are available, in an attempt to distance themselves from the child welfare system.
- **Medication Management:** Missing medications and the need for bridge prescriptions are common problems, as medications may not accompany youth from placement to placement.

Incomplete medication records and placement transitions increase risk that a youth may lack a necessary medication, experience an interruption of treatment, or receive an erroneous prescription.

- **Challenges for Parents/Caregivers:** Ensuring transportation to appointments, securing child care for other children in the home, and managing service costs can be substantial challenges for families, as many parents/caregivers care for multiple high-needs youth.
- **Cultural Issues:** Lack of cultural awareness and sensitivity in service settings may hinder engagement of youth and their parents/caregivers in services. Children of color are overrepresented in the child welfare system and although concerns over structural racism have led to some child welfare reforms, racism compounds trauma for adolescents in care.[12] In addition, refugee youth in out-of-home care who arrive without parents/caregivers need translation services as well as culturally appropriate community supports.

RECOMMENDATIONS

- **Care Delivery and Coordination:** Many adolescents in the child welfare system experience multiple placement moves. When these moves result in a change in clinician, the adolescent's medical records often do not accompany them. Therefore, it is important to gather as much medical, dental, and mental health history as possible on the initial visit and make every attempt to obtain prior records subsequently. For emancipating youth, trauma-informed anticipatory guidance should include a plan for accessing health services post emancipation. A longer appointment time may be needed for adolescents in out-of-home care to allow for discussion with their parents/caregiver or caseworker, and completion of any documentation required by placement agencies. Medical findings and treatment plans may need to be communicated with the multiple individuals involved with each youth, including the youth's attorney, probation officer, and court or legal professionals.
- **Out-of-Home Health Clinics:** Youth in out-of-home care are a special-needs population and several health care delivery models exist that address their specific needs. In any model, health care professionals should be experienced in issues of child abuse and neglect, be familiar with child welfare processes, and understand the impact of trauma and out-of-home placement on adolescents. A case manager is invaluable to ensure that necessary health information is obtained, recommended referrals and evaluations are completed, and treatment plans are disseminated. If youth do not receive recommended treatments, the child welfare caseworker should be notified so that they can intervene.
- **Establishing a Medical Record:** Child welfare departments are charged with ensuring the health and well-being of youth in out-of-home care. Strategies to accomplish this include ensuring that a caseworker gathers and shares all relevant information, especially immunization records and having a designated medical team charged with acquiring health records and developing a health record or health "passport" which can accompany the youth as they move in and out of the child welfare system. It is important that diagnostic and treatment information is well documented and available to the adolescent when they leave the child welfare system.
- **Monitoring Medication Use:** When prescribing a medication, clinicians must consider who can give consent for the medication, how the adolescent will access the medication, who will monitor the adolescent's adherence, and how the prescription will be refilled if the adolescent's placement changes. When a decision is made to prescribe medication, especially psychotropic medications, it is critical that the adolescent is informed about what they have been prescribed and why, the potential side effects and benefits, and the consequences of stopping the medication

suddenly. For older adolescents, it is important to ensure they will be able to obtain the medication once they leave the child welfare system.

- **Educating Parents/Caregivers:** Training for parents/caregivers through the child welfare system is not always consistent. Therefore, clinicians should offer education about typical adolescent reactions to trauma and out-of-home placement and other potential difficulties. Since many adolescents may not have had a regular source of medical care prior to placement, clinicians should also provide anticipatory guidance to both parents/caregivers and adolescents on issues such as sleep, nutrition, sexual health, and substance use. Discussion of normative adolescent development should include the teen's need for growth in autonomy as well as involvement in positive and healthy activities (e.g., sports, youth clubs).
- **Engaging Families of Origin:** As many adolescents will have ongoing contact with their biologic families, especially postemancipation, it is important that clinicians include families of origin in treatment decisions, when appropriate and feasible. Youth may seek input from their families of origin when making medical decisions, especially regarding the use of psychotropic medications and reproductive health services.
- **Relationship with the Child Welfare Agency:** It is important to develop mechanisms of communication with the child welfare agency to enhance information sharing and treatment coordination. Caseworkers need to be aware of health issues that can impact placement stability, and ideally the medical team will be involved when making placement decisions and developing treatment plans.
- **Consent for Treatment:** It is important for clinicians to educate themselves and abide by state statutes relating to who (e.g., birth parent, foster parent, caseworker, attorney for child, adolescent, or emancipated youth) can consent for treatment of adolescents in out-of-home care. Local clinics, agencies, and hospitals may differ in regard to consent practices, especially with regard to management of STIs, substance use and mental health problems, and access to testing results.
- **Confidentiality:** While coordination of care for adolescents in the child welfare system is of critical importance, clinicians should understand and respect laws that may limit the sharing of health information. It is also important that they clearly explain to the youth information they can and cannot keep confidential, so that clinician trust can be established.
- **Postemancipation:** When adolescents emancipate from out-of-home care and transition between clinicians, they should be provided comprehensive health records. Young adults who are eager to leave the system may focus on basic needs other than health care, which can lead to negative physical and behavioral health outcomes. The transition from out-of-home care should include: (1) securing access to health care coverage until age 26 through Medicaid or the Affordable Care Act for eligible young adults; (2) transfer of health care to a new medical home as needed; (3) access to reproductive health services; (4) resources for housing, education, and employment; (5) appropriate mental health services; and (6) substance abuse treatment resources, if needed.[13]
- **Positive Youth Development Approach:** There is often great focus on the multiple challenges or problem behaviors of youth in out-of-home care, but all adolescents and young adults have strengths. Clinicians should take an approach consistent with positive youth development principles by identifying strengths in multiple domains (e.g., physical, intellectual, social, and emotional) and encouraging young people to pursue interests in these areas.[14] Clinicians should also connect youth to community-based resources whenever possible (e.g., mentoring programs, youth groups, Boys and Girls Clubs, YMCA programs).
- **Empowering Youth:** Youth in out-of-home care and young adults who have emancipated from care report that positive interactions

with clinicians and having a voice in their treatment planning can empower them to take a more proactive role in their own care. Assisting youth in identifying and achieving their goals can help them establish a healthy trajectory throughout young adulthood.

SUMMARY

Providing comprehensive, continuous, and culturally competent care for youth and young adults in and emancipated from out-of-home care may be challenging. Common barriers can be addressed by collaborating with child welfare personnel, using a medical home approach that includes strong case management, developing a comprehensive medical record, working closely with all involved clinicians across multiple systems, engaging family members in treatment, proactively providing resources and referrals, and empowering youth and young adults to take ownership of their health care needs while they are in care and postemancipation.

REFERENCES

1. United States Department of Health and Human Services, Administration for Children and Families, Administration for Children, Youth, and Families. The AFCARS Report. https://www.acf.hhs.gov/sites/default/files/documents/cb/afcarsreport27.pdf
2. United States Department of Health and Human Services, Administration for Children and Families, Administration on Children, Youth, and Families. Child Maltreatment 2018. https://www.acf.hhs.gov/cb/report/child-maltreatment-2018
3. Courtney ME, Okpych NJ, Park K, et al. Findings from the California youth transitions to adulthood study (CalYOUTH): conditions of youth at age 21. Chapin Hall. 2020. https://www.chapinhall.org/research/calyouth/
4. Annie B. Casey Foundation. Fostering youth transitions: using data to drive policy and practice decisions. 2018. https://www.aecf.org/resources/fostering-youth-transitions/
5. Congressional Research Service. Medicaid coverage for former foster youth up to age 26. In Focus. 2018. https://fas.org/sgp/crs/misc/IF11010.pdf
6. Woodgate RL, Morakinyo O, Martin K. Interventions for youth aging out of care: a scoping review. *Child & Youth Serv Rev.* 2017;82:280–300.
7. American Academy of Pediatrics. *Physical Health Needs of Children in Foster Care.* 2021. https://www.aap.org/en/patient-care/foster-care/physical-health-needs-of-children-in-foster-care/#:%E2%88%BC:text=Fractures%2C%20infections%2C%20
8. Center for Mental Health Services and Center for Substance Use Treatment. *Diagnoses and Health Care Utilization of Children who are in Foster Care and Covered by Medicaid. HHS Publication No. (SAM) 13–4804.* Center for Mental Health Services and Center for Substance Use Treatment, Substance Abuse and Mental Health Services Administration; 2013. http://store.samhsa.gov/shin/content/SMA13-4804/SMA13-4804.pdf
9. Palmieri LE, La Salle TP. Supporting students in foster care. *Psych in the Sch.* 2017;54(2):117–126.
10. Szilagyi MA, Rosen DS, Rubin D, et al. Health care issues for children and adolescents in foster and kinship care (Policy Statement). *Pediatrics.* 2015;136(4):e1131–1140.
11. Szilagyi MA, Rosen DS, Rubin D, et al. Health care issues for children and adolescents in foster care and kinship care (Technical Report). *Pediatrics.* 2015;136(4):e1142–1166.
12. Jones VF, Schulte EE, Waite D, et al. Pediatrician guidance in supporting families of children who are adopted, fostered, or in kinship care. *Pediatrics.* 2020;146(6):e2020034629.
13. Keeshin B, Forkey HC, Fouras G, et al. Children exposed to maltreatment: Assessment and the role of psychotropic medication. *Pediatrics.* 2020;145(2):e20193751.
14. Font SA, Gershoff ET. Foster care: how we can, and should, do more for maltreated children. *Soc Policy Rep.* 2020;33(3):1–40.

ADDITIONAL RESOURCES AND WEBSITES

Additional Resources and Websites for Clinicians:
Council on Foster Care Adoption and Kinship Care (COFCAKC)—https://www.aap.org/cofcake
Healthy Foster Care America—https://www.aap.org/en/patient-care/foster-care/
Fostering Health: Health Care for Children and Adolescents in Foster Care—http://www.aap.org/en-us/advocacy-and-policy/aap-health-initiatives/healthy-foster-care-america/Pages/Fostering-Health.aspx
Health Issues and Needs—https://www.aap.org/en-us/advocacy-and-policy/aap-health-initiatives/healthy-foster-care-america/Pages/Health-Issues.aspx
The Resilience Project—https://www.aap.org/en-us/advocacy-and-policy/aap-health-initiatives/resilience/Pages/Training-Toolkit.aspx
National Child Traumatic Stress Network—www.nctsn.org

Additional Resources and Websites for Parents/Caregivers:
Helping Youth Transition to Adulthood: Guidance for Foster Parents—https://www.childwelfare.gov/pubPDFs/youth_transition.pdf
Grandparents Raising Grandchildren—http://www.raisingyourgrandchildren.com/grandparent_and_kinship_caregivers.htm
Child Welfare Information Gateway—https://www.childwelfare.gov/
National Child Traumatic Stress Network—www.nctsn.org
National Foster Parent Association—www.nfpaonline.org

Additional Resources and Websites for Adolescents and Young Adults:
Foster Care Alumni Resources—www.fostercarealumni.org
FosterClub—www.fosterclub.com
Health Care for Former Foster Youth—https://healthcareffy.org/

CHAPTER 83

Juvenile Detention and Incarcerated Youth and Young Adults

Matthew C. Aalsma
Allyson L. Dir
Rebecca M. Beyda
Katherine Schwartz

KEY WORDS

- Adult criminal justice system
- Detention
- Disproportionate minority contact
- Health care
- Health risk
- Incarceration
- Juvenile detention
- Juvenile justice
- Juvenile justice system

INTRODUCTION

The risk of involvement with the justice system increases in adolescence and young adulthood. In the United States, youth offenders under the age of 18 years are subject to the juvenile justice system, a process that is separate and distinct from that of adult criminals. For over 100 years, the juvenile justice system has been tasked with both protecting the community from delinquent youth through supervision and incarceration and aiding the rehabilitation of these youth. Over time, society may vacillate toward either end of this continuum—law enforcement versus rehabilitation—but the political climate since the late 90s has increasingly favored limiting the incarceration of youth. Contributions to this societal shift may include research findings that highlight procedural and racial/ethnic injustice within the system, the unique needs of youth offenders, and the health costs of incarceration to both individual youth and their communities. For example, much research has affirmed that youth of color are disproportionately involved in both the juvenile and adult criminal justice systems; a recent study found that Black adolescents and young adults (AYAs) were arrested seven times more frequently than White AYAs, even after controlling for behavioral and contextual factors.[1] In addition, increased health screening efforts have confirmed that justice system–involved youth face both physical and mental health issues at higher rates than their nondelinquent peers.[2] As such, juvenile justice policy reform efforts continue.

Young adult offenders (ages 18 to 26 years) are not typically afforded the protections, however limited, associated with the juvenile justice system. In contrast, they are subject to the adult criminal justice system, where their experiences and needs are rarely separated from those of older adult offenders. Research on the health of young adult offenders as a distinct group is limited, though their physical and mental health issues may be similar to the needs of older adolescent offenders, and the criminal behavior of young adults is frequently a continuation of adolescent delinquency. Young adult offenders are likely more similar to juvenile offenders than adults in both their physical and mental development as well as their criminal activity. This is reflected in policy recommendations to extend the jurisdiction of the juvenile justice system to include young adults.

EPIDEMIOLOGY OF JUSTICE SYSTEM INVOLVEMENT

Approximately 728,000 juveniles <18 years old were arrested in the United States in 2018, with 744,500 delinquency cases processed in juvenile courts; 54% of cases involved youth under age 16, 27% involved females, and 44% involved White youth.[3] Of the cases in which youth were adjudicated delinquent, 28% of dispositions resulted in out-of-home placements, while for 63% probation was the most restrictive disposition.[3] In 2018, approximately 3,600 delinquency cases were waived for prosecution in the adult criminal justice system, a 47% decrease from 2006 rates.[3] In terms of young adults, more than 2.52 million individuals between the ages of 18 and 24 were arrested in 2013. This age range represents nearly a third of arrests, though they make up only 10% of the general population.[4]

Recidivism

The repetition of criminal behavior, recidivism, is a common outcome among detained adolescents, with roughly a third recidivating within 1 year of release from detention.[5] Reported recidivism rates vary dramatically depending on the location and characteristics of the youth population, definition of recidivism (i.e., rearrest vs. readjudication), and length of study period.[5] Within the detained AYA populations, recidivism rates tend to be higher among males, racial and ethnic minorities, youth younger at their first offense, youth with prior criminal history, youth in unstable families, those with high rates of substance use, and those with a history of early childhood misbehavior or conduct problems.

Disproportionate Minority Contact

Racial and ethnic minority AYAs—particularly Black and Hispanic individuals—are overrepresented in the justice system, described as disproportionate minority contact. Over 60% of justice system–involved youth are minority youth, though they make up only a third of the general population.[6] Youth of color are also more likely than White youth to receive harsh treatment in the system, including stringent probation conditions, placement in adult prisons, and removal from their home environments.[7] Racial disparities are also prevalent throughout every stage of the adult criminal justice system.[8]

On May 25, 2020, public outrage over the disparate treatment of Black individuals by the justice system was revived when news and social media outlets widely distributed a recording of police killing George Floyd. Floyd, a Black man held on suspicion of using a counterfeit $20 bill in a Minneapolis grocery, died after nearly 9 minutes of the arresting officer's knee on his neck. In the months following Floyd's death, protests erupted across the country to oppose police brutality and support the Black Lives Matter movement, renewing national discourse over systemic racism and prompting reform efforts that may improve the health of racial and ethnic minority AYAs.

Mortality

Adolescents and young adults involved in the justice system die at greater rates than AYAs in the general public. In a formative longitudinal study of detained youth, the mortality rate among these youth was four times that of the general population for males and eight times for females.[9] Most of these deaths resulted from gunshot wounds post-release.[4] Black, male, young adults are at greatest risk for violent death.[9] A recent large-scale study found that the mortality rate differed by severity of justice system involvement, with arrested youth having the lowest rate of mortality and those transferred to the adult court having the highest mortality rate.[10]

Summary

It is likely that most clinicians will encounter patients involved in the justice system, especially clinicians who see racial/ethnic minority AYAs. These individuals face much more troubled futures than the general population. Knowledge of high recidivism and mortality rates can have a direct effect on improving health by identifying factors that could lead to reinvolvement and screening for nonaccidental trauma risks, such as access to firearms. Advocacy is another way to intervene on behalf of young people; clinicians are in a unique role to advocate for youth as they are most knowledgeable about healthy adolescent development and conditions, such as substance use disorder, which are associated with continued delinquent behavior.

HEALTH ISSUES OF YOUNG PEOPLE IN THE JUSTICE SYSTEM

Adolescents and young adults involved in the justice system exhibit significant acute and chronic medical problems, whether precursors to, causes of, or direct and indirect effects of their system involvement. As examples, problems resulting from dog bites or drug use can be related to the reason for an individual's involvement in the system; other medical problems, such as poor dentition, may manifest frequently among AYA offenders because this population is largely medically underserved. Young people in custody are more likely than the general population to suffer from asthma, sexually transmitted infections (STIs), substance use disorders, and other chronic conditions.[8]

Detention Conditions

The range of common health problems experienced by AYAs in the justice system presents unique challenges to clinicians, especially when their illnesses may arise as a direct result of confinement. Youth may experience somatic pain related to stress and adaption to a new environment. Gastrointestinal complaints may result from a set menu of food that differs significantly from predetention diet (e.g., menus high in lactose). Communicable diseases are also a concern for youth in custody, since detained youth are often housed together in conditions that facilitate disease spread (e.g., crowded quarters, communal eating and bathing) and because some diseases, such as tuberculosis and viral illnesses, occur at high rates in correctional facilities. During the coronavirus disease 2019 (COVID-19) global pandemic, juvenile facilities were charged to reduce the transmission of COVID-19 while mitigating the negative effects of practices that may be required to reduce the transmission.[11]

The 2016 Juvenile Residential Facility Census collected information from 1,772 facilities in the United States.[12] The census is performed biennially. This census reported a decrease in the number of youth in residential facilities with the lowest population recorded since 1975. Among the juvenile facilities, 55% were publicly operated and housed 71% of juvenile offenders. Mechanical restraints and isolation (defined as locking a youth in a room for more than 4 hours) were used in 44% of detention centers and just over 20% of all facilities. Use of mechanical restraints and/or isolation can exacerbate existing health conditions. In addition, this census collected information on acute health events in custody. One-third of facilities utilized emergency room visits (most commonly for sports-related injuries and illness). While deaths were rare, six were reported in 2016 (one was ruled a suicide).[12]

Mental Health and Substance Use

Adolescents and young adults involved in the justice system suffer from mental health and substance use disorders at higher rates than the general population.[8,13] Studies have consistently found that both externalizing (e.g., conduct disorder, attention deficit hyperactivity disorder) and internalizing disorders (e.g., major depression, anxiety, and posttraumatic stress disorder) are prevalent.[13] Substance use is also quite common among AYAs involved in the system, with approximately half of detained youth meeting the criteria for a substance use disorder.[13] Unfortunately, most detention centers are not equipped to address the mental health needs of young people; even 5 years after release, at least 45% of male and 30% of female detainees experience one or more psychiatric disorders with associated impairment.[2] Even for nondetained youth, access to and funding for services specifically for justice-involved AYA remains a concern. Recent efforts have been made to improve the behavioral health services among justice-involved youth from the point of initial identification of service needs at the justice system level to retention in behavioral health services.[14] Residential facilities are also improving screening procedures; as of 2016, the Juvenile Residential Facility Census reported that 65% of facilities screened all youth for mental health needs, 75% screened all youth for substance use needs, and 93% screened all youth for suicide risk.[12]

Physical Health

Few national studies have described detainee health issues or how detention conditions specifically affect AYAs in juvenile or adult facilities. The Survey of Youth in Residential Placement (SYRP),[15] which conducted periodically, and a seminal study by the National Commission on Correctional Health Care (NCCHC)[16] have both revealed higher rates of health problems among AYAs in detention when compared to the general population. The data regarding general health issues are reviewed in the following sections.

Preexisting Health Needs

The health needs of some youth in detention are related to neglected preexisting health conditions, which are common among this vulnerable population. Analysis using the 2009 to 2014 National Survey on Drug Use and Health found adolescents with juvenile justice involvement had a higher prevalence of asthma (12%), hypertension (2%), emergency department visits (39%), and hospitalizations (8%) within the preceding year compared to youth without justice involvement.[17] Again, physical health problems among detained youth are often a consequence of poor access to care before custody. Justice-involved youth experience longer gaps in Medicaid coverage and subsequently report lower rates of well-child visits.[18]

Injuries

Physical injuries are common among juvenile justice system–involved youth. Some youth present with injuries upon detention center intake, which may be related to the crime committed or sustained during the process of being arrested. Unfortunately, injuries also commonly occur in custody. The SYRP directly and anonymously interviewed a large, nationally representative sample of youth in custody.[15] Safety concerns and injuries were frequently reported by youth, with 38% fearing attack by someone, most often other residents or a staff member (25% and 22%, respectively). In addition, 22% of youth in the SYRP reported that they would not know what to do in case of a fire.[15] Two-thirds of incarcerated youth reported having physical health care needs while detained, including injuries.[15] Injuries may be sustained in sports, through altercations with other youth, or self-inflicted. One recent study found a lifetime prevalence of 25.7% for nonsuicidal self-injury among incarcerated youth.[19]

Sleep Disturbances

Youth in custody also experience sleep disturbances at higher rates than youth not in custody. In the SYRP survey, 34% of youth reported problems falling asleep while in custody compared to 11% of youth in the general population.[15] Lack of sleep exposes youth to the consequences of chronic sleep deprivation such as depression and school problems.

Sexually Transmitted Infections

Adolescents and young adults involved in the justice system have high rates of STIs due to a combination of uncontrollable demographic factors such as age and race, as well as increased rates of risk behaviors associated with STI acquisition. Regardless of involvement in the justice system, AYAs represent the age group with the highest STI rates, with almost half of all new STI diagnoses occurring in this age group.[20] Shared racial disparities between STI rates in the United States (see Chapters 36, 62, 64, and 65) and the justice system population also impact these rates.

Rates of chlamydia, gonorrhea, human immunodeficiency virus (HIV), syphilis, and trichomonas are higher among persons involved in the justice system. Based on these historically high rates of infection, the Centers for Disease Control and Prevention (CDC) recommends chlamydia and gonorrhea screening for both females <35 years old and males <30 years old admitted to detention facilities.[20] In one of the only nationally representative studies of incarcerated youth, youth offenders were more likely to be sexually active, used contraception at lower rates, and were more likely to report more than four lifetime partners when compared to their nondelinquent peers.[16] Young females involved in the juvenile justice system may have a history of minor sex trafficking victimization and/or childhood sexual abuse increasing their STI risk. A review of 26 cross-sectional studies revealed substance use is highly associated with HIV risk behaviors (e.g., inconsistent condom use, multiple partners, and anal sex) among justice-involved youth.[21] Risk for STI persists before and after justice system involvement. A large cohort study following over 200,000 individuals 1-year post incarceration found higher STI and HIV positivity rates among recent offenders compared to nonoffenders.[22] This study highlights the need for close follow-up after release from incarceration.

Other Reproductive Health Issues

In addition to the high rate of STIs among young offenders, detained youth often navigate other serious reproductive health issues. Many of these adolescents are parents/caregivers. The SYRP found that one in five reported either having had or that they were expecting a child.[15] Unknown pregnancy and delayed prenatal care are potential health issues for many young women in custody. Unintended pregnancy and chronic pelvic pain are consequences of nonconsensual sex for some youth in the justice system. While consensual sexual activity is common among teens, being a victim of sexual abuse is common among the juvenile justice population. Twelve percent of youth in the SYRP reported a history of sexual abuse, with more

females than males reporting.[15] Given the often unmet reproductive needs of youth in the community, detention provides an opportunity for contraception counseling and initiation.[23]

Dental

Dental problems and poor oral health have been well documented among juvenile justice system–involved youth.[24] In the SYRP, the need for dental, vision, or hearing care ranked the highest of all physical health care needs for youth with 40% reporting concerns.[15] Only 14% had evidence of dental care (preventive sealants) in a study of 400 youth detained between 1999 and 2003.[25]

Summary

Young individuals involved in the justice system are likely to have serious health conditions, with some of these health conditions being a consequence of their involvement. Familiarity with common conditions, such as reproductive health issues and substance use, is important to provide adequate care to AYAs in custody and after their release. Clinicians seeing these individuals should inquire about previous health care, including emergency room and dental visits, and be prepared to screen for substance use, STIs, and contraceptive needs. Since many justice system–involved AYAs carry mental health diagnoses, it is especially important to connect them with care once released; few resources for treatment are available in secure facilities, and untreated mental health issues can lead to criminal recidivism (**Table 83.1**).

🔵 ASSESSMENT AND TREATMENT ISSUES

While there are health care standards and recommendations for AYAs in custody, none are mandatory. Additionally, these standards are controlled and monitored by state and local government

---

TABLE 83.1

Recommended Health Services for Youth Involved in Juvenile Justice

At intake
- Complete health history, including physical, dental, and mental health histories and visits to clinicians, including emergency services, in the past 3 y
- Review vaccination history
- Screen for reproductive health needs; include STI testing and discussion of contraception
- Screen for acute and chronic mental health problems, such as suicidality and substance use
- Perform physical examination, with attention to potential preexisting and/or unmet health needs, traumatic injuries, and signs of substance use withdrawal
- Assess for dental health needs, preferably via examination by a dentist

During detention/incarceration
- Manage treatment for acute and chronic health care needs
- Utilize support and resources from mental clinicians
- Emphasize discharge planning for appointments and continuation of medications

After release from detention
- Review health insurance status
- Review services received where the youth was detained
- Assess adaptation, distress, and new health problems present as a consequence of juvenile justice system involvement
- Screen for STIs
- Refer to affordable dentistry
- Inquire into mental health and substance use treatment needs; refer if indicated
- Give anticipatory guidance on mortality risks for juvenile justice–involved youth

STI, sexually transmitted infection.

agencies, leading to significant system and geographic variability in services rendered. Variability in health services in secure facilities is also exacerbated by cost and access to services, since federal Medicaid services cannot be billed while an individual is detained or incarcerated. Federal Medicaid law prohibits payment "with respect to care or services for any individual who is an inmate of a public institution" (except as a patient in a medical institution; 42 C.F.R 441.33 (a)(1), 435.1008(a)(1)).

Detention Care Guidelines

The NCCHC was founded by the American Medical Association to address the lack of national standards for health care in all jails and prisons. These standards are supported by major health, law, and correctional organizations, including the American Academy of Pediatrics, American Bar Association, American Dental Association, and American Psychological Association. The most recent NCCHC Standards address nine general areas ranging from health services to medical–legal issues related to secure facilities. This document calls for a comprehensive health assessment (medical, mental health, and dental history), physical examination, as well as a mental health and oral health screening within 7 days of admission.[26] Recommended laboratory measurements include a pregnancy test for youth assigned female at birth, STI screening, and tuberculosis screening after entry. Immunizations, especially human papillomavirus and hepatitis A and B should be reviewed and updated for youth in secure facilities.[27] The NCCHC provides standards for addressing new health concerns in custody and discharge planning.[26] The NCCHC also offers voluntary accreditation, yet very few juvenile facilities are accredited.

In addition to the NCCH Standards, there are other standards for correctional health care services. The American Correctional Association, the largest correctional professional association, has published 25 different manuals of standards, including one for juvenile facilities.[28] These standards cover physical and mental health care along with other aspects of the correctional system, such as food service and security. The Juvenile Detention Alternatives Initiative, a project of the Annie E. Casey Foundation to reform juvenile justice, publishes standards to acknowledge and incorporate regulations that affect the full range of facility operations. These standards cover physical and mental health care, programming, restraints, safety, and more.[29] Additional recommendations include policy statements from the American Academy of Pediatrics and Society for Adolescent Health and Medicine.

Despite existing detention care guidelines, many juvenile justice facilities fall short of the published standards, especially in regard to mental health services.[30] For example, over one-third of facilities use correctional staff to administer mental health assessments and services, despite staff having little relevant training to do so.[30] For youth in juvenile detention facilities, mental health treatment options often consist of medication administration and management.

Insurance Coverage

In the United States, insurance status may pose significant obstacles to care once young people are released from secure facilities. Many young people in the justice system, and their families, are economically disadvantaged and living in poverty. As mentioned, Medicaid insurance may be terminated upon admission to detention facilities, jeopardizing inmate health care access once they are released. However, Medicaid rules do not state that individuals become ineligible or lose Medicaid once detained, just that Medicaid funds cannot pay for care while in custody. If suspended only, Medicaid can be quickly resumed once AYAs are released to cover health expenses, avoiding interruptions in care due to reenrollment and application times. Justice system programs serving AYAs may also have the ability to determine presumptive eligibility for Medicaid, allowing temporary Medicaid eligibility to cover health

TABLE 83.2
Clinical Summary

- Many juvenile justice–involved youth have poor or no access to health care prior to detention. Comprehensive screening for preexisting and chronic conditions should be performed with a full review of systems to identify unmet health needs.
- STIs are common. AYAs should be offered confidential and complete screening, testing, and treatment. Vaccination against STIs (human papillomavirus and hepatitis A and B) is an intervention with great benefits to this population.
- AYA parents/caregivers are often present in this population. Prenatal care, education on pregnancy prevention, parenting, and sexuality are necessary and valuable resources to employ.
- Dental problems are among the most commonly identified issues for this population and should be addressed while youth are in custody, as they are often the result of poor predetention access to care.
- The majority of detained AYAs have a mental health and/or a substance use disorder. Differential diagnosis is important, as are referral and coordination of behavioral health treatment.
- Free and paid policy statements and standards are available to guide care.
- Insurance status may be interrupted during detention; prompt reenrollment is important for care upon release.

AYAs, adolescents and young adults; STIs, sexually transmitted infections.

care pending final eligibility determinations. Finally, young offenders do not lose Medicaid eligibility upon involvement in the justice system and can be screened for eligibility and enrolled when entering the system, creating an opportunity to improve their health care access during detention. Justice system facilities can also help AYAs ineligible for Medicaid gain access to other health plans, many with subsidies to improve affordability of care.

SUMMARY

Young people receive no standard medical care while in custody, and services received vary greatly by geographic area, making it essential that clinicians know what care is available in their local jurisdiction. When centers are compliant with national standards, young people may receive very good care. However, most secure holding facilities are not in compliance, especially regarding mental health services standards. Medical coverage while AYAs are detained is often financed through the local court, as Medicaid cannot be billed for detention services in most cases. Unfortunately, as a result, health insurance coverage is sometimes canceled, creating significant barriers to these young people receiving care once they are released from detention into the community. Because most justice–involved AYAs are eligible for Medicaid subsidies, it is important to enroll or reenroll this population to connect them with regular and effective health care once released (**Table 83.2**).

REFERENCES

1. Schleiden C, Soloski KL, Milstead K, et al. Racial disparities in arrests: a race specific model explaining arrest rates across Black and white young adults. *Ch Adol Social Work J.* 2020;37(1):1–4.
2. Teplin LA, Welty LJ, Abram KM, et al. Prevalence and persistence of psychiatric disorders in youth after detention: a prospective longitudinal study. *Arch Gen Psychiatry.* 2012;69:1031–1043.
3. Hockenberry S, Puzzanchera C. *Juvenile Court Statistics 2018.* National Center for Juvenile Justice; 2020. Accessed February 23, 2020. https://www.ojjdp.gov/ojstatbb/ezajcs/
4. U.S. Department of Justice, Federal Bureau of Investigation, Criminal Justice Information Services Division. Crime in the United States 2013. Accessed December 17, 2014. http://www.fbi.gov/about-us/cjis/ucr/crime-in-the-u.s/2013/crime-in-the-u.s.-2013/persons-arrested/persons-arrested
5. Robertson AA, Fang Z, Weiland D, et al. Recidivism among justice-involved youth: findings from JJ-TRIALS. *Crim Justice Behav.* 2020;47(9):1059–1078.
6. Desai RA, Falzer PR, Chapman J, et al. Mental illness, violence risk, and race in juvenile detention: implications for disproportionate minority contact. *Am J Orthopsychiatry.* 2012;82:32–40.
7. Steinmetz KF, Anderson JO. A probation profanation: race, ethnicity, and probation in a Midwestern sample. *Race and Justice.* 2016;6(4):325–349.

8. Binswanger IA, Redmond N, Steiner JF, et al. Health disparities and the criminal justice system: an agenda for further research and action. *J Urban Health.* 2012;89(1):98–107.

9. Teplin LA, McClelland GM, Abram KM, et al. Early violent death among delinquent youth: a prospective longitudinal study. *Pediatrics.* 2005;115(6):1586–1593.

10. Aalsma MC, Lau KSL, Perkins AJ, et al. Mortality of youth offenders along a continuum of justice system involvement. *Am J Prev Med.* 2016;50(3):303–310.

11. American Academy of Pediatrics. Responding to the needs of youth involved with the justice system during the COVID-19 pandemic. *Clinical Guidance*; 2020. Accessed July 17, 2020. https://services.aap.org/en/pages/2019-novel-coronavirus-covid-19-infections/clinical-guidance/responding-to-the-needs-of-youth-involved-with-the-justice-system–during-the-covid-19-pandemic/

12. Hockenberry S, Sladky A. Juvenile residential facility census, 2016: selected findings. *OJJDP National Report Series.* Office of Juvenile Justice and Delinquency Prevention; 2018. Accessed June 22, 2020. https://ojjdp.ojp.gov/sites/g/files/xyckuh176/files/pubs/251785.pdf

13. Beaudry G, Yu R, Långström N, et al. An updated systematic review and meta-regression analysis: mental disorders among adolescents in juvenile detention and correctional facilities. *J Am Acad Child Adolesc Psychiatry.* 2021;60(1):46–60.

14. Belenko S, Knight D, Wasserman GA, et al. The juvenile justice behavioral health services cascade: a new framework for measuring unmet substance use treatment services needs among adolescent offenders. *J Subst Abuse Treat.* 2017;74:80–91.

15. Sedlak AJ. *Survey of Youth in Residential Placement Report.* Westat; 2016.

16. Morris RE, Harrison EA, Knox GW, et al. Health risk behavioral survey from 39 juvenile correctional facilities in the United States. *J Adolesc Health.* 1995;17(6):334–344.

17. Winkelman TNA, Frank JW, Binswanger IA, et al. Health conditions and racial differences among justice-involved adolescents, 2009 to 2014. *Acad Pediatr.* 2017;17(7):723–731.

18. Aalsma MC, Anderson VR, Schwartz K, et al. Preventive care use among justice-involved and non-justice involved youth. *Pediatrics.* 2017;140(5):e20171107.

19. McReynolds LS, Wasserman G, Ozbardakci E. Contributors to nonsuicidal self-injury in incarcerated youth. *Health Justice.* 2017;5(1):13.

20. Workowski KA, Bachmann LH, Chan PA, et al. Sexually transmitted infections treatment guidelines, 2021. *MMWR Recomm Rep.* 2021;70(4):1–187.

21. Tolou-Shams M, Harrison A, Hirschtritt ME, et al. Substance use and HIV among justice-involved youth: intersecting risks. *Curr HIV/AIDS Rep.* 2019;16(1):37–47.

22. Wiehe SE, Rosenman MB, Aalsma MC, et al. Epidemiology of sexually transmitted infections among offenders following arrest or incarceration. *Am J Public Health.* 2015;105(12):e26–e32.

23. Grubb LK, Beyda RM, Eissa MA, et al. A contraception quality improvement initiative with detained young women: counseling, initiation, and utilization. *J Pediatr Adolesc Gynecol.* 2018;31(4):405–410.

24. Barnert ES, Perry R, Morris RE. Juvenile incarceration and health. *Acad Pediatr.* 2016;16(2):99–109.

25. Bolin K, Jones D. Oral health needs of adolescents in a juvenile detention facility. *J Adolesc Health.* 2006;38(6):755–757.

26. National Commission on Correctional Health Care. *Standards for Health Services in Juvenile Detention and Confinement Facilities.* National Commission on Correctional Health Care; 2015.

27. Gaskin GL, Glanz JM, Binswanger IA, et al. Immunization coverage among juvenile justice detainees. *J Correct Health Care.* 2015;21(3):265–275.

28. American Correctional Association. Accessed February 23, 2021. https://aca.org/ACA_Member/ACA/ACA_Member/Standards_and_Accreditation/SAC.aspx

29. The Annie E. Casey Foundation. *Juvenile Detention Facility Assessment.* The Annie E. Casey Foundation; 2014. Accessed July 16, 2020. https://www.aecf.org/resources/juvenile-detention-facility-assessment/

30. Desai RA, Goulet JL, Robbins J, et al. Mental health care in juvenile detention facilities: a review. *J Am Acad Psychiatry Law.* 2006;34(2):204–214.

ADDITIONAL RESOURCES AND WEBSITES

Additional Resources and Websites for Clinicians:

Information exchange on all issues related to juvenile justice and reform efforts—https://jjic.org/

Juvenile Justice Geography, Policy, Practice and Statistics—Online repository for juvenile justice laws and practices by state—http://www.jjgps.org/

Nonprofit devoted to gathering articles and information criminal and juvenile justice system reform—https://www.themarshallproject.org/

Nonprofit devoted to equity reform within the juvenile justice system—https://burnsinstitute.org/

Owen MC, Wallace SB, Committee on Adolescence. Advocacy and collaborative health care for justice-involved youth. *Pediatrics.* 2020;145(6):e20201755.

Position statement for advocacy and health care for justice-involved youth from the American Academy of Pediatrics—https://pediatrics.aappublications.org/content/early/2020/06/25/peds.2020-1755?versioned=true

Position statement for health care funding for incarcerated youth from the National Commission on Correctional Health Care—https://www.ncchc.org/health-care-funding-for-incarcerated-youth

Position statement for promoting youth development and alternatives to incarceration from the Society for Adolescent Health and Medicine—https://www.sciencedirect.com/science/article/pii/S1054139X16302427

Society for Adolescent Health and Medicine. International Youth Justice Systems: promoting youth development and alternative approaches: a position paper of the Society for Adolescent Health and Medicine. *J Adolesc Health.* 2016;59(4):482–486.

Additional Resources and Websites for Parents/Caregivers:

Advocacy organization to promote parental involvement in juvenile justice reform—https://www.justice4families.org/

Parent advocacy network for improving systems, including juvenile justice—https://spanadvocacy.org/

Parent guide for navigating juvenile justice system—https://www.in.gov/ipdc/juvenile-justice/information-for-youth-and-parents/indiana-juvenile-justice-system/

Additional Resources and Websites for Adolescents and Young Adults:

Comic book detailing what to expect when involved in juvenile justice system—https://www.courtinnovation.org/sites/default/files/comic_book.pdf

XVI

CHAPTER 84

Immigrant Adolescents and Young Adults

Carol Lewis
Delma-Jean Watts

KEY WORDS

- Asylee
- Cultural competence
- Health screening
- Hepatitis B
- Immigrant
- Lead
- Legal permanent resident
- Malaria
- Mental health
- Parasitic infections
- Refugee
- Tuberculosis
- Unauthorized immigrants

INTRODUCTION

International migration has become increasingly fluid, diverse, and common. Immigrants and refugees have health burdens and face barriers to care, including linguistic, cultural, and legal issues, as well as those that accompany poverty. As a result, many clinicians do not feel adequately equipped to provide effective cross-cultural care.[1]

Worldwide, the migrant population has increased dramatically to more than 3.5% of the world's population.[2] The United States leads in countries welcoming foreign-born individuals.[2] It is estimated that over 44 million U.S. residents are foreign-born, representing just over 13% of the entire U.S. population, and more than half have noncitizen status.[3]. Over half of new immigrants reside in five states: California (23.7%), New York (10%), Florida (10%), Texas (11%), and New Jersey (4.6%).[3]

In 2019, 38 million migrants were less than 20 years of age, representing about one-seventh of migrants globally.[3] In the same year, over 30 million international migrants were adolescents and young adults (AYAs) (ages 15 to 24 years).[2] In addition, 72% of unaccompanied immigrant children (UIC) are over 14 years old.[4] This group is officially classified by U.S. customs as "unaccompanied alien children." However, we will use a more widely accepted term, "UIC." Unaccompanied immigrant children are referred to the Office of Refugee Resettlement by other federal agencies, often after being detained after crossing a border. Notably, the number of referrals for UIC has risen dramatically, with an increase of over 42% from fiscal year 2018 to fiscal year 2019.

The 2020 global coronavirus pandemic has led to dramatic decreases in migration. Economic and immigration policy changes are likely to continue to affect migration and it is unclear how long lasting those effects will be.[5]

Legal Status

The specific legal status of migrants may hinder them from obtaining medical insurance and make them wary of seeking medical care. It is useful to understand the different classifications of foreign-born individuals to better appreciate such barriers.

1. *Refugees* are individuals who are forced to leave their country of origin owing to a well-founded fear of being persecuted for reasons of race, religion, nationality, membership in a particular social group, or political opinion and are living outside the country of nationality.[6] They are given the status of "refugee" by the United Nations High Commissioner for Refugees when they are displaced within their own borders or across adjacent borders, but prior to being resettled into the United States. They typically are from countries experiencing significant violence and conflict. People with refugee status have benefits such as health insurance and permissions to work upon arrival and may apply for legal permanent resident (LPR) status after living in the United States for 1 year.

2. Legal permanent residents are individuals who come to the United States and are legally accorded the privilege of residing permanently.

3. *Unauthorized immigrants* arrive but do not have LPR status and face potential deportation and separation from family members.

4. *Asylees* meet the definition of refugees, but are already in the United States or are seeking admission at a port of entry.

Legal status has implications for access to health insurance. Refugees are provided with increased services, such as housing and job assistance, medical insurance, health care navigation and orientation to the community as well as other social services through the U.S. State Department in partnership with local Volunteer Resettlement Agencies (VOLAG). In addition to initial reception and placement, they are provided with medical assistance for the first 8 months after arrival in the United States. Application for change in legal status to LPR necessitates a specific medical examination as required by the U.S. Citizen and Immigration Service (USCIS). Unauthorized immigrants do not have access to health insurance and often do not seek medical care for fear of deportation. Unauthorized immigrants are not eligible for change in legal status to LPR under U.S. federal law. They are unique as compared to other marginalized young adults in that they are categorically excluded from programs, benefits, and services offered to other young adult groups.[7]

Cultural Competency

A clinician should:

- Learn about the different group(s) one is working with and/or develop relationships with medical interpreters or community health workers who can assist with cultural and linguistic interpretation.
- Use a medical interpreter for all encounters with limited English proficient (LEP) patients.

- Approach each encounter with humility and respect, recognizing that all medical clinicians have cultural biases that may affect their perception of patients from other cultures.
- Develop a comfort with differences that may exist between one's own personal culture and the cultural values and beliefs of others.
- Remember that most immigrant AYAs are forgiving of cultural "mistakes" as long as the clinician conveys a genuine sense of caring and respect.
- Understand and respect that family dynamics in immigrant and refugee families may be complicated by gaps in acculturation and language proficiency between AYAs and their parents/caregivers through the migration and resettlement process; this may disrupt the traditional roles held by the parent/caregiver and AYA.
- Avoid making assumptions about beliefs or values of an individual patient or family, based solely on family of origin or country of emigration.
- Ask about traditional healing practices and seek to understand the family's health belief system.

Interpretation

Poor communication can undermine health care experiences and decrease access to needed services.[8,9] Limited English proficient patients are at increased risk for medical errors. The U.S. federal law mandates "linguistic accessibility to health care" under Title VI of the Civil Rights Act. Clinicians who receive federal funding are required to provide language access to LEP individuals who cannot communicate with their clinician, but despite this, interpreters are often underutilized.[10,11] Useful tips for the effective use of medical interpreters can be found in **Table 84.1**.[12]

If an in-person interpreter is not available, the use of a telephone or video interpreter service may be an option. It is important to provide information to the telephone or video interpreter regarding the setting and circumstances of the encounter prior to initiating the interview. Adolescents and young adults have unique challenges with respect to confidentiality and sensitive health topics such as sexual and reproductive health and mental health, which can affect the type of interpreter they prefer. Preferences as to the gender of the interpreter and the modality used (e.g., video, phone, in-person) should be accommodated whenever possible.

Health Screenings
Overseas Medical Screening

Overseas medical screening is required for all immigrants and refugees before entering the United States. The purpose of this examination is to identify individuals with any diseases of public health concern that render the individual inadmissible. For refugees, the evaluation is performed by panel physicians designated by the local U.S. Embassy overseas. Guidelines for panel physicians are determined by the Centers for Disease Control and Prevention (CDC) Division of Global Migration and Quarantine.[13]

Excludable conditions of public health significance (Class A conditions) include:
- Active tuberculosis (TB)
- Syphilis

TABLE 84.1

Guidelines for Using Medical Interpreters

1. Use qualified interpreters trained in medical interpretation.
2. Do not depend on children or other relatives and friends to interpret.
3. Have a brief preinterview meeting with the interpreter.
4. Address yourself to the interviewee, not to the interpreter. Maintain eye contact with the interviewee.
5. Avoid jargon and technical terms.
6. Keep your utterances short, pausing to permit the interpretation.

Adapted from the Minnesota Department of Health Refugee Provider Guide.

- Chancroid
- Gonorrhea
- Hansen's disease (leprosy)
- Mental health disorders with associated harmful behaviors that could pose potential risk to others
- Substance-related disorders with associated harmful behaviors that could pose potential risk to others

The U.S. Medical Screening

The CDC recommends medical screening for all immigrants and refugees within 30 to 60 days of arrival in order to identify public health risks, promote and improve the health of the immigrant/refugee, prevent disease, and familiarize refugees with the U.S. health care system.[14]

The health burdens of refugees have been well documented,[15–17] and evidence-based screening recommendations for immigrant and refugee AYAs include the following:
- A complete history (including a detailed travel history)
- Review of all predeparture overseas documents and health records including chest x-ray and documentation of predeparture presumptive treatment for malaria, schistosomiasis, or strongyloides

Complete physical examination should include the following:
- Height/weight/body mass index/nutritional assessment
- Vision/hearing screen
- Oral heath screen
- Scars suggesting previous injury/torture
- Genitourinary examination for both males and females. The genital examination may be deferred until the patient–clinician relationship is further developed and cultural implications of sensitive examinations are considered.

Evaluation of immigrant and refugee AYAs should also include:
- Tuberculosis screening—tuberculin skin test (TST) or an interferon gamma-release assay (IGRA), such as QuantiFERON or T-SPOT, which may be preferred for those who have previously received Bacillus Calmette–Guérin vaccination
- Complete blood count (CBC) with differential and platelet count (to identify iron deficiency, thalassemias and other hemoglobinopathies, cell enzyme defects, or eosinophilia)
- Hepatitis B surface antigen testing
- Gonorrhea and chlamydia nucleic acid amplification testing (NAATs)
- Human immunodeficiency virus (HIV) antibody screening

Evaluation of refugees and targeted immigrants based on symptoms, physical findings, predeparture treatment or living conditions, and country of emigration should also include the following screening tests:
- Stool for complete ova and parasites
- Urinalysis—(schistosomiasis, renal disease)
- Lead level (adolescents 16 years or younger)
- Vitamin D
- Syphilis (treponemal or nontreponemal)
- Malaria smear
- Varicella, hepatitis A and B, and measles serologies
- Strongyloides serology
- Schistosomiasis serology

Screening for Adjustment of Legal Status

Application for LPR requires a specific medical examination by USCIS. Medical information for this adjudication of status (I 693 Form) may be supplied by the clinician, but should only be signed by an authorized civil surgeon.

Specific Health Issues
Immunizations

- Immunizations should be administered using the age-based immunization guidelines provided by the CDC's Advisory

Committee on Immunization Practices (https://www.cdc.gov/vaccines/schedules/downloads/child/0-18yrs-child-combined-schedule.pdf and http://www.cdc.gov/vaccines/schedules/hcp/imz/adult.html).

- Overseas immunizations are considered valid if given at appropriate ages and intervals and documented with specific dates of administration.
- Vaccination series do not need to be restarted due to delays between immunizations.
- If no written documentation is available, the youth is considered unvaccinated unless serum immunity is verified and must be immunized according to the "catch-up" schedule.
- Tuberculin skin test can be applied before or on the same day that live virus vaccines are given (measles, mumps, rubella, varicella, intranasal flu). However, if a live virus vaccine was given on the previous day or earlier, the TST should be delayed for at least 1 month. Live measles vaccine given prior to the application of a TST can reduce the reactivity of the skin test because of mild immunosuppression.
- Consider obtaining serologies for varicella, measles, hepatitis A, and hepatitis B to assess for immunity prior to immunizing.
- Proof of immunizations or positive serologies are required for adjustment of legal status (human papillomavirus recommended but not required).

Tuberculosis

Overall, tuberculosis rates have declined in the U.S. general population, and a majority of new cases are diagnosed among non-U.S. born individuals.[18]

- Review predeparture medical records for TB testing, including chest x-ray.
- Obtain information regarding any prior treatment for TB, symptoms suggestive of TB (fevers, night sweats, cough >3 weeks, weight loss), or TB exposures.
- Perform TST or IGRA if no reliable documentation of predeparture testing is available.
- Tuberculin skin test >5 mm is considered positive in a refugee with HIV or other immunosuppression, or if in close contact with someone with active TB, or if there are changes on chest x-ray consistent with prior TB. Induration >10 mm is positive for all other refugees.[19]
- Obtain a chest x-ray for all patients with a positive TST or IGRA.
- Encourage treatment for latent tuberculosis infection (LTBI).
- Prompt referral should be made to local departments of public health or infectious disease specialists for individuals with active pulmonary or extrapulmonary disease.

Parasitic Infections

- All refugees and at-risk immigrants should be screened for parasitic infections. Common parasites include *Giardia*, *Ascaris*, *Hookworm*, *Trichuris* (whipworm), *Entamoeba histolytica*, and *Schistosoma*.[20]
- Collect two stool specimens (for ova and parasites separated by 24 hours) and a CBC for eosinophilia (total eosinophil count >400/μL of blood).
- Confirm predeparture presumptive treatment, which will guide initial screening and treatment.[21]

Malaria

- Individuals from sub-Saharan Africa and other highly endemic regions should receive presumptive treatment on arrival (if no documented predeparture treatment) or have laboratory screening.
- There should be a high index of suspicion for malaria in individuals from tropical or subtropical areas if they have fever of unknown origin or other symptoms suggestive of malaria.
- Laboratory evaluation includes malaria blood films (thick and thin smears) and rapid antigen testing. Polymerase chain reaction is more sensitive particularly in asymptomatic individuals and should be used if available.

Hepatitis B

- Screen all refugees and at-risk immigrants for hepatitis B virus, and immunize all AYAs without documentation of prior vaccination or immunity.

Lead

Lead exposure and toxicity are common in many countries of origin in addition to risk for continued exposures after arrival.[22]

- All young adolescent refugees (16 years of age or less) should be tested for lead upon arrival in the United States.

Sexual Health

Sexual and reproductive health is an important aspect of care for all AYAs, but immigrant and refugee AYAs may have additional needs or challenges[23] including:

- A lack of sex education
- Cultural values that may discourage open discussion of sexual health with AYAs
- Greater risk of having experienced sexual violence prior to arrival, depending on the circumstances of their migration
- A history of female genital mutilation
- Cultural values and beliefs that marginalize and discriminate against sexual minorities

As with all AYAs, a portion of the visit should be conducted alone with the patient as confidential sexual and reproductive health care is standard of care.[24] Confidentiality needs to be discussed with the patient and family in a sensitive way, especially because AYA autonomy may be viewed differently across cultures.[25] "Western" societies such as the United States or Europe often value autonomy and individualism, while others value interdependence. Parenting styles and family structures often reflect these underlying cultural priorities, which can affect how families may perceive a clinician discussing sensitive topics with adolescent patients, especially alone. It is important for the clinician to respectfully work with the family to understand any cultural differences while providing appropriate confidential care to the adolescent.

Mental Health

Most refugee and immigrant AYAs display impressive resilience and the ability to adjust and adapt despite significant adversity and trauma. However, as many as half of AYAs exhibit significant symptoms of posttraumatic stress disorder (PTSD), and up to 30% experience significant depression.[26,27] Predictors include the following:

- Experience prior to migration—trauma, separation from family members, death of loved ones, personal injury
- Experiences postmigration—adjustment to language and cultural differences, discrimination, peer bullying, change in family hierarchy when the adolescent becomes a cultural broker for the parents/caregivers, isolation for those who come without family
- Lack of community social support, community violence, living arrangements

Common symptoms:
- Aggression and anger
- Depression
- Risky behaviors: illegal drug use, risky sexual behaviors
- Disturbing thoughts and images
- Concentration and school problems
- Somatic complaints

Interventions to support mental health and resilience:
- Helping with important tasks for family/community
- Peer group activities
- Validation of experiences
- Culturally informed mental health services

NONIMMIGRANT FOREIGN-BORN ADOLESCENTS AND YOUNG ADULTS

Nonimmigrant foreign-born individuals are granted temporary admission visas for a specific purpose such as academic and vocational study, temporary employment, business, and pleasure. Over a million students are actively attending academic or vocational institutions in the United States at the undergraduate as well as graduate levels. The most represented countries are China, South Korea, India, Saudi Arabia, and Canada.[28]

Guidelines for Nonimmigrant Foreign-born Adolescents and Young Adults

- All international students from areas with high rates of TB should be tested with TST or IGRA. High-incidence areas are those with 20 cases or more per 100,000 population and includes most countries in Africa, Asia, Central America, Eastern Europe, and South America. Updates on priority health topics including TB can be found in the World Health Organization (WHO) Global Health Observatory Data Repository, a publicly available interface for the WHO's health-related statistics (https://www.who.int/data/gho).
- American College Health Association (ACHA) guidelines for institutional prematriculation immunization may be found at the ACHA website (https://www.acha.org/documents/resources/guidelines/ACHA_Immunization_Recommendations_April2022.pdf).
- All nonimmigrant visas require proof of medical health insurance.
- International nonimmigrant AYA students who seek adjustment of legal status to LPR must undergo a medical examination as required by the USCIS.
- Interpreters should be used with all LEP nonimmigrant AYAs, and guidelines for cultural competency (see above) should be utilized.

SECOND-GENERATION IMMIGRANTS

Ambiguity surrounds the terminology used to describe different generations of immigrants and such terms must be interpreted through context. "First-generation" can refer to foreign-born individuals who migrate to the United States or to the first generation born in the United States. "Second-generation" immigrants are those born to first-generation immigrants and thus the ambiguity persists. The term "1.5 generation" is commonly used to describe individuals arriving prior to adolescence. U.S.-born children of immigrants represent 12% of the United States, a number that is expected to increase further.[3]

It should be noted that the health needs of immigrant foreign-born and U.S.-born AYAs differ. Issues to consider include the following:

- Newly arrived immigrants to the United States have increased acute illnesses such as infectious diseases, but in general have fewer chronic conditions and lower mortality. Mortality patterns for immigrants and for U.S.-born AYA vary considerably with immigrants experiencing lower mortality, particularly in young adulthood.[29] This health advantage seems to diminish with time and across generations. The reason for this is unclear, but it is thought that it might, in part, be that healthier individuals migrate and that access to healthy lifestyle choices diminishes once in the United States.
- Foreign-born immigrants and second-generation immigrants exhibit differences in health beliefs and behaviors.
  - Foreign-born young adults exhibit lower prevalence of smoking and tobacco use than U.S.-born young adults, especially among Latino women.[30]
  - U.S.-born Hispanic women are more likely to report having their first sexual experience under the age of 20 as compared

to foreign-born Hispanic women. They are also more likely to have their first live birth under the age of 20.[31]
- Knowledge, attitudes, and beliefs regarding tuberculosis varies between foreign-born and U.S.-born patients with LTBI. Foreign-born patients with LTBI are less likely to acknowledge that they have LTBI and are more likely to feel protected from the disease than U.S.-born patients with LTBI.[32] Since the majority of patients with LTBI are foreign-born, these differences are clinically meaningful.
- U.S.-born Latino youths are more likely to be enrolled in high school or college than their foreign-born counterparts.[33]
- Foreign-born Latinos (aged 16 to 25 years) are less likely to have been in a fight in the past year, know someone in a gang, carry a weapon during the last year, or be questioned by police.[33]

SUMMARY

Global migration is more prevalent than ever. Clinicians who care for AYAs need nuanced knowledge and skills to provide culturally appropriate medical care that addresses the specific needs of foreign-born young people. Sensitivity to their unique challenges as well as cultural humility are needed for clinicians to forge strong relationships with these patients and families and provide the comprehensive care they deserve.

REFERENCES

1. Greer JA, Park ER, Green AR, et al. Primary care resident perceived preparedness to deliver cross-cultural care: an examination of training and specialty differences. *J Gen Intern Med.* 2007;22(8):1107–1113.
2. Department of Economic and Social Affairs. International Migration 2019. United Nations. 2019. Accessed December 1, 2020. https://www.un.org/en/development/desa/population/migration/publications/migrationreport/docs/InternationalMigration2019_Report.pdf
3. Budiman A, Tamir C, Mora L, et al. *Facts on US Immigrants 2018.* Pew Research Center; 2020. Accessed December 1, 2020. https://www.pewresearch.org/hispanic/2020/08/20/facts-on-u-s-immigrants-current-data/
4. US Department of Health & Human Services; Office of Refugee Resettlement. Fact Sheet: Unaccompanied Alien Children (UAC) Program. Released August 11, 2020. Accessed December 1, 2020. https://www.hhs.gov/sites/default/files/unaccompanied-alien-children-program-fact-sheet-01-2020.pdf
5. Papademetriou DG. *Managing the Pandemic and its Aftermath: Economies, Jobs, and International Migration in the Age of COVID-19.* Migration Policy Institute; 2020. Accessed December 1 2020. https://www.migrationpolicy.org/sites/default/files/publications/tcm2020-papademetriou-migration-covid-19_final.pdf
6. Office of the United Nations High Commissioner for Refugees. Accessed December 1, 2020. http://www.unhcr.org/pages/49c3646c125.html
7. Bonnie RJ, Stroud C, Breiner H, eds. *Investing in the Health and Well-Being of Young Adults.* Institute of Medicine and National Research Council of the National Academies Press; 2014:312–313.
8. Flores G, Tomany-Korman SC. The language spoken at home and disparities in medical and dental health, access to care, and use of services in US children. *Pediatrics.* 2008;121(6):e1703–1714.
9. Cohen AL, Rivara F, Marcuse EK, et al. Are language barriers associated with serious medial events in hospitalized pediatric patients? *Pediatrics.* 2005;116(3):575–579.
10. Grubbs V, Chen AH, Bindman AB, et al. Effect of awareness of language law on language access in the health care setting. *J Gen Intern Med.* 2006;21(7):683–688.
11. Diamond LC, Schenker Y, Curry L, et al. Getting by: underuse of interpreters by resident physicians. *J Gen Intern Med.* 2009;24(2):256–262.
12. Minnesota Department of Health. Minnesota refugee health provider guide 2013: working with medical interpreters. Accessed December 1, 2020. https://www.health.state.mn.us/communities/rih/guide/11interpreters.pdf
13. Medical Examination of Immigrants and Refugees. Center for Disease Control and Prevention. Accessed December 1, 2020. https://www.cdc.gov/immigrantrefugeehealth/guidelines/overseas-guidelines.html
14. Center for Disease Control and Prevention. Refugee Health Guidance. Accessed December 1, 2020. http://www.cdc.gov/immigrantrefugeehealth/guidelines/refugee-guidelines.html
15. Museru OI, Vargas M, Kinyua M, et al. Hepatitis B virus infection among refugees resettled in the U.S.: high prevalence and challenges in access to health care. *J Immigr Minor Health.* 2010;12(6):823–827.
16. Lifson AR, Thai D, O'Fallon A, et al. Prevalence of tuberculosis, hepatitis B virus, and intestinal parasitic infections among refugees to Minnesota. *Public Health Rep.* 2002;117:69–77.
17. Barnett ED. Infectious disease screening for refugees resettled in the United States. *Clin Infect Dis.* 2004;39(6):833–841.
18. Deutsch-Feldman M, Pratt RH, Price SF, et al. Tuberculosis—United States, 2020. *MMWR Morb Mortal Wkly Rep.* 2021;70(12):409–414.
19. Center for Disease Control and Prevention. Accessed February 16, 2014. https://www.cdc.gov/immigrantrefugeehealth/guidelines/domestic/tuberculosis-guidelines.html

20. De Silva NR, Booker S, Hotez PJ, et al. Soil-transmitted helminth infections: updating the global picture. *Trends Parasitol.* 2003;19(12):547–551.

21. Center for Disease Control and Prevention. Overseas refugee health guidance. Accessed December 1, 2020. http://www.cdc.gov/immigrantrefugeehealth/guidelines/overseas/intestinal-parasites-overseas.html

22. Eisenberg KW, van Wijngaarden E, Fisher SG, et al. Blood lead levels of refugee children resettled in Massachusetts, 2000 to 2007. *Am J Public Health.* 2011;101:48–54.

23. Tirado V, Chu J, Hanson C, et al. Barriers and facilitators for the sexual and reproductive health and rights of young people in refugee contexts globally: a scoping review. *PLoS One.* 2020;15(7):e0236316.

24. Center for Adolescent Health and the Law. *General Policy Statements that Address Adolescents' Access to Confidential Health Care, Including the Roles of Parents and Guardians in Adolescent Health Care and Procedures to Safeguard Adolescents' Confidentiality.* Policy Compendium on Confidential Health Services for Adolescents, 2nd ed. 2005. Accessed February 12, 2021. http://www.cahl.org/PDFs/PolicyCompendium/General_Statements2_with_References.pdf

25. Johnson L, Radesky J, Zuckerman B. Cross-cultural parenting: reflections on autonomy and interdependence. *Pediatrics.* 2013;131(4):631–633.

26. Fazel M, Reed RV, Panter-brick C, et al. Mental health of displaced and refugee children resettled in high-income countries: risk and protective factors. *Lancet.* 2012;379(9812):266–282.

27. Bronstein L, Montgomery P. Psychological distress in refugee children: a systematic review. *Clin Child Fam Psychol Rev.* 2011;14:44–56.

28. Department of Homeland Security. Student and Exchange Visitor Program (SEVP) 2020 Student and Exchange Visitor Information System (SEVIS) by the Numbers Report. Accessed April 14, 2021. https://www.ice.gov/doclib/sevis/pdf/sevis-BTN2020.pdf

29. Singh GK, Siahpush M. All-cause and cause-specific mortality of immigrants and native-born in the United States. *Am J Public Health.* 2001;91(3):392–399.

30. Lariscy JT, Hummer RA, Rath JM, et al. Race/Ethnicity, nativity, and tobacco use among US young adults: results from a nationally representative survey. *Nicotine Tob Res.* 2013;15(8):1417–1426.

31. Tapales A, Douglas-Hall A, Whitehead H. The sexual and reproductive health of foreign-born women in the United States. *Contraception.* 2018; 98(1):47–51.

32. Colson PW, Franks J, Sondengam R, et al. Tuberculosis knowledge, attitudes, and beliefs in foreign-born and US-born patients with latent tuberculosis infection. *J Immigr Minor Health.* 2010;12(6):859–866.

33. Pew Research Center. *Between Two Worlds: How Young Latinos Come of Age in America.* Pew Research Center; 2013. Accessed December 1, 2020. http://www.pewhispanic.org/2009/12/11/between-two-worlds-how-young-latinos-come-of-age-in-america/

🛜 ADDITIONAL RESOURCES AND WEBSITES

Additional Resources and Websites for Clinicians:

American Academy of Pediatrics' Immigrant Child Health Toolkit—https://www.aap.org/en-us/advocacy-and-policy/aap-health-initiatives/Immigrant-Child-Health-Toolkit/Pages/Immigrant-Child-Health-Toolkit.aspx

American Psychological Association Committee on Sexual Orientation and Gender Diversity—https://www.apa.org/pi/lgbt/resources/lgbtq-asylum-seekers.pdf

Between Two Worlds: How Young Latinos Come of Age in America—https://www.pewresearch.org/hispanic/2009/12/11/between-two-worlds-how-young-latinos-come-of-age-in-america/

Bridging Refugee Youth and Children's Services—https://brycs.org/

Centers for Disease Control and Prevention Immigrant Refugee and Migrant Health Refugee Health Topics—https://www.cdc.gov/immigrantrefugeehealth/profiles/index.html

Ethnomed: Integrating Cultural Information into Clinical Practice—https://ethnomed.org

Minnesota Department of Health Refugee Topics—https://www.health.state.mn.us/communities/rih/topics/index.html

NIH U.S. National Library of Medicine Medline Plus—https://medlineplus.gov/languages/languages.html

Additional Resources and Websites for Parents/Caregivers:

Bridging Refugee Youth and Children's Services—https://brycs.org/refugee-portal/

Consumer Health Information in Many Languages Resources

Immigration Advocates Network—https://www.immigrationadvocates.org/legaldirectory/

NIH National Library of Medicine—https://www.immigrationadvocates.org/legaldirectory/

The UN Refugee Agency

Resources for Asylum-Seekers—https://www.unhcr.org/en-us/asylum-resources.html

U.S. Limited English Proficiency—https://www.lep.gov/education

Women's Refugee Commission—https://www.womensrefugeecommission.org/

Additional Resources and Websites for Adolescents and Young Adults:

Asylum Connect—https://asylumconnect.org/mission/

Asylum Connect Catalogue—http://catalog.asylumconnect.org/

Bridging Refugee Youth and Children's Services—https://brycs.org/refugee-portal/

Educational Resources for Immigrant, Refugees, Asylees and other New Americans—https://www2.ed.gov/about/overview/focus/immigration-resources.html

National Immigration Legal Services Directory—https://www.immigrationadvocates.org/legaldirectory

Women's Refugee Commission—https://www.womensrefugeecommission.org/

Health Care for Minoritized, Disenfranchised, and Marginalized Adolescent and Young Adults

Pamela A. Matson
Faye Korich

KEY WORDS

- Adverse childhood experiences
- Disenfranchised
- Opportunity youth
- Marginalized
- Minoritized
- Poverty
- Racism
- Resiliency
- Trauma

INTRODUCTION

During adolescence, many adverse health outcomes we seek to treat or prevent fall disproportionately to minoritized, marginalized, and disenfranchised youth–youth with the fewest resources, the least access to services, and the most stigmatized. Social, political, economic, and historical forces have created a vulnerability to individual, environmental, and societal factors that drive health disparities. Marginalization can result from economic or social status, identity, system involvement, or other factors. The needs of marginalized youth based on their sexual or gender identity, system involvement, and immigration status are addressed in other chapters in this text. Here we focus on youth who are marginalized due to their experiences of poverty, trauma, racism, and other forms of discrimination. While there are common concerns across all marginalized youth, there are also unique needs outlined below.

EPIDEMIOLOGY

Definitions and Terms

Marginalization is the treatment of a person or group as insignificant. Although youth, collectively, can be thought of as a marginalized group, we will refer to marginalized youth as racial or ethnic minorities or those living in poverty for the remainder of this chapter.[1]

Disenfranchised describes a person or group of people deprived of rights, privileges, or immunity. Typically, it is used in the context of criminal disenfranchisement or the deprivation of the right to vote resulting from a felony conviction. Disenfranchisement can also result from economic or social deprivations. Economic disenfranchisement is seen when communities do not receive the resources needed to create their wealth. For example, if a community is considered "unsafe," property developers may feel discouraged to build in this area, leading political leaders to decrease investments, further depleting community resources.[2] Social disenfranchisement is the exclusion from society or the feeling of isolation based on race or ethnicity. The unifying theme across different forms of disenfranchisement is the presence of a power differential resulting in the oppression of one individual or group.[3]

Opportunity youth are adolescents and young adults (AYAs) ages 16 to 24 years old who are disconnected from school and work.[4] Youth who are disconnected from both school and work will have difficulty achieving adult milestones, such as earning wages that can support a family. The term 'opportunity' is in reference to the opportunity to engage youth in education and training during this critical developmental period. In order to support opportunity youth, it is essential to understand the obstacles they face to engagement and connect them with resources to overcome these barriers.

The National Institutes of Health has defined *discrimination* as "a socially structured action that is unfair or unjustified and harms individuals and groups. Discrimination can be attributed to social interactions that occur to protect more powerful and privileged groups or institutions at the detriment of other groups." *Structural discrimination* refers to macro-level conditions (e.g., residential segregation) limiting less privileged groups' opportunities, resources, and well-being.[5] *Racism* refers to discrimination based on race or ethnicity. Racism is a social determinant of health that has a vast impact on the health of AYAs and is a significant driver of health inequities. In their recent policy statement, the American Academy of Pediatrics defines racism as "a system of structuring opportunity and assigning value based on the social interpretation of how one looks (which is what we call "race") that unfairly disadvantages some individuals and communities, unfairly advantages other individuals and communities, and saps the strength of the whole society through the waste of human resources."[6] Racism operates at multiple levels of influence including individual, interpersonal, community, and societal. Structural and personally mediated racism can lead to internalized racism or internalizing racial stereotypes about one's racial group.[6]

Prevalence and Demographics

Poverty

Poverty is one of the foremost social determinants of health.[7] The United States consistently ranks among the worst poverty rates among high-income countries.[8] Poverty is classified as an income below 100% of the federal poverty level based on family size. Deep poverty is an income below 50% of the federal poverty level. Families need an income twice the federal poverty level to meet their basic needs. Therefore, families with incomes less than 200% of the federal poverty level are considered low-income. In 2019, 8.6 million (35%) adolescents ages 12 to 17 lived in low-income families, 3.6 million (15%) lived in poverty, and 1.5 million (6%) lived in deep poverty.[9] Poverty often intersects with other social determinants of health, such that youth who live in poverty are more likely to live in neighborhoods with higher rates of violent crime and poorer educational and employment opportunities, to be exposed to environmental hazards as well as have reduced access to health-promoting resources. These conditions together lead to health-harming behaviors and poor physiologic functioning.[10] Black/African American, Hispanic/Latino, and American Indian/Alaska Native (AI/AN) youth are three times more likely to live in poverty than White or Asian youth.[11] These minoritized youth also grow up with higher rates of parental unemployment and lower household wealth compared to White youth, influencing access to opportunities and putting the subsequent generation at risk of poverty.[6]

There is an estimated 4.5 million opportunity youth in the United States, a significant reduction from 2010.[4] However, the declines have not been uniform. There has been an increase in the number of Black/African American opportunity youth. American Indian/Alaska Native youth have the highest rates of youth disconnected from school and work. Further, opportunity youth are disproportionately concentrated in the rural south. Opportunity youth are almost twice as likely to live in poverty as connected youth.[12]

Disenfranchisement

The 13th Amendment to the Constitution made slavery illegal in the United States. One exception to the amendment allowed for enslavement as punishment for a crime, leading several states to enact laws for formerly enslaved people. These Black Codes were used to control the labor force in a manner similar to pre-13th Amendment times. They were followed by Jim Crow laws which further legalized racial segregation and marginalization of African Americans. If one violated any of these laws, they risked being arrested, forced into unpaid labor, or losing their right to vote, which we still see today in the form of disenfranchisement. Criminal disenfranchisement laws prevent more than 5 million people from voting. These laws disproportionately affect Black/African Americans, with over 6% of the adult Black/African American population excluded from voting, compared to 1.2% of non-Black Americans.[13] Criminal disenfranchisement laws vary per state, with some states allowing individuals in prison to vote (e.g., Maine and Vermont), some requiring the payment of some or all fines, fees, and restitution in addition to fulfillment of their prison, parole, or probation sentences prior to re-enfranchisement, and others permanently disenfranchising individuals based on certain offenses.

Outside of criminal disenfranchisement laws, many Americans face voter disenfranchisement through voter suppression. For example, voter identification (ID) laws that require identification at the polls may seem unobstructive. Still, when over 21 million U.S. citizens lack a government-issued photo ID, these laws can lead to disenfranchisement due to cost or the expenses needed to obtain necessary documents. And for many minoritized youth, this ID requirement becomes a deterrent to voting. Further, prohibiting the use of student ID in states that require photo ID disproportionately impacts the participation of young voters.

Racism and Discrimination

The health of Black/African American, Hispanic/Latino, AI/AN, and Asian/Pacific Islander youth is impacted significantly by racism, which must be explicitly accounted for when addressing health disparities.[14] Experiences with discrimination are associated with numerous adverse health outcomes, including negative mental, physical, and behavioral health. English and colleagues found that Black/African American adolescents report experiencing over five episodes of discrimination a day. These experiences were either directed toward them personally in the form of bullying or indirectly by witnessing discrimination against someone of color, most commonly on the internet.[15]

Risk Behaviors and Morbidity

Behavioral Risk

Youth who live in poor or low-income families may be less likely to adhere to medical regimens or engage in preventative behaviors.[10]

Marginalized and minoritized youth are at increased risk of experiencing psychological stress leading to unsafe sexual behavior and substance misuse resulting from disproportionate exposure to neighborhood environments with high rates of violence and poverty. Similarly, alcohol outlet density (the number of physical locations in which alcoholic beverages are available for purchase per area or per population) and higher availability of tobacco, drug paraphernalia, and marketing of substances tend to be higher in minoritized and low-income communities.[16] Race-related stress, specifically personal experiences of racism, is associated with sexual risk and increased substance use among Black/African American adolescents.[17] Black/African American, Hispanic/Latino, and AI/AN youth experience disproportionate incarceration rates, which itself has a profound impact on the health and trajectories of youth.

Education

Educational achievement is critical for future economic well-being and healthy adulthood. Minoritized youth and those living in poverty experience greater chronic absenteeism rates and lower graduation rates resulting from disproportionate challenges, including poor health, family responsibilities, residential mobility, and inadequate or unsafe transportation options. Structural discrimination further impacts access to high-quality educational resources as school expenditures largely depend on neighborhood wealth. Non-White children are less likely to receive special education support services but more likely to receive disciplinary actions, including suspension.

Mental Health

One in four young adults has a mental illness (excluding substance use disorders).[18] Marginalized youth are at an increased risk of developing anxiety and depression.[19] Poverty may directly affect adolescent mental health. Youth are often aware of familial economic difficulties leading to increased stress, affecting mental health. In addition, exposure to violence in high-poverty neighborhoods has been associated with increased depressive symptoms, anxiety, and behavior problems. Finally, experiences of racism and discrimination are associated with emotional distress and poorer mental health outcomes.

Disenfranchised individuals are also at increased risk of anxiety and depression. They feel less control over decisions that may affect their lives, which can lead to this increased risk.[20] In addition, young people who live in poverty or experience discrimination or disenfranchisement are often required to mature at a faster pace.[21] As adolescence is an important time of development, the rapid transition into adulthood can negatively impact their emotional development, leading to a mental illness.[1]

Trauma

Trauma is an umbrella term that encompasses various experiences that can cause harm to one's emotional and physical well-being.

Definitions of Trauma Adverse Childhood Experiences (ACEs) are traumatic events that occur before the age of 18 and include emotional, physical, or sexual abuse, neglect, domestic violence, parental substance use or mental illness, parental separation or divorce, or incarceration of a household member (see **Table 85.1**).[22] The prevalence estimates of ACEs typically come from adult, retrospective cohort surveys. Early ACE studies found that nearly two-thirds of adults experienced at least one ACE before 18 years of age, but racial diversity was limited, with 75% of respondents identifying as White.[22] An updated estimate in a more diverse population found significantly higher ACE exposures reported in Black/African American, Hispanic/Latino, and multiracial respondents. Increased prevalence was also reported in respondents with less than a high school education, annual income less than $15,000, and those identifying as gay/lesbian or bisexual.[23] Data from surveys of youth also highlight the prevalence of ACEs. The 2011/12 National Survey of Children's Health (NSCH) found over 50% of adolescents aged 12 to

TABLE 85.1

Adverse Childhood Experiences[a]

1. Did a parent/caregiver or other adult in the household often or very often... Swear at you, insult you, put you down, or humiliate you? Or act in a way that made you afraid that you might be physically hurt?
2. Did a parent/caregiver or other adult in the household often or very often... Push, grab, slap, or throw something at you? Or ever hit you so hard that you had marks or were injured?
3. Did an adult or person at least 5 years older than you ever... Touch or fondle you or have you touch their body in a sexual way? Or attempt or actually have oral, anal, or vaginal intercourse with you?
4. Did you often or very often feel that... No one in your family loved you or thought you were important or special? Or your family didn't look out for each other, feel close to each other, or support each other?
5. Did you often or very often feel that... You didn't have enough to eat, had to wear dirty clothes, and had no one to protect you? Or your parents/caregivers were too drunk or high to take care of you or take you to the doctor if you needed it?
6. Were your parents/caregivers ever separated or divorced?
7. Was your parent or caregiver: Often or very often pushed, grabbed, slapped, or had something thrown at her? Or sometimes, often, or very often kicked, bitten, hit with a fist, or hit with something hard? Or ever repeatedly hit over at least a few minutes or threatened with a gun or knife?
8. Did you live with anyone who was a problem drinker or alcoholic, or who used street drugs?
9. Was a household member depressed or mentally ill, or did a household member attempt suicide?
10. Did a household member go to prison?

[a]10 types of trauma measured in CDC-Kaiser Permanente Adverse Childhood Experiences Study, Felitti VJ, Anda RF, Nordenberg D, et al. Relationship of childhood abuse and household dysfunction to many of the leading causes of death in adults: The adverse childhood experiences (ACE) study. *Am J Prev Med.* 1998;14(4):245–258.

17 have experienced at least one adverse childhood experience, and over 15% have experienced three or more.[24]

Psychological Trauma occurs when someone experiences an intense event that threatens or causes harm to their emotional or physical well-being.[25] Experiences may be acute or chronic in nature. Marginalized youth are at greater risk of experiencing trauma because of ongoing experiences of racism, including personally mediated discrimination and systemic racism that destabilize the communities in which they live.

Complex Trauma describes the exposure to multiple types of widespread and chronic traumatic events that involve violence, betrayal, exploitation, and loss, such as maltreatment and living in an unsafe family, community, or school settings.[26]

Posttraumatic Stress Disorder (PTSD) is a formal psychiatric diagnosis made when specific criteria about the number, duration, and intensity of symptoms are met after a person experienced or witnessed an event involving actual or threatened death or serious injury.[26] Marginalized AYAs who experience acute trauma may go on to develop PTSD.

Toxic Stress is a response that occurs after someone experiences strong, frequent, and prolonged adversity leading to prolonged activation of the stress response and disruption of the developing brain.[27] The developing brain can be affected by chronic exposure to stress due to marginalization, disenfranchisement, and poverty. The biologic stress response involves the hypothalamic–pituitary–adrenal (HPA) axis and the catecholamine system (see Fig. 85.1). Under acute stress, the HPA axis leads to the secretion of corticotrophin-releasing hormone (CRH), adrenocorticotrophic hormone (ACTH), and eventually cortisol in the adrenal glands. Cortisol regulates the release of CRH through negative feedback to bring the body back to a homeostatic state. In the presence of chronic and persistent stress, the body has difficulty reestablishing homeostasis. This dysregulation can lead to structural and neurochemical brain

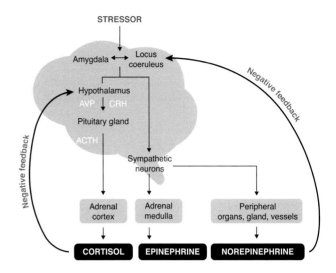

The HPA axis controls the body's response to stress and is a complex interplay of direct interactions. The HPA axis is composed of:

1. The **hypothalamus** which releases AVP and CRH to the pituitary gland
2. The **pituitary gland** which secretes ACTH when stimulated by AVP and CRH
3. The **adrenal cortex** which secretes glucocorticoids (cortisol) when stimulated by ACTH

The SAM axis mediates a rapid response to stress through interconnected neurons and regulates autonomic functions in multiple organ systems. The SAM axis is composed of:

1. The **sumpathetic neurons** which release epinephrine and norepinephrine and activate the body's fight-or-flight response
2. The **parasympathetic neurons** which withdraw the activity of the sympathetic neurons and promote the body's rest nad digest" response
3. The **adrenal medulla** which when triggered by the sympathetic neurons secretes cirulating epinephrine and activate the body's fight-or-flight response

FIGURE 85.1 Stress response pathway. (Bucci M, Marques SS, Oh D, Harris NB. From toxic stress in children and adolescents. *Adv Pediatr.* 2016;63(1):403–428.)

changes, weakened metabolic and immune systems, and changes to cardiovascular physiology.[20] This stress can also lead to unhealthy coping mechanisms (see behavioral risk above).

Minority Stress and Stress Proliferation

Minoritized youth are much more likely to experience poverty, amplifying the intersection of two great sources of stress—race and poverty.[14] Minority stress frameworks explain the relationships between additional stressors uniquely experienced by people of a minoritized status and race-related stress in youth. Stress proliferation theory articulates how stressors emanating from experiences of social disadvantage and racism spill over into other experiences of stress, including relationship stressors, magnifying the impact on health outcomes.[28] Figure 85.2 further illustrates the exposure–disease–stress framework incorporating both community- and individual-level vulnerabilities.

PRINCIPLES AND APPROACH TO CARE

Screening Considerations

History and Review of Systems

Exposure to trauma, marginalization, and poverty may present in various ways. Clinicians need to be aware of this and keep these diagnoses on the differential of many presenting symptoms.

Symptoms
• Sleeping disturbance
• Eating disturbance
• Functional abdominal pain
• Headaches
• Anxiety
• Depression

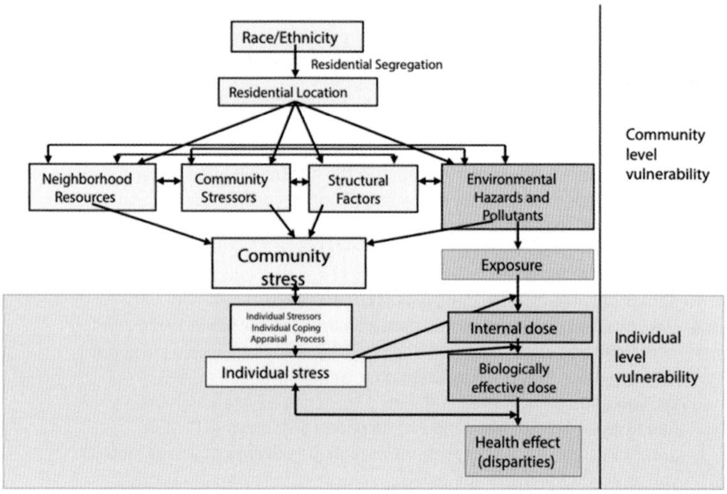

FIGURE 85.2 Exposure–disease–stress framework for environmental health disparities. (From National Academies of Sciences, Engineering, Medicine. Framing the dialogue on race and ethnicity to advance health equity. Proceedings of a workshop. National Academies Press; 2016.)

- Low mood or other depressive symptoms
- Difficulty with self-regulation
- Aggression
- Hypervigilance

Risk-taking behavioral assessment
- Any indicator of risk behavior or environment as identified using HEEADSSS/SSHADESS assessments (see Chapter 4).

Physical Assessment

- Blood pressure
- Overweight and obesity
- Bruises or other signs of trauma

Laboratory Assessment

Although there are no specific Laboratory
Although there are no specific labs to screen for exposure to trauma, marginalization, and poverty, sequelae (risk behaviors, eating disturbances, etc.) can help assess these diagnoses.
- Complete blood count (CBC)
- Comprehensive metabolic panel (CMP)
- Sexually transmitted infections (STI)/human immunodeficiency virus (HIV) screening (e.g., chlamydia/gonorrhea, syphilis)
- Nutritional deficiencies (e.g., iron, vitamin A, thiamine, folate)

Mental Health and Behavior Screening

- Depression (e.g., Patient Health Questionnaire-9 [PHQ-9]) (Chapter 74)
- Anxiety (e.g., General Anxiety Disorder-7 [GAD-7]) (Chapter 74)
- Substance use (e.g., CRAFFT, screening to brief intervention [S2BI], brief screener for tobacco [BSTAD]) (Chapter 69)

Psychosocial Screening

Trauma Screening/Adverse Childhood Experiences The seminal work by Felitti et al. on ACEs provides one framework to look at correlations between exposure of household dysfunction and health risk behaviors.[22] The since developed ACEs screening tool for children and adolescents has questions for young children and others directed toward 13- to 19-year-olds and can be used to assess for a history of or current toxic stress (see ACEs Table 85.1). Although this is not a validated tool, this assessment can be completed within 3 to 5 minutes and can identify an adolescent at risk.

Validated screening tools are available but are often too long to be performed by a clinician during a routine medical visit.[29] Alternatively, clinicians can utilize a previsit questionnaire that includes an assessment of stress (Table 85.2) and can be filled out prior to the start of the visit, followed by alone time with the clinician to review. If time allows, or with the help of ancillary staff, these validated tools may be helpful:

- *Center for Youth Wellness ACE-Questionnaire child, teen, and teen self-report*

 The Center for Youth Wellness ACE-Questionniare (CYW ACE-Q) highlights the connections between chronic, toxic stress and harm to the developing brain. They developed a questionnaire to be used as a clinical screening tool to assess cumulative exposure to ACEs. Questionnaires are available for children and adolescents up to 19 years of age.

- *Yale-Vermont Adversity in Childhood Scale*

 The Yale-Vermont Adversity in Childhood Scale (Y-VACS) is an extension of the ten-item ACEs questionnaire. It assesses for adverse experiences outside of the family and seeks information from multiple sources, including parents/caregivers and clinicians.

- *The University of California at Los Angeles (UCLA) Posttraumatic Stress Disorder Reaction Index for Diagnostic and Statistical Manual of Mental Disorders, Fifth Edition (DSM-5)*

 This instrument is used to comprehensively assess for a history of trauma in adolescents and children. Recently, an 11-item trauma

TABLE 85.2

Clinician Questions to Ask Youth During Well or Acute Care Visits

Assessment	Question
Housing Insecurity	During the past year, have there been any changes in the home (e.g., new people in the home, people leaving the home, moving to a new house)?
School Engagement	Are you having trouble in school (failing grades, trouble with peers, difficulty concentrating)?
Trauma	Has anything bad or scary happened to you recently?
Food Insecurity	Each day, do you feel that you have enough to eat?
Racism/Discrimination	Have you experienced discrimination or unfair treatment because of your skin color, language or accent, or your culture or country of origin?
Intimate Partner Violence	Do you feel safe in your relationship?
Resiliency	Do you know at least one person you can talk to about a problem?

screening tool was developed to briefly evaluate for trauma and PTSD symptoms.

Clinicians can also assess for trauma using simple questions during well-visits or acute care as indicated (see Table 85.2).

Basic Needs

Most tools used in clinical settings do not assess poverty directly but ask about basic material needs such as housing and food insecurity or financial strain (difficulty paying for basic needs). The harmful effects of poverty may be mitigated by connecting youth and families to available resources. Screening for basic needs in clinical settings helps identify patients who need help with food or stable housing, insurance, transportation, or necessary supplies, such as formula or diapers.[11] There are four widely used social health screening tools designed for pediatric settings, iHELP, Safe Environment for Every Kid (SEEK), The Survey of Well-being of Young Children (SWYC), and WE CARE.[30] All four screening tools assess food insecurity but vary with respect to determining other social needs. The iHELP tool screens for pediatric social histories and includes questions about financial strain, housing insecurity, and other needs, including insurance. However, each of these instruments is designed to be completed by the parent/caregiver. However, the clinician can assess the adolescent's experiences using routine HEEADSSS/SSHADES assessments, specifically when addressing the home environment and diet/eating.

Racism/Discrimination

Clinicians can assess patients for experiences of racism and assist youth with differentiating racism from other forms of unfair treatment. The Perceptions of Racism in Children and Youth (PRaCY) and the Index of Race-Related Stress for Adolescents (IRRS) are validated instruments to assess youths' experiences of discrimination and racism.[31,32] Clinicians can ask, "Have you experienced discrimination or unfair treatment because of your skin color, language or accent, or your culture or country of origin?"

School Engagement

Assess patients for school attendance and any academic issues to identify signs of disengagement, academic difficulties, or indicators of learning difficulties. For example, clinicians can ask, "Are you having trouble in school (failing grades, trouble with peers, difficulty concentrating)?" Clinicians can coordinate with schools to ensure patients meet their educational goals and milestones.

Healthy Relationships

Stress proliferation processes often result in stressors due to poverty and racism spilling over to impact relationships with family and romantic partners. Assess relationship functioning, sources of support, and any signs of intimate partner violence. There are several validated tools to assess intimate partner violence (see Resources). However, clinicians can also ask some basic questions to determine relationship safety, such as "Do you currently have a romantic or dating partner?" and if yes, then "Do you feel safe in your relationship?"

Resiliency Factors

Protective factors have the potential to counteract the negative impacts of ACEs.[33] These protective factors include positive relationships with friends both in school and in the community, family health, positive parenting, and positive parent/caregiver–child interaction. Protective factors play an important role in having the social and emotional support needed to succeed. This, in turn, potentially reduces the impact of the trauma, even if it is ongoing.[34] Although prevention of ACEs is ideal, asking about and understanding these protective factors gives clinicians an area to generate resilience within AYAs. For example, clinicians can ask patients, "Do you know at least one person you can talk to about a problem?" Fostering a positive racial identity can mitigate experiences of racism and discrimination. Clinicians can gauge youth's racial/ethnic pride and positive socialization.

SPECIAL CONSIDERATIONS

Insurance Issues

The U.S. health system differs from other industrialized countries with universal health care. In the United States, Medicaid is an excellent resource for physical health care coverage; however, mental health coverage can be challenging as many therapists do not accept Medicaid. The number of therapists available is limited, resulting in patients waiting weeks to months for mental health services. Medications to treat mental health and trauma are typically covered. Navigating the sign-up process and income thresholds for Medicaid eligibility can also be challenging. Clinicians should be aware that discontinuity in coverage is common. As periods without insurance can result in poor health outcomes, clinicians should ask about gaps in coverage.

Nutrition Support

Anticipatory guidance for overall health and many specific conditions involves recommending patients to follow a healthy diet. Unfortunately, the most nutritious foods (e.g., fresh fruits and vegetables, lean proteins) are the most expensive to purchase in the United States. In addition, poor and low-income families often live in food deserts, areas without nearby grocery stores or other outlets providing access to affordable healthy foods.[35] Clinicians should be aware of these challenges when evaluating and advising patients.

Neighborhood Safety

Poor and low-income youth and families are more likely to live in neighborhoods with high rates of violence and lack of sidewalks or inadequate lighting that create unsafe conditions in which to recreate or commute to school or care. Exercise is essential to good health and particularly important to prevent or address conditions such as for overweight and obesity. Clinicians should be aware of these neighborhood safety constraints when providing recommendations for outdoor activities and anticipatory guidance.

Transportation Barriers

Poor and low-income youth and families are less likely to own a car.[36] This limits their ability to control their transportation and requires them to rely on others to borrow a vehicle or use public transit. Poor and underserved communities often lack adequate and reliable public transportation. Patients may need to navigate multiple bus lines, unreliable schedules, and weather vulnerabilities to attend clinic appointments. Those who do have access to a car incur both clinic parking and gas costs, the latter of which may be particularly onerous for rural patients. These transportation issues are magnified for youth who may seek confidential care or otherwise attend clinic visits independently.

The increased use of virtual medical care may help assuage some of these transportation barriers and increase access to care. Virtual care has additional advantages, including increased cost-effectiveness, increased patient engagement, and overall convenience. However, these virtual care advantages need to be weighed against potential disadvantages, including the training required to use these services, inability to perform a comprehensive physical exam, and the digital divide (persons with disabilities and lower SES population with limited access to computers/phones or internet).

RECOMMENDATIONS

Recommendations to Clinicians

Trauma-Informed Care

- Utilize a trauma-informed care framework to identify, acknowledge, and manage the effects of trauma. It is an approach that assumes an individual has a history of trauma and strives to identify and sensitively address the trauma. For example, the American Academy of Pediatrics has an extensive 6-part trauma-informed care series that equips clinicians and practices with the tools to create a trauma-informed environment.

Mental Health Support

- Assess patients for stressors associated with experiences of both poverty and racism, with an awareness that stressors may result from interpersonal, academic, institutional, community, and other sources.
- Clinicians can use cognitive behavioral therapy focusing on trauma management to help AYAs who have experienced trauma. It can provide them with tools like breathing and relaxation techniques. It can also allow the young person to create their own story of the trauma, helping them understand this is a part of their story while reducing the power of the trauma to continue causing harm.

Medications

- Medications are often used in conjunction with mental health services and should not be considered for the sole management of trauma. It is important to explain to patients and families that medications such as selective serotonin reuptake inhibitors can support low mood. Still, it is also essential to use these medications in conjunction with mental health services to help manage trauma.

Racism/Discrimination

- During health visits, clinicians can ask about events in the community that may have impacted the patient, determine the need for counseling or other sources of support such as affinity groups, and provide anticipatory guidance on effective strategies to keep AYAs safe.[6]

Positive Youth Development/Empowering Youth

- Civic engagement, or any individual or collective action designed to identify or address the concerns or well-being of a community, social group, or society in general, is an important tool for youth empowerment for marginalized youth. It can encompass a range of activities, including political participation, volunteering and community service, sociopolitical action, belonging to a community or civic organization.
- Studies have found that adolescent civic engagement is predictive of future optimism, decreased depression, higher household income, higher personal earnings, and decreased risky health behaviors.[34,37]
- Youth who experience marginalization and alienation due to systemic racism and oppression can demonstrate their strengths and realize their rights as contributing community members through civic engagement.
- For youth who cannot vote due to age, immigration status, or previous incarceration, engaging in other forms of civic engagement is an important tool to fight stigmatization. For example, clinicians can encourage youth to volunteer at polls and promote voter registration and voting with friends and family.[38] Further, clinicians can encourage youth to optimize their school service-learning requirements as opportunities for community engagement.

Future Orientation

- Greater future orientation or envisioning aspects of one's future self, including education and career goals, family and other life milestones, is associated with better health and education outcomes and fewer risk behaviors as well as an important predictor of youths' ability to overcome adversity.[39]
- Ask patients about their education or employment goals.
- Discuss how they may overcome any personal or institutional barriers to achieving their goals.

Recommendations to Health Care Settings That Provide Care to Adolescents and Young Adults

- Train all staff to provide culturally competent care and create an environment sensitive to experiences of poverty and racism. Prioritize growing and maintaining a diverse workforce.
- Have an onsite social worker, community resources, or patient navigator supporting youth as they move through the medical system and providing support and connection to community resources.
- Maintain a list of resources and referral sources to meet basic needs (food banks, insurance support, shelters, diaper banks/formula [for youth with infants], food bags).
- Ensure health care policies minimize barriers to care, including accommodating late arrivals, rescheduling no-shows without penalty, and expanding access to telehealth for follow-up care when possible.
- Institute programs that overcome transportation barriers to care resulting from onerous public transportation routes or prohibitively expensive costs of onsite parking. These programs can include providing parking vouchers, bus passes, or ride-share services sponsored by the clinic.

Recommendations to Communities and Policy Makers

Advocacy

Continued advocacy is needed to preserve safety-net programs globally that bridge critical gaps for poor and low-income youth and families. Clinicians should be aware of the safety-net programs in their geographic areas to reduce poverty and inequality. For example, programs like the U.S. Child Health Insurance Program (CHIP) ensure access to health care by providing low-cost health coverage to low-income families who do not qualify for Medicaid. Others, such as the Supplemental Nutrition Assistance Program (SNAP), assist extremely impoverished families with meeting their basic needs. Continued advocacy is necessary to protect funding for existing programs and new public policies that expand programs and benefits (e.g., Medicaid expansion, child tax credit) to address the needs and improve social mobility for poor and low-income youth and families, including the working poor. Advocacy opportunities related to discrimination include support for supplemental funding to enhance and improve the quality of education and vocational training opportunities for youth in communities with less financial capital; promote multicultural curricula and teaching of critical race theory in schools, and advocate for access to mental health services and linkage to resources to reduce racial/ethnic disparities in school disciplinary actions. Similarly, advocacy is urgently needed for policies that move away from the incarceration of youth and other policies that advance social justice.

Major Strategic Investments in Child and Adolescent Health

Ultimately, to shift the trajectory for marginalized, minoritized, and disenfranchised youth and make fundamental improvements to their health and economic well-being requires making strategic and impactful investments in adolescent health. Examples include the *Harlem Children's Zone, North Carolina School of Science and Mathematics,* and the *Lebron James Family Foundation's I Promise School.* The I Promise School is a new model for public schools that provides support and resources to students already falling behind, promising a 4-year all-expenses–paid college scholarship at graduation. The *Harlem Children's Zone* aims to interrupt the cycle of intergenerational poverty by providing programs and services that build opportunities for youth and families, from early childhood and education programs to youth programs that support college and career readiness, all the while building a healthy and thriving neighborhood. States can also make impactful investments. For example, the *North Carolina School of Science and Mathematics* is a public high school that invites juniors and seniors from across the state of North Carolina to attend a residential program specializing in science, technology, engineering, and math. The school provides an unparalleled education to youth from rural and low-income communities who may not otherwise have access to similar resources. The return on investment is significant, and thus the program has expanded to a second campus in western North Carolina and has been duplicated in South Carolina and Illinois.

Justice Initiatives

The disproportionate incarceration and sentencing of minoritized youth in the United States warrants robust advocacy for criminal justice reform. Organizations such as *Equal Justice Initiative* and *The Sentencing Project* advocate for policies that minimize imprisonment and criminalization, particularly addressing racial disparities in youth incarceration, and advocating for developmentally appropriate and humane approaches to juvenile justice.

● SUMMARY

Clinicians and health care settings that evaluate AYAs should be aware of unique challenges poor and low-income AYAs face when seeking care and barriers to health-promoting behaviors. Non-White AYAs experience stressors resulting from racism and discrimination. Poverty is highly prevalent and often intersects with other social determinants of health that limit opportunities and resources and bring about chronic exposure to stress. Experiences of poverty and trauma are associated with a wide range of adverse physical, mental, and behavioral health outcomes. Clinicians can ask simple questions to assess basic needs, experiences of trauma and racism, and protective factors.

REFERENCES

1. Sapiro B, Ward A. Marginalized youth, mental health, and connection with others: a review of the literature. *Child Adolesc Social Work J.* 2019;37(4):343–357.
2. Burrell M, White AM, Frerichs L, et al. Depicting "the system": how structural racism and disenfranchisement in the United States can cause dynamics in community violence among males in urban black communities. *Soc Sci Med.* 2021;272:113469.
3. Birtles BE. Disenfranchisement breeds conflict. *InterAgency J.* 2018;9(3).
4. Youth.gov. Opportunity youth. 2021. https://youth.gov/youth-topics/opportunity-youth
5. Office of Disease Prevention and Health Promotion. Discrimination. Healthy People 2020. 2020. https://www.healthypeople.gov/2020/topics-objectives/topic/social-determinants-health/interventions-resources/discrimination
6. Trent M, Dooley DG, Dougé J, et al. The impact of racism on child and adolescent health. *Pediatrics.* 2019;144(2):e20191765.
7. World Health Organization. Poverty and social determinants. 2021. https://www.who.int/health-topics/social-determinants-of-health#tab=tab_1
8. OECD. Poverty rate (indicator). 2021. https://data.oecd.org/inequality/poverty-rate.htm. Accessed October 18, 2021.
9. Koball H, Moore A, Hernandez, J. *Basic Facts About Low-Income Children: Children Under 9 Years, 2019.* National Center for Children in Poverty, Bank Street College of Education; 2021.
10. Beck AF, Cohen AJ, Colvin JD, et al. Perspectives from the Society for Pediatric Research: interventions targeting social needs in pediatric clinical care. *Pediatr Res.* 2018;84(1):10–21.
11. Council on Community Pediatrics. Poverty and child health in the United States. *Pediatrics.* 2016;137(4):e20160339.
12. Mendelson T, Mmari K, Blum RW, et al. Opportunity youth: insights and opportunities for a public health approach to reengage disconnected teenagers and young adults. *Public Health Rep.* 2018;133(1_suppl):54S–64S.
13. Uggen C, Larson R, Shannon S, et al. Locked out 2020: estimates of people denied voting rights due to a felony conviction. 2020. https://www.sentencingproject.org/publications/locked-out-2020-estimates-of-people-denied-voting-rights-due-to-a-felony-conviction
14. National Academies of Sciences, Engineering, Medicine. Framing the dialogue on race and ethnicity to advance health equity: proceedings of a workshop. National Academies Press; 2016.
15. English D, Lambert SF, Tynes BM, et al. Daily multidimensional racial discrimination among Black U.S. American adolescents. *J Appl Dev Psychol.* 2020;66:101068.
16. Milam AJ, Furr-Holden CDM, Cooley-Strickland MC, et al. Risk for exposure to alcohol, tobacco, and other drugs on the route to and from school: the role of alcohol outlets. *Prevention Science.* 2014;15(1):12–21.
17. Sanders-Phillips K, Kliewer W, Tirmazi T, et al. Perceived racial discrimination, drug use, and psychological distress in african american youth: a pathway to child health disparities. *J Soc Issue.* 2014;70(2):279–297.
18. Substance Abuse and Mental Health Services Administration. *Key Substance use and Mental Health Indicators in the United States: Results From the 2018 National Survey on Drug Use and Health.* Center for Behavioral Health Statistics and Quality, Substance Abuse and Mental Health Services Administration; 2019.
19. Reiss F. Socioeconomic inequalities and mental health problems in children and adolescents: a systematic review. *Soc Sci Med.* 2013;90:24–31.
20. Purtle J. Felon disenfranchisement in the United States: a health equity perspective. *Am J Public Health.* 2013;103(4):632–637.
21. Kendig SM, Mattingly MJ, Bianchi SM. Childhood poverty and the transition to adulthood. *Fam Relat.* 2014;63(2):271–286.
22. Felitti VJ, Anda RF, Nordenberg D, et al. Relationship of childhood abuse and household dysfunction to many of the leading causes of death in adults: the adverse childhood experiences (ACE) study. *Am J Prev Med.* 1998;14(4):245–258.
23. Merrick MT, Ford DC, Ports KA, et al. Prevalence of adverse childhood experiences from the 2011–2014 behavioral risk factor surveillance system in 23 states. *JAMA Pediatr.* 2018;172(11):1038–1044.
24. Moore KA, Ramirez AN. Adverse childhood experience and adolescent well-being: do protective factors matter? *Child Indicators Research.* 2015;9(2):299–316.
25. The National Child Traumatic Stress Network. What is child traumatic stress? 2003.
26. The National Child Traumatic Stress Network (NCTSN) . Glossary of terms related to trauma-informed integrated healthcare. 2018. https://www.nctsn.org/sites/default/files/resources//glossary_of_terms_related_to_trauma-Informed_integrated_healthcare.pdf
27. Center on the Developing Child, Harvard University. Toxic stress. 2021. https://developingchild.harvard.edu/science/key-concepts/toxic-stress/
28. LeBlanc AJ, Frost DM, Wight RG. Minority stress and stress proliferation among same-sex and other marginalized couples. *J Marriage Fam.* 2015;77(1):40–59.
29. Racine N, Killam T, Madigan S. Trauma-informed care as a universal precaution: beyond the adverse childhood experiences questionnaire. *JAMA Pediatr.* 2020;174(1):5–6.
30. Social Interventions Research and Evaluation Network, University of San Francisco California. Social needs screening tools comparison table (pediatric settings). 2019. https://sirenetwork.ucsf.edu/tools-resources/resources/screening-tools-comparison/peds
31. Pachter LM, Szalacha LA, Bernstein BA, et al. Perceptions of racism in children and youth (PRaCY): properties of a self-report instrument for research on children's health and development. *Ethn Health.* 2010;15(1):33–46.
32. Seaton EK. An examination of the factor structure of the index of race-related stress among a sample of african american adolescents. *J Black Psychol.* 2003;29(3):292–307.
33. Balistreri KS, Alvira-Hammond M. Adverse childhood experiences, family functioning and adolescent health and emotional well-being. *Public Health.* 2016;132:72–78.
34. Bethell C, Jones J, Gombojav N, et al. Positive childhood experiences and adult mental and relational health in a statewide sample: associations across adverse childhood experiences levels. *JAMA Pediatr.* 2019;173(11):e193007.
35. ver Ploeg M, Breneman V, Farrigan T, et al. *Access to affordable and nutritious food: measuring and understanding food deserts and their consequences: report to congress.* 2009.
36. Klein NJ, Smart MJ. Life events, poverty, and car ownership in the United States: a mobility biography approach. *J Trans Land Use.* 2019;12(1):395–418.
37. Wray-Lake L, Shubert J, Lin L, et al. Examining associations between civic engagement and depressive symptoms from adolescence to young adulthood in a national U.S. sample. *Appl Dev Sci.* 2017;23(2):1–13.
38. Banales J, Hoffman AJ, Rivas-Drake D, et al. The development of ethnic-racial identity process and its relation to civic beliefs among latinx and black american adolescents. *J Youth Adolesc.* 2020;49(12):2495–2508.
39. Johnson SRL, Blum RW, Cheng TL. Future orientation: a construct with implications for adolescent health and well-being. *Int J Adolesc Med Health.* 2014;26(4):459–468.

🛜 ADDITIONAL RESOURCES AND WEBSITES

Additional Resources and Websites for Clinicians:

AAP Trauma Informed Toolkit—https://www.aap.org/en-us/advocacy-and-policy/aap-health-initiatives/healthy-foster-care-america/Pages/Trauma-Guide.aspx#trauma

Brief Screener for Tobacco, Alcohol, and other Drugs (BSTAD) Substance Use Screening Tool—https://www.drugabuse.gov/ast/bstad/#/

Center for Youth Wellness (CYW) ACE-Questionnaire Child, Teen and Teen Self-Report—https://centerforyouthwellness.org/aceq-pdf/

IHELP Pediatric Social History Tool—https://sirenetwork.ucsf.edu/tools-resources/resources/ihelp-pediatric-social-history-tool

Pediatric Social History Screening Tools—https://sirenetwork.ucsf.edu/tools-resources/resources/screening-tools-comparison/peds

Programs & Initiatives for Opportunity Youth—https://youth.gov/youth-topics/opportunity-youth

Screening to Brief Intervention (S2BI) Substance Use Screening Tool—https://www.drugabuse.gov/ast/s2bi/#/

UCLA Brief Screen for Child/Adolescent Trauma and PTSD—https://www.reactionindex.com/tools_measures/

Validated Screening Tools for Intimate Partner Violence—https://www.cdc.gov/violenceprevention/pdf/ipv/ipvandsvscreening.pdf

Yale-Vermont Adversity in Childhood Scale—https://www.kennedykrieger.org/sites/default/files/library/documents/faculty/Y-VACS_Child_Self-Report_4.2020.pdf

Additional Resources and Websites for Parents/Caregivers:

Futures Without Violence, How to Talk to Teens About Dating Violence—https://www.futureswithoutviolence.org/talk-teens-teen-dating-violence/

XVI

Futures Without Violence, The Amazing Brain—https://www.futureswithoutviolence.org/amazing-brain-what-every-parentcaregiver-needs-to-know/

Georgetown University, Anti-racism toolkit—https://guides.library.georgetown.edu/antiracism/parents

Healthy Children, Talking to your Children About Racial Bias—https://www.healthychildren.org/english/healthy-living/emotional-wellness/building-resilience/pages/talking-to-children-about-racial-bias.aspx

Love is Respect, Parent Tip Sheet—https://www.loveisrespect.org/wp-content/uploads/2019/01/Parent-toolkit.pdf

Partnership to End Addiction, Marijuana talk kit—https://drugfree.org/wp-content/uploads/2017/02/Marijuana_Talk_Kit.pdf

PBS, Talking to your children about race and racism—https://www.pbs.org/parents/talking-about-racism

SAMHSA's National Helpline—https://www.samhsa.gov/find-help/national-helpline

TulsaKids Dismantling Racism Toolkit: Resources for Parents—https://www.tulsakids.com/dismantling-racism-toolkit-resources-for-parents/

Well Being Trust Mental Health School Toolkits Resources for parents—https://wellbeingtrust.org/wp-content/uploads/2019/02/wellbeingtrustmentalhealthtoolkitforparents.pdf

Index

Note: Page number followed by f and t indicates figure and table respectively.

A

Abdominal migraine, 390t
Abdominal pain, 390t. *See also* Chronic abdominal pain
  ectopic pregnancy, 525
  infectious mononucleosis and, 321
Abetalipoproteinemia, 172
Abnormal keratinization, 256
Abnormal uterine bleeding (AUB), 484–487. *See also* Uterine bleeding, abnormal
Aborted suicide attempt, 671
Abortion, 417
  access to abortion services, 417
  clinicians, role of, 417–418
  complete, 419
  incomplete, 419
  induced, 418
  medical method, 418
  method for, selection of, 418
  rate, 417
  risks and complications, 418
  spontaneous, 419
  surgical method, 418
  threatened, 419
Abstinence-only education, school-based, 415
Abusive relationships, and unplanned pregnancy, 413
Acamprosate, for alcohol use disorder, 619
Acanthosis nigricans (AN), 273, 492, 492f
  clinical manifestations, 273
  HAIR-AN syndrome and, 273
  obesity and, 273
  treatment, 273
ACC/AHA Guideline on the Primary Prevention of Cardiovascular Disease, 174
Acceptance and commitment therapy, for anxiety disorders, 669
Accessory nipples/breasts, 539
Accountability, 118
Acellular pertussis vaccines (Tdap), 326
N-acetylcysteine, 635
ACHA-National College Health Assessment Survey (ACHA-NCHA), 707
Achieving a Better Life Experience Act account, 682
Acne, 256–261
  clinical manifestations, 256–257
  conglobata, 257
  differential diagnosis, 257–258
  etiology, 256
  evaluation, 257
  fulminans, 257
  history and physical examination, 257, 257t
  inflammatory lesions, 256–257, 256f, 257f
  management, 258–261
    azelaic acid, 260
    benzoyl peroxide, 259
    dapsone, 260
    hormonal therapy, 261
    isotretinoin, 261
    oral medications, 260–261
    patient education, 258–259
    salicylic acid, 260
    topical antibiotics, 259
    topical retinoids, 259–260, 260t
    treatment plan, 258t, 259t

  microcomedo, 256
  mild, 257, 258t
  moderate, 256f, 257, 259t
  obstructive lesions, 256, 256f
  oral contraceptives for, 452
  pomade, 257
  scars, 257, 257f
  severe, 257, 257f, 259t
  steroid, 257
  treatment follow-up, 261
  variants, 257
Acne vulgaris. *See* Acne
Acquaintance rape, 696
Acquired immunodeficiency syndrome (AIDS), 341. *See also* Human immunodeficiency virus (HIV) infection
Acromioclavicular joint sprain, 222
ACSM Guidelines for Exercise Prescription, 232
Actigraphy, 297
Action on Smoking and Health, 631
Activated charcoal, 638, 648
Activity and exercise, in ME/CFS, 384
Acupuncture, 94, 94f
  for headache management, 290
Acute residential treatment (ART), for substance use disorders, 655t
Acute treatment, for headache, 290, 291t. *See also* Headaches
Acyclovir, for genital herpes, 581, 581t
Adams forward-bend test, 223, 223f, 226
Adapalene, 260, 260t
Adapalene/benzoyl peroxide (Epiduo), 260t
Addiction, 609, 653
  nicotine, 624
Adenoma sebaceum, 258
Adequate intake (AI), 80, 81t
ADHD. *See* Attention deficit hyperactivity disorder (ADHD)
Adherence to treatment, 108–109
Adiposity rebound, 42
Adjustable gastric band (AGB), 360f, 361
Adjustment disorder, 375, 662
Adnexal torsion, 518, 518f
  diagnosis, 518
  treatment, 518
Adolescence, 10, 45, 127
  brain maturation during, 42–43, 609
  challenges of, 55
  close relationships in, 396
  early, 45, 46
  late, 45, 47
  middle, 45, 46–47
  phases and tasks of, 45
  process of, 45
Adolescent and young adult health, quality improvement in, 124t, 125, 125t
Adolescent Brain & Cognitive Development (ABCD Study), 133t
Adolescent brain development, 609, 653
  nicotine exposure, effects of, 624–625
  substance use and, 609
Adolescent community reinforcement approach, for alcohol use disorder, 619
Adolescent development, 551
Adolescent fertility rate, 4t, 5

Adolescent-friendly care, 4t, 29, 107–108, 107f, 108f
Adolescent idiopathic scoliosis (AIS), 226
Adolescent parents and children, interventions for, 413, 420
Adolescents and young adults (AYAs), 2
  acne vulgaris in, 256–261
  birth rates, 413, 414f
  chronic health conditions in, 105–110
  COVID-19 effect on, 8, 10
  demographics of, 11, 11f–16f
  eating habits and nutritional problems, 78–79
  enuresis in, 306–310
  evidence-based clinical preventive services for, 63t
  feeding and eating disorders in, 362–372
  health care services for, 29–30
  health care utilization, by age group and sex, 64t
  interviewing suggestions for, 52t
  interviewing techniques for, 53t
  interview structure, 51–54
  life-course influences on, 3f, 10–11
  with life-limiting conditions, 112–114, 113t (*See also* Palliative care)
  mortality in, 16–22
  physical growth and development, 35–43
  pregnancy rates, 413
  preventive health care for, 58–76
  preventive services for, 58–64
  principles to approach, 54–55
  psychosocial development in, 45–48
  racial and ethnic composition of, 11
  recommended dietary allowances for, 80, 80t
  renal and genitourinary tract infections in, 300–305
  social determinants of health of, 2–10, 3f
  suicide among, 17
  technology and social media use, 98–104
  transgender, 408–411
Adoption, 420
Adrenarche, 36, 39
  dehydroepiandrosterone sulfate (DHEA-S) level at, 256
Adrenergic storm, 637
Adult criminal justice system, 733. *See also* Justice system, involvement with
Advance care planning, 115–116
Advance Care Planning Readiness Assessment, 115
Adverse childhood experiences (ACEs), 744–745, 745t
  and hypertension, 197
  as risk factor for suicide, 672
Advertising, tobacco, 623, 624f–625f
Advocate, physician as, 54
Affirm VP III, 509, 510
Affordable Care Act (ACA), 88, 252, 617, 630, 636, 712, 729–730, 743
Agoraphobia, 668
Airway obstruction, infectious mononucleosis and, 321
Al-Anon, 620
Alateen, 620

Alcohol, 614
  among adolescents, 614–615
  among youth, 615
    alcohol use disorders, 617–619
    consequences of, 616–617
    drinking and driving, 616–617
    high-risk behaviors, 617
    neurotoxicity of, 617
  BAC levels and intoxication effects, 614t
  binge drinking, 614
  college students and, 615
  with energy drinks, 617
  heavy drinking, 614
  media/advertising of, 616
  during pregnancy, 419
  use, 27, 107
    early onset of, 607
    epidemiology of, 614–616
    media influences on, 616
    middle and high school youth, 605t, 606
    morbidity and mortality from, 616
    puberty and, 616
    risk factors for, 616
    screening for, 617–618
    sociodemographic trends of, 616
    young adult, 607
  withdrawal, 617, 619
Alcoholics Anonymous, 620
Alcohol intoxication, 614
Alcohol, marijuana, tobacco, and other illicit
    drugs (AMTOD), AYA use of, 602
Alcohol-related birth defects, 687. See also
    Fetal alcohol spectrum disorders
Alcohol-related neurodevelopmental disorder,
    687. See also Fetal alcohol spectrum
    disorders
Alcohol Screening and Brief Intervention Guide
    for Youth, 618
Alcohol, Smoking and Substance Involvement
    Screening Test (ASSIST), 618
Alcohol use disorder (AUD), 615, 616
  among youth, 617–620
  brief interventions and referrals to treatment,
    618–619
  diagnosis of, 619
    DSM-5 criteria for, 619, 619t
  screening for, 617–618
  treatment, 619–620
Alcohol Use Disorders Identification Test
    (AUDIT), 618, 652, 652t
All-cause mortality, 4t
Allergic contact dermatitis (ACD), 264–265
  metal (nickel) and, 265, 265f
  plants and, 264–265, 264f
  preservatives/fragrances and, 265
Allergic shiners, 204
Allergies, in ME/CFS patients, 382
Allopregnanolone, 480
Alopecia areata, 273
  alopecia totalis, 273
  alopecia universalis, 273
Alosetron, for diarrhea-predominant IBS
    (IBS-D), 393
Alport syndrome, 316
Aluminum chloride, for hyperhidrosis, 273
Amastia, 539–540
Ambulatory BP monitoring (ABPM), 198
Ambulatory ECG monitoring, 180
Amenorrhea, 488–494
  athletes with, 494
  definition, 488
  diagnosis, 490–493, 491f, 492f
  etiology, 488–490
  history, 490
  laboratory evaluation, 493
  physical examination, 492

  primary, 488, 491f
  secondary, 488, 492f
  treatment, 493–494
  with weight loss, 494
  weight loss and, 363
American Academy of Child and Adolescent
    Psychiatry (AACAP), 636
American Academy of Pediatrics (AAP), 51,
    173, 252, 391, 437, 460, 641, 651, 687,
    748
  Clinical Practice Guideline on High Blood
    Pressure in Children and Adolescents,
    196
  Policy Statement on Office-Based Care for
    Lesbian, Gay, Bisexual, Transgender,
    and Questioning Youth, 404, 405
  on racism, 743
  on universal screening of adolescents for
    substance use, 617
American Cancer Society, 630
American College Health Association (ACHA),
    706
American Gastroenterology Association (AGA),
    392
American Heart Association (AHA), 168, 169t,
    190, 192t, 196
American Lung Association, 630
American Psychiatric Association, 636
Americans for Nonsmokers' Rights, 631
Americans with Disabilities Act (ADA), 284
Amitriptyline, for AMPS, 379
Amoxicillin
  for acne, 261
  for genitourinary tract infections, 303
Amphetamines, 639–640
  in ADHD, 685
  adverse effects, 639, 639f
  chronic use, 640
  intoxication, effects of, 639
  "meth mouth", 639, 639f
  overdose and emergency treatment, 640
  physiology and metabolism, 639
  during pregnancy, 419
  preparation and dose, 639
  tolerance and withdrawal, 640
  use by young adults, 609
Ampicillin, for genitourinary tract infections, 303
Amplified musculoskeletal pain syndrome
    (AMPS), 376
  differential diagnosis, 378t
  diffuse, 376–377
  epidemiology, 377
  localized, 377–378
  management, 379
    education, 379
    multidisciplinary approach, 379
    nonpharmacologic therapies, 379
    pharmacotherapy, 379
  pathophysiology, 377
AMPS. See Amplified musculoskeletal pain
    syndrome (AMPS)
Amyl nitrite, 645
AN. See Anorexia nervosa (AN)
Anabolic–androgenic steroids (AAS), 649
Anal intraepithelial neoplasia (AIN), 584
Androgen
  and acne, 256, 257
  excess (See Polycystic ovary syndrome
    (PCOS))
  and hair loss, 272–273
  sources of, in females, 496, 496f
Androgenetic alopecia (AGA), 272–273
Androgen insensitivity
  and amenorrhea, 489, 494
  complete, 143
  partial, 143

Androgen-receptor defects, 143
Androstenedione, 495
Angiotensin-converting enzyme inhibitors, for
    hypertension, 201t
Angiotensin receptor blockers, for hypertension,
    201t
Angry patient, 54
Ankle, 216–218
  fractures, 217–218
  history of ankle symptoms, 216
  injuries treatment, 216
  Ottawa ankle rules, 216, 217f
  physical examination, 216
Ankle sprain, 216–217
  clinical manifestation, 216
  definition and etiology, 216, 217f
  diagnosis, 216
  epidemiology, 216
  prognosis, 217
  rehabilitation, 217
  treatment, 216–217
Annovera, 427
Anogenital warts, 268, 584
  clinical course, 585
  color, 585
  counseling, 588
  differential diagnosis, 586
  exacerbating factors, 585
  in pregnancy, 589
  sites for, 585
  symptoms, 585
  treatment, 587, 587t–588t
  types of, 585, 585f, 586f
Anorchism, 143
Anorectal–gonococcal infections, 559
Anorexia nervosa (AN), 106, 142, 362–368, 362t
  age at onset, 363
  and amenorrhea, 490
  binge-eating/purging subtype (AN-B/P), 362,
    362t
  clinical manifestations, 363–364
  comorbidity conditions with, 363
  diagnosis and differential diagnosis, 364, 366
  DSM-5 diagnostic criteria for, 362t
  epidemiology, 363
  etiology, 362–363
  evaluation, 366
  gender and, 363
  history in, 366
  instruments for diagnosis of, 366
  laboratory features, 364
  laboratory tests, 367
  medical complications, 365t–366t
  in middle adolescence, 47
  neurotransmitter abnormalities and, 362
  nutritional assessment, 366–367
  outcome, 368
  physical examination, 367
  prevalence and incidence, 363
  restricting type (AN-R), 362, 362t
  risk factors, 363
  societal emphasis on thinness and, 362–363
  treatment, 367–368
Anovulatory bleeding, 484, 485
Anterior cruciate ligament (ACL)
  injury prevention, 246
  tear, 218
Anthropometric measurements, 79–80
Antibiotics
  for acne, 260–261
  for atopic dermatitis, 264
  for folliculitis, 269
  for genitourinary tract infections, 303–305,
    304t
  for hidradenitis suppurativa, 273
  for mastitis, 541

for *Mycoplasma* infections, 325
for pelvic inflammatory disease, 565, 566t
for pertussis, 326
Antibody testing, in infectious mononucleosis, 321, 321t
Anticholinergics, 393
for enuresis, 309
for overactive bladder, 309
Anticonvulsants, hormonal contraceptives and, 454
Antidepressants, 664, 673
for bulimia nervosa, 370
for premenstrual disorders, 482
Antidiarrheals, 393
Antidiuretic hormone (ADH), 307
Antiemtics, for headache management, 291t
Antihistamine
for allergic contact dermatitis, 2645
for atopic dermatitis, 264
for exanthematous drug eruptions, 272
for pityriasis rosea, 269
for urticaria, 271
Antihypertensive medications, 200, 201, 201t
Antiretroviral therapy (ART), 341, 350–351, 351t
Antiseborrheic shampoo, 265
Antiseizure medication (ASM), 278, 281t, 282
congenital malformation with, 282
and hormonal birth control failure, 282
teratogenicity, 282
Antispasmodics, 393
Antithyroid therapy, 156
Antituberculosis agents, hormonal contraceptives and, 454
Anxiety, 106, 665. *See also* Anxiety disorders
epilepsy and, 283
and FGIDs in AYAs, 393–394
transgender youth and young adults, 409
transient, 665, 666
Anxiety disorders, 665–669
assessment, 666–667
comorbidity assessment, 666
confidentiality in, 666
cultural background, 666
illness characteristics, 666
interviews and collateral information, 666
causality, 666
course of illness, 665
in DSM-5, 667–668
in early childhood, 665
epidemiology, 665
generalized anxiety disorder, 667, 667t
panic disorder, 667t, 668
risk factors, 665
environmental factors, 666
genetic factors, 666
temperamental factors, 665
screening tools for, 666–667
selective mutism, 667t, 668
separation anxiety disorder, 667t, 668
social anxiety disorder, 667–668, 667t
specific phobias, 667, 667t
treatment, 668–669
general considerations, 668
medications, 669
mild anxiety disorders, 668
moderate to severe anxiety disorders, 668
psychoeducation, 668
psychotherapy, 668–669
safety consideration, 668
stressors and psychiatric comorbidities, 668
in youth experiencing homelessness, 725
Anxiolytics, for premenstrual disorders, 482
Anxious patient, 54
Aortic coarctation, 194, 194t

Aortic dissection, 139
Aortic valve disease, 194t
Apnea, 293, 295. *See also* Sleep disturbances and disorders
Apolipoprotein B, 172
Apolipoproteins, 171–172
Apophysitis, 216
Appendix testis, 531
Applications (Apps), 102
Appointments, 51
ARFID. *See* Avoidant restrictive food intake disorder (ARFID)
Argyll Robertson pupils, 572
Aripiprazole, for autism spectrum disorder, 686
Armed Forces Qualification Test (AFQT), 719
Armed services vocational aptitude battery (ASVAB), 717
Arterial switch for d-transposition, 194t
ASD. *See* Autism spectrum disorder (ASD)
Asexual, 401
Asherman syndrome, 490, 493
Ask Suicide-Screening Questions (ASQ), 673, 673f
ASQ Brief Suicide Safety Assessment (ASQ BSSA), 673
Assessment
developmental, 67
HIV infection, 347–348
nutritional, 79–81, 366–367
sleep disturbances and disorders, 297
Asthma, 204–206
diagnosis, 204
exacerbations, 206
history, 204
management, 205–206, 205f, 206f
physical examination, 204
risk factors, 204
symptoms, 204
Asylees, 738
Asymptomatic bacteriuria, 302
Asymptomatic proteinuria, 312–314. *See also* Proteinuria
Atenolol
for neurocardiogenic syncope, 181t
for orthostatic intolerance, 385t
Atherosclerosis, 169–171
atheroma, 169
atherosclerotic lesions, development of, 169, 171f
atherosclerotic plaques, 169
in childhood, 171
cholesterol and, 170–171
risk factors, 170
Athletes. *See also* Sport-related concussion (SRC)
with ADHD, 244
amenorrhea in, 489–490, 494
anorexia nervosa, 363
and blood pressure, 243
calories requirements, 83
carbohydrate loading, 83
daily recommended intake of protein and micronutrients in, 243t
with disability and special health care needs, 245
female athlete, 245
female athlete triad, 489
hematuria in, 316
hydration before and during activity, 83
iron and zinc deficiency risk in, 82–83
nutritional supplements, 83
overuse injuries, 246
relative energy deficiency in sport, 372, 489–490
sodium and potassium intake, 83
stimulants use, 244

sudden cardiac arrest in, 184
transgender/nonbinary athletes, 245
weight restriction, 83
Athlete's foot. *See* Tinea pedis
Athletics, 241, 244, 245. *See also* Athletes; Physical activity (PA); Sports participation
Atlantoaxial instability (AAI), 245
Atomoxetine, in ADHD, 685
Atopic dermatitis (AD), 263–264
clinical manifestations, 263, 263f
complications, 263
lichenification in, 263, 263f
in persons of color, 263
treatment, 264
variant, 263
Atrial septal defect (ASD), 187, 188t
Atrial switch for d-TGA, 194t
Attention deficit hyperactivity disorder (ADHD), 106, 107, 244, 677t, 683–685, 687, 713
ADHD care algorithm, 684f
associated features, 683
comorbidities with, 683
diagnosis of, 683
epilepsy and, 283
exercise and, 244
interventions, 686
medication, 683
nonstimulant medications, 685
nutrition, 685
physical exercise, 683
sleep regulation, 683
stimulant medications, 683–685
psychosocial treatment, 683
school supports, 683
Atypical anorexia nervosa (AAN), 368
Auricular acupuncture, 94, 94f
Authoritative parenting style, 55
Autism spectrum disorder (ASD), 677t, 681t, 685
associated features, 685–686
diagnosis, 685
early childhood screening for, 685
with gender nonconformity, 685
interventions, 686
medications, 686
prognosis, 685
sensory processing, 685–686
Autoimmune thyroiditis, 143, 152
AV canal defects, 194t
Avoidant restrictive food intake disorder (ARFID), 371
clinical presentation, 371
DSM-5 diagnostic criteria for, 371t
epidemiology, 371
evaluation, 371
medical complications, 365t–366t, 371
psychiatric comorbidities with, 371
treatment, 371
AYAs. *See* Adolescents and young adults (AYAs)
Azathioprine, for atopic dermatitis, 264
Azelaic acid, for acne, 260
Azithromycin, 535, 559
for acne, 261
for chancroid, 593t
for gonococcal infections, 560
for granuloma inguinale, 595t
for *Mycoplasma* infections, 325
for pertussis, 326
for syphilis treatment, 575

B
Bacille Calmette–Guérin (BCG) vaccine, 70
Back pain
discogenic, 224–225, 225f
low, 225–226

Baclofen, 644
Bacterial endocarditis, 190, 192t
Bacterial infections
  bullous impetigo, 268
  crusted (nonbullous) impetigo, 268
  folliculitis, 268–269
Bacterial vaginosis, 507, 508–510
  clinical manifestations, 509
  counseling, 510
  diagnosis, 509
    Amsel criteria, 509
    commercial tests, 509
    NAATs, 509
    Nugent scoring, 509
    Pap tests, 509
  epidemiology, 509
  etiology, 509
  predisposing factors, 509
  recurrent, 509
  therapy, 509–510
Balancing measures, 120
Baloxavir, for influenza, 327
Barbiturates, 642–643
  adverse effects, 642–643
  intoxication, effects of, 642
  medical use, 642
  overdose and emergency treatment, 643
  physiology and metabolism, 642
  tolerance and withdrawal, 643
Bardet–Biedl syndrome, 144
Bariatric surgery, 360–361, 360f
Barrier contraception, 436–448
  cervical cap and diaphragm, 444–447
  cervical shield, 444, 444f
  contraceptive sponge, 441, 443–444
  internal condoms (female condoms),
    440–441
  traditional condoms (male condoms),
    436–440
  vaginal spermicides, 447–448
Bartholin glands, 470
Bartholinitis, 559
Battlefield acupuncture, 94
Bayley–Pinneau method, 40
Bebtelovimab, for COVID-19, 329
Beck Anxiety Inventory (BAI), 666–667
Beck Depression Inventory-II (BDI-II), 662
Bedwetting. See Enuresis
Bedwetting alarms, 308–309
Behavioral change, for HIV prevention, 347
Behavioral counseling, for STI reduction, 551
Behavioral disorders, 106
Behavioral health, of adolescents in out-of-home
    care, 730
Behavioral inhibition, 665, 666. See also
    Anxiety disorders
Behaviors
  eating, 363, 369
  and health, 2, 9, 10, 58, 107 (See also Health
    behaviors)
Beighton score, for joint hypermobility, 383,
    383f
Bell clapper deformity, 530, 532f, 533
Benign cystic teratomas, 521–522, 522f
Benign mucinous cystadenomas, 522, 522f
Benzalkonium chloride, 447
Benzathine penicillin G, for syphilis treatment,
    575
Benzodiazepines, 643–644, 643t
  administration routes, 643
  adverse effects, 643
  chronic use, 644
  designer, 643
  intoxication, effects of, 643
  medical use, 643, 643t

  overdose and emergency treatment, 643–644
  physiology and metabolism, 643
  tolerance and withdrawal, 644
Benzoylmethylecgonine. See Cocaine
Benzoyl peroxide (BPO), for acne, 259
Bereavement, 116–117
Berger disease. See IgA nephropathy
Beta blockers
  for long QT syndrome, 184
  for neurocardiogenic syncope, 181t
Bilateral salpingo-oophorectomy, 482
Billing for confidential services, 51
Bimanual examination, 470, 472f
  ruptured ectopic pregnancy, 526
Binge drinking, 614–616. See also Alcohol
Binge-eating disorder, 370
  DSM-5 diagnostic criteria for, 370t
  prevalence, 370
  risk factors, 370
  treatment, 370
Biofeedback, 95
  for headache management, 290
Biologic agents, for SJS and TEN, 271
Biologic false-positive (BFP) tests, 573–574
Biopsychosocial assessment, 376
Bipolar depression, 662–663
Birth control, 437, 449. See Contraceptives;
    Traditional condoms
Birth rates among AYAs, 413, 414f
Birth weight, and hypertension, 198
Bisexual, 401
Bisphosphonates, in CRPS, 379
Blackheads, 256
Bladder and bowel dysfunction (BBD), 306–307
Bleach baths, 269
Bleeding
  abnormal uterine bleeding, 484–487
  hormonal contraceptives and, 453, 454t
Blood alcohol concentration (BAC), 614
Blood pressure (BP), 243, 243t
  classification of, 197t
  elevated BP, 196
  in hypertension, 196, 197t
  measurement, 69, 198
Blueprints for Healthy Youth Development
    website, 694
Body composition, pubertal changes in, 41, 43t
Body image, 46
  in early adolescence, 46
  in late adolescence, 47
  in middle adolescence, 47
  young adults, 48
Body mass index (BMI), 42, 79, 354, 357
  calculation, 69
  puberty and, 42
Body modifications
  piercing, 274–275
  tattooing, 274–275
Body stuffer syndrome, 639
Bodywork, 95
Bone age, 40, 139, 145
  delayed, 145
  normal, 145
Bone health, epilepsy and, 282–283
Bone mineral density (BMD), 41
  anorexia nervosa and, 364
Bordetella pertussis, 325
Borjeson–Forseeman–Lehman syndrome, 144
Botulinum toxin, for hyperhidrosis, 273
BP. See Blood pressure (BP)
Brain development, in AYAs, 42–43
  cerebellum, 43
  connections among regions, 43
  early and midadolescence, 43
  executive suite, 43
  gray matter, 43

  prefrontal cortex, 43
  rate of development, 43
  white matter, 43
  young adulthood, 43
Brain MRI, in epilepsy, 280
Breakthrough bleeding, 486
Breakthrough therapy, 640
Breast
  complaints, 539t
    key factors for evaluation of, 539t
  normal development, 539
  physical examination, 545
Breast abscesses, 541
Breast asymmetry, 540
Breast biopsy, 545
Breast Cancer and the Environment Research
    Program (BCERP), 37
Breast cancer, CHCs and risk of, 453
Breast cancer gene 1 (BRCA-1), 523
Breast cysts, 544
Breast disorders
  benign breast disease
    mastalgia, 541
    mastitis, 541, 541f
    nipple discharge, 541
  congenital anomalies, 539–540
    accessory nipples/breasts, 539
    breast tissue, absence of, 539–540
  disorders of development
    breast asymmetry, 540
    macromastia, 540
    tuberous breast deformity, 540, 540f
Breastfeeding, epilepsy and, 282
Breast imaging, 545
Breast infection. See Mastitis
Breast malignancy, 544–545
Breast masses, in females, 543–544, 543t
  breast cysts, 544
  evaluation, 543
  fibroadenomas, 543–544
  fibrocystic breast changes, 544
  juvenile papillomatosis, 544
  phyllodes tumors, 544
Breast overgrowth, 540
Breast pain. See Mastalgia
Breast self-examinations (BSE), 545
Breast tissue, absence of, 539–540
Breath tests, 392
Brief interventions, 652–653
Brief Screener for Tobacco, Alcohol, and
    Other Drugs (BSTAD), 66–67, 618,
    652, 652t
Brief suicide safety assessment (BSSA), 673
Bright Futures, 617
  guidelines, 58–60
Brivaracetam, for seizure treatment, 281t
Bromocriptine, for prolactinomas, 543
Bronchial provocation testing, 204
Bronchoconstriction, exercise-induced, 207
Brugada syndrome, 184
Bubo, 591, 592
BufferGel Duet, 447
Bulimia nervosa (BN), 106, 368–370
  age at onset, 369
  binge–purge activity, 369
  clinical manifestations, 369
  comorbidity conditions with, 369
  diagnosis and differential diagnosis, 369
  DSM-5 diagnostic criteria for, 368t
  epidemiology, 368–369
  evaluation, 370
  gender and, 369
  medical complications, 365t–366t
  outcome, 370
  prevalence, 368
  risk factors, 369

signs and symptoms, 369
    and suicidal behaviors, 370
    treatment, 370
Bullying, 107, 691
    of sexual minority youth, 403
Buprenorphine, for opioid use disorder, 641
Bupropion
    in ADHD, 685
    for tobacco cessation, 628
Burnout from sports participation, 246
Butterbur (*Petasites Hybridus*), 93
Bystanders, 120

C
CA-125, 523
Cabergoline, for prolactinomas, 543
Cabotegravir, for HIV prevention, 346
CAH. *See* Congenital adrenal hyperplasia (CAH)
Calcaneal apophysitis, 216
Calcineurin inhibitor, for vitiligo, 274
Calcipotriene, for psoriasis, 270
Calcium
    DRI for, 81, 81t
    inadequate intake, 81
    in PMS, 481
    during pregnancy, 82
    requirements for, 81
    supplements, 81
Calcium channel blockers, for hypertension,
        201t
California Health Interview Survey (CHIS), 133t
Campaign for Tobacco-Free Kids, 631
Candida albicans, 507, 510
Candidiasis, 267
Cannabidiol (CBD), 633
    for seizure treatment, 281t
Cannabimimetics. *See* Synthetic cannabinoids
Cannabinoid hyperemesis syndrome (CHS), 635
Cannabinoids
    for fibromyalgia, 379
    for sleep disorders, 294
Cannabis, 633
    for insomnia, 294
Cannabis-induced psychosis, 635
Cannabis use disorder, 635
Cantharidin, for molluscum contagiosum, 599t
Capacity, 86
    to consent, 86
Cape Area Panel Study (CAPS), 133t
Carbamazepine, for seizure treatment, 281t
Carbohydrate loading, 83
Carbohydrates, 80
    foods containing, 80
    glycemic index, 80
Cardiac murmurs. *See* Murmurs
Cardiopulmonary exercise testing, 204
Cardiovascular disease (CVD), 168
    cardiovascular health role, in prevention of
        (*See* Cardiovascular health)
    dietary choices and risk of, 79
    risk of (*See* Atherosclerosis; Dyslipidemia)
Cardiovascular health, 168–169, 169t
    causes of variation in trajectories of, 170f
    ideal, 168–169, 169t, 170f
    metrics, 168, 170f
Cardiovascular risk screening, 173–174
Cardiovascular syncope, 181–182
    cardiac disease on examination, 182
    differential diagnosis, 181t
    echocardiography, 182
    warning signs of, 181, 182t
Case-control studies, 131t
Catamenial disorders, combined hormonal
        contraceptives in, 452
Catamenial epilepsy, 282–283
Cataplexy, 295

Catch-up vaccines, 74
Catecholaminergic polymorphic ventricular
        tachycardia, 184
Cathine, 640
Cathinone ("bath salts" or "plant food"), 640
Cause-and-effect diagram. *See* Fishbone
        diagrams
CB1 receptor (CB1R), 633
CB2 receptor (CB2R), 633
CBT. *See* Cognitive behavioral therapy (CBT)
Cefotetan, 566
Cefoxitin, 566
Ceftriaxone, 536, 565
    chancroid, 593t
    for gonococcal infections, 560–561
    for gonococcal urogenital infections, 559
    for pyelonephritis, 303, 304t
    for syphilis treatment, 575
Celecoxib, for dysmenorrhea, 479
Celiac disease, 391
Celiac sprue. *See* Celiac disease
Cenobamate, for seizure treatment, 281t
Center for Medicare and Medicaid Services
        (CMS), 101, 125, 125t
Center for Youth Wellness (CYW)
    ACE-questionnaire child, teen, and teen
        self-report, 746
Centers for Disease Control and Prevention
        (CDC), 41, 70, 449
    adult immunization schedule, 72t
    child and adolescent immunization schedule
        for ages 18 years or younger, 71t
    on medical screening for immigrants and
        refugees, 739
    Sexually Transmitted Diseases Treatment
        Guidelines, 552
    Sexually Transmitted Disease (STD)
        Surveillance Report, 556
    weight-for-age and height-for-age charts, 79
Central nervous system (CNS), and seizures,
        277
Central sensitization, 378
Centre for Epidemiologic Studies Depression
        Scale for Children, 662
Cerebral palsy, 106, 677t
Cerebral venous sinus thrombosis (CVST),
        headaches related to, 289
Cerebrotendinous xanthomatosis, 173t
Certain Dri, for hyperhidrosis, 273
Certificates of Confidentiality (COCs), 129
Cervarix, 73
Cervical cancer, 73, 501
    cervical transformation zone, 502, 502f
    CHCs and risk of, 453
    human papillomavirus infection and,
        502–503
    risk factors, 502–503
    screening for (*See* Cervical cancer screening)
    tobacco exposure and, 503
Cervical cancer screening, 501–505, 586
    abnormal screening tests, management of, 504
    American Cancer Society guidelines for, 503
    follow-up evaluation for nonmalignant
        cytology findings, 503, 503t
    high-grade squamous intraepithelial lesions
        (HSILs), 501
    low-grade squamous intraepithelial lesions
        (LSILs), 501
    prevalence of abnormal cytology, 501–502
        HPV vaccination, impact of, 501–502
    primary HPV testing, 503, 504
        with reflex testing, 504
    recommendations for young adults, 504
    tests, 503–504
    triage test, 503
    USPSTF guidelines for, 503, 503t

Cervical cap, 444–447, 445f
    advantages, 447
    contraindications, 445
    disadvantages, 447
    effectiveness, 445
    insertion of, 446
    patient education, 446
    removal of, 446
    tips to improve success, 445
Cervical dysplasia, 349
    therapy for, 505
Cervical ectopy, 557
Cervical ectropion, 470
Cervical intraepithelial neoplasia (CIN), 584
Cervical intraepithelial neoplasia 1 (CIN 1), 504
Cervical intraepithelial neoplasia 2 (CIN 2),
        504–505
Cervical intraepithelial neoplasia 3 (CIN 3),
        504–505
Cervical shield, 444, 444f
    advantages, 444
    disadvantages, 444
    efficacy, 444
    insertion, 444
    one-way valve design, 444
    removal, 444
Cervical transformation zone (TZ), 502, 502f
Cervical venous hum, 187
Cervicitis, 558
Cervix
    chlamydial infections of, 558
    gonococcal infection of, 558
Cessation
    follow-up after, 629
    pharmacotherapy, 628
    tobacco, 627–629
Cetirizine, for urticaria, 271
CF. *See* Cystic fibrosis (CF)
CF transmembrane conductance regulator
        (CFTR) modulators, 209–210
Chamomile, 92
Champions, 120
Chancroid, 572, 591
    clinical manifestations, 591, 592f
    diagnosis, 591, 592t
    epidemiology, 591
    etiology, 591
    treatment, 593t
Change concepts, 120
Cheilitis, 261
Chemical depilatories, 497
Chemiluminescence immunoassay (CIA), 573
Chest dysphoria, 455
Chest examination, 70
Chewing tobacco, 626
Chief Student Affairs Officer, 712
Child abuse and neglect, 731
Child/Adolescent Anxiety Multimodal Study,
        669
Childhood apraxia of speech (CAS), 686
Children's Depression Inventory (CDI-2), 662
Children's Online Privacy Protection Act
        (COPPA), 129
Children with special health care needs
        (CSHCNs), 105
Chiropractic medicine, 95
Chlamydia screening, annual, 125
Chlamydia trachomatis, 503, 517, 535, 555,
        591
    chlamydial serovars, 555
    clinical manifestations, 558–559
        Bartholinitis, 559
        cervicitis, 558
        conjunctivitis, 559
        epididymitis, 559
        lymphogranuloma venereum, 559

Chlamydia trachomatis (Continued)
    pelvic inflammatory disease, 558–559
    pharyngitis, 559
    proctitis, 559
    reactive arthritis triad, 559
    urethritis, 558, 559
  etiology, 555
  expedited partner therapy, 560
  at extragenital sites, 557
  factors contributing to, 557
  female genital urinary tract and, 558–559
  incidence and prevalence, 556–557, 556f
  incubation period, 558
  infection with, 555–561
  male genital urinary tract and, 559
  prevention, 561
  retesting, 560
  screening for, 557–558
    guidelines on, 557–558
  screening test for, 468, 470
  special circumstances, 561
  treatment, 559–560
Cholesterol, 170–171, 173. *See also*
    Atherosclerosis; Lipoproteins
  elevated LDL cholesterol, 174
  HDL cholesterol, 171
  LDL cholesterol, 170
  screening, 174, 175t
Chronic abdominal pain, 388–394. *See also*
    Functional gastrointestinal disorders
    (FGIDs)
  altered bowel pattern and, 391
  causes of, 391
  definition, 388
  diagnosis, 391–393
  differential diagnosis, 388–391
  dyspepsia and, 391
  functional gastrointestinal disorders, 388
  paroxysmal abdominal pain, 391
  prevalence, 388–389
  treatment, 393–394
Chronic active EBV (CAEBV) disease, 321
Chronic fatigue syndrome, 379. *See* Myalgic
    encephalomyelitis/chronic fatigue
    syndrome (ME/CFS)
Chronic health conditions, 105–110
  adherence with treatment, 108–109
  categories of, 105
  confidential consultations with patient, 108
  elements of, 105
  and fertility, 109
  growth monitoring in adolescents with, 106
  health professionals, role of, 108–110
  health-related behaviors and states, 107
  illnesses and disorders in, 105
  impairments/disability and, 105
  incidence and prevalence of, 105–106
  interaction with adolescent development,
    106–107
  parents, role of, 108, 109
  quality health care to AYAs with, 107–108,
    107f (*See also* Adolescent-friendly care)
    elements of, 108–110, 108f
  school engagement and peer support groups,
    role of, 107
  sexual and reproductive health care, 109
  social determinants of health, influence of,
    107
  transition to adult health care, 109–110
Chronic illness, 105–106. *See also* Chronic
    health conditions
  and amenorrhea, 490
Chronic renal failure, 106
Chronic traumatic encephalopathy (CTE),
    253
Chylomicrons, 171, 172

Cigarettes
  effects of other compounds in, 626
  nicotine in, 626
  smoking of, 622
    among high school students, 622
    and cardiovascular disease, 200
Cigarillos, 622
Ciliostasis, 324
Cimetidine, for warts, 268
Ciprofloxacin, for chancroid, 593t
Citalopram, 367, 664, 664t
Civic engagement, 99, 748
Civilian, 720t, 721
Clarithromycin
  for *Mycoplasma* infections, 325
  for pertussis, 326
Classical orthostatic hypotension, 382
Clindamycin, 259
  for folliculitis, 269
  for hidradenitis suppurativa, 273
Clindamycin cream, 509
The Clinical Opiate Withdrawal Scale, 642
Clinic staff, 51
Clitoral index, 500
Clobazam, for seizure treatment, 281t
Clobetasol foam, for alopecia areata, 273
Clobetasol propionate, for psoriasis, 270
Clomiphene citrate, 497
Clonazepam, 646
  for seizure treatment, 281t
Clonidine, 642, 646
  in ADHD, 685
  for orthostatic intolerance, 385t
Clotrimazole, for tinea pedis, 267
Clue cells, 508, 508f
Cluster headaches, 288, 291t. *See also*
    Headaches
Cocaethylene, 639
Cocaine, 637–639
  adverse effects, 638, 638f
  alcohol with, 639
  chronic use, 639
  crack pipe smoker's callus, 638f
  intoxication, effects of, 638
  medical use, 637
  overdose and treatment, 638–639
  physiology and metabolism, 637–638
  during pregnancy, 419
  preparation and dose, 637
  tolerance and withdrawal, 639
  use by young adults, 609
Cocaine-associated chest pain, 638
Coccidioidomycosis, and erythema nodosum,
    271
Cognitive behavioral therapy (CBT)
  for alcohol use disorder, 619
  amplified musculoskeletal pain syndrome,
    379
  for anxiety disorders, 668–669
  for bulimia nervosa, 370
  for depression, 663
  for FGIDs, 394
  for headache management, 290
  for premenstrual disorders, 481
  for substance use disorders, 654t
  trauma management, 748
Cognitive development
  early adolescence, 46
  late adolescence, 47
  middle adolescence, 46
  young adults, 48
Cognitive impairments, in marijuana users,
    634
Cohort studies, 131t
Colchicine, for erythema nodosum, 272
Colitis, 391

College health, 706–715
  disease-specific considerations, 712–714
    ADHD, 713
    allergy immunotherapy, 713
    asthma, 713
    bipolar and psychotic disorders, 713
    chronic medical conditions, 714
    chronic pain, 713
    diabetes, 713
    disabilities, 713
    eating disorders, 713
    food allergies, 713
    infusion medications, 714
    NCAA athletes, 713
    physical therapy, 713
    substance use recovery, 713–714
  funding and student health insurance, 712
  health care services
    health promotion, wellness, prevention,
      708–709
    medical care, 708
    mental health care, 708
    public health and communicable disease
      control, 709
  on-campus student health service (SHS),
    706, 707, 712
  ongoing engagement with college student,
    714
    leave of absence, 715
    matriculated students, 715
    prematriculation, 714–715
College students, 706
  behavioral and other risk factors, 709
    alcohol, 709
    amphetamine use, 709
    injury prevention, 710
    international study, 711–712
    marijuana, 709
    nutrition and physical activity, 710
    opioids, 710
    prescription stimulants, 709
    sexual and gender minority students,
      710–711
    sexual and reproductive health, 710
    sexual assault, dating violence, and
      stalking, 710
    sleep, 711
    tobacco, 709
    vocational health risks, 711
  demographics, 707–708
  eating disorder in, 363, 710
  e-cigarettes use, 709
  health insurance issues for, 712
  impediments to academic success, 707,
    707t
  obesity in, 710
  relationship difficulties among, 710
Colorectal cancer, combined hormonal
    contraceptives in, 452
Columbia-Suicide Severity Rating Scale
    (C-SSRS), 66, 673
Combination oral contraceptive (COCs) pills,
    426–427, 450, 451
  advantages, 426–427
  availability, 427
  current use, 426
  dysmenorrhea, 479
  noncontraceptive benefits, 426–427
Combined estrogen/progestin hormonal
    contraceptives, for prolactinomas, 543
Combined hormonal contraceptives (CHCs),
    426–427, 449–450
  contraceptive ring and patch, 427
  drug–drug interactions, 454
    anticonvulsants, 454
    antiretroviral agents, 454

antituberculosis drugs and antibiotics, 454
drospirenone, 454
herbal medicines, 454
other interactions, 454
late or missed dose(s) of, recommendations for, 451t
noncontraceptive benefits of
menstrually related benefits, 452
nonmenstrually related benefits, 452
oral contraceptives, 426–427, 450–451
risks posed by
breast cancer, 453
cervical cancer and dysplasia, 453
thromboembolism, 452–453
side effects with, 453–454
bleeding changes, 453, 453t
commonly attributed effects, 453
depression and mood disorders, 454
dry eye, 453
hormones implicated with specific side effects, 453t
infectious diseases, 453–454
menstrual migraine symptoms, 453
skin changes, 453
special populations and, 456
transdermal patches, 452
vaginal contraceptive rings, 451
Combined oral contraceptives (COCs), for acne, 261
Comedones, 256, 256f
Common Rule, 127
Communication
adolescent and young adult–provider, optimization of, 55
and language disorders, 686
nonverbal, 54
Community-acquired pneumonia (CAP), 324–325
clinical manifestations, 324
complications, 324–325
diagnosis, 325
differential diagnosis, 325
epidemiology, 324
etiology and pathophysiology, 324
laboratory evaluation, 325
management, 325
Mycoplasma pneumoniae as cause of, 324
Community-acquired respiratory distress syndrome (CARDS), 325
Community-clinic linkages, 64
Complementary and integrative medicine, 90–96
acupuncture, 94, 94f
biofeedback, 95
butterbur, 93
chamomile, 92
chiropractic medicine, 95
commonly used products and practices, 90t
Echinacea, 92–93
education, 90
elderberry, 92
feverfew, 93
herbs/supplements, 91–94
conditions treated with, 92
dosing issues and active compounds, 91–92
drug interactions and toxicity, 91
long-term use, 92
in pregnancy and lactation, 92
homeopathy, 90
hypnosis, 95
inositol, 93–94
manual therapies, 95
massage therapy, 95–96
medical conditions treated with, 90
meditation, 94

melatonin, 93, 93f
mindfulness, 96
physician knowledge about, 91
research in, 90
St. John's wort, 91, 92
talking with AYAs about, 96t
use by adolescents and young adults, 90, 91f
valerian root, 92
yoga, 94–95
Complementary medicine, for premenstrual disorders, 481
Complex regional pain syndrome (CRPS), 376, 377
imaging studies, 377–378
type I, 377
type II, 377
Complex trauma, 745
Comprehensive educational evaluation, 680, 682f
Conceptual model, 132
Concussion, 249–254. *See also* Sport-related concussion (SRC)
Condoms
internal, 440–441
traditional, 436–440
Conduct disorder, 106
Condylomata acuminata, 585
penis, 585f
vaginal introitus, 585f
Condylomata lata (perineum), 586, 586f
Confidentiality, 52, 86–88
adolescent minors, protections for, 87
electronic health information, 87–88
HIPAA Privacy Rule, 87
HIPAA Security Rule, 87–88
in-person visit, 50–52
pregnant AYA, 417
in substance use screening, 651, 652
telehealth visits and, 56
21st Century Cures Act, 88
Confidentiality, universal education, empowerment, and support (CUES), 698
Confidential services, billing for, 51
Conflict, effects of, 9
Confluent and reticulated papillomatosis of Gougerot and Carteaud, 266
Congenital adrenal hyperplasia (CAH), 484, 497
Congenital heart disease, 193–194, 194t
of great complexity, 194
of moderate complexity, 194
simple, 194
transition to adult care for youth with, 193–194
Congenital syphilis, 572
early, 572
late, 572
Conjunctivitis, *C. trachomatis* infection and, 559
Connective tissue disease, and heart
Ehlers–Danlos syndromes, 190, 191f
fragile X syndrome, 190
Marfan syndrome, 190, 191f
Consent, 85
for ectopic pregnancy treatment, 527
for HIV testing, 343
for immunization, 73–74
informed, 86
for LARC insertion, 461t, 464
legal, 85, 86
for treatment of adolescents in out-of-home care, 730, 731
young adults and capacity to consent, 86
Constitutional delay of puberty, 141
and bone age, 145

criteria for provisional diagnosis of, 146t
short stature and, 139
Constitutional rights, 85
Contact dermatitis, 259
due to plants, 264, 264f
due to shoes, 266
of nipple, 541
Contingency management, in substance use disorders, 654t
Contraception, 29, 109, 422–434. *See also* Contraceptives
access to and adherence with, 414–415
barrier methods, 436–448
choosing method of, 428
counseling, 438
dual methods, 438
emergency, 428, 431 (*See also* Emergency contraception)
injectable hormonal, 454–455
long-acting reversible, 457–465
methods used, 414–415
obstacles to, 415
sexual activity and contraception use, 422–423
starting, 428
quick start method, 428
tier 1 methods, 423
tier 2 methods, 423
tier 3 methods, 423
and unintended pregnancies, 423, 424t
for youth living with HIV, 349
Contraceptive implants, 425–426
advantages, 426
availability in United States, 426
current use, 425–426
Nexplanon, 425–426
Contraceptive patches, 452
Contraceptives, 422–423
for AYAs with chronic medical conditions, 428
intellectual disabilities, 428
psychiatric disease, 428
clinical practices to enhance success, 449–450
combination oral contraceptive pills, 426–427
contraceptive ring and patch, 427
counseling, 423, 425–426
failure, 423
racial and ethnic differences, 423
hormonal, 450
injectables, 426
long-acting reversible, 423, 425–426
progestin-only pills, 427–428
U.S. Medical Eligibility Criteria (MEC) for Contraceptive Use, 428, 429f–430f, 449
Contraceptive shield. *See* Cervical shield
Contraceptive sponge, 441, 443–444
Contraceptive vaginal rings, 450, 451
"Contract for Life," 618
Conversion disorder, 376
Conversion/reparative therapy, 404
Copper intrauterine device (Paragard), 425, 425t, 457, 458, 458t
effectiveness, 459
indications for, 462
Core, 227, 227t
strengthening exercises, 227t
Coronary Artery Risk Development in Young Adults (CARDIA) study, 168
Coronavirus, 328. *See also* COVID-19 (Coronavirus disease 2019)
Corpus callosotomy, 280
Corpus luteal cysts, 519, 520–521, 520f
Corpus luteum, 475

Corticosteroids
for alopecia areata, 273
in CRPS, 379
for infectious mononucleosis, 322
for pityriasis rosea, 269
for psoriasis, 270
for urticaria, 271
for vitiligo, 274
Corynebacterium minutissimum, erythrasma
by, 267–268
Cotinine, 626
Couch surfing, 723, 723f. *See also* Youth
experiencing homelessness (YEH)
Cough, 207
Counseling
contraceptives, 423, 425–426
genital HSV, 582
pregnant AYA, 417
COVID-19 (Coronavirus disease 2019), 327–329
clinical manifestations, 328
colleges and universities, impact on, 709
complications, 328
long COVID, 328
multisystem inflammatory syndrome in
children, 328, 328t
diagnosis, 329
differential diagnosis, 328
effects of, 8, 10
etiology and pathophysiology, 328
immunization, 329
management, 329
myocardial inflammation after, 193
by SARS-CoV-2, 327–328
viral variants, 328
sleep, impact on, 296
Crack cocaine, 637
CRAFFT (behavioral health screening tool),
617–618
Cremasteric reflex, 532
Criminal disenfranchisement laws, 744
Crisaborole, for atopic dermatitis, 264
Crocus sativus (saffron), 481
Crohn disease, 391
Cross-sectional studies, 131t
CRPS. *See* Complex regional pain syndrome
(CRPS)
Cryotherapy
with liquid nitrogen, 588
molluscum contagiosum, 599t
for warts, 268
Cryptorchidism, 143, 531–532
complications
infertility, 532
malignancy, 532
diagnosis, 531–532
epidemiology, 531
therapy, 532
CSHCN Screener, 106
Cultural competence, 738–739
Cultural humility, 113
Curettage/needle extraction, molluscum
contagiosum, 599t
Cushing syndrome, 143, 497, 498, 500
Cyberbullying, 101, 103
Cyclobenzaprine, for AMPS, 379
Cyclooxygenase pathway, 477
COX-1 enzyme, 477
COX-2 enzyme, 477
Cyclosporine, for atopic dermatitis, 264
Cystic fibrosis (CF), 208–210
clinical manifestations, 209f, 209t
diagnosis, 209
physical examination, 209
prevalence, 209
pulmonary complications, 209
treatment, 209–210

Cystic fibrosis–related diabetes (CFRD), 159
Cystic fibrosis transmembrane conductance
regulator genetic analysis, 209
Cystitis, 300–302. *See also* Urinary tract
infection (UTI)
complicated, 303
diagnosis, 301–302
dysuria in, 301, 301t
epidemiology, 300
microbiology and resistance, 300–301
recurrent, 302
resistant organisms, risk factors for, 301
risk factors, 300
symptoms and signs, 301
treatment, 303, 304t
uncomplicated, 300–302
Cytology, 501. *See also* Cervical cancer
screening

D

Daily Record of Severity of Problems, 481
Daily requirements, 80
DALYs. *See* Disability-adjusted life years
(DALYs)
Dapsone, for acne, 260
DASH (Dietary Approaches to Stop
Hypertension) diet, 200
Data sources, 130, 132, 133t–134t
Date rape, 696
"Date rape" drug, 644
Dating violence, 423
Daytime incontinence, 306. *See also* Enuresis
Daytime sleepiness, 294
Deaf–blindness, 681t
Deafness, 681t
Decision making, 115
conflict in, 116
tools for, 115–116
Deep brain stimulation (DBS), for intractable
focal epilepsy, 280
Dehydroepiandrosterone (DHEA), 35, 490
Dehydroepiandrosterone-sulfate (DHEA-S), 35,
39, 495
Delayed development, 140. *See* Delayed puberty
Delayed orthostatic hypotension, 382
Delayed puberty, 140–148
boys, treatment for, 147–148
clues to other diagnoses, 146–147
constitutional delay of puberty, 141, 146,
146t
definition, 140
differential diagnosis, 140–144
females, treatment for, 147, 147t
breast development, induction of, 147,
147t
long-term estrogen replacement, 147
menses, induction of, 147
functional causes, 141–143
gonadal failure and, 143
history, 144–145
hypothalamic causes, 143
laboratory evaluation, 145–146
management, 147–149
patient education, 148
physical examination, 145
pituitary causes, 143
short stature without, 138–140
specific conditions, treatment of
chronic illness, 148
gonadal dysgenesis, 148
hypothyroidism, 148
Turner syndrome, 148
syndromes associated with, 144
workup of, 144–147
Delayed sleep phase syndrome (DSPS), 294
22q11.2 deletion syndrome, 688

Delta-like noncanonical Notch ligand 1 (DLK1),
36
Delta-9-tetrahydrocannabinol (THC), 633, 635
potency, 633
Demographic dividend, 4t
Demographics, of adolescents and young adults,
11, 11f–16f
Demographic transition, 4t, 10
Dennie–Morgan lines, 263
Dental dams, 551
Department of Health and Human Services'
Title X, 62
Dependent variables, 132
Deployment, 720–722
Depot medroxyprogesterone acetate (Depo-
Provera or DMPA), 426, 449, 454–455,
460
advantages, 426
availability in United States, 426
benefits of, 455
bleeding abnormalities with, 455
bone density loss with, 455
clinical pearls, 455t
current use, 426
disadvantages with, 455
formulations, 454
IM formulation, 454
sub-Q formulation, 454
practice considerations, 455, 455t
and weight gain, 455
Depression, 66, 106, 660–665
age of onset, 660
assessment, 661–662
cultural background, 661–662
illness characteristics, 661
interviews and collateral information, 661
causality, 661
course of illness, 660
depressive disorders and DSM-5
adjustment disorder, 662
bipolar depression, 662–663
major depressive episode, 662
persistent depression, 662
early-life stress and, 661
epidemiology, 660
epilepsy and, 283
and FGIDs in AYAs, 393–394
hormonal contraceptives and, 454
isotretinoin use and, 261
ME/CFS and, 382
in pregnant and parenting teens, 414, 419
risk factors, 660, 661t
biologic factors, 660–661
psychological factors, 661
social factors, 661
screening for, 66
screening tools for, 662
social isolation and, 661
St. John's wort for, 92
treatment
general considerations, 663
medications, 664–665, 664t
mild depression, 663
moderate to severe depression, 663
psychoeducation, 663
psychotherapy, 663–664
safety consideration, 663
stressors and psychiatric comorbidities,
663
Dermatitis, 263–265
allergic contact, 264–265, 264f, 265f
atopic, 263–264, 263f
seborrheic, 265, 265f
Dermoid cysts, 521–522, 522f
Desensitization therapy, for amplified
musculoskeletal pain syndrome, 379

Designated sex at birth, 408
Designer benzodiazepines (DBZD), 643
Desloratadine, for urticaria, 271
Desmopressin (DDAVP)
  enuresis, 309
  nocturnal polyuria, 308–309
Desmopressin acetate, for orthostatic
    intolerance, 385t
Desomorphine (krocodil), 641. *See also* Opioids
Detention, 735–736
Developmental assessment, in preventive health
    visit, 68
Developmental coordination disorder (DCD),
    686
Developmental Coordination Disorder
    Questionnaire (DCDQ), 686
Dextroamphetamine, for orthostatic
    intolerance, 385t
Dextromethorphan (DXM), 648
Diabetes. *See* Diabetes mellitus
Diabetes complications, 164–165
Diabetes mellitus, 106, 107, 159–166
  classification and etiology, 159–160, 160t
  complications and associated conditions,
      164–165
    alcohol use, 165
    autoimmune diseases, 164
    dyslipidemia, 165
    eating disorders, 165
    gluten sensitivity, 165
    hypertension, 165
    hypoglycemia, 165
    macrovascular complications, 165
    microvascular complications, 165
  diagnosis, 160, 160t
  epidemiology, 160
  evaluation and treatment, 161, 164
    diet, 161
    education, 161
    glycemic control, 161
    insulin therapy, 161, 164
    medications, 164
    physical activity, 164
  genetic disorders associated with, 159
  gestational, 159–160
  patient-centered care, 165–166
  prevention, 161
  screening, 161, 162f–163f
  transition to adult care, 166
  type 1, 159
  type 2, 159
Diabetes screen, 70
Diacetylmorphine, 641
*Diagnostic and Statistical Manual of Mental
    Disorders, 5th edition* (DSM-5), 375
  feeding and eating disorders in, 362
Dialectical behavior therapy (DBT), 664
  to reduce suicide attempts, 674
  for substance use disorders, 654t
Diaphragm, 444–447, 445f
  advantages, 447
  contraindications, 445
  correct fitting of, 445, 446f
  disadvantages, 447
  effectiveness, 445
  future developments, 447
  insertion and removal, 446
  Milex Wide Seal R diaphragm, 445, 445f
  patient education, 446
  SILCS diaphragm (Caya R), 445, 445f
  tips to improve success, 445
Diarrhea, 392
Dienogest, for dysmenorrhea, 480
Diet
  acne and, 258
  for headache treatment, 290

obesity and, 357–358
  for seizure treatment, 282
  vegetarian, 82
Dietary counseling, during pregnancy, 82
2015–2020 Dietary Guidelines for Americans, 78
Dietary reference intakes (DRIs), 80
Dietary Supplement Health and Education Act
    of 1994, 91
Diet Intervention Study in Children, 174
Diet therapies, in irritable bowel syndrome, 393
Differentiated thyroid cancers, 154
Diffuse amplified pain syndromes, 376–377
Diffuse pain, 377
DiGeorge syndrome. *See* 22q11.2 deletion
    syndrome
Digital health, 64–66
Digital technology, 98
  apps, 102
  benefits of, 99–100
  use, role of adolescent providers, 102–102
    balance, 102
    boundaries, 102, 103
    communication, 102, 103
    education, 103
    intervention, 103–104
    media multitasking, 103
    prevention, 102–103
    screening, 103
  use to access social media (*See* Social media)
Dihydrotestosterone (DHT), 496
Dilation and evacuation, 418
Dimethyltryptamine (DMT), 649
Diphenhydramine, for urticaria, 271
Diphtheria and tetanus toxoids and pertussis
    (DTP) vaccine, 73
Dipstick test, 314
Direct-acting antivirals (DAAs), for HCV
    treatment, 338
Disability, 105, 107, 109
Disability-adjusted life years (DALYs), 4t, 22
  causes of, 22, 24f–26f
  in OECD countries, 27f, 28f
Disability benefits, 682
Discrimination, 9, 743
Disease-specific mortality, 4t
Disease-specific surveys, 105–106
Disenfranchised, 743
Disenfranchisement, 744
Disorders of Gut–Brain Interaction (DGBI), 388.
    See also Functional gastrointestinal
    disorders (FGIDs)
Disparity, 729
Disproportionate minority contact, 733–734
Disulfiram, for alcohol use disorder, 619
Diuretics, for hypertension, 201t
Dix–Hallpike maneuver, 183
Documentation
  in electronic health records, 66
  of vaccination, 74
Dolutegravir, for HIV infection, 345
Domestic violence, during pregnancy, 419
Donovan bodies, 594
Donovanosis. *See* Granuloma inguinale
Dopamine agonists, for prolactinomas, 542
Downey cells, 319
Down syndrome, 245, 677t
Doxycycline, 535, 536, 565
  for acne, 260–261
  for hidradenitis suppurativa, 273
  lymphogranuloma venereum, 594t
  for *Mycoplasma* infections, 325
  for syphilis treatment, 575
  for urogenital chlamydial infections, 559
Driver diagram, 120, 121f
Drospirenone, 450–451, 454
  for PMDD, 481–482

Drug Abuse Screening Test (DAST-10), 618,
    652, 652t
Drug Abuse Screen Test (DAST), 67
Drug eruptions, 272
  drug-induced hypersensitivity syndrome, 272
  exanthematous (morbilliform), 272
  fixed drug eruption, 272
  photosensitivity eruptions, 272
Drug-induced hypersensitivity syndrome
    (DIHS), 272
Drug reaction with eosinophilia and systemic
    symptoms (DRESS). *See* Drug-induced
    hypersensitivity syndrome (DIHS)
Drug resistance, 301, 303, 305. *See also*
    Extended spectrum beta lactamase
    (ESBL)
Drug-resistant epilepsy. *See* Intractable epilepsy
Drugs
  and amenorrhea, 489
  interview questions about, 53
Drug testing, 656
Drug use, 602–603, 604t–605t
Drug use prevention, 612t
Drysol, for hyperhidrosis, 273
Dual-energy x-ray absorptiometry (DXA), 147,
    364
Ductal ectasia, 541
Duloxetine
  for fibromyalgia, 379
  for orthostatic intolerance, 385t
Dupilumab, for atopic dermatitis, 264
Dysgerminomas, 523, 523f
Dysgraphia, 686
Dyshidrotic eczema, 263
Dyslipidemia, 172
  and CVD risk, 171
  screening, 70
  in type 2 diabetes, 165
Dysmenorrhea, 477–480
  clinical manifestations, 478
  diagnosis, 478–479
  differential diagnosis, 478
  epidemiology, 478
  etiology, 477
  history in, 478
  imaging modalities, 479
  laboratory tests, 479
  laparoscopy, 479
  physical examination, 479
  primary, 477, 478
  prostaglandins and leukotrienes in, 477
  risk factors, 477
  secondary, 477, 478
  treatment, 479
    hormonal contraceptives, 452, 479
    nonhormonal modalities, 480
    nonsteroidal anti-inflammatory drugs, 479,
        479t
    other hormonal modalities, 479–480
    patient education, 479
Dyspepsia, 391, 392
Dysthymia, 662
Dysuria, 301, 301t. *See also* Genitourinary tract
    infections
  differential diagnosis of, 301
  signs and symptoms, in women, 301t

E
Early adolescence, 45, 46
  close relationships in, 396
Early Assessment Risk List (EARL), 693
Early Periodic Screening, Diagnosis, and
    Treatment Program (EPSDT), 62–63
Eating Attitudes Test (EAT-26), 79, 366
Eating Disorder Examination-ARFID module
    (EDE-ARFID), 371

Eating disorders. *See also* Feeding and eating disorders; specific disorder
  in athletes, 83
  in diabetes, 165
  family-based therapy for, 367, 370, 371
  familial predisposition to, 362
  hospitalization in, 367t
  instruments for diagnosis of, 366
  in males, 371–372
  medical complications of, 365t–366t
  sexual minority youth, 403
  transgender youth and young adults, 410
Eating Disorders Examination Questionnaire (EDE-Q), 366
Eating Disturbances in Youth Questionnaire (EDY-Q), 371
Eating habits, interview questions about, 52–53
Ebstein anomaly, 194t
EBV DNA nucleic acid amplification tests, serum-based, 322
EBV nuclear antigen (EBNA), 321
Echinacea, 92–93
E-cigarette or vaping use-associated lung injury (EVALI), 210–211, 635
  chest CT, 210, 210f
  definition, 210
  symptoms, 210
  treatment, 211
E-cigarettes, 622, 626, 628
E-cigarette Use among Youth and Young Adults (report), 622
Econazole, for tinea pedis, 267
Economic disenfranchisement, 743
Ecstasy. *See* Methylenedioxymethamphetamine (MDMA)
Ectopic pregnancy, 419, 525–529, 559
  β-hCG levels, 416, 526–527
  clinical presentation, 525–526
    acute, 525–526
    subacute, 526
  death from, 525
  differential diagnosis, 525
  in ethnic minorities, 525
  etiology and risk factors, 525
  fertility after treatment of, 529
  follow-up, 528–529
  incidence and prevalence, 525
  laboratory and imaging evaluation, 526
    β-human chorionic gonadotropin, 526
    ultrasound, 526
  management, 527–528
    access to care and follow-up, 527
    confidentiality and consent, 527
    contraception after, 528–529
    expectant management, 528
    medical therapy, 527, 528t
    Rh considerations, 529
    surgical approach, 527
  outpatient follow-up, 526–527
  persistent disease, 528
  ruptured, 525–526
  ultrasonography, 525–526
Ectopy, 502
Education
  amplified musculoskeletal pain syndrome, 379
  for AYAs with neurodevelopmental disorders, 678, 680–682
  and health status, 7
  for HIV/AIDS prevention, 347
  interview questions about, 52
  technology in, role of, 99
Educational materials, in office space, 51
Educational support, to AYAs with neurodevelopmental disorders, 680, 681t
  comprehensive educational evaluation, 680

definitions and eligibility categories for school service determination, 681t
    Section 504, 680
    special education, 680
Efavirenz, 454
Eflornithine hydrochloride 13.9% cream, 497
Ehlers–Danlos syndrome, 383
EHRs. *See* Electronic health records (EHRs)
EIB. *See* Exercise-induced bronchoconstriction (EIB)
EILO. *See* Exercise-induced laryngeal obstruction (EILO)
EIM *Healthcare Provider's Action Guide,* 232
Elbasvir, 454
Elderberry (Sambucus), 92
Electrocardiogram (ECG), 180
Electrodesiccation and curettage, for warts, 268
Electroencephalography (EEG), 277, 279, 280t
Electronic active gaming, 230
Electronic health information (EHI), 87–88
Electronic health records (EHRs), 51, 102
  for AYA preventive services, 64
    challenges to confidential care, 64
    health maintenance, 66
    patient portal, 66
    population health management, 66
    previsit questionnaires, 65–66, 66f
    provider documentation, 66
  confidentiality in, protection of, 51
  Health e-Check screening module, 65, 66f
Electronic nicotine delivery systems (ENDS), 709
Electronic personal health information (e-PHI), 87
Electronic records, of transgender youth and young adults, 411
Eluxadoline, for diarrhea-predominant IBS (IBS-D), 393
Emancipation, 729, 731. *See also* Out-of-home care
Emergency contraception (EC), 428, 431, 449
  advance prescription and access, 428, 431
  copper IUD for, 431–432
  counseling about, 431
  effectiveness of, 431
  ethical considerations around mechanism of action, 434
  levonorgestrel-intrauterine devices for, 432
  levonorgestrel pills for, 433
  pregnancy prevention after intercourse, 428
  repeated use, 434
  side effects, 433–434
  transgender or gender nonbinary (TGNB) AYA and, 428, 431
  ulipristal acetate (UPA) for, 432–433
  use of, data on, 428
  and weight, 433–434
Emergency contraceptive pills (ECPs), 431
Emerging adults, 47–48. *See also* Young adults
Emerging sexually transmitted infections, 598–599
Emotional distress, and somatic symptoms, 375
Emotional disturbance (ED), 681t
Employment
  and health status, 8
  interview questions about, 52
Emtricitabine, for HIV infection, 345, 346
Endocannabinoids (eCBs), 633
Endocannabinoid system (ECS), 633
Endocarditis, 190
  AHA guidelines on prevention of, 192t
  cardiac conditions associated with, 192t
  dental procedures and prophylaxis recommendations, 192t
  regimens for dental procedures, 192t

Endocrine axes, affecting pubertal maturation, 35
  hypothalamic–pituitary–adrenal axis, 35, 35f
  hypothalamic–pituitary–gonadal axis, 35, 35f
Endocrine causes of short stature, 139
Endocrine Society's Clinical Care Guidelines, 410, 411
End-of-life care, 116. *See also* Palliative care
Endometrial biopsy, 485
Endometrial cancer, COC in, 452
Endometrioma, 521, 521f
Endometriosis, 521
  clinical manifestations, 521
  common sites of, 478f
  and dysmenorrhea, 478, 478f
  laparoscopy, 521
  prevalence, 521
  symptoms of, 478
Endometrium, secretory, 475
Endoscopic bariatric procedures, 361
Energix-B, for hepatitis B, 335
Energy requirements, 80
  during pregnancy, 81t, 82
Engagement of AYAs in research, 129–130
Enteric-coated peppermint oil capsules, 393
Enuresis, 306–310
  and bladder and bowel dysfunction, 306–307
  definition, 306
  diagnosis and evaluation, 307, 308t
  history and physical examination, 307, 308t
  monosymptomatic, 306, 307
  nonmonosymptomatic, 306
  pathophysiology, 307
    bladder dysfunction, 307
    central nervous system abnormalities, 307
    genetic factors, 307
    nocturnal polyuria, 307
  primary, 306
  psychosocial burden, 307
  secondary, 306
  terminology related to, 306–307
  treatment, 307, 310f
    bedwetting alarms, 308–309
    lifestyle changes, 307
    medications, 309–310
    neuromodulation, 310
Environment, youth friendly, 66, 67t
Enzyme immunoassay test, for HIV infection, 344
Enzyme immunosorbent assay (EIA), 573
Enzyme-linked immunosorbent assay (ELISA), 416
Epidemiologic transition, 4t, 10
Epidemiology, youth violence, 691–692
Epidermophyton floccosum (E. floccosum)
  onychomycosis, 267
  tinea cruris, 267
  tinea pedis, 266
Epididymitis, 303, 304t, 531, 532, 534f, 535–536
  diagnosis, 536
  epidemiology, 536
  etiology, 535–536
  N. gonorrhoeae and *C. trachomatis* infection, 559, 560
  non–sexually transmitted, 535–536
  sexually transmitted, 535
  therapy, 536
  and torsion, 536t
Epigenetic mechanisms, and obesity, 355
Epilepsy, 277–284. *See also* Seizures
  comorbidities, 283
  definitions, 277
  epidemiology, 277–278
  etiologies, 278–279, 279t
  females with, 282

bone health, 282–283
breastfeeding, 282
catamenial epilepsy, 282–283
contraception, 282
polycystic ovary syndrome, 282
pregnancy, 282
International League Against Epilepsy (ILAE)
on, 277
intractable, 280
living with, 283
employment, 284
first aid for seizure, 284, 284t
general seizure precautions, 283, 283t
medication adherence, 283
recreational seizure precautions, 283t
Seizure Action Plan, 284
SUDEP prevention, 284
preconceptual counseling, 282
risk factors, 278
treatment, 280
dietary therapy, 280–282
medications, 280, 281t
surgical intervention, 280
Epstein-Barr virus (EBV), 319
associated conditions, 322–323
EBV antibody tests, 321, 321t
erythema nodosum, 271
and infectious mononucleosis, 319–323
routes of transmission, 319
Equal Justice Initiative, 749
Ertapenem, for pyelonephritis, 303, 304t
Erythema multiforme (EM), 270, 271. See also
Stevens–Johnson syndrome (SJS)
clinical manifestations, 271, 271f
treatment, 271
Erythema nodosum (EN), 271–272
clinical manifestations, 271–272, 272f
evaluation, 272
treatment, 272
Erythrasma, 267
Erythromycin, 259
for acne, 261
chancroid, 593t
for Mycoplasma infections, 325
for pertussis, 326
Escherichia coli, and cystitis, 300
Escitalopram, 664, 664t
for orthostatic intolerance, 385t
for PMDD, 482
Eslicarbazepine, for seizure treatment, 281t
Estetrol (E₄), 450
Estimated average requirement (EAR), 80
Estradiol, 475, 490
Estradiol patches, 147
Estradiol (E₂) valerate, 450
Estrogen, 35–36, 39, 475
in hormonal contraceptives, 450
Ethical principles, 87
Ethics, 86, 127–129
Ethinyl estradiol (EE), 427, 450, 451
Ethosuximide, for seizure treatment, 281t
Etonogestrel implants, 425–426.
See also Long-acting reversible
contraceptives (LARCs); Nexplanon
indications for, 462
insertion, 464
patient-centered counseling, 464
removal, 464
European School Survey Project on Alcohol and
Other Drugs (ESPAD), 606
Event-driven PrEP (ED-PrEP), 346
Evidence-based tobacco cessation treatment,
629
EVUSHELD (tixagevimab copackaged with
cilgavimab), 329
Examination room, 51

Exanthematous drug eruptions, 272
Excessive daytime sleepiness, 294, 295
Exercise, 229
and amenorrhea, 489–490
for amplified musculoskeletal pain syndrome,
379
for BP reduction, 200
for headache treatment, 290
and sudden cardiac arrest, 242–243
for weight loss, 358
Exercise-induced bronchoconstriction (EIB),
207
Exercise-induced laryngeal obstruction (EILO),
207
continuous laryngoscopy during exercise
(CLE), 207
treatment, 207
Exercise prescription, 231–232
action plan for physical activity, 232
establishing baseline of physical activity, 232
evaluating physical activity goals, 232
FITT principle, 231
motivational interviewing, 232
reaching physical activity goals, 232
Expected bladder capacity (EBC) for age, 307
Expected date of delivery, 417
Expected due-date calculators, 417
Expedited partner therapy (EPT), 552, 560
Experimental research, 131t
Explanation of Benefits (EOB), 62
Exposure–disease–stress framework, for
environmental health disparities, 745,
746f
Exposure-response–prevention (ERP) therapy.
See Exposure therapy
Exposure therapy, for anxiety disorders, 669
Exposure to HIV, 345. See also Human
immunodeficiency virus (HIV) infection
Extended spectrum beta lactamase (ESBL), 301,
305
External genital warts, 585, 585f
diagnosis of, 587
treatment options for, 587, 587t–588t
clinician-administered treatments,
587t–588t, 588
patient-applied treatments, 587t–588t,
588
Extragenital infections, 557. See also
Chlamydia trachomatis; Neisseria
gonorrhoeae
Extrauterine pregnancy, 419

F
Fabry disease, and proteinuria, 314
Facial angiofibromas, 258
Factitious disorder, 376
Fainting, 180
Famciclovir, for genital herpes, 581, 581t
Familial chylomicronemia syndrome, 173t
Familial dysbetalipoproteinemia, 172, 173t
Familial hypercholesterolemia (FH), 172–173,
173t
Familial hypertriglyceridemia, 173t
Families Medical Leave Act (FMLA), 680
Family (ies)
AYAs with disabilities and support to, 680
influence of, 9
military, 720–722
office visit, 50, 54–55
transgender youth and, 411
Family Acceptance Project, 402
Family-based treatment (FBT)
for adolescents with eating disorders, 367,
370
for anxiety disorders, 669
for substance use disorders, 654t

FAmily-CEntered Advance Care Planning
(FACE), 115
Family-centered care for mother and newborn,
417, 420
Family Educational Rights and Privacy Act
(FERPA), 88
Family history, 67–68, 469
Family Media Use Plan, 103
Family planning, 428. See also Contraception
male partner participation in, 439
Fanconi syndrome, 314
Fasting plasma glucose (FPG), 160
Fat, 80–81
Fatigue, 381. See also Myalgic
encephalomyelitis/chronic fatigue
syndrome (ME/CFS)
acute, 381
causes of, 381
Fatty acids, 171
Feeding and eating disorders, 362. See also
specific disorder
anorexia nervosa, 362–368
atypical anorexia nervosa, 368
avoidant restrictive food intake disorder, 371
binge-eating disorder, 370
bulimia nervosa, 368–370
in DSM-5, 362
familial predisposition to, 362
males and eating disorders, 371–372
relative energy deficiency in sport, 372
Felbamate, for seizure treatment, 281t
Female athlete triad, 242, 489, 494
Female Athlete Triad Cumulative Risk
Assessment, 242
Female contraception, 423. See also
Contraception; Emergency
contraception
Female patient, cystitis, 300–302, 301t
Female pubertal changes, 37–38
age at puberty, 38
biologic maturity in girls, 38f
events of puberty, 37
menarche, 38
sequence, 37–38
FemCap. See Cervical cap
Fenfluramine, for seizure treatment, 281t
Fentanyl, 641. See also Opioids
Fermentable oligosaccharides, disaccharides,
monosaccharides, and polyols
(FODMAP) diet, 393
low-FODMAP diets, 393
Ferriman–Gallwey hirsutism scoring system,
498, 499f
Fertility awareness method (FAM), 437
Fertility, chronic health conditions and, 109
Fertility rates, 4t, 5, 7f, 8f
Fesoterodine, for overactive bladder, 309
Fetal alcohol effect, 687. See also Fetal alcohol
spectrum disorders
Fetal alcohol spectrum disorders, 677t, 687,
688f
Fetal alcohol syndrome, 419, 687. See also Fetal
alcohol spectrum disorders
Feverfew, 93
Fexofenadine, for urticaria, 271
FGIDs. See Functional gastrointestinal disorders
(FGIDs)
Fibroadenomas, 543–544
Fibrocystic breast changes, 544
Fibroids, 519
Fibromyalgia, 376, 377, 377t
Fine-needle aspiration (FNA), 544, 545
Firearms use, 691
interventions for prevention of, 693–694
mortality related to, 691

Fishbone diagrams, 120, 121, 121f
FitBit® devices, 297
Fitz–Hugh–Curtis syndrome, 558–559, 564
Fixed drug eruption, 272
Fixed proteinuria, 313–314, 313t
Flat-topped macules, 585
Flat warts, 268
Flexibility exercises, 230. *See also* Physical
    activity (PA)
Flowchart, 120–121
Fluconazole, 511
    for onychomycosis, 267
    for tinea pedis, 267
    for tinea versicolor, 266
Fludrocortisone
    for neurocardiogenic syncope, 181t
    for orthostatic intolerance, 385t
Flumazenil, 643–644
FluMist, 73
Fluocinolone acetonide, for psoriasis, 270
Fluocinonide, for psoriasis, 270
Fluorescent Treponemal Antibody–Absorbed
    (FTA-ABS), 573
Fluoxetine, 367, 664, 664t, 673
    for bulimia nervosa, 370
    for neurocardiogenic syncope, 181t
    for PMDD, 482, 482t
Fluvoxamine, 367, 664, 664t
Focal segmental glomerulosclerosis (FSGS),
    313, 314
    and proteinuria, 313
Folate during pregnancy, 82
Follicle-stimulating hormone (FSH), 35, 146,
    474, 475
Follicular cysts, 519, 520, 520f
Follicular phase, 475
Follicular thyroid cancers (FTCs), 153, 154
Folliculitis, 268–269
    clinical manifestations, 268, 269f
    treatment, 268–269
Food sensitivities, in ME/CFS patients, 382
Forensic evaluation, 699–700
Foster care, 729
Fragile mental retardation protein (FMRP), 688
Fragile X syndrome, 190, 677t, 687–688
Friendly atmosphere for AYAs, creation of, 66, 67t
FSH. *See* Follicle-stimulating hormone (FSH)
Full and individual evaluation (FIE), 680, 681t
Functional abdominal pain, 389t, 390t, 393
Functional dyspepsia (FD), 389, 390t
Functional gastrointestinal disorders (FGIDs),
    388
    anxiety and, 393–394
    celiac disease and, 391
    depression and, 393–394
    diagnostic tests, 392
    diet therapies, 393
    etiology, 389
    evaluation approach, 392–393
    gut–brain axis in, pathophysiology of, 389
    history in, 391–392
    pharmacologic treatments, 393
    physical examination, 392
    prevalence, 388
    psychological factors and interventions,
      393–394
    Rome IV classification for, 389, 389t
    Rome IV diagnostic criteria, 390t
    stress and, 393–394
    treatment, 393–394
Functional neurologic symptom disorder.
    See Conversion disorder
Functional ovarian cysts, 519–521, 520f
    corpus luteal cysts, 519, 520–521, 520f
    follicular cysts, 519, 520, 520f
    theca lutein cysts, 519

Fungal infections, 265–268
    onychomycosis, 267, 267f
    tinea cruris, 267–268, 267f
    tinea pedis, 266–267, 266f
    tinea (pityriasis) versicolor, 265–266, 266f
Future planning, for AYAs with ID, 687

G
Gabapentin
    for AMPS, 379
    for seizure treatment, 281t
GAHs. *See* Gender-affirming hormones (GAHs)
Galactorrhea, 541–543. *See also* Prolactinomas
    diagnosis, 542
    etiology, 542
    hyperprolactinemia in, 542, 542t
    serum prolactin concentrations, 542, 542t
GamaSTAN, 332
Gamma-aminobutyric acid analog antiepileptics
    for AMPS, 379
γ-aminobutyric acid (GABA), 480
Gamma-hydroxybutyrate (GHB), 644
Gardasil, 73
Gardasil 9, 73
Gardnerella vaginalis, 509
Garmin® devices, 297
Garrulous patient, 54
Gastrointestinal disorders, and pelvic pain, 478
Gateway drugs, 27
Gay, 401
Gay, bisexual, and other men who have sex with
    men, STIs in, 557
Gay, Lesbian & Straight Education Network
    2019 National School Climate Survey,
    403
Gender-affirming hormones (GAHs), 408, 410
    estrogen and androgen blocker therapy,
      410–411
    side effects of, in transgender adolescents,
      410–411
    testosterone therapy, 411
Gender-affirming medical care, 408, 410
Gender diverse youth, 409
    preventive care for, 69
Gender dysphoria, 408, 409
Gender expression, 401, 408
Gender identity, 401, 408
Gender & Sexualities Alliances, 404
General Data Protection Regulation for children
    or "kids" (GDPR-K), 129
Generalized anxiety disorder (GAD), 665, 667,
    667t
Generalized Anxiety Disorder scale (GAD)-7, 66
Generational forgetting, 602, 605
Genetic syndromes. *See also* Fragile X
    syndrome; 22q11.2 deletion syndrome
    and obesity, 355
Genetic testing, in thyroid disease, 153
Genital dysphoria, 455
Genital examination, 70
    male, 530–531
Genital herpes, 572, 578–582
    causative agents, 578
    clinical manifestations, 579–580
    complications, 582
    counseling, 582
    diagnosis, 580
    differential diagnosis, 580
    epidemiology, 578
    first clinical episode, 579, 581
    infections by serologic type, 579, 579t
    laboratory evaluation, 580–581
    lesions, 579, 580f
    management of sex partners, 582
    pathogenesis, 579
    prevalence and incidence, 578

    primary infection, 579, 580f
    recurrent episodes
      episodic therapy for, 582
      suppressive therapy for, 582
    transmission, 578
    treatment, 581–582
Genital ulcer disease, 579, 580, 591. *See also*
    Genital herpes
Genital ulcers, 572
    differential diagnosis of, 592t
Genitourinary abnormalities, and pelvic pain,
    478
Genitourinary tract infections, 300–305
    asymptomatic bacteriuria, 302
    complicated, 303
    cystitis, 300–302, 301t
    epididymitis, 303
    future perspective, 305
    prostatitis, 303
    pyelonephritis, 303
    treatment of, 303–305, 304t
    uncomplicated, 300–302
    urethritis, 301t
    vaginitis, 301t
Genome-wide association studies (GWAS), 36
Gentamicin, for pyelonephritis, 303, 304t
Gepants, for headache management, 291t
Gestational age, 417
Gestational diabetes mellitus (GDM), 159–160
Gestational trophoblastic disease, 419
GH stimulation testing, 146
Giant fibroadenomas, 544
Gifted and talented (GT), 681t
Ginkgo biloba (ginkgo leaf extract), 481
Glenohumeral joint dislocations, 222
Global Burden of Disease (GBD) study 2019, 2,
    4t, 6f, 17f
Global health strategies and initiatives, 2
Global Initiative for Asthma (GINA), 206
Global School-based Student Health Survey
    (GSHS), 133t
Glomerular causes, proteinuria, 313–314, 313t
Glomerulopathies, and proteinuria, 313
Gluten-free diet, 393
Glutensensitive enteropathy. *See* Celiac disease
Gluten sensitivity, 165
Glycemic index (GI), 80
Glycopyrrolate, for hyperhidrosis, 273
GnRH analog stimulation test, 149
GnRH analog therapy, 149
GnRH pulse generator, 475
Goiter, 153
Gonadal disorders, 143, 146
    acquired, 143
    congenital, 143
Gonadal dysgenesis, 143
Gonadal failure
    with abnormal karyotype, 143
      gonadal dysgenesis, 143
      Klinefelter syndrome, 143
    with normal karyotype, 143
      acquired gonadal disorders, 143
      androgen-receptor defects, 143
      congenital gonadal disorders, 143
Gonadal steroids, 35–36
Gonadarche, 36, 474
Gonadectomy, 147
Gonadotropin deficiency, 146
Gonadotropin-releasing hormone (GnRH), 35,
    36, 141, 474, 475, 482
Gonadotropin-releasing hormone (GnRH)
    agonists, in dysmenorrhea, 479–480
Gonadotropin-releasing hormone analogs
    (GnRHa), 410
Gonadotropin-releasing hormone pulse
    generator, 36

Gonadotropins, 36. *See also* Follicle-stimulating hormone (FSH); Luteinizing hormone (LH)
Gonococcal conjunctivitis, 559, 560
Gonococcal Isolate Surveillance Project (GISP), 560
Gonococcal urethritis, 559
Got Transition program, 678
Got Transitions toolkit, 76
Gram-negative folliculitis, 257
Granuloma inguinale, 572, 594
    clinical manifestations, 594, 594f
    diagnosis, 594
    epidemiology, 594
    etiology, 594
    treatment, 594, 595t
Granulosa cell tumors, 522, 523f
Graves disease, 155–156, 157
Graves ophthalmopathy, 155, 155f
Grazoprevir, 454
Griseofulvin, for tinea pedis, 267
Group therapy, for substance use disorders, 654t
Growing Up Today Study (GUTS), 133t
Growth
    anorexia nervosa and, 364
    monitoring of, 106
Growth and development, abnormal, 138–150
    delayed puberty, 140–148
    precocious puberty, 148–149
    short stature without delayed puberty, 138–140
Growth and development, in AYAs, 35–43
Growth hormone (GH), 39, 146
    during puberty, 39
Growth hormone deficiency, 139
Growth plate, 216
    disorders, 216
Guanfacine, in ADHD, 685
Guardianship, 683
Guardianship alternatives, 683
Guided imagery, 394
Guidelines, on adolescent hypertension, 196
Guillain–Barré syndrome, 73
Gynecologic examination, 468–473
    bimanual examination, 470, 472f
    cervical cancer screening, 468
    complete pelvic examination, 468, 468t
    equipment, 469t
    external genitalia inspection, 470, 470f
    history, 469
    indications, 468, 468t
    office environment, 468
    postexamination discussion, 473
    privacy during, 469t
    rectovaginal–abdominal examination, 472–473
    sexually transmitted infection screening, 468
    speculum examination, 470
        insertion of speculum, 470, 472f
        size of speculum, 470, 471f
    steps in, 469–473
Gynecologic histories, 469
Gynecomastia, 38, 54, 70, 545–546
    androgen, decrease in, 545
    clinical manifestations, 546
    diagnosis, 546
    epidemiology, 545
    estrogen, increase in, 545
    etiology, 545
    management, 546
    medications causing, 546, 546t
    pathologic, 546
    physical examination, 546
    transient, 545

H
Habit cough, 207
Haemophilus ducreyi, 591. *See also* Chancroid
Haemophilus influenzae, 208
Hair loss, 272
    generalized, 272–273
    localized, 273
Hair-pulling disorder. *See* Trichotillomania (TTM)
Haller index, 208
Hallucinogen-persisting perception disorder (HPPD), 646
Hallucinogens, 615–619
    dextromethorphan, 648
    dimethyltryptamine, 649
    Jimson weed, 648
    ketamine, 647
    D-lysergic acid diethylamide, 647–648
    morning glory seeds, 649
    nutmeg, 649
    peyote and mescaline, 649
    phencyclidine, 646–647
    psilocybin, 648
    salvia, 649
    types of, 646t
Harlem Children's Zone, 748
Hashimoto disease, 156
HAVRIX for hepatitis A, 332
HCM. *See* Hypertrophic cardiomyopathy (HCM)
Headaches, 286
    chronic form, 286
    classification, 286
    epidemiology, 286
    episodic form, 286
    evaluation of, 289
    in females, 286
    headache diary, 290
    history and physical examination, 289
    imaging studies, 289
    International Classification of Headache Disorders (ICHD), 286
    primary, 286, 287t
        cluster headaches, 288
        migraine, 286–288, 287t
        new daily persistent headache, 288
        tension-type headache, 288
    "red flags" in evaluation of, 288, 288t
    secondary, 286, 287t, 288
        cerebral venous sinus thrombosis related, 289
        idiopathic intracranial hypertension, 289
        medication overuse headache, 288–289
        post-traumatic headache, 288
    treatment, 289–291, 291t
        goal of, 290
        hormone therapy, 290–291
        lifestyle modifications, 290
        medication, 290, 291t
        multitiered approach in, 290
        nonpharmacologic therapies, 290
        other procedures, 291
        prophylactic, 290
Head Start program, 10, 420
Health and Human Services (HHS), 127
Health behaviors, 2, 7, 10, 23, 27, 29, 58, 107
    alcohol use, 27
    AYAs with chronic health conditions and, 107
    illicit drug use, 27
    nutrition, 27, 29
    obesity/overweight, 27
    physical activity, 27
    screening for, 58
    sexual and reproductive health, 29
    smoking, 27
    substance use, 23, 27

Health Behaviours in School-Aged Children (HBSC), 23
Health care
    for justice–involved AYAs, 736t
    nutrition in, role of, 78–83
    organizations supporting quality and practice improvement in, 125, 125t
    quality in, 118 (*See also* Quality improvement (QI))
Healthcare Effectiveness Data and Information Set (HEDIS), 62, 124t, 125, 125t
Health care transitions (HCT), 4t, 10–11, 56, 76
    Got Transitions toolkit, 76
    readiness assessments, 76
Health care utilization, 29–30, 30f
Health conditions, chronic. *See* Chronic health conditions
The Health Consequences of Involuntary Exposure to Tobacco Smoke (report), 627
Health disparities, 5, 9. *See also* Social determinants of health
Health Insurance Portability and Accountability Act (HIPAA), 86, 128, 131
    HIPAA Privacy Rule, 87
    HIPAA Security Rule, 87–88
Health, of adolescents and young adults, 2
    health care services for, 29–30
    proximal determinants of, 9
        families, 9
        neighborhoods, 9
        new media, 10
        orphanhood, 9–10
        peers, 10
        school, 9
    structural determinants of, 5
        education, 7
        employment, 8
        income, 5, 7
        migration, 8–9
        racism, 9
        sex inequality, 9
        war and conflict, 9
    WHO on social determinants of health, 2, 5
Health professionals, role of, 108–110
Health promotion, 708
Health risk behaviors, as risk factor for suicide, 672
Health risk, of AYAs in detention, 734–735
Health screening, for immigrants and refugees, 739
Health services, 2, 9, 30, 107–108
Health status, 2, 3f
    factors impacting (*See* Social determinants of health)
    of youth experiencing homelessness, 725–726
Health visit, 50. *See also* Office visits
Healthy Campus 2020, 708
Healthy People 2030, 229, 399
Hearing impairment (HI), 681t
Hearing screening, 69
Heart
    connective tissue disease and
        Ehlers–Danlos syndromes, 190, 191f
        fragile X syndrome, 190
        Marfan syndrome, 190, 191f
        hypertension and, 196, 199, 202
Heart lesions, considerations in evaluation of, 193
Heart rate, measurement of, 69
Heated tobacco products, 626
Heavy drinking, 614. *See also* Alcohol
Heavy menstrual bleeding (HMB), 484
HEEADSSS (home, education/employment, eating, activities, drugs, sexuality, suicide/depression, safety), 52
    neurodevelopmental screening, 677, 678t
HEEADSSS/SSHADES assessments, 747

Height and weight assessment, 69
Height velocity, 39–40, 40f, 41f
Helpers, 120
Helping Patients Who Drink Too Much: A
   Clinician's Guide (NIAAA), 66
Hematocolpos, 515, 517f
Hematocrit, 70
Hematometra, 515, 517f
Hematuria, 314–315
   causes of, 315t
   diagnostic approach, 315–316
   differential diagnosis, 315
   epidemiology, 315
   glomerular, 315, 315t, 316
   gross, 314
   history and physical examination, 315–316
   microscopic, 314
   nonglomerular, 315, 315t, 316
   pathophysiology, 315
   screening for, 314
   specific conditions, 316
Hemiplegic migraine, 287–288
Hemispherectomy, 280
Hemoglobin A1c (HbA1c), 160
Hemoglobin screening, 70
Hemp, 633
HepaGam B, 335
Hepatitis, 331–339. See also specific type
Hepatitis A, 331
   antigens and antibodies, 331, 332f
   clinical course, 331
   epidemiology, 331
   human serum immunoglobulin, 332
   during pregnancy, 333
   prevention and prophylaxis, 331–332
   risk factors, 332t
   treatment, 331
   vaccine, 331–332
Hepatitis A virus (HAV). See Hepatitis A
Hepatitis B, 333
   antigens and antibodies, 333, 334f
   chronic HBV infection, 333, 334, 334f
   clinical course, 333
   epidemiology, 333
   hepatitis B immunoglobulin, 335
   laboratory screening for, 333t
   postexposure prophylaxis for health care
      workers, 336t
   during pregnancy, 335
   prevention and prophylaxis, 334–335
   recommendations for transmission reduction,
      334t
   risk factors, 333, 335t
   screening refugees and immigrants for, 740
   treatment, 333–334
   vaccine, 334
Hepatitis B immunoglobulin (HBIG), 335
Hepatitis B virus (HBV). See Hepatitis B
Hepatitis C, 336
   acute infection, 337
   antigens and antibodies, 336–337, 337f
   chronic HCV, 336–338
   clinical course, 336
   epidemiology, 336
   during pregnancy, 338
   prevention and prophylaxis, 338
   progression to cirrhosis, 336
   screening for, 70, 336
   serologic test results interpretation, 337t
   treatment, 337–338
Hepatitis C virus (HCV). See Hepatitis C
Hepatitis D, 338–339
   antigens and antibodies, 338
   clinical course, 338
   epidemiology, 338
   prevention and prophylaxis, 339

risk factors, 338
   with superinfection, 338
Hepatitis D virus (HDV). See Hepatitis D
Hepatitis E, 339
   antigens and antibodies, 339
   clinical course, 339
   epidemiology, 339
   in pregnancy, 339
   prevention and prophylaxis, 339
   treatment, 339
Hepatitis E virus (HEV). See Hepatitis E
Hepatosplenomegaly, 319
Heplisav-B, for hepatitis B, 335
Herbal medicines, hormonal contraceptives and,
   454
Herbal therapies, 91–94
   butterbur, 93
   chamomile, 92
   conditions treated with, 92
   dosing issues and active compounds, 91–92
   drug interactions and toxicity, 91
   Echinacea, 92–93
   elderberry, 92
   feverfew, 93
   long-term use, 92
   in pregnancy and lactation, 92
   St. John's wort, 91, 92
   valerian root, 92
Hereditary nephritis. See Alport syndrome
Herniated disk, 225, 225f
Heroin, 641. See also Opioids
   during pregnancy, 419
   use by young adults, 608
Herpes genitalis. See Genital herpes
Herpes simplex virus (HSV), 268, 578.
      See also Genital herpes
   erythema multiforme by, 271
   type 1 (HSV-1), 578
   type 2 (HSV-2), 578
Heterophile antibodies, 321, 321t, 322
Heterosexism, 402
   sexual minorities, impact on, 402
Heterosexual, 401
Heterotopic pregnancy, 525
Hidradenitis suppurativa, 273
   clinical manifestations, 273
   treatment, 273
High-density lipoprotein (HDL), 171
High-fiber diet, in IBS, 393
High-grade squamous intraepithelial lesion
   (HSIL), 584
High-intensity interval training (HIIT), 230
High School & Beyond (HSB), 133t
High-speed video microscopy analysis
   (HSVMA), 210
Hip, 220–221
   femoroacetabular impingement and labral
      tears, 220–221
   history of hip symptoms, 220
   imaging studies, 220
   physical examination, 220
   slipped capital femoral epiphysis, 221, 221f
   treatment, 220
Hirsutism, 488, 498–500. See also Polycystic
   ovary syndrome (PCOS)
   androgen excess in, 498, 500
   differential diagnosis, 498, 499t
   drug induced, 498
   Ferriman–Gallwey hirsutism scoring system,
      498, 499f
   indications for evaluation, 498
   laboratory evalu, 500
   nonandrogenic causes, 498
   PCOS and, 495, 496, 498
   physical examination, 498, 500
   therapy for, 497

Histoplasmosis, and erythema nodosum, 271
Historical Clinical Risk Management-20
   (HCR-20), 693
History
   in HIV infection, 347
   in preventive health visit, 67–69
      developmental assessment, 68
      family history, 67–68
      past medical history, 67
      psychosocial history, 68, 68t
      review of systems, 69
Home, interview questions about, 52
Homelessness
   sexual minority youth and, 403
   transgender youth and young adults, 409
Homeless youth, 723. See also Youth
      experiencing homelessness (YEH)
Homeopathy, 90
Home pregnancy testing (HPT), 416
Homicides, 691
Homophobia, 402
Hook effect, 542
Hormonal contraceptives, in dysmenorrhea,
   479
Hormonal implant, 457. See also Nexplanon
Hormone therapy
   for acne, 261
   for amenorrhea, 493–494
   for dysmenorrhea, 479–480
   for headache management, 290
Hospice, 115, 116
Host homes, 727
Hot tub folliculitis, 268–269
House rules, 55–56
H2-receptor antagonists, in dyspepsia, 393
Human chorionic gonadotropin (hCG), 416,
   475, 519
   after pregnancy, 416
   false-negative hCG test, 416–417
   false-positive test, 417
   immunometric tests, 416
   levels during pregnancy, 416
Human growth hormone (hGH), 147
Human immunodeficiency virus (HIV) infection,
   341
   acute HIV infection, 341, 341t
   antiretroviral therapy, 341, 350–351
      barriers to adherence, 351t
      initiation of, 350–351
   in AYAs, 29, 106
   contraception, 349
   cough in, 349
   diarrhea in, 350
   dysphagia in, 350
   epidemiology, 342
   ethnicity and, 342
   etiology, 341–342
   family planning, 349
   fever in, 349–350
   follow-up, 348
   gender and, 342
   history and physical examination, 347–348
   immunization recommendations, 348
   initial assessment, 347–348
   laboratory evaluation, 348
   long-term nonprogressors, 341
   management of, 347–351
   manifestations, 348t
   mother–child transmission risk, 349
   in MSM, 403
   neurocognitive function in adolescents with,
      342
   neurologic evaluation, 350
   opportunistic infections with, 348, 349, 349t
   pathogenesis and natural history, 341–342
   during pregnancy, 419

prevention, 345–347
  behavioral, 347
  educational intervention, 347
  primary, 345–347
  risk reduction counseling, 347
  secondary, 347
prophylaxis, 350
recommendations for clinicians, 351
screening for, 70, 71
sexually transmitted infections, management of, 349
shortness of breath in, 349
sports participation, 349
testing and counseling, 343
  consent and confidentiality, 343
  posttest counseling, 344–345
  pretest counseling, 344
  screening recommendations, 343–344
  testing methods, 344, 344t
  testing sites, 344
in transgender youth and young adults, 410
transmission, 342
  needle sharing, 343
  routes of, 342–343, 342t
  sexual transmission, 343
  vertical transmission, 343
treatment, 350–351
tuberculosis in, 350
in young adults, 342
in youth experiencing homelessness, 725
Human papillomavirus (HPV), 501, 584.
    See also Anogenital warts
  and cervical cancer, 502–503, 586
  clinical manifestations, 585, 585f, 586f
  counseling about, 589
  detection methods, 586
  diagnosis, 586–587
  differential diagnosis, 586
  epidemiology, 584
  genital HPV types, 584
  infection, 584–590
  natural history of, 502, 584–585
  pathophysiology, 584–585
  prevalence, 584
  primary HPV testing, 70
  risk factors, 584
  screening for, 70
  transmission, 584
  treatment, 587–589, 587t–588t
  vaccination in patients with HIV, 348
  vaccines against, 73, 109, 589, 590
  vulnerability of cervix to, 502
    metaplasia and HPV infection, 502
    pubertal metaplastic changes, 502
    in utero and prepuberty, 502
  and warts, 268
Human papillomavirus vaccines, 501–502, 589–590
Human Rights Campaign 2018 LGBTQ Youth Survey, 403
Human serum immunoglobulin (HSIG), 332
Humeral epiphysiolysis, 216, 223
Hydatidiform mole, 419
Hydration
  athletes and, 83
  for headache treatment, 290
Hydrocele, 532, 534f, 537
  communicating, 537
  diagnosis, 537
  etiology, 537
  therapy, 537
Hydrogen breath test, 391
Hydrosalpinx, 564
17α-hydroxylase deficiency, 488, 493, 494
Hydroxyzine, for urticaria, 271
Hyperandrogenism, in PCOS, 495, 496, 496f

Hyperfiltration renal injury, and proteinuria, 313
Hyperglycemia, 159–164. *See also* Diabetes mellitus
Hypergonadotropic hypogonadism, and amenorrhea, 488–489
Hyperhidrosis, 273–274
  clinical manifestations, 273
  primary, 273
  secondary, 273
  treatment, 273–274
Hyperprolactinemia, 542. *See also* Galactorrhea; Prolactinomas
  medication-induced, 542, 542t
Hypersensitivity reactions
  drug eruptions, 272
  erythema multiforme, 271, 271f
  erythema nodosum, 271–272
  urticaria, 270–271, 270f
Hypertension, 196–202
  asthma and, 202
  definition, 196
  diabetes and, 202
  diagnosis
    blood pressure measurement, 198
    confirmation of, 198
  diagnostic evaluation, 198
    history, 198, 199t
    imaging studies, 199
    laboratory testing, 199
    physical examination, 198–199, 199t
  elevated BP, 196
  etiology, 198
  factors influencing BP, 196, 197t
    age, 197
    birth weight and other perinatal factors, 198
    genetics, 198
    height and weight, 197
    race/ethnicity, 197
    sodium and other dietary constituents, 197
    stress and adverse childhood experiences, 197
  nonpharmacologic interventions, 200
  pharmacologic treatment, 200
    adolescents ≤ 18 years, 200, 200f, 201t
    special populations, 202
    young adults ≥ 18 years, 200–202
  in pregnancy, 202
  prevalence of, 196
  prevention, 199–200
  primary, 196, 198
  staging system, 196, 197t
  white coat, 198
Hypertensive emergencies, 202
Hyperthyroidism, 155–156
Hypertrophic cardiomyopathy (HCM), 183, 184, 188t, 189, 189f
  definition, 189
  evaluation, 189
  management, 189
  natural history, 189
  physical examination, 189
Hypertrophic scars, 257
Hypnagogic hallucinations, 295
Hypnosis, 95
Hypnotherapy, for FGIDs, 394
Hypogonadotropic hypogonadism, and amenorrhea, 489, 493
Hypokalemia, anorexia nervosa and, 364
Hyponatremia, anorexia nervosa and, 364
Hypotension, in ME/CFS patients, 382
Hypothalamic–pituitary–adrenal (HPA) axis, 35, 35f
Hypothalamic–pituitary–gonadal (HPG) axis
  maturation of, 35–36
  and pubertal maturation, 35, 35f

Hypothalamic–pituitary–ovarian (HPO) axis, 474
  immaturity of, 484
Hypothyroidism, 143, 147, 156

I

IBS. *See* Irritable bowel syndrome (IBS)
Ibuprofen (Motrin), for dysmenorrhea, 479, 479t
Ichthyosis vulgaris, 263
ICs. *See* Internal condoms (ICs)
Ideal cardiovascular health, 168–169, 169t, 170f
Identity development
  early adolescence, 46
  late adolescence, 47
  middle adolescence, 47
  social media use and, 99
  young adults, 48, 113
Idiopathic hypogonadotropic hypogonadism (IHH), 489
  and amenorrhea, 489
Idiopathic intracranial hypertension (IIH), 289
  cerebrospinal fluid (CSF) pressure in, 289
  lumbar puncture in, 289
  presentation and features, 289
IgA nephropathy, 316
iHELP tool, 747
Illicit drug use, 27
Illness anxiety disorder, 376
Imidazole
  for tinea cruris, 268
  for tinea pedis, 267
  for tinea versicolor, 266
Imipramine, for enuresis, 309
Immigrant, 738. *See* Immigrant adolescents and young adults
Immigrant adolescents and young adults, 738–741
  communication and interpreter use, 739, 739t
  cultural competency, 738–739
  health issues of
    hepatitis B, 740
    immunizations, 739–740
    lead exposure, 740
    malaria, 740
    mental health, 740
    parasitic infections, 740
    sexual health, 740
    tuberculosis, 740
  health screenings
    for adjustment of legal status, 739
    overseas medical screening, 739
    U.S. medical screening, 739
  legal status of, 738
  nonimmigrant foreign-born AYAs, 741
  second-generation immigrants, 741
Immunization, 71
  consent for, 73–74
  contraindications to, 74
  COVID-19, 329, 348
  hepatitis A, 331–332, 348
  hepatitis B, 335, 348
  HIV infection, 348
  human papillomavirus, 71–72
  immigrant and refugee AYAs, 739–740
  influenza, 72–73, 327, 348
  meningococcal disease, 71
  pertussis, 326
  polio, 348
  recommended schedule, 71–72
    adult, 72t
    for ages 18 years or younger, 71t
  varicella, 348

Immunoglobulin, in SJS and TEN, 271
Immunometric tests, 416
    false-negative hCG test, 416–417
    false-positive test, 417
Immunomodulators, for molluscum
        contagiosum, 599t
Immunosuppressants, for SJS and TEN, 271
Immunosuppression, 109
Imperforate hymen, 517, 517f
Impetigo
    bullous, 268
    crusted (nonbullous), 268
Implanon, 425
Implanon NXT, 425
Implantable cardioverter-defibrillators, 184
Inactivated influenza vaccine, 72–73
Incarceration, 733, 735
Incidence, 4t, 106
Income, and health status, 5, 7
Incontinence, 306
Independence, 45
    early adolescence, 46
    late adolescence, 47
    middle adolescence, 46–47
    young adults, 48
Independent educational evaluation (IEE), 681,
        681t
Independent variables, 132
Index of race-related stress for adolescents
        (IRRS), 747
Individual counseling, in substance use
        disorders, 654t
Individualized education plan (IEP), 252, 681t,
        683
Individuals with Disabilities Education Act
        (IDEA), 680, 681t
Inequality
    income, 5
    sex, 9
Infection(s)
    after abortion, 418
    as cause of pelvic mass, 517–518
    COVID-19, 327–329
    Epstein-Barr virus, 319–323
    hepatitis A, 331–333
    hepatitis B, 333–336
    hepatitis C, 336–338
    hepatitis D, 338–339
    hepatitis E, 339
    HIV, 341–352
    infectious mononucleosis, 319–323
    influenza, 326–327
    Mycoplasma pneumoniae, 324–325
    pertussis, 325–326
Infectious diseases, in youth experiencing
        homelessness, 725
Infectious mononucleosis (IM), 319–323
    clinical manifestations, 319–320
    complications of, 320–321, 320t
        airway obstruction, 321
        chronic active EBV disease, 321
        splenic rupture, 320–321
    diagnosis, 322
    differential diagnosis, 322
    EBV infection and, 319
    epidemiology, 319
    etiology and pathophysiology, 319
    laboratory evaluation, 321–322
        antibody testing, 321, 321f, 321t
        complete blood count, 321–322
        EBV viral load tests, 322
        hepatic transaminases, 322
        patterns of EBV serology, 321t
    management
        antimicrobials, 322
        corticosteroids, 322

    physical activity, recommendations on,
        322
    symptomatic care, 322
    signs and symptoms, 320, 320t
    skin rashes in, 320
Infectious respiratory illnesses, 324
    COVID-19, 327–329
    influenza, 326–327
    Mycoplasma pneumoniae, 324–325
    pertussis, 325–326
Infertility
    chronic health conditions and, 109
    pelvic inflammatory disease and, 564
Inflammatory bowel disease (IBD), 391, 392
Inflammatory heart disease
    Lyme carditis, 191
    myopericarditis, 191–193
Inflammatory lesions, acne, 256–257, 256f, 257f
Influenza, 326–327
    clinical manifestations, 327
    complications, 327
    diagnosis, 327
    differential diagnosis, 327
    epidemiology, 327
    etiology, 326–327
    laboratory evaluation, 327
    management, 327
    vaccine, 73, 327, 348
        inactivated vaccine, 73
        live attenuated vaccine, 73
Informational privacy, 128
Informed consent, 86
Inguinal syndromes, 559
Inhalants, 644–645, 644t, 645t
    adverse effects, 645, 645t
    chronic use, 645
    classes of, 644t
    diagnosis, 645
    identifying use of, 644–645
    intoxication, effects of, 645
    physiology and metabolism, 645
    preparation and administration routes, 644
    treatment, 645
Injectable hormonal contraception, 454–455.
        See also Depot medroxyprogesterone
        acetate
Injectable preexposure prophylaxis, 346
Injection drug use (IDU), among YEH, 725
Injuries among AYAs, 2, 5, 9, 16, 22
    deaths from, 2, 16, 17, 19f–21f
Injury prevention, 245–247
    anterior cruciate ligament injury prevention,
        246
    athletic organizations and facilities, role of,
        246–247
    guidelines and rules, 246
    overuse injuries, 246
    safety equipment, use of, 246
    sports injury epidemiology, 245–246
    sport specialization, 246
Innovative technology, in preventive health
        care, 58, 66
In-situ DNA hybridization (ISH), 586
Insomnia, 294. *See also* Sleep disturbances and
        disorders
Institute for Healthcare Improvement (IHI),
        125t
Institute of Medicine (IOM) report
    "Crossing the Quality Chasm," 118
    "To Err is Human," 118
Institutional review board (IRB), 127
Institutions of higher education (IHEs), 706,
        712. *See also* College health
Insulin, 161, 164
Insulin-like growth factor–binding protein 1
        (IGFBP1), 495

Insulin-like growth factors (IGFs), 39
Insulin resistance, 159–161, 164. *See also*
        Diabetes mellitus
Insulin-sensitizing agents, in PCOS, 497, 498
Integrated behavioral health (IBH) approach,
        678
Intellectual disability (ID), 677t, 681t, 686–687
Intensive outpatient program (IOP), for
        substance use disorders, 655t
Interdisciplinary care, for neurodevelopmental
        disorders, 678
Interdisciplinary team approach, for adolescents
        with eating disorders, 367, 370, 371,
        372
Interferon-gamma release assays (IGRAs), 70
Intermediate density lipoproteins (IDL), 171
Intermenstrual bleeding, 558
Internal condoms (ICs), 440–441, 442f
    advantages, 441
    Cupid FC condom, 441
    disadvantages, 441
    efficacy, 441
    failure rates, 441
    future developments, 441
    instructions for insertion and use, 442f–443f
    Natural Sensation Panty Condom, 441
    PATH's Woman's Condom, 441
    use of, data on, 440
International Association for the Study of Pain
        (IASP), 376
International Children's Continence Society
        (ICCS), 306
International Classification of Diseases, 11th
        edition (ICD-11), 376
International Olympic Committee (IOC), 244
Internet, 98, 101. *See also* Digital technology;
        Social media
Interpersonal therapy for adolescents (IPT-A),
        663
Interpersonal therapy (IPT), for depression,
        663–664
Interpersonal violence, 691, 710. *See also* Youth
        violence
Interrupted suicide attempt, 671
Intersectionality, 402
Intertrigo, 267
Interview format, 51–54
    closure, 53–54
    confidentiality, 52
    developmental orientation and, 54
    physical examination, 53
    previsit questionnaires, 51–52
    rapport, establishing, 52
    social history, structure of, 52–53
    suggestions for AYAs, 52t
Interviewing techniques, for AYAs, 53t
Intimate partner violence, sexual minority
        youth and, 403–404
Intractable epilepsy, 280. *See also* Epilepsy
Intraductal papilloma, 541
Intrauterine device (IUD), 415, 422, 423.
        See also Long-acting reversible
        contraceptives (LARCs)
    advantages, 425
    CHOICE study, 425
    copper 10 year intrauterine device
        (Paragard), 425, 425t
    current use, 423, 425
    insertion, 463, 465
        bimanual and speculum exam, 465
        verbal distraction techniques to, 465
    levonorgestrel-intrauterine devices, 425,
        425t
    myths and misconceptions about, 425
    names and characteristics, 425t
    removal, 463, 465

Intrauterine growth restriction
    growth hormone treatment, 140
    and short stature, 140
Intrauterine system, levonorgestrel-releasing, 457. *See also* Intrauterine devices (IUD)
Intravenous immunoglobulin (IVIG)
    in CRPS, 379
    in ME/CFS, 384
Invasive stereo-EEG (sEEG), 280
Iodine deficiency, 153
Ion channel defects, 184
IPLEDGE, 261
I Promise School, 748
Iron
    high-iron foods, 81
    need during adolescence, 81
    non-heme iron, 81
Iron deficiency, in athletes, 82–83
Irritable bowel syndrome (IBS), 388, 389, 390t
Ishikawa diagram. *See* Fishbone diagrams
Isotretinoin, for acne, 261
Itraconazole
    for onychomycosis, 267
    for tinea pedis, 267
    for tinea versicolor, 266
IUD. *See* Intrauterine device (IUD)
Ivabradine, for orthostatic intolerance, 385t
Ivermectin
    pediculosis pubis, 596t
    scabies, 597t
IVIG. *See* Intravenous immunoglobulin (IVIG)

J
Jarisch–Herxheimer reaction, 576
Jaundice
    in hepatitis A, 331
    in hepatitis C, 336
Jimson weed *(Datura stramonium)*, 648
Joint hypermobility
    Beighton score, 383f
    in ME/CFS patients, 383, 383f
Judicial bypass, 85
Justice initiatives, 749
Justice system, involvement with, 733–736
    assessment and treatment issues, 735–736
        detention care guidelines, 736
        insurance coverage, 736
    epidemiology of, 733–734
        disproportionate minority contact, 733–734
        mortality rate, 734
        recidivism, 733
    health care for justice–involved AYAs, 736t
    health issues of young people in, 734–735
        dental problems, 735
        detention conditions, 734
        injuries, 734–735
        mental health and substance use disorders, 734
        other reproductive health issues, 735
        physical health, 734–735
        preexisting health conditions, 734
        sexually transmitted infections, 735
        sleep disturbances, 735
    recommended health services for youth involved in juvenile justice, 735t
Juvenile detention. *See* Justice system, involvement with
Juvenile Detention Alternatives Initiative, 736
Juvenile fibromyalgia, 377
Juvenile justice, 736. *See also* Justice system, involvement with
Juvenile justice system, 733. *See also* Justice system, involvement with
Juvenile papillomatosis, 544
Juvenile plantar dermatosis, 266

K
Kabat-Zinn, Jon, 96
Kallmann syndrome, 146, 492
Karyotype, 139, 146
Keloids, 257
    piercings and, 275
Keratinization, abnormal, 256
Keratosis pilaris (KP), 257, 263
Keratotic warts, 585, 586f
Ketamine, 379, 647
Ketoconazole shampoo, for tinea versicolor, 266
Ketogenic diet (KD), for seizure control, 282
Ketosisprone atypical diabetes mellitus, 159
Khat. *See* Cathinone
Kidney
    hypertension and, 198, 199
    sodium reabsorption in, 197
    ultrasound, 199
Kidney biopsy, in proteinuria, 314
Kids Eating Disorders Survey (KEDS), 366
Kids' Inpatient Database (KID), 134t
Kinship care, 727, 729
KISS1/Kiss1 gene, 36
KISS1/KISS1R/Kisspeptin system, 36
Kisspeptins, 36
Klebsiella granulomatis, 594
Klinefelter syndrome, 143
    phenotypic traits of, 144f
Knee, 218–220
    anatomy, 218f
    effusion, 218, 218t
    history of knee symptoms, 218
        acute pain, 218
        chronic pain, 218
        traumatic knee pain, 218
        valgus knee injury, 218
    imaging studies, 218–219
    Osgood–Schlatter disease, 219–220
    osteochondritis dissecans, 220
    Ottawa knee rules, 218–219
    patellofemoral pain, 219
    physical examination, 218, 218t
    treatment, 218
Kyleena, 425, 425t, 457

L
Lacosamide, for seizure treatment, 281t
Lactobacilli, 509
Lactobacillus crispatus–dominated microbiome, 503
Lactose-free diet, 393
Lactose intolerance, 82, 391
Lactose intolerance test, 391
Lamotrigine, for seizure treatment, 281t
Language disorders, 686
Lanugo hair, 364
Laparoscopy, in dysmenorrhea, 479
LARCs. *See* Long-acting reversible contraceptives (LARCs)
Laryngeal obstruction, exercise-induced, 207
Laser treatment
    for tattoo removal, 275
    for warts, 268
Last menstrual period (LMP), 416, 417, 460
Late adolescence, 45, 47, 59
    close relationships in, 396
Latent syphilis, 572. *See also* Syphilis
    diagnosis, 574
    early, 572
    late, 572
    latent syphilis of unknown duration, 572
    treatment, 575
Laughing gas. *See* Nitrous oxide
Lead, testing refugees and immigrants for, 740
Lean, 119. *See also* Quality improvement (QI)
Lean body mass, 41

Learning disabilities (LD), 677t, 687
Learning disorders, in epilepsy, 283
Lea's Shield. *See* Cervical shield
Least restrictive environment (LRE), 680, 681t
Left cervical sympathectomy, 184
Left ventricular hypertrophy (LVH), 196
Legal framework, 85
    care through telehealth, 88
    consent, 86
    constitutional rights, 85
    electronic health information, 87–88
    health care in school settings, 88
    HIPAA Privacy Rule, 87, 88
    HIPAA Security Rule, 87–88
    "mature minor" doctrine, 86
    minors and confidentiality protections, 87
    payment, 87–88
    privacy and confidentiality, 86–87
    right to refuse treatment, 86
    state and federal laws, 85
    21st Century Cures Act, 88
    young adults and capacity to consent, 86
Legal information, for AYAs with neurodevelopmental disorders, 682–683
Legal permanent resident (LPR), 738
Lennox–Gastaut syndrome (LGS), 277–278
Leptin, 36, 490
Leptospirosis, and erythema nodosum, 271
Lesbian, 401
Lesbian, gay, bisexual (LGB), 401, 403, 436
Lesbian, gay, bisexual, transgender, and questioning (LGBTQ), 9
    preventive care for, 69
Lethal means safety counseling, 674
Leukotriene receptor antagonists (LTRAs), 207
Leukotriene receptors, in uterine tissue, 477
Leukotrienes, dysmenorrhea and, 477
Leuprolide acetate, 486
Levamisole, 637
Levetiracetam, 283
    mood and behavior disturbances by, 283
    for seizure treatment, 281t
Levocetirizine, for urticaria, 271
Levofloxacin, 559
    for *Mycoplasma* infections, 325
Levonorgestrel-intrauterine devices, 425, 425t, 432
Levonorgestrel pills, for emergency contraception, 433
    advantages, 433
    availability, 433
    cost, 433
    mechanism of action, 433
    side effects, 433–434
    types, 433
LGV. *See* Lymphogranuloma venereum (LGV)
LH. *See* Luteinizing hormone (LH)
Lichen planus, 267
Life-course perspective, 3f, 4t, 10–11
Life-limiting conditions (LLCs), 112. *See also* Palliative care
    mortality rate from, 112
    needs of clinicians, 114
    needs of close others, 113–114
    psychological needs, 113
    social needs, 113
    spiritual and cultural needs, 113
    types of, 113t
    in young people, 112–113
Life-limiting illness, 112. *See also* Life-limiting conditions (LLCs)
Life Skills Training, 612
Lifestyle modifications, 71
    for headache treatment, 290
    in hypertension, 200
    for PCOS, 497

Liletta, 425, 425t, 432, 457
Linaclotide, for constipation-predominant IBS (IBS-C), 393
Lindane 1%, for scabies, 597t
Lipid disorders, 172, 173t. *See also specific disorder*
 treatment of, 174–178
  bempedoic acid, 176t, 177–178
  bile acid sequestrants, 177
  evinacumab, 178
  ezetimibe, 176t, 177
  fibrates, 176t, 177
  lomitapide, 178
  mipomersen, 178
  niacin, 177
  omega-3 polyunsaturated fatty acids, 176t, 177
  PCSK9 inhibitors, 176t, 177
  statins, 174–177, 176t
  universal lipid screening, 174
Lipids, 171
 physiology, 171–172
Lipooligosaccharide (LOS) protein, 555
Lipoproteins, 171–172, 172f
Liquid nitrogen, for warts, 268
Liraglutide
 in type 2 diabetes, 164
 for weight loss, 358, 359t
Lisdexamfetamine, 639
Literacy rate, global, 7
Literally homeless youth, 723. *See also* Youth experiencing homelessness (YEH)
Little League Elbow, 216
Little League Shoulder. *See* Humeral epiphysiolysis
Live, attenuated influenza vaccine (LAIV), 73
LLCs. *See* Life-limiting conditions (LLCs)
Localized amplified pain syndromes, 377–378
Lofexidine, 642
Loin pain hematuria syndrome, 316
Lomitapide (Juxtapid), 172
Long-acting reversible contraception (LARC). *See* Long-acting reversible contraceptives (LARCs)
Long-acting reversible contraceptives (LARCs), 109, 415, 422, 423, 425–426, 457–465. *See also* Intrauterine devices (IUD)
 abnormal uterine bleeding with, 464
 advantages of, 423, 461–462
 continuation, 461
 contraindications to, 462
 counseling and consent, 460t, 463
 disadvantages to, 462–463
 failure rates, 423
 future developments, 465
 implants, 425–426, 457, 458t
  advantages, 426
  availability in United States, 426
  current use, 425–426
 indications for, 462
 initiation and insertion, 459–461
 intrauterine devices, 422, 423, 457–459, 458t, 459f
  advantages, 425
  copper intrauterine device (Paragard), 425, 425t
  current use, 423, 425
  levonorgestrel-intrauterine devices, 425, 425t
  names and characteristics, 425t
 lack of LARC use, reasons for, 423
 mechanism, efficacy, and insertion, 457–459, 459f
 patient-centered counseling, 460t
 pros and cons of, 460t
 STIs and PID risk, 463–464

 top-tiered contraceptive method, 423
 types of, 457
 use of
  data on, 423, 457
  factors associated with, 459–460
Long QT syndrome (LQTS), 183–184
 acquired, 183, 184t
 definition, 183
 diagnosis, 183
 familial, 183
 treatment, 183
Loperamide, 393
Loratadine, for urticaria, 271
Loss of consciousness (LOC), 249
Low back pain, 225–226
Low-density lipoproteins (LDL), 171, 172
Lower urinary tract symptoms (LUTS), 306. *See also* Enuresis
Low glycemic index treatment (LGIT), 282
Low-grade squamous intraepithelial lesion (LSIL), 584
Low orthostatic tolerance, 382
LQTS. *See* Long QT syndrome (LQTS)
Lubiprostone, for constipation, 393
Luteal phase, 475
Luteinizing hormone (LH), 35, 146, 474, 475, 490
Lyme carditis, 191
Lymphadenopathy, 319, 320
Lymphocytosis, 319
Lymphogranuloma venereum (LGV), 559, 560, 572, 591–594
 clinical manifestations, 592–593
  groove sign, 592, 593f
  primary stage, 592
  secondary/inguinal stage, 592–593
  tertiary/genito-anorectal syndrome, 593
 diagnosis, 593
 epidemiology, 592
 etiology, 591–592
 stages of, 559
 treatment, 593, 594t
D-lysergic acid diethylamide (LSD), 647–648
 adverse effects, 647–648
 chronic use, 648
 intoxication, effects of, 647
 overdose and emergency treatment, 648
 physiology and metabolism, 647
 during pregnancy, 419
 preparation and dose, 647
 tolerance and withdrawal, 648
Lysosomal acid lipase deficiency, 173t

M
Macromastia, 540
Macules, hyperpigmented, 257, 257f
Magnetic resonance imaging (MRI), in complex regional pain syndrome, 378
Major depressive disorder (MDD), 660
Makorin Ring Finger Protein 3 (MKRN3), 36
Malaria, 740
 screening refugees and immigrants for, 740
Malassezia
 seborrheic dermatitis, 265
 tinea versicolor, 265
Malathion 0.5% lotion, for pediculosis pubis, 596t
Male condoms. *See* Traditional condoms
Male genital examination
 inspection, 530, 531f
  bell clapper deformity, 530, 532f
  pearly penile papules, 530, 532f
  penis and scrotum, 530, 531f
  testes, 530
 palpation, 530–531
Male genitalia, 530, 530f

Male-identifying AYA patients, preventive care for, 68–69
Male patient, cystitis in, 300–302, 301t
Male pubertal changes, 38–39
 age at puberty, 38–39
 biologic maturity in boys, 38f
 events of puberty, 38
 sequence, 38, 38f
 testicular volume by sexual maturity rating, 39t
Males with eating disorders, 371–372
 clinical presentation, 371–372
 epidemiology, 371
 medical management, 372
Malignant germ cell tumors, 523
Malignant melanoma, 274
Malingering, 376
Malnutrition, physical signs of, 363
Mammary duct ectasia, 541
Mammography, 545
Management
 HPV infection, 587–590
 sport-related concussion, 251–252
Marathon runner's hematuria, 316
Marfan syndrome, 190, 191f
Marginalization, 743
Marginalized. *See* Minoritized, disenfranchised, and marginalized AYAs
Marijuana, 606, 633
 behavioral and physiologic effects
  acute, 634
  cannabinoid hyperemesis syndrome, 635
  cannabis-induced psychosis, 635
  chronic, 634–635, 634t
  impact on driving, 634
  marijuana-related lung injuries, 635
 cannabis use disorder, 635
 changing risk perceptions, 634
 clinical assessment, 635
 cognitive effects of use, 609
 medical, 635–636
 middle and high school youth, 606–607
 pharmacology and endocannabinoid system, 633
 during pregnancy, 419
 preparations, potency, and use, 633–634
 repeated use, 635
 withdrawal, 635
 young adult, 607
Massage therapy, 95–96, 95f
Mastalgia, 541
Mast cell activation syndrome, 382
Mastitis, 541, 541f
Masturbation
 partnered, 397
 solo, 397
Maternal mortality, 16
Maturity-onset diabetes of youth (MODY), 159
Mayer–Rokitansky–Küster–Hauser (MRKH) syndrome, 144, 489, 517
McCune–Albright syndrome, 149
McKinney-Vento Homeless Education Assistance Act, 723
MDMA. *See* Methylenedioxymethamphetamine (MDMA)
MDMA-assisted psychotherapy, 640
Measles, mumps, rubella (MMR), 73, 348
Measurement, 135
Measures of fidelity, 120
Media curfew, 102
Media-free times, 103
Media, influence of, 55
Medial epicondyle apophysitis, 216
Media multitasking, 101, 103
Media Time Calculator, 103
Media use, and AYA health, 10

Medicaid, 747
Medical clinic, 64
Medical comorbidity, as risk factor for suicide, 672
Medical complications, of eating disorders, 365t–366t
Medical eligibility, for physical activity, 241
Medical Expenditure Panel Survey (MEPS), 133t
Medical homes, 678, 715
Medical interpreters, use of, 739, 739t
Medically managed withdrawal, in substance use disorders, 655t
Medical marijuana, 635–636
Medication overuse headache (MOH), 288–289
    ICHD-3 diagnostic criteria, 289
    treatment for, 289
Meditation, 94
Medium-chain triglyceride ketogenic diet (MCTKD), 282
Medroxyprogesterone acetate (Provera), 493
    for orthostatic intolerance, 385t
    for PCOS, 497
Medullary thyroid cancer (MTC), 151, 154
Mefenamic acid, for dysmenorrhea, 479t
Melanocortin-4 receptor (MC4R) mutations, in obesity, 355
Melatonin, 93, 93f
MenACWY vaccine, 72–73
Menarche, 38, 41, 414, 474, 488
Meningococcal disease, 71
Meningococcal vaccines (MenACWY), 71
Meningovascular syphilis, 572
Menses, 474
Menstrual cycle, 484
    duration of, 474
    follicular phase, 475
    initiation of, 474
    luteal phase, 475
    normal physiology of, 474–475, 474f
    ovulatory phase, 475
    vaginal secretions, 507
Menstrual history, 469
    dysmenorrhea and, 478
Menstrual-related migraines, 288, 291t
Menstruation, 474. *See also* Menstrual cycle
Mental health, 23, 29f
    adolescents in out-of-home care, 729–730
    immigrants and refugees, 740
    marginalized and minoritized youth, 744
    sexual minority youth, 403
    youth experiencing homelessness, 725
    youth with AUD, 619
Mental health disorders, in adolescents, 106, 107
Mental health services, by IHEs, 708
Mental illness, as risk factor for suicide, 672
Men who have sex with men (MSM), 401
    screening for, 71
    screening for STIs in, 558
    STIs in, 557
    syphilis, 569
Meperidine, 641. *See also* Opioids
Mescaline, 649
Mestranol, 450
Metabolic equivalent of task (MET), 229
Metabolic testing, 70–71
Metformin
    in PCOS, 497, 498
    in type 2 diabetes, 164
    for weight loss, 358
Methadone, for opioid use disorder, 641
Methamphetamine, 639. *See also* Amphetamines
Methimazole (MMI), 156
Meth mouth, 639, 639f

Methotrexate
    for atopic dermatitis, 264
    for ectopic pregnancy, 527, 528t
Methylenedioxymethamphetamine (MDMA), 640–641
    adverse effects, 640
    chronic use, 641
    intoxication, effects of, 640
    medical use/current state of research, 640
    overdose and emergency treatment, 640–641
    physiology and metabolism, 640
    preparation and dose, 640
    withdrawal, 641
3,4-Methylenedioxy-N-methylamphetamine (MDMA) use, by young adults, 609
Methylphenidate, 639
    for ADHD, 685
    for orthostatic intolerance, 385t
Metoprolol, for neurocardiogenic syncope, 181t
Metronidazole, 509, 512, 565
Miconazole nitrate
    for onychomycosis, 267
    for tinea pedis, 267
Middle adolescence, 46–47
    close relationships in, 396
Midodrine
    for neurocardiogenic syncope, 181t
    for orthostatic intolerance, 385t
Midparental height calculation, 139
Midparental target height, 40
Mifepristone (RU-486), 418
Mifepristone-misoprostol, for abortion, 418
Migraine, 286–288, 287t. *See also* Headaches
    with aura, 286–287, 291
    with brainstem aura, 287
    hemiplegic, 287–288
    historical features, 287
    ICHD-3 diagnostic criteria for, 287t
    and menses, 288
    treatment, 291t
    without aura, 287
Migration
    definition of migrant, 4t, 8
    health risks, 8–9
    reasons for, 8
Mild traumatic brain injury (TBI). *See* Concussion
Military, 717–722
    AYAs in military families, 720–721
        health considerations for, 721, 721f
        recommendations for providers working with, 722
        screening considerations, 722
    demographics, 719
    new recruit in, 717–719
        anticipatory guidance for, 717
        recommendations for providers working with, 719
        requirements for service entry, 717–719, 718f, 718t
    ROTC students, 719
        recommendations for providers working with, 719
    young adult service members, 719
        active-duty service members, 719, 719f
        health considerations for, 719–720, 720t
        recommendations for providers working with, 720
        risk-taking behaviors in civilian *vs.* military members, comparison of, 719, 719f
        screening considerations, 720, 721t
Military-affiliated youth. *See* Military
Military anticipatory guidance, 717, 719
Military eligibility, 717–719
Military experiences, as risk factor for suicide, 672

Military service, 717. *See also* Military
Milnacipran, for fibromyalgia, 379
Mind–body therapies, for headache management, 290
Mindfulness, 96
Mindfulness-Based Stress Reduction (MBSR), 96
Mindfulness-based therapy, for anxiety disorders, 669
Mini-pill. *See* Progestin-only pills (POPs)
Minocycline
    for acne, 261
    for hidradenitis suppurativa, 273
Minoritized, disenfranchised, and marginalized AYAs, 743–748
    clinicians, recommendations to
        future orientation, 748
        medications, 748
        mental health support, 748
        positive youth development/empowering youth, 748
        racism/discrimination, 748
        trauma-informed care, 747–748
    communities and policy makers, recommendations to
        advocacy, 748
        justice initiatives, 749
        strategic investments in adolescent health, 748–749
    definitions and terms, 743
    disenfranchisement, 744
    health care settings, recommendations to, 748
    insurance issues, 747
    neighborhood safety, 747
    nutrition support, 747
    poverty, 743–744
        American Indian/Alaska Native (AI/AN) youth, 744
        Black/African American opportunity youth, 744
    prevalence and demographics, 743–744
    principles and approach to care
        basic material needs, 747
        healthy relationships, 747
        history and review of systems, 745–746
        mental health and behavior screening, 746
        physical assessment, 746
        psychosocial screening, 746–747
        racism/discrimination, 747
        resiliency factors, 747
        school engagement, 747
    racism and discrimination, 744
    risk behaviors and morbidity
        behavioral risk, 744
        education, 744
        mental health, 744
        minority stress and stress proliferation, 745
        trauma, 744–745
    transportation barriers, 747
Minority stress, 745
Minority stress theory, 402
Minors in state custody and consent, 86
Minors, rights of, 85
Minoxidil, for androgenetic alopecia, 273
Mirabegron, for overactive bladder, 309
Mirena IUD, 425, 425t, 432, 459f
    indications for, 462
Misoprostol, 418
Missing data, 135
Mitral valve prolapse (MVP), 188t, 189–190
    complications, 190
    malignant MVP, 190
    management, 190
Mitral valve regurgitation, 190
Mittelschmerz disease syndrome, 426

Model for Improvement, 119–120, 119f. *See also* Quality improvement (QI)
Moderna vaccine, for COVID-19, 329
Modified Atkin diet (MAD), for seizure control, 282
Modified Balance Error Scoring System (mBESS), 250
Molar pregnancy, 416, 419–420
Molluscum bodies, 598
Molluscum contagiosum, 598
　clinical manifestations, 598, 598f
　diagnosis, 598
　epidemiology, 598
　etiology, 598
　follow-up, 598
　HIV infection and, 598, 598f
　treatment, 598, 599t
Molly. *See* Methylenedioxymethamphetamine (MDMA)
Molnupiravir, for COVID-19, 329
Monitoring the Future (MTF), 133t
Monitoring the Future (MTF) survey, 622
　on alcohol use, 615
Monogenetic disorders, and proteinuria, 313–314
Monogenic mutations, and obesity, 355
Mononucleosis, 244
Monosymptomatic enuresis (ME), 306, 307. *See also* Enuresis
Montgomery tubercles, 541
Mood disorders, 106
　in epilepsy, 283
　transgender youth and young adults, 409
　in youth experiencing homelessness, 725
Morbidity
　global, 22, 24f–26f
　health behaviors and, 23, 27, 29
　HIV infections, 29
　mental health and, 23, 29f
　nutritional deficiencies, 27, 29
　obesity/overweight, 27
　sexual and reproductive health, 29
　sexually transmitted infections, 29
　substance use, 23, 27
　United States, 22–23, 24f–26f
Morbilliform drug eruptions, 269
Morning glory seeds, 649
Mortality, 4t, 5, 6f
　causes and number of deaths, 17f, 19f
　global, 16
　global burden of disease causes, 17t
　global risk factors by age group, 16, 21f
　global risk factors by sex, 16, 20f
　high-income countries, 17, 22f
　maternal, 16
　by race and ethnicity, 22, 23t
　suicide and, 17, 22
　trends in mortality rate, 19f
　United States, 17
Motivational enhancement therapy, for alcohol use disorder, 619
Motivational interviewing (MI), 664
　in sleep disorders, 297
　for substance use disorders, 654t
　techniques, 54
Motor vehicle collisions, alcohol-related, 616
Motor vehicle crashes (MVCs), 2, 16
Movement toward independence
　early adolescence, 46
　late adolescence, 47
　middle adolescence, 46–47
　young adults, 48
Moxifloxacin, 535
Mucociliary clearance, disorders of, 208
　cystic fibrosis, 208–210
　primary ciliary dyskinesia, 210

Müllerian anomalies, 514, 517
Müllerian duct remnants, 517, 517f
Müllerian inhibitory factor (MIF), 489, 493
The Multidimensional Anxiety Screen for Children Second Edition (MASC 2), 667
Multiple disabilities, 681t
Multiple-gestation pregnancy, 416
Multiple sleep latency test (MSLT), narcolepsy, 295
Multipurpose Prevention Technologies (MPTs), 439
Multisystem inflammatory syndrome in children (MIS-C), 328, 328t
Mumps orchitis, 536
Mupirocin
　for crusted (nonbullous) impetigo, 268
　for folliculitis, 269
　intranasal, 269
Murmurs, 186
　history, 186
　innocent (normal) murmurs
　　cervical venous hum, 187
　　diagnostic clues, 186
　　pulmonary flow murmur, 187
　　Still's murmur, 187
　　supraclavicular (carotid) bruit, 187
　pathologic murmurs, 187
　　types of, 187t
　physical examination, 186
　with structural heart disease, 187, 188t
　　atrial septal defect, 187, 188t
　　hypertrophic cardiomyopathy, 188t, 189, 189f
　　mitral valve prolapse, 188t, 189–190
　　mitral valve regurgitation, 188t, 190
　　patent ductus arteriosus, 187–188, 188t
　　valvular aortic stenosis, 188–189, 188t
　　valvular pulmonary stenosis, 188, 188t
　　ventricular septal defect, 187, 188t
Muscle relaxants, 644
Musculoskeletal care, 213. *See* Musculoskeletal problems
Musculoskeletal examination, 70
Musculoskeletal pain, 376. *See also* Syndromes of chronic musculoskeletal pain
Musculoskeletal problems, 213–228
　ankle injuries, 216–218
　core, 227
　growth plate disorders, 216
　hip pain, 220–221
　history, 213
　imaging, indications for, 213
　knee injuries and pain syndromes, 218–220
　musculoskeletal problems, by body part, 214t
　physical examination, 213, 215t
　referral to musculoskeletal specialist, indications for, 213–214
　shoulder injuries, 221–223
　spine abnormalities, 223–226
　stress fractures, 227
　treatment and rehabilitation of injuries, 214–216
　　phases of rehabilitation, 215
　　PRICE (Protection, Rest, Ice, Compression, Elevation), 215, 215t
　　return to participation in physical activities, 216
MVP. *See* Mitral valve prolapse (MVP)
Myalgic encephalomyelitis/chronic fatigue syndrome (ME/CFS), 381
　allergic inflammation in, 382
　behavioral Interventions, 384
　definition, 381
　educational accommodations, 384
　epidemiology, 381–382
　etiology, 382

　evaluation, 382–383
　history in, 382–383
　infection and, 382
　in-office passive standing tests, 383
　Institute of Medicine criteria, 381, 382t
　joint hypermobility in, 383, 383f
　laboratory head-up tilt table test, 383
　laboratory studies, 383–384
　mental health and, 382
　nonpharmacologic treatments, 384
　orthostatic intolerance, 382
　outcomes, 386
　pharmacologic treatment, 384–386, 385t
　physical examination, 383
　postural dysfunctions in, 383
　symptoms, 382
　treatment approach, 384
Mycophenolate, for atopic dermatitis, 264
Mycoplasma genitalium, 535, 552–553
Mycoplasma pneumoniae, 324–325
Myopericarditis, 191–193
My Plate site, 78, 78f

N

NAAT. *See* Nucleic acid amplification tests (NAAT)
Nabi-HB, 335
Nabothian cysts, 502
Naftifine, for tinea pedis, 267
Nägele rule, 417
Nail infections, fungal, 267. *See also* Onychomycosis
Naloxone, for opioid overdose, 641, 642
Naltrexone
　for alcohol use disorder, 619
　for fibromyalgia, 379
　for opioid use disorder, 641
Naltrexone combined with bupropion (Contrave), for weight loss, 358, 359t
Nanocoated condoms, 439
Naproxen, for dysmenorrhea, 479, 479t
Naproxen sodium, for dysmenorrhea, 479t
Narcolepsy, 295
　cataplexy, 295
　excessive daytime sleepiness in, 295
　hypnagogic and hypnopompic hallucinations, 295
　sleep attacks, 295
　sleep paralysis, 295
National Alliance to Advance Adolescent Health, 678
National Cancer Institute, 630
National Center for Complementary and Integrative Health (NCCIH), 90
National Center for Health Statistics (NCHS), 90
National College Health Assessment, 707, 709
National Collegiate Athletic Association (NCAA) athletes, 713
National Commission on Correctional Health Care (NCCHC), 734
National Committee for Quality Assurance (NCQA), 62, 125t, 630
National Health and Nutrition Examination Survey (NHANES), 78, 133t, 168
National Health and Nutrition Examination Survey (NHANES III), 38
National Health Interview Survey (NHIS), 134t
National Health Statistics Report (NHSR), 422
National Heart Lung and Blood Institute Asthma Management Program, 206
National Human Immunodeficiency Virus (HIV) Behavioral Surveillance (NHBS), 557
National Immunization Surveys (NIS), 134t
National Institute on Alcohol Abuse and Alcoholism (NIAAA), 652

National Institutes of Health (NIH), 127, 135, 743
National Longitudinal Study of Adolescent to Adult Health (Add Health), 133t
National Longitudinal Surveys (NLS), 134t
National Quality Forum (NQF), 125t
National Survey of Children's Health (NSCH), 134t
National Survey of Children with Special Health Care Needs (NS-CSHCN), 134t
National Survey of Family Growth (NSFG), 134t, 422, 423
National Survey on Drug Use and Health (NSDUH), 134t
  on alcohol use, 615
National Youth Tobacco Survey (NYTS), 622
NCD Risk Factor Collaboration (NCD-RisC), 134t
Needle exchange programs, 343
Neighborhood, 9
Neighborhood safety, 747
Neisseria gonorrhoeae, 535, 555
  antibiotic resistance, 560–561, 561f
  CDC's 2021 STI Treatment Guidelines, 557, 559
  clinical manifestations, 558–559
    Bartholinitis, 559
    cervicitis, 558
    conjunctivitis, 559
    epididymitis, 559
    pelvic inflammatory disease, 558–559
    pharyngitis, 559
    proctitis, 559
    urethritis, 558, 559
  etiology, 555
  expedited partner therapy, 560
  at extragenital sites, 557
  factors contributing to, 557
  female genital urinary tract and, 558–559
  incidence and prevalence, 555–556, 556f
  incubation period, 558
  infection with, 555–561
  male genital urinary tract and, 559
  pathogenesis, 555
  prevention, 561
  reinfection, 555
  retesting, 560
  screening for, 468, 470, 557–558
    guidelines on, 557–558
  special circumstances, 561
  treatment, 559–560
    for pregnant females, 560
Neisseria meningitidis, 72, 591
Neonatal abstinence syndrome, 419
Neonatal herpes, 582
Nephropathy, 165
Nephrotic range proteinuria, 312, 314
Nerve blocks, for headache management, 291, 291t
Neurally mediated hypotension, 382
Neuraminidase inhibitors, for influenza, 327
Neurocardiogenic syncope, 179–181
  diagnostic evaluation, 180
  management, 180, 181f
Neurocognitive maturation, 106
Neurodevelopmental differences, people with, 676, 678. *See also* Neurodevelopmental disorders
Neurodevelopmental disorder associated with prenatal alcohol exposure (ND-PAE), 687. *See also* Fetal alcohol spectrum disorders
Neurodevelopmental disorders, 106, 676–689
  educational support, 680, 681t
    comprehensive educational evaluation, 680

Section 504, 680
  special education, 680
etiologic considerations in, 687
  fetal alcohol spectrum disorders, 687, 688f
  fragile X syndrome, 687–688
  22q11.2 deletion syndrome, 688
evaluation, 676
  clinical interview, 676
  clinician toolkits and screening instruments, 679t
  HEEADSSS neurodevelopmental screening, 677, 678t
  past and current information, 676
  physical examination, 677
  psychosocial assessment, 677
health care delivery
  integrated behavioral health, 678
  medical home, 678
  reproductive health, 678, 680
legal support and planning, 680–682
  disability benefits and financial planning, 680–682
  guardianship and alternatives, 682–683
parents/caregivers and family support, 679–680
prevalence, 677t
prevalent disorders
  attention deficit hyperactivity disorder, 683–685
  autism spectrum disorder, 685
  communication and language disorders, 686
  developmental coordination disorder, 686
  intellectual disability, 686–687
  learning disabilities, 687
Neurodiversity, 683, 686
Neurologic examination, 677
Neurosyphilis, 572. *See also* Syphilis
  diagnosis, 574–575
  treatment, 575–576
New daily persistent headache (NDPH), 286, 288, 291t
Nexplanon, 425–426, 457. *See also* Contraceptive implants; Long-acting reversible contraceptives (LARCs)
  insertion of, 457, 459f
Nickel allergy, 265, 265f
Nicotine
  addiction, 624
  in cigarette, 626
  effects of early exposure to, 624, 626
  modes of action, 626
  pharmacology, 626
  during pregnancy, 419
Nicotine Anonymous, 629
Nicotine replacement products, 628
Nicotine vapes, 622, 628
Nightmares, 295
  and insomnia, 295
  and sleep terrors, 295t
Nine Item ARFID Screen (NIAS), 371
Nipple discharge, 541
Nitrites, 645
Nitrous oxide, 645
Nocturnal polyuria, 307
Nodules, acne, 257
Noncardiovascular syncope, 182–183
Nonceliac gluten sensitivity (NCGS), 392
Noncommunicable diseases (NCDs), 105
Nongonococcal urethritis (NGU), 301, 535
Nonmelanoma skin cancers (NMSCs), 274
Nonmonosymptomatic enuresis (NME), 306. *See also* Enuresis
Nonnarcotic central nervous system depressants, 642–644. *See also* Barbiturates, Benzodiazepines, Gamma-Hydroxybutyrate, Baclofen

Nonrapid eye movement (NREM) sleep, 293
Nonsteroidal anti-inflammatory drugs (NSAIDs), 215
  for dysmenorrhea, 479, 479t
  for erythema nodosum, 272
  for headache management, 291t
Nonstimulant medications, in ADHD, 685
Nonsuicidal self-injury (NSSI), 671, 672
Nontreponemal antibody tests, 573
Nontropical sprue. *See* Celiac disease
Nontuberculous mycobacterial (NTB) infection, 274
Nonverbal communication, 54
Noonan syndrome, 140, 189
Norethindrone acetate, for dysmenorrhea, 480
Norplant, 425
North Carolina School of Science and Mathematics, 748–749
Not in employment, education, or training (NEET), 4t, 8
Not On Tobacco (NOT) Teen Smoking and Vaping Cessation program, 629
Nucleic acid amplification tests (NAAT), 508, 535
  bacterial vaginosis, 509
  in COVID-19, 329
  for *N. gonorrhoeae* and *C. trachomatis* screening, 558
  Trichomonas vaginalis, 511
  vaginal swab, 468
  vulvovaginal candidiasis, 510
Nucleus accumbens (NAc), 640
Nummular eczema, 268, 269
Nurse Family Partnership, 612
Nutmeg (*Myristica fragrans*), 649
Nutraceuticals, for headache management, 290
Nutrition, 78
  adolescents and, 27, 29
  anthropometric measurements, 79–80
  assessment, 79–81
  athletes and, 82–83
  and bone mass, 41
  carbohydrates, 80
  deficiency, clinical signs of, 79t
  dietary data, 79
  2015–2020 Dietary Guidelines for Americans, 78
  energy needs and, 80
  fat, 80–81
  guidelines, 82–83
  laboratory tests for status assessment, 80
  lactose intolerance, 82
  minerals, 81
    calcium, 81
    iron, 81
    zinc, 81
  My Plate site, 78, 78f
  during pregnancy, 81t, 82, 419
  problems, 78–79
  protein requirements, 80
  recommended dietary allowances, 80, 80t, 81t
  requirements, 80
  risk factors, 78–79
  screening for, 79
  special conditions, 82–83
  vegetarian diets, 82
  vitamin requirements, 81
Nutritional counseling, 78, 82
Nutritional rehabilitation, in anorexia nervosa, 367–368
NuvaRing, 427
Nylen–Bárány test, 183

O

Obesity, 4t, 27, 106, 354, *See also* Overweight
  bariatric surgery, 360–361, 360f
  body mass index (BMI), 354
  definition of, 354
  dietary interventions, 357–358
  environmental and behavioral risk factors, 354–355
  epidemiology, 354, 355t
  exercise and activity recommendations, 358
  genetic risk factors, 355
  health risks of, 355–357, 357f
  hormonal causes, 355
  and hypertension, 196, 198
  inactivity and, 230
  and macromastia, 540
  medical evaluation, 358t
  medications associated with, 355, 356t
  pathogenesis, 354–355
  prevention of, 357
  psychosocial support, 358
  and puberty, 356
  racial and ethnic differences, 354
  screening tests for, 70–71
  severe, 354
  sleep recommendations, 358
  syndromic, 355
  tertiary interventions, 358–361
  transgender youth and young adults, 410
  treatment of, 357–358
    avoiding bias in, 357
    in primary care setting, 357–358
  weight-loss medications, 358–360, 359f, 359t
  weight management programs, 358
Obstructive lesions, acne, 256, 256f
Obstructive sleep apnea (OSA), 295
Office setup
  appointments, 51
  clinic staff, 51
  educational materials availability, 51
  electronic health records, 51
  sensitive services, billing for, 51
  space, 51
Office visits, 50–54
  comfort with adolescents and young adults, 50
  electronic health records, 51
  general guidelines for, 50–54
  initial visit, 50
    with adolescent alone, 50
    with adolescent and parent together, 50
    with parent alone, 50
    summarizing, 51
  interview structure, 51–54
  meeting adolescent and family, 50
  reason for, 54
  recommendations to parents, 55–56
  setup of office, 51
  young adult visit, 51
Olanzapine, for weight gain, 367
Online gaming, 101
Online-only friends, 99
Onychomycosis, 267
  clinical manifestations, 267
  differential diagnosis, 267
  subungual, 267, 267f
  superficial white, 267
  treatment, 267
Opioid receptors, 641
Opioids, 641–642
  administration routes, 641
  adverse effects, 642
  chronic use, 642
  intoxication, effects of, 641
  medical use, 641
  overdose and emergency treatment, 642

  physiology and metabolism, 641
  preparation and dose, 641
  synthetic, 641
  tolerance and withdrawal, 642
Opioid use disorder, 602, 608
Opioid use, in young adults, 608–609
Opium, 641. *See also* Opioids
Opportunity youth, 743
Opt-out model, 629
Oral contraceptives, 450–451, 451t
  combined oral contraceptives, 451
  missed pill rules, 450, 451t
  for orthostatic intolerance, 385t
  progestin-only pills, 450–451
Oral estrogen, 147
Oral glucose tolerance test (OGTT), 160
Oral human papillomavirus, 584
Oral iron therapy, 485
Oral sex, 397–398
  National Survey of Family Growth (NSFG), 398
Oral warts, 588–589
Orchitis, 536
Organic disorders, 388
  tests for, 392
Organisation for Economic Co-Operation and Development (OECD) countries, 4t
  morbidity in, 22, 27f, 28f
  mortality rates, 17, 22f
Orlistat, for weight loss, 358, 359t
Oropharyngeal infection, 560
Orphanhood, 9–10
Ortho Evra patch, 427
Orthopedic impairment (OH), 681t
Orthostatic hypotension, 181
Orthostatic intolerance, 382, 383
  medications for, 385t
  treatment of, 384
Orthostatic or benign positional proteinuria, 313
Oseltamivir, for influenza, 327
Osgood–Schlatter disease, 70, 216, 219–220
OSOM BVBlue, 509
Osteochondritis dissecans (OCD), 218, 220
Osteomyelitis, 257
Osteopathic manipulative treatment (OMT), 95
Other health impairment (OHI), 681t
Ottawa ankle rules, 216, 217f
Ottawa knee rules, 218–219
Outcome measures, 119
Out-of-home care
  epidemiology, 729–730
    emancipating youth, 729
    general out-of-home care statistics, 729
    health and associated problems, 729–730
  health assessments and treatment, 730
    behavioral health, 730
    comprehensive assessment, 730
    follow-up assessment and ongoing care, 730
    immunizations, 730
    initial assessment, 730
    laboratory studies, 730
  recommendations
    care delivery and coordination, 731
    confidentiality, 731
    consent for treatment, 731
    educating parents/caregivers, 731
    empowering youth, 731–732
    engaging families of origin, 731
    establishing medical record, 731
    monitoring medication use, 731
    out-of-home health clinics, 731
    positive youth development approach, 731
    postemancipation, 731
    relationship with child welfare agency, 731

  special considerations
    consent and confidentiality issues, 730
    cultural issues, 731
    health history taking, barriers to, 730
    inaccurate and missing records, 730
    medication management, 730–731
    parents/caregivers, challenges for, 731
    systems of care issues, 730
  youth in and emancipated from, 729–732
Outpatient treatment, for substance use disorders, 655t
Ovarian cancer, 523–524
  combined hormonal contraceptives in, 452
  genetic risk of, 523
  incidence, 523
  malignant epithelial tumors, 523
  malignant germ cell tumors, 523
Ovarian cyst, 519–521, 520f
Ovarian masses
  benign, 514t, 519–522
    benign ovarian neoplasms, 521–522
    endometriomas and endometriosis, 521
    functional ovarian cysts, 519–521
  malignant, 523–524
  minimizing risks of, 523–524
Ovarian neoplasms, benign, 521–522, 521f
  benign epithelial neoplasia, 522, 522f
  benign germ cell tumors, 521–522, 522f
  sex cord–stromal tumors, 522, 523f
Ovarian torsion, 518, 518f
Overactive bladder (OAB), 307, 309. *See also* Enuresis
Overflow proteinuria, 312, 313t, 314
Overuse injuries, 246
Overweight, 4t, 27, 106, 354. *See also* Obesity
  screening tests for, 70–71
Ovulation, 475
Ovulation inhibition, 426, 427, 434. *See also* Contraception
Oxcarbazepine, for seizure treatment, 281t
Oxybutynin, for overactive bladder, 309
Oxycodone, 641. *See also* Opioids
Oxycontin, 608, 641. *See also* Opioids

P

PA. *See* Physical activity (PA)
Pachyonychia congenita, 267
Pain amplification. *See* Amplified musculoskeletal pain syndrome (AMPS)
Pain counseling/therapy, for headache management, 290
Pain, dysmenorrhea, 477–480
Palliative care. *See also* Life-limiting conditions (LLCs)
  bereavement supports, 116–117
  concept of, 112, 112t
  decision making and advance care planning, 115–116
  definition of, 112
  end-of-life care, 116
  goal of, 112
  introduction of, 114–115, 115t
  multidisciplinary team approach, 112–113
  service provision and resources, 115
  symptom management in, 115
  teams, 113–115
  transition to adult health care system, 116
Palpitations, 182
Pancolitis, 391
Pancreatic enzyme replacement therapy (PERT), 209
Panel Study of Income Dynamics (PSID), 134t
Panic attacks, 668
  expected, 668
  unexpected, 668
Panic disorder, 667t, 668

Panniculitis, 271. *See also* Erythema nodosum (EN)
Pansexual, 401
Papaver somniferum, 641
Papillary thyroid cancer (PTC), 152–154
Pap smear screening, 70
Pap test (Papanicolaou test), 468, 469, 470
Papular warts, 585, 585f
Papules, acne, 256, 256f
Papulosquamous diseases, 269
    pityriasis rosea, 269
    psoriasis, 269–270
Paragard, 425, 425t, 431–432, 457, 458, 458t
Parasitic infections, screening refugees and immigrants for, 740
Parasomnias, 295
    nightmares, 295
    sleep terrors, 295–296, 295t
    sleepwalking, 295–296
Paratubal cysts, 517, 517f
Parenchymatous neurosyphilis, 572
Parental advice, 55
Parental alcohol use, 616
Parenting, 420
Parenting styles, impact of, 55
Parents
    of adolescents, recommendations to, 55–56
    authoritative, 55
    of AYAs with chronic health conditions, 108, 109
    consent of, 86
    health guidance to, 58–59
    proactive, 55
Paroxetine, 367, 664, 664t
    for PMDD, 482, 482t
Partial fetal alcohol syndrome, 687. *See also* Fetal alcohol spectrum disorders
Partial hospital program, for substance use disorders, 655t
Participatory research, 130
Partnered masturbation, 397
    2015 National Sexual Exploration in America Study, 397
Partner management, 551–552
Past medical history, 67
Patellofemoral pain (PFP), 218, 219
Patent ductus arteriosus, 187–188, 188t
Pathobiological Determinants of Atherosclerosis in Youth (PDAY) study, 171
Pathologic murmurs, 187, 187t
Patient
    approach to, 54–55
    interview challenges, 54
    nonverbal interaction, 54
Patient-centered care, 165–166
Patient-delivered partner treatment, 552
Patient Health Questionnaire (PHQ), 135, 662
Patient Health Questionnaire (PHQ-2), 66
Patient Health Questionnaire (PHQ-9), 51, 66
Patient portal, 66
Patient Protection and Affordable Care Act (ACA) of 2010, 60, 62
Patient–provider rapport, 52
Patient-Reported Outcomes Measurement Information System (PROMIS), 135
    PROMIS Pediatric measures, 135
Patients assigned-female-at-birth, preventive care for, 68
Paver nocturnus. *See* Sleep terrors
Paxlovid, in COVID-19, 329
Payment, 85, 88
PCD. *See* Primary ciliary dyskinesia (PCD)
PCOS. *See* Polycystic ovary syndrome (PCOS)
Peak weight velocity (PWV), 41
Pectus excavatum, 207–208
    Haller index, 208
    identification, 208, 208f

    management, 208
    Nuss procedure, 208
    open Ravitch procedure, 208
    symptoms, 208
    vacuum bell, 208
PEDIARIX, for hepatitis B, 335
Pediatric diabetes screening, 498
Pediatric Health Information System (PHIS), 134t
Pediatric Research in Office Settings (PROS) study, 37–38
Pediculosis pubis, 594–596
    clinical manifestations, 595
    diagnosis, 595, 595f
    epidemiology, 594–595
    etiology, 594, 595f
    management considerations, 595–596
    transmission, 594
    treatment, 595, 596t
Peer group
    early adolescence, 46
    late adolescence, 47
    middle adolescence, 47
    young adults, 48
Peers, influence of, 10
Peer support, 107, 113
Pegylated-interferon-α (IFN), for HCV treatment, 337
Pelvic examination
    dysmenorrhea, 479
    in pregnancy, 417
Pelvic inflammatory disease (PID), 349, 563–567
    abdominal/pelvic pain, 563, 564
    chlamydial and gonorrheal infections and, 558–559, 563, 564
    complications, 558–559
    differential diagnosis, 564t
    ectopic pregnancy, 564
    epidemiology, 563
    etiology, 563
    evaluation and diagnosis, 564–565
        CDC diagnostic criteria, 565t
    hospitalization in, 565–566
    infertility, 564
    microbiology, 564
    pathogenesis, 564
    PEACH study, 563, 564
    in pregnancy, 565
    presentation, 564
    prevention, 567
        primary, 567
        secondary, 567
        tertiary, 567
    risk factors, 563
    sequelae, 566
    signs of, 558
    subclinical, 564
    treatment, 560, 565–566, 566t
Pelvic kidney, 517, 517f
Pelvic masses, 514–524
    adnexal torsion, 518
    conditions diagnosed as, 514t
    congenital anomalies, 515–517
        müllerian duct remnants, 517, 517f
        urachal cysts and pelvic kidneys, 517, 517f
        uterine defects, incomplete lateral fusion, 515–517, 515f–517f
        uterovaginal agenesis, 517
    infection as cause of, 517–518
    malignant ovarian masses, 523–524
    management of, 519f
    ovarian masses, 514t, 519–522
    pregnancy presenting as, 517
    uterine neoplasms, 519

Pelvic pain
    ectopic pregnancy, 525–526
    pelvic inflammatory disease, 559, 563
Pelvic ultrasound, 558, 565
Penicillin, for syphilis treatment, 575
Penile-anal sex, 398
    2015 National Sexual Exploration in America Study, 398
    National Survey of Family Growth (NSFG), 398
Penile intraepithelial neoplasia (PeIN), 584
Penile-vaginal sex, 398
    2015 National Sexual Exploration in America Study, 398
    National Survey of Family Growth (NSFG), 398
People with epilepsy (PWE), 277. *See also* Epilepsy; Seizures
Perampanel
    mood and behavior disturbances by, 283
    for seizure treatment, 281t
Perceptions of racism in children and youth (PRaCY), 747
Percutaneous electrical nerve stimulation, for abdominal pain, 393
Perihepatitis, 558–559, 563, 564
Perimolysis, 369
Periorificial dermatitis, 257
Peripheral α-antagonists, for hypertension, 201t
Peritonitis, 564
Permethrin 1% cream, for pediculosis pubis, 596t
Permethrin cream 5%, for scabies, 597t
Persistent depression, 662
Persistent postconcussive symptoms (PPCS), 252
Pertussis, 325–326
    catarrhal stage, 325
    clinical manifestations, 325
    control measures, 326
    convalescent stage, 325
    diagnosis, 326
    differential diagnosis, 326
    epidemiology, 325
    etiology, 325
    immunization, 326
    laboratory evaluation
        complete blood count, 326
        culture, 326
        nucleic acid amplification tests, 326
        serologic testing, 326
    management, 326
    paroxysmal stage, 325
    transmission, 325
Peyote, 649
Pfizer-BioNTech vaccine, for COVID-19, 329
Pharmatex, 444
Pharyngitis, *N. gonorrhoeae* and *C. trachomatis* infection, 559
Phencyclidine (PCP), 646–647
    adverse effects, 646, 647t
    intoxication, effects of, 646, 646t
    medical use, 646
    overdose and emergency treatment, 646
        medication, 647
        recovery, 647
        reduction of stimuli, 646
        supportive care, 646–647
    physiology and metabolism, 646
    preparation and dose, 646
Phenobarbital, for seizure treatment, 281t
Phentermine combined with topiramate (Qsymia), for weight loss, 358, 359t
Phentermine, for weight loss, 360
Phenytoin, for seizure treatment, 281t
Phobias, 667

Photosensitivity eruptions, 272
    photoallergic, 272
    phototoxic reactions, 272
Phyllodes tumors, 544
Physical activity (PA). *See also* Preparticipation
        physical evaluation (PPE); Sports
        participation
    barriers and predictors of participation,
        230–231
        puberty and bone maturation, 231
    benefits of, 230
    clinicians' roles in promoting of, 230–231
    defined, 229
    electronic active gaming, 230
    epidemiology, 229
    evaluation, considerations in, 242–245
        attention deficit hyperactivity disorder,
            244
        blood-borne pathogens, 244–245
        cardiovascular considerations, 242–243
        COVID-19 screening, 245
        eating disorders and energy deficiency,
            242, 242t
        mental health considerations, 244
        micronutrients, supplements, and fluids,
            243–244, 243t
        mononucleosis, 244
        sport-related concussion, 244
    exercise prescription, 231–232
    guidance for clinicians, 231
    high-intensity interval training, 230
    intensity, 229
    light activity, 229
    medical eligibility for, 241
    moderate activity, 229
    moderate to vigorous physical activity
        (MVPA), 229, 230
    and nutrition, 78
    2018 Physical Activity Guidelines, 230
    during pregnancy, 245
    promoting inclusion for all AYAs in, 245
    recommendations for, 230, 230t
    resistance training and flexibility, 230
    safe activity, promotion of, 231
    sedentary activity, 229
    and sports participation, 229–247
    vigorous activity, 229
    as vital sign, 232
Physical examination, 53, 69
    abdomen, 70
    cardiopulmonary, 70
    chest, 70
    genital examination, 70
    in HIV infection, 347–348
    musculoskeletal, 70
    neck, 70
    neurologic, 70
    in pregnancy, 417
    sexual maturity rating, 70
    skin, 70
    teeth and gums, 70
Physical fitness (PF), 229
    components of, 229
Physical privacy, 129
Physical therapy, for headache management,
    290
Piaget's cognitive theory, 46
Pica, ARFID, and Rumination Disorder
    Interview (PARDI), 371
PID. *See* Pelvic inflammatory disease (PID)
Piercing, 274–275
    complications of, 275
    and infections, 275
    scarring due to, 275
    sensitivity to jewelry, 275
Pimecrolimus, for atopic dermatitis, 264

Pituitary/hypothalamic-gonadotropin
    insufficiency, 489
Pityriasis alba, 263
Pityriasis rosea (PR), 265, 269
    clinical manifestations, 269
    differential diagnosis, 269
    herald patch, 269
    oval plaques with scale on trunk, 269f
    in persons of color, 269
    treatment, 269
Pityrosporum folliculitis, 258
Plan-do-study-act (PDSA) cycle, 122–123, 123f
Planned Parenthood, 100
Plantar warts, 268
Plants, contact dermatitis due to, 264, 264f
Plant sterols, 172
Plecanatide, for constipation, 393
PMDs. *See* Premenstrual disorders (PMDs)
PMS. *See* Premenstrual syndrome (PMS)
Pneumococcal vaccine, 348
Pneumonia, community-acquired, 324–325
Podophyllotoxin, in molluscum contagiosum,
    599t
Point-of-care tests (POCTs), 508, 552
Poison ivy and contact dermatitis, 264, 264f
Poland syndrome, 540, 540f
Polio vaccine, 73
Polycystic ovaries, 495–496, 497
Polycystic ovary syndrome (PCOS), 484, 488,
    494–498
    anovulation in, 495
    cancer risk with, 496
    cardiovascular disease risk, 497
    clinical consequences, 495–497
    definition, 494–495
    diagnosis, 497
        criteria used in, 495
    differential diagnosis, 497
    disorder of hypothalamic– pituitary–ovarian
        system, 494
    epilepsy and, 282
    etiology, 495
    factors for development of, 495
    genetic factor in, 495
    hirsutism in, 495, 496
    hyperandrogenism in, 495, 496, 496f
    hyperinsulinemia in, 495
    impaired glucose tolerance and diabetes risk,
        497
    and infertility, 496
    insulin resistance and hyperinsulinemia,
        496–497
    lipoprotein profile elevated in, 496
    obesity and, 357, 496
    ovaries in, 495–496
    pathophysiology, 495
    prevalence, 494
    Rotterdam criteria, 495
    therapy, 497–498
        for hirsutism, 497
        for metabolic abnormalities, 498
Polyethylene glycol (PEG), 393
Polymastia, 539
Polymerase chain reaction (PCR), 574
    Mycoplasma infection, 325
    pertussis, 326
Polythelia, 539
Pomade acne, 257
Poppers, 645
POPs. *See* Progestin-only pills (POPs)
Population age structure, 11
    Brazil, 14f
    China, 13f
    France, 12f
    Germany, 12f
    global, 11f

    India, 15f
    Indonesia, 15f
    Mexico, 14f
    Nigeria, 16f
    Pakistan, 15f
    Russia, 13f
    South Africa, 14f
    United Kingdom, 12f
    United States, 13f
Population health management, 66
Postconcussion syndrome (PCS), 252
Postexposure prophylaxis, for HIV, 345, 551
Postpartum thyroid disorders, 157
Posttest counseling, HIV test, 344–345
Post-transplant lymphoproliferative disorder,
    322–323
Post-traumatic headache, 288, 291t. *See also*
    Headaches
Posttraumatic stress disorder (PTSD),
    marginalized AYAs and, 745
Postural orthostatic tachycardia syndrome
    (POTS), 181, 382
Postural proteinuria, 313
Potassium hydroxide aqueous solution, in
    molluscum contagiosum, 599t
Potassium hydroxide preparation, 508
Potassium iodide, for erythema nodosum, 272
Poverty, 2, 5, 9, 743–744
    adolescent and unplanned pregnancy, 413
    minoritized youth in, 744
    opportunity youth in, 744
PPE. *See* Preparticipation physical evaluation
    (PPE)
Prader–Willi syndrome, 140, 144
Prebiotics, 83, 393
Precocious puberty, 148–149
    causes, 148–149
    definition, 148
    history, 149
    incomplete forms
        premature adrenarche, 149
        premature thelarche, 149
    laboratory evaluation, 149
    physical examination, 149
    treatment, 149
Prediabetes, 160, 162f
Prednisone, for erythema nodosum, 272
Preexposure prophylaxis (PrEP), for HIV, 346,
    551
    in adolescents and young adults, 346–347
    injectable, 346
    lab monitoring, 346
    oral regimens for, 346
Pregabalin
    for fibromyalgia, 379
    for seizure treatment, 281t
Pregnancy, 396, 413–421
    adoption, 420
    among AYA females, 29
    asymptomatic bacteriuria during, 302
    and birth rates, trends in, 413, 414f
    cervical softening, 417
    child outcomes, 420
    in chronically ill patients, 419
    complications, 419–420
        ectopic pregnancy, 419
        hydatidiform mole, 419–420
        spontaneous abortion, 419
    counseling, 416, 417
    ectopic, 525–529
    education and socioeconomic issues, 420
    epilepsy and, 282
    evaluation and management, 413, 416–417
        common presentations of pregnancy,
            416
        gestational age, 417

practitioner, role of, 416
  pregnancy tests, 416–417
expected date of delivery, 417
factors contributing to, 413–415
  behavioral health, 414
  contraception, lack of access to, 414–415
  cultural and family values, 413–414
  early puberty and development, 414
  physical and sexual abuse, 413
  poverty, 413
  sexual activity rates, 413
and family-centered care for mother and newborn, 420
fundal height corresponding to gestational age, 518f
growth and development, 420
HAV infection, 333
hepatitis B during, 335
hepatitis C in, 338
hepatitis E in, 339
male AYA as father, 420
medical management, 418–419
nutrition during, 81t, 82
pelvic examination, 417
pelvic mass and, 517
prevention interventions, 413, 415–416
rates, 413, 414f
repeat, 415, 420
signs, 417
termination, 417–418
tests, 416–417
transgender youth and young adults, 410
Trichomonas vaginalis treatment in, 512
ultrasound in, 417
unplanned, 413
uterine enlargement, 415f, 417
Pregnancy kits, 416
Prehn sign, 532
Premarin pill, 493
Premature ovarian insufficiency, 489
  and amenorrhea, 489, 490
Premenstrual disorders (PMDs), 480–483
  approach to treatment of, 482–483
  clinical manifestations, 480
  core PMD, 481
  diagnosis, 480–481
  emotional symptoms, 480
  epidemiology, 480
  2011 International Society for Premenstrual Disorders (ISPMD) on, 481, 482
  pathophysiology, 480
  physical symptoms, 480
  risk factors, 480
  therapy, 481–482
    anxiolytics and antidepressants, 482
    nonpharmacologic/complementary medicine, 481
    prostaglandin inhibitors, 482
    selective serotonin reuptake inhibitors, 482, 482t
    spironolactone, 482
    suppression of ovulation, 481–482
  variant PMD, 481
Premenstrual dysphoric disorder (PMDD), 452, 477, 480, 481. See also Premenstrual disorders (PMDs)
Premenstrual Symptoms Screening Tool (PSST), 481
Premenstrual syndrome (PMS), 452, 477, 480. See also Premenstrual disorders (PMDs)
Premenstrual Tension Syndrome Rating Scale, 481
Prenatal care, 418–419
Prenatal visits, 419
Preparticipation examination, 184

Preparticipation physical evaluation (PPE), 232–242
  diagnostic tests and laboratory evaluation, 241
  effectiveness of, 242
  goals and context of, 232–233
  history, 233
    The Monograph's PPE History Form, 234f–235f
  medical eligibility for physical activity, 241
  medical–legal issues in exclusion from sports participation, 241–242
    The Monograph's Medical Eligibility Form, 242
  physical examination, 233, 235, 240–241
    The Monograph's PPE Physical Examination Form, 236f
Pretest counseling, HIV test, 344
Prevalence, 4t
Prevention
  of CVD (See Cardiovascular health)
  of youth violence, 693–694
The Prevention Access Campaign, 347
Prevention of HIV, 345–347
  behavioral prevention, 347
  educational intervention, 347
  postexposure prophylaxis, 345
  preexposure prophylaxis, 346
    in adolescents and young adults, 346–347
    injectable, 346
    lab monitoring, 346
    oral regimens, 346
  primary biomedical prevention, 345–347
  risk reduction counseling, 347
  secondary biomedical prevention, 347
Preventive counseling, 74–76. See also Preventive health counseling
Preventive health care, 58–76
  access to, 63
  barriers to, 63
  clinical guidelines, 58
    for adolescents, 58–59, 59–60t
    for young adults, 59–60, 61–62t
  clinical settings for, 64
  counseling, 58, 74–76
  digital health, 64–66
    benefits of technology use, 66
    electronic health record, 64–66
    technology domains, 66
  evidence-based clinical preventive services, 63t
  health care transitions, 76
  immunizations, 71–74
    catch-up vaccines, 74
    consent for vaccination, 74
    human papillomavirus, 71–72
    influenza vaccine, 72–73
    meningococcal vaccine, 71
    SARS-CoV-2 vaccines, 73–74
    schedule, 71–72, 72t, 73t
    vaccine delivery, improving, 74
  improving preventive service delivery, 63–64
  preventive services and insurance coverage in United States, 60, 62–63
  telemedicine services, 64
  training and screening tools, 64
  visit, 66–71
    blood pressure, 69
    hearing screening, 69
    height, weight, and BMI calculation, 69
    history in, 67–69
    physical examination, 69–70
    questionnaires and screening tools, 66–67
    screening tests, 70–71
    stage for preventive care, setting, 66, 67t

vision screening, 69
  vital signs, 69
Preventive health counseling, 75–76. See also Preventive counseling
  approaches to, 75–76
  brief office-based intervention model, 75
  Guidelines for Adolescent Preventive Services (GAPS), 75
    A (assess further), 75
    G (gather initial information), 75
    P (problem identification), 75
    S (specific solutions), 76
Preventive health guidelines, 58
  for adolescents, 58–59, 59–60t
  for young adults, 59–60, 61–62t
Previsit questionnaires, 51–52
  in EHR, 65–66, 65f
Previsit screeners, in EHR, 66
PRICE (Protection, Rest, Ice, Compression, Elevation), 215, 215t, 219, 222
Primary amenorrhea, 488, 491f. See also Amenorrhea
Primary ciliary dyskinesia (PCD), 210
Primary data collection, 132
Primary enuresis, 306. See also Enuresis
Primary headache, 286–288, 287t. See also Headaches
Primary human papillomavirus testing with reflex testing, 504
Primary ovarian insufficiency, 488–490
Primary syphilis, 570. See also Syphilis
  diagnosis, 574
  differential diagnosis, 572
  treatment, 575
  ulcer characteristics, 570–571, 570f
Privacy, 128
  breach of, 128, 129
  informational, 128
  physical, 129
  psychological, 129
  of research information, 128–129
Privacy and safety, for study participant, 128–129
Probiotics, 83, 393
Problematic and Risky Internet Use Screening Scale
  PRIUSS-3, 103
  PRIUSS-18, 103
Problematic Internet use (PIU), 101, 103
Process map, 120–122
  of pediatric emergency admissions, 122f
Process measures, 119–120
Proctitis, 391, 406, 559, 560, 561
Proctocolitis, 406, 559
Proctosigmoiditis, 391
Progesterone, 475
Progesterone vaginal rings, 427
Progesterone withdrawal test, 493
Progestin-only contraceptives. See Progestin-only pills (POPs)
Progestin-only injectables, 450
Progestin-only pills (POPs), 425, 427–428, 449, 450
  advantages, 428
  availability, 427
Progestins, mechanisms of action, 450
Prolactin, 497, 541, 542f
Prolactinomas, 143, 542
  classification of
    macroadenomas, 542
    microadenomas, 542
  monitoring of, 543
  treatment of, 542–543
Prophylactic treatment, headache and, 290, 291t
Propionibacterium acnes, 256

Propranolol, for orthostatic intolerance, 385t
Prostaglandin inhibitors, for PMS, 482
Prostaglandins, dysmenorrhea and, 477
Prostatitis, 303, 304t
Prostitution, 697
Protectaid, 444
Protective factors
  suicide, 673
  against youth violence, 692
Protein, 80
  requirements, 80
  supplements, 83
Proteinuria, 312
  causes of, 313–314
  definition, 312
  epidemiology, 313
  factitious, 313t
  fixed, 313–314, 313t
  glomerular, 313–314, 313t
  history and physical examination, 314
  laboratory testing, 314
  low-molecular-weight (LMW), 312
  nephrotic range, 312, 314
  overflow, 312, 313t, 314
  pathophysiology, 312, 313t
  persistent asymptomatic, 312
  postural, 313
  prognosis, 314
  screening, 312
  transient, 313, 313t
  in urine of AYAs, 312
Proton-pump inhibitors, in dyspepsia, 393
Pseudomonas aeruginosa, 208
  hot tub folliculitis by, 268
Pseudosyncope, 182–183
Psilocybin, 648
Psoriasis, 267, 269–270
  Auspitz sign, 270
  clinical manifestations, 269–270, 270f
  erythematous scaling papules and plaques in, 269, 270f
  Koebner phenomenon, 270
  treatment, 270
Psychiatric disorders, 106
Psychoactive substances, 637–649
  amphetamine, 639–640
  anabolic–androgenic steroids, 649
  baclofen, 644
  barbiturates, 642–643
  benzodiazepines, 643–644, 643t
  cocaine, 637–639
  dextromethorphan, 648
  dimethyltryptamine, 649
  gamma-hydroxybutyrate (GHB), 644
  hallucinogens, 645–649
  inhalants, 644–645, 644t, 645t
  Jimson weed, 648
  ketamine, 647
  D-lysergic acid diethylamide, 647–648
  mescaline, 649
  methylenedioxymethamphetamine, 640–641
  morning glory seeds, 649
  muscle relaxants, 644
  nitrites, 645
  nitrous oxide, 645
  nonnarcotic central nervous system depressants, 642–644
  nutmeg, 649
  opioids, 641–642
  peyote, 649
  phencyclidine, 646–647
  psilocybin, 648
  salvia, 649
Psychoeducation
  anxiety and anxiety disorders, 668
  depression treatment, 663

Psychogenic nonepileptic events (PNEE), convulsive, 279, 279t
Psychogenic syncope, 182–183
Psychological disorders, and fatigue, 381
Psychological distress, 114
  genital herpes and, 582
  marginalized and minoritized youth, 744
  somatic symptoms with, 375
Psychological needs, 113
Psychological privacy, 129
Psychological trauma, 745
Psychopharmacology
  anxiety disorders, 669
  depression, 664–665
Psychosocial development
  in adolescents and young adults, 45–48
  early adolescent, 46
  late adolescent, 47
  middle adolescent, 46–47
  young adults, 47–48
Psychosocial history, 68, 68t
Psychosocial support, 113
Psychotherapy
  for anxiety disorders, 668–669
  for depression, 663–664
  to reduce suicide reattempts, 674
Psychotropic medications, for AYAs with eating disorders, 367
Pthirus pubis, 594
Pubarche, 36, 474
Pubertal delay, anorexia nervosa and, 364
Puberty, 106, 138
  and alcohol use, 616
  breast asymmetry, 540
  breast development, 539
  delayed, 140–148
  female breast development, 37f
  female pubertal changes, 37–38
  female pubic hair development, 36f
  first sign, 474
  genetic influences on timing of, 36
  growth hormone axis and growth, 39, 40f
  growth hormone during, 39
  hypothalamic–pituitary–adrenal axis and, 35, 35f
  hypothalamic–pituitary–gonadal axis and, 35, 35f
  male genital and pubic hair development, 37f
  male pubertal changes, 38–39
  obesity and, 356
  origins of, 36
  physical growth during, 39–43
    body composition, 41, 43t
    body mass index, 42
    final height, prediction of, 40–41
    genetic influences on, 40–41
    height velocity, 39–40, 40f, 41f
    lean body mass, 41
    skeletal mass, 41–42
    weight growth, 41
  physical manifestations of, 36–39
  precocious, 148–149
  sexual maturity rating scales, 36–37, 36f, 37f
  type 2 diabetes during, 160
Puberty blockers, 408
Pubic lice. *See* Pediculosis pubis
Public health model, 693–694, 693f
Pulmonary flow murmur, 187
Pulse dye laser, in molluscum contagiosum, 599t
Purified protein derivative (PPD) tuberculin skin test, 70
Pustules, acne, 256f, 257
Pyelonephritis, 303
Pyosalpinx, 564
Pyrethrins with piperonyl butoxide, for pediculosis pubis, 596t

Pyridostigmine bromide, for orthostatic intolerance, 385t

Q
Qbrexa, for hyperhidrosis, 273
Q Chat Space, 404
Qi, 94
Qualitative studies, 131t
Quality health services, for AYAs with chronic health conditions, 107–110
Quality improvement (QI), 118
  in adolescent and young adult health, 124t, 125, 125t
  clinical importance of, 118–119
  displaying QI data, 123–124, 123f
  elements of quality care, 118
  in health care, 118
  identifying opportunities for, 119
  methods in practice, 119
  Model for Improvement, 119–120, 119f
  plan-do-study-act cycle, 122–123, 123f
  research and, differences between, 124–125
  stakeholder participation, 120–122
Quality indicators, 118
Quality, in health care, 118
Quality problems, 120–121
QuantiFERON, 70
Quantitative β-hCG immunoassay, 416
Quantitative β-hCG levels, 526–527
Queer, 401
Questionnaire of Pediatric Gastrointestinal Symptoms-Rome IV (QPGS-IV) to, 388
Questionnaires, previsit, 51–52
Quick Start (Same Day Start), 449
Quiet patient, 54

R
Race-related stress, 744
Racism, 743
  and discrimination, 744
  and health status, 9
Raltegravir, for HIV infection, 345
Rape, 696. *See also* Sexual violence (SV)
Rapid eye movement (REM) sleep, 293
Rapid human immunodeficiency virus testing, 344
Rapid Plasma Reagin (RPR), 573
Reactive Arthritis Triad (RAT), 559
Recidivism, 736
Recombivax HB, for hepatitis B, 335
Recommended dietary allowance (RDA), 80, 80t
Rectal douching, 557
Recurrent abdominal pain, 390t
Recurrent respiratory papillomatosis (RRP), 584
RED-S. *See* Relative energy deficiency in sport (RED-S)
RED-S Clinical Assessment Tool, 242
Refeeding syndrome, 368
Reflex sympathetic dystrophy (RSD), 377. *See also* Complex regional pain syndrome (CRPS)
Refugees, 738. *See also* Immigrant adolescents and young adults
Relationships, in adolescence and young adulthood, 396–397, 399
  developmental benefits in, 397
    behavioral skills, 397
    emotional skills, 397
  relationship types, 396–397
Relative energy deficiency in sport (RED-S), 83, 242, 372, 489–490, 494
  early diagnosis of, 372
  physical examination, 372
  risk factors, 372
  screening for, 372
  treatment, 372

Relative poverty, 4t
Relaxation therapy, for FGIDs, 394
Remdesivir, in COVID-19, 329
Repeat pregnancy, 415, 420
Replacement smokers, 623
Reproductive coercion, 403–404
Reproductive health
    sexual minority women, 403
    youth experiencing homelessness, 725–726
Reproductive health education, 415–416
    for AYAs with disabilities, 678, 680
Research methods, 130–132, 131t
Research with and about AYAs, 127–136
    assent and developmental status, 127–128
    balancing privacy and safety, 129
    certificates of confidentiality, 129
    engagement and representation of AYAs in, 129–130
    ethics and oversight, 127–129
    methodologic issues for, 132, 135
    privacy and safety for study participant, 128–129
    regulatory conditions for engaging AYAs in, 128t
    research design and methods, 130–132, 131t
        data collection and analysis, 130–132
        pre-existing and publicly available data sources, 133t–134t
        selection of study design, 132
Reserve members, military, 719, 720
Reserve Officer Training Corps (ROTC), 719
Residential treatment programs, for substance use disorders, 655t
Resilience, 720–722, 747
Resiliency factors, 747
Resistance training and flexibility, 230
Resisters, 120
Respiratory complaints, 204–211
    asthma, 204–206
    cough, 207
    cystic fibrosis, 208–210
    EVALI, 210–211
    exercise-induced bronchoconstriction, 207
    exercise-induced laryngeal obstruction, 207
    pectus excavatum, 207–208
    primary ciliary dyskinesia, 210
Responsive neurostimulation (RNS), 280
Retail clinics, 64
Retapamulin
    for crusted (nonbullous) impetigo, 268
    for folliculitis, 269
Retin A, in molluscum contagiosum, 599t
Retinoids, topical, for acne, 259–260, 260t
Retinopathy, 165
Rett syndrome, 685
Return to learn, 252, 253f
Return-to-play, 252, 252f
Reverse sequence syphilis screening, 573, 574f
Reverse T₃ (rT₃), 152
Reverse transcription-polymerase chain reaction (RT-PCR), for influenza, 327
Review of systems
    in HIV infection, 347
    in preventive health visit, 69
Reye syndrome, 327
Rey–Osterrieth Complex Figure test, 686
Ribavirin
    for HCV treatment, 338
    for hepatitis E infection, 339
Rifampin, hormonal contraceptives and, 454
Rifaximin, in IBS, 393
Right to refuse treatment, 86
Risk and protective factors, substance use, 610–611, 611t, 612t
Risk assessment, CVD, 173–174, 175t
Risk behavior, screening for, 58

Risk factors
    for suicide, 672
    for youth violence, 692
Risk reduction counseling, 347
Risperidone, for autism spectrum disorder, 686
Ritonavir-boosted protease inhibitors, 454
Romantic relationships, 396, 399
Rome IV criteria, for FGIDs, 388, 389, 389t, 390t
Rosacea, 257
Rough sleeping, 723, 723f. See also Youth experiencing homelessness (YEH)
Roux-en-Y gastric bypass (RYGB), 360f, 361
Rufinamide, for seizure treatment, 281t
Runaways, 723, 723f. See also Youth experiencing homelessness (YEH)
Run charts, 123–124, 123f
Runner's knee. See Patellofemoral pain (PFP) syndrome
Russell sign, 369
RxforChange, 630

S
Sacral neurostimulation (SNS), in enuresis, 310
SAD. See Social anxiety disorder (SAD)
Safe environment for every kid (SEEK), 747
Safe Exercise at Every Stage, 242
Safety, interview questions about, 53
Safety of athletes, 232, 245, 246. See also Preparticipation physical evaluation (PPE)
Safety planning, 674
Salicylic acid
    for acne, 260
    for warts, 268
Salicylic acid gel, in molluscum contagiosum, 599t
Salpingectomy, 527
Salpingostomy (tube-sparing), 527
Salter–Harris fractures, 216
Salvia (Salvia divinorum), 649
Same-gender loving, 401
Sarcoptes scabiei var hominis, 596. See also Scabies
Sarecycline, for acne, 261
Saturday night fever, 640
SCA. See Sudden cardiac arrest (SCA)
Scabies, 596–597
    clinical manifestations, 596, 596f
        burrows, 596, 597f
        lesions, 596, 596f
    crusted/Norwegian, 596
    diagnosis, 597
    epidemiology, 596
    etiology, 596
    management considerations, 597
    transmission, 596
    treatment, 597t
Scapular stabilizing muscles, 223
Scapular winging, 222, 222f, 223
Scars, acne, 257, 257f
SCFE. See Slipped capital femoral epiphysis (SCFE)
Scheuermann kyphosis, 226
School
    health care in, 88
    role of, 9, 107
School-based clinics, 64
School shootings, 691
Scoliosis, 226
Screen for child anxiety-related emotional disorders (SCARED), 667
Screen-free week, 103
Screening. See also Screening tests
    and counseling, 58, 60 (See also Preventive health care)
    for sleep disturbances and disorders, 296, 296t
    for substance use and substance use disorders, 652, 652t
    tools, 66–67

Screening and brief intervention, for alcohol use, 617–618
Screening, Brief Intervention, and Referral to Treatment (SBIRT), 67, 617, 651
Screening questionnaire, previsit, 66
Screening tests, 70–71
    chlamydia, 71
    dyslipidemia, 70
    gonorrhea, 71
    hemoglobin, 70
    metabolic testing, 70–71
    sexually transmitted infections, 71
    tuberculosis, 70
    universal screening, 70
Screening to Brief Intervention (S2BI), 66, 618, 652, 652t
Scrotal masses. See Scrotal swelling and masses
Scrotal swelling and masses, 532–533
    differential diagnosis, 533
    evaluation, 532, 533f
    history, 532
    laboratory evaluation, 533
    physical examination, 532–533
Scrotal ultrasound, 536
Seattle Social Development Project, 612
Seborrheic dermatitis, 265
    clinical manifestations, 265, 265f
    treatment, 265
Sebum production, increased, and acne, 256
Secnidazole, 509
Secondary amenorrhea, 488, 492f. See also Amenorrhea
Secondary data analyses, 132
Secondary enuresis, 306. See also Enuresis
Secondary headache, 286, 287t, 288–289. See also Headaches
Secondary syphilis, 266, 269, 571–572, 571f. See also Syphilis
    condyloma lata, 571, 571f
    diagnosis, 574
    differential diagnosis, 572–573
    moth eaten–appearing alopecia, 571, 571f
    mucous patches, 571
    rash of, 571, 571f
    signs and symptoms, 571–572
    treatment, 575
Secondhand smoke (SHS), 626–627
Second-impact syndrome (SIS), 250, 253
Section 504, 680, 681t, 683
Segesterone acetate, 451
Seizure clusters, 277
Seizure precautions, 283, 283t
Seizures. See also Epilepsy
    acute symptomatic, 277, 278t
    definition, 277
    diagnostic evaluation, 279–280
        brain MRI, 280
        genetic epilepsy panel, 280
        imaging studies, 280, 280t
    differential diagnosis, 279, 279t
    etiologies, 278–279, 278t
    ILAE 2017 classification of seizure types, 278t
    recurrence risk, 279
    traumatic brain injury (TBI) and, 277
    unprovoked, 277
Selective mutism (SM), 665, 667t, 668
Selective serotonin reuptake inhibitors (SSRIs)
    for AMPS, 379
    for anxiety disorders, 669
    for AYAs with eating disorders, 367
    for depression, 664–665, 664t
    for neurocardiogenic syncope, 181t
    for PMS/PMDD, 482, 482t
    for trichotillomania, 273
Selenium sulfide lotion, for tinea versicolor, 266

Self-disclosure on social media, 99
Self-efficacy, 76
Self-Report for Childhood Anxiety Related
    Disorders (SCARED), 51
Seminomas, 536
Semmes–Weinstein monofilament test, 165
Sensory processing disorder (SPD), 685–686
The Sentencing Project, 749
Separation anxiety disorder, 667t, 668
Serotonin, 362, 480
Serotonin–norepinephrine reuptake inhibitors
    (SNRIs), for fibromyalgia, 379
Serotonin syndrome, 664
Serous cystadenomas, 522, 522f
Sertoli–Leydig cell tumors, 522
Sertraline, 367, 664, 664t
    for binge-eating disorder, 370
    for neurocardiogenic syncope, 181t
    for orthostatic intolerance, 385t
    for PMDD, 482, 482t
Serum ferritin, 82
Serum sickness-like eruption, 271
Setmelanotide, 355
Sever disease, 216
Severe obesity, 354. *See also* Obesity
Sex cord–stromal tumors, 522, 523f
Sex hormone–binding globulin (SHBG), 495
Sex inequality, and health, 9
Sex-segregated facilities, for transgender people,
    411
Sex steroids, mechanisms of action of, 450
Sexting, 101, 103, 398
Sex trafficking, 696, 697. *See also* Sexual
    violence (SV)
Sexual abstinence, 397, 399
Sexual abuse, 696. *See also* Sexual violence
    (SV)
    childhood, 697
    indicators, 697
Sexual and reproductive health, 29
    of adolescents with chronic health
        conditions, 109
Sexual assault, 696. *See also* Sexual violence
    (SV)
    on college campus, 710
    youth experiencing homelessness, 726
Sexual assault nurse examiner (SANE)
    programs, 699
Sexual attraction, 401, 408
Sexual behavior, 401
    oral sex, 397–398
    outcomes with, 398
    partnered and solo, 397–398
    partnered masturbation, 397
    penile-anal sex, 398
    penile-vaginal sex, 398
    sexting, 398
    sexual abstinence, 397
    solo masturbation, 397
Sexual development, 36
Sexual exploitation, 696, 697
Sexual health, 396, 397. *See also* Sexuality
    of sexual minority youth, 403
Sexual history, 469
Sexual identity, 401
Sexuality, 396–400, 401
    clinician recommendations, 398–399
    close relationships, 396–397, 399
    interview questions about, 53
    outcomes with sexual behavior, 398
    sexual behavior, 397–398
Sexuality education, 415–416
Sexually active AYA, PID in, suspicion for, 563,
    564
Sexually transmitted diseases (STDs). *See*
    Sexually transmitted infections (STIs)

Sexually transmitted infections (STIs), 396,
    549–553, 563, 584. *See also specific
    infection*
    acquisition of, 551
    adolescent development and, 551
    in AYAs, 29
    by bacteria, 549
    burden of disease and incidence, 549–550
    clinical manifestations, 549, 550t
    diagnosis, 552
    emerging issues
        Mycoplasma genitalium, 552–553
        testing and treatment in nontraditional
            settings, 553
    management of, 349
    nonsexual modes of transmission, 549
    prevention, 551
        antimicrobial-based interventions, 551
        behavioral interventions, 551
        partner management, 551–552
        vaccines, 551
    screening for, 71
    screening for asymptomatic STIs, 552
    syndromes caused by, 549
    transgender youth and young adults, 410
    transmission, 550–551
    treatment, 552
    by viruses, 549
Sexual maturity rating (SMR), 36–37, 70, 139,
    367, 530, 677
    amenorrhea, 488, 492, 493
    females, 36f, 37, 37f
    males, 36–37, 37f
    transgender youth and young adults, 410,
        411
Sexual minority, 401–402, 404. *See also* Sexual
    minority youth (SMY)
Sexual minority youth (SMY), 9, 401
    bullying and victimization, 403
    caring for, 404–406
    combatting stigma and building resilience,
        404
    dating violence risk, 403
    eating disorders, 403
    family rejection, 403
    health and social disparities experienced by,
        403
    health concerns, 402–404
    homelessness and foster involvement, 403
    homophobia and heterosexism, 402
    human trafficking and survival sex, 403
    inclusive clinical environment for, 404
    intimate partner violence, 403
    mental and behavioral health needs, 404
    mental health and suicidality, 403
    minority stress, intersectionality, and health
        of, 402
    parents/caregivers of, support to, 406
    prevalence, 401–402
    preventive care for, 69
    racial/ethnic, 402
    reproductive coercion and stealthing,
        403–404
    reproductive health, 403, 404
    school environments for, 404
    screening and treatment recommendations,
        405–406
        ACIP guidelines for STIs, 406t
        CDC's STI screening guidelines, 406t
        HIV PrEP, 406
        HIV/STI screening, 405, 406
        vaccines, 405
    sex education to, 405
    sexual health, 403, 404
    sexual identity development, 402
    sexual orientation, 401

substance use disorders, 403
support for, 404
taking inclusive sexual history, 404–405,
    405t
Sexual orientation, 401
Sexual violence (SV), 696–703
    assessment and support
        healing-centered approaches to, 698–699
        trauma-informed, strength-based approach
            to, 698
    epidemiology, 696–697
    evaluation of sexual abuse and assault,
        699–702
        collection of specimens, 701
        genital, pelvic, and rectal examination,
            701
        interpretation of findings, 701–702
        laboratory tests, 701, 701t
        medical evaluation, 699–700
        medical history, 700, 700t
        photography, 700
        physical examination, 700–701
        rape kit, 700, 701
    incidence, 696–697
    legal investigative process and outcomes,
        702–703
    legal issues related to reporting of, 699
    male, 696
    management, 702–703
    marginalized populations exposure to,
        697–698
        AYAs with disabilities, 698
        gender diverse, 698
        gender nonconforming AYAs, 698
        homeless/street AYAs, 697
        lesbian, gay, and bisexual (LGB), 698
        transgender, 698
    physical and anogenital trauma
        females, 699–700
        males, 700
        transgender and gender diverse AYAs, 700
    rates of, 696
    risk factors for, 696
    screening and reporting, 698–699
    sequelae, 697
    terminology associated with, 696
"Shaking on a contract," 76
Sheehan syndrome, 490
Shigella flexeneri, 591
Short-acting beta agonist (SABA), 205
Short-acting contraceptives, 449–455. *See also*
    Combined hormonal contraceptives
    (CHCs)
Short QT syndrome, 184
Short stature, 138
    chronic illness and, 138, 139
    congenital syndromes and, 138
    constitutional delay of puberty and, 138,
        139
    criteria for evaluation, 138
    definition of, 138
    differential diagnosis, 138
    endocrine causes, 139
    genetic/familial, 138, 139
    growth hormone deficiency and, 139
    growth hormone treatment, 139–140
    history, 138–139
    laboratory/radiologic evaluation, 139
    physical examination, 139
    treatment, 139
    Turner syndrome and, 139–140
    without delayed puberty, 138–140
Shoulder
    acromioclavicular joint sprain, 222
    chronic shoulder instability with glenoid
        labrum injuries, 222

humeral epiphysiolysis, 223
imaging studies, 222
physical examination, 221–222
shoulder dislocation, 222
shoulder impingement syndrome, 222–223
treatment, 222
weak scapular stabilizing muscles, 223
Shoulder injuries, 221–223
history of shoulder symptoms, 221
Simmonds disease, 490
Single maintenance and reliever therapy (SMART), 205–206
Single ventricular-Fontan, 194t
Sitosterolemia, 172, 173t
Six Sigma, 119
Skeletal mass during puberty, 41–42
Skeletal maturation, 40
Skeletal scintigraphy (bone scan), in complex regional pain syndrome, 377
Skene glands, 470
Skin
acne, 256–261
anorexia nervosa and, 364
bacterial infections, 268–269
cancer, 274
dermatitis, 263–265
fungal infections, 265–268
hypersensitivity reactions, 270–272
pityriasis rosea, 269
popping, 641
psoriasis, 269–270
sun exposure, 274
warts, 268
Skinfold measurements, 79
Skin prick testing, 204
Skyla, 425, 425t, 457
Skyn Condoms, 439
Sleep, 293, 381
COVID-19 impact on, 296
duration, 294
for headache treatment, 290
importance of, 293
insufficient, 294
in ME/CFS, 381, 384
nonrapid eye movement, 293
and obesity, 355, 357
pattern and changes during adolescence, 293–294
physiology, 293
rapid eye movement, 293
Sleep arousal disorder, 307
Sleep attacks, 295
Sleep diary, 297
Sleep-disordered breathing (SDB), 295
Sleep disturbances and disorders, 294
assessment of, 297
delayed sleep phase syndrome, 294
epilepsy and, 283
excessive daytime sleepiness, 294
history taking, 296
insomnia, 294
narcolepsy, 295
parasomnias, 295–296
physical examination, 297
prevention and screening, 296
ABCs of SLEEPING, 296, 296t
BEARS screener, 296
Pediatric Sleep Quality Index, 296
referral for further assessment, 297
sleep deprivation, 294
sleep disorder clinics, 297
sleep-disordered breathing/obstructive sleep apnea, 295
sleep history tool, 296–297
sleep-tracking devices, 297
treatment, 297

Sleep habits, 296
Sleep paralysis, 295
Sleep terrors, 295–296, 295t
versus nightmares, 295t
Sleepwalking, 295–296
Sleep wearables, 297
Sleeve gastrectomy (SG), 360f, 361
Slipped capital femoral epiphysis (SCFE), 218, 221, 221f
Small fiber neuropathy, 378
SMART (mnemonic), 119
SMART treatment strategy, for asthma, 206
Smoked marijuana, 634
Smoking, 622
among AYAs, 27, 107
among high school students, 622
public health efforts, 622
Smoking cessation
for BP reduction, 200
medications for, 629f–630f
SMR. See Sexual maturity rating (SMR)
SMY. See Sexual minority youth (SMY)
Snellen chart, 69
Snuff (dipping tobacco), 626
Snus, 626
Social anxiety disorder (SAD), 665, 667–668, 667t
Social cognition, 107
Social determinants of health, 2, 3f, 4t, 5, 107
definition of, 2, 4t
life-course factors and, 3f, 10
proximal factors in, 5, 9
families, 9
neighborhood, 9
new media, 10
orphanhood, 9–10
peers, 10
school, 9
structural factors in, 5
education, 7
employment, 8
income, 5, 7
migration, 8–9
racism, 9
sex inequality, 9
war and conflict, 9
Social disenfranchisement, 743
Social health screening tools, 747
Social history, structure of, 52–53
activities, 53
drugs, 53
eating, 52–53
education/employment, 52
home, 52
safety, 53
sexuality, 53
suicide/depression, 53
Social media
AYAs' food choices, influence on, 79
benefits of, 99
education and civic engagement, 99
health access and illness support, 99–100
identity development, 99
social support and social capital, 99
Facebook, 98, 99
influence of, 99, 100t
Instagram, 98
as mechanism of empowerment for patients, 100
mental health, effect on, 10
overview, 98–99
platforms, 98
Reddit, 98
risks of, 100–101
posted content, risks related to, 101
problematic use and multitasking, 101

sites, use of, 99
Snapchat, 98
TikTok, 98
Twitter, 98, 99
use rates, 98
video games and online gaming, 101
Web 2.0 tools, 98
YouTube, 98
Social needs, 113
Social Security Administration (SSA), 682
Social transitions, 2, 5t, 10
Sodium chloride, for orthostatic intolerance, 385t
Sodium choate, 447
Sodium intake, and hypertension, 197
Sodium oxybate (gamma hydroxybutyrate) in AMPS, 379
Sodium sulfacetamide, 259
Solifenacin, for overactive bladder, 309
Solo masturbation, 397, 399
National Survey of Sexual Health Behavior (NSSHB), 397
Solving problems, 76
Somatic cough syndrome. See Habit cough
Somatic symptom disorder, 375–376
Somatic symptoms
adjustment disorder, 375
biopsychosocial assessment, 376
physical symptoms with psychological distress, 375
psychiatric diagnoses with, 375–376
and related disorders, 375–376
Somatostatin, 39
Somnambulism. See Sleepwalking
Special education, 680
Special health care needs, 105, 110
Special needs, nutritional
of athletes, 82–83
of vegetarians, 82
Special Olympics, 245
Specific learning disability (SLD), 681t
Specific phobias, 667, 667t
Speech or language impairment (SI), 681t
Spermatocele, 532, 534f, 537
Spermicide-coated condoms, 447
Spermicides, 447–448
active ingredient, 447
advantages, 447
contraindications, 447
disadvantages, 448
efficacy, 447
future developments, 448
mechanism of action, 447
types of, 447, 447t
Spine, 223–226
discogenic back pain, 224–225, 225f
history of spine symptoms, 223
imaging studies, 223
nonspecific low back pain, 225–226
physical examination, 223
Scheuermann kyphosis, 226
scoliosis, 226
spondylolysis/spondylolisthesis, 223–224, 224f
treatment, 223
Spiritual support, 113
Spirometry, 204
Spironolactone
for acne, 261
for androgenetic alopecia, 273
for hirsutism, 497
for PMS, 482
Splenic rupture, infectious mononucleosis and, 320–321
Spondylolysis/spondylolisthesis, 223–224, 224f

Sponge, contraceptive, 441, 443–444
　advantages, 443
　contraindications, 443
　disadvantages, 443–444
　efficacy, 441
　future developments, 444
　mechanism of action, 441
　patient education
　　insertion, 441, 443
　　removal, 443
　toxic shock syndrome risk, 441
Spontaneous abortion, 419
　hCG levels, 416
Sport concussion assessment tool (SCAT), 250
Sport concussion assessment tool 5 (SCAT5), 250
Sport-related concussion (SRC), 244, 249
　biologic fluid biomarkers, 250
　clinic assessment, 250
　complications and chronic effects, 252–253
　　chronic traumatic encephalopathy, 253
　　disqualification or retirement from sport, 253
　　mental health and wellness, 253
　　second-impact syndrome, 253
　definition, 249
　diagnosis, 250, 251t
　epidemiology, 249–250
　management, 251–252
　　pharmacologic therapy, 252
　　return to academics, 252, 253f
　　return-to-play, 252, 252f
　　targeted therapies, 252
　neurocognitive testing, 250–251
　neuroimaging studies, 250
　on-field assessment, 250
　pathophysiology, 249
　postconcussion symptom scale, 250, 251t
　prevention, 253
　sideline assessment, 250
Sports injury epidemiology, 245–246
Sports participation. *See also* Physical activity (PA); Preparticipation physical evaluation (PPE)
　anterior cruciate ligament injury prevention, 246
　athletes with disability and special health care needs, 245
　blood-borne pathogens and, 244–245
　burnout from, 246
　COVID-19 screening for, 245
　epidemiology, 229
　female athlete, 245
　injury prevention, 245–247
　medical conditions and, 237t–240t
　medical–legal issues in exclusion from, 241–242
　physical activity and, 229–247
　physical fitness for, 229
　preparticipation physical evaluation, 232–242
　sport defined, 229
　sports classified by contact level, 231t
　transgender/nonbinary athletes, 245
　by youth living with HIV, 349
Sport specialization, 246
Sport-specific safety equipment, use of, 246
Squamocolumnar junction (SCJ), 470, 502
Squamous metaplasia, 502
Squaric acid, for warts, 268
SRC. *See* Sport-related concussion (SRC)
SSHADESS (strengths, school, home, activities, drugs, emotions/eating/depression, sexuality, safety), 52
SSRIs. *See* Selective serotonin reuptake inhibitors (SSRIs)

Stakeholders, 120
　QI project and, 120
Standard operating procedures (SOPs), 131–132
Staphylococcus aureus, 208
　and atopic dermatitis, 263
　bullous impetigo, 268
　crusted (nonbullous) impetigo, 268
　folliculitis, 268
Staphylococcus saprophyticus, cystitis by, 300
Statistical process control (SPC) chart, 123–124, 123f
Statistical techniques, in medical research, 132
Status epilepticus, 277
Statutory rape, 696, 699
Stealthing, 404
Steroid acne, 257
Stevens–Johnson syndrome (SJS), 271
STI clinical services, 552
STI diagnosis. *See* Sexually transmitted infections (STIs)
STI laboratory services, 552
Still's murmur, 187
STI management. *See* Sexually transmitted infections (STIs)
Stimulants, in ADHD, 685
STI prevention. *See* Sexually transmitted infections (STIs)
STIs. *See* Sexually transmitted infections (STIs)
STI syndromes, 549. *See also* Sexually transmitted infections (STIs)
St. John's wort (SJW), 91, 92
　hormonal contraceptives and, 454
Stork test, 224
Stranger rape, 696
Strawberry cervix, 470
Street victimization, 725
Street youth, 723. *See also* Youth experiencing homelessness (YEH)
Strengthening Families and Guiding Good Choices programs, 612
Strength training, 230. *See also* Physical activity (PA)
Streptococcus pneumoniae, 208
Streptococcus pyogenes, erythema nodosum by, 271
Stress
　and amenorrhea, 489
　and FGIDs in AYAs, 393–394
　and hypertension, 197
　postabortion, 418
Stress fractures, 227
　clinical manifestations, 227
　definition/etiology, 227
　diagnosis, 227
　epidemiology, 227
　prognosis, 227
　treatment, 227
Stress management, for headache treatment, 290
Stress response pathway, 745, 745f
Structural discrimination, 743
Structured Assessment of Violence Risk in Youth (SAVRY), 693
Student affairs, 712
Student health, 706, 712. *See also* College health
Student health insurance, 712
Student health insurance benefit plan (SHIP), 712
Student health service (SHS), 706, 707, 712. *See also* College health
Subdural grid electrodes, 280
Subluxations, 95
Substance Abuse and Mental Health Services Administration (SAMHSA), 610, 618–619, 651

Substance use/Substance use disorders, 23, 27, 106, 602–612, 651
　approaches to, 651–657
　AYAs with chronic medical conditions, 653
　brain development and, 609
　brief interventions by clinicians, 652–653
　confidentiality policies with AYA patients, 651–652
　diagnostic criteria in *DSM-5,* 609, 651t
　drug testing, 656
　epidemiology, 602–609
　high risk for, 653
　long-term outcomes, 609
　lower risk for, 653
　medical conditions associated with substance use, 655–656
　mental health evaluation, 655
　middle and high school youth, 602–607, 604t–605t
　　alcohol, 606
　　illicit drug use, 602–603, 603f
　　marijuana, 606–607
　　nonmedical prescription drug use (NMPDU), 607
　　race and ethnic groups, 605–606
　　vaping, 607, 608f
　Monitoring the Future survey 2020 (2020 MTF) on, 602
　parents/caregivers, role of, 656
　physical examination, 656
　during pregnancy, 419
　prevention, 610–612, 612t
　　community or structural prevention interventions, 612
　　family-based prevention programs, 612
　　school interventions, 612
　primary care provider, role of, 651
　progression of, 609–610
　　drug use, 610
　　first opportunity to use, 610
　　initiation of use, 610
　　remission from substance use, 610
　　substance dependence, 610
　protective factors, 610–611, 612t
　referral to treatment, 653–654
　risk factors, 610, 611t
　screening for, 66–67, 652, 652t
　sexual minority youth, 403
　transgender youth and young adults, 410
　treatment
　　criteria for selection of program, 654, 656t
　　equity, diversity, inclusion in, 657
　　levels of care for, 655t
　　pharmacologic treatment, 655
　　psychosocial formats and counseling modalities for, 654t
　　referral to, 653–654
　　treatment settings, 653, 655t
　young adult, 607–609
　　alcohol, 607
　　cigarettes and vaping, 607
　　illicit drugs use, 607–609
　　marijuana, 607
　in youth experiencing homelessness, 725
Subungual onychomycosis, 267, 267f
Sudden cardiac arrest (SCA), 183–184, 242–243
　in athletes, 184
　ECG screening, 184
　etiologies, 183–184
　and genetic screening, 184
　myocarditis and, 193
　prevention, 184
Sudden sniffing death syndrome, 645
Sudden unexplained death in epilepsy (SUDEP), 277, 284
Sufentanil, 641. *See also* Opioids

Suicidal behaviors, 671–672
Suicidal ideation, 671
  active ideation, 671
  emotional distress and, 671
  isotretinoin use and, 261
  panic disorder and, 668
  passive ideation, 671
  prevalence, 671–672
  sexual minority youth, 403
  transgender youth and young adults, 409
Suicide, 9, 16, 17, 22, 671–674
  American Indians/Alaska Natives (AI/AN), 671
  AYAs at risk for, 672
    case example, 674
    clinical approach for, 674
    safety planning and lethal means safety counseling, 674
    treatment plan, development of, 674
    treatments and interventions for, 673–674
  definitions, 671
  depression and, 672
  epidemiology, 671, 672f
  protective factors, 673
  racial disparities, 671
  rates of, variation in, 671
  "Ring the Alarm" (report), 671
  risk assessment, 673
  screening tool, 66, 673, 673f
  warning signs, 672
Suicide assessment, 673
Suicide attempt, 671
  aborted, 671
  interrupted, 671
  by lesbian, gay, or bisexual (LGB) students, 672
  rates among transgender youth, 672
Suicide risk screening, 673
Sun exposure, 274
Sunscreen, 274
Supplemental Nutrition Assistance Program (SNAP), 748
Support in modifying behavior, 76
Supraclavicular (carotid) bruit, 187
Supraventricular tachycardia (SVT), 182
Survey of well-being of young children (SWYC), 747
Survey of Youth in Residential Placement (SYRP), 734, 735
Survival sex, 696, 725. See also Sexual violence (SV)
Sweat chloride testing, 209
Sweating, excessive. See Hyperhidrosis
Swedish Match snus, 626
Swiss cheese disease, 544
Symptom management, 115
Syncope, 179–183
  cardiovascular, 181–182
  categories, 179
  differential diagnosis, 179, 180t
  etiology, 179
  history and physical examination, 179
  mid-exertional, 179
  neurocardiogenic, 179–181
  noncardiovascular, 182–183
  of unknown origin, 179
  warning signs, 179
Syndromes of chronic musculoskeletal pain, 376–379
  differential diagnosis, 378t
  diffuse amplified pain syndromes, 376–377
  epidemiology, 377
  localized amplified pain syndromes, 377–378
  management, 379
  pathophysiology, 377
  terminology related to, 376

Synthetic cannabinoids, 633
Synthetic cathinones, 640
Syphilis, 569–576
  causative agent, 569
  clinical manifestations, 570–572
  congenital, 572
  dark-field examination, 573, 573f
  diagnosis, 573–575
  differential diagnosis, 572–573
  epidemiology, 569
  gender disparity, 569
  geographic disparity, 569
  and human immunodeficiency virus, 575, 576
  Jarisch–Herxheimer reaction, 576
  laboratory findings, 573–574
  latent, 572
  management of sex partners, 576
  neurosyphilis, 572
  pathogenesis, 570
  in pregnancy, 575, 576
  primary, 570–571, 570f
  racial disparity, 569
  reverse sequence syphilis screening algorithms, 573, 574f
  screening, 71, 573
  secondary, 571–572, 571f
  serologic tests, 573–574
  sex partner disparity, 569
  treatment, 575–576
Syphilis serologic screening, 573
  reverse sequence syphilis screening, 573, 574f
  traditional nontreponemal-treponemal syphilis screening, 573, 574f
Systemic disorders, and proteinuria, 313
Systemic lupus erythematosus (SLE), and proteinuria, 313

T
Tabes dorsalis, 572
Tacrolimus, for atopic dermatitis, 264
Tanner staging, 36–37
Tap-water iontophoresis, for hyperhidrosis, 273
TasP (HIV prevention method), 347
Tattooing, 274–275
  and infections, 274
  inflammatory reactions, 274
  tattoo removal, 275
Tazarotene, 260, 260t
  for psoriasis, 270
Technology. See also Digital technology; Social media
  use of, 98–104
Teenagers, enuresis and overactive bladder in, 307, 309. See also Enuresis
Teen birth rates, 413
Teen-tot medical homes, 415
Telehealth, 101–102, 656–657. See also Telemedicine
  advantages of, 102
  care through, 88
  definition of, 101
  use during COVID-19 pandemic, 101
Telemedicine, 56, 64
Telogen effluvium, 272
Temperature, measurement of, 69
Tenofovir alafenamide (TAF), for HIV infection, 346
Tenofovir disoproxil fumarate (TDF), for HIV infection, 345, 346
Tension-type headache (TTH), 286, 288, 291t. See also Headaches
Terbinafine
  for onychomycosis, 267
  for tinea pedis, 267
  for tinea versicolor, 266

Termination of pregnancy, 417–418
  access to abortion services, 417
  medical methods, 418
    advantages of, 418
    disadvantages of, 418
    first trimester, 418
    second trimester, 418
    types of, 418
  methods for, selection of, 418
  risks and complications, 418
  surgical methods, 418
    dilation and evacuation, 418
    vacuum aspiration, 418
Testes, inspection of, 530
Testicular cancer, 531
Testicular regression syndrome, 143
Testicular self-examination, 537
Testicular torsion, 532, 533–535, 534f
  clinical manifestations, 533, 535
  diagnosis, 535
  epidemiology, 533
  etiology, 533
  surgical treatment, 535
Testicular tumors, 536
  diagnosis, 536
  epidemiology, 536
  etiology, 536
  therapy, 536
Testifying, 703
Testing, HIV, 343, 344t
  antibody tests, 344
  CDC recommendations for, 343
  confidentiality and consent for, 343
  deferred in some situations, 343–344
  high risk groups and, 343
  rapid HIV tests, 344
  viral nucleic acid tests, 344
  viral p24 antigen tests, 344
  youth-specific testing, 344
Testis tumor, 534f
Testosterone, 36, 39, 495
Tetanus, diphtheria, and acellular pertussis (Tdap), 348
Tetracycline, for syphilis treatment, 575
Tetralogy of Fallot, 194, 194t
Theca-cell hyperplasia, 495
Theca cell tumors, 522
Thelarche, 36, 37, 474
Therapeutic boarding schools, for substance use disorders, 655t
Therapy, nutritional, 82–83. See also Nutrition
Thermodestruction of hair follicle, 497
Thin basement membrane disease (TBMD), 316
Third testicle. See Spermatocele
Threatened abortion, 419
Thromboembolism, CHCs and risk of, 452–453
Throwaways, 723, 723f. See also Youth experiencing homelessness (YEH)
Thyroglobulin, 154
Thyroglossal duct cysts, 151
Thyroid cancer, 151, 154
  differentiated, 154
  medullary, 154
  risk for, 151–152
Thyroid disorders, 151
  functional disorders, 151, 154–155
    hyperthyroidism, 155–156
    hypothyroidism, 156
    nonthyroidal illness, 156–157
  pregnancy and, 157
  structural disorders, 153–154
    thyroid cancers, 154
    thyroid nodules, 154
    thyromegaly, 153–154

Thyroid gland. *See also* Thyroid disorders
  development, 151
  focused medical history, 151–152
  function
    during development, 151
    laboratory evaluation of, 152
    radiologic evaluation of, 152–153
  functional symptoms associated with activity
    of, 152t
  genetic testing in thyroid disease, 153
  lingual thyroid, 151
  physical evaluation of structure, 152, 153f
  during puberty, 151
  size of, 153
Thyroid hormone, 151, 154–155
  clinical effects of, 152t
  excess, 155
  feedback loop for production of, 155, 155f
Thyroid nodules, 152, 154
  biopsy, 154
  cold nodule, 153
  during pregnancy, 157
  and risk of thyroid cancer, 154
  toxic nodule, 153, 154
  TSH measurement, 154
Thyroid peroxidase (TPO) antibody, 152
Thyroid-releasing hormone (TRH), 151, 155
Thyroid-stimulating antibody (TSAb), 152
Thyroid-stimulating hormone (TSH), 151, 152,
    155, 156
Thyroid ultrasound, 152
Thyromegaly, 153–154
Tibial tubercle apophysitis, 216
Tic cough. *See* Habit cough
Tilt table testing, 180
Tinea corporis, 269
Tinea cruris, 267–268, 267f
  clinical manifestations, 267, 267f
  differential diagnosis, 267–268
  treatment, 268
  wood's lamp examination, 268
Tinea pedis, 266–267, 266f
  clinical manifestations, 266, 266f
  differential diagnosis, 266
  inflammatory form, 266, 266f
  interdigital form, 266, 266f
  moccasin form, 266
  treatment, 267
Tinea unguium. *See* Onychomycosis
Tinea versicolor, 265–266
  clinical manifestations, 265, 266f
  differential diagnosis, 265–266
  hypopigmented lesions, 265, 266f
  potassium hydroxide preparation, 265
  treatment, 266
  Wood's lamp examination, 265
Tinidazole, 509, 512
Tissue plasminogen activator (tPA), 287
Title X family planning regulations, 87
Title X of the Public Health Services Act, 88
Title XVI disability support, 682
TOA. *See* Tubo-ovarian abscess (TOA)
Tobacco, Alcohol, Prescription medication, and
    other Substance use Tool (TAPS), 652,
    652t
Tobacco cessation programs, teen-specific,
    629
Tobacco use, 622–631
  advocacy issues, 630–631
  among America's youth, 622
    high school students, 623f
    middle school students, 623f
  factors associated with, 623–624
    psychological factors, 623–624
    tobacco industry marketing, 623,
      624f–625f

nicotine addiction and health consequences,
    624–627
office practices, 629–630
prevalence, 622, 623f
prevention and treatment, 627
  5-A framework, 627f
  clinical interventions, 627–629, 627f
  educational materials, 630
  health plans and billing, 630
quitting, 628
research areas, 631
secondhand smoke, 626–627
smokeless oral tobacco, 626
systemic effects, 626
Tolerable upper intake level (UL), 80
Tolnaftate, for onychomycosis, 267
Tolterodine, for overactive bladder, 309
Topical antibiotics, for acne, 259
Topical calcineurin inhibitors, for atopic
    dermatitis, 264
Topical corticosteroid
  for allergic contact dermatitis, 265
  for atopic dermatitis, 264
  for seborrheic dermatitis, 265
Topical phosphodiesterase inhibitor, for atopic
    dermatitis, 264
Topical retinoids, for acne, 259–260, 260t
Topiramate
  for binge-eating disorder, 370
  for seizure treatment, 281t
Torsion of the appendix testis, 532
Total body pain, 377
Total triiodothyronine (T₃), 152
Tourette syndrome, 677t
Toxic epidermal necrolysis (TEN), 271
Toxic stress, 745
Traction alopecia, 273
Traditional condoms, 436–440
  advantages, 439
  aesthetic packaging, 439
  CDC STI guidelines, 437
  contraceptive use, 437
  disadvantages, 439
  double bagging, 437
  effectiveness, 437–438
  failure rates, 438
  future developments, 439–440
  improving consistent and correct use of, 439,
    440f
  latex condoms, 437
  mechanism of action, 437
  National College Health Assessment (NCHA)
    data, 437
  natural and skin condoms, 437
  noncontraceptive uses, 437
  NSFG survey data on, 436
  patient information sheet, 440f
  polyurethane condoms, 437
  side effects, 439
  for STIs prevention, 437
  types of, 437
  use of, data on, 436–437
  Youth Risk Behavior Survey (YRBS), 436
Trafficked youth, 725
Trafficking, 697
Tramadol, for AMPS, 379
Tranexamic acid, 486
Transactional sex, 696. *See also* Sexual violence
    (SV)
Transcutaneous electrical neurostimulation
    (TENS), for enuresis, 310
Transdermal contraceptive patches, 427,
    452
Transdermal estrogen, 147, 490, 494
Transdermal estrogen patch, 493
Trans fatty acid (TFA), 81

Transgender adolescents and young adults,
    408–411
  approach to family and, 411
  coming out process, 409
  disclosure of transgender identity, 409
  electronic records, 411
  emotional and behavioral health
    homelessness, 409
    mood disorders and anxiety, 409
    suicide, 409–410
    violence, 409
  etiology, 409
  health concerns
    eating disorders, 410
    obesity, 410
    pregnancy, 410
    sexually transmitted infections, 410
    substance use, 410
  medical intervention
    hormones, 410
    hormone therapy risk, 410–411
    surgery, 411
  nonbinary, 409
  parental support, 411
  preintervention assessment, 411
  prevalence, 409
  sex-segregated facilities, 411
  terminology related to, 408–409
Transgender youth, 408. *See also* Transgender
    adolescents and young adults
Transient proteinuria, 313, 313t
Transitional living/housing, 727
Transition care, 731
Transition Readiness Assessment Questionnaire
    (TRAQ), 76
Transitions in adolescence and young
    adulthood, 10–11
  health correlates of, 11
Transition to adult health care
  AYAs with chronic health conditions,
    109–110
  AYAs with life-limiting conditions, 116
Transmission of HIV, 342
  condom use to prevent, 349
  intravenous drug use, 343
  mother–child transmission risk, 349
  routes of transmission, 342–343, 342t
  sexual transmission, 343
  vertical transmission, 343
Transportation barriers, 747
Transport injuries, 2, 16, 17t
Transsphenoidal surgery, 543
Transvaginal ultrasound (TVUS), 526
Trauma, 744
  adverse childhood experiences (ACEs),
    744–745, 745t
  complex, 745
  definitions of, 744–745
  posttraumatic stress disorder, 745
  psychological, 745
  screening, 746–747, 746t
  toxic stress, 745
  youth in out-of-home care, 730, 731
Trauma-informed care framework, 747–748
Traumatic brain injuries (TBIs), 681t, 720
Treatment
  for anogenital warts, 587–589, 587t–588t
  HIV infection, 350–351
Treatment goal weight (TGW), 368, 372
Treatment of adolescent depression (TADS)
    study, 673
T₄ (levothyroxine) replacement therapy, 156
Treponemal antibody tests, 573
Treponema pallidum, 569. *See also* Syphilis
Treponema pallidum particle agglutination
    (TP-PA) test, 573

Tretinoin, 260, 260t
for warts, 268
Tretinoin/clindamycin (Ziana, Veltin), 260t
Trevor Chat, 404
Triamcinolone acetonide, for psoriasis, 270
Trichloroacetic acid (TCA), molluscum
contagiosum, 599t
Trichomonas infections, 470
Trichomonas vaginalis, 507, 511, 535
Trichomoniasis, 511–512
clinical manifestations, 511
counseling, 512
diagnosis, 511–512
culture, 512
NAATs, 511
rapid/POCT, 512
wet prep, 511–512, 512f
epidemiology, 511
etiology, 511
strawberry cervix, 511, 511f
therapy, 512
Trichophyton mentagrophytes (T. mentagrophytes)
onychomycosis, 267
tinea cruris, 267
tinea pedis, 266
Trichophyton rubrum (T. rubrum)
onychomycosis, 267
tinea pedis, 266
Trichotillomania (TTM), 273
Tricyclic antidepressants (TCAs)
for abdominal pain, 393
for AMPS, 379
for FGIDs, 393
Trigeminal autonomic cephalalgias (TACs), 288
Trimethoprim-sulfamethoxazole
for acne, 261
for genitourinary tract infections, 303, 304t
for pertussis, 326
Triptans, for headache management, 291t
Truncus arteriosus, 194t
Truth Initiative, 631
TSH. *See* Thyroid-stimulating hormone (TSH)
T-SPOT, 70
Tubal infertility, 559
Tuberculosis
and erythema nodosum, 271
immigrant and refugee AYAs, 740
screening refugees and immigrants for, 740
testing for, 70
Tuberous breast deformity, 540, 540f
Tube-sparing surgery, 527
Tubo-ovarian abscess (TOA), 518, 518f, 558, 563, 564, 566
Tubulointerstitial kidney disease, and proteinuria, 314
Tumor markers, serum, 536
Turner syndrome, 139–140, 143, 488, 489f
and amenorrhea, 488
cardiac monitoring protocol, 142f
characteristics, 146
growth chart for children with, 141f
growth hormone treatment, 139
health screening recommendations in, 140t
hGH therapy, 147
21st Century Cures Act, 64, 88
Twinrix, for hepatitis A and B, 332, 335
Twirla patch, 427
Two-Spirit, 401
Type 1 diabetes, 159. *See also* Diabetes
mellitus
immune mediated (type 1A), 159
nonimmune mediated (type 1B), 159
Type 2 diabetes, 159. *See also* Diabetes
mellitus

U
Ulcerative colitis (UC), 391
Ulipristal acetate (UPA, Ella), 431, 449
advantages, 432–433
for emergency contraception, 432–433
mechanism of action, 432
side effects, 433
Ultrasound
breast masses, 545
for gestational age, 417
Unaccompanied immigrant children (UIC), 738
Unauthorized immigrants, 738
Underage drinking, 606, 616
Undescended testis, 530. *See also*
Cryptorchidism
Unintended pregnancy, 422–423, 424t
prevention for (*See* Contraception)
Unintentional injuries, 2, 16, 17t, 18, 58
United Nations Convention on the Rights of the
Child (CRC), 86
United Nations Educational, Scientific and
Cultural Organization (UNESCO), 7
United Nations International Children's
Emergency Fund (UNICEF), 7, 9
United States
confidential services, billing for, 51
preventive services and insurance coverage
in, 60, 62–63
United States Department of Agriculture
(USDA), 78
United States Medical Eligibility Criteria for
Contraceptive (U.S. MEC), 423
The University of California at Los Angeles
(UCLA) Posttraumatic Stress Disorder
Reaction Index for DSM-5, 746–747
Unplanned pregnancy, 413–414. *See also*
Pregnancy
Unspecified functional bowel disorder, 389
Unstably housed, 723. *See also* Youth
experiencing homelessness (YEH)
Urachal cysts, 517
Urethral meatus warts, 588
Urethritis, in females, 558
Urethritis, in males, 535, 559
clinical manifestations, 535
diagnosis, 535
epidemiology, 535
etiology, 535
gonococcal urethritis, 535
nongonococcal urethritis (NGU), 535
treatment, 535
Urinalysis, in enuresis, 307, 308t
Urinary tract infection (UTI), 300. *See also*
Cystitis; Genitourinary tract infections
recurrent, 302
treatment, 303–304, 304t
Urine culture, for cystitis, 302
Urine dipstick test
diagnosis of dysuria, 302
hematuria, 314
proteinuria, 312, 314
Urine test kits, 416
Uroflowmetry, 308t
Urticaria, 270–271, 270f
acute, 270
chronic, 270
clinical manifestations, 270, 270f
differential diagnosis, 270–271
evaluation, 271
prevalence, 270
treatment, 271
Urticarial vasculitis, 270
U.S. Child Health Insurance Program (CHIP), 748
U.S. Citizen and Immigration Service (USCIS), 738

U.S. Food and Drug Administration, 91, 419
U.S. Preventive Services Task Force (USPSTF), 58, 60, 651
U.S. Substance Abuse and Mental Health
Services Administration (SAMHSA), 66–67
Uterine bleeding, abnormal, 484–487
acute, 485–486, 485f
chronic, 486, 486t
coagulopathies, 486
evaluation in, 484–485
HPO axis in, immaturity of, 484
iatrogenic bleeding, 486–487
laboratory testing for, 485t
therapy, 485–487
Uterine neoplasms, 519
Uterine synechiae, 490, 493, 494
Uterovaginal agenesis, 517
Uterus
congenital absence of, 489, 494
development of, from paired
paramesonephric ducts, 515, 515f
fusion abnormalities, 515–517, 516f

V
Vaccine information sheets (VIS), 73
Vaccine-related myocarditis, 193
Vaccines
consent for, 73–74
contraindications to, 74
COVID-19, 327, 348
hepatitis A, 331–332
hepatitis B, 335
human papillomavirus, 71–72
improving delivery, 74
influenza, 72–73
meningococcal, 72
pertussis, 325, 326
refusal by patients and parents, 74
Vacuum aspiration, 418
Vagal nerve stimulator (VNS), 280
Vaginal contraceptive rings, 427, 450, 451
Vaginal discharge, 507, 512
in AYAs, 507, 508t
history of, 469
Vaginal flora, 507
Vaginal intraepithelial neoplasia (VaIN), 584
Vaginal spermicides, 447–448
Vagina, normal, 507
Vaginitis, 507. *See also* Bacterial vaginosis;
Trichomoniasis; Vulvovaginal
candidiasis
causes, 507, 508t
treatment, 508
work-up, 507
Valacyclovir, for genital herpes, 581, 581t
Valerian root, 92
Valproate, 495
in women with epilepsy, 282
Valproic acid, for seizure treatment, 281t
Valvular aortic stenosis, 188–189, 188t
Valvular pulmonary stenosis, 188, 188t
Vaping, 27, 602
middle and high school youth, 607, 608f
young adult, 607
VAQTA, for hepatitis A, 332
Varenicline (Chantix), for tobacco cessation, 628
Varicella vaccination, 348
Varicocele, 530, 532, 534f, 537
bag of worms appearance, 537
diagnosis, 537
epidemiology, 537
etiology, 537
grading system for, 537
therapy, 537

Vasodilators, for hypertension, 201t
Vasovagal syncope. *See* Neurocardiogenic syncope
Vegetarians, 82
　supplemental needs of, 82
Velocardiofacial syndrome. *See* 22q11.2 deletion syndrome
Venereal Diseases Research Laboratory, 573
Venlafaxine
　for fibromyalgia, 379
　for PMDD, 482
Venous thromboembolism (VTE), 450, 451
Ventricular septal defect (VSD), 187, 188t
Vertigo, 183
　causes, 183, 183t
　history, 183
　physical examination, 183
　treatment, 183
Very low density lipoproteins (VLDL), 171, 172
Vestibular/oculomotor screening (VOMS) tool, 250
Vicodin use, 608
Victimization, 697–699
Video games, 101
Vigabatrin, for seizure treatment, 281t
Viloxazine, in ADHD, 685
Violence, transgender youth as victim of, 409
Viral exanthems, 269
Viral hepatitis
　hepatitis A, 331–333
　hepatitis B, 333–336
　hepatitis C, 336–338
　hepatitis D, 338–339
　hepatitis E, 339
Viral infections, skin, 268
Viral nucleic acid tests, for HIV infection, 344
Viral p24 antigen (fourth-generation) tests, for HIV infection, 344
Virilization, signs of, 500
Virtual communities, role of, 99
Visceral hypersensitivity, 389
Vision screening, 69
Visits to clinician, 58. *See also* Office visits; Preventive health care
Visual Analogue Scales for Premenstrual Mood Symptoms, 481
Visual impairment (VI), 681t
Vital signs monitoring, 69
Vitamin D levels, in epilepsy, 282–283
Vitamin D supplementation, for AMPS, 379
Vitamin requirements, 81, 81t
Vitex agnus-castus (chasteberry), 481
Vitiligo, 266, 274
　clinical manifestations, 274
　differential diagnosis, 274
　generalized, 274
　segmental, 274
　treatment, 274
Vocal cord dysfunction (VCD), 207. *See also* Exercise-induced laryngeal obstruction (EILO)
Voicing My CHOiCES, 115
Voiding diary, 307, 308t
Voter disenfranchisement, 744
Vulvar intraepithelial neoplasia (VIN), 584
Vulvovaginal candidiasis, 507, 510–511
　clinical manifestations, 510
　complicated, 510
　counseling, 511
　diagnosis, 510
　epidemiology, 510
　etiology, 510
　predisposing factors, 510
　recurrent, 510
　therapy, 510–511
　uncomplicated, 510

Vulvovaginitis and vaginosis, in pubertal females, 507–508
　etiology, 507
　evaluation, 507–508
　　clue cells, 508, 508f
　　examination, 507, 508f
　　history, 507
　　laboratory evaluation, 507–508
Vulvovaginitis, in prepubertal females, 507

W

Waist–hip ratio, 79–80
War and conflict, structural determinants of health, 9
Warning signs, suicide, 672
Warts, 268
　anogenital, 268
　clinical manifestations, 268
　common, 268
　flat, 268
　plantar, 268
　treatment, 268
WBC differential, in infectious mononucleosis, 321–322
Weak scapular stabilizing muscles, 223
Web 2.0, 98
WE CARE, 747
Weight dissatisfaction, 46
Weight gain
　during pregnancy, 82
　pubertal, 41
Weight-gain promoting medications, 355, 356t
Weight loss
　and amenorrhea, 490
　in anorexia nervosa, 363, 364
　PCOS and, 497
Western blot, 344
Whiff test, 508
White coat hypertension (WCH), 198
Whiteheads, 256
Wolff–Parkinson–White (WPW) syndrome, 182, 182f
Women with epilepsy, 282. *See also* Epilepsy
World Anti-Doping Agency (WADA), 244
World Health Organization (WHO)
　Adolescent Data, 133t
　on adolescent-friendly health care, 29, 107
　on palliative care, 112
　on social determinants of health, 2, 5
　Tiered-Effectiveness Counseling, 438
　on youth violence, 691

X

Xerac AC, for hyperhidrosis, 273
X-linked lymphoproliferative syndrome, 322
Xulane, 427

Y

Yale-Vermont Adversity in Childhood Scale (Y-VACS), 746
Years lived with disability (YLDs), 5t, 22
Years of life lost from mortality (YLLs), 5t
YEH. *See* Youth experiencing homelessness (YEH)
Yersinia enterocolitica, erythema nodosum by, 271
Yoga, 94–95
　for anxiety disorders, 669
Young adulthood, close relationships in, 396
Young adult offenders, 733. *See also* Justice system, involvement with
Young adults, 45, 47–48. *See also* Adolescents and young adults (AYAs)
　body image, 48
　and capacity to consent, 86
　challenges of, 55

　cognitive development, 48
　identity development, 48
　moving toward independence, 48
　nutritional needs of, 78
　peer group, 48
　preventive health guidelines for, 59–60, 61–62t
Young parents, care of, 420
Youth engagement, 129–130
Youth experiencing homelessness (YEH), 723–727
　common medical problems, 726
　COVID-19 pandemic and challenges for, 725
　definitions and related terms, 723, 723f
　infectious diseases and STIs risk, 725
　mental health concerns, 725
　paths to streets, 723
　population size and demographics, 723–725, 724f
　principles and approach to care, 726
　　clinicians, guidelines for, 726
　　communities, guidelines for, 727
　　guidelines for clinics and other programs, 726–727
　　intensive case management, 726
　reproductive health, 725–726
　risky behaviors and health of, 725
　sexual assault, 726
　structural racism and homelessness, 723–724
　substance use, 725
　unintended pregnancy, 726
　violence and abuse, 725
Youth friendly environment, creation of, 66, 67t
Youth-friendly health care. *See* Adolescent-friendly care
Youth Risk Behavior Surveillance System (YRBSS), 133t, 606, 691
Youth Risk Behavior Survey (YRBS), 397
　on alcohol use among adolescents, 614–615
Youth shelters, 727
Youth violence, 691–694
　assessment of risk and protective factors, 692–693
　　general risk assessment, 692–693
　　targeted risk assessment, 693
　CDC on, 691
　definition, 691
　epidemiology, 691–692
　gang involvement, 694
　mass casualty violent events, 691
　physical assault and other violent crime, 691
　prevention and intervention, 693–694
　　community-based, 694
　　family-based, 694
　　indicated programs, 694
　　individual-based, 694
　　multisystemic therapy (MST), 694
　　public health model, 693–694, 693f
　　school-based, 694
　　selected programs, 694
　　universal prevention programs, 694
　protective factors, 692
　race and gender differences, 691–692
　risk factors, 692
　WHO on, 691

Z

Zanamivir, for influenza, 327
Zika virus, 599
Zinc, 81
　deficiency in athletes, 82–83
　food sources, 81
　RDA for, 81
Zonisamide, for seizure treatment, 281t

QUADM0123